11. **CONTRAINDICATIONS** Condi[...] patient populations in which us[...] avoided.

12. **WARNINGS/PRECAUTIONS** Conditions related to the use of the drug and disease states or patient populations where caution is advised.

13. **ADVERSE REACTIONS** Side effects and adverse reactions listed in the FDA-approved labeling that occur with greater frequency (generally at a rate of ≥3%) or that are deemed significant in the clinical judgment of the editors. Refer to the full FDA-approved labeling for a complete list of adverse reactions.

14. **DRUG INTERACTIONS** Effects and implications of other drugs and food on the drug based on FDA-approved labeling.

[...] that the patient must be assessed for or undergo prior to starting treatment with the drug.

16. **MONITORING** Information used for monitoring patients currently treated with the drug; may include specific lab tests and drug-related or condition-specific information.

17. **PATIENT COUNSELING** Important treatment information to discuss with the patient.

18. **STORAGE** Instructions for safe storage and disposal of the drug.

1 Not all fields described here are included in every monograph. Drug monographs in this handbook contain concise information. For more detailed information, please see the full FDA-approved labeling or visit PDR.net® for a complete drug summary and other listings.

2 Abbreviations used within monographs are defined in the *Abbreviations, Acronyms, and Symbols* table on page A1 of the appendix.

HOW SUPPLIED
Inj: 180mcg/0.5mL [prefilled syringe]; 180mcg/0.5mL, 135mcg/0.5mL [ProClick autoinjector]; 180mcg/mL [vial]

11 **CONTRAINDICATIONS**
Autoimmune hepatitis, hepatic decompensation (Child-Pugh score >6 [Class B and C]) in cirrhotic patients before treatment, hepatic decompensation with Child-Pugh score ≥6 in cirrhotic CHC patients coinfected with HIV before treatment, neonates, and infants (contains benzyl alcohol).

12 **WARNINGS/PRECAUTIONS**
Not recommended, alone or in combination with ribavirin without additional HCV antiviral drugs, in CHC patients who previously failed therapy with an interferon-alfa, and in CHC patients who have had a solid organ transplantation. Extreme caution with history of depression; d/c immediately in severe cases and institute psychiatric intervention.

13 **ADVERSE REACTIONS**
Inj-site reactions, fatigue/asthenia, diarrhea, pyrexia, rigors, N/V, anorexia, neutropenia, myalgia, headache, irritability/anxiety/nervousness, insomnia, depression, alopecia, dizziness.

14 **DRUG INTERACTIONS**
May inhibit CYP1A2 and increase exposure of theophylline; monitor theophylline serum levels and consider dose adjustments. May increase levels of methadone; monitor for toxicity.

NURSING CONSIDERATIONS

15 **Assessment:** Assess for neuropsychiatric, autoimmune, ischemic or infectious disorders, hepatic/renal impairment, risk of severe anemia, known hypersensitivity reactions, treatment failure with interferon alfa or solid organ transplantation in CHC patients, pregnancy/nursing status, possible drug interactions, or any other conditions where treatment is contraindicated or cautioned.

16 **Monitoring:** Monitor for signs/symptoms of neuropsychiatric, autoimmune, ischemic, infectious, cardiovascular, cerebrovascular, endocrine, and pulmonary disorders; bone marrow toxicities; colitis; pancreatitis.

17 **Patient Counseling:** Counsel on benefits and risks of therapy. Advise not to use drug in combination with ribavirin for pregnant women or men whose female partners are pregnant; perform monthly pregnancy tests.

18 **Storage:** 2-8°C (36-46°F). Do not leave out of the refrigerator for >24 hrs. Do not freeze or shake. Protect from light.

For more drug summaries, visit PDR.net 1

(Continued)

*FDA/DEA CLASS

OTC: Available over-the-counter.

RX: Requires a prescription.

CII: High potential for abuse. Use may lead to severe physical or psychological dependence.

CIII: Potential for abuse less than the drugs or other substances in CII. Use may lead to low-to-moderate physical dependence or high psychological dependence.

CIV: Low potential for abuse relative to drugs or other substances in CIII. Use may lead to limited physical or psychological dependence relative to the drugs or other substances in CIII.

CV: Low potential for abuse relative to drugs or other substances in CIV. Use may lead to limited physical or psychological dependence relative to the drugs or other substances in CIV.

PDR® 2016 EDITION NURSE'S DRUG HANDBOOK

THE INFORMATION STANDARD FOR PRESCRIPTION DRUGS AND NURSING CONSIDERATIONS

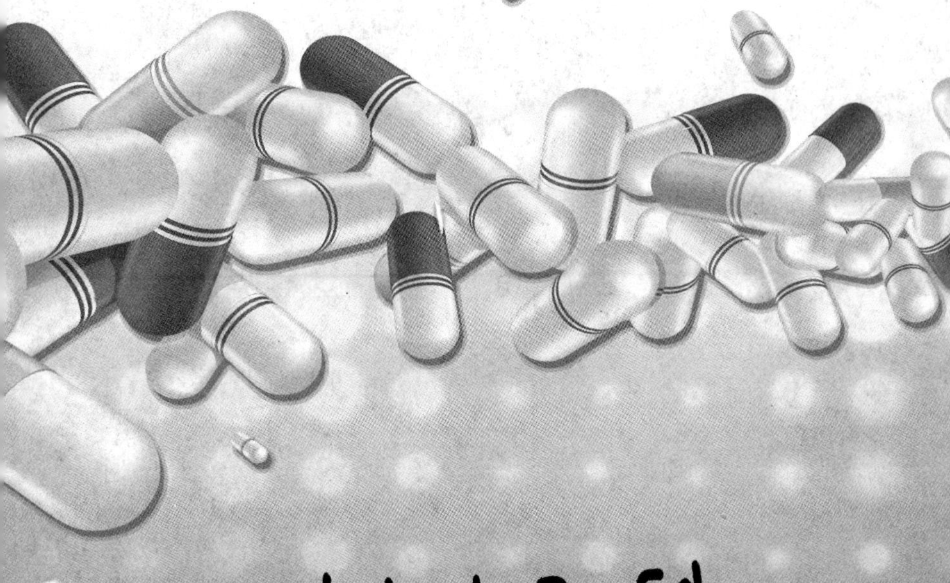

Diabetes Ed

PDR® Nurse's Drug Handbook

2016 EDITION

Vice President of Operations: Lisa Collins
Associate Vice President of Operations: Jeffrey D. Schaefer
Associate Director, Clinical Operations: Anila Patel, PharmD, RPh
Associate Manager, Clinical Content Development: Demyana Farag, PharmD, RPh
Associate Manager, Clinical Operations: Pauline Lee, PharmD, RPh
Senior Drug Information Specialist: Kristine Mecca, PharmD, RPh
Drug Information Specialists: Vanessa Azevedo, PharmD, RPh; Autri Sajedeen, PharmD
Managing Clinical Editor: Julia Tonelli, MD
Medical Editor: Christa Mary Kronick, MA
Director, Communications and Database Channel Lifecycle Management: David Weatherbee
Lead Project Manager: Gary Lew
Manager, Marketing Services: Livio Udina
Director, Manufacturing and Distribution: Thomas Westburgh

PDR, LLC

Chief Executive Officer: Mark Heinold
Chief Medical Officer: Salvatore Volpe, MD, FAAP, FACP, CHCQM
Executive Vice President and Chief Financial Officer: Gary Lubin
Chief Technology Officer: David Cheng
Senior Vice President, General Counsel and Corporate Secretary: Ruth Williams
Senior Vice President, Sales: Jeffrey Wiltrout, PhD
Vice President, Clinical and Regulatory Solutions: Mukesh Mehta, DPh, MBA, RPh
Senior Vice President, Product Marketing and Market Research: Barbara Senich, BSN, MBA, MPH
Senior Vice President, Digital Products: Eugene Lee
Senior Director, Digital Marketing: Lisa Damico

ISBN: 978-1-56363-833-6

Printed in Canada

Contents

Foreword

The 2016 *PDR® Nurse's Drug Handbook* is an essential volume for healthcare professionals who need to have important drug information at their fingertips. Following in the esteemed tradition of *Physicians' Desk Reference®*, the most highly trusted drug information reference available in the U.S., the *PDR Nurse's Drug Handbook* provides current and concise information concerning drug indications, dosages, interactions, and contraindications. Designed to be a primary resource for nurses, student nurses, and other healthcare professionals, its straightforward presentation delivers clear guidelines for administration of drugs, communication with patients, and nursing considerations. It is a trusted and invaluable guide to the latest updated and newly approved FDA-regulated drugs.

PDR values the insights of its readership and has restructured and streamlined the content within this edition in response to input obtained by surveying actual *PDR Nurse's Drug Handbook* readers. Under each alphabetically ordered drug monograph, indication and dosage information for adult and pediatric patients is succinctly presented in a new two-column format. Composed using current FDA-approved labeling, each entry includes the most pertinent information, covering a drug's brand and generic names, class, boxed warning, dose modifications, administration information, how supplied details, contraindications, relevant warnings and precautions, key adverse reactions, and drug interactions. Every monograph also has a special section devoted to nursing considerations, encompassing patient assessment, monitoring, and counseling, and details on safe storage and handling instructions.

In addition to drug summaries of top-prescribed medications, the *PDR Nurse's Drug Handbook* includes carefully chosen supplemental content, provided for easy reference to useful information. Among these are tables devoted to comparison of antiviral treatments, detailed treatment options for angina, heart failure, hypertension, and mental health, a comprehensive list of easily confused drug names (from ISMP), FDA-approved new drug products, a full-color Visual Identification Guide of commonly prescribed drugs, and more. To further this edition's functionality and ease of use, it also contains a set of indices cataloguing the drug monographs in two different ways to help navigate to the most useful drug information needed in any circumstance.

The 2016 *PDR Nurse's Drug Handbook* is a complete resource for healthcare professionals. For even more content, PDR.net® is also available for readers. The site provides online access to authoritative drug information, including full FDA-approved labeling as well as additional concise point-of-care drug information.

Concise Drug Monographs

ABELCET — amphotericin B lipid complex

RX

Class: Polyene antifungal

ADULT DOSAGE

Fungal Infections

Invasive fungal infections in patients who are refractory to or intolerant of conventional amphotericin B therapy

Usual: 5mg/kg given as a single IV infusion at a rate of 2.5mg/kg/hr

PEDIATRIC DOSAGE

Fungal Infections

Invasive fungal infections in patients who are refractory to or intolerant of conventional amphotericin B therapy

Usual: 5mg/kg given as a single IV infusion at a rate of 2.5mg/kg/hr

ADMINISTRATION

IV route

Do not dilute w/ saline sol or mix w/ other drugs or electrolytes

Existing IV lines should be flushed w/ D5 inj before infusion of therapy or a separate infusion line should be used

Do not use an in-line filter

Shake the infusion bag q2h if the infusion time exceeds 2 hrs

Preparation

Withdraw appropriate dose into 1 or more sterile syringes using an 18-gauge needle

Remove needle and use supplied 5-micron filter needle to empty contents of syringe in to an IV bag containing D5 inj

Final infusion concentration should be 1mg/mL (2mg/mL for pediatric patients and patients w/ cardiovascular disease)

Shake the bag until contents are thoroughly mixed; discard unused material

HOW SUPPLIED

Inj: 5mg/mL

WARNINGS/PRECAUTIONS

Anaphylaxis reported; d/c immediately infusion and avoid further infusions if severe respiratory distress occurs. Should be administered by medically trained personnel during the initial dosing of therapy. Acute reactions, including fever and chills, may occur 1-2 hrs after starting IV infusion. Infusion has been associated with hypotension, bronchospasm, arrhythmias, and shock (rare). Dose-dependent renal toxicity reported.

ADVERSE REACTIONS

Chills, fever, increased SrCr, multiple organ failure, N/V, hypotension, respiratory failure, dyspnea, sepsis, diarrhea, headache, cardiac arrest, HTN, hypokalemia, kidney failure.

DRUG INTERACTIONS

Caution with antineoplastic agents; may enhance the potential for renal toxicity, bronchospasm, and hypotension. Corticosteroids and corticotropin may potentiate hypokalemia; monitor serum electrolytes and cardiac function if used concomitantly. Concurrent initiation with cyclosporine A within several days of bone marrow ablation may be associated with increased nephrotoxicity. May induce hypokalemia and potentiate digitalis toxicity with digitalis glycosides; closely monitor serum K^+ levels. May increase flucytosine toxicity; use with caution. Antagonism with imidazole derivatives (eg, miconazole, ketoconazole, clotrimazole) reported. Acute pulmonary toxicity reported with leukocyte transfusions; avoid concurrent use. May enhance the potential for drug-induced renal toxicity with nephrotoxic agents (eg, aminoglycosides, pentamidine); use with caution and monitor renal function intensively. Amphotericin B-induced hypokalemia may enhance curariform effect of skeletal muscle relaxants (eg, tubocurarine) due to hypokalemia; closely monitor serum K^+ levels. Monitor renal and hematologic function with zidovudine.

NURSING CONSIDERATIONS

Assessment: Assess for previous hypersensitivity to the drug, pregnancy/nursing status, and possible drug interactions.

Monitoring: Monitor for signs and symptoms of anaphylaxis, severe respiratory distress, acute reactions, and other adverse reactions. Monitor for overall clinical condition. Frequently monitor SrCr. Regularly monitor LFTs, serum electrolytes (particularly Mg^{2+} and K^+), and CBCs.

Patient Counseling: Inform about the risks and benefits of therapy. Advise to seek medical attention if pregnant or nursing, and if any adverse reactions occur.

Storage: 2-8°C (36-46°F). Protect from light. Do not freeze. Diluted Ready-For-Use Admixture: Stable for up to 48 hrs at 2-8°C (36-46°F) and an additional 6 hrs at room temperature. Do not freeze. Discard any unused material.

ABILIFY – aripiprazole

RX

Class: Atypical antipsychotic

Elderly patients with dementia-related psychosis treated with antipsychotic drugs are at an increased risk of death; most deaths appeared to be either cardiovascular (CV) (eg, HF, sudden death) or infectious (eg, pneumonia) in nature. Not approved for treatment of patients with dementia-related psychosis. Antidepressants increased risk of suicidal thinking and behavior (suicidality) in children, adolescents, and young adults in short-term studies of major depressive disorder and other psychiatric disorders. Monitor and observe closely for clinical worsening, suicidality, or unusual changes in behavior in patients who are started on antidepressant therapy. Not approved for use in pediatric patients with depression.

OTHER BRAND NAMES

Abilify Discmelt

ADULT DOSAGE

Schizophrenia

Initial/Target: 10mg or 15mg qd
Titrate: Should not increase dose before 2 weeks
Usual: 10-30mg/day
Reassess periodically to determine the need for maint treatment

Bipolar I Disorder

Acute Treatment of Manic and Mixed Episodes, Both as Monotherapy and as an Adjunct to Lithium or Valproate:
Initial: 15mg qd (monotherapy), 10-15mg qd (adjunct)
Target: 15mg qd
Titrate: May increase to 30mg/day based on clinical response
Max: 30mg/day
Reassess periodically to determine the need for maint treatment

Major Depressive Disorder

Adjunctive Therapy to Antidepressants:
Initial: 2-5mg/day
Titrate: Dose adjustments of up to 5mg/day should occur gradually at intervals of no <1 week
Usual: 2-15mg/day
Reassess periodically to determine the need for maint treatment

Agitation

Acute Agitation Associated w/ Schizophrenia or Bipolar Disorder, Manic or Mixed:
Inj:
Usual: 9.75mg IM
Effective Range: 5.25-15mg
A lower dose of 5.25mg may be considered when clinical factors warrant. If agitation warranting a 2nd dose persists following the initial dose, cumulative doses of up to a total of 30mg/day may be given
Max: 30mg/day. Not more frequent than q2h
If ongoing treatment is clinically indicated, replace w/ PO at 10-30mg/day as soon as possible

PEDIATRIC DOSAGE

Schizophrenia

13-17 Years:
Initial: 2mg/day
Titrate: May increase to 5mg/day after 2 days and to the target dose of 10mg/day after 2 additional days. Subsequent dose increases, if needed, should be administered in 5mg increments
Max: 30mg/day
Reassess periodically to determine the need for maint treatment

Bipolar I Disorder

Acute Treatment of Manic and Mixed Episodes, Both as Monotherapy and as an Adjunct to Lithium or Valproate:
10-17 Years:
Initial: 2mg/day
Titrate: May increase to 5mg/day after 2 days and to the target dose of 10mg/day after 2 additional days. Subsequent dose increases, if needed, should be administered in 5mg increments
Max: 30mg/day
Reassess periodically to determine the need for maint treatment

Irritability

Associated w/ Autistic Disorder:
6-17 Years:
Initial: 2mg/day
Titrate: Increase to 5mg/day
May increase to 10mg or 15mg/day if needed
Dose adjustments of up to 5mg/day should occur gradually at intervals of no <1 week
Usual: 5-15mg/day
Reassess periodically to determine the need for maint treatment

DOSE MODIFICATION

Concomitant Medications

Strong CYP3A4 or Potential CYP2D6 Inhibitors:
Reduce to 1/2 the usual dose; when CYP3A4 or 2D6 inhibitor is withdrawn from combination therapy, increase the aripiprazole dose
Potential CYP2D6 Inhibitors in Patient w/ Major Depressive Disorder:
Administer w/o dose adjustment

Strong CYP3A4 and CYP2D6 Inhibitors:
Reduce to 1/4 of the usual dose; when CYP3A4 and CYP2D6 inhibitors are withdrawn from combination therapy, increase the aripiprazole dose
Strong, Moderate or Weak CYP3A4, and CYP2D6 Inhibitors:
Initial: Reduce to 1/4 of usual dose
Titrate: Adjust to achieve a favorable clinical response
Potential CYP3A4 Inducers:
Double aripiprazole dose and base additional dose increases on clinical evaluation; when CYP3A4 inducer is withdrawn from therapy, reduce aripiprazole dose to 10-15mg

Other Important Modifications
Poor CYP2D6 Metabolizer Patients:
Initial: Reduce to 1/2 or 1/4 (on strong CYP3A4 inhibitor) of usual dose
Titrate: Adjust to achieve a favorable clinical response

ADMINISTRATION
Oral/IM route

PO
Administer w/o regard to meals
Oral sol can be substituted for tabs on a mg-per-mg basis up to 25mg
Patients receiving 30mg tabs should receive 25mg of oral sol

Inj
Inject slowly, deep into the muscle mass

HOW SUPPLIED
Inj: 7.5mg/mL [1.3mL]; Sol: 1mg/mL [150mL]; Tab: 2mg, 5mg, 10mg, 15mg, 20mg, 30mg; Tab, Disintegrating: (Discmelt) 10mg, 15mg

WARNINGS/PRECAUTIONS
Initiate in pediatric patients only after a thorough diagnostic evaluation has been conducted and careful consideration given to the risks associated with therapy. Neuroleptic malignant syndrome (NMS) reported; d/c immediately, institute symptomatic treatment and monitor. May cause tardive dyskinesia (TD), especially in the elderly; d/c if this occurs. Hyperglycemia, in some cases extreme and associated with ketoacidosis or hyperosmolar coma or death, reported; monitor glucose control regularly in patients with diabetes mellitus (DM) and FPG in patients at risk for DM. Dyslipidemia and weight gain reported. May cause orthostatic hypotension; caution with known CV disease (history of myocardial infarction or ischemic heart disease, HF or conduction abnormalities), cerebrovascular disease, or conditions that would predispose patients to hypotension. Leukopenia, neutropenia, and agranulocytosis reported; monitor CBC frequently during 1st few months in patients with history of clinically significant low WBC counts or drug-induced leukopenia/neutropenia. D/C at 1st sign of a clinically significant decline in WBC counts in the absence of other causative factors. D/C therapy and follow WBC counts until recovery in patients with severe neutropenia (absolute neutrophil counts <1000/mm^3). Seizures reported; caution with history of seizures or with conditions that lower seizure threshold (eg, Alzheimer's dementia). May impair physical/mental abilities. May disrupt body's ability to reduce core body temperature; caution when exposed to conditions that may contribute to an elevation in core body temperature (eg, exercising strenuously, exposure to extreme heat, receiving concomitant medication with anticholinergic activity, or being subject to dehydration). May cause esophageal dysmotility and aspiration; caution in patients at risk for aspiration pneumonia.

ADVERSE REACTIONS
Headache, fatigue, tremor, anxiety, insomnia, increased appetite, N/V, somnolence, constipation, akathisia, extrapyramidal disorder, nasopharyngitis, dizziness, restlessness, weight increase.

DRUG INTERACTIONS
Caution with other centrally acting drugs. Avoid with alcohol. May potentiate the effect of certain antihypertensive agents. CYP3A4 inducers (eg, carbamazepine) may increase clearance and lower blood levels. CYP3A4 inhibitors (eg, ketoconazole, itraconazole) or CYP2D6 inhibitors (eg, quinidine, fluoxetine, paroxetine) may inhibit elimination and increase blood levels. (Inj) Greater intensity of sedation and greater orthostatic hypotension with lorazepam inj; monitor for excessive sedation and for orthostatic hypotension with parenteral benzodiazepines.

NURSING CONSIDERATIONS

Assessment: Assess for dementia-related psychosis, drug hypersensitivity, psychiatric disorders or any other conditions where treatment is cautioned, pregnancy/nursing status, and possible drug interactions. Obtain baseline FPG in patients with DM or at risk for DM. Obtain baseline CBC if at risk for leukopenia/neutropenia.

Monitoring: Monitor for clinical worsening of depression, suicidality, unusual changes in behavior, NMS, TD, hyperglycemia, orthostatic hypotension, seizures/convulsions, esophageal dysmotility, aspiration, and other adverse effects. Monitor CBC frequently in patients with preexisting low WBC counts or drug-induced leukopenia/neutropenia. Monitor for fever or other signs/symptoms of infection in patients with neutropenia. Monitor weight regularly and FPG in patients with DM or at risk for DM periodically during therapy. Periodically reassess to determine the continued need for maintenance treatment.

Patient Counseling: Inform about the risks and benefits of treatment. Instruct patients, families, and caregivers to be alert to the emergence of anxiety, agitation, panic attacks, insomnia, irritability, hostility, aggressiveness, impulsivity, akathisia, hypomania, mania, other unusual changes in behavior, worsening of depression, and suicidal ideation; advise to contact physician if these symptoms occur. Instruct to use caution when operating hazardous machinery and to avoid alcohol use while on therapy. Counsel to avoid overheating and dehydration. Advise to notify physician if patient becomes pregnant or intends to become pregnant during therapy, and if patient is taking or plans to take any prescription or OTC drugs. Instruct to not breastfeed during therapy. (Discmelt) Inform phenylketonurics that product contains phenylalanine. Instruct to not open blister until ready to administer. Instruct that drug is to be taken without liquid. However, if needed, drug can be taken with liquid. Advise not to split the tab. (Sol) Inform that sol contains sucrose and fructose.

Storage: 25°C (77°F); excursions permitted to 15-30°C (59-86°F). Oral Sol: May be used for ≤6 months after opening. Inj: Store in original container; protect from light.

Abilify Maintena – aripiprazole RX

Class: Atypical antipsychotic

Elderly patients with dementia-related psychosis treated with antipsychotic drugs are at an increased risk of death. Not approved for the treatment of patients with dementia-related psychosis.

ADULT DOSAGE

Schizophrenia

Initial/Maint: 400mg monthly (no sooner than 26 days after the previous inj); establish tolerability w/ oral aripiprazole prior to initiating treatment in naive patients

After the 1st inj, administer oral aripiprazole (10-20mg) or if already stable on another oral antipsychotic, continue treatment w/ the antipsychotic, for 14 consecutive days

Missed Dose

2nd or 3rd Doses are Missed:
>4 Weeks and <5 Weeks Since Last Inj: Administer inj as soon as possible
>5 Weeks Since Last Inj: Restart concomitant oral aripiprazole for 14 days w/ next administered inj

4th or Subsequent Doses are Missed:
>4 Weeks and <6 Weeks Since Last Inj: Administer inj as soon as possible
>6 Weeks Since Last Inj: Restart concomitant oral aripiprazole for 14 days w/ next administered inj

PEDIATRIC DOSAGE

Pediatric use may not have been established

DOSE MODIFICATION

Concomitant Medications

300mg:
Concomitant Use for >14 Days:
Strong CYP2D6 or CYP3A4 Inhibitors: 200mg
CYP2D6 and CYP3A4 Inhibitors: 160mg
CYP3A4 Inducers: Avoid use

400mg:
Concomitant Use for >14 Days:
Strong CYP2D6 or CYP3A4 Inhibitors: 300mg
CYP2D6 and CYP3A4 Inhibitors: 200mg
CYP3A4 Inducers: Avoid use

Adverse Reactions

If adverse reactions occur w/ the 400mg dose, consider reducing dose to 300mg once monthly

Other Important Modifications
CYP2D6 Poor Metabolizers: 300mg
CYP2D6 Poor Metabolizers Taking Concomitant CYP3A4 Inhibitors: 200mg

ADMINISTRATION

IM route

For deep IM gluteal inj by healthcare professionals only; do not administer by any other route
Use 21-gauge, 1.5-inch needle for non-obese patients; use 21-gauge, 2-inch needle for obese patients
Inject immediately following reconstitution; do not massage inj site
Rotate inj sites between the 2 gluteal muscles
To obtain 200mg and 160mg dosage adjustments, use 300mg or 400mg strength vials

Preparation
Prefilled Dual Chamber Syringe:
1. Reconstitute at room temperature
2. Push plunger rod slightly to engage threads, then rotate plunger rod until the rod stops rotating to release diluent. Middle stopper will be at the indicator line after plunger rod is at a complete stop
3. Vertically shake syringe vigorously for 20 sec until drug is uniform and milky white
4. Attach appropriate needle; hold syringe upright and advance plunger rod slowly to expel air until sus fills needle base
5. Inject slowly to appropriate site

Vial:
1. Reconstitute 400mg vial w/ 1.9mL sterile water for inj (SWFI) and 300mg vial w/ 1.5mL SWFI
2. Shake vigorously for 30 sec until sus appears uniform; if not injected immediately after reconstitution, keep at room temperature and shake vigorously for at least 60 sec to re-suspend prior to inj
3. Inject 2mL for 400mg dose (400mg vial only), 1.5mL for 300mg dose, 1mL for 200mg dose, and 0.8mg for 160mg dose

Refer to PI for further preparation and administration instructions

HOW SUPPLIED

Inj, Extended-Release: 300mg, 400mg [vial, prefilled dual chamber syringe]

WARNINGS/PRECAUTIONS

Do not substitute with other aripiprazole inj. Neuroleptic malignant syndrome (NMS) reported; d/c immediately and institute symptomatic treatment. May cause tardive dyskinesia (TD), especially in the elderly; consider discontinuation if this occurs. Hyperglycemia, in some cases extreme and associated with ketoacidosis or hyperosmolar coma or death, reported. Dyslipidemia and weight gain reported. May cause orthostatic hypotension. Leukopenia, neutropenia, and agranulocytosis reported; consider discontinuation at 1st sign of decline in WBC counts without causative factors. D/C therapy and follow WBC counts until recovery in patients with severe neutropenia (absolute neutrophil count [ANC] <1000/mm^3). Caution with history of seizures or with conditions that lower seizure threshold. May impair mental/physical abilities. May disrupt body's ability to reduce core body temperature. May cause esophageal dysmotility and aspiration; caution in patients at risk for aspiration pneumonia.

ADVERSE REACTIONS

Weight increase/decrease, akathisia, constipation, inj-site pain, sedation, dry mouth, URTI, arthralgia, back pain, myalgia, dizziness, diarrhea, vomiting, musculoskeletal pain.

DRUG INTERACTIONS

Strong CYP3A4 inducers may decrease exposure; avoid use with carbamazepine and other CYP3A4 inducers for >14 days. Concomitant use with strong CYP3A4 inhibitors (eg, ketoconazole) or strong CYP2D6 inhibitors (eg, paroxetine, fluoxetine) may increase exposure; reduce dose if using concomitantly for >14 days. May enhance effect of certain antihypertensives; monitor BP and adjust dose accordingly. Caution with benzodiazepines; monitor sedation and BP and adjust dose accordingly.

NURSING CONSIDERATIONS

Assessment: Assess for history of dementia-related psychosis, diabetes mellitus (DM), drug hypersensitivity, any other conditions where treatment is cautioned, pregnancy/nursing status, and possible drug interactions. Obtain baseline FPG in patients with DM or at risk for DM. Obtain baseline CBC if at risk for leukopenia/neutropenia.

Monitoring: Monitor for NMS, TD, hyperglycemia, orthostatic hypotension, seizures, weight gain, dyslipidemia, esophageal dysmotility, aspiration, and other adverse reactions. Monitor CBC frequently in patients with a history of a clinically significant low WBC count/ANC or drug-induced leukopenia/neutropenia. Monitor for fever or other symptoms/signs of infection in patients with neutropenia. Monitor for worsening of glucose control in patients with DM and FPG in patients at risk for DM.

Patient Counseling: Inform of the risks/benefits of therapy. Counsel about signs/symptoms of NMS. Instruct to notify physician if any movements that cannot be controlled in the face, tongue, or other body part develop. Advise to use caution when operating hazardous machinery. Counsel to avoid overheating and dehydration. Advise that breastfeeding is not recommended during therapy. Instruct to notify physician if taking/planning to take any prescription or OTC drugs.

Storage: Syringe: <30°C (86°F). Do not freeze. Protect from light. Vial: 25°C (77°F); excursions permitted to 15-30°C (59-86°F).

ABRAXANE – paclitaxel protein-bound RX

Class: Antimicrotubule agent

Do not administer to patients who have baseline neutrophil counts of <1500 cells/mm^3. Perform frequent peripheral blood cell counts to monitor occurrence of bone marrow suppression, primarily neutropenia. Do not substitute for or with other paclitaxel formulations.

ADULT DOSAGE

Non-Small Cell Lung Cancer

Locally Advanced or Metastatic:

100mg/m^2 IV infusion over 30 min on Days 1, 8, and 15 of each 21-day cycle
Give carboplatin on Day 1 of each 21-day cycle immediately after paclitaxel

Do not administer on Day 1 of a cycle until absolute neutrophil count (ANC) is at least 1500 cells/mm^3 and platelet count is at least 100,000 cells/mm^3

Pancreatic Adenocarcinoma

Metastatic:

125mg/m^2 IV infusion over 30-40 min on Days 1, 8, and 15 of each 28-day cycle
Give gemcitabine immediately after paclitaxel on Days 1, 8, and 15 of each 28-day cycle

Metastatic Breast Cancer

260mg/m^2 IV over 30 min every 3 weeks

PEDIATRIC DOSAGE

Pediatric use may not have been established

DOSE MODIFICATION

Hepatic Impairment

Metastatic Breast Cancer:
Moderate (AST <10X ULN and Bilirubin >1.5-≤3X ULN):
Initial: 200mg/m^2 for the 1st course of therapy
Titrate: May increase up to 260mg/m^2 in subsequent courses if reduced dose tolerated for 2 cycles
Severe (AST <10X ULN and Bilirubin >3-≤5X ULN):
Initial: 200mg/m^2 for the 1st course of therapy
Titrate: May increase up to 260mg/m^2 in subsequent courses if reduced dose tolerated for 2 cycles
Withhold if: AST >10X ULN or bilirubin >5X ULN

Non-Small Cell Lung Cancer:
Moderate (AST <10X ULN and Bilirubin >1.5-≤3X ULN):
Initial: 80mg/m^2 for the 1st course of therapy
Titrate: May increase up to 100mg/m^2 in subsequent courses if reduced dose tolerated for 2 cycles
Severe (AST <10X ULN and Bilirubin >3-≤5X ULN):
Initial: 80mg/m^2 for the 1st course of therapy
Titrate: May increase up to 100mg/m^2 in subsequent courses if reduced dose tolerated for 2 cycles
Withhold if: AST >10X ULN or bilirubin >5X ULN

Pancreatic Adenocarcinoma:
Moderate (AST <10X ULN and Bilirubin >1.5-≤3X ULN)/Severe Hepatic Impairment (AST <10X ULN and Bilirubin >3-≤5X ULN)/AST >10X ULN or Bilirubin >5X ULN: Not recommended

Adverse Reactions

Metastatic Breast Cancer:
Severe Neutropenia (Neutrophil <500 cells/mm^3 for a Week or Longer) or Severe Sensory Neuropathy: Reduce to 220mg/m^2
Recurrence of Severe Neutropenia or Severe Sensory Neuropathy: Additionally reduce to 180mg/m^2
Grade 3 Sensory Neuropathy: Hold treatment until resolution to Grade 1 or 2, followed by a dose reduction for all subsequent courses

Non-Small Cell Lung Cancer:
Severe Neutropenia or Thrombocytopenia: Withhold treatment until ANC at least 1500 cells/mm³ and platelet count at least 100,000 cells/mm³ on Day 1 or to ANC of at least 500 cells/mm³ and platelet count of at least 50,000 cells/mm³ on Days 8 or 15 of the cycle; upon resumption of dosing, permanently reduce as outlined below
Grade 3-4 Peripheral Neuropathy: Withhold; resume with improvement to Grade 1 or complete resolution
Peripheral Neuropathy Improves to Grade 1 or Completely Resolves: Resume at reduced doses

Neutropenic Fever (ANC <500/mm³ with Fever >38°C) or Delay of Next Cycle by >7 Days for ANC <1500/mm³ or ANC <500/mm³ for >7 Days:
First Occurrence: Reduce to 75mg/m² weekly
Second Occurrence: Reduce to 50mg/m² weekly
Third Occurrence: D/C treatment

Platelet Count <50,000/mm³:
First Occurrence: Reduce to 75mg/m² weekly
Second Occurrence: D/C treatment

Severe Sensory Neuropathy (Grade 3 or 4):
First Occurrence: Reduce to 75mg/m² weekly
Second Occurrence: Reduce to 50mg/m² weekly
Third Occurrence: D/C treatment

Pancreatic Adenocarcinoma:
Febrile Neutropenia (Grade 3 or 4): Withhold until fever resolves and ANC ≥ 1500; resume at 100mg/m²
Peripheral Neuropathy (Grade 3 or 4): Withhold until improvement to ≤Grade 1; resume at 100mg/m²
Cutaneous Toxicity (Grade 2 or 3): Reduce to 100mg/m²; d/c treatment if toxicity persists
Gastrointestinal Toxicity (Grade 3 Mucositis or Diarrhea): Withhold until improvement to ≤Grade 1; resume at 100mg/m²
Neutropenia and/or Thrombocytopenia at the Start of a Cycle or Within a Cycle: Refer to PI

ADMINISTRATION
IV route

If Abraxane (lyophilized cake or reconstituted sus) contacts the skin, wash the skin immediately and thoroughly with soap and water; if contact with mucous membranes, the membranes should be flushed thoroughly with water
Limit the infusion to 30 min

Preparation
Reconstitute each vial by injecting 20mL of 0.9% NaCl Inj onto the inside wall of the vial
Gently swirl and/or invert the vial slowly for at least 2 min; allow vial to sit for minimum of 5 min after inj into vial
Reconstituted Abraxane in the vial should be used immediately, but may be refrigerated at 2-8°C (36-46°F) for a max of 8 hrs if necessary
If not used immediately, each vial of reconstituted sus should be replaced in the original carton to protect it from bright light
Inject the appropriate amount of reconstituted Abraxane into an empty, sterile IV bag
Use of an in-line filter is not recommended
The sus for infusion when prepared in an infusion bag should be used immediately but may be refrigerated at 2-8°C (36-46°F) and protected from light for a max of 24 hrs

HOW SUPPLIED
Inj: 100mg

CONTRAINDICATIONS
Patients with baseline neutrophil counts of <1500 cells/mm³.

WARNINGS/PRECAUTIONS
Bone marrow suppression (primarily neutropenia) is dose-dependent and a dose-limiting toxicity. Resume treatment with every-3-week cycles after ANC recovers to >1500 cells/mm³ and platelets recover to >100,000 cells/mm³ in patients with metastatic breast cancer (MBC). Sensory neuropathy is dose- and schedule-dependent. Sepsis reported; initiate treatment with broad-spectrum antibiotics if patient becomes febrile (regardless of ANC). Pneumonitis reported; interrupt treatment and gemcitabine during evaluation of suspected pneumonitis. After ruling out infectious etiology and upon making a diagnosis of pneumonitis, permanently d/c combination therapy. Severe and sometimes fatal hypersensitivity reactions, including anaphylactic reactions, reported. Caution with hepatic impairment; not recommended in patients who have total bilirubin >5X ULN or AST >10X ULN and in patients with metastatic adenocarcinoma of the pancreas who have moderate to severe hepatic impairment (total bilirubin >1.5X ULN and AST ≤10X ULN). Contains human albumin; may carry a remote risk for transmission of viral diseases. May cause fetal harm. Men should be advised not to father a child while receiving treatment.

ADVERSE REACTIONS

Alopecia, neutropenia, thrombocytopenia, sensory/peripheral neuropathy, abnormal ECG, fatigue/asthenia, myalgia/arthralgia, AST elevation, alkaline phosphatase elevation, anemia, nausea, infections, diarrhea.

DRUG INTERACTIONS

Caution with medicines known to inhibit (eg, ketoconazole and other imidazole antifungals, erythromycin, fluoxetine, gemfibrozil, ritonavir) or induce (eg, rifampicin, carbamazepine, phenytoin, efavirenz, nevirapine) either CYP2C8 or CYP3A4.

NURSING CONSIDERATIONS

Assessment: Assess for previous hypersensitivity reactions to drug, pregnancy/nursing status, and possible drug interactions. Obtain baseline CBC, including neutrophil counts, and LFTs.

Monitoring: Monitor for neutropenia, sensory neuropathy, sepsis, pneumonitis, hypersensitivity reactions, and other adverse reactions. Frequently monitor CBC (including neutrophil counts); perform prior to dosing on Day 1 (for MBC) and Days 1, 8, and 15 (for NSCLC and pancreatic cancer).

Patient Counseling: Inform that drug may cause fetal harm; advise women of childbearing potential to avoid becoming pregnant. Advise men not to father a child while on therapy. Inform of the risk of low blood cell counts and severe and life-threatening infections; instruct to contact physician immediately for fever or evidence of infection. Advise to contact physician for persistent vomiting, diarrhea, or signs of dehydration. Inform that sensory neuropathy occurs frequently and to report to physician any numbness, tingling, pain, or weakness involving the extremities. Inform that alopecia, fatigue/asthenia, and myalgia/arthralgia occur frequently with therapy. Instruct to contact physician for signs of an allergic reaction and for sudden onset of dry, persistent cough or SOB.

Storage: 20-25°C (68-77°F). Retain in original packaging to protect from bright light. Reconstituted Sus in Vial: Use immediately or refrigerate at 2-8°C (36-46°F) for a max of 24 hrs if necessary and store in original carton to protect from bright light. Reconstituted Sus in Infusion Bag: Use immediately or refrigerate at 2-8°C (36-46°F) and protect from bright light for a max of 24 hrs. Total combined refrigerated storage time of reconstituted sus in the vial and in the infusion bag is 24 hrs; may be followed by storage in the infusion bag at ambient temperature (approximately 25°C [77°F]) and lighting conditions for a max of 4 hrs.

ABSORICA — isotretinoin RX

Class: Retinoid

Not for use by females who are or may become pregnant. Severe birth defects, including death, have been documented. Increased risk of spontaneous abortion and premature births reported. D/C immediately if pregnancy occurs during treatment and refer to an obstetrician-gynecologist experienced in reproductive toxicity for further evaluation and counseling. Available only through a restricted program under a Risk Evaluation and Mitigation Strategy called iPLEDGE. Prescribers, patients, pharmacies, and distributors must enroll and be registered in the program.

ADULT DOSAGE

Severe Recalcitrant Nodular Acne

Patients Who are Unresponsive to Conventional Therapy, Including Systemic Antibiotics:

0.5-1mg/kg/day given in 2 divided doses for 15-20 weeks

Titrate: May adjust dose according to response of disease and/or appearance of clinical side effects

Very Severe Disease w/ Scarring or Primarily Manifested on Trunk:

May adjust dose up to 2mg/kg/day, as tolerated

D/C if total nodule count has been reduced by >70% prior to completing 15-20 weeks; may initiate 2nd course of treatment w/ persistent or recurring severe nodular acne after a period of ≥2 months w/o therapy

PEDIATRIC DOSAGE

Severe Recalcitrant Nodular Acne

Patients Who are Unresponsive to Conventional Therapy, Including Systemic Antibiotics:

≥12 Years:

0.5-1mg/kg/day given in 2 divided doses for 15-20 weeks

Titrate: May adjust dose according to response of disease and/or appearance of clinical side effects

Very Severe Disease w/ Scarring or Primarily Manifested on Trunk:

May adjust dose up to 2mg/kg/day, as tolerated

D/C if total nodule count has been reduced by >70% prior to completing 15-20 weeks; may initiate 2nd course of treatment w/ persistent or recurring severe nodular acne after a period of ≥2 months w/o therapy

ADMINISTRATION
Oral route
Take w/o regard to meals
Swallow caps w/ a full glass of liquid

HOW SUPPLIED
Cap: 10mg, 20mg, 25mg, 30mg, 35mg, 40mg

CONTRAINDICATIONS
Pregnancy, vitamin A hypersensitivity.

WARNINGS/PRECAUTIONS
Avoid long-term use. Blood donation during therapy and for 1 month following discontinuation should be avoided. Micro-dosed progesterone preparations are an inadequate method of contraception during therapy. Hypersensitivity reactions reported; d/c therapy and institute appropriate management if severe allergic reactions occur. Acute pancreatitis, impaired hearing, inflammatory bowel disease, elevated TGs, decreased HDL, hepatotoxicity, premature epiphyseal closure, skeletal hyperostosis, dry eye, decreased night vision, corneal opacities, and impaired glucose control reported. May cause depression, psychosis, suicidal ideation/attempts, suicide, and aggressive and/or violent behaviors; d/c if symptoms occur. Associated with pseudotumor cerebri (benign intracranial HTN); d/c if papilledema present. D/C if significant decrease in WBC count, hearing or visual impairment, abdominal pain, rectal bleeding, severe diarrhea, hepatitis, or symptoms of pancreatitis occur, or if liver enzyme levels do not normalize or hypertriglyceridemia cannot be controlled at an acceptable level. Erythema multiforme and severe skin reactions reported; monitor for severe skin reactions and consider discontinuation of therapy if warranted. May have a negative effect on bone mineral density; caution with history of childhood osteoporosis, osteomalacia, other bone metabolism disorders, or anorexia nervosa. Osteoporosis, osteopenia, bone fractures, and/or delayed fracture healing reported; increased risk in patients participating in sports with repetitive impact.

ADVERSE REACTIONS
Allergic reactions, vascular thrombotic disease, stroke, palpitation, tachycardia, decreased appetite, weight fluctuation, lip dryness, N/V, anemia, thrombocytopenia, infections, headache, syncope, euphoria.

DRUG INTERACTIONS
Avoid use with tetracyclines or vitamin supplements containing vitamin A. Caution with drugs that cause drug-induced osteoporosis/osteomalacia and/or affect vitamin D metabolism (eg, systemic corticosteroids, any anticonvulsant).

NURSING CONSIDERATIONS

Assessment: Assess that females have had 2 (-) urine or serum pregnancy tests separated by at least 19 days, and are on 2 forms of effective contraception. Assess for hypersensitivity to the drug or vitamin A, history of psychiatric disorder, depression, risk of hyperlipidemia, pregnancy/nursing status, and possible drug interactions. Obtain blood lipids and LFTs.

Monitoring: Monitor for signs/symptoms of psychiatric disorders, pseudotumor cerebri, lipid abnormalities, acute pancreatitis, hearing/visual impairment, inflammatory bowel disease (regional ileitis), hepatotoxicity, premature epiphyseal closure, hyperostosis, musculoskeletal symptoms/abnormalities, hypersensitivity reactions, and other adverse reactions. Monitor lipid levels and LFTs (weekly or biweekly), glucose levels, and CPK levels until response is established. Monitor that females remain on 2 forms of contraception during and for 1 month following discontinuation of therapy.

Patient Counseling: Instruct to read the iPLEDGE and sign the Patient Information/Informed Consent form. Inform male and female patients, not of childbearing potential, the risks and benefits of the drug. Inform females of childbearing potential that 2 forms of contraception are required starting 1 month prior to initiation, during treatment, and for 1 month following discontinuation. Inform that monthly pregnancy tests are required before new prescription is issued. Instruct patients to d/c therapy if signs/symptoms of pseudotumor cerebri (eg, papilledema, headache, N/V) occur. Counsel not to share drug with anyone and not to donate blood during therapy and 1 month following discontinuation. Inform that transient exacerbation (flare) of acne may occur. Instruct to notify physician if depression, mood disturbances, psychosis, or aggression occurs. Instruct to avoid wax epilation and skin resurfacing procedures during and for at least 6 months thereafter. Instruct to avoid prolonged UV rays or sunlight exposure. Inform that dry eye, corneal opacities, and decreased night vision may be experienced, and decreased tolerance to contact lenses during and after therapy may occur. Inform that musculoskeletal symptoms, transient chest pain, back pain in pediatric patients, arthralgias, neutropenia, agranulocytosis, anaphylactic / allergic/severe skin reactions, and inflammatory bowel disease may occur. Inform adolescent patients who participate in sports with repetitive impact that medication may increase their risk of spondylolisthesis or hip growth plate injuries.

Storage: 20-25°C (68-77°F); excursions permitted to 15-30°C (59-86°F). Protect from light.

ABSTRAL – fentanyl CII

Class: Opioid analgesic

Fatal respiratory depression may occur. Contraindicated in the management of acute or postoperative pain (eg, headache/ migraine) and in opioid-nontolerant patients. Keep out of reach of children. Concomitant use with CYP3A4 inhibitors may increase plasma levels, and may cause fatal respiratory depression. Do not convert patients on a mcg-per-mcg basis from any other fentanyl products to Abstral or substitute for any fentanyl products; may result in fatal overdose. Contains fentanyl with abuse liability similar to other opioid analgesics. Available only through a restricted program called Transmucosal Immediate Release Fentanyl (TIRF) Risk Evaluation Mitigation Strategy (REMS) Access program due to risk of misuse, abuse, addiction, and overdose. Outpatients, healthcare professionals who prescribe to outpatients, pharmacies, and distributors must enroll in this program.

ADULT DOSAGE

Pain

Management of Breakthrough Pain in Cancer Patients Already Receiving and are Tolerant to Opioid Therapy for Their Underlying Persistent Cancer Pain:
≥18 Years:
Initial: 100mcg
Adequate Analgesia Obtained w/in 30 Min of Initial Dose: Continue to treat subsequent episodes of breakthrough pain with this dose
Adequate Analgesia Not Obtained After Initial Dose: Use 2nd dose (30 min after initial dose)
Titrate:
Continue dose escalation in a stepwise manner over consecutive breakthrough episodes until adequate analgesia with tolerable side effects is achieved
Increase dose by 100mcg multiples up to 400mcg prn
If adequate analgesia is not obtained w/ 400mcg dose, titrate to 600mcg
If adequate analgesia is not obtained w/ a 600mcg dose, titrate to 800mcg
During titration, patients may use multiples of 100mcg tabs and/or 200mcg tabs for any single dose
May repeat the same dose if adequate analgesia is not obtained 30 min after use
May use rescue medication if adequate analgesia not achieved
Do not use more than 4 tabs at one time

Maint:
Once an appropriate dose for pain management has been established, use only one tab of the appropriate strength per dose

Do not use more than 2 doses to treat an episode of breakthrough pain and wait at least 2 hrs before treating another episode

Conversions

Conversion from Actiq to Abstral:
200mcg: 100mcg
400mcg: 200mcg
600mcg: 200mcg
800mcg: 200mcg
1200mcg: 200mcg
1600mcg: 400mcg

PEDIATRIC DOSAGE

Pediatric use may not have been established

DOSE MODIFICATION

Discontinuation

Patients Who No Longer Require Opioid Therapy: Consider discontinuing w/ a gradual downward titration of other opioids
Patients Who No Longer Require Treatment for Breakthrough Pain: D/C immediately

ADMINISTRATION

SL route

Allow tabs to completely dissolve in the SL cavity; do not chew, suck, or swallow
Do not eat or drink until tab is completely dissolved
In patients who have dry mouth, water may be used to moisten buccal mucosa before taking dose

HOW SUPPLIED

Tab, SL: 100mcg, 200mcg, 300mcg, 400mcg, 600mcg, 800mcg

CONTRAINDICATIONS

Opioid-nontolerant patients, management of acute or postoperative pain (eg, headache/migraine, dental pain, or use in emergency room).

WARNINGS/PRECAUTIONS

May cause anaphylaxis and hypersensitivity reactions. Increased risk of respiratory depression in patients with underlying respiratory disorders and in elderly/debilitated. May impair mental/physical abilities. Caution with chronic obstructive pulmonary disease or preexisting medical conditions predisposing to hypoventilation; may further decrease respiratory drive to the point of respiratory failure. Extreme caution in patients who may be susceptible to intracranial effects of CO_2 retention (eg, with evidence of increased intracranial pressure or impaired consciousness). May obscure clinical course of head injuries. Caution with bradyarrhythmias. Caution with hepatic/renal impairment.

ADVERSE REACTIONS

Respiratory depression, nausea, somnolence, dizziness, headache, constipation, stomatitis, dry mouth, dysgeusia, fatigue, dyspnea, hyperhidrosis, bradycardia, asthenia, anxiety.

DRUG INTERACTIONS

See Boxed Warning. May produce increased depressant effects with other CNS depressants (eg, other opioids, sedatives or hypnotics, general anesthetics, phenothiazines, tranquilizers, skeletal muscle relaxants, sedating antihistamines, and alcoholic beverages); adjust dose if warranted. CYP3A4 inducers (eg, barbiturates, carbamazepine, efavirenz, glucocorticoids, modafinil, nevirapine, oxcarbazepine, phenobarbital, phenytoin, pioglitazone, rifabutin, rifampin, St. John's wort, troglitazone) may decrease levels and efficacy. Not recommended with MAOIs or within 14 days of discontinuation of MAOIs. Respiratory depression is more likely to occur when given with other drugs that depress respiration.

NURSING CONSIDERATIONS

Assessment: Assess for degree of opioid tolerance, previous opioid dose, level of pain intensity, type of pain, patient's general condition and medical status, and for any other conditions where treatment is contraindicated or cautioned. Assess for hypersensitivity to the drug, renal/hepatic function, pregnancy/nursing status, and possible drug interactions.

Monitoring: Monitor for signs/symptoms of respiratory depression, bradycardia, impairment of mental/physical abilities, drug abuse/addiction, hypersensitivity reactions, and other adverse reactions.

Patient Counseling: Inform outpatients to enroll in the TIRF REMS Access program. Counsel that therapy may be fatal in children, in individuals for whom it is not prescribed, and who are not opioid tolerant. Counsel on proper administration and disposal. Advise to take drug as prescribed and avoid sharing it with anyone else. Instruct not to take medication for acute or postoperative pain, pain from injuries, headache, migraine, or any other short-term pain. Instruct to notify physician if breakthrough pain is not alleviated or worsens after taking the drug. Inform that drug may impair mental/physical abilities; caution against performing activities that require high level of attention (eg, driving/using heavy machinery). Advise not to combine with alcohol, sleep aids, or tranquilizers except if ordered by the physician. Instruct to notify physician if pregnant or planning to become pregnant.

Storage: 20-25°C (68-77°F); excursions permitted between 15-30°C (59-86°F). Protect from moisture.

ACANYA — benzoyl peroxide/clindamycin phosphate RX

Class: Antibacterial/keratolytic

ADULT DOSAGE

Acne Vulgaris

Apply a pea-sized amount to face qd

PEDIATRIC DOSAGE

Acne Vulgaris

≥12 Years:

Apply a pea-sized amount to face qd

ADMINISTRATION
Topical route

HOW SUPPLIED
Gel: (Clindamycin-Benzoyl Peroxide) 1.2%-2.5% [50g]

CONTRAINDICATIONS
History of regional enteritis, ulcerative colitis, or antibiotic-associated colitis.

WARNINGS/PRECAUTIONS
Not for oral, ophthalmic, or intravaginal use. Diarrhea, bloody diarrhea, and colitis (including pseudomembranous colitis) reported; d/c if significant diarrhea occurs. Minimize sun exposure including use of tanning beds or sun lamps, following application.

ADVERSE REACTIONS
Erythema, scaling, itching, burning, stinging.

DRUG INTERACTIONS
Caution with topical acne therapy; possible cumulative irritancy effect may occur, especially with the use of peeling, desquamating, or abrasive agents. Caution with other neuromuscular blocking agents. Antiperistaltic agents (eg, opiates, diphenoxylate with atropine) may prolong and/or worsen severe colitis. Avoid with topical or oral erythromycin-containing products.

NURSING CONSIDERATIONS

Assessment: Assess for history of hypersensitivity to drug/lincomycin, regional enteritis, ulcerative colitis, antibiotic-associated colitis, pregnancy/nursing status, and possible drug interactions.

Monitoring: Monitor for local skin reactions, diarrhea, bloody diarrhea, colitis, and other adverse reactions.

Patient Counseling: Instruct to d/c use and contact physician immediately if allergic reactions (eg, severe swelling, SOB) develop. Inform that medication may cause irritation (eg, erythema, scaling, itching, burning), especially when used with other topical acne therapies. Instruct to limit excessive/prolonged exposure to sunlight by wearing a hat or other clothing and using sunscreen. Inform that medication may bleach hair or colored fabric.

Storage: Prior to Dispensing: 2-8°C (36-46°F). After Dispensing: Room temperature up to 25°C (77°F). Do not freeze.

ACCOLATE – zafirlukast RX

Class: Leukotriene receptor antagonist

ADULT DOSAGE
Asthma

Prophylaxis and Chronic Treatment:
20mg bid

PEDIATRIC DOSAGE
Asthma

Prophylaxis and Chronic Treatment:
5-11 Years:
10mg bid

≥12 Years:
20mg bid

ADMINISTRATION
Oral route

Take at least 1 hr ac or 2 hrs pc

HOW SUPPLIED
Tab: 10mg, 20mg

CONTRAINDICATIONS
Hepatic impairment, including hepatic cirrhosis.

WARNINGS/PRECAUTIONS
Life-threatening hepatic failure and liver injury reported. D/C if liver dysfunction is suspected based upon signs/symptoms. Measure LFTs (particularly serum ALT) immediately and manage patient accordingly. Not for use in the reversal of bronchospasm in acute asthma attacks, including status asthmaticus. May continue therapy during acute exacerbations of asthma. Eosinophilic conditions (eg, systemic eosinophilia, eosinophilic pneumonia, or clinical features of vasculitis consistent with Churg-Strauss syndrome) may occur (rare); vasculitic rash, cardiac complications, and/or neuropathy may present. Neuropsychiatric events (eg, insomnia, depression) reported; carefully evaluate risks and benefits of continuing treatment if such events occur.

ADVERSE REACTIONS
Headache, infection, nausea.

DRUG INTERACTIONS
Coadministration with warfarin results in a clinically significant increase in PT; monitor PT closely and adjust anticoagulant dose accordingly when given with oral warfarin. Caution with drugs metabolized by CYP2C9 (eg, tolbutamide, phenytoin, carbamazepine). Decreased levels with erythromycin and liquid theophylline. May increase theophylline levels (rare). Increased levels with aspirin and fluconazole. Moderate and strong CYP2C9 inhibitors may increase exposure. Monitor when coadministered with drugs metabolized by CYP3A4 (eg, dihydropyridine calcium channel blockers, cyclosporine, cisapride).

NURSING CONSIDERATIONS

Assessment: Assess for hypersensitivity to drug, hepatic impairment, hepatic cirrhosis, asthma status, pregnancy/nursing status, and possible drug interactions.

Monitoring: Monitor for signs/symptoms of eosinophilic conditions, vasculitic rash, worsening pulmonary symptoms, cardiac complications, neuropathy, neuropsychiatric events, and other adverse reactions. Monitor LFTs periodically. Closely monitor PT when given with oral warfarin.

Patient Counseling: Inform that hepatic dysfunction may occur; instruct to contact physician immediately if symptoms of hepatic dysfunction occur. Advise to take regularly as prescribed, even during symptom-free periods. Inform that it is not a bronchodilator and should not be used to treat acute episodes of asthma. Instruct not to decrease dose or stop taking any other antiasthma medications unless instructed by a physician. Instruct to notify physician if neuropsychiatric events occur. Instruct not to take the medication if breastfeeding.

Storage: 20-25°C (68-77°F). Protect from light and moisture.

AccuNeb – albuterol sulfate

RX

Class: Beta$_2$-agonist

PEDIATRIC DOSAGE

Bronchospasm

2-12 Years w/ Asthma:
Initial: 0.63mg or 1.25mg tid-qid prn

6-12 Years w/ More Severe Asthma (Baseline FEV$_1$ <60% Predicted), Weight >40kg, or 11-12 Years:
May achieve better initial response w/ 1.25mg dose

ADMINISTRATION
Inh route
Administer using a jet nebulizer connected to an air compressor w/ adequate air flow, equipped w/ a mouthpiece or suitable face mask
Use the entire contents of one unit-dose vial (3mL of 1.25mg or 0.63mg inh sol)
Adjust nebulizer flow rate to deliver over 5 to 15 min

HOW SUPPLIED
Sol, Inhalation: 0.63mg/3mL, 1.25mg/3mL

WARNINGS/PRECAUTIONS
Can produce paradoxical bronchospasm; d/c if this occurs. Consider adding anti-inflammatory agents (eg, corticosteroids) to adequately control asthma. Reevaluate patient and treatment regimen if deterioration of asthma observed. Can produce clinically significant cardiovascular (CV) effect (eg, ECG changes); caution with CV disorders (eg, coronary insufficiency, cardiac arrhythmias, HTN). Immediate hypersensitivity reactions reported. Aggravation of preexisting diabetes mellitus (DM) and ketoacidosis reported with large doses of IV albuterol. May cause hypokalemia. Has not been studied with acute attacks of bronchospasm.

ADVERSE REACTIONS
Asthma exacerbation, otitis media, allergic reaction, gastroenteritis, cold symptoms.

DRUG INTERACTIONS
Avoid other short-acting sympathomimetic aerosol bronchodilators and epinephrine. Extreme caution with MAOIs or TCAs, or within 2 weeks of discontinuation of such agents; action of albuterol may be potentiated. May decrease serum levels of digoxin; monitor levels. May worsen ECG changes and/or hypokalemia caused by non-K sparing diuretics (eg, loop/thiazide); caution is advised. Pulmonary effect blocked by β-blockers; caution with cardioselective β-blockers.

NURSING CONSIDERATIONS

Assessment: Assess for previous hypersensitivity to the drug, CV disorders, HTN, DM, pregnancy/nursing status, and possible drug interactions.

Monitoring: Monitor for signs/symptoms of CV effects (measured by pulse rate and BP), worsening of symptoms, paradoxical bronchospasm, deterioration of asthma, hypokalemia, and hypersensitivity reactions.

Patient Counseling: Instruct not to use more frequently than recommended. Advise not to increase dose or frequency without consulting physician. Counsel to seek medical attention if symptoms worsen, if therapy becomes less effective, or if there is need to use the drug more frequently than usual. Inform of the common effects (eg, palpitations, chest pain, rapid HR, tremor, nervousness). Advise not to use if the contents of vial change color or become cloudy. Inform that drug compatibility, clinical efficacy, and safety, when mixed with other drugs in nebulizer, have not been established.

Storage: 2-25°C (36-77°F). Protect from light and excessive heat. Store in protective foil pouch at all times. Once removed, use within 1 week. Discard if sol not colorless.

ACCUPRIL – quinapril hydrochloride — RX

Class: ACE inhibitor

D/C if pregnancy is detected. Drugs that act directly on the renin-angiotensin system (RAS) can cause injury/death to the developing fetus.

ADULT DOSAGE

Hypertension

Initial: 10mg or 20mg qd
Titrate: May adjust dosage at intervals of at least 2 weeks
Usual: 20mg, 40mg, or 80mg/day, given as single dose or in 2 equally divided doses

Heart Failure

Adjunctive therapy when added to conventional therapy, including diuretics and/or digitalis
Initial: 5mg bid
Titrate: Adjust weekly
Usual: 20-40mg/day given in 2 equally divided doses

PEDIATRIC DOSAGE

Pediatric use may not have been established

DOSE MODIFICATION

Concomitant Medications

HTN:
Concomitant Diuretics: 5mg qd
Titrate: Adjust to the optimal response
If possible, d/c diuretic 2-3 days prior to therapy to avoid hypotension. If BP is not controlled with quinapril alone, diuretic therapy should be resumed

Renal Impairment

HTN
CrCl >60mL/min:
Max Initial: 10mg/day
CrCl 30-60mL/min:
Max Initial: 5mg/day
CrCl 10-30mL/min:
Max Initial: 2.5mg/day

HF and Renal Impairment or Hyponatremia
CrCl >30mL/min:
Initial: 5mg/day
CrCl 10-30mL/min:
Initial: 2.5mg/day
Titrate: Increase dose at weekly intervals

Elderly

≥65 Years

HTN:
Initial: 10mg qd
Titrate: Adjust to the optimal response

ADMINISTRATION
Oral route

HOW SUPPLIED
Tab: 5mg*, 10mg, 20mg, 40mg *scored

CONTRAINDICATIONS
History of ACE inhibitor-associated angioedema. Coadministration with aliskiren in patients with diabetes.

WARNINGS/PRECAUTIONS
Less effect on BP and more reports of angioedema in blacks than nonblacks. Head/neck angioedema reported; d/c and administer appropriate therapy if laryngeal stridor or angioedema of the face, tongue, or glottis occurs. Intestinal angioedema reported; monitor for abdominal pain. Patients with history of angioedema unrelated to ACE inhibitor therapy may be at increased risk of angioedema during therapy. Anaphylactoid reactions reported during desensitization with hymenoptera venom, dialysis with high-flux membranes, and LDL apheresis with dextran sulfate absorption. Associated with syndrome that starts with cholestatic jaundice and progresses to fulminant hepatic necrosis and, sometimes, death; d/c if jaundice or marked hepatic enzyme elevations occur. Excessive hypotension sometimes associated with oliguria, azotemia, and (rarely) acute renal failure and/or death may occur. Risk factors for excessive hypotension include HF, hyponatremia, high-dose diuretic therapy, recent intensive diuresis, dialysis, or severe volume and/or salt depletion; eliminate or reduce the diuretic or cautiously increase salt intake (except with HF) prior to therapy and monitor closely. May cause agranulocytosis and bone marrow depression. May cause renal function changes. May increase BUN and SrCr levels with renal artery stenosis or without renal vascular disease. Risk of hyperkalemia with diabetes mellitus (DM) and renal dysfunction. Persistent nonproductive cough reported. Hypotension may occur with surgery or during anesthesia. Caution in elderly.

ADVERSE REACTIONS
Headache, dizziness, cough.

DRUG INTERACTIONS
See Contraindications. Dual blockade of the RAS is associated with increased risks of hypotension, hyperkalemia, and changes in renal function (including acute renal failure); avoid combined use of RAS inhibitors. Closely monitor BP, renal function, and electrolytes with concomitant agents that also affect the RAS. Avoid concomitant use of aliskiren in patients with renal impairment (GFR <60mL/min). Hypotension risk and increased BUN and SrCr with diuretics. Coadministration with NSAIDs, including selective COX-2 inhibitors, may attenuate antihypertensive effect of ACE inhibitors, and may further deteriorate renal function. Decreases tetracycline absorption (possibly due to Mg^{2+} content in quinapril); consider interaction with drugs that interact with Mg^{2+}. Increased risk of hyperkalemia with K^+-sparing diuretics (eg, spironolactone, amiloride, triamterene), K^+ supplements, or K^+-containing salt substitutes; use caution and monitor serum K^+. May increase lithium levels and risk of toxicity; use caution and monitor serum lithium levels. Nitritoid reactions reported rarely with injectable gold (eg, sodium aurothiomalate). Increased risk for angioedema with mammalian target of rapamycin inhibitor (eg, temsirolimus) therapy.

NURSING CONSIDERATIONS

Assessment: Assess for history of angioedema, hypersensitivity to drug, volume/salt depletion, collagen vascular disease, DM, renal artery stenosis, ischemic heart disease, cerebrovascular disease, renal function, pregnancy/nursing status, and possible drug interactions.

Monitoring: Monitor for signs/symptoms of hypotension, anaphylactoid or hypersensitivity reactions, head/neck/intestinal angioedema, agranulocytosis, neutropenia, bone marrow depression, cholestatic jaundice, fulminant hepatic necrosis, and hyperkalemia. Monitor BP and renal function. Monitor WBC count periodically in patients with collagen vascular disease and/or renal disease.

Patient Counseling: Inform of pregnancy risks and instruct to notify physician as soon as possible if pregnant/planning to become pregnant. Instruct to d/c therapy and immediately report signs/symptoms of angioedema. Caution about lightheadedness, especially during the 1st few days of therapy and advise to report to physician. Instruct to d/c and consult physician if syncope occurs. Caution that inadequate fluid intake or excessive perspiration, diarrhea, or vomiting may lead to an excessive fall in BP, resulting in lightheadedness or syncope. Instruct to inform physician about therapy if planning to undergo surgery/anesthesia. Instruct to avoid K^+ supplements or salt substitutes containing K^+ without consulting physician. Advise to report any symptoms of infection.

Storage: 15-30°C (59-86°F). Protect from light.

ACETAMINOPHEN AND CODEINE TABLETS – acetaminophen/codeine phosphate CIII

Class: Opioid analgesic

Associated with cases of acute liver failure, at times resulting in liver transplant and death. Most cases of liver injury are associated with acetaminophen (APAP) use at doses >4000mg/day, and often involve >1 APAP-containing product. Respiratory depression and death reported in children who received codeine following tonsillectomy and/or adenoidectomy and had evidence of being ultra-rapid metabolizers of codeine due to a CYP2D6 polymorphism.

OTHER BRAND NAMES

Tylenol with Codeine

ADULT DOSAGE

Mild to Moderately Severe Pain

Adjust dose according to severity of pain and response

Usual Range (Single Dose): 15mg-60mg codeine; 300mg-1000mg acetaminophen (APAP); may repeat doses up to q4h

Max: 360mg/24 hrs codeine; 4000mg/24 hrs APAP

PEDIATRIC DOSAGE

Pediatric use may not have been established

ADMINISTRATION

Oral route

HOW SUPPLIED

Tab: (APAP/Codeine) 300mg/15mg; (Tylenol with Codeine) 300mg/30mg, 300mg/60mg

CONTRAINDICATIONS

Postoperative pain management in children who have undergone tonsillectomy and/or adenoidectomy.

WARNINGS/PRECAUTIONS

Increased risk of acute liver failure in patients with underlying liver disease. May cause serious skin reactions (eg, acute generalized exanthematous pustulosis, Stevens-Johnson syndrome, toxic epidermal necrolysis), which can be fatal; d/c at the 1st appearance of skin rash or any other sign of hypersensitivity. Deaths reported in nursing infants exposed to high levels of morphine because their mothers were ultra-rapid metabolizers of codeine. Ultra-rapid metabolizers, due to specific CYP2D6 genotype (gene duplications denoted as *1/*1xN or *1/*2xN), may have life-threatening or fatal respiratory depression or experience signs of overdose (eg, extreme sleepiness, confusion, shallow breathing). Choose lowest effective dose for the shortest period of time. Hypersensitivity and anaphylaxis reported; d/c if signs/symptoms occur. Respiratory-depressant effects and capacity for elevating CSF pressure may be markedly enhanced in the presence of head injury or other intracranial lesions. May obscure diagnosis or clinical course of head injuries and acute abdominal conditions. Habit-forming and potentially abusable; extended use is not recommended. Caution with severe renal/hepatic impairment, head injuries, elevated intracranial pressure, acute abdominal conditions, hypothyroidism, urethral stricture, Addison's disease, prostatic hypertrophy, and in the elderly or debilitated. May increase serum amylase levels. Lab test interactions may occur. Avoid during labor if delivery of a premature infant is anticipated. (Tylenol with Codeine) Contains sodium metabisulfite; may cause allergic-type reactions in certain susceptible people.

ADVERSE REACTIONS

Acute liver failure, drowsiness, lightheadedness, dizziness, sedation, SOB, N/V.

DRUG INTERACTIONS

Increased risk of acute liver failure with alcohol ingestion. May enhance effects of other narcotic analgesics, alcohol, general anesthetics, tranquilizers (eg, chlordiazepoxide), sedative-hypnotics, or other CNS depressants; may increase CNS depression.

NURSING CONSIDERATIONS

Assessment: Assess for hypersensitivity to drug, hepatic/renal impairment, head injury, intracranial lesions, acute abdominal conditions, any other conditions where treatment is contraindicated or cautioned, pregnancy/nursing status, and possible drug interactions.

Monitoring: Monitor for signs/symptoms of hepatotoxicity, respiratory depression, skin reactions, hypersensitivity, anaphylaxis, elevation in CSF pressure, drug abuse, tolerance, dependence, and other adverse reactions. Monitor effects of therapy with serial LFTs and/or renal function tests in patients with severe hepatic/renal disease. Closely monitor newborn infants for signs of respiratory depression if the mother received the drug during labor.

Patient Counseling: Instruct to d/c therapy and contact physician immediately if signs of allergy develop. Instruct to look for APAP on package labels and not to use >1 APAP-containing product. Instruct to seek medical attention immediately upon ingestion of >4000mg/day APAP, even if patient is feeling well. Advise that drug may impair mental/physical abilities. Instruct to avoid performing potentially hazardous tasks (eg, driving, operating machinery), drinking alcohol, or taking other CNS depressants while on therapy. Inform that drug may be habit-forming; instruct to take ud.

Storage: 20-25°C (68-77°F).

ACIPHEX – rabeprazole sodium RX

Class: Proton pump inhibitor

OTHER BRAND NAMES

Aciphex Sprinkle

ADULT DOSAGE

***Helicobacter pylori* Eradication**

Treatment of *H. pylori* infection and duodenal ulcer disease (active or history w/in past 5 yrs) for *H. pylori* eradication to reduce the risk of duodenal ulcer recurrence

Usual: 20mg tab + clarithromycin 500mg + amoxicillin 1000mg, all bid w/ am and pm meals for 7 days

Pathological Hypersecretory Conditions

Treatment of pathological hypersecretory conditions, including Zollinger-Ellison syndrome

Initial: 60mg qd or in divided doses

Titrate: Adjust to individual needs and continue for as long as clinically indicated

Doses up to 100mg qd and 60mg bid have been administered. Some have been treated for up to 1 yr

Gastroesophageal Reflux Disease

Healing of Erosive or Ulcerative GERD:

20mg tab qd for 4-8 weeks; consider an additional 8 weeks if not healed after 8 weeks of treatment

Maint of Healing of Erosive or Ulcerative GERD:

20mg tab qd; controlled studies do not extend beyond 12 months

Symptomatic GERD:

Treatment of daytime and nighttime heartburn and other symptoms associated w/ GERD

20mg tab qd for 4 weeks; consider an additional course of treatment if symptoms do not resolve completely after 4 weeks

Duodenal Ulcers

Healing and Symptomatic Relief of Duodenal Ulcers:

20mg tab qd after am meal for up to 4 weeks; some patients may need additional therapy to achieve healing

PEDIATRIC DOSAGE

Gastroesophageal Reflux Disease

Treatment of GERD:

Cap:

1-11 Years:

<15kg: 5mg qd for up to 12 weeks w/ the option to increase to 10mg if inadequate response

≥15kg: 10mg qd for up to 12 weeks

Treatment of Symptomatic GERD:

Tab:

≥12 Years:

20mg qd for up to 8 weeks

ADMINISTRATION

Oral route

Tab

Swallow whole; do not chew, crush, or split

May be taken w/ or w/o food

Cap
Take 30 min ac
Open cap and sprinkle entire contents on a small amount of soft food (eg, applesauce, fruit or vegetable based baby food, yogurt) or empty contents into a small amount of liquid (eg, infant formula, apple juice, pediatric electrolyte sol); do not chew or crush granules
Take whole dose w/in 15 min of preparation
Food or liquid should be at or below room temperature; do not store mixture for future use

HOW SUPPLIED
Cap, Delayed-Release (Sprinkle): 5mg, 10mg; Tab, Delayed-Release: 20mg

WARNINGS/PRECAUTIONS
Symptomatic response does not preclude the presence of gastric malignancy. Acute interstitial nephritis reported; d/c if this develops. Cyanocobalamin (vitamin B12) deficiency may occur with daily long-term treatment (eg, >3 yrs) with any acid-suppressing medications. May increase risk of *Clostridium difficile*-associated diarrhea (CDAD), especially in hospitalized patients. May increase risk of osteoporosis-related fractures of the hip, wrist, or spine, especially with high-dose and long-term therapy. Use lowest dose and shortest duration appropriate to the condition being treated. Hypomagnesemia reported and may require Mg^{2+} replacement and discontinuation of therapy; consider monitoring Mg^{2+} levels prior to and periodically during therapy with prolonged treatment. Caution with severe hepatic impairment.

ADVERSE REACTIONS
Headache, flatulence, pain, pharyngitis, diarrhea, N/V, abdominal pain.

DRUG INTERACTIONS
May reduce absorption of drugs where gastric pH is an important determinant of their bioavailability; ketoconazole, atazanavir, iron salts, erlotinib, and mycophenolate mofetil (MMF) absorption can decrease, while digoxin absorption can increase. May substantially decrease atazanavir levels and reduce its therapeutic effect; concomitant use is not recommended. Caution in transplant patients receiving MMF. May inhibit cyclosporine metabolism. Increased INR and PT reported with warfarin. Combination with amoxicillin and clarithromycin may increase levels of rabeprazole and 14-hydroxyclarithromycin. May elevate and prolong levels of methotrexate (MTX) and/or its metabolite, possibly leading to MTX toxicities; consider temporary withdrawal of therapy with high-dose MTX. Caution with digoxin or with drugs that may cause hypomagnesemia (eg, diuretics).

NURSING CONSIDERATIONS

Assessment: Assess for hypersensitivity to the drug, hepatic impairment, risk for osteoporosis-related fractures, pregnancy/nursing status, and possible drug interactions. Obtain baseline Mg^{2+} levels.

Monitoring: Monitor for signs/symptoms of acute interstitial nephritis, cyanocobalamin deficiency, CDAD, bone fractures, hypersensitivity reactions, and other adverse reactions. Monitor Mg^{2+} levels periodically. Monitor INR and PT when given with warfarin.

Patient Counseling: Instruct to take ud. Advise to immediately report and seek care for diarrhea that does not improve.

Storage: 25°C (77°F); excursions permitted to 15-30°C (59-86°F). Protect from moisture.

ACTEMRA – tocilizumab

RX

Class: Interleukin-6 receptor antagonist

Increased risk for developing serious infections (eg, active tuberculosis (TB), invasive fungal infections, bacterial/viral infections due to opportunistic pathogens) that may lead to hospitalization or death. Most patients who developed these infections were taking concomitant immunosuppressants (eg, methotrexate [MTX], corticosteroids). If serious infection develops, interrupt treatment until infection is controlled. Test for latent TB prior to and during therapy; initiate latent TB treatment prior to therapy. Consider risks and benefits prior to initiating therapy in patients w/ chronic or recurrent infection. Monitor for development of signs/symptoms of infection during and after treatment.

ADULT DOSAGE

Rheumatoid Arthritis

Moderately to Severely Active:
IV:
Usual: 4mg/kg every 4 weeks; may increase to 8mg/kg every 4 weeks based on clinical response
Max: 800mg/infusion

PEDIATRIC DOSAGE

Juvenile Idiopathic Arthritis

≥2 Years:
IV:
Active Polyarticular Juvenile Idiopathic Arthritis:
<30kg: 10mg/kg every 4 weeks
≥30kg: 8mg/kg every 4 weeks

SQ:
<100kg: 162mg every other week, followed by an increase to every week based on response
≥100kg: 162mg every week
Transition from IV to SQ:
Administer 1st SQ dose instead of the next scheduled IV dose
May be used alone or in combination w/ methotrexate or other nonbiologic disease-modifying antirheumatic drugs

Active Systemic Juvenile Idiopathic Arthritis:
<30kg: 12mg/kg every 2 weeks
≥30 kg: 8mg/kg every 2 weeks
May be used alone or in combination w/ methotrexate
Do not change dose based on a single visit body weight measurement

DOSE MODIFICATION
Adverse Reactions
Rheumatoid Arthritis:
Liver Enzyme Abnormalities:
>1-3X ULN: Modify dose of concomitant disease-modifying antirheumatic drugs if appropriate. For persistent increases in this range, reduce dose to 4mg/kg or hold until ALT or AST have normalized if receiving IV. If receiving SQ, reduce inj frequency to every other week or hold dosing until ALT/AST have normalized and resume at every other week and increase frequency
>3-5X ULN: Hold until <3X ULN and follow recommendations above for >1-3X ULN. If persistent increases in this range, d/c therapy
>5X ULN: D/C
Low ANC:
ANC <500/mm^3: D/C
ANC 500-1000/mm^3: Hold dosing until ANC >1000/mm^3. If receiving IV, resume at 4mg/kg and increase to 8mg/kg; if receiving SQ, resume at every other week and increase to every week
Low Platelet Counts:
<50,000/mm^3: D/C
50,000-100,000/mm^3: Hold until >100,000/mm^3. If receiving IV, resume at 4mg/kg and increase to 8mg/kg. If receiving SQ, resume at every other week and increase to every week
Polyarticular/Systemic Juvenile Idiopathic Arthritis:
Dose reduction recommended for liver enzyme abnormalities, low neutrophil counts, and low platelet counts at levels similar to patients w/ rheumatoid arthritis
If appropriate, dose modify or stop methotrexate and/or other medications and hold therapy until clinical situation has been evaluated
Decision to d/c for a lab abnormality should be based on medical assessment of patient

ADMINISTRATION
IV/SQ route
Do not initiated therapy in patients w/ an ANC <2000/mm^3, platelet count <100,000/mm^3, or who have ALT or AST >1.5X ULN
Do not administer as IV bolus/push
IV
Preparation:
Polyarticular and Systemic Juvenile Idiopathic Arthritis:
<30kg: Use a 50mL infusion bag/bottle of 0.9% NaCl
≥30kg: Use a 100ml infusion bag/bottle of 0.9% NaCl
Rheumatoid Arthritis:
≥30kg: Use a 100mL infusion bag/bottle of 0.9% NaCl
Dilution:
Withdraw a volume of 0.9% NaCl inj, equal to volume of tocilizumab inj required for patient's dose from infusion bag/bottle
Withdraw amount of tocilizumab for IV infusion from vial(s) and add slowly into NaCl infusion bag/bottle; gently invert bag to avoid foaming to mix sol
Administration:
Administer infusion over 60 min, and must be administered w/ an infusion set
Do not infuse concomitantly in same IV line w/ other drugs
Fully diluted sol are compatible w/ polypropylene, polyethylene and polyvinyl chloride infusion bags and polypropylene, polyethylene, and glass infusion bottles
SQ
Inject full amount in syringe (0.9mL), which provides 162mg of tocilizumab
Rotate inj sites w/ each inj and never inj into moles, scars, or areas where the skin is tender, bruised, red, hard, or not intact

HOW SUPPLIED
Inj: 20mg/mL [4mL, 10mL, 20mL vials]; 162mg/0.9mL [prefilled syringe]

WARNINGS/PRECAUTIONS
Avoid w/ active infection, including localized infections. Caution in patients who have been exposed to TB, w/ history of serious/opportunistic infection, who resided or traveled in areas of endemic

TB/mycoses, or w/ underlying conditions that may predispose them to infection. Viral reactivation and herpes zoster exacerbation observed. GI perforation reported; caution in patients at risk for GI perforation. Neutropenia, thrombocytopenia, elevation of liver enzymes, and increase in lipid parameters reported; do not initiate treatment if ANC <2000/mm^3, platelets <100,000/mm^3, or ALT/AST >1.5X ULN. D/C treatment w/ ANC <500/mm^3, platelets <50,000/mm^3, or ALT/AST >5X ULN. May increase risk of malignancies. Hypersensitivity reactions, including anaphylaxis and death, reported; d/c immediately and permanently if anaphylaxis or other hypersensitivity reaction occurs. Should only be infused IV by a healthcare professional w/ appropriate medical support to manage anaphylaxis. MS and chronic inflammatory demyelinating polyneuropathy reported rarely in RA studies; caution w/ preexisting or recent onset demyelinating disorders. Not recommended in patients w/ active hepatic disease or hepatic impairment. Caution in elderly.

ADVERSE REACTIONS

URTIs, nasopharyngitis, headache, HTN, increased ALT/AST, dizziness, bronchitis, infusion reaction, neutropenia, diarrhea, inj-site reaction, total cholesterol elevation, increased LDL.

DRUG INTERACTIONS

See Boxed Warning. Avoid w/ live vaccines. May increase metabolism of CYP450 substrates (eg, 1A2, 2B6, 2C9, 2C19, 2D6, 3A4). Upon initiation or discontinuation of tocilizumab, monitor therapeutic effect (eg, warfarin) or drug concentrations (eg, cyclosporine, theophylline) and adjust dose prn. Caution w/ CYP3A4 substrates where decrease in effectiveness is undesirable (eg, oral contraceptives, lovastatin, atorvastatin). Avoid w/ biological DMARDs (eg, TNF antagonists, interleukin [IL]-1R antagonists, anti-CD20 monoclonal antibodies, selective costimulation modulators) due to increased immunosuppression and risk of infection. Increased frequency and magnitude of transaminase elevations w/ hepatotoxic drugs (eg, MTX). Decreased exposure of simvastatin and omeprazole.

NURSING CONSIDERATIONS

Assessment: Assess for infections (eg, bacteria, fungi, viruses), including latent TB. Assess for demyelinating disorders, risk of GI perforation, active hepatic disease or impairment, hypersensitivity to drug, pregnancy/nursing status, and possible drug interactions. Obtain baseline lipid levels and platelet, liver transaminases, and neutrophil counts.

Monitoring: Monitor for signs/symptoms of TB and other infections. Monitor for hypersensitivity reactions, GI perforation, malignancies, and demyelinating disorders. Monitor neutrophil counts, platelet counts, and LFTs, after 4-8 weeks after initiation and every 3 months thereafter in RA patients, or at the time of 2nd infusion and every 4-8 weeks thereafter in PJIA patients, or every 2-4 weeks thereafter in SJIA patients. Monitor lipid levels 4-8 weeks after initiation then at approx 24-week intervals.

Patient Counseling: Advise of the potential risks/benefits of therapy. Inform that therapy may lower resistance to infections and may cause serious GI side effects; instruct to contact physician if symptoms of infection or severe, persistent abdominal pain appear. Advise to inform physician of travel history, especially to places that are endemic for TB/mycoses. Inform that some patients have developed serious allergic reactions, including anaphylaxis. Advise to seek immediate medical attention if any symptoms of serious allergic reactions develop. Inform of inj techniques and procedures. Advise not to reuse needles/syringes and instruct on proper disposal procedures.

Storage: 2-8°C (36-46°F). Do not freeze. Protect from light; store in original package until time of use. Keep syringes dry. Diluted Sol for Infusion: 2-8°C (36-46°F) or room temperature for up to 24 hrs. Protect from light. Discard unused portion.

Actiq – fentanyl citrate **CII**

Class: Opioid analgesic

Fatal respiratory depression may occur. Contraindicated in the management of acute or postoperative pain (eg, headache/migraine) and in opioid-nontolerant patients. Death reported upon accidental ingestion in children; keep out of reach of children. Concomitant use with CYP3A4 inhibitors may increase plasma levels, and may cause fatal respiratory depression. Do not convert patients on a mcg-per-mcg basis from any other fentanyl products to Actiq. Do not substitute for any other fentanyl products; may result in fatal overdose. Contains fentanyl with abuse liability similar to other opioid analgesics. Available only through a restricted program called Transmucosal Immediate Release Fentanyl (TIRF) Risk Evaluation Mitigation Strategy (REMS) Access program due to risk of misuse, abuse, addiction, and overdose. Outpatients, healthcare professionals who prescribe to outpatients, pharmacies, and distributors must enroll in the program.

ADULT DOSAGE

Cancer Pain

Breakthrough Pain in Patients Already Receiving and Tolerant to Around-the-Clock Opioid Therapy:

Initial: 200mcg

Dispense no more than 6 units initially

PEDIATRIC DOSAGE

Cancer Pain

Breakthrough Pain in Patients Already Receiving and Tolerant to Around-the-Clock Opioid Therapy:

≥16 Years:

Initial: 200mcg

Titrate:
If signs of excessive opioid effects appear before unit is consumed, remove dosage unit, dispose properly, and decrease subsequent doses
If breakthrough pain is not relieved 15 min after completion of previous dose, give only 1 additional dose of the same strength
Maint: Once titrated to an effective dose, use only 1 unit of the appropriate strength per breakthrough pain episode; limit to ≤4 units/day
Max: 2 doses/breakthrough pain episode; wait ≥4 hrs before treating another breakthrough pain episode

Increase dose only when a single administration of current dose fails to adequately treat breakthrough pain episode for several consecutive episodes

If >4 breakthrough pain episodes/day are experienced, reevaluate maint dose (around-the-clock) used for persistent pain

Dispense no more than 6 units initially
Titrate:
If signs of excessive opioid effects appear before unit is consumed, remove dosage unit, dispose properly, and decrease subsequent doses
If breakthrough pain is not relieved 15 min after completion of previous dose, give only 1 additional dose of the same strength
Maint: Once titrated to an effective dose, use only 1 unit of the appropriate strength per breakthrough pain episode; limit to ≤4 units/day
Max: 2 doses/breakthrough pain episode; wait ≥4 hrs before treating another breakthrough pain episode

Increase dose only when a single administration of current dose fails to adequately treat breakthrough pain episode for several consecutive episodes

If >4 breakthrough pain episodes/day are experienced, reevaluate maint dose (around-the-clock) used for persistent pain

DOSE MODIFICATION
Discontinuation
Gradually titrate dose downward

ADMINISTRATION
Oral route

Place unit in mouth between cheek and lower gum, occasionally moving the drug matrix from one side to the other using the handle
Do not suck or chew
Consume unit over a 15-min period

HOW SUPPLIED
Loz: 200mcg, 400mcg, 600mcg, 800mcg, 1200mcg, 1600mcg

CONTRAINDICATIONS
Opioid-nontolerant patients, management of acute or postoperative pain, including headache/migraine and dental pain.

WARNINGS/PRECAUTIONS
Increased risk of respiratory depression in patients with underlying respiratory disorders and in elderly/debilitated. May impair mental/physical abilities. Caution with chronic obstructive pulmonary disease or preexisting medical conditions predisposing to respiratory depression; may further decrease respiratory drive to the point of respiratory failure. Extreme caution in patients who may be susceptible to the intracranial effects of CO_2 retention (eg, with evidence of increased intracranial pressure or impaired consciousness). May obscure clinical course of head injuries. Caution with bradyarrhythmias. Anaphylaxis and hypersensitivity reported. Avoid use during labor and delivery. Caution with renal/hepatic impairment.

ADVERSE REACTIONS
Respiratory depression, circulatory depression, hypotension, shock, N/V, headache, constipation, dizziness, dyspnea, anxiety, somnolence, asthenia, confusion, depression.

DRUG INTERACTIONS
See Boxed Warning. Respiratory depression is more likely to occur when given with other drugs that depress respiration. Increased depressant effects with other CNS depressants (eg, other opioids, sedatives, hypnotics, general anesthetics, phenothiazines, tranquilizers, skeletal muscle relaxants, sedating antihistamines, alcoholic beverages); adjust dose if warranted. Avoid with grapefruit and grapefruit juice. CYP3A4 inducers may decrease levels. Not recommended with MAOIs or within 14 days of discontinuation of MAOIs.

NURSING CONSIDERATIONS

Assessment: Assess for degree of opioid tolerance, previous opioid dose, level of pain intensity, type of pain, patient's general condition and medical status, and any other conditions where treatment is contraindicated or cautioned. Assess for hypersensitivity to the drug, renal/hepatic function, pregnancy/nursing status, and possible drug interactions.

Monitoring: Monitor for signs/symptoms of respiratory depression, impairment of mental/physical abilities, bradycardia, anaphylaxis/hypersensitivity, abuse/addiction, and other adverse reactions.

Patient Counseling: Advise to enroll in TIRF REMS Access program. Instruct to keep drug out of reach of children. Advise to take drug as prescribed and avoid sharing it with anyone else. Instruct to notify physician if breakthrough pain is not alleviated or worsens after taking the drug. Inform that drug may impair mental/physical abilities; caution against performing activities that require high level of attention (eg, driving/using heavy machinery). Advise not to combine with alcohol, sleep aids, or tranquilizers, except if ordered by the physician. Instruct to notify physician if pregnant or planning to become pregnant. Inform that frequent consumption may increase risk of dental decay; advise to consult dentist to ensure appropriate oral hygiene. Inform diabetics that drug contains approximately 2g sugar/U. Inform of proper storage, administration, and disposal.

Storage: 20-25°C (68-77°F); excursions permitted between 15-30°C (59-86°F). Protect from freezing and moisture.

ACTONEL – risedronate sodium — RX

Class: Bisphosphonate

ADULT DOSAGE

Osteoporosis

Treatment/Prevention of Postmenopausal Osteoporosis:
5mg qd, or 35mg once a week, or 75mg taken on 2 consecutive days for a total of 2 tabs/month, or 150mg once a month

Osteoporosis in Men:
35mg once a week

Treatment/Prevention of Glucocorticoid-Induced Osteoporosis:
5mg qd
Periodically reevaluate the need for continued therapy

Paget's Disease

30mg qd for 2 months

May consider retreatment (following post-treatment observation of at least 2 months) if relapse occurs, or if treatment fails to normalize serum alkaline phosphatase

Periodically reevaluate the need for continued therapy

Missed Dose

35mg Once a Week is Missed:
Take 1 tab on the am after remembering missed dose and return to taking 1 tab/week as originally scheduled on chosen day. Do not take 2 tabs on same day

One or Both 75mg Tabs (Taken on 2 Consecutive Days/Month) are Missed:
Next Month's Scheduled Doses are >7 Days Away:
If both tabs are missed, take one 75mg tab in the am after the day it is remembered, then take the other tab on the next consecutive am. If only one 75mg tab is missed, take the missed tab in the am after the day it is remembered. Return to taking 75mg tabs on 2 consecutive days per month as originally scheduled. Do not take more than two 75mg tabs w/in 7 days
Next Month's Scheduled Doses are w/in 7 Days:
Wait until the next month's scheduled doses and continue as originally scheduled

150mg Once a Month is Missed:
Next Month's Scheduled Dose is >7 Days

PEDIATRIC DOSAGE

Pediatric use may not have been established

Away:
Take missed tab in the am after the day it is remembered, then return to taking 150mg once a month as originally scheduled. Do not take more than one 150mg tab w/in 7 days
Next Month's Scheduled Doses are w/in 7 Days:
Wait until the next month's scheduled doses and continue as originally scheduled

ADMINISTRATION
Oral route
Take at least 30 min before the 1st food or drink of the day other than water, and before taking any oral medication or supplementation
Swallow tabs whole; do not chew or suck the tab
Swallow tabs w/ full glass of plain water (6-8 oz); avoid lying down for 30 min after taking medication

HOW SUPPLIED
Tab: 5mg, 30mg, 35mg, 150mg

CONTRAINDICATIONS
Esophageal abnormalities that delay esophageal emptying (eg, stricture or achalasia), inability to stand or sit upright for at least 30 min, and hypocalcemia.

WARNINGS/PRECAUTIONS
Consider discontinuation after 3-5 yrs of use in patients at low risk for fracture; periodically reevaluate risk for fracture in patients who d/c therapy. Contains same active ingredient as Atelvia; do not treat with Actonel if on concomitant therapy with Atelvia. May cause local irritation of the upper GI mucosa; caution with active upper GI problems (eg, Barrett's esophagus, dysphagia, esophageal diseases, gastritis, duodenitis, ulcers). Esophageal reactions (eg, esophagitis, esophageal ulcers/erosions) reported; d/c if dysphagia, odynophagia, retrosternal pain, or new/worsening heartburn develops. Use therapy under appropriate supervision in patients who cannot comply with dosing instructions due to mental disability. Gastric and duodenal ulcers reported. Hypocalcemia reported; treat hypocalcemia and other disturbances of bone and mineral metabolism before therapy, and ensure adequate Ca^{2+} and vitamin D intake. Osteonecrosis of the jaw (ONJ) reported; risk may increase with duration of exposure to drug. For patients requiring invasive dental procedures, discontinuation of treatment may reduce risk for ONJ. Consider discontinuation if ONJ develops. Severe and occasionally incapacitating bone, joint, and/or muscle pain reported; consider discontinuation if severe symptoms develop. Atypical, low-energy, or low-trauma fractures of the femoral shaft reported; evaluate any patient with a history of bisphosphonate exposure who presents with thigh/groin pain to rule out an incomplete femur fracture, and consider interruption of therapy. Not recommended with severe renal impairment (CrCl <30mL/min). Ascertain sex steroid hormonal status and consider appropriate replacement before initiating therapy for the treatment and prevention of glucocorticoid-induced osteoporosis. May interfere with the use of bone-imaging agents.

ADVERSE REACTIONS
Back pain, arthralgia, abdominal pain, dyspepsia, acute phase reaction, allergic reaction, arthritis, diarrhea, headache, infection, UTI, bronchitis, HTN, nausea, rash.

DRUG INTERACTIONS
Ca^{2+} supplements, antacids, or oral medications containing divalent cations will interfere with absorption; take such medications at a different time of the day.

NURSING CONSIDERATIONS

Assessment: Assess for esophageal abnormalities, ability to stand or sit upright for at least 30 min, active upper GI problems, mental disability, hypocalcemia, disturbances of bone and mineral metabolism, risk for ONJ, renal impairment, drug hypersensitivity, any other conditions where treatment is contraindicated or cautioned, pregnancy/nursing status, and possible drug interactions. For glucocorticoid-induced osteoporosis treatment/prevention, assess sex steroid hormonal status.

Monitoring: Monitor for signs/symptoms of ONJ, atypical femoral fracture, esophageal reactions, hypocalcemia, musculoskeletal pain, and other adverse events. Periodically reevaluate the need for continued therapy.

Patient Counseling: Instruct to carefully follow dosing instructions and on what to do if doses are missed. Advise to consult physician before continuing treatment if symptoms of esophageal disease develop. Advise that drug should be taken at least 30 min before the 1st food or drink of the day other than water. Advise to take with a full glass of plain water (6-8 oz) and to avoid the use of water with supplements (eg, mineral water). Advise to avoid lying down for 30 min after taking the drug. Instruct to take supplemental Ca^{2+} and vitamin D if dietary intake is inadequate. Counsel to consider weight-bearing exercise along with the modification of certain behavioral factors (eg, excessive cigarette smoking and/or alcohol consumption) if these factors exist. Advise to consult physician any time they have a medical problem they think may be from treatment.

Storage: 20-25°C (68-77°F).

ACTOPLUS MET XR – metformin hydrochloride/pioglitazone RX

Class: Biguanide/thiazolidinedione

Thiazolidinediones, including pioglitazone, cause or exacerbate congestive heart failure (CHF) in some patients. After initiation and dose increases, monitor carefully for signs and symptoms of heart failure (HF); manage accordingly and consider discontinuation or dose reduction if HF develops. Not recommended with symptomatic HF. Contraindicated with established NYHA Class III or IV HF. Lactic acidosis may occur due to metformin accumulation; risk increases with conditions such as sepsis, dehydration, excess alcohol intake, hepatic/renal impairment, and acute CHF. If acidosis is suspected, d/c therapy and hospitalize patient immediately.

OTHER BRAND NAMES

Actoplus Met

ADULT DOSAGE

Type 2 Diabetes Mellitus

Initial:

Tab:
15mg/500mg bid or 15mg/850mg qd

Tab, Extended-Release (ER):
15mg/1000mg or 30mg/1000mg qd

NYHA Class I or II CHF:

Tab:
15mg/500mg or 15mg/850mg qd

Tab, ER:
15mg/1000mg or 30mg/1000mg qd

Inadequately Controlled on Metformin Monotherapy:

Tab:
15mg/500mg bid or 15mg/850mg qd or bid, depending on metformin dose already being taken

Tab, ER:
15mg/1000mg bid or 30mg/1000mg qd, depending on metformin dose already being taken

Inadequately Controlled on Pioglitazone Monotherapy:

Tab:
15mg/500mg bid or 15mg/850mg qd

Tab, ER:
15mg/1000mg bid or 30mg/1000mg qd

Switching from Combination Therapy of Pioglitazone plus Metformin as Separate Tabs:

Tab/Tab, ER:
Take at doses that are as close as possible to the dose of pioglitazone and metformin already being taken

Titrate: Gradually adjust, as needed, after assessing adequacy of response and tolerability

Max:

Tab:
(45mg/2550mg)/day

Tab, ER:
(45mg/2000mg)/day

Metformin doses >2000mg may be better tolerated given tid

PEDIATRIC DOSAGE

Pediatric use may not have been established

DOSE MODIFICATION

Concomitant Medications

Insulin Secretagogue (eg, Sulfonylurea):
Reduce dose of insulin secretagogue if hypoglycemia occurs

Insulin:
Decrease insulin dose by 10-25% if hypoglycemia occurs; further insulin dose adjustments should be individualized based on glycemic response

Strong CYP2C8 Inhibitors (eg, Gemfibrozil):

Max:

Tab:
(15mg/850mg)/day

Tab, Extended-Release:
(15mg/1000mg)/day

Elderly

Generally, should not be titrated to max dose

ADMINISTRATION

Oral route

Take w/ meals

Tab, Extended-Release

Swallow whole; do not chew, cut, or crush

HOW SUPPLIED

(Pioglitazone/Metformin) Tab, ER (XR): 15mg/1000mg, 30mg/1000mg; (Actoplus Met) Tab: 15mg/500mg, 15mg/850mg

CONTRAINDICATIONS

NYHA Class III or IV HF, renal impairment (eg, SrCr ≥1.5mg/dL [males], ≥1.4mg/dL [females], or abnormal CrCl), metabolic acidosis, including diabetic ketoacidosis.

WARNINGS/PRECAUTIONS

Not for use in type 1 DM or for treatment of diabetic ketoacidosis. Dose-related edema reported; caution in patients with edema or at risk for CHF. Fatal and nonfatal hepatic failure reported; caution with abnormal LFTs. Measure LFTs promptly in patients who report symptoms that may indicate liver injury. D/C if ALT >3X ULN; do not restart if cause of abnormal LFTs not established or if ALT remains >3X ULN with total bilirubin >2X ULN without alternative etiologies. May use with caution in patients with lesser ALT or bilirubin elevations and with an alternate probable cause. Avoid with clinical or lab evidence of hepatic disease. Increased incidence of bone fracture reported in females. Not for use in patients with active bladder cancer; consider benefits versus risks in patients with a prior history of bladder cancer. Caution in patients susceptible to hypoglycemic effects, such as elderly, debilitated/malnourished patients, and those with adrenal/pituitary insufficiency, or alcohol intoxication. Macular edema reported; promptly refer to an ophthalmologist if visual symptoms occur. May result in ovulation in some premenopausal anovulatory women, which may increase risk for pregnancy; adequate contraception is recommended. Assess renal function before initiation of therapy and at least annually thereafter; d/c with evidence of renal impairment. D/C at the time of or prior to radiologic studies involving the use of intravascular iodinated contrast materials, withhold for 48 hrs subsequent to the procedure, and reinstitute only if renal function is normal. D/C in hypoxic states (eg, acute CHF, shock, acute myocardial infarction). Temporarily suspend for any surgical procedure (except minor procedures not associated with restricted food and fluid intake); restart when oral intake is resumed and renal function is normal. May decrease serum vitamin B12 levels; monitor hematologic parameters annually. Caution in elderly.

ADVERSE REACTIONS

Lactic acidosis, CHF, diarrhea, headache, edema, upper respiratory tract infection, weight gain.

DRUG INTERACTIONS

See Dosage. Risk for hypoglycemia with insulin or other antidiabetic medications (particularly insulin secretagogues [eg, sulfonylureas]); may require a reduction in the dose of the concomitant antidiabetic medication. May be difficult to recognize hypoglycemia with β-adrenergic blocking drugs. Caution with drugs that may affect renal function or result in significant hemodynamic change or may interfere with the disposition of metformin (eg, cationic drugs eliminated by renal tubular secretion). Alcohol potentiates the effect of metformin on lactate metabolism; avoid excessive alcohol intake. Increased exposure and $T_{1/2}$ with strong CYP2C8 inhibitors (eg, gemfibrozil). CYP2C8 inducers (eg, rifampin) may decrease exposure; if a CYP2C8 inducer is started or stopped during treatment, changes in diabetes treatment may be needed based on clinical response. Topiramate or other carbonic anhydrase inhibitors (eg, zonisamide, acetazolamide, dichlorphenamide) may induce metabolic acidosis; use with caution. Cationic drugs that are eliminated by renal tubular secretion (eg, cimetidine, amiloride, digoxin, morphine, procainamide) may potentially produce an interaction; monitor and adjust dose of therapy and/or the interfering drug. Observe for loss of blood glucose control with thiazides and other diuretics, corticosteroids, phenothiazines, thyroid products, estrogens, oral contraceptives, phenytoin, nicotinic acid, sympathomimetics, calcium channel blockers, and isoniazid; observe for hypoglycemia when such drugs are withdrawn during therapy. Pioglitazone: May cause dose-related fluid retention when used with other antidiabetic medications, most commonly with insulin.

NURSING CONSIDERATIONS

Assessment: Assess for HF or risk of HF, metabolic acidosis, risk factors for lactic acidosis, previous hypersensitivity to the drug, type of DM, diabetic ketoacidosis, edema, bone health, active/history of bladder cancer, inadequate vitamin B12 or Ca^{2+} intake/absorption, any other conditions where treatment is cautioned, pregnancy/nursing status, and possible drug interactions. Assess if patient is planning to undergo any surgical procedure or radiologic studies involving the use of intravascular iodinated contrast materials. Obtain baseline LFTs, renal function, FPG and HbA1c levels, and hematologic parameters.

Monitoring: Monitor for signs/symptoms of HF, liver injury, lactic acidosis, edema, fractures, visual symptoms, hypoxic states, and other adverse reactions. Monitor renal function, especially in elderly, at least annually. Monitor hematologic parameters annually. Perform routine serum vitamin B12 measurements at 2- to 3-yr intervals in patients predisposed to developing subnormal vitamin B12 levels. Monitor FPG and HbA1c. Periodically monitor LFTs in patients with liver disease.

Patient Counseling: Advise on the importance of adherence to dietary instructions and regular testing of blood glucose, HbA1c, renal function, and hematologic parameters. Advise to seek medical advice promptly during periods of stress, as medication requirements may change. Instruct to promptly report any signs/symptoms of bladder cancer or HF. Inform of the risk of lactic acidosis; instruct to d/c therapy immediately and notify physician if unexplained hyperventilation, myalgia, GI symptoms, malaise, unusual somnolence, or other nonspecific symptoms occur. Counsel against excessive alcohol intake while on therapy. Instruct to d/c use and seek medical advice promptly if signs/symptoms of hepatotoxicity occur. Counsel premenopausal women to use adequate contraception during treatment. Inform that hypoglycemia can occur; explain the risks, symptoms, and appropriate management. Instruct to take drug as prescribed and that any change in dosing should only be done if directed by physician. (Tab, ER) Inform that the inactive ingredients may occasionally be eliminated in the feces as a soft mass that may resemble the original tab.

Storage: 25°C (77°F); excursions permitted to 15-30°C (59-86°F). Protect from moisture and humidity.

ACTOS – pioglitazone RX

Class: Thiazolidinedione

Thiazolidinediones cause or exacerbate congestive heart failure (CHF) in some patients. After initiation and dose increases, monitor carefully for signs and symptoms of heart failure (HF) and manage accordingly; consider discontinuation or dose reduction. Not recommended in patients with symptomatic HF. Contraindicated with established NYHA Class III or IV HF.

ADULT DOSAGE

Type 2 Diabetes Mellitus

W/O CHF:
Initial: 15mg or 30mg qd
Titrate: In increments of 15mg
Max: 45mg qd

W/ CHF (NYHA Class I or II):
Initial: 15mg qd
Titrate: In increments of 15mg
Max: 45mg qd

PEDIATRIC DOSAGE

Pediatric use may not have been established

DOSE MODIFICATION

Concomitant Medications

Insulin Secretagogue:
Reduce dose of insulin secretagogue if hypoglycemia occurs

W/ Insulin:
Decrease insulin dose by 10-25% if hypoglycemia occurs
Further insulin dose adjustment should be individualized based on glycemic response

W/ Gemfibrozil/Other Strong CYP2C8 Inhibitors:
Max: 15mg qd

ADMINISTRATION

Oral route

Take w/o regard to meals

HOW SUPPLIED
Tab: 15mg, 30mg, 45mg

CONTRAINDICATIONS
Established NYHA Class III or IV HF.

WARNINGS/PRECAUTIONS
Not for use in treatment of type 1 DM or diabetic ketoacidosis. Fatal and nonfatal hepatic failure reported. May use with caution in patients with lesser ALT elevations or bilirubin and with an alternate probable cause. Obtain LFTs prior to initiation; caution with liver disease/abnormal LFTs. D/C if ALT >3X ULN; do not restart if cause of abnormal LFTs not established or if ALT remains >3X ULN with total bilirubin >2X ULN without alternative etiologies. Not for use in patients with active bladder cancer; consider benefits versus risks in patients with a prior history of bladder cancer. New onset or worsening of edema reported; caution in patients with edema and in patients at risk for CHF. Increased incidence of bone fractures reported in females. Macular edema reported; refer to an ophthalmologist if visual symptoms develop. Ovulation in premenopausal anovulatory patients may occur; use adequate contraception.

ADVERSE REACTIONS
CHF, URTI, hypoglycemia, edema, headache, cardiac failure, pain in extremity, sinusitis, back pain, myalgia, pharyngitis, chest pain.

DRUG INTERACTIONS
Increased exposure and $T_{1/2}$ with CYP2C8 inhibitors (eg, gemfibrozil). Decreased exposure with CYP2C8 inducers (eg, rifampin). Risk of fluid retention and hypoglycemia with insulin and other antidiabetic medications (eg, insulin secretagogues such as sulfonylureas).

NURSING CONSIDERATIONS

Assessment: Assess for previous hypersensitivity, HF, edema, risk factors for developing HF, liver disease, bone health, active/history of bladder cancer, pregnancy/nursing status, and possible drug interactions. Obtain baseline LFTs.

Monitoring: Monitor for signs and symptoms of HF, edema, weight gain, hematological changes (eg, decreases in Hgb, Hct), liver injury, macular edema, bone fractures, ovulation in premenopausal anovulatory women, and other adverse reactions. Perform periodic measurements of FPG and HbA1c. Periodically monitor LFTs in patients with liver disease. Perform periodic eye exams.

Patient Counseling: Advise to adhere to dietary instructions and have blood glucose and glycosylated Hgb levels tested regularly. Instruct to seek medical advice promptly during periods of stress and report rapid increase in weight or edema, SOB, or other symptoms of HF to physician. Instruct to d/c and consult physician if unexplained N/V, abdominal pain, anorexia, fatigue, or dark urine occurs. Advise to report any signs of macroscopic hematuria or other symptoms such as dysuria or urinary urgency. Advise to take qd with or without meals. If dose is missed, advise to not double the dose the following day. Inform about the risk of hypoglycemia when using with insulin or other antidiabetic medications. Inform that therapy may result in ovulation in some premenopausal anovulatory women; recommend adequate contraception for all premenopausal women.

Storage: 25°C (77°F); excursions permitted to 15-30°C (59-86°F). Protect from light, moisture, and humidity.

ACULAR – ketorolac tromethamine RX

Class: NSAID

ADULT DOSAGE

Seasonal Allergic Conjunctivitis

Ocular Itching:
1 drop qid to the affected eye(s)

Postoperative Inflammation

1 drop to affected eye(s) qid beginning 24 hrs after cataract surgery and continuing through the first 2 weeks of the postoperative period

PEDIATRIC DOSAGE

Seasonal Allergic Conjunctivitis

Ocular Itching:
≥2 Years:
1 drop qid to the affected eye(s)

Postoperative Inflammation

≥2 Years:
1 drop to affected eye(s) qid beginning 24 hrs after cataract surgery and continuing through the first 2 weeks of the postoperative period

DOSE MODIFICATION

Concomitant Medications

Topical Eye Medications: Give at least 5 min apart

ADMINISTRATION
Ocular route

HOW SUPPLIED
Sol: 0.5% [5mL]

WARNINGS/PRECAUTIONS
May slow or delay healing, or result in keratitis. Potential for cross-sensitivity to acetylsalicylic acid (ASA), phenylacetic acid derivatives, and other NSAIDs; caution with previous sensitivities to these agents. Bronchospasm or exacerbation of asthma reported with known hypersensitivity to ASA/NSAIDs or past history of asthma. Increased bleeding of ocular tissues (eg, hyphemas) reported in conjunction with ocular surgery; caution with known bleeding tendencies. Continued use may result in sight-threatening epithelial breakdown, corneal thinning, erosion, ulceration, or perforation; d/c if corneal epithelial breakdown occurs and monitor for corneal health. Caution with complicated ocular surgeries, corneal denervation, corneal epithelial defects, diabetes mellitus (DM), ocular surface diseases (eg, dry eye syndrome), rheumatoid arthritis (RA), or repeat ocular surgeries within a short period. Use for >1 day prior to surgery or beyond 14 days postsurgery may increase risk for occurrence and severity of corneal adverse events. Do not administer while patient is wearing contact lenses. Avoid in late pregnancy.

ADVERSE REACTIONS
Stinging, burning, superficial keratitis, ocular infections, allergic reactions, ocular inflammation/irritation, corneal edema, iritis.

DRUG INTERACTIONS
Caution with medications that may prolong bleeding time. May increase potential for healing problems with topical steroids.

NURSING CONSIDERATIONS

Assessment: Assess for previous hypersensitivity to the drug or cross-sensitivity to ASA, phenylacetic acid derivatives, and other NSAIDs, history of asthma, bleeding tendencies, complicated or repeated ocular surgeries, corneal denervation, corneal epithelial defects, DM, ocular surface diseases, RA, contact lens use, pregnancy/nursing status, and possible drug interactions.

Monitoring: Monitor for hypersensitivity reactions, healing problems, keratitis, increased bleeding of ocular tissues in conjunction with ocular surgery, and evidence of epithelial corneal breakdown.

Patient Counseling: Inform of the possibility that slow or delayed healing may occur. Instruct to avoid allowing the tip of the bottle to contact the eye or surrounding structures. Advise to use 1 bottle for ou following bilateral ocular surgery. Advise not to administer while wearing contact lenses and to seek physician's advice if an intercurrent ocular condition (eg, trauma, infection) develops, or in case of ocular surgery. Advise to administer at least 5 min apart if >1 ophthalmic medication is being used.

Storage: 15-25°C (59-77°F). Protect from light.

ACULAR LS – ketorolac tromethamine **RX**

Class: NSAID

ADULT DOSAGE

Corneal Refractive Surgery

Reduction of Ocular Pain and Burning/Stinging:
1 drop qid in the operated eye prn for up to 4 days following surgery

PEDIATRIC DOSAGE

Corneal Refractive Surgery

Reduction of Ocular Pain and Burning/Stinging:
≥3 Years:
1 drop qid in the operated eye prn for up to 4 days following surgery

ADMINISTRATION
Ocular route

HOW SUPPLIED
Sol: 0.4% [5mL]

WARNINGS/PRECAUTIONS
Potential cross-sensitivity to acetylsalicylic acid, phenylacetic acid derivatives, and other NSAIDs; caution with previous sensitivities to these drugs. May increase bleeding of ocular tissues (including hyphemas) in conjunction with ocular surgery; caution with known bleeding tendencies. May slow/delay healing or result in keratitis. Continued use may result in epithelial breakdown, corneal thinning, erosion, ulceration, or perforation; d/c if corneal epithelium breakdown occurs and closely monitor for corneal health. Caution with complicated ocular surgeries, corneal denervation, corneal epithelial defects, diabetes mellitus (DM), ocular surface diseases (eg, dry eye syndrome), rheumatoid arthritis (RA), or repeat ocular surgeries within a short period of time. Use for >24 hrs prior to surgery or beyond 14 days postsurgery may increase risk for occurrence and severity of corneal adverse events. Avoid in late pregnancy.

ADVERSE REACTIONS
Transient stinging/burning, allergic reactions, corneal edema, iritis, ocular inflammation/irritation/pain, superficial keratitis, superficial ocular infections.

DRUG INTERACTIONS
Concomitant use of topical NSAIDs and topical steroids may increase potential for healing problems. Caution with other medications that may prolong bleeding time.

NURSING CONSIDERATIONS

Assessment: Assess for drug hypersensitivity, cross-sensitivity reactions, bleeding tendencies, complicated ocular surgeries, corneal denervation, corneal epithelial defects, DM, ocular surface diseases, RA, and possible drug interactions.

Monitoring: Monitor for bleeding of ocular tissues, healing problems, keratitis, corneal epithelial breakdown, and corneal thinning/erosion/ulceration/perforation.

Patient Counseling: Advise not to use while wearing contact lenses.

Storage: 15-25°C (59-77°F).

ADCIRCA – tadalafil RX

Class: Phosphodiesterase type 5 inhibitor

ADULT DOSAGE

Pulmonary Arterial Hypertension

Treatment of pulmonary arterial HTN (WHO Group 1) to improve exercise ability

Usual: 40mg (two 20mg tabs) qd

PEDIATRIC DOSAGE

Pediatric use may not have been established

DOSE MODIFICATION

Concomitant Medications

Patients on Ritonavir (RTV) for at Least 1 Week:
Initial: 20mg qd
Titrate: Increase to 40mg qd based on individual tolerability

Adding RTV:
Avoid use of tadalafil during the initiation of RTV
Stop tadalafil at least 24 hrs prior to starting RTV
After at least 1 week following RTV initiation, resume tadalafil at 20mg qd
Increase to 40mg qd based on individual tolerability

Renal Impairment

Mild (CrCl 51-80mL/min) or Moderate (CrCl 31-50mL/min):
Initial: 20mg qd
Titrate: Increase to 40mg qd based on individual tolerability
Severe (CrCl <30mL/min and on Hemodialysis): Avoid use

Hepatic Impairment

Mild or Moderate Hepatic Cirrhosis (Child-Pugh Class A or B):
Initial: Consider 20mg qd
Severe Hepatic Cirrhosis (Child-Pugh Class C): Avoid use

ADMINISTRATION
Oral route
Take w/ or w/o food
Dividing the dose (40mg) over the course of the day is not recommended

HOW SUPPLIED
Tab: 20mg

CONTRAINDICATIONS
Patients using any form of organic nitrate, either regularly or intermittently, or guanylate cyclase (GC) stimulator (eg, riociguat).

WARNINGS/PRECAUTIONS
Patients who experience anginal chest pain after taking tadalafil should seek immediate medical attention. May cause a transient decrease in BP; caution w/ underlying cardiovascular disease (CVD). Patients w/ severely impaired autonomic control of BP or w/ left ventricular outflow obstruction may be particularly sensitive to vasodilatory effects. May significantly worsen cardiovascular status of patients w/ pulmonary veno-occlusive disease (PVOD); not recommended w/ veno-occlusive disease. Consider PVOD if signs of pulmonary edema occur. Nonarteritic anterior ischemic optic neuropathy (NAION) reported; seek immediate medical attention if sudden loss of vision in 1 or both eyes occurs. Not recommended in patients w/ hereditary degenerative retinal

disorders (eg, retinitis pigmentosa). Seek immediate medical attention in the event of sudden decrease or loss of hearing. Prolonged erections >4 hrs and priapism reported rarely; caution w/ conditions that might predispose to priapism (eg, sickle cell anemia, multiple myeloma, leukemia) or in patients w/ anatomical penile deformation (eg, angulation, cavernosal fibrosis, Peyronie's disease). Caution w/ bleeding disorders or significant active peptic ulceration.

ADVERSE REACTIONS

Headache, myalgia, nasopharyngitis, flushing, respiratory tract infection, pain in extremity, nausea, back pain, dyspepsia, nasal congestion.

DRUG INTERACTIONS

See Contraindications and Dose Modification. If nitrate administration is deemed medically necessary in a life-threatening situation, at least 48 hrs should elapse after the last dose of tadalafil before nitrate administration is considered; administer nitrates only under close medical supervision w/ appropriate hemodynamic monitoring. Additive hypotensive effects w/ α-adrenergic blockers, antihypertensives (eg, amlodipine, ARBs, bendroflumethiazide, enalapril, metoprolol), and alcohol. Avoid w/ potent CYP3A inhibitors (eg, ketoconazole, itraconazole) or chronic therapy of potent CYP3A inducers (eg, rifampin). Do not give w/ Cialis or other PDE-5 inhibitors.

NURSING CONSIDERATIONS

Assessment: Assess for CVD, PVOD, renal/hepatic impairment, history of NAION, hereditary degenerative retinal disorders, conditions that might predispose to priapism, anatomical deformation of the penis, bleeding disorders, active peptic ulceration, hypersensitivity to drug, pregnancy/nursing status, and possible drug interactions.

Monitoring: Monitor for signs/symptoms of anginal chest pain, pulmonary edema, NAION, hearing loss, prolonged erections >4 hrs, priapism, and other adverse reactions. Monitor BP.

Patient Counseling: Inform of contraindication of treatment w/ any use of organic nitrates or GC stimulators. Instruct not to take Cialis or other PDE-5 inhibitors. Advise to seek immediate medical attention if sudden loss of vision in 1 or both eyes, sudden decrease/loss of hearing, or erection lasting >4 hrs occurs. Counsel about appropriate action to take if anginal chest pain requiring nitroglycerin occurs following intake of therapy.

Storage: 25°C (77°F); excursions permitted to 15-30°C (59-86°F).

ADDERALL – amphetamine aspartate monohydrate/amphetamine sulfate/dextroamphetamine saccharate/dextroamphetamine sulfate CII

Class: Sympathomimetic amine

High potential for abuse; prolonged use may lead to drug dependence and must be avoided. Misuse of amphetamine may cause sudden death and serious cardiovascular (CV) adverse events.

ADULT DOSAGE

Narcolepsy

Individualize dose and administer at the lowest effective dose

Initial: 10mg/day

Titrate: May increase in increments of 10mg at weekly intervals until optimal response is obtained

Usual: 5-60mg/day in divided doses

Give 1st dose on awakening; additional doses (1 or 2) at intervals of 4-6 hrs

PEDIATRIC DOSAGE

Narcolepsy

Individualize dose and administer at the lowest effective dose

Usual: 5-60mg/day in divided doses

6-12 Years:

Initial: 5mg/day

Titrate: May increase in increments of 5mg at weekly intervals until optimal response is obtained

≥12 Years:

Initial: 10mg/day

Titrate: May increase in increments of 10mg at weekly intervals until optimal response is obtained

Give 1st dose on awakening; additional doses (1 or 2) at intervals of 4-6 hrs

Attention-Deficit Hyperactivity Disorder

Individualize dose and administer at the lowest effective dose

3-5 Years:

Initial: 2.5mg/day

Titrate: May increase in increments of 2.5mg

at weekly intervals until optimal response is obtained

≥6 Years:
Initial: 5mg qd or bid
Titrate: May increase in increments of 5mg at weekly intervals until optimal response is obtained. Only in rare cases will it be necessary to exceed a total of 40mg/day
Give 1st dose on awakening; additional doses (1 or 2) at intervals of 4-6 hrs

Interrupt occasionally to determine the need for continued therapy

DOSE MODIFICATION
Adverse Reactions
Narcolepsy:
Reduce dose if bothersome adverse reactions appear (eg, insomnia or anorexia)

ADMINISTRATION
Oral route

Give 1st dose on awakening; avoid late pm doses due to potential for insomnia

HOW SUPPLIED
Tab: 5mg*, 7.5mg*, 10mg*, 12.5mg*, 15mg*, 20mg*, 30mg* *scored

CONTRAINDICATIONS
Advanced arteriosclerosis, symptomatic CV disease, moderate to severe HTN, hyperthyroidism, glaucoma, agitated states, history of drug abuse, during or w/in 14 days of MAOI use.

WARNINGS/PRECAUTIONS
Sudden death reported in children and adolescents w/ structural cardiac abnormalities or other serious heart problems. Sudden death, stroke, and MI reported in adults. Avoid use in patients w/ serious structural cardiac abnormalities, cardiomyopathy, serious heart rhythm abnormalities, coronary artery disease, or other serious cardiac problems. May cause modest increase in average BP and HR. Perform prompt cardiac evaluation when symptoms suggestive of cardiac disease develop. May exacerbate symptoms of behavior disturbance and thought disorder in patients w/ preexisting psychotic disorder. Caution in patients w/ comorbid bipolar disorder; may induce mixed/manic episodes. May cause treatment-emergent psychotic/manic symptoms in children and adolescents w/o prior history of psychotic illness or mania; consider discontinuation if such symptoms occur. Aggressive behavior or hostility reported in children and adolescents w/ ADHD; monitor for appearance of or worsening. May cause long-term suppression of growth in children; may need to interrupt treatment if patients are not growing or gaining weight as expected. May lower convulsive threshold; d/c if seizures develop. Associated w/ peripheral vasculopathy, including Raynaud's phenomenon. Difficulties w/ accommodation and blurring of vision reported. May exacerbate motor and phonic tics and Tourette's syndrome. May cause a significant elevation in plasma corticosteroid levels or interfere w/ urinary steroid determinations.

ADVERSE REACTIONS
Palpitations, tachycardia, BP elevation, psychotic episodes, tremor, blurred vision, mydriasis, dry mouth, unpleasant taste, anorexia, urticaria, rash, libido changes, alopecia, rhabdomyolysis.

DRUG INTERACTIONS
See Contraindications. GI alkalinizing agents (eg, sodium bicarbonate, antacids) and urinary alkalinizing agents (eg, acetazolamide, some thiazides) may increase blood levels and potentiate effects; avoid w/ GI alkalinizing agents. GI acidifying agents (eg, guanethidine, reserpine, glutamic acid HCl) and urinary acidifying agents (eg, ammonium chloride, sodium acid phosphate) may lower blood levels and efficacy. May inhibit adrenergic blockers. May enhance activity of TCAs or sympathomimetic agents; caution w/ other sympathomimetic drugs. Increased d-amphetamine levels in the brain w/ desipramine or protriptyline and possibly other tricyclics. May counteract sedative effect of antihistamines. May antagonize the hypotensive effects of antihypertensives. Chlorpromazine and haloperidol may inhibit the central stimulant effects. Lithium carbonate may inhibit the anorectic and stimulatory effects. May delay intestinal absorption of ethosuximide, phenobarbital, and phenytoin; may produce a synergistic anticonvulsant action if coadministered w/ phenobarbital or phenytoin. May potentiate analgesic effect of meperidine. May enhance the adrenergic effect of norepinephrine. Use in cases of propoxyphene overdose may potentiate CNS stimulation and cause fatal convulsions. Monitor for changes in clinical effect when coadministered w/ proton pump inhibitors. May inhibit the hypotensive effect of veratrum alkaloids.

NURSING CONSIDERATIONS

Assessment: Assess for advanced arteriosclerosis, symptomatic CV disease, moderate to severe HTN, hyperthyroidism, hypersensitivity or idiosyncrasy to sympathomimetic amines, glaucoma, agitation, history of drug abuse, psychiatric history, history of seizure, tics or Tourette's syndrome, pregnancy/nursing status, and possible drug interactions. Prior to treatment, adequately screen patients to determine risk for bipolar disorder.

Monitoring: Monitor for CV abnormalities, exacerbations of behavior disturbances and thought disorder, psychotic or manic symptoms, aggressive behavior, hostility, seizures, visual disturbances, exacerbation of motor and phonic tics and Tourette's syndrome, and other adverse reactions. Monitor BP and HR. Monitor growth and weight in children. Periodically reevaluate long-term usefulness of therapy. Observe carefully for signs and symptoms of peripheral vasculopathy; further clinical evaluation (eg, rheumatology referral) may be appropriate for certain patients.

Patient Counseling: Inform about benefits and risks of treatment, appropriate use, and about the potential for abuse/dependence. Advise to avoid breastfeeding and to notify physician if pregnant/planning to become pregnant. Instruct to use caution when engaging in potentially hazardous activities (eg, operating machinery or vehicles). Inform about the risk of peripheral vasculopathy, including Raynaud's phenomenon; instruct to report to physician any new numbness, pain, skin color change, or sensitivity to temperature in fingers or toes, and to call physician immediately if any signs of unexplained wounds appear on fingers or toes while on therapy.

Storage: 20-25°C (68-77°F).

ADDERALL XR – amphetamine aspartate monohydrate/amphetamine sulfate/dextroamphetamine saccharate/dextroamphetamine sulfate CII

Class: Sympathomimetic amine

High potential for abuse; prolonged use may lead to drug dependence. Misuse may cause sudden death and serious cardiovascular (CV) adverse reactions.

ADULT DOSAGE

Attention-Deficit Hyperactivity Disorder

Individualize dose and administer at lowest effective dose

Amphetamine-Naive/Switching from Another Medication: 20mg qam

Switching from Amphetamine Immediate-Release: Give the same total daily dose, qd

Titrate at weekly intervals as indicated

PEDIATRIC DOSAGE

Attention-Deficit Hyperactivity Disorder

Individualize dose and administer at lowest effective dose

Amphetamine-Naive/Switching from Another Medication:

6-12 Years:

Initial: 10mg qam or 5mg qam when lower initial dose is appropriate

Titrate: Adjust daily dosage in increments of 5mg or 10mg at weekly intervals

Max: 30mg/day

13-17 Years:

Initial: 10mg qam

Titrate: May increase to 20mg/day after 1 week if symptoms are not controlled

Switching from Amphetamine Immediate-Release:

≥6 Years:

Give the same total daily dose, qd; titrate at weekly intervals as indicated

ADMINISTRATION

Oral route

Give upon awakening; avoid pm doses due to potential for insomnia

Take w/ or w/o food

Take caps whole or sprinkle entire contents on applesauce. Consume sprinkled applesauce immediately w/o chewing the sprinkled beads

Do not divide the dose of a single cap or take anything <1 cap/day

HOW SUPPLIED

Cap, Extended-Release: 5mg, 10mg, 15mg, 20mg, 25mg, 30mg

CONTRAINDICATIONS

Advanced arteriosclerosis, symptomatic CV disease, moderate to severe HTN, hyperthyroidism, glaucoma, agitated states, history of drug abuse, during or within 14 days following MAOI use.

WARNINGS/PRECAUTIONS

Sudden death, stroke, and MI reported in adults. Sudden death reported in children and adolescents with structural cardiac abnormalities or other serious heart problems. Avoid use in patients with known serious structural cardiac and heart rhythm abnormalities, cardiomyopathy, coronary artery disease (CAD), or other serious cardiac problems. May cause modest increase in BP and HR. May exacerbate symptoms of behavior disturbance and thought disorder in patients with preexisting psychotic disorder. Caution in patients with comorbid bipolar disorder; may cause induction of mixed/manic episode. May cause treatment-emergent psychotic/manic symptoms (eg, hallucinations, delusional thinking, mania) in children and adolescents without a prior history of psychotic illness or mania; consider discontinuation if such symptoms occur. Aggressive behavior or hostility reported; monitor for appearance or worsening. May cause long-term suppression of growth in children; may need to d/c if patients are not growing or gaining weight as expected. May lower convulsive threshold; d/c if seizures develop. Associated with peripheral vasculopathy, including Raynaud's phenomenon. Difficulties with accommodation and blurring of vision reported. Exacerbation of motor and phonic tics and Tourette's syndrome reported. May significantly elevate plasma corticosteroid levels or interfere with urinary steroid determinations. Where possible, interrupt occasionally to determine the need for continued therapy.

ADVERSE REACTIONS

Dry mouth, loss of appetite, insomnia, headache, abdominal pain, weight loss, agitation, anxiety, N/V, dizziness, tachycardia, nervousness, asthenia, diarrhea, UTI.

DRUG INTERACTIONS

See Contraindications. Avoid with GI alkalinizing agents (eg, sodium bicarbonate, antacids). Urinary alkalinizing agents (eg, acetazolamide, some thiazides) may increase blood levels and potentiate effects. GI acidifying agents (eg, guanethidine, reserpine, ascorbic acid) and urinary acidifying agents (eg, ammonium chloride, sodium acid phosphate, methenamine salts) may lower blood levels and efficacy. May reduce CV effects of adrenergic blockers. May counteract sedative effects of antihistamines. May antagonize effects of antihypertensives. May inhibit hypotensive effect of veratrum alkaloids. May delay intestinal absorption of phenobarbital, phenytoin, and ethosuximide. May enhance activity of TCAs or sympathomimetic agents. Increased d-amphetamine levels in the brain with desipramine or protriptyline and possibly other tricyclics. May potentiate analgesic effect of meperidine. May enhance the adrenergic effect of norepinephrine. Chlorpromazine and haloperidol may inhibit central stimulant effects. Lithium carbonate may inhibit anorectic and stimulatory effects. Norepinephrine may enhance the adrenergic effect. Use in cases of propoxyphene overdose may potentiate CNS stimulation and cause fatal convulsions. Monitor for changes in clinical effect when coadministered with proton pump inhibitors.

NURSING CONSIDERATIONS

Assessment: Assess for advanced arteriosclerosis, symptomatic CV disease, moderate to severe HTN, hyperthyroidism, hypersensitivity or idiosyncrasy to sympathomimetic amines, glaucoma, agitation, history of drug abuse, psychiatric history, history of seizure, tics or Tourette's syndrome, hepatic/renal dysfunction, pregnancy/nursing status, and possible drug interactions.

Monitoring: Monitor for CV abnormalities, exacerbations of behavior disturbances and thought disorder, psychotic or manic symptoms, aggressive behavior, hostility, seizures, visual disturbances, exacerbation of motor and phonic tics and Tourette's syndrome, and other adverse reactions. Monitor BP and HR. Monitor height and weight in children. Observe carefully for signs and symptoms of peripheral vasculopathy; further clinical evaluation (eg, rheumatology referral) may be appropriate for certain patients.

Patient Counseling: Inform about benefits and risks of treatment, appropriate use, and about the potential for abuse/dependence. Advise about serious CV risks. Inform that treatment-emergent psychotic or manic symptoms may occur. Instruct to report signs/symptoms of peripheral vasculopathy, including Raynaud's phenomenon. Advise parents or guardians of pediatric patients to monitor growth and weight during treatment. Advise to notify physician if pregnant or planning to become pregnant. Advise to avoid breastfeeding. Advise to use caution when engaging in potentially hazardous activities (eg, operating machinery or vehicles).

Storage: 25°C (77°F); excursions permitted to 15-30°C (59-86°F).

ADIPEX-P – phentermine hydrochloride

CIV

Class: Anorectic sympathomimetic amine

ADULT DOSAGE

Obesity

Short-term (few weeks) adjunctive therapy in weight reduction regimen based on exercise, behavioral modification, and caloric restriction in the management of exogenous obesity for patients w/ initial BMI ≥30kg/m², or ≥27kg/m² in the presence of other risk factors

>16 Years:

Usual: 37.5mg (cap or tab) qd or 18.75mg (1/2 tab) qd-bid; adjust dose to patient's needs

PEDIATRIC DOSAGE

Pediatric use may not have been established

DOSE MODIFICATION

Elderly

Start at lower end of dosing range

ADMINISTRATION

Oral route

Administer before breakfast or 1-2 hrs after breakfast; avoid late pm dosing

HOW SUPPLIED

Cap: 37.5mg; Tab: 37.5mg* *scored

CONTRAINDICATIONS

Hyperthyroidism, glaucoma, agitated states, pregnancy, nursing, history of cardiovascular disease (CVD) (eg, coronary artery disease, stroke, arrhythmias, CHF, uncontrolled HTN), history of drug abuse, and during or within 14 days after administration of MAOIs.

WARNINGS/PRECAUTIONS

Primary pulmonary HTN (PPH) reported (rare); d/c and evaluate for possible presence of pulmonary HTN if new, unexplained symptoms of dyspnea, angina pectoris, syncope or lower extremity edema develop. Valvular heart disease reported (rare). D/C when tolerance develops. May impair mental/physical abilities. Has the potential for abuse and dependence; prescribe or dispense the least amount feasible at one time to minimize possibility of overdosage. Caution with renal impairment, mild HTN, and in elderly.

ADVERSE REACTIONS

PPH, regurgitant cardiac valvular disease, palpitation, tachycardia, BP elevation, ischemic events, CNS overstimulation, insomnia, euphoria, psychosis, dry mouth, GI disturbances, urticaria, impotence, changes in libido.

DRUG INTERACTIONS

See Contraindications. Not recommended with other drug products for weight loss (eg, prescribed drugs, OTC preparations, and herbal products) or serotonergic agents such as SSRIs (eg, fluoxetine, sertraline, fluvoxamine, paroxetine). PPH and serious regurgitant cardiac valvular disease reported with fenfluramine or dexfenfluramine. Concomitant alcohol may cause an adverse drug reaction. Reduction in insulin or oral hypoglycemic medications in diabetes mellitus (DM) patients may be required. May decrease hypotensive effect of adrenergic neuron blockers.

NURSING CONSIDERATIONS

Assessment: Assess for hyperthyroidism, glaucoma, agitated states, HTN, DM, renal impairment, hypersensitivity/idiosyncrasy to sympathomimetic amines, history of CVD, drug abuse, pregnancy/nursing status, and possible drug interactions.

Monitoring: Monitor for signs/symptoms of PPH, valvular heart disease, tolerance, drug abuse/dependence, and other adverse reactions.

Patient Counseling: Inform that coadministration with other drugs for weight loss is not recommended. Instruct to take exactly ud; inform about the potential for developing tolerance, risk of dependence, and potential consequences of abuse. Inform about the risks and benefits of therapy; advise about the development of PPH and serious valvular heart disease, effects on ability to engage in potentially hazardous tasks, and risk of increase in BP and of interactions. Counsel to immediately report any deterioration in exercise tolerance. Advise not to use the drug in pregnant and nursing mothers.

Storage: 20-25°C (68-77°F).

ADOXA – doxycycline

RX

Class: Tetracyclines

ADULT DOSAGE

General Dosing

Treatment of the following infections caused by susceptible microorganisms: Rocky Mountain spotted fever, typhus fever and the typhus group, Q fever, rickettsialpox, tick fevers, respiratory tract infections, lymphogranuloma venereum, psittacosis (ornithosis), trachoma, inclusion conjunctivitis, relapsing fever, chancroid, plague, tularemia, cholera, *Campylobacter fetus* infections, brucellosis, bartonellosis, granuloma inguinale, UTIs, skin and skin structure infections, and anthrax. Treatment of infections caused by *Escherichia coli, Enterobacter aerogenes, Shigella* species, or *Acinetobacter* species. Treatment of uncomplicated gonorrhea, syphilis, yaws, listeriosis, Vincent's infection, actinomycosis, and *Clostridium* species infections when penicillin is contraindicated. Adjunct to amebicides in acute intestinal amebiasis. Adjunctive therapy in severe acne

Initial: 100mg q12h or 50mg q6h on 1st day
Maint: 100mg qd or 50mg q12h
More Severe Infections (eg, Chronic UTIs):
100mg q12h

Streptococcal Infections:
Continue therapy for 10 days

Gonococcal Infections

Uncomplicated Infections (Except Anorectal Infections in Men):
100mg bid for 7 days

Alternate Dosing:
Single visit dose of 300mg stat followed in 1 hr by a second 300mg dose

Acute Epididymo-Orchitis

Caused by *Neisseria gonorrhoeae/Chlamydia trachomatis*:
100mg bid for at least 10 days

Syphilis

Primary and Secondary:
300mg/day in divided doses for at least 10 days

Urethral Infections

Uncomplicated Infections Caused by *Chlamydia trachomatis*:
100mg bid for at least 7 days

Endocervical Infections

Uncomplicated Infections Caused by *Chlamydia trachomatis*:
100mg bid for at least 7 days

Rectal Infections

Uncomplicated Infections Caused by *Chlamydia trachomatis*:
100mg bid for at least 7 days

Nongonococcal Urethritis

Caused by *Chlamydia trachomatis* and *Ureaplasma urealyticum*:
100mg bid for at least 7 days

Inhalational Anthrax (Postexposure)

100mg bid for 60 days

PEDIATRIC DOSAGE

General Dosing

Treatment of the following infections caused by susceptible microorganisms: Rocky Mountain spotted fever, typhus fever and the typhus group, Q fever, rickettsialpox, tick fevers, respiratory tract infections, lymphogranuloma venereum, psittacosis (ornithosis), trachoma, inclusion conjunctivitis, relapsing fever, chancroid, plague, tularemia, cholera, *Campylobacter fetus* infections, brucellosis, bartonellosis, granuloma inguinale, UTIs, skin and skin structure infections, and anthrax. Treatment of infections caused by *Escherichia coli, Enterobacter aerogenes, Shigella* species, or *Acinetobacter* species. Treatment of uncomplicated gonorrhea, syphilis, yaws, listeriosis, Vincent's infection, actinomycosis, and *Clostridium* species infections when penicillin is contraindicated. Adjunct to amebicides in acute intestinal amebiasis. Adjunctive therapy in severe acne

>8 Years:
≤100 lbs:
2mg/lb divided into 2 doses on 1st day, followed by 1mg/lb qd or as 2 divided doses, on subsequent days
More Severe Infections: Up to 2mg/lb
>100 lbs:
Initial: 100mg q12h or 50mg q6h on 1st day
Maint: 100mg qd or 50mg q12h
More Severe Infections (eg, Chronic UTIs):
100mg q12h
Streptococcal Infections:
Continue therapy for 10 days

Inhalational Anthrax (Postexposure)

<100 lbs:
1mg/lb bid for 60 days
≥100 lbs:
100mg bid for 60 days

ADMINISTRATION

Oral route

Administer w/ adequate amounts of fluid

May be given w/ food if gastric irritation occurs

HOW SUPPLIED

Cap: 150mg

WARNINGS/PRECAUTIONS

May cause permanent discoloration of the teeth (yellow-gray-brown) if used during tooth development (last 1/2 of pregnancy, infancy, and childhood to 8 yrs of age); do not use in this age group, except for anthrax. Enamel hypoplasia reported. *Clostridium difficile*-associated diarrhea (CDAD) reported; may need to d/c if CDAD is suspected or confirmed. May decrease fibula growth rate in prematures. May cause an increase in BUN. Photosensitivity manifested by an exaggerated sunburn reaction reported; d/c at the 1st evidence of skin erythema. May result in bacterial resistance if used in the absence of proven or suspected bacterial infection, or a prophylactic indication; take appropriate measures if superinfection develops. Bulging fontanels in infants and benign intracranial HTN in adults reported. False elevations of urinary catecholamine levels may occur due to interference w/ the fluorescence test.

ADVERSE REACTIONS

Anorexia, N/V, diarrhea, hepatotoxicity, maculopapular/erythematous rash, Stevens-Johnson syndrome, toxic epidermal necrolysis, urticaria, anaphylaxis, pericarditis, hemolytic anemia, thrombocytopenia, neutropenia, eosinophilia.

DRUG INTERACTIONS

Depresses plasma prothrombin activity; may require downward adjustment of anticoagulant dose. May interfere w/ bactericidal action of PCN; avoid concurrent use. Impaired absorption w/ antacids containing aluminum, Ca^{2+}, or Mg^{2+}, and iron-containing preparations. Decreased $T_{1/2}$ w/ barbiturates, carbamazepine, and phenytoin. Fatal renal toxicity reported w/ methoxyflurane. May render oral contraceptives less effective.

NURSING CONSIDERATIONS

Assessment: Assess for hypersensitivity to drug or any tetracyclines, pregnancy/nursing status, and possible drug interactions. Perform culture and susceptibility tests. In venereal disease when coexistent syphilis is suspected, perform a dark-field examination and blood serology.

Monitoring: Monitor for signs/symptoms of CDAD, photosensitivity, skin erythema, superinfection, bulging fontanels in infants, intracranial HTN in adults, and other adverse reactions. In long-term therapy, perform periodic lab evaluations of organ systems, including hematopoietic, renal, and hepatic studies. In venereal disease when coexistent syphilis is suspected, repeat blood serology monthly for at least 4 months.

Patient Counseling: Apprise of the potential hazard to fetus if used during pregnancy; instruct to notify physician if pregnant. Advise to avoid excessive sunlight or artificial UV light and to d/c therapy if phototoxicity (eg, skin eruptions) occurs; advise to consider use of sunscreen or sunblock. Inform that absorption of drug is reduced when taken w/ bismuth subsalicylate and w/ foods, especially those that contain Ca^{2+}. Inform that drug may increase the incidence of vaginal candidiasis. Inform that diarrhea may be experienced and instruct to immediately contact physician if watery and bloody stools (w/ or w/o stomach cramps and fever) occur, even as late as ≥2 months after the last dose. Counsel that therapy should only be used to treat bacterial, not viral, infections. Instruct to take exactly ud even if the patient feels better early in the course of therapy. Inform that skipping doses or not completing the full course of therapy may decrease effectiveness of treatment and increase bacterial resistance.

Storage: 20-25°C (68-77°F).

ADRENACLICK — epinephrine RX

Class: Sympathomimetic catecholamine

ADULT DOSAGE

Allergic Reactions

Emergency treatment of allergic reactions (Type I) including anaphylaxis to stinging and biting insects, allergen immunotherapy, foods, drugs, diagnostic testing substances, and other allergens, as well as idiopathic anaphylaxis or exercise-induced anaphylaxis

15-30kg:
0.15mg IM/SQ

PEDIATRIC DOSAGE

Allergic Reactions

Emergency treatment of allergic reactions (Type I) including anaphylaxis to stinging and biting insects, allergen immunotherapy, foods, drugs, diagnostic testing substances, and other allergens, as well as idiopathic anaphylaxis or exercise-induced anaphylaxis

15-30kg:
0.15mg IM/SQ

≥30kg: 0.3mg IM/SQ **Severe Persistent Anaphylaxis:** Repeat inj may be necessary	**≥30kg:** 0.3mg IM/SQ **Severe Persistent Anaphylaxis:** Repeat inj may be necessary

ADMINISTRATION

IM/SQ route

Inject into the anterolateral aspect of the thigh, through clothing if necessary
Consider using other forms of injectable epinephrine if doses <0.15mg are deemed necessary

HOW SUPPLIED

Inj: 0.15mg/0.15mL, 0.3mg/0.3mL

WARNINGS/PRECAUTIONS

Intended for immediate administration in patients who are determined to be at increased risk for anaphylaxis, including those with a history of anaphylactic reactions. Intended for immediate administration as emergency supportive therapy only and is not a substitute for immediate medical care. More than 2 sequential doses should only be administered under direct medical supervision. Do not inject IV. Large doses or accidental IV inj may result in cerebral hemorrhage due to sharp rise in BP; rapidly acting vasodilators can counteract the marked pressor effects of epinephrine. Do not inject into buttock; may not provide effective treatment of anaphylaxis. Do not inject into digits, hands, or feet; may result in loss of blood flow to the affected area. Contains sodium bisulfite; should not deter administration of the drug for treatment of serious allergic or other emergency situations, even in certain susceptible persons. Caution in elderly, pregnant women, and patients with heart disease, hyperthyroidism, or diabetes mellitus (DM). May temporarily worsen symptoms of Parkinson's disease.

ADVERSE REACTIONS

Anxiety, apprehensiveness, restlessness, tremor, weakness, dizziness, sweating, palpitations, pallor, N/V, headache, respiratory difficulties.

DRUG INTERACTIONS

May precipitate/aggravate angina pectoris as well as produce ventricular arrhythmias with drugs that may sensitize the heart to arrhythmias; use with caution. Monitor for cardiac arrhythmias with antiarrhythmics, cardiac glycosides, and diuretics. Effects may be potentiated by TCAs, MAOIs, levothyroxine sodium, and certain antihistamines (eg, chlorpheniramine, tripelennamine, diphenhydramine). Cardiostimulating and bronchodilating effects are antagonized by β-adrenergic blockers (eg, propranolol). Vasoconstricting and hypertensive effects are antagonized by α-adrenergic blockers (eg, phentolamine). Ergot alkaloids may reverse pressor effects.

NURSING CONSIDERATIONS

Assessment: Assess for risk of anaphylaxis, heart disease, hyperthyroidism, DM, Parkinson's disease, pregnancy/nursing status, and for possible drug interactions.

Monitoring: Monitor for allergic-type reactions, angina pectoris, ventricular arrhythmias, cerebral hemorrhage, and other adverse reactions. Monitor HR and BP.

Patient Counseling: Review patient instructions and operation of drug with patient and caregiver. Advise that therapy may produce signs and symptoms that include increased HR, sensation of more forceful heartbeat, palpitations, sweating, N/V, difficulty breathing, pallor, dizziness, weakness or shakiness, headache, apprehension, nervousness, or anxiety; advise that these signs and symptoms usually subside rapidly, especially with rest, quiet, and recumbency. Inform that patients may develop more severe or persistent effects if they have HTN or hyperthyroidism. Inform that patient may experience angina if they have coronary artery disease. Advise that patients may develop increased blood glucose levels following administration if they have DM. Advise that a temporary worsening of symptoms may be noticed if patient has Parkinson's disease. Instruct to seek immediate medical care in case of accidental inj.

Storage: 20-25°C (68-77°F); excursions permitted to 15-30°C (59-86°F). Store in the carrying-case provided. Protect from light. Do not refrigerate.

ADVAIR DISKUS – fluticasone propionate/salmeterol RX

Class: Beta$_2$-agonist/corticosteroid

Long-acting β_2-adrenergic agonists (LABAs), such as salmeterol, increase the risk of asthma-related death. LABAs may increase the risk of asthma-related hospitalization in pediatric and adolescent patients. Use only for patients not adequately controlled on a long-term asthma control medication (eg, inhaled corticosteroid) or whose disease severity clearly warrants initiation of treatment with both an inhaled corticosteroid and a LABA. Do not use if asthma is adequately controlled on low- or medium-dose inhaled corticosteroids.

ADULT DOSAGE

Asthma

Usual: 1 inh bid, approximately 12 hrs apart
Titrate: May replace current strength with a higher strength if response to initial dose after 2 weeks is inadequate
Max: 500/50 bid

Chronic Obstructive Pulmonary Disease

Maint Treatment of Airflow Obstruction Associated with COPD, Including Chronic Bronchitis and Emphysema
Usual: 1 inh of 250/50 bid, approximately 12 hrs apart

PEDIATRIC DOSAGE

Asthma

4-11 Years:
Usual: 1 inh of 100/50 bid, approximately 12 hrs apart

≥12 Years:
Usual: 1 inh bid, approximately 12 hrs apart
Titrate: May replace current strength with a higher strength if response to initial dose after 2 weeks is inadequate
Max: 500/50 bid

ADMINISTRATION

Orally inhaled powder

After inhalation, rinse mouth with water without swallowing

HOW SUPPLIED

Disk: (Fluticasone-Salmeterol) (100/50) 100mcg-50mcg/inh, (250/50) 250mcg-50mcg/inh, (500/50) 500mcg-50mcg/inh [14, 60 blisters]

CONTRAINDICATIONS

Primary treatment of status asthmaticus or other acute episodes of asthma or COPD where intensive measures are required. Milk protein hypersensitivity.

WARNINGS/PRECAUTIONS

Not indicated for acute bronchospasm relief. Do not initiate during rapidly deteriorating or potentially life-threatening episodes of asthma or COPD; serious acute respiratory events reported. D/C regular use of oral/inhaled short-acting β_2-agonists (SABAs) when beginning treatment. Do not use more often or at higher doses than recommended; clinically significant cardiovascular (CV) effects and fatalities reported with excessive use. *Candida albicans* infections of mouth and pharynx reported; treat and if needed, interrupt therapy. Lower respiratory tract infections (eg, pneumonia) reported in patients with COPD. Increased susceptibility to infections. May lead to serious/fatal course of chickenpox or measles; avoid exposure and, if exposed, consider prophylaxis/treatment. Caution with active/quiescent tuberculosis (TB), systemic fungal, bacterial, viral, or parasitic infections, or ocular herpes simplex. Deaths due to adrenal insufficiency reported during and after transfer from systemic to inhaled corticosteroids; wean slowly from systemic corticosteroid use after transferring to therapy. Resume oral corticosteroids during periods of stress or a severe asthma attack in patients previously withdrawn from systemic corticosteroids. Transfer from systemic to inhaled corticosteroids may unmask allergic conditions previously suppressed by systemic therapy (eg, rhinitis, conjunctivitis, eczema). Monitor for systemic corticosteroid effects. Reduce dose slowly and consider other treatments if hypercorticism and adrenal suppression occur. May produce paradoxical bronchospasm; treat immediately with an inhaled, short acting bronchodilator; d/c and institute alternative therapy. Upper airway symptoms reported. Immediate hypersensitivity reactions, and CV and CNS effects may occur. Decreases in bone mineral density (BMD) reported with long-term use; caution with major risk factors for decreased bone mineral content, including chronic use of drugs that can reduce bone mass (eg, anticonvulsants, oral corticosteroids). Assess BMD prior to initiating therapy and periodically thereafter in patients with COPD; if significant reductions in BMD are seen and therapy is still considered medically important, use medicine to treat or prevent osteoporosis. May reduce growth velocity in pediatric patients; routinely monitor growth. Glaucoma, increased intraocular pressure (IOP), and cataracts reported with long-term use. Systemic eosinophilic conditions, and vasculitis consistent with Churg-Strauss syndrome may occur. Caution with CV disorders, convulsive disorders, thyrotoxicosis, diabetes mellitus (DM), ketoacidosis, hepatic disease, and in patients unusually responsive to sympathomimetic amines. Clinically significant changes in blood glucose and/or serum K^+ reported.

ADVERSE REACTIONS

Upper respiratory tract infection/inflammation, pharyngitis, hoarseness/dysphonia, bronchitis, cough, headache, N/V, sinusitis, throat irritation, viral respiratory infection, musculoskeletal pain, fever, dizziness.

DRUG INTERACTIONS

Do not use with other medicines containing LABA. Not recommended with strong CYP3A4 inhibitors (eg, ritonavir, clarithromycin, itraconazole); increased systemic corticosteroid and increased CV adverse effects may occur. Extreme caution with TCAs or MAOIs, or within 2 weeks of discontinuation of such agents; action on the vascular system may be potentiated. β-blockers may block pulmonary effects and produce severe bronchospasm; if such therapy is needed, consider cardioselective β-blockers and use with caution. Caution is advised when coadministered with non-K^+-sparing diuretics (eg, loop, thiazide).

NURSING CONSIDERATIONS

Assessment: Assess for hypersensitivity to milk proteins, status asthmaticus, acute asthma/COPD episodes, rapidly deteriorating asthma/COPD, active/quiescent TB, systemic infections, ocular herpes simplex, risk factors for decreased bone mineral content, CV disorders, convulsive disorders, thyrotoxicosis, DM, ketoacidosis, history of increased IOP, glaucoma, and/or cataracts, hepatic disease, pregnancy/nursing status, and possible drug interactions. Assess BMD in patients with COPD.

Monitoring: Monitor for deteriorating disease, localized oropharyngeal *C. albicans* infections, pneumonia, infections, systemic corticosteroid effects (eg, hypercorticism, adrenal suppression), paradoxical bronchospasm, upper airway symptoms, immediate hypersensitivity reactions, CV and CNS effects, glaucoma, cataracts, increased IOP, eosinophilic conditions, changes in blood glucose and/or serum K^+, and other adverse reactions. Periodically monitor BMD in patients with COPD. Monitor growth of pediatric patients routinely. Closely monitor patients with hepatic disease.

Patient Counseling: Counsel about the risks and benefits of therapy. Inform that drug is not meant to relieve acute asthma symptoms or exacerbations of COPD; advise to treat acute symptoms with an inhaled SABA (eg, albuterol). Instruct to seek medical attention immediately if experiencing a decrease in effectiveness of inhaled SABAs, a need for more inhalations than usual of inhaled SABAs, or a significant decrease in lung function. Advise not to d/c therapy without physician guidance and not to use other LABA. Instruct to contact physician if oropharyngeal candidiasis or symptoms of pneumonia develop. Advise to avoid exposure to chickenpox or measles, and, if exposed, to consult physician without delay. Inform about risk of immunosuppression, hypercorticism, adrenal suppression, reduction in BMD, reduced growth velocity in pediatric patients, ocular effects, and of adverse effects (eg, palpitations, chest pain, rapid HR, tremor, nervousness). Instruct to d/c therapy if immediate hypersensitivity reactions occur. Inform that the inhaler is not reusable and advise not to take the inhaler apart.

Storage: 20-25°C (68-77°F); excursions permitted from 15-30°C (59-86°F). Store in a dry place away from direct heat or sunlight. Store inside the unopened moisture-protective foil pouch and only remove from the pouch immediately before initial use. Discard 1 month after opening the foil pouch or when the counter reads "0," whichever comes 1st.

ADVAIR HFA – fluticasone propionate/salmeterol RX

Class: $Beta_2$-agonist/corticosteroid

Long-acting β_2-adrenergic agonists (LABAs), such as salmeterol, increase the risk of asthma-related death. LABAs may increase the risk of asthma-related hospitalization in pediatric and adolescent patients. Use only for patients not adequately controlled on a long-term asthma control medication (eg, inhaled corticosteroid) or whose disease severity clearly warrants initiation of treatment with both an inhaled corticosteroid and a LABA. Do not use if asthma is adequately controlled on low- or medium-dose inhaled corticosteroids.

ADULT DOSAGE

Asthma

Usual: 2 inh bid (q12h)
Titrate: Replace w/ higher strength if response to initial dose after 2 weeks is inadequate
Max: 2 inh of 230mcg-21mcg bid

PEDIATRIC DOSAGE

Asthma

≥12 Years:
Usual: 2 inh bid (q12h)
Titrate: Replace w/ higher strength if response to initial dose after 2 weeks is inadequate
Max: 2 inh of 230mcg-21mcg bid

DOSE MODIFICATION

Elderly

Start at lower end of dosing range

ADMINISTRATION

Oral inh route

Rinse mouth after inh
Shake well for 5 sec before each spray

Priming

Prime before using for the 1st time by releasing 4 test sprays into the air, shaking well for 5 sec before each spray
If the inhaler has not been used for more than 4 weeks or has been dropped, prime inhaler by releasing 2 sprays into the air, shaking well for 5 sec before each spray

HOW SUPPLIED

MDI: (Fluticasone-Salmeterol) (45/21) 45mcg-21mcg/inh, (115/21) 115mcg-21mcg/inh, (230/21) 230mcg-21mcg/inh [60, 120 inhalations]

CONTRAINDICATIONS

Primary treatment of status asthmaticus or other acute episodes of asthma where intensive measures are required.

WARNINGS/PRECAUTIONS

Not indicated for acute bronchospasm relief. May produce paradoxical bronchospasm; treat immediately with an inhaled, short-acting bronchodilator; d/c and institute alternative therapy. Upper airway symptoms reported. Immediate hypersensitivity reactions, including anaphylaxis, may occur. Salmeterol: Serious acute respiratory events reported when initiated during rapidly deteriorating or potentially life-threatening episodes of asthma. D/C regular use of oral/inhaled short-acting β_2-agonists (SABAs) when beginning treatment. Do not use more often or at higher doses than recommended; clinically significant cardiovascular (CV) effects and fatalities reported with excessive use. CV and CNS effects may occur. Caution with CV disorders (coronary insufficiency, cardiac arrhythmias, and HTN), convulsive disorders, thyrotoxicosis, diabetes mellitus (DM), ketoacidosis, and in patients unusually responsive to sympathomimetic amines. Clinically significant changes in blood glucose and/or serum K^+ reported infrequently. Fluticasone: *Candida albicans* infections of mouth and pharynx reported; treat and, if needed, interrupt therapy. Lower respiratory tract infections (eg, pneumonia) reported in patients with chronic obstructive pulmonary disease. Increased susceptibility to infections. May lead to serious/fatal course of chickenpox or measles; avoid exposure and, if exposed, consider prophylaxis/treatment. Caution with active/quiescent tuberculosis (TB), systemic fungal, bacterial, viral, or parasitic infections, or ocular herpes simplex. Deaths due to adrenal insufficiency reported during and after transfer from systemic to inhaled corticosteroids; wean slowly from systemic corticosteroid use after transferring to therapy. Resume oral corticosteroids during periods of stress or a severe asthma attack in patients previously withdrawn from systemic corticosteroids. Transfer from systemic corticosteroids may unmask allergic conditions previously suppressed by systemic therapy (eg, rhinitis, conjunctivitis, eczema). Monitor for systemic corticosteroid effects. Hypercorticism and adrenal suppression may occur in patients sensitive to these effects; if such effects occur, reduce therapy slowly and consider other treatments for management of asthma symptoms. Decreases in bone mineral density (BMD) reported with long-term use; caution with major risk factors for decreased bone mineral content, including chronic use of drugs that can reduce bone mass (eg, anticonvulsants, oral corticosteroids). May reduce growth velocity in pediatric patients; routinely monitor growth. Glaucoma, increased IOP, and cataracts reported with long-term use. Systemic eosinophilic conditions, and vasculitis consistent with Churg-Strauss syndrome may occur.

ADVERSE REACTIONS

URTI/inflammation, headache, throat irritation, musculoskeletal pain, N/V, dizziness, viral GI infection, hoarseness/dysphonia, GI signs and symptoms.

DRUG INTERACTIONS

Not recommended with strong CYP3A4 inhibitors (eg, ritonavir [RTV], atazanavir, clarithromycin, indinavir, itraconazole, nefazodone, nelfinavir, saquinavir, ketoconazole, telithromycin); increased systemic corticosteroid and CV adverse effects may occur. RTV and ketoconazole may increase exposure and reduce cortisol levels. Do not use with other medicines containing LABAs. Salmeterol: Extreme caution with TCAs or MAOIs, or within 2 weeks of discontinuation of such agents; action on the vascular system may be potentiated. β-blockers may block pulmonary effects and also produce severe bronchospasm in patients with asthma; if such therapy is needed, consider cardioselective β-blockers and use with caution. Use caution when coadministered with non-K^+-sparing diuretics (eg, loop, thiazide).

NURSING CONSIDERATIONS

Assessment: Assess for status asthmaticus, acute asthma episodes, rapidly deteriorating asthma, active/quiescent TB, systemic infections, ocular herpes simplex, risk factors for decreased bone mineral content, CV disorders, convulsive disorders, thyrotoxicosis, DM, ketoacidosis, history of increased IOP, glaucoma, and/or cataracts, hepatic disease, drug hypersensitivity, pregnancy/nursing status, and possible drug interactions.

Monitoring: Monitor for deteriorating asthma, localized oropharyngeal *C. albicans* infections, pneumonia, infections, systemic corticosteroid effects (eg, hypercorticism, adrenal suppression), paradoxical bronchospasm, upper airway symptoms, immediate hypersensitivity reactions, CV and CNS effects, decreases in BMD, glaucoma, cataracts, increased IOP, eosinophilic conditions, changes in blood glucose and/or serum K^+, and other adverse reactions. Monitor growth of pediatric patients routinely. Closely monitor patients with hepatic disease. Carefully monitor infants born of mothers receiving therapy during pregnancy for hypoadrenalism.

Patient Counseling: Counsel about the risks and benefits of therapy. Inform that drug is not meant to relieve acute asthma symptoms; advise to treat acute symptoms with an inhaled SABA (eg, albuterol). Instruct to seek medical attention immediately if experiencing a decrease in effectiveness of inhaled SABA, a need for more inhalations than usual of inhaled SABA, or a significant decrease in lung function. Advise not to d/c therapy without physician guidance and not to use other LABA. Instruct to contact physician if oropharyngeal candidiasis or symptoms of pneumonia develop. Advise to avoid exposure to chickenpox or measles, and, if exposed, to consult physician without delay. Advise to d/c therapy if immediate hypersensitivity reactions occur. Instruct to avoid spraying in eyes. Advise women to contact physician if they become pregnant while taking the drug.

Storage: 20-25°C (68-77°F); excursions permitted from 15-30°C (59-86°F). Store with the mouthpiece down. Do not puncture, use/store near heat or open flame, or throw into fire/incinerator. Exposure to temperatures >49°C (120°F) may cause bursting. Discard when the counter reads "000."

AFINITOR – everolimus

RX

Class: Kinase inhibitors

OTHER BRAND NAMES

Afinitor Disperz

ADULT DOSAGE

Subependymal Giant Cell Astrocytoma with Tuberous Sclerosis Complex

Requiring Therapeutic Intervention but Cannot be Curatively Resected:

Sus/Tab:

Initial: 4.5mg/m^2 qd

Titrate (Based on Trough Levels):

<5ng/mL: Increase daily dose by 2.5mg (Tab) or 2mg (Disperz)

>15ng/mL: Reduce daily dose by 2.5mg (Tab) or 2mg (Disperz)

Assess trough levels 2 weeks after initiation, a change in dose, a change in coadministration of CYP3A4/P-gp inducers/inhibitors, a change in hepatic function, or a change in dosage form

Once stable, monitor trough every 3-6 months in patients w/ changing BSA or every 6-12 months in patients w/ stable BSA

Breast Cancer

Treatment of postmenopausal women w/ advanced hormone receptor-positive, HER2-negative breast cancer in combination w/ exemestane, after failure of treatment w/ letrozole or anastrozole

Tab:

10mg qd

Advanced Renal Cell Carcinoma

After Failure of Treatment w/ Sunitinib or Sorafenib:

Tab:

10mg qd

Advanced Pancreatic Neuroendocrine Tumors

Progressive Neuroendocrine Tumors of Pancreatic Origin w/ Unresectable, Locally Advanced or Metastatic Disease:

Tab:

10mg qd

Renal Angiomyolipoma with Tuberous Sclerosis Complex

In Patients Not Requiring Immediate Surgery:

Tab:

10mg qd

Missed Dose

Missed doses may be taken up to 6 hrs after scheduled time; if >6 hrs, skip missed dose and resume at next scheduled time

PEDIATRIC DOSAGE

Subependymal Giant Cell Astrocytoma with Tuberous Sclerosis Complex

Requiring Therapeutic Intervention but Cannot be Curatively Resected:

≥1 Year:

Sus/Tab:

Initial: 4.5mg/m^2 qd

Titrate (Based on Trough Levels):

<5ng/mL: Increase daily dose by 2.5mg (Tab) or 2mg (Disperz)

>15ng/mL: Reduce daily dose by 2.5mg (Tab) or 2mg (Disperz)

Assess trough levels 2 weeks after initiation, a change in dose, a change in coadministration of CYP3A4/P-gp inducers/inhibitors, a change in hepatic function, or a change in dosage form

Once stable, monitor trough every 3-6 months in patients w/ changing BSA or every 6-12 months in patients w/ stable BSA

Missed Dose

Missed doses may be taken up to 6 hrs after scheduled time; if >6 hrs, skip missed dose and resume at next scheduled time

DOSE MODIFICATION

Concomitant Medications

Advanced Hormone Receptor (HR)-Positive, HER2-Negative Breast Cancer, Progressive Neuroendocrine Tumors of Pancreatic Origin (PNET), Renal Cell Carcinoma (RCC), Renal Angiomyolipoma w/ Tuberous Sclerosis Complex (TSC):
Strong CYP3A4/P-gp Inhibitors: Avoid use
If Moderate CYP3A4/P-gp Inhibitor is Necessary:
Reduce to 2.5mg qd; may increase to 5mg if tolerated
Return to dose used prior to initiating the inhibitor 2-3 days after discontinuation of the moderate inhibitor
Strong CYP3A4/P-gp Inducers: Avoid use
If Necessary:
Consider doubling daily dose by increments of ≤5mg
Return to dose used prior to initiating the inducer 3-5 days after discontinuation of the strong inducer
Subependymal Giant Cell Astrocytoma (SEGA) w/ TSC:
Strong CYP3A4/P-gp Inhibitors: Avoid use
If Moderate CYP3A4/P-gp Inhibitor is Necessary:
Initial: 2.5mg/m^2 qd
Reduce dose by 50% and administer qod if receiving the lowest available strength
Return to dose used prior to initiating the inhibitor 2-3 days after discontinuation of the moderate inhibitor
Strong CYP3A4/P-gp Inducers: Avoid use unless necessary
If Necessary:
Initial: 9mg/m^2 qd
Double the dose and assess tolerability
Return to dose used prior to initiating the inducer if the strong inducer is discontinued

Hepatic Impairment

Advanced HR-Positive, HER2-Negative Breast Cancer, PNET, RCC, Renal Angiomyolipoma w/ TSC:
Mild (Child-Pugh Class A): 7.5mg qd; reduce to 5mg qd if not tolerated
Moderate (Child-Pugh Class B): 5mg qd; reduce to 2.5mg qd if not tolerated
Severe (Child-Pugh Class C): 2.5mg qd if benefit outweighs the risk

SEGA w/ TSC:
Severe (Child-Pugh Class C):
Initial: 2.5mg/m^2 qd
Reduce starting dose by 50%

Adverse Reactions

Advanced HR-Positive, HER2-Negative Breast Cancer, PNET, RCC, Renal Angiomyolipoma w/ TSC:
If dose reduction is required, administer approx 50% lower than the previously administered daily dose

Noninfectious Pneumonitis:
Grade 2 (Symptomatic, Not Interfering w/ Activities of Daily Living [ADL]):
Consider interrupting therapy, rule out infection, and consider treatment w/ corticosteroids until symptoms improve to Grade ≤1
Reinitiate at lower dose
D/C if failure to recover w/in 4 weeks
Grade 3 (Symptomatic, Interfering w/ ADL; O_2 Indicated):
Interrupt therapy until symptoms resolve to Grade ≤1, rule out infection, and consider treatment w/ corticosteroids
Consider reinitiating at a lower dose
Consider discontinuation if toxicity recurs at Grade 3
Grade 4 (Life-Threatening, Ventilator Support Indicated):
D/C, rule out infection, and consider treatment w/ corticosteroids

Stomatitis:
Grade 2 (Symptomatic but Can Eat and Swallow Modified Diet):
Temporarily interrupt dose until recovery to Grade ≤1; reinitiate at the same dose
If stomatitis recurs at Grade 2, interrupt dose until recovery to Grade ≤1; reinitiate at a lower dose
Manage w/ topical oral analgesics (eg, benzocaine, butyl aminobenzoate, tetracaine, menthol, phenol) 3 topical corticosteroids (eg, triamcinolone)
Grade 3 (Symptomatic and Unable to Aliment or Hydrate Orally):
Temporarily interrupt dose until recovery to Grade ≤1
Reinitiate at a lower dose
Manage w/ topical oral analgesics (eg, benzocaine, butyl aminobenzoate, tetracaine, menthol, phenol) 3 topical corticosteroids (eg, triamcinolone)

Grade 4 (Symptoms Associated w/ Life-Threatening Consequences):
D/C and treat appropriately

Other Nonhematologic Toxicities (Excluding Metabolic Events):
Grade 2:
If toxicity becomes intolerable, temporarily interrupt dose until recovery to Grade ≤1; reinitiate at same dose
If toxicity recurs at Grade 2, interrupt until recovery to Grade ≤1; reinitiate at lower dose
Grade 3:
Temporarily interrupt dose until recovery to Grade ≤1
Initiate appropriate therapy and monitor
Consider reinitiating at a lower dose
If toxicity recurs at Grade 3, consider discontinuation
Grade 4:
D/C and treat appropriately

Metabolic Events (eg, Hyperglycemia, Dyslipidemia):
Grade 3:
Temporarily interrupt dose
Reinitiate at a lower dose
Manage w/ appropriate therapy and monitor
Grade 4:
D/C and treat appropriately

SEGA w/ TSC:
Temporarily interrupt or permanently d/c for severe or intolerable adverse reactions
If dose reduction is required when reinitiating therapy, reduce dose by 50%
If dose reduction is required for patients receiving the lowest available strength, administer qod

ADMINISTRATION

Oral route
Take consistently w/ or w/o food
Do not combine the 2 dosage forms to achieve the desired total dose

Tab
Swallow whole w/ a glass of water
Do not break or crush

Disperz
Wear gloves to avoid possible contact w/ drug when preparing sus for another person
Administer as sus only
Administer sus immediately after preparation and discard if not given w/in 60 min after preparation
Prepare sus in water only

HOW SUPPLIED

Sus (Tab): (Disperz) 2mg, 3mg, 5mg; Tab: 2.5mg, 5mg, 7.5mg, 10mg

WARNINGS/PRECAUTIONS

Not indicated for the treatment of functional carcinoid tumors. Noninfectious pneumonitis reported; opportunistic infections such as *Pneumocystis jiroveci* pneumonia (PJP) should be considered in the differential diagnosis. May continue therapy w/o dose alteration in patients who develop radiological changes and have few or no symptoms of noninfectious pneumonitis. For moderate symptoms, consider interrupting therapy until symptoms improve and consider corticosteroid use. Immunosuppressive properties may predispose patients to localized and systemic infections, including infections w/ opportunistic pathogens. Treat preexisting invasive fungal infections completely prior to therapy. Institute appropriate treatment if diagnosis of an infection is made and consider interruption or discontinuation of therapy. If a diagnosis of a fungal invasive systemic infection is made, d/c therapy. PJP reported; consider prophylaxis of PJP w/ concomitant use of corticosteroids or other immunosuppressive agents. Mouth ulcers, stomatitis, and oral mucositis reported. Cases of renal failure observed. May delay wound healing and increase the occurrence of wound-related complications (eg, wound dehiscence, wound infection, incisional hernia). Caution use in the perisurgical period. Elevated SrCr, proteinuria, hyperglycemia, hyperlipidemia, hypertriglyceridemia, and decreased Hgb, lymphocytes, neutrophils, and platelets reported. Exposure is increased in patients w/ hepatic impairment. Avoid close contact w/ those who have received live vaccines during treatment. In pediatric patients w/ SEGA who do not require immediate treatment, complete the recommended childhood series of live virus vaccinations prior to therapy; an accelerated vaccination schedule may be appropriate. May cause fetal harm. Caution in elderly.

ADVERSE REACTIONS

Stomatitis, infections, rash, fatigue, diarrhea, edema, abdominal pain, N/V, fever, headache, respiratory tract infection, asthenia, cough, decreased appetite.

DRUG INTERACTIONS

See Dose Modification. ACE inhibitor therapy may increase risk for angioedema. CYP3A4 and P-gp inhibitors increase levels. Avoid use w/ St. John's wort; may decrease levels. Avoid use w/

grapefruit, grapefruit juice, and other foods that are known to inhibit CYP450 and P-gp activity; may increase exposures. May increase midazolam and octreotide levels. Avoid use of live vaccines while on therapy. May alter exemestane levels. More frequent monitoring is recommended when coadministered w/ other drugs that may induce hyperglycemia.

NURSING CONSIDERATIONS

Assessment: Assess for hypersensitivity reactions, preexisting fungal infections, pregnancy/nursing status, and possible drug interactions. Assess renal/hepatic function. Obtain FPG, lipid profile, and CBC prior to start of therapy. Assess vaccination history in pediatric patients w/ SEGA.

Monitoring: Monitor for signs/symptoms of hypersensitivity reactions, noninfectious pneumonitis, infections, mouth ulcers, stomatitis, oral mucositis, and other adverse reactions. Monitor renal/hepatic function, FPG, lipid profile, and CBC periodically. Routine therapeutic drug monitoring is recommended.

Patient Counseling: Inform that noninfectious pneumonitis or infections may develop; advise to report new or worsening respiratory symptoms or any signs or symptoms of infection. Inform that patients are more susceptible to angioedema if concomitantly taking ACE inhibitors; advise to be aware of any signs/symptoms of angioedema and to seek prompt medical attention. Inform of the possibility of developing mouth ulcers, stomatitis, and oral mucositis; instruct to use topical treatments and mouthwashes (w/o alcohol, peroxide, iodine, or thyme) in such cases. Inform of the possibility of developing kidney failure and the need to monitor kidney function. Inform of the possibility of impaired wound healing or dehiscence during therapy. Inform of the need to monitor blood chemistry and hematology prior to therapy and periodically thereafter. Advise to notify physician of all concomitant medications, including OTC medications and dietary supplements. Advise of risk of fetal harm. Advise female patients of reproductive potential to avoid becoming pregnant and to use highly effective contraception while on treatment and for up to 8 weeks after ending treatment. Advise to avoid the use of live vaccines and close contact w/ those who have received live vaccines. Instruct to follow the dosing instructions ud and that if a dose is missed, to take it up to 6 hrs after the time they would normally take it. Advise to read and carefully follow the FDA-approved "Instructions for Use" to minimize unintended exposure.

Storage: 25°C (77°F); excursions permitted between 15-30°C (59-86°F). Store in the original container; protect from light and moisture.

AFLURIA – influenza vaccine RX

Class: Vaccine

ADULT DOSAGE

Influenza

Active Immunization Against Virus Subtypes A and Type B:

1 dose of 0.5mL

PEDIATRIC DOSAGE

Influenza

Active Immunization Against Virus Subtypes A and Type B:

5-8 Years:
1 or 2 doses (at least 1 month apart) of 0.5mL, depending on vaccination history

≥9 Years:
1 dose of 0.5mL

ADMINISTRATION

IM route

Available by needle and syringe (≥5 years) or by PharmaJet Stratis Needle-Free Injection System (18-64 years)

Inject preferably in the deltoid muscle of the upper arm
Shake thoroughly before use and administer dose immediately
Administer in separate syringes and use a separate arm if to be given at the same time as another injectable vaccine(s)

Refer to PI for further administration instructions

HOW SUPPLIED

Inj: 0.5mL [prefilled syringe], 5mL [multidose vial]

CONTRAINDICATIONS

Known severe allergic reactions to egg protein.

WARNINGS/PRECAUTIONS

Increased rates of fever and febrile seizures reported in children predominantly <5 yrs of age; febrile events were also reported in children 5-8 yrs of age. Caution if Guillain-Barre syndrome (GBS) has occurred within 6 weeks of previous influenza vaccination. Appropriate medical treatment and supervision must be available to manage possible anaphylactic reactions. Immune response may be diminished if vaccine is administered to immunocompromised persons. May not protect all individuals.

ADVERSE REACTIONS

Inj-site reactions (pain, redness, swelling, tenderness, induration), headache, myalgia, irritability, malaise, N/V, fever, cough, diarrhea, oropharyngeal pain.

DRUG INTERACTIONS

Corticosteroid or immunosuppressive therapies may diminish immunological response to vaccine.

NURSING CONSIDERATIONS

Assessment: Review vaccination history. Assess for known severe allergic reactions to any component of the vaccine (eg, egg protein) or to a previous influenza vaccine, development of GBS following a prior dose of influenza vaccine, immunosuppression, pregnancy/nursing status, and possible drug interactions.

Monitoring: Monitor for signs/symptoms of fever, febrile seizures, GBS, allergic reactions, and other adverse reactions.

Patient Counseling: Inform of the potential benefits and risks of immunization. Inform that vaccine cannot cause influenza but produces antibodies that protect against influenza and that the full effect of the vaccine is achieved approximately 3 weeks after vaccination. Instruct to report any severe or unusual adverse reactions to physician. Instruct that annual revaccination is recommended.

Storage: 2-8°C (36-46°F). Do not freeze; discard if it has been frozen. Protect from light. Discard vial within 28 days once stopper has been pierced.

AFREZZA — insulin human

RX

Class: Insulin

Acute bronchospasm reported in patients with asthma and COPD. Contraindicated with chronic lung disease (eg, asthma, COPD). Perform a detailed medical history, physical examination, and spirometry before initiating therapy.

ADULT DOSAGE

Diabetes Mellitus

Initial Mealtime Dose:

Insulin Naive:

4 U at each meal

From SQ Mealtime (Prandial) Insulin:

See Conversions

Using SQ Premixed Insulin:

Divide 1/2 of total daily premixed insulin dose equally among the 3 meals of the day and convert each estimated mealtime dose (see Conversions); administer 1/2 of total daily premixed dose as a basal insulin dose

Conversions

Mealtime Dose Conversion:

Up to 4 U SQ: 4 U
5-8 U SQ: 8 U
9-12 U SQ: 12 U
13-16 U SQ: 16 U
17-20 U SQ: 20 U
21-24 U SQ: 24 U

PEDIATRIC DOSAGE

Pediatric use may not have been established

DOSE MODIFICATION

Renal Impairment

Dose adjustment may be necessary

Hepatic Impairment

Dose adjustment may be necessary

ADMINISTRATION

Oral inh route

Administer using a single inh/cartridge
Administer at the beginning of the meal

Keep inhaler level and white mouthpiece on top and purple base on the bottom after a cartridge has been inserted into the inhaler; loss of drug effect can occur if the inhaler is turned upside down, held with the mouthpiece pointing down, or shaken (or dropped) after the cartridge has been inserted but before the dose has been administered. If any of the above occur, the cartridge should be replaced before use

Doses >8 U

Administer using a combination of 4 U and 8 U cartridges to achieve required total mealtime dose

HOW SUPPLIED

Powder, Inh: 4 U, 8 U

CONTRAINDICATIONS

During episodes of hypoglycemia, chronic lung disease (eg, asthma, COPD).

WARNINGS/PRECAUTIONS

Not a substitute for long-acting insulin; use in combination with long-acting insulin with type 1 DM. Not recommended for the treatment of diabetic ketoacidosis (DKA) or in patients who smoke or who have recently stopped smoking. Increase the frequency of glucose monitoring and consider alternative route of delivery of insulin in patients at risk for DKA. Changes in strength, manufacturer, type, or method of administration may affect glycemic control and predispose to hypo/hyperglycemia; these changes should be made under close medical supervision and with increased frequency of blood glucose monitoring. Hypoglycemia may occur; increased risk with renal/hepatic impairment. May cause a decline in lung function over time as measured by FEV_1; consider discontinuing therapy with decline of ≥20% in FEV_1. Consider more frequent monitoring of pulmonary function with pulmonary symptoms; d/c if symptoms persist. Consider benefits and potential risk in patients with active, prior history of, or at risk for lung cancer. Severe, life-threatening, generalized allergy, including anaphylaxis, may occur; if hypersensitivity reactions occur, d/c therapy, treat, and monitor until symptoms/signs resolve. May cause hypokalemia; monitor K^+ levels in patients at risk for hypokalemia. Patients with renal/hepatic impairment may require dose adjustment and more frequent blood glucose monitoring.

ADVERSE REACTIONS

Cough, throat pain/irritation, headache, hypoglycemia.

DRUG INTERACTIONS

Concomitant oral antidiabetic treatment may need to be adjusted. Thiazolidinediones (TZDs) may cause fluid retention and lead to or exacerbate HF; observe for signs and symptoms of HF and consider dose reduction or discontinuation of TZDs. Risk of hypoglycemia may be increased with antidiabetic agents, ACE inhibitors, ARBs, disopyramide, fibrates, fluoxetine, MAOIs, pentoxifylline, pramlintide, propoxyphene, salicylates, somatostatin analogues (eg, octreotide), and sulfonamide antibiotics. Glucose lowering effect may be decreased with atypical antipsychotics (eg, olanzapine, clozapine), corticosteroids, danazol, diuretics, estrogens, glucagon, isoniazid, niacin, oral contraceptives, phenothiazines, progestogens, protease inhibitors, somatropin, sympathomimetic agents (eg, albuterol, epinephrine, terbutaline), and thyroid hormones. Glucose lowering effect may be increased or decreased when coadministered with alcohol, β-blockers, clonidine, and lithium salts. Pentamidine may cause hypoglycemia, sometimes followed by hyperglycemia. Signs/symptoms of hypoglycemia may be blunted with β-blockers, clonidine, guanethidine, and reserpine. Dose adjustment and increased frequency of glucose monitoring may be required when administered with drugs that increase/decrease glucose lowering effect or increase hypoglycemia risk.

NURSING CONSIDERATIONS

Assessment: Assess for drug hypersensitivity, risk of hypoglycemia, chronic lung disease, lung cancer, renal/hepatic impairment, pregnancy/nursing status, and possible drug interactions. Obtain baseline blood glucose. Assess pulmonary function at baseline. Perform medical history, physical examination, and spirometry.

Monitoring: Monitor for signs/symptoms of hypoglycemia, hypokalemia, allergic reactions, decline in lung function, and other adverse reactions. Monitor for acute bronchospasm in patients with asthma or COPD. Monitor pulmonary function after first 6 months of therapy and annually thereafter. Increase frequency of glucose monitoring in patients at higher risk for hypoglycemia or who have reduced symptomatic awareness of hypoglycemia.

Patient Counseling: Inform of the potential risks and benefits and of alternative modes of therapy. Inform about the importance of adherence to dietary instructions, regular physical activity, periodic blood glucose monitoring and HbA1c testing, recognition and management of hypo/hyperglycemia, and assessment for diabetes complications. Instruct to promptly seek medical advice during periods of stress (eg, fever, trauma, infection, surgery) as medication requirements may change. Instruct to use only with inhaler. Instruct to inform physician of any history of lung disease, if any unusual symptom develops, or if any known symptom persists or worsens. Inform that the most common adverse reactions associated with therapy are hypoglycemia, cough, and throat pain/irritation. Advise women with diabetes to inform physician if pregnant or planning to become pregnant. Advise to immediately report to physician if any respiratory difficulty occurs after inhalation.

Instruct on self-management procedures and on handling of special situations. Inform that ability to concentrate and react may be impaired as a result of hypoglycemia; advise to use caution when driving or operating machinery. Inform that therapy may cause a decline in lung function. Instruct to promptly report any signs or symptoms potentially related to lung cancer. Instruct to monitor blood glucose during illness, infection, and other risk situations for DKA; advise to contact physician if blood glucose control worsens. Educate on the symptoms of hypersensitivity reactions.

Storage: Not in Use: 2-8°C (36-46°F). Use within 10 days if not refrigerated. In Use: 25°C (77°F); excursions permitted to 15-30°C (59-86°F). Sealed (Unopened) Blister Cards + Strips: Use within 10 days. Opened Strips: Use within 3 days. Inhaler: 2-25°C (36-77°F); excursions permitted. May refrigerate, but should be at room temperature before use. Handling: Before use, cartridges should be at room temperature for 10 min.

AGGRASTAT – tirofiban hydrochloride RX

Class: Glycoprotein IIb/IIIa inhibitor

ADULT DOSAGE

Acute Coronary Syndrome

To reduce the rate of thrombotic cardiovascular events (combined endpoint of death, MI, or refractory ischemia/repeat cardiac procedure) w/ non-ST elevation acute coronary syndrome

Usual: 25mcg/kg IV over 3 min, then 0.15mcg/kg/min for up to 18 hrs

Refer to PI for dosing by weight and CrCl

PEDIATRIC DOSAGE

Pediatric use may not have been established

DOSE MODIFICATION

Renal Impairment

CrCl ≤60mL/min: 25mcg/kg IV over 3 min, then 0.075mcg/kg/min for up to 18 hrs

Refer to PI for dosing by weight and CrCl

ADMINISTRATION

IV route

Do not administer through the same IV line as diazepam
May administer in the same IV line as atropine sulfate, dobutamine, dopamine, epinephrine HCl, famotidine inj, furosemide, lidocaine, midazolam HCl, morphine sulfate, nitroglycerin, potassium chloride, and propranolol HCl
Do not add other drugs or remove sol directly from the bag w/ a syringe
Do not use plastic containers in series connections; this can result in air embolism by drawing air from the 1st container if it is empty of sol

HOW SUPPLIED

Inj: 50mcg/mL [100mL, 250mL]

CONTRAINDICATIONS

Active internal bleeding, history of bleeding diathesis, major surgical procedure or severe physical trauma within the previous month, history of thrombocytopenia following prior drug exposure.

WARNINGS/PRECAUTIONS

Most bleeding associated with therapy occurs at the arterial access site for cardiac catheterization. Minimize the use of traumatic or potentially traumatic procedures (eg, arterial and venous punctures, IM inj, nasotracheal intubation). Fatal bleeding events reported. Profound thrombocytopenia reported; monitor platelet counts beginning about 6 hrs after treatment initiation and daily thereafter. Monitor platelet counts to exclude pseudothrombocytopenia if platelet count decreases to <90,000/mm^3; d/c therapy and heparin if thrombocytopenia is confirmed. Previous exposure to a glycoprotein (GP) IIb/IIIa receptor antagonist may increase the risk of developing thrombocytopenia.

ADVERSE REACTIONS

Bleeding, pelvic pain, bradycardia, coronary artery dissection, leg pain, dizziness.

DRUG INTERACTIONS

Concomitant use of antiplatelet agents, thrombolytics, oral anticoagulants, heparin, and aspirin increases the risk of bleeding.

NURSING CONSIDERATIONS

Assessment: Assess for drug hypersensitivity, active internal bleeding, history of bleeding diathesis, major surgical procedure or severe physical trauma within the previous month, history of thrombocytopenia following prior exposure to drug, pregnancy/nursing status, and possible drug interactions. Assess use of traumatic or potentially traumatic procedures. Obtain baseline platelet count.

Monitoring: Monitor for signs/symptoms of bleeding, hypersensitivity reaction (eg, anaphylaxis), thrombocytopenia, and other adverse reactions. Monitor platelet counts beginning about 6 hrs after treatment initiation and daily thereafter.

Patient Counseling: Advise to watch closely for any signs of bleeding or bruising and to report to physician if these occur. Advise to notify physician of use of any other medications, including OTC or herbal products prior to drug use.

Storage: 25°C (77°F); excursions permitted between 15-30°C (59-86°F). Protect from light. Do not freeze.

AGGRENOX – aspirin/dipyridamole RX

Class: Platelet aggregation inhibitor

ADULT DOSAGE

Stroke

Used to reduce risk of stroke in patients who have had transient ischemia of the brain or completed ischemic stroke due to thrombosis

Usual: 1 cap bid (1 in am and 1 in pm)

PEDIATRIC DOSAGE

Pediatric use may not have been established

DOSE MODIFICATION

Adverse Reactions

Intolerable Headaches During Initial Treatment:

Switch to 1 cap at hs and low-dose aspirin (ASA) in am

Return to usual regimen as soon as possible, usually w/in 1 week

ADMINISTRATION

Oral route

Take PO w/ or w/o food

Swallow whole; do not chew or crush

HOW SUPPLIED

Cap: (ASA/Dipyridamole Extended-Release) 25mg/200mg

CONTRAINDICATIONS

NSAID allergy, syndrome of asthma, rhinitis, and nasal polyps, and children or teenagers with viral infections.

WARNINGS/PRECAUTIONS

May increase risk of bleeding. Intracranial hemorrhage reported. Risk of GI side effects (eg, stomach pain, heartburn, N/V, gross GI bleeding, dyspepsia); monitor for signs of ulceration and bleeding. May cause fetal harm; avoid in 3rd trimester of pregnancy. Not interchangeable with individual components of ASA and dipyridamole tabs. ASA: Avoid with history of active peptic ulcer disease (PUD) or with severe hepatic or severe renal (GFR <10mL/min) dysfunction. Bleeding risks reported with chronic, heavy alcohol use (≥3 alcoholic drinks/day). May not provide adequate treatment for cardiac indications for stroke/transient ischemic attack patients for whom ASA is indicated to prevent recurrent MI or angina pectoris. Dipyridamole: Elevations of hepatic enzymes and hepatic failure reported. Has a vasodilatory effect; may precipitate/aggravate chest pain in patients with underlying coronary artery disease (CAD). May exacerbate preexisting hypotension.

ADVERSE REACTIONS

Headache, dyspepsia, abdominal pain, N/V, diarrhea, fatigue, arthralgia, pain, back pain, GI bleeding, hemorrhage.

DRUG INTERACTIONS

Increased risk of bleeding with other drugs that increase the risk of bleeding (eg, anticoagulants, antiplatelet agents, heparin, fibrinolytics, NSAIDs). Dipyridamole: May increase plasma levels and cardiovascular (CV) effects of adenosine. May counteract effect of cholinesterase inhibitors, potentially aggravating myasthenia gravis. ASA: May decrease effects of ACE inhibitors and β-blockers. Concurrent use with acetazolamide may lead to high serum concentrations of acetazolamide (and toxicity). May displace warfarin from protein binding sites, leading to prolongation of both PT and bleeding time. May decrease total concentration of phenytoin. May increase serum valproic acid levels. May decrease effects of diuretics in renal or CV disease. May inhibit renal clearance of methotrexate, leading to bone marrow toxicity (especially in elderly/renally impaired). Decreased renal function with NSAIDs. Moderate doses may increase effectiveness of oral hypoglycemics. May antagonize uricosuric agents (probenecid and sulfinpyrazone).

NURSING CONSIDERATIONS

Assessment: Assess for NSAID allergy, syndrome of asthma, rhinitis and nasal polyps, renal/hepatic dysfunction, history of active PUD, alcohol use, CAD, hypotension, hypersensitivity, pregnancy/nursing status, and possible drug interactions.

Monitoring: Monitor for signs/symptoms of allergic reactions, GI effects, elevated hepatic enzymes, hepatic failure, and for bleeding.

Patient Counseling: Inform of risk and signs/symptoms of bleeding (eg, occult bleeding). Instruct to notify physician of all medications and supplements being taken, especially drugs that may increase risk of bleeding. Counsel patients who consume ≥3 alcoholic drinks daily about the bleeding risks. Inform that transient headache may occur; instruct to notify physician if an intolerable headache develops. Inform about signs and symptoms of GI side effects and what steps to take if they occur. Advise that if a dose is missed, take next dose on regular schedule and not to take a double dose. Inform of potential hazard to fetus if used during pregnancy; instruct to notify physician if patient is pregnant or becomes pregnant.

Storage: 25°C (77°F); excursions permitted to 15-30°C (59-86°F). Protect from excessive moisture.

AKYNZEO – netupitant/palonosetron RX

Class: Substance P/neurokinin 1 receptor antagonist and 5-HT_3 receptor antagonist

ADULT DOSAGE

Chemotherapy-Associated Nausea/Vomiting

Highly Emetogenic Chemotherapy (Including Cisplatin Based):

Day 1: 1 cap approx 1 hr prior to the start of chemotherapy w/ dexamethasone 12mg PO 30 min prior to chemotherapy

Days 2-4: Dexamethasone 8mg PO qd

Anthracyclines and Cyclophosphamide Based/Non-Highly Emetogenic Chemotherapy:

Day 1: 1 cap approx 1 hr prior to the start of chemotherapy w/ dexamethasone 12mg PO 30 min prior to chemotherapy

Days 2-4: Administration of dexamethasone is not necessary

PEDIATRIC DOSAGE

Pediatric use may not have been established

ADMINISTRATION

Oral route

Take w/ or w/o food

HOW SUPPLIED

Cap: (Netupitant-Palonosetron) 300mg-0.5mg

WARNINGS/PRECAUTIONS

Hypersensitivity reactions, including anaphylaxis, reported. Serotonin syndrome reported; d/c and initiate supportive treatment if symptoms occur. Avoid with severe hepatic/renal impairment and end-stage renal disease. Caution in elderly.

ADVERSE REACTIONS

Dyspepsia, fatigue, constipation, erythema, headache, asthenia.

DRUG INTERACTIONS

Serotonin syndrome reported with concomitant use of other serotonergic drugs (eg, SSRIs, SNRIs, MAOIs); d/c and initiate supportive treatment if symptoms occur. May increase levels of CYP3A4 substrates; use with caution. Increased exposure of dexamethasone. Increased exposure to midazolam; consider the potential effects of increased levels of midazolam or other benzodiazepines metabolized via CYP3A4 (alprazolam, triazolam). May increase exposure of chemotherapy agents metabolized by CYP3A4 (eg, docetaxel, imatinib, vinblastine); use with caution and monitor for chemotherapeutic-related adverse reactions. Strong CYP3A4 inducers may decrease efficacy; avoid with chronic strong CYP3A4 inducers (eg, rifampin). Strong CYP3A4 inhibitors (eg, ketoconazole) may increase exposure.

NURSING CONSIDERATIONS

Assessment: Assess for hypersensitivity to drug, renal/hepatic impairment, pregnancy/nursing status, and possible drug interactions.

Monitoring: Monitor for hypersensitivity reactions, serotonin syndrome, and other adverse reactions.

Patient Counseling: Instruct to seek immediate medical attention if any signs/symptoms of a hypersensitivity reaction or serotonin syndrome (eg, changes in mental status, autonomic instability, neuromuscular symptoms, with or without GI symptoms) occur.

Storage: 20-25°C (68-77°F); excursions permitted from 15-30°C (59-86°F).

ALBUTEROL – albuterol sulfate RX

Class: Beta$_2$-agonist

ADULT DOSAGE

Bronchospasm

Syrup/Tab:
Initial: 2mg or 4mg tid or qid
Max: 8mg qid

0.5% Sol/0.083% Sol:
Usual: 2.5mg tid-qid

PEDIATRIC DOSAGE

Bronchospasm

Syrup:
2-5 Years:
Initial: 0.1mg/kg tid; not to exceed 2mg tid
Titrate: May increase to 0.2mg/kg tid
Max: 4mg tid

6-14 Years:
Initial: 2mg tid or qid
Max: 24mg/day in divided doses

>14 Years:
Initial: 2mg or 4mg tid or qid
Max: 8mg qid

Tab:
6-12 Years:
Initial: 2mg tid or qid
Max: 24mg/day in divided doses

>12 Years:
Initial: 2mg or 4mg tid or qid
Max: 8mg qid

0.5% Sol:
2-12 Years:
Initial: 0.1-0.15mg/kg/dose
Max: 2.5mg tid-qid

>12 Years:
Usual: 2.5mg tid-qid

0.083% Sol:
≥2 Years:
Usual:
≥15kg: 2.5mg tid-qid

DOSE MODIFICATION

Elderly
Syrup/Tab:
Initial: 2mg tid or qid
Individually adjust thereafter

Other Important Modifications
Syrup/Tab:
Patients Sensitive to β-Adrenergic Stimulators:
Initial: 2mg tid or qid
Individually adjust thereafter

ADMINISTRATION

Oral and inh route

0.5% Sol
To Administer 2.5mg of Albuterol:
1. Dilute 0.5mL of the sol w/ 2.5mL of sterile normal saline sol
2. Flow rate is regulated to suit the particular nebulizer so that sol will be delivered over approx 5-15 min

0.083% Sol
To Administer 2.5mg of Albuterol:
1. Administer the entire contents of one sterile unit dose vial (3mL)

NURSING CONSIDERATIONS

Assessment: Assess for renal/hepatic impairment, hyperkalemia, Addison's disease or other conditions associated with hyperkalemia, anuria, any other conditions where treatment is contraindicated or cautioned, pregnancy/nursing status, and for possible drug interactions.

Monitoring: Monitor for signs/symptoms of fluid/electrolyte imbalance, dilutional hyponatremia, BUN elevation, hyperchloremic metabolic acidosis, somnolence, dizziness, gynecomastia, and other adverse reactions. Monitor serum electrolytes periodically at appropriate intervals particularly in the elderly and with significant renal/hepatic impairment. Monitor serum K^+ and SrCr one week after initiation or dose increase, monthly for the first 3 months, then quarterly for a yr, and then every 6 months with severe HF.

Patient Counseling: Instruct to avoid K^+ supplements and foods containing high levels of K^+, including salt substitutes. Inform that somnolence and dizziness may occur; advise to use caution when driving or operating machinery, until response to initial treatment has been determined.

Storage: <25°C (77°F).

ALDARA – imiquimod

RX

Class: Immune response modifier

ADULT DOSAGE

Actinic Keratosis

Clinically Typical, Nonhyperkeratotic, Nonhypertrophic Actinic Keratoses on Face or Scalp:

Usual: Apply 2X/week (eg, Monday, Thursday) before hs for a full 16 weeks to defined treatment area (contiguous area 25cm^2 [eg, 5cm x 5cm]) on face (forehead or 1 cheek) or on scalp (but not both concurrently)

Max: 36 pkts for 16 weeks

Superficial Basal Cell Carcinomas

Biopsy-Confirmed, Primary Carcinoma, w/ a Max Tumor Diameter of 2cm, Located on Trunk (Excluding Anogenital Skin), Neck, or Extremities (Excluding Hands and Feet):

Use only when surgical methods are medically less appropriate and follow-up can be assured

Apply a sufficient amount before hs to cover treatment area including 1cm of skin surrounding tumor 5X/week for a full 6 weeks

Tumor Diameter:

0.5-<1cm: 4mm cre droplet (10mg)

1-<1.5cm: 5mm cre droplet (25mg)

1.5-2cm: 7mm cre droplet (40mg)

Max: 36 pkts for 6 weeks

External Genital and Perianal Warts

Usual: Apply a thin layer 3X/week before hs until warts are totally cleared

Max: 16 weeks

PEDIATRIC DOSAGE

External Genital and Perianal Warts

≥12 Years:

Usual: Apply a thin layer before hs and rub in until no longer visible 3X/week until warts are totally cleared

Max: 16 weeks

ADMINISTRATION

Topical route

Prior to application, wash treatment area w/ mild soap and water and allow to dry thoroughly for at least 10 min

Wash hands before and after application

Use 1 pkt/application

Rub in until no longer visible

Wash off w/ mild soap and water

Do not occlude treatment area

Actinic Keratosis

Wash off after 8 hrs

Superficial Basal Cell Carcinoma

Wash off after 8 hrs

External Genital and Perianal Warts/Condyloma Acuminata
Wash off after 6-10 hrs

HOW SUPPLIED
Cre: 5% [250mg, 12s]

WARNINGS/PRECAUTIONS
Caution in patients with preexisting autoimmune conditions. Not recommended for treatment of BCC subtypes other than sBCC. Not for oral, ophthalmic, or intravaginal use. Not recommended until completely healed from any previous drug/surgical treatment or sunburn. Avoid contact with eyes, lips, and nostrils. Local skin reactions are common; a rest period of several days may be taken if required by patient's discomfort or severity of local skin reaction. Do not extend treatment beyond 16 weeks due to missed doses or rest periods. Non-occlusive dressings (eg, cotton gauze, cotton underwear) may be used in the management of skin reactions. Early clinical clearance cannot be adequately assessed until resolution of local skin reactions (eg, 12 weeks post-treatment). Consider biopsy or other alternative interventions if there is evidence of persistent tumor. Carefully reevaluate treatment and reconsider management with lesions that do not respond to treatment. Avoid or minimize exposure to sunlight (including sunlamps); sunburn susceptibility may be heightened. Caution in patients with considerable sun exposure (eg, due to occupation) and in those with inherent sensitivity to sunlight. Intense local inflammatory reactions (eg, skin weeping or erosion, severe vulvar swelling that can lead to urinary retention) may occur and may be accompanied or preceded by flu-like signs/symptoms. May exacerbate inflammatory skin conditions, including chronic graft versus host disease. Interruption of dosing should be considered if systemic/local inflammatory reactions occur.

ADVERSE REACTIONS
Application-site reaction, local skin reactions, URTI, sinusitis, headache, squamous cell carcinoma, diarrhea, back pain, rhinitis, lymphadenopathy, influenza-like symptoms.

NURSING CONSIDERATIONS

Assessment: Assess for preexisting autoimmune conditions, immunosuppression, previous drug/surgical treatment, sunburn, inherent sensitivity to sunlight, and pregnancy/nursing status. For treatment of sBCC, perform biopsy to confirm diagnosis.

Monitoring: Monitor for local inflammatory reactions (eg, weeping or erosion, vulvar swelling), application-site reactions, systemic reactions (eg, flu-like symptoms), and other adverse reactions. For sBCC, monitor treatment site regularly; assess at 12 weeks post-treatment for clinical clearance.

Patient Counseling: Instruct on proper application technique and to use ud. Instruct to avoid contact with eyes, lips, and nostrils. Instruct not to bandage or occlude treatment area. Inform that local skin reactions may occur; instruct to contact physician promptly if experiencing any sign/symptom at application site that restricts/prohibits daily activities or makes continued application difficult. For patients being treated for actinic keratosis and sBCC, encourage using sunscreen and minimizing or avoiding exposure to natural or artificial sunlight (tanning beds, UVA/B treatment) while on therapy. Inform that subclinical lesions may appear in treatment area and may subsequently resolve. For patients being treated for external genital warts, instruct to avoid sexual (genital, anal, oral) contact while cream is on the skin. Advise female patients to avoid vaginal application and caution when applying cream at the vaginal opening. Instruct uncircumcised males treating warts under the foreskin to retract foreskin and clean area daily. Inform that new warts may develop during therapy, as drug is not a cure. Inform that drug may also weaken condoms and vaginal diaphragms and that concurrent use is not recommended.

Storage: 4-25°C (39-77°F). Do not freeze. Discard unused and partially used pkts; do not reuse partially used pkts.

Alimta – pemetrexed disodium — RX

Class: Antifolate

ADULT DOSAGE

Nonsquamous Non-Small Cell Lung Cancer

Initial treatment of locally advanced or metastatic nonsquamous non-small cell lung cancer (NSCLC) in combination w/ cisplatin. Maint treatment of patients w/ locally advanced or metastatic nonsquamous NSCLC whose disease has not progressed after 4 cycles of platinum-based first-line chemotherapy. Single-agent for the treatment of patients w/ locally advanced or metastatic nonsquamous NSCLC after prior chemotherapy

PEDIATRIC DOSAGE

Pediatric use may not have been established

Combination w/ Cisplatin:
Usual: 500mg/m^2 IV infused over 10 min on Day 1 of each 21-day cycle
Give cisplatin 75mg/m^2 infused over 2 hrs beginning 30 min after the end of administration

Single Agent:
Usual: 500mg/m^2 IV infused over 10 min on Day 1 of each 21-day cycle

Malignant Pleural Mesothelioma

Patients whose disease is unresectable or who are otherwise not candidates for curative surgery in combination w/ cisplatin

Combination w/ Cisplatin:
Usual: 500mg/m^2 IV infused over 10 min on Day 1 of each 21-day cycle
Give cisplatin 75mg/m^2 infused over 2 hrs beginning 30 min after the end of administration

Premedication

Initiate folic acid (400-1000mcg) PO qd beginning 7 days before the 1st dose; continue during the full course of therapy and for 21 days after the last dose of therapy
Administer vitamin B12 1mg IM 1 week prior to the 1st dose and every 3 cycles thereafter
Subsequent vitamin B12 inj may be given the same day as treatment
Give dexamethasone 4mg PO bid the day before, the day of, and the day after administration of therapy

DOSE MODIFICATION

Adverse Reactions

As a Single Agent or in Combination:
Hematologic Toxicities:
Nadir ANC <500/mm^3 and Nadir Platelets ≥50,000/mm^3: 75% of previous dose (pemetrexed and cisplatin)
Nadir Platelets <50,000/mm^3 w/o Bleeding Regardless of Nadir ANC: 75% of previous dose (pemetrexed and cisplatin)
Nadir Platelets <50,000/mm^3 w/ Bleeding Regardless of Nadir ANC: 50% of previous dose (pemetrexed and cisplatin)

Nonhematologic Toxicities:
≥Grade 3 (Excluding Neurotoxicity): Treatment should be withheld until resolution to ≤pre-therapy value
Any Grade 3 or 4 Toxicities Except Mucositis: 75% of previous dose (pemetrexed and cisplatin)
Any Diarrhea Requiring Hospitalization (Irrespective of Grade) or Grade 3 or 4 Diarrhea: 75% of previous dose (pemetrexed and cisplatin)
Grade 3 or 4 Mucositis: 50% of previous pemetrexed dose, 100% of previous cisplatin dose

Neurotoxicity:
CTC Grade 1: 100% of previous pemetrexed and cisplatin dose
CTC Grade 2: 100% of previous pemetrexed dose, 50% of previous cisplatin dose

Discontinuation

For Any of the Following:
Experiences any hematologic or nonhematologic Grade 3 or 4 toxicity after 2 dose reductions
Grade 3 or 4 neurotoxicity is observed

ADMINISTRATION

IV route
The use of gloves is recommended
If sol contacts the skin, wash the skin immediately and thoroughly w/ soap and water
If sol contacts the mucous membranes, flush thoroughly w/ water

Preparation

1. Calculate dose and determine the number of vials needed
2. Reconstitute each 100mg vial w/ 4.2mL of 0.9% NaCl (preservative free). Reconstitute each 500mg vial w/ 20mL of 0.9% NaCl (preservative free)

3. Gently swirl each vial until the powder is completely dissolved. The resulting sol is clear and ranges in color from colorless to yellow or green-yellow w/o adversely affecting product quality
4. An appropriate quantity of the reconstituted sol must be further diluted into a sol of 0.9% NaCl (preservative free), so that the total volume of sol is 100mL.
5. Administered as an IV infusion over 10 min

Stability and Compatibility

Chemical/physical stability of reconstituted and infusion sol were demonstrated for up to 24 hrs following initial reconstitution, when stored refrigerated
Compatible w/ standard polyvinyl chloride administration sets and IV sol bags

HOW SUPPLIED

Inj: 100mg, 500mg

WARNINGS/PRECAUTIONS

Not indicated for the treatment of patients with squamous cell NSCLC. Premedicate with folic acid and vitamin B12 to reduce hematologic/GI toxicity, and with dexamethasone. Do not substitute oral vitamin B12 for IM vitamin B12. Bone marrow suppression may occur; myelosuppression is usually the dose-limiting toxicity. Caution with renal/hepatic impairment and in elderly. Avoid in patients with CrCl <45mL/min. D/C if hematologic or nonhematologic Grade 3 or 4 toxicity after two dose reductions or immediately if Grade 3 or 4 neurotoxicity is observed. Do not start a cycle of treatment unless CrCl is ≥45mL/min, absolute neutrophil count is ≥1500 cells/mm^3, and platelet count is ≥100,000 cells/mm^3; obtain CBC and renal function tests at the beginning of each cycle and prn. May cause fetal harm; use effective contraception to prevent pregnancy.

ADVERSE REACTIONS

Anemia, anorexia, fatigue, leukopenia, N/V, stomatitis, neutropenia, rash/desquamation, thrombocytopenia, constipation, pharyngitis, diarrhea.

DRUG INTERACTIONS

Reduced clearance with ibuprofen. In patients with mild to moderate renal insufficiency (CrCl 45-79mL/min), caution with NSAIDs; avoid NSAIDs with short $T_{1/2}$ (eg, diclofenac, indomethacin) for 2 days before, the day of, and 2 days following therapy. Interrupt dosing of NSAIDs with longer $T_{1/2}$ (eg, meloxicam, nabumetone) for at least 5 days before, the day of, and 2 days following therapy. If concomitant NSAID administration is necessary, monitor for toxicity. Delayed clearance with nephrotoxic or tubularly secreted drugs (eg, probenecid).

NURSING CONSIDERATIONS

Assessment: Assess for drug hypersensitivity, renal/hepatic impairment, pregnancy/nursing status, and possible drug interactions. Obtain CBC and renal function tests at the beginning of each cycle.

Monitoring: Monitor for signs and symptoms of hematologic/nonhematologic toxicities, bone marrow suppression (eg, neutropenia, thrombocytopenia, anemia), GI toxicity, neurotoxicity, and other adverse events. Monitor CBC with platelet counts and for nadir and recovery. Perform renal and hepatic function tests periodically.

Patient Counseling: Inform about benefits and risks of therapy. Instruct on the need for folic acid and vitamin B12 supplementation to reduce treatment-related hematological and GI toxicities, and of the need for corticosteroids to reduce treatment-related dermatologic toxicity. Inform about risks of low blood cell counts and instruct to contact physician immediately if signs of infection (eg, fever, bleeding or symptoms of anemia) occur. Instruct to contact physician if persistent vomiting, diarrhea, or signs of dehydration appear. Instruct to inform physician of all concomitant prescription or OTC medications (eg, NSAIDs). Inform female patients of the potential hazard to fetus; advise to avoid pregnancy and to use effective contraceptive measures to prevent pregnancy during treatment.

Storage: Unreconstituted: 25°C (77°F); excursions permitted to 15-30°C (59-86°F). Reconstituted and Infusion Sol: Stable at 2-8°C (36-46°F) for up to 24 hrs.

ALOXI – palonosetron hydrochloride RX

Class: 5-HT_3 receptor antagonist

ADULT DOSAGE

Chemotherapy-Associated Nausea/Vomiting

Prevention of acute and delayed N/V associated w/ initial and repeat courses of moderately emetogenic cancer chemotherapy. Prevention of acute N/V associated w/ initial and repeat courses of highly emetogenic cancer chemotherapy

Usual: 0.25mg IV as a single dose over 30 sec; begin approx 30 min before the start of chemotherapy

PEDIATRIC DOSAGE

Chemotherapy-Associated Nausea/Vomiting

Prevention of Acute N/V Associated w/ Initial and Repeat Courses of Emetogenic Cancer Chemotherapy, Including Highly Emetogenic Cancer Chemotherapy:

1 Month-<17 Years:

Usual: 20mcg/kg IV as a single dose over 15 min; begin approx 30 min before the start of chemotherapy

Max Dose: 1.5mg

Postoperative Nausea/Vomiting

Prevention of Postoperative N/V for up to 24 Hrs Following Surgery:
0.075mg IV as single dose over 10 sec immediately before induction of anesthesia

ADMINISTRATION
IV route

Do not mix w/ other drugs
Flush infusion line w/ normal saline before and after administration

HOW SUPPLIED
Inj: 0.075mg/1.5mL, 0.25mg/5mL

WARNINGS/PRECAUTIONS
Hypersensitivity reactions, including anaphylaxis, reported with or without known hypersensitivity to other 5-HT_3 receptor antagonists. Routine prophylaxis is not recommended in patients who demonstrate low risk of PONV. Therapy is recommended in patients where N/V must be avoided during the postoperative period. Serotonin syndrome reported; d/c treatment and initiate supportive treatment if symptoms occur.

ADVERSE REACTIONS
Headache, constipation, QT prolongation, bradycardia.

DRUG INTERACTIONS
Serotonin syndrome reported with concomitant use of serotonergic drugs (eg, SSRIs, SNRIs, MAOIs, mirtazapine, fentanyl).

NURSING CONSIDERATIONS

Assessment: Assess for hypersensitivity to drug, risk/possibility of PONV, emetogenicity of cancer chemotherapy, pregnancy/nursing status, and possible drug interactions.

Monitoring: Monitor for hypersensitivity reactions, emergence of serotonin syndrome, and other adverse reactions.

Patient Counseling: Inform of the benefits/risks of therapy. Advise to report to physician all medical conditions, including any pain, redness, or swelling in and around infusion site. Advise of the possibility of serotonin syndrome, especially with concomitant use of other serotonergic agents; instruct to seek immediate medical attention if changes in mental status, autonomic instability, or neuromuscular symptoms with or without GI symptoms occur.

Storage: 20-25°C (68-77°F); excursions permitted to 15-30°C (59-86°F). Protect from light and freezing.

ALPHAGAN P – brimonidine tartrate RX

Class: Selective $alpha_2$ agonist

ADULT DOSAGE

Elevated Intraocular Pressure

Reduction of Elevated IOP in Patients w/ Open-Angle Glaucoma or Ocular HTN:
Instill 1 drop in affected eye(s) tid (8 hrs apart)

PEDIATRIC DOSAGE

Elevated Intraocular Pressure

Reduction of Elevated IOP in Patients w/ Open-Angle Glaucoma or Ocular HTN:
≥2 Years:
Instill 1 drop in affected eye(s) tid (8 hrs apart)

ADMINISTRATION
Ocular route

Space by at least 5 min if using >1 topical ophthalmic drug

HOW SUPPLIED
Sol: 0.1%, 0.15% [5mL, 10mL, 15mL]

CONTRAINDICATIONS
Neonates and infants <2 yrs of age.

WARNINGS/PRECAUTIONS
May potentiate syndromes associated with vascular insufficiency. Caution with severe cardiovascular disease (CVD), depression, cerebral or coronary insufficiency, Raynaud's phenomenon, orthostatic hypotension, or thromboangiitis obliterans. Bacterial keratitis reported with multidose containers.

ADVERSE REACTIONS
Allergic conjunctivitis, conjunctival hyperemia, eye pruritus, burning sensation, conjunctival folliculosis, HTN, oral dryness, ocular allergic reaction, visual disturbance, somnolence, decreased alertness.

DRUG INTERACTIONS
May potentiate effect with CNS depressants (alcohol, barbiturates, opiates, sedatives, anesthetics). Caution with antihypertensives, cardiac glycosides, and TCAs. May increase systemic side effects (eg, hypotension) with MAOIs; caution is advised.

NURSING CONSIDERATIONS

Assessment: Assess for hypersensitivity, severe CVD, depression, cerebral or coronary insufficiency, Raynaud's phenomenon, orthostatic hypotension, thromboangiitis obliterans, pregnancy/nursing, and possible drug interactions.

Monitoring: Monitor vascular insufficiency, bacterial keratitis, and other adverse reactions.

Patient Counseling: Advise to avoid touching tip of applicator to eye or surrounding areas. Instruct patient to notify physician if they have ocular surgery or develop an intercurrent ocular condition (eg, trauma or infection). Inform patients that fatigue and/or drowsiness may occur; may impair physical or mental abilities. Instruct to space by at least 5 min if using >1 topical ophthalmic drug.

Storage: 15-25°C (59-77°F).

ALREX – loteprednol etabonate — RX

Class: Corticosteroid

ADULT DOSAGE

Seasonal Allergic Conjunctivitis

1 drop into the affected eye(s) qid

PEDIATRIC DOSAGE

Pediatric use may not have been established

ADMINISTRATION
Ocular route

Shake well before use

HOW SUPPLIED
Sus: 0.2% [5mL, 10mL]

CONTRAINDICATIONS
Viral diseases of the cornea and conjunctiva, including epithelial herpes simplex keratitis (dendritic keratitis), vaccinia, and varicella. Mycobacterial infection of the eye and fungal diseases of the ocular structures.

WARNINGS/PRECAUTIONS
Prolonged use may result in glaucoma with optic nerve damage, visual acuity and visual field defects, and posterior subcapsular cataract formation. Caution with glaucoma. Prolonged use may increase the hazard of secondary ocular infections. Caution with diseases causing thinning of the cornea/sclera; perforations may occur. May mask/enhance existing infection in acute purulent conditions of the eye. May prolong the course or exacerbate severity of many viral infections of the eye. Caution with history of herpes simplex virus. Perform eye exam (eg, slit-lamp biomicroscopy, fluorescein staining) prior to therapy and renewal of medication order >14 days. Reevaluate if signs/symptoms fail to improve after 2 days. Monitor IOP if used >10 days. Fungal infections of the cornea may develop with long-term use; consider fungal invasion in any persistent corneal ulceration.

ADVERSE REACTIONS
Elevated IOP, abnormal vision/blurring, burning on instillation, chemosis, discharge, dry eyes, epiphora, foreign body sensation, itching, photophobia, headache, rhinitis, pharyngitis.

NURSING CONSIDERATIONS

Assessment: Assess for hypersensitivity to the drug, viral diseases of the cornea and conjunctiva, vaccinia varicella, mycobacterial eye infection, fungal diseases of the ocular structures, glaucoma, diseases causing thinning of the cornea/sclera, acute purulent conditions of the eye, and pregnancy/nursing status. Perform eye exam (eg, slit-lamp biomicroscopy, fluorescein staining) prior to therapy.

Monitoring: Monitor for signs and symptoms of glaucoma, optic nerve damage, visual acuity and visual field defects, posterior subcapsular cataracts, sclera/corneal perforations, masking or enhancement of existing infections in acute purulent conditions of the eye, and other adverse reactions. Monitor IOP and perform eye exams.

Patient Counseling: Advise not to touch dropper tip to any surface to avoid contamination. Instruct to contact physician if redness or itching becomes aggravated. Instruct not to wear contact lenses if eyes are red. Counsel not to use for contact lens-related irritation. Inform that the medication contains benzalkonium chloride that may be absorbed by soft contact lenses. Instruct to wait ≥10 min after administration before wearing soft contact lenses.

Storage: 15-25°C (59-77°F). Store upright. Do not freeze.

ALSUMA – sumatriptan RX

Class: 5-$HT_{1B/1D}$ agonist

ADULT DOSAGE

Migraine

W/ or w/o Aura:

Max Single Dose: 6mg SQ

Max Dose/24 Hrs: 2 doses separated by at least 1 hr; only consider 2nd dose if there was some response to the 1st inj

Cluster Headache

Acute Treatment:

Max Single Dose: 6mg SQ

Max Dose/24 Hrs: 2 doses separated by at least 1 hr; only consider 2nd dose if there was some response to the 1st inj

PEDIATRIC DOSAGE

Pediatric use may not have been established

DOSE MODIFICATION

Elderly

Use caution; start at lower end of dosing range

ADMINISTRATION

SQ route

HOW SUPPLIED

Inj: 6mg/0.5mL

CONTRAINDICATIONS

Ischemic coronary artery disease (CAD) (eg, angina pectoris, history of myocardial infarction [MI], or documented silent ischemia), coronary artery vasospasm (eg, Prinzmetal's angina), Wolff-Parkinson-White syndrome or arrhythmias associated with other cardiac accessory conduction pathway disorders, history of stroke or transient ischemic attack (TIA), hemiplegic/basilar migraine or history thereof, peripheral vascular disease, ischemic bowel disease, uncontrolled HTN, and severe hepatic impairment. Recent use (within 24 hrs) of ergotamine-containing or ergot-type medication (eg, dihydroergotamine, methysergide) or another 5-HT_1 agonist. Concurrent administration or recent use (within 2 weeks) of an MAO-A inhibitor.

WARNINGS/PRECAUTIONS

Reconsider the diagnosis of migraine before treating any subsequent attacks if patient has no response to the 1st dose of therapy. Serious cardiac adverse reactions (eg, acute MI) reported. May cause coronary artery vasospasm and sensations of tightness, pain, pressure, and heaviness in the precordium, throat, neck, and jaw, usually noncardiac in origin. Perform cardiovascular (CV) evaluation in triptan-naive patients with multiple CV risk factors (eg, increased age, diabetes, HTN, smoking, obesity, strong family history of CAD) prior to therapy; if (-), consider administering 1st dose under medical supervision and perform an ECG immediately following administration. Consider periodic CV evaluation in intermittent long-term users with risk factors for CAD. Life-threatening cardiac rhythm disturbances (eg, ventricular tachycardia, ventricular fibrillation leading to death) reported; d/c if these occur. Cerebral/subarachnoid hemorrhage and stroke reported; d/c therapy if a cerebrovascular event occurs. Exclude other potentially serious neurological conditions before therapy in patients not previously diagnosed as migraineurs, and in migraineurs who present with atypical symptoms. May cause noncoronary vasospastic reactions (eg, peripheral vascular ischemia, GI vascular ischemia/infarction, splenic infarction, Raynaud's syndrome); rule out a vasospastic reaction before giving additional doses. Transient/permanent blindness and significant partial vision loss reported. Overuse of acute migraine drugs may lead to exacerbation of headache; detoxification may be necessary. Serotonin syndrome may occur; d/c if suspected. Significant elevation in BP, including hypertensive crisis with acute impairment of organ systems, reported. Anaphylactic/anaphylactoid/hypersensitivity reactions and seizures reported. Caution in elderly.

ADVERSE REACTIONS

Inj-site reactions, tingling, warm/burning/pressure sensation, dizziness, feeling of heaviness/tightness, flushing, numbness, chest discomfort/tightness, throat discomfort, weakness, neck pain.

DRUG INTERACTIONS

See Contraindications. Serotonin syndrome reported with SSRIs, SNRIs, TCAs, or MAOIs.

NURSING CONSIDERATIONS

Assessment: Confirm diagnosis of migraine or cluster headache and exclude other potentially serious neurologic conditions prior to therapy. Assess for CV disease, HTN, hemiplegic/basilar migraine, hypersensitivity to drug, and any other conditions where treatment is cautioned or contraindicated. Assess hepatic function, pregnancy/nursing status, and for possible drug interactions.

Monitoring: Monitor for signs/symptoms of cardiac events, cerebrovascular events, noncoronary vasospastic reactions, serotonin syndrome, hypersensitivity reactions, HTN, ophthalmic changes, and other adverse reactions. Perform periodic CV evaluation in intermittent long-term users with risk factors for CAD.

Patient Counseling: Inform that therapy may cause serious CV side effects and anaphylactic/anaphylactoid reactions. Instruct to seek medical attention if signs/symptoms of chest pain, SOB, weakness, or slurring of speech occur. Caution about the risk of serotonin syndrome. Inform that use of acute migraine drugs for ≥10 days/month may lead to an exacerbation of headache; encourage to record headache frequency and drug use (eg, by keeping a headache diary). Inform that drug should not be used during pregnancy; instruct to notify physician if breastfeeding/planning to breastfeed. Inform that drug may cause somnolence and dizziness; instruct to evaluate ability to perform complex tasks during migraine attacks and after administration of drug. Instruct on proper use of product, to avoid IM or intravascular delivery, and to use inj sites with adequate skin and SQ thickness (eg, lateral thigh, upper arms) to accommodate the length of the needle.

Storage: 25°C (77°F); excursions permitted to 15-30°C (59-86°F). Protect from light. Do not refrigerate.

ALTACE – ramipril

RX

Class: ACE inhibitor

D/C when pregnancy is detected. Drugs that act directly on the renin-angiotensin system (RAS) can cause injury/death to the developing fetus.

ADULT DOSAGE

Hypertension

Not Receiving a Diuretic:
Initial: 2.5mg qd
Titrate: Adjust dose according to BP response
Maint: 2.5-20mg/day as single dose or in 2 equally divided doses
May add diuretic if BP is not controlled

≥55 Years:
Initial: 2.5mg qd for 1 week
Titrate: Increase to 5mg qd for next 3 weeks, then increase as tolerated
Maint: 10mg qd
May be given as a divided dose if hypertensive or recently post-MI

Initial: 2.5mg bid or may switch to 1.25mg bid if hypotensive at this dose
Titrate: If tolerated, increase to 5mg bid at 3-week intervals after 1 week of initial dose
After initial dose, observe for at least 2 hrs and until BP has stabilized for at least an additional hr

PEDIATRIC DOSAGE

Pediatric use may not have been established

DOSE MODIFICATION

Renal Impairment

CrCl ≤40mL/min:
HTN:
Initial: 1.25mg qd
Titrate: May increase dosage until BP is controlled
Max: 5mg/day

CHF Post MI:
Initial: 1.25mg qd
Titrate: May increase to 1.25mg bid
Max: 2.5mg bid

Other Important Modifications
Renal Artery Stenosis/Volume Depletion (eg, Past and Current Diuretic Use):
Initial: 1.25mg qd
Titrate: Adjust dosage according to BP response

ADMINISTRATION

Oral route

Swallow whole
May sprinkle contents on a small amount (about 4 oz) of applesauce or mix in 4 oz (120mL) of water or apple juice
Consume mixture in its entirety
May pre-prepare and store described mixtures for up to 24 hrs at room temperature or up to 48 hrs under refrigeration

HOW SUPPLIED

Cap: 1.25mg, 2.5mg, 5mg, 10mg

CONTRAINDICATIONS

History of ACE inhibitor-associated angioedema. Coadministration with aliskiren in patients with diabetes.

WARNINGS/PRECAUTIONS

Increased risk of angioedema in patients with history of angioedema unrelated to ACE inhibitor therapy. Head/neck angioedema reported; d/c and institute appropriate therapy if laryngeal stridor or angioedema of the face, tongue, or glottis occurs. Higher rate of angioedema in blacks than nonblacks. Intestinal angioedema reported; monitor for abdominal pain. Anaphylactoid reactions reported during desensitization with hymenoptera venom, dialysis with high-flux membranes, and LDL apheresis with dextran sulfate absorption. Rarely, associated with a syndrome that starts with cholestatic jaundice and progresses to fulminant hepatic necrosis and sometimes death; d/c if jaundice or marked hepatic enzyme elevations develop. May cause changes in renal function. Excessive hypotension associated with oliguria or azotemia and, rarely, with acute renal failure and death may occur in patients with CHF; closely monitor during first 2 weeks of therapy and whenever the dose is increased. Increases in BUN and SrCr may occur in hypertensive patients with renal artery stenosis or without preexisting renal vascular disease; dosage reduction of therapy and/or discontinuation of diuretic may be required. Agranulocytosis, pancytopenia, bone marrow depression, and mild reductions in RBC count and Hgb content, blood cell, or platelet counts may occur; consider monitoring WBCs in patients with collagen vascular disease (eg, systemic lupus erythematosus, scleroderma), especially with renal impairment. Symptomatic hypotension may occur and is most likely in patients with volume and/or salt depletion; correct depletion prior to therapy. Hypotension may occur with surgery or during anesthesia. Hyperkalemia reported; risk factors include renal insufficiency and diabetes mellitus (DM). Persistent nonproductive cough reported.

ADVERSE REACTIONS

Hypotension, cough increased, dizziness, angina pectoris, headache, asthenia, fatigue.

DRUG INTERACTIONS

See Contraindications. Dual blockade of the RAS is associated with increased risks of hypotension, hyperkalemia, and changes in renal function (including acute renal failure); avoid combined use of RAS inhibitors, or closely monitor BP, renal function, and electrolytes with concomitant agents that also affect the RAS. Avoid with aliskiren in patients with renal impairment (GFR <60mL/min). Hypotension risk, and increased BUN and SrCr with diuretics. Increased risk of hyperkalemia with K^+-sparing diuretics, K^+ supplements, and/or K^+-containing salt substitutes; use with caution and frequently monitor serum K^+. Not recommended with telmisartan; increased risk of renal dysfunction. Increased lithium levels and symptoms of lithium toxicity reported; frequently monitor serum lithium levels. Diuretics may further increase risk of lithium toxicity. Nitritoid reactions reported rarely with injectable gold (sodium aurothiomalate). Coadministration with NSAIDs, including selective COX-2 inhibitors, may deteriorate renal function and attenuate antihypertensive effect. Increased risk for angioedema with mammalian target of rapamycin inhibitor (eg, temsirolimus).

NURSING CONSIDERATIONS

Assessment: Assess for history of angioedema, CHF, renal artery stenosis, collagen vascular disease, volume/salt depletion, DM, hepatic impairment, hypersensitivity to drug, pregnancy/nursing status, and possible drug interactions. Obtain baseline renal function.

Monitoring: Monitor for signs/symptoms of angioedema, abdominal pain, anaphylactoid reactions, jaundice, hypotension, hyperkalemia, cough, and other adverse reactions. Consider monitoring WBCs in patients with collagen vascular disease, especially with renal impairment. Monitor BP and renal/hepatic function.

Patient Counseling: Instruct to d/c therapy and to immediately report any signs/symptoms of angioedema. Advise to promptly report any indication of infection. Instruct to report lightheadedness, especially during 1st days of therapy; advise to d/c and consult with a physician if syncope occurs. Inform that inadequate fluid intake or excessive perspiration, diarrhea, or vomiting may lead to an excessive fall in BP, with the same consequences of lightheadedness and possible syncope. Inform females of childbearing age about the consequences of exposure during pregnancy and discuss treatment options in women planning to become pregnant; instruct to report pregnancy to physician as soon as possible. Advise not to use salt substitutes containing K⁺ without consulting physician.

Storage: 15-30°C (59-86°F). Pre-prepared Mixtures: Up to 24 hrs at room temperature or up to 48 hrs under refrigeration.

ALVESCO – ciclesonide

RX

Class: Non-halogenated glucocorticoid

ADULT DOSAGE

Asthma

Previous Therapy:

Bronchodilators Alone:
Initial: 80mcg bid
Max: 160mcg bid

Inhaled Corticosteroids:
Initial: 80mcg bid
Max: 320mcg bid

Oral Corticosteroids:
Initial/Max: 320mcg bid
Titrate: Reduce to lowest effective dose once asthma stability is achieved. May increase to higher dose if response to initial dose is inadequate after 4 weeks

PEDIATRIC DOSAGE

Asthma

≥12 Years:

Previous Therapy:

Bronchodilators Alone:
Initial: 80mcg bid
Max: 160mcg bid

Inhaled Corticosteroids:
Initial: 80mcg bid
Max: 320mcg bid

Oral Corticosteroids:
Initial/Max: 320mcg bid
Titrate: Reduce to lowest effective dose once asthma stability is achieved. May increase to higher dose if response to initial dose is inadequate after 4 weeks

DOSE MODIFICATION

Elderly

Start at lower end of dosing range

ADMINISTRATION

Oral inh route

Refer to PI for further administration instructions

Priming

Prime inhaler before using for the 1st time or when inhaler has not been used for >10 days by actuating 3 times

HOW SUPPLIED

MDI: 80mcg/actuation, 160mcg/actuation [60 actuations]

CONTRAINDICATIONS

Primary treatment of status asthmaticus or other acute episodes of asthma where intensive measures are required.

WARNINGS/PRECAUTIONS

Localized *Candida albicans* infections of mouth and pharynx reported; treat appropriately while remaining on treatment, or interrupt treatment if needed. Not indicated for rapid relief of bronchospasm or other acute episodes of asthma. Increased susceptibility to infections (eg, chickenpox, measles); may lead to serious/fatal course. Avoid exposure to chickenpox and measles; if exposed, consider prophylaxis/treatment. Caution with active/quiescent tuberculosis (TB), untreated systemic fungal, bacterial, viral, or parasitic infections, or ocular herpes simplex. Deaths due to adrenal insufficiency reported with transfer from systemic to inhaled corticosteroids; if oral corticosteroid is required, wean slowly from systemic corticosteroid use after transferring to therapy. Resume oral corticosteroids immediately during periods of stress or a severe asthma attack if previously withdrawn from systemic corticosteroids. Transferring from systemic to inhalation therapy may unmask allergic conditions previously suppressed (eg, rhinitis, conjunctivitis, eczema, arthritis, eosinophilic conditions). Systemic corticosteroid withdrawal effects may occur during withdrawal from oral steroids. Reduce dose slowly if hypercorticism and adrenal suppression occur. Decreases in bone mineral density (BMD) reported with long-term use; caution with major risk factors for decreased bone mineral content (eg, prolonged immobilization, family history of osteoporosis, chronic use of drugs that can reduce bone mass [eg, anticonvulsants, corticosteroids]). May reduce growth velocity in pediatric patients; monitor growth of pediatric patients routinely (eg, via stadiometry). Glaucoma, increased intraocular pressure (IOP), and cataracts reported. Bronchospasm may occur; d/c use, treat immediately, and institute alternative treatment. Caution in elderly.

ADVERSE REACTIONS
Headache, nasopharyngitis, sinusitis, pharyngolaryngeal pain, upper respiratory infection, arthralgia, nasal congestion, pain in extremity, back pain.

DRUG INTERACTIONS
Oral ketoconazole may increase the exposure of the active metabolite des-ciclesonide.

NURSING CONSIDERATIONS

Assessment: Assess for status asthmaticus or other acute episodes of asthma, active/quiescent TB, untreated systemic infections, ocular herpes simplex, risk factors for decreased bone mineral content, previous hypersensitivity, pregnancy/nursing status, and possible drug interactions. Assess for history of increased IOP, glaucoma, and/or cataracts.

Monitoring: Monitor for infections, TB, chickenpox, measles, hypercorticism, adrenal suppression, decreased BMD, glaucoma, increased IOP, cataracts, bronchospasm, and other adverse events. Monitor growth routinely (eg, via stadiometry) in pediatric patients.

Patient Counseling: Advise that localized infections with *C. albicans* may occur in the mouth and pharynx; advise to rinse mouth after use and to notify physician if oropharyngeal candidiasis develops. Inform that drug is not a bronchodilator and is not for use as rescue medication for acute asthma exacerbations; instruct to contact physician immediately if deterioration of asthma occurs. Advise to avoid exposure to chickenpox or measles, and, if exposed, to consult physician immediately. Counsel on risks of immunosuppression, hypercorticism, adrenal suppression, and decreased BMD. Inform of risk of reduced growth velocity in pediatric patients. Advise to use medication at regular intervals, not to increase the prescribed dosage, not to stop use abruptly, and to contact physician if symptoms do not improve, condition worsens, or if use is discontinued. Inform to use only with the actuator supplied with the product.

Storage: 25°C (77°F); excursions permitted to 15-30°C (59-86°F). Do not puncture or use/store near heat or open flame. Exposure to temperatures >49°C (120°F) may cause bursting. Discard when dose indicator display window shows zero.

AMBIEN – zolpidem tartrate CIV

Class: Imidazopyridine hypnotic

ADULT DOSAGE

Insomnia

Difficulties w/ Sleep Initiation:
Initial:
Women: 5mg qhs
Men: 5mg or 10mg qhs
Titrate: May increase to 10mg if the 5mg dose is not effective
Max: 10mg qhs

PEDIATRIC DOSAGE

Pediatric use may not have been established

DOSE MODIFICATION

Concomitant Medications
CNS Depressants: May need to adjust dose of zolpidem

Hepatic Impairment
5mg qhs

Elderly
5mg qhs

Other Important Modifications
Debilitated: 5mg qhs

ADMINISTRATION
Oral route

Take immediately before hs w/ at least 7-8 hrs remaining before the planned time of awakening
Do not administer w/ or immediately after a meal

HOW SUPPLIED
Tab: 5mg, 10mg

WARNINGS/PRECAUTIONS
Increased risk of next-day psychomotor impairment if taken with less than a full night of sleep remaining (7-8 hrs). May impair mental/physical abilities. Initiate only after careful evaluation; failure of insomnia to remit after 7-10 days of treatment may indicate presence of a primary psychiatric and/or medical illness. Angioedema and anaphylaxis reported; do not rechallenge if such reactions develop. Abnormal thinking, behavior changes, and visual and

auditory hallucinations reported. Complex behaviors (eg, sleep-driving) while not fully awake reported; consider discontinuation if a sleep-driving episode occurs. Amnesia, anxiety, and other neuropsychiatric symptoms may occur. Worsening of depression and suicidal thoughts and actions (including completed suicides) reported primarily in depressed patients; prescribe the lowest feasible number of tabs at a time. Caution with compromised respiratory function; prior to prescribing, consider the risk of respiratory depression in patients with respiratory impairment (eg, sleep apnea, myasthenia gravis). Withdrawal signs and symptoms reported following rapid dose decrease or abrupt discontinuation; monitor for tolerance, abuse, and dependence. May cause drowsiness and a decreased level of consciousness, which may lead to falls and consequently to severe injuries (eg, hip fractures, intracranial hemorrhage).

ADVERSE REACTIONS
Drowsiness, dizziness, headache, diarrhea, drugged feeling, lethargy, dry mouth, back pain, pharyngitis, sinusitis, allergy.

DRUG INTERACTIONS
See Dosage. Increased risk of CNS depression and complex behaviors with other CNS depressants (eg, benzodiazepines, opioids, TCAs, alcohol). Use with other sedative-hypnotics (eg, other zolpidem products) at hs or the middle of the night is not recommended. Increased risk of next-day psychomotor impairment with other CNS depressants or drugs that increase zolpidem levels. May decrease peak levels of imipramine. Additive effect of decreased alertness with imipramine or chlorpromazine. Additive adverse effect on psychomotor performance with chlorpromazine or alcohol. Sertraline and CYP3A inhibitors may increase exposure. Fluoxetine may increase $T_{1/2}$. Rifampin (a CYP3A4 inducer) may reduce exposure, pharmacodynamic effects, and efficacy. Ketoconazole (a potent CYP3A4 inhibitor) may increase pharmacodynamic effects; consider lower dose of zolpidem.

NURSING CONSIDERATIONS

Assessment: Assess for physical and/or psychiatric disorder, depression, compromised respiratory function, sleep apnea, myasthenia gravis, hepatic impairment, history of drug/alcohol addiction or abuse, hypersensitivity to the drug, pregnancy/nursing status, and possible drug interactions.

Monitoring: Monitor for angioedema, anaphylaxis, emergence of any new behavioral signs/symptoms of concern, respiratory depression, withdrawal signs/symptoms, tolerance, abuse, dependence, drowsiness, decreased level of consciousness, and other adverse reactions.

Patient Counseling: Inform about the benefits and risks of treatment. Instruct to take only as prescribed; advise to wait at least 8 hrs after dosing before driving or engaging in other activities requiring full mental alertness. Instruct to contact physician immediately if any adverse reactions (eg, severe anaphylactic/anaphylactoid reactions, sleep-driving, other complex behaviors, suicidal thoughts) develop. Advise not to use the drug if patient drank alcohol that pm or before bed. Instruct not to increase the dose and to inform physician if it is believed that the drug does not work.

Storage: 20-25°C (68-77°F).

AMBIEN CR – zolpidem tartrate CIV

Class: Imidazopyridine hypnotic

ADULT DOSAGE

Insomnia

Difficulties w/ Sleep Onset and/or Sleep Maintenance:

Use lowest effective dose
Initial:
Women: 6.25mg qhs
Men: 6.25mg or 12.5mg qhs
Titrate: May increase to 12.5mg if the 6.25mg dose is not effective
Max: 12.5mg qhs

PEDIATRIC DOSAGE

Pediatric use may not have been established

DOSE MODIFICATION

Concomitant Medications
CNS Depressants: May need to adjust dose of zolpidem

Hepatic Impairment
Hepatic Insufficiency: 6.25mg qhs

Elderly

Elderly/Debilitated:
6.25mg qhs

ADMINISTRATION

Oral route

Swallow whole; do not divide, crush, or chew
Take immediately before hs w/ at least 7-8 hrs remaining before the planned time of awakening
Do not administer w/ or immediately after a meal

HOW SUPPLIED

Tab, Extended-Release: 6.25mg, 12.5mg

WARNINGS/PRECAUTIONS

May impair daytime function; monitor for excess depressant effects. May impair mental/physical abilities. Increased risk of next-day psychomotor impairment if taken with less than a full night of sleep remaining (7-8 hrs). Initiate only after careful evaluation; failure of insomnia to remit after 7-10 days of treatment may indicate presence of a primary psychiatric and/or medical illness. Angioedema and anaphylaxis reported; do not rechallenge if such reactions develop. Abnormal thinking, behavior changes, and visual and auditory hallucinations reported. Complex behaviors (eg, sleep-driving) while not fully awake reported; consider discontinuation if a sleep-driving episode occurs. Amnesia, anxiety, and other neuropsychiatric symptoms may occur. Worsening of depression and suicidal thoughts and actions (including completed suicides) reported primarily in depressed patients; prescribe the lowest feasible number of tabs at a time. Caution with compromised respiratory function; prior to prescribing, consider the risk of respiratory depression in patients with respiratory impairment (eg, sleep apnea, myasthenia gravis). Withdrawal signs and symptoms reported following rapid dose decrease or abrupt discontinuation; monitor for tolerance, abuse, and dependence. May cause drowsiness and a decreased level of consciousness, which may lead to falls and consequently to severe injuries (eg, hip fractures, intracranial hemorrhage).

ADVERSE REACTIONS

Headache, somnolence, dizziness, anxiety, nausea, influenza, hallucinations, back pain, myalgia, fatigue, disorientation, memory disorder, visual disturbance, nasopharyngitis.

DRUG INTERACTIONS

See Dosage. Additive effects with other CNS depressants (eg, benzodiazepines, opioids, TCAs, alcohol), including daytime use. Use with other sedative-hypnotics (eg, other zolpidem products) at hs or the middle of the night is not recommended. Increased risk of next-day psychomotor impairment with other CNS depressants or drugs that increase zolpidem levels. Increased risk of complex behaviors with alcohol and other CNS depressants. May decrease peak levels of imipramine. Additive effect of decreased alertness with imipramine or chlorpromazine. Additive adverse effect on psychomotor performance with chlorpromazine or alcohol. Sertraline and CYP3A inhibitors may increase exposure. Fluoxetine may increase $T_{1/2}$. Rifampin (a CYP3A4 inducer) may reduce exposure, pharmacodynamic effects, and efficacy. Ketoconazole (a potent CYP3A4 inhibitor) may increase pharmacodynamic effects; consider lower dose of zolpidem.

NURSING CONSIDERATIONS

Assessment: Assess for physical and/or psychiatric disorder, depression, compromised respiratory function, sleep apnea, myasthenia gravis, hepatic impairment, history of drug/alcohol addiction or abuse, hypersensitivity to the drug, pregnancy/nursing status, and possible drug interactions.

Monitoring: Monitor for angioedema, anaphylaxis, emergence of any new behavioral signs/symptoms of concern, respiratory depression, withdrawal signs/symptoms, tolerance, abuse, dependence, drowsiness, decreased level of consciousness, and other adverse reactions. Monitor for excess depressant effects.

Patient Counseling: Inform about the benefits and risks of treatment. Instruct to take only as prescribed. Caution against driving and other activities requiring complete mental alertness the day after use. Instruct to contact physician immediately if any adverse reactions (eg, severe anaphylactic/anaphylactoid reactions, sleep-driving, other complex behaviors, suicidal thoughts) develop. Advise not to use the drug if patient drank alcohol that pm or before bed. Instruct not to increase the dose and to inform physician if it is believed that the drug does not work.

Storage: 15-25°C (59-77°F); limited excursions permissible up to 30°C (86°F).

AmBisome – amphotericin B liposome

RX

Class: Polyene antifungal

ADULT DOSAGE

Fungal Infections

Empirical therapy for presumed fungal infection in febrile, neutropenic patients
Initial: 3mg/kg/day IV

Systemic Infections

Aspergillus species, *Candida* species, and/or *Cryptococcus* species infections refractory to amphotericin B deoxycholate, or in patients where renal impairment or unacceptable toxicity precludes the use of amphotericin B deoxycholate
Initial: 3-5mg/kg/day IV

Cryptococcal Meningitis

In HIV-Infected Patients:
Initial: 6mg/kg/day IV

Leishmaniasis

Visceral:
Immunocompetent:
Usual: 3mg/kg/day IV on Days 1-5, 14, 21; may repeat course if parasitic clearance is not achieved w/ recommended dose
Immunocompromised:
Usual: 4mg/kg/day IV on Days 1-5, 10, 17, 24, 31, 38

PEDIATRIC DOSAGE

Fungal Infections

Empirical therapy for presumed fungal infection in febrile, neutropenic patients

≥1 Month of Age:
Initial: 3mg/kg/day IV

Systemic Infections

Aspergillus species, *Candida* species, and/or *Cryptococcus* species infections refractory to amphotericin B deoxycholate, or in patients where renal impairment or unacceptable toxicity precludes the use of amphotericin B deoxycholate
≥1 Month of Age:
Initial: 3-5mg/kg/day IV

Cryptococcal Meningitis

In HIV-Infected Patients:
Initial: 6mg/kg/day IV

Leishmaniasis

≥1 Month of Age:
Visceral:
Immunocompetent:
Usual: 3mg/kg/day IV on Days 1-5, 14, 21; may repeat course if parasitic clearance is not achieved w/ recommended dose

Immunocompromised:
Usual: 4mg/kg/day IV on Days 1-5, 10, 17, 24, 31, 38

ADMINISTRATION

IV route

Infuse over 120 min; may reduce to 60 min if well tolerated or increase duration if experiencing discomfort
An in-line membrane filter may be used provided the mean pore diameter of the filter is not <1.0 micron
Flush existing IV line w/ D5W prior to infusion; if not feasible, administer through a separate line

Preparation

Reconstitute w/ 12mL of sterile water for inj and shake vial vigorously for 30 sec
Do not reconstitute w/ saline or add saline to reconstituted sol or mix w/ other drugs
Calculate appropriate volume of reconstituted sol to be further diluted and withdraw amount into syringe
Attach provided 5-micron filter to syringe and inject contents through filter into appropriate amount of D5 inj diluent for a final concentration of 1-2mg/mL (lower concentrations [0.2-0.5mg/mL] may be appropriate for infants and small children)
Use only 1 filter per vial and discard partially used vials

HOW SUPPLIED

Inj: 50mg

WARNINGS/PRECAUTIONS

Anaphylaxis reported; d/c immediately and do not give further infusions if severe anaphylactic reaction occurs. Should be administered by medically trained personnel; monitor closely during the initial dosing period. Significantly less toxic than amphotericin B deoxycholate. False elevations of serum phosphate seen with PHOSm assays.

ADVERSE REACTIONS

Hypokalemia, chills/rigors, SrCr elevation, anemia, N/V, diarrhea, hypomagnesemia, rash, dyspnea, bilirubinemia, BUN increased, headache, abdominal pain.

DRUG INTERACTIONS

Antineoplastic agents may enhance potential for renal toxicity, bronchospasm, and hypotension. Corticosteroids and adrenocorticotropic hormone may potentiate hypokalemia; closely monitor serum electrolytes and cardiac function. May induce hypokalemia and potentiate digitalis toxicity with digitalis glycosides; closely monitor serum K^+ levels. May increase flucytosine toxicity.

Imidazoles (eg, ketoconazole, miconazole, clotrimazole, fluconazole) may induce fungal resistance; use with caution, especially in immunocompromised patients. Acute pulmonary toxicity reported with simultaneous leukocyte transfusions. Nephrotoxic drugs may enhance drug-induced renal toxicity; intensive monitoring of renal function is recommended. Amphotericin B-induced hypokalemia may enhance curariform effect of skeletal muscle relaxants (eg, tubocurarine); closely monitor serum K^+ levels.

NURSING CONSIDERATIONS

Assessment: Assess for hypersensitivity, health status, pregnancy/nursing status, and possible drug interactions.

Monitoring: Monitor for severe anaphylactic and other adverse reactions. Monitor renal, hepatic and hematopoietic function, and serum electrolytes (particularly Mg^{2+} and K^+).

Patient Counseling: Inform of risks and benefits of therapy. Advise to seek medical attention if any adverse reactions occur.

Storage: Unopened Vials: ≤25°C (77°F). Reconstituted Concentrate: 2-8°C (36-46°F) for up to 24 hrs. Do not freeze. Diluted Product: Inj should commence within 6 hrs of dilution with D5W.

AMERGE – naratriptan hydrochloride RX

Class: 5-$HT_{1B/1D}$ agonist

ADULT DOSAGE

Migraine

W/ or w/o Aura:

Usual: 1mg or 2.5mg

May repeat once after 4 hrs if migraine returns or if patient has only partial response

Max: 5mg/24 hrs

Safety of treating an average of >4 migraine attacks in a 30-day period has not been established

PEDIATRIC DOSAGE

Pediatric use may not have been established

DOSE MODIFICATION

Renal Impairment

Mild-Moderate:

Initial: 1mg

Max: 2.5mg/24 hrs

Hepatic Impairment

Mild-Moderate:

Initial: 1mg

Max: 2.5mg/24 hrs

Elderly

Use caution; start at lower end of dosing range

ADMINISTRATION

Oral route

HOW SUPPLIED

Tab: 1mg, 2.5mg

CONTRAINDICATIONS

Ischemic coronary artery disease (CAD) (angina pectoris, history of MI, documented silent ischemia), or coronary artery vasospasm, including Prinzmetal's angina; Wolff-Parkinson-White syndrome or arrhythmias associated with other cardiac accessory conduction pathway disorders; history of stroke or transient ischemic attack or history of hemiplegic or basilar migraine; peripheral vascular disease; ischemic bowel disease; uncontrolled HTN, recent use (eg, within 24 hrs) of another 5-HT_1 agonist, ergotamine-containing medication, ergot-type medication (eg, dihydroergotamine, methysergide); severe renal/hepatic impairment.

WARNINGS/PRECAUTIONS

Rare reports of serious cardiac adverse reactions, including acute MI, occurring within a few hrs following administration. May cause coronary artery vasospasm (Prinzmetal's angina); caution in patients with CAD risk factors. Perform cardiovascular (CV) evaluation in triptan-naive patients. If patient has a negative CV evaluation, consider administering 1st dose in a medically supervised setting, performing an ECG immediately following administration, and consider periodic CV evaluation with long-term intermittent use. Life-threatening disturbances of cardiac rhythm, including ventricular tachycardia and ventricular fibrillation leading to death, reported; d/c if these disturbances occur. Sensations of tightness, pain, and pressure in the chest, throat, neck, and jaw may occur after treatment and are usually noncardiac in origin; perform a cardiac evaluation if these patients are at high cardiac risk. Cerebral hemorrhage, subarachnoid hemorrhage, and stroke reported; d/c if a cerebrovascular event occurs. Exclude other potentially serious neurological conditions before treating headaches in patients not previously diagnosed as migraineurs and in migraineurs who present with symptoms atypical for migraine. May cause noncoronary vasospastic reactions (eg, peripheral vascular ischemia, GI vascular ischemia and infarction, splenic infarction, Raynaud's syndrome); rule out a vasospastic reaction, before receiving additional doses. Transient and permanent blindness and significant partial vision loss reported. Overuse of acute migraine drugs may lead to exacerbation of headache; detoxification, including withdrawal of overused drugs, and treatment of withdrawal symptoms may be necessary. Serotonin syndrome may occur; d/c if suspected. Significant BP elevation, including hypertensive crisis with acute impairment of organ systems reported; monitor BP. Anaphylaxis/anaphylactoid/hypersensitivity reactions, including angioedema reported. Caution in elderly.

ADVERSE REACTIONS

Paresthesias, nausea, dizziness, drowsiness, malaise/fatigue, throat and neck symptoms.

DRUG INTERACTIONS

See Contraindications. Serotonin syndrome reported during coadministration of triptans and SSRIs, SNRIs, TCAs, and MAOIs.

NURSING CONSIDERATIONS

Assessment: Confirm diagnosis of migraine before therapy. Assess for CAD, uncontrolled HTN, history of hemiplegic/basilar migraine, ECG changes, renal/hepatic impairment, or any conditions where treatment is cautioned or contraindicated. Assess for pregnancy/nursing status and for possible drug interactions. Exclude other potentially serious neurological conditions before therapy. Perform a CV evaluation in triptan-naive patients who have multiple CV risk factors (eg, increased age, diabetes, HTN, smoking, obesity, strong family history of CAD).

Monitoring: Monitor for serious cardiac adverse reactions, arrhythmias, cerebrovascular events, noncoronary vasospastic reactions, exacerbation of headache, serotonin syndrome, increase in BP, anaphylactic/anaphylactoid reactions, and other adverse reactions. Perform ECG immediately after administration of 1st dose in patients with multiple CV risk factors. Consider periodic cardiac evaluation in patients who have multiple CV risk factors and are long-term intermittent users.

Patient Counseling: Inform that drug may cause serious CV effects (eg, MI, stroke); instruct to be alert for signs/symptoms of chest pain, SOB, irregular heartbeat, significant rise in BP, weakness, and slurring of speech, and ask for medical advice if any indicative sign/symptoms are observed. Inform that anaphylactic/anaphylactoid reactions may occur. Inform that use of drug within 24 hrs of another triptan or an ergot-type medication is contraindicated. Caution about the risk of serotonin syndrome, particularly during combined use with SSRIs, SNRIs, TCAs, and MAOIs. Inform that use of acute migraine drugs for ≥10 days/month may lead to an exacerbation of headache, and encourage to record headache frequency and drug use (eg, by keeping a headache diary). Inform that drug should not be used during pregnancy unless the potential benefit justifies the potential risk to the fetus. Advise to notify physician if breastfeeding or planning to breastfeed. Inform that treatment may cause somnolence and dizziness; instruct to evaluate the ability to perform complex tasks after drug administration.

Storage: 20-25°C (68-77°F).

AMIKACIN – amikacin sulfate **RX**

Class: Aminoglycoside

Potential for nephrotoxicity, neurotoxicity, and ototoxicity; adjust dose or d/c on evidence of ototoxicity/nephrotoxicity. Risk of nephrotoxicity is greater with impaired renal function and in those who receive high dose or prolonged therapy. Neurotoxicity (eg, vestibular and permanent bilateral auditory ototoxicity) can occur with preexisting renal damage and normal renal function treated at higher doses and/or longer treatment periods than recommended. Hearing loss may increase with the degree of exposure to either high peak or high trough serum concentrations. After the drug has been discontinued, total or partial irreversible bilateral deafness may occur. Neuromuscular blockade, respiratory paralysis reported following parenteral inj, topical instillation (as in orthopedic and abdominal irrigation or in local treatment of empyema), and oral use of therapy. Increased risk of neuromuscular blockade and respiratory paralysis with anesthetics, neuromuscular blockers or massive transfusions of citrate-anticoagulated blood. Closely monitor renal and 8th cranial nerve function. Examine urine for decreased specific gravity, increased protein excretion, and presence of cells/casts. Obtain serial audiograms in patients old enough to be tested. Avoid concurrent and/or sequential neurotoxic or nephrotoxic drugs and potent diuretics (eg, ethacrynic acid, furosemide). Advanced age and dehydration may increase risk of toxicity.

ADULT DOSAGE

General Dosing

Short-term treatment of serious infections due to susceptible strains of gram-negative bacteria; bacterial septicemia (including neonatal sepsis); serious infections of respiratory tract, bones and joints, CNS (including meningitis), skin and soft tissue; intra-abdominal infections (including peritonitis); burns and postoperative infections (including post-vascular surgery); serious complicated and recurrent UTIs due to susceptible strains of microorganisms; infections caused by gentamicin- and/or tobramycin-resistant strains of gram-negative organisms, particularly *Proteus rettgeri*, *Providencia stuartii*, *Serratia marcescens*, and *Pseudomonas aeruginosa*; staphylococcal infections; and severe infections in combination w/ a penicillin-type drug

Usual: 15mg/kg/day IM/IV divided into 2 or 3 equal doses given at equally divided intervals

Max: 15mg/kg/day

Max for Heavier Weight Patients: 1.5g/day

Urinary Tract Infections

Uncomplicated:

250mg bid

Treatment Duration

Usual: 7-10 days; d/c therapy if definite clinical response does not occur w/in 3-5 days

Reevaluate if considering therapy beyond 10 days in difficult and complicated infections

PEDIATRIC DOSAGE

General Dosing

Newborns:

LD: 10mg/kg IM/IV

Maint: 7.5mg/kg IM/IV q12h

Older Infants and Children:

15mg/kg/day IM/IV divided into 2 or 3 equal doses given at equally divided intervals

Max: 15mg/kg/day

Max for Heavier Weight Patients: 1.5g/day

Treatment Duration

Usual: 7-10 days; d/c therapy if definite clinical response does not occur w/in 3-5 days

Reevaluate if considering therapy beyond 10 days in difficult and complicated infections

DOSE MODIFICATION

Renal Impairment

Reduce dose or prolong intervals

Normal Dosage at Prolonged Intervals:

If CrCl is unavailable and patient's condition is stable, may calculate dosage interval in hrs by multiplying patient's SrCr by 9 (eg, if SrCr is 2mg/100mL, dosing interval is q18h)

Reduced Dosage at Fixed Intervals:

Initial LD: 7.5mg/kg

Maint Dose q12h: (Observed CrCl [mL/min]/Normal CrCl [mL/min]) x Calculated LD (mg)

Alternatively, may determine reduced q12h dose (if steady state SrCr known) by dividing normal recommended dose by SrCr

ADMINISTRATION

IM/IV route

IV

Add contents of a 500mg vial to 100 or 200mL of sterile diluent (eg, 0.9% NaCl inj, D5 inj)

Infuse over a period of 30-60 min; infuse over 1-2 hrs in infants

Do not physically premix w/ other drugs; administer separately

Stability:

Stable for 24 hrs at room temperature (at concentrations of 0.25 and 5mg/mL) in D5 inj, D5 and 0.2% or 0.45% NaCl inj, 0.9% NaCl inj, Lactated Ringer's inj, Normosol M in D5 inj (or Plasma-Lyte 56 inj in D5W), and Normosol R in D5 inj (or Plasma-Lyte 148 in D5W)

At same concentrations, sol frozen and aged for 30 days at -15°C, thawed, and stored at 25°C had utility times of 24 hrs

HOW SUPPLIED

Inj: 250mg/mL [2mL, 4mL]

WARNINGS/PRECAUTIONS

Avoid peak levels >35mcg/mL and trough levels >10mcg/mL. Not for uncomplicated initial episodes of UTI unless the causative organisms are not susceptible to antibiotics having less potential for toxicity. May cause fetal harm. Contains sodium metabisulfite; allergic-type reactions may occur more frequently in asthmatics. *Clostridium difficile*-associated diarrhea (CDAD) reported; d/c if CDAD is suspected or confirmed. May result in overgrowth of nonsusceptible organisms with prolonged use; take appropriate measures if superinfection develops. Use in the absence of a proven or strongly suspected bacterial infection or prophylactic indication is unlikely to provide benefit and increases the risk of the development of drug-resistant bacteria. Signs of renal irritation may occur (casts, white/red cells/albumin); increase hydration. D/C therapy if azotemia increases or if a progressive decrease in urinary output occurs. May aggravate muscle weakness. Cross-allergenicity among aminoglycosides demonstrated. Caution in elderly, and premature and neonatal infants.

ADVERSE REACTIONS
Ototoxicity, neurotoxicity, nephrotoxicity, skin rash, drug fever, headache, paresthesia, tremor, N/V, eosinophilia, arthralgia, anemia, hypotension, hypomagnesemia.

DRUG INTERACTIONS
See Boxed Warning. Increased nephrotoxicity with parenteral administration of aminoglycosides, antibiotics, and cephalosporins. Significant mutual inactivation may occur with β-lactam antibiotics.

NURSING CONSIDERATIONS

Assessment: Assess for history of hypersensitivity to drug, other aminoglycosides, or to sulfites. Assess for muscular disorders, renal impairment, pregnancy/nursing status, and possible drug interactions. Obtain pretreatment body weight for calculation of correct dosage. Assess and document bacterial infection using culture and susceptibility techniques.

Monitoring: Monitor for signs/symptoms of nephrotoxicity, neurotoxicity, ototoxicity, neuromuscular blockade, respiratory paralysis, and other adverse reactions. Monitor 8th cranial nerve function, hydration status, and drug serum concentrations, and perform urinalysis.

Patient Counseling: Inform about potential risks/benefits of therapy. Inform that drug only treats bacterial, not viral, infections. Instruct to take exactly ud; explaining that skipping doses or not completing full course of therapy may decrease effectiveness and increase the likelihood of bacterial resistance. Inform that diarrhea may occur and will usually end if therapy is discontinued. Instruct to contact physician as soon as possible if watery/bloody stools (with/without stomach cramps, fever) develop even as late as 2 months after having taken the last dose of therapy.

Storage: 20-25°C (68-77°F).

AMITIZA — lubiprostone RX

Class: Chloride channel activator

ADULT DOSAGE

Chronic Idiopathic Constipation

Usual: 24mcg bid

Opioid-Induced Constipation

Chronic Non-Cancer Pain:
Usual: 24mcg bid

Irritable Bowel Syndrome with Constipation

Women:
Usual: 8mcg bid

PEDIATRIC DOSAGE

Pediatric use may not have been established

DOSE MODIFICATION
Hepatic Impairment
Chronic Idiopathic Constipation/Opioid-Induced Constipation:
Moderate (Child-Pugh Class B):
Initial: 16mcg bid
Severe (Child-Pugh Class C):
Initial: 8mcg bid
Titrate: If dose is tolerated but adequate response not obtained, may escalate to full dose w/ appropriate monitoring
Irritable Bowel Syndrome w/ Constipation:
Severe (Child-Pugh Class C):
Initial: 8mcg qd
Titrate: If dose is tolerated but adequate response not obtained, may escalate to full dose w/ appropriate monitoring

ADMINISTRATION
Oral route

Take w/ food and water
Swallow caps whole; do not break or chew

HOW SUPPLIED
Cap: 8mcg, 24mcg

CONTRAINDICATIONS
Known or suspected mechanical GI obstruction.

WARNINGS/PRECAUTIONS
Effectiveness not established in treatment of OIC in patients taking diphenylheptane opioids (eg, methadone). May cause nausea; give with food to reduce symptoms of nausea. Diarrhea may occur; avoid in patients with severe diarrhea and d/c therapy if severe diarrhea occurs. Dyspnea reported; resolves within a few hrs after dose but may recur with subsequent doses. Thoroughly evaluate patients with symptoms suggestive of mechanical GI obstruction prior to initiation of therapy.

ADVERSE REACTIONS
N/V, diarrhea, headache, abdominal pain/distention, flatulence, loose stools, dizziness, edema, dyspnea, abdominal discomfort.

DRUG INTERACTIONS
Diphenylheptane opioids (eg, methadone) may cause dose-dependent decrease in efficacy.

NURSING CONSIDERATIONS

Assessment: Assess for known or suspected mechanical GI obstruction, severe diarrhea, pregnancy/nursing status, and possible drug interactions.

Monitoring: Monitor for nausea, dyspnea, severe diarrhea, and other adverse reactions. Periodically assess the need for continued therapy.

Patient Counseling: Instruct to notify physician if experiencing severe nausea, diarrhea, or dyspnea during treatment. Inform that dyspnea may occur within an hr after 1st dose and resolves within 3 hrs, but may recur with repeat dosing. Advise lactating women to monitor their breastfed infants for diarrhea while on therapy.

Storage: 25°C (77°F); excursions permitted to 15-30°C (59-86°F). Protect from light and extreme temperatures.

AMNESTEEM – isotretinoin RX

Class: Retinoid

Not for use by females who are or may become pregnant. Severe birth defects, including death, have been documented. Increased risk of spontaneous abortion and premature births reported. D/C immediately if pregnancy occurs during treatment and refer to an obstetrician-gynecologist experienced in reproductive toxicity for evaluation and counseling. Approved only under special restricted distribution program called iPLEDGE™. Prescribers, patients, pharmacies, and distributors must be registered and activated with the program.

OTHER BRAND NAMES
Claravis, Sotret

ADULT DOSAGE

Severe Recalcitrant Nodular Acne

Patients Who are Unresponsive to Conventional Therapy, Including Systemic Antibiotics:
0.5-1mg/kg/day given in 2 divided doses for 15-20 weeks
Titrate: Adjust dose according to response and/or tolerability
Very Severe Disease with Scarring or Primarily Manifested on Trunk:
May adjust dose up to 2mg/kg/day, as tolerated

D/C if total nodule count has been reduced by >70% prior to completing 15-20 weeks; may initiate 2nd course of treatment after a period of ≥2 months off therapy

PEDIATRIC DOSAGE

Severe Recalcitrant Nodular Acne

≥12 Years:
Patients Who are Unresponsive to Conventional Therapy, Including Systemic Antibiotics:
0.5-1mg/kg/day given in 2 divided doses for 15-20 weeks

Titrate: Adjust dose according to response and/or tolerability

Very Severe Disease with Scarring or Primarily Manifested on Trunk:
May adjust dose up to 2mg/kg/day, as tolerated

D/C if total nodule count has been reduced by >70% prior to completing 15-20 weeks; may initiate 2nd course of treatment after a period of ≥2 months off therapy

ADMINISTRATION
Oral route

Take with food

HOW SUPPLIED
Cap: 10mg, 20mg, 40mg, (Claravis, Sotret) 10mg, 20mg, 30mg, 40mg

CONTRAINDICATIONS
Pregnancy, paraben sensitivity (Sotret).

WARNINGS/PRECAUTIONS
Avoid long-term use. Blood donation during therapy and for 1 month following discontinuation should be avoided. Do not initiate 2nd course of therapy until at least 8 weeks after completion of 1st course. Hypersensitivity reactions reported; d/c therapy and institute appropriate management if severe allergic reactions occur. Acute pancreatitis, impaired hearing, inflammatory bowel disease, elevated TGs, decreased HDL, hepatotoxicity, premature epiphyseal closure, skeletal hyperostosis, corneal opacities, decreased night vision, and impaired glucose control reported. May cause depression, psychosis, suicidal ideation/attempts, suicide, and aggressive and/or violent behaviors. Associated with pseudotumor cerebri (benign intracranial HTN). D/C if significant decrease in WBC count, hearing or visual impairment, abdominal pain, rectal bleeding, severe diarrhea, or hepatitis occurs, or if liver enzyme levels do not normalize. Spontaneous osteoporosis, osteopenia, bone fractures, and delayed fracture healing reported; caution with genetic predisposition for osteoporosis, history of childhood osteoporosis conditions, osteomalacia, other bone metabolism disorders, anorexia nervosa, and in patients participating in sports with repetitive impact. Micro-dosed progesterone preparations may be an inadequate method of contraception during therapy. (Amnesteem/Claravis) Erythema multiforme and severe skin reactions (eg, Stevens-Johnson syndrome, toxic epidermal necrolysis) reported; closely monitor for severe skin reactions and consider discontinuation of therapy.

ADVERSE REACTIONS
Cheilitis, hypertriglyceridemia, allergic reactions, inflammatory bowel disease, skeletal hyperostosis, pseudotumor cerebri, suicidal ideation/attempt, abnormal menses, bronchospasms, hearing impairment, corneal opacities.

DRUG INTERACTIONS
Avoid use with tetracyclines or vitamin supplements containing vitamin A. Caution with drugs that cause drug-induced osteoporosis/osteomalacia and/or affect vitamin D metabolism (eg, systemic corticosteroids, any anticonvulsant).

NURSING CONSIDERATIONS

Assessment: Assess that females have had 2 (-) urine or serum pregnancy tests separated by at least 19 days, and are on 2 forms of effective contraception. Assess for hypersensitivity to parabens, history of psychiatric disorder, depression, risk of hyperlipidemia, pregnancy/nursing status, and possible drug interactions. Obtain blood lipids and LFTs.

Monitoring: Monitor for signs/symptoms of psychiatric disorders, pseudotumor cerebri, lipid abnormalities, acute pancreatitis, hearing impairment, hepatotoxicity, inflammatory bowel disease (regional ileitis), decreased bone mineral density, hyperostosis, premature epiphyseal closure, and other adverse reactions. Monitor lipid levels and LFTs (weekly or biweekly), glucose levels, and CPK levels until response to drug is established. Monitor that females remain on 2 forms of contraception during and for 1 month following discontinuation of therapy.

Patient Counseling: Instruct to read the Medication Guide/iPLEDGE and sign the Patient Information/Informed Consent form. Inform females of childbearing potential that 2 forms of effective contraception are required starting 1 month prior to initiation, during treatment, and for 1 month following discontinuation. Inform that monthly pregnancy tests are required before new prescription is issued. Instruct patients to d/c therapy if signs/symptoms of pseudotumor cerebri (eg, papilledema, headache, N/V) occur. Counsel not to share drug with anyone and not to donate blood during therapy and for 1 month following discontinuation. Instruct to take with a meal and swallow cap with a full glass of liquid. Inform that transient exacerbation (flare) of acne may occur. Advice to notify physician if depression, mood disturbances, psychosis, or aggression occurs. Instruct to avoid wax epilation and skin resurfacing procedures during and for at least 6 months following therapy; instruct to avoid prolonged exposure to UV rays or sunlight. Inform that decreased tolerance to contact lenses during and after therapy may occur. Inform that musculoskeletal symptoms, transient pain in chest, back pain in pediatrics, arthralgias, neutropenia, agranulocytosis, anaphylactic reactions, allergic vasculitis, purpura of the extremities, and extraneous involvement may occur. (Amnesteem/Claravis) Advise that severe skin reactions may occur.

Storage: 20-25°C (68-77°F). Protect from light.

AMOXICILLIN – amoxicillin

RX

Class: Semisynthetic ampicillin derivative

ADULT DOSAGE

Helicobacter pylori Eradication

W/ *Helicobacter pylori* Infection and Duodenal Ulcer Disease:
Dual Therapy: 1g + 30mg lansoprazole, each q8h for 14 days
Triple Therapy: 1g + 30mg lansoprazole + 500mg clarithromycin, all q12h for 14 days

Ear/Nose/Throat Infection

Mild/Moderate: 500mg q12h or 250mg q8h
Severe: 875mg q12h or 500mg q8h

Usual Duration:
Continue for a minimum of 48-72 hrs beyond the time the patient becomes asymptomatic or evidence of bacterial eradication has been obtained
***Streptococcus pyogenes* Infections:** Treat at least 10 days

Genitourinary Tract Infections

Mild/Moderate: 500mg q12h or 250mg q8h
Severe: 875mg q12h or 500mg q8h

Usual Duration:
Continue for a minimum of 48-72 hrs beyond the time that patient becomes asymptomatic or evidence of bacterial eradication has been obtained

Skin and Skin Structure Infections

Mild/Moderate: 500mg q12h or 250mg q8h
Severe: 875mg q12h or 500mg q8h
Usual Duration:
Continue for a minimum of 48-72 hrs beyond the time the patient becomes asymptomatic or evidence of bacterial eradication has been obtained
***Streptococcus pyogenes* Infections:** Treat at least 10 days

Lower Respiratory Tract Infections

875mg q12h or 500mg q8h
Usual Duration:
Continue for a minimum of 48-72 hrs beyond the time that patient becomes asymptomatic or evidence of bacterial eradication has been obtained
***Streptococcus pyogenes* Infections:** Treat at least 10 days

Gonorrhea

Acute, Uncomplicated Ano-Genital and Urethral Infections:
3g as single dose

PEDIATRIC DOSAGE

Lower Respiratory Tract Infections

≤12 Weeks of Age:
Max: 30mg/kg/day divided q12h
>3 Months of Age:
<40kg:
45mg/kg/day divided q12h or 40mg/kg/day divided q8h
≥40kg:
875mg q12h or 500mg q8h

Usual Duration:
Continue for a minimum of 48-72 hrs beyond the time that patient becomes asymptomatic or evidence of bacterial eradication has been obtained
***Streptococcus pyogenes* Infections:** Treat at least 10 days

Gonorrhea

Acute, Uncomplicated Ano-Genital and Urethral Infections:
>2 Years:
Prepubertal Children:
<40kg: 50mg/kg combined w/ 25mg/kg probenecid as a single dose
≥40kg: 3g as single dose

Ear/Nose/Throat Infection

≤12 Weeks of Age:
Max: 30mg/kg/day divided q12h
>3 Months of Age:
<40kg:
Mild/Moderate: 25mg/kg/day divided q12h or 20mg/kg/day divided q8h
Severe: 45mg/kg/day divided q12h or 40mg/kg/day divided q8h
≥40kg:
Mild/Moderate: 500mg q12h or 250mg q8h
Severe: 875mg q12h or 500mg q8h

Usual Duration:
Continue for a minimum of 48-72 hrs beyond the time that patient becomes asymptomatic or evidence of bacterial eradication has been obtained
***Streptococcus pyogenes* Infections:** Treat at least 10 days

Genitourinary Tract Infections

≤12 Weeks of Age:
Max: 30mg/kg/day divided q12h
>3 Months of Age:
<40kg:
Mild/Moderate: 25mg/kg/day divided q12h or 20mg/kg/day divided q8h
Severe: 45mg/kg/day divided q12h or 40mg/kg/day divided q8h
≥40kg:
Mild/Moderate: 500mg q12h or 250mg q8h
Severe: 875mg q12h or 500mg q8h

Usual Duration:
Continue for a minimum of 48-72 hrs beyond the time that patient becomes asymptomatic or evidence of bacterial eradication has been obtained

Skin and Skin Structure Infections
≤12 Weeks of Age:
Max: 30mg/kg/day divided q12h
>3 Months of Age:
<40kg:
Mild/Moderate: 25mg/kg/day divided q12h or 20mg/kg/day divided q8h
Severe: 45mg/kg/day divided q12h or 40mg/kg/day divided q8h
≥40kg:
Mild/Moderate: 500mg q12h or 250mg q8h
Severe: 875mg q12h or 500mg q8h

Usual Duration:
Continue for a minimum of 48-72 hrs beyond the time that patient becomes asymptomatic or evidence of bacterial eradication has been obtained
***Streptococcus pyogenes* Infections:** Treat at least 10 days

DOSE MODIFICATION

Renal Impairment
GFR <30mL/min: Should not receive a 875mg dose
GFR 10-30mL/min: 250mg or 500mg q12h, depending on severity of infection
GFR <10mL/min: 250mg or 500mg q24h, depending on severity of infection
Hemodialysis: 250 or 500mg q24h, depending on severity of infection; give an additional dose during and at end of dialysis

ADMINISTRATION

Oral route

Sus
125mg/5mL: Reconstitute 80mL, 100mL, or 150mL bottle size w/ 62mL, 77mL, or 113mL of water respectively
200mg/5mL: Reconstitute 50mL, 75mL, or 100mL bottle size w/ 39mL, 57mL, or 75mL of water respectively
250mg/5mL: Reconstitute 80mL, 100mL, or 150mL bottle size w/ 47mL, 60mL, or 90mL of water respectively
400mg/5mL: Reconstitute 50mL, 75mL, or 100mL bottle size w/ 35mL, 51mL, or 67mL of water respectively
Add approximately 1/3 of the total amount of water to wet powder then shake vigorously
Add the remainder of the water and shake vigorously
Place directly on tongue for swallowing
Can be added to formula, milk, fruit juice, water, ginger ale, or cold drinks; take immediately
Shake well before use

HOW SUPPLIED

Cap: 250mg, 500mg; Sus: 125mg/5mL [80mL, 100mL, 150mL], 200mg/5mL [50mL, 75mL, 100mL], 250mg/5mL [80mL, 100mL, 150mL], 400mg/5mL [50mL, 75mL, 100mL]; Tab: 500mg, 875mg*; Tab, Chewable: 125mg, 250mg *scored

WARNINGS/PRECAUTIONS

Serious and occasionally fatal, hypersensitivity (anaphylactic) reactions reported with penicillin (PCN) therapy. *Clostridium difficile*-associated diarrhea (CDAD) reported; d/c if CDAD is suspected or confirmed. Avoid use with mononucleosis; erythematous skin rash may develop in these patients. May result in bacterial resistance if used in the absence of a proven/suspected bacterial indication; d/c and institute appropriate therapy if superinfection develops. Lab test interactions may occur. Caution in elderly; monitor renal function.

ADVERSE REACTIONS

N/V, diarrhea, rash.

DRUG INTERACTIONS

Decreased renal tubular secretion and increased/prolonged levels with probenecid. May reduce efficacy of combined oral estrogen/progesterone contraceptives. Chloramphenicol, macrolides, sulfonamides, and tetracyclines may interfere with bactericidal effects of PCN. PT prolongation (increased INR) reported with oral anticoagulants; dose adjustment of oral anticoagulant may be necessary. Increased incidence of rashes with allopurinol.

NURSING CONSIDERATIONS

Assessment: Assess for history of allergic reaction to PCNs, cephalosporins, or other allergens, mononucleosis, renal function, pregnancy/nursing status, and possible drug interactions.

Monitoring: Monitor for serious anaphylactic reactions, erythematous skin rash, development of drug-resistant bacteria or superinfection, and CDAD. Monitor renal function. Monitor PT and INR if coadministered with an oral anticoagulant.

Patient Counseling: Inform that drug treats only bacterial, not viral (eg, common colds), infections. Instruct to take exactly ud; inform that skipping doses or not completing full course of therapy may decrease effectiveness and increase resistance. Instruct to notify physician as soon as possible if watery and bloody stools (with/without stomach cramps and fever) develop, even as late as ≥2 months after having last dose. Advise patients that drug may cause allergic reactions.

Storage: 20-25°C (68-77°F). (Sus) Discard any unused portion after 14 days. Refrigeration preferable but not required.

AMPHOTEC – amphotericin B cholesteryl sulfate complex RX

Class: Polyene antifungal

ADULT DOSAGE

Aspergillosis

Invasive aspergillosis in patients where renal impairment or unacceptable toxicity precludes the use of amphotericin B deoxycholate in effective doses, and in patients w/ invasive aspergillosis where prior amphotericin B deoxycholate therapy has failed

Test Dose:

Infuse small amount (eg, 10mL of the final preparation containing between 1.6-8.3mg) over 15-30 min; carefully observe for next 30 min

Usual:

3-4mg/kg as required, qd, at infusion rate of 1mg/kg/hr

PEDIATRIC DOSAGE

Aspergillosis

Invasive aspergillosis in patients where renal impairment or unacceptable toxicity precludes the use of amphotericin B deoxycholate in effective doses, and in patients w/ invasive aspergillosis where prior amphotericin B deoxycholate therapy has failed

Test Dose:

Infuse small amount (eg, 10mL of the final preparation containing between 1.6-8.3mg) over 15-30 min; carefully observe for next 30 min

Usual:

3-4mg/kg as required, qd, at infusion rate of 1mg/kg/hr

ADMINISTRATION

IV route

May shorten infusion time to a minimum of 2 hrs if no evidence of intolerance or infusion-related reactions
If acute reactions or intolerance to infusion volume occurs, may extend infusion time
Do not reconstitute w/ saline or dextrose sol, or admix reconstituted liquid w/ saline or electrolytes
Avoid addition of sol containing a bacteriostatic agent (eg, benzyl alcohol)
Do not mix infusion admixture w/ other drugs; if administered through existing IV line, flush w/ D5 for inj prior to and following infusion of therapy
Do not filter or use an in-line filter

Preparation

Reconstitute w/ 10mL or 20mL of sterile water for inj in 50mg or 100mg vial, respectively, using a sterile syringe and a 20-gauge needle
Further dilute reconstituted liquid to final concentration of 0.6mg/mL (range 0.16-0.83mg/mL) by adding appropriate reconstituted volume to D5 for inj infusion bag

HOW SUPPLIED

Inj: 50mg [20mL], 100mg [50mL]

WARNINGS/PRECAUTIONS

Anaphylaxis reported; administer epinephrine, oxygen, IV steroids, and airway management as indicated. D/C if severe respiratory distress occurs; do not give further infusions. Acute infusion-related reactions may occur 1-3 hrs after starting IV infusion; manage by pretreatment with antihistamines and corticosteroids and/or by reducing the rate of infusion and by prompt administration of antihistamines and corticosteroids. Avoid rapid IV infusion. Monitor renal and hepatic function, serum electrolytes, CBC, and PT as medically indicated.

ADVERSE REACTIONS

Chills, fever, tachycardia, N/V, increased creatinine, hypotension, HTN, headache, thrombocytopenia, hypokalemia, hypomagnesemia, hypoxia, abnormal LFTs, dyspnea.

DRUG INTERACTIONS

Caution with antineoplastic agents; may enhance potential for renal toxicity, bronchospasm, hypotension. Corticosteroids and corticotropin may potentiate hypokalemia; monitor serum electrolytes and cardiac function. Cyclosporine and tacrolimus may cause renal toxicity. Concurrent use with digitalis glycosides may induce hypokalemia and may potentiate digitalis toxicity of digitalis glycosides; closely monitor serum K^+ levels. May increase flucytosine toxicity; use with caution. Antagonism with imidazole derivatives (eg, miconazole, ketoconazole) reported.

Nephrotoxic agents (eg, aminoglycosides, pentamidine) may enhance the potential for drug-induced renal toxicity; use with caution and intensively monitor renal function. Amphotericin B-induced hypokalemia may enhance curariform effect of skeletal muscle relaxants (eg, tubocurarine) due to hypokalemia; closely monitor serum K^+ levels.

NURSING CONSIDERATIONS

Assessment: Assess for previous hypersensitivity to the drug, pregnancy/nursing status, and for possible drug interactions. Assess renal function.

Monitoring: Monitor for anaphylaxis, respiratory distress, and acute infusion-related reactions. Monitor renal and hepatic function, serum electrolytes, CBC, and PT. Monitor patients for 30 min after administering the test dose.

Patient Counseling: Inform of risks and benefits of therapy. Advise to seek medical attention if any adverse reactions occur.

Storage: Unopened Vials: 15-30°C (59-86°F). Retain in carton until time of use. Reconstituted: 2-8°C (36-46°F). Use within 24 hrs. Do not freeze. Further Diluted with D5W for Inj: 2-8°C (36-46°F). Use within 24 hrs.

AMPHOTERICIN B – amphotericin B RX

Class: Polyene antifungal

Used primarily for treatment of progressive and potentially life-threatening fungal infections; do not use to treat noninvasive forms of fungal disease (eg, oral thrush, vaginal and esophageal candidiasis) in patients with normal neutrophil counts. Do not give in doses >1.5mg/kg. Exercise caution to prevent inadvertent overdosage; may result in potentially fatal cardiac or cardiopulmonary arrest. Verify product name and dosage preadministration, especially if dose exceeds 1.5mg/kg.

ADULT DOSAGE

Fungal Infections

Potentially life-threatening fungal infections: aspergillosis, cryptococcosis (torulosis), North American blastomycosis, systemic candidiasis, coccidioidomycosis, histoplasmosis, zygomycosis including mucormycosis due to susceptible species of the genera *Absidia*, *Mucor*, and *Rhizopus*, and infections due to related susceptible species of *Conidiobolus* and *Basidiobolus*, and sporotrichosis; may be useful for treatment of American mucocutaneous leishmaniasis, but not the drug of choice as primary therapy

Test Dose:
1mg in 20mL of D5W over 20-30 min

Initial Treatment Dose:

Good Cardio-Renal Function and Well-Tolerated Test Dose: 0.25mg/kg/day

Severe and Rapidly Progressive Infection:
0.3mg/kg/day

Impaired Cardio-Renal Function or Severe Reaction to Test Dose: Initiate w/ smaller daily dose (eg, 5-10mg)

Titrate:
May increase by 5-10mg/day to final dose of 0.5-0.7mg/kg/day, depending on cardio-renal status

Total Daily Dose:
May range up to 1mg/kg/day or up to 1.5mg/kg/day when given on alternate days

Max:
1.5mg/kg/day

Sporotrichosis:
Total dose up to 2.5g for up to 9 months

Aspergillosis:
Total dose up to 3.6g for up to 11 months

Rhinocerebral Phycomycosis:
Cumulative dose of at least 3g is recommended; if there is evidence of deep tissue invasion, may use total dose of 3-4g

PEDIATRIC DOSAGE

Pediatric use may not have been established

ADMINISTRATION

IV route

Administer by slow IV infusion over a period of approx 2-6 hrs (depending on dose) observing the usual precautions for IV therapy

Recommended concentration for IV infusion is 0.1mg/mL (1mg/10mL)

Preparation

Reconstitute vial w/ 10mL sterile water for inj (w/o a bacteriostatic agent) directly into the lyophilized cake, using a needle w/ a minimum diameter of 20 gauge

Shake vial immediately until sol is clear

Obtain infusion sol, providing 0.1mg/mL, by further dilution (1:50) w/ D5W (pH >4.2)

Do not reconstitute w/ saline sol or use any diluent other than the ones recommended

May use an in-line membrane filter for IV infusion; however, the mean pore diameter of the filter should not be <1.0 micron

HOW SUPPLIED

Inj: 50mg

WARNINGS/PRECAUTIONS

Balance possible life-saving benefit against untoward and dangerous side effects. Administer IV under close clinical observation by medically trained personnel. Acute reactions, including fever, shaking chills, hypotension, anorexia, N/V, headache, tachypnea may occur 1-3 hrs after starting IV infusion. Avoid rapid IV infusion; may cause hypotension, hypokalemia, arrhythmias, and shock. Caution with reduced renal function; frequently monitor renal function. Hydration and Na^+ repletion prior to administration may reduce the risk of developing nephrotoxicity. Supplemental alkali medication may decrease renal tubular acidosis complications. Leukoencephalopathy reported; total body irradiation may be a predisposition.

ADVERSE REACTIONS

Fever, malaise, weight loss, hypotension, tachypnea, anorexia, N/V, diarrhea, dyspepsia, cramping epigastric pain, normochromic normocytic anemia, inj-site pain, generalized pain, headache, decreased renal function.

DRUG INTERACTIONS

Antineoplastic agents (eg, nitrogen mustard) may enhance potential for renal toxicity, bronchospasm, hypotension; use with great caution. Corticosteroids and corticotropin may potentiate drug-induced hypokalemia; avoid use unless necessary to control side effects of the drug; if used concomitantly, closely monitor serum electrolytes and cardiac function. Drug-induced hypokalemia may potentiate digitalis toxicity with digitalis glycosides; closely monitor serum K^+ levels and cardiac function, and promptly correct any deficit. May increase flucytosine toxicity. Imidazoles (eg, ketoconazole, miconazole, clotrimazole) may induce fungal resistance; use with caution, especially in immunocompromised patients. Nephrotoxic agents (eg, aminoglycosides, cyclosporine, pentamidine) may enhance the potential for drug-induced renal toxicity; use with great caution and intensively monitor renal function. Drug-induced hypokalemia may enhance curariform effect of skeletal muscle relaxants (eg, tubocurarine); monitor serum K^+ levels and correct deficiencies. Acute pulmonary reactions/toxicity reported with leukocyte transfusions; separate infusions as far as possible and monitor pulmonary function.

NURSING CONSIDERATIONS

Assessment: Assess for type of fungal disease, previous hypersensitivity to the drug, reduced renal function, pregnancy/nursing status, and possible drug interactions.

Monitoring: Monitor clinical status, and for overdosage, acute reactions, nephrotoxicity, and other adverse reactions. Monitor temperature, pulse, respiration, and BP every 30 min for 2-4 hrs after test dose. Frequently monitor renal function. Regularly monitor LFTs, serum electrolytes (particularly Mg^{2+} and K^+), blood counts, and Hgb concentrations.

Patient Counseling: Inform of risks and benefits of therapy. Advise to seek medical attention if any adverse reactions occur.

Storage: Prior to Reconstitution: 2-8°C (36-46°F). Protect against exposure to light. Concentrate (5mg/mL after reconstitution with 10mL Sterile Water for Inj USP): May be stored in the dark, at room temperature for 24 hrs, or refrigerate for 1 week with minimal loss of potency and clarity. Sol for IV Infusion (≤0.1mg/mL): Use promptly after preparation and protect from light during administration.

AMPICILLIN INJECTION – ampicillin sodium

RX

Class: Semisynthetic penicillin derivative

ADULT DOSAGE

Respiratory Tract/Soft Tissue Infections

<40kg:
25-50mg/kg/day in equally divided doses q6-8h
≥40kg:
250-500mg q6h

Gastrointestinal Infections

Including *Neisseria gonorrhoeae* Infections in Females:
<40kg:
50mg/kg/day given in equally divided doses q6-8h
≥40kg:
500mg q6h
Use higher doses for stubborn or severe infections; stubborn infections may require therapy for several weeks

Genitourinary Tract Infections

Including *Neisseria gonorrhoeae* Infections in Females:
<40kg:
50mg/kg/day given in equally divided doses q6-8h
≥40kg:
500mg q6h
Use higher doses for stubborn or severe infections; stubborn infections may require therapy for several weeks

Urethral Infections

Urethritis in Males Caused by *Neisseria gonorrhoeae*:
2 doses of 500mg at an interval of 8-12 hrs; may be repeated if necessary or extended if required
Prolonged and intensive therapy recommended for gonorrheal urethritis (eg, prostatitis, epididymitis)

Bacterial Meningitis

150-200mg/kg/day in equally divided doses q3-4h; may initiate w/ IV drip and continued w/ IM inj

Septicemia

150-200mg/kg/day; start w/ IV administration for at least 3 days and continue w/ IM route q3-4h

Treatment Duration

Continue for a minimum of 48-72 hrs beyond the time the patient becomes asymptomatic or evidence of bacterial eradication has been obtained
Group A β-Hemolytic Streptococci Infections:
Treatment recommended for a minimum of 10 days

PEDIATRIC DOSAGE

Bacterial Meningitis

150-200mg/kg/day in equally divided doses q3-4h; may initiate w/ IV drip and continued w/ IM inj

Septicemia

150-200mg/kg/day; start w/ IV administration for at least 3 days and continue w/ IM route q3-4h

Treatment Duration

Continue for a minimum of 48-72 hrs beyond the time the patient becomes asymptomatic or evidence of bacterial eradication has been obtained

Group A β-Hemolytic Streptococci Infections:
Treatment recommended for a minimum of 10 days

ADMINISTRATION

IM/IV routes
Use only freshly prepared sol
Administer w/in 1 hr after preparation
IM
125mg/mL: Reconstitute 125mg vial w/ 1.2mL of sterile water for inj (SWFI) or bacteriostatic water for inj

250mg/mL: Reconstitute 250mg, 500mg, 1g, or 2g vials w/ 1mL, 1.8mL, 3.5mL, or 6.8mL, respectively, w/ SWFI or bacteriostatic water for inj

IV

Direct IV Use:

Dissolve 125mg, 250mg, or 500mg vial w/ 5mL of SWFI or bacteriostatic water for inj and administer slowly over 3-5 min

Dissolve 1g or 2g vial w/ 7.4mL or 14.8mL of SWFI or bacteriostatic water for inj, respectively, and administer slowly over at least 10-15 min to avoid convulsive seizures

IV Drip:

Reconstitute as directed above prior to diluting w/ compatible IV sol

IV Diluents

SWFI, bacteriostatic water for inj, 0.9% NaCl inj, D5 inj, D5 and 0.45% NaCl inj, lactated Ringer's inj

Refer to PI for additional administration and storage instructions

HOW SUPPLIED

Inj: 125mg, 250mg, 500mg, 1g, 2g. Refer to individual package insert for more information.

WARNINGS/PRECAUTIONS

Reserve this drug for moderately severe and severe infections and for patients unable to take the oral forms; change to oral form may be made as soon as appropriate. Serious and occasionally fatal hypersensitivity (anaphylactoid) reactions w/ penicillin (PCN) therapy reported. Prior to therapy, assess for previous hypersensitivity reactions to PCNs, cephalosporins, and other allergens. D/C and institute appropriate therapy if an allergic reaction occurs. *Clostridium difficile*-associated diarrhea (CDAD) reported; d/c therapy if CDAD is suspected/confirmed. Avoid in infectious mononucleosis; skin rash reported. Use in the absence of a proven or strongly suspected bacterial infection or a prophylactic indication is unlikely to provide benefit and increases the risk of development of drug-resistant bacteria; d/c and substitute appropriate treatment if superinfection occurs. Lab test interactions may occur. More rapid administration may result in convulsive seizures.

ADVERSE REACTIONS

Skin rashes, urticaria, glossitis, N/V, diarrhea, black hairy tongue, stomatitis, enterocolitis, anemia, thrombocytopenia, eosinophilia, leukopenia, agranulocytosis.

DRUG INTERACTIONS

Increased incidence of skin rash w/ allopurinol.

NURSING CONSIDERATIONS

Assessment: Assess for hypersensitivity to PCNs/cephalosporins or other allergens, infectious mononucleosis, pregnancy/nursing status, and possible drug interactions. Conduct culture and susceptibility testing prior to therapy. In gonorrhea w/ a suspected primary lesion of syphilis, perform a dark-field exam before therapy.

Monitoring: Monitor for signs/symptoms of hypersensitivity reactions, CDAD, superinfection, skin rashes, and other adverse reactions. Perform periodic monitoring of organ system function, including renal, hepatic, and hematopoietic function w/ prolonged therapy. Where concomitant syphilis is suspected, perform serological tests monthly for at least 4 months.

Patient Counseling: Inform that drug treats bacterial, not viral, infections. Instruct to take exactly ud; skipping dose or not completing full course of therapy may decrease effectiveness and increase the likelihood of bacterial resistance. Instruct to contact physician as soon as possible if watery and bloody stools (w/ or w/o stomach cramps, fever) develop even as late as 2 or more months after having taken the last dose of therapy.

AMPICILLIN ORAL – ampicillin sodium

RX

Class: Semisynthetic penicillin derivative

ADULT DOSAGE

Genitourinary Tract Infections

Other Than Gonorrhea in Men and Women:

500mg qid in equally spaced doses; severe or chronic infections may require larger doses

Prolonged intensive therapy is needed for complications (eg, prostatitis, epididymitis)

Gonorrhea

3.5g single dose w/ 1g probenecid; use no less than the recommended dosage

Gastrointestinal Disorders

500mg qid in equally spaced doses; severe or chronic infections may require larger doses

PEDIATRIC DOSAGE

Genitourinary Tract Infections

≤20kg:

100mg/kg/day total, qid in equally divided and spaced doses

>20kg:

500mg qid in equally spaced doses

Severe or chronic infections may require larger doses

Prolonged intensive therapy is needed for complications (eg, prostatitis, epididymitis)

Respiratory Tract Infections

250mg qid in equally spaced doses; severe or chronic infections may require larger doses

Treatment Duration

Except for single dose regimen of gonorrhea, continue therapy for a minimum of 48-72 hrs after patient becomes asymptomatic or evidence of bacterial eradication has been obtained; stubborn infections may require treatment for several weeks

Hemolytic Strains of Streptococci: Treat for a minimum of 10 days

Gastrointestinal Infections

≤20kg:
100mg/kg/day total, qid in equally divided and spaced doses
>20kg:
500mg qid in equally spaced doses
Severe or chronic infections may require larger doses

Gonorrhea

>20kg:
3.5g single dose w/ 1g probenecid; use no less than the recommended dosage

Respiratory Tract Infections

≤20kg:
50mg/kg/day total, in equally divided and spaced doses tid-qid
Max: Do not exceed adult doses
>20kg:
250mg qid in equally spaced doses
Severe or chronic infections may require larger doses

Treatment Duration

Except for single dose regimen of gonorrhea, continue therapy for a minimum of 48-72 hrs after patient becomes asymptomatic or evidence of bacterial eradication has been obtained; stubborn infections may require treatment for several weeks
Hemolytic Strains of Streptococci: Treat for a minimum of 10 days

ADMINISTRATION
Oral route
Take at least 30 min before or 2 hrs pc w/ a full glass of water
Preparation
125mg/5mL: Reconstitute 100mL and 200mL package sizes w/ 86mL and 170mL of water respectively
250mg/5mL: Reconstitute 100mL and 200mL package sizes w/ 70mL and 139mL of water respectively
Add water in 2 portions; shake well after each addition

HOW SUPPLIED
Cap: 250mg, 500mg; Sus: 125mg/5mL, 250mg/5mL [100mL, 200mL]

CONTRAINDICATIONS
Infections caused by penicillinase-producing organisms.

WARNINGS/PRECAUTIONS
Serious and fatal hypersensitivity reactions reported w/ penicillin (PCN) therapy; anaphylactoid reactions require immediate treatment w/ epinephrine, oxygen, IV steroids, and airway management. Possible cross-sensitivity w/ cephalosporins. Pseudomembranous colitis reported; initiate therapeutic measures if diagnosed and consider discontinuation of treatment. May result in bacterial resistance w/ prolonged use or use in the absence of a proven or suspected bacterial infection or a prophylactic indication; take appropriate measures if superinfection develops. Give additional parenteral PCN in patients w/ gonorrhea who also have syphilis. Treatment does not preclude the need for surgical procedures, particularly in staphylococcal infections. Lab test interactions may occur.

ADVERSE REACTIONS
Stomatitis, N/V, diarrhea, rash, SGOT elevation, agranulocytosis, anemia, eosinophilia, leukopenia, thrombocytopenia, thrombocytopenic purpura, hypersensitivity reactions.

DRUG INTERACTIONS
Increased risk of rash w/ allopurinol. Bacteriostatic antibiotics (eg, chloramphenicol, erythromycins, sulfonamides, tetracyclines) may interfere w/ bactericidal activity. May increase breakthrough bleeding with oral contraceptives and decrease oral contraceptive effectiveness. Increased blood levels and toxicity w/ probenecid.

NURSING CONSIDERATIONS

Assessment: Assess for previous hypersensitivity reactions to PCNs, cephalosporins, or other allergens; history of allergy, asthma, hay fever, or urticaria; pregnancy/nursing status, syphilis, and possible drug interactions. Conduct susceptibility testing as guide to therapy.

Monitoring: Monitor for hypersensitivity reactions, pseudomembranous colitis, and overgrowth of nonsusceptible organisms. Evaluate renal/hepatic/hematopoietic systems periodically w/ prolonged therapy. Upon completion, obtain cultures to determine organism eradication. Monitor for masked syphilis; perform follow-up serologic test for each month for 4 months for syphilis in patients w/o suspected lesions of syphilis.

Patient Counseling: Instruct to notify physician of history of hypersensitivity to PCNs, cephalosporins, or other allergens. Inform diabetics to consult w/ physician prior to changing diet or dosage of diabetic medication. Inform to take exactly ud; skipping doses or not completing full course decreases effectiveness and increases bacterial resistance. Instruct to d/c and notify physician if side effects occur. Inform that therapy only treats bacterial, and not viral, infections.

Storage: 20-25°C (68-77°F). (Sus) Store reconstituted sus in the refrigerator; discard unused portion after 14 days.

AMPYRA – dalfampridine

RX

Class: Potassium channel blocker

ADULT DOSAGE

Multiple Sclerosis

To Improve Walking in Patients w/ Multiple Sclerosis:

Usual/Max: 10mg bid (approx 12 hrs apart)

PEDIATRIC DOSAGE

Pediatric use may not have been established

ADMINISTRATION

Oral route

Take w/ or w/o food

Take tab whole; do not divide, crush, chew, or dissolve

HOW SUPPLIED

Tab, Extended-Release: 10mg

CONTRAINDICATIONS

History of seizure, moderate or severe renal impairment (CrCl ≤50mL/min).

WARNINGS/PRECAUTIONS

May cause seizures; d/c and do not restart in patients who experience a seizure while on therapy. Caution with mild renal impairment (CrCl 51-80mL/min). Avoid with other forms of 4-aminopyridine; d/c use of any product containing 4-aminopyridine prior to initiating therapy. May cause anaphylaxis and severe allergic reactions; d/c if signs and symptoms occur. Urinary tract infections (UTIs) reported; evaluate and treat patients as clinically indicated.

ADVERSE REACTIONS

UTI, insomnia, dizziness, headache, nausea, asthenia, back pain, balance disorder, MS relapse, paresthesia, nasopharyngitis, constipation.

NURSING CONSIDERATIONS

Assessment: Assess for hypersensitivity to the drug or 4-aminopyridine, history of seizures, and pregnancy/nursing status. Obtain baseline CrCl.

Monitoring: Monitor for seizures, anaphylaxis, severe allergic reactions, UTIs, and other adverse reactions. Monitor CrCl at least annually.

Patient Counseling: Inform that therapy may cause seizures and to d/c treatment if seizure is experienced. Instruct to take exactly ud and not take a double dose if a dose is missed. Instruct not to take more than 2 tabs in a 24-hr period and to make sure that there is an approximate 12-hr interval between doses. Inform of the signs/symptoms of anaphylaxis; instruct to d/c therapy and seek medical care if anaphylaxis develops.

Storage: 25°C (77°F); excursions permitted to 15-30°C (59-86°F).

AMRIX – cyclobenzaprine hydrochloride RX

Class: Skeletal muscle relaxant (central-acting)

ADULT DOSAGE

Muscle Spasms

Adjunct to rest and physical therapy for relief of muscle spasm associated with acute, painful musculoskeletal conditions

Usual: 15mg qd; may require up to 30mg qd

PEDIATRIC DOSAGE

Pediatric use may not have been established

ADMINISTRATION

Oral route

Take at the same time each day

HOW SUPPLIED

Cap, Extended-Release: 15mg, 30mg

CONTRAINDICATIONS

Concomitant use of MAOIs or within 14 days after their discontinuation. During the acute recovery phase of MI. Arrhythmias, heart block or conduction disturbances, CHF, hyperthyroidism.

WARNINGS/PRECAUTIONS

Use for periods longer than 2 or 3 weeks is not recommended. Not effective in the treatment of spasticity associated with cerebral or spinal cord disease or in children with cerebral palsy. May produce arrhythmias, sinus tachycardia, and conduction time prolongation leading to MI and stroke; consider discontinuation if clinically significant CNS symptoms develop. Not recommended with hepatic impairment and in elderly. Caution with history of urinary retention, angle-closure glaucoma, and increased IOP. Consider certain withdrawal symptoms; abrupt cessation after prolonged administration rarely may produce nausea, headache, and malaise.

ADVERSE REACTIONS

Dry mouth, dizziness, somnolence, fatigue, constipation, nausea, dyspepsia.

DRUG INTERACTIONS

See Contraindications. Serotonin syndrome reported when used with SSRIs, SNRIs, TCAs, tramadol, bupropion, meperidine, verapamil, or MAOIs; d/c immediately if this occurs. Observe carefully, particularly during treatment initiation or dose increases, if concomitant use with other serotonergic drugs is warranted. May enhance effects of alcohol, barbiturates, and other CNS depressants. Caution with anticholinergics. May block the antihypertensive action of guanethidine and similarly acting compounds. May enhance seizure risk with tramadol.

NURSING CONSIDERATIONS

Assessment: Assess for arrhythmias, heart block or conduction disturbances, CHF, hyperthyroidism, acute recovery phase of MI, history of urinary retention, angle-closure glaucoma, increased IOP, hepatic impairment, drug hypersensitivity, pregnancy/nursing status, and possible drug interactions.

Monitoring: Monitor for arrhythmias, sinus tachycardia, conduction time prolongation, CNS symptoms, withdrawal symptoms, and other adverse reactions.

Patient Counseling: Advise to d/c use and notify physician immediately if experiencing symptoms of an allergic reaction (eg, difficulty breathing, hives, swelling of face/tongue, itching), arrhythmias, or tachycardia. Caution about the risk of serotonin syndrome; instruct to seek medical care immediately if signs/symptoms occur. Inform that drug may enhance impairment effects of alcohol and other CNS depressants. Caution about operating an automobile or other hazardous machinery until accustomed to effects of medication.

Storage: 25°C (77°F); excursions permitted to 15-30°C (59-86°F).

AMTURNIDE – aliskiren/amlodipine/hydrochlorothiazide RX

Class: Calcium channel blocker (dihydropyridine)/renin inhibitor/thiazide diuretic

D/C when pregnancy is detected. Drugs that act directly on the renin-angiotensin system can cause injury/death to the developing fetus.

ADULT DOSAGE

Hypertension

Usual: Dose qd

Titrate: May increase after 2 weeks of therapy

Max: 300mg/10mg/25mg

PEDIATRIC DOSAGE

Pediatric use may not have been established

Add-On/Switch Therapy:
Use if not adequately controlled w/ any 2 of the following: aliskiren, dihydropyridine calcium channel blockers, and thiazide diuretics
W/ dose-limiting adverse reactions to any component on dual therapy, switch to triple therapy at a lower dose of that component
Replacement Therapy:
Substitute for individually titrated components

DOSE MODIFICATION

Renal Impairment
Consider lower doses

Hepatic Impairment
Consider lower doses

Elderly
Consider lower initial doses

ADMINISTRATION

Oral route

Establish a routine pattern for taking the drug, either w/ or w/o a meal; high-fat meals decrease absorption substantially

HOW SUPPLIED

Tab: (Aliskiren/Amlodipine/Hydrochlorothiazide [HCTZ]) 150mg/5mg/12.5mg, 300mg/5mg/12.5mg, 300mg/5mg/25mg, 300mg/10mg/12.5mg, 300mg/10mg/25mg

CONTRAINDICATIONS

Anuria, sulfonamide-derived drug hypersensitivity. Concomitant use w/ ARBs or ACE inhibitors in patients w/ diabetes.

WARNINGS/PRECAUTIONS

Not indicated for initial therapy of HTN. Symptomatic hypotension may occur in patients w/ marked volume depletion or w/ salt depletion; correct volume/salt depletion prior to administration, or start treatment under close medical supervision. May cause changes in renal function, including acute renal failure; caution in patients whose renal function depend in part on the activity of the renin-angiotensin-aldosterone system (RAAS) (eg, renal artery stenosis, severe heart failure [HF], post-MI, or volume depletion. Consider withholding or discontinuing therapy if significant decrease in renal function develops. May cause serum electrolyte abnormalities (eg, hyper/hypokalemia, hyponatremia, hypomagnesemia); correct hypokalemia and any coexisting hypomagnesemia prior to initiation. D/C if hypokalemia is accompanied by clinical signs (eg, muscular weakness, paresis, ECG alterations). Aliskiren: Hypersensitivity reactions and head/neck angioedema reported; d/c therapy immediately and do not readminister if anaphylactic reactions or angioedema develop. Amlodipine: May cause symptomatic hypotension, particularly in patients w/ severe aortic stenosis. May develop worsening of angina and acute MI after starting or increasing the dose, particularly w/ severe obstructive coronary artery disease (CAD). HCTZ: May cause hypersensitivity reactions and exacerbation or activation of systemic lupus erythematosus (SLE). Minor alterations of fluid and electrolyte balance may precipitate hepatic coma in patients w/ hepatic impairment or progressive liver disease. May cause idiosyncratic reaction, resulting in transient myopia and acute angle-closure glaucoma; d/c as rapidly as possible. May alter glucose tolerance, increase serum cholesterol/TG levels, and cause hypercalcemia. May cause or exacerbate hyperuricemia and precipitate gout in susceptible patients.

ADVERSE REACTIONS

Peripheral edema, dizziness, headache.

DRUG INTERACTIONS

See Contraindications. Aliskiren: Cyclosporine or itraconazole may increase levels; avoid concomitant use w/ such drugs. NSAIDs, including selective COX-2 inhibitors, may deteriorate renal function and attenuate antihypertensive effect. Dual blockade of the RAAS is associated w/ increased risk of hypotension, hyperkalemia, and changes in renal function (including acute renal failure); in general, avoid combined use w/ ACE inhibitors or ARBS, particularly in patients w/ CrCl <60mL/min. Oral coadministration w/ furosemide reduced exposure to furosemide; monitor diuretic effects when coadministered. May develop hyperkalemia w/ NSAIDs, K^+ supplements, or K^+-sparing diuretics. Amlodipine: May increase simvastatin exposure; limit simvastatin dose to 20mg/day. Increased systemic exposure w/ CYP3A inhibitors (moderate and strong) warranting dose reduction; monitor for symptoms of hypotension and edema w/ CYP3A4 inhibitors to determine the need for dose adjustment. Monitor BP when coadministered w/ CYP3A4 inducers. HCTZ: Dosage adjustment of antidiabetic drugs (insulin or oral hypoglycemic agents) may be required. Space dosing ≥4 hrs before or 4-6 hrs after the administration of ion-exchange resins (eg, cholestyramine, colestipol). May increase risk of lithium toxicity; monitor serum lithium levels.

NURSING CONSIDERATIONS

Assessment: Assess for diabetes, sulfonamide derived drug hypersensitivity, hepatic/renal impairment, anuria, CAD, renal artery stenosis, HF, post-MI status, history of penicillin allergy, volume/salt depletion, SLE, severe aortic stenosis, bronchial asthma, pregnancy/nursing status, and possible drug interactions. Correct electrolyte imbalances (eg, hypokalemia, hypomagnesemia) prior to initiation of therapy.

Monitoring: Monitor for hypersensitivity/anaphylactic reactions, head/neck angioedema, airway obstruction, worsening of angina and MI, exacerbation of SLE, idiosyncratic reaction, transient myopia, acute angle-closure glaucoma, and other adverse reactions. Monitor BP, hepatic/renal function, serum uric acid, serum electrolytes, and glucose/cholesterol/TG levels.

Patient Counseling: Advise female patients of childbearing age about consequences of exposure during pregnancy and discuss the treatment options w/ women planning to become pregnant. Advise to report pregnancy to physician as soon as possible. Caution that lightheadedness may occur, especially during the 1st days of therapy; instruct to contact physician if lightheadedness occurs. Advise to d/c treatment and to consult physician if syncope occurs. Caution that inadequate fluid intake, excessive perspiration, diarrhea, or vomiting can lead to excessive fall in BP. Advise to d/c and immediately report any signs/symptoms of severe allergic reaction or angioedema. Inform that angioedema, including laryngeal edema, may occur anytime during treatment. Instruct not to use K^+ supplements or salt substitutes containing K^+ w/o consulting physician.

Storage: 25°C (77°F); excursions permitted to 15-30°C (59-86°F). Protect from heat and moisture.

ANAGRELIDE – anagrelide hydrochloride RX

Class: Platelet-reducing agent

OTHER BRAND NAMES

Agrylin

ADULT DOSAGE

Thrombocythemia

Secondary to myeloproliferative neoplasms, to reduce the elevated platelet count and risk of thrombosis and to ameliorate associated symptoms including thrombo-hemorrhagic events

Initial: 0.5mg qid or 1mg bid for ≥1 week
Titrate: Adjust to reduce and maintain platelet count to <600,000/µL, and ideally between 150,000-400,000/µL
Increase by not more than 0.5mg/day in any 1 week
Usual Range: 1.5-5mg/day
Max: 10mg/day or 2.5mg/dose

PEDIATRIC DOSAGE

Thrombocythemia

Secondary to myeloproliferative neoplasms, to reduce the elevated platelet count and risk of thrombosis and to ameliorate associated symptoms including thrombo-hemorrhagic events

Initial: 0.5mg qd for ≥1 week
Titrate: Adjust to reduce and maintain platelet count to <600,000/µL, and ideally between 150,000-400,000/µL
Increase by not more than 0.5mg/day in any 1 week
Usual Range: 1.5-5mg/day
Max: 10mg/day or 2.5mg/dose

DOSE MODIFICATION

Hepatic Impairment

Moderate (Child-Pugh 7-9):
Initial: 0.5mg/day
Titrate: May increase in patients who have tolerated initial dose for 1 week; increase by not more than 0.5mg/day in any 1 week

Severe: Avoid use

ADMINISTRATION

Oral route

HOW SUPPLIED

Cap: 1mg; (Agrylin) 0.5mg

WARNINGS/PRECAUTIONS

Torsades de pointes and ventricular tachycardia reported. Increases QTc interval and HR; do not use in patients with risk factors for QT interval prolongation (eg, congenital long QT syndrome, known history of acquired QTc prolongation). Hepatic impairment increases exposure and could increase the risk of QTc prolongation. Consider periodic monitoring with ECGs in patients with heart failure (HF), bradyarrhythmias, or electrolyte abnormalities. May cause vasodilation, tachycardia, palpitations, and congestive heart failure; use only when benefits outweigh the risks in cardiac disease. Interstitial lung diseases (eg, allergic alveolitis, eosinophilic pneumonia, interstitial pneumonitis) reported; if suspected, d/c therapy and evaluate.

ADVERSE REACTIONS

Headache, palpitations, diarrhea, asthenia, edema, N/V, abdominal pain, dizziness, pain, dyspnea, flatulence, fever, peripheral edema, rash.

DRUG INTERACTIONS

Do not use with medications that may prolong QTc interval (eg, chloroquine, clarithromycin, haloperidol). Concomitant use with aspirin (ASA) increased major hemorrhagic events; assess potential risks and benefits for concomitant use, and monitor for bleeding, including with other drugs known to cause bleeding (eg, anticoagulants, PDE3 inhibitors, NSAIDs, antiplatelet agents, SSRIs). Avoid the effects of drug products with similar properties such as inotropes and other PDE3 inhibitors (eg, cilostazol, milrinone). CYP1A2 inhibitors (eg, fluvoxamine, ciprofloxacin) may increase exposure; monitor for cardiovascular (CV) events and titrate doses accordingly. CYP1A2 inducers (eg, omeprazole) may decrease exposure; may need to titrate dose of CYP1A2 inducers. May alter exposure of CYP1A2 substrates (eg, theophylline, fluvoxamine, ondansetron).

NURSING CONSIDERATIONS

Assessment: Assess for risk factors for QT interval prolongation, pregnancy/nursing status, and possible drug interactions. Assess hepatic/renal function and electrolytes. Perform CV exam, including ECG.

Monitoring: Monitor for CV effects, interstitial lung diseases, and other adverse reactions. Consider periodic monitoring with ECGs in patients with HF, bradyarrhythmias, or electrolyte abnormalities. Monitor for bleeding with ASA or other drugs known to cause bleeding. Monitor hepatic/renal function and electrolytes. Monitor CBCs; monitor platelet counts every 2 days during the 1st week of treatment and at least weekly thereafter until the maintenance dosage is reached, then monthly or as necessary.

Patient Counseling: Inform patients that their dose will be adjusted on a weekly basis until they are on a dose that lowers their platelets to an appropriate level; advise to contact physician if tolerability issues develop. Instruct to contact physician immediately if chest pain, palpitations, or irregular heartbeat occurs. Inform of the risk of bleeding with concomitant ASA; advise to contact physician immediately if signs/symptoms of bleeding or unexplained bruising/bruise more easily than usual occurs.

Storage: 20-25°C (68-77°F). (Agrylin) 25°C (77°F); excursions permitted to 15-30°C (59-86°F).

ANDRODERM – testosterone CIII

Class: Androgen

ADULT DOSAGE

Testosterone Replacement Therapy

Congenital/Acquired Primary Hypogonadism or Hypogonadotropic Hypogonadism in Males:

Initial: One 4mg/day system applied nightly for 24 hrs

Titrate: Measure early am serum testosterone concentrations, approx 2 weeks after starting therapy

If outside the range of 400-930ng/dL, increase daily dose to 6mg (one 4mg/day and one 2mg/day system) or decrease to 2mg (one 2mg/day system), maintaining nightly application

Patients currently maintained on 2.5mg/day, 5mg/day, or 7.5mg/day systems may be switched to 2mg/day, 4mg/day, or 6mg/day (2mg/day and 4mg/day) systems respectively, at the next scheduled dose

Measure early am serum testosterone concentration approx 2 weeks after switching to ensure proper dosing

PEDIATRIC DOSAGE

Pediatric use may not have been established

ADMINISTRATION

Transdermal route

Immediately apply adhesive side of the system to a clean, dry area of the skin on the back, abdomen, upper arms, or thighs

Avoid swimming, showering, or washing the administration site for a minimum of 3 hrs after application

Rotate application site w/ an interval of 7 days between applications to the same site

Refer to PI for further application instructions

HOW SUPPLIED

Patch: 2mg/day [60^s], 4mg/day [30^s]

CONTRAINDICATIONS

Men with breast carcinoma or known/suspected prostate carcinoma; women who are or may become pregnant, or who are breastfeeding.

WARNINGS/PRECAUTIONS

Monitor patients with BPH for worsening of signs/symptoms of BPH. May increase risk for prostate cancer. Increases in Hct/RBC mass may increase risk for thromboembolic events; lower dose or d/c therapy until Hct decreases to acceptable level. Venous thromboembolic events (VTE) (eg, deep vein thrombosis, pulmonary embolism) reported; d/c treatment and initiate appropriate workup and management if VTE is suspected. Suppression of spermatogenesis may occur at large doses. Risk of edema with or without CHF in patients with preexisting cardiac/renal/hepatic disease. Gynecomastia may develop and persist. May potentiate sleep apnea. Changes in serum lipid profile may require dose adjustment or discontinuation of therapy. Caution in cancer patients at risk of hypercalcemia (and associated hypercalciuria); monitor serum Ca^{2+} concentrations regularly. May decrease concentrations of thyroxine-binding globulin, resulting in decreased total T4 serum concentrations and increased resin uptake of T3 and T4. Skin burns reported at application site in patients wearing an aluminized transdermal system during a magnetic resonance imaging scan (MRI); remove the system before patient undergoes an MRI.

ADVERSE REACTIONS

Application-site reactions (eg, pruritus, blistering, erythema, vesicles, burning, induration), back pain, prostate abnormalities, headache, contact dermatitis, depression.

DRUG INTERACTIONS

Changes in insulin sensitivity or glycemic control may occur; may decrease blood glucose and therefore, decrease insulin requirements in diabetic patients. Changes in anticoagulant activity may occur; frequently monitor INR and PT in patients taking anticoagulants, especially at initiation and termination of androgen therapy. Concurrent use with adrenocorticotropic hormone or corticosteroids may increase fluid retention; caution in patients with cardiac/renal/hepatic disease. Pretreatment with triamcinolone oint formulation significantly reduced testosterone absorption.

NURSING CONSIDERATIONS

Assessment: Assess for breast/prostate cancer, BPH, cardiac/renal/hepatic disease, risk factors for sleep apnea, cancer patients at risk for hypercalcemia, upcoming MRI exam, any other conditions where treatment is contraindicated or cautioned, and possible drug interactions. Obtain baseline Hct, lipid, and serum testosterone levels.

Monitoring: Monitor for signs/symptoms of edema with or without CHF, VTE, gynecomastia, sleep apnea, worsening of BPH and other adverse reactions. Monitor Hct, prostate-specific antigen, serum lipid profile, liver function, and serum testosterone levels periodically. In cancer patients at risk for hypercalcemia, regularly monitor serum Ca^{2+} levels. Reevaluate for prostate cancer 3-6 months after initiation, and then in accordance with prostate cancer screening practices. Reevaluate Hct 3-6 months after start of therapy, then annually. Monitor PT/INR more frequently with concomitant anticoagulants.

Patient Counseling: Inform that men with known or suspected prostate/breast cancer should not use androgen therapy. Inform about potential adverse reactions. Instruct to apply ud. Advise not to apply to the scrotum, over a bony prominence, or any part of the body that could be subject to prolonged pressure during sleep or sitting. Advise not to remove during sexual intercourse, nor while taking a shower or bath. Inform that strenuous exercise or excessive perspiration may loosen a patch or cause it to fall off; if patch falls off, advise not to tape to skin. Advise to avoid swimming or showering until 3 hrs following application. Instruct to use OTC topical hydrocortisone cream after system removal in order to ameliorate mild skin irritation. Advise to remove the patch before undergoing MRI. Advise not to cut the patches.

Storage: 20-25° (68-77°F). Do not store outside the pouch provided. Drug reservoir may be burst by excessive pressure or heat.

ANDROGEL – testosterone

CIII

Class: Androgen

Virilization reported in children secondarily exposed to testosterone gel. Children should avoid contact w/ unwashed or unclothed application sites in men using testosterone gel. Advise to strictly adhere to recommended instructions for use.

ADULT DOSAGE

Testosterone Replacement Therapy

Congenital/Acquired Primary Hypogonadism or Hypogonadotropic Hypogonadism in Males:

1%:

Initial: Apply 50mg (4 pump actuations, two 25mg pkts, or one 50mg pkt) qd in am (preferably at the same time every day)

Titrate: May increase to 75mg qd and then to 100mg qd as instructed by physician if serum testosterone is below normal range

May decrease daily dose if serum testosterone exceeds normal range

D/C therapy if serum testosterone consistently exceeds the normal range at a daily dose of 50mg

Assess serum testosterone concentrations periodically

Refer to PI for specific dosing guidelines using the multidose pump

1.62%:

Initial: Apply 40.5mg (2 pump actuations or a single 40.5mg pkt) qd in am

Titrate: May adjust dose between a minimum of 20.25mg (1 pump actuation or a single 20.25mg pkt) and a max of 81mg (4 pump actuations or two 40.5mg pkts)

Titrate based on the predose am serum testosterone concentration from a single blood draw at approximately 14 days and 28 days after starting treatment or following dose adjustment

Titration Based on Predose AM Serum Testosterone:

Serum Testosterone > 750ng/dL: Decrease daily dose by 20.25mg (1 pump actuation or a single 20.25 mg packet)

Serum Testosterone 350-750ng/dL: Continue current dose

Serum Testosterone <350ng/dL: Increase daily dose by 20.25mg (1 pump actuation or a single 20.25 mg packet)

Assess serum testosterone concentrations periodically

PEDIATRIC DOSAGE

Pediatric use may not have been established

ADMINISTRATION

Topical route

Apply to clean, dry, healthy, intact skin

Refer to PI for additional administration and priming instructions

1%

Apply to right and left upper arms/shoulders and/or right and left abdomen; do not apply to any other parts of the body (eg, genitals, chest)

Avoid swimming or showering for at least 5 hrs after application

1.62%

Apply to upper arms and shoulders; do not apply to any other parts of the body (eg, abdomen, genitals)

Avoid swimming, showering, or washing the administration site for a minimum of 2 hrs after application

HOW SUPPLIED

Gel: 1% [2.5g, 5g pkt; 75g pump], 1.62% [1.25g, 2.5g pkt; 88g pump]

CONTRAINDICATIONS

Breast carcinoma or known/suspected prostate carcinoma in men; women who are or may become pregnant, or are breastfeeding.

WARNINGS/PRECAUTIONS

Topical testosterone products may have different doses, strengths, or application instructions that may result in different systemic exposure. Application site and dose are not interchangeable w/ other topical testosterone products. Patients w/ BPH treated w/ androgens, may be at increased risk for worsening of signs/symptoms of BPH. May increase risk for prostate cancer. Increases in Hct, reflective of increases in RBC mass, may require lowering or discontinuation of therapy; increase in RBC mass may increase risk for thromboembolic events. Venous thromboembolic events (eg, DVT, pulmonary embolism) reported; d/c and initiate appropriate workup and management if a venous thromboembolic event is suspected. Suppression of spermatogenesis may occur w/ large doses. Edema w/ or w/o CHF may be a serious complication in patients w/ preexisting cardiac, renal, or hepatic disease. Gynecomastia may develop and persist. May potentiate sleep apnea. Changes in serum lipid profile may require dose adjustment or discontinuation of therapy. Caution in cancer patients at risk of hypercalcemia and associated hypercalciuria. May decrease levels of thyroxin-binding globulins, resulting in decreased total T4 serum concentrations and increased resin uptake of T3 and T4. Flammable; avoid fire, flame, or smoking until the gel has dried.

ADVERSE REACTIONS

(1.62%) Prostate specific antigen (PSA) increase. (1%) Acne, application-site reactions, prostatic/urinary/testicular disorders, abnormal lab tests, headache, emotional lability, gynecomastia, HTN, nervousness, asthenia, decreased libido.

DRUG INTERACTIONS

Changes in insulin sensitivity or glycemic control may occur; may decrease blood glucose and, therefore, may decrease insulin requirements in diabetic patients. Changes in anticoagulant activity may occur; frequently monitor INR and PT in patients taking anticoagulants, especially at initiation and termination of androgen therapy. Adrenocorticotropic hormone or corticosteroids may increase fluid retention; caution in patients w/ cardiac, renal, or hepatic disease.

NURSING CONSIDERATIONS

Assessment: Assess for BPH, breast/prostate cancer, cardiac/renal/hepatic disease, risk factors for sleep apnea, cancer patients at risk for hypercalcemia, any conditions where treatment is contraindicated or cautioned, and possible drug interactions. Obtain baseline Hct and serum testosterone levels.

Monitoring: Monitor for prostate cancer, edema w/ or w/o CHF, venous thromboembolic events, gynecomastia, sleep apnea, worsening of signs/symptoms of BPH, and other adverse reactions. Perform periodic monitoring of Hgb, PSA, serum lipid profile, LFTs, and serum testosterone concentrations. In cancer patients at risk for hypercalcemia, regularly monitor serum Ca^{2+} levels. Reevaluate Hct 3-6 months after start of therapy, then annually. Frequently monitor PT/INR w/ anticoagulants.

Patient Counseling: Inform that men w/ known or suspected prostate/breast cancer should not use androgen therapy. Advise to report signs and symptoms of secondary exposure in children and women to the physician. Instruct women and children to avoid contact w/ unwashed or unclothed application sites of men. Instruct to apply qd and to wash hands w/ soap and water after application, cover application site w/ clothing after gel dries, and wash application site w/ soap and water prior to direct skin-to-skin contact w/ others. Counsel about possible adverse reactions. Advise to read Medication Guide before therapy and reread each time prescription is renewed. Inform that drug is flammable; instruct to avoid fire, flame, or smoking until the gel has dried. Advise not to share the medication w/ anyone. Inform patients about importance of adhering to all the recommended monitoring, to report changes in their state of health, and to wait 5 hrs (1%) or 2 hrs (1.62%) before swimming or bathing.

Storage: (1%) 25°C (77°F); excursions permitted to 15-30°C (59-86°F). (1.62%) 20-25°C (68-77°F); excursions permitted to 15-30°C (59-86°F).

ANORO ELLIPTA – umeclidinium/vilanterol RX

Class: Anticholinergic/beta$_2$-agonist

Long-acting β_2-adrenergic agonists (LABAs) increase the risk of asthma-related death. Not indicated for the treatment of asthma.

ADULT DOSAGE

Chronic Obstructive Pulmonary Disease

Long-Term Maint Treatment of Airflow Obstruction in Patients w/ COPD (eg, Chronic Bronchitis, Emphysema):

1 inh qd; do not use >1 time q24h

PEDIATRIC DOSAGE

Pediatric use may not have been established

ADMINISTRATION

Oral inh route

Take at the same time every day

HOW SUPPLIED

Powder, Inhalation: (Umeclidinium/Vilanterol) (62.5mcg/25mcg)/blister [7, 30 blisters]

CONTRAINDICATIONS

Milk protein hypersensitivity.

WARNINGS/PRECAUTIONS

Not indicated for acute bronchospasm relief. Do not initiate during rapidly deteriorating or potentially life-threatening episodes of COPD. D/C regular use of oral/inhaled short acting β_2-agonist when beginning treatment. Do not use more often or at higher doses than recommended; clinically significant cardiovascular (CV) effects and fatalities reported with excessive use. May produce paradoxical bronchospasm; treat immediately with an inhaled, short acting bronchodilator; d/c and institute alternative therapy. Hypersensitivity reactions and CV effects may occur. Caution with CV disorders, convulsive disorders, thyrotoxicosis, diabetes mellitus (DM), ketoacidosis, narrow-angle glaucoma, urinary retention, and in patients unusually responsive to sympathomimetic amines. Monitor for signs and symptoms of acute narrow-angle glaucoma and urinary retention (especially in those with prostatic hyperplasia or bladder-neck obstruction). May produce significant hypokalemia or transient hyperglycemia.

ADVERSE REACTIONS

Pharyngitis, diarrhea, pain in extremity, sinusitis, lower respiratory tract infection, constipation, muscle spasms, neck pain, chest pain, productive cough, dry mouth, dyspepsia, abdominal pain, gastroesophageal reflux disease, vomiting.

DRUG INTERACTIONS

Do not use with other medicines containing LABAs. Caution with long-term ketoconazole and other strong CYP3A4 inhibitors (eg, ritonavir, clarithromycin, conivaptan); increased CV adverse effects may occur. Extreme caution with MAOIs, TCAs, or drugs known to prolong the QTc interval or within 2 weeks of discontinuation of such agents; effect on CV system may be potentiated. β-blockers may block pulmonary effects and produce severe bronchospasm in patients with COPD; if such therapy is needed, consider cardioselective β-blockers and use with caution. Caution is advised when coadministered with non-K^+-sparing diuretics (eg, loop, thiazide). Avoid with other anticholinergics; may increase anticholinergic adverse effects.

NURSING CONSIDERATIONS

Assessment: Assess for hypersensitivity to milk proteins, COPD status, CV/convulsive disorders, thyrotoxicosis, DM, ketoacidosis, narrow-angle glaucoma, urinary retention, prostatic hyperplasia, bladder-neck obstruction, pregnancy/nursing status, and possible drug interactions.

Monitoring: Monitor for deteriorating disease, paradoxical bronchospasm, hypersensitivity reactions, CV effects, narrow-angle glaucoma, urinary retention, hypokalemia, hyperglycemia, and other adverse reactions.

Patient Counseling: Inform that drug is not for treatment of asthma or to relieve acute symptoms of COPD. Advise that acute symptoms should be treated with a rescue inhaler (eg, albuterol). Instruct to seek medical attention immediately if experiencing worsening of symptoms, or a need for more inhalations than usual of the rescue inhaler. Advise not to d/c therapy without physician guidance and not to use an additional LABA. Instruct to d/c therapy if paradoxical bronchospasm occurs. Inform about adverse effects (eg, palpitations, chest pain, rapid HR, tremor, nervousness) and other risks (eg, narrow-angle glaucoma, urinary retention) associated with therapy; instruct to consult physician immediately if any signs/symptoms develop. Advise to contact physician if pregnancy occurs while on therapy. Inform that the inhaler is not reusable and advise not to take the inhaler apart.

Storage: 20-25°C (68-77°F); excursions permitted from 15-30°C (59-86°F). Store in a dry place away from direct heat or sunlight. Store inside the unopened moisture-protective foil tray and only remove from the tray immediately before initial use. Discard 6 weeks after opening the foil tray or when the counter reads "0" (after all blisters have been used), whichever comes 1st.

ANTARA – fenofibrate **RX**

Class: Fibric acid derivative

ADULT DOSAGE

Primary Hypercholesterolemia/Mixed Dyslipidemia

Initial/Max: 90mg/day
Titrate: May consider dose reduction if lipid levels fall significantly below the targeted range

D/C if no adequate response after 2 months of therapy with max dose

Severe Hypertriglyceridemia

Initial: 30-90mg/day
Titrate: Adjust dose if necessary following repeat lipid determinations at 4- to 8-week intervals; may consider dose reduction if lipid levels fall significantly below the targeted range
Max: 90mg/day

D/C if no adequate response after 2 months of therapy with max dose

PEDIATRIC DOSAGE

Pediatric use may not have been established

DOSE MODIFICATION
Renal Impairment
Mild to Moderate:
Initial: 30mg/day
Titrate: Increase only after evaluation of effects on renal function and lipid levels

ADMINISTRATION
Oral route

May be taken without regard to meals
Swallow cap whole; do not open, crush, dissolve, or chew

HOW SUPPLIED
Cap: 30mg, 90mg

CONTRAINDICATIONS
Severe renal impairment (including dialysis), active liver disease (including primary biliary cirrhosis and unexplained persistent liver function abnormalities), preexisting gallbladder disease, and nursing mothers.

WARNINGS/PRECAUTIONS
Not shown to reduce coronary heart disease morbidity and mortality in patients with type 2 diabetes mellitus (DM). Increased risk of myopathy and rhabdomyolysis; risk increased with diabetes, renal failure, hypothyroidism, and in elderly. D/C therapy if markedly elevated CPK levels occur or myopathy/myositis is suspected or diagnosed. Increases in serum transaminases, hepatocellular, chronic active and cholestatic hepatitis, and cirrhosis (extremely rare) reported; perform baseline and regular monitoring of LFTs, and d/c therapy if enzyme levels persist >3X the normal limit. Elevations in SrCr reported; monitor renal function in patients with renal impairment or at risk for renal insufficiency. May cause cholelithiasis; d/c if gallstones are found. Acute hypersensitivity reactions and pancreatitis reported. Mild to moderate decreases in Hgb, Hct, and WBCs, thrombocytopenia, and agranulocytosis reported; periodically monitor RBC and WBC counts during the first 12 months of therapy. May cause venothromboembolic disease (eg, pulmonary embolism [PE], deep vein thrombosis [DVT]). Severe decreases in HDL levels reported; check HDL levels within the 1st few months after initiation of therapy. If a severely depressed HDL level is detected, withdraw therapy, monitor HDL level until it has returned to baseline, and do not reinitiate therapy. Estrogen therapy, thiazide diuretics, and β-blockers may be associated with massive rises in plasma TG levels; discontinuation of the specific etiologic agent may obviate the need for specific drug therapy of hypertriglyceridemia.

ADVERSE REACTIONS
Abdominal pain, back pain, headache, abnormal LFTs, respiratory disorder, increased AST/ALT/CPK.

DRUG INTERACTIONS
May potentiate coumarin anticoagulant effects; use with caution, reduce anticoagulant dose, and monitor PT/INR frequently. Increased risk of rhabdomyolysis with HMG-CoA reductase inhibitors

(statins); avoid combination unless benefits outweigh risks. Bile acid-binding resins may bind other drugs given concurrently; take at least 1 hr before or 4-6 hrs after the bile acid-binding resin. Immunosuppressants (eg, cyclosporine, tacrolimus) may produce nephrotoxicity; consider benefits and risks of use with immunosuppressants and other potentially nephrotoxic agents, and use lowest effective dose. Cases of myopathy, including rhabdomyolysis, reported when coadministered with colchicine; caution when prescribing with colchicine.

NURSING CONSIDERATIONS

Assessment: Assess for hypersensitivity to the drug, renal impairment, active liver disease, preexisting gallbladder disease, other medical conditions (eg, DM, hypothyroidism), pregnancy/nursing status, and for possible drug interactions. Obtain baseline LFTs.

Monitoring: Monitor for cholelithiasis, pancreatitis, hypersensitivity reactions, PE, and DVT. Monitor renal function, LFTs, CBC, and lipid levels. Monitor for signs/symptoms of myositis, myopathy, or rhabdomyolysis; measure CPK levels in patients reporting such symptoms. Monitor PT/INR frequently with coumarin anticoagulants.

Patient Counseling: Advise of potential risks and benefits of therapy and medications to avoid during treatment. Instruct to continue to follow appropriate lipid-modifying diet during therapy and to take drug ud. Instruct to inform physician of all medications, supplements, and herbal preparations being taken; any changes in medical condition; development of muscle pain, tenderness, or weakness; onset of abdominal pain; or any other new symptoms. Advise to return to the physician's office for routine monitoring.

Storage: 25°C (77°F); excursions permitted to 15-30°C (59-86°F).

ANZEMET — dolasetron mesylate **RX**

Class: 5-HT_3 receptor antagonist

ADULT DOSAGE

Postoperative Nausea/Vomiting

Inj:

Prevention/Treatment:

12.5mg IV as a single dose approx 15 min before cessation of anesthesia (prevention) or as soon as N/V presents (treatment)

Chemotherapy-Associated Nausea/Vomiting

Tab:

Prevention of N/V Associated w/ Moderately Emetogenic Cancer Chemotherapy, Including Initial and Repeat Courses:

Usual: 100mg w/in 1 hr before chemotherapy

PEDIATRIC DOSAGE

Postoperative Nausea/Vomiting

Inj:

2-16 Years:

Prevention/Treatment:

0.35mg/kg IV as a single dose approx 15 min before cessation of anesthesia or as soon as N/V presents

Max Dose: 12.5mg

Oral Administration of the IV Product:

May mix inj sol into apple or apple-grape juice for oral dosing

Usual: 1.2mg/kg up to a max 100mg dose given w/in 2 hrs before surgery

Chemotherapy-Associated Nausea/Vomiting

Tab:

2-16 Years:

Prevention of N/V Associated w/ Moderately Emetogenic Cancer Chemotherapy, Including Initial and Repeat Courses:

Usual: 1.8mg/kg w/in 1 hr before chemotherapy

Max: 100mg

In children for whom the 100mg tab is not appropriate based on weight or ability to swallow tabs, dolasetron inj sol may be mixed into apple or apple-grape juice for oral dosing

DOSE MODIFICATION

Elderly

Inj:

Start at lower end of dosing range

ADMINISTRATION

IV/oral route

Inj

Administration:

May be safely infused IV as rapidly as 30 sec or diluted in a compatible IV sol to 50mL and infused over a period of up to 15 min

Do not mix w/ other drugs
Flush infusion line before and after administration

Stability:
After dilution, inj is stable under normal lighting conditions at room temperature for 24 hrs or under refrigeration for 48 hrs w/ the following compatible IV fluids:
0.9% NaCl inj
D5 inj
D5 and 0.45% NaCl inj
D5 and lactated Ringer's inj
Lactated Ringer's inj
10% mannitol inj

Oral Administration of the IV Product:
Diluted product may be kept up to 2 hrs at room temperature before use

HOW SUPPLIED

Inj: 20mg/mL [0.625mL, 5mL, 25mL]; Tab: 50mg, 100mg

CONTRAINDICATIONS

(Inj) Prevention of N/V associated with initial and repeat courses of emetogenic cancer chemotherapy in adults and pediatric patients due to dose-dependent QT prolongation.

WARNINGS/PRECAUTIONS

May prolong QT interval; avoid in patients with congenital long QT syndrome, hypokalemia, or hypomagnesemia. Correct hypokalemia and hypomagnesemia prior to administration and monitor these electrolytes after administration. Monitor ECG in patients with CHF, bradycardia, or renal impairment, and in elderly. May cause dose dependent prolongation of the PR and QRS interval and reports of 2nd- or 3rd-degree atrioventricular block, cardiac arrest, and serious ventricular arrhythmias including fatalities. Use caution in patients with underlying structural heart disease and preexisting conduction system abnormalities, sick sinus syndrome, atrial fibrillation with slow ventricular response, or myocardial ischemia; monitor ECG in these patients. Avoid in patients with or at risk for complete heart block, unless implanted pacemaker is present. Serotonin syndrome reported; d/c and initiate supportive treatment if symptoms occur. (Inj) When prophylaxis has failed, a repeat dose should not be initiated as rescue therapy.

ADVERSE REACTIONS

Headache, dizziness. (Tab) fatigue, diarrhea, bradycardia, pain, tachycardia, dyspepsia.

DRUG INTERACTIONS

Caution with drugs that prolong QT interval, PR interval (eg, verapamil), and QRS interval (eg, flecainide, quinidine), diuretics with potential for inducing electrolyte abnormalities, antiarrhythmics, cumulative high-dose anthracycline therapy, and/or drugs that cause hypokalemia or hypomagnesemia. May cause serotonin syndrome with other serotonergic drugs (eg, SSRIs, SNRIs, MAOIs, mirtazapine, fentanyl). (Inj) Atenolol may decrease clearance. (PO) Cimetidine may increase levels. Rifampin may decrease levels.

NURSING CONSIDERATIONS

Assessment: Assess for presence or possibility of cardiac conduction interval prolongation, renal impairment, pregnancy/nursing status, possible drug interactions, and other conditions where treatment is cautioned or contraindicated. Correct hypokalemia and hypomagnesemia prior to administration.

Monitoring: Monitor for QT/PT/QRS interval prolongation, torsades de pointes, serotonin syndrome, and other adverse reactions. Monitor ECG in patients with CHF, bradycardia, renal impairment, and those at risk for cardiac conduction interval prolongation. Monitor serum electrolytes (K^+, Mg^{2+}).

Patient Counseling: Inform about potential benefits/risks of therapy. Inform that drug may cause serious cardiac arrhythmias; instruct patients to contact physician immediately if they perceive a change in their HR, if they feel lightheaded, or have a syncopal episode. Inform that chances of developing severe cardiac arrhythmias are higher in patients with a personal/family history of abnormal heart rhythms; personal history of sick sinus syndrome; atrial fibrillation with slow ventricular response or myocardial ischemia; patients taking medications that may prolong PR interval, QRS interval, or that may cause electrolyte abnormalities; patients with hypokalemia or hypomagnesemia, and in elderly patients. Advise of the possibility of serotonin syndrome with concomitant use with another serotonergic agent such as medications to treat depression and migraines; instruct to seek immediate medical attention if changes in mental status, autonomic instability, and neuromuscular symptoms with or without GI symptoms occur.

Storage: (Inj) 20-25°C (68-77°F) with excursions permitted to 15-30°C (59-86°F). Protect from light. Diluted IV Sol: Room temperature for 24 hrs or under refrigeration for 48 hrs. Diluted Sol with Apple or Apple-grape Juice: Room temperature for up to 2 hrs before use. Refer to PI for further information on stability. (Tab) 20-25°C (68-77°F). Protect from light.

APIDRA – insulin glulisine (rDNA origin) RX

Class: Insulin

OTHER BRAND NAMES
Apidra Solostar

ADULT DOSAGE
Diabetes Mellitus
Total Daily Insulin Requirement:
Usual: 0.5-1 U/kg/day; give SQ w/in 15 min ac or w/in 20 min after starting a meal
IV:
Use at concentrations of 0.05-1 U/mL in infusion systems using polyvinyl chloride bags

PEDIATRIC DOSAGE
Type 1 Diabetes Mellitus
≥4 Years:
Total Daily Insulin Requirement:
Usual: 0.5-1 U/kg/day; give SQ w/in 15 min ac or w/in 20 min after starting a meal

DOSE MODIFICATION
Renal Impairment
May require dose reduction
Hepatic Impairment
May require dose reduction

ADMINISTRATION
SQ/IV route
SQ
Inject SQ in the abdominal wall, thigh, or upper arm; rotate inj sites w/in the same region
Use w/ an intermediate or long-acting insulin
Do not mix w/ insulin preparations other than NPH insulin; if mixed w/ NPH insulin, draw Apidra into syringe 1st, and inject mixture immediately after mixing
Continuous SQ Insulin Infusion by External Pump
Read the pump label to make sure the pump has been evaluated w/ Apidra
Administer by continuous SQ infusion in the abdominal wall by an external insulin pump; rotate infusion sites w/in the same region
Must have an alternative insulin delivery system in case of pump system failure
Do not mix w/ other insulins
IV
Do not mix w/ other insulins
Stable only in 0.9% NaCl

HOW SUPPLIED
Inj: 100 U/mL [3mL, SoloStar; 10mL, vial]

CONTRAINDICATIONS
During episodes of hypoglycemia.

WARNINGS/PRECAUTIONS
Insulin pens must never be shared between patients; poses a risk for transmission of blood-borne pathogens. Any change in insulin regimen should be made cautiously and only under medical supervision. Changes in insulin strength, manufacturer, type, or method of administration may result in the need for a change in dosage or adjustment in concomitant oral antidiabetic treatment. Insulin requirements may be altered during stress, major illness, or w/ changes in exercise, meal patterns, or coadministered drugs. Hypoglycemia may occur and may impair ability to concentrate and react; caution in patients w/ hypoglycemia unawareness and in those predisposed to hypoglycemia. Severe, life-threatening, generalized allergy, including anaphylaxis, may occur. Hypokalemia may occur; caution in patients who may be at risk. May be administered IV under medical supervision w/ close monitoring of glucose and K^+ levels to avoid potentially fatal hypoglycemia and hypokalemia. Malfunction of insulin pump or infusion set, handling errors, or insulin degradation can rapidly lead to hyperglycemia, ketosis, and diabetic ketoacidosis; prompt identification/correction of the cause is necessary and interim SQ inj may be required. Train patients using CSII pump therapy how to administer by inj and have alternate insulin therapy available. Caution in elderly.

ADVERSE REACTIONS
Allergic reactions, infusion-site reactions, hypoglycemia, influenza, nasopharyngitis, URTI, arthralgia, HTN, headache, peripheral edema.

DRUG INTERACTIONS
Dose adjustment and close monitoring may be necessary w/ drugs that may increase blood-glucose-lowering effect and susceptibility to hypoglycemia (eg, oral antidiabetic products, pramlintide, ACE inhibitors), drugs that may reduce blood-glucose-lowering effect (eg, corticosteroids, danazol, niacin), or drugs that may either increase or decrease

blood-glucose-lowering effect (eg, β-blockers, clonidine, lithium salts, alcohol). Pentamidine may cause hypoglycemia, sometimes followed by hyperglycemia. Hypoglycemic signs may be reduced or absent w/ antiadrenergic drugs (eg, β-blockers, clonidine, guanethidine, reserpine). Caution w/ K^+-lowering drugs and drugs sensitive to serum K^+ levels. Concomitant use w/ thiazolidinediones (TZDs) may cause dose-related fluid retention and heart failure (HF); observe for signs/symptoms of HF and consider dose reduction or discontinuation of TZDs if HF occurs.

NURSING CONSIDERATIONS

Assessment: Assess for predisposition to hypoglycemia, risk of hypokalemia, hypersensitivity to drug or to any of its excipients, renal/hepatic impairment, pregnancy/nursing status, and possible drug interactions. Obtain baseline blood glucose and HbA1c levels.

Monitoring: Monitor for signs/symptoms of hypoglycemia, hypokalemia, allergic reactions, and other adverse reactions. Monitor blood glucose, HbA1c levels, and renal/hepatic function. Frequent glucose monitoring may be required w/ renal/hepatic impairment. Monitor glucose and K^+ levels frequently during IV administration.

Patient Counseling: Advise never to share insulin pen w/ another person, even if needle is changed. Counsel on self-management procedures including glucose monitoring, proper inj technique, and management of hypo/hyperglycemia. Instruct on handling of special situations (eg, intercurrent conditions, inadequate or skipped dose, inadvertent administration of increased dose, inadequate food intake, skipped meals). Advise to inform physician if pregnant or contemplating pregnancy. Instruct to always check the label before each inj to avoid medication errors. Instruct on how to use an external infusion pump.

Storage: Unopened: 2-8°C (36-46°F). Do not freeze; discard if frozen. Protect from light. Must be used within 28 days if not stored in a refrigerator. Open (In-Use): <25°C (77°F). Discard after 28 days. Protect from direct heat and light. Do not refrigerate opened (in-use) SoloStar. Discard infusion sets and insulin in reservoir after 48 hrs of use or after exposure to temperatures >37°C (98.6°F). Prepared Infusion Bags: Room temperature for 48 hrs.

APLENZIN — bupropion hydrobromide — RX

Class: Aminoketone

Antidepressants increased the risk of suicidal thinking and behavior (suicidality) in children, adolescents, and young adults in short-term studies of major depressive disorder (MDD) and other psychiatric disorders. Monitor and observe closely for clinical worsening, suicidality, or unusual changes in behavior. Serious neuropsychiatric reactions reported in patients taking bupropion for smoking cessation; not approved for smoking cessation.

ADULT DOSAGE

Major Depressive Disorder

Initial: 174mg qam
Titrate: After 4 days, may increase to target dose of 348mg qam

Periodically reassess need for maint treatment

Seasonal Affective Disorder

Initial: 174mg qam
Titrate: After 7 days, may increase to target dose of 348mg qam

Prevention of Seasonal Major Depressive Episodes in Patients w/ Seasonal Affective Disorder:
Initiate in the autumn, prior to the onset of depressive symptoms. Continue through the winter season; taper and d/c in early spring
Treated w/ 348mg/day: Decrease to 150mg qd before discontinuing

Individualize timing of initiation and treatment duration

Conversions

Equivalent Daily Doses of Bupropion HBr and Bupropion HCl:
522mg: 450mg bupropion HCl
348mg: 300mg bupropion HCl
174mg: 150mg bupropion HCl

PEDIATRIC DOSAGE

Pediatric use may not have been established

DOSE MODIFICATION

Renal Impairment

Consider reducing dose and/or frequency

Hepatic Impairment

Mild to Moderate:

Consider reducing dose and/or frequency

Severe:

Initial/Max: 174mg qod

Discontinuation

Treated w/ 348mg qd: Decrease to 174mg qd prior to discontinuation

ADMINISTRATION

Oral route

Swallow whole; do not crush, divide, or chew
Administer in the am
May be taken w/ or w/o regard to meals

HOW SUPPLIED

Tab, Extended-Release: 174mg, 348mg, 522mg

CONTRAINDICATIONS

Seizure disorder or conditions that increase the risk of seizure (eg, arteriovenous malformation, severe head injury, CNS tumor/infection, severe stroke, anorexia nervosa/bulimia, or abrupt discontinuation of alcohol, benzodiazepines, barbiturates, antiepileptic drugs). Concurrent use of MAOIs or initiation of treatment within 14 days of discontinuation of an MAOI.

WARNINGS/PRECAUTIONS

Dose-related risk of seizures; do not exceed 522mg qd and gradually increase dose. D/C and do not restart treatment if seizure occurs. May result in elevated BP and HTN. May precipitate a manic, mixed, or hypomanic manic episode; risk appears to be increased in patients with bipolar disorder or who have risk factors for bipolar disorder. Neuropsychiatric signs and symptoms (eg, delusions, hallucinations, psychosis, concentration disturbance, paranoia, confusion) reported; d/c if these reactions occur. Pupillary dilation that occurs following use may trigger an angle-closure attack in a patient with anatomically narrow angles who does not have a patent iridectomy. D/C treatment if anaphylactoid/anaphylactic reactions occur. Arthralgia, myalgia, fever with rash, and other symptoms of serum sickness suggestive of delayed hypersensitivity reported. Caution with renal/hepatic impairment and in elderly. False (+) urine immunoassay screening tests for amphetamines reported.

ADVERSE REACTIONS

Dry mouth, sweating, headache/migraine, insomnia, anxiety, agitation, weight loss, N/V, constipation, dizziness, pharyngitis, tinnitus, rash.

DRUG INTERACTIONS

See Contraindications. CYP2B6 inhibitors (eg, ticlopidine, clopidogrel) may increase exposure; may need to reduce bupropion dose. CYP2B6 inducers (eg, ritonavir, lopinavir, efavirenz) may decrease exposure; may need to increase bupropion dose. Other CYP inducers (eg, carbamazepine, phenobarbital, phenytoin) may decrease exposure; may need to increase bupropion dose. May increase exposure of CYP2D6 substrates (eg, antidepressants, antipsychotics, β-blockers, type 1C antiarrhythmics [eg, propafenone, flecainide]); may need to decrease the dose of CYP2D6 substrates, particularly for drugs with a narrow therapeutic index. May reduce efficacy of drugs that require metabolic activation by CYP2D6 to be effective (eg, tamoxifen); may require increase doses of the drug. Extreme caution with drugs that lower seizure threshold (eg, other bupropion products, antipsychotics, antidepressants, theophylline, systemic corticosteroids); use low initial doses and increase the dose gradually. Increased risk of seizure with use of illicit drugs (eg, cocaine), abuse or misuse of prescription drugs (eg, CNS stimulants), oral hypoglycemic drugs or insulin, use of anorectic drugs, excessive use of alcohol, benzodiazepines, sedative/hypnotics, or opiates. CNS toxicity reported when coadministered with levodopa or amantadine; use with caution. Altered PT and/or INR, associated with hemorrhagic or thrombotic complication, reported with warfarin.

NURSING CONSIDERATIONS

Assessment: Assess for seizure disorders or conditions that may increase risk of seizure, susceptibility to angle-closure glaucoma, hypersensitivity to the drug, bipolar disorder, hepatic/renal impairment, any other conditions where treatment is contraindicated or cautioned, pregnancy/nursing status, and possible drug interactions. Obtain baseline BP.

Monitoring: Monitor for clinical worsening, suicidality, or unusual changes in behavior, seizures, neuropsychiatric signs/symptoms, angle-closure glaucoma, anaphylactoid/anaphylactic reactions, delayed hypersensitivity reactions, HTN, activation of mania or hypomania, and other adverse reactions. Monitor hepatic/renal function and BP.

Patient Counseling: Inform about benefits/risks of therapy. Advise patients and caregivers of need for close observation for clinical worsening and suicidal risks. Educate on the symptoms of hypersensitivity and to d/c if a severe allergic reaction occurs. Instruct to d/c and not restart if a seizure occurs while on therapy. Inform that excessive use or abrupt discontinuation of alcohol or sedatives may alter seizure threshold; advise to minimize or avoid alcohol use. Caution about risk of angle-closure glaucoma. Inform that therapy may impair mental/physical abilities; advise to use caution while operating hazardous machinery/driving. Instruct to notify physician if taking/planning to take any prescription or OTC medications. Advise to contact physician if become/intend to be pregnant during therapy. Inform that it is normal to notice something that looks like a tab in the stool.

Storage: 25°C (77°F); excursions permitted to 15-30°C (59-86°F).

APOKYN – apomorphine hydrochloride

RX

Class: Non-ergoline dopamine agonist

ADULT DOSAGE

Parkinson's Disease

Acute, Intermittent Treatment of Hypomobility, "Off" Episodes ("End-of-Dose Wearing Off" and Unpredictable "On/Off" Episodes) in Patients w/ Advanced Parkinson's Disease:

Initial Test Dose:
0.2mL (2mg); begin dosing when patients are in an "off" state
Check both supine and standing BP and pulse pre-dose and at 20, 40, and 60 min post-dose (and after 60 min, if there is significant hypotension at 60 min)
If significant orthostatic hypotension develops in response to test dose, do not consider patients candidates for treatment
If Initial Test Dose Tolerated:
Initial: 0.2mL (2mg) prn to treat recurring "off" episodes
Titrate: Increase in increments of 0.1mL (1mg) every few days, if needed, on an outpatient basis
Subsequent Dosing:
Determine that patient needs and tolerates a higher test dose (0.3mL [3mg] or 0.4mL [4mg]), under close medical supervision; outpatient dosing trial may follow using a 0.1mL (1mg) dose lower than the tolerated test dose
If Patient Tolerates 0.2mL (2mg) Test Dose but Responds Inadequately:
May administer 0.4mL (4mg) at the next observed "off" period (at least 2 hrs after initial test dose)
If Patient Tolerates and Responds to 0.4mL (4mg) Test Dose:
Initial Maint: 0.3mL (3mg) prn to treat recurring "off" episodes
Titrate: May increase in 0.1mL (1mg) increments every few days, if needed, on an outpatient basis
If Patient Does Not Tolerate 0.4mL (4mg) Test Dose:
May administer 0.3mL (3mg) during a separate "off" period (at least 2 hrs after the previous dose)
If Patient Tolerates 0.3mL (3mg) Test Dose:
Initial Maint: 0.2mL (2mg) prn to treat existing "off" episodes
Titrate: May increase to 0.3mL (3mg) after a few days, if needed and the 0.2mL (2mg) dose is tolerated; do not increase to 0.4mL (4mg) on an outpatient basis in such patients

PEDIATRIC DOSAGE

Pediatric use may not have been established

Max Dose: 0.6mL (6mg)

Premedication and Concomitant Medication:
Initiate therapy w/ a concomitant antiemetic; oral trimethobenzamide (300mg tid) should be started 3 days prior to initial dose and continued at least during the first 2 months of therapy

Re-treatment and Interruption in Therapy:
If a single dose of therapy is ineffective for a particular "off" period, do not give a 2nd dose for that "off" episode
Do not administer a repeat dose sooner than 2 hrs after last dose
If therapy is interrupted for >1 week, restart on 0.2mL (2mg) dose and gradually titrate to effect and tolerability

DOSE MODIFICATION

Renal Impairment

Mild/Moderate: Reduce test dose and starting dose to 0.1mL (1mg)

ADMINISTRATION

SQ route

Administer only by a multiple-dose pen w/ supplied cartridges
Initial dose and dose titrations should be performed by a healthcare provider
Rotate inj site

HOW SUPPLIED

Inj: 10mg/mL [3mL]

CONTRAINDICATIONS

Concomitant use with $5HT_3$ antagonists, including antiemetics (eg, ondansetron, granisetron, dolasetron, palonosetron) and alosetron.

WARNINGS/PRECAUTIONS

Serious adverse reactions (eg, thrombus formation, pulmonary embolism) following IV use reported; not for IV administration. N/V, syncope, orthostatic hypotension, and falling reported. Falling asleep during activities of daily living may occur; d/c if daytime sleepiness or episodes of falling asleep develop. May impair mental/physical abilities. Hallucinations/psychotic-like behavior reported; avoid with major psychotic disorder. May cause or worsen dyskinesias. May cause intense urges to gamble, increased sexual urges, intense urges to spend money uncontrollably, and other intense urges and the inability to control these urges while on therapy; consider dose reduction or discontinuation of therapy. Coronary events (eg, angina, myocardial infarction [MI], cardiac arrest, sudden death) reported; caution with known cardiovascular (CV)/cerebrovascular disease. May prolong the QT interval and increase potential for proarrhythmic effects; caution with hypokalemia, hypomagnesemia, bradycardia, or genetic predisposition (eg, congenital prolongation of the QT interval). Monitor for withdrawal-emergent hyperpyrexia and confusion, fibrotic complications (eg, retroperitoneal fibrosis, pulmonary infiltrates, pleural effusion/thickening, cardiac valvulopathy), and melanoma. May cause priapism. Patients with sulfite sensitivity (eg, sodium bisulfite) may experience various allergic-type reactions. Potential for abuse. Caution with hepatic/renal impairment.

ADVERSE REACTIONS

Yawning, dyskinesia, N/V, somnolence, dizziness, rhinorrhea, hallucinations, edema, chest pain, inj-site reaction, fall, arthralgia, insomnia, headache, depression.

DRUG INTERACTIONS

See Contraindications. Antihypertensives and vasodilators may increase risk of hypotension, MI, serious pneumonia, serious falls, and bone and joint injuries. Dopamine antagonists, such as neuroleptics (eg, phenothiazines, butyrophenones, thioxanthenes) or metoclopramide, may diminish effectiveness. Caution with drugs that prolong QT/QTc interval. May increase drowsiness with sedating medications. Avoid with alcohol.

NURSING CONSIDERATIONS

Assessment: Assess for hypersensitivity to the drug, sulfite sensitivity, asthma, risk for QT prolongation, history of psychotic disorders, CV/cerebrovascular disease, dyskinesia, hepatic/renal impairment, pregnancy/nursing status, and possible drug interactions. Obtain baseline BP (supine and standing position).

Monitoring: Monitor for N/V, syncope, QT/QTc interval prolongation and other proarrhythmic effects, hypotension, hallucinations/psychotic-like behavior, coronary/cerebral ischemia, dyskinesia (or exacerbation), impulse control/compulsive behaviors, hepatic/renal impairment, withdrawal-emergent hyperpyrexia and confusion, fibrotic complications, priapism, and other adverse reactions. Perform periodic skin exams to monitor for melanomas. Monitor BP closely.

Patient Counseling: Instruct to use only as prescribed. Instruct to rotate the inj site and observe proper aseptic technique. Inform of the potential risks and benefits of therapy. Inform that hypersensitivity/allergic reaction may occur; advise patients to avoid taking the drug again if a reaction occurs. Advise not to drive a car or engage in any other potentially dangerous activities while on treatment. Advise to limit alcohol intake. Alert patients that they may have increased risk for falling when using the drug. Inform of the potential for hallucinations, psychotic-like behavior, hypotension, sedating effects including somnolence, and the possibility of falling asleep, coronary events, dyskinesias, and other adverse events. Instruct to rise slowly after sitting or lying down after taking the drug. Advise to inform physician if new or increased gambling urges, increased sexual urges, or other intense urges develop while on treatment. Instruct to notify physician if pregnancy occurs, or if intending to become pregnant and/or breastfeed.

Storage: 25°C (77°F); excursions permitted to 15-30°C (59-86°F).

APRISO – mesalamine RX

Class: 5-aminosalicylic acid derivative

ADULT DOSAGE

Ulcerative Colitis

Maintenance of Remission:
1.5g (4 caps) qam

PEDIATRIC DOSAGE

Pediatric use may not have been established

ADMINISTRATION

Oral route

HOW SUPPLIED

Cap, Extended Release: 0.375g

WARNINGS/PRECAUTIONS

Renal impairment, including minimal change nephropathy, acute and chronic interstitial nephritis, and, rarely, renal failure reported; caution with renal dysfunction or history of renal disease. Evaluate renal function prior to therapy and periodically thereafter. May cause acute intolerance syndrome (eg, acute abdominal pain, cramping, bloody diarrhea); d/c if suspected. Hepatic failure reported in patients with preexisting liver disease; caution with liver disease. Caution with sulfasalazine hypersensitivity and in elderly.

ADVERSE REACTIONS

Headache, diarrhea, upper abdominal pain, nausea, nasopharyngitis, influenza/influenza-like illness, sinusitis.

DRUG INTERACTIONS

Avoid with antacids.

NURSING CONSIDERATIONS

Assessment: Assess for previous hypersensitivity to sulfasalazine or salicylates, history of or known renal/hepatic dysfunction, phenylketonuria, pregnancy/nursing status, and possible drug interactions. Evaluate renal function prior to initiation of therapy.

Monitoring: Monitor for renal impairment, hepatic failure, acute intolerance syndrome, and hypersensitivity reactions. Perform periodic monitoring of renal function and blood cell counts (in elderly).

Patient Counseling: Inform patients with phenylketonuria that each cap contains aspartame. Instruct not to take with antacids. Instruct to contact a healthcare provider if symptoms of ulcerative colitis worsen.

Storage: 20-25°C (68-77°F); excursions permitted between 15-30°C (59-86°F).

APTIOM – eslicarbazepine acetate RX

Class: Dibenzazepine

ADULT DOSAGE

Partial Onset Seizures

Adjunctive Treatment:
Initial: 400mg qd; may initiate at 800mg qd if need for additional seizure reduction outweighs increased risk of adverse reactions during initiation

PEDIATRIC DOSAGE

Pediatric use may not have been established

Titrate: Increase to recommended maint dose of 800mg qd after 1 week
Max: 1200mg qd; initiate only after patient has tolerated 800mg/day for at least a week

DOSE MODIFICATION

Concomitant Medications
Oxcarbazepine: Do not coadminister
Carbamazepine: Dose of eslicarbazepine or carbamazepine may need to be adjusted
Other Enzyme-Inducing Antiepileptic Drugs: May need higher doses of eslicarbazepine

Renal Impairment
Moderate and Severe (CrCl <50mL/min):
Initial: 200mg qd
Titrate: Increase to recommended maint dose of 400mg qd after 2 weeks
Max: 600mg qd

Hepatic Impairment
Severe: Not recommended for use

Discontinuation
Reduce dose gradually and avoid abrupt discontinuation

ADMINISTRATION

Oral route

Administer as whole or crushed tabs
Take w/ or w/o food

HOW SUPPLIED

Tab: 200mg*, 400mg, 600mg*, 800mg* *scored

WARNINGS/PRECAUTIONS

Increased risk of suicidal thoughts or behavior; monitor for emergence/worsening of depression, suicidal thoughts or behavior, and/or any unusual changes in mood or behavior. Serious dermatological reactions (eg, Stevens-Johnson syndrome) reported; d/c use if dermatologic reaction develops, unless the reaction is not drug-related. Drug reaction with eosinophilia and systemic symptoms (DRESS), also known as multiorgan hypersensitivity, reported; evaluate immediately if signs/symptoms of hypersensitivity (eg, fever, lymphadenopathy) are present and d/c if alternative etiology cannot be established. Anaphylaxis and angioedema reported; d/c if any of these reactions develop. Avoid in patients with prior DRESS reaction or anaphylactic-type reaction with either the drug or oxcarbazepine. Consider measuring serum Na^+ and Cl^- levels during maintenance treatment; clinically significant hyponatremia with concurrent hypochloremia may develop, requiring dose reduction/discontinuation. Associated with dose-related increases in adverse reactions related to dizziness and disturbance in gait and coordination, somnolence and fatigue, cognitive dysfunction, and visual changes. May impair mental/physical abilities. Withdraw gradually due to risk of increased seizure frequency and status epilepticus. Hepatic effects reported; d/c in patients with jaundice or other evidence of significant liver injury. Dose-dependent decreases in serum T3 and T4 (free and total) observed. Not recommended with severe hepatic impairment. Caution in elderly.

ADVERSE REACTIONS

Dizziness, somnolence, N/V, headache, diplopia, fatigue, vertigo, ataxia, blurred vision, tremor, diarrhea.

DRUG INTERACTIONS

See Dosage. Greater incidence of dizziness reported with the concomitant use of carbamazepine. Do not use as an adjunctive therapy with oxcarbazepine. Several antiepileptic drugs (eg, carbamazepine, phenobarbital, phenytoin, primidone) can induce enzymes that metabolize eslicarbazepine and can cause decreased plasma concentrations. May increase levels of CYP2C19 substrates (eg, phenytoin, clobazam, omeprazole). Monitor plasma phenytoin concentration; in epilepsy, dose adjustment may be needed based on clinical response and serum levels of phenytoin. May decrease levels of CYP3A4 substrates (eg, simvastatin). Adjust dose of simvastatin or rosuvastatin if a clinically significant change in lipids is noted. May decrease levels of oral contraceptives (eg, ethinyl estradiol, levonorgestrel); use additional or alternative nonhormonal birth control. Monitor to maintain INR in patients on warfarin.

NURSING CONSIDERATIONS

Assessment: Assess for history of hypersensitivity to the drug or oxcarbazepine, renal/hepatic impairment, pregnancy/nursing status, and possible drug interactions.

Monitoring: Monitor for suicidal thoughts or behavior, any unusual changes in mood or behavior, dermatologic reactions, multiorgan hypersensitivity reaction, hyponatremia, anaphylaxis, angioedema, dizziness, disturbance in gait and coordination, somnolence, fatigue, cognitive dysfunction, visual changes, and other adverse reactions. Monitor Na^+ and Cl^- levels. Monitor to maintain INR in patients on warfarin.

Patient Counseling: Inform of the availability of a Medication Guide and instruct to read the Medication Guide prior to treatment. Instruct to take ud. Advise of the need to be alert for the emergence/worsening of symptoms of depression, any unusual changes in mood/behavior, or the emergence of suicidal thoughts, behavior, or thoughts about self-harm; instruct to immediately report behaviors of concern to physician. Educate about signs/symptoms of a skin reaction; instruct to consult physician immediately if a skin reaction occurs. Inform that a fever associated with signs of other organ system involvement may be drug-related; instruct to contact physician immediately if such signs/symptoms occur. Instruct to d/c and contact physician immediately if signs/symptoms suggesting angioedema develop. Advise to report symptoms of low Na^+ to physician. Inform that drug may cause dizziness, gait disturbance, somnolence/fatigue, cognitive function, and visual changes; advise not to drive or operate machinery until effects have been determined. Instruct not to d/c use without consulting physician. Recommend female patients of childbearing age to use additional nonhormonal forms of contraception during treatment and after treatment has been discontinued for at least 1 menstrual cycle or until otherwise instructed by physician. Encourage to enroll in the North American Antiepileptic Drug Pregnancy Registry if patient becomes pregnant.

Storage: 20-25°C (68-77°F); excursions permitted to 15-30°C (59-86°F).

Aptivus – tipranavir

RX

Class: Protease inhibitor

Both fatal and nonfatal intracranial hemorrhage (ICH) reported. Clinical hepatitis and hepatic decompensation, including some fatalities, reported. Extra vigilance is warranted in patients w/ chronic hepatitis B or hepatitis C coinfection due to an increased risk of hepatotoxicity.

ADULT DOSAGE

HIV-1 Infection

Coadministered w/ ritonavir (RTV) in treatment-experienced patients infected w/ HIV-1 strains resistant to >1 protease inhibitor

Cap:
500mg (two 250mg caps) + 200mg RTV bid

Sol:
500mg (5mL) + 200mg RTV bid

PEDIATRIC DOSAGE

HIV-1 Infection

Coadministered w/ ritonavir (RTV) in treatment-experienced patients infected w/ HIV-1 strains resistant to >1 protease inhibitor

2-18 Years:
14mg/kg + 6mg/kg RTV (or 375mg/m^2 + 150mg/m^2 RTV) bid
Max: 500mg + 200mg RTV bid

DOSE MODIFICATION

Adverse Reactions

Pediatrics:

Development of Intolerance/Toxicity: Decrease dose to 12mg/kg + 5mg/kg ritonavir (RTV) (or 290mg/m^2 + 115mg/m^2 RTV) bid

ADMINISTRATION

Oral route

Coadministered w/ Ritonavir (RTV) Caps/Sol

May be taken w/ or w/o meals

Coadministered w/ RTV Tabs

Must only be taken w/ meals

HOW SUPPLIED

Cap: 250mg; Sol: 100mg/mL [95mL]

CONTRAINDICATIONS

Moderate or severe (Child-Pugh Class B or C) hepatic impairment. Coadministration w/ drugs that are highly dependent on CYP3A for clearance or are potent CYP3A inducers (eg, amiodarone, bepridil, flecainide, propafenone, quinidine, rifampin, dihydroergotamine, ergonovine, ergotamine, methylergonovine, cisapride, St. John's wort, lovastatin, simvastatin, pimozide, oral midazolam, triazolam, alfuzosin, and sildenafil [for treatment of pulmonary arterial HTN]). Refer to the individual monograph for RTV.

WARNINGS/PRECAUTIONS

Not recommended for treatment-naive patients. Caution w/ elevated transaminases, hepatitis B or C coinfection, mild hepatic impairment (Child-Pugh Class A), supplemental high doses of vitamin E, known sulfonamide allergy, patients at risk of increased bleeding from trauma, surgery, or other medical conditions, and in elderly. D/C if signs and symptoms of clinical hepatitis develop. D/C if asymptomatic elevations in AST or ALT >10X the ULN or if asymptomatic elevations in AST or ALT between 5-10X the ULN and increases in total bilirubin >2.5X the ULN occur. Rash (eg, urticarial, maculopapular, possible photosensitivity) accompanied by joint pain/stiffness, throat tightness, or generalized pruritus reported; d/c and initiate appropriate treatment if severe skin rash develops. New onset diabetes mellitus (DM), exacerbation of preexisting DM, hyperglycemia, and diabetic ketoacidosis reported. Increased total cholesterol and TG levels reported. Immune reconstitution syndrome reported; autoimmune disorders (eg, Graves' disease, polymyositis, and Guillain-Barre syndrome) have also been reported in the setting of immune reconstitution. Redistribution/accumulation of body fat may occur. Increased bleeding in patients w/ hemophilia type A and B reported; additional factor VIII may be given. (Sol) Avoid supplemental vitamin E greater than a standard multivitamin as oral sol contains 116 IU/mL of vitamin E, which is higher than the Reference Daily Intake (adults 30 IU, pediatrics approx 10 IU). Refer to individual monograph for RTV.

ADVERSE REACTIONS

ICH, clinical hepatitis, hepatic decompensation, diarrhea, N/V, abdominal pain, pyrexia, fatigue, headache, cough, rash, anemia, weight decreased, hypertriglyceridemia, bleeding.

DRUG INTERACTIONS

See Contraindications. Not recommended w/ other protease inhibitors, boceprevir, telaprevir, salmeterol, and fluticasone. Concomitant colchicine is contraindicated in renally/hepatically impaired patients. Avoid w/ atorvastatin and etravirine. Caution w/ medications known to increase the risk of bleeding (eg, antiplatelets, anticoagulants, or high doses of vitamin E). May increase levels of rilpivirine, SSRIs (eg, fluoxetine, paroxetine, sertraline), atorvastatin, rosuvastatin, trazodone, desipramine, colchicine, bosentan, itraconazole, ketoconazole, clarithromycin, rifabutin, quetiapine, parenteral midazolam, normeperidine, and PDE-5 inhibitors. May decrease levels of etravirine, abacavir, atazanavir, didanosine, zidovudine, amprenavir, lopinavir, saquinavir, raltegravir, valproic acid, methadone, meperidine, and omeprazole. Increased levels w/ fluconazole, enfuvirtide, clarithromycin, and atazanavir. Decreased levels w/ buprenorphine/naloxone, carbamazepine, phenobarbital, and phenytoin. May alter levels of voriconazole, calcium channel blockers, and immunosuppressants. May decrease levels of ethinyl estradiol by 50%; use alternative methods of nonhormonal contraception. Monitor glucose w/ hypoglycemic agents. Monitor INR w/ warfarin. (Cap) May produce disulfiram-like reactions w/ disulfiram or other drugs that produce the reaction (eg, metronidazole). See Prescribing Information for detailed information.

NURSING CONSIDERATIONS

Assessment: Assess for hepatitis B or C infection, hepatic impairment, increased bleeding risk, hemophilia, sulfonamide allergy, DM, pregnancy/nursing status, and possible drug interactions. Assess LFTs and lipid levels. Assess the ability to swallow caps in pediatric patients.

Monitoring: Monitor for signs and symptoms of clinical hepatitis, hepatic decompensation, ICH, rash, DM, hyperglycemia, diabetic ketoacidosis, bleeding, immune reconstitution syndrome, autoimmune disorders, fat redistribution, and other adverse reactions. Monitor for LFTs and lipid levels periodically during treatment. Monitor INR w/ warfarin.

Patient Counseling: Inform of the risks and benefits of therapy. Advise to seek medical attention for symptoms of hepatitis (eg, fatigue, malaise, anorexia, nausea), any unusual/unexplained bleeding, and rash. Advise to report use of all medications, including prescription or nonprescription medications (eg, St. John's wort). Instruct to avoid vitamin E supplements greater than a standard multivitamin when taking oral sol. Instruct to report any history of sulfonamide allergy. Instruct to use additional or alternative contraceptive measures for patients taking estrogen-based hormonal contraceptives. Inform that redistribution/accumulation of body fat may occur. Instruct to take medication ud. Inform that therapy is not a cure for HIV-1 infection and that illness associated w/ HIV-1 infection may continue, including opportunistic infection; advise to remain under the care of a physician during therapy. Advise to avoid doing things that can spread HIV-1 infection to others.

Storage: Must be used w/in 60 days after 1st opening the bottle. (Cap) Prior to Opening the Bottle: 2-8°C (36-46°F). After Opening the Bottle: 25°C (77°F); excursions permitted to 15-30°C (59-86°F). (Sol) 25°C (77°F); excursions permitted to 15-30°C (59-86°F). Do not refrigerate or freeze.

ARANESP — darbepoetin alfa

RX

Class: Erythropoiesis stimulator

Increased risk of death, MI, stroke, venous thromboembolism (VTE), thrombosis of vascular access, and tumor progression or recurrence. Use the lowest dose sufficient to reduce/avoid the need for RBC transfusions. Chronic Kidney Disease (CKD): Greater risks for death, serious adverse cardiovascular (CV) reactions, and stroke when administered erythropoiesis-stimulating agents (ESAs) to target Hgb level of >11g/dL. Cancer: Shortened overall survival and/or increased risk of tumor progression or recurrence in patients w/ breast, non-small cell lung, head and neck, lymphoid, and cervical cancers. Must enroll in and comply w/ the ESA APPRISE Oncology Program to prescribe and/or dispense drug to patients. Use only for anemia from myelosuppressive chemotherapy. Not indicated for patients receiving myelosuppressive chemotherapy when anticipated outcome is cure. D/C following completion of chemotherapy course.

ADULT DOSAGE

Anemia Due to Chronic Kidney Disease

On Dialysis:
Initiate when Hgb is <10g/dL
Initial: 0.45mcg/kg IV/SQ weekly or 0.75mcg/kg IV/SQ once every 2 weeks
Titrate: Adjust dose based on Hgb levels. If Hgb approaches or exceeds 11g/dL, reduce or interrupt dose

Not on Dialysis:
Initiate when Hgb is <10g/dL, the rate of Hgb decline indicates likelihood of a RBC transfusion, and when reducing the risk of alloimmunization and/or other RBC transfusion-related risks is a goal
Initial: 0.45mcg/kg IV/SQ once every 4 weeks
Titrate: Adjust dose based on Hgb levels. If Hgb exceeds 10g/dL, reduce or interrupt dose and use lowest dose sufficient to reduce RBC transfusion

All Patients:
Titrate:
Do not increase dose more frequently than once every 4 weeks; decreases may occur more frequently
Rapid Increase in Hgb (>1g/dL in Any 2-Week Period): Reduce by ≥25% prn to reduce rapid responses
Hgb Has Not Increased by >1g/dL After 4 Weeks of Therapy: Increase by 25%
No Adequate Response Over a 12-Week Escalation Period: Further dose increase is unlikely to improve response and may increase risks. Use lowest dose to maintain Hgb level sufficient to reduce the need of RBC transfusion; d/c if responsiveness does not improve

Anemia Due to Chemotherapy

Initiate when Hgb is <10g/dL and if there is a minimum of 2 additional months of chemotherapy
Initial: 2.25mcg/kg SQ weekly or 500mcg SQ every 3 weeks until completion of chemotherapy course
Titrate:
Hgb Increases >1g/dL in Any 2-Week Period/Hgb Reaches a Level Needed to Avoid RBC Transfusion: Reduce dose by 40%
Hgb Exceeds Level Needed to Avoid RBC Transfusion: Withhold until Hgb approaches a level where RBC transfusions may be required; reinitiate at a dose 40% below previous dose
Hgb Increases by <1g/dL and Remains <10g/dL After 6 Weeks of Therapy: Increase dose to 4.5mcg/kg/week (weekly schedule) or no dose adjustment (3-week schedule)
No Response in Hgb Levels/Still Require RBC Transfusions After 8 Weeks of Therapy/Following Completion of Chemotherapy Course: D/C therapy

Conversions

Adults w/ CKD on Dialysis:
Conversion from Epoetin Alfa:
Administer less frequently than epoetin alfa; estimate the starting weekly dose based on weekly epoetin alfa dose at the time of substitution

PEDIATRIC DOSAGE

Anemia Due to Chronic Kidney Disease

>1 Year w/ CKD on Dialysis:
Conversion from Epoetin Alfa:
Administer less frequently than epoetin alfa; estimate the starting weekly dose based on weekly epoetin alfa dose at the time of substitution
Epoetin Alfa Dose (U/week):
1500-2499: 6.25mcg/week
2500-4999: 10mcg/week
5000-10,999: 20mcg/week
11,000-17,999: 40mcg/week
18,000-33,999: 60mcg/week
34,000-89,999: 100mcg/week
≥90,000: 200mcg/week

Administer once weekly or every 2 weeks in patients who were receiving epoetin alfa 2-3X weekly or once weekly, respectively

Epoetin Alfa Dose (U/week):
<1500: 6.25mcg/week
1500-2499: 6.25mcg/week
2500-4999: 12.5mcg/week
5000-10,999: 25mcg/week
11,000-17,999: 40mcg/week
18,000-33,999: 60mcg/week
34,000-89,999: 100mcg/week
≥90,000: 200mcg/week
Administer once weekly or every 2 weeks in patients who were receiving epoetin alfa 2-3X weekly or once weekly, respectively

ADMINISTRATION
IV/SQ route
IV route is recommended for hemodialysis patients
Do not shake
Do not use if it has been frozen or shaken
Do not dilute and do not administer in conjunction w/ other drug sol
Discard any unused portion in vials or prefilled syringes; do not re-enter vial
Maintain route of administration when converting from epoetin alfa

HOW SUPPLIED
Inj: 25mcg/mL, 40mcg/mL, 60mcg/mL, 100mcg/mL, 150mcg/0.75mL, 200mcg/mL, 300mcg/mL [single-dose vial]; 10mcg/0.4mL, 25mcg/0.42mL, 40mcg/0.4mL, 60mcg/0.3mL, 100mcg/0.5mL, 150mcg/0.3mL, 200mcg/0.4mL, 300mcg/0.6mL, 500mcg/mL [single-dose prefilled syringe]

CONTRAINDICATIONS
Uncontrolled HTN, pure red cell aplasia (PRCA) that begins after treatment w/ darbepoetin alfa or other erythropoietin protein drugs.

WARNINGS/PRECAUTIONS
Not indicated for use in patients w/ cancer receiving hormonal agents, biologic products, or radiotherapy, unless also receiving concomitant myelosuppressive chemotherapy, or as a substitute for RBC transfusions in patients requiring immediate correction of anemia. Evaluate transferrin saturation and serum ferritin prior to and during treatment; administer supplemental iron when serum ferritin is <100mcg/L or serum transferrin saturation is <20%. Correct/exclude other causes of anemia (eg, vitamin deficiency, metabolic/chronic inflammatory conditions, bleeding) before initiating therapy. Caution in patients w/ coexistent CV disease and stroke. Not approved for reduction of RBC transfusions in patients scheduled for surgical procedures. Hypertensive encephalopathy and seizures reported in patients w/ CKD. Appropriately control HTN prior to initiation of and during treatment; reduce/withhold therapy if BP becomes difficult to control. Cases of PRCA and severe anemia, w/ or w/o other cytopenias that arise following development of neutralizing antibodies to erythropoietin reported. Withhold and evaluate for neutralizing antibodies to erythropoietin if severe anemia and low reticulocyte count develop; d/c permanently if PRCA develops, and do not switch to other ESAs. Serious allergic reactions may occur; immediately and permanently d/c treatment and administer appropriate therapy if a serious allergic/anaphylactic reaction occurs. Patients may require adjustments in dialysis prescriptions after initiation of therapy, or require increased anticoagulation w/ heparin to prevent clotting of extracorporeal circuit during hemodialysis. Needle cover of the prefilled syringe contains dry natural rubber (a derivative of latex), which may cause allergic reactions.

ADVERSE REACTIONS
MI, stroke, VTE, thrombosis of vascular access, tumor progression/recurrence, HTN, dyspnea, peripheral edema, cough, procedural hypotension, angina pectoris, fluid overload, rash/erythema.

NURSING CONSIDERATIONS

Assessment: Assess for uncontrolled HTN, previous hypersensitivity to the drug, latex allergy, causes of anemia, pregnancy/nursing status, and other conditions where treatment is cautioned/contraindicated. Obtain baseline Hgb levels, transferrin saturation, and serum ferritin.

Monitoring: Monitor for signs/symptoms of an allergic reaction, CV/thromboembolic events, stroke, PRCA, severe anemia, progression/recurrence of tumor, HTN, and other adverse reactions. Monitor BP, transferrin saturation, and serum ferritin. Monitor closely for premonitory neurologic symptoms during the 1st several months following initiation of treatment. Following initiation of therapy and after each dose adjustment, monitor Hgb weekly until Hgb is stable and sufficient to minimize need for RBC transfusion, and then monitor Hgb less frequently, provided Hgb levels remain stable.

Patient Counseling: Inform of the risks/benefits of therapy and of the increased risks of mortality, serious CV reactions, thromboembolic reactions, stroke, and tumor progression. Advise of the need to have regular lab tests for Hgb. Inform cancer patients that they must sign the patient-physician acknowledgment form prior to the start of each treatment course. Instruct to undergo regular BP monitoring, adhere to prescribed antihypertensive regimen, and follow recommended dietary restrictions. Advise to contact physician for new-onset neurologic symptoms or change in seizure frequency. Instruct regarding proper disposal and caution against reuse of needles, syringes, or unused portions of single-dose vials.

Storage: 2-8°C (36-46°F). Do not freeze. Protect from light.

ARAVA – leflunomide **RX**

Class: Pyrimidine synthesis inhibitor

Exclude pregnancy before start of treatment. Avoid pregnancy during treatment or prior to completion of drug elimination procedure after treatment. Severe liver injury, including fatal liver failure, reported; not for use with preexisting acute or chronic liver disease, or those with serum ALT >2X ULN before initiating treatment. Caution with other potentially hepatotoxic drugs. Monitor ALT levels at least monthly for 6 months after starting therapy, and thereafter every 6-8 weeks. Interrupt therapy if ALT elevation >3X ULN occurs; if likely leflunomide-induced, start cholestyramine washout and monitor liver tests weekly until normalized. If leflunomide-induced liver injury is unlikely, may consider resumption of therapy.

ADULT DOSAGE

Rheumatoid Arthritis

LD: 100mg qd for 3 days
Maint: 20mg qd; if not well tolerated, may reduce to 10mg qd
Max: 20mg qd

PEDIATRIC DOSAGE

Pediatric use may not have been established

DOSE MODIFICATION

Hepatic Impairment

Not recommended

ADMINISTRATION

Oral route

HOW SUPPLIED

Tab: 10mg, 20mg, 100mg

CONTRAINDICATIONS

Women who are or may become pregnant.

WARNINGS/PRECAUTIONS

Not recommended with severe immunodeficiency, bone marrow dysplasia, or severe, uncontrolled infections; interruption of therapy and administration of cholestyramine or charcoal may be necessary if a serious infection occurs. May cause immunosuppression, increased susceptibility to infections, including opportunistic infections, especially *Pneumocystis jiroveci* pneumonia, tuberculosis (TB), and aspergillosis, or increase risk of malignancy. Pancytopenia, agranulocytosis, and thrombocytopenia reported (rare). D/C therapy with evidence of bone marrow suppression. Monitor for hematologic toxicity if switching to another antirheumatic agent with a known potential for hematologic suppression. Serious toxicity (eg, hypersensitivity), peripheral neuropathy, rare cases of Stevens-Johnson syndrome and toxic epidermal necrolysis, and drug reaction with eosinophilia and systemic symptoms reported; d/c therapy, and a drug elimination procedure is recommended if any of these occur. Age >60 yrs and diabetes may increase risk for peripheral neuropathy. Interstitial lung disease (ILD) reported. New onset or worsening of pulmonary symptoms (eg, cough, dyspnea), with or without associated fever, may be a reason for discontinuation of therapy; consider initiation of washout procedures if discontinuation is necessary. Screen for latent TB infection with a tuberculin skin test prior to initiating therapy. Caution with renal impairment. Has uricosuric effect and a separate effect of hypophosphaturia seen in some patients. Men wishing to father a child should consider discontinuing use and taking cholestyramine 8g tid for 11 days.

ADVERSE REACTIONS

Severe liver injury, diarrhea, upper respiratory infection, abnormal liver enzymes, alopecia, headache, N/V, rash, HTN, joint disorder, bronchitis, abdominal/back/GI pain, asthenia.

DRUG INTERACTIONS

See Boxed Warning. Coadministration with teriflunomide is not recommended. Vaccination with live vaccines is not recommended; consider long $T_{1/2}$ when contemplating administration of live vaccine after stopping therapy. Decreased plasma levels of M1 with cholestyramine or activated charcoal. Multiple doses of rifampin may increase levels; use with caution. May increase levels of diclofenac, ibuprofen, or tolbutamide. May increase risk of hepatotoxicity with methotrexate or peripheral neuropathy with neurotoxic medications. Increased INR with warfarin (rare). Concomitant immunosuppressant therapy may increase susceptibility to infections.

NURSING CONSIDERATIONS

Assessment: Assess for hypersensitivity to drug or to teriflunomide, severe immunodeficiency, bone marrow dysplasia, severe uncontrolled infections, hepatic/renal impairment, comorbid illnesses, latent TB infection, any other conditions where treatment is cautioned or contraindicated, pregnancy/nursing status, and possible drug interactions. Obtain baseline BP, platelet, WBC count, Hgb or Hct, and ALT levels.

Monitoring: Monitor for signs/symptoms of immunosuppression and opportunistic infections, sepsis, pancytopenia, agranulocytosis, thrombocytopenia, severe liver injury, skin/hypersensitivity reactions, ILD, malignancy, and other adverse reactions. Monitor BP periodically. Monitor platelets, WBC count, Hgb/Hct, and ALT levels monthly for 6 months following initiation of therapy and every 6-8 weeks thereafter. Monitor carefully after dose reduction. Monitor for hematologic toxicity when switching to another antirheumatic agent with known potential for hematologic suppression. Monitor for bone marrow suppression monthly if used concomitantly with immunosuppressants.

Patient Counseling: Advise women of childbearing potential of the increased risk of birth defects if used during pregnancy, if they become pregnant while on therapy, or do not wait to become pregnant until they have stopped taking the drug and followed the drug elimination procedure; instruct to use reliable form of contraception while on therapy. Advise of the possibility of rare, serious skin reactions; instruct to inform physician promptly if skin rash or mucous membrane lesions develop. Advise of the potential hepatotoxic effects and of the need for monitoring liver enzymes; instruct to notify physician if symptoms such as unusual tiredness, abdominal pain, or jaundice develop. Advise that lowering of blood counts may develop; instruct to have frequent hematologic monitoring, particularly in patients who are receiving other concurrent immunosuppressive therapy, or who have had a history of significant hematologic abnormality, and to notify physician if symptoms of pancytopenia (eg, easy bruising/bleeding, recurrent infections, fever, paleness, unusual tiredness) develop. Inform about the early warning signs of ILD and instruct to contact physician as soon as possible if these symptoms appear/worsen during therapy.

Storage: 25°C (77°F); excursions permitted to 15-30°C (59-86°F). Protect from light.

ARCAPTA – indacaterol

Class: Beta$_2$-agonist

RX

Long-acting β_2-adrenergic agonists (LABAs) may increase the risk of asthma-related death. Not indicated for treatment of asthma.

ADULT DOSAGE

Chronic Obstructive Pulmonary Disease

Long-term, maintenance treatment of airflow obstruction in patients w/ COPD (eg, chronic bronchitis, emphysema)

1 inh (75mcg) qd via Neohaler device

PEDIATRIC DOSAGE

Pediatric use may not have been established

ADMINISTRATION

Oral inh route

Use only w/ Neohaler device
Do not swallow caps
Administer at the same time every day
Remove cap from blister immediately before use

HOW SUPPLIED

Cap, Inh: 75mcg

CONTRAINDICATIONS

Asthma without use of a long-term asthma control medication. Not indicated for treatment of asthma.

WARNINGS/PRECAUTIONS

Not for acutely deteriorating COPD, or relief of acute symptoms (eg, as rescue therapy for treatment of acute episodes of bronchospasm). Cardiovascular (CV) effects and fatalities reported with excessive use; do not use excessively or with other LABA. D/C if paradoxical bronchospasm or CV effects occur. ECG changes reported. Caution with CV disorders (eg, coronary insufficiency, cardiac arrhythmias, HTN), convulsive disorders, thyrotoxicosis, and in patients unusually responsive to sympathomimetic amines. Hypokalemia, hyperglycemia, and immediate hypersensitivity reactions may occur. D/C immediately and institute alternative therapy if signs suggesting allergic reactions occur.

ADVERSE REACTIONS

Cough, nasopharyngitis, headache, COPD exacerbation, pneumonia, angina pectoris, A-fib.

DRUG INTERACTIONS

Adrenergic drugs may potentiate effects; use with caution. Xanthine derivatives, steroids, or diuretics may potentiate any hypokalemic effect. ECG changes or hypokalemia that may result from non-K^+-sparing diuretics (eg, loop/thiazide diuretics) can be acutely worsened; use with caution. MAOIs, TCAs, and drugs known to prolong QTc interval may potentiate effect on CV system; use with extreme caution. Drugs that are known to prolong the QTc interval may increase risk of ventricular arrhythmias. β-blockers may block effects and produce severe bronchospasm in COPD patients; if needed, consider cardioselective β-blocker with caution. May result in overdose if used in conjunction with other medications containing LABAs. Increased plasma levels with ketoconazole, verapamil, erythromycin, and ritonavir.

NURSING CONSIDERATIONS

Assessment: Assess for previous hypersensitivity to the drug, acute COPD deteriorations, asthma and use of control medication, CV disorders, convulsive disorders, thyrotoxicosis, diabetes mellitus, pregnancy/nursing status, and possible drug interactions. Assess use in patients unusually responsive to sympathomimetic amines. Obtain baseline serum K^+ and blood glucose levels.

Monitoring: Monitor lung function periodically. Monitor for signs of worsening asthma, CV effects, paradoxical bronchospasm, and immediate hypersensitivity reactions. Monitor pulse rate, BP, ECG changes, and serum K^+ and glucose levels.

Patient Counseling: Inform of the risks and benefits of therapy. Instruct on proper administration of caps using the inhaler device and not to swallow caps. Caution that inhaler cannot be used more than once a day. Advise to d/c the regular use of short acting β_2-agonist (SABA) and use them only for the symptomatic relief of acute symptoms. Instruct to notify physician immediately if worsening of symptoms, decreasing effectiveness of inhaled SABA, need for more inhalations than usual of inhaled SABA, and significant decrease in lung function occur. Instruct not to stop therapy without physician's guidance. Inform patients not to use other inhaled medications containing LABAs. Inform about associated adverse effects, such as palpitations, chest pain, rapid HR, tremor, or nervousness.

Storage: 25°C (77°F); excursions permitted to 15-30°C (59-86°F). Protect from light and moisture.

ARICEPT – donepezil hydrochloride — RX

Class: Acetylcholinesterase inhibitor

ADULT DOSAGE

Alzheimer's Disease

Dementia of the Alzheimer's type

Mild to Moderate:
Initial: 5mg qd
Titrate: May increase to 10mg qd after 4-6 weeks
Usual: 5-10mg qd

Moderate to Severe:
Initial: 5mg qd
Titrate: May increase to 10mg qd after 4-6 weeks, then to 23mg qd after at least 3 months
Usual: 10-23mg qd

PEDIATRIC DOSAGE

Pediatric use may not have been established

ADMINISTRATION

Oral route

Take qhs
Take w/ or w/o food

23mg Tab
Do not split, crush, or chew

ODT
Dissolve on the tongue and follow w/ water

HOW SUPPLIED

Tab: 5mg, 10mg, 23mg; Tab, Disintegrating: (ODT) 5mg, 10mg

WARNINGS/PRECAUTIONS

May exaggerate succinylcholine-type muscle relaxation during anesthesia. May have vagotonic effects on sinoatrial (SA) and atrioventricular (AV) nodes, manifesting as bradycardia or heart block. Syncopal episodes reported. May produce diarrhea, N/V; observe closely at initiation of treatment and after dose increases. May increase gastric acid secretion; monitor for active or occult GI bleeding. Caution patients with increased risk for developing ulcers (eg, history of ulcer disease). May cause weight loss, generalized convulsions, and bladder outflow obstruction. Caution with history of asthma or obstructive pulmonary disease.

ADVERSE REACTIONS

N/V, diarrhea, insomnia, muscle cramps, fatigue, anorexia, headache, dizziness, weight decrease, infection, HTN, back pain, abnormal dreams, ecchymosis.

DRUG INTERACTIONS

Monitor closely for GI bleeding with concurrent NSAID use. Ketoconazole and quinidine, inhibitors of CYP3A4 and CYP2D6, respectively, inhibit metabolism in vitro. Increased concentrations with ketoconazole. CYP3A4 inducers (eg, phenytoin, dexamethasone, rifampin) may increase elimination rate. May interfere with activity of anticholinergic medications. Synergistic effect with neuromuscular blocking agents (eg, succinylcholine) or cholinergic agonists (eg, bethanechol).

NURSING CONSIDERATIONS

Assessment: Assess for hypersensitivity to the drug or piperidine derivatives, underlying cardiac conduction abnormalities, risks for developing ulcers, history of asthma or obstructive pulmonary disease, pregnancy/nursing status, and possible drug interactions.

Monitoring: Monitor for vagotonic effects on SA and AV nodes, syncopal episodes, diarrhea, N/V, active/occult GI bleeding, weight loss, bladder outflow obstruction, generalized convulsions, and other possible adverse reactions.

Patient Counseling: Instruct to take as prescribed. Advise that N/V, diarrhea, insomnia, muscle cramps, fatigue, and decreased appetite may occur.

Storage: 15-30°C (59-86°F).

ARIMIDEX – anastrozole — RX

Class: Nonsteroidal aromatase inhibitor

ADULT DOSAGE

Breast Cancer

In postmenopausal women for adjuvant treatment of hormone receptor-positive early breast cancer; 1st-line treatment of hormone receptor-positive or hormone receptor unknown locally advanced or metastatic breast cancer; and treatment of advanced breast cancer w/ disease progression following tamoxifen therapy

Advanced Breast Cancer:
1mg qd; continue until tumor progression

Adjuvant Treatment of Early Breast Cancer:
1mg qd; administered for 5 years in a clinical trial

PEDIATRIC DOSAGE

Pediatric use may not have been established

ADMINISTRATION

Oral route

Take w/ or w/o food

HOW SUPPLIED

Tab: 1mg

CONTRAINDICATIONS

Women who are or may become pregnant, premenopausal women.

WARNINGS/PRECAUTIONS

Increased incidence of ischemic cardiovascular (CV) events in women with preexisting ischemic heart disease reported. Decreases in bone mineral density (BMD) may occur. Elevated serum cholesterol reported.

ADVERSE REACTIONS

Hot flashes, asthenia, arthritis, pain, pharyngitis, HTN, depression, N/V, rash, osteoporosis, fractures, headache, bone pain, peripheral edema.

DRUG INTERACTIONS

Tamoxifen may decrease levels; avoid concomitant use. Avoid with estrogen-containing therapies.

NURSING CONSIDERATIONS

Assessment: Assess for hypersensitivity to drug, preexisting ischemic cardiac disease, premenopausal status, pregnancy/nursing status, and possible drug interactions.

Monitoring: Monitor for hypersensitivity reactions and other adverse reactions. Monitor BMD and serum cholesterol levels.

Patient Counseling: Inform that drug may cause fetal harm and is not for use in premenopausal women; instruct to d/c therapy if patient becomes pregnant and to immediately contact physician. Instruct to seek medical attention immediately if serious allergic reactions occur. Inform patients with preexisting ischemic heart disease that an increased incidence of CV events has been observed; advise to seek medical attention immediately if new or worsening chest pain or SOB occurs. Inform that drug may lower estrogen level, which may lead to a loss of the mineral content of bones, possibly decreasing the bone strength, leading to an increased risk of fractures. Inform that an increased level of cholesterol might be seen while receiving therapy. Instruct to notify physician if tickling, tingling, or numbness is experienced. Advise not to take drug with tamoxifen.

Storage: 20-25°C (68-77°F).

ARIXTRA – fondaparinux sodium

RX

Class: Selective factor Xa inhibitor

Epidural or spinal hematomas may occur in patients who are anticoagulated with low molecular weight heparins (LMWHs), heparinoids, or fondaparinux sodium and who are receiving neuraxial anesthesia or undergoing spinal puncture; long-term or permanent paralysis may result. Increased risk of developing epidural or spinal hematomas in patients using indwelling epidural catheters, concomitant use of other drugs that affect hemostasis (eg, NSAIDs, platelet inhibitors, other anticoagulants), history of traumatic or repeated epidural or spinal puncture, history of spinal deformity or spinal surgery, or unknown optimal timing between the administration of therapy and neuraxial procedures. Monitor frequently for signs/symptoms of neurologic impairment; if neurologic compromise noted, urgent treatment is necessary. Consider benefit and risks before neuraxial intervention in patients anticoagulated or to be anticoagulated for thromboprophylaxis.

ADULT DOSAGE

Deep Vein Thrombosis/Pulmonary Embolism

DVT Prophylaxis Following Hip Fracture Surgery, Hip Replacement Surgery, Knee Replacement Surgery, or Abdominal Surgery (in Patients at Risk for Thromboembolic Complications):

≥50kg: 2.5mg SQ qd after hemostasis has been established; administer initial dose no earlier than 6-8 hrs after surgery

Usual Duration: 5-9 days (administered up to 11 days following hip replacement or knee replacement surgery and administered up to 10 days following abdominal surgery in clinical trials); extended prophylaxis course of up to 24 additional days recommended for patients undergoing hip fracture surgery (total of 32 days administered in clinical trials)

DVT/PE Treatment:

Treatment of acute DVT w/ warfarin sodium, and treatment of acute PE w/ warfarin sodium when initial therapy is administered in the hospital

<50kg: 5mg SQ qd

50-100kg: 7.5mg SQ qd

>100kg: 10mg SQ qd

Initiate concomitant treatment w/ warfarin sodium as soon as possible, usually w/in 72 hrs

Continue fondaparinux for at least 5 days and until therapeutic oral anticoagulant effect is established (INR 2-3)

Usual Duration: 5-9 days (administered up to 26 days in clinical trials)

PEDIATRIC DOSAGE

Pediatric use may not have been established

DOSE MODIFICATION

Renal Impairment

CrCl 30-50mL/min: Use caution

ADMINISTRATION

SQ route

Do not mix w/ other medications or sol

Do not expel air bubble from syringe before the inj

Administer in fatty tissue, alternating inj sites

Refer to PI for further instructions for use

HOW SUPPLIED

Inj: 2.5mg/0.5mL, 5mg/0.4mL, 7.5mg/0.6mL, 10mg/0.8mL

CONTRAINDICATIONS

Severe renal impairment (CrCl <30mL/min), active major bleeding, bacterial endocarditis, thrombocytopenia associated with a (+) in vitro test for antiplatelet antibody in the presence of fondaparinux sodium, body weight <50kg (venous thromboembolism prophylaxis only).

WARNINGS/PRECAUTIONS

Extreme caution in conditions with increased risk of hemorrhage (eg, congenital or acquired bleeding disorders, active ulcerative and angiodysplastic GI disease, hemorrhagic stroke, uncontrolled arterial HTN, diabetic retinopathy, or shortly after brain, spinal, or ophthalmological surgery). Elevated activated PTT temporally associated with bleeding events reported. Administration of initial dose earlier than 6 hrs after surgery increases risk of major bleeding. Increased risk of bleeding in patients with impaired renal function; d/c therapy immediately if severe renal impairment develops. Caution with CrCl 30-50mL/min. Increased risk of bleeding in patients who weigh <50kg; caution in treatment of PE and DVT. Thrombocytopenia reported. D/C if platelet count falls <100,000/mm^3. D/C if unexpected changes in coagulation parameters or major bleeding occur during therapy. Needle guard of the prefilled syringe contains dry natural latex rubber that may cause allergic reactions in latex-sensitive individuals. Caution with moderate hepatic impairment (Child-Pugh Category B) and in elderly.

ADVERSE REACTIONS

Bleeding complications, thrombocytopenia, local irritation (eg, inj-site bleeding, rash, pruritus), anemia, insomnia, increased wound drainage, hypokalemia, dizziness, purpura, hypotension, confusion.

DRUG INTERACTIONS

See Boxed Warning. Agents that may enhance the risk of hemorrhage should be discontinued prior to initiation of therapy unless these agents are essential; if coadministration is necessary, monitor closely for hemorrhage.

NURSING CONSIDERATIONS

Assessment: Assess for history of serious hypersensitivity reaction to the drug, conditions that increase the risk of hemorrhage, or any other conditions where treatment is cautioned or contraindicated, renal/hepatic impairment, latex sensitivity, pregnancy/nursing status, and for possible drug interactions.

Monitoring: Monitor for signs/symptoms of bleeding, thrombocytopenia, and other adverse reactions. In patients undergoing neuraxial anesthesia or spinal puncture, monitor for epidural or spinal hematomas and neurologic impairment. Perform periodic CBC (including platelet count), stool occult blood tests, and SrCr level tests.

Patient Counseling: Advise patients who have had neuraxial anesthesia or spinal puncture to watch for signs and symptoms of spinal/epidural hematoma, especially if concomitantly taking NSAIDs, platelet inhibitors, or other anticoagulants; instruct to contact physician immediately if symptoms occur. Advise that the use of aspirin and other NSAIDs may enhance the risk of hemorrhage. Instruct on proper administration technique. Counsel on signs/symptoms of possible bleeding. Inform patients that it may take longer than usual to stop bleeding and that they may bruise and/or bleed more easily while on therapy. Instruct to report any unusual bleeding, bruising, or signs of thrombocytopenia to the physician. Instruct to notify physician or dentist of all prescription and nonprescription medications currently being taken.

Storage: 25°C (77°F); excursions permitted to 15-30°C (59-86°F).

ARMOUR THYROID – thyroid RX

Class: Thyroid replacement hormone

Do not use for the treatment of obesity or weight loss; doses within range of daily hormonal requirements are ineffective for weight reduction in euthyroid patients. Serious or life-threatening manifestations of toxicity may occur when given in larger doses, particularly when given in association with sympathomimetic amines.

ADULT DOSAGE

Hypothyroidism

Replacement/supplemental therapy in hypothyroidism of any etiology, except transient hypothyroidism during the recovery phase of subacute thyroiditis

Initial: 30mg/day; 15mg/day in patients w/ long-standing myxedema
Titrate: Increase by 15mg every 2-3 weeks
Readjust dose w/in the first 4 weeks
Maint: 60-120mg/day

Myxedema Coma: Resume oral therapy when clinical situation has been stabilized after IV administration and patient is able to take oral medications

PEDIATRIC DOSAGE

Hypothyroidism

Congenital:
0-6 Months of Age: 4.8-6mg/kg/day
6-12 months of Age: 3.6-4.8mg/kg/day
1-5 Years: 3-3.6mg/kg/day
6-12 Years: 2.4-3mg/kg/day
>12 Years: 1.2-1.8mg/kg/day

Pituitary TSH Suppressant

Used to treat/prevent various types of euthyroid goiters (eg, thyroid nodules, subacute or chronic lymphocytic thyroiditis [Hashimoto's], multinodular goiter) and to manage thyroid cancer

Thyroid Suppression Therapy:
1.56mcg/kg/day T4 for 7-10 days

Thyroid Cancer:
Give larger doses than those used for replacement therapy

ADMINISTRATION
Oral route

HOW SUPPLIED
Tab: 15mg, 30mg, 60mg, 90mg, 120mg, 180mg*, 240mg, 300mg* *scored

CONTRAINDICATIONS
Uncorrected adrenal cortical insufficiency, untreated thyrotoxicosis.

WARNINGS/PRECAUTIONS
Use is unjustified for the treatment of male or female infertility unless accompanied by hypothyroidism. Caution with cardiovascular (CV) disorders (eg, angina pectoris) and elderly with risk of occult cardiac disease; initiate at low doses (eg, 15-30mg/day) and reduce dose if euthyroid state can only be reached at the expense of aggravation of CV disease. May aggravate diabetes mellitus (DM), diabetes insipidus (DI), and adrenal cortical insufficiency. Treatment of myxedema coma requires simultaneous administration of glucocorticoids. Excessive doses in infants may cause craniosynostosis. Caution with strong suspicion of thyroid gland autonomy. Androgens, corticosteroids, estrogens, iodine-containing preparations, and salicylates may interfere with lab tests.

DRUG INTERACTIONS
See Boxed Warning. Closely monitor PT in patients on oral anticoagulants; dose reduction of anticoagulant may be required. May increase insulin or oral hypoglycemic requirements. Impaired absorption with cholestyramine and colestipol; space dosing by 4-5 hrs. Estrogens may increase thyroxine-binding globulin and may decrease free T4; increase in thyroid dose may be needed.

NURSING CONSIDERATIONS

Assessment: Assess for adrenal cortical insufficiency, thyrotoxicosis, previous hypersensitivity to the drug, CV disorders (eg, coronary artery disease, angina pectoris), DM, DI, myxedema coma, nursing status, and possible drug interactions.

Monitoring: Monitor response to treatment, urinary glucose levels in patients with DM, PT in patients receiving anticoagulants, and aggravation of diabetes or CV disease. Monitor thyroid function periodically.

Patient Counseling: Inform that replacement therapy is to be taken essentially for life, except in transient hypothyroidism. Instruct to immediately report any signs/symptoms of thyroid hormone toxicity. Inform about the importance of frequent/close monitoring of PT and urinary glucose and the need for dose adjustment of antidiabetic and/or oral anticoagulant medication. Inform that partial hair loss may be seen in children in 1st few months of therapy. Inform that drug is not for treatment of obesity or weight loss.

Storage: 15-30°C (59-86°F). Protect from light and moisture.

ARNUITY ELLIPTA – fluticasone furoate RX

Class: Corticosteroid

ADULT DOSAGE

Asthma

Prophylactic Maint Treatment:
Administer as 1 inh qd; do not use >1X q24h

Initial:
Not on an Inhaled Corticosteroid: 100mcg qd
All Other Patients: Dose based on previous asthma drug therapy and disease severity
Titrate: May replace w/ 200mcg in patients who do not respond to 100mcg after 2 weeks of therapy

PEDIATRIC DOSAGE

Asthma

Prophylactic Maint Treatment:
Administer as 1 inh qd; do not use >1X q24h

>12 Years:

Initial:
Not on an Inhaled Corticosteroid: 100mcg qd
All Other Patients: Dose based on previous asthma drug therapy and disease severity
Titrate: May replace w/ 200mcg in patients who do not respond to 100mcg after 2 weeks of therapy

Max: 200mcg/day After asthma stability is achieved, titrate to the lowest effective dose	**Max:** 200mcg/day After asthma stability is achieved, titrate to the lowest effective dose

DOSE MODIFICATION

Elderly

Start at lower end of dosing range

ADMINISTRATION

Oral inh route

Rinse mouth w/ water w/o swallowing after each dose

Use at the same time every day

HOW SUPPLIED

Powder, Inhalation: 100mcg/blister, 200mcg/blister [14, 30 blisters]

CONTRAINDICATIONS

Primary treatment of status asthmaticus or other acute episodes of asthma where intensive measures are required. Milk protein hypersensitivity.

WARNINGS/PRECAUTIONS

Not indicated for acute bronchospasm relief. *Candida albicans* infections of mouth and pharynx reported; treat and, if needed, interrupt therapy. Increased susceptibility to infections. May lead to serious/fatal course of chickenpox or measles; avoid exposure and if exposed, consider prophylaxis/treatment. Caution with active/quiescent tuberculosis (TB), untreated systemic fungal, bacterial, viral or parasitic infections, or ocular herpes simplex. Deaths due to adrenal insufficiency reported during and after transfer from systemic to inhaled corticosteroids; wean slowly from systemic corticosteroid use after transferring to therapy. Resume oral corticosteroids during periods of stress or a severe asthma attack in patients previously withdrawn from systemic corticosteroids. Transfer from systemic to inhaled corticosteroids may unmask allergic conditions previously suppressed by systemic therapy (eg, rhinitis, conjunctivitis, eczema). Monitor for systemic corticosteroid effects. Reduce dose slowly if hypercorticism and adrenal suppression occur. Bronchospasm may occur with an immediate increase in wheezing after dosing; treat immediately with an inhaled, short acting bronchodilator; d/c and institute alternative therapy. Hypersensitivity reactions may occur; d/c if such reactions occur. Decreases in bone mineral density (BMD) reported with long-term use; caution with major risk factors for decreased bone mineral content, including chronic use of drugs that can reduce bone mass (eg, anticonvulsants, oral corticosteroids). May reduce growth velocity in children and adolescents; routinely monitor growth. Glaucoma, increased intraocular pressure (IOP), and cataracts reported with long-term use. Caution with moderate or severe hepatic impairment and in elderly.

ADVERSE REACTIONS

Nasopharyngitis, bronchitis, upper respiratory tract infection, headache, pharyngitis, sinusitis, toothache, viral gastroenteritis, oral candidiasis, oropharyngeal candidiasis/pain, influenza, back pain, dysphonia, rhinitis.

DRUG INTERACTIONS

Caution with long-term ketoconazole and other known strong CYP3A4 inhibitors (eg, ritonavir, clarithromycin, itraconazole); increased systemic corticosteroid adverse effects may occur.

NURSING CONSIDERATIONS

Assessment: Assess for status asthmaticus; acute episodes of asthma; hypersensitivity to drug or to milk proteins; active/quiescent TB; untreated systemic infections; ocular herpes simplex; risk factors for decreased bone mineral content; history of increased IOP, glaucoma, and/or cataracts; hepatic impairment; pregnancy/nursing status; and possible drug interactions.

Monitoring: Monitor for localized oropharyngeal infections with *C. albicans*, infections, systemic corticosteroid effects (eg, hypercorticism, adrenal suppression), bronchospasm, hypersensitivity reactions, decreases in BMD, glaucoma, cataracts, increased IOP, and other adverse reactions. Monitor growth of children and adolescents routinely (eg, via stadiometry). Closely monitor patients with moderate to severe hepatic disease.

Patient Counseling: Inform that drug is not meant to relieve acute asthma symptoms; advise to treat acute symptoms with an inhaled short-acting β_2-agonist (SABA). Instruct to seek medical attention immediately if experiencing worsening of symptoms, a significant decrease in lung function, or a need for more inhalations than usual of inhaled SABAs. Advise to use at regular intervals, not to increase the dose or frequency of therapy, and not to d/c or reduce therapy without physician guidance. Instruct to contact physician if oropharyngeal candidiasis develops, if symptoms do not improve after 2 weeks, or if patient becomes pregnant while on therapy. Advise to avoid exposure to chickenpox or measles, and, if exposed, to consult physician without delay. Inform about risk of immunosuppression, hypercorticism, adrenal suppression, reduction in BMD, reduced growth velocity in pediatric patients, ocular effects, and hypersensitivity reactions, including anaphylaxis; instruct to d/c if hypersensitivity reactions occur. Inform that the inhaler is not reusable and advise not to take the inhaler apart.

Storage: 20-25°C (68-77°F); excursions permitted from 15-30°C (59-86°F). Store in a dry place away from direct heat or sunlight. Store inside the unopened moisture-protective foil tray and only remove from the tray immediately before initial use. Discard 6 weeks after opening the foil tray or when the counter reads "0" (after all blisters have been used), whichever comes 1st.

AROMASIN – exemestane

RX

Class: Aromatase inactivator

ADULT DOSAGE

Estrogen-Receptor Positive Early Breast Cancer

Adjuvant treatment of postmenopausal women who have received 2-3 years of tamoxifen and are switched to exemestane for completion of a total of 5 consecutive years of adjuvant hormonal therapy

25mg qd

Advanced Breast Cancer

In postmenopausal women whose disease has progressed following tamoxifen therapy

25mg qd

PEDIATRIC DOSAGE

Pediatric use may not have been established

DOSE MODIFICATION

Concomitant Medications

Strong CYP3A4 Inducers: 50mg qd

ADMINISTRATION

Oral route

Take after a meal

HOW SUPPLIED

Tab: 25mg

CONTRAINDICATIONS

Women who are or may become pregnant, premenopausal women.

WARNINGS/PRECAUTIONS

Lymphocytopenia (common toxicity criteria [CTC] Grade 3 or 4) reported with advanced breast cancer; most had a preexisting lower grade lymphopenia. Elevations of serum levels of AST, ALT, alkaline phosphatase, and gamma-glutamyl transferase >5X ULN (eg, ≥CTC Grade 3) have been rarely reported with advanced breast cancer, but appear mostly attributable to the underlying presence of liver and/or bone metastases. Elevations in bilirubin, alkaline phosphatase, and creatinine reported with early breast cancer. Reductions in bone mineral density (BMD) over time reported. During adjuvant treatment, assess BMD in women with osteoporosis or at risk of osteoporosis at the commencement of treatment. Monitor patients for BMD loss and treat as appropriate. Perform routine assessment of 25-hydroxy vitamin D levels prior to treatment; give vitamin D supplementation in women with vitamin D deficiency.

ADVERSE REACTIONS

Hot flushes, fatigue, arthralgia, headache, insomnia, increased sweating, HTN, dizziness, limb/back pain, nausea, depression, osteoarthritis, visual disturbances, alopecia.

DRUG INTERACTIONS

See Dosage. Avoid coadministration with estrogen-containing agents. CYP3A4 inducers (eg, rifampicin, phenytoin, carbamazepine, phenobarbital, St. John's wort) may significantly decrease exposure; dose modification is recommended with a strong CYP3A4 inducer.

NURSING CONSIDERATIONS

Assessment: Assess for hypersensitivity, preexisting lower grade lymphopenia, liver and/or bone metastases, osteoporosis/at risk of osteoporosis, pregnancy/nursing status, and for possible drug interactions. Perform routine assessment of 25-hydroxy vitamin D levels prior to treatment. Assess BMD in women with osteoporosis/at risk of osteoporosis.

Monitoring: Monitor for hematological abnormalities, BMD loss, osteoporosis, and other adverse reactions. Monitor LFTs, creatinine, alkaline phosphatase, and bilirubin levels.

Patient Counseling: Advise that drug is not for use in premenopausal women. Inform not to take concomitant estrogen-containing agents. Counsel that drug lowers estrogen level in the body, which may lead to reduction in BMD over time, and that the lower the BMD, the greater the risk of osteoporosis and fracture.

Storage: 25°C (77°F); excursions permitted to 15-30°C (59-86°F).

ARZERRA – ofatumumab

Class: Monoclonal antibody/CD20-blocker

RX

Hepatitis B virus (HBV) reactivation may occur, in some cases resulting in fulminant hepatitis, hepatic failure, and death. Progressive multifocal leukoencephalopathy (PML) resulting in death may occur.

ADULT DOSAGE

Chronic Lymphocytic Leukemia

Previously Untreated:

In combination w/ chlorambucil, for the treatment of patients for whom fludarabine-based therapy is considered inappropriate

300mg on Day 1, followed 1 week later by 1000mg on Day 8 (Cycle 1), followed by 1000mg on Day 1 of subsequent 28-day cycles for a minimum of 3 cycles until best response or a max of 12 cycles

Infusion Rates:

Cycle 1, Day 1 (300mg Dose):

0-30 Min After Start of Infusion: 12mL/hr
31-60 Min After Start of Infusion: 25mL/hr
61-90 Min After Start of Infusion: 50mL/hr
91-120 Min After Start of Infusion: 100mL/hr
121-150 Min After Start of Infusion: 200mL/hr
151-180 Min After Start of Infusion: 300mL/hr
>180 Min After Start of Infusion: 400mL/hr

Cycle 1, Day 8 and Cycles 2-12 (1000mg Doses):

0-30 Min After Start of Infusion: 25mL/hr; initiate at 12mg/hr if ≥Grade 3 infusion-related adverse event is experienced during previous infusion
31-60 Min After Start of Infusion: 50mL/hr
61-90 Min After Start of Infusion: 100mL/hr
91-120 Min After Start of Infusion: 200mL/hr
>121 Min After Start of Infusion: 400mL/hr

Refractory to Fludarabine and Alemtuzumab:

300mg initially (Dose 1), followed 1 week later by 2000mg weekly for 7 doses (Doses 2 through 8), followed 4 weeks later by 2000mg every 4 weeks for 4 doses (Doses 9-12)

Infusion Rates:

Dose 1 (300mg Dose) and Dose 2 (2000mg Dose):

0-30 Min After Start of Infusion: 12mL/hr
31-60 Min After Start of Infusion: 25mL/hr
61-90 Min After Start of Infusion: 50mL/hr
91-120 Min After Start of Infusion: 100mL/hr
121-150 Min After Start of Infusion: 200mL/hr

Doses 3-12 (2000mg Doses):

0-30 Min After Start of Infusion: 25mL/hr
31-60 Min After Start of Infusion: 50mL/hr
61-90 Min After Start of Infusion: 100mL/hr
91-120 Min After Start of Infusion: 200mL/hr
121-150 Min After Start of Infusion: 400mL/hr

Premedication

Administer 30 min to 2 hrs prior to each infusion

Previously Untreated Chronic Lymphocytic Leukemia:

Oral acetaminophen 1000mg (or equivalent) + oral/IV antihistamine (diphenhydramine 50mg, cetirizine 10mg, or equivalent) + IV corticosteroid (prednisolone 50mg or equivalent)

PEDIATRIC DOSAGE

Pediatric use may not have been established

If patient does not experience ≥Grade 3 infusion-related adverse event during the first 2 infusions, the corticosteroid dose may be reduced or omitted for subsequent infusions

Refractory Chronic Lymphocytic Leukemia: Oral acetaminophen 1000mg (or equivalent) + oral/IV antihistamine (diphenhydramine 50mg, cetirizine 10mg, or equivalent) + IV corticosteroid (prednisolone 100mg or equivalent)

Do not reduce corticosteroid dose for Doses 1, 2, and 9. Corticosteroid dose may be reduced as follows:

Doses 3-8: Corticosteroid may be reduced or omitted w/ subsequent infusions if ≥Grade 3 infusion reaction did not occur w/ the preceding dose

Doses 10-12: Administer prednisolone 50-100mg or equivalent if ≥Grade 3 infusion reaction did not occur w/ Dose 9

DOSE MODIFICATION

Infusion Reactions

Interrupt infusion for reactions of any severity

If infusion reaction resolves/remains ≤Grade 2, resume infusion according to initial grade of reaction:

Grade 1 or 2: Infuse at 1/2 of the previous infusion rate

Grade 3 or 4: Infuse at a rate of 12mL/hr

After resuming infusion, increase infusion rate as specified in Dosing, based on patient tolerance

Consider permanent discontinuation if severity of infusion reaction does not resolve to ≤Grade 2 despite adequate clinical intervention; permanently d/c therapy if anaphylactic reaction develops

ADMINISTRATION

IV route

Do not administer as IV push or bolus, or as SQ inj

Do not shake

Preparation of Sol

300mg Dose:

1. Withdraw and discard 15mL from a 1000mL bag of 0.9% NaCl inj
2. Withdraw 5mL from each of 3 single-use 100mg vials and add to the bag
3. Mix diluted sol by gentle inversion

1000mg Dose:

1. Withdraw and discard 50mL from a 1000mL bag of 0.9% NaCl inj
2. Withdraw 50mL from 1 single-use 1000mg vial and add to the bag
3. Mix diluted sol by gentle inversion

2000mg Dose:

1. Withdraw and discard 100mL from a 1000mL bag of 0.9% NaCl inj
2. Withdraw 50mL from each of 2 single-use 1000mg vials and add to the bag
3. Mix diluted sol by gentle inversion

Administration Instructions

Do not mix w/, or administer as an infusion w/, other medicinal products

Administer using an infusion pump and an administration set

Flush the IV line w/ 0.9% NaCl inj before and after each dose

Start infusion w/in 12 hrs of preparation

Discard prepared sol after 24 hrs

HOW SUPPLIED

Inj: 20mg/mL [5mL, 50mL]

WARNINGS/PRECAUTIONS

Administer in an environment where facilities to adequately monitor and treat infusion reactions are available. May cause serious, including fatal, infusion reactions; interrupt for infusion reactions of any severity and institute medical management for severe reactions. Permanently d/c if an anaphylactic reaction occurs. Screen for HBV infection before initiating treatment. Monitor patients with evidence of current or prior HBV infection for clinical and laboratory signs of hepatitis or HBV reactivation during and for several months following treatment. Immediately d/c therapy and any concomitant chemotherapy, and institute appropriate treatment if HBV reactivation develops. Fatal infection due to hepatitis B in patients who have not been previously infected reported. Consider PML in any patient with new onset of or changes in preexisting neurological signs/symptoms; if PML is suspected, d/c therapy and initiate evaluation for PML. Tumor lysis syndrome (TLS), including the need for hospitalization, reported; increased risk with high tumor burden and/or high circulating lymphocyte counts (>25X 10^9/L). Consider tumor lysis prophylaxis with antihyperuricemics and hydration beginning 12-24 hrs prior to infusion. Severe cytopenias, including neutropenia, thrombocytopenia, and anemia, may occur.

ADVERSE REACTIONS
HBV reactivation, fulminant hepatitis, hepatic failure, PML, neutropenia, pneumonia, pyrexia, cough, diarrhea, anemia, fatigue, dyspnea, rash, nausea, bronchitis, infusion reactions.

DRUG INTERACTIONS
Do not administer live viral vaccines to recently treated patients.

NURSING CONSIDERATIONS

Assessment: Assess for current/prior HBV infection, risk for TLS, pregnancy/nursing status, and possible drug interactions.

Monitoring: Monitor for signs/symptoms of HBV reactivation, hepatitis, PML, infusion reactions, TLS, and other adverse reactions. Monitor CBC at regular intervals during and after conclusion of therapy, and at increased frequency in patients who develop Grade 3 or 4 cytopenias.

Patient Counseling: Instruct to inform physician of signs/symptoms of infusion reactions; symptoms of hepatitis (eg, worsening fatigue, yellow discoloration of skin/eyes); new neurological symptoms (eg, confusion, dizziness or loss of balance); bleeding, easy bruising, petechiae, pallor, worsening weakness, or fatigue; or signs of infections. Advise to notify physician if pregnant/nursing. Advise of the need for monitoring and possible need for treatment if patient has a history of hepatitis B infection, for periodic monitoring of blood counts, and for avoiding vaccination with live viral vaccines.

Storage: 2-8°C (36-46°F). Do not freeze. Protect from light. Discard prepared solution after 24 hrs.

ASACOL HD – mesalamine RX

Class: 5-aminosalicylic acid derivative

ADULT DOSAGE
Ulcerative Colitis
Moderately Active:
Usual: Two 800mg tabs tid for 6 weeks

PEDIATRIC DOSAGE
Pediatric use may not have been established

ADMINISTRATION
Oral route

Swallow tab whole; do not cut, break, or chew
Take with or without food

HOW SUPPLIED
Tab, Delayed-Release: 800mg

WARNINGS/PRECAUTIONS
Renal impairment, including minimal change nephropathy, acute and chronic interstitial nephritis, and, rarely, renal failure reported; evaluate renal function prior to therapy and periodically thereafter. Has been associated with an acute intolerance syndrome that may be difficult to distinguish from an exacerbation of UC. Exacerbation of symptoms of colitis reported; symptoms usually abate when therapy is discontinued. Patients with sulfasalazine hypersensitivity may have similar reaction to therapy. Mesalamine-induced cardiac hypersensitivity reactions (myocarditis and pericarditis) reported; caution with conditions that predispose to the development of myocarditis or pericarditis. Hepatic failure reported in patients with preexisting liver disease; caution with liver disease. Organic or functional obstruction in the upper GI tract may cause prolonged gastric retention of the drug, which could delay the release of mesalamine in the colon. Caution in elderly.

ADVERSE REACTIONS
Headache.

DRUG INTERACTIONS
Known nephrotoxic agents, including NSAIDs, may increase the risk of renal reactions. Azathioprine or 6-mercaptopurine may increase the risk for blood disorders.

NURSING CONSIDERATIONS

Assessment: Assess for hypersensitivity to sulfasalazine, salicylates, or aminosalicylates; conditions that predispose to the development of myocarditis or pericarditis; organic or functional obstruction in the upper GI tract; hepatic impairment; pregnancy/nursing status; and possible drug interactions. Evaluate renal function prior to initiation of therapy.

Monitoring: Monitor for acute intolerance syndrome, exacerbation of symptoms of colitis, myocarditis, pericarditis, hepatic failure, hypersensitivity reactions, and other adverse reactions. Perform periodic monitoring of renal function. Monitor blood cell counts in elderly patients.

Patient Counseling: Instruct to swallow tabs whole and not to break, cut, or chew tabs. Advise to d/c previous oral mesalamine therapy and follow dosing instructions if switching therapy. Instruct to contact physician if intact, partially intact, and/or tab shells are seen in stool repeatedly. Advise pregnant and breastfeeding women, or women of childbearing potential that the medication contains dibutyl phthalate, which is excreted in breast milk and could possibly cause fetal malformations. Instruct to leave any desiccant pouches present in the bottle.

Storage: 20-25°C (68-77°F); excursions permitted 15-30°C (59-86°F). Protect from moisture.

ASMANEX – mometasone furoate — RX

Class: Corticosteroid

ADULT DOSAGE

Asthma

Maint Treatment of Asthma as Prophylactic Therapy:

Previous Therapy:
Bronchodilators Alone or Inhaled Corticosteroids:
Initial: 220mcg qpm
Titrate: Higher doses may provide additional control if inadequate response after 2 weeks of therapy; adjust to lowest effective dose once asthma stability is achieved
Max: 440mcg qpm or 220mcg bid

Oral Corticosteroids:
Initial: 440mcg bid
Titrate: Higher doses may provide additional control if inadequate response after 2 weeks of therapy; adjust to lowest effective dose once asthma stability is achieved
Max: 880mcg/day

PEDIATRIC DOSAGE

Asthma

Maint Treatment of Asthma as Prophylactic Therapy:

4-11 Years:
Initial/Max: 110mcg qpm

≥12 Years:
Previous Therapy:
Bronchodilators Alone or Inhaled Corticosteroids:
Initial: 220mcg qpm
Titrate: Higher doses may provide additional control if inadequate response after 2 weeks of therapy; adjust to lowest effective dose once asthma stability is achieved
Max: 440mcg qpm or 220mcg bid

Oral Corticosteroids:
Initial: 440mcg bid
Titrate: Higher doses may provide additional control if inadequate response after 2 weeks of therapy; adjust to lowest effective dose once asthma stability is achieved
Max: 880mcg/day

ADMINISTRATION

Orally inhaled powder

When administered qd, Asmanex should be taken only in the pm
Inhale rapidly and deeply
Rinse mouth after inh

HOW SUPPLIED

Powder, Inhalation: 110mcg/actuation, 220mcg/actuation

CONTRAINDICATIONS

Primary treatment of status asthmaticus or other acute episodes of asthma where intensive measures are required. Hypersensitivity to milk proteins.

WARNINGS/PRECAUTIONS

Not for the relief of acute bronchospasm. Localized *Candida albicans* infections of the mouth and pharynx reported; treat accordingly or interrupt therapy if needed. D/C if hypersensitivity reactions occur. Contains small amount of lactose that contains milk proteins; anaphylactic reactions with milk protein allergy reported. May increase susceptibility to infections; caution with active or quiescent tuberculosis (TB) infection, untreated systemic fungal, bacterial, viral, or parasitic infections, or ocular herpes simplex. Avoid exposure to chickenpox and measles. Deaths due to adrenal insufficiency have occurred with transfer from systemic to inhaled corticosteroids; wean slowly from systemic corticosteroid therapy. Resume oral corticosteroids immediately during periods of stress or severe asthma attack. Transferring from systemic corticosteroid may unmask allergic conditions (eg, rhinitis, conjunctivitis, eczema, arthritis, eosinophilic conditions). Monitor for systemic corticosteroid effects, such as hypercorticism and adrenal suppression; reduce dose slowly when the effects occur. Prolonged use may result in decrease of bone mineral density (BMD); caution in patients at risk (eg, prolonged immobilization, family history of osteoporosis, chronic use of drugs that reduce bone mass [eg, anticonvulsants, corticosteroids]). May cause reduction in growth velocity in pediatric patients; monitor growth routinely. Glaucoma, increased IOP, and cataracts reported. Bronchospasm may occur with an increase in wheezing after dosing; d/c treatment and institute alternative therapy.

ADVERSE REACTIONS

Headache, allergic rhinitis, pharyngitis, URTI, sinusitis, oral candidiasis, dysmenorrhea, musculoskeletal pain, back pain, dyspepsia, myalgia, abdominal pain, nausea.

DRUG INTERACTIONS

Ketoconazole may increase plasma levels.

NURSING CONSIDERATIONS

Assessment: Assess for status asthmaticus, acute asthma episodes, known hypersensitivity to milk proteins or to any drug component, risk factors for decreased BMD, history of increased IOP/glaucoma/cataracts, active or quiescent pulmonary TB, ocular herpes simplex, untreated systemic infections, chickenpox, measles, pregnancy/nursing status, and possible drug interactions.

Monitoring: Monitor for localized infections of mouth and pharynx with *C. albicans*, decreased BMD, asthma instability, growth in pediatrics routinely, development of glaucoma, increased IOP, cataracts, change in vision, hypercorticism, signs and symptoms of adrenal insufficiency, paradoxical bronchospasm, hypersensitivity reactions, and immunosuppression. Monitor for lung function, β-agonist use, and asthma symptoms during withdrawal of oral corticosteroids

Patient Counseling: Advise that localized infection with *C. albicans* may occur in mouth and pharynx; instruct to rinse mouth after inhalation. Inform that therapy should not be used to treat status asthmaticus or to relieve acute asthma symptoms. Counsel to d/c if hypersensitivity reactions occur. Advise to avoid exposure to chickenpox or measles and to seek medical attention if exposed. Inform of potential worsening of existing TB, other infections, or ocular herpes simplex. Inform that drug may cause systemic corticosteroid effects of hypercorticism and adrenal suppression, may reduce BMD, and may cause reduction in growth rate (pediatrics). Advise to take ud, to use medication at regular intervals, and to contact physician if symptoms do not improve or if condition worsens. Instruct on proper administration procedures and on when to discard inhaler.

Storage: 25°C (77°F); excursions permitted to 15-30°C (59-86°F). Store in dry place. Discard inhaler 45 days after opening foil pouch or when dose counter reads "00," whichever comes 1st.

ASTELIN – azelastine hydrochloride **RX**

Class: H_1-antagonist

ADULT DOSAGE

Vasomotor Rhinitis

2 sprays/nostril bid

Seasonal Allergic Rhinitis

1-2 sprays/nostril bid

PEDIATRIC DOSAGE

Vasomotor Rhinitis

≥12 Years:
2 sprays/nostril bid

Seasonal Allergic Rhinitis

5-11 Years:
1 spray/nostril bid

≥12 Years:
1-2 sprays/nostril bid

DOSE MODIFICATION

Elderly

Start at lower end of dosing range

ADMINISTRATION

Intranasal route

Priming

Prime before initial use by releasing 4 sprays or until a fine mist appears
When not used for ≥3 days, reprime w/ 2 sprays or until a fine mist appears

HOW SUPPLIED

Spray: 137mcg/spray [30mL]

WARNINGS/PRECAUTIONS

Occurrence of somnolence reported. May impair physical/mental abilities. Caution in elderly.

ADVERSE REACTIONS

Bitter taste, headache, somnolence, dysesthesia, rhinitis, cough, conjunctivitis, asthma, epistaxis, sinusitis, nasal burning, pharyngitis, paroxysmal sneezing.

DRUG INTERACTIONS
Avoid alcohol or other CNS depressants; additional reductions in alertness and CNS performance impairment may occur.

NURSING CONSIDERATIONS

Assessment: Assess for pregnancy/nursing status and possible drug interactions.

Monitoring: Monitor for somnolence and other adverse reactions.

Patient Counseling: Instruct to use only as prescribed. Caution patients against engaging in hazardous occupations requiring complete mental alertness and motor coordination (eg, driving a car or operating machinery). Instruct to avoid concurrent use with alcohol or other CNS depressants because additional reductions in alertness or CNS performance impairment may occur. Inform that therapy may lead to adverse reactions (eg, bitter taste, headache, somnolence). Instruct to consult physician if pregnant/nursing or planning to become pregnant. Instruct to keep out of reach of children and to seek medical help or call a poison control center immediately if a child accidentally ingests the medication.

Storage: 20-25°C (68-77°F). Store upright. Protect from freezing.

ASTEPRO – azelastine hydrochloride RX

Class: H_1-antagonist

ADULT DOSAGE

Seasonal/Perennial Allergic Rhinitis

Seasonal Allergic Rhinitis:
0.1%, 0.15%:
Usual: 1 or 2 sprays/nostril bid or 2 sprays (0.15%)/nostril qd

Perennial Allergic Rhinitis:
0.15%:
Usual: 2 sprays/nostril bid

PEDIATRIC DOSAGE

Seasonal/Perennial Allergic Rhinitis

Seasonal Allergic Rhinitis:
2-5 Years:
0.1%:
Usual: 1 spray/nostril bid
6-11 Years:
0.1%, 0.15%:
Usual: 1 spray/nostril bid

≥12 Years:
0.1%, 0.15%:
Usual: 1 or 2 sprays/nostril bid or 2 sprays (0.15%)/nostril qd

Perennial Allergic Rhinitis:
6 Months-5 Years:
0.1%:
Usual: 1 spray/nostril bid
6-11 Years:
0.1%, 0.15%:
Usual: 1 spray/nostril bid

≥12 Years:
0.15%:
Usual: 2 sprays/nostril bid

DOSE MODIFICATION
Elderly
Start at lower end of dosing range

ADMINISTRATION
Intranasal route
Avoid spraying into eyes
Discard after 200 sprays have been used

Priming
Prime before initial use by releasing 6 sprays or until a fine mist appears
When not used for ≥3 days, reprime w/ 2 sprays or until a fine mist appears

HOW SUPPLIED
Spray: 0.1%, 0.15% [30mL]

WARNINGS/PRECAUTIONS
Somnolence reported. May impair mental/physical abilities. Caution in elderly.

ADVERSE REACTIONS
Bitter taste, nasal discomfort, headache, sinusitis, epistaxis, dysgeusia, URI, sneezing, cough, rhinalgia, vomiting, otitis media, contact dermatitis, oropharyngeal pain.

DRUG INTERACTIONS

Avoid w/ alcohol or other CNS depressants; additional reductions in alertness and additional impairment of CNS performance may occur. Cimetidine increased levels of orally administered azelastine.

NURSING CONSIDERATIONS

Assessment: Assess pregnancy/nursing status and for possible drug interactions.

Monitoring: Monitor for somnolence and other adverse reactions.

Patient Counseling: Caution against engaging in hazardous occupations requiring complete mental alertness and motor coordination (eg, driving, operating machinery). Advise to avoid alcohol or other CNS depressants. Inform that treatment may lead to adverse reactions, the most common of which include pyrexia, dysgeusia, nasal discomfort, epistaxis, headache, sneezing, fatigue, somnolence, URI, cough, rhinalgia, vomiting, otitis media, contact dermatitis, and oropharyngeal pain. Advise to avoid spraying into eyes.

Storage: 20-25°C (68-77°F). Protect from freezing.

ASTRAMORPH PF – morphine sulfate CII

Class: Opioid analgesic

Risk of severe adverse effects with epidural or intrathecal route; observe patients in a fully equipped and staffed environment for at least 24 hrs after initial dose. Naloxone inj and resuscitative equipment should be immediately available in case of life-threatening or intolerable side effects and whenever therapy is initiated. Intrathecal dosage is usually 1/10 that of epidural dosage. Remove any contaminated clothing and rinse affected area with water if accidental dermal exposure occurs. Associated with risk of overdosage, diversion, and abuse; special measures must be taken to control this product within the hospital/clinic. Do not use if color is darker than pale yellow, discolored in any other way, or if it contains a precipitate.

ADULT DOSAGE

Pain

Unresponsive to Non-Narcotic Analgesics:
IV:
Initial: 2-10mg/70kg

Epidural:
Initial: 5mg in the lumbar region
If adequate pain relief is not achieved w/in 1 hr, may give incremental doses of 1-2mg at intervals sufficient to assess effectiveness
Max: 10mg/24 hrs

Continuous Infusion:
Initial: 2-4mg/24 hrs
May give additional 1-2mg if pain is not relieved initially

Intrathecal:
Usual: Single 0.2-1mg dose
Do not inject more than 2mL of the 5mg/10mL ampule or 1mL of the 10mg/10mL ampule
Repeat intrathecal inj not recommended; use alternative routes if pain recurs

PEDIATRIC DOSAGE

Pediatric use may not have been established

ADMINISTRATION

IV/Epidural/Intrathecal route

Proper placement of a needle or catheter in the epidural space should be verified before inj
Limit administration by epidural/intrathecal routes to lumbar area

Intrathecal
May administer a constant IV infusion of 0.6mg/hr naloxone for 24 hrs after intrathecal inj to reduce incidence of potential side effects

HOW SUPPLIED

Inj: 0.5mg/mL [2mL, 10mL], 1mg/mL [2mL, 10mL]

CONTRAINDICATIONS

Medical conditions that would preclude the administration of opioids by the IV route (acute bronchial asthma, upper airway obstruction).

WARNINGS/PRECAUTIONS

May be habit-forming. Administration should be limited to use by those familiar with respiratory depression management. Rapid IV administration may result in chest wall rigidity. Prior to any epidural or intrathecal administration, assess for patient conditions (eg, infection at the inj site, bleeding diathesis, anticoagulant therapy) that call for special evaluation of the benefit versus risk potential. Should be administered by or under the direction of a physician experienced in the techniques and familiar with the patient management problems associated with epidural or intrathecal administration. Severe respiratory depression up to 24 hrs following epidural/intrathecal administration reported. Unusual acceleration of neuraxial morphine requirements may occur, which may cause concern regarding systemic absorption and the hazards of large doses; patients may benefit from hospitalization and detoxification. Myoclonic-like spasm of the lower extremities reported with intrathecal doses of >20mg/day; after detoxification, it might be possible to resume treatment at lower doses. Intrathecal route has higher incidence of respiratory depression than epidural route. Seizures may result from high doses; caution with known seizure disorders. Extreme caution with head injury or increased intracranial pressure; pupillary changes (miosis) may obscure the existence, extent, and course of intracranial pathology. High neuraxial doses may produce myoclonic events. Maintain a high index of suspicion for adverse drug reactions when evaluating altered mental status or movement abnormalities. Caution with decreased respiratory reserve. Avoid with chronic asthma, upper airway obstruction, or in any other chronic pulmonary disorder. Use caution when administering epidurally to patients with reduced metabolic rates and with hepatic and/or renal dysfunction. Smooth muscle hypertonicity may result in biliary colic. Initiation of neuraxial opiate analgesia is frequently associated with micturition disturbances, especially in males with prostatic enlargement. Monitor patients with reduced circulating blood volume or impaired myocardial function for possible occurrence of orthostatic hypotension. May cause severe hypotension when ability to maintain BP has already been compromised by a depleted blood volume. Avoid abrupt withdrawal. Caution in elderly.

ADVERSE REACTIONS

Respiratory depression/arrest, convulsions, dysphoric reactions, toxic psychoses, pruritus, urinary retention, constipation, lumbar puncture-type headache.

DRUG INTERACTIONS

CNS depressants (eg, alcohol, sedatives, antihistamines, psychotropic drugs) potentiate depressant effects. Neuroleptics may increase risk of respiratory depression. Monitor for possible occurrence of orthostatic hypotension in patients on sympatholytic drugs. May cause severe hypotension with concurrent administration of drugs such as phenothiazines or general anesthetics.

NURSING CONSIDERATIONS

Assessment: Assess for patient's general condition and medical status, renal/hepatic impairment, hypersensitivity to drug, any other conditions where treatment is contraindicated or cautioned, pregnancy/nursing status, and possible drug interactions.

Monitoring: Monitor for signs/symptoms of respiratory depression, seizures, myoclonic events, biliary colic, urinary retention, orthostatic hypotension, drug abuse/dependence, and other adverse reactions.

Patient Counseling: Inform about risks and benefits of therapy. Inform of adverse reactions that may occur. Instruct to inform physician of other medications being taken. Inform that medication has potential for abuse and dependence.

Storage: 20-25°C (68-77°F). Protect from light. Do not freeze. Do not heat-sterilize.

ATACAND – candesartan cilexetil **RX**

Class: Angiotensin II receptor antagonist

D/C when pregnancy is detected. Drugs that act directly on the renin-angiotensin system (RAS) can cause injury/death to the developing fetus.

ADULT DOSAGE

Hypertension

Initial: 16mg qd
Usual: 8-32mg/day given qd or bid
May add diuretic if BP not controlled

Heart Failure

Heart failure (NYHA Class II-IV) w/ Left Ventricular Systolic Dysfunction (Ejection Fraction <40):
Initial: 4mg qd
Titrate: Double the dose at 2-week intervals, as tolerated, to the target dose of 32mg qd

PEDIATRIC DOSAGE

Hypertension

1-<6 Years:
Initial: 0.20mg/kg (Sus)
Usual: 0.05-0.4mg/kg/day
6-<17 Years:
<50kg:
Initial: 4-8mg
Usual: 2-16mg/day
>50kg:
Initial: 8-16mg
Usual: 4-32mg/day
May be administered qd or divided into 2 equal doses

DOSE MODIFICATION

Hepatic Impairment

Moderate:

Initial: 8mg

Other Important Modifications

Intravascular Volume Depletion in Pediatric Patients:

Consider initiating at a lower dose

ADMINISTRATION

Oral route

Take w/ or w/o food

For children who cannot swallow tabs, sus may be substituted

Sus

Use w/in 30 days after 1st opening

Shake well before each use

Preparation of Sus

The number of tabs and volume of vehicle specified below will yield 160mL of a 1mg/mL sus

1. Prepare the vehicle by adding equal volumes of Ora-Plus (80mL) and Ora-Sweet SF (80mL) or, alternatively, use Ora-Blend SF (160mL)
2. Add a small amount of vehicle to the required number of Atacand tabs (five 32mg tabs) and grind into a smooth paste using a mortar and pestle
3. Add the paste to a preparation vessel of suitable size
4. Rinse the mortar and pestle clean using the vehicle and add this to the vessel. Repeat, if necessary
5. Prepare the final volume by adding the remaining vehicle
6. Mix thoroughly and dispense into suitably sized amber PET bottles
7. Label with an expiration date of 100 days

HOW SUPPLIED

Tab: 4mg*, 8mg*, 16mg*, 32mg* *scored

CONTRAINDICATIONS

Coadministration w/ aliskiren in patients w/ diabetes.

WARNINGS/PRECAUTIONS

Symptomatic hypotension may occur in patients who have been volume- and/or salt-depleted (eg, prolonged diuretic therapy, dietary salt restriction, dialysis, diarrhea, vomiting); correct volume and/or salt depletion prior to therapy and temporary dose reduction of candesartan, diuretic, or both may be required. Hypotension may occur during major surgery and anesthesia. Renal function changes may occur. Oliguria, progressive azotemia or acute renal failure may occur in patients whose renal function is dependent on the RAS (eg, severe HF, renal artery stenosis, volume depletion); consider withholding or discontinuing therapy if clinically significant decrease in renal function develops. May cause hyperkalemia. Do not give to pediatric patients w/ GFR <30mL/min.

ADVERSE REACTIONS

URTI, dizziness, back pain.

DRUG INTERACTIONS

See Contraindications. Dual blockade of the RAS is associated w/ increased risk of hypotension, hyperkalemia, and changes in renal function (eg, acute renal failure); closely monitor BP, renal function, and electrolytes w/ concomitant agents that also affect the RAS. Do not coadminister aliskiren in patients w/ renal impairment (GFR <60mL/min). NSAIDs, (eg, selective COX-2 inhibitors), may deteriorate renal function and attenuate the antihypertensive effect; monitor renal function periodically. Increased lithium levels and toxicity reported; monitor serum lithium levels.

NURSING CONSIDERATIONS

Assessment: Assess for hypersensitivity to drug, volume/salt depletion, HF, hepatic/renal impairment, pregnancy/nursing status, and possible drug interactions.

Monitoring: Monitor for signs/symptoms of hypotension, renal function changes, and other adverse reactions. Monitor serum K^+ periodically and BP during dose escalation and periodically thereafter.

Patient Counseling: Inform of risks/benefits of therapy. Inform of pregnancy risks; instruct to notify physician as soon as possible if pregnant.

Storage: 25°C (77°F); excursions permitted to 15-30°C (59-86°F). (Sus) <30°C (86°F). Do not freeze.

ATACAND HCT – candesartan cilexetil/hydrochlorothiazide RX

Class: Angiotensin II receptor antagonist/thiazide diuretic

D/C when pregnancy is detected. Drugs that act directly on the renin-angiotensin system (RAS) can cause injury/death to developing fetus.

ADULT DOSAGE

Hypertension

Usual:

16-32mg candesartan/12.5-25mg HCTZ PO qd

Replacement Therapy:

May be substituted for its titrated components

PEDIATRIC DOSAGE

Pediatric use may not have been established

ADMINISTRATION

Oral route

Take w/ or w/o food

HOW SUPPLIED

Tab: (Candesartan-HCTZ) 16mg-12.5mg*, 32mg-12.5mg*, 32mg-25mg* *scored

CONTRAINDICATIONS

Anuria, hypersensitivity to other sulfonamide-derived drugs. Coadministration with aliskiren in patients with diabetes.

WARNINGS/PRECAUTIONS

Not for initial therapy. Not recommended for initiation with moderate to severe hepatic impairment. Symptomatic hypotension may occur in patients who have been volume- and/or Na^+-depleted (eg, prolonged diuretic therapy, dietary salt restriction, dialysis, diarrhea, vomiting); correct volume and/or salt depletion prior to therapy and may require temporary dose reduction. May cause excessive hypotension leading to oliguria, azotemia, and (rarely) with acute renal failure and death in patients with heart failure (HF); monitor closely for the first 2 weeks of therapy and whenever dose is increased. Oliguria, progressive azotemia, or acute renal failure may occur in patients whose renal function is dependent on the RAS (eg, severe HF, renal artery stenosis, chronic kidney disease, volume depletion); consider withholding or discontinuing therapy if clinically significant decrease in renal function develops. Caution with severe renal disease; dosing recommendations in patients with CrCl <30mL/min cannot be provided. Caution with hepatic impairment or progressive liver disease; may precipitate hepatic coma. HCTZ: May cause hypokalemia and hyponatremia; monitor serum electrolytes periodically. May cause idiosyncratic reaction, resulting in acute transient myopia and acute angle-closure glaucoma; d/c as rapidly as possible. May cause hypersensitivity reactions (with or without history of allergy or bronchial asthma), alter glucose tolerance, raise serum levels of cholesterol/TG/uric acid, cause/exacerbate hyperuricemia and precipitate gout, and exacerbate/activate systemic lupus erythematosus (SLE). May decrease urinary Ca^{2+} excretion and cause mild elevation of serum Ca^{2+}; avoid with hypercalcemia.

ADVERSE REACTIONS

Upper respiratory tract infection, back pain.

DRUG INTERACTIONS

See Contraindications. NSAIDs, including selective COX-2 inhibitors, may deteriorate renal function and attenuate the antihypertensive effect; monitor renal function periodically. May increase lithium levels and risk of lithium toxicity; monitor serum lithium levels. Candesartan: Dual blockade of the RAS is associated with increased risk of hypotension, hyperkalemia, and changes in renal function (including acute renal failure); closely monitor BP, renal function, and electrolytes with concomitant agents that also affect the RAS. Avoid with aliskiren in patients with renal impairment (GFR <60mL/min). HCTZ: Alcohol, barbiturates, or narcotics may potentiate orthostatic hypotension. Dose adjustment of antidiabetic drugs (oral agents and insulin) may be required. Single doses of either cholestyramine or colestipol resins may impair absorption; administer therapy at least 4 hrs before or 4-6 hrs after administration of resins. May increase responsiveness to nondepolarizing skeletal muscle relaxants (eg, tubocurarine). Thiazide-induced hypokalemia or hypomagnesemia may predispose to digoxin toxicity.

NURSING CONSIDERATIONS

Assessment: Assess for hypersensitivity to the drugs and their components, anuria, sulfonamide-derived drug hypersensitivity, history of penicillin allergy, volume/salt depletion, SLE, diabetes, HF, hepatic/renal impairment, renal artery stenosis, pregnancy/nursing status, and possible drug interactions.

Monitoring: Monitor for signs/symptoms of fluid/electrolyte imbalance, exacerbation or activation of SLE, hypotension, hypersensitivity reactions, idiosyncratic reaction, renal function changes, and other adverse reactions. Monitor BP and serum electrolytes periodically.

Patient Counseling: Inform females of childbearing potential of the consequences of exposure during pregnancy and of the treatment options for women planning to become pregnant; instruct to notify physician as soon as possible if pregnant. Inform that lightheadedness may occur, especially during the 1st days of therapy; instruct to d/c therapy if syncope occurs and seek consult. Caution that inadequate fluid intake, excessive perspiration, diarrhea, or vomiting may lead to an excessive fall in BP, with the same consequences of lightheadedness and possible syncope. Instruct not to use K^+ supplements or salt substitutes containing K^+ without consulting physician.

Storage: 25°C (77°F); excursions permitted to 15-30°C (59-86°F).

ATELVIA – risedronate sodium RX

Class: Bisphosphonate

ADULT DOSAGE

Postmenopausal Osteoporosis

1 tab once a week

Periodically reevaluate the need for continued therapy

PEDIATRIC DOSAGE

Pediatric use may not have been established

ADMINISTRATION

Oral route

Take in the am immediately following breakfast

Swallow tabs whole in upright position with ≥4 oz. of plain water. Avoid lying down for 30 min after taking medication

Do not chew, cut, or crush

Instruct patient to supplement Ca^{2+} and vitamin D if dietary intake is inadequate

HOW SUPPLIED

Tab, Delayed-Release: 35mg

CONTRAINDICATIONS

Esophageal abnormalities that delay esophageal emptying (eg, stricture, achalasia), inability to stand or sit upright for at least 30 min, hypocalcemia.

WARNINGS/PRECAUTIONS

Consider discontinuation after 3-5 yrs of use in patients at low-risk for fracture; periodically reevaluate risk for fracture in patients who d/c therapy. Contains same active ingredient as Actonel; do not treat with Atelvia if on concomitant therapy with Actonel. May cause local irritation of the upper GI mucosa; caution with active upper GI problems (eg, Barrett's esophagus, dysphagia, other esophageal diseases, gastritis, duodenitis, ulcers). Esophageal reactions (eg, esophagitis, esophageal ulcers/erosions) reported; d/c if dysphagia, odynophagia, retrosternal pain, or new/worsening heartburn develops. Use therapy under appropriate supervision in patients who cannot comply with dosing instructions due to mental disability. Gastric and duodenal ulcers reported. Hypocalcemia reported; treat hypocalcemia and other disturbances of bone and mineral metabolism before therapy, and ensure adequate Ca^{2+} and vitamin D intake. Osteonecrosis of the jaw (ONJ) reported; risk may increase with duration of exposure to drug. If invasive dental procedures are required, discontinuation of treatment may reduce risk for ONJ. Consider discontinuation if ONJ develops. Severe and occasionally incapacitating bone, joint, and/or muscle pain reported; consider discontinuing use if severe symptoms develop. Atypical, low-energy, or low-trauma fractures of the femoral shaft reported; evaluate any patient with a history of bisphosphonate exposure who presents with thigh/groin pain to rule out incomplete femur fracture, and consider interruption of therapy. Not recommended with severe renal impairment (CrCl <30mL/min). May interfere with the use of bone-imaging agents.

ADVERSE REACTIONS

Diarrhea, influenza, arthralgia, back pain, abdominal pain, constipation, N/V, dyspepsia, bronchitis, upper respiratory tract infection, pain in extremity.

DRUG INTERACTIONS

Ca^{2+} supplements, antacids, Mg^{2+}-based supplements or laxatives, and iron preparations interfere with absorption; take such medications at a different time of the day. Drugs that raise stomach pH (eg, proton pump inhibitors [PPIs], H_2 blockers) may cause faster drug release from the enteric coating. Increased bioavailability with esomeprazole. Not recommended with H_2 blockers or PPIs. Upper GI adverse reactions reported with NSAIDs.

NURSING CONSIDERATIONS

Assessment: Assess for esophageal abnormalities, ability to stand or sit upright for at least 30 min, active upper GI problems, mental disability, hypocalcemia, disturbances of bone and mineral metabolism, risk for ONJ, renal impairment, drug hypersensitivity, any other conditions where treatment is contraindicated or cautioned, pregnancy/nursing status, and possible drug interactions.

Monitoring: Monitor for signs/symptoms of esophageal reactions, hypocalcemia, ONJ, musculoskeletal pain, atypical femoral fractures, and other adverse events. Periodically reevaluate the need for continued therapy.

Patient Counseling: Instruct to pay particular attention to the dosing instructions. Advise to take in the am with at least 4 oz. of plain water immediately following breakfast. Advise to avoid lying down for 30 min after taking the drug. Advise to consult physician before continuing treatment if symptoms of esophageal disease develop. Instruct that if the once-weekly dose is missed, to take 1 tab on the am after they remember and to return to taking the dose, as originally scheduled on their chosen day; instruct not to take 2 tabs on the same day. Instruct to take supplemental Ca^{2+} and vitamin D if dietary intake is inadequate. Advise to consult physician any time they have a medical problem they think may be from treatment.

Storage: 20-25°C (68-77°F).

ATIVAN INJECTION – lorazepam CIV

Class: Benzodiazepine

ADULT DOSAGE

Status Epilepticus

4mg IV (given slowly at 2mg/min); may repeat 1 dose after 10-15 min if seizures recur or fail to cease

Preanesthetic

To produce sedation, anxiety relief, and to decrease ability to recall events related to the day of surgery

Usual:

IM:

0.05mg/kg given at least 2 hrs prior to anticipated operative procedure

IV:

2mg or 0.044mg/kg IV (whichever is smaller) 15-20 min prior to anticipated operative procedure

Max (IM/IV): 4mg

PEDIATRIC DOSAGE

Pediatric use may not have been established

DOSE MODIFICATION

Concomitant Medications

Probenecid or Valproate: Reduce lorazepam dose by 50%

Oral Contraceptives: May be necessary to increase lorazepam dose

Elderly

Start at the low end of the dosing range

ADMINISTRATION

IM/IV route

Can be used w/ atropine sulfate, narcotic analgesics, other parenterally used analgesics, commonly used anesthetics, and muscle relaxants

IM

Inject undiluted deep in muscle mass

IV

Must be diluted w/ an equal volume of compatible sol (Sterile Water for Inj, NaCl Inj, D5 Inj)

Mix thoroughly by gently inverting container repeatedly until a homogenous solution results; do not shake vigorously

When properly diluted, the drug may be injected directly into a vein or into the tubing of an existing IV infusion

Rate of inj should not exceed 2.0mg/min

HOW SUPPLIED

Inj: 2mg/mL, 4mg/mL [1mL, 10mL]

CONTRAINDICATIONS

Acute narrow-angle glaucoma, sleep apnea syndrome, severe respiratory insufficiency. Not for intra-arterial inj.

WARNINGS/PRECAUTIONS

May produce heavy sedation. Airway obstruction and respiratory depression may occur; ensure airway patency and monitor respiration. May impair mental/physical abilities. Avoid in patients with hepatic and/or renal failure; caution in patients with hepatic and/or renal impairment. May cause fetal damage during pregnancy. When used for peroral endoscopic procedures, adequate topical/regional anesthesia is recommended to minimize reflex activity. Extreme caution when administering inj to elderly, very ill, or to patients with limited pulmonary reserve; hypoventilation and/or hypoxic cardiac arrest may occur. Paradoxical reaction, propylene glycol toxicity (eg, lactic acidosis, hyperosmolality, hypotension) and polyethylene glycol toxicity (eg, acute tubular necrosis) reported; premature and low birth weight infants as well pediatric patients receiving high-doses may be at higher risk. Pediatric patients may exhibit sensitivity to benzyl alcohol; "gasping syndrome" associated with administration of IV sol containing benzyl alcohol in neonates. Repeated doses over a prolonged period may result in physical and psychological dependence and withdrawal symptoms following abrupt discontinuation.

ADVERSE REACTIONS

Respiratory depression/failure, hypotension, somnolence, headache, hypoventilation, inj-site reactions, paradoxical excitement.

DRUG INTERACTIONS

Additive CNS depression with other CNS depressants (eg, ethyl alcohol, phenothiazines, barbiturates, MAOIs, antidepressants). Increased sedation, hallucinations, and irrational behavior with scopolamine. Reduce dose by 50% when given in combination with valproate or probenecid due to decreased clearance. Increased clearance with oral contraceptives. Severe adverse effects with clozapine, loxapine, and haloperidol reported. Prolonged and profound effect with concomitant sedatives, tranquilizers, narcotic analgesics.

NURSING CONSIDERATIONS

Assessment: Perform a comprehensive review of benefits/risks in status epilepticus. Assess for hypersensitivity to benzodiazepine or its vehicle, acute-angle glaucoma, preexisting respiratory impairment, hepatic/renal impairment, pregnancy/nursing status, and possible drug interactions.

Monitoring: Monitor for respiratory depression, airway obstruction, heavy sedation, drowsiness, excessive sleepiness, hypoglycemia and hyponatremia in status epilepticus, seizures, myoclonus, somnolence, inj-site reactions, and paradoxical reactions. Monitor for signs of toxicity to the vehicle's components (eg, lactic acidosis, hyperosmolarity, hypotension, acute tubular necrosis). Monitor for hypersensitivity reactions.

Patient Counseling: Inform of risks/benefits. Advise to use caution with hazardous tasks. Instruct to not get out of bed unassisted. Advise to avoid alcoholic beverages for at least 24-48 hrs after receiving drug. Advise about potential for physical/psychological dependence and withdrawal symptoms.

Storage: Refrigerate; protect from light.

ATRIPLA – efavirenz/emtricitabine/tenofovir disoproxil fumarate RX

Class: Non-nucleoside reverse transcriptase inhibitor/nucleoside analogue combination

Lactic acidosis and severe hepatomegaly w/ steatosis, including fatal cases, reported w/ the use of nucleoside analogues. Not approved for the treatment of chronic hepatitis B virus (HBV) infection. Severe acute exacerbations of hepatitis B reported in patients coinfected w/ HBV upon discontinuation of therapy; closely monitor hepatic function for at least several months. If appropriate, initiation of antihepatitis B therapy may be warranted.

ADULT DOSAGE

HIV-1 Infection

Alone/Combination w/ Other Antiretrovirals:
1 tab qd

PEDIATRIC DOSAGE

HIV-1 Infection

Alone/Combination w/ Other Antiretrovirals:
≥12 Years and ≥40kg:
1 tab qd

DOSE MODIFICATION

Concomitant Medications

Rifampin:
≥50kg: Additional 200mg/day of efavirenz is recommended

Renal Impairment

Moderate or Severe (CrCl <50mL/min): Not recommended for use

Hepatic Impairment

Moderate or Severe: Not recommended for use

ADMINISTRATION
Oral route
Take on an empty stomach
Bedtime dosing may improve tolerability of nervous system symptoms

HOW SUPPLIED
Tab: (Efavirenz-Emtricitabine-Tenofovir Disoproxil Fumarate [TDF]) 600mg-200mg-300mg

CONTRAINDICATIONS
Coadministration w/ voriconazole.

WARNINGS/PRECAUTIONS
Immune reconstitution syndrome and autoimmune disorders (eg, Graves' disease, polymyositis, Guillain-Barre syndrome) in the setting of immune reconstitution reported. Redistribution/accumulation of body fat has been observed. Caution in elderly. Efavirenz: Serious psychiatric adverse events and CNS symptoms reported. May impair mental/physical abilities. May cause fetal harm if administered during 1st trimester of pregnancy; avoid pregnancy during use. Use adequate contraceptive measures for 12 weeks after discontinuation. Skin rash reported; d/c if severe rash associated w/ blistering, desquamation, mucosal involvement, or fever develops. Consider alternative therapy in patients who have had a life-threatening cutaneous reaction (eg, Stevens-Johnson syndrome). Convulsions reported; caution w/ history of seizures. TDF: Obesity and prolonged nucleoside exposure may be risk factors for lactic acidosis and severe hepatomegaly w/ steatosis. Caution w/ known risk factors for liver disease. D/C if lactic acidosis or pronounced hepatotoxicity occurs. Renal impairment reported. Decreased bone mineral density (BMD), increased biochemical markers of bone metabolism, and osteomalacia reported; consider assessment of BMD in patients w/ history of pathologic bone fracture or other risk factors for osteoporosis or bone loss. Arthralgias and muscle pain/weakness reported in cases of proximal renal tubulopathy. Consider hypophosphatemia and osteomalacia secondary to proximal renal tubulopathy in patients at risk of renal dysfunction who present w/ persistent or worsening bone or muscle symptoms.

ADVERSE REACTIONS
Lactic acidosis, severe hepatomegaly w/ steatosis, diarrhea, nausea, fatigue, depression, dizziness, sinusitis, URTI, rash, headache, insomnia, abnormal dreams, anxiety, nasopharyngitis.

DRUG INTERACTIONS
See Contraindications. Avoid w/ adefovir dipivoxil, atazanavir, drugs containing same component or lamivudine, other NNRTIs, boceprevir, posaconazole, or nephrotoxic agents (eg, high dose or multiple NSAIDs). Potential additive CNS effects w/ alcohol or psychoactive drugs. May increase levels of didanosine and ritonavir (RTV). May decrease levels of amprenavir, lopinavir, saquinavir, raltegravir, telaprevir, bupropion, sertraline, itraconazole, ketoconazole, clarithromycin, rifabutin, diltiazem or other calcium channel blockers, atorvastatin, pravastatin, simvastatin, indinavir, maraviroc, carbamazepine, anticonvulsants, norelgestromin, levonorgestrel, etonogestrel, immunosuppressants, and methadone. May decrease levels of artemether, dihydroartemisinin, and/or lumefantrine resulting in a decrease antimalarial efficacy of arthemether/lumefantrine; use w/ caution. May alter levels of warfarin and substrates of CYP2C9, 2C19, 3A4, or 2B6. Efavirenz: RTV may increase levels. Telaprevir, carbamazepine, anticonvulsants, rifabutin, and rifampin may decrease levels. CYP3A substrates, inhibitors, or inducers may alter levels. May alter plasma levels of drugs metabolized by CYP3A or CYP2B6. TDF/Emtricitabine: Coadministration of drugs that reduce renal function or compete for active tubular secretion (eg, acyclovir, adefovir dipivoxil, cidofovir, ganciclovir, valacyclovir, valganciclovir, aminoglycosides [eg, gentamicin], and high-dose or multiple NSAIDs) may increase levels of emtricitabine, TDF, and/or other renally eliminated drugs. Darunavir w/ RTV and lopinavir/RTV may increase TDF levels. An increase in absorption may be observed when TDF is coadministered w/ an inhibitor of P-gp or breast cancer resistance protein. Refer to PI for further information on drug interactions.

NURSING CONSIDERATIONS

Assessment: Assess for obesity, prolonged nucleoside exposure, liver dysfunction or risk factors for liver disease, renal dysfunction, HBV infection, psychiatric history, history of injection drug use/seizures/cutaneous reaction, drug hypersensitivity, pregnancy/nursing status, and possible drug interactions. Assess BMD in patients w/ a history of pathological bone fracture or w/ other risk factors for osteoporosis or bone loss. Assess estimated CrCl, serum P, urine glucose and urine protein in patients at risk for renal dysfunction.

Monitoring: Monitor for signs/symptoms of lactic acidosis, severe hepatomegaly w/ steatosis, psychiatric/nervous system symptoms, new onset/worsening renal impairment, decreased BMD, increased biochemical markers for bone metabolism, osteomalacia, convulsions, immune reconstitution syndrome (eg, opportunistic infections), fat redistribution/accumulation, skin rash, and other adverse reactions. Monitor for acute exacerbations of hepatitis B in patients w/ coinfection upon discontinuation of therapy. Monitor LFTs. Monitor estimated CrCl, serum P, urine glucose, and urine protein periodically in patients at risk for renal dysfunction.

Patient Counseling: Inform that therapy is not a cure for HIV-1 infection and illnesses associated w/ HIV-1 infection may still be experienced. Advise to practice safe sex, use latex or polyurethane condoms, not to share personal items (eg, toothbrush, razor blades), needles, or other inj equipment, and not to breastfeed. Instruct to contact physician if N/V, unusual stomach discomfort, weakness, aggressive behavior, severe depression, suicide attempts, delusions, paranoia, psychosis-like symptoms, dizziness, insomnia, impaired concentration, drowsiness, abnormal dreams, or skin rash develops. Advise that fat redistribution/accumulation and decreases in BMD may occur. Counsel to avoid pregnancy while on therapy and use adequate contraceptive measures for 12 weeks after discontinuation; instruct that barrier contraception must always be used in combination w/ other methods of contraception. Advise to avoid potentially hazardous tasks if experiencing CNS/psychiatric symptoms or taking alcohol or psychoactive drugs. Advise that severe acute exacerbation of hepatitis B may occur if coinfected. Advise to report use of any prescription, nonprescription medication, vitamins and herbal supplements.

Storage: 25°C (77°F); excursions permitted to 15-30°C (59-86°F).

ATROVENT HFA – ipratropium bromide — RX

Class: Anticholinergic bronchodilator

ADULT DOSAGE

Chronic Obstructive Pulmonary Disease

Maint Treatment of Bronchospasm (eg, Chronic Bronchitis, Emphysema):
Initial: 2 inh qid; may take additional inh as required
Max: 12 inh/24 hrs

PEDIATRIC DOSAGE

Pediatric use may not have been established

ADMINISTRATION

Oral inh route

Priming

Prime inhaler before using for the 1st time or if inhaler has not been used for >3 days by releasing 2 test sprays into the air, away from the face

HOW SUPPLIED

MDI: 17mcg/inh [200 inhalations]

CONTRAINDICATIONS

Hypersensitivity to atropine or any of its derivatives.

WARNINGS/PRECAUTIONS

Not for initial treatment of acute episodes of bronchospasm. Hypersensitivity reactions and/or paradoxical bronchospasm may occur; d/c therapy and consider alternative treatment if these occur. May increase IOP, which may result in precipitation/worsening of narrow-angle glaucoma; caution with narrow-angle glaucoma. Avoid spraying in eyes. May cause urinary retention; caution with prostatic hyperplasia or bladder neck obstruction.

ADVERSE REACTIONS

Bronchitis, COPD exacerbation, sinusitis, UTI, influenza-like symptoms, dyspnea, back pain, dyspepsia, headache, dizziness, nausea, dry mouth.

DRUG INTERACTIONS

Avoid with other anticholinergic-containing drugs; may lead to an increase in anticholinergic adverse effects.

NURSING CONSIDERATIONS

Assessment: Assess for hypersensitivity to drug or to atropine or any of its derivatives, narrow-angle glaucoma, prostatic hyperplasia, bladder neck obstruction, pregnancy/nursing status, and possible drug interactions.

Monitoring: Monitor for hypersensitivity reactions, paradoxical bronchospasm, increased IOP, urinary retention, and other adverse reactions.

Patient Counseling: Inform that drug is not for initial treatment of acute episodes of bronchospasm where rescue therapy is required for rapid response. Instruct to d/c use if paradoxical bronchospasm occurs. Instruct to avoid spraying the aerosol into the eyes; advise to consult physician immediately if ocular effects develop. Inform that dizziness, accommodation disorder, mydriasis, and blurred vision may occur; caution about engaging in activities requiring balance and visual acuity (eg, driving, operating appliances/machinery). Advise to consult physician if experiencing difficulty with urination. Instruct to use consistently as prescribed throughout the course of therapy. Counsel not to increase the dose or frequency without consulting physician, and to seek immediate medical attention if treatment becomes less effective for symptomatic relief, symptoms become worse, and/or there is a need to use the product more frequently than usual. Advise on the use of medication in relation to other inhaled drugs.

Storage: 25°C (77°F); excursions permitted to 15-30°C (59-86°F). Do not puncture, use/store near heat or open flame, or throw into fire/incinerator. Exposure to temperatures >49°C (120°F) may cause bursting. Discard when indicator displays "0."

ATROVENT NASAL – ipratropium bromide RX

Class: Anticholinergic

ADULT DOSAGE

Rhinorrhea

Associated w/ Allergic and Nonallergic Perennial Rhinitis:
0.03%:
2 sprays/nostril bid-tid

Associated w/ Common Cold:
0.06%:
2 sprays/nostril tid-qid for ≤4 days

Associated w/ Seasonal Allergic Rhinitis:
0.06%:
2 sprays/nostril qid for ≤3 weeks

PEDIATRIC DOSAGE

Rhinorrhea

Associated w/ Allergic and Nonallergic Perennial Rhinitis:
0.03%:
≥6 Years:
2 sprays/nostril bid-tid

Associated w/ Common Cold:
0.06%:
5-11 Years:
2 sprays/nostril tid for ≤4 days
≥12 Years:
2 sprays/nostril tid-qid for ≤4 days

Associated w/ Seasonal Allergic Rhinitis:
0.06%:
≥5 Years:
2 sprays/nostril qid for ≤3 weeks

ADMINISTRATION

Intranasal route

Priming

Initially prime w/ 7 sprays
When not used for > 24 hrs, reprime w/ 2 sprays
When not used for >7 days, reprime w/ 7 sprays

HOW SUPPLIED

Spray: (0.03%) 21mcg/spray [31.1g], (0.06%) 42mcg/spray [16.6g]

CONTRAINDICATIONS

Hypersensitivity to atropine or its derivatives.

WARNINGS/PRECAUTIONS

Immediate hypersensitivity reactions reported; d/c at once if reaction occurs and consider alternative treatment. Caution with narrow-angle glaucoma, prostatic hyperplasia, bladder neck obstruction, and hepatic or renal insufficiency.

ADVERSE REACTIONS

Epistaxis, pharyngitis, URTI, nasal dryness, dry mouth/throat, headache, taste perversion.

DRUG INTERACTIONS

May produce additive effects with other anticholinergic agents.

NURSING CONSIDERATIONS

Assessment: Assess for hypersensitivity to atropine or its derivatives, narrow-angle glaucoma, prostatic hyperplasia, bladder-neck obstruction, hepatic/renal insufficiency, pregnancy/nursing status, and possible drug interactions.

Monitoring: Monitor for signs and symptoms of hypersensitivity reactions (eg, urticaria, angioedema, rash, bronchospasm, anaphylaxis, oropharyngeal edema). Monitor visual changes and nasal symptoms.

Patient Counseling: Advise not to alter size of nasal spray opening. Instruct to avoid spraying medication into the eyes. Inform that temporary blurring of vision, precipitation or worsening of narrow-angle glaucoma, mydriasis, increased IOP, acute eye pain or discomfort, visual halos, or colored images in association with red eyes from conjunctival and corneal congestion may occur if medication comes into direct contact with the eyes. Instruct to contact physician if eye pain, blurred vision, excessive nasal dryness, or episodes of nasal bleeding occur. Caution about engaging in activities requiring balance and visual acuity (eg, driving or operating machines).

Storage: 25°C (77°F); excursions permitted to 15-30°C (59-86°F). Avoid freezing.

AUBAGIO – teriflunomide

RX

Class: Pyrimidine synthesis inhibitor

Severe liver injury, including fatal liver failure, reported in patients treated with leflunomide; similar risk would be expected because recommended doses of teriflunomide and leflunomide result in a similar range of plasma concentrations of teriflunomide. Concomitant use with other potentially hepatotoxic drugs may increase risk of severe liver injury. Obtain transaminase and bilirubin levels within 6 months before initiation of therapy. Monitor ALT levels at least monthly for 6 months after starting therapy. D/C therapy and start an accelerated elimination procedure with cholestyramine or charcoal if drug-induced liver injury is suspected. Contraindicated in patients with severe hepatic impairment. Increased risk of developing elevated serum transaminases in patients with preexisting liver disease. May cause major birth defects if used during pregnancy. Contraindicated in pregnant women or women of childbearing potential who are not using reliable contraception. Avoid pregnancy during treatment or before completion of an accelerated elimination procedure after treatment.

ADULT DOSAGE

Multiple Sclerosis

Relapsing Forms:

Usual: 7mg or 14mg qd

PEDIATRIC DOSAGE

Pediatric use may not have been established

ADMINISTRATION

Oral route

May take w/ or w/o food

HOW SUPPLIED

Tab: 7mg, 14mg

CONTRAINDICATIONS

Severe hepatic impairment, women who are pregnant or of childbearing potential not using reliable contraception, concomitant use of leflunomide.

WARNINGS/PRECAUTIONS

Not for use with preexisting acute or chronic liver disease, or those with serum ALT >2X ULN before initiating therapy. Consider discontinuing therapy if serum transaminase >3X ULN. Consider additional monitoring if given with other potentially hepatotoxic drugs. Eliminated slowly from the plasma. An accelerated elimination procedure can be used at any time after discontinuation of therapy; refer to PI. Decrease in WBC count and platelet count reported; obtain CBC within 6 months before initiation of treatment, and base further monitoring on signs and symptoms of bone marrow suppression. Do not start treatment until the infection(s) is resolved with active acute or chronic infections. Consider suspending treatment and using an accelerated elimination procedure if serious infection develops. Not recommended with severe immunodeficiency, bone marrow disease, or severe, uncontrolled infections. May cause immunosuppression and increased susceptibility to infections. May increase risk of malignancy. Peripheral neuropathy reported; increased risk with age >60 yrs of age, concomitant neurotoxic medications, and diabetes. Consider discontinuing and performing an accelerated elimination procedure if peripheral neuropathy symptoms develop. Stevens-Johnson syndrome and toxic epidermal necrolysis may occur; d/c and perform an accelerated elimination procedure. HTN was reported. Interstitial lung disease (ILD) and worsening of preexisting ILD reported. New onset or worsening of pulmonary symptoms, with or without associated fever, may be a reason for discontinuation; consider initiation of an accelerated elimination procedure. Monitor for hematologic toxicity if switching to another agent with a known potential for hematologic suppression.

ADVERSE REACTIONS

Severe liver injury, headache, diarrhea, alopecia, nausea, ALT increased, paresthesia, arthralgia, neutropenia, HTN.

DRUG INTERACTIONS

See Boxed Warning and Contraindications. May increase exposure of drugs metabolized by CYP2C8 (eg, paclitaxel, pioglitazone, repaglinide, rosiglitazone). May decrease exposure of drugs metabolized by CYP1A2 substrates (eg, alosetron, duloxetine, theophylline, tizanidine). May increase exposure of organic anion transporter 3 (OAT3) substrates (eg, cefaclor, cimetidine, ciprofloxacin, furosemide, zidovudine). Monitor and adjust the dose of OAT3 substrates and drugs metabolized by CYP2C8/CYP1A2 as required. Vaccination with live vaccines is not recommended. Coadministration with warfarin requires close monitoring of the INR; may decrease peak INR of warfarin. May increase the systemic exposures of ethinyl estradiol and levonorgestrel; consider the type or dose of contraceptives to be used. Do not exceed rosuvastatin dose to 10mg qd if used concomitantly. Consider reducing the dose of other breast cancer resistance protein substrates (eg, mitoxantrone) and drugs in the organic anion transporting polypeptide family (eg, methotrexate, rifampin), especially HMG-CoA reductase inhibitors (eg, atorvastatin, nateglinide, pravastatin); monitor closely for signs and symptoms of increased exposures to the drugs while on therapy.

NURSING CONSIDERATIONS

Assessment: Assess for severe immunodeficiency, bone marrow disease, severe uncontrolled infections, ILD, hepatic impairment, diabetes, any other conditions where treatment is cautioned or contraindicated, pregnancy/nursing status, and for possible drug interactions. Obtain transaminase levels, bilirubin levels, and CBC within 6 months before initiation of therapy. Obtain BP. Screen for latent tuberculosis (TB) infection with a tuberculin skin test or blood test for mycobacterium TB infection.

Monitoring: Monitor for signs/symptoms of immunosuppression and infections, bone marrow suppression, severe liver injury, peripheral neuropathy, skin reactions, ILD, new onset or worsening of pulmonary symptoms, malignancy, and other adverse reactions. Monitor ALT levels at least monthly for 6 months after starting therapy. Monitor BP periodically thereafter.

Patient Counseling: Instruct to contact physician if unexplained N/V, abdominal pain, fatigue, anorexia, jaundice, dark urine, or symptoms of infection develop. Advise women of childbearing potential and men and their female partners to use effective contraception during and until completion of an accelerated elimination procedure. Instruct to immediately report pregnancy if suspected or confirmed. Advise that therapy may stay in the blood for up to 2 yrs after the last dose and that accelerated elimination procedure may be used if needed. Instruct to avoid some vaccines during treatment and for at least 6 months after discontinuation. Advise to contact physician if symptoms of peripheral neuropathy develop. Inform that treatment may increase BP. Advise to either d/c breastfeeding or d/c therapy.

Storage: 20-25°C (68-77°F); excursions permitted between 15-30°C (59-86°F).

AUGMENTIN — amoxicillin/clavulanate potassium **RX**

Class: Aminopenicillin/beta lactamase inhibitor

ADULT DOSAGE

General Dosing

Tab:
One 500mg tab q12h or one 250mg tab q8h

Severe Infections

Tab:
One 875mg tab q12h or one 500mg tab q8h

Respiratory Tract Infections

Tab:
One 875mg tab q12h or one 500mg tab q8h

PEDIATRIC DOSAGE

General Dosing

<12 Weeks of Age:
30mg/kg/day divided q12h (125mg/5mL sus)

Severe Infections

≥12 Weeks of Age:
45mg/kg/day q12h (200mg/5mL or 400mg/5mL sus; 200mg or 400mg chewable tab) or 40mg/kg/day q8h (125mg/5mL or 250mg/5mL sus; 125mg or 250mg chewable tab)

≥40kg:
Use adult dose

Less Severe Infections

≥12 Weeks of Age:
25mg/kg/day q12h (200mg/5mL or 400mg/5mL sus; 200mg or 400mg chewable tab) or 20mg/kg/day q8h (125mg/5mL or 250mg/5mL sus; 125mg or 250mg chewable tab)

≥40kg:
Use adult dose

Otitis Media

≥12 Weeks of Age:
45mg/kg/day q12h (200mg/5mL or 400mg/5mL sus; 200mg or 400mg chewable tab) or 40mg/kg/day q8h (125mg/5mL or 250mg/5mL sus; 125mg or 250mg chewable tab) for 10 days

≥40kg:
Use adult dose

Sinusitis

≥12 Weeks of Age:
45mg/kg/day q12h (200mg/5mL or 400mg/5mL sus; 200mg or 400mg chewable tab) or 40mg/kg/day q8h (125mg/5mL or

250mg/5mL sus; 125mg or 250mg chewable tab)

≥40kg:
Use adult dose

Lower Respiratory Tract Infections

≥12 Weeks of Age:
45mg/kg/day q12h (200mg/5mL or 400mg/5mL sus; 200mg or 400mg chewable tab) or 40mg/kg/day q8h (125mg/5mL or 250mg/5mL sus; 125mg or 250mg chewable tab)

≥40kg:
Use adult dose

DOSE MODIFICATION

Renal Impairment

GFR <30mL/min: Do not give the 875mg dose
GFR 10-30mL/min: 500mg or 250mg q12h
GFR <10mL/min: 500mg or 250mg q24h
Hemodialysis: 500mg or 250mg q24h; give additional dose during and at the end of dialysis

ADMINISTRATION

Oral route

Doses are based on amoxicillin component
Take w/ or w/o food
Take at start of a meal to reduce GI intolerance

Sus

Shake well before use
Refer to PI for mixing directions

Adults:
May use 125mg/5mL or 250mg/5mL sus in place of 500mg tab
May use 200mg/5mL or 400mg/5mL sus in place of 875mg tab

HOW SUPPLIED

(Amoxicillin-Clavulanic Acid) Sus: 125mg-31.25mg/5mL, 250mg-62.5mg/5mL [75mL, 100mL, 150mL], 200mg-28.5mg/5mL, 400mg-57mg/5mL [50mL, 75mL, 100mL]; Tab: 250mg-125mg, 500mg-125mg, 875mg-125mg*; Tab, Chewable: 125mg-31.25mg, 200mg-28.5mg, 250mg-62.5mg, 400mg-57mg *scored

CONTRAINDICATIONS

History of amoxicillin/clavulanate-associated cholestatic jaundice/hepatic dysfunction.

WARNINGS/PRECAUTIONS

Serious and occasionally fatal hypersensitivity (anaphylactic) reactions reported; d/c if an allergic reaction occurs and institute appropriate therapy. Hepatic dysfunction, including hepatitis and cholestatic jaundice, may occur. *Clostridium difficile*-associated diarrhea (CDAD) reported; d/c if CDAD is suspected or confirmed. Avoid with mononucleosis. May result in bacterial resistance with prolonged use in the absence of a proven/suspected bacterial infection; take appropriate measures if superinfection develops. The 200mg and 400mg chewable tabs and 200mg/5mL and 400mg/5mL sus contain phenylalanine; avoid with phenylketonurics. The 250mg tab and 250mg chewable tab are not interchangeable due to unequal clavulanic acid amounts; do not use 250mg tab in pediatric patients until child weighs at least 40kg. Do not substitute two 250mg tabs for one 500mg tab. May decrease estrogen levels in pregnant women. Lab test interactions may occur. Caution in elderly.

ADVERSE REACTIONS

Diarrhea/loose stools, nausea, skin rashes, urticaria

DRUG INTERACTIONS

Probenecid may increase/prolong levels of amoxicillin; coadministration not recommended. Abnormal prolongation of PT (increased INR) reported with oral anticoagulants; may require oral anticoagulant dose adjustment. Allopurinol may increase incidence of rashes. May reduce efficacy of combined oral estrogen/progesterone contraceptives.

NURSING CONSIDERATIONS

Assessment: Assess for history of serious hypersensitivity reactions to other β-lactam antibacterial drugs (eg, PCN, cephalosporins) or other allergens, history of amoxicillin/clavulanate-associated cholestatic jaundice/hepatic dysfunction, hepatic/renal impairment, mononucleosis, phenylketonuria, pregnancy/nursing status, and possible drug interactions.

Monitoring: Monitor for anaphylactic reactions, superinfection, skin rash, CDAD, and other adverse reactions. Periodically monitor renal (especially in elderly) and hepatic function. Monitor PT/INR with oral anticoagulants.

Patient Counseling: Instruct to take each dose with a meal or snack to reduce possibility of GI upset. Counsel that drug only treats bacterial, not viral (eg, common cold), infections. Instruct to take ud; inform that skipping doses or not completing the full course of therapy may decrease effectiveness of the drug and increase resistance of bacteria. Advise to consult physician if severe diarrhea or watery/bloody stools occur (even as late as ≥2 months after treatment). Instruct to use a dosing spoon or medicine dropper when dosing a child with sus, and rinse measuring device after each use. Instruct to discard any unused medicine.

Storage: ≤25°C (77°F). Reconstituted Sus: Refrigerate; discard after 10 days.

AUGMENTIN XR – amoxicillin/clavulanate potassium — RX

Class: Aminopenicillin/beta lactamase inhibitor

ADULT DOSAGE

Acute Bacterial Sinusitis

2 tabs q12h for 10 days

Community-Acquired Pneumonia

2 tabs q12h for 7-10 days

PEDIATRIC DOSAGE

Acute Bacterial Sinusitis

≥40kg (Able to Swallow Tab):
2 tabs q12h for 10 days

Community-Acquired Pneumonia

≥40kg (Able to Swallow Tab):
2 tabs q12h for 7-10 days

DOSE MODIFICATION

Hepatic Impairment

Caution and monitor hepatic function at regular intervals

ADMINISTRATION

Oral route

Take at the start of a meal; not recommended w/ a high-fat meal

HOW SUPPLIED

Tab, Extended-Release: (Amoxicillin/Clavulanic Acid) 1000mg/62.5mg* *scored

CONTRAINDICATIONS

Severe renal impairment (CrCl <30mL/min), hemodialysis, history of amoxicillin/clavulanate-associated cholestatic jaundice/hepatic dysfunction.

WARNINGS/PRECAUTIONS

Serious, occasionally fatal, hypersensitivity reactions reported with PCN therapy; d/c if allergic reaction occurs and institute appropriate therapy. *Clostridium difficile*-associated diarrhea (CDAD) reported; d/c if CDAD is suspected or confirmed. Caution with hepatic dysfunction. Avoid with mononucleosis. May result in bacterial resistance with prolonged use or use in the absence of a proven/suspected bacterial infection or a prophylactic indication; take appropriate measures if superinfection develops. May decrease estrogen levels in pregnant women. Lab test interactions may occur.

ADVERSE REACTIONS

Diarrhea, vaginal mycosis.

DRUG INTERACTIONS

Probenecid may increase/prolong levels; coadministration not recommended. Abnormal prolongation of PT (increased INR) reported with oral anticoagulants; may require anticoagulant dose adjustment. Allopurinol may increase incidence of rashes. May reduce efficacy of oral contraceptives.

NURSING CONSIDERATIONS

Assessment: Assess for history of serious hypersensitivity reactions to other β-lactam antibacterial drugs (eg, PCN, cephalosporins) or other allergens, history of amoxicillin/clavulanate-associated cholestatic jaundice/hepatic dysfunction, hepatic/renal impairment, mononucleosis, pregnancy/nursing status, and possible drug interactions.

Monitoring: Monitor for anaphylactic reactions, hepatic toxicity, superinfection, skin rash, diarrhea, CDAD, and other adverse reactions. Monitor PT/INR with oral anticoagulants. Monitor renal function in elderly. Monitor renal, hepatic, and hematopoietic functions with prolonged use.

Patient Counseling: Instruct to take q12h with a meal or snack to reduce possibility of GI upset. Advise to consult physician if severe diarrhea or watery/bloody stools occur (even as late as ≥2 months after treatment). Instruct to take ud; skipping doses or not completing the full course of therapy may decrease effectiveness of the drug and increase resistance of bacteria. Instruct to discard any unused medicine.

Storage: ≤25°C (77°F).

AURODEX – antipyrine/benzocaine RX

Class: Analgesic combination

ADULT DOSAGE

Acute Otitis Media

Relief of pain and reduction of inflammation in congestive and serous stages. Adjuvant therapy during systemic antibiotic administration for resolution of infection

Instill permitting sol to run along the wall of canal until it is filled
Then moisten cotton pledget w/ sol and insert into meatus
Repeat every 1-2 hrs until pain and congestion relieved

Cerumen Removal

Excessive/Impacted Cerumen:
Before: Instill tid for 2-3 days; moisten cotton pledget w/ sol and insert into meatus following instillation
After: Use to dry out canal or relieve discomfort; moisten cotton pledget w/ sol and insert into meatus following instillation

PEDIATRIC DOSAGE

Pediatric use may not have been established

ADMINISTRATION

Otic route

Avoid touching ear w/ dropper

HOW SUPPLIED

Sol: (Antipyrine-Benzocaine) 54mg-14mg/mL [10mL]

CONTRAINDICATIONS

Spontaneous perforation of the tympanic membrane, discharge.

WARNINGS/PRECAUTIONS

For otic use only; not for use in eyes. D/C promptly if sensitization or irritation occurs.

ADVERSE REACTIONS

Sensitization, irritation.

NURSING CONSIDERATIONS

Assessment: Assess for hypersensitivity to drug, tympanic membrane perforation, ear discharge, and pregnancy/nursing status.

Monitoring: Monitor for sensitization or irritation, and other possible adverse reactions.

Patient Counseling: Inform that drug is for otic use only. Instruct to avoid contaminating dropper tip with material from the ear, fingers, or other source. Advise not to rinse dropper tip after use and not to use drug if sol turns brown or contains precipitate.

Storage: 20-25°C (68-77°F); excursions permitted to 15-30°C (59-86°F). Protect from light and heat. Discard 6 months after opening.

AVALIDE – hydrochlorothiazide/irbesartan RX

Class: Angiotensin II receptor antagonist/thiazide diuretic

D/C when pregnancy is detected. Drugs that act directly on the renin-angiotensin system (RAS) can cause injury/death to the developing fetus.

ADULT DOSAGE

Hypertension

Add-On Therapy:
Use if not controlled on monotherapy w/ irbesartan or HCTZ
150mg-12.5mg, 300mg-12.5mg, and 300mg-25mg

PEDIATRIC DOSAGE

Pediatric use may not have been established

Replacement Therapy:
May be substituted for titrated components

Initial Therapy:
Usual: 150mg-12.5mg qd
Titrate: May increase after 1-2 weeks of therapy
Max: 300mg-25mg qd

ADMINISTRATION
Oral route
Take w/ or w/o food

HOW SUPPLIED
Tab: (Irbesartan-HCTZ) 150mg-12.5mg, 300mg-12.5mg

CONTRAINDICATIONS
Anuria, sulfonamide-derived drug hypersensitivity. Coadministration with aliskiren in patients with diabetes.

WARNINGS/PRECAUTIONS
Not for initial therapy with intravascular volume depletion. Not recommended with severe renal impairment (CrCl ≤30mL/min). Symptomatic hypotension may occur in intravascular volume- or Na^+-depleted patients (eg, patients treated vigorously with diuretics or on dialysis); correct volume depletion prior to therapy. Hypokalemia and hyperkalemia reported. Irbesartan: May increase BUN or SrCr levels in patients with renal artery stenosis. Oliguria and/or progressive azotemia and (rarely) acute renal failure and/or death may occur in patients whose renal function may depend on the renin-angiotensin-aldosterone system activity (eg, severe congestive heart failure [CHF]). HCTZ: May cause hypersensitivity reactions, exacerbation or activation of systemic lupus erythematosus (SLE), hyponatremia, hypomagnesemia, and hyperuricemia or precipitation of frank gout. May alter glucose tolerance and increase cholesterol, TG, and Ca^{2+} levels. D/C before testing for parathyroid function. May cause idiosyncratic reaction, resulting in transient myopia and acute angle-closure glaucoma; d/c as rapidly as possible. Enhanced effects in postsympathectomy patients. Caution with hepatic impairment or progressive liver disease; may precipitate hepatic coma. May precipitate azotemia in patients with renal disease.

ADVERSE REACTIONS
Dizziness, hypokalemia, fatigue, musculoskeletal pain, influenza, edema, N/V, headache.

DRUG INTERACTIONS
See Contraindications. NSAIDs, including selective COX-2 inhibitors, may decrease effects of diuretics and angiotensin II receptor antagonists and may deteriorate renal function. Increases in lithium concentrations and lithium toxicity reported; monitor lithium levels. Irbesartan: Dual blockade of the RAS is associated with increased risks of hypotension, hyperkalemia, and changes in renal function (including acute renal failure); avoid combined use of RAS inhibitors, or closely monitor BP, renal function, and electrolytes with concomitant agents that also affect the RAS. Avoid with aliskiren in patients with renal impairment (GFR <60mL/min). Concomitant use with K^+-sparing diuretics, K^+ supplements, or salt substitutes containing K^+ may increase serum K^+. HCTZ: Alcohol, barbiturates, and narcotics may potentiate orthostatic hypotension. Dosage adjustment of antidiabetic drugs (oral agents and insulin) may be required. Anionic exchange resins (eg, cholestyramine, colestipol) may impair absorption; take at least 1 hr before or 4 hrs after these medications. Additive effect or potentiation with other antihypertensive drugs. Corticosteroids and adrenocorticotropic hormone may intensify electrolyte depletion, particularly hypokalemia. May decrease response to pressor amines (eg, norepinephrine). May increase responsiveness to nondepolarizing skeletal muscle relaxants (eg, tubocurarine). Risk of symptomatic hyponatremia with carbamazepine; monitor electrolytes.

NURSING CONSIDERATIONS

Assessment: Assess for hypersensitivity to drug and its components, anuria, sulfonamide-derived drug hypersensitivity, diabetes, volume/salt depletion, SLE, CHF, renal/hepatic impairment, renal artery stenosis, postsympathectomy status, pregnancy/nursing status, and possible drug interactions.

Monitoring: Monitor for hypersensitivity/idiosyncratic reactions, exacerbation/activation of SLE, hyperuricemia, precipitation of gout, myopia, angle-closure glaucoma, and other adverse reactions. Monitor BP, serum electrolytes, cholesterol and TG levels, and renal/hepatic function.

Patient Counseling: Inform females of childbearing age about the consequences of exposure during pregnancy. Discuss treatment options with women planning to become pregnant. Instruct to report pregnancies to physician as soon as possible. Inform that lightheadedness may occur, especially during 1st days of use; instruct to d/c use and contact physician if fainting occurs. Inform that dehydration, which may occur with excessive sweating, diarrhea, vomiting, and not drinking enough liquids, may lower BP too much and lead to lightheadedness and possible fainting.

Storage: 25°C (77°F); excursions permitted to 15-30°C (59-86°F).

AVANDAMET – metformin hydrochloride/rosiglitazone maleate RX

Class: Biguanide/thiazolidinedione

Thiazolidinediones, including rosiglitazone, cause or exacerbate CHF in some patients. After initiation and dose increases, observe for signs and symptoms of heart failure (HF); manage accordingly and consider discontinuation or dose reduction if signs/symptoms develop. Not recommended in patients with symptomatic HF. Contraindicated with established NYHA Class III or IV HF. Lactic acidosis may occur due to metformin accumulation; risk increases with conditions such as sepsis, dehydration, excess alcohol intake, hepatic/renal impairment, and acute CHF. If acidosis is suspected, d/c therapy and hospitalize patient immediately.

ADULT DOSAGE

Type 2 Diabetes Mellitus

Initial: 2mg/500mg qd or bid; may consider a starting dose of 2mg/500mg bid w/ HbA1c >11% or FPG >270mg/dL
Titrate: May increase in increments of (2mg/500mg)/day given in divided doses if inadequately controlled after 4 weeks
Max: (8mg/2000mg)/day

Start the rosiglitazone component at the lowest recommended dose

Inadequately Controlled on Rosiglitazone or Metformin Monotherapy:
Initial:
On Metformin 1000mg/day: 2mg/500mg bid
On Metformin 2000mg/day: 2mg/1000mg bid
On Rosiglitazone 4mg/day: 2mg/500mg bid
On Rosiglitazone 8mg/day: 4mg/500mg bid
Individualize therapy if on metformin 1000-2000mg/day
Titrate:
If additional glycemic control is needed, may increase daily dose by increments of 4mg rosiglitazone and/or 500mg metformin
After an increase in metformin dose, if inadequately controlled, titrate after 1-2 weeks
After an increase in rosiglitazone dose, if inadequately controlled, titrate after 8-12 weeks
Max: (8mg/2000mg)/day taken in divided doses bid

PEDIATRIC DOSAGE

Pediatric use may not have been established

DOSE MODIFICATION

Hepatic Impairment

Active Liver Disease/Increased Serum Transaminase Levels (ALT >2.5X ULN): Do not initiate therapy

Elderly

Elderly/Debilitated/Malnourished: Dose conservatively; do not titrate to max dose

ADMINISTRATION

Oral route

Take in divided doses w/ meals

HOW SUPPLIED

Tab: (Rosiglitazone/Metformin) 2mg/500mg, 4mg/500mg, 2mg/1000mg, 4mg/1000mg

CONTRAINDICATIONS

NYHA Class III or IV HF, renal disease or dysfunction (eg, SrCr ≥1.5mg/dL [males], ≥1.4mg/dL [females], abnormal CrCl), acute/chronic metabolic acidosis including diabetic ketoacidosis with or without coma. Use in patients undergoing radiologic studies involving intravascular administration of iodinated contrast materials.

WARNINGS/PRECAUTIONS

Assess renal function before initiation of therapy and at least annually thereafter; d/c with evidence of renal impairment. Promptly withhold in the presence of any condition associated with hypoxemia, dehydration, or sepsis. Temporarily d/c at the time of or prior to radiologic studies involving the use of intravascular iodinated contrast materials, withhold for 48 hrs subsequent to the procedure, and reinstitute only if renal function is normal. Temporarily suspend for any surgical procedure (except minor procedures not associated with restricted food and fluid intake); restart when oral intake is resumed and renal function is normal. Evaluate patients previously well-controlled on therapy who develop laboratory abnormalities or clinical illness for evidence of ketoacidosis or lactic acidosis; d/c if acidosis occurs. Increased risk of cardiovascular events in patients with CHF NYHA Class I and II. Treatment initiation is not recommended for patients experiencing an acute coronary event; consider discontinuation during this acute phase. Increased risk for myocardial infarction (MI) reported. Caution in patients with edema or at risk for HF. Edema and dose-related weight gain reported. Macular edema reported; promptly refer to an ophthalmologist if visual symptoms develop. Increased incidence of bone fracture, particularly in females. Dose-related decreases in Hgb and Hct reported. May decrease serum vitamin B12 levels. Temporary loss of glycemic control may occur when exposed to stress (eg, fever, trauma, infection, surgery); may be necessary to withhold therapy and temporarily administer insulin. Caution in patients susceptible to hypoglycemic effects, such as elderly, debilitated/malnourished patients, and those with adrenal/pituitary insufficiency, or alcohol intoxication. May result in ovulation in some premenopausal anovulatory women, which may increase risk for pregnancy; adequate contraception is recommended. Review benefits of continued therapy if unexpected menstrual dysfunction occurs. Do not initiate in patients ≥80 yrs of age unless renal function is not reduced. Not recommended for use in pregnancy. Avoid with active liver disease or if ALT levels >2.5X ULN. Caution in patients with mild LFT elevations (ALT levels ≤2.5X ULN). If ALT levels increase to >3X ULN during therapy, recheck LFTs as soon as possible; d/c if ALT levels remain >3X ULN. Check LFTs if symptoms suggesting hepatic dysfunction develop; d/c if jaundice is observed.

ADVERSE REACTIONS

CHF, lactic acidosis, N/V, upper respiratory tract infection, headache, diarrhea, arthralgia, dyspepsia, dizziness, edema, nasopharyngitis, abdominal pain, loose stools, constipation, anemia.

DRUG INTERACTIONS

Caution with drugs that may affect renal function or result in significant hemodynamic change or may interfere with the disposition of metformin, such as cationic drugs eliminated by renal tubular secretion (eg, cimetidine, amiloride, digoxin, morphine, procainamide); monitor and adjust dose of Avandamet and/or the interfering drug. Alcohol potentiates the effects of metformin on lactate metabolism; avoid excessive alcohol intake. Increased risk of CHF with insulin; coadministration is not recommended. Hypoglycemia may occur with other hypoglycemic agents (eg, sulfonylureas, insulin) or ethanol; may need to reduce dose of the concomitant agent. May be difficult to recognize hypoglycemia with β-adrenergic blocking drugs. CYP2C8 inhibitors (eg, gemfibrozil) may increase exposure and CYP2C8 inducers (eg, rifampin) may decrease exposure; if an inhibitor or an inducer of CYP2C8 is started or stopped during treatment, changes in diabetes treatment may be needed based upon clinical response. Observe for loss of glycemic control with drugs that produce hyperglycemia.

NURSING CONSIDERATIONS

Assessment: Assess for HF or risk of HF, metabolic acidosis, diabetic ketoacidosis, risk factors for lactic acidosis, previous hypersensitivity to the drug, presence of an acute coronary event, cardiac status, edema, bone health, inadequate vitamin B12 or Ca^{2+} intake/absorption, any other conditions where treatment is cautioned, pregnancy/nursing status, and possible drug interactions. Assess if patient is planning to undergo any surgical procedure, radiologic studies involving the use of intravascular iodinated contrast materials, or is under any form of stress. Assess baseline renal function, LFTs, FPG, and HbA1c levels, and hematologic parameters.

Monitoring: Monitor for signs/symptoms of HF, lactic acidosis, hypoxic states, MI, edema, weight gain, visual symptoms, fractures, menstrual dysfunction, and other adverse reactions. Monitor for changes in clinical status. Monitor renal function, especially in elderly, at least annually. Monitor hematologic parameters annually. Perform routine serum vitamin B12 measurements at 2- to 3-yr intervals in patients predisposed to developing subnormal vitamin B12 levels. Periodically monitor LFTs, FPG, and HbA1c levels.

Patient Counseling: Inform of the risks and benefits of therapy. Inform of the risk of lactic acidosis; instruct to d/c therapy immediately and notify physician if unexplained hyperventilation, myalgia, malaise, unusual somnolence, or other nonspecific symptoms occur. Counsel against excessive alcohol intake. Advise on the importance of adherence to dietary instructions and regular testing of blood glucose, HbA1c, renal/hepatic function, and hematologic parameters. Instruct to immediately report any signs/symptoms of hepatotoxicity or HF to physician. Counsel premenopausal women to use adequate contraception during treatment.

Storage: 25°C (77°F); excursions permitted to 15-30°C (59-86°F).

AVANDARYL – glimepiride/rosiglitazone maleate

RX

Class: Sulfonylurea/thiazolidinedione

Thiazolidinediones, including rosiglitazone, cause or exacerbate CHF in some patients. After initiation and dose increases, observe for signs and symptoms of heart failure (HF); manage accordingly and consider discontinuation or dose reduction if signs/symptoms develop. Not recommended in patients w/ symptomatic HF. Contraindicated w/ established NYHA Class III or IV HF.

ADULT DOSAGE

Type 2 Diabetes Mellitus

Initial: 4mg/1mg qd w/ 1st meal of the day; may consider 4mg/2mg for patients already treated w/ a sulfonylurea or rosiglitazone
Max: (8mg/4mg)/day

Start the rosiglitazone component at the lowest recommended dose; if hypoglycemia occurs, may consider dose reduction of glimepiride component

Switching from Combination Therapy of Rosiglitazone Plus Glimepiride as Separate Tablets:
Initial: Start at the dose of rosiglitazone and glimepiride already being taken

Conversions

Switching to Avandaryl in Patients Currently Treated w/ Rosiglitazone:
If not adequately controlled after 1-2 weeks, may increase glimepiride component of Avandaryl in no >2mg increments; afterwards, may titrate Avandaryl if not adequately controlled after 1-2 weeks

Switching to Avandaryl in Patients Currently Treated w/ Sulfonylurea:
If not adequately controlled after 8-12 weeks, may titrate rosiglitazone component of Avandaryl; afterwards, may titrate Avandaryl if not adequately controlled after 2-3 months

PEDIATRIC DOSAGE

Pediatric use may not have been established

DOSE MODIFICATION

Concomitant Medications

Colesevelam: Administer therapy at least 4 hrs prior to colesevelam

Renal Impairment

Dose conservatively and carefully titrate

Hepatic Impairment

Dose conservatively and carefully titrate

Elderly

Elderly/Debilitated/Malnourished:
Dose conservatively and carefully titrate

Other Important Modifications

Adrenal Insufficiency: Dose conservatively and carefully titrate

ADMINISTRATION

Oral route

Take w/ the 1st meal of the day

HOW SUPPLIED

Tab: (Rosiglitazone/Glimepiride) 4mg/1mg, 4mg/2mg, 4mg/4mg, 8mg/2mg, 8mg/4mg

CONTRAINDICATIONS

NYHA Class III or IV HF.

WARNINGS/PRECAUTIONS

Not for use in patients w/ type 1 DM or for the treatment of diabetic ketoacidosis. Treatment initiation is not recommended in patients experiencing an acute coronary event; consider discontinuation during this acute phase. May cause severe hypoglycemia; caution in patients susceptible to hypoglycemic action, such as elderly, debilitated, or malnourished patients, and those w/ adrenal, pituitary, renal, or hepatic insufficiency. Temporary loss of glycemic control may occur when exposed to stress (eg, fever, trauma, infection, surgery); may be necessary to withhold therapy and temporarily administer insulin. Should not be used during pregnancy. Rosiglitazone: Increased risk of CHF w/ insulin; coadministration is not recommended. Caution in patients w/ edema or at risk for HF. Edema and dose-related weight gain reported. Elevation of LFTs may occur; hepatic impairment and hepatitis reported. Do not initiate in patients w/ increased baseline LFTs (ALT levels >2.5X ULN). Caution in patients w/ mild LFT elevations (ALT levels ≤2.5X ULN). If ALT levels increase to >3X ULN during therapy, recheck LFTs as soon as possible; d/c if ALT levels remain >3X ULN. Check LFTs if symptoms suggesting hepatic dysfunction develop; d/c if jaundice is observed. Increased risk of cardiovascular (CV) events in patients w/ CHF NYHA Class I and II. Increased risk for MI reported. Macular edema reported; promptly refer to an ophthalmologist if visual symptoms develop. Increased incidence of bone fracture, particularly in females. Dose-related decreases in Hgb and Hct reported. May result in ovulation in some premenopausal anovulatory women, which may increase risk for pregnancy; adequate contraception is recommended. Review benefits of continued therapy if unexpected menstrual dysfunction occurs. Glimepiride: May be associated w/ increased CV mortality. Hypersensitivity reactions (eg, anaphylaxis, angioedema, Stevens-Johnson syndrome) reported; if suspected, promptly d/c therapy, assess for other potential causes for the reaction, and institute alternative treatment. May cause hemolytic anemia; caution w/ G6PD deficiency and consider the use of a non-sulfonylurea alternative.

ADVERSE REACTIONS

CHF, headache, hypoglycemia, nasopharyngitis, HTN, edema.

DRUG INTERACTIONS

See Dose Modification. May require dose adjustment and close monitoring for hypoglycemia or worsening glycemic control w/ drugs that may increase glucose-lowering effect (eg, ACE inhibitors, fibrates, somatostatin analogues, highly protein-bound drugs), drugs that may reduce glucose-lowering effect (eg, protease inhibitors, corticosteroids, oral contraceptives), or drugs that may either increase or decrease glucose-lowering effect (eg, β-blockers, clonidine, reserpine). Signs of hypoglycemia may be reduced or absent w/ sympatholytic drugs (eg, β-blockers, clonidine, guanethidine, reserpine). Glimepiride: Alcohol may also potentiate or weaken glucose-lowering action. Colesevelam may reduce levels. Potential interaction leading to severe hypoglycemia reported w/ oral miconazole. Potential interaction may occur w/ other drugs metabolized by CYP2C9 (eg, phenytoin, ibuprofen, mefenamic acid), and w/ CYP2C9 inhibitors (eg, fluconazole) or inducers (eg, rifampin). Rosiglitazone: CYP2C8 inhibitors (eg, gemfibrozil) may increase AUC and CYP2C8 inducers (eg, rifampin) may decrease AUC; if an inhibitor or an inducer of CYP2C8 is started or stopped during treatment, changes in diabetes treatment may be needed based upon clinical response. Refer to PI for additional drug interactions.

NURSING CONSIDERATIONS

Assessment: Assess for HF or risk of HF, presence of acute coronary event, cardiac status, susceptibility to hypoglycemia, edema, bone health, G6PD deficiency, previous hypersensitivity to the drug or sulfonamide derivatives, pregnancy/nursing status, and possible drug interactions. Assess if patient is under any form of stress. Obtain baseline renal function, LFTs, FPG, and HbA1c levels.

Monitoring: Monitor for signs/symptoms of HF, MI, hypoglycemia, edema, weight gain, visual symptoms, fractures, hypersensitivity reactions, hematologic effects, menstrual dysfunction, and other adverse reactions. Periodically monitor LFTs, FPG, and HbA1c levels.

Patient Counseling: Inform of the risks and benefits of therapy. Advise on the importance of adherence to dietary instructions and regular testing of blood glucose, HbA1c, and liver function. Inform about the risk of hypoglycemia, its symptoms and treatment, and conditions that predispose to its development. Instruct to immediately report to physician any symptoms of HF or hepatic dysfunction. Counsel premenopausal women to use adequate contraception during treatment.

Storage: 25°C (77°F); excursions permitted to 15-30°C (59-86°F).

AVANDIA — rosiglitazone maleate RX

Class: Thiazolidinedione

Thiazolidinediones, including rosiglitazone, cause or exacerbate congestive heart failure (CHF) in some patients. After initiation and dose increases, observe for signs and symptoms of heart failure (HF); manage accordingly and consider discontinuation or dose reduction if signs/symptoms develop. Not recommended in patients with symptomatic HF. Contraindicated with established NYHA Class III or IV HF.

ADULT DOSAGE

Type 2 Diabetes Mellitus

Initial: 4mg as qd dose or in 2 divided doses

Titrate: May increase to 8mg/day if response is inadequate after 8-12 weeks

Max: 8mg/day

PEDIATRIC DOSAGE

Pediatric use may not have been established

DOSE MODIFICATION

Concomitant Medications

Other Hypoglycemic Agents: May need to reduce dose of the concomitant agent

Hepatic Impairment

Do not initiate therapy in patients w/ clinical evidence of active liver disease or increased serum transaminase levels (ALT >2.5X ULN at start of therapy)

ADMINISTRATION

Oral route

Take w/ or w/o food

HOW SUPPLIED

Tab: 2mg, 4mg, 8mg

CONTRAINDICATIONS

NYHA Class III or IV HF.

WARNINGS/PRECAUTIONS

Not for use in patients with type 1 DM or for the treatment of diabetic ketoacidosis. Increased risk of cardiovascular events in patients with CHF NYHA Class I and II. Treatment initiation is not recommended for patients experiencing an acute coronary event; consider discontinuation during this acute phase. Increased risk for myocardial infarction (MI) reported. Caution in patients with edema or at risk for HF. Edema and dose-related weight gain reported. Do not initiate in patients with active liver disease or increased baseline LFTs (ALT levels >2.5X ULN). Caution in patients with mild LFT elevations (ALT levels ≤2.5X ULN). If ALT levels increase to >3X ULN during therapy, recheck LFTs as soon as possible; d/c if ALT levels remain >3X ULN. Check LFTs if symptoms suggesting hepatic dysfunction develop; d/c if jaundice is observed. Macular edema reported; promptly refer to an ophthalmologist if visual symptoms develop. Increased incidence of bone fracture, particularly in females. Dose-related decreases in Hgb and Hct reported. May result in ovulation in some premenopausal anovulatory women, which may increase risk for pregnancy; adequate contraception is recommended. Review benefits of continued therapy if unexpected menstrual dysfunction occurs.

ADVERSE REACTIONS

CHF, upper respiratory tract infection, headache, back pain, hyperglycemia, fatigue, sinusitis, edema.

DRUG INTERACTIONS

See Dosage. Risk for hypoglycemia when given with other hypoglycemic agents; a reduction in the dose of concomitant agent may be necessary. CYP2C8 inhibitors (eg, gemfibrozil) may increase exposure and CYP2C8 inducers (eg, rifampin) may decrease exposure; if an inhibitor or an inducer of CYP2C8 is started or stopped during treatment, changes in diabetes treatment may be needed based upon clinical response. Increased risk of CHF with insulin; coadministration is not recommended.

NURSING CONSIDERATIONS

Assessment: Assess for HF or risk factors for HF, presence of an acute coronary event, cardiac status, edema, drug hypersensitivity, pregnancy/nursing status, and possible drug interactions. Obtain baseline LFTs, FPG and HbA1c levels, and bone health.

Monitoring: Monitor for signs/symptoms of HF, MI, edema, weight gain, macular edema, fractures, hematologic effects, menstrual dysfunction, and other adverse reactions. Periodically monitor LFTs, FPG, and HbA1c levels.

Patient Counseling: Inform of the risks and benefits of therapy. Advise on the importance of adherence to dietary instructions and regular testing of blood glucose, HbA1c, and liver function. Instruct to immediately report to physician any symptoms of HF or hepatic dysfunction. Inform about the risk of hypoglycemia, its symptoms and treatment, and conditions that predispose to its development when using in combination with other hypoglycemic agents. Counsel premenopausal women to use adequate contraception during treatment.

Storage: 25°C (77°F); excursions permitted to 15-30°C (59-86°F).

AVAPRO — irbesartan RX

Class: Angiotensin II receptor antagonist

D/C when pregnancy is detected. Drugs that act directly on the renin-angiotensin system (RAS) can cause injury/death to the developing fetus.

ADULT DOSAGE

Hypertension

Initial: 150mg qd

Titrate: May increase to 300mg qd

Max: 300mg qd

A low dose diuretic may be added if BP is not controlled

PEDIATRIC DOSAGE

Pediatric use may not have been established

Diabetic Nephropathy **Elevated SrCr/Proteinuria (>300mg/day) in Patients w/ Type 2 Diabetes and HTN:** **Maint:** 300mg qd	

DOSE MODIFICATION

Other Important Modifications

Intravascular Volume and Salt Depleted Patients:

Initial: 75mg qd

ADMINISTRATION

Oral route

Take w/ or w/o food

HOW SUPPLIED

Tab: 75mg, 150mg, 300mg

CONTRAINDICATIONS

Coadministration with aliskiren in patients with diabetes.

WARNINGS/PRECAUTIONS

Symptomatic hypotension may occur in patients with intravascular volume or Na^+ depletion (eg, patients treated vigorously with diuretics or on dialysis); correct volume depletion prior to therapy or use low starting dose. Changes in renal function may occur. Oliguria and/or progressive azotemia and (rarely) acute renal failure and/or death may occur in patients whose renal function may depend on the renin-angiotensin-aldosterone system activity (eg, severe congestive heart failure [CHF]). May increase SrCr or BUN in patients with renal artery stenosis.

ADVERSE REACTIONS

Hyperkalemia, dizziness, orthostatic dizziness, orthostatic hypotension, fatigue, diarrhea.

DRUG INTERACTIONS

See Contraindications. Increases in serum lithium concentrations and lithium toxicity reported; monitor lithium levels. CYP2C9 substrates/inhibitors sulphenazole, tolbutamide, and nifedipine significantly inhibited metabolism in vitro. Concomitant use with K^+-sparing diuretics, K^+ supplements, or salt substitutes containing K^+ may increase serum K^+. NSAIDs, including selective COX-2 inhibitors, may attenuate antihypertensive effect and may deteriorate renal function. Dual blockade of the RAS is associated with increased risks of hypotension, hyperkalemia, and changes in renal function (including acute renal failure); avoid combined use of RAS inhibitors, or closely monitor BP, renal function, and electrolytes with concomitant agents that also affect the RAS. Avoid with aliskiren in patients with renal impairment (GFR <60mL/min).

NURSING CONSIDERATIONS

Assessment: Assess for hypersensitivity, volume/salt depletion, renal impairment, CHF, renal artery stenosis, diabetes, pregnancy/nursing status, and possible drug interactions.

Monitoring: Monitor for signs/symptoms of hypotension, renal dysfunction, and other adverse reactions.

Patient Counseling: Inform about the consequences of exposure during pregnancy in females of childbearing age. Discuss treatment options with women planning to become pregnant. Instruct to report pregnancies to physician as soon as possible.

Storage: 25°C (77°F); excursions permitted to 15-30°C (59-86°F).

AVASTIN – bevacizumab **RX**

Class: Vascular endothelial growth factor (VEGF) inhibitor

GI perforation reported; d/c with GI perforation. Increased incidence of wound-healing and surgical complications; d/c at least 28 days prior to elective surgery. Do not initiate for at least 28 days after surgery and until surgical wound is fully healed. D/C in patients with wound dehiscence. Severe or fatal hemorrhage, including hemoptysis, GI bleeding, CNS hemorrhage, epistaxis, and vaginal bleeding may occur; do not administer to patients with serious hemorrhage or recent hemoptysis.

ADULT DOSAGE

Metastatic Colorectal Cancer

1st- or 2nd-line treatment of metastatic colorectal cancer (mCRC) in combination w/ IV 5-fluorouracil-based chemotherapy

2nd-line treatment of patients with mCRC, in combination w/ fluoropyrimidine-irinotecan- or fluoropyrimidine-oxaliplatin-based

PEDIATRIC DOSAGE

Pediatric use may not have been established

chemotherapy, who have progressed on a 1st-line bevacizumab-containing regimen

In Combination w/ Bolus-IFL:
5mg/kg every 2 weeks

In Combination w/ FOLFOX4:
10mg/kg every 2 weeks

In Combination w/ Fluoropyrimidine-Irinotecan- or Fluoropyrimidine-Oxaliplatin-Based Chemotherapy:
5mg/kg every 2 weeks or 7.5mg/kg every 3 weeks

Nonsquamous Non-Small Cell Lung Cancer

1st-line treatment of unresectable, locally advanced, recurrent, or metastatic nonsquamous non-small cell lung cancer in combination w/ carboplatin and paclitaxel

15mg/kg every 3 weeks

Glioblastoma

Treatment of glioblastoma w/ progressive disease in adults following prior therapy as a single agent

10mg/kg every 2 weeks

Metastatic Renal Cell Carcinoma

Treatment of metastatic renal cell carcinoma in combination w/ interferon alfa

10mg/kg every 2 weeks

Cervical Cancer

Treatment of persistent, recurrent, or metastatic carcinoma of the cervix in combination w/ paclitaxel and cisplatin or paclitaxel and topotecan

15mg/kg every 3 weeks

Ovarian, Fallopian Tube, or Peritoneal Cancer

Treatment of patients w/ platinum-resistant recurrent epithelial ovarian, fallopian tube, or primary peritoneal cancer who received no more than 2 prior chemotherapy regimens in combination w/ paclitaxel, pegylated liposomal doxorubicin, or topotecan

10mg/kg every 2 weeks w/ one of the following IV chemotherapy regimens: paclitaxel, pegylated liposomal doxorubicin, or topotecan (weekly); or 15mg/kg every 3 weeks in combination w/ topotecan (every 3 weeks)

Treatment Duration

Continue treatment until disease progression or unacceptable toxicity

ADMINISTRATION

IV route

Do not administer as an IV push/bolus; administer only as an IV infusion
Do not initiate until ≥28 days following major surgery and after surgical incision has fully healed
Give 1st infusion over 90 min
Give 2nd infusion over 60 min if 1st infusion is tolerated
Give all subsequent infusions over 30 min if infusion over 60 min is tolerated

Preparation

Withdraw necessary amount and dilute in a total volume of 100mL of 0.9% NaCl Inj
Discard any unused portion left in a vial, as the product contains no preservatives
Do not administer or mix w/ dextrose sol

HOW SUPPLIED

Inj: 100mg/4mL, 400mg/16mL

WARNINGS/PRECAUTIONS

Not indicated for adjuvant treatment of colon cancer. Avoid use in patients with ovarian cancer with evidence of recto-sigmoid involvement by pelvic examination or bowel involvement on CT scan or clinical symptoms of bowel obstruction. GI fistula reported. Serious and sometimes fatal non-GI fistula formation involving tracheoesophageal (TE), bronchopleural, biliary, vaginal, renal, and bladder sites may occur; d/c therapy in patients with fistula formation involving an internal organ and d/c permanently in patients with TE fistula or any Grade 4 fistula. D/C in patients with wound-healing complications requiring medical intervention. Necrotizing fasciitis, usually secondary to wound-healing complications, GI perforation, or fistula formation, reported; d/c therapy if necrotizing fasciitis develops. D/C if hemorrhage occurs. Arterial thromboembolic events (ATEs) (eg, cerebral infarction, transient ischemic attacks, MI, angina) reported; increased risk with history of arterial thromboembolism, diabetes, or age >65 yrs. D/C if severe ATE develops. Increased risk of VTE in patients treated for persistent, recurrent, or metastatic cervical cancer; permanently d/c in patients with life-threatening (Grade 4) VTE, including pulmonary embolism. Increased incidence of severe HTN; d/c if hypertensive crisis or hypertensive encephalopathy occurs and temporarily suspend for severe uncontrolled HTN. Posterior reversible encephalopathy syndrome (PRES) reported; d/c if PRES develops. Increased incidence and severity of proteinuria; suspend therapy for ≥2g proteinuria/24 hrs and resume when proteinuria is <2g/24 hrs. Nephrotic syndrome may occur; d/c in patients with nephrotic syndrome. Infusion reactions (eg, HTN, hypertensive crisis with neurologic signs/symptoms, wheezing, oxygen desaturation, Grade 3 hypersensitivity, chest pain, headaches, rigors, diaphoresis) reported; stop infusion if a severe infusion reaction occurs and administer appropriate medical therapy. Increases the risk of ovarian failure and may impair fertility.

ADVERSE REACTIONS

GI perforation, wound-healing and surgical complications, hemorrhage, epistaxis, headache, HTN, rhinitis, proteinuria, taste alteration, dry skin, rectal hemorrhage, lacrimation disorder, back pain, exfoliative dermatitis, diarrhea.

DRUG INTERACTIONS

May decrease paclitaxel exposure with paclitaxel/carboplatin.

NURSING CONSIDERATIONS

Assessment: Assess for recent hemoptysis, serious hemorrhage, HTN, proteinuria, history of ATEs, diabetes, pregnancy/nursing status, and possible drug interactions. Assess for prior surgical history and for any scheduled elective surgeries. Assess for evidence of recto-sigmoid involvement in patients with ovarian cancer.

Monitoring: Monitor for GI perforation, fistula formation, wound-healing complications, hemorrhage, ATEs, VTEs, hypertensive crisis, hypertensive encephalopathy, PRES, nephrotic syndrome, severe infusion reactions, and other adverse reactions. Monitor BP every 2-3 weeks, treat with appropriate anti-hypertensive therapy, and monitor BP regularly; continue to monitor BP at regular intervals with drug-induced or -exacerbated HTN after drug discontinuation. Monitor for proteinuria by dipstick urine analysis for the development or worsening of proteinuria with serial urinalyses.

Patient Counseling: Advise to undergo routine BP monitoring and to contact physician if BP is elevated. Instruct to immediately seek medical attention for unusual bleeding, high fever, rigors, sudden onset of worsening neurological function, persistent/severe abdominal pain, severe constipation, or vomiting. Inform of pregnancy risks and the need to continue adequate contraception for at least 6 months after therapy. Inform of the increased risk of wound-healing complications, ovarian failure, and ATE.

Storage: 2-8°C (36-46°F). Protect from light. Do not freeze. Diluted Sol: May be stored at 2-8°C (36-46°F) for up to 8 hrs. Store in original carton until time of use.

AVELOX – moxifloxacin hydrochloride

RX

Class: Fluoroquinolone

Fluoroquinolones are associated with an increased risk of tendinitis and tendon rupture in all ages. Risk is further increased in patients >60 yrs of age, patients taking corticosteroids, and with kidney, heart, or lung transplants. May exacerbate muscle weakness with myasthenia gravis; avoid in patients with known history of myasthenia gravis.

ADULT DOSAGE

Skin and Skin Structure Infections

Uncomplicated:
400mg PO/IV q24h for 7 days

Complicated:
400mg PO/IV q24h for 7-21 days

PEDIATRIC DOSAGE

Pediatric use may not have been established

Intra-Abdominal Infections

Complicated:
400mg PO/IV q24h for 5-14 days

Acute Bacterial Sinusitis

400mg PO/IV q24h for 10 days

Acute Bacterial Exacerbation of Chronic Bronchitis

400mg PO/IV q24h for 5 days

Community-Acquired Pneumonia

400mg PO/IV q24h for 7-14 days

ADMINISTRATION

Oral/IV route

Oral

May take w/ or w/o food
Drink fluids liberally
Administer at least 4 hrs before or 8 hrs after multivitamins containing iron or zinc, antacids containing Mg^{2+} or aluminum, sucralfate, and Videx (didanosine) chewable/buffered tabs or the pediatric powder for oral sol

Inj

Avoid rapid or bolus IV infusion
Infuse IV over 60 min by direct infusion or through a Y-type IV infusion set
Do not add other IV substances, additives, or other medications to inj or infuse simultaneously through same IV line
Refer to complete directions that have been provided w/ the administration set

Compatible IV Sol

0.9% NaCl inj
1M NaCl inj
5% dextrose inj
Sterile water for inj
10% dextrose for inj
Lactated Ringer's for inj

HOW SUPPLIED

Inj: 400mg/250mL; Tab: 400mg

WARNINGS/PRECAUTIONS

D/C if pain, swelling, inflammation, or rupture of a tendon occurs. May prolong QT interval; avoid with QT interval prolongation or uncorrected hypokalemia. Caution with ongoing proarrhythmic conditions (eg, clinically significant bradycardia, acute myocardial ischemia) and liver cirrhosis. Serious anaphylactic reactions and other serious and sometimes fatal events reported; d/c immediately and institute supportive measures if skin rash, jaundice, or any other signs of hypersensitivity occur. Convulsions, increased intracranial pressure (eg, pseudotumor cerebri), and other CNS events reported; d/c and institute appropriate measures if CNS events (eg, dizziness, confusion, tremors, hallucinations, depression, and rarely, suicidal thoughts/acts) occur. Caution with CNS disorders (eg, severe cerebral arteriosclerosis, epilepsy) or risk factors that may predispose to seizures or lower seizure threshold. *Clostridium difficile*-associated diarrhea (CDAD) reported; may need to d/c if CDAD is suspected or confirmed. Cases of sensory or sensorimotor axonal polyneuropathy, resulting in paresthesias, hypoesthesias, dysesthesias, and weakness reported; d/c if symptoms of peripheral neuropathy occur. Blood glucose disturbances (eg, hypo/hyperglycemia) in diabetics reported; d/c therapy and immediately initiate appropriate therapy if hypoglycemic reaction occurs. May cause photosensitivity/phototoxicity reactions; d/c if phototoxicity occurs. Avoid excessive exposure to sun/UV light. May result in bacterial resistance if used in the absence of a proven/strongly suspected bacterial infection or a prophylactic indication. Caution in elderly and with hepatic impairment.

ADVERSE REACTIONS

Tendinitis, tendon rupture, nausea, diarrhea, headache, dizziness.

DRUG INTERACTIONS

See Boxed Warning. May prolong QT interval; avoid with Class IA (eg, quinidine, procainamide) or Class III (eg, amiodarone, sotalol) antiarrhythmics. Caution with other drugs that prolong the QT interval (eg, cisapride, erythromycin, antipsychotics, TCAs). NSAIDs may increase risk of CNS stimulation and convulsions. May enhance anticoagulant effects of warfarin or its derivatives; monitor PT and INR. Disturbances of blood glucose in diabetic patients receiving a concomitant antidiabetic agent reported; monitor glucose levels. (PO) Antacids containing Mg^{2+} or aluminum, sucralfate, metal cations (eg, iron), multivitamins containing iron or zinc, or formulations containing divalent and trivalent cations such as Videx (didanosine) chewable/buffered tabs or the pediatric powder for oral sol, may substantially interfere with absorption and lower systemic concentrations; take at least 4 hrs before or 8 hrs after these agents.

NURSING CONSIDERATIONS

Assessment: Assess for risk factors for developing tendinitis and tendon rupture, history of myasthenia gravis, drug hypersensitivity, QT interval prolongation, uncorrected hypokalemia, ongoing proarrhythmic conditions, liver cirrhosis, CNS disorders or risk factors that may predispose to seizures or lower seizure threshold, diabetes, hepatic impairment, pregnancy/nursing status, and possible drug interactions. Obtain baseline culture and susceptibility tests.

Monitoring: Monitor for ECG changes (eg, QT interval prolongation), signs/symptoms of anaphylactic reactions, CNS events, drug resistance, CDAD, peripheral neuropathy, tendon rupture, tendinitis, photosensitivity/phototoxicity reactions, and other adverse reactions. Monitor for muscle weakness in patients with myasthenia gravis. Monitor blood glucose levels in diabetic patients. Monitor PT and INR if administered with warfarin or its derivatives.

Patient Counseling: Inform that drug treats only bacterial, not viral, infections. Instruct to take exactly ud; skipping doses or not completing full course may decrease effectiveness and increase bacterial resistance. Instruct to notify physician if pain, swelling, or inflammation of a tendon, or weakness or inability to move joints occurs; advise to rest and refrain from exercise and to d/c therapy. Instruct to notify physician if experiencing worsening muscle weakness or breathing problems, palpitations or fainting spells, sunburn-like reaction or skin eruption, or if watery and bloody stools (even ≥2 months after last dose) develop. Advise to notify physician of all medications and supplements currently being used. Instruct to inform physician of any personal or family history of QT prolongation, proarrhythmic conditions, convulsions, or psychiatric illness. Instruct diabetic patients being treated with antidiabetic agents to d/c therapy and notify physician if hypoglycemia occurs. Instruct to d/c and notify physician if an allergic reaction, skin rash, and symptoms of peripheral neuropathy develop. Inform that drug may cause dizziness, lightheadedness, and vision disorders; instruct to use caution with activities requiring mental alertness or coordination. Advise to minimize or avoid exposure to natural or artificial light (eg, tanning beds or UVA/B treatment).

Storage: 25°C (77°F); excursions permitted to 15-30°C (59-86°F). (Tab) Avoid high humidity. (Inj) Do not refrigerate.

AVINZA – morphine sulfate CII

Class: Opioid analgesic

Exposes users to risks of addiction, abuse, and misuse, leading to overdose and death; assess each patient's risk prior to prescribing, and monitor regularly for development of these behaviors/conditions. Serious, life-threatening, or fatal respiratory depression may occur; monitor during initiation or following a dose increase. Crushing, chewing, or dissolving can cause rapid release and absorption of a potentially fatal dose; instruct to swallow caps whole or sprinkle contents on applesauce. Accidental ingestion, especially by children, can result in fatal overdose. Prolonged use during pregnancy can result in neonatal opioid withdrawal syndrome; advise pregnant women of the risk and ensure availability of appropriate treatment. Avoid alcohol consumption or medications containing alcohol; may result in increased plasma levels and potentially fatal overdose of morphine.

ADULT DOSAGE

Severe Pain (Daily, Around-the-Clock Management)

1st Opioid Analgesic:
Initial: 30mg q24h
Titrate: Adjust dose in increments of ≥30mg every 3-4 days

Opioid Intolerant:
Initial: 30mg q24h

Titration/Maint:
Individually titrate to a dose that provides adequate analgesia and minimizes adverse reactions; dose adjustments may be dose every 3-4 days
Max Daily Dose: 1600mg/day

Breakthrough Pain:
May require a dose increase or may need rescue medication w/ an appropriate dose of an immediate-release analgesic

Conversions

From Other Opioids:
Initial: 30mg q24h; d/c all other around-the-clock opioids

PEDIATRIC DOSAGE

Pediatric use may not have been established

From Other Oral Morphine Formulations:
Administer total daily oral morphine dose once daily; do not give more frequently than q24h

From Parenteral Morphine:
Between 2-6mg of oral morphine may be required to provide analgesia equivalent to 1mg of parenteral morphine

From Other Non-Morphine Opioids (Parenteral or Oral):
Initial: 1/2 the estimated daily morphine requirement

DOSE MODIFICATION

Discontinuation

Do not abruptly d/c; use a gradual downward titration of dose every 2-4 days to prevent signs/symptoms of withdrawal

ADMINISTRATION

Oral route

Take caps whole; do not crush, chew, or dissolve the pellets in the caps

Alternative Administration

Sprinkle over applesauce and consume immediately w/o chewing
Rinse mouth to ensure all pellets have been swallowed
Discard any unused portion of caps after contents have been sprinkled on applesauce

Do not administer through a NG or gastric tubes

HOW SUPPLIED

Cap, Extended-Release: 30mg, 45mg, 60mg, 75mg, 90mg, 120mg

CONTRAINDICATIONS

Significant respiratory depression, acute or severe bronchial asthma in an unmonitored setting or in the absence of resuscitative equipment, known/suspected paralytic ileus.

WARNINGS/PRECAUTIONS

Reserve use in patients for whom alternative treatment options are ineffective, not tolerated, or would be otherwise inadequate to provide sufficient management of pain. Should be prescribed only by healthcare professionals knowledgeable in the use of potent opioids for management of chronic pain. 90mg and 120mg caps are for use in opioid-tolerant patients only. Doses >1600mg/day contain a quantity of fumaric acid that may cause serious renal toxicity. Life-threatening respiratory depression is more likely to occur in elderly, cachectic, or debilitated patients. Consider alternative nonopioid analgesics in patients with significant chronic obstructive pulmonary disease (COPD) or cor pulmonale, and in patients having a substantially decreased respiratory reserve, hypoxia, hypercapnia, or preexisting respiratory depression. May cause severe hypotension, including orthostatic hypotension and syncope; increased risk in patients whose ability to maintain BP has already been compromised by a reduced blood volume or concurrent administration of certain CNS depressants. Avoid with circulatory shock, impaired consciousness, coma, or GI obstruction. Monitor patients who may be susceptible to intracranial effects of carbon dioxide retention (eg, those with evidence of increased intracranial pressure, brain tumors) for signs of sedation and respiratory depression, particularly when initiating therapy. May obscure clinical course in patients with head injury. May cause spasm of sphincter of Oddi and increases in serum amylase; monitor patients with biliary tract disease, including acute pancreatitis, for worsening symptoms. May aggravate convulsions and induce/aggravate seizures. May impair mental/physical abilities. Not recommended for use during and immediately prior to labor.

ADVERSE REACTIONS

Respiratory depression, constipation, N/V, somnolence, headache, peripheral edema, diarrhea, abdominal pain, infection, urinary tract infection, flu syndrome, back pain, rash, insomnia, depression, dyspnea.

DRUG INTERACTIONS

See Boxed Warning. Concomitant use with other CNS depressants (eg, sedatives, anxiolytics, neuroleptics) may increase risk of respiratory depression, profound sedation, hypotension, coma and death; if coadministration is required, consider dose reduction of one or both agents. Monitor use in elderly, cachectic, and debilitated patients when coadministered with other drugs that depress respiration. Mixed agonist/antagonists (eg, pentazocine, nalbuphine, butorphanol) and partial agonist (buprenorphine) analgesics may reduce analgesic effect or precipitate withdrawal symptoms; avoid coadministration. May enhance neuromuscular blocking action of skeletal muscle relaxants and produce an increased degree of respiratory depression. MAOIs may potentiate effects of morphine; avoid use with MAOIs or within 14 days of stopping such treatment. Cimetidine may potentiate morphine-induced respiratory depression. Confusion and severe respiratory depression in a patient undergoing hemodialysis reported with concurrent cimetidine. May reduce efficacy of diuretics and lead to acute urinary retention. Anticholinergics or other medications with anticholinergic activity may increase risk of urinary retention and/or severe constipation and lead to paralytic ileus. Absorption/exposure may be increased with p-glycoprotein inhibitors (eg, quinidine).

NURSING CONSIDERATIONS

Assessment: Assess for abuse/addiction risk, pain intensity, prior opioid therapy, opioid tolerance, respiratory depression, drug hypersensitivity, pregnancy/nursing status, possible drug interactions, or any other condition where treatment is contraindicated or cautioned.

Monitoring: Monitor for respiratory depression (especially within first 24-72 hrs of initiation), hypotension, seizures/convulsions, and other adverse reactions. Monitor BP and serum amylase levels. Routinely monitor for signs of misuse, abuse, and addiction. Periodically reassess the continued need for therapy.

Patient Counseling: Inform that use of drug can result in addiction, abuse, and misuse; instruct not to share with others and to take steps to protect from theft or misuse. Inform about risk of respiratory depression and advise to seek medical attention if breathing difficulties develop. Advise to store securely and dispose unused caps by flushing down the toilet. Inform female patients of reproductive potential that prolonged use during pregnancy may result in neonatal opioid withdrawal syndrome and instruct to inform physician if pregnant or planning to become pregnant. Inform that potentially serious additive effects may occur when used with alcohol or other CNS depressants, and not to use such drugs unless supervised by physician. Instruct about proper administration instructions. Inform that drug may cause orthostatic hypotension, syncope, and impair the ability to perform potentially hazardous activities; advise to not perform such tasks until patients know how they will react to medication. Advise of potential for severe constipation, including management instructions. Advise how to recognize anaphylaxis and when to seek medical attention.

Storage: 25°C (77°F); excursions permitted to 15-30°C (59-86°F). Protect from light and moisture.

AVITA – tretinoin

RX

Class: Retinoid

ADULT DOSAGE

Acne Vulgaris

Apply qpm where acne lesions appear; use enough to cover the entire affected area lightly

If therapy is temporarily discontinued or frequency of application is reduced, may resume therapy/increase frequency as tolerated

May require >6 weeks therapy before beneficial effects seen

PEDIATRIC DOSAGE

Pediatric use may not have been established

DOSE MODIFICATION

Adverse Reactions

If the degree of local irritation warrants, temporarily decrease frequency, d/c use temporarily, or d/c use altogether

ADMINISTRATION

Topical route

Thoroughly cleanse areas to be treated before medication is applied

HOW SUPPLIED

Cre/Gel: 0.025% [20g, 45g]

WARNINGS/PRECAUTIONS

D/C if sensitivity reaction or chemical irritation occurs. Minimize exposure to sunlight, including sunlamps, or artificial sunlight. Caution in patients w/ sun exposure due to occupation, and sensitivity to sun. Use sunscreen products and protective clothing over treated areas when exposure to sun cannot be avoided. Extreme weather may increase skin irritation. Keep away from eyes, mouth, paranasal creases, mucous membranes, and sunburned skin. May exacerbate acne during early weeks of therapy. May cause transitory feeling of warmth or stinging. May induce severe local erythema and application-site peeling. May cause severe irritation w/ eczematous skin; use w/ utmost caution. (Gel) Flammable; keep away from heat and flame.

ADVERSE REACTIONS

Local skin reactions (red, edematous, blistered, crusted), photosensitivity, temporary skin pigmentation changes.

DRUG INTERACTIONS
Caution w/ topical medications, medicated/abrasive soaps and cleansers, soaps and cosmetics w/ strong drying effect, and products w/ high concentrations of alcohol/astringents/spices/lime; possible interaction w/ tretinoin. Caution w/ preparations containing sulfur, resorcinol, or salicylic acid; allow effects of these agents to subside before application.

NURSING CONSIDERATIONS

Assessment: Assess for hypersensitivity to any ingredients of the drug, presence of sunburn, presence of eczematous skin, pregnancy/nursing status, and for possible drug interactions.

Monitoring: Monitor for signs/symptoms of sensitivity or chemical irritation, skin tolerance, severe local erythema, peeling at the application site, and other adverse reactions. Closely monitor alterations of dose frequency.

Patient Counseling: Instruct to wash w/ a mild soap and then dry gently, waiting 20-30 min before applying medication. Inform that it is important for skin to be completely dry before applying medication to minimize irritation. Instruct to use caution in the sun; advise to use effective sunscreen when outside and to use protective clothing (eg, hat) if extended sun exposure is expected. Counsel to avoid excessive exposure to wind or cold. Advise to d/c use and contact physician if experiencing severe/persistent irritation. Instruct to keep medication away from the mouth, eyes, open wounds, and corners of the nose. Counsel to notify physician if pregnant/nursing. Advise that cosmetics may be used, but areas to be treated should be cleansed thoroughly before treatment. Advise that gel is flammable; advise to keep away from heat and flame.

Storage: <30°C (86°F); avoid freezing.

AVODART – dutasteride RX

Class: Type I and II 5 alpha-reductase inhibitor (2nd generation)

ADULT DOSAGE

Benign Prostatic Hyperplasia

Monotherapy:
1 cap (0.5mg) qd

W/ Tamsulosin:
1 cap (0.5mg) qd and tamsulosin 0.4mg qd

PEDIATRIC DOSAGE
Pediatric use may not have been established

ADMINISTRATION
Oral route

Swallow whole; do not chew or open
Take w/ or w/o food

HOW SUPPLIED
Cap: 0.5mg

CONTRAINDICATIONS
Pregnancy, women of childbearing potential, pediatric patients.

WARNINGS/PRECAUTIONS
Not approved for the prevention of prostate cancer. May decrease serum prostate specific antigen (PSA) concentration during therapy or in the presence of prostate cancer; establish a new baseline PSA at least 3 months after starting treatment and monitor PSA periodically thereafter. Any confirmed increase from lowest PSA value during treatment may signal presence of prostate cancer. May increase risk of high-grade prostate cancer. Prior to treatment initiation, consider other urological conditions that may cause similar symptoms; BPH and prostate cancer may coexist. Risk to male fetus; cap should not be handled by pregnant women or women who could become pregnant. Avoid donating blood until at least 6 months after last dose. Reduced total sperm count, semen volume, and sperm motility reported.

ADVERSE REACTIONS
Impotence, decreased libido, breast disorders, ejaculation disorders.

DRUG INTERACTIONS
Caution with potent, chronic CYP3A4 inhibitors (eg, ritonavir). CYP3A4/5 inhibitors (eg, ritonavir, ketoconazole, verapamil, diltiazem, cimetidine, troleandomycin, ciprofloxacin) may increase levels.

NURSING CONSIDERATIONS

Assessment: Assess for urological conditions that may cause similar symptoms, previous hypersensitivity to the drug, and for possible drug interactions.

Monitoring: Monitor for signs/symptoms of prostate cancer and other urological diseases. Obtain new PSA baseline at least 3 months after starting treatment and monitor PSA periodically thereafter.

Patient Counseling: Inform of the importance of periodic PSA monitoring. Advise that therapy may increase risk of high-grade prostate cancer. Counsel that drug should not be handled by women who are pregnant or who could become pregnant, due to potential fetal risks; advise to wash area immediately with soap and water if contact is made. Instruct not to donate blood until at least 6 months after last dose.

Storage: 25°C (77°F); excursions permitted to 15-30°C (59-86°F).

AXIRON – testosterone CIII

Class: Androgen

Virilization reported in children secondarily exposed to topical testosterone. Children should avoid contact with unwashed or unclothed application sites in men using topical testosterone. Advise patients to strictly adhere to recommended instructions for use.

ADULT DOSAGE

Testosterone Replacement Therapy

Congenital/Acquired Primary Hypogonadism or Hypogonadotropic Hypogonadism in Males:

Initial: Apply 60mg (2 pump actuations) qam
Titrate: May adjust dose based on serum testosterone concentration from a single blood draw 2-8 hrs after application, and at least 14 days after starting treatment or following dose adjustment
If Serum Testosterone Concentration <300ng/dL: May increase from 60mg to 90mg or from 90mg to 120mg
If Serum Testosterone Concentration >1050ng/dL: Decrease from 60mg to 30mg

D/C if serum testosterone concentration is consistently >1050ng/dL at lowest daily dose of 30mg

PEDIATRIC DOSAGE

Pediatric use may not have been established

ADMINISTRATION

Topical route

Apply to clean, dry, intact skin of axilla, preferably at the same time each am
Do not apply to other parts of the body, including the scrotum, penis, abdomen, shoulders, or upper arms
Prime pump in upright position, depress actuator 3 times prior to first use
Refer to PI for administration instructions

HOW SUPPLIED

Sol: 30mg/actuation [110mL]

CONTRAINDICATIONS

Breast carcinoma or known/suspected prostate carcinoma in men, women who are or may become pregnant, or are breastfeeding.

WARNINGS/PRECAUTIONS

Application site and dose are not interchangeable with other topical testosterone products. Monitor patients with BPH for worsening of signs and symptoms of BPH. May increase risk for prostate cancer; evaluate for prostate cancer prior to initiating treatment and reevaluate 3-6 months after initiation of therapy. Risk of virilization in women due to secondary exposure. Increases in Hct/RBC mass may increase risk for thromboembolic events; lower dose or d/c therapy until Hct decreases to acceptable level. Venous thromboembolic events (eg, deep vein thrombosis, pulmonary embolism) reported; d/c treatment and initiate appropriate workup and management if suspected. Suppression of spermatogenesis may occur with large doses. Prolonged use of high doses of orally active 17-α-alkyl androgens has been associated with serious hepatic effects (eg, peliosis hepatis, hepatic neoplasms, cholestatic hepatitis, jaundice). May cause edema with preexisting cardiac, renal, or hepatic disease. Gynecomastia may develop and persist. May potentiate sleep apnea, especially with risk factors such as obesity or chronic lung disease. Changes in serum lipid profile may require dose adjustment or discontinuation. Caution in cancer patients at risk of hypercalcemia and associated hypercalciuria. May decrease concentrations of thyroxin-binding globulins, resulting in decreased total T4 serum concentrations and increased resin uptake of T3 and T4. Flammable; avoid fire, flame, or smoking until applied dose has dried.

ADVERSE REACTIONS

Application-site irritation, application-site erythema, headache, Hct increase, diarrhea, vomiting, prostate-specific antigen (PSA) increase.

DRUG INTERACTIONS

Changes in insulin sensitivity or glycemic control may occur; may decrease blood glucose and insulin requirements in diabetic patients. Changes in anticoagulant activity may occur; frequently monitor INR and PT in patients taking anticoagulants, especially at initiation and termination of androgen therapy. Adrenocorticotropic hormone or corticosteroids may increase fluid retention; caution in patients with cardiac, renal, or hepatic disease.

NURSING CONSIDERATIONS

Assessment: Assess for prostate cancer, breast carcinoma, BPH, cardiac/renal/hepatic disease, risk factors for sleep apnea, and any other conditions where treatment is contraindicated or cautioned, and possible drug interactions. Obtain baseline Hct level, lipid levels, and serum testosterone levels.

Monitoring: Monitor for prostate cancer, worsening of BPH, edema, gynecomastia, sleep apnea, venous thromboembolic events, and other adverse reactions. Perform periodic monitoring of Hct, Hgb, PSA, serum lipid profile, and serum testosterone levels. In cancer patients at risk for hypercalcemia, regularly monitor serum Ca^{2+} levels. Reevaluate Hct 3-6 months after start of therapy, then annually.

Patient Counseling: Inform that men with known or suspected prostate/breast cancer should not use androgen therapy. Advise to report signs/symptoms of secondary exposure in children (eg, penis/clitoris enlargement, premature development of pubic hair, increased erections) and in women (eg, changes in hair distribution, increase in acne). Inform that children and women should avoid contact with unwashed or unclothed application sites of men using topical testosterone. Instruct to apply only to axilla and not to any other part of the body, to wash hands immediately with soap and water after application, and to cover application site with clothing after waiting 3 min for the sol to dry. Instruct to wash application site with soap and water prior to any situation in which direct skin-to-skin contact is anticipated, and to immediately wash area of contact if unwashed/unclothed skin comes in direct contact with skin of another person. Inform of the potential adverse reactions. Instruct to prime the pump by depressing 3X prior to 1st use; advise that no priming is needed with subsequent uses of the pump. Inform not to apply to the stratum, penis, abdomen, shoulders, or upper arms. Instruct patient to allow the sol to dry after the 1st application before the 2nd. Instruct to apply to clean, dry skin at approximately the same time each day. Inform that antiperspirant or deodorant may be used before applying the medication. Counsel to avoid swimming or washing application site until 2 hrs following application. Advise to avoid splashing in the eyes; instruct to flush thoroughly with water in case of contact and to seek medical advice if irritation persists.

Storage: 25°C (77°F); excursions permitted to 15-30°C (59-86°F). Discard used bottles and applicators in household trash in a manner that prevents accidental exposure of children or pets.

AZACTAM – aztreonam

RX

Class: Monobactam

ADULT DOSAGE

Urinary Tract Infections

500mg or 1g q8h or q12h
Max: 8g/day

Systemic Infections

Lower respiratory tract infections (eg, pneumonia, bronchitis), septicemia, skin and skin-structure infections (eg, postoperative wounds, ulcers, burns), intra-abdominal infections (eg, peritonitis), and gynecologic infections (eg, endometritis, pelvic cellulitis) caused by susceptible gram-negative microorganisms; adjunctive therapy to surgery in the management of infections caused by susceptible organisms (eg, abscesses, hollow viscus perforation infections, cutaneous infections, infections of serous

PEDIATRIC DOSAGE

General Dosing

9 Months-16 Years:
IV:
Mild to Moderate Infections: 30mg/kg q8h
Max: 120mg/kg/day
Moderate to Severe Infections: 30mg/kg q6h or q8h
Max: 120mg/kg/day
Patients w/ cystic fibrosis may require higher doses

Treatment Duration

Continue treatment for at least 48 hrs after the patient becomes asymptomatic or evidence of bacterial eradication has been obtained; persistent infections may require treatment for several weeks

surfaces); and concurrent initial therapy w/ other antimicrobial agents before causative organism(s) is known in seriously ill patients who are also at risk of having gram-positive aerobic/anaerobic infection
Moderately Severe: 1g or 2g q8h or q12h
Max: 8g/day
Severe or Life-Threatening: 2g q6h or q8h
Max: 8g/day
IV route is recommended for single doses >1g or w/ bacterial septicemia, localized parenchymal abscess, peritonitis, or other severe systemic or life-threatening infections

***Pseudomonas aeruginosa* Infections**

2g q6h or q8h, at least upon initiation of therapy
Max: 8g/day

Treatment Duration

Continue treatment for at least 48 hrs after the patient becomes asymptomatic or evidence of bacterial eradication has been obtained; persistent infections may require treatment for several weeks

DOSE MODIFICATION

Renal Impairment
CrCl 10-30mL/min:
Initial LD: 1g or 2g
Maint: 50% of dose
CrCl <10mL/min (eg, Hemodialysis):
Initial: 500mg, 1g, or 2g
Maint: 25% of initial dose given at fixed intervals of 6, 8, or 12 hrs; for serious/life-threatening infections, in addition to the maint doses, give 1/8 of the initial dose after each hemodialysis session

ADMINISTRATION

IM/IV route

Aztreonam sol (at concentrations >2% w/v) prepared w/ sterile water for inj (SWFI) or NaCl inj must be used w/in 48 hrs (stored at room temperature) or w/in 7 days (refrigerated); all other prepared sol must be used promptly after preparation

IM
Reconstitute 15mL vial w/ at least 3mL of appropriate diluent
Appropriate diluents are SWFI, Sterile Bacteriostatic Water for inj, 0.9% NaCl inj, or Bacteriostatic NaCl inj
Inject deep into a large muscle mass (eg, gluteus maximus)

IV
Reconstitute 15mL vial w/ 6-10mL of SWFI for a bolus inj; if contents of 15mL vial are to be transferred to an appropriate infusion sol, each gram of aztreonam should be initially constituted w/ at least 3mL of SWFI
Refer to PI for appropriate diluents for further dilution
Inject bolus slowly over 3-5 min
Infuse aztreonam infusion over 20-60 min
If administering multiple drug sol, do not deliver simultaneously; flush delivery tube before and after delivery w/ any appropriate infusion sol compatible w/ both drug sol

Galaxy
Intermittent IV infusion only
Thaw frozen container; do not force thawing by immersion in water baths or by microwave irradiation
Do not add supplementary medication
Do not freeze thawed antibiotics
Do not use plastic containers in series connects
Aztreonam infusion should be completed w/in 20-60 min; discard any unused portion
Refer to PI for compatible infusion sol

Refer to PI for further preparation/administration instructions and compatibility information

HOW SUPPLIED

Inj: 1g, 2g; 1g/50mL, 2g/50mL [Galaxy]

WARNINGS/PRECAUTIONS
Hypersensitivity reactions may occur; d/c and institute appropriate supportive treatment. Caution w/ history of hypersensitivity to β-lactams (eg, penicillins, cephalosporins, carbapenems). *Clostridium difficile*-associated diarrhea (CDAD) reported; d/c if CDAD is suspected or confirmed. Toxic epidermal necrolysis (TEN) reported (rare) in patients undergoing bone marrow transplant w/ multiple risk factors (eg, sepsis, radiation therapy, concomitant drugs associated w/ TEN). May result in bacterial resistance w/ prolonged use in the absence of proven or suspected bacterial infection, or a prophylactic indication; take appropriate measures if superinfection develops. Caution w/ renal/hepatic impairment and in elderly.

ADVERSE REACTIONS
ALT/AST elevation, rash, eosinophilia, neutropenia, pain at inj site, increased SrCr, thrombocytosis.

DRUG INTERACTIONS
Avoid w/ β-lactamase inducing antibiotics (eg, cefoxitin, imipenem). Potential nephrotoxicity and ototoxicity w/ aminoglycosides; monitor renal function.

NURSING CONSIDERATIONS

Assessment: Assess for drug hypersensitivity (eg, β-lactams), hypersensitivity to any allergens, hepatic/renal impairment, pregnancy/nursing status, and for possible drug interactions. Assess use in patients undergoing bone marrow transplant w/ multiple risk factors. Confirm diagnosis of causative organisms.

Monitoring: Monitor for signs/symptoms of hypersensitivity reactions, CDAD, superinfection, TEN in patients undergoing bone marrow transplant, and hepatic/renal function.

Patient Counseling: Inform that therapy should only be used to treat bacterial and not viral infections (eg, common cold). Advise to take exactly ud; inform that skipping doses or not completing full course may decrease effectiveness and increase resistance. Inform that diarrhea is a common problem caused by therapy and will usually end upon discontinuation of therapy. Inform that diarrhea may occur, even as late as ≥2 months after last dose of therapy; instruct to notify physician as soon as possible if watery/bloody stools (w/ or w/o stomach cramps and fever) occur.

Storage: Vial: Room temperature. Avoid excessive heat. Galaxy Container: ≤-20°C (-4°F). Thawed Sol: Stable for 14 days at 2-8°C (36-46°F) or 48 hrs at 25°C (77°F). Do not refreeze. Refer to PI for diluted/reconstituted sol storage information.

AZASITE — azithromycin RX

Class: Macrolide

ADULT DOSAGE
Bacterial Conjunctivitis
Instill 1 drop in affected eye(s) bid, 8-12 hrs apart for the first 2 days, then 1 drop qd for the next 5 days

PEDIATRIC DOSAGE
Bacterial Conjunctivitis
≥1 Year:
Instill 1 drop in affected eye(s) bid, 8-12 hrs apart for the first 2 days, then 1 drop qd for the next 5 days

ADMINISTRATION
Ocular route

HOW SUPPLIED
Sol: 1% [2.5mL]

WARNINGS/PRECAUTIONS
Not for inj. Do not administer systemically, inject subconjunctivally, or introduce directly into the anterior chamber of the eye. Serious allergic reactions, including angioedema, anaphylaxis, and dermatologic reactions (eg, Stevens-Johnson syndrome, toxic epidermal necrolysis), rarely reported when administered systemically. May result in bacterial resistance with prolonged use; take appropriate measures if superinfection develops. Avoid wearing contact lenses if signs or symptoms of bacterial conjunctivitis exist.

ADVERSE REACTIONS
Eye irritation, blurred vision, burning/stinging upon instillation, contact dermatitis, corneal erosion, dry eye, eye pain, ocular discharge, dysgeusia, facial swelling, hives, nasal congestion, periocular swelling, rash.

NURSING CONSIDERATIONS

Assessment: Assess for hypersensitivity, proper diagnosis of causative organisms, use of contact lenses, and pregnancy/nursing status.

Monitoring: Monitor for hypersensitivity reactions, superinfection, eye irritation, and other adverse reactions.

Patient Counseling: Advise to avoid contaminating the applicator tip by allowing it to touch the eye, fingers, or other sources. Instruct to d/c and contact physician if any signs of allergic reaction occur. Instruct to use exactly ud; skipping doses or not completing full course may decrease effectiveness of treatment and increase bacterial resistance. Advise not to wear contact lenses if patient has signs/symptoms of bacterial conjunctivitis. Advise to wash hands thoroughly before instillation. Counsel on proper administration; shake bottle once before each use.

Storage: Unopened Bottle: 2-8°C (36-46°F). Opened Bottle: 2-25°C (36-77°F) for up to 14 days. Discard after 14 days.

Azelex – azelaic acid — RX

Class: Dicarboxylic acid antimicrobial

ADULT DOSAGE

Acne Vulgaris

Mild to Moderate Inflammatory Acne:
Massage gently but thoroughly into affected area bid (am and pm)

PEDIATRIC DOSAGE

Acne Vulgaris

Mild to Moderate Inflammatory Acne:
≥12 Years:
Massage gently but thoroughly into affected area bid (am and pm)

ADMINISTRATION

Topical route

Wash and pat dry skin prior to application
Wash hands following application

HOW SUPPLIED

Cre: 20% [30g, 50g]

WARNINGS/PRECAUTIONS

For dermatologic use only; not for ophthalmic use. Hypopigmentation reported; monitor for signs of hypopigmentation in patients with dark complexion. D/C if sensitivity or severe irritation occurs and institute appropriate therapy.

ADVERSE REACTIONS

Pruritus, burning, stinging, tingling.

NURSING CONSIDERATIONS

Assessment: Assess for hypersensitivity and pregnancy/nursing status.

Monitoring: Monitor for signs/symptoms of hypopigmentation, sensitivity reactions, and severe skin irritation.

Patient Counseling: Counsel to use medication for the full prescribed treatment period. Instruct not to use occlusive dressings or wrappings. Advise to keep medication away from mouth, eyes, and mucous membranes; if contact occurs with eyes, instruct to wash eyes with large amounts of water and consult physician if problem persists. Counsel patients with dark complexions to notify physician if they notice skin color changes. Instruct that temporary skin irritation may occur when applied to broken or inflamed skin; if irritation persists, advise to consult physician immediately.

Storage: 15-30°C (59-86°F). Protect from freezing.

Azilect – rasagiline mesylate — RX

Class: Monoamine oxidase inhibitor (type B)

ADULT DOSAGE

Parkinson's Disease

Monotherapy or Adjunctive Therapy in Patients Not Taking Levodopa:
Initial: 1mg qd

Patients Taking Levodopa w/ or w/o Other Parkinson's Disease Drugs:
Initial: 0.5mg qd
Titrate: May increase to 1mg qd if a sufficient clinical response is not achieved. May consider dose reduction of concomitant levodopa based upon individual response

PEDIATRIC DOSAGE

Pediatric use may not have been established

DOSE MODIFICATION

Concomitant Medications

Ciprofloxacin or Other CYP1A2 Inhibitors:

Max: 0.5mg qd

Hepatic Impairment

Mild:

Max: 0.5mg qd

ADMINISTRATION

Oral route

May be administered w/ or w/o food

HOW SUPPLIED

Tab: 0.5mg, 1mg

CONTRAINDICATIONS

Concomitant use with any other MAOI, meperidine, tramadol, methadone, or propoxyphene; at least 14 days should elapse between discontinuation of rasagiline and initiation of treatment with these medications. Concomitant use with St. John's wort, cyclobenzaprine, or dextromethorphan.

WARNINGS/PRECAUTIONS

Avoid with moderate/severe hepatic impairment. Exacerbation of HTN may occur; medication adjustment may be necessary if BP elevation is sustained. Falling asleep during activities of daily living and somnolence reported; d/c therapy if significant daytime sleepiness or episodes of falling asleep during activities that require active participation (eg, driving a motor vehicle, conversations, eating) develop. May potentiate dopaminergic side effects and cause/exacerbate dyskinesia when used as an adjunct to levodopa; reducing levodopa dose may mitigate effect. Hypotension (eg, orthostatic hypotension) and hallucinations reported. New/worsening mental status and behavioral changes, which may be severe, including psychotic-like behavior, may occur; consider dose reduction or discontinuation if these symptoms develop. Do not use in patients with a major psychotic disorder. Increased sexual urges, binge eating, intense urges to gamble or spend money, and/or other intense urges, and the inability to control these urges may occur; consider dose reduction or discontinuation if such urges develop. A symptom complex resembling neuroleptic malignant syndrome reported with rapid dose reduction, withdrawal of, or changes in drugs that increase central dopaminergic tone. Patients with PD have a higher risk of developing melanoma.

ADVERSE REACTIONS

Headache, arthralgia, dyspepsia, depression, fall, flu syndrome, conjunctivitis, fever, gastroenteritis, rhinitis, dyskinesia, weight loss, N/V, dizziness, abdominal pain.

DRUG INTERACTIONS

See Contraindications and Dosage. Not recommended with antidepressants; serotonin syndrome reported. At least 14 days should elapse between discontinuation of therapy and initiation of an SSRI, SNRI, TCA, tetracyclic, or triazolopyridine antidepressant. At least 5 weeks (longer with chronic/high-dose fluoxetine) should elapse between discontinuation of fluoxetine and initiation of rasagiline due to the long $T_{1/2}$ of fluoxetine and its active metabolite. Ciprofloxacin and other CYP1A2 inhibitors may increase levels. Hypertensive crisis/reactions reported with sympathomimetics or tyramine-rich foods; caution with sympathomimetics (eg, nasal/oral/ophthalmic decongestants, cold remedies), and avoid foods containing a very large amount of tyramine (eg, aged cheese). Dopamine antagonists (eg, antipsychotics, metoclopramide) may diminish effectiveness.

NURSING CONSIDERATIONS

Assessment: Assess for hepatic impairment, HTN, dyskinesia, major psychotic disorder, pregnancy/nursing status, and possible drug interactions.

Monitoring: Monitor for HTN, drowsiness/sleepiness, dyskinesia, hypotension, hallucinations, new/worsening mental status and behavioral changes, psychotic-like behavior, intense urges, and other adverse reactions. Monitor for melanomas frequently and on a regular basis.

Patient Counseling: Inform of the risk of using higher than recommended daily doses; provide a brief description of the tyramine-associated hypertensive reaction. Advise to avoid foods containing a very large amount of tyramine while on therapy. Instruct to inform physician if taking or planning to take any prescription or OTC drugs. Instruct not to drive a car or engage in other potentially dangerous activities until patient has gained sufficient experience with therapy and other dopaminergic medications; advise to exercise caution when taking alcohol. Inform that orthostatic hypotension may develop; caution against standing up rapidly after sitting or lying down for prolonged periods and at the initiation of treatment. Instruct to contact physician if discontinuation of therapy is desired, or if BP elevation, hallucinations, new/increased gambling urges, increased sexual urges, or other intense urges develop. Instruct to take drug as prescribed. Advise to undergo periodic skin examinations.

Storage: 25°C (77°F); excursions permitted to 15-30°C (59-86°F).

Azopt – brinzolamide RX

Class: Carbonic anhydrase inhibitor

ADULT DOSAGE

Elevated Intraocular Pressure

Ocular HTN/Open-Angle Glaucoma:
1 drop in the affected eye(s) tid

PEDIATRIC DOSAGE

Pediatric use may not have been established

DOSE MODIFICATION

Concomitant Medications

Space dosing by at least 10 min if using >1 topical ophthalmic drug

ADMINISTRATION

Ocular route

Shake well before use

HOW SUPPLIED

Sus: 1% [10mL, 15mL]

WARNINGS/PRECAUTIONS

Systemically absorbed. Fatalities occurred (rarely) due to severe reactions to sulfonamides including Stevens-Johnson syndrome, toxic epidermal necrolysis, fulminant hepatic necrosis, agranulocytosis, aplastic anemia, and other blood dyscrasias. Sensitization may recur when a sulfonamide is readministered irrespective of route. D/C if signs of serious reactions or hypersensitivity occur. Caution with low endothelial cell counts; increased potential for corneal edema. Not recommended with severe renal impairment (CrCl <30mL/min). Contains benzalkonium chloride, which may be absorbed by soft contact lenses; contact lenses should be removed during instillation, but may be reinserted 15 min after instillation.

ADVERSE REACTIONS

Blurred vision, bitter/sour/unusual taste, blepharitis, dermatitis, dry eye, foreign body sensation, headache, hyperemia, ocular discharge/discomfort/keratitis/pain/pruritus, rhinitis.

DRUG INTERACTIONS

Potential additive systemic effects with oral carbonic anhydrase inhibitors; coadministration is not recommended. Acid-base alterations reported with high-dose salicylate therapy in patients treated with oral carbonic anhydrase inhibitors.

NURSING CONSIDERATIONS

Assessment: Assess for hypersensitivity to drug or to sulfonamides, low endothelial cell counts, renal impairment, contact lens use, pregnancy/nursing status, and possible drug interactions.

Monitoring: Monitor for sulfonamide/hypersensitivity reactions, and other adverse reactions.

Patient Counseling: Advise to d/c use and consult physician if serious or unusual ocular or systemic reactions or signs of hypersensitivity occur. Inform that vision may be temporarily blurred following administration; instruct to use caution in operating machinery or driving a motor vehicle. Instruct to avoid allowing the container tip to contact the eye or surrounding structures or other surfaces. Instruct to consult physician about the continued use of the present multidose container if undergoing ocular surgery or if an intercurrent ocular condition (eg, trauma, infection) develops. Instruct that if using >1 topical ophthalmic drug, to administer the drugs at least 10 min apart. Advise that contact lenses should be removed during instillation, but may be reinserted 15 min after instillation.

Storage: 4-30°C (39-86°F).

Azor – amlodipine/olmesartan medoxomil RX

Class: ARB/calcium channel blocker (dihydropyridine)

D/C when pregnancy is detected. Drugs that act directly on the renin-angiotensin system (RAS) can cause death/injury to the developing fetus.

ADULT DOSAGE

Hypertension

Initial Therapy:
Initial: 5mg-20mg qd
Titrate: May increase dose after 1-2 weeks
Max: 10mg-40mg qd

PEDIATRIC DOSAGE

Pediatric use may not have been established

Replacement Therapy:
May substitute for individually titrated components
When substituting for individual components, the dose of 1 or both components may be increased if BP is not adequately controlled

Add-On Therapy:
May be used to provide additional BP lowering when not adequately controlled on amlodipine (or another dihydropyridine calcium channel blocker) or olmesartan (or another ARB) alone

DOSE MODIFICATION

Hepatic Impairment
Initial Therapy: Not recommended

Elderly
≥75 Years:
Initial Therapy: Not recommended

ADMINISTRATION
Oral route

Take w/ or w/o food
May be administered w/ other antihypertensive agents

HOW SUPPLIED
Tab: (Amlodipine-Olmesartan) 5mg-20mg, 5mg-40mg, 10mg-20mg, 10mg-40mg

CONTRAINDICATIONS
Coadministration with aliskiren in patients with diabetes.

WARNINGS/PRECAUTIONS
Not recommended for use as initial therapy in patients ≥75 yrs of age or with hepatic impairment. May decrease Hct and Hgb levels. Amlodipine: Acute hypotension reported (rare); caution with severe aortic stenosis. May develop increased frequency, duration, or severity of angina or acute MI with dosage initiation or increase, particularly in patients with severe obstructive coronary artery disease (CAD). May cause hepatic enzyme elevation. Caution with severe hepatic impairment and in elderly. Olmesartan: Symptomatic hypotension, especially in patients with an activated RAS (eg, volume- and/or salt-depleted patients treated with high doses of diuretics), may occur after initiation of treatment; initiate treatment under close medical supervision. May cause changes in renal function. Oliguria or progressive azotemia and (rare) acute renal failure and/or death may occur in patients whose renal function may depend upon the activity of the RAS (eg, severe CHF). May increase BUN or SrCr levels in patients with renal artery stenosis. Sprue-like enteropathy with symptoms of severe, chronic diarrhea with substantial weight loss reported; exclude other etiologies if these symptoms develop, and consider discontinuation in cases where no other etiology is identified. Hyperkalemia may occur.

ADVERSE REACTIONS
Edema, headache, palpitation, dizziness, flushing.

DRUG INTERACTIONS
See Contraindications. Amlodipine: May increase simvastatin exposure; limit simvastatin dose to 20mg/day. Olmesartan: Dual blockade of the RAS is associated with increased risks of hypotension, hyperkalemia, and changes in renal function (including acute renal failure); avoid combined use of RAS inhibitors, or closely monitor BP, renal function, and electrolytes with concomitant agents that affect the RAS. Avoid with aliskiren in patients with renal impairment (GFR <60mL/min). NSAIDs, including selective COX-2 inhibitors, may deteriorate renal function and attenuate antihypertensive effect; monitor renal function periodically. Colesevelam may decrease levels; administer at least 4 hrs before colesevelam dose. Increases in serum lithium levels and lithium toxicity reported; monitor lithium levels.

NURSING CONSIDERATIONS

Assessment: Assess for severe obstructive CAD, CHF, severe aortic stenosis, volume/salt depletion, diabetes, renal/hepatic impairment, pregnancy/nursing status, and possible drug interactions.

Monitoring: Monitor for signs/symptoms of hypotension, sprue-like enteropathy, and other adverse reactions. Monitor for symptoms of angina or MI, particularly in patients with severe obstructive CAD, after dosage initiation or increase. Monitor for decrease in Hct/Hgb, increase in SrCr, BUN, K^+ levels, and hepatic enzymes.

Patient Counseling: Inform about the consequences of exposure during pregnancy and of the treatment options in women if planning to become pregnant; instruct to report pregnancy to the physician as soon as possible.

Storage: 25°C (77°F); excursions permitted to 15-30°C (59-86°F).

BACTROBAN NASAL – mupirocin calcium

RX

Class: Bacterial protein synthesis inhibitor

ADULT DOSAGE

Methicillin-Resistant *Staphylococcus aureus*

Eradication of nasal colonization w/ MRSA as part of a comprehensive infection control program to reduce risk of infection among patients at high risk of MRSA infection during institutional outbreaks of infections w/ this pathogen

Apply 1/2 tube into each nostril bid (am and pm) for 5 days

PEDIATRIC DOSAGE

Methicillin-Resistant *Staphylococcus aureus*

Eradication of nasal colonization w/ MRSA as part of a comprehensive infection control program to reduce risk of infection among patients at high risk of MRSA infection during institutional outbreaks of infections w/ this pathogen

≥12 Years:

Apply 1/2 tube into each nostril bid (am and pm) for 5 days

ADMINISTRATION

Intranasal route

Spread oint by pressing together and releasing the sides of the nose repetitively for 1 min

HOW SUPPLIED

Oint: 2% [1g]

WARNINGS/PRECAUTIONS

Avoid contact w/ eyes; rinse well w/ water in case of accidental contact. D/C if sensitization or severe local irritation occurs. *Clostridium difficile*-associated diarrhea (CDAD) reported; may need to d/c if CDAD is suspected/confirmed. Prolonged use may result in overgrowth of nonsusceptible microorganisms, including fungi.

ADVERSE REACTIONS

Headache, rhinitis, respiratory disorder, pharyngitis, taste perversion.

DRUG INTERACTIONS

Avoid use w/ any other intranasal products.

NURSING CONSIDERATIONS

Assessment: Assess for drug hypersensitivity and possible drug interactions.

Monitoring: Monitor for sensitization, severe local irritation, CDAD, and other adverse reactions.

Patient Counseling: Instruct to avoid contact w/ eyes; advise to rinse thoroughly w/ water if therapy gets in or near the eyes. Advise to take ud and to d/c use and contact physician if sensitization or severe local irritation occurs.

Storage: 20-25°C (68-77°F); excursions permitted to 15-30°C (59-86°F). Do not refrigerate.

BACTROBAN TOPICAL – mupirocin

RX

Class: Bacterial protein synthesis inhibitor

ADULT DOSAGE

Secondarily Infected Traumatic Skin Lesions

Lesions up to 10cm in length or 100cm^2 in area due to *Staphylococcus aureus* and *Streptococcus pyogenes*

Cre:

Apply a small amount to the affected area tid for 10 days; reevaluate if no clinical response w/in 3-5 days

Impetigo

Due to *Staphylococcus aureus* and *Streptococcus pyogenes*

Oint:

Apply a small amount to the affected area tid; reevaluate if no clinical response w/in 3-5 days

PEDIATRIC DOSAGE

Secondarily Infected Traumatic Skin Lesions

Lesions up to 10cm in length or 100cm^2 in area due to *Staphylococcus aureus* and *Streptococcus pyogenes*

3 Months-16 Years:

Cre:

Apply a small amount to the affected area tid for 10 days; reevaluate if no clinical response w/in 3-5 days

Impetigo

Due to *Staphylococcus aureus* and *Streptococcus pyogenes*

2 Months-16 Years:

Oint:

Apply a small amount to the affected area tid; reevaluate if no clinical response w/in 3-5 days

ADMINISTRATION
Topical route

May be covered w/ gauze dressing if desired

HOW SUPPLIED
Cre: 2% [15g, 30g]; Oint: 2% [22g]

WARNINGS/PRECAUTIONS
Avoid contact w/ eyes; rinse well w/ water in case of accidental contact. D/C and institute appropriate alternative therapy if sensitization or severe local irritation occurs. *Clostridium difficile*-associated diarrhea (CDAD) reported; may need to d/c if CDAD is suspected/confirmed. Prolonged use may result in overgrowth of nonsusceptible organism, including fungi. Not for use on mucosal surfaces. (Oint) Contains polyethylene glycol; avoid use in conditions where absorption of large quantities is possible, especially if there is evidence of moderate or severe renal impairment. Avoid use w/ IV cannulae or at central IV sites; may promote fungal infections and antimicrobial resistance.

ADVERSE REACTIONS
Systemic allergic reactions, rash, nausea, burning at application site, dermatitis, dry skin. (Cre) Headache, pruritus. (Oint) Stinging, pain, itching.

NURSING CONSIDERATIONS

Assessment: Assess for hypersensitivity to the drug and pregnancy/nursing status.

Monitoring: Monitor for sensitization, severe local irritation, CDAD, and other adverse reactions.

Patient Counseling: Instruct to use only ud. Inform that medication is for external use only. Instruct to avoid contact w/ eyes; advise to rinse thoroughly w/ water if therapy gets in or near the eyes. Counsel that treated area can be covered w/ a gauze dressing if desired. Advise to d/c medication and contact physician if irritation, severe itching, or rash occurs. Instruct to notify physician if no improvement is seen in 3-5 days.

Storage: (Cre) At or below 25°C (77°F). Do not freeze. (Oint) 20-25°C (68-77°F).

BANZEL – rufinamide RX

Class: Triazole derivative

ADULT DOSAGE
Seizures
Associated w/ Lennox-Gastaut Syndrome:
Initial: 400-800mg/day given bid; initiate at <400mg/day if taking concomitant valproate
Titrate: Increase by 400-800mg qod until max dose is reached
Max: 3200mg/day

PEDIATRIC DOSAGE
Seizures
Associated w/ Lennox-Gastaut Syndrome:
1-<17 Years:
Initial: 10mg/kg/day given bid; initiate at <10mg/kg/day if taking concomitant valproate
Titrate: Increase by 10mg/kg increments qod
Max: 45mg/kg/day, not to exceed 3200mg/day

DOSE MODIFICATION
Renal Impairment
Hemodialysis:
May reduce systemic exposure; consider dosage adjustment during dialysis process

Hepatic Impairment
Not recommended w/ severe (Child-Pugh score 10-15) hepatic impairment. Caution w/ mild (Child-Pugh score 5-6) to moderate (Child-Pugh score 7-9) hepatic impairment

Elderly
Start at lower end of dosing range

ADMINISTRATION
Oral route
Take w/ food

Tab
May be administered whole, as 1/2 tabs, or crushed

Sus
Shake well before every administration
Provided adapter and calibrated oral dosing syringe should be used to administer oral sus
Adapter should be firmly inserted into the neck of the bottle before use and remain in place for the duration of the usage of the bottle
Dosing syringe should be inserted into the adapter and the dose withdrawn from inverted bottle
Replace cap after each use

HOW SUPPLIED

Sus: 40mg/mL [460mL]; Tab: 200mg*, 400mg* *scored

CONTRAINDICATIONS

Familial short QT syndrome.

WARNINGS/PRECAUTIONS

May increase risk of suicidal thoughts or behavior. CNS-related adverse effects (eg, somnolence, coordination abnormalities, dizziness), QT interval shortening, and leukopenia reported. Multiorgan hypersensitivity syndrome, drug reaction w/ eosinophilia and systemic symptoms (DRESS), and Stevens-Johnson syndrome (SJS) reported; d/c if suspected and start alternative treatment. Withdraw gradually to minimize risk of precipitating seizures, seizure exacerbation, or status epilepticus. If abrupt discontinuation is necessary, transition to another antiepileptic drug should be made under close medical supervision. Not recommended w/ severe hepatic impairment (Child-Pugh 10-15). Caution w/ mild (Child-Pugh 5-6) to moderate (Child-Pugh 7-9) hepatic impairment and in elderly.

ADVERSE REACTIONS

Somnolence, N/V, headache, fatigue, dizziness, constipation, cough, decreased appetite, rash, otitis media, pneumonia, decreased weight, diplopia, bronchitis, blurred vision.

DRUG INTERACTIONS

See Dosage. Potent CYP450 inducers (eg, carbamazepine, phenytoin, primidone, phenobarbital) may increase clearance and decrease levels. Valproate may increase levels. May increase phenytoin or phenobarbital levels. May decrease levels of lamotrigine or carbamazepine. Concurrent use w/ hormonal contraceptives may render this method of contraception less effective; additional forms of nonhormonal contraception are recommended during coadministration. Caution w/ other drugs that shorten QT interval.

NURSING CONSIDERATIONS

Assessment: Assess for familial short QT syndrome, depression, hepatic/renal impairment, pregnancy/nursing status, and possible drug interactions.

Monitoring: Monitor for CNS reactions, QT interval shortening, multiorgan hypersensitivity syndrome, DRESS, SJS, leukopenia, emergence or worsening of depression, suicidal thoughts/behavior, unusual changes in mood/behavior, and other adverse reactions. Upon withdrawal of therapy, monitor for precipitation/exacerbation of seizures, and status epilepticus.

Patient Counseling: Inform patients, caregivers, and families of the increased risk of suicidal thoughts/behavior; advise to be alert for emergence or worsening of signs/symptoms of depression, any unusual changes in mood/behavior, or emergence of suicidal thoughts, behavior, or thoughts about self-harm. Instruct to immediately report behaviors of concern to healthcare provider. Inform of the potential for somnolence or dizziness; advise not to drive or operate machinery until the effects of drug are known. Advise to notify physician if rash associated w/ fever develops. Inform females of childbearing age that concurrent use w/ hormonal contraceptives may render this method of contraception less effective and recommend using additional nonhormonal forms of contraception during therapy. Inform that alcohol may cause additive CNS effects. Advise to notify physician if pregnant or intend to become pregnant; encourage to enroll in the North American Antiepileptic Drug Pregnancy Registry. Advise to notify physician if breastfeeding or intending to breastfeed.

Storage: 25°C (77°F); excursions permitted to 15-30°C (59-86°F). (Tab) Protect from moisture. (Sus) Store in an upright position. Use w/in 90 days of 1st opening bottle.

BARACLUDE – entecavir RX

Class: Guanosine nucleoside analogue

Severe acute exacerbations of hepatitis B reported upon discontinuation of therapy; monitor liver function for at least several months after discontinuation. If appropriate, may initiate antihepatitis B therapy. Potential for development of resistance to HIV nucleoside reverse transcriptase inhibitors if entecavir is used to treat chronic hepatitis B virus (HBV) infection in patients with untreated HIV infection. Not recommended for HIV/HBV coinfected patients not receiving highly active antiretroviral therapy (HAART). Lactic acidosis and severe hepatomegaly with steatosis, including fatal cases, have been reported with the use of nucleoside analogue inhibitors.

ADULT DOSAGE

Chronic Hepatitis B

In patients w/ evidence of active viral replication and either evidence of persistent elevations in serum aminotransferases (ALT/AST) or histologically active disease

PEDIATRIC DOSAGE

Chronic Hepatitis B

In patients w/ evidence of active viral replication and either evidence of persistent elevations in serum aminotransferases (ALT/AST) or histologically active disease

Compensated Liver Disease:
Nucleoside-Inhibitor Treatment-Naive:
0.5mg qd

History of Hepatitis B Viremia While Receiving Lamivudine or Known Lamivudine- or Telbivudine-Resistant Substitutions:
1mg qd

Decompensated Liver Disease:
1mg qd

≥2 Years:
Treatment-Naive:
10-11kg: 3mL qd
>11-14kg: 4mL qd
>14-17kg: 5mL qd
>17-20kg: 6mL qd
>20-23kg: 7mL qd
>23-26kg: 8mL qd
>26-30kg: 9mL qd
>30kg: 10mL or 0.5mg tab qd

Lamivudine-Experienced:
10-11kg: 6mL qd
>11-14kg: 8mL qd
>14-17kg: 10mL qd
>17-20kg: 12mL qd
>20-23kg: 14mL qd
>23-26kg: 16mL qd
>26-30kg: 18mL qd
>30kg: 20mL or 1mg tab qd

Compensated Liver Disease:
Nucleoside-Inhibitor Treatment-Naive:
≥16 Years:
0.5mg qd

History of Hepatitis B Viremia While Receiving Lamivudine or Known Lamivudine- or Telbivudine-Resistant Substitutions:
≥16 Years:
1mg qd

DOSE MODIFICATION

Renal Impairment

CrCl 30-<50mL/min:
Usual: 0.25mg qd or 0.5mg q48h
Lamivudine-Refractory or Decompensated Liver Disease: 0.5mg qd or 1mg q48h

CrCl 10-<30mL/min:
Usual: 0.15mg qd or 0.5mg q72h
Lamivudine-Refractory or Decompensated Liver Disease: 0.3mg qd or 1mg q72h

CrCl <10mL/min or CAPD:
Usual: 0.05mg qd or 0.5mg every 7 days
Lamivudine-Refractory or Decompensated Liver Disease: 0.1mg qd or 1mg every 7 days

Hemodialysis:
Usual: 0.05mg qd or 0.5mg every 7 days (after session if administered on hemodialysis day)
Lamivudine-Refractory or Decompensated Liver Disease: 0.1mg qd or 1mg every 7 days (after session if administered on hemodialysis day)

ADMINISTRATION

Oral route

Take on an empty stomach (at least 2 hrs pc and 2 hrs before the next meal)

HOW SUPPLIED

Sol: 0.05mg/mL [210mL]; Tab: 0.5mg, 1mg

WARNINGS/PRECAUTIONS

Dosage adjustment is recommended in renal dysfunction (CrCl <50mL/min), including patients on hemodialysis or continuous ambulatory peritoneal dialysis. May require HIV antibody testing prior to treatment. Caution with known risk factors for liver disease. D/C if lactic acidosis or pronounced hepatotoxicity occurs. Caution in elderly.

ADVERSE REACTIONS

Hepatitis B exacerbation, lactic acidosis, hepatomegaly, headache, fatigue, dizziness, nausea, ALT/lipase/total bilirubin elevation, hyperglycemia, glycosuria, hematuria.

DRUG INTERACTIONS

May increase levels of either entecavir or concomitant drugs that reduce renal function or compete for active tubular secretion; closely monitor for adverse events.

NURSING CONSIDERATIONS

Assessment: Assess for hepatic/renal impairment, pregnancy/nursing status, and possible drug interactions. Perform HIV antibody testing before initiating therapy.

Monitoring: Monitor for signs/symptoms of lactic acidosis, hepatotoxicity, renal/hepatic impairment, and other adverse reactions.

Patient Counseling: Advise to remain under care of physician during therapy and report any new symptoms or concurrent medications. Advise that treatment has not been shown to reduce risk of transmission of HBV to others through sexual contact or blood contamination. Advise to take the missed dose as soon as remembered unless it is almost time for the next dose and not to take 2 doses at the same time. Inform that treatment may lower the amount of HBV in the body and improve the condition of the liver, but will not cure HBV. Counsel that it is not known whether treatment will reduce risk of liver cancer or cirrhosis. Inform that deterioration of liver disease may occur in some cases if treatment is discontinued, and instruct to discuss any change in regimen with physician. Inform that drug may increase the chance of HIV resistance to HIV medication if HIV-infected patient is not receiving effective HIV treatment.

Storage: 25°C (77°F); excursions permitted between 15-30°C (59-86°F). Protect from light.

BELVIQ – lorcaserin hydrochloride CIV

Class: Serotonin 2C receptor agonist

ADULT DOSAGE

Weight Loss

Adjunct to reduced-calorie diet and increased physical activity for chronic weight management in patients w/ initial BMI ≥30kg/m², or ≥27kg/m² in the presence of ≥1 weight-related comorbid condition

Usual: 10mg bid

Evaluate response to therapy by Week 12; d/c therapy if patient has not lost at least 5% of baseline weight

PEDIATRIC DOSAGE

Pediatric use may not have been established

ADMINISTRATION

Oral route

Take w/ or w/o food

HOW SUPPLIED

Tab: 10mg

CONTRAINDICATIONS

Pregnancy.

WARNINGS/PRECAUTIONS

Potentially life-threatening serotonin syndrome or neuroleptic malignant syndrome (NMS)-like reactions reported; monitor for emergence of serotonin syndrome or NMS-like signs/symptoms. Regurgitant cardiac valvular disease reported; evaluate and consider discontinuation of therapy if signs/symptoms of valvular heart disease develop. Caution with chronic heart failure (CHF). May impair mental/physical abilities. Monitor for emergence or worsening of depression, suicidal thoughts or behavior, and/or any unusual changes in mood or behavior; d/c in patients who experience suicidal thoughts or behaviors. Hypoglycemia reported; measure blood glucose levels prior to and during therapy in patients with type 2 diabetes. Caution in men who have conditions that might predispose them to priapism, or in men with anatomical deformation of the penis. Caution with bradycardia or history of heart block >1st degree, moderate renal impairment, and severe hepatic impairment. Not recommended with severe renal impairment or ESRD. Decrease in WBCs and RBCs reported; consider monitoring CBC periodically during therapy. May elevate prolactin levels. May increase risk for pulmonary HTN.

ADVERSE REACTIONS

Nasopharyngitis, headache, constipation, diarrhea, hypoglycemia, cough, dizziness, fatigue, back pain, N/V, dry mouth, URTI, peripheral edema, UTI, muscle spasms.

DRUG INTERACTIONS

Use extreme caution, particularly during initiation and dose increases, with drugs that may affect the serotonergic neurotransmitter system (eg, triptans, drugs that impair metabolism of serotonin including MAOIs [eg, linezolid], SSRIs, SNRIs, dextromethorphan, TCAs, bupropion, lithium, tramadol, tryptophan, St. John's wort, antipsychotics, other dopamine antagonists); d/c lorcaserin and any concomitant serotonergic or antidopaminergic agents immediately if serotonin syndrome occurs. Consider decreasing dose of non-glucose dependent antidiabetic medications in order to mitigate risk of hypoglycemia. Caution with CYP2D6 substrates. Avoid with serotonergic and dopaminergic drugs that are potent 5-HT_{2B} receptor agonists and are known to increase the risk for cardiac valvulopathy (eg, cabergoline). Caution with medications indicated for erectile dysfunction (eg, PDE-5 inhibitors).

NURSING CONSIDERATIONS

Assessment: Assess for CHF, bradycardia or history of heart block >1st degree, renal/hepatic impairment, pregnancy/nursing status, and possible drug interactions. Assess for conditions in men that might predispose them to priapism and assess for anatomical deformities of the penis. Assess baseline body weight and CBC. Assess baseline blood glucose levels in patients with type 2 diabetes.

Monitoring: Monitor for signs/symptoms of serotonin syndrome or NMS-like reactions, valvular heart disease, emergence or worsening of depression, suicidal thoughts or behavior, any unusual changes in mood or behavior, and other adverse reactions. Monitor CBC periodically during therapy. Monitor blood glucose levels in patients with type 2 diabetes. Evaluate response to treatment by Week 12 of therapy.

Patient Counseling: Inform about the risk and benefits of the drug. Inform that therapy is indicated for chronic weight management only in conjunction with a reduced-calorie diet and increased physical activity. Instruct to d/c therapy if patient has not achieved 5% weight loss by 12 weeks of therapy. Inform of the possibility of serotonin or NMS-like reactions. Instruct to use caution when operating hazardous machinery, including automobiles, until aware of the effects of the medication. Instruct not to increase the dose. Instruct to notify physician if signs/symptoms of valvular heart disease, emergence or worsening of depression, suicidal thoughts or behavior, or if any unusual changes in mood or behavior develop. Instruct men who have an erection lasting >4 hrs to immediately d/c and seek emergency medical attention. Advise to avoid pregnancy/breastfeeding while on therapy and to inform physician if planning to get pregnant/breastfeed. Instruct to inform physician about all medications, nutritional supplements, and vitamins that patient is taking while on therapy.

Storage: 25°C (77°F); excursions permitted to 15-30°C (59-86°F).

BENAZEPRIL – benazepril hydrochloride

RX

Class: ACE inhibitor

D/C when pregnancy is detected. Drugs that act directly on the renin-angiotensin system (RAS) can cause injury/death to the developing fetus.

OTHER BRAND NAMES

Lotensin

ADULT DOSAGE

Hypertension

Not Receiving a Diuretic:
Initial: 10mg qd
Maint: 20-40mg/day as single dose or in 2 equally divided doses
Adjust dose based on measurement of peak (2-6 hrs after dosing) and trough responses
Max: 80mg/day
May add diuretic if BP is not controlled

PEDIATRIC DOSAGE

Hypertension

≥6 Years:
Initial: 0.2mg/kg qd
Max: 0.6mg/kg (or 40mg/day)

DOSE MODIFICATION

Concomitant Medications

Concomitant Diuretics:
Initial: 5mg qd
If possible, d/c diuretic 2-3 days prior to therapy to avoid hypotension. If BP is not controlled w/ benazepril alone, diuretic therapy should be resumed

Renal Impairment

CrCl <30mL/min (SrCr >3mg/dL):
Initial: 5mg qd
Titrate: May increase until BP is controlled
Max: 40mg/day

ADMINISTRATION

Oral route

Sus

Preparation of Sus (for 150mL of a 2mg/mL sus):
1. Add 75mL of Ora-Plus oral suspending vehicle to an amber polyethylene terephthalate bottle containing 15 benazepril 20mg tablets, and shake for at least 2 min
2. Allow the sus to stand for a minimum of 1 hr
3. After the standing time, shake the sus for a minimum of 1 additional min
4. Add 75mL of Ora-Sweet oral syrup vehicle to the bottle and shake the sus to disperse the ingredients
5. Shake the sus before each use

HOW SUPPLIED

Tab: 5mg, 10mg; (Lotensin) 20mg, 40mg

CONTRAINDICATIONS

History of angioedema. Coadministration w/ aliskiren in patients w/ diabetes.

WARNINGS/PRECAUTIONS

Not recommended in pediatric patients w/ GFR <30mL/min. Head/neck angioedema reported; d/c and institute appropriate therapy immediately. Higher incidence of angioedema in blacks than nonblacks. Intestinal angioedema reported; monitor for abdominal pain. Anaphylactoid reactions reported during desensitization w/ hymenoptera venom, dialysis w/ high-flux membranes, and LDL apheresis w/ dextran sulfate absorption. Symptomatic hypotension may occur, most likely in patients w/ volume and/or salt depletion; correct depletion before initiating therapy. Excessive hypotension, which may be associated w/ oliguria or azotemia and, rarely, w/ acute renal failure and death, may occur in patients w/ CHF; monitor closely during first 2 weeks of therapy and whenever dose is increased. Associated w/ syndrome that starts w/ cholestatic jaundice and progresses to fulminant hepatic necrosis and sometimes death (rare); d/c if jaundice or marked hepatic enzyme elevations develop. May cause changes in renal function. Increases in BUN and SrCr reported in patients w/ renal artery stenosis or w/ no preexisting renal vascular disease; monitor renal function during the 1st few weeks of therapy, and reduce dose and/or d/c the diuretic if needed. Hyperkalemia and persistent nonproductive cough reported. Hypotension may occur w/ surgery or during anesthesia. Caution in elderly.

ADVERSE REACTIONS

Headache, dizziness.

DRUG INTERACTIONS

See Contraindications. Hypotension risk and increased BUN and SrCr w/ diuretics. Increased risk of hyperkalemia w/ K^+-sparing diuretics, K^+-containing salt substitutes, or K^+ supplements; use w/ caution and periodically monitor K^+. Increased lithium levels and symptoms of lithium toxicity reported; monitor lithium levels. Nitritoid reactions reported w/ injectable gold. Hypoglycemia may develop w/ insulin or oral antidiabetics. NSAIDs, including selective COX-2 inhibitors, may attenuate antihypertensive effect and may cause deterioration of renal function. Dual blockade of the RAS is associated with increased risks of hypotension, hyperkalemia, and changes in renal function (including acute renal failure); avoid combined use and closely monitor BP, renal function, and electrolytes w/ concomitant agents that also affect the RAS. Avoid w/ aliskiren in patients w/ renal impairment (GFR <60mL/min).

NURSING CONSIDERATIONS

Assessment: Assess for history of angioedema, diabetes, volume/salt depletion, CHF, renal artery stenosis, risk factors for hyperkalemia, renal impairment, drug hypersensitivity, pregnancy/nursing status, and possible drug interactions.

Monitoring: Monitor for angioedema, anaphylactoid reactions, hyperkalemia, and other adverse reactions. Monitor BP, LFTs, and renal function.

Patient Counseling: Inform about fetal risks if taken during pregnancy and discuss treatment options in women planning to become pregnant; instruct to report pregnancy as soon as possible. Instruct to d/c therapy and to immediately report signs/symptoms of angioedema. Instruct to report lightheadedness, especially during the 1st days of therapy; advise to d/c and consult w/ a physician if syncope occurs. Inform that inadequate fluid intake or excessive perspiration, diarrhea, or vomiting may lead to excessive fall in BP, w/ the same consequences of lightheadedness and possible syncope. Advise not to use K^+ supplements or salt substitutes containing K^+ w/o consulting physician. Advise to promptly report any indication of infection.

Storage: 20-25°C (68-77°F); excursions permitted to 15-30°C (59-86°F). Protect from moisture. (Lotensin) ≤30°C (86°F). Protect from moisture. (Sus) 2-8°C (36-46°F) for up to 30 days.

BENICAR – olmesartan medoxomil

RX

Class: Angiotensin II receptor antagonist

D/C when pregnancy is detected. Drugs that act directly on the renin-angiotensin system (RAS) can cause injury/death to the developing fetus.

ADULT DOSAGE
Hypertension
Initial: 20mg qd
Titrate: May increase to 40mg qd after 2 weeks if needed
May add diuretic if BP is not controlled

PEDIATRIC DOSAGE
Hypertension
6-16 Years:
20-<35kg:
Initial: 10mg qd
Titrate: May increase to 20mg qd after 2 weeks if needed
Max: 20mg qd
≥35kg:
Initial: 20mg qd
Titrate: May increase to 40mg qd after 2 weeks if needed
Max: 40mg qd

DOSE MODIFICATION
Other Important Modifications
Intravascular Volume Depleted Patients:
Consider a lower initial dose and monitor closely

ADMINISTRATION
Oral route

May be administered w/ or w/o food.
May administer same dose as sus if unable to swallow tabs

Preparation of Sus (for 200mL of a 2mg/mL Sus):
1. Add 50mL of purified water to an amber polyethylene terephthalate bottle containing twenty Benicar 20mg tabs and allow to stand for a minimum of 5 min
2. Shake the container for at least 1 min and allow the sus to stand for at least 1 min
3. Repeat 1 min shaking and 1 min standing for 4 additional times
4. Add 100mL of Ora-Sweet and 50mL of Ora-Plus to the sus and shake well for at least 1 min
5. The sus should be refrigerated at 2-8°C (36-46°F) and can be stored for up to 4 weeks
6. Shake the sus well before each use and return promptly to the refrigerator

HOW SUPPLIED
Tab: 5mg, 20mg, 40mg

CONTRAINDICATIONS
Coadministration with aliskiren in patients with diabetes.

WARNINGS/PRECAUTIONS
Symptomatic hypotension may occur after treatment initiation in patients with an activated renin-angiotensin-aldosterone system (RAAS) (eg, volume- and/or salt-depleted patients [eg, those being treated with high doses of diuretics]). Changes in renal function may occur. Oliguria and/or progressive azotemia and (rare) acute renal failure and/or death may occur in patients whose renal function may depend on the RAAS activity (eg, severe CHF). May increase SrCr or BUN levels in patients with renal artery stenosis. Sprue-like enteropathy with symptoms of severe, chronic diarrhea with substantial weight loss reported; exclude other etiologies if these symptoms develop, and consider discontinuation in cases where no other etiology is identified.

ADVERSE REACTIONS
Dizziness.

DRUG INTERACTIONS
See Contraindications. NSAIDs, including selective COX-2 inhibitors, may attenuate antihypertensive effect and may deteriorate renal function. Dual blockade of the RAS is associated with increased risks of hypotension, hyperkalemia, and changes in renal function (including acute renal failure); avoid combined use of RAS inhibitors, or closely monitor BP, renal function, and electrolytes with concomitant agents that also affect the RAS. Avoid with aliskiren in patients with renal impairment (GFR <60mL/min). Reduced levels with colesevelam; administer at least 4 hrs before colesevelam dose. Increases in serum lithium concentrations and lithium toxicity reported; monitor lithium levels.

NURSING CONSIDERATIONS

Assessment: Assess for diabetes, CHF, renal artery stenosis, and volume/salt depletion, renal function, pregnancy/nursing status, and for possible drug interactions.

Monitoring: Monitor for signs/symptoms of hypotension, renal dysfunction, sprue-like enteropathy, and other adverse reactions.

Patient Counseling: Inform females of childbearing potential of the consequences of exposure to drug during pregnancy and of the treatment options for women planning to become pregnant. Instruct to report pregnancy to the physician as soon as possible.

Storage: (Tab) 20-25°C (68-77°F). (Sus) 2-8°C (36-46°F) for up to 4 weeks.

BENICAR HCT – hydrochlorothiazide/olmesartan medoxomil RX

Class: Angiotensin II receptor antagonist/thiazide diuretic

D/C when pregnancy is detected. Drugs that act directly on the renin-angiotensin system (RAS) can cause injury/death to the developing fetus.

ADULT DOSAGE

Hypertension

Uncontrolled BP on Olmesartan or HCTZ Alone:
Switch to once-daily combination therapy
Usual: 1 tab qd
Titrate: May adjust at intervals of 2-4 weeks
Max: 1 tab/day

Replacement Therapy:
May be substituted for its titrated components

PEDIATRIC DOSAGE

Pediatric use may not have been established

DOSE MODIFICATION

Elderly
Start at lower end of dosing range

ADMINISTRATION

Oral route

HOW SUPPLIED

Tab: (Olmesartan-HCTZ) 20mg-12.5mg, 40mg-12.5mg, 40mg-25mg

CONTRAINDICATIONS

Anuria, sulfonamide-derived drug hypersensitivity. Coadministration with aliskiren in patients with diabetes.

WARNINGS/PRECAUTIONS

Not indicated for initial therapy. Symptomatic hypotension may occur after treatment initiation in patients with an activated RAS (eg, volume- or salt-depleted patients [eg, those being treated with high doses of diuretics]). Sprue-like enteropathy with symptoms of severe, chronic diarrhea with substantial weight loss reported; exclude other etiologies if these symptoms develop, and consider discontinuation where no other etiology is identified. Hypo/hyperkalemia reported. Not recommended with severe renal impairment (CrCl ≤30mL/min). Oliguria and/or progressive azotemia and (rare) acute renal failure and/or death may occur in patients whose renal function may depend on the renin-angiotensin-aldosterone system activity (eg, severe CHF). May increase SrCr or BUN levels in patients with renal artery stenosis. Caution with severe renal disease; may precipitate azotemia. Caution in elderly. HCTZ: Caution with hepatic impairment or progressive liver disease; may precipitate hepatic coma. May cause hypersensitivity reactions (with or without a history of allergy or bronchial asthma), exacerbation or activation of systemic lupus erythematosus (SLE), hyperuricemia or precipitation of frank gout, hyperglycemia, hypomagnesemia, hypercalcemia, and manifestations of latent diabetes mellitus (DM). May cause idiosyncratic reaction, resulting in acute transient myopia and acute angle-closure glaucoma; d/c as rapidly as possible. Observe for signs of fluid or electrolyte imbalance (eg, hyponatremia, hypochloremic alkalosis, hypokalemia). Hypokalemia may sensitize/exaggerate the response of the heart to toxic effects of digitalis. D/C before testing for parathyroid function. Enhanced effects in postsympathectomy patients. D/C or withhold if progressive renal impairment becomes evident. Increased cholesterol and TG levels reported.

ADVERSE REACTIONS

Dizziness, URTI, hyperuricemia, nausea.

DRUG INTERACTIONS

See Contraindications. NSAIDs, including selective COX-2 inhibitors, may decrease antihypertensive effects and may deteriorate renal function. Increases in serum lithium concentrations and lithium toxicity reported; monitor lithium levels. Olmesartan: Dual blockade of the RAS is associated with increased risks of hypotension, hyperkalemia, and changes in renal function (including acute renal failure); avoid combined use of RAS inhibitors, or closely monitor BP, renal function, and electrolytes with concomitant agents that also affect the RAS. Avoid with aliskiren in patients with renal impairment (GFR <60mL/min). Reduced levels with colesevelam; administer at least 4 hrs before colesevelam dose. HCTZ: Alcohol, barbiturates, or narcotics may potentiate orthostatic hypotension. Dose adjustment of antidiabetic drugs (eg, oral agents and insulin) may be required. Additive effect or potentiation with other antihypertensives. Anionic exchange resins (eg, cholestyramine, colestipol) may impair absorption. Corticosteroids and adrenocorticotropic hormone may intensify electrolyte depletion, particularly hypokalemia. May decrease response to pressor amines (eg, norepinephrine). May increase responsiveness to nondepolarizing skeletal muscle relaxants (eg, tubocurarine).

NURSING CONSIDERATIONS

Assessment: Assess for hypersensitivity to the drug and its components, anuria, sulfonamide-derived drug hypersensitivity, volume/salt depletion, SLE, DM, CHF, hepatic/renal impairment, postsympathectomy status, renal artery stenosis, pregnancy/nursing status, and possible drug interactions.

Monitoring: Monitor for signs/symptoms of fluid/electrolyte imbalance, sprue-like enteropathy, exacerbation/activation of SLE, idiosyncratic reaction, latent DM, hyperuricemia, precipitation of gout, hypersensitivity reactions, and other adverse reactions. Monitor BP, serum electrolytes, cholesterol, and TG levels, and renal/hepatic function.

Patient Counseling: Inform females of childbearing potential of the consequences of exposure during pregnancy and of the treatment options for women planning to become pregnant. Instruct to report pregnancy to the physician as soon as possible. Counsel that lightheadedness may occur, especially during the 1st days of therapy; instruct to report to physician. Instruct to d/c therapy and consult physician if syncope occurs. Advise that inadequate fluid intake, excessive perspiration, diarrhea, or vomiting may lead to an excessive fall in BP, with the same consequences of lightheadedness and possible syncope.

Storage: 20-25°C (68-77°F).

BEPREVE – bepotastine besilate RX

Class: H_1-antagonist

ADULT DOSAGE

Allergic Conjunctivitis

Itching:

1 drop into the affected eye(s) bid

PEDIATRIC DOSAGE

Allergic Conjunctivitis

Itching:

≥2 Years:

1 drop into the affected eye(s) bid

ADMINISTRATION

Ocular route

HOW SUPPLIED

Sol: 1.5% [5mL, 10mL]

WARNINGS/PRECAUTIONS

For topical ophthalmic use only. Avoid touching the eyelids or surrounding areas with dropper tip of the bottle. Not for the treatment of contact lens-related irritation. Contains benzalkonium chloride, which may be absorbed by soft contact lenses; remove contact lenses prior to instillation and may reinsert 10 min after administration.

ADVERSE REACTIONS

Mild taste, eye irritation, headache, nasopharyngitis.

NURSING CONSIDERATIONS

Assessment: Assess for previous hypersensitivity to the drug, contact lens use, and pregnancy/nursing status.

Monitoring: Monitor for hypersensitivity and other adverse reactions.

Patient Counseling: Counsel that therapy is not for the treatment of lens-related irritation and advise not to instill while wearing contact lenses; inform that they may reinsert contact lenses 10 min after instillation. Advise not to touch the dropper tip to any surface, as this may contaminate the contents. Inform that sol is for topical ophthalmic use only.

Storage: 15-25°C (59-77°F). Keep bottle tightly closed when not in use.

BESIVANCE – besifloxacin

Class: Fluoroquinolone

RX

ADULT DOSAGE

Bacterial Conjunctivitis

1 drop in affected eye(s) tid, 4-12 hrs apart for 7 days

PEDIATRIC DOSAGE

Bacterial Conjunctivitis

≥1 Year:
1 drop in affected eye(s) tid, 4-12 hrs apart for 7 days

ADMINISTRATION

Ocular route

Invert closed bottle and shake once before use

HOW SUPPLIED

Sus: 0.6% [5mL]

WARNINGS/PRECAUTIONS

For topical ophthalmic use only; should not be injected subconjunctivally, nor should it be introduced directly into the anterior chamber of the eye. May result in overgrowth of nonsusceptible organisms (eg, fungi) with prolonged use; d/c and institute alternative therapy if superinfection occurs. Avoid wearing contact lenses if signs or symptoms of bacterial conjunctivitis occur and avoid wearing contact lenses during the course of therapy.

ADVERSE REACTIONS

Conjunctival redness.

NURSING CONSIDERATIONS

Assessment: Assess for previous hypersensitivity to the drug, use of contact lenses, and pregnancy/nursing status. Assess for proper diagnosis of causative organisms.

Monitoring: Monitor for superinfection; examine with magnification (eg, slit-lamp biomicroscopy) and fluorescein staining, where appropriate. Monitor for hypersensitivity reactions and other adverse reactions.

Patient Counseling: Advise to avoid contaminating applicator tip with material from the eye, fingers, or other source. Advise to d/c use immediately and contact physician at first sign of a rash or allergic reaction. Instruct to use medication exactly ud. Inform that skipping doses or not completing the full course of therapy may decrease effectiveness and increase bacterial resistance. Advise to avoid wearing contact lenses if having signs or symptoms of bacterial conjunctivitis and avoid wearing during the course of therapy. Advise to thoroughly wash hands before use. Instruct to invert closed bottle and shake once before each use. Instruct to remove cap with bottle still in inverted position. Instruct to tilt head back, and with bottle inverted, gently squeeze bottle to instill 1 drop into the affected eye(s).

Storage: 15-25°C (59-77°F). Protect from light.

BETAPACE – sotalol hydrochloride

Class: Beta-blocker (group II/III antiarrhythmic)

RX

To minimize risk of arrhythmia, for a minimum of 3 days, place patients initiated or reinitiated on therapy in a facility that can provide cardiac resuscitation and continuous ECG monitoring. Calculate CrCl prior to dosing. Not approved for A-fib or A-flutter; do not substitute for Betapace AF.

OTHER BRAND NAMES

Sorine

ADULT DOSAGE

Ventricular Arrhythmias

Documented Ventricular Arrhythmias (eg, Sustained Ventricular Tachycardia):

Initial: 80mg bid
Titrate: May increase after appropriate evaluation to 240 or 320mg/day (120-160mg bid); adjust dose gradually, allowing 3 days between dosing increments
Usual: 160-320mg/day in 2 or 3 divided doses

PEDIATRIC DOSAGE

Ventricular Arrhythmias

Documented Ventricular Arrhythmias (eg, Sustained Ventricular Tachycardia):

<2 Years:
Refer to PI for dosing chart

≥2 Years:
Initial: $30mg/m^2$ tid ($90mg/m^2$ total daily dose)
Titrate: Allow at least 36 hrs between dose increments; guide titration by response, HR, and QTc

Refractory Ventricular Arrhythmia:
480-640mg/day when benefit outweighs risk

Transferring to Betapace/Sorine:
Withdraw previous antiarrhythmic therapy for a minimum of 2-3 plasma half-lives before initiating therapy
After discontinuation of amiodarone, do not initiate therapy until QT interval is normalized

Max: 60mg/m^2
Reduce dose or d/c if QTc >550 msec

Transferring to Betapace/Sorine:
Withdraw previous antiarrhythmic therapy for a minimum of 2-3 plasma half-lives before initiating therapy
After discontinuation of amiodarone, do not initiate therapy until QT interval is normalized

DOSE MODIFICATION

Renal Impairment

Adults:
CrCl >60mL/min: Dose q12h
CrCl 30-59mL/min: Dose q24h
CrCl 10-29mL/min: Dose q36-48h
CrCl <10mL/min: Dose should be individualized

Pediatrics:
Lower doses or increase intervals between doses

ADMINISTRATION

Oral route

Preparation of Extemporaneous Oral Sol

1. Measure 120mL of simple syrup containing 0.1% sodium benzoate
2. Transfer the syrup to a 6-oz amber plastic (polyethylene terephthalate) prescription bottle
3. Add 5 sotalol 120mg tabs to the bottle. These tabs are added intact; it is not necessary to crush the tabs
4. Shake the bottle to wet the entire surface of the tabs. If the tabs have been crushed, shake the bottle until the endpoint is achieved
5. Allow the tabs to hydrate for at least 2 hrs. After at least 2 hrs have elapsed, shake the bottle intermittently over the course of at least another 2 hrs until the tabs are completely disintegrated
6. The procedure results in a sol containing 5mg/mL of sotalol HCl

HOW SUPPLIED

Tab: (Betapace) 80mg*, 120mg*, 160mg*; (Sorine) 80mg*, 120mg*, 160mg*, 240mg* *scored

CONTRAINDICATIONS

Bronchial asthma, sinus bradycardia, 2nd- and 3rd-degree AV block (unless a functioning pacemaker is present), congenital or acquired long QT syndromes, cardiogenic shock, uncontrolled CHF.

WARNINGS/PRECAUTIONS

May provoke new or worsen ventricular arrhythmias (eg, sustained ventricular tachycardia or ventricular fibrillation). Torsades de pointes, QT interval prolongation, and new or worsened CHF reported. Anticipate proarrhythmic events upon initiation and every upward dose adjustment. Caution in patients with QTc >500 msec on-therapy and consider reducing dose or discontinuing therapy when QTc >550 msec. Avoid with uncorrected hypokalemia or hypomagnesemia. Give special attention to electrolyte and acid-base balance in patients with severe/prolonged diarrhea or with concomitant diuretic drugs. May cause further depression of myocardial contractility and precipitate more severe failure; caution with CHF controlled by digitalis and/or diuretics. Caution with left ventricular dysfunction, sick sinus syndrome associated with symptomatic arrhythmias, and renal impairment (especially with hemodialysis). Caution during the first 2 weeks post-MI; careful dose titration is especially important (eg, in patients with markedly impaired ventricular function). Exacerbation of angina pectoris, arrhythmias, and MI reported after abrupt discontinuation; reduce dose gradually over 1-2 weeks. May unmask latent coronary insufficiency in patients with arrhythmias. Avoid in patients with bronchospastic diseases; use lowest effective dose. Impaired ability of the heart to respond to reflex adrenergic stimuli may augment the risks of general anesthesia and surgical procedures; chronically administered therapy should not be routinely withdrawn prior to major surgery. Patients with a history of anaphylactic reaction to various allergens may have a more severe reaction on repeated challenge and may be unresponsive to usual doses of epinephrine. Caution in patients with diabetes (especially labile diabetes) or with a history of episodes of spontaneous hypoglycemia; may mask premonitory signs of acute hypoglycemia (eg, tachycardia). May mask certain clinical signs (eg, tachycardia) of hyperthyroidism.

ADVERSE REACTIONS

Torsades de pointes, dyspnea, fatigue, dizziness, bradycardia, chest pain, palpitation, asthenia, abnormal ECG, hypotension, headache, light-headedness, edema, N/V, pulmonary problems.

DRUG INTERACTIONS

Avoid with Class Ia (eg, disopyramide, quinidine, procainamide) and Class III (eg, amiodarone) antiarrhythmics. Additive Class II effects with other β-blockers. Proarrhythmic events were more common with digoxin. May increase risk of bradycardia with digitalis glycosides. Possible additive effects on AV conduction or ventricular function and BP with calcium-blocking agents. May produce excessive reduction of resting sympathetic nervous tone with catecholamine-depleting drugs (eg, reserpine, guanethidine). Hyperglycemia may occur; may require dose adjustment of insulin or antidiabetic agents. β_2-agonists (eg, salbutamol, terbutaline, isoprenaline) may need dose increase. May potentiate rebound HTN with clonidine withdrawal. Avoid administration within 2 hrs of antacids containing aluminum oxide and magnesium hydroxide; may reduce levels. Caution with drugs that prolong QT interval (eg, Class I and III antiarrhythmics, phenothiazines, TCAs, astemizole, bepridil, certain oral macrolides, certain quinolone antibiotics).

NURSING CONSIDERATIONS

Assessment: Assess for hypersensitivity to drug, bronchial asthma, sinus bradycardia, sick sinus syndrome, 2nd- and 3rd-degree AV block, pacemaker, long QT syndromes, cardiogenic shock, left ventricular dysfunction or uncontrolled CHF, recent MI, ischemic heart disease, hypokalemia or hypomagnesemia, bronchospastic disease, diabetes, episodes of hypoglycemia, upcoming major surgery, hyperthyroidism, renal impairment, any other conditions where treatment is contraindicated or cautioned, pregnancy/nursing status, and possible drug interactions.

Monitoring: Monitor for ECG changes, tachycardia, arrhythmias, depressed myocardial contractility, severe CHF, anaphylaxis, hypoglycemia, electrolyte imbalance, hyperthyroidism, and other adverse reactions.

Patient Counseling: Inform of the benefits/risks of therapy. Advise not to d/c therapy without consulting physician. Instruct to report any adverse reactions to physician.

Storage: (Betapace) 25°C (77°F); excursions permitted to 15-30°C (59-86°F). (Sorine) 15-30°C (59-86°F). Sus: Stable for 3 months at 15-30°C (59-86°F) and ambient humidity.

BETAPACE AF – sotalol hydrochloride RX

Class: Beta-blocker (group II/III antiarrhythmic)

To minimize risk of induced arrhythmia, for a minimum of 3 days, place patients initiated or reinitiated on therapy in a facility that can provide cardiac resuscitation, continuous ECG monitoring, and calculations of CrCl. Do not substitute Betapace for Betapace AF.

ADULT DOSAGE

Atrial Fibrillation/Flutter

Maint of Normal Sinus Rhythm in Symptomatic A-Fib/Flutter:
Start only if baseline QT interval is ≤450 msec
Individualize dose according to calculated CrCl

Initial: 80mg qd (CrCl 40-60mL/min) or bid (CrCl >60mL/min)
Monitor QT interval 2-4 hrs after each dose; reduce or d/c if QT interval prolongs to ≥500 msec
May discharge patient if QT <500 msec after at least 3 days (after 5th or 6th dose if patient receiving qd dosing)
Alternatively, may increase dose to 120mg bid during hospitalization, and monitor for 3 days (monitor for 5 or 6 doses if receiving qd doses); if 120mg is inadequate, may increase to 160mg qd or bid depending on CrCl
Maint: Reduce dose if QT interval is ≥520 msec and monitor until QT returns to <520 msec; d/c if QT is ≥520 msec while on 80mg dose
Max: 160mg bid (CrCl >60mL/min)

Transfer to Betapace AF from Other Antiarrhythmic Agents:
Withdraw previous antiarrhythmic therapy for a minimum of 2-3 plasma half-lives if patient's condition permits before initiating Betapace AF
After discontinuing amiodarone, do not initiate Betapace AF until QT interval is normalized

PEDIATRIC DOSAGE

Atrial Fibrillation/Flutter

Maint of Normal Sinus Rhythm in Symptomatic A-Fib/Flutter:
Individualize dose
<2 Years:
See dosing chart in PI
Reduce dose or d/c if QTc >550 msec

≥2 Years:
Initial: 30mg/m² tid
Titrate: Wait ≥36 hrs between dose increases; guide dose by response, HR, and QTc
Max: 60mg/m²

Transfer to Betapace AF from Other Antiarrhythmic Agents:
Withdraw previous antiarrhythmic therapy for a minimum of 2-3 plasma half-lives if patient's condition permits before initiating Betapace AF
After discontinuing amiodarone, do not initiate Betapace AF until QT interval is normalized

DOSE MODIFICATION

Renal Impairment

Adults:

If renal function deteriorates, reduce daily dose in 1/2 by administering the drug qd

Pediatrics:

Reduce dose or increase intervals between doses

ADMINISTRATION

Oral route

Take PO w/ or w/o food

Initiate/titrate sotalol therapy in presence of continuous ECG monitoring and personnel trained in management of serious ventricular arrhythmias

Preparation of Extemporaneous Oral Sol for Betapace AF Syrup 5mg/mL

1. Measure 120mL of simple syrup
2. Transfer the syrup to a 6-oz amber plastic (polyethylene terephthalate) prescription bottle.
3. Add 5 Betapace AF 120mg tabs to the bottle. These tabs are added intact; it is not necessary to crush the tabs. The tabs can also be crushed if preferred. If the tabs are crushed, care should be taken to transfer the entire quantity of tab powder into the bottle containing the syrup
4. Shake the bottle to wet the entire surface of the tabs. If the tabs have been crushed, shake the bottle until the endpoint is achieved
5. Allow the tabs to hydrate for approx 2 hrs
6. After at least 2 hrs have elapsed, shake the bottle intermittently over the course of at least another 2 hrs until the tabs are completely disintegrated. The tabs can be allowed to hydrate overnight to simplify the disintegration process

HOW SUPPLIED

Tab: 80mg*, 120mg*, 160mg* *scored

CONTRAINDICATIONS

Sinus bradycardia (<50bpm during waking hrs), sick sinus syndrome or 2nd- or 3rd-degree atrioventricular (AV) block (unless a functioning pacemaker is present), congenital or acquired long QT syndromes, baseline QT interval >450 msec, cardiogenic shock, uncontrolled heart failure (HF), hypokalemia (<4mEq/L), CrCl <40mL/min, bronchial asthma.

WARNINGS/PRECAUTIONS

May cause serious ventricular arrhythmias, primarily torsades de pointes. QT interval prolongation, bradycardia, and new/worsened congestive HF reported. Avoid with hypokalemia or hypomagnesemia; correct electrolyte imbalances before therapy. May cause depression of myocardial contractility and precipitate more severe failure in patients with congestive HF. Caution with HF controlled by digitalis and/or diuretics, left ventricular dysfunction, renal impairment, recent acute MI, and sick sinus syndrome associated with symptomatic arrhythmias. Exacerbation of angina pectoris, arrhythmias, and MI reported after abrupt discontinuation; reduce dose gradually over a period of 1-2 weeks. May unmask latent coronary insufficiency in patients with arrhythmias. Avoid in patients with bronchospastic diseases; use lowest effective dose. Impaired ability of heart to respond to reflex adrenergic stimuli may augment the risks of general anesthesia and surgical procedures; chronically administered therapy should not be routinely withdrawn prior to major surgery. Patients with a history of anaphylactic reaction to various allergens may have a more severe reaction on repeated challenge and may be unresponsive to usual doses of epinephrine. Caution in patients with diabetes (especially labile diabetes) or with a history of episodes of spontaneous hypoglycemia; may mask premonitory signs of acute hypoglycemia (eg, tachycardia). May mask certain clinical signs (eg, tachycardia) of hyperthyroidism.

ADVERSE REACTIONS

Bradycardia, dyspnea, fatigue, abnormal ECG, chest pain, abdominal pain, disturbance rhythm subjective, diarrhea, N/V, cough, hyperhidrosis, weakness, dizziness, headache, insomnia.

DRUG INTERACTIONS

Avoid with Class Ia (eg, disopyramide, quinidine, procainamide) and Class III (eg, amiodarone) antiarrhythmics. Not recommended with drugs that prolong the QT interval (eg, many antiarrhythmics, some phenothiazines, TCAs, bepridil, certain oral macrolides). Proarrhythmic events more common with digoxin. Increased risk of bradycardia with digitalis glycosides. Possible additive effects on AV conduction or ventricular function and BP with calcium-blocking agents. May produce an excessive reduction of resting sympathetic nervous tone with catecholamine-depleting drugs (eg, reserpine, guanethidine). Hyperglycemia may occur; may require dose adjustment of insulin or antidiabetic agents. β_2-agonists (eg, salbutamol, terbutaline, isoprenaline) may need dose increase. May potentiate rebound HTN with clonidine withdrawal. Avoid administration of therapy within 2 hrs of antacids containing aluminum oxide and magnesium hydroxide; may reduce levels.

NURSING CONSIDERATIONS

Assessment: Assess for hypersensitivity to drug, sinus bradycardia, sick sinus syndrome, 2nd- and 3rd-degree AV block, pacemaker, long QT syndromes, baseline QT interval >450 msec, cardiogenic shock, uncontrolled HF, hypokalemia, bronchial asthma, recent MI, ischemic heart disease, hypomagnesemia, bronchospastic disease, diabetes, hypoglycemia, upcoming major surgery, hyperthyroidism, renal impairment, or any other conditions where treatment is contraindicated or cautioned. Assess for pregnancy/nursing status and possible drug interactions.

Monitoring: Monitor for ECG changes, tachycardia, arrhythmias, depressed myocardial contractility, HF, anaphylaxis, hypoglycemia, electrolyte imbalance, hyperthyroidism, and other adverse reactions.

Patient Counseling: Inform of benefits/risks of therapy. Instruct to take exactly ud. Advise not to d/c therapy without consulting physician. Instruct to inform physician if taking any other medications, supplements, or OTC drugs and to report immediately if experiencing symptoms that may be associated with electrolyte imbalance. Instruct not to double next dose if a dose is missed and to take next dose at the usual time.

Storage: 25°C (77°F); excursions permitted to 15-30°C (59-86°F). Sus: Stable for 3 months at 15-30°C (59-86°F) and ambient humidity.

BETHKIS – tobramycin RX

Class: Aminoglycoside

ADULT DOSAGE

Pseudomonas aeruginosa **Infections**

In Cystic Fibrosis Patients:
300mg bid by oral inh (as close to 12 hrs apart as possible; not <6 hrs apart) in repeated cycles of 28 days on drug, followed by 28 days off drug

PEDIATRIC DOSAGE

Pseudomonas aeruginosa **Infections**

In Cystic Fibrosis Patients:
≥6 Years:
300mg bid by oral inh (as close to 12 hrs apart as possible; not <6 hrs apart) in repeated cycles of 28 days on drug, followed by 28 days off drug

ADMINISTRATION

Oral inh route

Administer by using a hand-held Pari LC Plus reusable nebulizer w/ a Pari Vios air compressor over approx 15 min and until sputtering from the output of the nebulizer has occurred for at least 1 min
Do not mix w/ other medicines in the nebulizer
Administer other inhaled medicines (eg, bronchodilators) before administration of therapy
Refer to PI for further preparation and administration instructions

HOW SUPPLIED

Sol, Inhalation: 300mg/4mL

WARNINGS/PRECAUTIONS

Ototoxicity (eg, tinnitus) may occur; caution with auditory or vestibular dysfunction. Nephrotoxicity may occur; caution with renal dysfunction. If nephrotoxicity occurs, d/c therapy until serum concentrations fall <2mcg/mL. If an increase in SrCr develops, closely monitor renal function. May aggravate muscle weakness; caution with muscular disorders (eg, myasthenia gravis, Parkinson's disease). Bronchospasm and wheezing reported. Consider an audiogram for patients with any evidence of or at increased risk for auditory dysfunction. May cause fetal harm.

ADVERSE REACTIONS

Decreased forced expiratory volume, rales, increased RBC sedimentation rate, dysphonia, wheezing, epistaxis, pharyngolaryngeal pain, bronchitis.

DRUG INTERACTIONS

Avoid concurrent and/or sequential use with other drugs with neurotoxic or ototoxic potential. Some diuretics may enhance toxicity by altering concentrations in serum and tissue; do not administer with ethacrynic acid, furosemide, urea, or mannitol.

NURSING CONSIDERATIONS

Assessment: Assess for auditory, vestibular, or renal dysfunction, muscular disorders, drug hypersensitivity, pregnancy/nursing status, and possible drug interactions. Consider a baseline audiogram for patients at increased risk for auditory dysfunction.

Monitoring: Monitor for ototoxicity, nephrotoxicity, muscle weakness, bronchospasm, wheezing, and other adverse reactions. Consider an audiogram for patients who show any evidence of auditory dysfunction.

Patient Counseling: Instruct to take drug ud, and to complete a full 28-day course of therapy even if feeling better. Inform of the adverse reactions associated with therapy, such as ototoxicity, bronchospasm, nephrotoxicity, and neuromuscular disorders. Inform of the need to monitor hearing, serum concentrations, and renal function during treatment. Advise to inform physician if pregnant/nursing or planning to become pregnant. Counsel on proper storage of the drug.

Storage: 2-8°C (36-46°F). Upon removal from the refrigerator, or if refrigeration is unavailable, may be stored at room temperature (up to 25°C [77°F]) for up to 28 days. Do not expose to intense light.

BEXSERO – meningococcal group B vaccine RX

Class: Vaccine

ADULT DOSAGE

Meningococcal Vaccine

Active Immunization to Prevent Invasive Disease Caused by *Neisseria meningitidis* Serogroup B:

≤25 Years:

2 doses (0.5mL/dose) at least 1 month apart

Sufficient data not available on the safety and effectiveness of using interchangeably w/ other meningococcal group B vaccines to complete vaccination series

PEDIATRIC DOSAGE

Meningococcal Vaccine

Active Immunization to Prevent Invasive Disease Caused by *Neisseria meningitidis* Serogroup B:

≥10 Years:

2 doses (0.5mL/dose) at least 1 month apart

Sufficient data not available on the safety and effectiveness of using interchangeably w/ other meningococcal group B vaccines to complete vaccination series

ADMINISTRATION

IM route

Shake syringe immediately before use; do not use if vaccine cannot be resuspended

Administer into the deltoid muscle of upper arm

HOW SUPPLIED

Inj: 0.5mL

WARNINGS/PRECAUTIONS

Appropriate observation and medical treatment should always be readily available in case of an anaphylactic event. Syncope may occur; procedures should be in place to avoid injury from falling. Tip caps of prefilled syringes contain natural rubber latex; may cause allergic reactions in latex sensitive individuals. May not protect all vaccine recipients. May not provide protection against all meningococcal serogroup B strains. Individuals w/ altered immunocompetence may have reduced immune responses to therapy.

ADVERSE REACTIONS

Inj-site pain, myalgia, erythema, fatigue, headache, induration, nausea, arthralgia.

NURSING CONSIDERATIONS

Assessment: Assess for hypersensitivity, vaccination history, latex sensitivity, altered immunocompetence, and pregnancy/nursing status.

Monitoring: Monitor for allergic/anaphylactic reactions, syncope, and other adverse reactions. Monitor immune response to vaccine.

Patient Counseling: Inform patients and parents/guardians about the importance of completing the immunization series. Instruct to report any adverse reactions to physician. Inform women who receive therapy while pregnant that they will need to be registered in the vaccine's pregnancy registry.

Storage: 2-8°C (36-46°F). Do not freeze; discard if the vaccine has been frozen. Protect from light.

BEYAZ – drospirenone/ethinyl estradiol/levomefolate calcium RX

Class: Estrogen/progestogen combination

Cigarette smoking increases the risk of serious cardiovascular events from combination oral contraceptive (COC) use. Risk increases with age (>35 yrs) and with the number of cigarettes smoked. Should not be used by women who are >35 yrs of age and smoke.

ADULT DOSAGE

Contraception

1 tab qd at the same time each day for 28 days, then repeat

Start 1st Sunday after menses begin or 1st day of menses

PEDIATRIC DOSAGE

Contraception

Not indicated for use premenarche; refer to adult dosing

Premenstrual Dysphoric Disorder

Not indicated for use premenarche; refer to adult dosing

Premenstrual Dysphoric Disorder

1 tab qd at the same time each day for 28 days, then repeat

Start 1st Sunday after menses begin or 1st day of menses

Acne Vulgaris

Moderate Acne in Women Who Desire Oral Contraception:
1 tab qd at the same time each day for 28 days, then repeat

Start 1st Sunday after menses begin or 1st day of menses

Other Indications

May be used to raise folate levels for the purpose of reducing the risk of neural tube defect in a pregnancy conceived while taking the product or shortly after discontinuation

Conversions

Switching from Another Oral Contraceptive: Start on the same day that a new pack of the previous oral contraceptive would have been started

Switching from a Method Other than an Oral Contraceptive:
Transdermal Patch/Vaginal Ring/Inj: Start when the next application/inj would have been due
Intrauterine Contraceptive/Implant: Start on day of removal

Missed Dose

Miss 1 Pink Pill: Take as soon as dose is remembered; take next pill at regular time (may take 2 pills in 1 day). No backup birth control method is needed
Miss 2 Pink Pills in a Row in Week 1 or 2: Take 2 pills on day it is remembered and 2 pills the next day, then take 1 pill qd until the pack is finished
Miss 2 Pink Pills in a Row in Week 3 or Miss ≥3 Pink Pills in a Row During the 1st 3 Weeks: (Day 1 starter) Throw out rest of the pack and start new pack the same day. (Sunday starter) Continue to take 1 pill qd until Sunday, then throw out the rest of the pack and start a new pack of pills that same day
Miss Any of Light Orange Pills in Week 4: Throw away missed dose and continue to take 1 pill qd until pack is empty. No backup birth control method is needed

Acne Vulgaris

Moderate Acne in Postpubertal Women ≥14 Years Who Desire Oral Contraception:
1 tab qd at the same time each day for 28 days, then repeat
Start 1st Sunday after menses begin or 1st day of menses

DOSE MODIFICATION

Adverse Reactions
GI Disturbances: If vomiting occurs w/in 3-4 hrs after taking tab, may regard as missed dose

ADMINISTRATION

Oral route

Take preferably pm pc or hs
Take tabs in the order directed on the package
Use a nonhormonal contraceptive as backup during the 1st 7 days of therapy of initiating therapy or restarting after ≥2 missed doses

HOW SUPPLIED

Tab: (Drospirenone [DRSP]-Ethinyl Estradiol [EE]-Levomefolate calcium) 3mg-0.02mg-0.451mg; Tab: (Levomefolate calcium) 0.451mg

CONTRAINDICATIONS

Renal impairment, adrenal insufficiency, high risk of arterial/venous thrombotic disease (eg, smoking if >35 yrs of age, history/presence of deep vein thrombosis/pulmonary embolism, cerebrovascular disease, coronary artery disease, thrombogenic valvular or thrombogenic rhythm diseases of the heart [eg, subacute bacterial endocarditis with valvular disease, atrial fibrillation], inherited/acquired hypercoagulopathies, uncontrolled HTN, diabetes mellitus [DM] with vascular disease, headaches with focal neurological symptoms or migraine with/without aura if >35 yrs of age), undiagnosed abnormal uterine bleeding, history/presence of breast or other estrogen-/progestin-sensitive cancer, benign/malignant liver tumors, liver disease, pregnancy.

WARNINGS/PRECAUTIONS

Increased risk of venous thromboembolism and arterial thromboses (eg, stroke, myocardial infarction). D/C if arterial/deep venous thrombotic events, unexplained loss of vision, proptosis, diplopia, papilledema, or retinal vascular lesions occur; evaluate for retinal vein thrombosis immediately. Caution in women with cardiovascular disease (CVD) risk factors. D/C at least 4 weeks before and through 2 weeks after major surgery or other surgeries known to have an elevated risk of thromboembolism. Avoid use in patients predisposed to hyperkalemia. May increase risk of breast cancer, cervical cancer, intraepithelial neoplasia, and gallbladder disease. Hepatic adenoma and increased risk of hepatocellular carcinoma reported; d/c if jaundice or acute/chronic disturbances of liver function occur. Cholestasis may occur with history of pregnancy-related cholestasis. Increased BP reported; d/c if BP rises significantly. May decrease glucose tolerance; monitor prediabetic and diabetic patients. Consider alternative contraception with uncontrolled dyslipidemia. Increased risk of pancreatitis with hypertriglyceridemia or family history thereof. May increase frequency/severity of migraine; d/c if new headaches that are recurrent, persistent, or severe develop. Unscheduled bleeding and spotting may occur; rule out pregnancies or malignancies. Caution with history of depression; d/c if depression recurs to serious degree. May change results of lab tests. Folate may mask vitamin B12 deficiency. May induce/exacerbate angioedema in patients with hereditary angioedema. Chloasma may occur, especially with history of chloasma gravidarum; avoid sun exposure or UV radiation. Women who do not breastfeed may start therapy no earlier than 4 weeks postpartum.

ADVERSE REACTIONS

Menstrual irregularities, N/V, headache/migraine, breast pain/tenderness, fatigue.

DRUG INTERACTIONS

Risk of hyperkalemia with ACE inhibitors, angiotensin II receptor antagonists, K^+-sparing diuretics, K^+ supplementation, heparin, aldosterone antagonists, and NSAIDs. Reduced effectiveness or increased breakthrough bleeding with enzyme inducers, including CYP3A4, (eg, phenytoin, barbiturates, carbamazepine, bosentan, felbamate, griseofulvin, oxcarbazepine, rifampicin, topiramate, St. John's wort). Significant changes (increase/decrease) in plasma estrogen and progestin levels with HIV/hepatitis C virus protease inhibitors or non-nucleoside reverse transcriptase inhibitors. Pregnancy reported with use of hormonal contraceptives and antibiotics. Increased levels with atorvastatin, ascorbic acid, acetaminophen, and CYP3A4 inhibitors (eg, itraconazole, ketoconazole). May decrease plasma concentrations of lamotrigine and reduce seizure control; adjust dose of lamotrigine. Increases thyroid-binding globulin; may need to increase dose of thyroid hormone in patients on thyroid hormone replacement therapy. May decrease pharmacological effect of antifolate drugs (eg, antiepileptics [phenytoin], methotrexate, pyrimethamine). Reduced folate levels via inhibition of dihydrofolate reductase enzyme (eg, methotrexate, sulfasalazine), reduced folate absorption (eg, cholestyramine), or unknown mechanism (eg, antiepileptics [carbamazepine, phenytoin, phenobarbital, primidone, valproic acid]).

NURSING CONSIDERATIONS

Assessment: Assess for renal impairment, abnormal uterine bleeding, adrenal insufficiency, known or suspected pregnancy, and other conditions where treatment is cautioned or contraindicated. Assess use in women who are >35 yrs of age and smoke, have CVD and arterial/venous thrombosis risk factors, predisposition to hyperkalemia, pregnancy-related cholestasis, HTN, DM, uncontrolled dyslipidemia, history of hypertriglyceridemia, history of depression, hereditary angioedema, and history of chloasma. Assess for possible drug interactions.

Monitoring: Monitor for bleeding irregularities, venous/arterial thrombotic and thromboembolic events, cervical cancer or intraepithelial neoplasia, retinal vein thrombosis or any other ophthalmic changes, jaundice, acute/chronic disturbances in liver function, new/worsening headaches or migraines, serious depression, cholestasis with history of pregnancy-related cholestasis, and pancreatitis. Monitor K^+ levels, thyroid function if receiving thyroid replacement therapy, glucose levels in DM or prediabetes, lipids with dyslipidemia, and check BP annually.

Patient Counseling: Counsel that cigarette smoking increases the risk of serious CV events from COC use and to avoid use in women who are >35 yrs old and smoke. Inform that drug does not protect against HIV infection and other sexually transmitted diseases. Instruct to take at the same time every day, preferably pm pc or hs. Instruct on what to do if pills are missed or vomiting occurs within 3-4 hrs after taking tab. Inform that COCs may reduce breast milk production. Inform that amenorrhea may occur and pregnancy should be ruled out if amenorrhea occurs in ≥2 consecutive cycles. Counsel to report if taking folate supplements and advise to maintain folate supplementation upon discontinuation due to pregnancy. Advise to inform physician of preexisting medical conditions and/or drugs currently being taken. Counsel to use additional method of contraception when enzyme inducers are used with COCs. Counsel women who start COCs postpartum and have not yet had a period to use additional method of contraception until drug taken for 7 consecutive days. Instruct to d/c if pregnancy occurs during treatment.

Storage: 25°C (77°F); excursions permitted to 15-30°C (59-86°F).

BIAXIN – clarithromycin RX

Class: Macrolide

OTHER BRAND NAMES

Biaxin XL

ADULT DOSAGE

Mycobacterial Infections

Prophylaxis of disseminated *Mycobacterium avium* disease in patients w/ advanced HIV infection. Treatment of disseminated infection due to *M. avium* complex

Tab/Sus:

500mg bid; continue therapy if clinical response is observed

D/C when the patient is considered at low risk of disseminated infection

Pharyngitis/Tonsillitis

Due to *Streptococcus pyogenes*:

Tab/Sus:

250mg q12h for 10 days

Acute Maxillary Sinusitis

Due to *Haemophilus influenzae, Moraxella catarrhalis*, or *Streptococcus pneumoniae*:

Tab/Sus:

500mg q12h for 14 days

XL Tab:

1000mg q24h for 14 days

Community-Acquired Pneumonia

Tab/Sus:

***Haemophilus influenzae*:**

250mg q12h for 7 days

***Streptococcus pneumoniae, Chlamydophila pneumoniae*, or *Mycoplasma pneumoniae*:**

250mg q12h for 7-14 days

XL Tab:

***H. influenzae, Haemophilus parainfluenzae, Moraxella catarrhalis, S. pneumoniae, C. pneumoniae*, or *M. pneumoniae*:**

1000mg q24h for 7 days

Skin and Skin Structure Infections

Uncomplicated Infections Due to *Staphylococcus aureus* or *Streptococcus pyogenes*:

Tab/Sus:

250mg q12h for 7-14 days

***Helicobacter pylori* Eradication**

Tab:

Triple Therapy:

500mg + 1g amoxicillin + 20mg omeprazole, all q12h for 10 days; give additional 20mg omeprazole qd for 18 days for ulcer healing/symptom relief if an ulcer was present at the time of initiation

or

PEDIATRIC DOSAGE

General Dosing

Pharyngitis/tonsillitis due to *Streptococcus pyogenes*; community-acquired pneumonia due to *Mycoplasma pneumoniae, S. pneumoniae*, or *Chlamydophila pneumoniae*; acute maxillary sinusitis or acute otitis media due to *Haemophilus influenzae, Moraxella catarrhalis*, or *S. pneumoniae*; or uncomplicated skin and skin structure infections due to *Staphylococcus aureus* or *S. pyogenes*

Tab/Sus:

≥6 Months of Age: 15mg/kg/day divided q12h for 10 days

Mycobacterial Infections

Prophylaxis of disseminated *Mycobacterium avium* disease or treatment of disseminated infection due to *M. avium* complex

Tab/Sus:

≥20 Months of Age: 7.5mg/kg bid, up to 500mg bid

Continue therapy if clinical response is observed; d/c when the patient is considered at low risk of disseminated infection

500mg + 1g amoxicillin + 30mg lansoprazole, all q12h for 10 or 14 days

Dual Therapy:
500mg q8h + 40mg omeprazole qam for 14 days; give additional 20mg omeprazole qd for 14 days for ulcer healing/symptom relief
or
500mg q8h or q12h + 400mg ranitidine bismuth citrate q12h for 14 days; give additional 400mg ranitidine bismuth citrate bid for 14 days for ulcer healing/symptom relief

Acute Bacterial Exacerbation of Chronic Bronchitis

Tab/Sus:
***Moraxella catarrhalis* or *Streptococcus pneumoniae*:**
250mg q12h for 7-14 days
***Haemophilus influenzae*:**
500mg q12h for 7-14 days
***Haemophilus parainfluenzae*:**
500mg q12h for 7 days
XL Tab:
***H. influenzae, H. parainfluenzae, M. catarrhalis*, or *S. pneumoniae*:**
1000mg q24h for 7 days

DOSE MODIFICATION

Concomitant Medications

Ranitidine Bismuth Citrate: Not recommended if CrCl <25mL/min or w/ history of acute porphyria

Renal Impairment

Severe (CrCl <30mL/min): Reduce dose by 50%

Concomitant Atazanavir or Ritonavir:
CrCl 30-60mL/min: Reduce dose by 50%
CrCl <30mL/min: Reduce dose by 75%

ADMINISTRATION

Oral route

Tab/Sus

Take w/ or w/o food; may be taken w/ milk

Sus

Shake well before each use
Reconstitute 50mL bottle sizes w/ 27mL of water and 100mL bottle sizes w/ 55mL of water
Add water in 2 portions and shake after each aliquot
Use w/in 14 days

XL Tab

Take w/ food
Swallow whole; do not chew, crush, or break

HOW SUPPLIED

Sus: 125mg/5mL, 250mg/5mL [50mL, 100mL]; Tab: 250mg, 500mg; Tab, Extended-Release (XL): 500mg

CONTRAINDICATIONS

History of cholestatic jaundice/hepatic dysfunction associated w/ prior use of clarithromycin. History of QT prolongation or ventricular cardiac arrhythmia, including torsades de pointes. Concomitant use w/ cisapride, pimozide, astemizole, terfenadine, ergotamine, or dihydroergotamine, and w/ HMG-CoA reductase inhibitors that are extensively metabolized by CYP3A4 (lovastatin or simvastatin). Concomitant use w/ colchicine in patients w/ renal/hepatic impairment.

WARNINGS/PRECAUTIONS

Avoid in pregnancy, except in clinical circumstances where no alternative therapy is appropriate. Hepatic dysfunction, including increased liver enzymes, and hepatocellular and/or cholestatic hepatitis, w/ or w/o jaundice, reported; d/c immediately if signs/symptoms of hepatitis occur. QT interval prolongation, arrhythmia (infrequent), and torsades de pointes reported; avoid w/ ongoing proarrhythmic conditions (eg, uncorrected hypokalemia, hypomagnesemia) and clinically significant bradycardia. *Clostridium difficile*-associated diarrhea (CDAD) reported; may need to d/c if CDAD is suspected or confirmed. D/C therapy immediately and initiate prompt treatment if severe acute hypersensitivity reactions (eg, Stevens-Johnson syndrome, toxic epidermal necrolysis, drug rash w/ eosinophilia and systemic symptoms, Henoch-Schonlein purpura) occur. May result in bacterial resistance w/ prolonged use in the absence of a proven/suspected bacterial infection or a prophylactic indication. Exacerbation of symptoms of myasthenia gravis and new onset of symptoms of myasthenic syndrome reported. Caution in elderly.

ADVERSE REACTIONS

Diarrhea, N/V, dysgeusia, abdominal pain.

DRUG INTERACTIONS

See Contraindications and Dose Modification. Avoid Class IA (quinidine, procainamide) or Class III (dofetilide, amiodarone, sotalol) antiarrhythmic agents. May increase serum theophylline, carbamazepine, omeprazole, and digoxin, drugs metabolized by CYP3A, colchicine, saquinavir, tolterodine, and itraconazole levels. Bradyarrhythmias and lactic acidosis observed w/ verapamil. Hypotension and acute kidney injury may occur w/ calcium channel blockers metabolized by CYP3A4 (eg, verapamil, amlodipine, diltiazem). Increased levels w/ fluconazole, itraconazole, and saquinavir. Avoid doses of >1000mg/day w/ protease inhibitors. May potentiate oral anticoagulant effects. Risk of serious hemorrhage and significant elevations in PT/INR w/ warfarin; monitor PT/INR frequently. Caution w/ other drugs known to be CYP3A enzyme substrates, especially if substrate has a narrow safety margin (eg, carbamazepine) and/or substrate is extensively metabolized by this enzyme. Decreased levels w/ CYP3A inducers (eg, efavirenz, rifampicin, rifapentine); caution use. May increase levels of rifabutin. Etravirine may decrease exposure; consider alternative for treatment of MAC. Concomitant use w/ phosphodiesterase inhibitors (sildenafil, tadalafil, vardenafil) is not recommended. Consider reduction of sildenafil dose. CNS effects, increased sedation, and prolongation of sedation reported w/ concomitant triazolobenzodiazepines (eg, triazolam, midazolam); monitor for additive CNS effects and consider appropriate dose adjustments. May increase AUC of midazolam; possible prolongation and intensity of effect should be anticipated. Occurrence of torsades de pointes w/ quinidine or disopyramide reported; monitor serum levels and for QT prolongation. Interactions may occur w/ cyclosporine, tacrolimus, alfentanil, rifabutin, methylprednisolone, cilostazol, bromocriptine, vinblastine, phenobarbital, St. John's wort, hexobarbital, phenytoin, and valproate. Significant hypoglycemia may occur w/ oral hypoglycemic agents (eg, nateglinide, pioglitazone, repaglinide) and/or insulin. Caution when prescribing w/ statins; if concomitant use w/ atorvastatin or pravastatin cannot be avoided, do not exceed 20mg/day of atorvastatin and 40mg/day of pravastatin. Consider use of a statin that is not dependent on CYP3A metabolism (eg, fluvastatin); prescribe the lowest registered dose if concomitant use cannot be avoided. (Tab) May decrease levels of zidovudine; separate zidovudine administration by at least 2 hrs.

NURSING CONSIDERATIONS

Assessment: Assess for history of cholestatic jaundice/hepatic dysfunction associated w/ prior use of clarithromycin, hepatic/renal impairment, history of QT prolongation, ongoing proarrhythmic conditions, clinically significant bradycardia, ventricular cardiac arrhythmia, torsades de pointes, myasthenia gravis, history of acute porphyria, pregnancy/nursing status, possible drug interactions, and hypersensitivity to the drug, any of its ingredients, erythromycin, or any of the macrolide antibiotics.

Monitoring: Monitor for development of drug-resistant bacteria, CDAD, hepatitis, QT prolongation, severe acute hypersensitivity reactions, exacerbation of myasthenia gravis, new onset of symptoms of myasthenic syndrome, and other adverse reactions. Monitor LFTs and renal function. Frequently monitor INR/PT w/ oral anticoagulants.

Patient Counseling: Inform about potential benefits/risks of therapy. Counsel that therapy should only be used to treat bacterial, not viral, infections. Instruct to take exactly ud; inform that skipping doses or not completing full course may decrease effectiveness and increase antibiotic resistance. Instruct to notify physician if watery/bloody diarrhea (w/ or w/o stomach cramps) develops; inform that this may occur up to 2 or more months after treatment. Instruct to notify physician if pregnant/nursing and of all medications currently being taken.

Storage: (250mg tab) 15-30°C (59-86°F). Protect from light. (500mg tab) 20-25°C (68-77°F). (Sus) <25°C (77°F). Do not refrigerate. (XL) 20-25°C (68-77°F); excursions permitted 15-30°C (59-86°F).

BINOSTO – alendronate sodium RX

Class: Bisphosphonate

ADULT DOSAGE

Osteoporosis

In Postmenopausal Women:

Usual: One 70mg effervescent tab once weekly

To Increase Bone Mass in Men w/ Osteoporosis:

Usual: One 70mg effervescent tab once weekly

Periodically reevaluate the need for continued therapy

Ca^{2+} and Vitamin D Supplementation:

Instruct patients to take supplemental calcium and vitamin D if dietary intake is inadequate

Patients at increased risk for vitamin D insufficiency (eg, >70 years of age, nursing home-bound, or chronically ill) may need vitamin D supplementation

Patients w/ GI malabsorption syndromes may require higher doses of vitamin D supplementation and measurement of 25-hydroxyvitamin D should be considered

Missed Dose

If the once-weekly dose is missed, instruct patients to take 1 dose on the morning after they remember

Patient should not take 2 doses on the same day but should return to taking 1 dose once a week, as originally scheduled on their chosen day

PEDIATRIC DOSAGE

Pediatric use may not have been established

ADMINISTRATION

Oral route

Take upon arising for the day and at least 30 min before the 1st food, beverage, or medication of the day

Dissolve the effervescent tab in 4 oz room temperature plain water only (not mineral water or flavored water)

HOW SUPPLIED

Tab, Effervescent: 70mg

CONTRAINDICATIONS

Esophageal abnormalities that delay esophageal emptying (eg, stricture, achalasia), inability to stand or sit upright for at least 30 min, hypocalcemia, patients at increased risk of aspiration.

WARNINGS/PRECAUTIONS

Consider discontinuation after 3-5 yrs of use in patients at low risk for fracture; periodically reevaluate risk for fracture in patients who d/c therapy. May cause local irritation of the upper GI mucosa; caution with active upper GI problems (eg, Barrett's esophagus, dysphagia, gastritis). Esophageal reactions (eg, esophagitis, esophageal ulcers/erosions) reported; d/c if dysphagia, odynophagia, retrosternal pain, or new/worsening heartburn develops. Use therapy under appropriate supervision in patients who cannot comply with dosing instructions due to mental disability. Gastric and duodenal ulcers reported. Treat hypocalcemia and other disorders affecting mineral metabolism (eg, vitamin D deficiency) prior to therapy; monitor serum Ca^{2+} and for symptoms of hypocalcemia during therapy. Asymptomatic decreases in serum Ca^{2+} and phosphate may occur; ensure adequate Ca^{2+} and vitamin D intake. Severe and occasionally incapacitating bone, joint, and/or muscle pain reported; d/c if severe symptoms develop. Osteonecrosis of the jaw (ONJ) reported; risk may increase with duration of exposure to drug. If invasive dental procedures are required, discontinuation of treatment may reduce risk for ONJ. Consider discontinuation if ONJ develops. Atypical, low-energy, or low-trauma fractures of the femoral shaft reported; evaluate any patient with a history of bisphosphonate exposure who presents with thigh/groin pain to rule out incomplete femur fracture, and consider interruption of therapy. Not recommended with CrCl <35mL/min. Contains 650mg of Na^+; caution in patients who have Na^+-intake restrictions.

ADVERSE REACTIONS

Nausea, abdominal pain, musculoskeletal pain, acid regurgitation, dyspepsia, constipation, diarrhea.

DRUG INTERACTIONS

Ca^{2+} supplements, antacids, or oral medications containing multivalent cations will interfere with absorption; wait at least 1/2 hr after taking alendronate before taking any other oral medications. Increased incidence of upper GI adverse events in patients receiving concomitant therapy with daily doses of alendronate >10mg and aspirin-containing products. NSAID use is associated with GI irritation; use with caution.

NURSING CONSIDERATIONS

Assessment: Assess for esophageal abnormalities, ability to stand or sit upright for at least 30 min, hypocalcemia, risk for aspiration or ONJ, active upper GI problems, mental disability, Na^{+}-intake restriction, renal impairment, drug hypersensitivity, any other conditions where treatment is contraindicated or cautioned, pregnancy/nursing status, and possible drug interactions.

Monitoring: Monitor for signs/symptoms of ONJ, atypical fractures, esophageal reactions, musculoskeletal pain, hypocalcemia, and other adverse events. Monitor serum Ca^{2+} levels. Periodically reevaluate the need for continued therapy.

Patient Counseling: Instruct to take supplemental Ca^{2+} and vitamin D if daily dietary intake is inadequate. Counsel to consider weight-bearing exercise along with modification of certain behavioral factors (eg, cigarette smoking, excessive alcohol use), if these factors exist. Instruct to take upon arising for the day and at least 30 min before the 1st food, beverage, or medication of the day. Advise to avoid lying down for at least 30 min after taking the drug and until after 1st food of the day. Instruct to follow all dosing instructions, and inform that failure to follow them may increase risk of esophageal problems. Instruct not to attempt to swallow, chew, or suck on the tab because of a potential for oropharyngeal ulceration. Advise to d/c and consult physician if symptoms of esophageal disease develop. Instruct that if the once-weekly dose is missed, to take 1 dose on the am after they remember and to return to taking the dose, as originally scheduled on their chosen day; instruct not to take 2 doses on the same day. Inform patients on Na^{+}-restricted diet that each tab contains 650mg Na^{+}, equivalent to 1650mg NaCl.

Storage: 20-25°C (68-77°F); excursions permitted to 15-30°C (59-86°F). Protect from moisture.

BLINCYTO – blinatumomab RX

Class: CD19-directed CD3 T-cell engager

Cytokine release syndrome (CRS), which may be life-threatening or fatal, reported; interrupt or d/c therapy as recommended. Neurological toxicities, which may be severe, life-threatening, or fatal, reported; interrupt or d/c therapy as recommended.

ADULT DOSAGE

Acute Lymphoblastic Leukemia

Philadelphia Chromosome-Negative: Relapsed or Refractory B-Cell Precursor:

≥45kg:
Cycle 1: 9mcg/day on Days 1-7, and 28mcg/day on Days 8-28
Subsequent Cycles: 28mcg/day on Days 1-28

Single cycle of treatment consists of 4 weeks of continuous IV infusion followed by a 2-week treatment-free interval
Treatment course consists of up to 2 cycles for induction followed by 3 additional cycles for consolidation treatment (up to a total of 5 cycles)

PEDIATRIC DOSAGE

Acute Lymphoblastic Leukemia

Philadelphia Chromosome-Negative: Relapsed or Refractory B-Cell Precursor:

Limited experience in pediatric patients
Evaluated in a dose-escalation study of 41 pediatric patients with relapsed or refractory B-precursor acute lymphoblastic leukemia (median age was 6 yrs [range: 2-17 yrs]). Administered at doses of 5-30mcg/m^2/day. Recommended phase 2 regimen was 5mcg/m^2/day on Days 1-7 and 15mcg/m^2/day on Days 8-28 for cycle 1, and 15mcg/m^2/day on Days 1-28 for subsequent cycles

Steady-state concentrations were comparable in adult and pediatric patients at the equivalent dose levels based on BSA-based regimens

DOSE MODIFICATION

Adverse Reactions

If interruption after an adverse event is no longer than 7 days, continue same cycle to a total of 28 days of infusion inclusive of days before and after the interruption in that cycle. If an interruption due to an adverse event is >7 days, start a new cycle

Cytokine Release Syndrome:
Grade 3: Withhold until resolved, then restart at 9mcg/day. Escalate to 28mcg/day after 7 days if the toxicity does not recur
Grade 4: D/C permanently

Neurological Toxicity:
Seizure: D/C permanently if >1 seizure occurs
Grade 3: Withhold until no more than Grade 1 (mild) for at least 3 days, then restart at 9mcg/day. Escalate to 28mcg/day after 7 days if the toxicity does not recur. If the toxicity occurred at 9mcg/day, or if the toxicity takes >7 days to resolve, d/c permanently
Grade 4: D/C permanently
Other Clinically Relevant Adverse Reactions:
Grade 3: Withhold until no more than Grade 1 (mild), then restart at 9mcg/day. Escalate to 28mcg/day after 7 days if the toxicity does not recur. If the toxicity takes >14 days to resolve, d/c permanently
Grade 4: Consider discontinuing permanently

ADMINISTRATION
IV route

Premedicate with dexamethasone 20mg IV 1 hr prior to the 1st dose of each cycle, prior to a step dose (eg, Cycle 1 day 8), or when restarting an infusion after an interruption of ≥4 hrs
Administer as a continuous IV infusion at a constant flow rate using an infusion pump that is programmable, lockable, non-elastomeric, and has an alarm

Infusion bags should be infused over 24 hrs or 48 hrs
Infuse the total 240mL sol according to the instructions on the pharmacy label on the bag at 1 of the following constant infusion rates:
Infusion rate of 10mL/hr for a duration of 24 hrs, or 5mL/hr for a duration of 48 hrs
Refer to PI for further administration, reconstitution, and preparation instructions

HOW SUPPLIED
Inj: 35mcg

WARNINGS/PRECAUTIONS
Hospitalization is recommended for the first 9 days of the 1st cycle and the first 2 days of the 2nd cycle. For all subsequent cycle starts and reinitiation (eg, if treatment is interrupted for ≥4 hrs), supervision by a healthcare professional or hospitalization is recommended. Infusion reactions may occur and may be clinically indistinguishable from manifestations of CRS. Disseminated intravascular coagulation (DIC), capillary leak syndrome (CLS), and hemophagocytic lymphohistiocytosis/macrophage activation syndrome (HLH/MAS) reported in the setting of CRS. Serious infections (eg, sepsis, pneumonia, bacteremia, opportunistic infections, catheter-site infections) reported; administer prophylactic antibiotics and employ surveillance testing during treatment as appropriate. Tumor lysis syndrome (TLS) reported; use appropriate prophylactic measures, including pretreatment nontoxic cytoreduction and on-treatment hydration; may require either temporary interruption or discontinuation of therapy. Neutropenia and febrile neutropenia, including life-threatening cases, reported; interrupt therapy if prolonged neutropenia occurs. Risk for loss of consciousness. Associated with transient elevations in liver enzymes; interrupt therapy if the transaminases rise to >5X ULN or if bilirubin rises to >3X ULN. Cranial magnetic resonance imaging changes showing leukoencephalopathy observed, especially in patients with prior treatment with cranial irradiation and antileukemic chemotherapy (including systemic high-dose methotrexate or intrathecal cytarabine); clinical significance of this is unknown. Preparation and administration errors reported; follow instructions strictly to minimize medication errors. Potential for immunogenicity. Caution in elderly.

ADVERSE REACTIONS
CRS, neurological toxicities, pyrexia, headache, peripheral edema, febrile neutropenia, nausea, hypokalemia, constipation, anemia, diarrhea, fatigue, bacterial infections, tremor, cough.

DRUG INTERACTIONS
May suppress CYP450 enzymes; highest risk during the first 9 days of the 1st cycle and the first 2 days of the 2nd cycle in patients receiving concomitant CYP450 substrates, particularly those with a narrow therapeutic index; monitor for toxicity (eg, warfarin) or drug concentrations (eg, cyclosporine) and adjust dose of concomitant drug PRN.

NURSING CONSIDERATIONS

Assessment: Assess for known hypersensitivity to drug or to any component of the formulation, prior treatment with cranial irradiation and antileukemic chemotherapy, pregnancy/nursing status, and possible drug interactions. Obtain baseline WBC count, absolute neutrophil count (ANC), ALT, AST, gamma-glutamyl transferase (GGT), and total bilirubin.

Monitoring: Monitor for signs/symptoms of CRS, DIC, CLS, HLH/MAS, neurological toxicities, infections, TLS, loss of consciousness, and other adverse reactions. Monitor for neutropenia/febrile neutropenia; monitor lab parameters (eg, WBC count, ANC) during infusion. Monitor ALT, AST, GGT, and total blood bilirubin during therapy.

Patient Counseling: Advise to contact physician for any signs/symptoms of CRS or infusion reactions, neurological toxicities, or infections (eg, pneumonia). Advise to refrain from driving and engaging in hazardous occupations/activities (eg, operating heavy/potentially dangerous machinery) while on therapy and inform that neurological events may be experienced. Inform that it is very important to keep area around the IV catheter clean to reduce the risk of infection. Advise to not adjust setting on the infusion pump; inform that any changes to pump function may result in dosing errors. Instruct to contact physician or nurse immediately if there is a problem with the infusion pump or the pump alarms.

Storage: 2-8°C (36-46°F). Protect from light until time of use. Do not freeze. May store lyophilized vial and IV sol stabilizer for a max of 8 hrs at room temperature. Reconstituted Vial: 23-27°C (73-81°F) for 4 hrs, or 2-8°C (36-46°F) for 24 hrs. Protect from light. Prepared IV Bag Containing Sol for Infusion: 23-27°C (73-81°F) for 48 hrs (storage time includes infusion time; if not administered within the time frames and temperatures indicated, discard and do not refrigerate again), or 2-8°C (36-46°F) for 8 days. Ship in packaging that has been validated to maintain temperature of the contents at 2-8°C (36-46°F). Do not freeze.

BONIVA – ibandronate — RX

Class: Bisphosphonate

ADULT DOSAGE

Osteoporosis

Inj:
Treatment in Postmenopausal Women:
3mg IV over 15-30 sec every 3 months

Tab:
Treatment and Prevention in Postmenopausal Women:
150mg once monthly on the same date each month

Inj/Tab:
Periodically reevaluate the need for continued therapy

Missed Dose

Inj:
If dose is missed, administer as soon as it can be rescheduled
Thereafter, schedule every 3 months from date of last inj

Tab:
If next scheduled ibandronate day is >7 days away, take one 150mg tab in am following date that it is remembered
If next scheduled ibandronate day is 1-7 days away, wait until subsequent month's scheduled ibandronate day to take tab
For both scenarios, return to original schedule by taking one 150mg tab every month on previous chosen day for subsequent doses

PEDIATRIC DOSAGE

Pediatric use may not have been established

DOSE MODIFICATION

Renal Impairment
Severe (CrCl <30mL/min): Not recommended

ADMINISTRATION

IV/Oral route

Recommendations for Ca^{2+} and Vitamin D Supplementation
If dietary intake is inadequate, patients should take supplemental Ca^{2+} and vitamin D

Administration Instructions

Inj:
Do not mix w/ Ca^{2+}-containing sol or other IV administered drugs
Do not use prefilled syringes w/ particulate matter or discoloration
Administer only w/ the enclosed needle
Do not administer more frequently than once every 3 months

Tab:
Take at least 60 min before the 1st food or drink of the day other than water or before taking any oral medication or supplementation
Swallow tabs whole; do not chew or suck

Swallow tabs w/ full glass of plain water (6-8 oz) while standing or sitting in upright position; avoid lying down for 60 min after taking medication
Do not eat, drink anything except plain water, or take other medications for at least 60 min after taking ibandronate

HOW SUPPLIED

Inj: 3mg/3mL [prefilled syringe]; Tab: 150mg

CONTRAINDICATIONS

Hypocalcemia. (Tab) Esophageal abnormalities that delay esophageal emptying (eg, stricture or achalasia), and inability to stand or sit upright for at least 60 min.

WARNINGS/PRECAUTIONS

Consider discontinuation after 3-5 yrs of use in patients at low-risk for fracture; periodically reevaluate risk for fracture in patients who d/c therapy. Hypocalcemia reported; treat hypocalcemia and other disturbances of bone and mineral metabolism before therapy. Osteonecrosis of the jaw (ONJ) reported; risk may increase w/ duration of exposure to drug or w/ concomitant administration of drugs associated w/ ONJ. Consider a dental examination w/ appropriate preventive dentistry prior to treatment in patients w/ a history of concomitant risk factors (eg, cancer, chemotherapy, angiogenesis inhibitors, radiotherapy, corticosteroids, poor oral hygiene) and if possible, avoid invasive dental procedures while on treatment. For patients requiring invasive dental procedures, discontinuation of treatment may reduce risk for ONJ. Consider discontinuation if ONJ develops. Severe and occasionally incapacitating bone, joint, and/or muscle pain reported; d/c if severe symptoms develop. Atypical, low-energy, or low-trauma fractures of the femoral shaft reported; evaluate any patient w/ a history of bisphosphonate exposure who presents w/ thigh/groin pain to rule out an incomplete femur fracture, and consider interruption of therapy. (Inj) Caution not to administer intra-arterially or paravenously as this could lead to tissue damage. Anaphylaxis reported; d/c and initiate appropriate treatment if anaphylactic or other severe hypersensitivity/allergic reactions occur. (Tab) May cause local irritation of the upper GI mucosa; caution w/ active upper GI problems (eg, Barrett's esophagus, dysphagia, esophageal diseases, gastritis, duodenitis, ulcers). Esophageal reactions (eg, esophagitis, esophageal ulcers/erosions) reported; d/c if dysphagia, odynophagia, retrosternal pain, or new/worsening heartburn develops. Use therapy under appropriate supervision in patients who cannot comply w/ dosing instructions due to mental disability. Gastric and duodenal ulcers reported.

ADVERSE REACTIONS

Influenza, nasopharyngitis, abdominal pain, dyspepsia, constipation, arthralgia, back pain, pain in extremity, headache, diarrhea, UTI, myalgia.

DRUG INTERACTIONS

May interfere w/ the use of bone-imaging agents. (Tab) Products containing Ca^{2+} and other multivalent cations (eg, aluminum, Mg^{2+}, iron) may interfere w/ absorption; do not take these products w/in 60 min of dosing. Caution w/ aspirin or NSAIDs due to GI irritation.

NURSING CONSIDERATIONS

Assessment: Assess for hypocalcemia, disturbances of bone and mineral metabolism, risk for ONJ, renal impairment, drug hypersensitivity, any other conditions where treatment is contraindicated or cautioned, pregnancy/nursing status, and possible drug interactions. (Inj) Obtain SrCr before each dose. Perform routine oral exam, and consider appropriate preventive dentistry in patients w/ history of concomitant risk factors for ONJ. (Tab) Assess for esophageal abnormalities, ability to stand or sit upright for at least 60 min, active upper GI problems, and mental disability.

Monitoring: Monitor for signs/symptoms of ONJ, musculoskeletal pain, hypocalcemia, atypical femoral fracture, and other adverse reactions. Monitor renal function and periodically reevaluate the need for continued therapy. (Tab) Monitor for esophageal reactions. (Inj) Monitor for severe hypersensitivity/allergic reactions.

Patient Counseling: Inform about benefits/risks of therapy. Instruct to take supplemental Ca^{2+} and vitamin D if dietary intake is inadequate. (Tab) Instruct to carefully follow dosing instructions and on what to do if doses are missed. Advise to d/c and seek medical attention if symptoms of esophageal irritation develop. Instruct on appropriate administration of drug.

Storage: 25°C (77°F); excursions permitted to 15-30°C (59-86°F).

BOOSTRIX – tetanus toxoid, reduced diphtheria toxoid and acellular pertussis vaccine, adsorbed RX

Class: Toxoid/vaccine combination

ADULT DOSAGE

Active Booster Immunization Against Tetanus, Diphtheria, and Pertussis

0.5mL IM single dose

Wound Management:

May be given as a tetanus prophylaxis if no previous dose of any tetanus toxoid, reduced diphtheria toxoid, and acellular pertussis vaccine, adsorbed (Tdap) has been administered

PEDIATRIC DOSAGE

Active Booster Immunization Against Tetanus, Diphtheria, and Pertussis

≥10 Years:

0.5mL IM single dose

Wound Management:

May be given as a tetanus prophylaxis if no previous dose of any tetanus toxoid, reduced diphtheria toxoid, and acellular pertussis vaccine, adsorbed (Tdap) has been administered

ADMINISTRATION

IM route

5 years should have elapsed since last dose of recommended series of diphtheria and tetanus toxoids and acellular pertussis vaccine adsorbed (DTaP) and/or tetanus and diphtheria toxoids adsorbed for adult use (Td) vaccine

Shake well before use

Inject into the deltoid muscle of the upper arm

Do not administer IV, intradermally, or SQ

Do not mix w/ any other vaccine in the same syringe or vial

HOW SUPPLIED

Inj: 0.5mL [vial, prefilled syringe]

CONTRAINDICATIONS

Encephalopathy (eg, coma, decreased level of consciousness, prolonged seizures) within 7 days of administration of a previous dose of a pertussis antigen-containing vaccine that is not attributable to another identifiable cause.

WARNINGS/PRECAUTIONS

Administer 5 yrs after last dose of recommended series of diphtheria and tetanus toxoids and acellular pertussis vaccine adsorbed and/or tetanus and diphtheria toxoids adsorbed for adult use vaccine. Tip caps of prefilled syringes may contain natural rubber latex; allergic reactions may occur in latex-sensitive individuals. May cause brachial neuritis and Guillain-Barre syndrome. Risk of Guillain-Barre syndrome may increase if Guillain-Barre syndrome occurred within 6 weeks of receipt of a prior tetanus toxoid-containing vaccine. Syncope may occur and can be accompanied by transient neurological signs (eg, visual disturbance, paresthesia, tonic-clonic limb movements). Defer vaccination in patients with progressive/unstable neurologic conditions (eg, cerebrovascular events, acute encephalopathic conditions). Avoid if experienced an Arthus-type hypersensitivity reaction following a prior dose of tetanus toxoid-containing vaccine unless at least 10 yrs have elapsed since last dose of tetanus toxoid-containing vaccine. Expected immune response may not be obtained in immunosuppressed persons. Review immunization history for possible vaccine sensitivity and previous vaccination-related adverse reactions; epinephrine and other appropriate agents should be immediately available for control of allergic reactions.

ADVERSE REACTIONS

Inj-site reactions (eg, pain, redness, swelling, increased arm circumference), headache, fatigue, fever, GI symptoms.

DRUG INTERACTIONS

Lower postvaccination geometric mean antibody concentrations (GMCs) to pertactin observed following concomitant administration with meningococcal conjugate vaccine as compared to Boostrix administered 1st. Lower GMCs for antibodies to the pertussis antigens filamentous hemagglutinin and pertactin observed when concomitantly administered with influenza virus vaccine as compared with Boostrix alone. Immunosuppressive therapies, including irradiation, antimetabolites, alkylating agents, cytotoxic drugs, and corticosteroids (used in greater than physiologic doses), may reduce the immune response to vaccine.

NURSING CONSIDERATIONS

Assessment: Assess for history of encephalopathy, latex hypersensitivity, development of Guillain-Barre syndrome following a prior vaccine containing tetanus toxoid, progressive/unstable neurologic conditions, immunosuppression, pregnancy/nursing status, and for possible drug interactions. Review immunization history for possible vaccine sensitivity and previous vaccination-related adverse reactions.

Monitoring: Monitor for signs and symptoms of Guillain-Barre syndrome, brachial neuritis, allergic reactions, syncope, neurological signs, and other adverse reactions. Monitor immune response.

Patient Counseling: Inform about benefits/risks of immunization. Advise about the potential for adverse reactions. Instruct to notify physician if any adverse reactions occur, if pregnant, or planning to become pregnant. Encourage pregnant women receiving the vaccine to contact the pregnancy registry.

Storage: 2-8°C (36-46°F). Do not freeze; discard if has been frozen.

BOSULIF – bosutinib RX

Class: Kinase inhibitors

ADULT DOSAGE

Chronic Myelogenous Leukemia

Chronic, accelerated, or blast phase Philadelphia chromosome-positive chronic myelogenous leukemia w/ resistance or intolerance to prior therapy

Usual: 500mg qd until disease progression or patient intolerance

Titrate: Consider escalation to 600mg qd who do not reach complete hematological response by Week 8 or a complete cytogenetic response by Week 12, who did not have Grade 3 or higher adverse reactions, and who are currently taking 500mg qd

PEDIATRIC DOSAGE

Pediatric use may not have been established

DOSE MODIFICATION

Concomitant Medications

CYP3A Strong or Moderate Inducers/Inhibitors: Avoid use

Renal Impairment

CrCl 30-50mL/min: 400mg qd

CrCl <30mL/min: 300mg qd

Declining Renal Function/Not Tolerating 500mg: Follow recommendations for

Hepatic Impairment

Mild (Child-Pugh A), Moderate (Child-Pugh B), or Severe (Child-Pugh C): 200mg qd

Adverse Reactions

Nonhematologic:

Elevated Liver Transaminases:

≥3X ULN w/ Bilirubin elevations >2X ULN and Alkaline Phosphatase <2X ULN: D/C therapy

>5X ULN: Withhold therapy until recovery to ≤2.5X ULN and resume at 400mg qd thereafter; if recovery takes longer than 4 weeks, d/c therapy

Diarrhea:

Grade 3-4: Withhold therapy until recovery to Grade ≤1; may resume at 400mg qd

Other Significant, Moderate/Severe Toxicity:

Withhold until toxicity has resolved, then consider 400mg qd; if clinically appropriate, consider re-escalating to 500mg qd

Myelosuppression:

ANC <1000 x 10^6/L or Platelets <50,000 x 10^6/L:

Withhold therapy until ANC ≥1000 x 10^6/L and platelets ≥50,000 x 10^6/L; resume therapy at the same dose if recovery occurs w/in 2 weeks Reduce to 100mg and resume treatment if blood counts remain low for >2 weeks upon recovery

Reduce dose by an additional 100mg upon recovery, if cytopenia recurs and resume treatment

ADMINISTRATION

Oral route

Take w/ food

Do not crush or cut tab; do not touch or handle crushed or broken tabs

HOW SUPPLIED

Tab: 100mg, 500mg

WARNINGS/PRECAUTIONS

Diarrhea, N/V, and abdominal pain reported; monitor and manage patients using standards of care. Thrombocytopenia, anemia, and neutropenia reported; withhold, reduce dose, or d/c therapy as necessary. Hepatic toxicity reported. Fluid retention reported and may manifest as pericardial effusion, pleural effusion, pulmonary edema, and/or peripheral edema; monitor and manage patients using standards of care. Consider dose adjustment w/ baseline and treatment emergent renal impairment. May cause fetal harm.

ADVERSE REACTIONS
Diarrhea, N/V, thrombocytopenia, abdominal pain, rash, anemia, pyrexia, fatigue, neutropenia, edema, asthenia, respiratory tract infection, decreased appetite, headache, dyspnea.

DRUG INTERACTIONS
Avoid concomitant use w/ strong CYP3A inhibitors (eg, ritonavir, ketoconazole, clarithromycin), moderate CYP3A inhibitors (eg, fluconazole, imatinib, grapefruit products), or P-gp inhibitors as increase in bosutinib concentration is expected. Avoid concomitant use w/ strong CYP3A inducers (eg, rifampin, phenytoin, carbamazepine) or moderate CYP3A inducers (eg, bosentan, nafcillin, efavirenz) as a large reduction in exposure is expected. Lansoprazole may decrease levels; consider using short-acting antacids or H_2-blockers instead of proton pump inhibitors, but separate dosing by >2 hrs. May increase concentrations of drugs that are P-gp substrates (eg, digoxin).

NURSING CONSIDERATIONS

Assessment: Assess for hypersensitivity to drug, hepatic/renal impairment, pregnancy/nursing status, and possible drug interactions.

Monitoring: Monitor for signs/symptoms of GI toxicity, fluid retention, and other adverse reactions. Perform CBC weekly for the 1st month and then monthly thereafter, or as clinically indicated. Perform monthly LFTs for the first 3 months and as clinically indicated; monitor more frequently in patients w/ transaminase elevations. Monitor renal function during therapy w/ particular attention to patients w/ preexisting renal impairment or risk factors for renal dysfunction.

Patient Counseling: Instruct to take medication exactly as prescribed and not to change the dose or d/c unless directed by physician. Instruct that if a dose is missed beyond 12 hrs, to skip the dose and take the usual prescribed dose on the following day. Advise to seek medical attention promptly if symptoms of GI problems or fluid retention develop, developing renal problems or if symptoms of other adverse reactions (eg, respiratory tract infections, rash, fatigue) are significant. Instruct to immediately report fever, any suggestion of infection, signs/symptoms of bleeding or easy bruising, or jaundice. Inform that drug may cause fetal harm; counsel females of reproductive potential to use effective contraceptive measures to prevent pregnancy during and for at least 30 days after completing treatment. Instruct to contact physician immediately if pregnancy occurs during treatment. Advise not to breastfeed or provide breast milk to infants while on therapy; if a patient wishes to restart breastfeeding after treatment, advise to discuss the appropriate timing w/ physician. Inform that drug and certain other medicines, including OTC drugs and herbal supplements (eg, St. John's wort), can interact w/ each other and may alter the effects of treatment.

Storage: 20-25°C (68-77°F); excursions permitted to 15-30°C (59-86°F).

BREO ELLIPTA – fluticasone furoate/vilanterol — RX

Class: Beta$_2$-agonist/corticosteroid

Long-acting β_2-adrenergic agonists (LABAs) increase the risk of asthma-related death. Not indicated for the treatment of asthma.

ADULT DOSAGE

Chronic Obstructive Pulmonary Disease

Long-Term Maint Treatment of Airflow Obstruction in Patients w/ COPD (eg, Chronic Bronchitis, Emphysema):
1 inh qd; do not use >1 time q24h

Also indicated to reduce exacerbations of COPD in patients w/ history of exacerbations

PEDIATRIC DOSAGE

Pediatric use may not have been established

ADMINISTRATION
Oral inh route

After inh, rinse mouth w/ water w/o swallowing
Take at the same time every day

HOW SUPPLIED
Powder, Inhalation: (Fluticasone-Vilanterol) (100mcg/25mcg)/blister [14, 30 blisters]

CONTRAINDICATIONS
Milk protein hypersensitivity.

WARNINGS/PRECAUTIONS

Not indicated for acute bronchospasm relief. Do not initiate during rapidly deteriorating or potentially life-threatening episodes of COPD. D/C regular use of oral/inhaled short-acting β_2-agonist when beginning treatment. Do not use more often or at higher doses than recommended; clinically significant cardiovascular (CV) effects and fatalities reported with excessive use. *Candida albicans* infections of mouth and pharynx reported; treat and if needed, interrupt therapy. Increased incidence of pneumonia reported. Increased susceptibility to infections. May lead to serious/fatal course of chickenpox or measles; avoid exposure and if exposed, consider prophylaxis/treatment. Caution in patients with active/quiescent tuberculosis (TB), systemic fungal, bacterial, viral, or parasitic infections, or ocular herpes simplex. Deaths due to adrenal insufficiency reported during and after transfer from systemic to inhaled corticosteroids; wean slowly from systemic corticosteroid use after transferring to therapy. Resume oral corticosteroids during periods of stress or a severe COPD exacerbation in patients previously withdrawn from systemic corticosteroids. Transferring from systemic to inhaled corticosteroid may unmask allergic conditions previously suppressed by systemic therapy (eg, rhinitis, conjunctivitis, eczema). Monitor for systemic corticosteroid effects. Reduce dose slowly and consider other treatments if hypercorticism and adrenal suppression occur. May produce paradoxical bronchospasm; treat immediately, d/c therapy, and institute alternative therapy. Hypersensitivity reactions may occur; d/c if such reactions occur. CV effects may occur; may need to discontinue if such effects occur. Decreases in bone mineral density (BMD) reported with long-term use; caution with major risk factors for decreased bone mineral content, including chronic use of drugs that can reduce bone mass (eg, anticonvulsants, oral corticosteroids). If significant reductions in BMD are seen and therapy is still considered medically important, use medicine to treat or prevent osteoporosis. Glaucoma, increased intraocular pressure (IOP), and cataracts reported with long-term use. Caution with convulsive disorders, thyrotoxicosis, diabetes mellitus (DM), ketoacidosis, moderate/severe hepatic impairment, and in patients unusually responsive to sympathomimetic amines. May produce significant hypokalemia or transient hyperglycemia.

ADVERSE REACTIONS

Nasopharyngitis, upper respiratory tract infection, oropharyngeal candidiasis, headache, back pain, sinusitis, cough, oropharyngeal pain, arthralgia, HTN, influenza, pharyngitis, diarrhea, peripheral edema, pyrexia.

DRUG INTERACTIONS

Do not use with other medicines containing a LABA. Caution with long-term ketoconazole and other strong CYP3A4 inhibitors (eg, ritonavir, clarithromycin, conivaptan); increased systemic corticosteroid and increased CV adverse effects may occur. Extreme caution with MAOIs, TCAs, or drugs known to prolong the QTc interval or within 2 weeks of discontinuation of such agents; effect on CV system may be potentiated by these agents. β-blockers may block pulmonary effects and produce severe bronchospasm in patients with reversible obstructive airways disease; if such therapy is needed, consider cardioselective β-blockers and use with caution. Caution is advised when coadministered with non-K^+-sparing diuretics (eg, loop, thiazide diuretics).

NURSING CONSIDERATIONS

Assessment: Assess for hypersensitivity to drug or to milk proteins, COPD status, active/quiescent TB, systemic infections, ocular herpes simplex, CV disorders, risk factors for decreased bone mineral content, convulsive disorders, thyrotoxicosis, DM, ketoacidosis, history of increased IOP, glaucoma, and/or cataracts, hepatic impairment, pregnancy/nursing status, and possible drug interactions. Assess BMD.

Monitoring: Monitor for deteriorating disease, localized oropharyngeal *C. albicans* infections, pneumonia, infections, systemic corticosteroid effects (eg, hypercorticism, adrenal suppression), paradoxical bronchospasm, hypersensitivity reactions, CV effects, glaucoma, cataracts, increased IOP, hypokalemia, hyperglycemia, and other adverse reactions. Periodically monitor BMD.

Patient Counseling: Inform that drug is not for treatment of asthma or to relieve acute COPD symptoms; advise that acute symptoms should be treated with a rescue inhaler (eg, albuterol). Instruct to notify physician immediately if experiencing worsening of symptoms, a need for more inhalations than usual of the rescue inhaler, or a significant decrease in lung function. Advise not to d/c therapy without physician guidance and not to use additional LABA. Instruct to contact physician if oropharyngeal candidiasis or symptoms of pneumonia develop. Advise to avoid exposure to chickenpox or measles, and, if exposed, to consult physician without delay. Inform about risk of immunosuppression, hypercorticism, adrenal suppression, reduction in BMD, ocular effects, and of adverse effects (eg, palpitations, chest pain, rapid HR, tremor, nervousness). Advise that hypersensitivity reactions may occur; instruct to d/c therapy if such reactions occur. Inform that the inhaler is not reusable and advise not to take the inhaler apart.

Storage: 20-25°C (68-77°F); excursions permitted from 15-30°C (59-86°F). Store in a dry place away from direct heat or sunlight. Store inside the unopened moisture-protective foil tray and only remove from the tray immediately before initial use. Discard 6 weeks after opening the foil tray or when the counter reads "0" (after all blisters have been used), whichever comes 1st.

BRILINTA – ticagrelor

RX

Class: Platelet aggregation inhibitor

May cause significant, sometimes fatal, bleeding. Do not use in patients w/ active pathological bleeding or a history of intracranial hemorrhage. Do not start therapy in patients planned to undergo urgent CABG; when possible, d/c therapy at least 5 days prior to any surgery. Suspect bleeding in any patient who is hypotensive and has recently undergone coronary angiography, percutaneous coronary intervention (PCI), CABG, or other surgical procedures in the setting of ticagrelor. If possible, manage bleeding w/o discontinuing therapy; stopping therapy increases the risk of subsequent cardiovascular (CV) events. Maintenance doses of aspirin (ASA) >100mg reduce the effectiveness of ticagrelor and should be avoided; after any initial dose, use w/ ASA 75-100mg/day.

ADULT DOSAGE

Acute Coronary Syndrome

Reduction in Rate of Thrombotic Cardiovascular Events in Patients w/ Acute Coronary Syndrome (Unstable Angina, Non-ST Elevation MI, or ST Elevation MI):

LD: 180mg w/ aspirin (ASA) (usually 325mg)
Maint: 90mg bid w/ ASA (75-100mg/day)

Patients who have received a LD of clopidogrel may be started on therapy

Missed Dose

If a dose is missed, take one 90mg tab (next dose) at its scheduled time

PEDIATRIC DOSAGE

Pediatric use may not have been established

ADMINISTRATION

Oral route
Take w/ or w/o food

Administration Options

If unable to swallow tab(s) whole, tab can be crushed, mixed w/ water, and drunk immediately; the glass should be refilled w/ water, stirred, and the contents drunk
The mixture can be also administered via a NG tube (≥CH8); it is important to flush the NG tube through w/ water after administration of the mixture

HOW SUPPLIED

Tab: 90mg

CONTRAINDICATIONS

History of intracranial hemorrhage, active pathological bleeding (eg, peptic ulcer, intracranial hemorrhage), severe hepatic impairment.

WARNINGS/PRECAUTIONS

Risk factors for bleeding include older age, history of bleeding disorders, performance of PCI procedures, and concomitant use of medications that increase risk of bleeding (eg, anticoagulant and fibrinolytic therapy, higher doses of ASA, chronic NSAIDS). Consider the risks and benefits of treatment in patients w/ moderate hepatic impairment. Dyspnea reported; exclude underlying diseases that may require treatment if a patient develops new, prolonged, or worsened dyspnea. If dyspnea is determined to be related to therapy, no specific treatment is required; continue therapy w/o interruption. In the case of intolerable dyspnea requiring discontinuation of therapy, consider another antiplatelet agent. Avoid interruption of treatment; if it must be temporarily discontinued, restart as soon as possible.

ADVERSE REACTIONS

Bleeding, dyspnea, headache, cough, dizziness, nausea, atrial fibrillation, HTN, noncardiac chest pain, diarrhea, back pain, hypotension, fatigue, chest pain.

DRUG INTERACTIONS

See Boxed Warning. Avoid w/ strong CYP3A inhibitors (eg, atazanavir, clarithromycin, ketoconazole). Avoid w/ potent CYP3A inducers (eg, rifampin, phenytoin, carbamazepine). May increase concentrations of simvastatin and lovastatin (CYP3A4 substrates); avoid simvastatin and lovastatin doses >40mg. Inhibits P-glycoprotein transporter; monitor digoxin levels w/ initiation of or any change in ticagrelor therapy.

NURSING CONSIDERATIONS

Assessment: Assess for history of intracranial hemorrhage, active pathological bleeding, risk factors for bleeding, hepatic impairment, hypersensitivity to drug, pregnancy/nursing status, and possible drug interactions.

Monitoring: Monitor for bleeding, dyspnea, and other adverse reactions.

Patient Counseling: Instruct to take drug exactly as prescribed, not to d/c therapy w/o consulting physician, not to exceed 100mg/day ASA, and to avoid taking any other medications that contain ASA. Inform that patient will bleed and bruise more easily and will take longer than usual to stop bleeding. Advise to report any unanticipated, prolonged or excessive bleeding, or blood in stool or urine. Inform that drug can cause SOB; advise to contact physician if experiencing unexpected SOB, especially if severe. Instruct patients to inform physicians and dentists that they are taking the drug before any surgery or dental procedure, and to tell the physician performing any surgery or dental procedure to talk to the prescribing physician before stopping therapy. Advise patient to inform physician of all prescription/OTC medications or dietary supplements that he or she is taking or plans to take.

Storage: 25°C (77°F); excursions permitted to 15-30°C (59-86°F).

BRINTELLIX – vortioxetine

Class: Miscellaneous antidepressant

RX

Antidepressants increased the risk of suicidal thoughts and behavior in children, adolescents, and young adults in short-term studies. Monitor closely for worsening and for emergence of suicidal thoughts and behaviors in patients who are started on antidepressant therapy. Not evaluated for use in pediatric patients.

ADULT DOSAGE

Major Depressive Disorder

Initial: 10mg/day

Titrate: Increase to 20mg/day, as tolerated. May consider decreasing dose to 5mg/day for patients who do not tolerate higher doses

Max: 20mg/day

Maint: Acute episodes of major depression should be followed by several months or longer of sustained therapy to decrease risk of recurrence

Dosing Considerations with MAOIs

Switching to/from an MAOI for Psychiatric Disorders:

Allow at least 14 days between discontinuation of an MAOI and initiation of treatment, and allow at least 21 days between discontinuation of treatment and initiation of an MAOI

Use w/ Other MAOIs (eg, Linezolid, IV Methylene Blue):

Do not start vortioxetine in a patient being treated w/ linezolid or IV methylene blue

In patients already receiving vortioxetine, if acceptable alternatives are not available and benefits outweigh risks, d/c vortioxetine and administer linezolid or IV methylene blue; monitor for serotonin syndrome for 21 days or until 24 hrs after the last dose of linezolid or IV methylene blue, whichever comes 1st. May resume vortioxetine therapy 24 hours after the last dose of linezolid or IV methylene blue

PEDIATRIC DOSAGE

Pediatric use may not have been established

DOSE MODIFICATION

Concomitant Medications

Use w/ Strong CYP2D6 Inhibitors:

Reduce vortioxetine dose by 1/2; increase dose to original level when CYP2D6 inhibitor is discontinued

Use w/ Strong CYP Inducers:
Consider increasing vortioxetine dose when a strong CYP inducer is coadministered for >14 days; max recommended dose should not exceed 3X original dose
Reduce dose to original level w/in 14 days, when the inducer is discontinued

Hepatic Impairment
Severe: Not recommended
Discontinuation
Decrease dose to 10mg/day for 1 week before full discontinuation of 15mg/day or 20mg/day

Other Important Modifications
CYP2D6 Poor Metabolizers:
Max: 10mg/day

ADMINISTRATION
Oral route

Take w/o regard to meals

HOW SUPPLIED
Tab: 5mg, 10mg, 15mg, 20mg

CONTRAINDICATIONS
Use of an MAOI for psychiatric disorders either concomitantly or within 21 days of stopping treatment. Treatment within 14 days of stopping an MAOI for psychiatric disorders. Starting treatment in patients being treated with other MAOIs (eg, linezolid, IV methylene blue).

WARNINGS/PRECAUTIONS
May increase likelihood of precipitation of a mixed/manic episode in patients at risk for bipolar disorder. Screen patient to determine if at risk for bipolar disorder; not approved for treatment of bipolar depression. Serotonin syndrome reported; d/c immediately and initiate supportive symptomatic treatment. May increase risk of bleeding events. Activation of mania/hypomania reported. Pupillary dilation that occurs following use may trigger an angle-closure attack in a patient with anatomically narrow angles who does not have a patent iridectomy. Transient adverse reactions (eg, headache, muscle tension) reported following abrupt discontinuation of doses of 15mg/day or 20mg/day. Hyponatremia reported; caution in the elderly and in volume-depleted patients. D/C in patients with symptomatic hyponatremia and institute appropriate medical intervention. Not recommended with severe hepatic impairment.

ADVERSE REACTIONS
N/V, constipation, diarrhea, dry mouth, dizziness, flatulence, abnormal dreams, pruritus, sexual dysfunction.

DRUG INTERACTIONS
See Dosage and Contraindications. May cause serotonin syndrome when coadministered with other serotonergic drugs (eg, SSRIs, triptans, TCAs, fentanyl, lithium) and with drugs that impair metabolism of serotonin; d/c immediately if this occurs and initiate supportive symptomatic treatment. Increased risk of bleeding with ASA, NSAIDs, warfarin, and other anticoagulants; monitor patients receiving other drugs that interfere with hemostasis when vortioxetine is initiated or discontinued. Increased risk of hyponatremia with diuretics. Consider increasing vortioxetine dose when coadministered with a strong CYP inducer. Coadministration with another drug that is highly protein bound may increase free concentrations of the other drug.

NURSING CONSIDERATIONS

Assessment: Assess for history or family history of bipolar disorder, mania, or hypomania. Assess for hypersensitivity to drug or any of its components, syndrome of inappropriate antidiuretic hormone secretion, volume depletion, susceptibility to angle-closure glaucoma, hepatic dysfunction, pregnancy/nursing status, and for possible drug interactions.

Monitoring: Monitor for clinical worsening, suicidality, unusual changes in behavior, serotonin syndrome, abnormal bleeding, activation of mania/hypomania, angle-closure glaucoma, hyponatremia, hypersensitivity reactions, and other adverse reactions. If discontinuing therapy (particularly if abrupt), monitor for discontinuation symptoms.

Patient Counseling: Inform of risks, benefits, and appropriate use of therapy. Advise patients and caregivers to look for the emergence of suicidality, especially early during treatment and when the dose is adjusted up or down. Inform that if taking 15mg/day or 20mg/day, patient may experience headache, muscle tension, mood swings, sudden outburst of anger, dizziness, and runny nose if therapy is abruptly discontinued; advise not to d/c without notifying physician. Advise to inform physician if taking or planning to take any prescription or OTC drugs. Caution about risk of bleeding with NSAIDs, ASA, warfarin, or other drugs that affect hemostasis. Advise to look for signs of activation of mania/hypomania. Inform that drug may cause mild pupillary dilation, which in susceptible individuals may lead to an episode of angle-closure glaucoma. Inform of the greater risk of hyponatremia if treated with diuretics, if volume depleted, or if elderly. Inform that nausea is the most common adverse reaction, and is dose related. Instruct to notify physician if an allergic reaction occurs, if pregnant/planning to become pregnant, or if breastfeeding/planning to breastfeed.

Storage: 25°C (77°F); excursions permitted to 15-30°C (59-86°F).

BROMDAY – bromfenac RX

Class: NSAID

ADULT DOSAGE

Postoperative Inflammation/Ocular Pain

Instill 1 drop qd in affected eye(s), starting 1 day prior to cataract surgery, continued on day of surgery, and through first 14 days of postoperative period

PEDIATRIC DOSAGE

Pediatric use may not have been established

DOSE MODIFICATION

Concomitant Medications

Space dosing ≥5 min apart with other topical ophthalmic medications

ADMINISTRATION

Ocular route

HOW SUPPLIED

Sol: 0.09% [1.7mL]

WARNINGS/PRECAUTIONS

Contains sodium sulfite; may cause allergic-type reactions (eg, anaphylactic symptoms, asthmatic episodes). Sulfite sensitivity is seen more frequently in asthmatics. May slow or delay healing. Potential cross-sensitivity to acetylsalicylic acid, phenylacetic acid derivatives, and other NSAIDs. Caution when treating individuals who previously exhibited sensitivity to these drugs. May increase bleeding of ocular tissues (eg, hyphemas) in conjunction with ocular surgery. Caution in patients with known bleeding tendencies. May result in keratitis. Continued use may lead to sight-threatening epithelial breakdown, corneal thinning, corneal erosion, corneal ulceration, or corneal perforation; d/c if corneal epithelium breakdown occurs. Caution in patients with complicated ocular surgeries, corneal denervation, corneal epithelial defects, diabetes mellitus (DM), ocular surface diseases (eg, dry eye syndrome), rheumatoid arthritis (RA), or repeat ocular surgeries within a short period of time. Increased risk for occurrence and severity of corneal adverse events if used >24 hrs prior to surgery or use beyond 14 days postsurgery. Avoid use with contact lenses. Avoid use during late pregnancy because of the known effects on the fetal cardiovascular system (closure of ductus arteriosus).

ADVERSE REACTIONS

Abnormal sensation in eye, conjunctival hyperemia, eye irritation (burning/stinging), eye pain, eye pruritus, eye redness, headache, iritis.

DRUG INTERACTIONS

Concomitant use of topical NSAIDs and topical steroids may increase potential for healing problems. Caution with other medications that may prolong bleeding time.

NURSING CONSIDERATIONS

Assessment: Assess for hypersensitivity (eg, sodium sulfite) or cross-sensitivity (eg, aspirin) reactions, history of complicated or repeated ocular surgeries, corneal denervation, corneal epithelial defects, DM, ocular surface diseases (eg, dry eye syndrome), RA, bleeding tendencies, pregnancy/nursing status, and possible drug interactions.

Monitoring: Monitor for anaphylactic symptoms, severe asthma attacks, wound-healing problems, keratitis, corneal epithelial breakdown, corneal thinning/erosion/ulceration/perforation, increased bleeding time, and bleeding of ocular tissues (hyphemas) in conjunction with ocular surgery.

Patient Counseling: Advise not to wear contact lenses during therapy. Advise of the possibility of slow or delayed healing that may occur while using this product. Advise not to touch the dropper tip to any surface, as this may contaminate the contents. If >1 topical ophthalmic medication is used, instruct to administer 5 min apart.

Storage: 15-25°C (59-77°F).

BROVANA – arformoterol tartrate

RX

Class: $Beta_2$-agonist

Long-acting β_2-adrenergic agonists (LABAs) increase the risk of asthma-related death. Contraindicated in asthma without use of a long-term asthma control medication.

ADULT DOSAGE

Chronic Obstructive Pulmonary Disease

Bronchoconstriction:
Usual: 15mcg bid (am and pm) by nebulization
Max: 30mcg/day (15mcg bid)

PEDIATRIC DOSAGE

Pediatric use may not have been established

ADMINISTRATION

Oral inhalation route

Administer via a standard jet nebulizer connected to an air compressor
Refer to PI for further administration instructions

HOW SUPPLIED

Sol, Inhalation: 15mcg base/2mL [30[s], 60[s]]

CONTRAINDICATIONS

Asthma without use of a long-term asthma control medication.

WARNINGS/PRECAUTIONS

Not indicated to treat asthma, acute deteriorations of COPD, or acute episodes of bronchospasm (eg, as rescue therapy). D/C regular use of inhaled short-acting β_2-agonist (SABA) when beginning treatment; use only for symptomatic relief of acute respiratory symptoms. Do not use more often or at higher doses than recommended; fatalities reported with excessive use. May produce paradoxical bronchospasm; d/c therapy immediately and institute alternative therapy. Cardiovascular (CV) effects may occur; d/c if such effects occur. Caution with CV disorders, convulsive disorders, thyrotoxicosis, diabetes mellitus (DM), ketoacidosis, hepatic impairment, and in patients unusually responsive to sympathomimetic amines. May produce significant hypokalemia or transient hyperglycemia. Immediate hypersensitivity reactions may occur.

ADVERSE REACTIONS

Pain, chest/back pain, diarrhea, sinusitis, leg cramps, dyspnea, rash, flu syndrome, peripheral edema.

DRUG INTERACTIONS

Do not use with other medications containing LABAs. Adrenergic drugs may potentiate sympathetic effects; use with caution. Methylxanthine (aminophylline, theophylline), steroids, or diuretics may potentiate hypokalemic effect. Increased HR and systolic BP with theophylline. ECG changes and/or hypokalemia that may result from non-K^+-sparing diuretics (eg, loop or thiazide diuretics) may be acutely worsened; use with caution. Extreme caution with MAOIs, TCAs, or drugs known to prolong the QTc interval; effect on CV system may be potentiated by these agents. Drugs known to prolong the QTc interval have an increased risk of ventricular arrhythmias. β-blockers and arformoterol may inhibit the effect of each other when administered concurrently. β-blockers may block therapeutic effects and produce severe bronchospasm in COPD patients; if such therapy is needed, consider cardioselective β-blockers and use with caution.

NURSING CONSIDERATIONS

Assessment: Assess for asthma and use of control medication, acutely deteriorating COPD, CV disorders, convulsive disorders, thyrotoxicosis, DM, ketoacidosis, hepatic impairment, history of hypersensitivity to drug, pregnancy/nursing status, and possible drug interactions. Assess use in patients unusually responsive to sympathomimetic amines.

Monitoring: Monitor for deteriorating disease, paradoxical bronchospasm, CV effects, hypokalemia, hyperglycemia, immediate hypersensitivity reactions, and other adverse reactions.

Patient Counseling: Inform that drug is not for treatment of asthma. Advise not to use to relieve acute respiratory symptoms; inform that acute symptoms should be treated with an inhaled SABA. Instruct to seek medical attention if symptoms worsen despite recommended doses, if treatment becomes less effective, or if experiencing a need for more inhalations of a SABA than usual. Advise not to stop therapy unless directed by physician, not to inhale >1 dose at any 1 time, and not to exceed recommended daily dosage. Instruct to d/c the regular use of inhaled SABAs (eg, levalbuterol) when beginning treatment. Counsel not to use with other inhaled medications containing a LABA, and not to stop or change the dose of other concomitant COPD therapy without medical advice, even if symptoms improve after initiating treatment. Inform of the common adverse reactions with therapy. Instruct on how to properly use the medication. Advise to contact physician if pregnancy occurs, or if nursing.

Storage: 2-8°C (36-46°F). Store in the protective foil pouch. Protect from light and excessive heat. After opening the pouch, unused vials should be returned to, and stored in, the pouch. Use opened vial immediately; discard if sol is not colorless. Unopened foil pouches can also be stored at 20-25°C (68-77°F) for up to 6 weeks.

BUMETANIDE – bumetanide RX

Class: Loop diuretic

May lead to profound diuresis with water and electrolyte depletion if given in excessive amounts; careful medical supervision required and dose and dosage schedule must be adjusted to individual patient's needs.

ADULT DOSAGE

Edema

Associated w/ CHF, Hepatic/Renal Disease (Nephrotic Syndrome):

Tab:

Usual: 0.5-2mg/day as single dose; may give a 2nd or 3rd dose at 4- to 5-hr intervals if response is not adequate

Maint: Give on alternate days or for 3-4 days w/ rest periods of 1-2 days in between

Max: 10mg/day

Inj:

Initial: 0.5-1mg IV/IM (give IV over 1-2 min); may give a 2nd or 3rd dose at 2- to 3-hr intervals if response is insufficient

Max: 10mg/day

Initiate oral treatment as soon as possible

PEDIATRIC DOSAGE

Pediatric use may not have been established

DOSE MODIFICATION

Hepatic Failure

Tab:

Give minimum dose, and if necessary, increase dose very carefully

Elderly

Tab/Inj:

Start at lower end of dosing range

ADMINISTRATION

Oral/IV/IM route

Compatibility

5% dextrose sol; 0.9% NaCl; Lactated Ringer's inj

HOW SUPPLIED

Inj: 0.25mg/mL [4mL, 10mL]; Tab: 0.5mg*, 1mg*, 2mg* *scored

CONTRAINDICATIONS

Anuria, hepatic coma, severe electrolyte depletion.

WARNINGS/PRECAUTIONS

Excessive doses may cause dehydration, blood volume reduction, and circulatory collapse with possible vascular thrombosis and embolism, particularly in elderly. Hypokalemia may occur; caution with hepatic cirrhosis and ascites, states of aldosterone excess with normal renal function, K^+-losing nephropathy, certain diarrheal states, other states where hypokalemia represents added risks, or in patients receiving digitalis and diuretics for CHF. Sudden alterations of electrolyte balance may precipitate hepatic encephalopathy and coma in patients with hepatic cirrhosis and ascites; initiate therapy in hospital. Ototoxicity, thrombocytopenia, hypocalcemia, hypomagnesemia, and hyperuricemia may occur. May affect glucose metabolism; monitor glucose levels in patients with diabetes or suspected latent diabetes. Monitor for blood dyscrasias, hepatic damage, or idiosyncratic reactions. Caution with sulfonamide allergy. Reversible elevations of BUN and creatinine may occur; d/c if marked increase in BUN or creatinine occurs, or if oliguria develops in patients with progressive renal disease. Tab may be substituted at approximately a 1:40 ratio of bumetanide tabs to furosemide in patients allergic to furosemide.

ADVERSE REACTIONS

Muscle cramps, dizziness, hypotension, headache, nausea, encephalopathy, hyperuricemia, hypochloremia, hypokalemia, hyponatremia, hyperglycemia, azotemia, increased SrCr.

DRUG INTERACTIONS

Avoid with drugs known to have a nephrotoxic potential. Not recommended for use with indomethacin. High risk of lithium toxicity; avoid coadministration. Pretreatment with probenecid reduces effects; do not administer concurrently. May potentiate the effect of various antihypertensives; reduction in the dose of these drugs may be necessary. (Inj) Avoid with aminoglycosides (except in life-threatening situations).

NURSING CONSIDERATIONS

Assessment: Assess for progressive renal disease, severe electrolyte depletion, anuria, diabetes or suspected latent diabetes, sulfonamide allergy, liver disease (hepatic coma), any other conditions where treatment is contraindicated or cautioned, pregnancy/nursing status, and possible drug interactions.

Monitoring: Monitor for ototoxicity, blood dyscrasias, liver damage or idiosyncratic reactions, hypersensitivity reactions, hyperuricemia, oliguria, thrombocytopenia, and other adverse reactions. Periodically monitor serum K^+, serum electrolytes, blood glucose, and renal function.

Patient Counseling: Inform of the risks/benefits of therapy. Advise to seek medical attention if adverse reactions occur.

Storage: 20-25°C (68-77°F). Protect from light. (Inj) Excursions permitted to 15-30°C (59-86°F).

BUPRENEX – buprenorphine hydrochloride

CIII

Class: Partial opioid agonist

ADULT DOSAGE

Moderate to Severe Pain

0.3mg IM/IV q6h PRN; repeat once (up to 0.3mg) if needed, 30-60 min after initial dose

May use single doses up to 0.6mg IM if not at high risk

PEDIATRIC DOSAGE

Moderate to Severe Pain

2-12 Years:

2-6mcg/kg IM/IV q4-6h

≥13 Years:

0.3mg IM/IV q6h PRN; repeat once (up to 0.3mg) if needed, 30-60 min after initial dose

May use single doses up to 0.6mg IM if not at high risk

DOSE MODIFICATION

Concomitant Medications

≥13 Years:

Concomitant CNS Depressants:

Reduce dose by approximately 50%

Other Important Modifications

≥13 Years:

High-Risk Patients (eg, Elderly, Debilitated, Presence of Respiratory Disease):

Reduce dose by approximately 50%

ADMINISTRATION

Deep IM or slow (over at least 2 min) IV route

HOW SUPPLIED

Inj: 0.3mg/mL

WARNINGS/PRECAUTIONS

Clinically significant respiratory depression may occur; caution with compromised respiratory function. Naloxone may not be effective in reversing respiratory depression. May increase CSF pressure; caution with head injury, intracranial lesions, and other circumstances where cerebrospinal pressure may be increased. Can produce miosis and changes in level of consciousness. May impair mental or physical abilities; caution in ambulatory patients. May result in withdrawal effects in physically dependent patients. Caution in elderly, debilitated, and pediatric patients. Caution with hepatic/renal/pulmonary impairment, myxedema or hypothyroidism, adrenal cortical insufficiency, CNS depression or coma, toxic psychoses, prostatic hypertrophy or urethral stricture, acute alcoholism, delirium tremens, kyphoscoliosis, or biliary tract dysfunction.

ADVERSE REACTIONS

Sedation, N/V, dizziness, sweating, hypotension, headache, miosis, hypoventilation.

DRUG INTERACTIONS

Caution with MAOIs and CNS and respiratory depressants. Increased CNS depression with other narcotic analgesics, general anesthetics, antihistamines, benzodiazepines, phenothiazines, other tranquilizers, sedative-hypnotics, or other CNS depressants (eg, alcohol); reduce dose of one or both agents. Respiratory and cardiovascular collapse reported with diazepam. Suspected interaction with phenprocoumon resulting in purpura. Decreased clearance with CYP3A4 inhibitors (eg, macrolides, azole antifungals, protease inhibitors). Increased clearance with CYP3A4 inducers (eg, rifampin, carbamazepine, phenytoin).

NURSING CONSIDERATIONS

Assessment: Assess for compromised respiratory function (eg, chronic obstructive pulmonary disease, hypoxia), head injury, intracranial lesions, hepatic/renal function, any condition where treatment is cautioned, pregnancy/nursing status, and possible drug interactions.

Monitoring: Monitor for signs/symptoms of respiratory depression, CNS depression, elevation of CSF pressure, increased intracholedochal pressure, drug abuse/dependence, and withdrawal effects.

Patient Counseling: Counsel that effects (eg, drowsiness) may be potentiated by other centrally acting agents (eg, alcohol); advise not to drive/operate machinery under these circumstances. Advise that medication may lead to dependence. Counsel to not exceed prescribed dosage. Advise to notify physician of all medications currently being taken.

Storage: 20-25°C (68-77°F); excursions permitted between 15-30°C (59-86°F). Protect from prolonged exposure to light.

BUTRANS – buprenorphine CIII

Class: Partial opioid agonist

Exposes users to risks of addiction, abuse, and misuse, leading to overdose and death; assess each patient's risk prior to prescribing, and monitor regularly for development of these behaviors/conditions. Serious, life-threatening, or fatal respiratory depression may occur; monitor during initiation or following a dose increase. Chewing, swallowing, snorting, or injecting buprenorphine extracted from the transdermal system will result in uncontrolled delivery and pose risk of overdose and death. Accidental exposure, especially in children, can result in a fatal overdose. Prolonged use during pregnancy can result in neonatal opioid withdrawal syndrome; advise pregnant women of the risk and ensure availability of appropriate treatment.

ADULT DOSAGE

Severe Pain (Daily, Around-the-Clock Management)

Long-Term Opioid Treatment for Which Alternative Treatment Options are Inadequate:

First Opioid Analgesic:

Initial: 5mcg/hr

Titrate: Individualize dose

Minimum Titration Interval: 72 hrs; may adjust dose every 3 days

Max: 20mcg/hr

Dose adjustments may be made in 5mcg/hr, 7.5mcg/hr, or 10mcg/hr increments by using no more than 2 patches of the 5mcg/hr, 7.5mcg/hr, or 10mcg/hr systems

Conversions

From Other Opioids to Buprenorphine Transdermal System:

Discontinue all other around-the-clock opioid drugs when therapy is initiated

Prior Total Daily Dose of Opioid <30mg of Oral Morphine Equivalents/Day:

Initiate treatment w/ 5mcg/hr at the next dosing interval

Prior Total Daily Dose of Opioid Between 30mg to 80mg of Oral Morphine Equivalents/Day:

Taper the patient's current around-the-clock opioids for up to 7 days to no more than 30mg of morphine or equivalent/day before beginning treatment

Then initiate treatment w/ 10mcg/hr at the next dosing interval

Patients may use short-acting analgesics prn until efficacy is attained

PEDIATRIC DOSAGE

Pediatric use may not have been established

Prior Total Daily Dose of Opioid >80mg of Oral Morphine Equivalents/Day:
20mcg/hour may not provide adequate analgesia for patients requiring >80mg/day oral morphine equivalents
Consider the use of an alternate analgesic

DOSE MODIFICATION

Hepatic Impairment

Severe: Consider use of an alternate analgesic that may permit more flexibility w/ dosing

Discontinuation

Use gradual downward titration every 7 days
Consider introduction of an appropriate immediate-release opioid medication

ADMINISTRATION

Transdermal route

Each patch is intended to be worn for 7 days
Do not cut patch
Apply immediately after removal from individually sealed pouch
Apply to intact skin on upper outer arm, upper chest, upper back, or side of chest; rotate application site w/ a minimum of 21 days before reapplying to the same skin site
For use of 2 patches, remove current patch and apply the 2 new patches at the same time, adjacent to one another at a different application site
Refer to PI for further administration and disposal instructions

HOW SUPPLIED

Patch: 5mcg/hr, 7.5mcg/hr, 10mcg/hr, 15mcg/hr, 20mcg/hr

CONTRAINDICATIONS

Significant respiratory depression, acute or severe bronchial asthma in an unmonitored setting or in the absence of resuscitative equipment, known or suspected paralytic ileus.

WARNINGS/PRECAUTIONS

Reserve use in patients for whom alternative treatment options are ineffective, not tolerated, or would be otherwise inadequate to provide sufficient management of pain. Should only be prescribed by healthcare professionals who are knowledgeable in the use of potent opioids for management of chronic pain. Doses of 7.5, 10, 15, and 20mcg/hr are for opioid-experienced patients only. Life-threatening respiratory depression is more likely to occur in elderly, cachectic, or debilitated patients. Consider alternative nonopioid analgesics in patients with significant chronic obstructive pulmonary disease or cor pulmonale, and in patients who have a substantially decreased respiratory reserve, hypoxia, hypercapnia, or preexisting respiratory depression. QTc interval prolongation observed at dose of 40mcg/hr; caution with hypokalemia or clinically unstable cardiac disease. Avoid use with history/immediate family history of long QT syndrome. May cause severe hypotension, orthostatic hypotension, and syncope; increased risk in patients whose ability to maintain BP has already been compromised by a reduced blood volume or concurrent administration of certain CNS depressants. Monitor patients who may be susceptible to intracranial effects of carbon dioxide retention for signs of sedation and respiratory depression when initiating therapy. Therapy may obscure clinical course in patients with head injury. Avoid with impaired consciousness or coma. Obtain baseline liver enzyme levels and monitor periodically during treatment in patients at increased risk of hepatotoxicity (eg, history of excessive alcohol intake, IV drug abuse). Application-site skin reactions with signs of marked inflammation reported; d/c if severe application-site reactions develop. Cases of acute and chronic hypersensitivity, bronchospasm, angioneurotic edema, and anaphylactic shock reported. Potential for temperature-dependent increases in drug release, resulting in possible overdose and death; avoid exposure of application site and surrounding area to direct external heat sources. If fever or increased core body temperature due to strenuous exertion develops, monitor for side effects and adjust dose if signs of respiratory/CNS depression occur. Avoid with GI obstruction. May cause spasm of sphincter of Oddi and increase in serum amylase; monitor patients with biliary tract disease. May aggravate convulsions and induce/aggravate seizures. May impair mental/physical abilities. Not approved for management of addictive disorders. Not for use during and immediately prior to labor. Caution in elderly.

ADVERSE REACTIONS

Respiratory depression, N/V, dizziness, headache, application-site pruritus/irritation/erythema/rash, constipation, somnolence, dry mouth, fatigue, hyperhidrosis, peripheral edema.

DRUG INTERACTIONS

Respiratory depression, hypotension, profound sedation, or coma may occur with alcohol and other CNS depressants (eg, sedatives, anxiolytics, neuroleptics); if coadministration is required, consider dose reduction of one or both agents. Monitor use in elderly, cachectic, and debilitated patients when coadministered with other drugs that depress respiration. Monitor closely with benzodiazepines. CYP3A4 inhibitors may increase levels and prolong opioid effects; these effects could be more pronounced with concomitant use of CYP2D6 and 3A4 inhibitors; if coadministration is necessary, monitor for respiratory depression and sedation at frequent intervals and consider dose adjustments. CYP3A4 inducers may decrease levels and cause lack of efficacy or development of abstinence syndrome; if coadministration or discontinuation of a CYP3A4 inducer is necessary, monitor for signs of opioid withdrawal and consider dose adjustments. May enhance neuromuscular blocking action of skeletal muscle relaxants and increase respiratory depression. Avoid with Class IA antiarrhythmics (eg, quinidine, procainamide, disopyramide) or Class III antiarrhythmics (eg, sotalol, amiodarone, dofetilide). Anticholinergics or other drugs with anticholinergic activity may increase risk of urinary retention and/or severe constipation and lead to paralytic ileus.

NURSING CONSIDERATIONS

Assessment: Assess for abuse/addiction risk, pain intensity, prior opioid therapy, opioid tolerance, respiratory depression, drug hypersensitivity, pregnancy/nursing status, possible drug interactions, or any other conditions where treatment is contraindicated or cautioned. Obtain baseline liver enzyme levels in patients at increased risk of hepatotoxicity.

Monitoring: Monitor for respiratory depression (especially within first 24-72 hrs of initiation), hypotension, application-site skin reactions, seizures/convulsions, and other adverse reactions. Monitor BP and serum amylase levels. Regularly monitor for signs of misuse, abuse, and addiction. Periodically reassess the continued need for therapy. Monitor liver enzyme levels periodically in patients at increased risk of hepatotoxicity.

Patient Counseling: Inform that use of drug can result in addiction, abuse, and misuse; instruct not to share with others and to take steps to protect from theft or misuse. Inform patients about risk of respiratory depression. Advise to store securely and dispose unused patch by folding the patch in 1/2 and flushing down the toilet. Inform women of reproductive potential that prolonged use during pregnancy may result in neonatal opioid withdrawal syndrome and instruct to inform physician if pregnant or planning to become pregnant. Inform that potentially serious additive effects may occur when used with alcohol or CNS depressants, and not to use such drugs unless supervised by healthcare provider. Instruct about proper application, removal, and disposal instructions. Inform that drug may cause orthostatic hypotension, syncope, impair the ability to perform potentially hazardous activities; advise to not perform such tasks until patients know how they will react to medication. Advise of potential for severe constipation, including management instructions. Advise how to recognize anaphylaxis and when to seek medical attention.

Storage: 25°C (77°F); excursions permitted between 15-30°C (59-86°F).

BYDUREON – exenatide

RX

Class: Glucagon-like peptide-1 receptor agonist

Causes an increased incidence in thyroid C-cell tumors at clinically relevant exposures in animal studies. It is unknown whether drug causes thyroid C-cell tumors (eg, medullary thyroid carcinoma [MTC]) in humans. Contraindicated in patients w/ a personal/family history of MTC and w/ multiple endocrine neoplasia syndrome type 2 (MEN 2). Counsel patients on the potential risk for MTC w/ exenatide use and inform them of symptoms of thyroid tumors (eg, mass in the neck, dysphagia, dyspnea, persistent hoarseness). Routine monitoring of serum calcitonin or using thyroid ultrasound is of uncertain value for detection of MTC in patients treated w/ exenatide.

ADULT DOSAGE

Type 2 Diabetes Mellitus

Usual: 2mg/dose SQ once every 7 days, at any time of day

Changing Weekly Dosing Schedule:
May change the day of weekly administration if necessary as long as the last dose was given ≥3 days before

Changing from Byetta to Bydureon:
D/C Byetta
Prior treatment w/ Byetta is not required when initiating therapy
Patients changing from Byetta may experience transient (approx 2 weeks) elevations in blood glucose concentrations

Missed Dose

Administer as soon as noticed, provided the next regularly scheduled dose is due at least 3 days later

PEDIATRIC DOSAGE

Pediatric use may not have been established

Thereafter, may resume usual dosing schedule of once every 7 days (weekly)

If a dose is missed and the next regularly scheduled dose is due 1 or 2 days later, do not administer the missed dose and instead resume therapy w/ the next regularly scheduled dose

DOSE MODIFICATION

Renal Impairment

Moderate (CrCl 30-50mL/min): Use w/ caution
Severe (CrCl <30mL/min) or ESRD: Not recommended for use
Patients w/Renal Transplantation: Use w/ caution

Elderly

Caution when initiating treatment

ADMINISTRATION

SQ route

Administer w/ or w/o meals
Inject in the abdomen, thigh, or upper arm region; use a different inj site each week when injecting in the same region
Do not administer IV or IM
Intended for patient self-administration
Administer immediately after powder is suspended in diluent
Refer to PI for further administration instructions

HOW SUPPLIED

Inj, Extended-Release: 2mg [vial, pen]

CONTRAINDICATIONS

MEN 2, personal/family history of MTC.

WARNINGS/PRECAUTIONS

Not recommended as 1st-line therapy for patients who have inadequate glycemic control on diet and exercise. Not a substitute for insulin; do not use in type 1 DM or for treatment of diabetic ketoacidosis. Not studied and cannot be recommended w/ insulin. Acute pancreatitis, including fatal and nonfatal hemorrhagic or necrotizing pancreatitis, reported; d/c promptly if suspected, and do not restart therapy if confirmed. Consider other antidiabetic therapies in patients w/ history of pancreatitis. Patients w/ elevated calcitonin levels and those w/ thyroid nodules noted on physical examination or neck imaging should be further evaluated. Altered renal function, including increased SrCr, renal impairment, worsened chronic renal failure, and acute renal failure reported. Avoid w/ severe GI disease. May develop antibodies; consider alternative antidiabetic therapy if there is worsening glycemic control or failure to achieve targeted glycemic control. Serious hypersensitivity reactions reported; d/c if a hypersensitivity reaction occurs. Serious inj-site reactions (eg, abscess, cellulitis, necrosis), w/ or w/o subcutaneous nodules reported; isolated cases required surgical intervention.

ADVERSE REACTIONS

Constipation, diarrhea, dyspepsia, headache, N/V, inj-site nodule, fatigue, decreased appetite, inj-site pruritus, viral gastroenteritis, GERD, inj-site erythema, inj-site hematoma.

DRUG INTERACTIONS

Increased risk of hypoglycemia w/ a sulfonylurea or other glucose-independent insulin secretagogues (eg, meglitinides); may require a lower dose of the sulfonylurea. May reduce the rate of absorption of orally administered drugs; caution w/ oral medications. May increase INR w/ warfarin, sometimes associated w/ bleeding; monitor INR more frequently after initiation of exenatide. Should not be used w/ other drugs containing the same active ingredient (eg, Byetta).

NURSING CONSIDERATIONS

Assessment: Assess for previous hypersensitivity reactions, MEN 2, personal/family history of MTC, history of pancreatitis, type of DM, diabetic ketoacidosis, renal impairment, severe GI disease, pregnancy/nursing status, and possible drug interactions. Assess glucose and HbA1c levels.

Monitoring: Monitor for signs/symptoms of thyroid tumor, pancreatitis, elevated serum calcitonin levels, hypoglycemia, GI events, immunogenicity, hypersensitivity reactions, inj-site reactions, and other adverse reactions. Monitor renal function, blood glucose levels, and HbA1c levels. Monitor INR more frequently after initiation of therapy in patients receiving warfarin.

Patient Counseling: Counsel on potential risks/benefits of therapy and alternative modes of therapy. Inform of importance of adhering to dietary instructions, regular physical activity, periodic blood glucose monitoring and HbA1c testing, recognition/management of hypo/hyperglycemia, and assessment for diabetes complications. Advise to report symptoms of thyroid tumors (eg, lump in the neck, hoarseness, dysphagia, dyspnea) to physician. Inform of potential risk for pancreatitis, worsening of renal function, and serious hypersensitivity reactions. Instruct to d/c therapy promptly and contact physician if persistent severe abdominal pain and/or symptoms of a hypersensitivity reaction occur. Inform that serious inj-site reactions w/ or w/o subcutaneous nodules may occur; advise to seek medical advice if symptomatic nodules occur, or for any signs/symptoms of abscess, cellulitis, or necrosis. Instruct to never share a prefilled syringe/pen w/ another person, even if the needle is changed. Advise that if a dose is missed, administer as soon as noticed, provided that the next regularly scheduled dose is due at least 3 days later. Instruct to then resume the usual dosing schedule thereafter. Inform that if a dose is missed and the next regularly scheduled dose is due in 1 or 2 days, to not administer the missed dose and instead resume w/ the next regularly scheduled dose. Advise to inform physician if pregnant or intending to become pregnant. Inform about the importance of proper storage, inj technique, and dosing.

Storage: 2-8°C (36-46°F). May store at room temperature not exceeding 25°C (77°F) for ≤4 weeks, if needed. Do not freeze; do not use if product has been frozen. Protect from light.

Byetta – exenatide

RX

Class: Glucagon-like peptide-1 receptor agonist

ADULT DOSAGE

Type 2 Diabetes Mellitus

Initial: 5mcg SQ bid, at any time w/in 60 min before am and pm meals (or before the 2 main meals of the day, approx 6 hrs or more apart)
Titrate: May increase to 10mcg bid after 1 month based on response

PEDIATRIC DOSAGE

Pediatric use may not have been established

DOSE MODIFICATION

Renal Impairment

Moderate (CrCl 30-50mL/min): Caution when initiating or escalating doses from 5mcg to 10mcg
Severe (CrCl <30mL/min) or ESRD: Not recommended
Renal Transplantation: Use w/ caution

ADMINISTRATION

SQ route

Inject into thigh, abdomen, or upper arm
Do not mix w/ insulin
Do not transfer from the pen to a syringe or a vial

HOW SUPPLIED

Inj: 5mcg/dose, 10mcg/dose [60 doses]

WARNINGS/PRECAUTIONS

Not a substitute for insulin; do not use in type 1 DM or for the treatment of diabetic ketoacidosis. Not studied and cannot be recommended w/ prandial insulin. Evaluate dose of insulin if used in combination; consider dose reduction in patients at risk of hypoglycemia. Do not share pens between patients, even if needle is changed; risk of transmission of blood-borne pathogens. Acute pancreatitis, including fatal and nonfatal hemorrhagic or necrotizing pancreatitis, reported; observe for signs/symptoms of pancreatitis after initiation of therapy and dose increases, d/c promptly if suspected, and do not restart therapy if confirmed. Consider other antidiabetic therapies in patients w/ history of pancreatitis. Altered renal function, including increased SrCr, renal impairment, worsened chronic renal failure, and acute renal failure, reported. Not recommended w/ severe GI disease. May develop antibodies; consider alternative antidiabetic therapy if there is worsening glycemic control or failure to achieve targeted glycemic control. Serious hypersensitivity reactions (eg, anaphylaxis, angioedema) reported; d/c if a hypersensitivity reaction occurs.

ADVERSE REACTIONS

Hypoglycemia, N/V, immunogenicity, dyspepsia, diarrhea, feeling jittery, dizziness, headache, constipation, asthenia, GERD, hyperhidrosis, abdominal distension, decreased appetite.

DRUG INTERACTIONS

Increased risk of hypoglycemia w/ a sulfonylurea or other glucose-independent insulin secretagogues (eg, meglitinides); may require a lower dose of the sulfonylurea. May reduce the extent and rate of absorption of orally administered drugs; caution w/ oral medications w/ narrow therapeutic index or that require rapid GI absorption. Oral medications that are dependent on threshold concentrations for efficacy (eg, contraceptives, antibiotics) should be taken at least 1 hr before inj. May increase INR w/ warfarin, sometimes associated w/ bleeding; monitor PT more frequently after initiation or alteration of therapy.

NURSING CONSIDERATIONS

Assessment: Assess for history of hypersensitivity to drug or any product components, type of DM, diabetic ketoacidosis, history of pancreatitis, renal impairment, severe GI disease, pregnancy/nursing status, and possible drug interactions.

Monitoring: Monitor for signs/symptoms of hypoglycemia, pancreatitis, GI events, immunogenicity, hypersensitivity reactions, and other adverse reactions. Monitor renal function, blood glucose levels, and HbA1c levels. Monitor PT more frequently after initiation or alteration of therapy in patients receiving warfarin.

Patient Counseling: Counsel on the potential risks/benefits of therapy and alternative modes of therapy. Inform of importance of proper storage of drug, inj technique, timing of dosage and concomitant oral drugs, adherence to meal planning, regular physical activity, periodic blood glucose monitoring and HbA1c testing, recognition/management of hypo/hyperglycemia, and assessment for diabetes complications. Advise to never share inj pen w/ another person, even if needle is changed. Inform that pen needles are purchased separately and advise on proper needle selection and disposal. Inform that if a dose is missed, treatment regimen should be resumed as prescribed w/ the next scheduled dose. Instruct to inform physician if pregnant or intending to become pregnant. Advise that treatment may result in reduction in appetite, food intake, and/or body weight, and that there is no need to modify the dosing regimen due to such effects. Inform that nausea, particularly upon initiation of therapy, may occur. Instruct to contact a physician if signs/symptoms of acute pancreatitis (eg, severe abdominal pain), renal dysfunction, or hypersensitivity reactions develop.

Storage: Prior to 1st Use: 2-8°C (36-46°F). After 1st Use: <25°C (77°F). Do not freeze. Do not use if it has been frozen. Protect from light. Discard pen 30 days after 1st use.

BYSTOLIC – nebivolol

RX

Class: Selective $beta_1$-blocker

ADULT DOSAGE

Hypertension

Initial: 5mg qd
Titrate: May increase at 2-week intervals
Max: 40mg

PEDIATRIC DOSAGE

Pediatric use may not have been established

DOSE MODIFICATION

Renal Impairment

Severe (CrCl <30mL/min):
Initial: 2.5mg qd; titrate up slowly if needed

Hepatic Impairment

Moderate:
Initial: 2.5mg qd; titrate up slowly if needed

ADMINISTRATION

Oral route

Take with or without food

HOW SUPPLIED

Tab: 2.5mg, 5mg, 10mg, 20mg

CONTRAINDICATIONS

Severe bradycardia, heart block >1st degree, cardiogenic shock, decompensated cardiac failure, sick sinus syndrome (unless permanent pacemaker in place), severe hepatic impairment (Child-Pugh >B).

WARNINGS/PRECAUTIONS

Severe exacerbation of angina, myocardial infarction, and ventricular arrhythmias reported in patients with coronary artery disease (CAD) following abrupt discontinuation; taper over 1-2 weeks when possible. Restart therapy promptly, at least temporarily, if angina worsens or acute coronary insufficiency develops. Caution patients without overt CAD against interruption or abrupt discontinuation of therapy. Avoid with bronchospastic disease. Treatment should generally be continued throughout perioperative period. If therapy is to be continued perioperatively, monitor closely when anesthetic agents that depress myocardial function (eg, ether, cyclopropane, trichloroethylene) are used. If therapy is withdrawn prior to major surgery, impaired ability of the heart to respond to reflex adrenergic stimuli may augment the risks of general anesthesia and surgical procedures; difficulty in restarting and maintaining heartbeat reported. May mask manifestations of hypoglycemia/hyperthyroidism, particularly tachycardia; abrupt withdrawal may be followed by exacerbation of the symptoms of hyperthyroidism or may precipitate a thyroid storm. May precipitate/aggravate symptoms of arterial insufficiency with peripheral vascular disease (PVD). Patients with history of severe anaphylactic reactions to variety of allergens may be more reactive to repeated accidental/diagnostic/therapeutic challenge; may be unresponsive to usual doses of epinephrine. Initiate an α-blocker prior to use of any β-blocker in patients with known/suspected pheochromocytoma.

ADVERSE REACTIONS

Headache, fatigue, dizziness, diarrhea, nausea.

DRUG INTERACTIONS

Avoid with other β-blockers. D/C for several days before the gradual tapering of clonidine. Caution with CYP2D6 inhibitors (eg, quinidine, propafenone, paroxetine, fluoxetine); may need to reduce dose of nebivolol. May produce excessive reduction of sympathetic activity with catecholamine-depleting drugs (eg, reserpine, guanethidine). May increase risk of bradycardia with digitalis glycosides. May exacerbate effects of myocardial depressants/inhibitors of atrioventricular conduction (eg, antiarrhythmics, certain Ca^{2+} antagonists). May potentiate hypoglycemic effect of insulin and oral hypoglycemics. Significant negative inotropic and chronotropic effects may occur with verapamil and diltiazem type; monitor ECG and BP.

NURSING CONSIDERATIONS

Assessment: Assess for CAD, bronchospastic disease, diabetes mellitus, hypoglycemia, hyperthyroidism, PVD, pheochromocytoma, hepatic/renal impairment, pregnancy/nursing status, any other conditions where treatment is contraindicated or cautioned, and possible drug interactions.

Monitoring: Monitor for precipitation/aggravation of arterial insufficiency, hypersensitivity, and other adverse reactions. Monitor ECG, BP, and serum glucose levels.

Patient Counseling: Inform of the risks and benefits of therapy. Advise to take drug regularly and continuously, ud. Instruct to take only the next scheduled dose, without doubling it, if a dose is missed, and not to interrupt or d/c without consulting physician. Advise to consult physician if any difficulty in breathing occurs, or signs/symptoms of worsening congestive heart failure develop. Caution about operating automobiles, using machinery, or engaging in tasks requiring alertness. Caution patients subject to spontaneous hypoglycemia, or diabetic patients receiving insulin or oral hypoglycemics, that the drug may mask some of the manifestations of hypoglycemia, particularly tachycardia.

Storage: 20-25°C (68-77°F).

CADUET – amlodipine besylate/atorvastatin calcium RX

Class: Calcium channel blocker/HMG-CoA reductase inhibitor

ADULT DOSAGE

Hypertension

Individualize dose based on effectiveness and tolerance for each individual component; select doses of amlodipine and atorvastatin independently

Amlodipine:
Initial: 5mg qd
Max: 10mg qd

Adjust dose according to BP goals usually waiting 7-14 days between titration steps; titration may proceed more rapidly if clinically warranted

Angina

Individualize dose based on effectiveness and tolerance for each individual component; select doses of amlodipine and atorvastatin independently

Amlodipine:
Usual: 5-10mg qd

Coronary Artery Disease

Individualize dose based on effectiveness and tolerance for each individual component; select doses of amlodipine and atorvastatin independently

PEDIATRIC DOSAGE

Hypertension

Individualize dose based on effectiveness and tolerance for each individual component; select doses of amlodipine and atorvastatin independently

Amlodipine:
6-17 Years:
Usual: 2.5-5mg qd
Max: 5mg qd

Individualize dose based on effectiveness and tolerance for each individual component; select doses of amlodipine and atorvastatin independently

Atorvastatin:
Heterozygous Familial Hypercholesterolemia:
10-17 Years:
Initial: 10mg/day
Max: 20mg/day
Dose adjustments should be made at intervals of ≥4 weeks

Amlodipine:
Usual: 5-10mg qd

Hyperlipidemia/Mixed Dyslipidemia

Individualize dose based on effectiveness and tolerance for each individual component; select doses of amlodipine and atorvastatin independently

Atorvastatin:
Hyperlipidemia (Heterozygous Familial and Nonfamilial) and Mixed Dyslipidemia (Fredrickson Types 2a and 2b):
Initial: 10 or 20mg qd; patients who require ≥45% reduction in LDL-C may be started at 40mg qd
Titrate: Analyze lipid levels w/in 2-4 weeks and adjust dose accordingly
Usual Range: 10-80mg qd
Homozygous Familial Hypercholesterolemia:
Usual Range: 10-80mg qd
Atorvastatin should be used as an adjunct to other lipid-lowering treatments (eg, LDL apheresis)

DOSE MODIFICATION

Concomitant Medications

Antihypertensives: Start w/ 2.5mg qd amlodipine
Cyclosporine or HIV Protease Inhibitors (Tipranavir Plus Ritonavir) or Telaprevir: Avoid therapy w/ atorvastatin
Lopinavir Plus Ritonavir: Use lowest necessary dose of atorvastatin
Clarithromycin, Itraconazole, Fosamprenavir, or Combination of Saquinavir/Darunavir/ Fosamprenavir Plus Ritonavir: Limit therapy w/ atorvastatin to 20mg and ensure lowest dose needed is employed
Nelfinavir or Boceprevir: Limit therapy w/ atorvastatin to 40mg and ensure lowest dose needed is employed

Hepatic Impairment

May require lower amlodipine dose

Elderly

May require lower amlodipine dose

Other Important Modifications

Small Adult or Fragile: Start w/ 2.5mg qd amlodipine

ADMINISTRATION

Oral route

Take w/ or w/o food

HOW SUPPLIED

Tab: (Amlodipine/Atorvastatin) 2.5mg/10mg, 2.5mg/20mg, 2.5mg/40mg, 5mg/10mg, 5mg/20mg, 5mg/40mg, 5mg/80mg, 10mg/10mg, 10mg/20mg, 10mg/40mg, 10mg/80mg

CONTRAINDICATIONS

Active liver disease, which may include unexplained persistent elevations in hepatic transaminases, women who are pregnant or may become pregnant, and nursing mothers.

WARNINGS/PRECAUTIONS

Amlodipine: Worsening angina and acute MI may develop after starting or increasing the dose, particularly w/ severe obstructive CAD. Symptomatic hypotension may occur, particularly in patients w/ severe aortic stenosis. Atorvastatin: Rare cases of rhabdomyolysis w/ acute renal failure secondary to myoglobinuria reported. Increased risk of rhabdomyolysis in patients w/ history of renal impairment; closely monitor for skeletal muscle effects. Myopathy (including immune-mediated necrotizing myopathy [IMNM]) reported; predisposing factor includes advanced age (≥65 yrs of age). D/C if markedly elevated CPK levels occur or if myopathy is diagnosed or suspected. Withhold or d/c if an acute, serious condition suggestive of a myopathy occurs or if there is a risk factor predisposing to development of renal failure secondary to rhabdomyolysis. Persistent increases in serum transaminases reported; perform LFTs prior to initiation and repeat as clinically indicated. Fatal and nonfatal hepatic failure (rare) reported; promptly interrupt therapy if serious liver injury w/ clinical symptoms and/or hyperbilirubinemia or jaundice occurs and do not restart if no alternate etiology found. Increases in HbA1c and FPG levels reported. May blunt adrenal and/ or gonadal steroid production. Increased risk of hemorrhagic stroke in patients w/ recent stroke or transient ischemic attack (TIA).

ADVERSE REACTIONS

Edema, palpitations, dizziness, fatigue, nasopharyngitis, nausea, insomnia, diarrhea, arthralgia, pain in extremities, UTI, dyspepsia, myalgia, muscle spasms.

DRUG INTERACTIONS

Amlodipine: Diltiazem increased systemic exposure in elderly hypertensive patients. Strong inhibitors of CYP3A4 (eg, ketoconazole, itraconazole, ritonavir, clarithromycin) may increase plasma concentrations; monitor for symptoms of hypotension and edema. Closely monitor BP if coadministered w/ CYP3A4 inducers. Risk of increased tacrolimus blood levels; monitor blood levels and adjust dose of tacrolimus when appropriate. May increase cyclosporine levels in renal transplant patients. Atorvastatin: Avoid w/ cyclosporine, telaprevir, gemfibrozil, tipranavir plus ritonavir, and drugs that decrease levels or activity of endogenous steroid hormones (eg, ketoconazole, spironolactone, cimetidine). Increased risk of myopathy w/ fibric acid derivatives, erythromycin, lipid-modifying doses of niacin, strong CYP3A4 inhibitors, clarithromycin, combinations of HIV protease inhibitors, and azole antifungals; consider lower initial and maintenance doses. Strong CYP3A4 inhibitors (eg, clarithromycin, several combinations of HIV protease inhibitors, telaprevir, itraconazole, boceprevir) and grapefruit juice may increase levels. CYP3A4 inducers (eg, efavirenz, rifampin) may decrease levels; simultaneous coadministration w/ rifampin recommended. May increase digoxin levels; monitor appropriately. May increase AUC of norethindrone and ethinyl estradiol. Myopathy, including rhabdomyolysis, reported w/ colchicine; use w/ caution. OATP1B1 inhibitors (eg, cyclosporine) may increase bioavailability.

NURSING CONSIDERATIONS

Assessment: Assess for active liver disease, unexplained and persistent elevations in serum transaminase levels, history of renal impairment, risk factors for developing renal failure secondary to rhabdomyolysis, recent stroke or TIA, hypersensitivity to the drug, pregnancy/nursing status, and possible drug interactions. Obtain baseline lipid profile (total-C, LDL, HDL, TG), liver function (eg, AST, ALT) parameters, and BP.

Monitoring: Monitor for signs/symptoms of rhabdomyolysis, myopathy (eg, IMNM), worsening angina, MI, and other adverse reactions. Monitor lipid profile, and CPK levels. Monitor LFTs as clinically indicated, and for increases in HbA1c and FPG levels. Monitor BP.

Patient Counseling: Advise to adhere to medication, along w/ the National Cholesterol Education Program-recommended diet, a regular exercise program, and periodic fasting lipid panel testing. Inform of the substances that should not be taken concomitantly w/ the drug. Advise patients to inform other healthcare professionals that they are taking the drug. Inform of the risk of myopathy; instruct to report promptly any unexplained muscle pain, tenderness, or weakness, particularly if accompanied by malaise or fever, or if muscle signs and symptoms persist after discontinuation. Instruct to report promptly any symptoms that may indicate liver injury. Instruct women of childbearing potential to use effective contraceptive methods to prevent pregnancy and to d/c therapy and contact physician if pregnancy occurs. Instruct not to use the drug if breastfeeding.

Storage: 25°C (77°F); excursions permitted to 15-30°C (59-86°F).

CALAN – verapamil hydrochloride RX

Class: Calcium channel blocker (nondihydropyridine)

ADULT DOSAGE

Hypertension

Initial (Monotherapy): 80mg tid (240mg/day)
Usual Range: 360-480mg/day; no evidence that dosages >360mg/day provided added effect
Titrate: Based upward titration on therapeutic efficacy, assessed at the end of the dosing interval

Angina

Angina at rest including vasospastic (Prinzmetal's variant) angina and unstable (crescendo, pre-infarction) angina/chronic stable angina (classic effort-associated angina)
Usual Range: 80-120mg tid
Titrate: Base upward titration on therapeutic efficacy and safety evaluated approx 8 hrs after dosing; may increase daily (eg, patients w/ unstable angina) or at weekly intervals until optimum response is obtained

PEDIATRIC DOSAGE

Pediatric use may not have been established

Arrhythmias

In association w/ digitalis, for the control of ventricular rate at rest and during stress in patients w/ chronic A-flutter/A-fib
Usual Range: 240-320mg/day in divided doses tid or qid

Paroxysmal Supraventricular Tachycardia

Prophylaxis (Non-Digitalized):
Usual: 240-480mg/day in divided doses tid or qid
Max effects for any given dosage will be apparent during the first 48 hrs of therapy

DOSE MODIFICATION

Hepatic Impairment
Severe Dysfunction: Give 30% of normal dose

Other Important Modifications
Patients Who May Respond to Lower Doses (eg, Elderly, People of Small Stature):
HTN: Consider beginning titration at 40mg tid
Angina: 40mg tid may be warranted

ADMINISTRATION

Oral route

HOW SUPPLIED

Tab: 40mg, 80mg*, 120mg* *scored

CONTRAINDICATIONS

Severe left ventricular dysfunction, hypotension (systolic pressure <90mmHg) or cardiogenic shock, sick sinus syndrome or 2nd- or 3rd-degree atrioventricular (AV) block (except with functioning ventricular artificial pacemaker), A-fib/flutter and an accessory bypass tract (eg, Wolff-Parkinson-White, Lown-Ganong-Levine syndromes).

WARNINGS/PRECAUTIONS

Has negative inotropic effect; avoid with severe left ventricular dysfunction (eg, ejection fraction <30%) or moderate to severe symptoms of cardiac failure. Patients with milder ventricular dysfunction should, if possible, be controlled with optimum doses of digitalis and/or diuretics before treatment. May cause congestive heart failure (CHF), pulmonary edema, hypotension, asymptomatic 1st-degree AV block, transient bradycardia, and PR interval prolongation. Marked 1st-degree AV block or progressive development to 2nd- or 3rd-degree AV block requires dose reduction, or in rare instances, discontinuation and institution of appropriate therapy. Hepatocellular injury as well as elevated transaminases with or without concomitant elevations in alkaline phosphatase and bilirubin reported; monitor LFTs periodically. Sinus bradycardia, 2nd-degree AV block, pulmonary edema, severe hypotension, and sinus arrest reported in patients with hypertrophic cardiomyopathy. Caution with renal/hepatic impairment; monitor for abnormal PR interval prolongation or other signs of overdosage. 30% of normal dose should be given to patients with severe hepatic dysfunction. May decrease neuromuscular transmission in patients with Duchenne muscular dystrophy and may cause worsening of myasthenia gravis; may be necessary to decrease dose when administered to patients with attenuated neuromuscular transmission. Caution in elderly.

ADVERSE REACTIONS

Constipation, dizziness.

DRUG INTERACTIONS

CYP3A4 inhibitors (eg, erythromycin, ritonavir) and grapefruit juice may increase levels. CYP3A4 inducers (eg, rifampin) may decrease levels. May cause myopathy/rhabdomyolysis with HMG-CoA reductase inhibitors that are CYP3A4 substrates and may increase levels of such drugs; limit dose of simvastatin to 10mg/day and lovastatin to 40mg/day, and lower starting/maintenance doses of other CYP3A4 substrates (eg, atorvastatin) may be required. Increased bleeding times with aspirin. Additive negative effects on HR, AV conduction, and/or cardiac contractility with β-blockers; monitor closely and avoid with any degree of ventricular dysfunction. Combined therapy with propranolol should usually be avoided in patients with AV conduction abnormalities and those with depressed left ventricular function. May produce asymptomatic bradycardia with a wandering atrial pacemaker with timolol eye drops. Decreased metoprolol and propranolol clearance and variable effect with atenolol reported. Chronic treatment may increase digoxin levels, which may result in digitalis toxicity; reduce maintenance and digitalization doses and monitor carefully to avoid over-/under-digitalization. May reduce total body/extra renal clearance of digitoxin. Additive effects with other oral antihypertensives (eg, vasodilators, ACE inhibitors, diuretics); monitor appropriately. Coadministration with agents that attenuate α-adrenergic function (eg, prazosin) may excessively reduce BP. Avoid disopyramide within 48 hrs before or 24 hrs after administration. Coadministration with flecainide may result in additive negative inotropic effect and AV conduction prolongation. May counteract effects of quinidine on AV conduction and increase levels of quinidine; avoid concomitant use in patients with hypertrophic cardiomyopathy. Reduced or unchanged clearance with cimetidine. Increased sensitivity to effects of lithium (neurotoxicity) when used concomitantly; monitor carefully. May increase carbamazepine, theophylline, cyclosporine, and alcohol levels. Increased clearance with phenobarbital. Rifampin may reduce oral bioavailability. Titrate both verapamil and inhalation anesthetics carefully, in order to avoid excessive cardiovascular depression. May potentiate neuromuscular blockers (eg, curare-like and depolarizing); verapamil or both agents may need dose reduction. Hypotension and bradyarrhythmias reported with telithromycin. Sinus bradycardia resulting in hospitalization and pacemaker insertion reported with clonidine; monitor HR.

NURSING CONSIDERATIONS

Assessment: Assess for known hypersensitivity to the drug, cardiac failure, severe left ventricular dysfunction, hypertrophic cardiomyopathy, hepatic/renal impairment, attenuated neuromuscular transmission (eg, Duchenne muscular dystrophy), any conditions where treatment is contraindicated or cautioned, pregnancy/nursing status, and possible drug interactions.

Monitoring: Monitor for CHF, hypotension, AV block, abnormal prolongation of the PR interval, transient bradycardia, and other adverse reactions. Monitor LFTs periodically.

Patient Counseling: Inform of the risks/benefits of therapy. Advise to seek medical attention if any adverse reactions occur.

Storage: 15-25°C (59-77°F). Protect from light.

CALAN SR – verapamil hydrochloride RX

Class: Calcium channel blocker (nondihydropyridine)

ADULT DOSAGE

Hypertension

Initial: 180mg qam

Titrate: If response is inadequate, increase to 240mg qam, then 180mg bid (am and pm) or 240mg qam plus 120mg qpm, then 240mg q12h

Upward titration should be based on therapeutic efficacy and safety evaluated weekly and approx 24 hrs after the previous dose

Switching from IR Calan to Calan SR: Total daily dose in mg may remain the same

PEDIATRIC DOSAGE

Pediatric use may not have been established

DOSE MODIFICATION

Hepatic Impairment

Severe Dysfunction: Give 30% of normal dose

Other Important Modifications

Increased Response to Verapamil (eg, Elderly, Small Stature):
Initial: 120mg qam may be warranted

ADMINISTRATION

Oral route

Take w/ food

HOW SUPPLIED

Tab, ER: 120mg, 180mg*, 240mg* *scored

CONTRAINDICATIONS

Severe left ventricular dysfunction, hypotension (systolic pressure <90mmHg) or cardiogenic shock, sick sinus syndrome or 2nd- or 3rd-degree AV block (except with functioning artificial ventricular pacemaker), A-flutter/A-fib and an accessory bypass tract (eg, Wolff-Parkinson-White, Lown-Ganong-Levine syndromes).

WARNINGS/PRECAUTIONS

Has negative inotropic effect; avoid with severe left ventricular dysfunction (eg, ejection fraction <30%) or moderate to severe symptoms of cardiac failure. Patients with milder ventricular dysfunction should, if possible, be controlled with optimum doses of digitalis and/or diuretics before treatment. May cause hypotension, CHF, pulmonary edema, asymptomatic 1st-degree AV block, transient bradycardia, and PR-interval prolongation. Marked 1st-degree AV block or progressive development to 2nd- or 3rd-degree AV block requires dose reduction, or in rare instances, discontinuation and institution of appropriate therapy. Sinus bradycardia, pulmonary edema, severe hypotension, 2nd-degree AV block, and sinus arrest reported in patients with hypertrophic cardiomyopathy. Hepatocellular injury as well as elevated transaminases with or without concomitant elevations in alkaline phosphatase and bilirubin reported; monitor LFTs periodically. Caution with renal/hepatic impairment; monitor for abnormal PR interval prolongation or other signs of overdosage. 30% of normal dose should be given to patients with severe hepatic dysfunction. May decrease neuromuscular transmission in patients with Duchenne muscular dystrophy; may be necessary to decrease dose when administered to patients with attenuated neuromuscular transmission. Caution in elderly.

ADVERSE REACTIONS

Constipation, dizziness.

DRUG INTERACTIONS

May cause myopathy/rhabdomyolysis with HMG-CoA reductase inhibitors that are CYP3A4 substrates and may increase levels of such drugs; limit dose of simvastatin to 10mg/day or lovastatin to 40mg/day, and consider lower starting/maintenance doses of other CYP3A4 substrates (eg, atorvastatin). Additive negative effects on HR, AV conduction, and/or cardiac contractility with β-blockers; monitor closely and avoid with any degree of ventricular dysfunction. May produce asymptomatic bradycardia with a wandering atrial pacemaker with timolol eye drops. Decreased metoprolol and propranolol clearance and variable effect with atenolol reported. Additive effects with other oral antihypertensives (eg, vasodilators, ACE inhibitors, diuretics); monitor appropriately. Coadministration with agents that attenuate α-adrenergic function (eg, prazosin) may excessively reduce BP. May increase carbamazepine, theophylline, and cyclosporine levels. Chronic treatment may increase digoxin levels, which may result in digitalis toxicity; reduce maintenance and digitalization doses and monitor carefully to avoid over-/under-digitalization. May reduce total body/extrarenal clearance of digitoxin. Avoid disopyramide within 48 hrs before or 24 hrs after administration. Coadministration with flecainide may result in additive negative inotropic effect and AV conduction prolongation. May counteract effects of quinidine on AV conduction and increase levels of quinidine; avoid concomitant use in patients with hypertrophic cardiomyopathy. May increase ethanol concentrations that may prolong the intoxicating effects of alcohol. Increased sensitivity to effects of lithium (neurotoxicity) when used concomitantly; monitor carefully. Increased clearance with phenobarbital. Rifampin may reduce oral bioavailability. May potentiate neuromuscular blockers (eg, curare-like and depolarizing); verapamil or both agents may need dose reduction. Titrate both verapamil and inhalation anesthetics carefully to avoid excessive cardiovascular depression. Hypotension and bradyarrhythmias reported with telithromycin. Sinus bradycardia resulting in hospitalization and pacemaker insertion reported with clonidine; monitor HR. Reduced or unchanged clearance with cimetidine.

NURSING CONSIDERATIONS

Assessment: Assess for known hypersensitivity to drug, severe left ventricular dysfunction, attenuated neuromuscular transmission (eg, Duchenne muscular dystrophy), cardiac failure, hypertrophic cardiomyopathy, hepatic/renal impairment, and for any other conditions where treatment is contraindicated or cautioned. Assess pregnancy/nursing status and for possible drug interactions.

Monitoring: Monitor for abnormal prolongation of PR-interval, hypotension, CHF, pulmonary edema, AV block, transient bradycardia, and other adverse reactions. Monitor LFTs periodically.

Patient Counseling: Inform of the risks/benefits of therapy. Advise to seek medical attention if any adverse reactions occur.

Storage: 15-25°C (59-77°F). Protect from light and moisture.

CAMPATH – alemtuzumab

RX

Class: Monoclonal antibody/CD52-blocker

Serious, including fatal, pancytopenia/marrow hypoplasia, autoimmune idiopathic thrombocytopenia, and autoimmune hemolytic anemia may occur; single doses >30mg or cumulative doses >90mg/week increase the incidence of pancytopenia. May result in serious, including fatal, infusion reactions; monitor during infusion and withhold therapy for Grade 3 or 4 infusion reactions. Gradually escalate therapy to the recommended dose at the initiation of therapy and after interruption of therapy for ≥7 days. Serious, including fatal, bacterial, viral, fungal, and protozoan infections may occur; administer prophylaxis against *Pneumocystis jiroveci* pneumonia (PCP) and herpes virus infections.

ADULT DOSAGE

B-Cell Chronic Lymphocytic Leukemia

Recommended Dosing Regimen:

Gradually escalate to max recommended single dose of 30mg

Escalation ordinarily accomplished in 3-7 days

PEDIATRIC DOSAGE

Pediatric use may not have been established

Escalation Strategy:
1. Administer 3mg/day until infusion reactions are ≤Grade 2
2. Then administer 10mg/day until infusion reactions are ≤Grade 2
3. Then administer 30mg/day 3X/week on alternate days

Total duration of therapy, including escalation, is 12 weeks

DOSE MODIFICATION

Concomitant Medications

Premedication:
50mg diphenhydramine and 500-1000mg acetaminophen 30 min prior to first infusion and each dose escalation

***Pneumocystis jiroveci* Pneumonia Prophylaxis:**
Trimethoprim/sulfamethoxazole DS bid 3X/week

Herpetic Prophylaxis:
Famciclovir 250mg bid or equivalent

Adverse Reactions

ANC <250/µL and/or Platelets ≤25,000/µL:
1st Occurrence: Withhold therapy, then resume at 30mg when ANC ≥500/µL and platelets ≥50,000/µL
2nd Occurrence: Withhold therapy, then resume at 10mg when ANC ≥500/µL and platelets ≥50,000/µL
3rd Occurrence: D/C therapy

≥50% Decrease From Baseline in Patients Initiating Therapy with Baseline ANC ≤250/µL and/or Baseline Platelets ≤25,000/µL:
1st Occurrence: Withhold therapy, then resume at 30mg upon return to baseline value(s)
2nd Occurrence: Withhold therapy, then resume at 10mg upon return to baseline value(s)
3rd Occurrence: D/C therapy

ADMINISTRATION

IV route

Administer as an IV infusion over 2 hrs
Do not administer as IV push or bolus
Do not add or simultaneously infuse other drugs through the same IV line
Refer to PI for further preparation and administration instructions

HOW SUPPLIED

Inj: 30mg/mL [1mL]

WARNINGS/PRECAUTIONS

Prolonged myelosuppression and pure red cell/bone marrow aplasia reported; withhold therapy for severe cytopenias (except lymphopenia) and d/c for autoimmune cytopenias or recurrent/persistent severe cytopenias (except lymphopenia). Severe and prolonged lymphopenia with increased incidence of opportunistic infections reported; administer PCP and herpes viral prophylaxis during therapy and for a minimum of 2 months after completion of therapy or until the CD4+ count is ≥200 cells/µL, whichever occurs later. Monitor for cytomegalovirus (CMV) infection during treatment and for at least 2 months after completion of treatment; withhold therapy for serious infections and during CMV infection treatment or confirmed CMV viremia. Administer only irradiated blood products to avoid transfusion-associated graft versus host disease unless emergent circumstances dictate immediate transfusion.

ADVERSE REACTIONS

Cytopenias, infusion reactions, CMV and other infections, immunosuppression, nausea, emesis, abdominal pain, insomnia, anxiety, cardiac dysrhythmias, HTN, headache, dyspnea, diarrhea.

DRUG INTERACTIONS

Do not administer live viral vaccines to patients who have recently received therapy.

NURSING CONSIDERATIONS

Assessment: Assess pregnancy/nursing status and for possible drug interactions. Obtain baseline CBCs and platelet counts.

Monitoring: Monitor CBCs weekly and more frequently if worsening anemia, neutropenia, or thrombocytopenia occurs. Assess CD4+ counts after treatment until recovery to ≥200 cells/µL. Monitor for CMV infection during treatment and for at least 2 months after completion of treatment. Monitor for cytopenias, infusion reactions, immunosuppression, infection, and other adverse reactions.

Patient Counseling: Advise to report any signs/symptoms of cytopenias, infusion reactions, and infection. Counsel of the need to take premedications and prophylactic anti-infectives as prescribed. Advise that irradiation of blood products is required. Inform not to be immunized with live viral vaccines if recently treated with the drug. Advise to use effective contraceptive methods during treatment and for a minimum of 6 months following therapy.

Storage: 2-8°C (36-46°F). Do not freeze. If accidentally frozen, thaw at 2-8°C (36-46°F) before administration. Protect from direct sunlight. Diluted Sol: 2-8°C (36-46°F) or 15-30°C (59-86°F). Protect from light. Use within 8 hrs.

CAMPTOSAR – irinotecan hydrochloride RX

Class: Topoisomerase I inhibitor

Early and late forms of diarrhea can occur. Early diarrhea may be accompanied by cholinergic symptoms; may be prevented or ameliorated by atropine. Late diarrhea can be life-threatening; treat properly w/ loperamide. Monitor patients w/ diarrhea; give fluid/electrolytes PRN or institute antibiotic therapy if ileus, fever, or severe neutropenia develops. Interrupt therapy and reduce subsequent doses if severe diarrhea occurs. Severe myelosuppression may occur.

ADULT DOSAGE

Metastatic Carcinoma of the Colon/Rectum

1st-line therapy in combination w/ 5-fluorouracil (5-FU) and leucovorin (LV) for metastatic carcinoma of the colon or rectum, and for patients w/ metastatic carcinoma of the colon or rectum whose disease has recurred or progressed following initial 5-FU therapy

Combination w/ 5-FU and LV:
Administer as 90-min infusion followed by LV and 5-FU
Regimen 1 (6-Week Cycle w/ Bolus 5-FU/LV):
125mg/m² IV over 90 min on Days 1, 8, 15, and 22
Modified Dose Levels:
Starting Dose: 125mg/m²
Dose Level-1: 100mg/m²
Dose Level-2: 75mg/m²
Regimen 2 (6-Week Cycle w/ Infusional 5-FU/LV): 180mg/m² IV over 90 min on Days 1, 15, and 29
Modified Dose Levels:
Starting Dose: 180mg/m²
Dose Level-1: 150mg/m²
Dose Level-2: 120mg/m²
Both Regimens:
Begin next cycle on Day 43
Refer to PI for doses of 5-FU/LV

Single Therapy:
Regimen 1 (Weekly): 125mg/m² IV over 90 min on Days 1, 8, 15, and 22 followed by 2-week rest
Titrate: Subsequent doses may be adjusted as high as 150mg/m² or to as low as 50mg/m² in 25-50mg/m² decrements, depending upon individual tolerance
Modified Dose Levels:
Starting Dose: 125mg/m²
Dose Level-1: 100mg/m²
Dose Level-2: 75mg/m²

Regimen 2 (Every 3 Weeks): 350mg/m² IV over 90 min once every 3 weeks
Titrate: Subsequent doses may be adjusted as low as 200mg/m² in 50mg/m² decrements, depending upon individual tolerance
Modified Dose Levels:
Starting Dose: 350mg/m²
Dose Level-1: 300mg/m²
Dose Level-2: 250mg/m²

PEDIATRIC DOSAGE

Pediatric use may not have been established

DOSE MODIFICATION

Renal Impairment

Dialysis: Not recommended

Other Important Modifications

Reduced UGT1A1 Activity

Consider reducing starting dose by at least one level for known homozygous UGT1A1*28 allele
Subsequent dose modifications are based on individual tolerance; refer to PI

Prior Pelvic or Abdominal Radiotherapy/Performance Status of 2/Increased Bilirubin

Consider reducing starting dose by one level

Refer to PI for Subsequent Dose Modifications for Single-Agent Schedules
All dose modifications should be based on worst preceding toxicity

Elderly

In patients ≥70 years, the once-every-3-week-dosage schedule should be 300mg/m²

ADMINISTRATION

IV route

Dilute in D5 Inj or 0.9% NaCl Inj to a final concentration of 0.12-2.8mg/ml
Do not add other drugs to the infusion sol

Stability

Use immediately after reconstitution, since it contains no antibacterial preservative
Use admixture prepared w/ D5 Inj w/in 24 hrs if refrigerated (2-8°C or 36-46°F)
Use admixture prepared w/ D5 Inj or NaCl w/in 4 hrs if kept at room temperature
If reconstitution and dilution are performed under strict aseptic conditions (eg, Laminar Air Flow bench), use sol w/in 12 hrs at room temperature or 24 hrs if refrigerated (2-8°C or 36-46°F)

HOW SUPPLIED

Inj: 20mg/mL [2mL, 5mL, 15mL]

WARNINGS/PRECAUTIONS

Not recommended in patients on dialysis or w/ bilirubin >2mg/dL. If late diarrhea occurs, delay subsequent weekly therapy until return of pretreatment bowel function for at least 24 hrs w/o antidiarrheals; decrease subsequent doses if late diarrhea is Grade 2, 3, or 4. Avoid diuretics or laxatives in patients w/ diarrhea. Deaths due to sepsis following severe neutropenia reported; d/c if neutropenic fever occurs, or if absolute neutrophil count <1000/mm³. Increased risk for neutropenia in patients homozygous for the UGT1A1*28 allele. Severe anaphylactic/anaphylactoid reactions reported; d/c if anaphylactic reaction occurs. Renal impairment/acute renal failure reported, usually in patients who became volume depleted from severe vomiting and/or diarrhea. Interstitial pulmonary disease (IPD) events reported; d/c therapy if IPD is diagnosed and institute appropriate treatment. Should not be used w/ a regimen of 5-FU/LV administered for 4-5 consecutive days every 4 weeks due to increased toxicity. Increased toxicity in patients w/ performance status 2 at baseline. May cause fetal harm. Caution to avoid extravasation and monitor for inflammation at infusion site. Premedicate w/ antiemetics at least 30 min prior to therapy. Consider prophylactic/therapeutic administration of atropine if cholinergic symptoms develop. Caution in patients w/ deficient glucuronidation of bilirubin (eg, Gilbert's syndrome), renal/hepatic impairment, previous pelvic/abdominal irradiation, and in elderly. Avoid in unresolved bowel obstruction.

ADVERSE REACTIONS

N/V, diarrhea, neutropenia, abdominal pain, anemia, asthenia, anorexia, alopecia, fever, constipation, leukopenia, decreased body weight.

DRUG INTERACTIONS

Avoid concurrent irradiation therapy. Greater incidence of akathisia reported w/ prochlorperazine. Exposure is substantially reduced w/ CYP3A4 enzyme-inducing anticonvulsants phenytoin, phenobarbital, carbamazepine, or St. John's wort; consider substituting non-enzyme-inducing therapies at least 2 weeks prior to initiation of treatment. Ketoconazole (a CYP3A4 and UGT1A1 inhibitor) increased exposure; coadministration w/ other inhibitors of CYP3A4 (eg, clarithromycin, lopinavir, itraconazole) or UGT1A1 (eg, atazanavir, gemfibrozil, indinavir) may increase exposure. D/C strong CYP3A4 inhibitors at least 1 week prior to starting therapy. Do not administer w/ strong CYP3A4 inducers or strong CYP3A4 or UGT1A1 inhibitors unless there are no therapeutic alternatives. May prolong neuromuscular-blocking effects of suxamethonium, and the neuromuscular blockade of nondepolarizing drugs may be antagonized.

NURSING CONSIDERATIONS

Assessment: Assess for unresolved bowel obstruction, UGT1A1 status, deficient glucuronidation of bilirubin (Gilbert's syndrome), pelvic/abdominal irradiation, preexisting lung disease, renal/hepatic impairment, pregnancy/nursing status, and possible drug interactions. Obtain baseline CBC.

Monitoring: Monitor for diarrhea, signs/symptoms of neutropenia, neutropenic complications (eg, neutropenic fever), ileus, respiratory symptoms, inflammation and/or extravasation of infusion site, cholinergic symptoms, hypersensitivity reactions, and other adverse reactions. For patients w/ diarrhea, monitor for signs/symptoms of dehydration, electrolyte imbalance, ileus, fever, or severe neutropenia. Monitor CBC w/ differential.

Patient Counseling: Instruct to seek medical attention if experiencing diarrhea for 1st time during treatment, black or bloody stools, dehydration, inability to take fluids by mouth due to N/V, or inability to get diarrhea under control w/in 24 hrs. Inform about potential for dizziness or visual disturbances, which may occur w/in 24 hrs. Explain importance of routine blood cell counts. Instruct to report any occurrence of fever or infection. Inform that therapy may cause fetal harm, and advise to avoid becoming pregnant while on therapy. Explain about the possibility of alopecia. Inform that the product contains sorbitol.

Storage: 15-30°C (59-86°F). Protect from light. Keep in carton until time of use. Avoid freezing.

CANASA – mesalamine

RX

Class: 5-aminosalicylic acid derivative

ADULT DOSAGE

Ulcerative Proctitis

Mild to Moderately Active:
Usual: 1 sup rectally qhs for 3-6 weeks depending on symptoms and sigmoidoscopic findings. Retain sup for at least 1-3 hrs

PEDIATRIC DOSAGE

Pediatric use may not have been established

DOSE MODIFICATION

Elderly
Start at lower end of dosing range

ADMINISTRATION

Rectal route

HOW SUPPLIED

Sup: 1000mg

CONTRAINDICATIONS

Hypersensitivity to sup vehicle (saturated vegetable fatty acid esters).

WARNINGS/PRECAUTIONS

Renal impairment, including minimal change nephropathy, acute and chronic interstitial nephritis, and renal failure (rare), reported; evaluate renal function prior to initiation and periodically during therapy. Caution with known renal dysfunction or history of renal disease. Associated with acute intolerance syndrome (eg, cramping, acute abdominal pain and bloody diarrhea, fever, headache, rash); observe closely for worsening of these symptoms, and promptly d/c therapy if acute intolerance syndrome is suspected. Patients with sulfasalazine hypersensitivity may have similar reaction to therapy. Drug-induced cardiac hypersensitivity reactions (myocarditis, pericarditis) reported. Hepatic failure in patients with preexisting liver disease reported; caution with liver disease. Possible interference with measurements, by liquid chromatography, of urinary normetanephrine observed in patients exposed to sulfasalazine or its metabolite, mesalamine/mesalazine. Caution in elderly.

ADVERSE REACTIONS

Dizziness, rectal pain, fever, rash, acne, colitis, headache, flatulence, abdominal pain, diarrhea, nausea.

DRUG INTERACTIONS

Concurrent use with nephrotoxic agents (eg, NSAIDs) may increase risk of renal reactions. Concurrent use with azathioprine or 6-mercaptopurine may increase risk for blood disorders.

NURSING CONSIDERATIONS

Assessment: Assess for hypersensitivity to drug, sup vehicle, salicylates, or sulfasalazine. Assess renal/hepatic function, pregnancy/nursing status, and possible drug interactions.

Monitoring: Monitor for acute intolerance syndrome, hypersensitivity reactions (eg, myocarditis, pericarditis), hepatic failure, and other adverse reactions. Monitor renal function periodically. Monitor blood cell counts in elderly.

Patient Counseling: Instruct to notify physician of all medications being taken and if patient is allergic to sulfasalazine, salicylates, or mesalamine; experiences cramping, abdominal pain, bloody diarrhea, fever, headache, or rash; has a history of myocarditis/pericarditis or stomach blockage; has kidney/liver disease; or is pregnant, intends to become pregnant, or is breastfeeding. Inform that sup will cause staining of direct contact surfaces (eg, fabrics, flooring, painted surfaces, marble, granite, vinyl, enamel).

Storage: <25°C (77°F). May be refrigerated. Keep away from direct heat, light, or humidity.

CAPEX – fluocinolone acetonide

RX

Class: Corticosteroid

ADULT DOSAGE

Seborrheic Dermatitis

Apply up to 1 oz. to scalp qd

PEDIATRIC DOSAGE

Pediatric use may not have been established

ADMINISTRATION

Topical route

Work into lather, rinse after 5 min

Pharmacist should empty contents of enclosed cap into shampoo base prior to dispensing

Shake well before use

HOW SUPPLIED

Shampoo: 0.01% [6 oz.]

WARNINGS/PRECAUTIONS

Not proven to be effective in other corticosteroid-responsive dermatoses. May produce reversible hypothalamic pituitary adrenal (HPA)-axis suppression with potential for glucocorticosteroid insufficiency; when noted, gradually withdraw the drug, reduce frequency of application, or substitute a less potent steroid. Evaluate periodically for evidence of HPA-axis suppression when applying to a large surface area or to areas under occlusion. May produce Cushing's syndrome, hyperglycemia, and glucosuria. Infrequently, signs/symptoms of glucocorticoid insufficiency may occur. Pediatrics may be more susceptible to systemic toxicity. D/C and institute appropriate treatment if irritation develops. Allergic contact dermatitis may occur; confirm via patch testing. Use appropriate antifungal or antibacterial agent with skin infections; d/c until infection has been adequately controlled.

ADVERSE REACTIONS

Allergic contact dermatitis, secondary infection, skin atrophy, striae, miliaria, burning, itching, irritation, hypopigmentation, perioral dermatitis, dryness, folliculitis, acneiform eruptions.

NURSING CONSIDERATIONS

Assessment: Assess for hypersensitivity reactions, concomitant skin infections, and pregnancy/nursing status.

Monitoring: Monitor for HPA-axis suppression, manifestation of Cushing's syndrome, hyperglycemia, glucosuria, irritation at treatment site, allergic contact dermatitis (eg, failure to heal) and skin infections. If applying medication to large surface area or to occluded areas, periodically monitor for HPA-axis suppression using adrenocorticotropic stimulation, AM plasma cortisol, and urinary free cortisol tests. Monitor for glucocorticoid insufficiency following end of therapy.

Patient Counseling: Instruct to use exactly as directed and externally only. Avoid contact with eyes; if contact occurs, wash eyes liberally with water. Advise patients that this medication should not be used for any disorder other than for which it was prescribed. Inform that treated scalp area should not be bandaged, covered, or wrapped unless directed by physician. Advise to report signs of adverse reactions. Inform that medication contents should be discarded after 3 months.

Storage: 15-30°C (59-86°F).

CAPRELSA – vandetanib

RX

Class: Kinase inhibitors

May prolong the QT interval. Torsades de pointes and sudden death reported. Avoid with hypocalcemia, hypokalemia, hypomagnesemia, or long QT syndrome; correct hypocalcemia, hypokalemia, and/or hypomagnesemia prior to therapy. Monitor electrolytes periodically. Avoid drugs known to prolong QT interval. Only prescribers and pharmacies certified through the restricted distribution program are able to prescribe and dispense this therapy.

ADULT DOSAGE

Medullary Thyroid Cancer

Symptomatic or progressive cancer in patients w/ unresectable locally advanced or metastatic disease

300mg qd until disease progression or unacceptable toxicity occurs

Missed Dose

Do not take a missed dose w/in 12 hrs of the next dose

PEDIATRIC DOSAGE

Pediatric use may not have been established

DOSE MODIFICATION

Renal Impairment

Moderate (CrCl ≥30-<50mL/min) and Severe (CrCl <30mL/min):

Initial: 200mg qd

Hepatic Impairment

Moderate and Severe: Not recommended for use

Adverse Reactions

Corrected QT Interval, Fridericia (QTcF) >500 ms:

Interrupt therapy, then resume at a reduced dose when the QTcF returns to <450 ms

CTCAE Grade ≥3 Toxicities:

Interrupt therapy, then resume at 200mg (two 100mg tabs) when toxicity resolves or improves to CTCAE Grade 1

For recurrent toxicities, reduce the dose to 100mg after resolution or improvement to CTCAE Grade 1 severity, if continued treatment is warranted

ADMINISTRATION

Oral route

Take w/ or w/o food
Do not crush

If Unable to Swallow Whole Tab

1. Disperse in 2 oz of water; do not use other liquids for dispersion
2. Stir for approx 10 min (will not completely dissolve)
3. Swallow immediately after dispersion
4. Mix any remaining residue w/ additional 4 oz of water and swallow

The dispersion can also be administered through nasogastric or gastrostomy tubes

HOW SUPPLIED

Tab: 100mg, 300mg

CONTRAINDICATIONS

Congenital long QT syndrome.

WARNINGS/PRECAUTIONS

Caution in patients with indolent, asymptomatic, or slowly progressing disease. Do not start therapy with QTcF interval >450 ms. Avoid with history of torsades de pointes, bradyarrhythmias, or uncompensated heart failure (HF). Severe skin reactions (eg, Stevens-Johnson syndrome) reported; consider permanent discontinuation if any develop. Photosensitivity reactions may occur during treatment and up to 4 months after discontinuation. Interstitial lung disease (ILD) or pneumonitis reported; interrupt treatment for acute/worsening pulmonary symptoms and d/c if ILD is confirmed. Ischemic cerebrovascular events and serious hemorrhagic events reported; d/c if severe. Avoid with recent history of hemoptysis of ≥1/2 tsp of red blood. HF reported; monitor for signs/symptoms of HF and consider discontinuation in patients with HF. Diarrhea of ≥Grade 3 reported; interrupt therapy for severe diarrhea and resume at a reduced dose upon improvement. HTN, including hypertensive crisis, may occur; monitor for HTN. Reduce dose or interrupt therapy if HTN occurs; do not resume therapy if BP cannot be controlled. Reversible posterior leukoencephalopathy syndrome (RPLS) reported; d/c in patients with RPLS. Not recommended for use in patients with moderate and severe hepatic impairment. May cause fetal harm. Women of childbearing potential should avoid pregnancy; use effective contraception during treatment and for at least 4 months following the last dose.

ADVERSE REACTIONS

QT interval prolongation, torsades de pointes, diarrhea/colitis, rash, acneiform dermatitis, HTN, N/V, headache, upper respiratory tract infections, decreased appetite, abdominal pain, fatigue, hypocalcemia, corneal abnormalities, proteinuria.

DRUG INTERACTIONS

See Boxed Warning. Rifampicin, a strong CYP3A4 inducer, decreased levels. Avoid use with strong CYP3A4 inducers, St. John's wort, antiarrhythmic drugs (eg, amiodarone, disopyramide, procainamide), and other drugs that may prolong QT interval (eg, chloroquine, clarithromycin, dolasetron). Increased plasma levels of metformin that is transported by organic cation transporter type 2 (OCT2); use caution and closely monitor for toxicities when administering with drugs that are transported by OCT2. Increased digoxin levels; use caution and closely monitor for toxicities. May require dose increase of thyroid replacement therapy; if signs or symptoms of hypothyroidism occur, examine thyroid hormone levels and adjust thyroid replacement therapy accordingly.

NURSING CONSIDERATIONS

Assessment: Assess for congenital long QT syndrome, history of torsades de pointes or hemoptysis, bradyarrhythmias, uncompensated HF, renal/hepatic impairment, pregnancy/nursing status, and possible drug interactions. Obtain baseline ECG, serum K^+, Ca^{2+}, Mg^{2+}, and TSH levels.

Monitoring: Monitor for QT interval prolongation, torsades de pointes, skin/photosensitivity reactions, ILD, ischemic cerebrovascular events, hemorrhage, HF, diarrhea, hypothyroidism, HTN,

RPLS, and other adverse reactions. Monitor ECG, serum K^+, Ca^{2+}, Mg^{2+}, and TSH levels at 2-4 weeks and 8-12 weeks after initial therapy, every 3 months thereafter, and following any dose reduction for QT prolongation, or any dose interruptions >2 weeks. Monitor renal function.

Patient Counseling: Instruct to contact physician in the event of syncope, pre-syncopal symptoms, and cardiac palpitations. Inform patients that the physician will monitor electrolytes and ECGs during treatment. Advise to contact physician in the event of skin reactions or rash, sudden onset or worsening of breathlessness, persistent cough or fever, diarrhea, seizures, headaches, visual disturbances, confusion, or difficulty thinking. Advise patients of reproductive potential to use effective contraception during therapy and for at least 4 months after the last dose and to immediately contact physician if pregnancy is suspected or confirmed. Advise to d/c nursing while on therapy. Instruct to use appropriate sun protection due to the increased susceptibility to sunburn while on therapy and for at least 4 months after drug discontinuation.

Storage: 25°C (77°F); excursions permitted to 15-30°C (59-86°F).

CARAFATE – sucralfate RX

Class: Duodenal ulcer adherent complex

ADULT DOSAGE

Active Duodenal Ulcer

1g qid on an empty stomach; continue for 4-8 weeks unless healing has been demonstrated by x-ray or endoscopic exam

Antacids may be prescribed prn for relief of pain but should not be taken w/in 1/2 hr before or after administration

Tab:
Maint: 1g bid

PEDIATRIC DOSAGE

Pediatric use may not have been established

DOSE MODIFICATION

Elderly

Start at the lower end of dosing range

ADMINISTRATION

Oral route

Sus

Shake well before use

HOW SUPPLIED

Sus: 1g/10mL [14 fl oz]; Tab: 1g* *scored

WARNINGS/PRECAUTIONS

DU is a chronic, recurrent disease; a successful course of treatment should not be expected to alter post healing frequency or severity of duodenal ulceration. May impair excretion of absorbed aluminum with chronic renal failure or those receiving dialysis; aluminum accumulation and toxicity (aluminum osteodystrophy, osteomalacia, encephalopathy) reported with renal impairment. Caution with chronic renal failure and in elderly. (Sus) Episodes of hyperglycemia reported in diabetic patients; may need to adjust dose of antidiabetic treatment during therapy. (Tab) Aspiration with accompanying respiratory complications reported; caution with known conditions that may impair swallowing (eg, recent or prolonged intubation, tracheostomy, prior history of aspiration, dysphagia), or any other conditions that may alter gag and cough reflexes, or diminish oropharyngeal coordination or motility.

ADVERSE REACTIONS

Constipation, diarrhea, N/V, pruritus, rash, dizziness, insomnia, back pain, headache, dry mouth, flatulence, gastric discomfort, indigestion, sleepiness, vertigo.

DRUG INTERACTIONS

Simultaneous administration may reduce the extent of absorption of single doses of cimetidine, digoxin, fluoroquinolone antibiotics, ketoconazole, l-thyroxine, phenytoin, quinidine, ranitidine, tetracycline, and theophylline; administer separately when alterations in bioavailability are felt to be critical and monitor patients appropriately. Subtherapeutic PT with concomitant warfarin reported. Concomitant use with other products that contain aluminum (eg, aluminum-containing antacids) may increase the total body burden of aluminum.

NURSING CONSIDERATIONS

Assessment: Assess for drug hypersensitivity or to any of the excipients, chronic renal failure or receiving dialysis, pregnancy/nursing status, and possible drug interactions. (Sus) Assess for diabetes mellitus. (Tab) Assess for known conditions that may impair swallowing or any other conditions that may alter gag and cough reflexes, or diminish oropharyngeal coordination or motility.

Monitoring: Monitor for aluminum accumulation and toxicity in patients with renal impairment and other adverse reactions. Monitor renal function. (Sus) Monitor for episodes of hyperglycemia. (Tab) Monitor for aspiration with accompanying respiratory complications.

Patient Counseling: Inform about the risks/benefits of treatment. Instruct to take exactly ud. Advise to contact physician if any side effects develop. Counsel about the possible drug interactions. Advise to notify physician if pregnant/nursing or planning to become pregnant.

Storage: (Sus) 20-25°C (68-77°F). Avoid freezing. (Tab) 15-30°C (59-86°F).

CARBAMAZEPINE – carbamazepine RX

Class: Carboxamide

Serious and sometimes fatal dermatologic reactions, including toxic epidermal necrolysis (TEN) and Stevens-Johnson syndrome (SJS) reported; increased risk with presence of HLA-B*1502 allele. Screen patients with ancestry in genetically at risk populations for the presence of HLA-B*1502 prior to initiation of therapy. Avoid in patients testing (+) for the allele unless benefits clearly outweigh risks. Aplastic anemia and agranulocytosis reported; obtain complete pretreatment hematological testing as a baseline and monitor closely if a patient exhibits low/decreased WBC or platelet counts during treatment. Consider discontinuation if evidence of significant bone marrow depression develops.

OTHER BRAND NAMES

Tegretol, Tegretol-XR, Epitol

ADULT DOSAGE

Trigeminal Neuralgia

Initial (Day 1): 100mg bid (tab/tab, ER) or 1/2 tsp qid sus (200mg/day)
Titrate: May increase by up to 200mg/day using increments of 100mg q12h (tab/tab, ER) or 50mg (1/2 tsp) qid sus prn
Maint: 400-800mg/day. Attempt to reduce dose to minimum effective level or even to d/c therapy at least once every 3 months
Max: 1200mg/day
Beneficial results have also been reported in glossopharyngeal neuralgia

Epilepsy

Partial Seizures w/ Complex Symptomatology (Psychomotor, Temporal Lobe), Generalized Tonic-Clonic Seizures (Grand Mal), and Mixed Seizure Patterns of These, or Other Partial or Generalized Seizures:
Initial: 200mg bid (tab/tab, ER) or 1 tsp qid sus (400mg/day)
Titrate: Increase at weekly intervals by adding up to 200mg/day bid (tab, ER) or tid or qid (all other formulations)
Maint: 800-1200mg/day
Max: 1200mg/day; doses up to 1600mg/day have been used

Combination Therapy:
When added to existing anticonvulsant therapy, add gradually while other anticonvulsants are maintained or gradually decreased (except phenytoin, which may have to be increased)

Conversions

From Oral Carbamazepine Tabs to Carbamazepine Sus:
Patients should be converted by administering the same number of mg per day in smaller, more frequent doses

From Carbamazepine Conventional Tabs to Carbamazepine Extended-Release Tabs:
The same total daily mg dose of carbamazepine ER tabs should be administered

PEDIATRIC DOSAGE

Epilepsy

<6 Years:
Initial: 10-20mg/kg/day bid or tid (tab) or qid (sus)
Titrate: Increase weekly to tid or qid (tab/sus)
Maint: Optimal clinical response is achieved at daily doses <35mg/kg
Max: 35mg/kg/day

6-12 Years:
Initial: 100mg bid (tab/tab, ER) or 1/2 tsp qid (200mg/day) (sus)
Titrate: Increase at weekly intervals by adding up to 100mg/day bid (tab, ER) or tid or qid (all other formulations)
Maint: 400-800mg/day
Max: 1000mg/day

>12 Years:
Initial: 200mg bid (tab/tab, ER) or 1 tsp qid (400mg/day) (sus)
Titrate: Increase at weekly intervals by adding up to 200mg/day bid (tab, ER) or tid or qid (all other formulations)
Maint: 800-1200mg/day
Max:
12-15 Years: 1000mg/day
>15 Years: 1200mg/day

Combination Therapy:
When added to existing anticonvulsant therapy, add gradually while other anticonvulsants are maintained or gradually decreased (except phenytoin, which may have to be increased)

Conversions

From Oral Carbamazepine Tabs to Carbamazepine Sus:
Patients should be converted by administering the same number of mg per day in smaller, more frequent doses

From Carbamazepine Conventional Tab to Carbamazepine Extended-Release Tabs:
The same total daily mg dose of carbamazepine ER tabs should be administered

ADMINISTRATION
Oral route
Take w/ meals

Sus
Do not administer simultaneously w/ other liquid medications or diluents
Shake well before using

Tab, ER
Swallow whole; do not chew or crush

HOW SUPPLIED
Tab, Chewable: 200mg*, (Tegretol) 100mg*; Sus: (Tegretol) 100mg/5mL [450mL]; Tab: (Tegretol, Epitol) 200mg*; Tab, ER: (Tegretol-XR) 100mg, 200mg, 400mg *scored

CONTRAINDICATIONS
History of previous bone marrow depression, sensitivity to any of the tricyclic compounds (eg, amitriptyline, desipramine, imipramine, protriptyline, nortriptyline), coadministration with nefazodone. Concomitant use of an MAOI or within 14 days after discontinuing an MAOI.

WARNINGS/PRECAUTIONS
D/C at 1st sign of rash; do not resume treatment and consider alternative therapy if signs/symptoms suggest SJS/TEN. Consider risks and benefits of therapy in patients known to be (+) for HLA-A*3101. Drug reaction with eosinophilia and systemic symptoms (DRESS), also known as multiorgan hypersensitivity, reported; evaluate immediately if signs/symptoms (eg, fever, lymphadenopathy) are present and d/c if an alternative etiology cannot be established. Caution in patients with history of hypersensitivity reactions to anticonvulsants (eg, phenytoin, primidone, phenobarbital). Increased risk of suicidal thoughts or behavior reported. Has mild anticholinergic activity; closely observe patients with increased intraocular pressure. Consider the possibility of activation of latent psychosis, and confusion or agitation in the elderly. Avoid in patients with history of hepatic porphyria (eg, acute intermittent porphyria, variegate porphyria, porphyria cutanea tarda); acute attacks reported. Withdraw gradually to minimize potential of increased seizure frequency. May cause fetal harm and symptoms representing neonatal withdrawal syndrome. Caution in patients with history of cardiac conduction disturbance, cardiac/hepatic/renal damage, adverse hematologic reactions to drugs, interrupted courses of carbamazepine, and mixed seizure disorder; atrioventricular heart block, hepatic effects, and increased frequency of generalized convulsions reported. D/C if new or worsening clinical/lab evidence of liver dysfunction/hepatic damage, or active liver disease develop. Interference with some pregnancy tests, decreased values of thyroid function tests, hyponatremia, renal dysfunction, and eye changes reported. Higher prevalence of teratogenic effects with the use of anticonvulsants in combination therapy; if therapy is to be continued, monotherapy may be preferable for pregnant women. (Sus/Tab, Chewable 200mg) Contains sorbitol; avoid with rare hereditary problems of fructose intolerance. (Tab, ER) Coating is not absorbed and is excreted in the feces; may be noticeable in the stool.

ADVERSE REACTIONS
Dermatologic reactions, aplastic anemia, agranulocytosis, bone marrow depression, dizziness, drowsiness, unsteadiness, N/V.

DRUG INTERACTIONS
See Contraindications. Close monitoring of carbamazepine levels is indicated and dosage adjustment may be required when given with drugs that increase/decrease levels. CYP3A4 inhibitors (eg, azole antifungals, erythromycin, protease inhibitors) may increase levels. Coadministration of inhibitors of human microsomal epoxide hydrolase may result in increased carbamazepine-10,11 epoxide levels; adjust dose and/or monitor levels of carbamazepine when used with loxapine, quetiapine, or valproic acid. CYP3A4 inducers (eg, cisplatin, doxorubicin, rifampin) may decrease levels. May decrease levels of CYP1A2, 2B6, 2C9/19, and 3A4 substrates; monitoring of concentrations or dosage adjustment of the concomitant agents may be necessary. When added to aripiprazole therapy, double aripiprazole dose and if carbamazepine is later withdrawn, reduce aripiprazole dose. When used with tacrolimus, monitoring of tacrolimus levels and appropriate dosage adjustments are recommended. Avoid with temsirolimus; consider dose adjustment of temsirolimus if coadministration is a must. Avoid with lapatinib; gradually titrate up dose of lapatinib if carbamazepine is started in a patient already taking lapatinib and reduce lapatinib dose when carbamazepine is discontinued. Monitor concentrations of valproate when carbamazepine is introduced or withdrawn in patients using valproic acid. May cause, or would be expected to cause, decreased levels of the following drugs, for which monitoring of concentrations or dosage adjustment may be necessary: acetaminophen, albendazole, alprazolam, aprepitant, buprenorphine, bupropion, citalopram, clonazepam, clozapine, corticosteroids (eg, prednisolone, dexamethasone), cyclosporine, dicumarol, dihydropyridine calcium channel blockers (eg, felodipine), doxycycline, ethosuximide, everolimus, haloperidol, imatinib, itraconazole, lamotrigine, levothyroxine, methadone, methsuximide, mianserin, midazolam, olanzapine, oxcarbazepine, paliperidone, phensuximide, phenytoin, praziquantel, protease inhibitors, risperidone, sertraline, sirolimus, tadalafil, theophylline, tiagabine, topiramate, tramadol, trazodone, TCAs (eg,

imipramine, amitriptyline, nortriptyline), valproate, warfarin, ziprasidone, zonisamide. May increase cyclophosphamide toxicity. May increase risk of neurotoxic side effects with lithium. Increased isoniazid-induced hepatotoxicity reported with isoniazid. May lead to symptomatic hyponatremia with some diuretics (eg, HCTZ, furosemide). Alterations of thyroid function reported with other anticonvulsant medications. May decrease levels of hormonal contraceptive products (eg, oral and levonorgestrel subdermal implant contraceptives) that may render contraceptives less effective; consider alternative or back-up method of contraception. Resistance to the neuromuscular blocking action of the nondepolarizing neuromuscular blocking agents (eg, pancuronium, vecuronium, rocuronium) reported with chronic carbamazepine administration; monitor closely for more rapid recovery from neuromuscular blockade than expected, and infusion rate requirements may be higher. (Sus) Occurrence of stool precipitate reported with liquid chlorpromazine or thioridazine; avoid simultaneous administration with other liquid medicinal agents or diluents.

NURSING CONSIDERATIONS

Assessment: Assess for hypersensitivity to the drug, known sensitivity to any of the tricyclic compounds, mixed seizure disorder, history of cardiac conduction disturbance, renal/hepatic impairment, any other conditions where treatment is contraindicated or cautioned, pregnancy/nursing status, and possible drug interactions. Perform detailed history and physical exam prior to treatment. Screen for HLA-B*1502 and HLA-A*3101 allele in suspected populations. Obtain baseline CBC with platelet and reticulocyte counts, serum iron, LFTs, complete urinalysis, BUN determinations, and eye examination (eg, including slit-lamp exam, funduscopy, and tonometry).

Monitoring: Monitor for signs/symptoms of dermatologic reactions, DRESS, bone marrow depression, aplastic anemia, agranulocytosis, increase in seizure frequency, emergence or worsening of depression, suicidal thoughts/behavior, unusual changes in mood/behavior, latent psychosis, confusion or agitation in elderly patients, hepatic effects, and other adverse reactions. Periodically monitor WBC and platelet counts, LFTs, serum drug levels, complete urinalysis, BUN determinations, and eye examinations.

Patient Counseling: Inform of the early toxic signs and symptoms of a potential hematologic problem, dermatologic, hypersensitivity, or hepatic reactions; advise to report to physician even if the signs and symptoms are mild or when occurring after extended use. Instruct to immediately contact physician if a skin reaction occurs. Counsel about the increased risk of suicidal thoughts and behavior; advise to report behaviors of concern immediately and to be alert for the emergence/worsening of symptoms of depression, any unusual changes in mood or behavior, the emergence of suicidal thoughts, or behavior/thoughts about self-harm. Advise to report the use of any other prescription or nonprescription medications or herbal products. Instruct to exercise caution when taken with alcohol due to a possible additive sedative effect. Inform that drowsiness or dizziness may occur; caution against hazardous tasks. Encourage patients to enroll in the North American Antiepileptic Drug (NAAED) Pregnancy Registry.

Storage: Tab, Chewable: 20-25°C (68-77°F). Protect from light/moisture. (Tegretol) Tab, Chewable: ≤30°C (86°F). Protect from light/moisture. Sus: ≤30°C (86°F). Tab: ≤30°C (86°F). Protect from moisture. Tab, ER: 25°C (77°F); excursions permitted to 15-30°C (59-86°F). Protect from moisture. (Epitol) Tab: 20-25°C (68-77°F). Protect from moisture.

CARDENE IV – nicardipine hydrochloride — RX

Class: Calcium channel blocker (dihydropyridine)

OTHER BRAND NAMES

Cardene IV Premixed

ADULT DOSAGE

Hypertension

Short-term treatment when PO therapy is not feasible or not desirable

Patients Not Receiving Oral Nicardipine:
Initial: 5mg/hr (50mL/hr) IV infusion
Titrate: May increase by 2.5mg/hr (25mL/hr) every 5 min (for rapid titration) to 15 min (for gradual titration) if desired BP reduction is not achieved
Max: 15mg/hr (150mL/hr)
Decrease infusion rate to 3mg/hr (30mL/hr) after BP goal achieved w/ rapid titration
IV Dosage as a Substitute for Oral Nicardipine Therapy:
20mg q8h=0.5mg/hr

PEDIATRIC DOSAGE

Pediatric use may not have been established

30mg q8h=1.2mg/hr
40mg q8h=2.2mg/hr
Transition to Oral Antihypertensives:
Switch to Oral Nicardipine: Give 1st dose 1 hr prior to discontinuation of infusion
Switch to Oral Antihypertensive Other Than Nicardipine: Initiate therapy upon discontinuation of IV nicardipine

DOSE MODIFICATION

Renal Impairment

Titrate gradually

Hepatic Impairment

Impaired Function/Reduced Hepatic Blood Flow: Consider lower dosages

Elderly

Use low initial doses

Other Important Modifications

Heart Failure: Titrate gradually
Premixed:
Impending Hypotension/Tachycardia: D/C then restart at 3-5mg/hr when BP has stabilized and adjust to maintain desired BP

ADMINISTRATION

IV route

Premixed Sol

Do not combine Cardene IV Premixed Inj w/ any product in the same IV line or premixed container
No further dilution is required

Ampules

Administered by slow continuous infusion at a concentration of 0.1mg/mL
Each ampul (25mg) should be diluted w/ 240mL of compatible IV fluid (yielding 250mL of sol at a concentration of 0.1mg/mL

IV Compatibilities

Compatible and stable in glass or polyvinyl chloride containers for 24 hrs at controlled room temperature w/:
D5 inj; D5 and NaCl 0.45% inj; D5 and NaCl 0.9% inj; D5 w/ 40mEq potassium; NaCl 0.45% inj, NaCl 0.9% inj

IV Incompatibilities

Sodium bicarbonate (5%) inj, USP or lactated Ringer's inj, USP

HOW SUPPLIED

Inj: 2.5mg/mL [10mL], 0.1mg/mL [200mL], 0.2mg/mL [200mL]

CONTRAINDICATIONS

Advanced aortic stenosis.

WARNINGS/PRECAUTIONS

May induce or exacerbate angina in coronary artery disease (CAD) patients. Caution with heart failure (HF) or significant left ventricular dysfunction. To reduce possibility of venous thrombosis, phlebitis, local irritation, swelling, extravasation, and occurrence of vascular impairment, administer through large peripheral or central veins; change IV site q12h to minimize risk of peripheral venous irritation. May occasionally produce symptomatic hypotension or tachycardia. Avoid systemic hypotension when administering in sustained acute cerebral infarction or hemorrhage. Caution in hepatic/renal impairment, reduced hepatic blood flow, and in elderly.

ADVERSE REACTIONS

Headache, hypotension, tachycardia, N/V.

DRUG INTERACTIONS

Titrate slowly with β-blockers in HF or significant left ventricular dysfunction due to possible negative inotropic effects. Increased nicardipine levels when oral nicardipine is given with cimetidine; frequently monitor response. Elevated cyclosporine levels reported with oral nicardipine; closely monitor cyclosporine levels and reduce its dose accordingly.

NURSING CONSIDERATIONS

Assessment: Assess for advanced aortic stenosis, HF, CAD, left ventricular dysfunction, sustained acute cerebral infarction or hemorrhage, hepatic/renal impairment, pregnancy/nursing status, and possible drug interactions.

Monitoring: Monitor for symptomatic hypotension, tachycardia, induction or exacerbation of angina, and other adverse reactions. Monitor BP and HR during administration. Closely monitor responses with impaired liver function or reduced hepatic blood flow.

Patient Counseling: Advise to seek medical attention if adverse reactions occur.

Storage: 20-25°C (68-77°F). Avoid excessive heat. Protect from light. Diluted Sol: Stable at room temperature for 24 hrs. Premixed: Protect from freezing.

CARDENE SR – nicardipine hydrochloride RX

Class: Calcium channel blocker (dihydropyridine)

ADULT DOSAGE

Hypertension

Initial: 30mg bid
Titrate: Adjust according to BP response
Effective Dose Range: 30-60mg bid

Currently on Nicardipine Immediate-Release (IR):
Titrate w/ Cardene SR starting at current total daily dose of IR; reexamine adequacy of BP control

PEDIATRIC DOSAGE

Pediatric use may not have been established

DOSE MODIFICATION

Renal Impairment
Carefully titrate dose

Elderly
Start at lower end of dosing range

ADMINISTRATION

Oral route

HOW SUPPLIED

Cap, Sustained-Release (SR): 30mg, 60mg

CONTRAINDICATIONS

Advanced aortic stenosis.

WARNINGS/PRECAUTIONS

Increased frequency, duration, or severity of angina reported with nicardipine IR. Caution with congestive heart failure (CHF), particularly in combination with β-blocker and during dose titration. Not a β-blocker and therefore gives no protection against dangers of abrupt β-blocker withdrawal; reduce dose of β-blocker gradually (preferably over 8-10 days). May occasionally produce symptomatic hypotension. Avoid systemic hypotension when administering in patients who have sustained an acute cerebral infarction or hemorrhage. Measure BP 2-4 hrs after the 1st dose or dose increase and at the end of a dosing interval. Caution with hepatic/renal impairment, reduced hepatic blood flow, and in elderly.

ADVERSE REACTIONS

Headache, pedal edema, vasodilatation, dizziness, asthenia.

DRUG INTERACTIONS

May increase levels with cimetidine; monitor carefully. May elevate plasma cyclosporine levels; closely monitor cyclosporine levels and reduce its dose accordingly. May increase serum digoxin levels; evaluate serum digoxin levels after concomitant therapy is initiated. Caution with fentanyl anesthesia.

NURSING CONSIDERATIONS

Assessment: Assess for advanced aortic stenosis, angina, CHF, acute cerebral infarction or hemorrhage, hepatic/renal impairment, reduced hepatic blood flow, pregnancy/nursing status, and possible drug interactions.

Monitoring: Monitor for signs/symptoms of increased angina, symptomatic hypotension, and other adverse reactions. Monitor BP during the initiation and titration.

Patient Counseling: Inform of the risks/benefits of therapy. Advise to seek medical attention if adverse reactions occur.

Storage: 15-30°C (59-86°F).

Cardizem CD – diltiazem hydrochloride RX

Class: Calcium channel blocker (nondihydropyridine)

OTHER BRAND NAMES
Cartia XT, Cardizem LA

ADULT DOSAGE

Hypertension

Cardizem CD, Cartia XT:
Initial (Monotherapy): 180-240mg qd
Titrate: Adjust to individual patient needs (schedule accordingly)
Usual Range: 240-360mg qd
Max: 480mg qd
Cardizem LA:
Initial (Monotherapy): 180-240mg qd (am or hs)
Titrate: Adjust to individual patient needs (schedule accordingly)
Usual Range: 120-540mg qd
Max: 540mg/day

Angina

Chronic Stable Angina and Angina Due to Coronary Artery Spasm:
Cardizem CD, Cartia XT:
Initial: 120mg or 180mg qd
Titrate: Adjust to each patient's needs; may be carried out over a 7- to 14-day period when necessary
Max: 480mg qd
Chronic Stable Angina:
Cardizem LA:
Initial: 180mg qd (am or pm)
Titrate: Increase at 1- to 2-week intervals
Max: 360mg

PEDIATRIC DOSAGE
Pediatric use may not have been established

DOSE MODIFICATION

Concomitant Medications

Other Antihypertensives:
Diltiazem HCl or the concomitant antihypertensives may need to be adjusted when adding one to the other

Elderly
Start at lower end of dosing range

ADMINISTRATION
Oral route

Cardizem LA
Swallow whole; do not chew or crush

HOW SUPPLIED
Cap, ER (Cardizem CD, Cartia XT) 120mg, 180mg, 240mg, 300mg, (Cardizem CD) 360mg; Tab, ER: (Cardizem LA) 120mg, 180mg, 240mg, 300mg, 360mg, 420mg

CONTRAINDICATIONS
Sick sinus syndrome and 2nd- or 3rd-degree AV block (except with functioning ventricular pacemaker), hypotension (<90mmHg systolic), acute MI, and pulmonary congestion documented by x-rays on admission.

WARNINGS/PRECAUTIONS
Prolongs AV node refractory periods without significantly prolonging sinus node recovery time. Periods of asystole reported in a patient with Prinzmetal's angina. Worsening of congestive heart failure reported in patients with preexisting ventricular dysfunction. Symptomatic hypotension may occur. Mild transaminase elevation with or without concomitant alkaline phosphatase and bilirubin elevation reported. Significant enzyme elevations and other phenomena consistent with acute hepatic injury reported in rare instances. Caution with renal/hepatic dysfunction. Dermatologic reactions (eg, erythema multiforme, exfoliative dermatitis) may occur; d/c if such reaction persists. Caution in elderly.

ADVERSE REACTIONS
Dizziness, bradycardia, 1st-degree AV block. (CD, Cartia XT) Headache, edema. (LA) Edema lower limb, fatigue.

DRUG INTERACTIONS

May increase levels of propranolol, carbamazepine, quinidine, midazolam, triazolam, buspirone, and lovastatin. Increased levels with cimetidine. Monitor digoxin and cyclosporine levels. Depression of cardiac contractility, conductivity, automaticity, and vascular dilation potentiated with anesthetics. Additive cardiac conduction effects with digitalis or β-blockers. Potential additive effects with agents known to affect cardiac contractility and/or conduction; caution and careful titration warranted. May have significant impact on efficacy and side effect profile with CYP450 3A4 substrates, inducers, and inhibitors. Avoid with CYP3A4 inducers (eg, rifampin). (CD, LA) Sinus bradycardia resulting in hospitalization and pacemaker insertion reported with clonidine; monitor HR. Increased exposure of simvastatin; limit daily doses of both agents. Risk of myopathy and rhabdomyolysis with statins metabolized by CYP3A4 may be increased; monitor closely.

NURSING CONSIDERATIONS

Assessment: Assess for sick sinus syndrome, 2nd- or 3rd-degree AV block, hypotension, acute MI and pulmonary congestion, ventricular dysfunction, hepatic/renal impairment, pregnancy/nursing status, and possible drug interactions.

Monitoring: Monitor for bradycardia, AV block, symptomatic hypotension, and dermatological reactions. Perform regular monitoring of liver and renal function.

Patient Counseling: Counsel to report any adverse reactions to physician and to notify physician if pregnant or nursing. Instruct to swallow tab whole; do not chew or crush.

Storage: 25°C (77°F); excursions permitted to 15-30°C (59-86°F) (CD, LA); 20-25°C (68-77°F) (Cartia XT). Avoid excessive humidity and (LA) temperature >30°C (86°F).

CARDURA — doxazosin mesylate

RX

Class: Alpha$_1$-blocker (quinazoline)

ADULT DOSAGE

Hypertension

Initial: 1mg qd (am or pm)
Titrate: May increase to 2mg and thereafter if necessary to 4mg, 8mg, and 16mg qd depending on standing BP response

Benign Prostatic Hyperplasia

Initial: 1mg qd (am or pm)
Titrate: May increase to 2mg and thereafter to 4mg, and 8mg qd in 1- to 2-week intervals, depending on urodynamics and BPH symptomatology
Max: 8mg qd

PEDIATRIC DOSAGE

Pediatric use may not have been established

DOSE MODIFICATION

Elderly

Start at lower end of dosing range

ADMINISTRATION

Oral route

HOW SUPPLIED

Tab: 1mg*, 2mg*, 4mg*, 8mg* *scored

WARNINGS/PRECAUTIONS

May cause syncope and orthostatic hypotension (eg, dizziness, lightheadedness, vertigo), especially with 1st dose, dose increase, or if therapy is interrupted for more than a few days; restart using initial dosing regimen if therapy was discontinued for several days. Rule out carcinoma of the prostate prior to therapy. Priapism (rare) and leukopenia/neutropenia reported. Intraoperative floppy iris syndrome (IFIS) observed during cataract surgery. Caution with hepatic impairment and in the elderly.

ADVERSE REACTIONS

Dizziness, headache, fatigue/malaise, somnolence, edema, nausea, rhinitis.

DRUG INTERACTIONS

Caution with additional antihypertensive agents and drugs known to influence hepatic metabolism. Additive BP-lowering effects and symptomatic hypotension with PDE-5 inhibitors.

NURSING CONSIDERATIONS

Assessment: Assess for previous sensitivity to drug/quinazolines, hepatic impairment, prostate cancer, pregnancy/nursing status, and possible drug interactions.

Monitoring: Monitor for signs/symptoms of orthostatic hypotension, syncope, priapism, IFIS during cataract surgery, and other adverse reactions. Measure BP periodically, particularly 2-6 hrs after the 1st dose and with each increase in dose.

Patient Counseling: Inform of the possibility of syncopal and orthostatic symptoms, especially at the initiation of therapy; urge to avoid driving or hazardous tasks for 24 hrs after the 1st dose, dose increase, and interruption of therapy when treatment is resumed. Caution to avoid situations where injury could result should syncope occur. Advise to sit or lie down when symptoms of low BP occur. Instruct to report to physician if dizziness, lightheadedness, or palpitations are bothersome. Advise of possibility of priapism and to seek immediate medical attention if this occurs. Counsel to inform surgeon of drug use prior to cataract surgery.

Storage: 25°C (77°F); excursions permitted to 15-30°C (59-86°F).

CASODEX – bicalutamide

RX

Class: Nonsteroidal antiandrogen

ADULT DOSAGE

D_2 Metastatic Prostate Carcinoma

Combination w/ Luteinizing Hormone-Releasing Hormone (LHRH) Analogue:
50mg qd (am or pm) at the same time as LHRH analogue

Missed Dose

If a dose is missed, take the next dose at the scheduled time; do not take the missed dose and do not double the next dose

PEDIATRIC DOSAGE

Pediatric use may not have been established

ADMINISTRATION

Oral route
Take w/ or w/o food
Take at the same time each day

HOW SUPPLIED

Tab: 50mg

CONTRAINDICATIONS

Women, pregnancy.

WARNINGS/PRECAUTIONS

Death or hospitalization due to severe liver injury (hepatic failure) reported. Hepatitis or marked increases in liver enzymes leading to discontinuation reported. Measure serum ALT immediately if signs/symptoms of liver dysfunction occur; d/c immediately w/ close follow-up of liver function if jaundice occurs or ALT rises >2X ULN. Reduction in glucose tolerance reported. Regularly assess serum prostate-specific antigen (PSA) to monitor response; evaluate for clinical progression if PSA levels rise during therapy. For patients w/ objective disease progression w/ an elevated PSA, consider a treatment period free of antiandrogen while continuing the LHRH analogue. Caution w/ moderate-severe hepatic impairment.

ADVERSE REACTIONS

Pain, hot flashes, asthenia, infection, back pain, constipation, nausea, diarrhea, anemia, peripheral edema, dizziness, dyspnea, rash, nocturia, hematuria.

DRUG INTERACTIONS

Can displace coumarin anticoagulants from binding sites; closely monitor PT and consider anticoagulant dose adjustment. Caution w/ CYP3A4 substrates. May increase levels of midazolam.

NURSING CONSIDERATIONS

Assessment: Assess for drug hypersensitivity, diabetes, hepatic impairment, and possible drug interactions. Measure serum transaminase levels.

Monitoring: Measure serum transaminase levels at regular intervals for the first 4 months of treatment, then periodically thereafter. Measure serum ALT for signs/symptoms of liver dysfunction. Monitor LFTs in hepatically impaired patients on long-term therapy. Regularly monitor serum PSA levels. Monitor blood glucose levels.

Patient Counseling: Advise not to interrupt or d/c medication w/o consulting physician. Inform that somnolence may occur; advise to use caution when driving or operating machinery. Advise to monitor blood glucose levels while on therapy. Inform that photosensitivity has been reported during treatment; advise to avoid direct exposure to excessive sunlight or UV-light exposure and to consider using sunscreen.

Storage: 20-25°C (68-77°F).

CATAFLAM – diclofenac potassium

RX

Class: NSAID

NSAIDs may cause an increased risk of serious cardiovascular (CV) thrombotic events, MI, stroke, and serious GI adverse events, including bleeding, ulceration, and perforation of the stomach or intestines. Contraindicated for the treatment of perioperative pain in the setting of CABG surgery.

ADULT DOSAGE

Osteoarthritis

100-150mg/day in divided doses, 50mg bid or tid

Rheumatoid Arthritis

150-200mg/day in divided doses, 50mg tid or qid

Mild to Moderate Pain

50mg tid; may give initial dose of 100mg followed by 50mg doses in some

Primary Dysmenorrhea

50mg tid; may give initial dose of 100mg followed by 50-mg doses in some

PEDIATRIC DOSAGE

Pediatric use may not have been established

ADMINISTRATION

Oral route

HOW SUPPLIED

Tab: 50mg

CONTRAINDICATIONS

Aspirin (ASA) or other NSAID allergy that precipitates asthma, urticaria, or allergic reactions. Treatment of perioperative pain in the setting of CABG surgery.

WARNINGS/PRECAUTIONS

May lead to onset of new HTN or worsening of preexisting HTN; monitor BP closely. Fluid retention and edema reported; caution in patients with fluid retention or heart failure (HF). Caution with history of ulcer disease or GI bleeding. Caution in patients with considerable dehydration. Renal papillary necrosis and other renal injury reported after long-term use. Caution with impaired renal function, HF, liver dysfunction, and the elderly. Not recommended for use with advanced renal disease; if therapy must be initiated, monitor renal function. May cause elevations of LFTs; d/c if liver disease develops or systemic manifestations occur. Anaphylactoid reactions may occur. May cause serious skin adverse events (eg, exfoliative dermatitis, Stevens-Johnson syndrome, toxic epidermal necrolysis). Avoid in late pregnancy; may cause premature closure of ductus arteriosus. Not a substitute for corticosteroids or for the treatment of corticosteroid insufficiency. Anemia may occur; with long-term use, monitor Hgb/Hct if signs or symptoms of anemia develop. May inhibit platelet aggregation and prolong bleeding time; monitor with coagulation disorders. Caution with asthma and avoid with ASA-sensitive asthma.

ADVERSE REACTIONS

Dyspepsia, constipation, diarrhea, GI ulceration/perforation, N/V, flatulence, abnormal renal function, anemia, dizziness, edema, elevated liver enzymes, headache, increased bleeding time, rash, tinnitus.

DRUG INTERACTIONS

Avoid use with ASA. May enhance methotrexate toxicity; caution when coadministering. May increase nephrotoxicity of cyclosporine; caution when coadministering. May diminish antihypertensive effect of ACE inhibitors. May reduce natriuretic effect of furosemide and thiazides; monitor for renal failure. May increase lithium levels; monitor for toxicity. Synergistic effects on GI bleeding with warfarin. Caution with hepatotoxic drugs (eg, antibiotics, antiepileptics). Increased risk of GI bleeding with concomitant oral corticosteroids, anticoagulants, or alcohol. ACE inhibitors and diuretics may increase the risk of overt renal decompensation.

NURSING CONSIDERATIONS

Assessment: Assess for history of a hypersensitivity reaction to ASA or other NSAIDs, asthma, cardiovascular disease (CVD) (eg, preexisting HTN, congestive heart failure) or risk factors for CVD, risk factors for a GI event (eg, prior history of ulcer disease or GI disease, smoking), fluid retention, renal/hepatic dysfunction, coagulation disorders, pregnancy/nursing status, and for possible drug interactions. Assess baseline LFTs, renal function, and CBC.

Monitoring: Monitor for signs/symptoms of CV thrombotic events, new onset or worsening of preexisting HTN, GI events (eg, inflammation, bleeding, ulceration, perforation), fluid retention and edema, renal effects (eg, renal papillary necrosis), hepatic effects (eg, jaundice, liver necrosis, liver failure), anaphylactoid reactions, skin reactions (eg, exfoliative dermatitis, Stevens-Johnson syndrome, toxic epidermal necrolysis), hematological effects (eg, anemia, prolongation of bleeding time), and for bronchospasm. Monitor BP. Perform periodic monitoring of CBC, renal function, and LFTs.

Patient Counseling: Instruct to seek medical attention for symptoms of hepatotoxicity (eg, nausea, fatigue, jaundice), anaphylactic reactions (eg, difficulty breathing, swelling of the face/throat), rash, CV events (eg, chest pain, SOB, weakness, slurring of speech), or if unexplained weight gain or edema occurs. Inform of risks if used during pregnancy.

Storage: Do not store at >30°C (86°F). Dispense in tight container.

CATAPRES – clonidine

RX

Class: Alpha-adrenergic agonist

OTHER BRAND NAMES

Catapres-TTS

ADULT DOSAGE

Hypertension

Tab:
Initial: 0.1mg bid (am and hs)
Maint: May increase by 0.1mg/day at weekly intervals prn until desired response is achieved
Usual: 0.2-0.6mg/day in divided doses
Max: 2.4mg/day

Patch:
Initial: Apply 1 patch every 7 days; start w/ TTS-1
Titrate: If inadequate reduction in BP after 1-2 weeks, increase dosage by adding another TTS-1 or changing to a larger system

No usual additional efficacy w/ dose increase above 2 TTS-3

When substituting for PO clonidine or other antihypertensives, gradually reduce prior drug dose; effect of patch may not commence until 2-3 days after initial application

PEDIATRIC DOSAGE

Pediatric use may not have been established

DOSE MODIFICATION

Renal Impairment
Patch/Tab:
May benefit from lower initial dose

Elderly
Tab:
May benefit from lower initial dose

ADMINISTRATION

Tab
Oral route

Patch
Transdermal route
Apply to hairless area of intact skin of upper outer arm or chest once every 7 days
Apply each new patch on different skin site from previous location
If the system loosens during 7-day wearing, the adhesive cover should be applied directly over the system to ensure good adhesion

HOW SUPPLIED

Patch, Extended-Release (TTS): (TTS-1) 0.1mg, (TTS-2) 0.2mg, (TTS-3) 0.3mg; Tab: 0.1mg, 0.2mg, 0.3mg

WARNINGS/PRECAUTIONS

Sudden cessation of treatment may cause nervousness, agitation, headache, confusion, and tremor accompanied or followed by a rapid rise in BP and elevated catecholamine concentrations; if discontinuing therapy, reduce dose gradually over 2 to 4 days to avoid withdrawal symptoms. Rare instances of hypertensive encephalopathy, cerebrovascular accidents (CVAs), and death reported after withdrawal. Continuation of clonidine transdermal system or substitution to PO may cause generalized skin rash and elicit an allergic reaction if with localized contact sensitization or allergic reaction to clonidine transdermal system. Monitor BP during surgery; additional measures to control BP should be available. No therapeutic effect can be expected in HTN caused by pheochromocytoma. May worsen sinus node dysfunction and atrioventricular (AV) block, especially with other sympatholytic drugs; patients with conduction abnormalities and/or taking other sympatholytic drugs may develop severe bradycardia. (Tab) Continue administration to within 4 hrs of surgery and resume as soon as possible thereafter. (Patch) Loss of BP control reported (rare). Do not remove during surgery. Remove before defibrillation or cardioversion due to potential for altered electrical conductivity, and before undergoing an MRI due to the occurrence of skin burns.

ADVERSE REACTIONS

Dry mouth, drowsiness, dizziness, constipation, sedation.

DRUG INTERACTIONS

May potentiate CNS depressive effects of alcohol, barbiturates, or other sedating drugs. Hypotensive effect may be reduced by TCAs; may need to increase clonidine dose. Neuroleptics may induce or exacerbate orthostatic regulation disturbances (eg, orthostatic hypotension, dizziness, fatigue). Monitor HR with agents that affect sinus node function or AV nodal conduction (eg, digitalis, calcium channel blockers, β-blockers). D/C concurrent β-blockers several days before the gradual withdrawal of clonidine. Reports of sinus bradycardia and pacemaker insertion with diltiazem or verapamil. High IV doses of clonidine may increase the arrhythmogenic potential (QT prolongation, ventricular fibrillation) of high IV doses of haloperidol as observed in patients in a state of alcoholic delirium.

NURSING CONSIDERATIONS

Assessment: Assess for pheochromocytoma, renal impairment, allergic reactions/contact sensitization, pregnancy/nursing status, and for possible drug interactions.

Monitoring: Monitor BP and renal function periodically. Monitor for withdrawal signs/symptoms (eg, hypertensive encephalopathy, CVA), presence of generalized skin rash, and allergic reactions.

Patient Counseling: Caution patients against interrupting therapy without physician's advice and engaging in hazardous activities (eg, driving, operating appliances/machinery). Inform that sedative effect may be increased by concomitant use of alcohol, barbiturates, or other sedating drugs. Caution patients who wear contact lenses that drug may cause dryness of eyes. (Patch) Instruct to consult physician promptly about possible need to remove or replace patch if skin reactions develop. Inform that if patch begins to loosen, place adhesive cover directly over the patch to ensure adhesion for 7 days total. Advise to keep used and unused patch out of reach of children; instruct to fold in half with adhesive sides together and discard.

Storage: (Patch) Below 30°C (86°F). (Tab) 25°C (77°F); excursions permitted to 15-30°C (59-86°F).

CEFACLOR – cefaclor

RX

Class: Cephalosporin (2nd generation)

ADULT DOSAGE

General Dosing

Otitis media, pharyngitis, tonsillitis, and lower respiratory tract/urinary tract/skin and skin structure infections caused by susceptible strains of microorganisms

Usual: 250mg q8h

May double the dose for more severe infections (eg, pneumonia) or those caused by less susceptible organisms

β-Hemolytic Streptococcal Infections:

Administer for at least 10 days

PEDIATRIC DOSAGE

General Dosing

≥1 Month of Age:

20mg/kg/day q8h in divided doses

For pharyngitis total daily dosage may be divided and administered q12h

β-Hemolytic Streptococcal Infections:

Administer for at least 10 days

Acute Otitis Media

≥1 Month of Age:

40mg/kg/day q8h in divided doses

Max: 1g/day

Alternatively, total daily dosage may be divided and administered q12h

Serious Infections

≥1 Month of Age:

40mg/kg/day q8h in divided doses

Max: 1g/day

ADMINISTRATION

Oral route

Sus

Shake well before using

Add appropriate water volume in 2 portions to dry mixture in bottle; shake well after each addition
Refer to PI for appropriate water volume

HOW SUPPLIED

Cap: 250mg, 500mg; Sus: 125mg/5mL [75mL, 150mL], 187mg/5mL [50mL, 100mL], 250mg/5mL [75mL, 150mL], 375mg/5mL [50mL, 100mL]

WARNINGS/PRECAUTIONS

Caution in penicillin (PCN)-sensitive patients; cross-hypersensitivity among β-lactam antibiotics may occur. D/C if an allergic reaction occurs; serious acute hypersensitivity reactions may require treatment with epinephrine and other emergency measures as clinically indicated. *Clostridium difficile*-associated diarrhea (CDAD) (Sus)/Pseudomembranous colitis (Cap) reported. Consider CDAD/pseudomembranous colitis if diarrhea occurs. Institute appropriate fluid and electrolyte management, protein supplementation, antibiotic treatment of *C. difficile*, and surgical evaluation, as clinically indicated. Use in the absence of a proven or strongly suspected bacterial infection or prophylactic indication is unlikely to provide benefit and increases the risk of development of drug-resistant bacteria. May result in overgrowth of nonsusceptible organisms with prolonged use; take appropriate measures if superinfection develops. Lab test interactions may occur. Caution with markedly impaired renal function, history of GI disease particularly colitis, and in elderly. (Sus) If CDAD is suspected or confirmed, ongoing antibiotic use not directed against *C. difficile* may need to be discontinued.

ADVERSE REACTIONS

GI symptoms, hypersensitivity reactions, eosinophilia, genital pruritus, moniliasis, vaginitis, serum-sickness-like reactions.

DRUG INTERACTIONS

Renal excretion inhibited by probenecid. May increase anticoagulant effect of oral anticoagulants. (Cap) Concomitant use with warfarin may increase PT.

NURSING CONSIDERATIONS

Assessment: Assess for hypersensitivity to cephalosporins/PCNs/other drugs, history of GI disease (particularly colitis), renal impairment, pregnancy/nursing status, and possible drug interactions. Perform appropriate culture and susceptibility tests to determine susceptible causative organisms.

Monitoring: Monitor for hypersensitivity reactions, CDAD/pseudomembranous colitis, development of superinfection or drug resistance, and other adverse reactions. Monitor renal function in the elderly and those with markedly impaired renal function. Monitor PT with warfarin.

Patient Counseling: Inform that drug only treats bacterial, not viral infections. Instruct to take exactly ud and that skipping doses or not completing full course of therapy may decrease effectiveness and increase the likelihood of bacterial resistance. (Sus) Instruct to contact physician as soon as possible if watery/bloody stools (with/without stomach cramps and fever) develop, even as late as 2 months after discontinuation.

Storage: 20-25°C (68-77°F). Diluted Sol: Store in refrigerator after mixing. Discard unused portion after 14 days.

CEFACLOR ER – cefaclor

RX

Class: Cephalosporin (2nd generation)

ADULT DOSAGE

Acute Bacterial Exacerbation of Chronic Bronchitis

Due to *Haemophilus influenzae* (non-β-lactamase-producing strains only), *Moraxella catarrhalis* (including β-lactamase-producing strains), or *Streptococcus pneumoniae*

≥16 Years:
500mg q12h for 7 days

Bronchitis

Secondary bacterial infection of acute bronchitis due to *Haemophilus influenzae* (non-β-lactamase producing strains only), *Moraxella catarrhalis* (including β-lactamase-producing strains), or *Streptococcus pneumoniae*

≥16 Years:
500mg q12h for 7 days

PEDIATRIC DOSAGE

Pediatric use may not have been established

Pharyngitis/Tonsillitis

Due to *Streptococcus pyogenes*:
≥16 Years:
375mg q12h for 10 days

Skin and Skin Structure Infections

Uncomplicated Infections Due to *Staphylococcus aureus* (Methicillin-Susceptible):
≥16 Years:
375mg q12h for 7-10 days

ADMINISTRATION
Oral route

Take w/ meals (at least w/in 1 hr of eating)
Do not crush, cut, or chew tab

HOW SUPPLIED
Tab, Extended-Release: 500mg

WARNINGS/PRECAUTIONS
Cross-sensitivity among β-lactam antibiotics reported; caution with penicillin (PCN) allergy. D/C if allergic reaction occurs and institute appropriate therapy. *Clostridium difficile*-associated diarrhea (CDAD) reported. May result in bacterial resistance with prolonged use or use in the absence of a proven/suspected bacterial infection or a prophylactic indication; take appropriate measures if superinfection develops. Lab test interactions may occur.

ADVERSE REACTIONS
Headache, rhinitis, diarrhea, nausea

DRUG INTERACTIONS
Decreased absorption with magnesium or aluminum hydroxide-containing antacids. Renal excretion inhibited by probenecid. Concomitant use with warfarin may increase PT.

NURSING CONSIDERATIONS

Assessment: Assess for hypersensitivity reactions to the drug, cephalosporins, PCNs, other drugs, pregnancy/nursing status, and possible drug interactions. Perform appropriate culture and susceptibility tests for diagnosis and identification of causative organisms.

Monitoring: Monitor for allergic reactions, CDAD, superinfection, and drug resistance.

Patient Counseling: Instruct to take ud and that skipping doses or not completing full course may decrease effectiveness and increase resistance. Inform that diarrhea may occur but that it usually ends once treatment is completed. Instruct to notify physician as soon as possible if watery and bloody stools (with/without stomach cramps and fever) develop, even as late as ≥2 months after taking last dose.

Storage: 20-25°C (68-77°F). Store in a tight, light-resistant container.

CEFADROXIL – cefadroxil RX

Class: Cephalosporin (1st generation)

ADULT DOSAGE

Urinary Tract Infections

Uncomplicated Lower UTIs (eg, Cystitis):
Usual: 1 or 2g/day given qd or bid

Other UTIs:
Usual: 2g/day given bid

Skin and Skin Structure Infections

Usual: 1g/day given qd or bid

Tonsillitis and/or Pharyngitis

Caused by Group A β-Hemolytic Streptococci:
1g/day given qd or bid for 10 days

PEDIATRIC DOSAGE

Urinary Tract Infections

Usual: 30mg/kg/day in divided doses q12h

Skin and Skin Structure Infections

Impetigo:
Usual: 30mg/kg/day given qd or in equally divided doses q12h

Other SSSIs:
Usual: 30mg/kg/day in divided doses q12h

Tonsillitis and/or Pharyngitis

Usual: 30mg/kg/day given qd or in equally divided doses q12h

Streptococcal Infections

β-Hemolytic Infections:
Administer for at least 10 days

DOSE MODIFICATION

Renal Impairment

Adults:

Initial: 1g

Maint:

CrCl 25-50mL/min: 500mg q12h

CrCl 10-25mL/min: 500mg q24h

CrCl 0-10mL/min: 500mg q36h

ADMINISTRATION

Oral route

Take w/o regard to meals

Sus

Suspend 50mL bottle size in a total of 34mL water, 75mL bottle size in a total of 51mL water, 100mL bottle size in a total of 67mL water; add water in two portions and shake well after each addition

Shake well before using

Refer to PI for daily dosage of oral sus

HOW SUPPLIED

Cap: 500mg; Sus: 250mg/5mL [50mL, 100mL], 500mg/5mL [50mL, 75mL, 100mL]; Tab: 1000mg*
*scored

WARNINGS/PRECAUTIONS

Caution in penicillin (PCN)-sensitive patients; cross-sensitivity among β-lactam antibiotics may occur. D/C if an allergic reaction occurs. *Clostridium difficile*-associated diarrhea (CDAD) reported; may need to d/c if CDAD is suspected or confirmed. Caution w/ renal impairment (CrCl <50mL/min); monitor prior to and during therapy. May result in bacterial resistance if used in the absence of proven or suspected bacterial infection, or a prophylactic indication. May result in overgrowth of nonsusceptible organisms w/ prolonged use; take appropriate measures if superinfection develops. Caution w/ history of GI disease, particularly colitis. Lab test interactions may occur. D/C if seizures associated w/ drug therapy occur. Caution in elderly.

ADVERSE REACTIONS

Diarrhea, allergies, hepatic dysfunction, genital moniliasis, vaginitis, moderate transient neutropenia, fever, toxic epidermal necrolysis, abdominal pain, superinfection, renal dysfunction, toxic nephropathy, aplastic anemia, hemolytic anemia, hemorrhage.

NURSING CONSIDERATIONS

Assessment: Assess for allergy to other cephalosporins, PCN, or to other drugs, renal impairment, history of GI disease, and pregnancy/nursing status. Initiate culture and susceptibility tests prior to therapy.

Monitoring: Monitor for signs/symptoms of an allergic reaction, CDAD, seizure, and superinfection. Carefully observe patients w/ known or suspected renal impairment.

Patient Counseling: Inform that therapy only treats bacterial, not viral, infections. Instruct to take exactly ud; inform that skipping doses or not completing full course of therapy may decrease effectiveness and increase risk of bacterial resistance. Inform that diarrhea is a common problem that usually ends upon discontinuation. Instruct to notify physician as soon as possible if watery and bloody stools (w/ or w/o stomach cramps/fever) occur, even as late as ≥2 months after last dose.

Storage: (Cap/Tab) 20-25°C (68-77°F). (Sus) Before Reconstitution: 25°C (77°F); excursions permitted to 15-30°C (59-86°F). After Reconstitution: Store in refrigerator; discard unused portion after 14 days.

CEFAZOLIN – cefazolin — RX

Class: Cephalosporin (1st generation)

ADULT DOSAGE

Moderate to Severe Infections

Respiratory tract, skin and skin structure, biliary tract, bone and joint, and genital infections caused by susceptible strains of microorganisms

500mg-1g IV/IM q6-8h

Mild Infections

Caused by Gram-Positive Cocci:

250-500mg IV/IM q8h

PEDIATRIC DOSAGE

General Dosing

>1 Month of Age:

Mild to Moderately Severe Infections:

25-50mg/kg/day IV/IM, divided tid or qid in equal doses

Severe Infections:

May increase to 100mg/kg/day IV/IM

Urinary Tract Infections

Acute/Uncomplicated:
1g IV/IM q12h

Pneumonia

Pneumococcal Pneumonia:
500mg IV/IM q12h

Severe Infections

Severe/Life-Threatening Infections (eg, Endocarditis, Septicemia):
1-1.5g IV/IM q6h; doses up to 12g/day have been used in rare instances

Prophylaxis of Postoperative Infections

Preoperative:
1g IV/IM or 2g IV, 0.5-1 hr prior to surgery
Lengthy Procedures (eg, ≥2 Hrs):
500mg-1g IV/IM during surgery
Postoperative:
500mg-1g IV/IM q6-8h for 24 hrs
D/C w/in 24 hrs after the surgical procedure; continue for 3-5 days after the completion of surgery where occurrence of infection may be particularly devastating (eg, open-heart surgery, prosthetic arthroplasty)

DOSE MODIFICATION

Renal Impairment
Apply reduced dosage recommendations after initial LD is given
Adults:
CrCl 35-54mL/min: Full dose q8h or longer
CrCl 11-34mL/min: 1/2 usual dose q12h
CrCl ≤10mL/min: 1/2 usual dose q18-24h
Pediatrics:
CrCl 41-70mL/min: 60% of usual dose given in equally divided doses q12h
CrCl 21-40mL/min: 25% of usual dose given in equally divided doses q12h
CrCl ≤5-20mL/min: 10% of usual dose given in equally divided doses q24h

ADMINISTRATION

IV/IM route
Shake well

Preparation
Reconstitute 500mg or 1g vial size w/ 2mL or 2.5mL of sterile water for inj (SWFI) respectively, for a concentration of 225mg/mL (500g vial) or 330mg/mL (1g vial)

IM
Shake well until dissolved
Inject into a large muscle mass

IV
Direct (Bolus) Inj:
Further dilute reconstituted sol w/ 5mL SWFI
Inject sol slowly over 3-5 min directly or through tubing in patients receiving parenteral fluids
Intermittent/Continuous Infusion:
Dilute reconstituted sol in 50-100mL of a compatible IV sol

Compatible IV Sol
NaCl inj, D5 or D10 inj, D5 in lactated Ringer's inj, D5 and 0.9% NaCl inj, D5 and 0.45% NaCl inj, D5 and 0.2% NaCl inj, lactated Ringer's inj, invert sugar 5% or 10% in SWFI, Ringer's inj, 5% sodium bicarbonate inj

HOW SUPPLIED

Inj: 500mg, 1g

WARNINGS/PRECAUTIONS

Caution with penicillin (PCN)-sensitive patients; cross-hypersensitivity among β-lactam antibiotics may occur. D/C if an allergic reaction occurs. *Clostridium difficile*-associated diarrhea (CDAD) reported; d/c if CDAD suspected or confirmed. Institute appropriate fluid and electrolyte management, protein supplementation, antibacterial drug treatment of *C. difficile*, and surgical evaluation as clinically indicated. Use in the absence of a proven or strongly suspected bacterial infection or prophylactic indication is unlikely to provide benefit and increases the risk of the development of drug-resistant bacteria. May result in overgrowth of nonsusceptible microorganisms with prolonged use; take appropriate measures if superinfection develops. Lab test interactions may occur. Caution with renal impairment, overt/known subclinical diabetes mellitus (DM) or carbohydrate intolerance for any reason, and in elderly. Not recommended for premature infants and neonates.

ADVERSE REACTIONS

Diarrhea, oral candidiasis, N/V, stomach cramps, anorexia, anaphylaxis, leukopenia, thrombocytopenia, renal failure, hepatitis, pruritus, dizziness, fainting, confusion, weakness.

DRUG INTERACTIONS

Probenecid may decrease renal tubular secretion.

NURSING CONSIDERATIONS

Assessment: Assess for hypersensitivity to cephalosporin class of antibacterial drugs/PCN/other β-lactams, DM, carbohydrate intolerance, renal impairment, pregnancy/nursing status, and possible drug interactions. Perform appropriate culture and susceptibility tests to determine susceptible causative organisms.

Monitoring: Monitor for hypersensitivity reactions, CDAD, development of superinfection, drug resistance, and other adverse reactions. Monitor renal function in elderly. Monitor for seizures in patients with renal dysfunction.

Patient Counseling: Advise that allergic reactions, including serious allergic reactions may occur and require immediate treatment and discontinuation of therapy. Instruct to notify physician of any previous allergic reactions to the drug, cephalosporins, PCNs, or other similar antibacterials. Advise that diarrhea is a common problem that usually ends when therapy is discontinued; however, if watery and bloody stools (with/without stomach cramps and fever) occur, even as late as 2 or more months after last dose, instruct to contact physician as soon as possible. Inform that therapy only treats bacterial, not viral, infections. Instruct to take exactly ud even if the patient feels better early in the course of therapy. Inform that skipping doses or not completing the full course of therapy may decrease effectiveness and increase risk of bacterial resistance.

Storage: Before Reconstitution: 20-25°C (68-77°F). Protect from light. After Reconstitution: Stable for 24 hrs at room temperature or for 10 days if stored under refrigeration (5°C [41°F]).

CEFDINIR – cefdinir

RX

Class: Cephalosporin (3rd generation)

ADULT DOSAGE

Community-Acquired Pneumonia

Cap:
300mg q12h for 10 days

Acute Bacterial Exacerbation of Chronic Bronchitis

Cap:
300mg q12h for 5-10 days or 600mg q24h for 10 days

Acute Maxillary Sinusitis

Cap:
300mg q12h or 600mg q24h for 10 days

Pharyngitis/Tonsillitis

Cap:
300mg q12h for 5-10 days or 600mg q24h for 10 days

Skin and Skin Structure Infections

Uncomplicated:
Cap:
300mg q12h for 10 days

PEDIATRIC DOSAGE

Skin and Skin Structure Infections

Uncomplicated:
Sus:
6 Months-12 Years:
7mg/kg q12h for 10 days
≥43kg: 600mg/day
Max: 600mg/day
Cap:
≥13 Years:
300mg q12h for 10 days

Acute Otitis Media

Sus:
6 Months of Age-12 Years:
7mg/kg q12h for 5-10 days or 14mg/kg q24h for 10 days
≥43kg: 600mg/day
Max: 600mg/day

Community-Acquired Pneumonia

Cap:
≥13 Years:
300mg q12h for 10 days

Acute Bacterial Exacerbation of Chronic Bronchitis

Cap:
≥13 Years:
300mg q12h for 5-10 days or 600mg q24h for 10 days

Acute Maxillary Sinusitis

Sus:
6 Months of Age-12 Years:
7mg/kg q12h or 14mg/kg q24h for 10 days
≥43kg: 600mg/day
Max: 600mg/day
Cap:
≥13 Years:
300mg q12h or 600mg q24h for 10 days

Pharyngitis/Tonsillitis

Sus:
6 Months of Age-12 Years:
7mg/kg q12h for 5-10 days or 14mg/kg q24h for 10 days
≥43kg: 600mg/day
Max: 600mg/day
Cap:
≥13 Years:
300mg q12h for 5-10 days or 600mg q24h for 10 days

DOSE MODIFICATION

Renal Impairment
Adults:
CrCl <30mL/min: 300mg qd
Hemodialysis:
Initial: 300mg or 7mg/kg qod; give 300mg or 7mg/kg at the end of each hemodialysis session
Usual: 300mg or 7mg/kg qod

Pediatrics:
CrCl <30mL/min/1.73m²: 7mg/kg qd
Max: 300mg qd
Hemodialysis:
Initial: 300mg or 7mg/kg qod; give 300mg or 7mg/kg at the end of each hemodialysis session
Usual: 300mg or 7mg/kg qod

ADMINISTRATION

Oral route

Take without regard to food

Sus
Shake well before use
Reconstitute with 37mL of water (final volume of 60mL) or add 62mL of water (final volume of 100mL); add water in 2 portions, shake well after each aliquot

HOW SUPPLIED

Cap: 300mg; Sus: 125mg/5mL, 250mg/5mL [60mL, 100mL]

WARNINGS/PRECAUTIONS

Caution in PCN-sensitive patients; cross-hypersensitivity among β-lactam antibiotics may occur. D/C use if an allergic reaction occurs. Serious acute hypersensitivity reactions may require the use of SQ epinephrine and other emergency measures. *Clostridium difficile*-associated diarrhea (CDAD) reported. May result in bacterial resistance with prolonged use in the absence of a proven or suspected bacterial infection, or a prophylactic indication; take appropriate measures if superinfection develops. Reduce dose in patients with transient or persistent renal insufficiency (CrCl <30mL/min). Caution in patients with a history of colitis. Lab test interaction may occur.

ADVERSE REACTIONS

Diarrhea, vaginal moniliasis, nausea, rash.

DRUG INTERACTIONS

Iron-fortified foods (except iron-fortified infant formula), iron supplements, and aluminum- or magnesium-containing antacids reduce absorption; take dose at least 2 hrs before or after these medications. Inhibited renal excretion with probenecid. Reddish stools reported with iron-containing products. Possible interaction with diclofenac reported.

NURSING CONSIDERATIONS

Assessment: Assess for allergy to other cephalosporins, PCN, or to other drugs, history of colitis, renal impairment, and for possible drug interactions. Assess for diabetes if planning to use sus formulation.

Monitoring: Monitor for signs/symptoms of hypersensitivity reactions, CDAD, and development of superinfection.

Patient Counseling: Inform that therapy only treats bacterial, not viral, infections. Instruct to take ud; skipping doses or not completing full course may decrease drug effectiveness and increase risk of bacterial resistance. Instruct to take dose at least 2 hrs before or after antacid or iron supplements. Inform diabetic patients and caregivers that sus contains 2.86g of sucrose/tsp. Inform that diarrhea (watery/bloody stools) may be experienced as late as 2 months or more after last dose and instruct to contact physician as soon as possible if this occurs.

Storage: Cap: 25°C (77°F); excursions permitted to 15-30°C (59-86°F). Unsuspended Powder: 20-25°C (68-77°F). Reconstituted Sus: Can be stored at controlled room temperature for 10 days.

CEFOXITIN – cefoxitin sodium RX

Class: Cephalosporin (2nd generation)

ADULT DOSAGE

General Dosing

Lower respiratory tract/urinary tract/intra-abdominal/gynecological/skin and skin structure/bone and joint infections and septicemia caused by susceptible strains of microorganisms

Usual:
1-2g IV q6-8h

Uncomplicated Infections (eg, Pneumonia, UTI, Cutaneous):
1g IV q6-8h

Moderately Severe/Severe Infections:
1g IV q4h or 2g IV q6-8h

Gas Gangrene/Other Infections Requiring Higher Dose:
2g IV q4h or 3g IV q6h

Group A β-Hemolytic Streptococcal Infections:
Administer for at least 10 days

Prophylaxis of Postoperative Infections

For Uncontaminated GI Surgery, Abdominal/Vaginal Hysterectomy:
2g IV prior to surgery (0.5-1 hr before initial incision), then 2g IV q6h after 1st dose for ≤24 hrs

Cesarean Section:
Single dose of 2g IV as soon as umbilical cord is clamped, or 2g IV as soon as umbilical cord is clamped, followed by 2g IV at 4 and 8 hrs after initial dose

PEDIATRIC DOSAGE

General Dosing

≥3 Months of Age:
80-160mg/kg/day divided into 4-6 equal doses; use higher doses for more severe/serious infections
Max: 12g/day

Group A β-Hemolytic Streptococcal Infections:
Administer for at least 10 days

Prophylaxis of Postoperative Infections

≥3 Months of Age:
For Uncontaminated GI Surgery, Abdominal/Vaginal Hysterectomy:
30-40mg/kg IV prior to surgery (0.5-1 hr before initial incision) and q6h after 1st dose for ≤24 hrs

DOSE MODIFICATION

Renal Impairment

Adults:
LD: 1-2g IV
Maint:
CrCl 30-50mL/min: 1-2g IV q8-12h
CrCl 10-29mL/min: 1-2g IV q12-24h
CrCl 5-9mL/min: 0.5-1g IV q12-24h
CrCl <5mL/min: 0.5-1g q24-48h

Hemodialysis:
LD: 1-2g IV after each hemodialysis
Maint: See renal impairment maintenance dose above

Pediatrics:
Modify dosage and frequency of dosage consistent w/ recommendations for adults

ADMINISTRATION

IV route

Preparation

1g vial should be constituted w/ at least 10mL of diluent, and 2g vial w/ 10mL or 20mL of diluent
May use sterile water for inj (SWFI), bacteriostatic water for inj, 0.9% NaCl inj, or D5 inj for initial dilution
Further dilute in 50-1000mL of compatible diluents

IV

Intermittent IV:

May inject 1g or 2g sol in 10mL of SWFI over 3-5 min

May give over a longer period of time through the tubing system if receiving other IV sol

D/C administration of any other sol at the same site

Higher Doses by Continuous Infusion:

May add to an IV bottle containing D5 inj, 0.9% NaCl inj, or D5 and 0.9% NaCl inj; butterfly or scalp vein-type needles are preferred

Do not add to aminoglycoside sol; administer separately

Compatibility

0.9% NaCl, D5 or D10 inj, D5 and 0.9% NaCl inj, D5 inj w/ 0.2% or 0.45% saline sol, lactated Ringer's inj, D5 in lactated Ringer's inj, 5% sodium bicarbonate inj, M/6 sodium lactate sol, mannitol 5% and 10%

HOW SUPPLIED

Inj: 1g, 2g

WARNINGS/PRECAUTIONS

Caution with previous hypersensitivity to cephalosporins, penicillins (PCNs), or other drugs. D/C if allergic reaction occurs. *Clostridium difficile*-associated diarrhea (CDAD) reported; d/c if CDAD suspected or confirmed. May result in overgrowth of nonsusceptible organisms with prolonged use or use in the absence of a proven or strongly suspected bacterial infection or prophylactic indication; take appropriate measures if superinfection develops. Appropriate anti-chlamydial coverage should be added when used in the treatment of pelvic inflammatory disease and *Chlamydia trachomatis* is the suspected pathogen. Lab test interactions may occur. Caution with impaired renal function, history of GI disease (particularly colitis), and in elderly.

ADVERSE REACTIONS

Local reactions, rash, pruritus, fever, dyspnea, hypotension, diarrhea, pseudomembranous colitis, exacerbation of myasthenia gravis, eosinophilia, leukopenia, thrombocytopenia, bone marrow depression, elevated LFTs, SrCr elevation.

DRUG INTERACTIONS

Increased nephrotoxicity with aminoglycoside antibiotics.

NURSING CONSIDERATIONS

Assessment: Assess for previous hypersensitivity reactions to cephalosporins, PCNs, or other drugs, renal impairment, GI disease (eg, colitis), pregnancy/nursing status, and possible drug interactions. Perform appropriate culture and susceptibility studies to determine susceptible causative organisms.

Monitoring: Monitor for signs/symptoms of an allergic reaction, CDAD, development of superinfection or drug resistance, and other adverse reactions. Periodically monitor renal/hepatic/hematopoietic functions, especially with prolonged therapy.

Patient Counseling: Inform that drug only treats bacterial, not viral, infections. Instruct to take exactly ud; skipping doses or not completing full course of therapy may decrease effectiveness and increase the likelihood of bacterial resistance. Inform that diarrhea may occur and will usually end if therapy is discontinued. Instruct to contact physician as soon as possible if watery/bloody stools (with/without stomach cramps, fever) develop even as late as 2 or more months after discontinuation.

Storage: Dry State: 2-25°C (36-77°F). Avoid >50°C [122°F]. Reconstituted Sol: Maintains satisfactory potency at room temperature for 6 hrs or for 1 week under refrigeration (<5°C [41°F]). Further Diluted Sol: Room temperature for additional 18 hrs or additional 48 hrs under refrigeration.

CEFPODOXIME – cefpodoxime proxetil RX

Class: Cephalosporin (3rd generation)

ADULT DOSAGE

Tonsillitis and/or Pharyngitis

100mg q12h for 5-10 days

Community-Acquired Pneumonia

200mg q12h for 14 days

Acute Bacterial Exacerbation of Chronic Bronchitis

Tab:

200mg q12h for 10 days

PEDIATRIC DOSAGE

Acute Otitis Media

2 Months-12 Years:

Sus:

5mg/kg q12h for 5 days

Max: 200mg/dose

Tonsillitis and/or Pharyngitis

2 Months-12 Years:

Sus:

5mg/kg/dose q12h for 5-10 days

Gonorrhea

Uncomplicated Gonorrhea (Men and Women):
Single 200mg dose

Rectal Infections

Gonococcal Infections (Women):
Single 200mg dose

Skin and Skin Structure Infections

400mg q12h for 7-14 days

Acute Maxillary Sinusitis

200mg q12h for 10 days

Urinary Tract Infections

Uncomplicated:
100mg q12h for 7 days

Max: 100mg/dose
≥12 Years:
100mg q12h for 5-10 days

Acute Maxillary Sinusitis

2 Months-12 Years:
Sus:
5mg/kg q12h for 10 days
Max:
200mg/dose
≥12 Years:
200mg q12h for 10 days

Community-Acquired Pneumonia

≥12 Years:
200mg q12h for 14 days

Gonorrhea

Uncomplicated (Men and Women):
≥12 Years:
Single 200mg dose

Rectal Infections

Gonococcal Infections (Women):
≥12 Years:
Single 200mg dose

Skin and Skin Structure Infections

≥12 Years:
400mg q12h for 7-14 days

Urinary Tract Infections

Uncomplicated:
≥12 Years:
100mg q12h for 7 days

Acute Bacterial Exacerbation of Chronic Bronchitis

≥12 Years:
200mg q12h for 10 days

DOSE MODIFICATION

Renal Impairment
Severe (CrCl <30mL/min): Increase dosing interval to q24h
Hemodialysis: Dose 3X/week after hemodialysis

ADMINISTRATION

Oral route

Tab
Take w/ food

Sus
May be given w/o regard to food
Shake well before using

Preparation of Sus
50mL of 50mg/5mL: Suspend in 32mL of distilled water
100mL of 50mg/5mL: Suspend in 63mL of distilled water
50mL of 100mg/5mL: Suspend in 32mL of distilled water
100mL of 100mg/5mL: Suspend in 63mL of distilled water
Add water in approx 2 equal portions, shaking vigorously after each aliquot

HOW SUPPLIED

Sus: 50mg/5mL, 100mg/5mL [50mL, 100mL]; Tab: 100mg, 200mg

WARNINGS/PRECAUTIONS

Cross hypersensitivity among β-lactam antibiotics reported; caution in patients with penicillin (PCN) sensitivity. D/C if an allergic reaction occurs. Serious acute hypersensitivity reactions may require treatment with epinephrine and other emergency measures. *Clostridium difficile*-associated diarrhea (CDAD) reported; d/c if CDAD is suspected or confirmed. Pseudomembranous colitis reported. May result in bacterial resistance with prolonged use or in the absence of proven or suspected bacterial infection, or a prophylactic indication; take appropriate measures if superinfection develops. Lab test interactions may occur.

ADVERSE REACTIONS

Diarrhea, nausea.

DRUG INTERACTIONS

High doses of antacids (sodium bicarbonate and aluminum hydroxide) or H_2 blockers reduce C_{max} and the extent of absorption. Oral anticholinergics (eg, propantheline) delay C_{max}. Probenecid inhibits renal excretion; monitor renal function with nephrotoxic agents. Caution with potent diuretics.

NURSING CONSIDERATIONS

Assessment: Assess for history of hypersensitivity to cephalosporins, PCNs, or other drugs, renal impairment, pregnancy/nursing status, and possible drug interactions. Perform culture and susceptibility testing.

Monitoring: Monitor for signs/symptoms of hypersensitivity reactions, CDAD, pseudomembranous colitis, development of superinfection, and other adverse reactions.

Patient Counseling: Inform that therapy should only be used to treat bacterial, not viral (eg, common cold), infections. Instruct to take exactly ud even if the patient feels better early in the course of therapy. Inform that skipping doses or not completing the full course of therapy may decrease effectiveness of immediate treatment and increase bacterial resistance. Inform that diarrhea is a common problem caused by therapy, which usually ends when therapy is discontinued. Instruct to immediately contact physician if watery and bloody stools (with or without stomach cramps and fever) occur, even as late as ≥2 months after the last dose. (Sus) Inform that drug contains phenylalanine.

Storage: 20-25°C (68-77°F). (Sus) After Constitution: 2-8°C (36-46°F). Discard unused portion after 14 days.

CEFPROZIL — cefprozil

RX

Class: Cephalosporin (2nd generation)

ADULT DOSAGE

Pharyngitis/Tonsillitis

500mg q24h for 10 days; administer for >10 days for *Streptococcus pyogenes* infections

Acute Bacterial Sinusitis

250mg or 500mg q12h for 10 days; use the higher dose for moderate to severe infections

Lower Respiratory Tract Infections

Secondary Bacterial Infection of Acute Bronchitis/Acute Bacterial Exacerbation of Chronic Bronchitis:
500mg q12h for 10 days

Skin and Skin Structure Infections

Uncomplicated:
250mg or 500mg q12h or 500mg q24h for 10 days

PEDIATRIC DOSAGE

Acute Otitis Media

6 Months-12 Years:
15mg/kg q12h for 10 days
Do not exceed recommended adult doses

Acute Bacterial Sinusitis

6 Months-12 Years:
7.5mg/kg or 15mg/kg q12h for 10 days
≥13 Years:
250mg or 500mg q12h for 10 days; use the higher dose for moderate to severe infections
Do not exceed recommended adult doses

Pharyngitis/Tonsillitis

2-12 Years:
7.5mg/kg q12h for 10 days
≥13 Years:
500mg q24h for 10 days
Administer for >10 days for *Streptococcus pyogenes* infections
Do not exceed recommended adult doses

Skin and Skin Structure Infections

Uncomplicated:
2-12 Years:
20mg/kg q24h for 10 days
≥13 Years:
250mg or 500mg q12h or 500mg q24h for 10 days

Lower Respiratory Tract Infections

Acute Bacterial Exacerbation of Chronic Bronchitis/Secondary Bacterial Infection of Acute Bronchitis:
≥13 Years:
500mg q12h for 10 days

DOSE MODIFICATION

Renal Impairment

CrCl 0-29mL/min: Give 50% of standard dose

ADMINISTRATION
Oral route
Shake sus well before use
Administer after completion of hemodialysis

Reconstitution

Final Concentration of 125mg/5mL:
Add 36mL, 54mL, or 72mL of water to the 50mL, 75mL, or 100mL bottle size respectively

Final Concentration of 250mg/5mL:
Add 36mL, 54mL, or 72mL of water to the 50mL, 75mL, or 100mL bottle size respectively

HOW SUPPLIED
Sus: 125mg/5mL, 250mg/5mL [50mL, 75mL, 100mL]; Tab: 250mg, 500mg

WARNINGS/PRECAUTIONS
Caution with previous hypersensitivity to cephalosporins, penicillins (PCNs), or other drugs; cross-sensitivity may occur with history of PCN allergy. D/C if allergic reaction occurs. *Clostridium difficile*-associated diarrhea (CDAD) reported. May result in bacterial resistance with prolonged use or use in the absence of a proven/suspected bacterial infection or a prophylactic indication; take appropriate measures if superinfection develops. Caution with GI disease, particularly colitis. Caution with renal impairment and elderly. Lab test interactions may occur.

ADVERSE REACTIONS
Diarrhea, N/V, ALT/AST elevation, eosinophilia, genital pruritus, vaginitis, superinfection, diaper rash, dizziness, abdominal pain.

DRUG INTERACTIONS
Nephrotoxicity with aminoglycosides reported. Probenecid may increase plasma levels. Caution with potent diuretics.

NURSING CONSIDERATIONS

Assessment: Assess for previous hypersensitivity reactions to PCNs/cephalosporins or other drugs, renal/hepatic function, GI disease, pregnancy/nursing status, and possible drug interactions. Perform appropriate culture and susceptibility studies to determine susceptible causative organisms.

Monitoring: Periodically monitor renal/hepatic/hematopoietic functions. Monitor for CDAD (may range from mild diarrhea to fatal colitis), development of superinfections or drug resistance, allergic reactions, and other adverse reactions.

Patient Counseling: Inform that the oral sus contains phenylalanine. Inform that drug only treats bacterial, not viral, infections. Instruct to take ud and that skipping doses or not completing full course may decrease effectiveness and increase resistance. Inform about potential benefits/risks. Notify physician if watery/bloody stools (with/without stomach cramps/fever) occur even ≥2 months after therapy. Notify if pregnant/nursing.

Storage: Tab/Dry Powder: 20-25°C (68-77°F). Reconstituted Sus: Refrigerate after mixing and discard unused portion after 14 days.

CEFTIN – cefuroxime axetil RX

Class: Cephalosporin (2nd generation)

ADULT DOSAGE

Pharyngitis/Tonsillitis
Tab:
250mg bid for 10 days

Acute Maxillary Sinusitis
Tab:
250mg bid for 10 days

Bronchitis
Tab:
Acute Bacterial Exacerbations of Chronic Bronchitis: 250mg or 500mg bid for 10 days
Secondary Bacterial Infections of Acute Bronchitis: 250mg or 500mg bid for 5-10 days

Skin and Skin Structure Infections
Tab:
Uncomplicated: 250mg or 500mg bid for 10 days

PEDIATRIC DOSAGE

Skin and Skin Structure Infections
Tab:
≥13 Years:
Uncomplicated: 250mg or 500mg bid for 10 days

Urinary Tract Infections
Tab:
≥13 Years:
Uncomplicated: 250mg bid for 7-10 days

Gonorrhea
Tab:
≥13 Years:
Uncomplicated: 1g as a single dose

Lyme Disease
Early Lyme disease (Erythema Migrans):
Tab:
≥13 Years: 500mg bid for 20 days

Urinary Tract Infections

Tab:
Uncomplicated: 250mg bid for 7-10 days

Gonorrhea

Tab:
Uncomplicated: 1g as a single dose

Lyme Disease

Early Lyme disease (Erythema Migrans):
Tab:
500mg bid for 20 days

Pharyngitis/Tonsillitis

Sus:
3 Months-12 Years:
20mg/kg/day divided bid for 10 days
Max: 500mg/day

Tab:
≥13 Years:
250mg bid for 10 days

Acute Otitis Media

Sus:
3 Months-12 Years:
30mg/kg/day divided bid for 10 days
Max: 1g/day

Tab:
Patients Who Can Swallow Tabs Whole:
250mg bid for 10 days

Acute Maxillary Sinusitis

Sus:
3 Months-12 Years:
30mg/kg/day divided bid for 10 days
Max: 1g/day

Tab:
≥13 Years or Pediatric Patients Who Can Swallow Tabs Whole: 250mg bid for 10 days

Impetigo

Sus:
3 Months-12 Years:
30mg/kg/day divided bid for 10 days
Max: 1g/day

Bronchitis

Tab:
≥13 Years:
Acute Bacterial Exacerbations of Chronic Bronchitis: 250mg or 500mg bid for 10 days

Secondary Bacterial Infections of Acute Bronchitis: 250mg or 500mg bid for 5-10 days

DOSE MODIFICATION

Renal Impairment
CrCl 10-<30mL/min: Standard individual dose given q24h
CrCl <10mL/min (w/o Hemodialysis): Standard individual dose given q48h
Hemodialysis: Give a single additional standard dose at the end of each dialysis

ADMINISTRATION

Oral route

Tabs and sus are not bioequivalent and are not substitutable on a mg-per-mg basis

Sus:
Reconstitute 125mg/5mL w/ 37mL (for a volume of 100mL after reconstitution) of water
Reconstitute 250mg/5mL w/ 19mL (for a volume of 50mL after reconstitution) or 35mL (for a volume of 100mL after reconstitution) of water
Take w/ food
Shake well before each use

Tab:
Take w/ or w/o regard to meals

HOW SUPPLIED

Sus: 125mg/5mL [100mL], 250mg/5mL [50mL, 100mL]; Tab: 250mg, 500mg

WARNINGS/PRECAUTIONS

Tab and sus are not bioequivalent and are therefore not a substitutable on mg-per-mg basis. Cross-hypersensitivity among β-lactam antibiotics reported; caution in penicillin-sensitive patients. D/C if a significant allergic reaction occurs. *Clostridium difficile*-associated diarrhea (CDAD) reported; may need to d/c if CDAD is suspected or confirmed. May result in bacterial resistance with prolonged use in the absence of proven or suspected bacterial infection, or a prophylactic indication; take appropriate measures if superinfection develops. Caution with history of colitis. May cause a fall in prothrombin activity; those at risk include patients with renal/hepatic impairment, poor nutritional state, patients receiving a protracted course of therapy, and patients previously stabilized on anticoagulant therapy. Monitor PT in patients at risk and administer exogenous vitamin K as indicated. Lab test interactions may occur. (Sus) Contains phenylalanine.

ADVERSE REACTIONS

Diarrhea/loose stools, N/V, vaginitis, (sus) dislike of taste, diaper rash.

DRUG INTERACTIONS

Probenecid increases plasma levels. May result in lower bioavailability with drugs that reduce gastric acidity. Caution with potent diuretics; suspected of adversely affecting renal function. May affect the gut flora, leading to lower estrogen reabsorption and reduced efficacy of combined oral estrogen/progesterone contraceptives.

NURSING CONSIDERATIONS

Assessment: Assess for hypersensitivity reactions to cephalosporins, PCNs, or other drugs, renal/hepatic impairment, nutritional status, history of colitis, pregnancy/nursing status, and possible drug interactions. For patients planning on using sus formulation, assess for phenylketonuria.

Monitoring: Monitor for signs/symptoms of an allergic reaction, CDAD, development of superinfection, and other adverse reactions. Monitor PT and renal function.

Patient Counseling: Advise of potential benefits/risks of therapy. Inform that drug only treats bacterial, not viral, infections. Instruct to take exactly ud; skipping doses or not completing full course of therapy may decrease effectiveness and increase the likelihood of bacterial resistance. Inform that diarrhea may occur and will usually end if therapy is discontinued. Instruct to contact physician as soon as possible if watery and bloody stools (with/without stomach cramps, fever) develop even as late as 2 or more months after having taken the last dose. Inform that pediatric patients who cannot swallow tab whole should receive oral sus. Inform that crushed tab has a strong, persistent, bitter taste and should not be administered to pediatric patients in this manner.

Storage: Tab: 15-30°C (59-86°F). Dry Powder: 2-30°C (36-86°F). Reconstituted Sus: 2-8°C (36-46°F) in a refrigerator immediately; discard after 10 days.

CEFTRIAXONE – ceftriaxone sodium RX

Class: Cephalosporin (3rd generation)

OTHER BRAND NAMES

Rocephin

ADULT DOSAGE

General Dosing

Lower respiratory tract infections, acute bacterial otitis media, skin and skin structure infections, UTIs, pelvic inflammatory disease, bacterial septicemia, bone and joint infections, intra-abdominal infections, and meningitis caused by susceptible strains of microorganisms

Usual: 1-2g IV/IM qd or in equally divided doses bid depending on the type and severity of infection
Max: 4g/day
Usual Duration of Therapy: 4-14 days; complicated infections may require longer therapy
Continue for ≥2 days after signs and symptoms of infection have disappeared

***Streptococcus pyogenes* Infections:** Continue therapy for ≥10 days

Appropriate coverage should be added for *Chlamydia trachomatis* infections

Gonococcal Infections
Uncomplicated:
250mg IM single dose

Prophylaxis of Postoperative Infections

Single dose of 1g IV, 0.5-2 hrs before surgery

PEDIATRIC DOSAGE

Skin and Skin Structure Infections

Usual: 50-75mg/kg IV/IM qd or in equally divided doses bid
Max: 2g/day

Acute Otitis Media

Usual: Single dose of 50mg/kg IM
Max: 1g

Serious Infections

Usual: 50-75mg/kg IV/IM in divided doses q12h
Max: 2g/day

Meningitis

Initial: 100mg/kg IV/IM, then 100mg/kg/day IV/IM qd or in equally divided doses q12h for 7-14 days
Max: 4g/day

DOSE MODIFICATION

Hepatic Impairment

Hepatic Dysfunction w/ Significant Renal Disease Max Dose: 2g/day

ADMINISTRATION

IV/IM route

Do not use diluents containing Ca^{2+} (eg, Ringer's sol or Hartmann's sol) to reconstitute or to further dilute a reconstituted vial for IV administration

Do not simultaneously administer w/ Ca^{2+}-containing IV sol; may administer sequentially of another if the infusion lines are thoroughly flushed between infusions in patients other than neonates

Compatible w/ metronidazole hydrochloride; do not exceed 5-7.5mg/mL of metronidazole hydrochloride w/ ceftriaxone w/ 10mg/mL as an admixture

Physically incompatible w/ vancomycin, amsacrine, aminoglycosides, and fluconazole; when administered concomitantly by intermittent IV infusion, give sequentially, w/ thorough flushing of the IV lines between administrations

Avoid physically mixing w/ or piggybacking into sol containing other antimicrobial drugs

IM

Reconstitute 250mg, 500mg, 1g, or 2g vial w/ 0.9mL, 1.8mL, 3.6mL, or 7.2mL (respectively) of compatible diluent for a concentration of approx 250mg/mL

Reconstitute 500mg, 1g, or 2g vial w/ 1mL, 2.1mL, or 4.2mL (respectively) of compatible diluent for a concentration of approx 350mg/mL

Inject well w/in the body of a relatively large muscle; avoid unintentional inj into a blood vessel

Compatible IM Diluents:

Sterile water for inj (SWFI), 0.9% NaCl sol, D5 sol, bacteriostatic water + 0.9% benzyl alcohol, or 1% lidocaine sol (w/o epinephrine)

IV

Infuse over a 30-min period

Concentrations of 10-40mg/mL are recommended; lower concentrations may be used if desired

Reconstitute 250mg, 500mg, 1g, or 2g vial w/ 2.4mL, 4.8mL, 9.6mL, or 19.2mL (respectively) of compatible IV diluent for a concentration of approx 100mg/mL

Withdraw entire contents of vial and dilute to desired concentration w/ appropriate IV diluent

Compatible IV Diluents:

SWFI, 0.9% NaCl sol, D5 sol, D10 sol, D5 + 0.9% or 0.45% NaCl sol (incompatible when refrigerated), sodium lactate sol, 10% invert sugar sol, 5% sodium bicarbonate sol, Freamine III sol, Normosol-M in D5 sol, Ionosol-B in D5 sol, 5% mannitol sol, or 10% mannitol sol

Refer to PI for further administration and stability instructions

HOW SUPPLIED

Inj: 250mg, 2g; (Rocephin) 500mg, 1g

CONTRAINDICATIONS

Hyperbilirubinemic neonates (≤28 days), especially if premature; concurrent use of Ca^{2+}-containing IV sol used in neonates.

WARNINGS/PRECAUTIONS

Caution in penicillin (PCN)-sensitive patients; serious acute hypersensitivity reactions may require the use of SQ epinephrine and other emergency measures. Anaphylactic reactions reported. *Clostridium difficile*-associated diarrhea (CDAD) reported; may need to d/c therapy if CDAD is suspected/confirmed. Severe cases of hemolytic anemia reported; consider if the diagnosis is associated w/ therapy and d/c until cause is determined. May result in overgrowth of nonsusceptible organisms w/ prolonged use or use in the absence of a proven or strongly suspected bacterial infection or prophylactic indication; take appropriate measures if superinfection develops. Transient BUN and SrCr elevations may occur. Alterations in PT may occur rarely; monitor w/ impaired vitamin K synthesis or low vitamin K stores during treatment (eg, chronic hepatitis disease, malnutrition). Caution w/ history of GI disease, especially colitis. Gallbladder sonographic abnormalities reported; d/c if signs and symptoms of gallbladder disease develop. Pancreatitis reported rarely.

ADVERSE REACTIONS

Inj-site reactions (eg, warmth, tightness, induration), eosinophilia, thrombocytosis, AST/ALT elevation.

DRUG INTERACTIONS

See Contraindications and Administration.

NURSING CONSIDERATIONS

Assessment: Assess for hyperbilirubinemic neonates, especially if premature, hypersensitivity to cephalosporins/PCNs/other drugs, presence of both hepatic dysfunction and significant renal disease, impaired vitamin K synthesis or low vitamin K stores, history of GI disease (eg, colitis), pregnancy/nursing status, and possible drug interactions. Obtain appropriate specimens for isolation of the causative organism and for determination of susceptibility to the drug.

Monitoring: Monitor for signs/symptoms of hypersensitivity reactions, CDAD, hemolytic anemia, overgrowth of nonsusceptible organisms (eg, superinfection), gallbladder disease, pancreatitis, and other adverse reactions. Periodically monitor BUN and SrCr levels. Monitor PT levels in patients w/ impaired vitamin K synthesis or low vitamin K stores (eg, chronic hepatic disease, malnutrition).

Patient Counseling: Inform that therapy only treats bacterial, not viral, infections. Instruct to take exactly ud even if feeling better early in the course of therapy; inform that skipping doses or not completing full course may decrease drug effectiveness and increase the likelihood of bacteria resistance. Instruct to contact physician as soon as possible if watery and bloody stools (w/ or w/o stomach cramps, fever) develop even as late as 2 or more months after having taken the last dose of therapy.

Storage: 20-25°C (68-77°F). Protect from light. Do not refreeze. Rocephin: ≤25°C (77°F).

CELEBREX – celecoxib

RX

Class: COX-2 inhibitor

May increase risk of serious cardiovascular (CV) thrombotic events, MI, and stroke, which can be fatal; increased risk with duration of use and with CV disease (CVD) or risk factors for CVD. Increased risk of serious GI adverse events (eg, bleeding, ulceration, perforation of stomach/intestines) that can be fatal and occur anytime during use, without warning symptoms; elderly patients are at a greater risk. Contraindicated for treatment of perioperative pain in the setting of CABG surgery.

ADULT DOSAGE

Osteoarthritis

200mg qd or 100mg bid

Rheumatoid Arthritis

100-200mg bid

Ankylosing Spondylitis

Usual: 200mg qd or 100mg bid
Titrate: May increase to 400mg/day if no effect is observed after 6 weeks; consider alternative treatment if no effect is observed after 6 weeks on 400mg/day

Acute Pain

Initial: 400mg initially, then 200mg if needed on 1st day
Maint: 200mg bid prn on subsequent days

Primary Dysmenorrhea

Initial: 400mg initially, then 200mg if needed on 1st day
Maint: 200mg bid prn on subsequent days

PEDIATRIC DOSAGE

Juvenile Rheumatoid Arthritis

≥2 Years:
10-25kg:
50mg bid
>25kg:
100mg bid

DOSE MODIFICATION

Renal Impairment
Severe: Not recommended

Hepatic Impairment
Moderate (Child-Pugh Class B): Reduce daily dose by 50%
Severe: Not recommended

Elderly
<50kg:
Initial: Lowest recommended dose

Other Important Modifications
Poor Metabolizers of CYP2C9 Substrates:
Initial: Consider 1/2 the lowest recommended dose; consider alternative management in JRA patients

ADMINISTRATION

Oral route

May be given w/o regard to timing of meals
For patients w/ difficulty swallowing caps, contents may be added to applesauce; entire cap contents should be emptied onto a level tsp of cool or room temperature applesauce and ingested immediately w/ water

HOW SUPPLIED
Cap: 50mg, 100mg, 200mg, 400mg

CONTRAINDICATIONS
History of allergic-type reactions to sulfonamides, history of asthma, urticaria, or other allergic-type reactions with aspirin (ASA) or other NSAIDs, active GI bleeding. Treatment of perioperative pain in the setting of CABG surgery.

WARNINGS/PRECAUTIONS
Use lowest effective dose for the shortest duration possible. Not recommended with severe hepatic impairment. May lead to onset of new HTN or worsening of preexisting HTN; caution with HTN, and monitor BP closely. Fluid retention and edema reported; caution with fluid retention or HF. Caution with history of ulcer disease, GI bleeding, and other risk factors for GI bleeding (eg, prolonged NSAID therapy, older age, poor general health status); monitor for GI ulceration/bleeding. May cause elevations of LFTs or severe hepatic reactions (eg, jaundice, fatal fulminant hepatitis, liver necrosis, hepatic failure); d/c if liver disease develops or systemic manifestations occur, or if abnormal LFTs persist/worsen. Renal injury reported with long-term use; increased risk with renal/hepatic impairment, HF, and in elderly. Not recommended with advanced renal disease; if therapy must be initiated, closely monitor renal function. D/C if abnormal renal tests persist/worsen. Anaphylactoid/anaphylactic reactions and angioedema reported. Caution with asthma and avoid with ASA-sensitive asthma and the ASA triad. May cause serious skin adverse events (eg, exfoliative dermatitis, Stevens-Johnson syndrome, toxic epidermal necrolysis); d/c at 1st appearance of skin rash or any other sign of hypersensitivity. Avoid in late pregnancy (starting at 30 weeks gestation); may cause premature closure of ductus arteriosus. Not a substitute for corticosteroids or for the treatment of corticosteroid insufficiency. Anemia reported; monitor Hgb/Hct if signs/symptoms of anemia or blood loss develop with long-term use. Caution in pediatric patients with systemic onset JRA due to risk of disseminated intravascular coagulation. Monitor CBC and chemistry profile periodically with long-term treatment. May mask signs of inflammation and fever. Caution with poor CYP2C9 metabolizers. Not a substitute for ASA for CV prophylaxis.

ADVERSE REACTIONS
CV thrombotic events, MI, stroke, GI adverse events, headache, HTN, diarrhea, fever, dyspepsia, URI, abdominal pain, N/V, cough, nasopharyngitis.

DRUG INTERACTIONS
Avoid with non-ASA NSAIDs. Caution with CYP2C9 inhibitors. Potential interaction with CYP2D6 substrates. Warfarin or similar agents may increase risk of bleeding complications; monitor anticoagulant activity. May increase lithium levels; monitor closely. ASA may increase rate of GI ulceration or other complications. May diminish the antihypertensive effect of ACE inhibitors and ARBs. Fluconazole may increase levels. May reduce the natriuretic effect of loop diuretics (eg, furosemide) and thiazides. Oral corticosteroids, anticoagulants, smoking, or alcohol may increase risk of GI bleeding. Risk of renal toxicity with diuretics, ACE inhibitors, and ARBs. Aluminum- and magnesium-containing antacids may reduce plasma concentrations.

NURSING CONSIDERATIONS

Assessment: Assess for history of allergic-type reactions to sulfonamides, history of asthma, urticaria, other allergic-type reactions with ASA or other NSAIDs, active GI bleeding, CVD, risk factors for CVD, renal/hepatic impairment, HTN, history of ulcer disease or GI bleeding, risk factors for GI bleeding, asthma, ASA triad, other conditions where treatment is contraindicated or cautioned, pregnancy/nursing status, and possible drug interactions.

Monitoring: Monitor for signs/symptoms of CV thrombotic events, GI events, anaphylactoid/hypersensitivity reactions, and other adverse reactions. Monitor BP, renal function, LFTs, CBC, and chemistry profile periodically. Monitor for development of abnormal coagulation tests in patients with systemic onset JRA.

Patient Counseling: Advise to seek medical attention if signs/symptoms of CV events (eg, chest pain, SOB, weakness, slurring of speech), GI ulceration/bleeding (eg, epigastric pain, dyspepsia, melena, hematemesis), hepatotoxicity (eg, nausea, fatigue, lethargy, pruritus, jaundice, right upper quadrant tenderness, and flu-like symptoms), skin/hypersensitivity reactions (eg, rash, blisters, fever, itching), unexplained weight gain or edema, or anaphylactoid reactions (eg, difficulty breathing, swelling of the face/throat) occur. Instruct to d/c the drug immediately if any type of rash or if signs/symptoms of hepatotoxicity occur. Instruct patients with preexisting asthma to seek immediate medical attention if asthma worsens after taking the medication. Inform that medication should be avoided in late pregnancy.

Storage: 25°C (77°F); excursions permitted to 15-30°C (59-86°F). Sprinkled contents on applesauce are stable for up to 6 hrs at 2-8°C (35-45°F).

CellCept – mycophenolate mofetil

RX

Class: Inosine monophosphate dehydrogenase inhibitor

Use during pregnancy is associated with increased risks of 1st trimester pregnancy loss and congenital malformations; counsel females of reproductive potential regarding pregnancy prevention and planning. Immunosuppression may lead to increased susceptibility to infection and possible development of lymphoma. Should only be prescribed by physicians experienced in immunosuppressive therapy and management of organ transplant patients. Manage patients in facilities equipped and staffed with adequate lab and supportive medical resources.

ADULT DOSAGE

Renal Transplant

Prophylaxis of organ rejection in patients receiving allogeneic renal transplants; use concomitantly w/ cyclosporine and corticosteroids

1g PO/IV bid

Cardiac Transplant

Prophylaxis of organ rejection in patients receiving allogeneic cardiac transplants; use concomitantly w/ cyclosporine and corticosteroids

1.5g PO/IV bid

Hepatic Transplant

Prophylaxis of organ rejection in patients receiving allogeneic hepatic transplants; use concomitantly w/ cyclosporine and corticosteroids

1.5g PO bid or 1g IV bid

PEDIATRIC DOSAGE

Renal Transplant

Prophylaxis of organ rejection in patients receiving allogeneic renal transplants; use concomitantly w/ cyclosporine and corticosteroids

3 Months-18 Years of Age:
Sus:
Usual: 600mg/m^2 bid
Max: 2g/10mL/day

Cap:
BSA 1.25m^2-1.5m^2: 750mg bid

Cap/Tab:
BSA >1.5m^2: 1g bid

DOSE MODIFICATION

Renal Impairment
Renal Transplant:
Severe Chronic Renal Impairment (GFR <25mL/min) Outside the Immediate Post-Transplant Period: Avoid doses >1g bid

No dose adjustments needed in renal transplant patients experiencing delayed graft function postoperatively

ADMINISTRATION

Oral/IV route

Exercise caution in handling; refer to PI

Cap/Tab/Sus:
Start as soon as possible after transplant
Administer on an empty stomach; may administer w/ food if necessary in stable renal transplant patients
Do not crush tab; do not open or crush cap
Sus may be given via NG tube (minimum size of 8 French)

IV:
Administer by slow IV infusion over no less than 2 hrs
Administer w/in 24 hrs following transplant
Can administer for up to 14 days; switch to oral therapy as soon as patient can tolerate oral medication
Start administration w/in 4 hrs from reconstitution and dilution
Do not mix or administer concurrently via same infusion catheter w/ other IV drugs or infusion admixtures

Preparation
Sus:
1. Measure 94mL of water in a graduated cylinder
2. Add approximately half the total amount of water to bottle and shake closed bottle well for about 1 min
3. Add remainder of water and shake closed bottle well for about 1 min
4. Remove child-resistant cap and push bottle adapter into neck of bottle; close bottle w/ child-resistant cap tightly

IV:
Reconstitution:
2 vials are needed to prepare for 1g dose; 3 vials are needed for 1.5g dose
Reconstitute contents of each vial by injecting 14mL of 5% dextrose inj; gently shake vials to dissolve

Dilution:
For 1g dose, further dilute contents of the 2 reconstituted vials into 140mL of 5% dextrose inj
For 1.5g dose, further dilute contents of the 3 reconstituted vials into 210mL of 5% dextrose inj
Final concentration of both sol is 6mg/mL

HOW SUPPLIED
Cap: 250mg; Inj: 500mg/20mL; Sus: 200mg/mL; Tab: 500mg

CONTRAINDICATIONS
(Inj) Hypersensitivity to Polysorbate 80.

WARNINGS/PRECAUTIONS
Do not administer IV sol by rapid or bolus inj. Limit exposure to sunlight and UV light due to increased risk for skin cancer. Polyomavirus-associated nephropathy (PVAN), JC virus associated progressive multifocal leukoencephalopathy (PML), cytomegalovirus infections, and reactivation of hepatitis B virus (HBV) or hepatitis C virus (HCV) reported; consider dose reduction if new or reactivated viral infection develops. PVAN, especially due to BK virus infection, may lead to deteriorating renal function and renal graft loss. Consider PML in differential diagnosis in patients reporting neurological symptoms and consider consultation with a neurologist. Severe neutropenia reported; interrupt or reduce dose if neutropenia (absolute neutrophil count <1.3 x $10^3/\mu L$) develops. Cases of pure red cell aplasia (PRCA) reported when used with other immunosuppressive agents. Acceptable birth control must be used during therapy and for 6 weeks after discontinuation. GI bleeding, ulceration, and perforation reported; caution with active serious digestive system disease. Avoid doses >1g bid in renal transplant patients with severe chronic renal impairment (GFR <25mL/min); caution with delayed renal graft function post-transplant. More reports of opportunistic/herpes virus infections in cardiac transplant patients in comparison with azathioprine. Avoid with rare hereditary deficiency of hypoxanthine-guanine phosphoribosyl-transferase (HGPRT) (eg, Lesch-Nyhan and Kelley-Seegmiller syndromes). Oral sus contains 0.56mg phenylalanine/mL; caution with phenylketonurics. Caution in elderly.

ADVERSE REACTIONS
Infection, diarrhea, leukopenia, sepsis, N/V, HTN, peripheral edema, abdominal pain, fever, headache, constipation, hyperglycemia, anemia, insomnia.

DRUG INTERACTIONS
Avoid with azathioprine, drugs that interfere with enterohepatic recirculation (eg, cholestyramine), and norfloxacin-metronidazole combination. Vaccinations may be less effective; avoid live, attenuated vaccines. Decreased exposure with rifampin; concomitant use not recommended unless benefit outweighs risk. Increased levels of both drugs with drugs that compete with renal tubular secretion (eg, acyclovir/valacyclovir, ganciclovir/valganciclovir, probenecid). Oral ciprofloxacin and amoxicillin plus clavulanic acid may decrease levels. Mean mycophenolic acid (MPA) exposure may be 30-50% greater when mycophenolate mofetil is administered without cyclosporine compared to when coadministered with cyclosporine. May decrease levels and effectiveness of hormonal contraceptives; use with caution and must use additional barrier contraceptive methods. Drugs that alter GI flora may reduce levels available for absorption. Decreased levels with proton pump inhibitors (eg, lansoprazole, pantoprazole), Mg^{2+}- and aluminum-containing antacids, and Ca^{2+} free phosphate binders (eg, sevelamer). Do not administer simultaneously with antacids containing aluminum and magnesium hydroxides. Do not administer Ca^{2+} free phosphate binders simultaneously; may give 2 hrs after intake. Combination immunosuppressant therapy should be used with caution.

NURSING CONSIDERATIONS

Assessment: Assess for hypersensitivity to the drug or its components, hepatic/renal impairment, delayed renal graft function post-transplant, phenylketonuria, hereditary deficiency of HGPRT (eg, Lesch-Nyhan and Kelley-Seegmiller syndromes), active digestive disease, vaccination history, nursing status, and possible drug interactions. Assess pregnancy status using serum or urine test of at least 25 mIU/mL sensitivity, immediately before starting therapy.

Monitoring: Monitor for signs/symptoms of lymphomas, skin cancer, and other malignancies, infections, HCV/HBV reactivation, neutropenia, PRCA, GI bleeding/perforation/ulceration, and other adverse reactions. Monitor CBC weekly during the 1st month, twice monthly for the 2nd and 3rd months of therapy, and then monthly through the 1st yr. Monitor pregnancy status by obtaining pregnancy test 8-10 days after initiation of therapy and repeatedly during follow-up visits.

Patient Counseling: Inform that use during pregnancy is associated with an increased risk of 1st trimester pregnancy loss and congenital malformations; discuss pregnancy testing, prevention (including acceptable contraception methods), and planning. Discuss appropriate alternative immunosuppressants with less potential for embryofetal toxicity if patient is considering pregnancy. Advise of complete dosage instructions and inform about increased risk of lymphoproliferative disease and certain other malignancies. Inform of the need for repeated appropriate lab tests during therapy. Instruct patients to report immediately any evidence of infection, unexpected bruising, bleeding, or any other manifestation of bone marrow depression. Advise not to breastfeed during therapy. Encourage to enroll in the pregnancy registry if patient becomes pregnant while on medication.

Storage: 25°C (77°F); excursions permitted to 15-30°C (59-86°F). Constituted Sus: Stable up to 60 days; may also be refrigerated at 2-8°C (36-46°F). Do not freeze.

CEPHALEXIN – cephalexin

Class: Cephalosporin (1st generation)

RX

OTHER BRAND NAMES

Keflex

ADULT DOSAGE

Respiratory Tract Infections

Usual: 250mg q6h
Range: 1-4g/day in divided doses

>15 Years:
Streptococcal Pharyngitis: 500mg q12h

May need larger doses in more severe infections or those caused by less susceptible organisms; if doses >4g/day are required, consider parenteral cephalosporins

Skin and Skin Structure Infections

Usual: 250mg q6h
Range: 1-4g/day in divided doses

>15 Years:
500mg q12h

May need larger doses in more severe infections or those caused by less susceptible organisms; if doses >4g/day are required, consider parenteral cephalosporins

Bone Infections

Usual: 250mg q6h
Range: 1-4g/day in divided doses

May need larger doses in more severe infections or those caused by less susceptible organisms; if doses >4g/day are required, consider parenteral cephalosporins

Genitourinary Tract Infections

Usual: 250mg q6h
Range: 1-4g/day in divided doses

>15 Years:
Uncomplicated Cystitis: 500mg q12h for 7-14 days

May need larger doses in more severe infections or those caused by less susceptible organisms; if doses >4g/day are required, consider parenteral cephalosporins

PEDIATRIC DOSAGE

Respiratory Tract Infections

Usual: 25-50mg/kg/day in divided doses
β-Hemolytic Streptococcal Infections:
Administer for at least 10 days
May double the dosage in severe infections
>1 Year:
Streptococcal Pharyngitis: May divide total daily dose and give q12h

Skin and Skin Structure Infections

Usual: 25-50mg/kg/day in divided doses
May divide total daily dose and give q12h
May double the dosage in severe infections

Otitis Media

75-100mg/kg/day in 4 divided doses
May double the dosage in severe infections

Bone Infections

Usual: 25-50mg/kg/day in divided doses
May double the dosage in severe infections

Genitourinary Tract Infections

Usual: 25-50mg/kg/day in divided doses
May double the dosage in severe infections

ADMINISTRATION

Oral route

Take PO w/o regard to meals

Sus
Shake well before use
Directions for mixing are included on the label
After mixing, store in refrigerator; may be kept for 14 days w/o significant loss of potency

HOW SUPPLIED

Cap: 250mg, 500mg, (Keflex) 250mg, 500mg, 750mg; Sus: 125mg/5mL [100mL, 200mL], 250mg/5mL [100mL, 200mL]; Tab: 250mg*, 500mg* *scored

WARNINGS/PRECAUTIONS

Caution in penicillin (PCN)-sensitive patients; cross-hypersensitivity among β-lactam antibiotics may occur. D/C use if an allergic reaction occurs and institute appropriate therapy. *Clostridium difficile*-associated diarrhea (CDAD) reported; d/c if CDAD is suspected or confirmed. May result in bacterial resistance with prolonged use or use in the absence of a proven/suspected bacterial infection or a prophylactic indication; take appropriate measures if superinfection develops. Perform indicated surgical procedures in conjunction with antibiotic therapy. Caution in patients with markedly impaired renal function or history of GI disease, particularly colitis. May cause a fall in prothrombin activity; monitor PT in patients at risk (eg, hepatic/renal impairment, poor nutritional state, patients on protracted course of antimicrobial therapy, patients previously stabilized on anticoagulant therapy) and administer vitamin K as indicated. Lab test interactions may occur. Caution in elderly.

ADVERSE REACTIONS
Diarrhea, allergic reactions, dyspepsia, gastritis, abdominal pain.

DRUG INTERACTIONS
Probenecid inhibits renal excretion. Concomitant use with metformin may increase concentrations of metformin and produce adverse effects; monitor patient closely and adjust dose of metformin accordingly.

NURSING CONSIDERATIONS

Assessment: Assess for previous hypersensitivity to cephalosporins, PCNs, or other drugs. Assess renal/hepatic function, for a history of GI disease, pregnancy/nursing status, and for possible drug interactions. Obtain baseline culture and susceptibility tests.

Monitoring: Monitor for signs/symptoms of hypersensitivity reactions, CDAD, superinfection, and other adverse reactions. Monitor PT and renal function when indicated. Perform culture and susceptibility tests.

Patient Counseling: Inform that drug only treats bacterial, not viral (eg, common cold), infections. Instruct to take exactly ud; inform that skipping doses or not completing full course of therapy may decrease effectiveness and increase bacterial resistance. Inform that diarrhea may be experienced as late as 2 or more months after last dose; counsel to contact physician if watery/bloody stools (with/without stomach cramps and fever) occur.

Storage: 20-25°C (68-77°F). (Sus) Store in refrigerator after mixing. May be kept for 14 days without significant loss of potency. Keep tightly closed. (Keflex) 25°C (77°F); excursions permitted to 15-30°C (59-86°F).

CERVARIX – human papillomavirus bivalent (types 16, 18) vaccine, recombinant RX

Class: Vaccine

ADULT DOSAGE

Prevention of Cervical Cancer

Prevention of cervical cancer, cervical intraepithelial neoplasia (CIN) Grade 2 or worse and adenocarcinoma in situ, and CIN Grade 1 caused by oncogenic human papillomavirus (HPV) types 16 and 18

≤25 Years:
3 IM doses (0.5mL each) at 0, 1, and 6 months

PEDIATRIC DOSAGE

Prevention of Cervical Cancer

Prevention of cervical cancer, cervical intraepithelial neoplasia (CIN) Grade 2 or worse and adenocarcinoma in situ, and CIN Grade 1 caused by oncogenic human papillomavirus (HPV) types 16 and 18

≥9 Years:
3 IM doses (0.5mL each) at 0, 1, and 6 months

ADMINISTRATION
IM route

Inject preferably in the deltoid region of the upper arm
Do not mix w/ any other vaccine in the same syringe or vial
Shake well before withdrawal and use

HOW SUPPLIED
Inj: 0.5mL

WARNINGS/PRECAUTIONS
Does not provide protection against disease due to all HPV types or from vaccine and non-vaccine HPV types to which a woman has previously been exposed through sexual activity. May not result in protection in all vaccine recipients. Females should continue to adhere to recommended cervical cancer screening procedures. Syncope sometimes associated w/ falling w/ injury, tonic-clonic movements, and other seizure-like activity reported; observe for 15 min after administration. Tip cap of prefilled syringe may contain natural rubber latex; may cause allergic reactions in latex-sensitive individuals. Review immunization history for possible vaccine hypersensitivity and previous vaccination-related adverse reactions; appropriate treatment and supervision must be available for possible anaphylactic reactions. Immunocompromised individuals may have diminished immune response.

ADVERSE REACTIONS
Inj-site reactions (eg, pain, redness, swelling), fatigue, headache, myalgia, GI symptoms, arthralgia, fever, rash, urticaria, nasopharyngitis, influenza.

DRUG INTERACTIONS
Immunosuppressive therapies, including irradiation, antimetabolites, alkylating agents, cytotoxic drugs, and corticosteroids (used in greater than physiologic doses), may reduce immune response to vaccine.

NURSING CONSIDERATIONS

Assessment: Assess for latex hypersensitivity, immunosuppression, pregnancy/nursing status, and possible drug interactions. Review immunization history for possible vaccine hypersensitivity and for previous vaccination-related adverse reactions.

Monitoring: Monitor for syncope, tonic-clonic movements, seizure-like activity, anaphylactic reactions, and other adverse reactions.

Patient Counseling: Inform that vaccine does not substitute for routine cervical cancer screening; advise women who receive the vaccine to continue to undergo cervical screening per standard of care. Counsel that vaccine does not protect against disease from HPV types to which a woman has previously been exposed through sexual activity. Inform that since syncope has been reported following vaccination in young females, observation for 15 min after administration is recommended.

Storage: 2-8°C (36-46°F). Do not freeze; discard if frozen.

CHANTIX – varenicline **RX**

Class: Nicotinic acetylcholine receptor agonist

Serious neuropsychiatric events including, but not limited to, depression, suicidal ideation, suicide attempt, and completed suicide reported. Some reported cases might have been complicated by nicotine withdrawal symptoms in patients who stopped smoking. Monitor for neuropsychiatric symptoms, including changes in behavior, hostility, agitation, depressed mood, and suicide-related events. Worsening of preexisting psychiatric illness and completed suicide reported in some patients attempting to quit smoking while on therapy. Advise patients and caregivers that the patient should stop taking therapy and contact a healthcare provider immediately if agitation, hostility, depressed mood, changes in behavior or thinking, suicidal ideation, or suicidal behavior occurs. Weigh risks against benefits of use.

ADULT DOSAGE

Smoking Cessation Aid

Set quit date and start 1 week before quit date. Alternatively, may begin therapy and then quit smoking between Days 8 and 35 of treatment

Days 1-3: 0.5mg qd
Days 4-7: 0.5mg bid
Day 8-End of Treatment: 1mg bid
Treat for 12 weeks
If patient has successfully stopped smoking at end of 12 weeks, additional course of 12-week treatment is recommended to ensure long-term abstinence

If patient is motivated to quit and not successful in stopping smoking during prior therapy for reasons other than intolerability due to adverse events, or if relapse occurs after treatment, should make another attempt once factors contributing to failed attempt are identified and addressed

PEDIATRIC DOSAGE

Pediatric use may not have been established

DOSE MODIFICATION

Renal Impairment

Severe (CrCl <30mL/min):
Initial: 0.5mg qd
Titrate: May titrate prn to a max dose of 0.5mg bid

ESRD w/ Hemodialysis:
Max: 0.5mg qd if tolerated

Adverse Reactions

Consider a temporary/permanent dose reduction in patients who cannot tolerate adverse effects

ADMINISTRATION

Oral route

Take pc and w/ a full glass of water
Provide patients w/ appropriate educational materials and counseling to support the quit attempt

HOW SUPPLIED

Tab: 0.5mg, 1mg

WARNINGS/PRECAUTIONS

Seizures reported; caution w/ history of seizures or other factors that can lower the seizure threshold. Somnolence, dizziness, loss of consciousness, and difficulty concentrating reported; may impair physical/mental abilities. Cardiovascular (CV) events reported in patients w/ stable CV disease. Hypersensitivity reactions, including angioedema, and rare but serious skin reactions (eg, Stevens-Johnson syndrome, erythema multiforme) reported. Nausea reported; consider dose reduction for patients w/ intolerable nausea. Caution in elderly.

ADVERSE REACTIONS
N/V, headache, insomnia, somnolence, abnormal dreams, flatulence, constipation, dysgeusia, fatigue, upper respiratory tract disorder, abdominal pain, dyspepsia, dry mouth, sleep disorder, increased appetite.

DRUG INTERACTIONS
May increase intoxicating effects of alcohol. Nicotine replacement therapy (transdermal nicotine) may increase incidence of adverse events. Physiological changes resulting from smoking cessation may alter pharmacokinetics or pharmacodynamics of certain drugs (eg, theophylline, warfarin, insulin) for which dosage adjustment may be necessary.

NURSING CONSIDERATIONS

Assessment: Assess for preexisting psychiatric illness, history of seizures or other factors that can lower the seizure threshold, CV disease, history of hypersensitivity to the drug, renal impairment, pregnancy/nursing status, and for possible drug interactions.

Monitoring: Monitor for neuropsychiatric symptoms or worsening of preexisting psychiatric illness, seizures, somnolence, dizziness, loss of consciousness, difficulty concentrating, CV events, skin reactions, hypersensitivity reactions, nausea, and other adverse reactions. Monitor renal function.

Patient Counseling: Inform about risks and benefits of treatment. Instruct to set a date to quit smoking and initiate treatment 1 week before quit date. Encourage to continue to attempt to quit even w/ early lapses after quit day. Encourage patients who are motivated to quit and who did not succeed in stopping smoking during prior therapy for reasons other than intolerability due to adverse events, or who relapsed after treatment to make another attempt w/ therapy once factors contributing to the failed attempt have been identified and addressed. Provide educational materials and necessary counseling to support attempt at quitting smoking. Instruct to notify physician if persistent nausea or insomnia develops. Advise to d/c and notify physician if agitation, hostility, depressed mood, or changes in behavior/thinking develop. Advise to notify physician prior to treatment of any history of psychiatric illness. Inform that quitting smoking may be associated w/ nicotine withdrawal symptoms or exacerbation of preexisting psychiatric illness. Advise to inform physician of any history of seizures or other factors that can lower seizure threshold; instruct patient to d/c treatment and contact physician immediately if seizure is experienced. Instruct patient to reduce amount of alcohol they consume while on therapy until they know whether therapy affects their tolerance for alcohol. Advise to use caution when driving or operating machinery until patients know how quitting smoking and/or therapy may affect them. Advise to notify physician if symptoms of new or worsening CV events develop and to seek immediate medical attention if signs/symptoms of a MI or stroke are experienced. Instruct to d/c and seek immediate medical care if angioedema or a skin reaction occurs. Inform that vivid, unusual, or strange dreams may occur. If patient is pregnant, planning to become pregnant, or breastfeeding, advise about the risks of smoking, the potential risks of therapy, and the benefits of smoking cessation.

Storage: 25°C (77°F); excursions permitted to 15-30°C (59-86°F).

CIALIS – tadalafil

RX

Class: Phosphodiesterase type 5 inhibitor

ADULT DOSAGE

Erectile Dysfunction

PRN Use:
Initial: 10mg prior to sexual activity
Titrate: May increase to 20mg or decrease to 5mg, based on individual efficacy and tolerability
Max Dosing Frequency: Once daily

Once-Daily Use:
Initial: 2.5mg qd
Titrate: May increase to 5mg qd based on individual efficacy and tolerability

Benign Prostatic Hyperplasia

W/ or w/o Erectile Dysfunction (ED): 5mg qd

Initiated w/ Finasteride: 5mg qd for ≤26 weeks

PEDIATRIC DOSAGE

Pediatric use may not have been established

DOSE MODIFICATION

Concomitant Medications

α-Blockers:
Erectile Dysfunction (ED):
Initial: Use lowest recommended dose; should be stable on α-blocker therapy prior to initiating treatment

BPH:
Not recommended
Potent CYP3A4 Inhibitors (eg, Ketoconazole, Ritonavir):
PRN Use:
Max: 10mg/72 hrs
Once-Daily Use:
Max: 2.5mg

Renal Impairment
PRN Use:
CrCl 30-50mL/min:
Initial: 5mg qd
Max: 10mg/48 hrs
CrCl <30mL/min or Hemodialysis:
Max: 5mg/72 hrs
Once-Daily Use:
ED:
CrCl <30mL/min or Hemodialysis:
Not recommended
BPH or ED/BPH:
CrCl 30-50mL/min:
Initial: 2.5mg
Titrate: May increase to 5mg based on individual response
CrCl <30mL/min or Hemodialysis:
Not recommended

Hepatic Impairment
PRN Use:
Mild/Moderate (Child-Pugh Class A/B):
Max: 10mg qd
Severe (Child-Pugh Class C):
Not recommended
Once-Daily Use:
Mild/Moderate (Child-Pugh Class A/B): Use caution
Severe (Child-Pugh Class C): Not recommended

ADMINISTRATION

Oral route

May be taken w/o regard to food
Do not split; entire dose should be taken

Once-Daily Use
Take at approx the same time every day

HOW SUPPLIED

Tab: 2.5mg, 5mg, 10mg, 20mg

CONTRAINDICATIONS

Any form of organic nitrate, either regularly and/or intermittently used.

WARNINGS/PRECAUTIONS

Cardiac risk associated with sexual activity may occur; avoid in men for whom sexual activity is inadvisable due to underlying cardiovascular (CV) status. Patients with severely impaired autonomic control of BP and with left ventricular outflow obstruction (eg, aortic stenosis, idiopathic hypertrophic subaortic stenosis) may be sensitive to vasodilators, including therapy. Avoid with MI (within last 90 days), unstable angina or angina occurring during sexual intercourse, NYHA Class 2 or greater HF (in the last 6 months), uncontrolled arrhythmias, hypotension (<90/50mmHg), uncontrolled HTN, and stroke (within the last 6 months). Mild systemic vasodilatory properties may result in transient decreases in BP. Prolonged erections (>4 hrs) and priapism (painful erections >6 hrs in duration) reported; caution in patients who have conditions predisposing to priapism (eg, sickle cell anemia, multiple myeloma, leukemia), or with anatomical deformation of the penis (eg, angulation, cavernosal fibrosis, Peyronie's disease). Non-arteritic anterior ischemic optic neuropathy (NAION) rarely reported; d/c if sudden loss of vision is experienced in one or both eyes. Caution in patients with underlying NAION risk factors, individuals who have experienced NAION, and individuals with "crowded" optic disc. Sudden decrease or loss of hearing reported which may be accompanied by tinnitus and dizziness; d/c if this occurs. Avoid qd use in patients with CrCl <30mL/min or on hemodialysis. Avoid use with severe hepatic impairment (Child-Pugh Class C) and hereditary degenerative retinal disorders, including retinitis pigmentosa. Caution with mild to moderate hepatic impairment (Child-Pugh Class A/B), bleeding disorders, or significant active peptic ulceration. Consider other urological conditions that may cause similar symptoms prior to initiating treatment for BPH.

ADVERSE REACTIONS

Headache, dyspepsia, back pain, myalgia, nasal congestion, flushing, limb pain, nasopharyngitis, URTI, gastroenteritis, cough, GERD, HTN.

DRUG INTERACTIONS

See Contraindications. Avoid concomitant use with other PDE-5 inhibitors, including Adcirca. Avoid concomitant use with nitrates within 48 hrs. Caution with α-blockers. Concomitant use not recommended with α-blockers for the treatment of BPH. BP-lowering effects of each individual compound may be increased with alcohol. Additive hypotensive effects with selected antihypertensive medications (amlodipine, ARBs, bendrofluazide, enalapril, metoprolol). Antacids (magnesium hydroxide/aluminum hydroxide) may reduce the apparent rate of absorption. CYP3A4 inhibitors (eg, ketoconazole, erythromycin, itraconazole, grapefruit juice), ritonavir, and other HIV protease inhibitors may increase exposure. CYP3A4 inducers (eg, rifampin, carbamazepine, phenytoin, phenobarbital) may decrease exposure. A small increase in HR reported with theophylline.

NURSING CONSIDERATIONS

Assessment: Assess for previous hypersensitivity to drug, CV disease, hereditary degenerative retinal disorders, bleeding disorders, significant active peptic ulceration, anatomical deformation of the penis or presence of conditions that would predispose to priapism, underlying NAION risk factors, "crowded" optic disc, potential underlying causes of ED, other urological conditions, renal/hepatic impairment, pregnancy/nursing status, and possible drug interactions.

Monitoring: Monitor for hypersensitivity reactions, BP decrease, decrease/loss of hearing or vision, prolonged erection, priapism, and other adverse reactions.

Patient Counseling: Instruct to seek emergency medical attention if erection persists >4 hrs. Advise of potential BP-lowering effect of α-blockers, antihypertensive medications, and alcohol. Inform of the potential cardiac risk of sexual activity in patients with preexisting CV disease; instruct patients who experience symptoms upon initiation of sexual activity to refrain from further sexual activity and seek immediate medical attention. Counsel about the protective measures necessary to guard against sexually transmitted disease, including HIV, that should be considered. Inform about contraindication with regular and/or intermittent use of organic nitrates and potential interactions with medications. Instruct to d/c and seek medical attention if sudden decrease or loss of vision or hearing occurs. Inform of the increased risk of NAION in individuals who have already experienced NAION in one eye and in patients with a "crowded" optic disc. Counsel to take one tab at least 30 min before anticipated sexual activity for prn use in men with ED, and at approximately the same time every day without regard to timing of sexual activity for qd use in men with ED, BPH, or ED/BPH.

Storage: 25°C (77°F); excursions permitted to 15-30°C (59-86°F).

CICLOPIROX – ciclopirox RX

Class: Broad-spectrum antifungal

OTHER BRAND NAMES

Loprox

ADULT DOSAGE

Tinea Cruris

Cre/Sus:
Gently massage into the affected/surrounding skin areas
bid (am and pm)

Review diagnosis if no clinical improvement after 4 weeks of therapy

Tinea Pedis

Cre/Sus:
Gently massage into the affected/surrounding skin areas
bid (am and pm)

Gel:
Interdigital Tinea Pedis:
Gently massage into the affected/surrounding skin areas
bid (am and pm) for 4 weeks

Review diagnosis if no clinical improvement after 4 weeks of therapy

Tinea Corporis

Cre/Sus:
Gently massage into the affected/surrounding skin areas
bid (am and pm)

PEDIATRIC DOSAGE

Tinea Cruris

≥10 Years:
Cre/Sus:
Gently massage into the affected/surrounding skin areas bid (am and pm)

Review diagnosis if no clinical improvement after 4 weeks of therapy

Tinea Pedis

≥10 Years:
Cre/Sus:
Gently massage into the affected/surrounding skin areas bid (am and pm)

≥16 Years:
Gel:
Interdigital Tinea Pedis:
Gently massage into the affected/surrounding skin areas bid (am and pm) for 4 weeks

Review diagnosis if no clinical improvement after 4 weeks of therapy

Tinea Corporis

≥10 Years:
Cre/Sus:
Gently massage into the affected/surrounding skin areas bid (am and pm)

Gel:
Gently massage into the affected/surrounding skin areas
bid (am and pm) for 4 weeks

Review diagnosis if no clinical improvement after 4 weeks of therapy

Cutaneous Candidiasis

Cre/Sus:
Gently massage into the affected/surrounding skin areas bid (am and pm)

Review diagnosis if no clinical improvement after 4 weeks of therapy

Tinea Versicolor

Cre/Sus:
Gently massage into the affected/surrounding skin areas bid (am and pm)

Review diagnosis if no clinical improvement after 4 weeks of therapy

Seborrheic Dermatitis

Seborrheic Dermatitis of the Scalp:
Shampoo:
Wet hair and apply 1 tsp (5mL) to scalp; may use up to 2 tsp (10mL) for long hair
Lather and leave on scalp for 3 min; rinse off
Repeat treatment 2X/week for 4 weeks, w/ a minimum of 3 days between applications
Gel:
Apply to affected scalp areas bid (am and pm) for 4 weeks

Review diagnosis if no clinical improvement after 4 weeks of therapy

≥16 Years:
Gel:
Gently massage into the affected/surrounding skin areas bid (am and pm) for 4 weeks

Review diagnosis if no clinical improvement after 4 weeks of therapy

Cutaneous Candidiasis

≥10 Years:
Cre/Sus:
Gently massage into the affected/surrounding skin areas bid (am and pm)

Review diagnosis if no clinical improvement after 4 weeks of therapy

Tinea Versicolor

≥10 Years:
Cre/Sus:
Gently massage into the affected/surrounding skin areas bid (am and pm)

Review diagnosis if no clinical improvement after 4 weeks of therapy

Seborrheic Dermatitis

Seborrheic Dermatitis of the Scalp:
≥16 Years:
Shampoo:
Wet hair and apply 1 tsp (5mL) to scalp; may use up to 2 tsp (10mL) for long hair
Lather and leave on hair for 3 min; rinse off
Repeat treatment 2X/week for 4 weeks, w/ a minimum of 3 days between applications

Gel:
Apply to affected scalp areas bid (am and pm) for 4 weeks

Review diagnosis if no clinical improvement after 4 weeks of therapy

ADMINISTRATION
Topical route

Gel
Clean/wash affected areas before application for treatment of interdigital tinea pedis and tinea corporis

Sus
Shake vigorously before use

Shampoo
Lather, leave on hair and scalp for 3 min, and then rinse off

HOW SUPPLIED
Cre: 0.77% [15g, 30g, 90g]; Gel: 0.77% [30g, 45g, 100g]; Sus (Lot): 0.77% [30mL, 60mL]; (Loprox) Shampoo: 1% [120mL]

WARNINGS/PRECAUTIONS
For dermatologic use only; not for ophthalmic, oral, or intravaginal use. Avoid contact w/ eyes. D/C and institute appropriate therapy if a reaction suggesting sensitivity or chemical irritation occurs. (Gel) Transient burning sensation may occur, especially in sensitive areas. (Shampoo) Hair discoloration reported in patients w/ lighter hair color.

ADVERSE REACTIONS
Application-site reactions (eg, pruritus, burning). (Gel) Contact dermatitis.

NURSING CONSIDERATIONS

Assessment: Assess for hypersensitivity to drug and pregnancy/nursing status.

Monitoring: Monitor for signs/symptoms of sensitivity or irritation and other adverse reactions. Review diagnosis if no clinical improvement seen after 4 weeks of treatment.

Patient Counseling: Instruct to use medication ud and to use for full treatment period even if signs/symptoms have improved. Inform that medication is for external use only; advise to avoid contact w/ eyes and mucous membranes. Advise not to use medication for any disorder other than that for which it is prescribed. Instruct to notify physician if no improvement seen after 4 weeks of therapy, or if treatment area shows signs of increased irritation (eg, redness, itching, burning) indicative of possible sensitization. (Cre/Gel/Sus) Instruct to avoid use of occlusive wrappings or dressings. (Gel) Counsel that transient burning/stinging sensation may occur when used to treat seborrheic dermatitis of the scalp. (Shampoo) Instruct to use on the scalp only and not to swallow. Instruct to rinse thoroughly w/ water if contact w/ eyes occurs.

Storage: (Shampoo) 15-30°C (59-86°F). Discard unused product after initial treatment duration. (Cre/Sus/Gel) 20-25°C (68-77°F).

CILOXAN – ciprofloxacin hydrochloride

RX

Class: Fluoroquinolone

ADULT DOSAGE

Bacterial Conjunctivitis

Sol:
1-2 drops into the conjunctival sac q2h while awake for 2 days, then 1-2 drops q4h while awake for the next 5 days

Oint:
Apply 1/2-inch ribbon into the conjunctival sac tid on the first 2 days, then 1/2-inch ribbon bid for the next 5 days

Corneal Ulcers

Sol:
Day 1: 2 drops into the affected eye every 15 min for the first 6 hrs, then 2 drops every 30 min for the remainder of the day
Day 2: 2 drops every hr
Days 3-14: 2 drops q4h

May continue treatment after 14 days if reepithelialization has not occurred

PEDIATRIC DOSAGE

Bacterial Conjunctivitis

Sol:
≥1 Year:
1-2 drops into the conjunctival sac q2h while awake for 2 days, then 1-2 drops q4h while awake for the next 5 days

Oint:
≥2 Years:
Apply 1/2-inch ribbon tid into the conjunctival sac on the first 2 days, then bid for the next 5 days

Corneal Ulcers

Sol:
≥1 Year:
Day 1: 2 drops into the affected eye every 15 min for the first 6 hrs, then 2 drops every 30 min for the remainder of the day
Day 2: 2 drops every hr
Days 3-14: 2 drops q4h

May continue treatment after 14 days if reepithelialization has not occurred

ADMINISTRATION

Ocular route

HOW SUPPLIED

Oint: 0.3% [3.5g]; Sol: 0.3% [2.5mL, 5mL, 10mL]

WARNINGS/PRECAUTIONS

For topical ophthalmic use only; do not inject into eye. Serious and occasionally fatal hypersensitivity (anaphylactic) reactions reported in patients receiving systemic therapy; immediate emergency treatment with epinephrine and other resuscitation measures may be required as clinically indicated. Prolonged use may result in overgrowth of nonsusceptible organisms, including fungi; initiate appropriate therapy if superinfection occurs. D/C at 1st appearance of skin rash or other signs of hypersensitivity reaction. Remove contact lenses before use; avoid wearing contact lenses when signs/symptoms of bacterial conjunctivitis are present. (Oint) May retard corneal healing and cause visual blurring. (Sol) May form a white crystalline precipitate in the superficial portion of the corneal defect.

ADVERSE REACTIONS

Local discomfort, keratopathy, allergic reactions, corneal staining, foreign body sensation. (Oint) Blurred vision, irritation, lid margin hyperemia. (Sol) Local burning, white crystalline precipitate formation, lid margin crusting, conjunctival hyperemia, crystals/scales, itching, bad taste.

DRUG INTERACTIONS

Systemic quinolone therapy may increase theophylline levels, interfere with caffeine metabolism, enhance effects of warfarin and its derivatives, and elevate SrCr with cyclosporine.

NURSING CONSIDERATIONS

Assessment: Assess for previous hypersensitivity to the drug and other quinolones, use of contact lenses, pregnancy/nursing status, and possible drug interactions.

Monitoring: Monitor for signs/symptoms of hypersensitivity/anaphylactic reactions, and other adverse reactions. Monitor for superinfection; examine with magnification (eg, slit-lamp biomicroscopy) and fluorescein staining, where appropriate.

Patient Counseling: Instruct to use as prescribed. Instruct not to touch dropper tip to any surface because it may contaminate sol. Advise to contact physician if hypersensitivity reaction occurs (eg, rash). Instruct to remove contact lenses before use and not to wear contact lenses if signs/symptoms of bacterial conjunctivitis are present.

Storage: 2-25°C (36-77°F). (Sol) Protect from light.

CIMZIA – certolizumab pegol

RX

Class: TNF-blocker

Increased risk for developing serious infections (eg, active tuberculosis [TB], latent TB reactivation, invasive fungal infections, bacterial/viral and other opportunistic infections) leading to hospitalization or death, mostly with concomitant use with immunosuppressants (eg, methotrexate [MTX] or corticosteroids). D/C if serious infection or sepsis develops. Active TB/reactivation of latent TB may present with disseminated or extrapulmonary disease; test for latent TB before and during therapy and initiate treatment for latent TB prior to therapy. Invasive fungal infections reported; consider empiric antifungal therapy in patients at risk who develop severe systemic illness. Consider risks and benefits prior to therapy in patients with chronic or recurrent infection. Monitor patients for development of infection during and after treatment, including development of TB in patients who tested negative for latent TB infection prior to therapy. Lymphoma and other malignancies, some fatal, reported in children and adolescents.

ADULT DOSAGE

Crohn's Disease

Moderately to Severely Active Disease w/ Inadequate Response to Conventional Therapy:
Initial: 400mg (given as 2 SQ inj of 200mg) initially, and at Weeks 2 and 4
Maint: 400mg every 4 weeks

Rheumatoid Arthritis

Moderately to Severely Active:
Initial: 400mg (given as 2 SQ inj of 200mg) initially and at Weeks 2 and 4, followed by 200mg every other week
Maint: Consider 400mg every 4 weeks

Psoriatic Arthritis

Active:
Initial: 400mg (given as 2 SQ inj of 200mg) initially and at Weeks 2 and 4, followed by 200mg every other week
Maint: Consider 400mg every 4 weeks

Ankylosing Spondylitis

Active:
Initial: 400mg (given as 2 SQ inj of 200mg) initially and at Weeks 2 and 4, followed by 200mg every 2 weeks or 400mg every 4 weeks

PEDIATRIC DOSAGE

Pediatric use may not have been established

ADMINISTRATION

SQ route

Rotate inj sites; avoid areas where the skin is tender, bruised, red, or hard

Lyophilized Powder for Inj

Preparation:

1. Reconstitute vial(s) w/ 1mL of sterile water for inj (SWFI) using 20-gauge needle provided
2. Gently swirl each vial w/o shaking, assuring that all of the powder comes in contact w/ SWFI
3. Leave the vial(s) undisturbed to fully reconstitute, which may take approx 30 min
4. Final reconstituted sol contains 200mg/mL

Administration:

1. Prior to injecting, reconstituted sol should be at room temperature (not >2 hrs prior to administration)
2. Withdraw reconstituted sol into a separate syringe for each vial using a new 20-gauge needle for each vial so that each syringe contains 1mL of sol (200mg of certolizumab pegol)
3. Replace 20-gauge needle(s) on syringes w/ a 23-gauge(s) for administration
4. Inject full contents of syringe(s) SQ into thigh or abdomen; when a 400mg dose is needed (given as 2 SQ inj of 200mg), inj should occur at separate sites in the thigh or abdomen

Prefilled Syringe

After proper training in SQ inj technique, a patient may self-inject w/ a prefilled syringe if a physician determines that it is appropriate

Patients using prefilled syringes should be instructed to inject full amount in syringe (1mL), according to the directions provided in Instructions for Use booklet

HOW SUPPLIED

Inj: 200mg/mL [prefilled syringe, vial]

WARNINGS/PRECAUTIONS

May be used as monotherapy or concomitantly with non-biological disease modifying antirheumatic drugs (DMARDs). Do not initiate with an active infection. Increased risk of infection in elderly patients and in patients with comorbid conditions; consider the risks prior to therapy for those who have resided or traveled in areas of endemic TB or mycoses, and with any underlying conditions predisposing to infection. Postmarketing cases of aggressive and fatal hepatosplenic T-cell lymphoma (HSTCL) reported in patients with CD or ulcerative colitis and the majority were in adolescent and young adult males; almost all of these patients were treated concomitantly with azathioprine or 6-mercaptopurine (6-MP). Carefully consider the potential risk of HSTCL with the combination of azathioprine or 6-MP. Cases acute and chronic leukemia reported. Perform periodic skin examination, particularly in patients with risk factors for skin cancer. New onset and worsening of congestive heart failure (CHF) reported; caution in patients with heart failure (HF) and monitor carefully. Hypersensitivity reactions reported (rare); d/c and institute appropriate therapy if such reactions occur. Hepatitis B virus (HBV) reactivation reported; if reactivation occurs, d/c and initiate antiviral therapy with appropriate supportive treatment. Monitor patients closely and exercise caution when considering resumption of therapy. Associated with rare cases of new onset or exacerbation of clinical symptoms and/or radiographic evidence of CNS and peripheral demyelinating disease; caution with preexisting or recent-onset central or peripheral nervous system demyelinating disorders. Rare cases of neurological disorders (eg, seizure disorder, optic neuritis, peripheral neuropathy) reported. Hematological reactions (eg, leukopenia, pancytopenia, thrombocytopenia) reported; caution in patients with ongoing, or a history of, significant hematologic abnormalities, and consider discontinuation in patients with confirmed significant hematologic abnormalities. May result in the formation of autoantibodies and rarely, in the development of a lupus-like syndrome; d/c if lupus-like syndrome develops. Lab test interactions may occur. Caution in elderly.

ADVERSE REACTIONS

Infections, lymphoma and other malignancies, upper respiratory tract infections, rash, urinary tract infections, arthralgia, headache, HTN, nasopharyngitis, back pain, pyrexia, pharyngitis, acute bronchitis, fatigue.

DRUG INTERACTIONS

See Boxed Warning. Avoid concurrent use with live (eg, attenuated) vaccines. Concomitant administration with other biological DMARDs (eg, anakinra, abatacept, rituximab), other TNF blockers or natalizumab is not recommended; may increase risk of serious infections.

NURSING CONSIDERATIONS

Assessment: Assess for active/chronic/recurrent infection (eg, TB, HBV), TB exposure, history of an opportunistic infection, recent travel to areas of endemic TB or endemic mycoses, underlying conditions that may predispose to infection, HF, presence or history of significant hematologic abnormalities, neurologic disorders, risk factors for skin cancer, pregnancy/nursing status, and possible drug interactions. Assess vaccination history in pediatric patients. Perform test for latent TB infection.

Monitoring: Monitor for sepsis, TB (active, reactivation, or latent), invasive fungal infections, bacterial/viral/other infections, lymphoma/other malignancies, new onset/worsening of CHF, active HBV infection, hematological events, hypersensitivity reactions, CNS demyelinating disorders, lupus-like syndrome, and other adverse reactions. Perform periodic skin examination, particularly in patients with risk factors for skin cancer and test for latent TB infection.

Patient Counseling: Advise of potential risks and benefits of therapy. Inform that therapy may lower the ability of the immune system to fight infections; instruct to immediately contact physician if any signs/symptoms of an infection develop, including TB and HBV reactivation. Counsel about the risks of lymphoma and other malignancies while on therapy. Advise to seek immediate medical attention if any symptoms of severe allergic reactions occur. Advise to report to physician signs of new or worsening medical conditions (eg, heart disease, neurological diseases, autoimmune disorders) and symptoms of a cytopenia (eg, bruising, bleeding, persistent fever). Instruct about proper administration techniques.

Storage: 2-8°C (36-46°F). Do not freeze. Protect sol from light. Reconstituted Sol: 2-8°C (36-46°F) for up to 24 hrs. Do not freeze.

CIPRO HC – ciprofloxacin hydrochloride/hydrocortisone RX

Class: Antibacterial/corticosteroid combination

ADULT DOSAGE

Acute Otitis Externa

Caused by Susceptible Strains of Microorganisms of *Pseudomonas aeruginosa, Staphylococcus aureus,* and *Proteus mirabilis*:
3 drops into affected ear bid for 7 days

PEDIATRIC DOSAGE

Acute Otitis Externa

Caused by Susceptible Strains of Microorganisms of *Pseudomonas aeruginosa, Staphylococcus aureus,* and *Proteus mirabilis*:

≥1 Year:
3 drops into affected ear bid for 7 days

ADMINISTRATION

Otic route

Shake well before use

Warm bottle in hand for 1-2 min to avoid dizziness (due to instillation of a cold sol in the ear canal)

Lie w/ affected ear upward, then instill drops; maintain position for 30-60 sec and repeat, if necessary, for the opposite ear

Discard unused portion after therapy is completed

HOW SUPPLIED

Sus: (Ciprofloxacin/Hydrocortisone) 0.2%/1% [10mL]

CONTRAINDICATIONS

Perforated tympanic membrane, viral infections of external ear canal, including varicella and herpes simplex infections.

WARNINGS/PRECAUTIONS

Not for inj or ophthalmic use. D/C at 1st appearance of skin rash or any other sign of hypersensitivity. Serious and occasionally fatal hypersensitivity (anaphylactic) reactions reported; may require immediate emergency treatment. May result in overgrowth of nonsusceptible organisms (eg, fungi). Reevaluate if no improvement after 1 week.

ADVERSE REACTIONS

Headache, pruritus.

NURSING CONSIDERATIONS

Assessment: Assess for history of drug hypersensitivity, perforated tympanic membrane, viral infections of external ear canal, (including varicella and herpes simplex infections) and pregnancy/nursing status.

Monitoring: Monitor for hypersensitivity reactions, overgrowth of nonsusceptible organisms (eg, fungi), and possible adverse reactions.

Patient Counseling: Instruct to d/c immediately and consult physician if rash or allergic reaction occurs. Advise not to use in the eyes. Advise to avoid contaminating the dropper with material from the ear, fingers, or other sources. Instruct to protect product from light. Instruct to shake well before using and to discard unused portion after therapy is completed.

Storage: Below 25°C (77°F). Avoid freezing. Protect from light.

CIPRO XR – ciprofloxacin RX

Class: Fluoroquinolone

Fluoroquinolones are associated w/ an increased risk of tendinitis and tendon rupture in all ages. Risk is further increased in patients >60 yrs of age, patients taking corticosteroids, and w/ kidney, heart, or lung transplants. May exacerbate muscle weakness w/ myasthenia gravis; avoid in patients w/ known history of myasthenia gravis.

ADULT DOSAGE

Urinary Tract Infections

Uncomplicated (Acute Cystitis):
500mg q24h for 3 days

Complicated UTI/Acute Uncomplicated Pyelonephritis:
1000mg q24h for 7-14 days
May switch from IV to Cipro XR at discretion of physician

PEDIATRIC DOSAGE

Pediatric use may not have been established

DOSE MODIFICATION

Renal Impairment

Hemodialysis/Peritoneal Dialysis: Give after procedure is completed

Max: 500mg q24h

Continuous Ambulatory Peritoneal Dialysis:

Max: 500mg q24h

Complicated UTI/Acute Uncomplicated Pyelonephritis:

CrCl ≤30mL/min: Reduce dose from 1000mg to 500mg qd; use of 1000mg tab is not recommended in this population

ADMINISTRATION

Oral route

Swallow tab whole; do not split, crush, or chew

Take w/ or w/o food

Space Ca^{2+} intake (>800mg) by 2 hrs

Administer ≥2 hrs before or 6 hrs after antacids containing Mg^{2+} or aluminum, polymeric phosphate binders, sucralfate, didanosine, chewable/buffered tabs or pediatric powder, other highly buffered drugs, metal cations such as iron, and multivitamin preparations w/ zinc.

HOW SUPPLIED

Tab, Extended-Release: 500mg, 1000mg

CONTRAINDICATIONS

Concomitant administration w/ tizanidine.

WARNINGS/PRECAUTIONS

Caution w/ history of tendon disorders; d/c if patient experiences pain, swelling, inflammation, or rupture of tendon. Serious and occasionally fatal hypersensitivity (anaphylactic) reactions reported; d/c immediately at the 1st appearance of a skin rash, jaundice, or any other sign of hypersensitivity, and institute supportive measures. Severe hepatotoxicity, including hepatic necrosis, life-threatening hepatic failure, and fatal events, reported; d/c immediately if signs and symptoms of hepatitis occur. Convulsions, status epilepticus, increased intracranial pressure (including pseudotumor cerebri), toxic psychosis, and other CNS events reported; d/c and institute appropriate measures if CNS events occur. Caution w/ epilepsy and CNS disorders (eg, severe cerebral arteriosclerosis, history of convulsion, reduced cerebral blood flow) or other risk factors that may predispose to seizures or lower seizure threshold; d/c if seizures occur. *Clostridium difficile*-associated diarrhea (CDAD) reported; may need to d/c if CDAD is suspected or confirmed. Cases of sensory or sensorimotor axonal polyneuropathy resulting in paresthesias, hypoesthesias, dysesthesias, and weakness reported; d/c immediately if symptoms of peripheral neuropathy occur. May prolong QT interval; avoid w/ known QT interval prolongation and w/ risk factors for QT prolongation/torsades de pointes (eg, congenital long QT syndrome, uncorrected hypokalemia/hypomagnesemia, cardiac disease). Crystalluria reported; maintain hydration and avoid alkalinity of urine. May cause photosensitivity/phototoxicity reactions; d/c if phototoxicity occurs. Avoid excessive exposure to sun/UV light. May result in bacterial resistance if used in the absence of a proven or strongly suspected bacterial infection or a prophylactic indication. Has not been shown to be effective in the treatment of syphilis; antimicrobial agents used in high dose for short periods to treat gonorrhea may mask or delay symptoms of incubating syphilis. Caution in elderly. Not interchangeable w/ immediate-release tabs.

ADVERSE REACTIONS

Tendinitis, tendon rupture, nausea, headache.

DRUG INTERACTIONS

See Boxed Warning and Contraindications. Avoid concomitant administration w/ dairy products (eg, milk, yogurt), or Ca^{2+}-fortified products alone; absorption may be reduced. May increase levels of CYP1A2 substrates (eg, theophylline, methylxanthines, olanzapine), duloxetine, or sildenafil. Increased theophylline levels may increase the risk of developing CNS or other adverse reactions; if coadministration cannot be avoided, monitor theophylline levels and adjust dose. May inhibit the formation of paraxanthine after caffeine administration (or pentoxifylline-containing products); monitor for xanthine toxicity and adjust dose as necessary. Avoid use w/ duloxetine; monitor for duloxetine toxicity if coadministration is unavoidable. Monitor for clozapine- or ropinirole-related adverse reactions and adjust dose of clozapine or ropinirole during and shortly after coadministration. Monitor for sildenafil toxicity. Avoid w/ Class IA (eg, quinidine, procainamide) and Class III (eg, amiodarone, sotalol) antiarrhythmics, TCAs, macrolides, and antipsychotics; may further prolong the QT interval. Hypoglycemia reported w/ oral antidiabetic agents, mainly sulfonylureas (eg, glyburide, glimepiride); monitor blood glucose. May alter serum levels of phenytoin; monitor phenytoin therapy, including phenytoin levels during and shortly after coadministration. Transient SrCr elevations w/ cyclosporine; monitor renal function. May increase effects of oral anticoagulants; monitor PT and INR frequently during and shortly after coadministration. May increase levels and toxic reactions of methotrexate; carefully monitor w/ concomitant use. High-dose quinolones in combination w/ NSAIDs (not acetyl salicylic acid) may provoke convulsions. Antacids, sucralfate, multivitamins, and other multivalent cation-containing products (eg, Mg^{2+}/aluminum antacids, polymeric phosphate binders, chewable/buffered tab or pediatric powder) may decrease absorption, resulting in lower serum and urine levels lower than desired; administer ≥2 hrs before or 6 hrs after these drugs. Probenecid may increase levels. Caution w/ drugs that may lower seizure threshold.

NURSING CONSIDERATIONS

Assessment: Assess for risk factors for developing tendinitis and tendon rupture, history of myasthenia gravis, drug hypersensitivity, epilepsy, CNS disorders or other risk factors that may predispose to seizures or lower seizure threshold, QT interval prolongation, renal/hepatic dysfunction, pregnancy/nursing status, and possible drug interactions. Obtain baseline culture and susceptibility tests. Perform serologic test for syphilis in patients w/ gonorrhea.

Monitoring: Monitor for tendinitis or tendon rupture, exacerbation of myasthenia gravis, signs/symptoms of hypersensitivity reactions, ECG changes, arrhythmias, CNS effects, CDAD, hepatotoxicity, peripheral neuropathy, crystalluria, photosensitivity/phototoxicity reactions, and other adverse reactions. Monitor PT and INR if coadministered w/ an oral anticoagulant (eg, warfarin). Monitor renal function. Perform periodic culture and susceptibility testing. Perform follow-up serologic test for syphilis 3 months after treatment.

Patient Counseling: Inform that drug treats only bacterial, not viral, infections. Advise to take exactly ud; inform that skipping doses or not completing full course of therapy may decrease effectiveness and increase likelihood of drug resistance. Advise to drink fluids liberally. Counsel to avoid concomitant use w/ dairy products or Ca^{2+}-fortified juices alone. Advise to contact physician of any tendon disorder symptoms; instruct to d/c therapy and rest/refrain from exercise. Instruct to notify physician if experiencing symptoms of myasthenia gravis, photosensitivity/phototoxicity, or liver injury. Instruct to notify physician of any history of convulsions. Advise to assess reaction to therapy before engaging in activities that require mental alertness or coordination; instruct to notify physician if persistent headache w/ or w/o blurred vision occurs. Advise to contact physician as soon as possible if watery and bloody stools (w/ or w/o stomach cramps and fever) develop even as late as ≥2 months after last dose. Instruct to d/c and notify physician if hypersensitivity reactions or symptoms of peripheral neuropathy develop. Inform physician of any personal or family history of QT prolongation or proarrhythmic conditions and if symptoms of prolongation of the QT interval occur. Advise to seek medical help immediately if experiencing seizures, palpitations, or breathing difficulty. Counsel to minimize or avoid exposure to natural/artificial sunlight (tanning beds or UVA/B treatment). Instruct to contact physician if low blood sugar occurs.

Storage: 25°C (77°F); excursions permitted to 15-30°C (59-86°F).

CIPRODEX – ciprofloxacin/dexamethasone RX

Class: Antibacterial/corticosteroid combination

ADULT DOSAGE

Acute Otitis Externa

4 drops into the affected ear(s) bid for 7 days

PEDIATRIC DOSAGE

Acute Otitis Media

≥6 Months of Age w/ Tympanostomy Tubes:
4 drops into the affected ear(s) bid for 7 days

Acute Otitis Externa

≥6 Months of Age:
4 drops into the affected ear(s) bid for 7 days

ADMINISTRATION

Otic route

1. Warm bottle by holding in hand for 1 or 2 min prior to use and shake well before using
2. Lie w/ affected ear upward, and then instill drops
3. For otitis media, pump the tragus 5X by pushing inward to facilitate penetration of the drops into the middle ear
4. Maintain position for 60 sec and repeat, if necessary, for the opposite ear

HOW SUPPLIED

Sus: (Ciprofloxacin-Dexamethasone) 0.3%-0.1% [7.5mL]

CONTRAINDICATIONS

Viral infections of external canal, including herpes simplex infections.

WARNINGS/PRECAUTIONS

For otic use only; not for ophthalmic use. D/C at 1st appearance of skin rash or any other sign of hypersensitivity. Serious and occasionally fatal hypersensitivity/anaphylactic reactions reported; may require immediate emergency treatment. May result in overgrowth of nonsusceptible organisms (eg, yeast, fungi); perform culture testing if infection is not improved after 1 week. If otorrhea persists after full course of therapy, or if ≥2 episodes of otorrhea occur within 6 months, evaluate to exclude underlying condition such as cholesteatoma, foreign body, or tumor.

ADVERSE REACTIONS

Ear discomfort/pain/precipitate/pruritus/debris/congestion, irritability, taste perversion, superimposed ear infection, erythema.

NURSING CONSIDERATIONS

Assessment: Assess for history of drug hypersensitivity, viral infection of the external canal (eg, herpes simplex virus infection), and pregnancy/nursing status.

Monitoring: Monitor for hypersensitivity/anaphylactic reactions, skin rash, overgrowth of nonsusceptible organisms (eg, yeast, fungi), otorrhea, and other adverse reactions. Perform culture testing if infection is not improved after 1 week of treatment.

Patient Counseling: Inform that drug is for otic use only. Advise to avoid contaminating the tip with material from the ear, fingers, or other sources. Instruct to d/c immediately and consult physician if rash or allergic reaction occurs. Instruct to take as prescribed, even if symptoms improve. Advise to discard unused portion after therapy is completed.

Storage: 20-25°C (68-77°F); excursions permitted to 15-30°C (59-86°F). Avoid freezing. Protect from light.

Ciprofloxacin Injection – ciprofloxacin RX

Class: Fluoroquinolone

Fluoroquinolones are associated w/ an increased risk of tendinitis and tendon rupture in all ages. Risk is further increased in patients >60 yrs of age, patients taking corticosteroids, and patients w/ kidney, heart, or lung transplants. May exacerbate muscle weakness w/ myasthenia gravis; avoid in patients w/ known history of myasthenia gravis.

OTHER BRAND NAMES

Cipro IV

ADULT DOSAGE

Intra-Abdominal Infections

Complicated:
400mg q12h for 7-14 days, concomitantly w/ metronidazole

Sinusitis

Acute:
400mg q12h for 10 days

Chronic Bacterial Prostatitis

400mg q12h for 28 days

Febrile Neutropenia

Empirical Therapy:
400mg q8h + piperacillin 50mg/kg q4h for 7-14 days

Inhalational Anthrax (Postexposure)

400mg q12h for 60 days

Urinary Tract Infections

200-400mg q8-12h for 7-14 days

Lower Respiratory Tract Infections

400mg q8-12h for 7-14 days

Pneumonia

Nosocomial:
400mg q8h for 10-14 days

Skin and Skin Structure Infections

400mg q8-12h for 7-14 days

Bone/Joint Infections

400mg q8-12h for 4-8 weeks

Plague

400mg q8-12h for 14 days

Conversions

IV to Oral:
200mg IV q12h: 250mg tab q12h
400mg IV q12h: 500mg tab q12h
400mg IV q8h: 750mg tab q12h

PEDIATRIC DOSAGE

Urinary Tract Infections

Complicated UTI/Pyelonephritis:
1-17 Years:
6-10mg/kg q8h for 10-21 days
Max: 400mg/dose; even in >51kg

Inhalational Anthrax (Postexposure)

10mg/kg q12h for 60 days
Max: 400mg/dose

Plague

10mg/kg q8-12h for 10-21 days
Max: 400mg/dose

DOSE MODIFICATION

Renal Impairment

Adults:

CrCl 5-29mL/min: 200-400mg q18-24h

ADMINISTRATION

IV route

Infuse IV over 60 min; slow infusion into larger vein will minimize discomfort and reduce risk of venous irritation

If Y-type method is used, temporarily d/c administration of other sol during the infusion (ciprofloxacin inj)

If concomitant use w/ another drug is necessary, give separately (ciprofloxacin inj)

Cipro IV Vials (Inj Concentrate)

Should be diluted to a final concentration of 1-2mg/mL

Flexible Containers

Do not need to be diluted

Infuse directly or through a Y-type IV infusion set that may already be in place (ciprofloxacin inj)

HOW SUPPLIED

Inj: 200mg/100mL (0.2%); (Cipro) 400mg/200mL (0.2%)

CONTRAINDICATIONS

Concomitant administration w/ tizanidine.

WARNINGS/PRECAUTIONS

Not a drug of 1st choice in the treatment of presumed or confirmed pneumonia secondary to *Streptococcus pneumoniae*. Caution w/ history of tendon disorders; d/c if patient experiences pain, swelling, inflammation, or rupture of tendon. Serious and occasionally fatal hypersensitivity (anaphylactic) reactions reported; d/c immediately at the 1st appearance of a skin rash, jaundice, or any other sign of hypersensitivity, and institute supportive measures. Severe hepatotoxicity, including hepatic necrosis, life-threatening hepatic failure, and fatal events, reported; d/c immediately if signs and symptoms of hepatitis occur. Convulsions, status epilepticus, increased intracranial pressure (including pseudotumor cerebri), toxic psychosis, and other CNS events reported; d/c and institute appropriate measures if CNS events occur. Caution w/ epilepsy and CNS disorders (eg, severe cerebral arteriosclerosis, history of convulsion, reduced cerebral blood flow) or other risk factors that may predispose to seizures or lower seizure threshold; d/c if seizures occur. *Clostridium difficile*-associated diarrhea (CDAD) reported; may need to d/c if CDAD is suspected or confirmed. Sensory or sensorimotor axonal polyneuropathy resulting in paresthesias, hypoesthesias, dysesthesias, and weakness reported; d/c immediately if symptoms of peripheral neuropathy occur. May prolong QT interval; avoid w/ known QT interval prolongation and risk factors for QT prolongation/torsades de pointes (eg, congenital long QT syndrome, uncorrected hypokalemia/hypomagnesemia, cardiac disease). Increased incidence of musculoskeletal disorders in pediatric patients. Crystalluria reported; maintain hydration and avoid alkalinity of urine. May cause photosensitivity/phototoxicity reactions; d/c if phototoxicity occurs. Avoid excessive exposure to sun/UV light. May result in bacterial resistance if used in the absence of a proven or strongly suspected bacterial infection or a prophylactic indication. Caution in elderly.

ADVERSE REACTIONS

Tendinitis, tendon rupture, N/V, diarrhea, abnormal LFTs, restlessness, rash.

DRUG INTERACTIONS

See Boxed Warning and Contraindications. May increase levels of CYP1A2 substrates (eg, theophylline, methylxanthines, olanzapine), duloxetine, or sildenafil. Use w/ caution w/ concomitant sildenafil; monitor for sildenafil toxicity. Avoid use w/ duloxetine; if unavoidable, monitor for duloxetine toxicity. Increased theophylline levels may increase the risk of developing CNS, or other adverse reactions; if coadministration cannot be avoided, monitor theophylline levels and adjust dose. May inhibit the formation of paraxanthine after caffeine administration (or pentoxifylline-containing products); monitor for xanthine toxicity and adjust dose as necessary. Monitor for clozapine- or ropinirole-related adverse reactions and adjust dose of clozapine or ropinirole during and shortly after coadministration. Avoid w/ Class IA (eg, quinidine, procainamide) and Class III (eg, amiodarone, sotalol) antiarrhythmics, TCAs, macrolides, and antipsychotics; may further prolong QT interval. Hypoglycemia reported w/ oral antidiabetic agents, mainly sulfonylureas (eg, glyburide, glimepiride); monitor blood glucose. May alter serum levels of phenytoin; monitor phenytoin therapy, including phenytoin levels during and shortly after coadministration. Transient SrCr elevations w/ cyclosporine; monitor renal function. May increase effects of oral anticoagulants; monitor PT and INR frequently during and shortly after coadministration. May increase levels and toxic reactions of methotrexate (MTX); carefully monitor w/ MTX therapy. High-dose quinolones in combination w/ NSAIDs (not acetyl salicylic acid) may provoke convulsions. Probenecid may increase levels; use w/ caution. Caution w/ drugs that may lower seizure threshold.

NURSING CONSIDERATIONS

Assessment: Assess for risk factors for developing tendinitis and tendon rupture, history of myasthenia gravis, drug hypersensitivity, epilepsy, CNS disorders or other risk factors that may predispose to seizures or lower seizure threshold, QT interval prolongation, pregnancy/nursing status, and possible drug interactions. Assess renal/hepatic/hematopoietic function. Obtain baseline culture and susceptibility test.

Monitoring: Monitor for tendinitis or tendon rupture, exacerbation of myasthenia gravis, signs/symptoms of hypersensitivity reactions, QT prolongations, CNS effects, CDAD, hepatotoxicity, peripheral neuropathy, musculoskeletal disorders (pediatric patients), crystalluria, photosensitivity/phototoxicity reactions, and other adverse reactions. Monitor PT and INR if coadministered w/ an oral anticoagulant (eg, warfarin). Perform periodic culture and susceptibility testing. Periodically monitor organ system function (eg, renal/hepatic/hematopoietic function), particularly during prolonged therapy.

Patient Counseling: Inform that drug treats only bacterial, not viral, infections. Advise to take exactly ud; inform that skipping doses or not completing full course of therapy may decrease effectiveness and increase bacterial resistance. Advise to drink fluids liberally. Advise to notify physician if tension disorder symptoms occur; instruct to d/c therapy and rest/refrain from exercise. Instruct to notify physician if myasthenia gravis, liver injury, or photosensitivity/phototoxicity symptoms occur. Instruct to notify physician of any history of convulsions. Advise to assess reaction to therapy before engaging in activities that require mental alertness or coordination; instruct to notify physician if persistent headache w/ or w/o blurred vision occurs. Advise to contact physician as soon as possible if watery and bloody stools (w/ or w/o stomach cramps and fever) develop even as late as ≥2 months after last dose. Instruct to d/c and notify physician if hypersensitivity reactions or symptoms of peripheral neuropathy develop. Inform physician of any personal or family history of QT prolongation or proarrhythmic conditions and if symptoms of prolongation of the QT interval occur. Counsel caregiver to inform physician if child has joint-related problems prior to, during, or after therapy. Advise to seek medical help immediately if experiencing seizures, palpitations, or breathing difficulty. Counsel to minimize or avoid exposure to natural/artificial sunlight (tanning beds or UVA/B treatment). Instruct to contact physician if low blood sugar occurs. (Cipro IV) Inform that efficacy studies of ciprofloxacin could not be conducted in humans w/ plague and anthrax for feasibility reasons; therefore approval for these conditions was based on an efficacy study conducted in animals.

Storage: 5-25°C (41-77°F). Protect from light and freezing. Avoid excessive heat.

CIPROFLOXACIN ORAL – ciprofloxacin RX

Class: Fluoroquinolone

Fluoroquinolones are associated w/ an increased risk of tendinitis and tendon rupture in all ages. Risk is further increased in patients >60 yrs of age, patients taking corticosteroids, and patients w/ kidney, heart, or lung transplants. May exacerbate muscle weakness w/ myasthenia gravis; avoid in patients w/ known history of myasthenia gravis.

OTHER BRAND NAMES

Cipro

ADULT DOSAGE

Urinary Tract Infections

250mg q12h for 7-14 days

Uncomplicated Cystitis

Acute:
250mg q12h for 3 days

Chronic Bacterial Prostatitis

500mg q12h for 28 days

Lower Respiratory Tract Infections

500-750mg q12h for 7-14 days

Acute Bacterial Sinusitis

500mg q12h for 10 days

Skin and Skin Structure Infections

500-750mg q12h for 7-14 days

Bone/Joint Infections

500-750mg q12h for 4-8 weeks

Intra-Abdominal Infections

Complicated:
500mg q12h for 7-14 days, in conjunction w/ metronidazole

PEDIATRIC DOSAGE

Urinary Tract Infections

Complicated UTIs or Pyelonephritis:

1-17 Years:
10-20mg/kg q12h for 10-21 days
Max: 750mg/dose; not to be exceeded even if >51kg

Inhalational Anthrax (Postexposure)

15mg/kg q12h for 60 days
Max: 500mg/dose
Begin as soon as possible after suspected or confirmed exposure

Plague

15mg/kg q8-12h for 10-21 days
Max: 500mg/dose
Begin as soon as possible after suspected or confirmed exposure

Diarrhea

Infectious:
500mg q12h for 5-7 days

Typhoid Fever
500mg q12h for 10 days

Gonococcal Infections

Uncomplicated Urethral and Cervical:
250mg single dose

Inhalational Anthrax (Postexposure)
500mg q12h for 60 days
Begin as soon as possible after suspected or confirmed exposure

Plague
500-750mg q12h for 14 days
Begin as soon as possible after suspected or confirmed exposure

Conversions

Switching from IV to Oral:
200mg IV q12h: 250mg tab q12h
400mg IV q12h: 500mg tab q12h
400mg IV q8h: 750mg tab q12h

DOSE MODIFICATION

Renal Impairment

Adults:
CrCl 30-50mL/min: 250-500mg q12h
CrCl 5-29mL/min: 250-500mg q18h
Hemodialysis/Peritoneal Dialysis: 250-500mg q24h (after dialysis)
Severe Impairment w/ Severe Infection: Unit dose of 750mg may be administered at intervals noted above

ADMINISTRATION

Oral route
Take w/ or w/o meals
Administer ≥2 hrs before or 6 hrs after Mg^{2+}/aluminum antacids; polymeric phosphate binders or sucralfate; Videx (didanosine) chewable/buffered tabs or pediatric powder for oral sol; other highly buffered drugs; or other products containing Ca^{2+}, iron, or zinc
Avoid concomitant administration w/ dairy products or Ca^{2+}-fortified juices alone; may take w/ a meal that contains these products
Assure adequate hydration

Reconstitution

Pour the microcapsules completely into the larger bottle of diluent; do not add water to the sus
Close the larger bottle completely and shake vigorously for about 15 sec

HOW SUPPLIED

Sus: (Cipro) 250mg/5mL, 500mg/5mL [100mL]; Tab: 100mg, 750mg; (Cipro) 250mg, 500mg

CONTRAINDICATIONS

Concomitant administration w/ tizanidine.

WARNINGS/PRECAUTIONS

Not a drug of choice in the treatment of presumed or confirmed pneumonia secondary to *Streptococcus pneumoniae*. Caution w/ history of tendon disorders; d/c if patient experiences pain, swelling, inflammation, or rupture of tendon. Serious and occasionally fatal hypersensitivity (anaphylactic) reactions reported; d/c immediately at the 1st appearance of a skin rash, jaundice, or any sign of hypersensitivity, and institute supportive measures. Severe hepatotoxicity, including hepatic necrosis, life-threatening hepatic failure, and fatal events, reported; d/c immediately if signs and symptoms of hepatitis occur. Convulsions, status epilepticus, increased intracranial pressure (including pseudotumor cerebri), toxic psychosis, and other CNS events reported; d/c and institute appropriate measures if CNS events occur. Caution w/ epilepsy and CNS disorders (eg, severe cerebral arteriosclerosis, history of convulsion, reduced cerebral blood flow) or other risk factors that may predispose to seizures or lower the seizure threshold; d/c if seizures occur. *Clostridium difficile*-associated diarrhea (CDAD) reported; may need to d/c if CDAD is suspected or confirmed. Cases of sensory or sensorimotor axonal polyneuropathy resulting in paresthesias, hypoesthesias, dysesthesias, and weakness reported; d/c immediately if symptoms of peripheral neuropathy occur. May prolong QT interval; avoid w/ known QT interval prolongation and risk factors for QT prolongation/torsades de pointes (eg, congenital long QT syndrome, uncorrected electrolyte imbalance, cardiac disease). Increased incidence of adverse reactions related to joints and/or surrounding tissues observed in pediatric patients. Crystalluria reported; maintain hydration and avoid alkalinity of urine. May cause photosensitivity/phototoxicity reactions; d/c if phototoxicity occurs. Avoid excessive exposure to sun/UV light. May result in bacterial resistance if used in the absence of a proven or strongly suspected bacterial infection or a prophylactic indication. Has not been shown to be effective in the treatment of syphilis; antimicrobial agents used in high dose for short periods to treat gonorrhea may mask or delay symptoms of incubating syphilis. Caution in elderly.

ADVERSE REACTIONS

Tendinitis, tendon rupture, N/V, diarrhea, abdominal pain, neurological events, abnormal LFTs, rash.

DRUG INTERACTIONS

See Boxed Warning and Contraindications. Avoid concomitant administration w/ dairy products (eg, milk, yogurt), or Ca^{2+}-fortified juices alone; absorption may be reduced. May increase levels of CYP1A2 substrates (eg, theophylline, methylxanthines, olanzapine), duloxetine, or sildenafil. Use w/ caution and monitor for sildenafil toxicity. Avoid use w/ duloxetine; if unavoidable, monitor for duloxetine toxicity. Increased theophylline levels may increase the risk of developing CNS, or other adverse reactions; if coadministration cannot be avoided, monitor theophylline levels and adjust dose. May inhibit the formation of paraxanthine after caffeine administration (or pentoxifylline containing products); monitor for xanthine toxicity and adjust dose as necessary. Monitor for clozapine- or ropinirole-related adverse reactions and adjust dose of clozapine or ropinirole during and shortly after coadministration. Avoid w/ Class IA (eg, quinidine, procainamide) and Class III (eg, amiodarone, sotalol) antiarrhythmics, TCAs, macrolides, and antipsychotics; may further prolong QT interval. Hypoglycemia reported w/ oral antidiabetic agents, mainly sulfonylureas (eg, glyburide, glimepiride); monitor blood glucose. May alter serum levels of phenytoin; monitor phenytoin therapy, including phenytoin levels during and shortly after coadministration. Transient SrCr elevations w/ cyclosporine; monitor renal function. May increase effects of oral anticoagulants; monitor PT and INR frequently during and shortly after coadministration. May increase levels and toxic reactions of methotrexate; carefully monitor w/ concomitant use. High-dose quinolones in combination w/ NSAIDs (not acetyl salicylic acid) may provoke convulsions. Antacids, sucralfate, multivitamins, and other multivalent cation-containing products (eg, Mg^{2+}/aluminum antacids, polymeric phosphate binders, Videx [didanosine] chewable/buffered tab or pediatric powder) may decrease absorption, resulting in lower serum and urine levels than desired; administer ≥2 hrs before or 6 hrs after these drugs. Probenecid may increase levels; use w/caution. Caution w/ drugs that may lower seizure threshold.

NURSING CONSIDERATIONS

Assessment: Assess for risk factors for developing tendinitis and tendon rupture, history of myasthenia gravis, drug hypersensitivity, epilepsy, CNS disorders or other risk factors that may predispose to seizures or lower seizure threshold, QT interval prolongation, renal dysfunction, previous liver damage, pregnancy/nursing status, and possible drug interactions. Obtain baseline culture and susceptibility tests. Perform serologic test for syphilis in patients w/ gonorrhea.

Monitoring: Monitor for tendinitis or tendon rupture, exacerbation of myasthenia gravis, signs/symptoms of hypersensitivity reactions, QT prolongations, CNS effects, CDAD, hepatotoxicity, peripheral neuropathy, musculoskeletal disorders (pediatric patients), crystalluria, photosensitivity/phototoxicity reactions, and other adverse reactions. Monitor PT and INR if coadministered w/ an oral anticoagulant (eg, warfarin). Monitor renal function. Perform periodic culture and susceptibility testing. Perform follow-up serologic test for syphilis after 3 months in patients w/ gonorrhea.

Patient Counseling: Inform that drug treats only bacterial, not viral, infections. Counsel to take exactly ud; inform that skipping doses or not completing full course of therapy may decrease effectiveness and increase bacterial resistance. Advise to drink fluids liberally. Counsel to avoid concomitant use w/ dairy products or Ca^{2+}-fortified juices alone; may take w/ a meal that contains these products. Advise to notify physician if tension disorder symptoms occur; instruct to d/c therapy and rest/refrain from exercise. Instruct to notify physician if myasthenia gravis, liver injury, or photosensitivity/phototoxicity symptoms occur. Instruct to notify physician of any history of convulsions. Advise to assess reaction to therapy before engaging in activities that require mental alertness or coordination; instruct to notify physician if persistent headache w/ or w/o blurred vision occurs. Advise to contact physician as soon as possible if watery and bloody stools (w/ or w/o stomach cramps and fever) develop even as late as ≥2 months after last dose. Instruct to d/c and notify physician if hypersensitivity reactions or symptoms of peripheral neuropathy develop. Instruct to inform physician of any personal or family history of QT prolongation or proarrhythmic conditions and if symptoms of prolongation of the QT interval occur. Counsel caregiver to inform physician if child has joint-related problems prior to, during, or after therapy. Advise to seek medical help immediately if experiencing seizures, palpitations, or breathing difficulty. Instruct to minimize or avoid exposure to natural/artificial sunlight (tanning beds or UVA/B treatment). Instruct to contact physician if low blood sugar occurs. Inform that efficacy studies of ciprofloxacin could not be conducted in humans w/ plague and anthrax for feasibility reasons and that approval for these conditions was therefore based on an efficacy studies conducted in animals.

Storage: Tab: (Generic) <30°C (86°F); (Cipro) 20-25°C (68-77°F), excursions permitted to 15-30°C (59-86°F). Microcapsules and Diluent/Reconstituted Sus: 25°C (77°F); excursions permitted from 15-30°C (59-86°F). Store reconstituted product for 14 days. Protect from freezing.

CITALOPRAM – citalopram hydrobromide

RX

Class: Selective serotonin reuptake inhibitor

Antidepressants increased the risk of suicidal thinking and behavior (suicidality) in children, adolescents, and young adults in short-term studies of major depressive disorder and other psychiatric disorders. Monitor and observe closely for clinical worsening, suicidality, or unusual changes in behavior. Not approved for use in pediatric patients.

OTHER BRAND NAMES
Celexa

ADULT DOSAGE

Depression

Initial Treatment:
Initial: 20mg qd
Titrate: Increase dose to 40mg/day at an interval of no less than 1 week
Max: 40mg/day

Maint Treatment:
Consider decreasing dose to 20mg/day if adverse reactions are bothersome

Periodically reevaluate long-term usefulness of drug if used for extended periods

Dosing Considerations with MAOIs

Switching to/from an MAOI for Psychiatric Disorders:
Allow at least 14 days between discontinuation of an MAOI and initiation of treatment, and allow at least 14 days between discontinuation of treatment and initiation of an MAOI

W/ Other MAOIs (eg, Linezolid, IV Methylene Blue):
Do not start citalopram in patient being treated w/ linezolid or IV methylene blue
In patients already receiving citalopram, if acceptable alternatives are not available and benefits outweigh risks, d/c citalopram and administer linezolid or IV methylene blue; monitor for serotonin syndrome for 2 weeks or until 24 hrs after the last dose of linezolid or IV methylene blue, whichever comes 1st. May resume citalopram therapy 24 hrs after the last dose of linezolid or IV methylene blue

PEDIATRIC DOSAGE
Pediatric use may not have been established

DOSE MODIFICATION

Concomitant Medications

Cimetidine or Another CYP2C19 Inhibitor:
Max: 20mg/day

Hepatic Impairment
Max: 20mg/day

Elderly
>60 Years:
Max: 20mg/day

Discontinuation
Gradually reduce dose to d/c; if intolerable symptoms occur following a decrease in dose or upon discontinuation of treatment, may consider resuming previously prescribed dose or continue decreasing dose at a more gradual rate

Other Important Modifications
CYP2C19 Poor Metabolizers:
Max: 20mg/day

ADMINISTRATION
Oral route

Administer qd, in am or pm, w/ or w/o food

HOW SUPPLIED

Sol: 10mg/5mL [240mL]; Tab: (Celexa) 10mg, 20mg*, 40mg* *scored

CONTRAINDICATIONS

Use of an MAOI for psychiatric disorders either concomitantly or w/in 14 days of stopping treatment. Treatment w/in 14 days of stopping an MAOI for psychiatric disorders. Starting treatment in a patient being treated w/ MAOIs (eg, linezolid, IV methylene blue). Concomitant use w/ pimozide.

WARNINGS/PRECAUTIONS

Not approved for the treatment of bipolar depression. May cause dose-dependent QTc prolongation. Avoid in patients w/ congenital long QT syndrome, bradycardia, hypokalemia or hypomagnesemia, recent acute MI (AMI), or uncompensated HF; monitor ECG if therapy is needed. Correct hypokalemia and/or hypomagnesemia prior to initiation of therapy and monitor periodically. D/C therapy w/ persistent QTc measurements >500 msec. May precipitate mixed/manic episode in patients at risk for bipolar disorder; screen for risk for bipolar disorder prior to initiating treatment. Serotonin syndrome reported; d/c immediately and initiate supportive symptomatic treatment. Pupillary dilation that occurs following use may trigger an angle-closure attack in a patient w/ anatomically narrow angles who does not have a patent iridectomy. Adverse events reported upon discontinuation; gradually reduce dose. May increase risk of bleeding events. Hyponatremia may occur; caution in elderly and volume-depleted patients. Consider discontinuation in patients w/ symptomatic hyponatremia and institute appropriate medical intervention. Activation of mania/hypomania reported; caution w/ history of mania. Seizures reported; caution w/ history of seizure disorder. Caution w/ hepatic impairment, severe renal impairment, and in pregnancy (3rd trimester). May impair mental/physical abilities.

ADVERSE REACTIONS

N/V, dyspepsia, diarrhea, dry mouth, somnolence, insomnia, increased sweating, ejaculation disorder, fatigue, URTI, rhinitis, anxiety, anorexia, tremor, agitation.

DRUG INTERACTIONS

See Contraindications and Dosage. Avoid w/ alcohol and drugs that prolong the QTc interval (eg, Class 1A [eg, quinidine, procainamide] or Class III [eg, amiodarone, sotalol] antiarrhythmic medications, antipsychotic medications [eg, chlorpromazine, thioridazine], antibiotics [eg, gatifloxacin, moxifloxacin], pentamidine, levomethadyl acetate, methadone). Caution w/ other centrally acting drugs or TCAs (eg, imipramine). Risk of QT prolongation w/ CYP2C19 inhibitors (eg, cimetidine). May cause serotonin syndrome w/ other serotonergic drugs (eg, triptans, TCAs, fentanyl) and w/ drugs that impair metabolism of serotonin; d/c immediately if this occurs. Risk of bleeding may be increased w/ aspirin, NSAIDs, warfarin, and other drugs that affect coagulation. May increase PT w/ warfarin. Monitor lithium levels and adjust its dose appropriately. Rare reports of weakness, hyperreflexia, and incoordination w/ sumatriptan. Possible increased clearance w/ carbamazepine. May decrease levels of ketoconazole. May increase levels of metoprolol. Increased risk of hyponatremia w/ diuretics.

NURSING CONSIDERATIONS

Assessment: Assess for drug hypersensitivity, risk for bipolar disorder, history of mania, history of seizures, susceptibility to angle-closure glaucoma, volume depletion, congenital long QT syndrome, hypokalemia, hypomagnesemia, bradycardia, recent AMI, uncompensated HF, hepatic/renal impairment, pregnancy/nursing status, and possible drug interactions. Obtain baseline serum K^+ and Mg^{2+} measurements for patients being considered for therapy who are at risk for significant electrolyte disturbances.

Monitoring: Monitor for signs/symptoms of clinical worsening, suicidality, unusual changes in behavior, serotonin syndrome, bleeding events, hyponatremia, seizures, angle-closure glaucoma, activation of mania/hypomania, discontinuation symptoms, and other adverse reactions. Monitor electrolytes in patients w/ diseases or conditions that cause hypokalemia or hypomagnesemia. Monitor ECG in patients w/ cardiac conditions/disorders and in patients on concomitant QTc interval prolonging agents. Periodically reevaluate long-term usefulness.

Patient Counseling: Inform about risks, benefits, and appropriate use of therapy. Caution about operating hazardous machinery, including automobiles, until reasonably certain that therapy does not affect ability to engage in such activities. Inform about serotonin syndrome and bleeding risks. Caution about risk of angle-closure glaucoma. Instruct to avoid alcohol. Advise to notify physician if taking or planning to take any prescription or OTC drugs. Instruct to notify physician if pregnant, intending to become pregnant, or breastfeeding. Encourage to be alert to unusual changes in behavior, worsening of depression, and suicidal ideation, especially early during treatment and when dose is adjusted up/down; instruct to report such symptoms, especially if severe, abrupt in onset, or not part of presenting symptoms.

Storage: (Tab) 25°C (77°F); excursions permitted to 15-30°C (59-86°F). (Sol) 20-25°C (68-77°F); excursions permitted to 15-30°C (59-86°F).

CLEOCIN – clindamycin

RX

Class: Lincomycin derivative

***Clostridium difficile*-associated diarrhea (CDAD) reported and may range in severity from mild diarrhea to fatal colitis. Due to association w/ severe colitis, reserve use for serious infections where less toxic agents are inappropriate. Not for use w/ nonbacterial infections such as most URIs. CDAD must be considered in all patients w/ diarrhea following antibiotic use. Careful medical history is necessary since CDAD has been reported to occur over 2 months after the administration of antibacterial agents. If CDAD is suspected or confirmed, ongoing antibiotic use not directed against *C. difficile* may need to be discontinued. Appropriate fluid and electrolyte management, protein supplementation, antibiotic treatment of *C. difficile* and surgical evaluation may be instituted as clinically indicated.**

OTHER BRAND NAMES

Cleocin Pediatric

ADULT DOSAGE

Serious Infections

Respiratory tract/skin and skin structure/intra-abdominal/gynecological infections and septicemia; (IV) bone and joint infections and adjunctive therapy in the surgical treatment of chronic bone and joint infections

Cap:
150-300mg PO q6h
More Severe: 300-450mg PO q6h
Inj:
Aerobic Gram-Positive Cocci and More Susceptible Anaerobes:
600-1200mg/day IV/IM given in 2, 3 or 4 equal doses
More Severe (Particularly Due to *Bacteroides fragilis, Peptococcus* species, or *Clostridium* species other than *Clostridium perfringens*):
1200-2700mg/day IV/IM given in 2, 3 or 4 equal doses
More Serious/Life-Threatening:
May have to increase dose; as much as 4800mg/day IV have been given

Single IM inj >600mg are not recommended

Alternative Administration:
Administer 1st dose as a single rapid infusion, followed by continuous IV infusion
To Maintain Serum Clindamycin Levels >4mcg/mL:
Rapid Infusion Rate: 10mg/min for 30 min
Maint Infusion Rate: 0.75mg/min
To Maintain Serum Clindamycin Levels >5mcg/mL:
Rapid Infusion Rate: 15mg/min for 30 min
Maint Infusion Rate: 1mg/min
To Maintain Serum Clindamycin Levels >6mcg/mL:
Rapid Infusion Rate: 20mg/min for 30 min
Maint Infusion Rate: 1.25mg/min

β-hemolytic Streptococcal Infection:
Treat for at least 10 days

PEDIATRIC DOSAGE

Serious Infections

Cap:
8-16mg/kg/day (4-8mg/lb/day) PO divided into 3 or 4 equal doses
More Severe: 16-20mg/kg/day (8-10mg/lb/day) PO divided into 3 or 4 equal doses
Sol:
8-12mg/kg/day (4-6mg/lb/day) PO divided into 3 or 4 equal doses
Severe: 13-16mg/kg/day (6.5-8mg/lb/day) PO divided into 3 or 4 equal doses
More Severe: 17-25mg/kg/day (8.5-12.5mg/lb/day) PO divided into 3 or 4 equal doses
≤10kg:
Minimum Dose: 1/2 tsp (37.5mg) tid
Inj:
Neonates (<1 Month of Age):
15-20mg/kg/day given in 3-4 equal doses; lower dosage may be adequate for small prematures
1 Month-16 Years:
20-40mg/kg/day IV/IM given in 3 or 4 equal doses; use higher dose for more severe infections
Alternative Dosing:
350mg/m²/day
More Severe: 450mg/m²/day

β-hemolytic Streptococcal Infection:
Treat for at least 10 days

ADMINISTRATION

Oral/IM/IV route

Cap

Take w/ full glass of water to avoid esophageal irritation

Sol

Reconstitute 100mL bottles w/ 75mL of water

Reconstitution Instructions:
1. Add a large portion of water and shake vigorously
2. Add remainder of the water and shake until sol is uniform

Inj
IM: Administer undiluted
IV: Administer diluted

IV Dilution and Infusion Rates:
Concentration of clindamycin in diluent should not exceed 18mg/mL
Infusion rates should not exceed 30mg/min
300mg Dose: Dilute w/ 50mL; infuse over 10 min
600mg Dose: Dilute w/ 50mL; infuse over 20 min
900mg Dose: Dilute w/ 50-100mL; infuse over 30 min
1200mg Dose: Dilute w/ 100mL; infuse over 40 min
Administration of >1200mg in a single 1-hr infusion is not recommended

Physical Incompatibilities:
Ampicillin sodium, phenytoin sodium, barbiturates, aminophylline, calcium gluconate, and magnesium sulfate
Do not add supplementary medication to Galaxy Container

HOW SUPPLIED
Cap: (HCl) 75mg, 150mg, 300mg; Inj: (Phosphate) 150mg/mL [2mL, 4mL, 6mL vial]; 150mg/mL [4mL, 6mL ADD-Vantage vial]; 300mg/50mL, 600mg/50mL, 900mg/50mL [Galaxy plastic container]; (Pediatric) Sol: (Palmitate) 75mg/5mL [100mL]

WARNINGS/PRECAUTIONS
D/C use if significant diarrhea occurs during therapy. Reserve use for penicillin (PCN)-allergic patients or other patients for whom a PCN is inappropriate. May increase bacterial resistance if used in the absence of a proven/strongly suspected bacterial infection or a prophylactic indication; take appropriate measures if superinfection develops. Not for treatment of meningitis. Caution w/ severe liver disease, history of GI disease (eg, colitis), and in atopic or elderly patients. (75mg/150mg Caps) Contains tartrazine, which may cause allergic-type reactions (eg, bronchial asthma); caution w/ aspirin hypersensitivity. (Inj) Do not inject IV undiluted as bolus. Contains benzyl alcohol; has been associated w/ serious adverse events, including "gasping syndrome" and death in pediatric patients. Premature infants and low birth weight infants may be more likely to develop benzyl alcohol toxicity. (Cap/Inj) Severe skin reactions (eg, toxic epidermal necrolysis) reported; permanently d/c treatment in case of such an event.

ADVERSE REACTIONS
CDAD, abdominal pain, pseudomembranous colitis, N/V, maculopapular skin rash, pruritus, vaginitis, jaundice, abnormal LFTs, transient neutropenia, eosinophilia, drug reaction w/ eosinophilia and systemic symptoms, azotemia, oliguria, polyarthritis.

DRUG INTERACTIONS
May enhance the action of neuromuscular blockers; use w/ caution. Antagonism reported between clindamycin and erythromycin; avoid use concurrently.

NURSING CONSIDERATIONS
Assessment: Assess for history of hypersensitivity to drug or lincomycin, history of GI disease, presence of meningitis, atopy, and possible drug interactions. Assess hepatic function and pregnancy/nursing status. Obtain baseline culture and susceptibility tests.

Monitoring: Monitor for CDAD, superinfection, allergic reactions, severe skin reactions, and other adverse reactions. Monitor for changes in bowel frequency in older patients. If available, consider culture and susceptibility information when modifying antibacterial therapy. If on prolonged therapy, perform periodic LFTs, renal function tests, and blood counts. Perform periodic liver enzyme determinations in patients w/ severe liver disease.

Patient Counseling: Inform about potential benefits/risks of therapy. Inform that therapy only treats bacterial, not viral, infections. Instruct to take exactly ud and inform that skipping doses or not completing full course may decrease effectiveness and increase antibiotic resistance. Instruct to contact physician if an allergic reaction develops. Advise that watery and bloody stools (w/ or w/o stomach cramps and fever) may occur as late as ≥2 months after therapy; instruct to notify physician if this occurs. Advise to notify physician if pregnant/nursing.

Storage: 20-25°C (68-77°F). (Inj) Galaxy Container: 25°C (77°F); avoid temperatures >30°C (86°F). Refer to PI for stability information regarding diluted solutions. (Sol) Do not refrigerate the reconstituted sol; stable at room temperature for 2 weeks.

CLINDAGEL – clindamycin phosphate RX

Class: Lincomycin derivative

ADULT DOSAGE

Acne Vulgaris

Apply thin film qd; cover entire affected area lightly

PEDIATRIC DOSAGE

Acne Vulgaris

≥12 Years:

Apply thin film qd; cover entire affected area lightly

ADMINISTRATION

Topical route

HOW SUPPLIED

Gel: 1% [40mL, 75mL]

CONTRAINDICATIONS

Hypersensitivity to lincomycin. History of regional enteritis, ulcerative colitis, or antibiotic-associated colitis.

WARNINGS/PRECAUTIONS

D/C if significant diarrhea occurs. Caution in atopic individuals.

ADVERSE REACTIONS

Peeling, pruritus, pseudomembranous colitis (rare).

DRUG INTERACTIONS

May potentiate neuromuscular blockers.

NURSING CONSIDERATIONS

Assessment: Assess for hypersensitivity to lincomycin, history of regional or ulcerative colitis, antibiotic-associated colitis, nursing status. Assess use in atopic individuals and for possible drug interactions.

Monitoring: Monitor for signs/symptoms of colitis (pseudomembranous colitis), diarrhea, and bloody diarrhea. In patients with diarrhea, consider stool culture for *Clostridium difficile* and stool assay for *C. difficile* toxin. In patients with significant diarrhea, consider large bowel endoscopy.

Patient Counseling: Instruct to notify physician of significant diarrhea during therapy or up to several weeks following end of therapy.

Storage: Controlled room temperature, 20-25°C (68-77°F); excursions permitted to 15-30°C (59-86°F). Keep container tightly closed, out of direct sunlight.

CLOMID – clomiphene citrate RX

Class: Ovulatory stimulant

OTHER BRAND NAMES

Serophene

ADULT DOSAGE

Ovulatory Dysfunction

Initial: 50mg qd for 5 days

If progestin-induced bleeding is planned, or if spontaneous uterine bleeding occurs prior to therapy, start on 5th day of cycle; may start at any time if w/o recent uterine bleeding

Titrate: Increase to 100mg qd for 5 days only in patients who do not ovulate in response to cyclic 50mg after the 1st course of therapy; may start as early as 30 days after 1st course

Max: 100mg/day for 5 days

Long-term cyclic therapy beyond a total of 6 cycles is not recommended

If ovulation does not occur after 3 courses of therapy or if 3 ovulatory responses occur but pregnancy is not achieved, further treatment is not recommended

If menses does not occur after an ovulatory response, reevaluate patient

PEDIATRIC DOSAGE

Pediatric use may not have been established

DOSE MODIFICATION

Other Important Modifications

Polycystic Ovary Syndrome (PCOS)/Unusual Pituitary Gonadotropin Sensitivity:
Use lowest recommended dose and shortest treatment duration for the 1st course of therapy

ADMINISTRATION

Oral route

HOW SUPPLIED

Tab: 50mg* *scored

CONTRAINDICATIONS

Pregnancy, liver disease or history of liver dysfunction, abnormal uterine bleeding of undetermined origin, ovarian cysts or enlargement not due to PCOS, uncontrolled thyroid or adrenal dysfunction or in the presence of an organic intracranial lesion (eg, pituitary tumor).

WARNINGS/PRECAUTIONS

Workup and treatment should be supervised by physician experienced in management of gynecologic or endocrine disorders. Visual symptoms (eg, blurring, spots, flashes), some occurring after discontinuation of therapy, reported; d/c treatment and perform complete ophthalmological evaluation promptly if visual symptoms develop. Visual disturbances may be irreversible, especially w/ increased dosage or duration of therapy. Ovarian hyperstimulation syndrome (OHSS), which may progress rapidly (w/in 24 hrs to several days) reported; monitor for abdominal pain/distention, N/V, diarrhea, weight gain, and for other warning signs. If conception results, rapid progression to severe form of the syndrome may occur. Use lowest effective dose consistent w/ expected clinical results to minimize the hazard of abnormal ovarian enlargement. If ovarian enlargement occurs, do not give additional therapy until the ovaries have returned to pretreatment size, and reduce the dosage or duration of the next course. Ovarian enlargement and cyst formation usually regresses spontaneously w/in a few days or weeks after discontinuing treatment; manage cystic enlargement conservatively unless surgical indication for laparotomy exists. Perform a thorough evaluation to rule out ovarian neoplasia if ovarian cysts do not regress spontaneously. Prolonged use may increase risk of borderline/invasive ovarian tumor. Perform pelvic exam prior to initiating therapy and before each subsequent course. Carefully evaluate to exclude pregnancy, ovarian enlargement, or ovarian cyst formation between each treatment cycle. Caution w/ uterine fibroids; potential for further enlargement.

ADVERSE REACTIONS

Ovarian enlargement, vasomotor flushes, abdominal-pelvic discomfort/distention/bloating.

NURSING CONSIDERATIONS

Assessment: Assess for hypersensitivity to drug, ovarian cysts/enlargement, abnormal vaginal/uterine bleeding, presence of organic intracranial lesion, primary pituitary/ovarian failure, endometriosis/endometrial carcinoma, liver disease or history of liver dysfunction, impediments to pregnancy (eg, thyroid/adrenal disorders, hyperprolactinemia, male factor infertility), uterine fibroids, preexisting or family history of hyperlipidemia, and pregnancy/nursing status. Perform pelvic exam prior to treatment. Assess estrogen levels.

Monitoring: Monitor for signs/symptoms of visual symptoms (eg, blurring, spots, flashes), OHSS, ovarian neoplasia, and other adverse reactions. Monitor plasma TG levels periodically in patients w/ preexisting or family history of hyperlipidemia. Exclude pregnancy, ovarian enlargement, or ovarian cyst formation between each treatment cycle. Perform pelvic exam before each subsequent course.

Patient Counseling: Advise that blurring or other visual symptoms may occur during or shortly after therapy and inform that in some instances, visual disturbances may be prolonged, and possibly irreversible, especially w/ increased dosage or duration of therapy. Advise that visual symptoms may render such activities as driving a car or operating machinery more hazardous than usual, particularly under conditions of variable lighting. Instruct to inform physician whenever any unusual visual symptoms occur and to d/c therapy. Advise that ovarian enlargement may occur during or shortly after therapy; instruct to inform physician if any abdominal/pelvic pain, weight gain, discomfort, or distention occurs after taking therapy. Inform that preexisting or family history of hyperlipidemia and use of higher than recommended dose and/or longer duration of treatment may increase risk of hypertriglyceridemia. Inform of the increased chance of multiple pregnancy (eg, bilateral tubal pregnancy, coexisting tubal and intrauterine pregnancy), and the potential complications/hazards of multiple pregnancy.

Storage: 15-30°C (59-86°F). Protect from heat, light, and excessive humidity.

CLONAZEPAM – clonazepam CIV

Class: Benzodiazepine

OTHER BRAND NAMES

Klonopin

ADULT DOSAGE

Seizures

Treatment of Lennox-Gastaut syndrome (petit mal variant), akinetic, and myoclonic seizures. May be useful in patients w/ absence seizures (petit mal) who have failed to respond to succinimides

Initial: Not to exceed 1.5mg/day divided into 3 doses

Titrate: May increase in increments of 0.5-1mg every 3 days until seizures are controlled or until side effects preclude any further increase

Maint: Individualize dose

Max: 20mg/day

Panic Disorder

Initial: 0.25mg bid

Titrate: May increase to target dose of 1mg/day after 3 days; for some, may increase in increments of 0.125-0.25mg bid every 3 days until panic disorder is controlled or until side effects make further increases undesired

Max: 4mg/day

PEDIATRIC DOSAGE

Seizures

Treatment of Lennox-Gastaut syndrome (petit mal variant), akinetic, and myoclonic seizures. May be useful in patients w/ absence seizures (petit mal) who have failed to respond to succinimides

≤10 Years or ≤30kg:

Initial: 0.01-0.03mg/kg/day up to 0.05mg/kg/day given in 2 or 3 divided doses

Titrate: May increase by no more than 0.25-0.5mg every 3 days until daily maintenance dose is reached, unless seizures are controlled or until side effects preclude further increase

Maint: 0.1-0.2mg/kg/day divided into 3 doses. Whenever possible, divide daily dose into 3 equal doses; give the largest dose qhs if doses are not equally divided

ADMINISTRATION

Oral route

To reduce somnolence, may give 1 dose at hs

Tab, Disintegrating

Peel back foil on blister; do not push tab through foil

Using dry hands, remove tab and place it in mouth

Tab

Swallow whole w/ water

HOW SUPPLIED

Tab, Disintegrating: 0.125mg, 0.25mg, 0.5mg, 1mg, 2mg; (Klonopin) Tab: 0.5mg*, 1mg, 2mg *scored

CONTRAINDICATIONS

Significant liver disease, acute narrow angle glaucoma.

WARNINGS/PRECAUTIONS

May be used with treated open angle glaucoma. May impair mental/physical abilities. May increase risk of suicidal thoughts/behavior. Caution with use in pregnancy and women of childbearing potential; may increase risk of congenital malformations. Avoid use during the 1st trimester of pregnancy. May increase incidence or precipitate the onset of generalized tonic-clonic seizures in patients in whom several different types of seizure disorders coexist; addition of appropriate anticonvulsants or increase in their dosages may be required. Withdrawal symptoms reported after discontinuation. Abrupt withdrawal of therapy may precipitate status epilepticus; gradual withdrawal is essential, and simultaneous substitution of another anticonvulsant may be indicated while therapy is being gradually withdrawn. May produce an increase in salivation; caution with chronic respiratory diseases. Caution with renal impairment, addiction-prone individuals, and in elderly. (Tab, Disintegrating) Contains phenylalanine.

ADVERSE REACTIONS

CNS depression, ataxia, drowsiness, abnormal coordination, depression, somnolence, behavior problems, dizziness, URTI, memory disturbance, dysmenorrhea, fatigue, influenza, nervousness, sinusitis.

DRUG INTERACTIONS

CYP450 inducers (eg, phenytoin, carbamazepine, phenobarbital), and propantheline may decrease levels. Caution with CYP3A inhibitors (eg, oral antifungals). Alcohol, narcotics, barbiturates, nonbarbiturate hypnotics, antianxiety agents, phenothiazines, thioxanthene and butyrophenone antipsychotics, MAOIs, TCAs, other anticonvulsant drugs, and other CNS depressant drugs may potentiate CNS-depressant effects. May produce absence status with valproic acid.

NURSING CONSIDERATIONS

Assessment: Assess for drug/benzodiazepine hypersensitivity, significant liver disease, acute narrow angle glaucoma, mental depression, history of drug or alcohol addiction, renal/hepatic impairment, chronic respiratory diseases, pregnancy/nursing status, and possible drug interactions.

Monitoring: Monitor for CNS depression, emergence or worsening of depression, suicidal thoughts/behavior, unusual changes in mood or behavior, worsening of seizures, withdrawal symptoms upon discontinuation, and other adverse reactions. Periodically monitor blood counts and LFTs during long-term therapy.

Patient Counseling: Instruct to take only as prescribed. Inform that therapy may produce psychological and physical dependence; instruct to consult physician before either increasing the dose or abruptly discontinuing the drug. Caution about operating hazardous machinery, including automobiles. Counsel that drug may increase risk of suicidal thoughts and behavior; advise of the need to be alert for the emergence/worsening of symptoms of depression, any unusual changes in mood or behavior, or the emergence of suicidal thoughts, behavior, or thoughts of self-harm and immediately report to physician behaviors of concern. Advise to notify physician if becomes pregnant or intends to become pregnant during therapy; encourage enrollment in the North American Antiepileptic Drug Pregnancy Registry. Advise not to breastfeed while on therapy. Advise to inform physician if taking, or planning to take, any prescription or OTC drugs and to avoid alcohol while on therapy. (Tab, Disintegrating) Inform that drug contains phenylalanine.

Storage: (Tab, Disintegrating) 20-25°C (68-77°F). (Tab) 25°C (77°F); excursions permitted to 15-30°C (59-86°F).

CLOZAPINE – clozapine

RX

Class: Atypical antipsychotic

May cause agranulocytosis that can lead to serious infection and death. Absolute neutrophil count (ANC) must be ≥2000/mm³ and WBC count must be ≥3500/mm³ for a patient to begin treatment. D/C and do not rechallenge if ANC is <1000/mm³ or WBC count is <2000mm³. Available only through a restricted program. Orthostatic hypotension, bradycardia, syncope, and cardiac arrest may occur and the risk is highest during initial titration period, particularly with rapid dose escalation; caution with cardiovascular (CV)/cerebrovascular disease or conditions predisposing to hypotension (eg, dehydration, use of antihypertensives). Seizures may occur and risk is dose-related; caution with history or other predisposing risk factors for seizure (eg, CNS pathology, medications that lower seizure threshold, alcohol abuse). Caution about engaging in any activity where sudden loss of consciousness could cause serious risk to patient or others. Fatal myocarditis and cardiomyopathy reported; d/c and obtain cardiac evaluation upon suspicion of these reactions. Do not rechallenge in patients with clozapine-related myocarditis or cardiomyopathy. Elderly patients with dementia-related psychosis treated with antipsychotic drugs are at an increased risk for death. Not approved for use in patients with dementia-related psychosis.

OTHER BRAND NAMES

Clozaril

ADULT DOSAGE

Schizophrenia

Treatment of severely ill patients who fail to respond adequately to standard antipsychotic treatment. Reduction in risk of recurrent suicidal behavior in patients w/ schizophrenia or schizoaffective disorder who are judged to be at chronic risk for reexperiencing suicidal behavior

Initial: 12.5mg qd or bid
Titrate: May increase total daily dose in increments of 25-50mg/day, if well-tolerated
Target Dose: 300-450mg/day by the end of 2 weeks
Subsequent Dosing: May increase in increments of up to 100mg, once or twice weekly
Max: 900mg/day
Maint: Continue on the effective dose beyond the acute episode

Reinitiation (≥2 Days Since Last Dose): Reinitiate w/ 12.5mg qd or bid; if well-tolerated, may increase to previous therapeutic dose more quickly than recommended for initial treatment

PEDIATRIC DOSAGE

Pediatric use may not have been established

DOSE MODIFICATION

Concomitant Medications

Strong CYP1A2 Inhibitors (eg, Fluvoxamine, Ciprofloxacin, Enoxacin):
During coadministration, use 1/3 of clozapine dose; when discontinuing comedication, increase clozapine dose based on clinical response

Moderate or Weak CYP1A2 Inhibitors (eg, Oral Contraceptives, Caffeine) or CYP2D6/CYP3A4 Inhibitors (eg, Cimetidine, Escitalopram, Erythromycin):
During coadministration, monitor for adverse reactions and consider reducing clozapine dose if necessary; when discontinuing comedication, monitor for lack of effectiveness and increase clozapine dose if necessary

Strong CYP3A4 Inducers (eg, Phenytoin, Carbamazepine, St. John's Wort, Rifampin):
Concomitant use is not recommended; if the inducer is necessary, may need to increase clozapine dose and monitor for decreased effectiveness
When discontinuing comedication, reduce clozapine dose based on clinical response

Moderate or Weak CYP1A2 or CYP3A4 Inducers:
During coadministration, monitor for decreased effectiveness and consider increasing clozapine dose if necessary; when discontinuing comedication, monitor for adverse reactions and consider reducing clozapine dose if necessary

Renal Impairment

May need to reduce dose w/ significant renal impairment

Hepatic Impairment

May need to reduce dose w/ significant hepatic impairment

Discontinuation

Reduce gradually over 1-2 weeks

Other Important Modifications

CYP2D6 Poor Metabolizers:
May need to reduce dose

ADMINISTRATION

Oral route

Administer in divided doses
Take w/ or w/o food

HOW SUPPLIED

Tab: 50mg*, 200mg*; (Clozaril) 25mg*, 100mg* *scored

CONTRAINDICATIONS

History of clozapine-induced agranulocytosis or severe granulocytopenia.

WARNINGS/PRECAUTIONS

Eosinophilia reported and may be associated with myocarditis, pancreatitis, hepatitis, colitis, and nephritis. Evaluate promptly for signs/symptoms of systemic reactions if eosinophilia develops and d/c immediately if clozapine-related systemic disease is suspected. QT prolongation, torsades de pointes, and other life-threatening ventricular arrhythmias, cardiac arrest, and sudden death reported. D/C if QTc interval exceeds 500msec or symptoms consistent with torsades de pointes or other arrhythmias develop. Caution in patients at risk for significant electrolyte disturbance, particularly hypokalemia; correct electrolyte abnormalities before initiating treatment. Associated with metabolic changes (eg, hyperglycemia sometimes associated with ketoacidosis or hyperosmolar coma, dyslipidemia, weight gain) that may increase CV and cerebrovascular risk. Neuroleptic malignant syndrome (NMS) reported; d/c therapy immediately and institute symptomatic treatment. Transient fever may occur and may necessitate discontinuing treatment; rule out agranulocytosis, infection, or NMS. Pulmonary embolism (PE), deep vein thrombosis (DVT), and tardive dyskinesia (TD) reported; consider discontinuation if TD occurs. Has potent anticholinergic effects. Treatment can result in CNS and peripheral anticholinergic toxicity; caution in the presence of narrow-angle glaucoma, prostatic hypertrophy, or other conditions in which anticholinergic effects can lead to significant adverse reactions. May result in GI adverse reactions; ensure adequate hydration and use of ancillary therapy (eg, bulk laxatives) if constipation occurs. Consider dose reduction if sedation, or impairment of cognitive/motor performance occurs. Caution in patients with risk factors for cerebrovascular adverse reactions. If abrupt discontinuation is necessary, monitor carefully for the recurrence of psychotic symptoms and adverse reactions related to cholinergic rebound. Refer to PI for frequency of monitoring based on stage of therapy, WBC count, and ANC. Caution in elderly.

ADVERSE REACTIONS

Agranulocytosis, seizure, myocarditis, cardiomyopathy, orthostatic hypotension, hypersalivation, somnolence, sedation, syncope, dizziness/vertigo, constipation, bradycardia, N/V, tachycardia, sweating, visual disturbance, fever.

DRUG INTERACTIONS

See Boxed Warning and Dose Modifications. Not recommended with strong CYP3A4 inducers (eg, carbamazepine, phenytoin, St. John's wort). Caution with medications that prolong the QT interval (eg, ziprasidone, erythromycin, quinidine). CYP1A2, CYP2D6, or CYP3A4 inhibitors may increase levels and lead to adverse reactions. CYP3A4 or CYP1A2 inducers (eg, tobacco) may decrease levels, resulting in decreased effectiveness of therapy. May increase levels of drugs metabolized by CYP2D6 (eg, phenothiazines, carbamazepine, propafenone). Caution with anticholinergics. NMS reported with CNS-active medications (eg, lithium).

NURSING CONSIDERATIONS

Assessment: Assess for history of clozapine-induced agranulocytosis or severe granulocytopenia, previous hypersensitivity to the drug, history of seizures or other predisposing factors for seizure, renal/hepatic impairment, pregnancy/nursing status, possible drug interactions, and other conditions where treatment is cautioned. Obtain baseline CBC with differential (WBC count, ANC), FPG, lipid evaluations, ECG, and electrolytes (serum K^+ and Mg^{2+} levels).

Monitoring: Monitor for signs/symptoms of agranulocytosis, myocarditis, cardiomyopathy, orthostatic hypotension, bradycardia, syncope, seizures, cognitive/motor impairment, eosinophilia, NMS, recurrence of psychosis and cholinergic rebound after abrupt discontinuation, metabolic changes (hyperglycemia, diabetes mellitus [DM], dyslipidemia, weight gain), QT interval prolongation, fever, PE, DVT, TD, cerebrovascular adverse reactions, and other adverse reactions. Monitor serum electrolyte levels, glucose control in patients with DM and periodic FPG levels if at risk for hyperglycemia. Monitor WBC count and ANC regularly; refer to PI for frequency of monitoring based on stage of therapy, WBC count, and ANC.

Patient Counseling: Counsel about the significant risks of developing agranulocytosis. Advise to report immediately the appearance of signs or symptoms consistent with agranulocytosis or infection. Inform that drug is available only through a special program designed to ensure the required blood monitoring. Inform about the risk of orthostatic hypotension and syncope, especially during the period of initial dose titration; instruct to strictly follow the instructions of the physician for dosage and administration. Inform about the significant risk of seizure during treatment; caution about driving and any other potentially hazardous activity while on treatment. Advise to contact physician immediately if patient feels faint, loses consciousness, or has signs/symptoms suggestive of bradycardia or arrhythmia. Counsel about the risk of metabolic changes and the need for specific monitoring. If dose was missed for >2 days, instruct not to restart medication at same dose but to contact physician for dosing instructions. Instruct to notify physician if pregnant/intending to become pregnant during therapy. Advise not to breastfeed if taking the drug. Instruct to notify physician if taking/planning to take any prescription or OTC drugs.

Storage: 20-25°C (68-77°F). (Clozaril) Should not exceed 30°C (86°F).

Colcrys – colchicine

RX

Class: Miscellaneous gout agent

ADULT DOSAGE

Gout Flares

Prophylaxis:
> 16 Years:
Usual: 0.6mg qd or bid
Max: 1.2mg/day

Treatment:
Usual: 1.2mg at the 1st sign of flare followed by 0.6mg 1 hr later
Max: 1.8mg over a 1-hr period
May administer for treatment of gout flare during prophylaxis at doses not to exceed 1.2mg at the 1st sign of the flare followed by 0.6mg 1 hr later; wait 12 hrs, then resume prophylactic dose

Familial Mediterranean Fever

Usual Range: 1.2-2.4mg/day in 1 to 2 divided doses
Titrate: Increase or decrease dose in 0.3mg increments based on disease control or intolerable side effects

PEDIATRIC DOSAGE

Familial Mediterranean Fever

4-6 Years: 0.3-1.8mg/day
6-12 Years: 0.9-1.8mg/day
>12 Years: 1.2-2.4mg/day

May be given qd or bid

DOSE MODIFICATION

Concomitant Medications

Strong CYP3A4 Inhibitors:

Gout Flare Prophylaxis:

Original Dose 0.6mg bid: Adjust to 0.3mg qd
Original Dose 0.6mg qd: Adjust to 0.3mg qod

Gout Flare Treatment:

0.6mg for 1 dose, followed by 0.3mg 1 hr later; repeat dose no earlier than 3 days

Familial Mediterranean Fever:

Max: 0.6mg/day (may be given as 0.3mg bid)

Moderate CYP3A4 Inhibitors:

Gout Flare Prophylaxis:

Original Dose 0.6mg bid: Adjust to 0.3mg bid or 0.6mg qd
Original Dose 0.6mg qd: Adjust to 0.3mg qd

Gout Flare Treatment:

1.2mg for 1 dose; repeat dose no earlier than 3 days

Familial Mediterranean Fever:

Max: 1.2mg/day (may be given as 0.6mg bid)

P-gp Inhibitors:

Gout Flare Prophylaxis:

Original Dose 0.6mg bid: Adjust to 0.3mg qd
Original Dose 0.6mg qd: Adjust to 0.3mg qod

Gout Flare Treatment:

0.6mg for 1 dose; repeat dose no earlier than 3 days

Familial Mediterranean Fever:

Max: 0.6mg/day (may be given as 0.3mg bid)

Renal Impairment

Gout Flare Prophylaxis:

Severe Impairment:

Initial: 0.3mg/day
Titrate: Increase dose w/ close monitoring

Dialysis:

Initial: 0.3mg twice a week w/ close monitoring

Gout Flare Treatment:

Severe Impairment: Repeat treatment course no more than once every 2 weeks; consider alternate therapy if repeat treatment courses are required
Dialysis: Reduce to 0.6mg single dose; do not repeat treatment course more than once every 2 weeks

Familial Mediterranean Fever:

Mild (CrCl 50-80mL/min) to Moderate (CrCl 30-50mL/min): Consider reducing dose

Severe (CrCl <30mL/min)/Dialysis:

Initial: 0.3mg/day
Titrate: Increase dose w/ close monitoring

Hepatic Impairment

Gout Flare Prophylaxis:

Severe Impairment: Consider reducing dose

Gout Flare Treatment:

Severe Impairment: Repeat treatment course no more than once every 2 weeks; consider alternate therapy if repeat treatment courses are required

Familial Mediterranean Fever:

Severe Impairment: Consider reducing dose

ADMINISTRATION

Oral route

Take w/o regard to meals

HOW SUPPLIED

Tab: 0.6mg* *scored

CONTRAINDICATIONS

Concomitant use with P-gp or strong CYP3A4 inhibitors (includes all protease inhibitors, except fosamprenavir) in patients with renal/hepatic impairment.

WARNINGS/PRECAUTIONS

Not an analgesic medication and should not be used to treat pain from other causes. Fatal overdoses (accidental/intentional), myelosuppression, leukopenia, granulocytopenia, thrombocytopenia, pancytopenia, and aplastic anemia reported. Drug-induced neuromuscular toxicity and rhabdomyolysis reported with chronic use; increased risk in elderly and in patients with renal dysfunction. Treatment of gout flare with Colcrys is not recommended in patients with renal/hepatic impairment who are receiving Colcrys for prophylaxis. Caution with renal/hepatic impairment and in elderly.

ADVERSE REACTIONS

Diarrhea, pharyngolaryngeal pain, cramping, abdominal pain, N/V, fatigue.

DRUG INTERACTIONS

See Contraindications. Significant increase in plasma levels reported with strong CYP3A4 inhibitors (eg, atazanavir, clarithromycin, itraconazole), moderate CYP3A4 inhibitors (eg, amprenavir, aprepitant, diltiazem, erythromycin), and P-gp inhibitors (eg, cyclosporine, ranolazine); see PI for dose adjustments. Fatal toxicity reported with clarithromycin and cyclosporine. Neuromuscular toxicity reported with diltiazem and verapamil. May potentiate the development of myopathy and rhabdomyolysis when used with HMG-CoA reductase inhibitors (eg, atorvastatin, simvastatin), gemfibrozil, and fibrates. May potentiate the development of myopathy when used with cyclosporine. Rhabdomyolysis reported with digoxin.

NURSING CONSIDERATIONS

Assessment: Assess for renal/hepatic impairment, pregnancy/nursing status, and possible drug interactions.

Monitoring: Monitor for myelosuppression, leukopenia, granulocytopenia, thrombocytopenia, pancytopenia, aplastic anemia, neuromuscular toxicity, rhabdomyolysis, and other adverse reactions.

Patient Counseling: Instruct to take medication ud. If a dose is missed for treatment of gout flare, instruct to take missed dose as soon as possible. If a dose is missed for treatment of gout flare during prophylaxis, instruct to take missed dose immediately, wait 12 hrs, then resume previous schedule. If a dose is missed for prophylaxis without treatment of gout flares or FMF, instruct to take next dose as soon as possible, then return to normal dosing schedule, and not to double the next dose. Inform that fatal overdoses were reported. Counsel to avoid grapefruit/grapefruit juice consumption during treatment. Inform that bone marrow depression with agranulocytosis, aplastic anemia, and thrombocytopenia may occur. Advise to notify physician of all medications currently being taken and to notify physician before starting any new medications, particularly antibiotics. Advise to d/c therapy and notify physician if muscle pain/weakness, and/or tingling/numbness of fingers/toes occur.

Storage: 20-25°C (68-77°F). Protect from light.

COLLAGENASE SANTYL – *collagenase* RX

Class: Debriding agent

ADULT DOSAGE

Debridement of Chronic Dermal Ulcers and Severely Burned Areas

Apply qd (or more frequently if dressing becomes soiled, as from incontinence)

Whenever infection is present, apply appropriate topical antibiotic powder before oint; if no response, d/c therapy until remission of infection

Terminate use when debridement of necrotic tissue is complete and granulation tissue is well established

PEDIATRIC DOSAGE

Pediatric use may not have been established

ADMINISTRATION

Topical route

Clean and debride wound prior to application

May be applied directly to the wound or to a sterile gauze pad which is then applied to the wound and properly secured

HOW SUPPLIED

Oint: 250 U/g [15g, 30g, 90g]

WARNINGS/PRECAUTIONS

Optimal pH range is 6-8; lower or higher pH conditions may decrease enzyme activity. Closely monitor debilitated patients for systemic bacterial infections; may increase risk of bacteremia. Slight transient erythema in surrounding tissue noted particularly when oint was not confined to the wound; apply carefully.

DRUG INTERACTIONS

Avoid soaks containing metal ions or acidic sol. Enzyme activity may be adversely affected by certain detergents and heavy metal ions (eg, mercury, silver) which are used in some antiseptics; when use is suspected, carefully cleanse site by repeated washings with normal saline prior to application. Systemic manifestations of hypersensitivity to collagenase with cortisone reported.

NURSING CONSIDERATIONS

Assessment: Assess for previous local or systemic hypersensitivity to drug, higher/lower pH conditions, presence of wound infection, pregnancy/nursing status, and possible drug interactions.

Monitoring: Monitor for erythema and other adverse reactions. Monitor for systemic bacterial infections in debilitated patients.

Patient Counseling: Instruct on how to apply medication.

Storage: ≤25°C (77°F).

COMBIGAN – brimonidine tartrate/timolol maleate RX

Class: Alpha$_2$-agonist/beta-blocker

ADULT DOSAGE

Elevated Intraocular Pressure

Glaucoma/Ocular HTN:
Adjunctive or Replacement Therapy:
Instill 1 drop in affected eye(s) bid q12h

PEDIATRIC DOSAGE

Elevated Intraocular Pressure

Glaucoma/Ocular HTN:
Adjunctive or Replacement Therapy:
≥2 Years:
Instill 1 drop in affected eye(s) bid q12h

DOSE MODIFICATION

Concomitant Medications

Space by at least 5 min if using >1 topical ophthalmic drug

ADMINISTRATION

Ocular route

HOW SUPPLIED

Sol: (Brimonidine-Timolol) 0.2%-0.5% [5mL, 10mL]

CONTRAINDICATIONS

Bronchial asthma, history of bronchial asthma, severe chronic obstructive pulmonary disease (COPD), sinus bradycardia, 2nd- or 3rd-degree atrioventricular (AV) block, overt cardiac failure, cardiogenic shock, neonates, and infants (<2 yrs of age).

WARNINGS/PRECAUTIONS

Absorbed systemically; severe respiratory reactions in patients with asthma reported. May precipitate more severe failure in patients with diminished myocardial contractility; sympathetic stimulation may be essential for support of the circulation. D/C at the 1st sign/symptom of cardiac failure in patients without a history of cardiac failure. Avoid with bronchospastic disease, history of bronchospastic disease and/or mild to moderate COPD (eg, chronic bronchitis, emphysema). May potentiate syndromes associated with vascular insufficiency; caution with depression, cerebral or coronary insufficiency, Raynaud's phenomenon, orthostatic hypotension, or thromboangiitis obliterans. May increase reactivity to allergens. May potentiate muscle weakness consistent with certain myasthenic symptoms (eg, diplopia, ptosis, generalized weakness). May mask signs/symptoms of acute hypoglycemia; caution in patients subject to spontaneous hypoglycemia and in diabetic patients receiving insulin or hypoglycemic agents. May mask certain clinical signs of hyperthyroidism (eg, tachycardia); carefully manage patients suspected of developing thyrotoxicosis to avoid abrupt withdrawal that may precipitate a thyroid storm. Ocular hypersensitivity reactions reported. Bacterial keratitis reported with use of multiple-dose containers of topical ophthalmic products. May impair the ability of the heart to respond to β-adrenergically mediated reflex stimuli during surgery; gradual withdrawal of β-blocking agents is recommended in patients undergoing elective surgery.

ADVERSE REACTIONS

Allergic conjunctivitis, conjunctival folliculosis, conjunctival hyperemia, eye pruritus, ocular burning/stinging.

DRUG INTERACTIONS

May reduce BP; caution with antihypertensives and/or cardiac glycosides. Monitor for potentially additive effects, both systemic and on IOP with concomitant oral β-blockers; concomitant use of 2 topical β-blocking agents is not recommended. Possible AV conduction disturbances, left ventricular failure, and hypotension may occur with oral or IV calcium antagonists; use with caution and avoid use with impaired cardiac function. Closely observe patients receiving catecholamine-depleting drugs (eg, reserpine) because of possible additive effects and the production of hypotension and/or marked bradycardia. Possibility of additive or potentiating effect with CNS depressants (eg, alcohol, barbiturates, opiates, sedatives, anesthetics). Concomitant use of β-blockers with digitalis or calcium antagonists may have additive effects in prolonging AV-conduction time. Potentiated systemic β-blockade (eg, decreased HR, depression) reported with concomitant CYP2D6 inhibitors (eg, quinidine, SSRIs). May affect the metabolism and uptake of circulating amines with TCAs and/or MAOIs; caution with TCAs and MAOIs.

NURSING CONSIDERATIONS

Assessment: Assess for bronchial asthma, history of bronchial asthma, severe COPD, or any other conditions where treatment is contraindicated or cautioned. Assess for pregnancy/nursing status, and possible drug interactions.

Monitoring: Monitor for potentiation of respiratory reactions, vascular insufficiency, muscle weakness, increased reactivity to allergens, masking of signs/symptoms of hypoglycemia or hyperthyroidism, ocular hypersensitivity reactions, bacterial keratitis, and other adverse reactions.

Patient Counseling: Inform that ocular infections may occur if handled improperly or if the tip of dispensing container contacts the eye or surrounding structures. Advise that using contaminated sol may result in serious eye damage and subsequent loss of vision. Instruct to always replace cap after using. Advise not to use if sol changes color or becomes cloudy. Advise to immediately consult physician concerning continued use of multidose container if undergoing ocular surgery or if an intercurrent ocular condition (eg, trauma, infection) develops. Instruct to space dosing by at least 5 min apart if >1 topical ophthalmic drug is being used. Inform that drug contains benzalkonium chloride, which may be absorbed by soft contact lenses; instruct to remove contact lenses prior to administration and reinsert 15 min following administration. Inform that drug may cause fatigue and/or drowsiness in some patients; advise to use caution in engaging in hazardous activities because of the potential for a decrease in mental alertness.

Storage: 15-25°C (59-77°F). Protect from light.

COMBIPATCH – estradiol/norethindrone acetate RX

Class: Estrogen/progestogen combination

Should not be used for prevention of cardiovascular (CV) disease or dementia. Increased risk of myocardial infarction (MI), stroke, invasive breast cancer, pulmonary embolism (PE), and deep vein thrombosis (DVT) in postmenopausal women (50-79 yrs of age) reported. Increased risk of developing probable dementia in postmenopausal women ≥65 yrs of age reported. Increased risk of endometrial cancer in women with a uterus who use unopposed estrogens. Perform adequate diagnostic measures to rule out malignancy in postmenopausal women with undiagnosed persistent or recurrent abnormal vaginal bleeding. Should be prescribed at the lowest effective dose and for the shortest duration consistent with treatment goals and risks.

ADULT DOSAGE

Menopause

Severe Vasomotor Symptoms and/or Vulvar/Vaginal Atrophy:

Initiation of Therapy:
Start at lowest dose

Women Not Currently Using Continuous Estrogen or Combination Estrogen/Progestin Therapy:
May start therapy at any time

Women Currently Using Continuous Estrogen or Combination Estrogen/Progestin Therapy:
Complete current cycle of therapy prior to initiating estradiol-norethindrone acetate patch

Continuous Combined Regimen:
Apply 0.05mg-0.14mg patch
Apply twice weekly during 28-day cycle

Continuous Sequential Regimen:
Wear estradiol-only patch for first 14 days of 28-day cycle, replace twice weekly
Apply 0.05mg-0.14mg patch for remaining 14 days, replace twice weekly

For both regimens, use 0.05mg-0.25mg patch if greater progestin is required
Reevaluate at 3- to 6-month intervals

PEDIATRIC DOSAGE

Pediatric use may not have been established

Hypoestrogenism

Due to Hypogonadism, Castration, or Primary Ovarian Failure:

Initiation of Therapy:

Start at lowest dose

Women Not Currently Using Continuous Estrogen or Combination Estrogen/Progestin Therapy:

May start w/ CombiPatch at any time

Women Currently Using Continuous Estrogen or Combination Estrogen/Progestin Therapy:

Complete current cycle of therapy prior to initiating CombiPatch

Continuous Combined Regimen:

Apply 0.05mg-0.14mg patch
Apply twice weekly during 28-day cycle

Continuous Sequential Regimen:

Wear estradiol-only patch for first 14 days of 28-day cycle, replace twice weekly
Apply 0.05mg-0.14mg patch for remaining 14 days, replace twice weekly

For both regimens, use 0.05mg-0.25mg patch if greater progestin is required
Reevaluate at 3- to 6-month intervals

ADMINISTRATION

Transdermal route

Apply to a smooth (fold-free), clean, dry area of the lower abdomen
Do not apply to or near the breasts; avoid application to waistline as tight clothing may modify drug delivery
Rotate site of application, w/ an interval of at least 1 week between applications to the same site

Application

Remove 1 side of the protective liner and immediately apply to skin of lower abdomen
Remove 2nd side of the protective liner and press the system firmly in place for at least 10 sec
Only 1 system should be worn at any 1 time during the 3- to 4-day dosing interval

Refer to PI for further administration instructions

HOW SUPPLIED

Patch: (Estradiol-Norethindrone Acetate) 0.05-0.14mg/day, 0.05-0.25mg/day [8[s]]

CONTRAINDICATIONS

Undiagnosed abnormal genital bleeding, known/suspected/history of breast cancer, known/suspected estrogen-dependent neoplasia, active/history of DVT/PE, active/history of arterial thromboembolic disease (eg, stroke, MI), known liver impairment or disease, known protein C/protein S/antithrombin deficiency or other known thrombophilic disorders, known/suspected pregnancy.

WARNINGS/PRECAUTIONS

D/C immediately if stroke, DVT, PE, or MI occurs or is suspected. Caution with risk factors for arterial vascular disease and/or venous thromboembolism. If feasible, d/c at least 4-6 weeks before surgery of the type associated with an increased risk of thromboembolism, or during periods of prolonged immobilization. May increase risk of ovarian cancer and gallbladder disease. May lead to severe hypercalcemia in patients with breast cancer and bone metastases; d/c and take appropriate measures if hypercalcemia occurs. Retinal vascular thrombosis reported; d/c pending exam if sudden partial/complete loss of vision or sudden onset of proptosis, diplopia, or migraine occurs. D/C permanently if exam reveals papilledema or retinal vascular lesions. May elevate BP and thyroid-binding globulin levels. May elevate plasma TGs, leading to pancreatitis in patients with preexisting hypertriglyceridemia. Caution with history of cholestatic jaundice associated with past estrogen use or with pregnancy; d/c in case of recurrence. May cause fluid retention. Caution with hypoparathyroidism as estrogen-induced hypocalcemia may occur. May exacerbate symptoms of angioedema in women with hereditary angioedema. May exacerbate endometriosis, asthma, diabetes mellitus, epilepsy, migraine, porphyria, systemic lupus erythematosus, and hepatic hemangiomas. May affect certain endocrine and blood components in lab tests.

ADVERSE REACTIONS

Abdominal pain, back pain, asthenia, flu syndrome, headache, application-site reaction, diarrhea, nausea, nervousness, pharyngitis, respiratory disorder, breast pain, dysmenorrhea, menstrual disorder, vaginitis.

DRUG INTERACTIONS

CYP3A4 inducers (eg, St. John's wort preparations, phenobarbital, carbamazepine) may decrease levels and may decrease therapeutic effects and/or change uterine bleeding profile. CYP3A4 inhibitors (eg, erythromycin, clarithromycin, ketoconazole) may increase levels, which may result in side effects. Patients concomitantly receiving thyroid hormone replacement therapy and estrogens may require increased doses of their thyroid replacement therapy; monitor thyroid function.

NURSING CONSIDERATIONS

Assessment: Assess for undiagnosed abnormal genital bleeding, presence/history of breast cancer, estrogen-dependent neoplasia, active/history of DVT/PE/arterial thromboembolic disease, liver impairment/disease, thrombophilic disorders, drug hypersensitivity, pregnancy/nursing status, and for any other conditions where treatment is contraindicated or cautioned. Assess for possible drug interactions.

Monitoring: Monitor for signs/symptoms of CV disease, malignant neoplasms, dementia, gallbladder disease, hypercalcemia, visual abnormalities, BP and plasma TG elevations, pancreatitis, cholestatic jaundice, fluid retention, exacerbation of endometriosis and other conditions, and other adverse reactions. Perform annual breast exam; schedule mammography based on age, risk factors, and prior mammogram results. Periodically reevaluate (every 3-6 months) to determine need for therapy. Perform adequate diagnostic measures (eg, endometrial sampling) to rule out malignancies in cases of undiagnosed, persistent, or recurring abnormal genital bleeding. Regularly monitor thyroid function if on thyroid hormone replacement therapy.

Patient Counseling: Inform of the importance of reporting abnormal vaginal bleeding to physician as soon as possible. Inform of possible serious adverse reactions of therapy (eg, CV disorders, malignant neoplasms, probable dementia) and of possible less serious, but common adverse reactions (eg, headache, breast pain and tenderness, nausea). Instruct to have yearly breast exams by a healthcare provider and to perform monthly breast self-exams.

Storage: Prior to Dispensing: 2-8°C (36-46°F). After Dispensing: 20-25°C (66-77°F) for up to 6 months. Store the systems in the sealed foil pouch. Do not store in areas where extreme temperatures may occur.

COMBIVENT RESPIMAT – albuterol/ipratropium bromide RX

Class: Anticholinergic/beta$_2$-agonist

ADULT DOSAGE

Chronic Obstructive Pulmonary Disease

Bronchospasm Requiring a 2nd Bronchodilator:
Usual: 1 inh qid. May take additional inh as required
Max: 6 inh/24 hrs

PEDIATRIC DOSAGE

Pediatric use may not have been established

ADMINISTRATION

Oral inh route

Priming

Prior to 1st use, insert cartridge into the inhaler and prime the unit; actuate the inhaler toward the ground until an aerosol cloud is visible and then repeat the process 3 more times
If not used for >3 days, actuate the inhaler once
If not used for >21 days, actuate the inhaler until an aerosol cloud is visible and then repeat the process 3 more times

HOW SUPPLIED

Spray, Inhalation: (Albuterol-Ipratropium) 100mcg-20mcg/actuation [60, 120 actuations]

CONTRAINDICATIONS

Hypersensitivity to atropine or any of its derivatives.

WARNINGS/PRECAUTIONS

May produce paradoxical bronchospasm; d/c and institute alternative therapy if this occurs. Albuterol: May produce significant cardiovascular (CV) effects (eg, ECG changes); may need to d/c if symptoms occur. Caution with CV disorders (eg, coronary insufficiency, cardiac arrhythmias, HTN). Fatalities reported with excessive use of inhaled sympathomimetic drugs in patients with asthma. Caution with convulsive disorders, hyperthyroidism, diabetes mellitus (DM), and in patients who are unusually responsive to sympathomimetic amines. May produce significant but usually transient hypokalemia. Hypersensitivity reactions may occur; d/c and consider alternative treatment if such a reaction occurs. Ipratropium: May increase IOP and result in precipitation/worsening of narrow-angle glaucoma. May cause urinary retention; caution with prostatic hyperplasia or bladder-neck obstruction.

ADVERSE REACTIONS

Nasopharyngitis, cough, headache, bronchitis, URI, dyspnea.

DRUG INTERACTIONS

Potential for an additive interaction with other anticholinergic-containing drugs; avoid coadministration. Increased risk of adverse CV effects with other sympathomimetic agents; use with caution. β-blockers and albuterol inhibit the effect of each other; use β-blockers with caution in patients with hyperreactive airways. ECG changes and/or hypokalemia that may result from non-K^+-sparing diuretics (eg, loop or thiazide diuretics) may be acutely worsened; use with caution and consider monitoring K^+ levels. Administration with MAOIs or TCAs, or within 2 weeks of discontinuation of such agents may potentiate the action of albuterol on CV system; use with extreme caution and consider alternative therapy.

NURSING CONSIDERATIONS

Assessment: Assess for hypersensitivity to drug or to atropine or any of its derivatives, CV disorders, narrow-angle glaucoma, prostatic hyperplasia, bladder-neck obstruction, convulsive disorders, hyperthyroidism, DM, pregnancy/nursing status, and possible drug interactions. Assess if unusually responsive to sympathomimetic amines.

Monitoring: Monitor for signs/symptoms of hypersensitivity reactions, paradoxical bronchospasm, CV effects (measured by pulse rate and BP), hypokalemia, unexpected development of severe acute asthmatic crisis, hypoxia, and other adverse reactions.

Patient Counseling: Instruct to use caution to avoid spraying the product into eyes. Instruct to consult physician if ocular symptoms or difficulty with urination develops. Instruct to exercise caution when engaging in activities requiring balance and visual acuity (eg, driving a car, operating appliances/machinery). Instruct not to increase dose or frequency without consulting physician. Instruct to seek immediate medical attention if therapy lessens in effectiveness, symptoms worsen, and/or product is needed more frequently than usual. Counsel to take other inhaled drugs only ud by physician. Counsel to d/c if paradoxical bronchospasm occurs. Inform of possible adverse effects (eg, palpitations, chest pain, rapid HR, tremor, nervousness). Instruct to contact physician if pregnant/nursing.

Storage: 25°C (77°F); excursions permitted to 15-30°C (59-86°F). Avoid freezing.

COMPLERA – emtricitabine/rilpivirine/tenofovir disoproxil fumarate RX

Class: Non-nucleoside reverse transcriptase inhibitor/nucleoside analogue combination

Lactic acidosis and severe hepatomegaly with steatosis, including fatal cases, reported with the use of nucleoside analogues. Not approved for the treatment of chronic hepatitis B virus (HBV) infection. Severe acute exacerbations of hepatitis B reported in patients coinfected with HBV upon discontinuation of therapy; closely monitor hepatic function for at least several months. If appropriate, initiation of antihepatitis B therapy may be warranted.

ADULT DOSAGE

HIV-1 Infection

Antiretroviral Treatment-Naive w/ HIV-1 RNA ≤100,000 copies/mL at Initiation:
1 tab qd

HIV-1 RNA <50 copies/mL on Stable Antiretroviral Treatment at Initiation:
1 tab qd

PEDIATRIC DOSAGE

Pediatric use may not have been established

DOSE MODIFICATION

Concomitant Medications

Rifabutin: Add 25mg of rilpivirine qd to therapy

Renal Impairment

Moderate or Severe (CrCl <50mL/min): Not recommended for use

ADMINISTRATION

Oral route

Take w/ food

HOW SUPPLIED

Tab: (Emtricitabine-Rilpivirine-Tenofovir Disoproxil Fumarate [TDF]) 200mg-25mg-300mg

CONTRAINDICATIONS

Coadministration with CYP3A inducers or agents that increase gastric pH causing decreased plasma concentrations, which may result in loss of virologic response and possible resistance (eg, carbamazepine, oxcarbazepine, phenobarbital, phenytoin, rifampin, rifapentine, proton pump inhibitors [eg, dexlansoprazole, esomeprazole, lansoprazole, omeprazole, pantoprazole, rabeprazole], systemic dexamethasone [more than a single dose], St. John's wort).

WARNINGS/PRECAUTIONS

When considering replacing the current regimen in virologically-suppressed adults, patients should have no history of virologic failure, have been stably suppressed for at least 6 months prior to switching therapy, currently be on the 1st or 2nd antiretroviral regimen prior to switching therapy, and have no current/past history of resistance to any of the 3 drug components. Additional monitoring of HIV-1 RNA and regimen tolerability is recommended after replacing therapy to assess for potential virologic failure or rebound. Not for patients requiring dose reduction (eg, moderate or severe renal impairment [estimated CrCl <50mL/min], dialysis). Immune reconstitution syndrome, autoimmune disorders (eg, Graves' disease, polymyositis, Guillain-Barre syndrome) in the setting of immune reconstitution, and redistribution/accumulation of body fat reported. Caution in elderly. Rilpivirine: Depressive disorders reported; immediate medical evaluation is recommended if severe depressive symptoms occur. Hepatic adverse events reported; increased risk for worsening/ development of liver-associated test elevations in patients with underlying hepatitis B or C, or marked liver-associated test elevations prior to treatment. Consider liver-associated test monitoring for patients without preexisting hepatic dysfunction or other risk factors. TDF: Obesity and prolonged nucleoside exposure may be risk factors for lactic acidosis and severe hepatomegaly with steatosis. Caution with known risk factors for liver disease. D/C if lactic acidosis or pronounced hepatotoxicity occurs. Renal impairment (eg, acute renal failure, Fanconi syndrome) reported. Decreased bone mineral density (BMD), increased biochemical markers of bone metabolism, and osteomalacia reported. Consider assessment of BMD in patients with history of pathologic bone fracture or other risk factors for osteoporosis or bone loss. Arthralgias and muscle pain/weakness reported in cases of proximal renal tubulopathy. Consider hypophosphatemia and osteomalacia secondary to proximal renal tubulopathy in patients at risk of renal dysfunction who present with persistent or worsening bone or muscle symptoms.

ADVERSE REACTIONS

Lactic acidosis, severe hepatomegaly with steatosis, nausea, headache, dizziness, depressive disorders, insomnia, abnormal dreams, rash, diarrhea, fatigue.

DRUG INTERACTIONS

See Contraindications and Dosage. Avoid with concurrent or recent use of nephrotoxic agents (eg, high dose or multiple NSAIDs), other antiretrovirals, adefovir dipivoxil, or drugs containing any of the same active components or lamivudine. Avoid with rilpivirine unless needed for dose adjustment (eg, with rifabutin). Rilpivirine: Caution with drugs that may reduce exposure or drugs with a known risk of torsades de pointes. Decreased levels, loss of virologic response, and possible resistance with CYP3A inducers or drugs increasing gastric pH (eg, antacids, H2-receptor antagonists [H2-RAs]). Administer antacids at least 2 hrs before or at least 4 hrs after dosing, and H2-RAs at least 12 hrs before or at least 4 hrs after dosing. Decreased levels with rifabutin. CYP3A inhibitors, azole antifungals, clarithromycin, erythromycin, or telithromycin may increase levels. May decrease levels of ketoconazole and methadone. Emtricitabine and TDF: Drugs that reduce renal function or compete for active tubular secretion (eg, acyclovir, aminoglycosides [eg, gentamicin], high dose or multiple NSAIDs) may increase levels. Cases of acute renal failure after initiation of high dose or multiple NSAIDs reported in HIV-infected patients with risk factors for renal dysfunction who appeared stable on TDF; consider alternatives to NSAIDs, if needed.

NURSING CONSIDERATIONS

Assessment: Assess for history of virologic failure, current/past history of resistance to any of the drug components, obesity, prolonged nucleoside exposure, liver dysfunction or risk factors for liver disease, renal impairment, HBV infection, pregnancy/nursing status, and possible drug interactions. Assess BMD in patients with a history of pathological bone fracture or with other risk factors for osteoporosis/bone loss. Assess estimated CrCl, serum phosphorus (P), urine glucose, and urine protein in patients at risk for renal dysfunction.

Monitoring: Monitor for signs/symptoms of lactic acidosis, severe hepatomegaly with steatosis, depressive symptoms, hepatotoxicity, decreased BMD, increased biochemical markers for bone metabolism, osteomalacia, fat redistribution/accumulation, immune reconstitution syndrome (eg, opportunistic infections), autoimmune disorders, renal impairment, and other adverse reactions. Monitor patients coinfected with HBV and HIV-1 with clinical and lab follow-up for acute exacerbations of hepatitis B for at least several months upon discontinuation of therapy. Monitor estimated CrCl, serum P, urine glucose, and urine protein periodically in patients at risk for renal dysfunction. Additional monitoring of HIV-1 RNA and regimen tolerability is recommended after replacing therapy to assess for potential virologic failure or rebound.

Patient Counseling: Inform that therapy is not a cure for HIV infection; continuous therapy is necessary to control HIV infection and decrease HIV-related illnesses. Advise to practice safe sex and use latex or polyurethane condoms. Instruct to never reuse or share needles. Advise not to breastfeed. Counsel to take on a regular dosing schedule with food and avoid missing doses. Inform that a protein drink is not a substitute for food. Counsel patients on missed dose instructions. Inform not to take more or less than the prescribed dose at any one time. Instruct to contact physician if symptoms of lactic acidosis or severe hepatomegaly with steatosis, depression, or infection occurs. Inform that hepatotoxicity has been reported during treatment. Inform that fat redistribution/

accumulation, renal impairment, and decreases in BMD may occur. Advise to inform physician if taking any other prescription or nonprescription medications or herbal products (eg, St. John's wort). Instruct to take ud.

Storage: 25°C (77°F); excursions permitted to 15-30°C (59-86°F).

COMPRO – prochlorperazine RX

Class: Phenothiazine derivative

Elderly patients with dementia-related psychosis treated with antipsychotic drugs are at an increased risk of death; most deaths appeared to be cardiovascular (CV) (eg, heart failure, sudden death) or infectious (eg, pneumonia) in nature. Treatment with conventional antipsychotic drugs may similarly increase mortality. Not approved for the treatment of patients with dementia-related psychosis.

ADULT DOSAGE

Nausea/Vomiting

Control of Severe N/V:
Usual: 25mg bid; begin w/ lowest recommended dosage and adjust according to individual response

PEDIATRIC DOSAGE

Pediatric use may not have been established

DOSE MODIFICATION

Elderly

Start at lower end of dosing range and increase more gradually

Other Important Modifications

Debilitated or Emaciated Patients:
Increase dosage more gradually

ADMINISTRATION

Rectal route

HOW SUPPLIED

Sup: 25mg

CONTRAINDICATIONS

Comatose states, concomitant large doses of CNS depressants (eg, alcohol, barbiturates, narcotics), pediatric surgery, children <2 yrs of age or <20 lbs.

WARNINGS/PRECAUTIONS

Secondary extrapyramidal symptoms may occur. Tardive dyskinesia (TD) may develop, especially in elderly and during long-term use. Neuroleptic malignant syndrome (NMS) reported; d/c if it occurs and institute appropriate treatment. Caution during reintroduction of therapy as NMS recurrence reported. Avoid in patients with bone marrow depression, previous hypersensitivity reaction, and in pregnant women. May impair mental and/or physical abilities, especially during the 1st few days of therapy. May mask symptoms of overdose of other drugs, and obscure diagnosis of intestinal obstruction, brain tumor, and Reye's syndrome; avoid in children/adolescents whose signs and symptoms suggest Reye's syndrome. May cause hypotension; caution with large doses and parenteral administration in patients with impaired CV systems. Deep sleep and coma reported. May interfere with thermoregulation; caution in patients exposed to extreme heat. Evaluate therapy periodically in patients with history of long-term use. Leukopenia/neutropenia/agranulocytosis reported; monitor CBC frequently during 1st few months of therapy, and d/c at 1st sign of a decline in WBC in patients with preexisting low WBC or a history of drug induced leukopenia/neutropenia. D/C and monitor WBC until recovery in patients with severe neutropenia (absolute neutrophil count <1000/mm^3). Aspiration of vomitus has occurred in postsurgical patients. Caution with glaucoma, in children with dehydration or acute illness, and in elderly. May produce α-adrenergic blockade, lower seizure threshold, elevate prolactin levels, or cause false-positive phenylketonuria test results. D/C at least 48 hrs before myelography and should not resume for at least 24 hrs postprocedure.

ADVERSE REACTIONS

Drowsiness, dizziness, amenorrhea, blurred vision, skin reactions, hypotension, cholestatic jaundice, leukopenia, agranulocytosis, NMS, extrapyramidal symptoms, motor restlessness, dystonia, pseudoparkinsonism, TD.

DRUG INTERACTIONS

See Contraindications. May intensify and prolong action of CNS depressants (eg, opiates, analgesics, antihistamines, barbiturates, alcohol, anesthetics, narcotics), atropine, and organophosphorus insecticides. May decrease oral anticoagulant effects. Thiazide diuretics may accentuate orthostatic hypotension. May counteract antihypertensive effects of guanethidine and related compounds. Increased levels of both drugs with propranolol. Anticonvulsants may need dosage adjustment; may lower convulsive threshold. May interfere with metabolism of phenytoin and precipitate phenytoin toxicity. Avoid use prior to myelography with metrizamide. May reverse effect of epinephrine. May cause paradoxical further lowering of BP with epinephrine and other pressor agents (excluding norepinephrine bitartrate and phenylephrine hydrochloride); avoid concomitant use.

NURSING CONSIDERATIONS

Assessment: Assess for Reye's syndrome, TD, impaired CV systems, breast cancer, glaucoma, bone marrow depression, preexisting low WBC count, history of drug induced leukopenia/ neutropenia, history of psychosis, seizure disorder, pregnancy/nursing status, and possible drug interactions. Assess use in children with acute illness or dehydration, elderly, debilitated, or emaciated patients.

Monitoring: Monitor for extrapyramidal symptoms, signs/symptoms of TD, NMS, hypotension, fever, sore throat, infection, jaundice, motor restlessness, dystonia, pseudoparkinsonism, and hypersensitivity reactions. Monitor CBC, WBC, and prolactin levels. Conduct liver studies if fever with grippe-like symptoms occurs.

Patient Counseling: Inform of the risks and benefits of therapy. Instruct to avoid engaging in hazardous activities (eg, operating vehicles or machinery) and exposure to extreme heat. Counsel to seek medical attention if symptoms of TD, NMS, hypotension, mydriasis, encephalopathic syndrome, sore throat, infection, or hypersensitivity reactions occur.

Storage: 20-25°C (68-77°F). Do not remove from wrapper until ready to use.

CONCERTA – methylphenidate hydrochloride CII

Class: Sympathomimetic amine

Caution with history of drug dependence or alcoholism. Chronic abusive use may lead to marked tolerance and psychological dependence with varying degrees of abnormal behavior. Frank psychotic episodes may occur, especially with parenteral abuse. Careful supervision is required during withdrawal from abusive use since severe depression may occur. Withdrawal following chronic use may unmask symptoms of underlying disorder that may require follow-up.

ADULT DOSAGE

Attention-Deficit Hyperactivity Disorder

18-65 Years:
New to Methylphenidate:
Initial: 18mg or 36mg qam
Range: 18-72mg/day

Currently on Methylphenidate:
Initial:
18mg qam if previous dose 5mg bid-tid
36mg qam if previous dose 10mg bid-tid
54mg qam if previous dose 15mg bid-tid
72mg qam if previous dose 20mg bid-tid
Conversion dosage should not exceed 72mg/day

Titrate: May increase in 18mg increments at weekly intervals if optimal response is not achieved at a lower dose

Max: 72mg/day

Maint/Extended Treatment:
Periodically reevaluate the long-term usefulness of the drug

D/C if no improvement observed after appropriate dosage adjustment over 1 month

PEDIATRIC DOSAGE

Attention-Deficit Hyperactivity Disorder

New to Methylphenidate:
6-12 Years:
Initial: 18mg qam
Range: 18-54mg/day

13-17 Years:
Initial: 18mg qam
Range: 18-72mg/day not to exceed 2mg/kg/day

Currently on Methylphenidate:
≥6 Years:
Initial:
18mg qam if previous dose 5mg bid-tid
36mg qam if previous dose 10mg bid-tid
54mg qam if previous dose 15mg bid-tid
72mg qam if previous dose 20mg bid-tid
Conversion dosage should not exceed 72mg/day

Titrate: May increase in 18mg increments at weekly intervals if optimal response is not achieved at a lower dose

Max:
6-12 Years: 54mg/day
13-17 Years: 72mg/day

Maint/Extended Treatment:
Periodically reevaluate the long-term usefulness of the drug

D/C if no improvement observed after appropriate dosage adjustment over 1 month

DOSE MODIFICATION

Adverse Reactions

Reduce dose or, if necessary, d/c if paradoxical aggravation of symptoms or other adverse events occur

ADMINISTRATION
Oral route
Take w/ or w/o food
Swallow tab whole w/ the aid of liquids; do not chew, divide, or crush

HOW SUPPLIED
Tab, Extended-Release: 18mg, 27mg, 36mg, 54mg

CONTRAINDICATIONS
Marked anxiety, tension, agitation, glaucoma, motor tics, or family history or diagnosis of Tourette's syndrome. Treatment with MAOIs or within a minimum of 14 days following discontinuation of an MAOI.

WARNINGS/PRECAUTIONS
Avoid with known serious structural cardiac abnormalities, cardiomyopathy, serious heart rhythm abnormalities, coronary artery disease, or other serious cardiac problems. Sudden death reported in children and adolescents with structural cardiac abnormalities or other serious heart problems. Sudden deaths, stroke, and MI reported in adults. May increase BP and HR; caution with conditions that might be compromised by increases in BP/HR (eg, preexisting HTN, heart failure, recent MI, ventricular arrhythmia). Prior to treatment, obtain medical history (including assessment for family history of sudden death or ventricular arrhythmia) and perform physical exam to assess for presence of cardiac disease. Promptly perform cardiac evaluation if symptoms of cardiac disease develop. May exacerbate symptoms of behavior disturbance and thought disorder in patients with preexisting psychotic disorder. Caution in patients with comorbid bipolar disorder; may induce mixed/manic episode. May cause treatment-emergent psychotic or manic symptoms (eg, hallucinations, delusional thinking, mania) in patients without prior history of psychotic illness or mania; consider discontinuation if such symptoms occur. Aggressive behavior or hostility reported. May lower convulsive threshold; d/c if seizures occur. Priapism reported; seek immediate medical attention if abnormally sustained or frequent and painful erections develop. Associated with peripheral vasculopathy, including Raynaud's phenomenon; carefully observe for digital changes. May cause long-term suppression of growth in children; monitor growth, and may need to interrupt treatment in patients not growing or gaining height or weight as expected. Difficulties with accommodation and blurring of vision reported. Tab is nondeformable and does not appreciably change in shape in the GI tract; avoid with preexisting severe GI narrowing (pathologic or iatrogenic).

ADVERSE REACTIONS
Decreased appetite, headache, dry mouth, nausea, insomnia, anxiety, dizziness, decreased weight, irritability, upper abdominal pain, hyperhidrosis, palpitations, tachycardia, depressed mood, nervousness.

DRUG INTERACTIONS
See Contraindications. Caution with vasopressor agents. May inhibit metabolism of coumarin anticoagulants, anticonvulsants (eg, phenobarbital, phenytoin, primidone), and some antidepressants (eg, TCAs, SSRIs); downward dose adjustment and monitoring of plasma drug concentrations (or coagulation times for coumarin) of these drugs may be necessary when initiating or discontinuing methylphenidate.

NURSING CONSIDERATIONS

Assessment: Assess for hypersensitivity to the drug, marked anxiety, tension, agitation, glaucoma, motor tics, family history or diagnosis of Tourette's syndrome, cardiovascular conditions, history of drug dependence or alcoholism, psychotic disorder, comorbid bipolar disorder, severe GI narrowing, any other conditions where treatment is contraindicated or cautioned, pregnancy/nursing status, and possible drug interactions.

Monitoring: Monitor for changes in HR and BP, signs/symptoms of cardiac disease, exacerbation of behavior disturbance and thought disorder, psychosis, mania, appearance of or worsening of aggressive behavior or hostility, seizures, priapism, peripheral vasculopathy (including Raynaud's phenomenon), visual disturbances, and other adverse reactions. In pediatric patients, monitor growth. Perform periodic monitoring of CBC, differential, and platelet counts during prolonged therapy. Periodically reevaluate long-term usefulness of drug.

Patient Counseling: Inform about risks, benefits, and appropriate use of the medication. Advise of the possibility of priapism; instruct to seek immediate medical attention in the event of priapism. Inform about the risk of peripheral vasculopathy, including Raynaud's phenomenon; instruct to report to physician any new numbness, pain, skin color change, sensitivity to temperature in fingers or toes, or any signs of unexplained wounds appearing on fingers/toes. Advise that the tab shell, along with insoluble core components, is eliminated from the body; inform not to be concerned if something that looks like a tab is noticed in the stool. Inform that therapy may impair mental/physical abilities; advise to use caution with hazardous tasks (eg, operating machinery, driving).

Storage: 25°C (77°F); excursions permitted to 15-30°C (59-86°F). Protect from humidity.

CONSTULOSE – lactulose

RX

Class: Osmotic laxative

ADULT DOSAGE

Constipation

Usual: 15-30mL qd

Titrate: May increase to 60mL/day if necessary

24-48 hrs may be required to produce a normal bowel movement

PEDIATRIC DOSAGE

Pediatric use may not have been established

ADMINISTRATION

Oral route

May mix w/ fruit juice, water, or milk

HOW SUPPLIED

Sol: 10g/15mL (237mL, 946mL)

CONTRAINDICATIONS

Patients who require a low-galactose diet.

WARNINGS/PRECAUTIONS

Contains galactose and lactose; caution with diabetes. Monitor electrolytes periodically in elderly or debilitated if used >6 months. Potential for explosive reaction with electrocautery procedures during proctoscopy or colonoscopy; patients on therapy undergoing such procedures should have a thorough bowel cleansing with a non-fermentable solution.

ADVERSE REACTIONS

Flatulence, intestinal cramps, diarrhea, N/V.

DRUG INTERACTIONS

Nonabsorbable antacids may decrease effects.

NURSING CONSIDERATIONS

Assessment: Assess for diabetes, patients requiring a low-galactose diet, pregnancy/nursing, and possible drug interactions. Assess use in electrocautery procedures during proctoscopy or colonoscopy.

Monitoring: Monitor serum electrolytes (K^+, Cl^-, carbon dioxide) if used >6 months in elderly and debilitated patients. Monitor for diarrhea, vomiting, and other adverse reactions.

Patient Counseling: Instruct to contact physician if unusual diarrheal condition occurs. Advise to report any potential adverse effects.

Storage: 2-30°C (36-86°F). Do not freeze. Prolonged exposure >30°C (86°F) or to direct light may cause extreme darkening and turbidity; do not use if this condition develops. Prolonged exposure to freezing temperature may cause change to a semi-solid, too viscous to pour; viscosity will return to normal upon warming to room temperature.

COPAXONE – glatiramer acetate injection

RX

Class: Immunomodulatory agent

ADULT DOSAGE

Multiple Sclerosis

Relapsing Forms:

20mg/mL: Administer SQ qd

40mg/mL: Administer SQ 3X/week and at least 48 hrs apart

PEDIATRIC DOSAGE

Pediatric use may not have been established

ADMINISTRATION

SQ route

Allow to stand at room temperature for 20 min before administration

Areas for SQ self-inj include arms, abdomen, hips, and thighs

HOW SUPPLIED

Inj: 20mg/mL, 40mg/mL

CONTRAINDICATIONS

Hypersensitivity to mannitol.

WARNINGS/PRECAUTIONS

20mg/mL and 40mg/mL are not interchangeable. Immediate post-inj reaction (eg, flushing, chest pain, palpitations, anxiety, dyspnea, throat constriction, urticaria) reported. Transient chest pain reported. Localized lipoatrophy at inj sites and inj-site skin necrosis may occur; follow proper inj technique and rotate inj sites with each inj. May interfere with immune functions. Continued alteration of cellular immunity due to chronic treatment may result in untoward effects.

ADVERSE REACTIONS

Inj-site reactions, vasodilatation, rash, dyspnea, chest pain, nasopharyngitis, infection, asthenia, pain, N/V, influenza, anxiety, back pain, palpitations, edema.

NURSING CONSIDERATIONS

Assessment: Assess for hypersensitivity to drug or mannitol, and pregnancy/nursing status.

Monitoring: Monitor for immediate post-inj reactions, chest pain, lipoatrophy, inj-site skin necrosis, and other adverse reactions.

Patient Counseling: Advise to inform physician if pregnant, planning to become pregnant, or breastfeeding. Inform that drug may cause an immediate post-inj reaction and that symptoms are generally transient and self-limited and do not require specific treatment; inform that these symptoms may occur early or may have their onset several months after treatment initiation. Inform that transient chest pain (either as part of the immediate post-inj reaction or in isolation) may occur; advise to seek medical attention if chest pain of unusual duration or intensity occurs. Instruct to follow proper inj technique and to rotate inj areas and sites with each inj to help minimize localized lipoatrophy and inj-site necrosis. Inform that 20mg/mL and 40mg/mL are not interchangeable. Caution to use aseptic technique. Caution against the reuse of needles or syringes. Inform of safe disposal procedures.

Storage: 2-8°C (36-46°F). If needed, may store at 15-30°C (59-86°F) for up to 1 month, but refrigeration is preferred; avoid exposure to higher temperatures or intense light. Do not freeze; discard if frozen.

CORDARONE – amiodarone hydrochloride RX

Class: Class III antiarrhythmic

Use only in patients with the indicated life-threatening arrhythmias because of potentially fatal toxicities, including pulmonary toxicity (hypersensitivity pneumonitis or interstitial/alveolar pneumonitis). Liver injury is common, usually mild, and evidenced only by abnormal liver enzymes. Overt liver disease may occur, and has been fatal. May exacerbate arrhythmia. Significant heart block or sinus bradycardia reported. Patients must be hospitalized while LD is given, and a response generally requires at least 1 week, usually 2 or more. Maintenance-dose selection is difficult and may require dosage decrease or discontinuation of treatment.

ADULT DOSAGE

Ventricular Tachycardia

Documented, life-threatening recurrent hemodynamically unstable ventricular arrhythmia that has not responded to documented adequate doses of other available antiarrhythmics or when alternative agents could not be tolerated

LD: 800-1600mg/day for 1-3 weeks; give in divided doses w/ meals for total daily dose ≥1000mg or if GI intolerance occurs
Titrate: After control is achieved or w/ prominent side effects, reduce to 600-800mg/day for 1 month
Maint: 400mg/day; up to 600mg/day

Use lowest effective dose

Ventricular Fibrillation

Documented, life-threatening recurrent ventricular arrhythmia that has not responded to documented adequate doses of other available antiarrhythmics or when alternative agents could not be tolerated

LD: 800-1600mg/day for 1-3 weeks; give in divided doses w/ meals for total daily dose ≥1000mg or if GI intolerance occurs
Titrate: After control is achieved or w/ prominent side effects, reduce to 600-800mg/day for 1 month
Maint: 400mg/day; up to 600mg/day

Use lowest effective dose

PEDIATRIC DOSAGE

Pediatric use may not have been established

DOSE MODIFICATION

Elderly

Start at the lower end of dosing range

ADMINISTRATION

Oral route

Give LD in the hospital
Administer consistently w/ or w/o food
May be administered as a single dose, or in patients w/ severe GI intolerance, as a bid dose

HOW SUPPLIED

Tab: 200mg* *scored

CONTRAINDICATIONS

Cardiogenic shock; severe sinus-node dysfunction, causing marked sinus bradycardia; 2nd- or 3rd-degree AV block; when episodes of bradycardia have caused syncope (except when used with a pacemaker).

WARNINGS/PRECAUTIONS

D/C and institute steroid therapy if hypersensitivity pneumonitis occurs. Reduce dose if interstitial/alveolar pneumonitis occurs and institute appropriate treatment. Chronic administration may affect pacing and defibrillating thresholds. Amiodarone-induced hyperthyroidism may result in thyrotoxicosis and/or the possibility of arrhythmia breakthrough or aggravation. D/C or reduce dose if LFTs are >3X normal or double in patients with elevated baseline. Optic neuropathy and/or optic neuritis usually resulting in visual impairment reported. May cause fetal harm in pregnancy and neonatal hypo/hyperthyroidism. May develop reversible corneal microdeposits (eg, visual halos, blurred vision), photosensitivity, and peripheral neuropathy (rare). May cause hypo/hyperthyroidism and myxedema coma; monitor particularly in elderly and with history of thyroid nodules, goiter, or other thyroid dysfunction. Thyroid nodules/cancer reported. Hypotension reported upon discontinuation of cardiopulmonary bypass during open-heart surgery (rare). Adult respiratory distress syndrome (ARDS) reported with either cardiac or noncardiac surgery. May be ineffective or arrhythmogenic in patients with hypokalemia. Lab test interactions may occur. May be contraindicated with corneal refractive laser surgery devices. Caution with severe left ventricular dysfunction and in elderly.

ADVERSE REACTIONS

Pulmonary toxicity, arrhythmia exacerbation, liver injury, overt liver disease, heart block/sinus bradycardia, malaise, fatigue, involuntary movements, peripheral neuropathy, constipation, poor coordination and gait, N/V, anorexia, photosensitivity.

DRUG INTERACTIONS

Risk of interactions exists after discontinuation of therapy due to long and variable $T_{1/2}$. May increase sensitivity to myocardial depressant and conduction effects of halogenated inhalation anesthetics. CYP3A4 inhibitors increase serum levels (eg, protease inhibitors, loratadine, trazodone). Avoid with grapefruit juice. Consider monitoring for toxicity when used with protease inhibitors. QT interval prolongation and torsades de pointes (TdP) reported with loratadine and trazodone. May cause QTc prolongation, with or without TdP, when used with disopyramide, fluoroquinolones, macrolides, and azoles. Inhibits P-gp, CYP1A2, CYP2C9, CYP2D6, and CYP3A4 and may increase levels of their substrates. Rhabdomyolysis/myopathy reported with HMG-CoA reductase inhibitors that are CYP3A4 substrates; limit simvastatin dose to 20mg/day, lovastatin to 40mg/day, and lower initial/maintenance doses of other CYP3A4 substrates (eg, atorvastatin) may be required. Elevated SrCr reported with cyclosporine. May increase levels of cyclosporine, quinidine, procainamide, flecainide, and phenytoin. May increase levels of digoxin; d/c or reduce dose by 50% upon amiodarone initiation. Quinidine and procainamide doses should be reduced by 1/3 if coadministered. Initiate added antiarrhythmic drug at a lower than usual dose with monitoring. Caution with β-blockers and calcium channel blockers; if necessary, amiodarone can continue to be used after insertion of a pacemaker in patients with severe bradycardia or sinus arrest. Reduce warfarin dose by 1/3-1/2 and monitor PT closely. Ineffective inhibition of platelet aggregation reported with clopidogrel. CYP3A4 inducers (eg, St. John's wort, rifampin) decrease levels. Fentanyl may cause hypotension, bradycardia, and decreased cardiac output. Sinus bradycardia reported with lidocaine; seizure associated with increased lidocaine concentrations reported with IV amiodarone. Cholestyramine increases enterohepatic elimination and may decrease levels and $T_{1/2}$. Hemodynamic and electrophysiologic interactions observed with propranolol, diltiazem, and verapamil. May impair metabolism of dextromethorphan, MTX, and phenytoin with chronic use (>2 weeks). Antithyroid drugs' action may be delayed in amiodarone-induced thyrotoxicosis. Radioactive iodine is contraindicated with amiodarone-induced hyperthyroidism. Caution with drugs that may induce hypokalemia and/or hypomagnesemia.

NURSING CONSIDERATIONS

Assessment: Assess for cardiogenic shock, severe sinus node dysfunction causing marked sinus bradycardia, 2nd- or 3rd-degree AV block, life-threatening arrhythmias, renal/hepatic impairment, thyroid dysfunction, hypersensitivity to the drug (including iodine), pregnancy/nursing status, and possible drug interactions. Correct K^+ or Mg^{2+} deficiency prior to initiation. Assess pacing and defibrillation thresholds in patients with implanted defibrillators or pacemakers. Obtain chest x-ray, pulmonary function tests (including diffusion capacity), and physical exam.

Monitoring: Monitor for pulmonary toxicities, worsened arrhythmia, sinus bradycardia, heart block, photosensitivity, and other adverse reactions. Perform history, physical exam, and chest x-ray every 3-6 months. Monitor LFTs and thyroid function tests. Monitor pacing and defibrillation thresholds in patients with implanted defibrillators or pacemakers. Correct K^+ or Mg^{2+} deficiency. Peri/postoperative monitoring for patients undergoing general anesthesia and for patients with ARDS recommended. Perform regular ophthalmic examination, including funduscopy and slit-lamp examination.

Patient Counseling: Inform about benefits and risks of therapy. Advise to report any adverse reactions to physician. Counsel to take ud and not to take with grapefruit juice. Advise to avoid prolonged sunlight exposure and to use sun-barrier cre or protective clothing. Advise that corneal refractive laser surgery is contraindicated with concurrent use. Instruct to notify physician if pregnant/nursing.

Storage: 20-25°C (68-77°F). Protect from light.

Coreg CR – carvedilol RX

Class: Alpha$_1$/beta-blocker

OTHER BRAND NAMES

Coreg

ADULT DOSAGE

Heart Failure

Tab, Immediate-Release:
Initial: 3.125mg bid for 2 weeks
Titrate: If tolerated, may increase dose to 6.25mg, 12.5mg, and 25mg bid over successive intervals of at least 2 weeks
Max: 50mg bid in patients w/ mild to moderate heart failure weighing >85kg
Cap, Extended-Release:
Initial: 10mg qd for 2 weeks
Titrate: If tolerated, may increase dose to 20mg, 40mg, and 80mg qd over successive intervals of at least 2 weeks

Left Ventricular Dysfunction Post-Myocardial Infarction

Tab, Immediate-Release:
Initial: 6.25mg bid
Titrate: Increase after 3-10 days, based on tolerability, to 12.5mg bid, then again to target dose of 25mg bid
May use lower starting dose and/or slower titration
Cap, Extended-Release:
Initial: 20mg qd
Titrate: Increase after 3-10 days, based on tolerability, to 40mg qd, then again to target dose of 80mg qd
May use lower starting dose and/or slower titration

Hypertension

Tab, Immediate-Release:
Initial: 6.25mg bid
Titrate: If needed, based on blood pressure control, may increase to 12.5mg bid, then to 25mg bid over intervals of 7-14 days
Max: 50mg/day
Cap, Extended-Release:
Initial: 20mg qd
Titrate: If needed, based on blood pressure control, may increase to 40mg qd, then to 80mg qd, over intervals of 7-14 days
Max: 80mg/day

PEDIATRIC DOSAGE

Pediatric use may not have been established

Conversions

Daily Dose of Immediate-Release (IR) Tabs to Extended-Release (ER) Caps:
6.25mg (3.125mg bid): 10mg qd
12.5mg (6.25mg bid): 20mg qd
25mg (12.5mg bid): 40mg qd
50mg (25mg bid): 80mg qd

Elderly:
Initial:
Switching from 12.5mg bid IR Tabs: 20mg qd
Switching from 25mg bid IR Tabs: 40mg qd
Titrate: Increase doses, as appropriate, after an interval of at least 2 weeks

Patients at Increased Risk of Hypotension, Dizziness, or Syncope:
Initial:
Switching from 12.5mg bid IR Tabs: 20mg qd
Switching from 25mg bid IR Tabs: 40mg qd
Titrate: Increase doses, as appropriate, after an interval of at least 2 weeks

DOSE MODIFICATION

Hepatic Impairment

Not for use in severe hepatic impairment

ADMINISTRATION

Oral route

Take w/ food

Cap, Extended-Release

Take in am
Swallow caps whole
Cap may be opened and beads sprinkled over a spoonful of applesauce and consumed immediately, and may not be stored for future use
Applesauce should not be warm
Do not crush, chew, or divide cap and/or its contents

HOW SUPPLIED

Cap, ER (CR): (Phosphate) 10mg, 20mg, 40mg, 80mg; Tab: 3.125mg, 6.25mg, 12.5mg, 25mg

CONTRAINDICATIONS

Bronchial asthma or related bronchospastic conditions, 2nd- or 3rd-degree atrioventricular (AV) block, sick sinus syndrome, severe bradycardia (without permanent pacemaker), cardiogenic shock, decompensated HF requiring IV inotropic therapy, severe hepatic impairment.

WARNINGS/PRECAUTIONS

Minimize fluid retention prior to initiation of treatment. Severe exacerbation of angina and occurrence of MI and ventricular arrhythmias reported in angina patients following abrupt discontinuation; d/c therapy over 1-2 weeks whenever possible. If angina worsens or acute coronary insufficiency develops, promptly reinstitute therapy, at least temporarily. Avoid abrupt discontinuation even in patients treated only for HTN or HF. Bradycardia reported; reduce dose if HR drops <55 beats/min. Hypotension, postural hypotension, and syncope reported; highest risk during the first 30 days of dosing. May impair mental/physical abilities. Worsening HF or fluid retention may occur during up-titration; if such symptoms occur, increase dose of diuretics. If deemed necessary, use with caution in patients with bronchospastic disease who do not respond to, or cannot tolerate, other antihypertensives. May mask signs of hypoglycemia and hyperthyroidism (eg, tachycardia). May exacerbate symptoms of hyperthyroidism or precipitate thyroid storm with abrupt withdrawal. May lead to worsening hyperglycemia in HF patients with diabetes. May precipitate or aggravate symptoms of arterial insufficiency in patients with peripheral vascular disease. Rarely, use in patients with HF resulted in deterioration of renal function; d/c or reduce dosage if worsening of renal function occurs. Chronically administered therapy should not be routinely withdrawn prior to major surgery; may augment risks of general anesthesia and surgical procedures. Caution with pheochromocytoma and Prinzmetal's variant angina. Patients with history of severe anaphylactic reaction to a variety of allergens may be more reactive to repeated challenge and may be unresponsive to usual doses of epinephrine. Intraoperative floppy iris syndrome observed during cataract surgery.

ADVERSE REACTIONS

Bradycardia, fatigue, hypotension, dizziness, headache, diarrhea, N/V, hyperglycemia, weight increase, increased cough, asthenia, angina pectoris, syncope, edema, rales.

DRUG INTERACTIONS

Potent CYP2D6 inhibitors (eg, quinidine, fluoxetine, propafenone) may increase levels. Monitor closely for signs of hypotension and/or severe bradycardia with drugs that can deplete catecholamines (eg, reserpine, MAOIs). Potentiated BP- and HR-lowering effects with clonidine; when coadministration is to be terminated, d/c therapy several days before clonidine is withdrawn. May increase cyclosporine levels; monitor concentrations and adjust dose of cyclosporine as appropriate. Increased risk of bradycardia with digitalis glycosides. May increase digoxin levels; monitor digoxin. Rifampin may reduce levels. Cimetidine may increase exposure. Amiodarone and its metabolite desethyl amiodarone, CYP2C9 inhibitors, and P-gp inhibitors may increase levels. Amiodarone or other CYP2C9 inhibitors (eg, fluconazole) may enhance β-blocking properties; monitor for signs of bradycardia or heart block. Conduction disturbance reported with diltiazem; monitor ECG and BP with calcium channel blockers of the verapamil or diltiazem type. May enhance blood glucose-reducing effect of insulin and oral hypoglycemics; regularly monitor blood glucose. If treatment is to be continued perioperatively, use caution when anesthetic agents that depress myocardial function (eg, ether, cyclopropane, trichloroethylene) are used. Additive effects and exaggerated orthostatic component with diuretics.

NURSING CONSIDERATIONS

Assessment: Assess for bronchial asthma, 2nd- or 3rd-degree AV block, sick sinus syndrome, severe bradycardia, cardiogenic shock, hepatic/renal impairment, angina, fluid retention, diabetes, hyperthyroidism, any other conditions where treatment is contraindicated or cautioned, pregnancy/nursing status, and possible drug interactions.

Monitoring: Monitor for bradycardia, worsening HF/fluid retention, masking of signs of hypoglycemia/hyperthyroidism, and other adverse reactions. Monitor BP. Monitor blood glucose during dose initiation, adjustment, or discontinuation. Monitor renal function during up-titration in patients with risk factors for renal function deterioration.

Patient Counseling: Instruct not to interrupt or d/c therapy without consulting physician. Instruct patients with HF to consult physician if signs/symptoms of worsening HF occur. Inform that a drop in BP when standing, resulting in dizziness and, rarely, fainting, may occur; advise to sit or lie down when these symptoms occur. Advise to avoid driving or hazardous tasks if experiencing dizziness or fatigue, and to notify physician if dizziness or faintness occurs. Inform contact lens wearers that decreased lacrimation may be experienced, and diabetic patients to report any changes in blood sugar levels.

Storage: (Cap, ER) 25°C (77°F); excursions permitted to 15-30°C (59-86°F). (Tab) <30°C (86°F). Protect from moisture.

COSENTYX — secukinumab RX

Class: Monoclonal antibody/IL-17A antagonist

ADULT DOSAGE

Plaque Psoriasis

In Patients Who Are Candidates for Systemic/Phototherapy:

Moderate to Severe:

Usual: 300mg at Weeks 0, 1, 2, 3, and 4 followed by 300mg every 4 weeks; a dose of 150mg may be acceptable for some patients

Each 300mg dose is given as two 150mg inj

PEDIATRIC DOSAGE

Pediatric use may not have been established

ADMINISTRATION

SQ route

Administer each inj at a different anatomic location (eg, upper arms, thighs, any quadrant of abdomen) than previous inj

Do not inject into areas where the skin is tender, bruised, erythematous, indurated, or affected by psoriasis

Preparation

Pen and Prefilled Syringe:

Before inj, remove from refrigerator and allow to reach room temperature (15-30 min) without removing needle cap

Administer within 1 hr after removal from refrigerator and discard any unused product remaining in the pen/prefilled syringe

Single Use Vial:

Preparation time from piercing the stopper until end of reconstitution should not exceed 90 min

1. Remove vial from refrigerator and allow to stand for 15-30 min to reach room temperature; ensure SWFI is at room temperature

2. Slowly inject 1mL of SWFI into vial
3. Tilt vial at a 45° angle and gently rotate between fingertips for 1 min; do not shake/invert vial
4. Allow vial to stand for 10 min at room temperature, then tilt vial at a 45° angle and gently rotate between fingertips for 1 min; do not shake/invert vial
5. Allow vial to stand undisturbed at room temperature for 5 min
6. Prepare the required number for vials and may use immediately; if stored in refrigerator, allow to reach room temperature (15-30 min) before administration

HOW SUPPLIED

Inj: 150mg/mL [prefilled syringe, Sensoready pen], 150mg [vial]

WARNINGS/PRECAUTIONS

May increase risk of infections; exercise caution when considering use in patients with a chronic infection or a history of recurrent infection. If serious infection develops, closely monitor and d/c until infection resolves. Evaluate for tuberculosis (TB) infection prior to initiating treatment; do not administer to patients with active TB infection. Initiate treatment of latent TB prior to administering therapy; consider anti-TB therapy prior to initiation in patients with a past history of latent or active TB in whom an adequate course of treatment cannot be confirmed. Exacerbations of Crohn's disease reported; caution with active Crohn's disease. Anaphylaxis and urticaria reported; d/c immediately and initiate appropriate therapy if an anaphylactic or other serious allergic reaction occurs. Removable cap of the Sensoready pen and prefilled syringe contains natural rubber latex, which may cause an allergic reaction in latex-sensitive individuals. Prior to initiating therapy, consider completion of all age appropriate immunizations according to current immunization guidelines.

ADVERSE REACTIONS

Nasopharyngitis, diarrhea, upper respiratory tract infection.

DRUG INTERACTIONS

Avoid with live vaccines. Non-live vaccinations received during a course of therapy may not elicit an immune response sufficient to prevent disease. May normalize formation of CYP450 enzymes; upon initiation or discontinuation of therapy in patients who are receiving concomitant CYP450 substrates, particularly those with a narrow therapeutic index, consider monitoring for therapeutic effect (eg, warfarin) or drug concentration (eg, cyclosporine) and consider dosage modification of the CYP450 substrate.

NURSING CONSIDERATIONS

Assessment: Assess for previous hypersensitivity to the drug, chronic infection or history of recurrent infection, TB infection, active Crohn's disease, latex sensitivity, immunization status, pregnancy/nursing status, and possible drug interactions.

Monitoring: Monitor for signs/symptoms of infection, exacerbation of Crohn's disease, anaphylactic/allergic reactions, and other adverse reactions. Monitor for signs/symptoms of active TB during and after treatment.

Patient Counseling: Advise of the potential benefits and risks of therapy. Inform that drug may lower the ability of immune system to fight infections; instruct to contact physician if any symptoms of infection develop. Advise to seek immediate medical attention if any symptoms of a serious hypersensitivity reaction occur. Instruct in inj techniques, as well as proper syringe and needle disposal, and caution against reuse of needles and syringes.

Storage: 2-8°C (36-46°F). Protect from light. Do not freeze. To avoid foaming, do not shake. (Vial) Reconstituted Sol: Use immediately or store at 2-8°C (36-46°F) for up to 24 hrs. Do not freeze.

COSOPT – dorzolamide hydrochloride/timolol maleate RX

Class: Carbonic anhydrase inhibitor/nonselective beta-blocker

OTHER BRAND NAMES

Cosopt PF

ADULT DOSAGE

Elevated Intraocular Pressure

Open-Angle Glaucoma/Ocular HTN: Insufficiently Responsive to β-Blockers:

1 drop in the affected eye(s) bid

PEDIATRIC DOSAGE

Elevated Intraocular Pressure

Open-Angle Glaucoma/Ocular HTN: Insufficiently Responsive to β-Blockers:

≥2 Years:

1 drop in the affected eye(s) bid

DOSE MODIFICATION

Concomitant Medications

Cosopt PF:

If >1 topical ophthalmic drug is being used, administer at least 5 min apart

Cosopt:
If >1 topical ophthalmic drug is being used, administer at least 10 min apart

ADMINISTRATION
Ocular route

Refer to PI for instructions for use

HOW SUPPLIED
Sol: (Dorzolamide-Timolol) (Cosopt) 2%-0.5% [10mL]; (Cosopt PF) 2%-0.5% [0.2mL, 60[s] 180[s]]

CONTRAINDICATIONS
Bronchial asthma or history thereof, severe COPD, sinus bradycardia, 2nd- or 3rd-degree AV block, overt cardiac failure, cardiogenic shock. (Cosopt) Reactive airway disease, sinoatrial block.

WARNINGS/PRECAUTIONS
Absorbed systemically; severe respiratory and cardiac reactions reported. Fatalities reported (rare) due to severe reactions to sulfonamides; sensitization may recur if readministered irrespective of the route of administration. D/C if signs of hypersensitivity or other serious reactions occur. Withdrawal of therapy before surgery is controversial. May impair the ability of the heart to respond to β-adrenergically mediated reflex stimuli; gradual withdrawal of β-blocking agents is recommended in patients undergoing elective surgery. Caution w/ cardiac failure or hepatic impairment. May mask signs/symptoms of acute hypoglycemia; caution in patients subject to spontaneous hypoglycemia and in diabetic patients receiving insulin or hypoglycemic agents. May mask certain clinical signs of hyperthyroidism (eg, tachycardia); carefully manage patients suspected of developing thyrotoxicosis to avoid abrupt withdrawal that may precipitate a thyroid storm. May precipitate more severe failure in patients w/ diminished myocardial contractility; sympathetic stimulation may be essential for support of the circulation. D/C therapy at 1st sign/symptom of cardiac failure. Avoid w/ mild to moderate COPD (eg, chronic bronchitis, emphysema), bronchospastic disease, or history of bronchospastic disease. Not recommended w/ severe renal impairment (CrCl <30mL/min). Patients w/ a history of atopy or a history of severe anaphylactic reaction to a variety of allergens may be more reactive to repeated challenge and may be unresponsive to usual doses of epinephrine. May potentiate muscle weakness. Caution w/ low endothelial cell counts; increased potential for developing corneal edema. (Cosopt) Adequately control cardiac failure before beginning therapy; monitor for signs of deterioration in patients w/ history of cardiovascular disease, including cardiac failure, and check pulse rates. Caution w/ 1st degree heart block or w/ severe peripheral circulatory disturbance/disorders (eg, severe forms of Raynaud's disease/syndrome). Bacterial keratitis reported w/ the use of multiple-dose containers. Local ocular adverse effects (conjunctivitis and lid reactions) reported w/ chronic administration; d/c and evaluate before considering restarting therapy. Choroidal detachment after infiltration procedures reported.

ADVERSE REACTIONS
Taste perversion, ocular burning, conjunctival hyperemia, blurred vision, superficial punctate keratitis, eye itching, abdominal pain, back pain, blepharitis, bronchitis, cloudy vision, HTN, pharyngitis, sinusitis, nausea.

DRUG INTERACTIONS
Not recommended w/ oral carbonic anhydrase inhibitors. Monitor for potentially additive effects, both systemic and on IOP w/ concomitant oral β-blockers; concomitant use of 2 topical β-blocking agents is not recommended. Possible AV conduction disturbances, left ventricular failure, and hypotension may occur w/ oral or IV calcium antagonists; use w/ caution and avoid use w/ impaired cardiac function. Closely observe patients receiving catecholamine-depleting drugs (eg, reserpine) because of possible additive effects and the production of hypotension and/or marked bradycardia. Concomitant use of β-blockers w/ digitalis or calcium antagonists may have additive effects in prolonging AV-conduction time. Potentiated systemic β-blockade (eg, decreased HR, depression) reported w/ concomitant CYP2D6 inhibitors (eg, quinidine, SSRIs).

NURSING CONSIDERATIONS

Assessment: Assess for hypersensitivity to any component of product or to sulfonamides, reactive airway disease, bronchial asthma or history thereof, COPD, sinus bradycardia, sinoatrial block, 2nd- or 3rd-degree AV block, cardiac failure, severe peripheral circulatory disturbance/disorders, diabetes mellitus, renal/hepatic impairment, any other conditions where the treatment is contraindicated or cautioned, pregnant/nursing status, and possible drug interactions.

Monitoring: Monitor for signs/symptoms of cardiac failure, muscle weakness, bacterial keratitis, hypersensitivity reactions, hypoglycemia, hyperthyroidism, corneal edema, and other adverse reactions.

Patient Counseling: Advise patients w/ reactive airway disease, bronchial asthma or history thereof, severe COPD, sinus bradycardia, sinoatrial block, and 2nd- or 3rd-degree AV block, not to take this product. Inform that medication contains dorzolamide (a sulfonamide) and is absorbed systemically; instruct to d/c use if serious/unusual reactions or signs of hypersensitivity develop. Instruct to avoid allowing the tip of the dispensing container to contact eye or surrounding structures; inform that contamination may result in serious damage to the eye and subsequent loss of vision. Advise to immediately contact physician concerning the continued use of the product if undergoing ocular surgery or if an intercurrent ocular condition (eg, trauma, infection) develops. (Cosopt PF) Counsel that if using >1 topical ophthalmic drug, to administer at least 5 min apart. Inform that drug does not contain preservative; instruct to use immediately after opening, and to discard remaining contents. (Cosopt) Counsel that if using >1 topical ophthalmic drug, to administer at least 10 min apart. Instruct to d/c use and seek advice if any ocular reactions (particularly conjunctivitis and lid reactions) develop. Inform that medication contains benzalkonium chloride, which may be absorbed by soft contact lenses. Instruct to remove contact lenses prior to administration; may be reinserted 15 min after.

Storage: (Cosopt) 15-30°C (59-86°F). Protect from light. (Cosopt PF) 20-25°C (68-77°F). Do not freeze. Store in original pouch; after pouch is opened, store remaining containers in foil pouch to protect from light. Discard any unused containers 15 days after 1st opening the pouch.

COUMADIN – warfarin sodium RX

Class: Vitamin K-dependent coagulation factor inhibitor

May cause major or fatal bleeding; monitor INR regularly. Drugs, dietary changes, and other factors affect INR levels achieved with therapy. Instruct patients about prevention measures to minimize risk of bleeding and to report signs/symptoms of bleeding.

OTHER BRAND NAMES

Jantoven

ADULT DOSAGE

Venous Thromboembolism

Including Deep Vein Thrombosis (DVT) and Pulmonary Embolism (PE):
Target INR: 2.5 (INR Range, 2-3) for all treatment durations

Duration of Therapy:
DVT/PE Secondary to Transient Risk Factor: 3 months
Unprovoked DVT/PE: At least 3 months; evaluate risk-benefit ratio of long-term treatment after 3 months of therapy
2 Episodes of Unprovoked DVT/PE: Long-term treatment recommended

Nonvalvular Atrial Fibrillation

Target INR: 2.5 (INR Range, 2-3)

Duration of Therapy:
Persistent/Paroxysmal A-Fib and High Risk of Stroke: Long-term treatment recommended
Persistent/Paroxysmal A-Fib and Intermediate Risk of Ischemic Stroke: Long-term treatment recommended
A-Fib and Mitral Stenosis: Long-term treatment recommended
A-Fib and Prosthetic Heart Valves: Long-term treatment recommended; target INR may be increased and aspirin added depending on valve type and position, and on patient factors

Mechanical/Bioprosthetic Heart Valves

Bileaflet Mechanical Valve/Medtronic Hall Tilting Disk Valve in the Aortic Position in Sinus Rhythm and w/o Left Atrial Enlargement:
Target INR: 2.5 (INR Range, 2-3)

Tilting Disk Valves and Bileaflet Mechanical Valves in the Mitral Position:
Target INR: 3 (INR Range, 2.5-3.5)

Caged Ball or Caged Disk Valves:
Target INR: 3 (INR Range, 2.5-3.5)

Bioprosthetic Valve in the Mitral Position:
Target INR: 2.5 (INR Range, 2-3) for the first 3 months after valve insertion. If additional risk factors for thromboembolism present, target INR 2.5 (INR Range, 2-3)

PEDIATRIC DOSAGE

Pediatric use may not have been established

Post-Myocardial Infarction

High Risk Patients w/ MI:
Treat w/ combined moderate-intensity (INR Range, 2.0-3.0) warfarin plus low-dose aspirin (≤100 mg/day) for at least 3 months after MI

Recurrent Systemic Embolism

Unknown Etiology:
Use a moderate dose regimen (INR Range, 2-3)

Dosing Based on Genotype Consideration

Expected Maint Daily Doses Based on CYP2C9 and VKORC1 Genotypes:

VKORC1-GG:
CYP2C9 *1/*1: 5-7mg
CYP2C9 *1/*2: 5-7mg
CYP2C9 *1/*3: 3-4mg
CYP2C9 *2/*2: 3-4mg
CYP2C9 *2/*3: 3-4mg
CYP2C9 *3/*3: 0.5-2mg

VKORC1-AG:
CYP2C9 *1/*1: 5-7mg
CYP2C9 *1/*2: 3-4mg
CYP2C9 *1/*3: 3-4mg
CYP2C9 *2/*2: 3-4mg
CYP2C9 *2/*3: 0.5-2mg
CYP2C9 *3/*3: 0.5-2mg

VKORC1-AA:
CYP2C9 *1/*1: 3-4mg
CYP2C9 *1/*2: 3-4mg
CYP2C9 *1/*3: 0.5-2mg
CYP2C9 *2/*2: 0.5-2mg
CYP2C9 *2/*3: 0.5-2mg
CYP2C9 *3/*3: 0.5-2mg

CYP2C9 *1/*3, *2/*2, *2/*3, and *3/*3:
May require more prolonged time (>2-4 weeks) to achieve max INR effect

If CYP2C9 and VKORC1 Genotypes are Unknown:
Initial: 2-5mg qd
Maint: 2-10mg qd

Other Indications

Mitral Stenosis/Valvular Disease Associated w/ A-Fib:
Use a moderate dose regimen (INR Range, 2-3)

Conversions

From Heparin:
Conversion may begin concomitantly w/ heparin therapy or may be delayed 3-6 days
Continue full dose heparin therapy and overlap warfarin therapy for 4-5 days; D/C heparin once warfarin has produced the desired therapeutic response as determined by INR

Patients receiving both heparin and warfarin should have INR monitoring at least:
5 hrs after the last IV bolus heparin dose, or
4 hrs after cessation of continuous IV heparin infusion, or
24 hrs after the last SQ heparin inj

Warfarin may increase the aPTT test, even in the absence of heparin; severe elevation (>50 sec) in aPTT w/ INR in desired range has been identified as an indication of increased risk of postoperative hemorrhage

From Other Anticoagulants:
Consult the labeling of other anticoagulants for conversion instructions

DOSE MODIFICATION

Elderly

Elderly/Debilitated: Consider lower initial and maint doses

Other Important Modifications

Asian Patients: Consider lower initial and maint doses

Treatment During Dentistry or Surgery: Some procedures may necessitate an interruption or change in dose

ADMINISTRATION

(Coumadin, Jantoven) Oral or (Coumadin) IV route

Coumadin

IV dose is the same as oral dose

IV:

Reconstitute vial w/ 2.7mL of sterile water for inj; resulting yield is 2.5mL of a 2mg/mL sol

After reconstitution, administer as a slow bolus inj into a peripheral vein over 1-2 min

HOW SUPPLIED

Inj: (Coumadin) 5mg; Tab: (Coumadin, Jantoven) 1mg*, 2mg*, 2.5mg*, 3mg*, 4mg*, 5mg*, 6mg*, 7.5mg*, 10mg* *scored

CONTRAINDICATIONS

Pregnancy, except in pregnant women with mechanical heart valves, who are at high risk of thromboembolism. Hemorrhagic tendencies or blood dyscrasias. Recent or contemplated surgery of the CNS, eye, or traumatic surgery resulting in large open surfaces. Bleeding tendencies associated with active ulceration or overt bleeding of GI/genitourinary/respiratory tract, CNS hemorrhage, cerebral aneurysms, dissecting aorta, pericarditis and pericardial effusions, or bacterial endocarditis. Threatened abortion, eclampsia, and preeclampsia. Unsupervised patients with conditions associated with potential high level of noncompliance. Spinal puncture and other diagnostic/therapeutic procedures with potential for uncontrollable bleeding. Major regional, lumbar block anesthesia. Malignant HTN.

WARNINGS/PRECAUTIONS

Has no direct effect on established thrombus, nor does it reverse ischemic tissue damage. Some dental/surgical procedures may need interruption or change in the dose; determine INR immediately prior to procedure. Has a narrow therapeutic range (index) and its action may be affected by endogenous factors, other drugs, and dietary vitamin K; perform periodic INR monitoring. Risk of necrosis and/or gangrene of skin and other tissues; d/c if necrosis occurs and consider alternative therapy. May enhance the release of atheromatous plaque emboli, and systemic atheroemboli and cholesterol microemboli may occur. D/C if distinct syndrome resulting from microemboli to the feet ("purple toes syndrome") occurs. Do not use as initial therapy with heparin-induced thrombocytopenia (HIT) and with heparin-induced thrombocytopenia with thrombosis syndrome (HITTS); limb ischemia, necrosis, and gangrene reported when heparin was discontinued and warfarin started or continued. Can cause fetal harm in pregnant women. Increased risks of therapy in patients with hepatic impairment, infectious diseases/disturbances of intestinal flora, indwelling catheter, severe/moderate HTN, deficiency in protein C-mediated anticoagulant response, polycythemia vera, vasculitis, diabetes, and those undergoing eye surgery. Caution in elderly and hepatic impairment.

ADVERSE REACTIONS

Hemorrhage, necrosis of the skin and other tissues, systemic atheroemboli, cholesterol microemboli, hypersensitivity/allergic reactions, vasculitis, hepatitis, elevated liver enzymes, N/V, diarrhea, rash, dermatitis, tracheal/tracheobronchial calcifications, chills.

DRUG INTERACTIONS

May increase effect (increase INR) with CYP2C9, 1A2, and/or 3A4 inhibitors. May decrease effect (decrease INR) with CYP2C9, 1A2, and/or 3A4 inducers. Increased risk of bleeding with anticoagulants (argatroban, dabigatran, bivalirudin, desirudin, heparin, lepirudin), antiplatelet agents (ASA, cilostazol, clopidogrel, dipyridamole, prasugrel, ticlopidine), NSAIDs (celecoxib, diclofenac, diflunisal, fenoprofen, ibuprofen, indomethacin, ketoprofen, ketorolac, mefenamic acid, naproxen, oxaprozin, piroxicam, sulindac), serotonin reuptake inhibitors (eg, citalopram, desvenlafaxine, duloxetine, escitalopram, fluoxetine, fluvoxamine, milnacipran, paroxetine, sertraline, venlafaxine, vilazodone). Changes in INR reported with antibiotics or antifungals; closely monitor INR when starting or stopping any antibiotics or antifungals. Use caution with botanical (herbal) products. May potentiate anticoagulant effects with some botanicals (eg, garlic, Ginkgo biloba). May decrease effects with some botanicals (eg, coenzyme Q10, St. John's wort, ginseng). Some botanicals and foods can interact through CYP450 interactions (eg, echinacea, grapefruit juice, ginkgo, goldenseal, St. John's wort). Cholestatic hepatitis has been associated with coadministration of warfarin and ticlopidine.

NURSING CONSIDERATIONS

Assessment: Assess for risk factors for bleeding (eg, age ≥65 yrs, history of highly variable INR, GI bleeding, HTN, cerebrovascular disease, malignancy, anemia, trauma, renal impairment, certain genetic factors), factors affecting INR (eg, diarrhea, hepatic disorders, poor nutritional state, steatorrhea, vitamin K deficiency, increased vitamin K intake, hereditary warfarin resistance), pregnancy/nursing status, other conditions where treatment is contraindicated or cautioned, and drug-drug/drug-disease interactions. Assess INR. Obtain platelet counts in patients with HIT or HITTS.

Monitoring: Monitor for signs/symptoms of bleeding, necrosis/gangrene of skin and other tissues, systemic atheroemboli, cholesterol microemboli, "purple toes syndrome," and other adverse reactions. Perform periodic INR testing.

Patient Counseling: Instruct to inform physician if patient falls often as this may increase risk for complications. Counsel to maintain strict adherence to dosing regimen. Advise not to start or stop other medications, including salicylates (eg, ASA, topical analgesics), OTC drugs, or herbal medications, except on advice of physician. Instruct to inform physician if pregnancy is suspected (to discuss pregnancy planning) or if considering breastfeeding. Counsel to avoid any activity or sport that may result in traumatic injury. Instruct that regular PT tests and visits to physician are required during therapy. Advise patient to carry ID card stating drug is being taken. Instruct to eat a normal, balanced diet to maintain consistent intake of vitamin K and to avoid drastic changes in diet, such as eating large amounts of leafy, green vegetables. Advise to take ud. Advise to immediately report unusual bleeding or symptoms or any serious illness, such as severe diarrhea, infection, or fever. Inform that anticoagulant effects may persist for about 2 to 5 days after discontinuation.

Storage: Tab: (Coumadin) 15-30°C (59-86°F). (Jantoven) 20-25°C (68-77°F); excursions permitted 15-30°C (59-86°F). Protect from light and moisture. Inj: (Coumadin) 15-30°C (59-86°F). Protect from light. Use reconstituted sol within 4 hrs. Do not refrigerate. Discard any unused sol.

COZAAR — losartan potassium RX

Class: Angiotensin II receptor antagonist

D/C when pregnancy is detected. Drugs that act directly on the renin-angiotensin system (RAS) can cause injury/death to the developing fetus.

ADULT DOSAGE

Hypertension

Initial: 50mg qd
Usual Range: 25-100mg/day given qd or bid
May add a low dose diuretic if BP not controlled

Hypertension with Left Ventricular Hypertrophy

Reduction in Risk of Stroke:
Initial: 50mg qd
Titrate: Add HCTZ 12.5mg qd and/or increase losartan to 100mg qd, followed by an increase in HCTZ to 25mg qd based on BP response

This may not apply to black patients

Diabetic Nephropathy

Elevated SrCr/Proteinuria (Urinary Albumin to Creatinine Ratio ≥300mg/g) in Patients w/ Type 2 Diabetes and a History of HTN
Initial: 50mg qd
Titrate: Increase to 100mg qd based on BP response

PEDIATRIC DOSAGE

Hypertension

≥6 Years:
Initial: 0.7mg/kg qd (up to 50mg total) administered as a tab or sus
Titrate: Adjust dose according to BP response
Max: 1.4mg/kg/day (or 100mg/day)

DOSE MODIFICATION

Hepatic Impairment
Initial: 25mg qd

Other Important Modifications
Patients w/ Intravascular Volume Depletion
Initial: 25mg qd

ADMINISTRATION

Oral route

Take w/ or w/o food

Preparation of Sus (for 200mL of a 2.5mg/mL sus)

1. Add 10mL of Purified Water USP to an 8 oz (240mL) amber polyethylene terephthalate (PET) bottle containing ten 50mg Cozaar tabs. Immediately shake for at least 2 min
2. Let the concentrate stand for 1 hr and then shake for 1 min to disperse the tab contents
3. Separately prepare a 50/50 volumetric mixture of Ora-Plus and Ora-Sweet SF
4. Add 190mL of the 50/50 Ora-Plus/Ora-Sweet SF mixture to the tab and water slurry in the PET bottle and shake for 1 min to disperse the ingredients
5. The sus should be refrigerated at 2-8°C (36-46°F) and can be stored for up to 4 weeks
6. Shake the sus prior to each use and return promptly to the refrigerator

HOW SUPPLIED

Tab: 25mg, 50mg*, 100mg *scored

CONTRAINDICATIONS

Coadministration with aliskiren in patients with diabetes.

WARNINGS/PRECAUTIONS

Symptomatic hypotension may occur in patients who are intravascularly volume-depleted (eg, treated with diuretics); correct volume depletion before therapy or start therapy at a lower dose. Hypersensitivity, including angioedema, reported. Consider a lower dose in patients with hepatic dysfunction. Changes in renal function reported. Oliguria and/or progressive azotemia and (rarely) acute renal failure and/or death may occur in patients whose renal function is dependent on the RAS (eg, severe CHF). Increases in SrCr or BUN reported in patients with unilateral/bilateral renal artery stenosis. Electrolyte imbalances reported with renal impairment, with or without DM. Hyperkalemia reported in type 2 diabetics with proteinuria. Not recommended in pediatric patients with GFR <30mL/min.

ADVERSE REACTIONS

Dizziness, cough, URI, diarrhea, asthenia/fatigue, chest pain, hypotension, hypoglycemia, anemia, back pain, UTI, cataract, diabetic vascular disease, cellulitis, influenza-like disease.

DRUG INTERACTIONS

See Contraindications. Increases in lithium levels and lithium toxicity reported; monitor lithium levels. Dual blockade of the RAS is associated with increased risks of hypotension, syncope, hyperkalemia, and changes in renal function (including acute renal failure); closely monitor BP, renal function, and electrolytes with concomitant agents that affect the RAS. Avoid with aliskiren in patients with renal impairment (GFR <60mL/min). May increase serum K^+ with K^+-sparing diuretics (eg, spironolactone, triamterene, amiloride), K^+ supplements, or salt substitutes containing K^+. NSAIDs, including selective COX-2 inhibitors, may attenuate antihypertensive effect and deteriorate renal function. Rifampin may decrease levels. Fluconazole may decrease levels of the active metabolite and increase levels of losartan.

NURSING CONSIDERATIONS

Assessment: Assess for history of hypersensitivity, volume depletion, CHF, DM, unilateral or bilateral renal artery stenosis, hepatic/renal impairment, pregnancy/nursing status, and possible drug interactions.

Monitoring: Monitor for signs/symptoms of electrolyte imbalance, hypotension, hypersensitivity reactions, oliguria, azotemia, hepatic dysfunction, and other adverse reactions. Monitor BP, serum electrolytes, and renal function periodically.

Patient Counseling: Inform of pregnancy risks and discuss treatment options with women planning to become pregnant; instruct to report pregnancy to physician as soon as possible. Instruct not to use K^+ supplements or salt substitutes containing K^+ without consulting physician.

Storage: (Tab) 25°C (77°F); excursions permitted to 15-30°C (59-86°F). Protect from light. (Sus) 2-8°C (36-46°F) for up to 4 weeks.

CREON – pancrelipase RX

Class: Pancreatic enzyme supplement

ADULT DOSAGE

Exocrine Pancreatic Insufficiency

Due to Cystic Fibrosis, Chronic Pancreatitis, Pancreatectomy, or Other Conditions:
Start at the lowest recommended dose and increase gradually
Initial: 500 lipase U/kg/meal
Max: 2500 lipase U/kg/meal (or ≤10,000 lipase U/kg/day) or <4000 lipase U/g fat ingested/day

PEDIATRIC DOSAGE

Exocrine Pancreatic Insufficiency

Due to Cystic Fibrosis, Chronic Pancreatitis, Pancreatectomy, or Other Conditions:
Start at the lowest recommended dose and increase gradually

≤12 Months of Age:
3000 lipase U/120mL of formula or per breastfeeding; administer immediately prior to each feeding

Half of the dose used for meals should be given w/ each snack
Refer to PI for dosing limitations

>12 Months-<4 Years:
Initial: 1000 lipase U/kg/meal
Max: 2500 lipase U/kg/meal (or ≤10,000 lipase U/kg/day) or <4000 lipase U/g fat ingested/day

≥4 Years:
Initial: 500 lipase U/kg/meal
Max: 2500 lipase U/kg/meal (or ≤10,000 lipase U/kg/day) or <4000 lipase U/g fat ingested/day
Half of the dose used for meals should be given w/ each snack
Refer to PI for dosing limitations

DOSE MODIFICATION

Elderly

Reduce dose

ADMINISTRATION

Oral route

Take during meals or snacks, w/ sufficient fluid
Swallow whole; do not crush or chew caps/cap contents
Do not retain in mouth
Do not mix directly into formula or breast milk
For patients who are unable to swallow intact capsules, open the contents and add to a small amount of acidic soft food w/ a pH of 4.5 or less, such as applesauce. The mixture should be swallowed immediately and followed w/ water or juice to ensure complete ingestion

HOW SUPPLIED

Cap, Delayed-Release: (Lipase-Protease-Amylase) 3000 U-9500 U-15,000 U; 6000 U-19,000 U-30,000 U; 12,000 U-38,000 U-60,000 U; 24,000 U-76,000 U-120,000 U; 36,000 U-114,000 U-180,000 U

WARNINGS/PRECAUTIONS

Not interchangeable with other pancrelipase products. Fibrosing colonopathy reported; monitor closely for progression to stricture formation. Caution with doses >2500 lipase U/kg/meal (or >10,000 lipase U/kg/day); use only if these doses are documented to be effective by 3-day fecal fat measures indicating significant improvement. Examine patients receiving >6000 lipase U/kg/meal; immediately decrease or titrate dose downward to a lower range. Ensure that no drug is retained in the mouth. Should not be crushed or chewed, or mixed in foods with pH >4.5; may disrupt enteric coating of cap, resulting in early release of enzymes, irritation of oral mucosa, and/or loss of enzyme activity. Caution in patients with gout, renal impairment, or hyperuricemia; may increase blood uric acid levels. Risk for transmission of viral diseases. Caution with known allergy to proteins of porcine origin; severe allergic reactions reported.

ADVERSE REACTIONS

Vomiting, flatulence, abdominal pain, headache, cough, dizziness, frequent bowel movements, abnormal feces, hyperglycemia, hypoglycemia, nasopharyngitis, decreased appetite, irritability.

NURSING CONSIDERATIONS

Assessment: Assess for known allergy to porcine proteins, gout, renal impairment, hyperuricemia, and pregnancy/nursing status.

Monitoring: Monitor for fibrosing colonopathy, stricture formation, oral mucosa irritation, viral diseases, and allergic reactions. Monitor serum uric acid levels.

Patient Counseling: Instruct to take ud and with food and fluids. Inform that if a dose is missed, take the next dose with the next meal/snack ud; instruct not to double doses. Inform that cap contents can also be sprinkled on soft acidic foods (eg, applesauce), if necessary. Instruct to notify physician if pregnant/breastfeeding or planning to become pregnant/breastfeed during treatment. Advise to contact physician immediately if allergic reactions develop.

Storage: Room temperature up to 25°C (77°F); excursions permitted between 25-40°C (77-104°F) for up to 30 days. Discard if exposed to higher temperature and moisture conditions >70%. Protect from moisture. Store in original container.

CRESTOR – rosuvastatin calcium RX

Class: HMG-CoA reductase inhibitor

ADULT DOSAGE

Hypercholesterolemia

Hyperlipidemia and Mixed Dyslipidemia/Hypertriglyceridemia/Primary Dysbetalipoproteinemia (Type III Hyperlipoproteinemia)/Slowing of the Progression of Atherosclerosis:

General Dose:
Initial: 10-20mg qd
Range: 5-40mg qd

When initiating treatment or switching from another HMG-CoA reductase inhibitor, use the appropriate starting dose 1st, then titrate according to patient's response and individualized goal of therapy

Analyze lipid levels w/in 2-4 weeks and adjust dose accordingly

Use 40mg dose only if LDL goal is not achieved w/ 20mg dose

Homozygous Familial Hypercholesterolemia

Initial: 20mg qd

Prevention of Cardiovascular Disease

Reduce the risk of stroke, MI, arterial revascularization procedures in patients w/o clinically evident coronary heart disease but w/ an increased risk of cardiovascular disease based on age (≥50 yrs old men and ≥60 yrs women) hsCRP ≥2mg/L, and the presence of at least one additional cardiovascular disease risk factor

PEDIATRIC DOSAGE

Heterozygous Familial Hypercholesterolemia

10-17 Years (At Least 1-Year Postmenarche):
Individualize dose
Usual: 5-20mg/day
Titrate: Adjust dose at intervals of ≥4 weeks
Max: 20mg/day

DOSE MODIFICATION

Concomitant Medications

Cyclosporine:
Max: 5mg qd

Lopinavir/Ritonavir or Atazanavir/Ritonavir or Gemfibrozil:
Initial: 5mg qd
Max: 10mg qd

Renal Impairment

Severe (CrCl <30mL/min) Not on Hemodialysis:
Initial: 5mg qd
Max: 10mg qd

Other Important Modifications

Asian Patients:
Initial: 5mg qd

ADMINISTRATION

Oral route
Take PO w/ or w/o food
Swallow tab whole
Do not take 2 doses w/in 12 hrs of each other

HOW SUPPLIED

Tab: 5mg, 10mg, 20mg, 40mg

CONTRAINDICATIONS

Active liver disease including unexplained persistent elevations of hepatic transaminase levels, women who are pregnant or may become pregnant, nursing mothers.

WARNINGS/PRECAUTIONS

Myopathy (including immune-mediated necrotizing myopathy [IMNM]) and rhabdomyolysis reported with increased risk at 40mg; caution in patients with predisposing factors for myopathy (eg, age ≥65 yrs, inadequately treated hypothyroidism, renal impairment). D/C if markedly elevated

CPK levels occur or myopathy is diagnosed or suspected. Temporarily withhold in any patient with an acute, serious condition suggestive of myopathy or predisposing to the development of renal failure secondary to rhabdomyolysis. Increases in serum transaminases reported. Fatal and nonfatal hepatic failure reported (rare); promptly interrupt therapy if serious liver injury with clinical symptoms and/or hyperbilirubinemia or jaundice occurs, and do not restart if no alternate etiology is found. Caution in patients who consume substantial quantities of alcohol and/or have a history of chronic liver disease, severe renal impairment, are Asian, or are elderly. Dipstick-positive proteinuria and microscopic hematuria reported; consider dose reduction for patients with unexplained persistent proteinuria and/or hematuria. Increases in HbA1c and FPG levels reported.

ADVERSE REACTIONS

Headache, myalgia, nausea, dizziness, arthralgia, constipation, asthenia, abdominal pain.

DRUG INTERACTIONS

See dosage. Cyclosporine, gemfibrozil, lopinavir/ritonavir, and atazanavir/ritonavir may increase levels. Increased risk of myopathy with some other lipid-lowering therapies (fibrates or niacin), gemfibrozil, cyclosporine, lopinavir/ritonavir, atazanavir/ritonavir, OATP1B1 inhibitors, or breast cancer resistance protein inhibitors. Avoid with gemfibrozil. Caution with coumarin anticoagulants. May enhance the risk of skeletal muscle effects with ≥1g/day of niacin. Caution with drugs that may decrease levels or activity of endogenous steroid hormones (eg, ketoconazole, spironolactone, cimetidine), fenofibrates, or protease inhibitors in combination with ritonavir. Caution with colchicine; cases of myopathy, including rhabdomyolysis, reported.

NURSING CONSIDERATIONS

Assessment: Assess for active liver disease (including chronic alcohol liver disease), unexplained persistent elevations in serum transaminases, risk factors for developing myopathy or rhabdomyolysis, pregnancy/nursing status, and possible drug interactions. Obtain baseline lipid profile, LFTs, and evaluate renal function. Check INR with coumarin anticoagulants.

Monitoring: Monitor for signs/symptoms of myopathy (including IMNM), rhabdomyolysis, endocrine dysfunction, proteinuria, hematuria, and other adverse reactions. Monitor lipid levels, CPK, and LFTs. Monitor INR with coumarin anticoagulants frequently during early therapy.

Patient Counseling: Advise to report promptly any unexplained muscle pain, tenderness, or weakness, particularly if accompanied by malaise or fever or if muscle signs/symptoms persist after discontinuing therapy. Advise to wait at least 2 hrs if taking an antacid containing a combination of aluminum and magnesium hydroxide. Inform of potential hazard to fetus if patient becomes pregnant while on therapy. Advise to promptly report any symptoms that may indicate liver injury (eg, fatigue, anorexia, right upper abdominal discomfort, dark urine, jaundice).

Storage: 20-25°C (68-77°F). Protect from moisture.

CRIXIVAN – indinavir sulfate — RX

Class: Protease inhibitor

ADULT DOSAGE

HIV-1 Infection

Combination w/ Other Antiretrovirals:
800mg q8h

PEDIATRIC DOSAGE

Pediatric use may not have been established

DOSE MODIFICATION

Concomitant Medications

Delavirdine:
Consider dose reduction to 600mg q8h when administering delavirdine 400mg tid

Didanosine:
Administer at least 1 hr apart on an empty stomach

Itraconazole:
Reduce dose to 600mg q8h when administering itraconazole 200mg bid

Ketoconazole:
Reduce dose to 600mg q8h when administering ketoconazole

Rifabutin:
Reduce rifabutin dose to half the standard dose and increase indinavir dose to 1000mg q8h

Hepatic Insufficiency

Mild-to-Moderate Insufficiency Due to Cirrhosis:
Reduce dose to 600mg q8h

Adverse Reactions

Nephrolithiasis/Urolithiasis:
May temporarily interrupt (eg, 1-3 days) or d/c therapy

ADMINISTRATION

Oral route

Administer w/o food but w/ water 1 hr ac or 2 hrs pc

May administer w/ other liquids (eg, skim milk, juice, coffee, tea) or w/ a light meal

Drink at least 1.5L of liquids during the course of 24 hrs to ensure adequate hydration

HOW SUPPLIED

Cap: 200mg, 400mg

CONTRAINDICATIONS

Coadministration w/ CYP3A4 substrates for which elevated concentrations potentially cause serious or life-threatening reactions (eg, alfuzosin, amiodarone, dihydroergotamine, ergonovine, ergotamine, methylergonovine, cisapride, lovastatin, simvastatin, pimozide, sildenafil [for treatment of pulmonary arterial HTN], oral midazolam, triazolam, alprazolam).

WARNINGS/PRECAUTIONS

Nephrolithiasis/urolithiasis reported. Ensure adequate hydration in all patients. Acute hemolytic anemia, including cases resulting in death, reported; once a diagnosis is apparent, institute appropriate measures, including discontinuation of therapy. Hepatitis, including cases resulting in hepatic failure and death, reported. New onset or exacerbation of diabetes mellitus (DM), hyperglycemia, and diabetic ketoacidosis reported; initiation or dose adjustments of insulin or oral hypoglycemic agents may be required. Indirect hyperbilirubinemia reported frequently during treatment, and infrequently associated w/ increases in serum transaminases. Tubulointerstitial nephritis w/ medullary calcification and cortical atrophy observed in patients w/ asymptomatic severe leukocyturia (>100 cells/high power field); closely follow patients w/ asymptomatic severe leukocyturia and monitor frequently w/ urinalyses. Consider discontinuation of therapy in all patients w/ severe leukocyturia. Immune reconstitution syndrome reported. Autoimmune disorders (eg, Graves' disease, polymyositis, Guillain-Barre syndrome) reported in the setting of immune reconstitution and can occur many months after initiation of treatment. Spontaneous bleeding in patients w/ hemophilia A and B reported. Redistribution/accumulation of body fat reported. Caution in elderly.

ADVERSE REACTIONS

Nephrolithiasis/urolithiasis, hyperbilirubinemia, abdominal pain, headache, N/V, dizziness, pruritus, diarrhea, back pain.

DRUG INTERACTIONS

See Contraindications and Dose Modification. Caution w/ atorvastatin, rosuvastatin, parenteral midazolam, sildenafil (for treatment of erectile dysfunction), tadalafil, or vardenafil. Do not coadminister w/ rifampin. Not recommended w/ St. John's wort, atazanavir, salmeterol, or fluticasone (when indinavir is coadministered w/ a potent CYP3A4 inhibitor [eg, ritonavir]). Avoid w/ colchicine in patients w/ renal/hepatic impairment. May increase levels of CYP3A/CYP3A4 substrates, ritonavir, saquinavir, antiarrhythmics, trazodone, colchicine, quetiapine, dihydropyridine calcium channel blockers, clarithromycin, bosentan, atorvastatin, rosuvastatin, immunosuppressants, salmeterol, fluticasone, parenteral midazolam, rifabutin, sildenafil, tadalafil, and vardenafil. CYP3A/CYP3A4 inducers, St. John's wort, efavirenz, nevirapine, anticonvulsants, rifabutin, and venlafaxine may decrease levels. CYP3A/CYP3A4 inhibitors, delavirdine, nelfinavir, ritonavir, clarithromycin, itraconazole, and ketoconazole may increase levels. Refer to PI for dosing modifications when used w/ certain concomitant therapies.

NURSING CONSIDERATIONS

Assessment: Assess for hypersensitivity to drug, hepatic insufficiency, DM, hemophilia, pregnancy/nursing status, and possible drug interactions.

Monitoring: Monitor for nephrolithiasis/urolithiasis, hemolytic anemia, hepatitis, new onset or exacerbation of DM, hyperglycemia, diabetic ketoacidosis, hyperbilirubinemia, serum transaminase elevations, immune reconstitution syndrome, autoimmune disorders, fat redistribution/accumulation, and other adverse reactions. Closely follow patients w/ asymptomatic severe leukocyturia and monitor frequently w/ urinalyses. In patients w/ hemophilia, monitor for bleeding events.

Patient Counseling: Instruct to take drug ud. Inform that drug is not a cure for HIV-1 infection and that illnesses associated w/ HIV may continue. Advise to avoid doing things that can spread HIV to others. Instruct not to modify or d/c therapy w/o consulting physician. Instruct to report to physician the use of any other prescription/nonprescription medication or herbal products (eg, St. John's wort). Inform that fat redistribution/accumulation may occur. Instruct to notify physician if pregnant or nursing.

Storage: 15-30°C (59-86°F). Protect from moisture.

CYCLOBENZAPRINE – cyclobenzaprine hydrochloride RX

Class: Skeletal muscle relaxant (central-acting)

OTHER BRAND NAMES
Flexeril

ADULT DOSAGE

Muscle Spasms

Adjunct to rest and physical therapy for relief of muscle spasm associated w/ acute, painful musculoskeletal conditions

Usual: 5mg tid
Titrate: May increase to 10mg tid

Use for periods longer than 2 or 3 weeks is not recommended

PEDIATRIC DOSAGE

Muscle Spasms

Adjunct to rest and physical therapy for relief of muscle spasm associated w/ acute, painful musculoskeletal conditions

≥15 Years:
Usual: 5mg tid
Titrate: May increase to 10mg tid

Use for periods longer than 2 or 3 weeks is not recommended

DOSE MODIFICATION

Hepatic Impairment

Mild:
Initial: 5mg dose
Titrate: Increase slowly and consider less frequent dosing

Moderate to Severe:
Not recommended

Elderly

Initial: 5mg dose
Titrate: Increase slowly and consider less frequent dosing

ADMINISTRATION
Oral route

HOW SUPPLIED
Tab: 5mg, 7.5mg, 10mg

CONTRAINDICATIONS
Concomitant use of MAOIs or w/in 14 days after their discontinuation. Arrhythmias, heart block or conduction disturbances, CHF, hyperthyroidism, acute recovery phase of MI.

WARNINGS/PRECAUTIONS
Not effective in the treatment of spasticity associated w/ cerebral or spinal cord disease or in children w/ cerebral palsy. May produce arrhythmias, sinus tachycardia, and conduction time prolongation leading to MI and stroke. Caution w/ history of urinary retention, angle-closure glaucoma, increased IOP, mild hepatic impairment, and in elderly. Not recommended w/ moderate to severe hepatic impairment. Consider certain withdrawal symptoms; abrupt cessation after prolonged administration rarely may produce nausea, headache, and malaise.

ADVERSE REACTIONS
Drowsiness, dry mouth, fatigue, headache, dizziness.

DRUG INTERACTIONS
See Contraindications. Serotonin syndrome reported when used w/ SSRIs, SNRIs, TCAs, tramadol, bupropion, meperidine, verapamil, or MAOIs; d/c immediately if this occurs. Observe carefully, particularly during treatment initiation or dose increases, if concomitant use w/ other serotonergic drugs is warranted. May enhance effects of alcohol, barbiturates, and other CNS depressants. Caution w/ anticholinergics. May block the antihypertensive action of guanethidine and similarly acting compounds. May enhance seizure risk w/ tramadol.

NURSING CONSIDERATIONS

Assessment: Assess for arrhythmias, heart block or conduction disturbances, CHF, hyperthyroidism, acute recovery phase of MI, history of urinary retention, angle-closure glaucoma, increased IOP, hepatic impairment, drug hypersensitivity, pregnancy/nursing status, and possible drug interactions.

Monitoring: Monitor for arrhythmias, sinus tachycardia, conduction time prolongation, stroke, withdrawal symptoms, and other adverse reactions.

Patient Counseling: Inform that the drug, especially when used w/ alcohol or other CNS depressants, may impair mental and/or physical abilities required to perform hazardous tasks (eg, operating machinery, driving). Caution about the risk of serotonin syndrome; instruct to seek medical care immediately if signs/symptoms occur.

Storage: 20-25°C (68-77°F).

CYMBALTA – duloxetine

Class: Serotonin and norepinephrine reuptake inhibitor

RX

Antidepressants increased the risk of suicidal thoughts and behavior in children, adolescents, and young adults in short-term studies. Monitor and observe closely for worsening, and for emergence of suicidal thoughts and behaviors in all patients started on antidepressant therapy.

ADULT DOSAGE

Musculoskeletal Pain

Chronic:
Initial: 30mg qd for 1 week before increasing to 60mg qd
Maint: 60mg qd
Max: 60mg/day

Major Depressive Disorder

Initial: 40mg/day (given as 20mg bid) to 60mg/day (given qd or as 30mg bid); may start at 30mg qd for 1 week before increasing to 60mg qd in some patients
Maint: 60mg qd
Max: 120mg/day

Generalized Anxiety Disorder

Initial: 60mg qd; may start at 30mg qd for 1 week before increasing to 60mg qd in some patients
Maint: 60mg qd
Titrate: Dose increases beyond 60mg qd should be in increments of 30mg qd
Max: 120mg/day

Diabetic Peripheral Neuropathy

Initial: 60mg qd. May lower starting dose if tolerability is a concern
Max: 60mg qd

Fibromyalgia

Initial: 30mg qd for 1 week before increasing to 60mg qd; some patients may respond to the starting dose
Maint: 60mg qd
Max: 60mg/day

PEDIATRIC DOSAGE

Generalized Anxiety Disorder

7-17 Years:
Initial: 30mg qd for 2 weeks before considering an increase to 60mg
Maint: 30-60mg qd
Titrate: Dose increases beyond 60mg qd should be in increments of 30mg qd
Max: 120mg/day

DOSE MODIFICATION

Concomitant Medications

Other MAOIs (eg, Linezolid, IV Methylene Blue):
Do not start duloxetine in patients being treated with linezolid or IV methylene blue. Consider other interventions (eg, hospitalization) in patients who require more urgent treatment of a psychiatric condition

If acceptable alternatives are not available, d/c duloxetine and administer linezolid or IV methylene blue. Monitor for serotonin syndrome for 5 days or until 24 hrs after the last dose of linezolid or IV methylene blue, whichever comes first. May resume duloxetine therapy 24 hrs after last dose of linezolid or IV methylene blue

Renal Impairment

Avoid in patients with severe renal impairment (GFR <30mL/min)

Diabetic Peripheral Neuropathy:
Consider lower starting dose and gradual increase

Hepatic Impairment

Avoid in patients with chronic liver disease or cirrhosis

Elderly

Generalized Anxiety Disorder:
Initial: 30mg qd for 2 weeks before considering increasing to target dose of 60mg
Maint: 60mg qd
Titrate: Dose increases beyond 60mg qd should be in increments of 30mg qd
Max: 120mg/day

Discontinuation
Gradually reduce dose

Other Important Modifications
Switching to/from an MAOI for Psychiatric Disorders:
Allow at least 14 days between discontinuation of an MAOI and initiation of treatment, and allow at least 5 days between discontinuation of treatment and initiation of an MAOI

ADMINISTRATION
Oral route
Swallow cap whole; do not chew, crush, or open to sprinkle on food or mix with liquids
Take without regard to meals

HOW SUPPLIED
Cap, Delayed-Release: 20mg, 30mg, 60mg

CONTRAINDICATIONS
Use of an MAOI for psychiatric disorders either concomitantly or within 5 days of stopping treatment. Treatment within 14 days of stopping an MAOI for psychiatric disorders. Starting treatment in patients being treated with other MAOIs (eg, linezolid, IV methylene blue).

WARNINGS/PRECAUTIONS
Not approved for the treatment of bipolar depression; may precipitate mixed/manic episode for those at risk for bipolar disorder. Hepatic failure (sometimes fatal) and cholestatic jaundice with minimal elevation of serum transaminases reported; d/c if jaundice or other evidence of clinically significant hepatic dysfunction occurs. Avoid with substantial alcohol use or evidence of chronic liver disease or cirrhosis. Orthostatic hypotension, falls, and syncope reported; increased risk with doses >60mg/day. Consider dose reduction or discontinuation in patients who experience symptomatic orthostatic hypotension, falls, and/or syncope during therapy. Serotonin syndrome reported; d/c immediately if symptoms occur and initiate supportive symptomatic treatment. May increase risk of bleeding events. Severe skin reactions (eg, erythema multiforme, Stevens-Johnson syndrome [SJS]) may occur; d/c at the 1st appearance of blisters, peeling rash, mucosal erosions, or any other signs of hypersensitivity if no other etiology can be identified. Adverse events reported upon discontinuation. Activation of mania or hypomania reported in patients with MDD; caution with history of mania. Seizures/convulsions reported; caution with history of seizure disorder. Pupillary dilation that occurs following use may trigger an angle-closure attack in a patient with anatomically narrow angles who does not have a patent iridectomy. May increase BP. Hyponatremia may occur; caution in elderly and volume-depleted patients. Consider discontinuation and institute appropriate medical intervention in patients with symptomatic hyponatremia. Urinary hesitation and retention reported. Caution with conditions that may slow gastric emptying and with diabetes; worsening glycemic control observed in some patients with diabetes. Avoid in severe renal impairment (GFR <30mL/min).

ADVERSE REACTIONS
Nausea, dry mouth, somnolence, constipation, decreased appetite, hyperhidrosis, diarrhea, fatigue, dizziness, headache, insomnia, abdominal pain.

DRUG INTERACTIONS
See Contraindications. Greater risk of hypotension with concomitant use of medications that induce orthostatic hypotension (eg, antihypertensives) and potent CYP1A2 inhibitors. May cause serotonin syndrome with other serotonergic drugs (eg, triptans, TCAs, fentanyl) and with drugs that impair metabolism of serotonin; d/c immediately if this occurs. Caution with NSAIDs, aspirin (ASA), warfarin, or other drugs that affect coagulation due to potential increased risk of bleeding. Avoid use with thioridazine, potent CYP1A2 inhibitors (eg, fluvoxamine, cimetidine, some quinolone antibiotics), and substantial alcohol use. CYP2D6 inhibitors (eg, paroxetine, fluoxetine, quinidine) may increase levels. Caution with drugs metabolized by CYP2D6 having a narrow therapeutic index (eg, TCAs, phenothiazines, type 1C antiarrhythmics); may need to monitor levels/reduce dose of TCA. Caution with CNS-acting drugs, including those with a similar mechanism of action. Increased risk of hyponatremia with diuretics. Potential for interaction with drugs that affect gastric acidity. May increase theophylline and desipramine exposure. May increase free concentrations of highly protein-bound drugs.

NURSING CONSIDERATIONS

Assessment: Assess for bipolar disorder risk, history of mania, history of seizures, substantial alcohol use, diseases/conditions that slow gastric emptying (eg, diabetes mellitus), risk factors for hyponatremia, susceptibility to angle-closure glaucoma/urinary retention, hepatic/renal impairment, pregnancy/nursing status, and possible drug interactions. Assess BP.

Monitoring: Monitor for signs/symptoms of clinical worsening (eg, suicidality, unusual changes in behavior), activation of mania/hypomania, serotonin syndrome, hepatotoxicity, bleeding events, skin reactions (eg, erythema multiforme, SJS), hyponatremia, seizures, orthostatic hypotension, falls, worsened glycemic control, urinary hesitation/retention, angle-closure glaucoma, and other adverse reactions. Periodically monitor BP. Carefully monitor patients receiving concomitant warfarin therapy when duloxetine is initiated or discontinued. Periodically reassess need for maintenance treatment and appropriate dose.

Patient Counseling: Inform about benefits, risks, and appropriate use of therapy. Advise to avoid substantial alcohol use. Instruct to seek medical attention for clinical worsening, signs/symptoms of manic episodes, and symptoms of serotonin syndrome. Inform that abnormal bleeding (especially with the use of NSAIDs, ASA, warfarin), orthostatic hypotension, falls, syncope, hepatotoxicity, urinary hesitation/retention, seizures, BP increase, or discontinuation symptoms may occur. Caution about risk of angle-closure glaucoma. Advise of the signs/symptoms of hyponatremia. Counsel to immediately contact physician if skin blisters, peeling rash, mouth sores, hives, or any other allergic reactions occur. Advise to inform physician if taking/planning to take any prescription or OTC medications, if pregnant, intending to become pregnant, or if breastfeeding. Inform that therapy may impair judgment, thinking, or motor skills; instruct to use caution when operating hazardous machinery, including automobiles. Inform that improvement may be noticed within 1-4 weeks; instruct to continue therapy ud. Advise not to alter dosing regimen or d/c treatment without consulting physician.

Storage: 25°C (77°F); excursions permitted to 15-30°C (59-86°F).

CYRAMZA – ramucirumab RX

Class: Monoclonal antibody/VEGFR2 blocker

Increased risk of hemorrhage, including severe and sometimes fatal hemorrhagic events; permanently d/c if severe bleeding occurs.

ADULT DOSAGE

Advanced or Metastatic, Gastric or Gastroesophageal Junction Adenocarcinoma

W/ Disease Progression on or After Prior Fluoropyrimidine- or Platinum-Containing Chemotherapy:

As a Single Agent, or in Combination w/ Paclitaxel:

Usual: 8mg/kg every 2 weeks administered as an IV infusion over 60 min. Continue until disease progression or unacceptable toxicity

When given in combination, administer prior to administration of paclitaxel

Metastatic Non-Small Cell Lung Cancer

W/ Disease Progression:

On or After Platinum-Based Chemotherapy:

Usual: 10mg/kg IV over approx 60 min on Day 1 of a 21-day cycle prior to docetaxel infusion. Continue until disease progression or unacceptable toxicity

PEDIATRIC DOSAGE

Pediatric use may not have been established

DOSE MODIFICATION

Adverse Reactions

Infusion Related Reactions (IRRs):

Reduce infusion rate by 50% for Grade 1 or 2 IRRs
Permanently d/c for Grade 3 or 4 IRRs

HTN:

Interrupt for severe HTN until controlled w/ medical management
Permanently d/c for severe HTN that cannot be controlled w/ antihypertensive therapy

Proteinuria:

Interrupt for urine protein levels ≥2g/24 hrs
Reinitiate at a reduced dose (6mg/kg, if initial dose was 8mg/kg; or 8mg/kg, if initial dose was 10mg/kg) once the urine protein level returns to <2g/24 hrs. If protein level ≥2g/24 hrs reoccurs, interrupt and reduce dose (5mg/kg, if initial dose was 8mg/kg; or 6mg/kg, if initial dose was 10mg/kg) once the urine protein level returns to <2 g/24 hrs
Permanently d/c for urine protein level >3g/24 hrs or in the setting of nephrotic syndrome

Wound Healing Complications:
Interrupt prior to scheduled surgery until the wound is fully healed

Arterial Thromboembolic Events, Gastrointestinal Perforation, or Grade 3 or 4 Bleeding:
Permanently d/c

ADMINISTRATION
IV route

Prior to each infusion, premedicate all patients w/ an IV histamine H1 antagonist (eg, diphenhydramine)
For patients who have experienced a Grade 1 or 2 infusion-related reaction, also premedicate w/ dexamethasone (or equivalent) and acetaminophen prior to each infusion
Calculate dose and required volume of ramucirumab needed to prepare the infusion sol
Withdraw required volume of ramucirumab and further dilute w/ only 0.9% NaCl Inj in an IV infusion container to a final volume of 250mL
Do not use dextrose containing sol
Gently invert container to ensure adequate mixing
Do not dilute w/ other solutions or coinfuse w/ other electrolytes or medications
Administer diluted ramucirumab infusion via infusion pump over 60 min through a separate infusion line. Use of a protein sparing 0.22-micron filter is recommended. Flush line w/ sterile NaCl 0.9% sol for inj at the end of infusion
Do not administer as an IV push or bolus
Refer to PI for further administration and preparation instructions

HOW SUPPLIED
Inj: 10mg/mL [10mL, 50mL]

WARNINGS/PRECAUTIONS
Patients with epidermal growth factor receptor or anaplastic lymphoma kinase genomic tumor aberrations should have disease progression on FDA-approved therapy for these aberrations prior to receiving therapy. Increased risk of GI hemorrhage. Serious, sometimes fatal, arterial thromboembolic events (ATEs) (eg, myocardial infarction, cardiac arrest, cerebrovascular accident, cerebral ischemia) reported. Increased incidence of severe HTN reported; control HTN prior to initiation of treatment. Permanently d/c treatment in patients with hypertensive crisis or hypertensive encephalopathy. IRRs reported; monitor during infusion for signs and symptoms of IRRs in a setting with available resuscitation equipment. May increase risk of GI perforation. May adversely affect wound healing. If wound healing complications develop during therapy, d/c until wound is fully healed. Clinical deterioration, manifested by new onset or worsening encephalopathy, ascites, or hepatorenal syndrome, reported in patients with Child-Pugh B or C cirrhosis. Use in patients with Child-Pugh B or C cirrhosis only if potential benefits of treatment are judged to outweigh risks of clinical deterioration. Reversible posterior leukoencephalopathy syndrome (RPLS) reported; confirm diagnosis of RPLS with MRI and d/c if RPLS develops. May impair fertility of female patients. May cause fetal harm; avoid pregnancy during treatment and for at least 3 months after the last dose of treatment.

ADVERSE REACTIONS
Hemorrhage, HTN, diarrhea, hyponatremia, headache, neutropenia, epistaxis, proteinuria, fatigue/asthenia, stomatitis/mucosal inflammation, peripheral edema, thrombocytopenia, lacrimation increased.

NURSING CONSIDERATIONS

Assessment: Assess for HTN, presence of wound, upcoming surgery, Child-Pugh B or C cirrhosis, and pregnancy/nursing status.

Monitoring: Monitor for hemorrhage, ATEs, IRRs, GI perforation, wound healing complications, clinical deterioration (in Child-Pugh B or C cirrhosis patients), RPLS, and other adverse reactions. Monitor BP (every 2 weeks or more frequently as indicated) and urine protein levels.

Patient Counseling: Inform of the risks and benefits of therapy. Instruct to contact physician for bleeding or symptoms of bleeding, BP elevation or symptoms of HTN, severe diarrhea, vomiting, or severe abdominal pain. Advise to undergo routine BP monitoring. Inform that drug has the potential to impair wound healing; instruct not to undergo surgery without first discussing this potential risk with physician. Advise females of reproductive potential that drug may impair fertility, and to avoid getting pregnant while receiving treatment and for at least 3 months after the last dose of treatment. Counsel to d/c nursing during treatment.

Storage: 2-8°C (36-46°F). Protect from light. Do not freeze or shake. Diluted Sol: 2-8°C (36-46°F) for no >24 hrs or <25°C (77°F) for 4 hrs. Do not freeze or shake.

DALIRESP – roflumilast RX

Class: Selective phosphodiesterase 4 (PDE4) inhibitor

ADULT DOSAGE

Chronic Obstructive Pulmonary Disease

Reduce risk of exacerbations in patients w/ severe chronic obstructive pulmonary disease associated w/ chronic bronchitis and a history of exacerbations
500mcg qd

PEDIATRIC DOSAGE

Pediatric use may not have been established

ADMINISTRATION

Oral route

Take w/ or w/o food

HOW SUPPLIED

Tab: 500mcg

CONTRAINDICATIONS

Moderate to severe liver impairment (Child-Pugh B or C).

WARNINGS/PRECAUTIONS

Not a bronchodilator; not indicated for the relief of acute bronchospasm. Psychiatric adverse reactions, including suicidality, reported; carefully evaluate the risks and benefits of treatment in patients with history of depression and/or suicidal thoughts or behavior, and of continuing treatment if such reactions occur. Weight loss reported; evaluate and consider discontinuation if unexplained or clinically significant weight loss occurs. Do not use during labor and delivery. Caution with mild liver impairment (Child-Pugh A).

ADVERSE REACTIONS

Diarrhea, weight loss, nausea, headache, back pain.

DRUG INTERACTIONS

Strong CYP450 inducers (eg, rifampicin, phenobarbital, carbamazepine, phenytoin) decrease exposure and may reduce therapeutic effectiveness; concomitant use is not recommended. CYP3A4 inhibitors or dual inhibitors that inhibit both CYP3A4 and CYP1A2 simultaneously (eg, erythromycin, ketoconazole, fluvoxamine, enoxacin, cimetidine) and oral contraceptives containing gestodene and ethinyl estradiol may increase exposure and may result in increased adverse reactions; use with caution.

NURSING CONSIDERATIONS

Assessment: Assess for liver impairment, history of depression and/or suicidal thoughts or behavior, pregnancy/nursing status, and possible drug interactions.

Monitoring: Monitor for psychiatric events (including suicidality), and other adverse reactions. Monitor weight regularly.

Patient Counseling: Inform that drug is not a bronchodilator and should not be used for the relief of acute bronchospasm. Advise of the need to be alert for the emergence or worsening of insomnia, anxiety, depression, suicidal thoughts, or other mood changes; instruct to contact physician if such changes occur. Counsel to monitor weight regularly, and to consult physician if unexplained or clinically significant weight loss occurs. Instruct to notify physician of all medications being taken.

Storage: 20-25°C (68-77°F); excursions permitted to 15-30°C (59-86°F).

DAYTRANA – methylphenidate CII

Class: Sympathomimetic amine

Caution with history of drug dependence or alcoholism. Chronic abuse may lead to marked tolerance and psychological dependence with varying degrees of abnormal behavior. Frank psychotic episodes may occur, especially with parenteral abuse. Careful supervision is required during withdrawal from abusive use since severe depression may occur. Withdrawal following chronic use may unmask symptoms of underlying disorder that may require follow-up.

PEDIATRIC DOSAGE

Attention-Deficit Hyperactivity Disorder

≥6 Years:

Apply to hip area 2 hrs before effect is needed and remove 9 hrs after application

Titration Schedule:
Week 1: 10mg/9 hrs
Week 2: 15mg/9 hrs
Week 3: 20mg/9 hrs
Week 4: 30mg/9 hrs

Maint/Extended Treatment: Periodically reevaluate long-term usefulness w/ periods off medication

Dose/Wear Time Reduction and Discontinuation: May remove patch earlier than 9 hrs if a shorter duration of effect is desired or late day side effects appear

ADMINISTRATION

Transdermal route

Apply patch immediately upon removal from the individual protective pouch; press firmly for 30 sec
Apply to clean, dry area of the hip; area should not be oily, damaged, or irritated
Avoid application to waistline
Alternate sides when applying the next am
Do not cut patches
Avoid exposing patch application site to direct external heat sources while wearing the patch
Refer to PI for further application, removal, and disposal instructions

HOW SUPPLIED

Patch: 10mg/9 hrs, 15mg/9 hrs, 20mg/9 hrs, 30mg/9 hrs [30[s]]

CONTRAINDICATIONS

Marked anxiety, tension, agitation, glaucoma, motor tics, or family history or diagnosis of Tourette's syndrome. Treatment with MAOIs or within a minimum of 14 days following discontinuation of an MAOI.

WARNINGS/PRECAUTIONS

Reduce dose/wear time or, if necessary, d/c if aggravation of symptoms or other adverse events occur. Avoid with known serious structural cardiac abnormalities, cardiomyopathy, serious heart rhythm abnormalities, coronary artery disease, or other serious cardiac problems. Sudden death reported in children and adolescents with structural cardiac abnormalities or other serious heart problems. Sudden deaths, stroke, and MI reported in adults. May increase BP and HR; caution with conditions that might be compromised by increases in BP/HR (eg, preexisting HTN, heart failure, recent MI, ventricular arrhythmia). Prior to treatment, obtain medical history (including assessment for family history of sudden death or ventricular arrhythmia) and perform physical exam to assess for presence of cardiac disease. Promptly perform cardiac evaluation if symptoms of cardiac disease develop. May exacerbate symptoms of behavior disturbance and thought disorder in patients with preexisting psychotic disorder. Caution in patients with comorbid bipolar disorder; may induce mixed/manic episode. May cause treatment-emergent psychotic or manic symptoms (eg, hallucinations, delusional thinking, mania) in children and adolescents without prior history of psychotic illness or mania; consider discontinuation if such symptoms occur. Aggressive behavior or hostility reported in children and adolescents. May lower convulsive threshold; d/c if seizures occur. Priapism, sometimes requiring surgical intervention, reported. Associated with peripheral vasculopathy, including Raynaud's phenomenon; carefully observe for digital changes. May cause long-term suppression of growth in children; monitor growth, and may need to interrupt treatment in patients not growing or gaining height or weight as expected. Difficulties with accommodation and blurring of vision reported. May lead to contact sensitization; d/c if suspected. Patients who develop contact sensitization to therapy and require oral treatment with methylphenidate should be initiated on oral medication under close medical supervision. Avoid exposing application site to direct external heat sources while wearing the patch.

ADVERSE REACTIONS

Decreased appetite, headache, insomnia, N/V, decreased weight, irritability, tic, affect lability, anorexia, abdominal pain, dizziness.

DRUG INTERACTIONS

See Contraindications. Caution with pressor agents. May decrease effectiveness of drugs used to treat HTN. May inhibit metabolism of coumarin anticoagulants, anticonvulsants (eg, phenobarbital, phenytoin, primidone), and some TCAs (eg, imipramine, clomipramine, desipramine) and SSRIs; downward dose adjustments and monitoring of plasma drug concentrations (or coagulation times for coumarin) of these drugs may be necessary when initiating or discontinuing methylphenidate.

NURSING CONSIDERATIONS

Assessment: Assess for hypersensitivity to the drug, marked anxiety, tension, agitation, glaucoma, motor tics, family history or diagnosis of Tourette's syndrome, cardiovascular conditions, history of drug dependence or alcoholism, psychotic disorder, comorbid bipolar disorder, any other conditions where treatment is contraindicated or cautioned, pregnancy/nursing status, and possible drug interactions.

Monitoring: Monitor for changes in HR and BP, signs/symptoms of cardiac disease, exacerbation of behavior disturbance and thought disorder, psychosis, mania, appearance of or worsening of aggressive behavior or hostility, seizures, priapism, peripheral vasculopathy (including Raynaud's phenomenon), visual disturbances, contact sensitization, and other adverse reactions. In pediatric patients, monitor growth. Perform periodic monitoring of CBC, differential, and platelet counts during prolonged therapy. Periodically reevaluate long-term usefulness of drug.

Patient Counseling: Inform about the benefits and risks of therapy. Counsel on the appropriate use of the medication. Instruct to seek immediate medical attention in the event of priapism. Instruct to report to physician any new numbness, pain, skin color change, or sensitivity to temperature in fingers or toes; instruct to contact physician immediately with any signs of unexplained wounds appearing on fingers or toes while taking the drug. Advise to avoid exposing application site to direct external heat sources (eg, hair dryers, heating pads, electric blankets, heated water beds) while wearing the patch. Instruct to avoid touching the adhesive side of the patch during application, and to immediately wash hands after application if adhesive side is touched. Advise to take patch off earlier if there is an unacceptable duration of appetite loss or insomnia in the pm. Counsel to not wear the patch and to consult physician if any swelling or blistering occurs. Instruct not to apply hydrocortisone or other sol, cre, oint, or emollients immediately prior to patch application. Caution against operating potentially hazardous machinery or vehicles until accustomed to effects of medication.

Storage: 25°C (77°F); excursions permitted to 15-30°C (59-86°F). Do not store patches unpouched. Do not refrigerate or freeze patches. Once the sealed tray or outer pouch is opened, use contents within 2 months.

DDAVP Nasal – desmopressin acetate — RX

Class: Synthetic vasopressin analogue

OTHER BRAND NAMES
DDAVP Rhinal Tube

ADULT DOSAGE
Central Cranial Diabetes Insipidus

Usual: 0.1-0.4mL/day, as single dose or divided into 2 or 3 doses; separately adjust am and pm dose

PEDIATRIC DOSAGE
Central Cranial Diabetes Insipidus

3 Months of Age-12 Years:
Usual: 0.05-0.3mL/day, as single dose or divided into 2 doses; separately adjust am and pm dose

DOSE MODIFICATION
Elderly
Start at lower end of dosing range

ADMINISTRATION
Intranasal route

Nasal Spray
Pump must be primed prior to 1st use
To Prime Pump:
1. Press down 4 times
2. The bottle will now deliver 10mcg/spray

Discard after 50 sprays

HOW SUPPLIED
Sol: 10mcg/0.1mL [2.5mL (Rhinal Tube), 5mL (Nasal Spray)]

CONTRAINDICATIONS
Moderate to severe renal impairment (CrCl <50mL/min), hyponatremia, or history of hyponatremia.

WARNINGS/PRECAUTIONS
For intranasal use only. Use only when oral formulations are not feasible. May use inj if intranasal route is compromised. May cause water intoxication and/or hyponatremia; fluid restriction is recommended. May decrease plasma osmolality, resulting in seizures or coma. Caution with habitual or psychogenic polydipsia, conditions associated with fluid and electrolyte imbalance (eg, cystic fibrosis, HF, renal disorders), coronary artery insufficiency, and/or hypertensive cardiovascular disease (CVD). Severe allergic reactions reported (rare). Estimate response by adequate duration of sleep and adequate, not excessive, water turnover. Caution in elderly.

ADVERSE REACTIONS
Headache, rhinitis, epistaxis, dizziness.

DRUG INTERACTIONS

Carefully monitor with other pressor agents. Caution with drugs that may increase the risk of water intoxication with hyponatremia (eg, TCAs, SSRIs, chlorpromazine, opiate analgesics, NSAIDs, lamotrigine, carbamazepine). Hyponatremic convulsions (rare) reported with concomitant oxybutynin and imipramine.

NURSING CONSIDERATIONS

Assessment: Assess for renal function, hyponatremia, history of hyponatremia, compromised intranasal route, habitual or psychogenic polydipsia, coronary artery insufficiency, hypertensive CVD, fluid/electrolyte imbalance disorders, hypersensitivity to drug, pregnancy/nursing status, and possible drug interactions.

Monitoring: Monitor for signs/symptoms of hyponatremia, water intoxication, compromised intranasal route, and allergic reactions. Monitor BP, fluid and electrolyte levels, renal function, urine volume and osmolality periodically, and plasma osmolality.

Patient Counseling: Inform that administration in children should be under adult supervision. Instruct to seek medical attention if symptoms of hyponatremia or allergic reactions occur. Inform physician if symptoms of nasal blockage, discharge, congestion, and other adverse events occur.

Storage: (Nasal Spray) 20-25°C (68-77°F). Store bottle in upright position. (Rhinal Tube) 2-8°C (36-46°F). When traveling, closed bottles stable for 3 weeks at 20-25°C (68-77°F).

DEMEROL INJECTION – meperidine hydrochloride **CII**

Class: Opioid analgesic

ADULT DOSAGE

Moderate to Severe Pain

Usual: 50-150mg IM/SQ q3-4h prn
Adjust dose according to severity of pain and patient's response

Preoperative Medication

Usual: 50-100mg IM/SQ 30-90 min before beginning of anesthesia

Support of Anesthesia

Use repeated slow IV inj of fractional doses (eg, 10mg/mL) or continuous IV infusion of a more dilute sol (eg, 1mg/mL)
Titrate: Dependent on the premedication and type of anesthesia being employed, patient characteristics, and nature/duration of operative procedure

Obstetrical Anesthesia

Usual: 50-100mg IM/SQ when pain is regular; may repeat at 1- to 3-hr intervals

PEDIATRIC DOSAGE

Moderate to Severe Pain

Usual: 0.5-0.8mg/lb IM/SQ, up to the adult dose, q3-4h prn
Adjust dose according to severity of pain and patient's response

Preoperative Medication

Usual: 0.5-1mg/lb IM/SQ, up to the adult dose, 30-90 min before beginning of anesthesia

DOSE MODIFICATION

Concomitant Medications

Phenothiazines/Other Tranquilizers: Reduce dose by 25-50%

Elderly

Start at lower end of dosage range and observe closely

ADMINISTRATION

IM, IV, SQ route

SQ

Suitable for occasional use

IM

Preferred if repeated doses are required
Inj should be injected well into the body of a large muscle

IV

Dosage should be decreased and inj should be made very slowly, preferably utilizing a diluted sol

HOW SUPPLIED

Inj: 2.5% [1 mL, Carpuject], 5% [1mL, Carpuject; 0.5mL, 1mL, 1.5mL, 2mL, Uni-Amp; 30mL, multiple-dose vial], 7.5% [1mL, Carpuject], 10% [1mL, Carpuject; 1mL, Uni-Amp; 20mL, multiple-dose vial]

CONTRAINDICATIONS
During or w/in 14 days of MAOI use.

WARNINGS/PRECAUTIONS
May produce drug dependence and tolerance and has potential for abuse; prescribe and administer w/ caution. Respiratory depressant effects and capacity to elevate CSF pressure may be markedly exaggerated in the presence of head injury, other intracranial lesions, or a preexisting increase in intracranial pressure. May obscure the clinical course of patients w/ head injuries; use w/ extreme caution and only if deemed essential. Rapid IV inj increases the incidence of adverse reactions; do not administer IV unless a narcotic antagonist and the facilities for assisted/controlled respiration are immediately available. Extreme caution w/ acute asthmatic attack, COPD or cor pulmonale, substantially decreased respiratory reserve, preexisting respiratory depression, hypoxia, or hypercapnia. May cause severe hypotension in postoperative patients or individual whose ability to maintain BP has been compromised by a depleted blood volume. May impair mental/physical abilities. May produce orthostatic hypotension in ambulatory patients. Not for use in pregnant women prior to labor. Caution w/ A-flutter and other supraventricular tachycardias; may produce a significant increase in the ventricular response rate. May aggravate convulsions w/ convulsive disorders. May obscure the diagnosis or clinical course in patients w/ acute abdominal conditions. Caution and reduce initial dose w/ severe renal/hepatic impairment, hypothyroidism, Addison's disease, prostatic hypertrophy or urethral stricture, and in elderly or debilitated.

ADVERSE REACTIONS
Lightheadedness, dizziness, sedation, N/V, sweating, respiratory depression, circulatory depression.

DRUG INTERACTIONS
See Contraindications and Dose Modifications. Respiratory depression, hypotension, and profound sedation or coma may occur w/ other narcotic analgesics, general anesthetics, phenothiazines, other tranquilizers, sedative-hypnotics (eg, barbiturates), TCAs, and other CNS depressants (eg, alcohol); use w/ great caution and in reduced dosages.

NURSING CONSIDERATIONS

Assessment: Assess for level of pain intensity, patient's general condition and medical status, hypersensitivity to the drug, renal/hepatic impairment, respiratory depression, any other conditions where treatment is contraindicated or cautioned, pregnancy/nursing status, and possible drug interactions.

Monitoring: Monitor for respiratory depression, elevations in CSF pressure, hypotension, convulsions/seizures, drug abuse/tolerance/dependence, and other adverse reactions.

Patient Counseling: Inform of the risks/benefits of therapy. Inform that medication may impair mental/physical abilities required to perform hazardous tasks (eg, driving, operating machinery). Advise about potential for dependence upon repeated administration.

Storage: 20-25°C (68-77°F).

DENAVIR — penciclovir RX

Class: Nucleoside analogue

ADULT DOSAGE

Herpes Labialis (Cold Sores)

Recurrent:
Apply q2h during waking hours for a period of 4 days
Start treatment as early as possible (eg, during the prodrome or when lesions appear)

PEDIATRIC DOSAGE

Herpes Labialis (Cold Sores)

Recurrent:
≥12 Years:
Apply q2h during waking hours for a period of 4 days
Start treatment as early as possible (eg, during the prodrome or when lesions appear)

ADMINISTRATION
Topical route

HOW SUPPLIED
Cre: 1% [1.5g, 5g]

WARNINGS/PRECAUTIONS
Should only be used on herpes labialis on the lips and face. Avoid application in mucous membranes and/or near the eyes. Evaluate for secondary bacterial infection if lesions worsen or do not improve on therapy. Effect has not been established in immunocompromised patients.

ADVERSE REACTIONS
Application-site reaction, hypesthesia, local anesthesia, taste perversion, rash (erythematous).

NURSING CONSIDERATIONS

Assessment: Assess for bacterial infection, drug hypersensitivity, and pregnancy/nursing status.

Monitoring: Monitor for clinical response and improvement of symptoms. Evaluate for secondary bacterial infection if lesions worsen or do not improve.

Patient Counseling: Inform that drug is not a cure for cold sores and not all patients respond to treatment. Instruct not to use if allergic to the drug or any of its ingredients. Instruct to notify physician if pregnant, planning to become pregnant, or breastfeeding. Instruct to use ud. Instruct to wash hands with soap and water before and after applying product. Inform that face should be clean and dry. Instruct to apply a layer to cover only the cold sore area or area of tingling before the cold sore appears, and to rub in the cre until it disappears. Inform of possible adverse effects (eg, application-site reactions, local anesthesia, taste perversion, rash).

Storage: 20-25°C (68-77°F); excursions permitted to 15-30°C (59-86°F).

DEPAKOTE – divalproex sodium RX

Class: Valproate compound

Fatal hepatic failure reported, usually during first 6 months of treatment. Serious/fatal hepatotoxicity may be preceded by nonspecific symptoms (eg, malaise, weakness, lethargy, facial edema, anorexia, vomiting) or a loss of seizure control in patients with epilepsy; monitor closely. Monitor LFTs prior to therapy and at frequent intervals thereafter, especially during first 6 months of treatment. Increased risk of developing fatal hepatotoxicity in children <2 yrs of age, especially if on multiple anticonvulsants, with congenital metabolic disorders, with severe seizure disorders accompanied by mental retardation, and with organic brain disease; use with extreme caution and as a sole agent. Increased risk of drug-induced acute liver failure and resultant death in patients with hereditary neurometabolic syndromes caused by DNA mutations of the mitochondrial DNA polymerase gamma (POLG) gene (eg, Alpers-Huttenlocher syndrome). Contraindicated in patients known to have mitochondrial disorders caused by POLG mutations and in children <2 yrs of age who are clinically suspected of having a mitochondrial disorder. In patients >2 yrs of age who are clinically suspected of having a hereditary mitochondrial disease, drug should only be used after other anticonvulsants have failed; closely monitor for the development of acute liver injury with regular clinical assessments and serum liver testing. May cause major congenital malformations, particularly neural tube defects (eg, spina bifida). May cause decreased IQ scores following in utero exposure. Contraindicated in pregnant women treated for migraine prophylaxis (tab). Should only be used to treat pregnant women with epilepsy or bipolar disorder if other medications have failed to control their symptoms or are otherwise unacceptable. Do not administer to a woman of childbearing potential unless the drug is essential to the management of her medical condition; use effective contraception. Life-threatening pancreatitis reported; d/c if pancreatitis is diagnosed and initiate alternative treatment.

OTHER BRAND NAMES

Depakote Sprinkle

ADULT DOSAGE

Epilepsy

Monotherapy and Adjunctive Therapy for Complex Partial and Simple and Complex Seizures; Adjunctive Therapy w/ Multiple Seizure Types (eg, Absence Seizures):

Cap/Tab:

Complex Partial Seizures:
Initial: 10-15mg/kg/day
Titrate: Increase by 5-10mg/kg/week
Max: 60mg/kg/day

Simple and Complex Absence Seizures:
Initial: 15mg/kg/day
Titrate: Increase weekly by 5-10mg/kg/day
Max: 60mg/kg/day

If daily dose >250mg/day, give in divided doses

Mania

Associated w/ Bipolar Disorder:
Tab:
Initial: 750mg/day in divided doses
Titrate: Increase dose as rapidly as possible to achieve lowest therapeutic dose
Max: 60mg/kg/day

Migraine

Prophylaxis:
Tab:
Initial: 250mg bid
Max: 1000mg/day

PEDIATRIC DOSAGE

Epilepsy

Monotherapy and Adjunctive Therapy for Complex Partial and Simple and Complex Seizures; Adjunctive Therapy w/ Multiple Seizure Types (eg, Absence Seizures):

Cap/Tab:

Simple and Complex Absence Seizure:
Initial: 15mg/kg/day
Titrate: Increase weekly by 5-10mg/kg/day
Max: 60mg/kg/day

Complex Partial Seizures:
≥10 Years:
Initial: 10-15mg/kg/day
Titrate: Increase by 5-10mg/kg/week
Max: 60mg/kg/day

If daily dose >250mg/day, give in divided doses

DOSE MODIFICATION

Concomitant Medications

Complex Partial Seizures:

Conversion to Monotherapy: Reduce concomitant antiepilepsy drug dosage by approximately 25% every 2 weeks; reduction may be started at initiation of divalproex therapy, or delayed by 1-2 weeks if seizures are likely to occur w/ a reduction

Elderly

Reduce initial dose and titrate slowly; consider dose reductions or discontinuation in patients w/ decreased food/fluid intake or excessive somnolence

Adverse Reactions

Thrombocytopenia: Probability appears to increase significantly at total valproate concentrations of ≥110mcg/mL (females) or ≥135mcg/mL (males)

Other Important Modifications

In epileptic patients previously receiving divalproex, initiate at the same daily dose and frequency; once the patient is stabilized, the frequency of divalproex may be adjusted to bid-tid

ADMINISTRATION

Oral route

Give w/ food or slowly titrate from initial dose in patients w/ GI irritation

Cap

May be swallowed whole or the contents may be sprinkled on small amount of soft food

To Administer w/ Food:

1. Hold the cap so that the end marked "THIS END UP" is straight up and the arrow on the cap is up
2. To open the cap, gently twist it apart to separate the top from the bottom. It may be helpful to hold the cap over the food to which you will add the sprinkles. If you spill any of the cap contents, start over w/ a new cap and a new portion of food
3. Place all the sprinkles onto a small amount (about a tsp) of soft food such as applesauce or pudding
4. Make sure that all of the sprinkle/food mixture is swallowed right away. Do not chew the sprinkle/food mixture
5. Drinking water right after taking the sprinkle/food mixture will help make sure all sprinkles are swallowed
6. Throw away any unused sprinkle/food mixture; do not store any for future use

Tab

Swallow whole; do not crush, or chew

HOW SUPPLIED

Cap, Delayed-Release: (Sprinkle) 125mg; Tab, Delayed-Release: 125mg, 250mg, 500mg

CONTRAINDICATIONS

Hepatic disease, significant hepatic dysfunction, known urea cycle disorders (UCDs). Mitochondrial disorders caused by mutations in mitochondrial DNA POLG (eg, Alpers-Huttenlocher syndrome) and children <2 yrs of age who are suspected of having a POLG-related disorder. (Tab) Prophylaxis of migraine headaches in pregnant women.

WARNINGS/PRECAUTIONS

D/C immediately if significant hepatic dysfunction (suspected or apparent) occurs. Hyperammonemic encephalopathy reported in patients with UCDs; d/c and initiate treatment if symptoms develop. Increased risk of suicidal thoughts or behavior reported. Dose-related thrombocytopenia and decreases in other cell lines and myelodysplasia reported; reduce dose or d/c if hemorrhage, bruising, or a disorder of hemostasis/coagulation occurs. Hyperammonemia reported and may be present despite normal LFTs. Measure ammonia levels if unexplained lethargy, vomiting, or mental status changes occur; hyperammonemic encephalopathy should be considered. Hypothermia with and in absence of hyperammonemia reported; consider discontinuation. Drug reaction with eosinophilia and systemic symptoms (DRESS), also known as multiorgan hypersensitivity, reported; evaluate immediately if signs/symptoms (eg, fever, lymphadenopathy) are present, and d/c and do not resume if an alternative etiology cannot be established. Caution in elderly; monitor for fluid/nutritional intake, dehydration, somnolence, and other adverse reactions. Altered thyroid function tests and urine ketone tests reported. May stimulate replication of HIV and cytomegalovirus. Avoid abrupt discontinuation. Medication residue in stool reported; check valproate levels and monitor clinical condition, and consider alternative treatment if clinically indicated.

ADVERSE REACTIONS

Hepatotoxicity, pancreatitis, diarrhea, N/V, somnolence, dizziness, dyspepsia, thrombocytopenia, asthenia, abdominal pain, tremor, headache, anorexia, diplopia, blurred vision.

DRUG INTERACTIONS

Drugs that affect the level of expression of hepatic enzymes (eg, phenytoin, carbamazepine, phenobarbital, primidone) may increase or double valproate clearance; monitor valproate and concomitant drug concentrations whenever enzyme-inducing drugs are introduced or withdrawn.

Concomitant use with ASA decreases protein binding and inhibits metabolism of valproate; use with caution. Carbapenem antibiotics may reduce serum concentrations to subtherapeutic levels, resulting in loss of seizure control. Concomitant use with felbamate increases valproate C_{max}; may require decrease in valproate dosage. Rifampin increases oral clearance; may require valproate dosage adjustment. Reduces the clearance of amitriptyline and nortriptyline. May decrease levels of carbamazepine. Inhibits metabolism of diazepam, ethosuximide, phenobarbital, and phenytoin; monitor drug serum concentrations and adjust dose appropriately. Monitor for neurological toxicity with concomitant barbiturate therapy. Breakthrough seizures reported with concomitant use with phenytoin. Use with clonazepam may induce absence status in patients with absence seizures. Increases $T_{1/2}$ of lamotrigine; serious skin reactions reported. Monitor coagulation tests when coadministered with anticoagulants. May decrease zidovudine clearance in HIV-seropositive patients. Concomitant use with topiramate associated with hypothermia and hyperammonemia, with or without encephalopathy.

NURSING CONSIDERATIONS

Assessment: Assess for hepatic dysfunction, history of hepatic disease, pancreatitis, history of hypersensitivity to the drug, mitochondrial disorders caused by mutations in mitochondrial POLG, children <2 yrs of age who are suspected of having a POLG-related disorder, other conditions where treatment is contraindicated or cautioned, pregnancy/nursing status, and possible drug interactions. Assess LFTs, CBC, and coagulation parameters. Evaluate for UCDs, especially in high-risk patients (eg, history of unexplained encephalopathy or coma).

Monitoring: Monitor for hypersensitivity reactions, pancreatitis, hepatotoxicity, hyperammonemia, hypothermia, DRESS, drug-induced acute liver failure, acute liver injury, emergence/worsening of depression, suicidality or unusual changes in behavior, medication residue in stool, and other adverse reactions. Monitor LFTs frequently, especially during first 6 months. Monitor fluid/nutritional intake, ammonia levels, CBC, and coagulation parameters. Perform periodic plasma concentration determinations of valproate and concomitant drugs during the early course of therapy.

Patient Counseling: Instruct to take ud. Inform pregnant women and women of childbearing potential about the risk in pregnancy (eg, birth defects, decreased IQ); advise to use effective contraception while on therapy and counsel about alternative therapeutic options. Instruct to notify physician if pregnant or intending to become pregnant. Encourage patients to enroll in the North American Antiepileptic Drug Pregnancy Registry. Advise to notify physician if depression, suicidal thoughts/behavior, or thoughts about self-harm emerge; instruct to report behaviors of concern. Counsel about signs/symptoms of pancreatitis, hepatotoxicity, hyperammonemia, or hyperammonemic encephalopathy; advise to notify physician if any symptoms or adverse effects occur. Advise not to engage in hazardous activities (eg, driving/operating machinery) until the effects of the drug are known. Inform that a fever associated with other organ system involvement (eg, rash, lymphadenopathy) may be drug-related; instruct to report to physician. Instruct patients to notify their healthcare provider if they notice medication residue in the stool.

Storage: (Cap) <25°C (77°F). (Tab) <30°C (86°F).

DEPAKOTE ER – divalproex sodium

RX

Class: Valproate compound

Fatal hepatic failure may occur, usually during first 6 months of treatment. Serious/fatal hepatotoxicity may be preceded by nonspecific symptoms (eg, malaise, weakness, lethargy, facial edema, anorexia, vomiting) or loss of seizure control in patients with epilepsy; monitor closely. Monitor LFTs prior to therapy and at frequent intervals thereafter, especially during first 6 months of treatment. Increased risk of developing fatal hepatotoxicity in children <2 yrs of age, especially if on multiple anticonvulsants, with congenital metabolic disorders, severe seizure disorders with mental retardation, and organic brain disease; use with extreme caution and as a sole agent. Increased risk of drug-induced acute liver failure and resultant death in patients with hereditary neurometabolic syndromes caused by DNA mutations of the mitochondrial DNA polymerase gamma (POLG) gene (eg, Alpers-Huttenlocher syndrome). Contraindicated in patients known to have mitochondrial disorders caused by POLG mutations and children <2 yrs of age who are clinically suspected of having a mitochondrial disorder. In patients >2 yrs of age who are clinically suspected of having a hereditary mitochondrial disease, drug should only be used after other anticonvulsants have failed; closely monitor for the development of acute liver injury with regular clinical assessments and serum liver testing. May cause major congenital malformations, particularly neural tube defects (eg, spina bifida). May cause decreased IQ scores following in utero exposure. Contraindicated in pregnant women treated for prophylaxis of migraine; should only be used to treat pregnant women with epilepsy or bipolar disorder if other medications have failed to control their symptoms or are otherwise unacceptable. Do not administer to a woman of childbearing potential unless the drug is essential to the management of her medical condition; use effective contraception. Life-threatening pancreatitis reported; d/c if pancreatitis is diagnosed and initiate appropriate treatment.

ADULT DOSAGE

Mania

Initial: 25mg/kg qd
Max: 60mg/kg/day

Epilepsy

Complex Partial Seizures:
Initial: 10-15mg/kg/day
Titrate: Increase by 5-10mg/kg/week
Max: 60mg/kg/day

Simple/Complex Absence Seizures:
Initial: 15mg/kg/day
Titrate: Increase weekly by 5-10mg/kg/day
Max: 60mg/kg/day

Migraine

Prophylaxis:
Initial: 500mg qd for 1 week
Titrate: Increase to 1000mg qd

Conversions

Conversion from Depakote to Depakote ER:
Depakote 500-625mg/day: 750mg Depakote ER
Depakote 750-875mg/day: 1000mg Depakote ER
Depakote 1000-1125mg/day: 1250mg Depakote ER
Depakote 1250-1375mg/day: 1500mg Depakote ER
Depakote 1500-1625mg/day: 1750mg Depakote ER
Depakote 1750mg/day: 2000mg Depakote ER
Depakote 1875-2000mg/day: 2250mg Depakote ER
Depakote 2125-2250mg/day: 2500mg Depakote ER
Depakote 2375mg/day: 2750mg Depakote ER
Depakote 2500-2750mg/day: 3000mg Depakote ER
Depakote 2875mg/day: 3250mg Depakote ER
Depakote 3000-3125mg/day: 3500mg Depakote ER

PEDIATRIC DOSAGE

Epilepsy

≥10 Years:
Complex Partial Seizures:
Initial: 10-15mg/kg/day
Titrate: Increase by 5-10mg/kg/week
Max: 60mg/kg/day

Simple/Complex Absence Seizures:
Initial: 15mg/kg/day
Titrate: Increase weekly by 5-10mg/kg/day
Max: 60mg/kg/day

Conversions

Conversion from Depakote to Depakote ER:
Depakote 500-625mg/day: 750mg Depakote ER
Depakote 750-875mg/day: 1000mg Depakote ER
Depakote 1000-1125mg/day: 1250mg Depakote ER
Depakote 1250-1375mg/day: 1500mg Depakote ER
Depakote 1500-1625mg/day: 1750mg Depakote ER
Depakote 1750mg/day: 2000mg Depakote ER
Depakote 1875-2000mg/day: 2250mg Depakote ER
Depakote 2125-2250mg/day: 2500mg Depakote ER
Depakote 2375mg/day: 2750mg Depakote ER
Depakote 2500-2750mg/day: 3000mg Depakote ER
Depakote 2875mg/day: 3250mg Depakote ER
Depakote 3000-3125mg/day: 3500mg Depakote ER

DOSE MODIFICATION

Concomitant Medications

Complex Partial Seizures:
Conversion to Monotherapy: Reduce concomitant antiepilepsy drugs by 25% every 2 weeks; begin reduction at initiation of Depakote ER, or delay by 1-2 weeks

Elderly

Reduce initial dose and titrate slowly

Adverse Reactions

Thrombocytopenia: Probability increases significantly at total valproate concentrations of ≥110mcg/mL (females) or ≥135mcg/mL (males)

ADMINISTRATION

Oral route

Swallow whole; do not crush or chew

HOW SUPPLIED

Tab, Extended-Release: 250mg, 500mg

CONTRAINDICATIONS

Hepatic disease, significant hepatic dysfunction, known urea cycle disorder (UCD). Mitochondrial disorders caused by mutations in mitochondrial POLG (eg, Alpers-Huttenlocher syndrome) and children <2 yrs of age who are suspected of having a POLG-related disorder. Prophylaxis of migraine headaches in pregnant women.

WARNINGS/PRECAUTIONS

Caution with prior history of hepatic disease. D/C immediately if significant hepatic dysfunction (suspected or apparent) occurs. Reversible and irreversible cerebral and cerebellar atrophy reported; routinely monitor motor and cognitive functions, and evaluate continued use in the presence of suspected or apparent signs of brain atrophy. Cerebral atrophy reported in children exposed in utero. Increased risk of suicidal thoughts or behavior reported. Dose-related thrombocytopenia reported. Hyperammonemic encephalopathy reported in UCD patients; d/c and initiate treatment if symptoms develop. Prior to initiation of therapy, evaluate for UCD in high-risk patients (eg, history of unexplained encephalopathy, coma). Hyperammonemia reported and may be present despite normal LFTs. Measure ammonia levels if unexplained lethargy, vomiting, or mental status changes occur. Caution in elderly; monitor fluid/nutritional intake, and for dehydration, somnolence, and other adverse reactions. Altered thyroid function tests and urine ketone tests reported. Avoid abrupt discontinuation. May stimulate replication of HIV and cytomegalovirus. Multiorgan hypersensitivity reactions (rare) and hypothermia reported. Medication residue in stool reported; check valproate levels and monitor clinical condition, and consider alternative treatment if clinically indicated.

ADVERSE REACTIONS

Hepatotoxicity, pancreatitis, N/V, somnolence, dizziness, abdominal pain, dyspepsia, amblyopia/blurred vision, diarrhea, tremor, weight gain, back pain, alopecia, headache.

DRUG INTERACTIONS

Drugs that affect the level of expression of hepatic enzymes (eg, phenytoin, carbamazepine, phenobarbital, primidone) may increase valproate clearance; monitor valproate and concomitant drug concentrations whenever enzyme-inducing drugs are introduced or withdrawn. Concomitant use with aspirin decreases protein binding and inhibits metabolism of valproate; use with caution. Carbapenem antibiotics may reduce serum concentrations to subtherapeutic levels, resulting in loss of seizure control. Rifampin increases oral clearance; may require valproate dosage adjustment. Concomitant use with felbamate leads to an increase in valproate C_{max}; may require decrease in valproate dosage. Reduces the clearance of amitriptyline and nortriptyline. Induces metabolism of carbamazepine. Inhibits metabolism of diazepam, ethosuximide, phenobarbital, and phenytoin; monitor drug serum concentrations and adjust dose appropriately. Breakthrough seizures reported with concomitant use with phenytoin. Use with clonazepam may induce absence status in patients with absence seizures. Increases $T_{1/2}$ of lamotrigine; serious skin reactions reported. Concomitant use with topiramate has been associated with hyperammonemia, with or without encephalopathy, and hypothermia. May displace protein-bound drugs (eg, phenytoin, carbamazepine, tolbutamide, warfarin); monitor coagulation tests when coadministered with warfarin. May decrease clearance of zidovudine in HIV-seropositive patients.

NURSING CONSIDERATIONS

Assessment: Assess for hepatic dysfunction, history of hepatic disease, UCD, pancreatitis, history of hypersensitivity to the drug, mitochondrial disorders caused by mutations in mitochondrial POLG, children <2 yrs of age who are suspected of having a POLG-related disorders, other conditions where treatment is cautioned, pregnancy/nursing status, and possible drug interactions. Assess LFTs, CBC with platelet counts, and coagulation parameters.

Monitoring: Monitor for hypersensitivity reactions, multiorgan hypersensitivity reactions, pancreatitis, hepatotoxicity, hyperammonemia, hypothermia, drug-induced acute liver failure, acute liver injury, brain atrophy, emergence/worsening of depression, suicidality or unusual changes in behavior, medication residue in stool, and other adverse reactions. Monitor LFTs frequently, especially during first 6 months. Monitor fluid/nutritional intake, ammonia levels, CBC with platelets, and coagulation parameters in patients on warfarin.

Patient Counseling: Inform to take ud. Inform pregnant women and women of childbearing potential about the risk in pregnancy; advise to use effective contraception while on therapy and counsel about alternative therapeutic options. Advise to read medication guide. Instruct to notify physician if pregnant or intending to become pregnant. Encourage patients to enroll in North American Antiepileptic Drug Pregnancy Registry. Advise to notify physician if depression, suicidal thoughts, behavior, or thoughts about self-harm emerge; instruct to report behaviors of concern. Counsel about signs/symptoms of pancreatitis, hepatotoxicity, hyperammonemia, or hyperammonemic encephalopathy; advise to notify physician if any symptoms or adverse effects occur. Advise not to engage in hazardous activities (eg, driving/operating machinery) until the effects of the drug are known. Inform that a fever associated with other organ system involvement (eg, rash, lymphadenopathy) may be drug related; instruct to report to physician. Instruct patients to notify their physician if they notice a medication residue in the stool.

Storage: 25°C (77°F); excursions permitted to 15-30°C (59-86°F).

DEPO-PROVERA – medroxyprogesterone acetate

RX

Class: Progestogen

ADULT DOSAGE

Inoperable, Recurrent, and Metastatic Endometrial or Renal Carcinoma

Adjunctive Therapy and Palliative Treatment:

Initial: 400-1000mg/week

If improvement is noted w/in a few weeks or months and the disease appears stabilized, may be possible to maintain improvement w/ as little as 400mg/month

PEDIATRIC DOSAGE

Pediatric use may not have been established

ADMINISTRATION

IM route

Cleanse the vial top prior to aspiration of contents of multidose vial

HOW SUPPLIED

Inj: 400mg/mL [2.5mL]

CONTRAINDICATIONS

Known or suspected pregnancy or as a diagnostic test for pregnancy, undiagnosed vaginal bleeding, known or suspected malignancy of the breast, active thrombophlebitis, current or past history of thromboembolic disorders or cerebral vascular disease, liver dysfunction or disease.

WARNINGS/PRECAUTIONS

D/C if early manifestations of thrombotic disorder (thrombophlebitis, cerebrovascular disorder, pulmonary embolism, retinal thrombosis) occur or are suspected. D/C, pending examination, if there is a sudden partial or complete loss of vision, or a sudden onset of proptosis, diplopia, or migraine. If examination reveals papilledema or retinal vascular lesions, withdraw therapy. Avoid contamination of multidose vials. Perform annual history and physical examination. Physical examination should include special reference to BP, breasts, abdomen and pelvic organs, including cervical cytology and relevant lab tests. In cases of undiagnosed, persistent, or recurrent vaginal bleeding, perform adequate diagnostic measures to rule out malignancies. Monitor women who have a family history of breast cancer and those who develop breast nodules. May cause fluid retention; caution with epilepsy, migraine, asthma, and cardiac/renal dysfunction. Perform adequate diagnostic measures in cases of breakthrough bleeding. Caution with history of psychic depression; d/c if depression recurs to a serious degree. May mask the onset of climacteric. Use with estrogen may produce adverse effects on carbohydrate and lipid metabolism. Decrease in glucose tolerance reported in patients on estrogen-progestin combination treatment; caution in diabetic patients on estrogen-progestin combination treatment. May affect certain endocrine, hepatic, and blood components in lab tests.

ADVERSE REACTIONS

Menstrual irregularities, nervousness, dizziness, edema, weight gain/loss and cervical erosion/secretion changes, cholestatic jaundice, breast tenderness, rash, alopecia, hirsutism, depression, pyrexia, fatigue, insomnia.

DRUG INTERACTIONS

Decreased levels with aminoglutethimide.

NURSING CONSIDERATIONS

Assessment: Assess for drug hypersensitivity and for any other conditions where treatment is contraindicated or cautioned. Assess pregnancy/nursing status and for possible drug interactions.

Monitoring: Monitor for thrombotic disorders, loss of vision, proptosis, diplopia, migraine, papilledema, retinal vascular lesions, breakthrough bleeding, recurrence of depression, fluid retention, and other adverse reactions. Perform annual history and physical examination. If undiagnosed, persistent or recurrent abnormal vaginal bleeding occurs, take appropriate measures to rule out malignancy. Monitor for adverse effects on carbohydrate and lipid metabolism if used with estrogen therapy.

Patient Counseling: Inform of risks/benefits of treatment. Instruct to notify physician if pregnant, pregnancy occurs, or if any adverse reactions occur while on treatment.

Storage: 20-25°C (68-77°F) in upright position.

Depo-Provera Contraceptive Injection – RX

medroxyprogesterone acetate

Class: Progestin contraceptive

May lose significant bone mineral density (BMD); bone loss is greater w/ increasing duration of use and may not be completely reversible. Unknown if use during adolescence or early adulthood will reduce peak bone mass and increase risk for osteoporotic fractures in later life. Should not be used as long-term birth control (eg, >2 yrs) unless other birth control methods are considered inadequate.

ADULT DOSAGE

Contraception

Usual: 150mg deep IM every 3 months (13 weeks)

Dosage does not need to be adjusted for body weight

Conversions

Switching from Other Methods of Contraception:

Give in a manner that ensures continuous contraceptive coverage based upon the mechanism of action of both methods (eg, switching from oral contraceptives should have the 1st inj on the day after the last active tab or at the latest, on the day following the final inactive tab)

PEDIATRIC DOSAGE

Contraception

Not indicated for use premenarche; refer to adult dosing

ADMINISTRATION

IM route

Shake vigorously before use

Administer in the gluteal or deltoid muscle

Give the 1st inj only during the first 5 days of a normal menstrual period, only w/in the first 5 days postpartum if not breastfeeding, or only at the 6th postpartum week if exclusively nursing

If the interval between inj is >13 weeks, determine that patient is not pregnant before administering

HOW SUPPLIED

Inj: 150mg/mL [1mL, vial, prefilled syringe]

CONTRAINDICATIONS

Known or suspected pregnancy or as a diagnostic test for pregnancy, active thrombophlebitis, current or past history of thromboembolic disorders, cerebral vascular disease, known or suspected malignancy of the breast, significant liver disease, undiagnosed vaginal bleeding.

WARNINGS/PRECAUTIONS

May pose additional risk of BMD loss in patients w/ risk factors for osteoporosis (eg, chronic alcohol and/or tobacco use, anorexia nervosa, chronic use of drugs that can reduce bone mass [eg, anticonvulsants, corticosteroids]); consider other birth control methods. Serious thrombotic events reported; d/c if thrombosis develops while on therapy unless there are no other acceptable options for birth control. Do not readminister therapy pending examination if there is sudden partial/complete loss of vision, or sudden onset of proptosis/diplopia/migraine; if examination reveals papilledema or retinal vascular lesions, do not readminister. May increase risk of breast cancer; monitor women w/ strong family history of breast cancer carefully. Be alert to possibility of ectopic pregnancy in patients who become pregnant or complain of severe abdominal pain. Anaphylaxis/anaphylactoid reactions reported; institute emergency medical treatment if an anaphylactic reaction occurs. D/C if jaundice or acute/chronic disturbances of liver function develop; do not resume use until markers of liver function return to normal and medroxyprogesterone acetate causation has been excluded. Convulsions and weight gain reported. Monitor patients who have history of depression; do not readminister if depression recurs. May cause disruption of menstrual bleeding patterns (eg, amenorrhea, irregular or unpredictable bleeding/spotting, prolonged spotting/bleeding, heavy bleeding); rule out possibility of organic pathology if abnormal bleeding persists or is severe, and institute appropriate treatment. Decrease in glucose tolerance reported; monitor diabetic patients carefully. May cause fluid retention. Return to ovulation and fertility after discontinuation of therapy may be delayed. Does not protect against HIV infection and other STDs. May change results of some lab tests (eg, coagulation factors, lipids, glucose tolerance, binding proteins).

ADVERSE REACTIONS

BMD loss, menstrual irregularities, increased weight, abdominal pain/discomfort, dizziness, headache, asthenia/fatigue, nervousness, decreased libido, nausea, leg cramps.

DRUG INTERACTIONS

Drugs or herbal products that induce enzymes, including CYP3A4 that metabolize contraceptive hormones (eg, barbiturates, bosentan, St. John's wort) may decrease levels and effectiveness; use additional contraception or a different method of contraception. HIV protease inhibitors and non-nucleoside reverse transcriptase inhibitors may alter levels. Pregnancy reported w/ antibiotics.

NURSING CONSIDERATIONS

Assessment: Assess for active thrombophlebitis, current/past history of thromboembolic disorders or cerebral vascular disease, known or suspected malignancy of the breast, drug hypersensitivity, significant liver disease, undiagnosed vaginal bleeding, osteoporosis risk factors, family history of breast cancer, history of depression, diabetes mellitus (DM), conditions that may be influenced by fluid retention (eg, epilepsy, migraine, asthma, cardiac/renal dysfunction), pregnancy/nursing status, and possible drug interactions.

Monitoring: Monitor for thrombosis, loss of BMD, breast cancer, sudden/partial loss of vision, proptosis, diplopia, migraine, papilledema, retinal vascular lesions, anaphylaxis/anaphylactoid reactions, jaundice or acute/chronic disturbances in liver function, ectopic pregnancy, convulsions, weight gain, fluid retention, disruption of menstrual bleeding patterns, and other adverse reactions. Monitor patients w/ DM. Monitor for recurrence of depression w/ history of depression. Perform annual exam for a BP check and for other indicated healthcare.

Patient Counseling: Counsel about the risks/benefits of therapy. Advise at the beginning of treatment that the menstrual cycle may be disrupted and that irregular and unpredictable bleeding or spotting may occur; inform that this usually decreases to the point of amenorrhea as treatment continues w/o other therapy being required. Inform about the possible increased risk of breast cancer in women who use the drug. Inform that drug does not protect against HIV infection and other STDs. Counsel to use a back-up method or alternative method of contraception when enzyme inducers are used w/ the drug. Advise to take adequate Ca^{2+} and vitamin D. Advise to have a yearly visit w/ healthcare provider for a BP check and for other indicated healthcare.

Storage: 20-25°C (68-77°F). Store vials upright.

DEPO-TESTOSTERONE – testosterone cypionate CIII

Class: Androgen

ADULT DOSAGE

Testosterone Replacement Therapy

Congenital/Acquired Primary Hypogonadism or Hypogonadotropic Hypogonadism in Males:

Individualize dose based on age, sex, and diagnosis
50-400mg every 2-4 weeks

PEDIATRIC DOSAGE

Testosterone Replacement Therapy

Congenital/Acquired Primary Hypogonadism or Hypogonadotropic Hypogonadism in Males:

≥12 Years:
Individualize dose based on age, sex, and diagnosis
50-400mg every 2-4 weeks

ADMINISTRATION

IM route

Administer deep into gluteal muscle
Warm and shake the vial to redissolve any crystals that may have formed during storage at temperatures lower than recommended.

HOW SUPPLIED

Inj: 100mg/mL [10mL], 200mg/mL [1mL, 10mL]

CONTRAINDICATIONS

Males w/ carcinoma of the breast or known/suspected carcinoma of the prostate gland. Serious cardiac, hepatic, or renal disease. Women who are or may become pregnant.

WARNINGS/PRECAUTIONS

May cause hypercalcemia in immobilized patients; d/c if this occurs. Peliosis hepatis, hepatocellular carcinoma, and hepatic adenomas reported w/ prolonged use of high doses. May increase risk of prostatic hypertrophy and prostatic carcinoma in elderly. Venous thromboembolic events reported; evaluate patients who report symptoms of pain, edema, warmth, and erythema in the lower extremity for deep vein thrombosis and those who present w/ acute SOB for pulmonary embolism. D/C treatment and initiate appropriate workup and management if venous thromboembolic event is suspected. Increased risk of major adverse cardiovascular events (MACE) reported. Edema w/ or w/o CHF may be a serious complication in patients w/ preexisting cardiac, renal, or hepatic disease. Gynecomastia may develop and persist. Contains benzyl alcohol; has been associated w/ serious adverse events, including gasping syndrome and death, in pediatric patients. Caution in healthy males w/ delayed puberty; monitor bone maturation by assessing bone age of wrist and hand every 6 months. May accelerate bone maturation w/o producing compensatory gain in linear growth in children; compromised adult stature may result. Acute urethral obstruction in patients w/ benign prostatic hypertrophy (BPH), priapism or excessive sexual stimulation, and oligospermia after prolonged use or excessive dosage may develop; if these effects appear d/c therapy and if restarted, use a lower dose. Do not use interchangeably w/ testosterone propionate and for enhancement of athletic performance. May increase serum cholesterol. May decrease levels of thyroxin-binding globulins, resulting in decreased total T4 serum concentrations and increased resin uptake of T3 and T4.

ADVERSE REACTIONS

Gynecomastia, excessive frequency/duration of penile erections, oligospermia (if at high doses), male pattern baldness, increased/decreased libido, hirsutism, acne, MI, stroke, nausea, clotting factor suppression, polycythemia, altered LFTs, headache, anxiety.

DRUG INTERACTIONS

May increase sensitivity to oral anticoagulants; may require dose reduction in anticoagulants. May increase levels of oxyphenbutazone. May decrease blood glucose and insulin requirements in diabetic patients.

NURSING CONSIDERATIONS

Assessment: Assess for breast carcinoma in males, prostate carcinoma, cardiac/hepatic/renal disease, delayed puberty, BPH, drug hypersensitivity, any other conditions where treatment is contraindicated/cautioned, and possible drug interactions. Confirm diagnosis of hypogonadism by measuring testosterone levels on at least 2 separate days prior to initiation.

Monitoring: Monitor for signs/symptoms of hypercalcemia, edema w/ or w/o CHF, prostatic hypertrophy/carcinoma in elderly, venous thromboembolic events, MACE and other adverse reactions. Monitor bone maturation by assessing bone age of wrist and hand every 6 months. Periodically check Hgb and Hct in patients receiving long-term androgen therapy. Monitor serum cholesterol levels and LFTs.

Patient Counseling: Instruct to report to physician if N/V, changes in skin color, ankle swelling, or too frequent or persistent penile erections occurs. Inform of the possible risk of MACE when deciding whether to use or continue to use drug.

Storage: 20-25°C (68-77°F). Protect from light.

DETROL LA – tolterodine tartrate

RX

Class: Muscarinic antagonist

OTHER BRAND NAMES

Detrol

ADULT DOSAGE

Overactive Bladder

Cap, ER:

Usual: 4mg qd; may be lowered to 2mg qd based on response and tolerability

Tab:

Usual: 2mg bid; may be lowered to 1mg bid based on response and tolerability

PEDIATRIC DOSAGE

Pediatric use may not have been established

DOSE MODIFICATION

Concomitant Medications

Potent CYP3A4 Inhibitors:

Cap, ER:

Usual: 2mg qd

Tab:

Usual: 1mg bid

Renal Impairment

Cap, ER:

CrCl 10-30mL/min:

Usual: 2mg qd

CrCl <10mL/min: Not recommended

Tab:

Significantly Reduced Renal Function:

Usual: 1mg bid

Hepatic Impairment
Cap, ER:
Mild to Moderate (Child-Pugh Class A or B):
Usual: 2mg qd
Severe (Child-Pugh Class C): Not recommended

Tab:
Significantly Reduced Hepatic Function:
Usual: 1mg bid

ADMINISTRATION
Oral route

Cap, ER
Take with water and swallow whole

HOW SUPPLIED
Cap, ER: (Detrol LA) 2mg, 4mg; Tab: (Detrol) 1mg, 2mg

CONTRAINDICATIONS
Urinary/gastric retention, uncontrolled narrow-angle glaucoma, hypersensitivity to fesoterodine fumarate ER tab.

WARNINGS/PRECAUTIONS
Anaphylaxis/angioedema requiring hospitalization and emergency treatment occurred with 1st or subsequent doses; d/c and provide appropriate therapy if difficulty in breathing, upper airway obstruction, or fall in BP occurs. Risk of urinary retention; caution in patients with clinically significant bladder outflow obstruction. Risk of gastric retention; caution in patients with GI obstructive disorders (eg, pyloric stenosis). Caution with decreased GI motility (eg, intestinal atony), myasthenia gravis, known history of QT prolongation, hepatic/renal impairment, and in patients being treated for narrow-angle glaucoma. CNS anticholinergic effects (eg, dizziness, somnolence) reported; may impair physical/mental abilities. Monitor for signs of anticholinergic CNS effects (particularly after beginning treatment and increasing the dose); consider dose reduction or d/c if such effects occur.

ADVERSE REACTIONS
Dry mouth, dizziness, headache, abdominal pain, constipation.

DRUG INTERACTIONS
Caution with Class IA (eg, quinidine, procainamide) or Class III (eg, amiodarone, sotalol) antiarrhythmics. May aggravate dementia symptoms when initiating therapy in patients taking cholinesterase inhibitors. Increased concentrations with ketoconazole or other potent CYP3A4 inhibitors (eg, itraconazole, miconazole, clarithromycin). Increased levels with fluoxetine reported with IR tolterodine. May increase the frequency and/or severity of anticholinergic effects with other anticholinergic (antimuscarinic) agents.

NURSING CONSIDERATIONS

Assessment: Assess for hypersensitivity to the drug or fesoterodine fumarate, urinary/gastric retention, bladder outflow obstruction, GI obstructive disorders, decreased GI motility, narrow-angle glaucoma, myasthenia gravis, history of QT prolongation, hepatic/renal impairment, pregnancy/nursing status, and possible drug interactions.

Monitoring: Monitor for anaphylaxis, angioedema, difficulty breathing, upper airway obstruction, fall in BP, urinary retention, gastric retention, CNS anticholinergic effects, QT prolongation, hypersensitivity reactions, and other adverse reactions.

Patient Counseling: Inform patients that drug may produce blurred vision, dizziness, or drowsiness. Advise to exercise caution against potentially dangerous activities until drug's effects have been determined.

Storage: (Tab): 25°C (77°F); excursions permitted to 15-30°C (59-86°F). (Cap, ER): 20-25°C (68-77°F); excursions permitted to 15-30°C (59-86°F). Protect from light.

DEXAMETHASONE ORAL – dexamethasone RX

Class: Glucocorticoid

ADULT DOSAGE
Steroid-Responsive Disorders
Initial: 0.75-9mg/day depending on disease
Maint: Decrease in small amounts at appropriate time intervals to lowest effective dose; may need to increase dose for a period of time in stressful situations

PEDIATRIC DOSAGE
Steroid-Responsive Disorders
Sol/Tab:
Initial: 0.02-0.3mg/kg/day in 3 or 4 divided doses (0.6-9mg/m2BSA/day) depending on the disease

Upon discontinuation after long-term therapy, withdraw gradually

Cushing's Syndrome Test:
1mg at 11pm; draw blood at 8 am next morning
Alternatively, may give 0.5mg q6h for 48 hrs for greater accuracy

Test to Distinguish Cushing's Syndrome Due to Pituitary ACTH Excess from Cushing's Syndrome Due to Other Causes:
2mg q6h for 48 hrs; obtain 24-hr urine collections

Elixir:
Less Severe Diseases: Doses <0.75mg may suffice
Severe Diseases: >9mg may be required

D/C and transfer to other therapy, if satisfactory clinical response does not occur

Sol/Tab:
Acute Exacerbations of Multiple Sclerosis:
30mg/day for 1 week, then 4-12mg qod for 1 month

Acute, Self-Limited Allergic Disorders/Acute Exacerbations of Chronic Allergic Disorders:
Day 1: 1 or 2mL of 4mg/mL dexamethasone sodium phosphate IM
Day 2-3: Four 0.75mg tabs in 2 divided doses
Day 4: Two 0.75mg tabs in 2 divided doses
Day 5-6: One 0.75mg tab/day
Day 7: No treatment
Day 8: Follow-up visit

Palliative Management of Recurrent or Inoperable Brain Tumors:
Maint: 2mg bid or tid

Maint: Decrease in small amounts at appropriate time intervals to lowest effective dose; may need to increase dose for a period of time in stressful situations

Upon discontinuation after long-term therapy, withdraw gradually

Cushing's Syndrome Test:
1mg at 11 pm; draw blood at 8 am next morning
Alternatively, may give 0.5mg q6h for 48 hrs for greater accuracy

Test to Distinguish Cushing's Syndrome Due to Pituitary ACTH Excess from Cushing's Syndrome Due to Other Causes:
2mg q6h for 48 hrs; obtain 24-hr urine collections

DOSE MODIFICATION

Elderly

Start at lower end of dosing range

ADMINISTRATION

Oral route

Intensol

Mixed w/ liquid or semi-solid food (eg, water, juices, soda or soda-like beverages
Use only calibrated dropper provided
Refer to PI for proper use

Elixir

When large doses are given, may take w/ meals and antacids in between meals to help prevent peptic ulcers

HOW SUPPLIED

Elixir: 0.5mg/5mL [237mL]; Sol: 0.5mg/5mL [240mL, 500mL], (Intensol) 1mg/mL [30mL]; Tab: 0.5mg*, 0.75mg*, 1mg*, 1.5mg*, 2mg*, 4mg*, 6mg* *scored

CONTRAINDICATIONS

Systemic fungal infections.

WARNINGS/PRECAUTIONS

May cause BP elevation, Na^+/water retention, and increased K^+ and Ca^{2+} excretion. May cause left ventricular free-wall rupture after a recent myocardial infarction; use with caution. May mask signs of current infection. May increase susceptibility to infections. Rule out latent or active amebiasis before initiating therapy. Use lowest possible dose to control treatment condition; reduce gradually if dosage reduction is possible. Caution with active/latent tuberculosis or tuberculin reactivity, active/latent peptic ulcers, diverticulitis, fresh intestinal anastomoses, nonspecific ulcerative colitis, HTN, and renal insufficiency. May have negative effects on pediatric growth; monitor growth and development of pediatric patients on prolonged use. May increase or decrease motility and number of spermatozoa in some patients. Enhanced effect in patients with cirrhosis. More serious/fatal course of chickenpox and measles reported; avoid exposure in patients who have not had these diseases. May produce posterior subcapsular cataracts, glaucoma with possible optic nerve damage, and enhance establishment of secondary ocular infections. Drug-induced secondary adrenocortical insufficiency may be minimized by gradual dose reduction. Psychic derangements, and emotional instability or psychotic tendencies aggravation may occur. Fat embolism reported. May suppress reactions to skin tests. False (-) dexamethasone suppression test results in patients being treated with indomethacin reported. (Elixir) Prolongation of coma and high incidence of pneumonia and GI bleeding in patients with cerebral malaria reported. Enhanced effect in patients with hypothyroidism. Caution with ocular herpes simplex, osteoporosis, myasthenia gravis. Withdrawal syndrome reported following prolonged use. May affect the nitroblue-tetrazolium test for bacterial infection and produce false-negative results. (Sol/Tab) Anaphylactoid reactions may occur. Caution with congestive heart failure (CHF). May produce reversible hypothalamic-pituitary-adrenal axis suppression with the potential for corticosteroid insufficiency after withdrawal. Changes in thyroid status may necessitate dose adjustment. May activate latent disease or exacerbate intercurrent infections. May exacerbate systemic fungal infections; avoid use unless needed to control life-threatening drug reactions. May increase risk of GI perforation with certain GI disorders. Caution with known or suspected *Strongyloides* infestation and in the elderly. Not for use in cerebral malaria and active ocular herpes simplex. Not recommended in optic neuritis treatment. Kaposi's sarcoma reported. Acute myopathy reported with use of high doses. Creatinine kinase elevation may occur. May elevate intraocular pressure (IOP); monitor IOP if used for >6 weeks.

ADVERSE REACTIONS

Fluid retention, Na^+ retention, muscle weakness, osteoporosis, peptic ulcer, pancreatitis, ulcerative esophagitis, impaired wound healing, headache, psychic disturbances, growth suppression (pediatrics), glaucoma, weight gain, nausea, malaise.

DRUG INTERACTIONS

Live or live, attenuated vaccines are contraindicated with immunosuppressive doses. May diminish response to toxoids and live or inactivated vaccines. Observe closely for hypokalemia with K^+-depleting agents (eg, amphotericin B, diuretics). Dose adjustment of antidiabetic agents may be required. Barbiturates, phenytoin, and rifampin may enhance metabolism; may need to increase corticosteroid dose. Caution with aspirin (ASA) in patients with hypoprothrombinemia. Ephedrine may enhance metabolic clearance; may require an increase in corticosteroid dose. (Elixir) Phenobarbital may enhance the metabolic clearance; may require adjustment of corticosteroid dose. Monitor PT frequently with coumarin anticoagulants. (Sol/Tab) May potentiate replication of some organisms contained in live, attenuated vaccines. D/C anticholinesterase agents at least 24 hrs before start of therapy. Monitor coagulation indices with warfarin. Hepatic enzyme inducers (eg, carbamazepine) may enhance metabolism; may need to increase corticosteroid dose. CYP3A4 inhibitors may increase plasma concentrations. May decrease plasma concentrations of CYP3A4 substrates (eg, indinavir). Convulsions and increased activity of both drugs reported with cyclosporine. May increase risk of arrhythmias due to hypokalemia with digitalis glycosides. Estrogens and ketoconazole may decrease metabolism. ASA or other NSAIDs may increase risk of GI side effects. May increase clearance of salicylates. Acute myopathy reported with neuromuscular-blocking drugs (eg, pancuronium). May decrease concentrations of isoniazid. Cholestyramine may increase clearance. Cardiac enlargement and CHF reported when hydrocortisone is used with amphotericin B. Aminoglutethimide may diminish adrenal suppression. Macrolide antibiotics may decrease clearance. May increase and decrease levels of phenytoin, leading to alterations in seizure control. Caution with thalidomide; toxic epidermal necrolysis reported.

NURSING CONSIDERATIONS

Assessment: Assess for vaccination history, current infections, systemic fungal infections, thyroid status, latent/active amebiasis, cerebral malaria, ocular herpes simplex, cirrhosis, emotional instability or psychotic tendencies, any condition where treatment is cautioned, pregnancy/nursing status, and possible drug interactions.

Monitoring: Monitor for Na^+/water retention, infections/secondary ocular infections, changes in thyroid status, posterior subcapsular cataracts, glaucoma, optic nerve damage, Kaposi's sarcoma, development of osteoporosis, acute myopathy, creatinine kinase elevation, psychic derangements, emotional instability or psychotic tendencies aggravation, and other adverse effects. Monitor IOP, BP, and serum K^+ and Ca^{2+} levels. Monitor bone growth and development in pediatric patients.

Patient Counseling: Instruct not to d/c therapy abruptly or without medical supervision. Advise to inform any medical attendants about current corticosteroid therapies. Instruct to seek medical advice if an acute illness including fever or other signs of infection develop. Advise to avoid exposure to chickenpox or measles; if exposed, instruct to seek medical advice without delay.

Storage: 20-25°C (68-77°F). (Tab) Protect from moisture. (Intensol) Do not freeze. Discard opened bottle after 90 days.

DEXILANT – dexlansoprazole

RX

Class: Proton pump inhibitor

ADULT DOSAGE

Erosive Esophagitis

Healing:
60mg qd for up to 8 weeks

Maint of Healed Erosive Esophagitis and Relief of Heartburn:
30mg qd for up to 6 months

Symptomatic Nonerosive Gastroesophageal Reflux Disease
30mg qd for 4 weeks

PEDIATRIC DOSAGE

Pediatric use may not have been established

DOSE MODIFICATION

Hepatic Impairment

Moderate (Child-Pugh Class B):
Max Dose: 30mg qd

ADMINISTRATION

Oral route

Take w/o regard to food
Swallow cap whole; do not chew

Administration w/ Applesauce
Open cap and sprinkle intact granules on 1 tbsp of applesauce
Swallow immediately; do not chew granules

Administration w/ Water in an Oral Syringe
Open the cap and empty the granules into 20mL of water
Withdraw the entire mixture into a syringe and gently swirl the syringe
Administer immediately
Refill the syringe 2 more times w/ 10mL of water, swirl gently, and administer

Administration w/ Water Via a Nasogastric Tube (≥16 French)
Open the cap and empty the granules into 20mL of water
Withdraw the entire mixture into a catheter-tip syringe
Swirl the syringe gently and immediately inject the mixture through the NG tube into the stomach
Refill the syringe w/ 10mL of water, swirl gently, and flush the tube
Refill the syringe again w/ 10mL of water, swirl gently, and administer

HOW SUPPLIED

Cap, Delayed-Release: 30mg, 60mg

WARNINGS/PRECAUTIONS

Symptomatic response does not preclude the presence of gastric malignancy. Acute interstitial nephritis reported; d/c if this develops. Cyanocobalamin (vitamin B12) deficiency may occur due to malabsorption with daily long-term treatment (eg, >3 yrs) with any acid-suppressing medications. May increase risk of *Clostridium difficile*-associated diarrhea (CDAD), especially in hospitalized patients. May increase risk for osteoporosis-related fractures of the hip, wrist, or spine, especially with high-dose and long-term therapy. Use lowest dose and shortest duration appropriate to the conditions being treated. Hypomagnesemia reported and may require Mg^{2+} replacement and discontinuation of therapy; consider monitoring Mg^{2+} levels prior to and periodically during therapy with prolonged treatment.

ADVERSE REACTIONS

Diarrhea, abdominal pain, nausea, URTI.

DRUG INTERACTIONS

May reduce absorption of drugs where gastric pH is an important determinant of their bioavailability; ampicillin esters, ketoconazole, atazanavir, iron salts, erlotinib, and mycophenolate mofetil (MMF) absorption can decrease, while digoxin absorption can increase. May substantially decrease atazanavir concentrations; avoid concurrent use. Caution in transplant patients receiving MMF. Monitor for increases in INR and PT with warfarin. May increase tacrolimus levels. Caution with digoxin or other drugs that may cause hypomagnesemia (eg, diuretics). May elevate and prolong levels of MTX and/or its metabolite, possibly leading to toxicities; consider temporary withdrawal of therapy with high-dose MTX.

NURSING CONSIDERATIONS

Assessment: Assess for hypersensitivity to the drug, risk for osteoporosis-related fractures, hepatic impairment, pregnancy/nursing status, and possible drug interactions. Obtain baseline Mg^{2+} levels.

Monitoring: Monitor for signs/symptoms of acute interstitial nephritis, cyanocobalamin deficiency, CDAD, bone fractures, hypersensitivity reactions, and other adverse reactions. Monitor Mg^{2+} levels periodically. Monitor INR and PT when given with warfarin.

Patient Counseling: Instruct to watch for signs of an allergic reaction, as these could be serious and may require discontinuation. Advise to immediately report and seek care for diarrhea that does not improve, and for any cardiovascular/neurological symptoms (eg, palpitations, dizziness, seizures, tetany). Instruct to take ud and to inform physician of any other medication use.

Storage: 25°C (77°F); excursions permitted to 15-30°C (59-86°F).

DiaBeta – glyburide

RX

Class: Sulfonylurea (2nd generation)

ADULT DOSAGE

Type 2 Diabetes Mellitus

Initial: 2.5-5mg qd; 1.25mg qd if more sensitive to hypoglycemic drugs

Titrate: Increase by ≤2.5mg at weekly intervals

Maint: 1.25-20mg/day as single dose or in divided doses

Max: 20mg/day

Transferring from Other Oral Antidiabetic Agents:

Initial: 2.5-5mg qd

No transition period or initial priming dose necessary

Monitor carefully during 1st two weeks when transitioning from chlorpropamide, due to overlapping drug effects

Transferring from Insulin:

Insulin Dose <20 U/Day:
2.5-5mg qd

Insulin Dose 20-40 U/Day:
5mg qd

Insulin Dose >40 U/Day:
Decrease insulin dose by 50% and start w/ 5mg qd

Progressively withdraw insulin and increase dose in increments of 1.25-2.5mg every 2-10 days

PEDIATRIC DOSAGE

Pediatric use may not have been established

DOSE MODIFICATION

Renal Impairment

Initial/Maint: Dose conservatively

Hepatic Impairment

Initial/Maint: Dose conservatively

Concomitant Medications

Colesevelam: Administer at least 4 hrs prior to colesevelam

Elderly

Elderly/Debilitated/Malnourished:

Initial/Maint: Dose conservatively

ADMINISTRATION

Oral route

Take w/ breakfast or 1st main meal

HOW SUPPLIED

Tab: 1.25mg*, 2.5mg*, 5mg* *scored

CONTRAINDICATIONS

Type 1 DM or diabetic ketoacidosis, with or without coma. Coadministration with bosentan.

WARNINGS/PRECAUTIONS

Caution during the first 2 weeks of therapy if transferring from chlorpropamide. May be associated with increased cardiovascular (CV) mortality. May produce severe hypoglycemia; increased risk when caloric intake is deficient, after severe/prolonged exercise, with severe renal/hepatic insufficiency, with adrenal/pituitary insufficiency, or in elderly, debilitated, or malnourished patients.

Loss of glycemic control may occur when exposed to stress (eg, fever, trauma, infection, surgery); may be necessary to d/c therapy and administer insulin. Secondary failure may occur over a period of time. May cause hemolytic anemia; caution with G6PD deficiency and consider a non-sulfonylurea alternative. Caution in elderly. Not bioequivalent to Glynase PresTab and therefore not substitutable.

ADVERSE REACTIONS

Hypoglycemia, nausea, epigastric fullness, heartburn, hyponatremia, LFT abnormalities, photosensitivity reactions, leukopenia, agranulocytosis, thrombocytopenia, porphyria cutanea tarda, blurred vision, changes in accommodation, angioedema, arthralgia.

DRUG INTERACTIONS

See Contraindications and Dosage. Hypoglycemic effects may be potentiated by NSAIDs, ACE-inhibitors, disopyramide, fluoxetine, clarithromycin, fluoroquinolones, other highly protein-bound drugs, salicylates, sulfonamides, chloramphenicol, probenecid, MAOIs, and β-adrenergic blocking drugs; monitor closely for hypoglycemia during coadministration and for loss of glycemic control when such drugs are withdrawn. Increased risk of hypoglycemia with alcohol or use of >1 glucose-lowering drug. May be difficult to recognize hypoglycemia with β-adrenergic blocking drugs or other sympatholytics. Potential interaction leading to severe hypoglycemia reported with oral miconazole. Potentiates or weakens effects of coumarin derivatives. Rifampin may worsen glucose control. Thiazides and other diuretics, corticosteroids, phenothiazines, thyroid products, estrogens, oral contraceptives, phenytoin, nicotinic acid, sympathomimetics, calcium channel blockers, and isoniazid may produce hyperglycemia and may lead to loss of glycemic control; monitor closely for loss of control during coadministration and for hypoglycemia when such drugs are withdrawn. May increase cyclosporine plasma levels and toxicity; monitor and adjust dosage of cyclosporine. Colesevelam may decrease levels. Caution with inducers/inhibitors of CYP2C9.

NURSING CONSIDERATIONS

Assessment: Assess for previous hypersensitivity to drug or other sulfonamide derivatives, type of DM, risk factors of hypoglycemia, renal/hepatic impairment, G6PD deficiency, pregnancy/nursing status, and possible drug interactions. Obtain baseline FPG and HbA1c levels.

Monitoring: Monitor for CV effects, hypoglycemia, loss of glycemic control when exposed to stress, hypersensitivity reactions, secondary failure, hemolytic anemia, and other adverse reactions. Monitor FPG and HbA1c levels periodically.

Patient Counseling: Inform of the potential risks, benefits, and alternative modes of therapy. Counsel about importance of adherence to dietary instructions, regular exercise program, and regular testing of blood glucose. Inform about the symptoms, treatment, and predisposing conditions of hypoglycemia, as well as primary and secondary failure. During the insulin withdrawal period, instruct patients to test blood glucose and acetone in urine at least tid and report results to physician.

Storage: 25°C (77°F); excursions permitted to 15-30°C (59-86°F).

DICLEGIS — doxylamine succinate/pyridoxine hydrochloride RX

Class: Antihistamine/vitamin B6 analogue

ADULT DOSAGE

Nausea/Vomiting

Treatment of N/V of Pregnancy in Women Who Do Not Respond to Conservative Management:

Initial: 2 tabs hs (Day 1)

Titrate: If this dose adequately controls symptoms the next day, continue taking 2 tabs/day hs; if symptoms persist into the afternoon of Day 2, take the usual dose of 2 tabs hs that night then take 3 tabs starting on Day 3 (1 tab in the am and 2 tabs hs)

If dose adequately controls symptoms on Day 4, continue taking 3 tabs/day; otherwise take 4 tabs starting on Day 4 (1 tab in the am, 1 tab mid-afternoon, and 2 tabs hs)

Max: 4 tabs/day (1 tab in the am, 1 tab mid-afternoon, and 2 tabs hs)

Reassess for continued need as pregnancy progresses

PEDIATRIC DOSAGE

Pediatric use may not have been established

ADMINISTRATION

Oral route

Take on an empty stomach w/ a glass of water
Swallow tab whole; do not crush, chew, or split
Take as a daily prescription and not prn

HOW SUPPLIED

Tab, Delayed Release: (Doxylamine-Pyridoxine) 10mg-10mg

CONTRAINDICATIONS

Concomitant MAIOs.

WARNINGS/PRECAUTIONS

Not studied in women with hyperemesis gravidarum. May cause somnolence and impair physical/mental abilities. Caution with asthma, increased intraocular pressure (IOP), narrow-angle glaucoma, stenosing peptic ulcer, pyloroduodenal obstruction, and urinary bladder-neck obstruction.

ADVERSE REACTIONS

Somnolence, dyspnea, vertigo, visual disturbances, abdominal pain, fatigue, dizziness, anxiety, dysuria, pruritus, palpitation, constipation, malaise, paresthesia, rash.

DRUG INTERACTIONS

See Contraindications. Not recommended with alcohol and other CNS depressants (eg, hypnotic sedatives, tranquilizers).

NURSING CONSIDERATIONS

Assessment: Assess for hypersensitivity reaction to the drug or to its components, hyperemesis gravidarum, asthma, IOP, narrow-angle glaucoma, stenosing peptic ulcer, pyloroduodenal obstruction, urinary bladder-neck obstruction, nursing status, and possible drug interactions.

Monitoring: Monitor for somnolence and other adverse reactions. Reassess for continued need as pregnancy progresses.

Patient Counseling: Instruct to avoid engaging in activities requiring complete mental alertness (eg, driving, operating heavy machinery), until cleared to do so. Inform of the importance of not taking the medication with alcohol or sedating medications including other antihistamines, opiates, and sleep aids.

Storage: 20-25°C (68-77°F); excursions permitted between 15-30°C (59-86°F). Protect from moisture.

Dicyclomine HCl – dicyclomine hydrochloride RX

Class: Anticholinergic

OTHER BRAND NAMES

Bentyl

ADULT DOSAGE

Functional Bowel/Irritable Bowel Syndrome

PO:

Initial: 20mg qid

Titrate: May increase to 40mg qid after 1 week of initial dose, unless side effects limit dose escalation. D/C if efficacy not achieved w/in 2 weeks or side effects require doses below 80mg/day

Inj:

Initial: 10-20mg IM qid for 1-2 days if unable to take oral medication

PEDIATRIC DOSAGE

Pediatric use may not have been established

DOSE MODIFICATION

Elderly

Start at lower end of dosing range

ADMINISTRATION

Oral, IM route

Aspirate the syringe before injecting to avoid intravascular inj

HOW SUPPLIED

Sol: 10mg/5mL [473mL]; (Bentyl) Cap: 10mg; Inj: 10mg/mL; Tab: 20mg

CONTRAINDICATIONS

GI tract obstructive disease, obstructive uropathy, severe ulcerative colitis, reflux esophagitis, glaucoma, myasthenia gravis, unstable cardiovascular status in acute hemorrhage, nursing mothers, infants <6 months of age.

WARNINGS/PRECAUTIONS

Caution in conditions characterized by tachyarrhythmia (eg, thyrotoxicosis, CHF, in cardiac surgery). Caution with coronary heart disease; ischemia and infarction may worsen. Peripheral effects (eg, dryness of mouth with difficulty in swallowing/talking) and CNS signs/symptoms (eg, confusional state, disorientation, amnesia) reported. Psychosis and delirium reported in sensitive individuals (eg, elderly patients and/or in patients with mental illness) given anticholinergic drugs. Heat prostration may occur in high environmental temperatures; d/c if symptoms occur and institute supportive measures. May impair mental abilities. Diarrhea may be the early symptom of incomplete intestinal obstruction, especially with ileostomy/colostomy patients; treatment would be inappropriate and possibly harmful. Caution with ulcerative colitis; large doses may suppress intestinal motility and produce paralytic ileus, and use of this drug may precipitate or aggravate the serious complication of toxic megacolon. Caution in patients with HTN, fever, autonomic neuropathy, prostatic enlargement, hepatic/renal impairment, and in the elderly. (Cap/Tab/Inj) Avoid with myasthenia gravis except to reduce adverse muscarinic effects of an anticholinesterase. Ogilvie's syndrome (colonic pseudo-obstruction) rarely reported. Caution with Salmonella dysentery; toxic dilation of intestine and intestinal perforation may occur. (Inj) For IM use only; inadvertent IV use may result in thrombosis, thrombophlebitis, and inj-site reactions. (Sol) Caution with hyperthyroidism and hiatal hernia.

ADVERSE REACTIONS

Dry mouth, dizziness, blurred vision, nausea, somnolence, asthenia, nervousness.

DRUG INTERACTIONS

May antagonize the effect of antiglaucoma agents and drugs that alter GI motility (eg, metoclopramide). Avoid concomitant use with corticosteroids in glaucoma patients. Potentiated by amantadine, Class I antiarrhythmics (eg, quinidine), antihistamines, antipsychotics (eg, phenothiazines), benzodiazepines, MAOIs, narcotic analgesics (eg, meperidine), nitrates/nitrites, sympathomimetics, TCAs, and other drugs with anticholinergic activity. Antacids may interfere with absorption; avoid simultaneous use. May affect GI absorption of various drugs by affecting GI motility; increased serum digoxin concentration may result with slowly dissolving forms of digoxin. Inhibiting effects on gastric hydrochloric acid secretion are antagonized by drugs used to treat achlorhydria and those used to test gastric secretion.

NURSING CONSIDERATIONS

Assessment: Assess for cardiovascular conditions, myasthenia gravis, glaucoma, intestinal obstruction, psychosis, ulcerative colitis, tachycardia, or any other conditions where treatment is contraindicated or cautioned. Assess for history of hypersensitivity, pregnancy/nursing status, renal/hepatic dysfunction, and for possible drug interactions.

Monitoring: Monitor for increased HR, worsening of ischemia/infarction, heat prostration, drowsiness, blurred vision, confusion, disorientation, hallucinations, paralytic ileus with large doses, urinary retention, hypersensitivity reactions, and for other adverse reactions. Monitor renal function.

Patient Counseling: Counsel on proper administration. Advise not to breastfeed while on therapy and not to administer to infants <6 months of age. Advise not to engage in activities requiring mental alertness (eg, operating motor vehicle or other machinery) or to perform hazardous work while taking the drug. Inform of risk of heat prostration in high environmental temperature; instruct to d/c if symptoms occur and to consult a physician.

Storage: (Cap/Tab/Inj) Room temperature <30°C (86°F). Sol: 20-25°C (68-77°F). Inj: Protect from freezing. Tab: Avoid exposure to direct sunlight.

DIFFERIN – adapalene

RX

Class: Naphthoic acid derivative (retinoid-like)

ADULT DOSAGE

Acne Vulgaris

Cre:

Apply a thin film qpm

0.1% Gel:

Apply a thin film qpm after washing

0.3% Gel:

Apply a thin film qpm after washing

Reevaluate if therapeutic results are not noticed after 12 weeks of treatment

Lot:

Apply a thin film (3-4 actuations of the pump) qd after washing

PEDIATRIC DOSAGE

Acne Vulgaris

≥12 Years:

Cre:

Apply a thin film qpm

0.1% Gel:

Apply a thin film qpm after washing

0.3% Gel:

Apply a thin film qpm after washing

Reevaluate if therapeutic results are not noticed after 12 weeks of treatment

Lot:

Apply a thin film (3-4 actuations of the pump) qd after washing

ADMINISTRATION
Topical route

Apply enough to cover the entire face or other affected areas completely and lightly

HOW SUPPLIED
Cre: 0.1% [45g]; Gel: 0.1% [45g], 0.3% [15g, 45g tube; 45g pump]; Lot: 0.1% [2 oz.]

WARNINGS/PRECAUTIONS
Not for ophthalmic, oral, or intravaginal use. Avoid exposure to sunlight, including sunlamps; caution in patients with high levels of sun exposure and those with inherent sensitivity to sun. Extreme weather (eg, wind, cold) may cause irritation. Local skin irritation may be experienced; depending on severity, may use moisturizer, reduce frequency of application, or d/c use. (Cre/Gel) Apparent exacerbation of acne may occur. (Cre/0.1% Gel) D/C if reaction suggesting sensitivity or chemical irritation occurs. (Cre/0.3% Gel) A mild transitory sensation of warmth or slight stinging may occur shortly after application. (0.1% Gel) Avoid in patients with sunburn until fully recovered. (0.3% Gel) Reactions characterized by pruritus, face edema, eyelid edema, and lip swelling, requiring medical treatment reported; d/c use if experiencing allergic or anaphylactoid/anaphylactic reactions during therapy.

ADVERSE REACTIONS
Local cutaneous irritation. (0.3% Gel) Skin discomfort.

DRUG INTERACTIONS
Caution with preparations containing sulfur, resorcinol, or salicylic acid. (Cre/Gel) Do not start therapy until effects of such preparations in the skin have subsided. Caution with other potentially irritating topical products (medicated/abrasive soaps and cleansers, soaps and cosmetics that have a strong drying effect, and products with high concentrations of alcohol, astringents, spices, or lime). (Lot) Caution with concomitant topical acne therapy, especially with peeling, desquamating, or abrasive agents. Avoid with other potentially irritating topical products.

NURSING CONSIDERATIONS

Assessment: Assess for excessive sun exposure, sun sensitivity, hypersensitivity to any of the components of the drug, pregnancy/nursing status, and for possible drug interactions. Assess for presence of cuts, abrasions, eczematous, or sunburned skin at the treatment site.

Monitoring: Monitor for sensitivity or chemical irritation, cutaneous signs/symptoms, and other adverse reactions.

Patient Counseling: Advise to cleanse area with mild or soapless cleanser before applying the medication. Instruct to avoid or minimize exposure to sunlight and sunlamps. Instruct to use sunscreen products and protective clothing when exposure cannot be avoided. Instruct not to use more than the recommended amount. Instruct to avoid contact with eyes, lips, angles of the nose, and mucous membranes. Advise not to apply medication to cuts, abrasions, eczematous, or sunburned skin. Counsel to avoid use of waxing as depilatory method. Advise to use moisturizers if necessary and to avoid products containing α-hydroxyl or glycolic acids. Instruct to use externally and ud. Inform that an apparent exacerbation of acne may occur during the early weeks of therapy and that it should not be considered a reason for discontinuation. Instruct to contact the physician if signs of allergy or hypersensitivity develop. (Cre/0.3% Gel/Lot) Avoid waxing as a depilatory method.

Storage: 20-25°C (68-77°F); excursions permitted to 15-30°C (59-86°F). Protect from freezing. (Lot) Do not refrigerate. Protect from light. Keep away from heat.

DIFICID – fidaxomicin — RX

Class: Macrolide

ADULT DOSAGE

***Clostridium difficile*-Associated Diarrhea**

200mg bid for 10 days

PEDIATRIC DOSAGE

Pediatric use may not have been established

ADMINISTRATION
Oral route

Take w/ or w/o food

HOW SUPPLIED
Tab: 200mg

WARNINGS/PRECAUTIONS
Not effective for treatment of systemic infections. Acute hypersensitivity reactions (eg, dyspnea, rash, pruritus) reported; d/c therapy if severe hypersensitivity reaction occurs. May increase the risk of the development of drug resistant bacteria when prescribed in the absence of a proven or strongly suspected *C. difficile* infection.

ADVERSE REACTIONS
N/V, abdominal pain, GI hemorrhage.

NURSING CONSIDERATIONS

Assessment: Assess for hypersensitivity to the drug, macrolide allergy, and pregnancy/nursing status.

Monitoring: Monitor for development of drug resistant bacteria, hypersensitivity reactions, and other adverse reactions.

Patient Counseling: Inform that drug only treats CDAD infections, not other bacterial or viral infections. Instruct to take exactly ud; inform that skipping doses or not completing full course may decrease effectiveness and increase antibiotic resistance.

Storage: 20-25°C (68-77°F); excursions permitted 15-30°C (59-86°F).

DIFLUCAN ORAL – fluconazole

RX

Class: Azole antifungal

ADULT DOSAGE

Prophylaxis in Bone Marrow Transplant

Decrease Incidence of Candidiasis:
400mg qd
Start prophylaxis several days before the anticipated onset of neutropenia in patients who are anticipated to have severe granulocytopenia (<500 neutrophils/mm^3); continue for 7 days after the neutrophil count rises >1000 cells/mm^3

Cryptococcal Meningitis
400mg on 1st day, followed by 200mg qd for 10-12 weeks after the CSF becomes culture (-); a dose of 400mg qd may be used

Suppression of Cryptococcal Meningitis Relapse in AIDS:
200mg qd

Vaginal Candidiasis

PO Single Dose:
150mg

Oropharyngeal Candidiasis
200mg on 1st day, followed by 100mg qd for ≥2 weeks

Esophageal Candidiasis
200mg on 1st day, followed by 100mg qd for a minimum of 3 weeks and for ≥2 weeks following resolution of symptoms
Doses up to 400mg/day may be used

***Candida* Infections**

Systemic Infections:
Max: 400mg qd

UTIs/Peritonitis:
50-200mg/day

PEDIATRIC DOSAGE

Cryptococcal Meningitis
12mg/kg on 1st day, followed by 6mg/kg qd for 10-12 weeks after the CSF becomes culture (-); a dose of 12mg/kg qd may be used (not to exceed 600mg/day)

Suppression of Cryptococcal Meningitis Relapse in AIDS:
6mg/kg qd

***Candida* Infections**

Systemic:
6-12mg/kg/day (not to exceed 600mg/day)

Esophageal Candidiasis
6mg/kg on 1st day, followed by 3mg/kg qd for a minimum of 3 weeks and for ≥2 weeks following resolution of symptoms; doses up to 12mg/kg/day may be used (not to exceed 600mg/day)

Oropharyngeal Candidiasis
6mg/kg on 1st day, followed by 3mg/kg qd for ≥2 weeks

DOSE MODIFICATION

Renal Impairment

Multiple Doses:
Initial LD: 50-400mg
Maint:
CrCl ≤50mL/min (No Dialysis): Give 50% of recommended dose
Regular Dialysis: Give 100% of recommended dose after each dialysis; on non-dialysis days, administer a reduced dose based on CrCl

ADMINISTRATION
Oral route

Take w/ or w/o food
Shake sus well before using

Sus
To reconstitute, add 24mL of distilled or purified water to bottle

HOW SUPPLIED
Sus: 10mg/mL, 40mg/mL [35mL]; Tab: 50mg, 100mg, 150mg, 200mg

CONTRAINDICATIONS
Coadministration with terfenadine (with multiple doses ≥400mg of fluconazole), other drugs known to prolong the QT interval and that are metabolized via the enzyme CYP3A4 (eg, cisapride, astemizole, erythromycin, pimozide, quinidine).

WARNINGS/PRECAUTIONS
Associated with rare cases of serious hepatic toxicity; monitor for more severe hepatic injury if abnormal LFTs develop. D/C if clinical signs and symptoms consistent with liver disease develop. Anaphylaxis reported (rare). Exfoliative skin disorders reported; closely monitor patients with deep seated fungal infections who develop rashes during treatment and d/c if lesions progress. D/C therapy if rash develops in patients treated for superficial fungal infection. QT prolongation and torsades de pointes reported (rare); caution with potentially proarrhythmic conditions. Caution in elderly or with renal/hepatic dysfunction. May impair mental/physical abilities. (Sus) Contains sucrose; do not use in patients with hereditary fructose, glucose/galactose malabsorption, and sucrase-isomaltase deficiency. (Tab) Consider risk versus benefits of single dose oral tab versus intravaginal agent therapy for the treatment of vaginal yeast infections.

ADVERSE REACTIONS
Headache, N/V, abdominal pain, diarrhea.

DRUG INTERACTIONS
See Contraindications. Carefully monitor coadministration of fluconazole at doses <400mg/day with terfenadine. Avoid with voriconazole. Risk of increased plasma concentration of compounds metabolized by CYP2C9 and CYP3A4; caution when coadministered and monitor patients carefully. May precipitate clinically significant hypoglycemia with oral hypoglycemics; monitor blood glucose and adjust dose of sulfonylurea as necessary. May increase PT with coumarin-type anticoagulants; monitor PT and, if necessary, adjust warfarin dose. May increase levels of phenytoin, cyclosporine, theophylline, rifabutin, oral tacrolimus, triazolam, celecoxib, halofantrine, flurbiprofen, racemic ibuprofen, methadone, saquinavir, sirolimus, and vinca alkaloids (eg, vincristine, vinblastine). May increase exposure of ethinyl estradiol and levonorgestrel. May reduce the metabolism and increase levels of tolbutamide, glyburide, and glipizide. Monitor SrCr with cyclosporine. Rifampin may enhance metabolism. May increase levels and psychomotor effects of oral midazolam; consider dose reduction of short-acting benzodiazepines metabolized by CYP450, and monitor appropriately. May increase systemic exposure to tofacitinib; reduce tofacitinib dose when given concomitantly. HCTZ may increase levels. May reduce clearance/distribution volume and prolong $T_{1/2}$ of alfentanil. May increase effect of amitriptyline and nortriptyline. May increase levels of zidovudine; consider dose reduction. May potentially increase systemic exposure of other NSAIDs that are metabolized by CYP2C9 (eg, naproxen, lornoxicam, meloxicam, diclofenac), and calcium channel antagonists. Risk of carbamazepine toxicity. May increase serum bilirubin and SrCr with cyclophosphamide. May significantly delay elimination of fentanyl, leading to respiratory depression. May increase risk of myopathy and rhabdomyolysis with HMG-CoA reductase inhibitors metabolized through CYP3A4 (eg, atorvastatin, simvastatin) or through CYP2C9 (eg, fluvastatin); monitor for symptoms and d/c statin if a marked increase in creatinine kinase is observed or myopathy/rhabdomyolysis is diagnosed or suspected. May inhibit the metabolism of losartan; monitor BP continuously. Acute adrenal cortex insufficiency reported after discontinuation of a 3-month therapy with fluconazole in a liver-transplanted patient treated with prednisone. CNS-related undesirable effects reported with all-trans-retinoid acid (an acid form of vitamin A).

NURSING CONSIDERATIONS

Assessment: Assess for hypersensitivity to the drug, renal/hepatic impairment, AIDS, malignancies, risk factors for QT prolongation, any other conditions where treatment is contraindicated or cautioned, pregnancy/nursing status, and possible drug interactions. Obtain specimens for fungal culture and other relevant lab studies (serology, histopathology) to isolate and identify causative organisms. (Sus) Assess for hereditary fructose, glucose/galactose malabsorption, and sucrase-isomaltase deficiency.

Monitoring: Monitor for signs/symptoms of liver disease, rash, and other adverse reactions. Monitor LFTs and renal function. Monitor PT when used with coumarin-type anticoagulants.

Patient Counseling: Inform about risks/benefits of therapy. Advise to notify physician if pregnant/nursing and counsel about potential hazard to the fetus if pregnant or pregnancy occurs. Instruct to inform physician of all medications currently being taken.

Storage: Tab: <30°C (86°F). Sus: Dry Powder: <30°C (86°F). Reconstituted: 5-30°C (41-86°F); discard unused portion after 2 weeks. Protect from freezing.

DIGOXIN ORAL – digoxin

Class: Cardiac glycoside

RX

OTHER BRAND NAMES

Lanoxin

ADULT DOSAGE

Atrial Fibrillation

Control of Ventricular Response Rate in Chronic A-Fib:

Dosing can be either initiated with LD followed by maint dosing if rapid titration is desired or initiated w/ maint dosing w/o LD

Sol:

LD: 10-15mcg/kg

Maint: 3-4.5mcg/kg/dose qd

Tab:

Initial: Give 1/2 the total LD, then 1/4 the LD every 6-8 hrs, twice, w/ careful assessment of clinical response and toxicity before each dose

LD: 10-15mcg/kg

Starting Maint: 3.4-5.1mcg/kg/day qd

Titrate: May be increased every 2 weeks according to clinical response, serum drug levels, and toxicity

Heart Failure

Mild to Moderate:

Dosing can be either initiated w/ LD followed by maint dosing if rapid titration is desired or initiated w/ maint dosing w/o LD

Sol:

LD: 10-15mcg/kg

Maint: 3-4.5mcg/kg/dose qd

Tab:

Initial: Give 1/2 the total LD, then 1/4 the LD every 6-8 hrs, twice, w/ careful assessment of clinical response and toxicity before each dose

LD: 10-15mcg/kg

Starting Maint: 3.4-5.1mcg/kg/day qd

Titrate: May be increased every 2 weeks according to clinical response, serum drug levels, and toxicity

Where possible, use in combination with a diuretic and an ACE inhibitor

Conversions

IV to PO Conversion:

50mcg inj = 62.5mcg tab

100mcg inj = 125mcg tab

200mcg inj = 250mcg tab

400mcg inj = 500mcg tab

PEDIATRIC DOSAGE

Heart Failure

Increase Myocardial Contractility:

Dosing can be either initiated w/ LD followed by maint dosing if rapid titration is desired or initiated w/ maint dosing w/o LD

Sol:

LD (If needed):

Give 1/2 the total as the 1st dose

Additional fractions of planned total dose may be given at 4- to 8-hr intervals, w/ careful assessment of clinical response before each additional dose

Premature Infants: 20-30mcg/kg

Full-Term Infants: 25-35mcg/kg

1-24 Months: 35-60mcg/kg

2-5 Years: 30-45mcg/kg

5-10 Years: 20-35mcg/kg

>10 Years: 10-15mcg/kg

Maint:

Premature Infants: 2.3-3.9mcg/kg/dose bid

Full-Term Infants: 3.8-5.6mcg/kg/dose bid

1-24 Months: 5.6-9.4mcg/kg/dose bid

2-5 Years: 4.7-6.6mcg/kg/dose bid

5-10 Years: 2.8-5.6mcg/kg/dose bid

>10 Years: 3-4.5mcg/kg/dose qd

Tab:

Initial: Give 1/2 the total LD, then 1/4 the LD every 6-8 hrs twice, w/ careful assessment of clinical response and toxicity before each dose

LD:

5-10 Years: 20-45mcg/kg

>10 Years: 10-15mcg/kg

Starting Maint:

5-10 Years: 3.2-6.4mcg/kg/dose bid

>10 Years: 3.4-5.1mcg/kg/day qd

Titrate: May be increased every 2 weeks according to clinical response, serum drug levels, and toxicity

DOSE MODIFICATION

Renal Impairment

Sol/Tab:

Refer to PI for recommended maint dose according to lean body weight and renal function

ADMINISTRATION

Oral route

Sol

The calibrated dropper supplied w/ the 60mL bottle is not appropriate to measure doses <0.2mL.

HOW SUPPLIED

Sol: 0.05mg/mL [60mL]; (Lanoxin) Tab: 62.5mcg, 125mcg*, 187.5mcg, 250mcg* *scored

CONTRAINDICATIONS

Ventricular fibrillation.

WARNINGS/PRECAUTIONS

Increased risk of ventricular fibrillation in patients with Wolff-Parkinson-White syndrome who develop A-fib. May cause severe sinus bradycardia or sinoatrial block with preexisting sinus node disease and may cause advanced or complete heart block in patients with preexisting incomplete atrioventricular (AV) block; consider insertion of a pacemaker before treatment. Avoid in patients with HF associated with preserved left ventricular ejection fraction (eg, restrictive cardiomyopathy, constrictive pericarditis, amyloid heart disease, acute cor pulmonale), idiopathic hypertrophic subaortic stenosis, and myocarditis. May be desirable to reduce dose or d/c therapy 1-2 days prior to electrical cardioversion of A-fib. If digitalis toxicity is suspected, delay elective cardioversion and if it is not prudent to delay cardioversion, select the lowest possible energy level to avoid provoking ventricular arrhythmias. Hypocalcemia may nullify the effects of treatment. Hypothyroidism may reduce the requirements for therapy. HF and/or atrial arrhythmias resulting from hypermetabolic or hyperdynamic states (eg, hyperthyroidism, hypoxia, arteriovenous shunt) are best treated by addressing the underlying condition. Signs/symptoms of digoxin toxicity may be mistaken for worsening symptoms of CHF. May increase myocardial oxygen demand and ischemia in patients with acute MI (AMI); not recommended in patients with AMI. Caution with impaired renal function and in the elderly. Endogenous substances of unknown composition (digoxin-like immunoreactive substances) may interfere with standard radioimmunoassays for digoxin. (Sol) May result in potentially detrimental increases in coronary vascular resistance. (Tab) Avoid with acute cor pulmonale. Patients with low body weight, advanced age or impaired renal function, hypokalemia, hypercalcemia, or hypomagnesia may be predisposed to digoxin toxicity; assess serum electrolytes and renal function periodically. Patients with beri beri heart disease may fail to respond adequately to therapy if the underlying thiamine deficiency is not treated concomitantly.

ADVERSE REACTIONS

Cardiac arrhythmias, N/V, abdominal pain, intestinal ischemia, hemorrhagic necrosis of the intestines, headache, weakness, dizziness, apathy, mental disturbances.

DRUG INTERACTIONS

Potential to alter digoxin pharmacokinetics with drugs that induce/inhibit P-glycoprotein in the intestine/kidney. May increase risk of arrhythmias with rapid IV calcium administration, sympathomimetics (epinephrine, norepinephrine, dopamine), and succinylcholine. Increased digoxin dose requirement with thyroid supplements. Calcium channel blockers and β-adrenergic blockers produce additive effects on AV node conduction, which can result in bradycardia and advanced or complete heart block. Higher rate of torsades de pointes with dofetilide. Teriparatide transiently increases serum calcium. Increased levels with amiodarone, captopril, clarithromycin, erythromycin, itraconazole, nitrendipine, propafenone, quinidine, ranolazine, ritonavir, tetracycline, verapamil, carvedilol, diltiazem, indomethacin, nifedipine, propantheline, spironolactone, telmisartan, alprazolam, azithromycin, cyclosporine, diclofenac, diphenoxylate, epoprostenol, esomeprazole, ketoconazole, lansoprazole, metformin, omeprazole, rabeprazole. Decreased levels with acarbose, activated charcoal, albuterol, antacids, cholestyramine, colestipol, exenatide, kaolin-pectin, meals high in bran, metoclopramide, miglitol, neomycin, rifampin, St. John's wort, sucralfate, sulfasalazine. Proarrhythmic events reported to be more common in patients receiving concomitant therapy with sotalol. Refer to PI for dose adjustment information when used with certain concomitant therapies. (Sol) Increased PR interval and QRS duration reported with moricizine. Decreased levels with anti-cancer drugs, salbutamol. (Tab) Increased levels with dronedarone, gentamicin, atorvastatin, nefazodone, quinine, saquinavir, tolvaptan, trimethoprim, ibuprofen. Decreased levels with certain cancer chemotherapy or radiation therapy, penicillamine, and phenytoin. ACE inhibitors, ARBs, NSAIDs, and COX-2 inhibitors may impair digoxin excretion. Sudden death reported to be more common in patients receiving concomitant therapy with dronedarone.

NURSING CONSIDERATIONS

Assessment: Assess for known hypersensitivity to the drug or other digitalis preparations, ventricular fibrillation, myocarditis, hypermetabolic or hyperdynamic states, sinus node disease, AV block, pregnancy/nursing status, possible drug interactions, and any other conditions where treatment is cautioned. Assess serum electrolytes and renal function. Obtain a baseline digoxin level.

Monitoring: Monitor for signs/symptoms of severe sinus bradycardia, sinoatrial block, advanced or complete heart block, digoxin toxicity, vasoconstriction, and other adverse reactions. Monitor serum electrolytes and renal function periodically. Obtain serum digoxin concentrations just before the next dose or at least 6 hrs after the last dose. Monitor for clinical response.

Patient Counseling: Advise that therapy is a cardiac glycoside used to treat HF and heart arrhythmias. Instruct to take the drug ud by physician. Advise to notify physician if taking any OTC medications, including herbal medication, or if started on a new prescription. Inform that blood tests will be necessary to ensure the appropriate digoxin dose. Instruct to contact physician if N/V, persistent diarrhea, confusion, weakness, or visual disturbances occur. Advise parents or caregivers that symptoms of having too high doses may be difficult to recognize in infants and pediatric patients; symptoms such as weight loss, failure to thrive in infants, abdominal pain, and behavioral disturbances may be indications of digoxin toxicity. Suggest to monitor and record HR and BP daily. Instruct women of childbearing potential who become or are planning to become pregnant to consult physician prior to initiation or continuing therapy with digoxin. (Sol) Instruct to use calibrated dropper to measure the dose and to avoid less precise measuring tools (eg, tsp).

Storage: 25°C (77°F); excursions permitted to 15-30°C (59-86°F). Protect from light. (Tab) Store in dry place.

DILANTIN – phenytoin RX

Class: Hydantoin

OTHER BRAND NAMES

Dilantin Infatabs, Dilantin-125

ADULT DOSAGE

Epilepsy

Tonic-Clonic (Grand Mal) and Psychomotor (Temporal Lobe) Seizure:

Sus:

Initial: 125mg (1 tsp) tid

Titrate: May increase to 625mg (5 tsp) daily

Generalized Tonic-Clonic (Grand Mal) and Complex Partial (Psychomotor/Temporal Lobe) Seizures and Prevention/Treatment of Neurosurgery-Associated Seizures:

Cap, ER:

Divided Daily Dosing:

Initial: 100mg tid

Maint: 100mg tid-qid

Titrate: May increase up to 200mg tid, if necessary

QD Dosing:

May consider 300mg qd if seizure is controlled on divided doses of three 100mg caps daily

LD (Clinic/Hospital):

Initial: 1g in 3 divided doses (400mg, 300mg, 300mg) at 2-hr intervals

Maint: Start maint dose 24 hrs after LD

Do not give oral loading regimen in patients w/ history of renal/liver disease

Tab, Chewable:

Initial: 100mg (2 tabs) tid

Maint: 300-400mg (6-8 tabs) daily

Titrate: May increase to 600mg (12 tabs) daily

Do not change dose at intervals <7-10 days

PEDIATRIC DOSAGE

Epilepsy

Tonic-Clonic (Grand Mal) or Psychomotor (Temporal Lobe) Seizure:

Sus:

Initial: 5mg/kg/day in 2 or 3 equally divided doses

Maint: 4-8mg/kg/day

Max: 300mg/day

Generalized Tonic-Clonic (Grand Mal) and Complex Partial (Psychomotor/Temporal Lobe) Seizures and Prevention/Treatment of Neurosurgery-Associated Seizures:

Cap, ER/Tab, Chewable:

Initial: 5mg/kg/day in 2 or 3 equally divided doses

Maint: 4-8mg/kg/day

Max: 300mg/day

>6 Years: May require the minimum adult dose (300mg/day)

Do not change dose at intervals <7-10 days

DOSE MODIFICATION

Elderly

May require lower or less frequent dosing

Other Important Modifications

May require dose adjustment when switching from product formulated w/ free acid to product formulated w/ Na^+ salt and vice versa

ADMINISTRATION

Oral route

Tab, Chewable

May chew or swallow tab whole

Not for once-a-day dosing

If daily dose cannot be divided equally, give larger dose hs

Sus

Use an accurately calibrated measuring device to ensure accurate dosing

HOW SUPPLIED

Cap, ER: 30mg, 100mg; (Dilantin-125) Sus: 125mg/5mL [237mL]; (Infatabs) Tab, Chewable: 50mg*

*scored

CONTRAINDICATIONS

Coadministration with delavirdine.

WARNINGS/PRECAUTIONS

Caution in the interpretation of total phenytoin plasma concentrations with renal/hepatic disease, or in those with hypoalbuminemia. Avoid abrupt withdrawal; may precipitate status epilepticus. May increase risk of suicidal thoughts/behavior; monitor for emergence/worsening of depression, suicidal thoughts/behavior, and/or any unusual changes in mood/behavior. Serious and sometimes fatal dermatologic reactions, including toxic epidermal necrolysis (TEN) and Stevens-Johnson syndrome (SJS), reported; d/c at 1st sign of rash, unless the rash is clearly not drug-related. Do not resume therapy, and consider alternative therapy if signs/symptoms suggest SJS/TEN. Avoid use as an alternative for carbamazepine in patients positive for HLA-B*1502. Drug reaction with eosinophilia and systemic symptoms (DRESS)/multiorgan hypersensitivity reported; evaluate immediately if signs and symptoms (eg, rash, fever, lymphadenopathy) are present and d/c if an alternative etiology cannot be established. Caution with history of hypersensitivity to structurally similar drugs (eg, carboxamides, barbiturates, succinimides, oxazolidinediones); consider alternatives to therapy. Acute hepatotoxicity (eg, acute hepatic failure) reported; d/c immediately and do not readminister. Hematopoietic complications and lymphadenopathy reported; extended follow-up observation is indicated and every effort should be made to achieve seizure control using alternative antiepileptic drugs in all cases of lymphadenopathy. Decreased bone mineral density and bone fractures reported during chronic use; consider screening and initiating treatment plans as appropriate. Caution with porphyria, hepatic impairment, and in elderly or gravely ill patients. Bleeding disorder in newborns may occur; give vitamin K to mother before delivery and to neonate after birth. Check plasma levels immediately if early signs of dose-related CNS toxicity develop. Hyperglycemia reported; may increase serum glucose levels in diabetics. Not indicated for seizures due to hypoglycemia or other metabolic causes. Not effective for absence (petit mal) seizures; if tonic-clonic (grand mal) and absence (petit mal) seizures are present, combined drug therapy is needed. May produce confusional states at levels sustained above optimal range; reduce dose if plasma levels are excessive, or d/c if symptoms persist. Lab test interactions may occur. (Cap, ER) Do not use if discolored. (Tab, Chewable) Not for qd dosing.

ADVERSE REACTIONS

Rash, nystagmus, ataxia, slurred speech, decreased coordination, somnolence, mental confusion, dizziness, insomnia, transient nervousness, motor twitching, N/V, thrombocytopenia, altered taste sensation, Peyronie's disease.

DRUG INTERACTIONS

See Contraindications. Acute alcohol intake, amiodarone, antiepileptic agents (eg, ethosuximide, felbamate, oxcarbazepine, topiramate), azoles (eg, fluconazole, ketoconazole, itraconazole), capecitabine, chloramphenicol, chlordiazepoxide, disulfiram, estrogens, fluorouracil, fluoxetine, fluvastatin, fluvoxamine, H_2-antagonists (eg, cimetidine), halothane, isoniazid, methylphenidate, omeprazole, phenothiazines, salicylates, sertraline, succinimides, sulfonamides (eg, sulfamethizole, sulfadiazine, sulfamethoxazole-trimethoprim), ticlopidine, tolbutamide, trazodone, and warfarin may increase levels. Anticancer drugs (eg, bleomycin, carboplatin, cisplatin, doxorubicin, methotrexate), carbamazepine, chronic alcohol abuse, diazepam, diazoxide, folic acid, fosamprenavir, nelfinavir, reserpine, rifampin, ritonavir (RTV), St. John's wort, sucralfate, vigabatrin, and theophylline may decrease levels. Administration with preparations that increase gastric pH (eg, supplements or antacids containing calcium carbonate, aluminum hydroxide, and magnesium hydroxide) may affect absorption; do not take at the same time of day. Phenobarbital, sodium valproate, and valproic acid may increase or decrease levels. May impair efficacy of azoles (eg, fluconazole, ketoconazole, voriconazole), corticosteroids, doxycycline, estrogens, furosemide, irinotecan, oral contraceptives, paclitaxel, paroxetine, quinidine, rifampin, sertraline, teniposide, theophylline, and vitamin D. Increased and decreased PT/INR responses reported with warfarin. May decrease levels of active metabolites of albendazole, certain HIV antivirals (eg, efavirenz, lopinavir/RTV, indinavir), anti-epileptic agents (eg, felbamate, topiramate, quetiapine), atorvastatin, chlorpropamide, clozapine, cyclosporine, digoxin, fluvastatin, folic acid, methadone, mexiletine, nifedipine, nimodipine, nisoldipine, praziquantel, simvastatin, and verapamil. May decrease levels of amprenavir (active metabolite) when given with fosamprenavir alone. May increase levels of amprenavir when given with the combination of fosamprenavir and RTV. Resistance to the neuromuscular blocking action of pancuronium, vecuronium, rocuronium, and cisatracurium reported in patients chronically administered phenytoin; monitor closely for more rapid recovery from neuromuscular blockade than expected and for higher infusion rate requirements. Avoid with enteral feeding preparations and/or nutritional supplements.

NURSING CONSIDERATIONS

Assessment: Assess for hypersensitivity to the drug, its inactive ingredients, or other hydantoins, alcohol use, hepatic/renal impairment, porphyria, grave illness, seizures due to hypoglycemia or other metabolic causes, absence seizures, any other conditions where treatment is contraindicated or cautioned, pregnancy/nursing status, and possible drug interactions.

Monitoring: Monitor for hypersensitivity reactions, dermatologic reactions, DRESS/multiorgan hypersensitivity, hepatotoxicity, hematopoietic complications, lymphadenopathy, decreased bone mineral density, bone fractures, exacerbation of porphyria, hyperglycemia, and other adverse reactions. Monitor for emergence/worsening of depression, suicidal thoughts/behavior, and/or any unusual changes in mood/behavior. Monitor serum levels when switching from Na^+ salt to free acid form and vice versa.

Patient Counseling: Instruct to read medication guide and to take ud. Advise of the importance of adhering strictly to the prescribed dosage regimen, and of informing the physician of any clinical condition in which it is not possible to take the drug orally as prescribed (eg, surgery). Counsel about the early toxic signs and symptoms of potential hematologic, dermatologic, hypersensitivity, or hepatic reactions; instruct to immediately contact physician if these develop. Caution on the use of other drugs or alcoholic beverages without first seeking physician's advice. Stress the importance of good dental hygiene to minimize the development of gingival hyperplasia and its complications. Advise to notify physician immediately if depression, suicidal thoughts/behavior, or thoughts about self-harm emerge. Encourage patients to enroll in the North American Antiepileptic Drug Pregnancy Registry.

Storage: 20-25°C (68-77°F). Protect from moisture. (Cap, ER) Preserve in tight, light-resistant containers. (Sus) Protect from freezing and light.

DILAUDID INJECTION — hydromorphone hydrochloride CII

Class: Opioid analgesic

Contains hydromorphone, a Schedule II controlled opioid agonist with an abuse liability similar to other opioid analgesics. May be abused in a manner similar to other opioid agonists, legal or illicit; consider these risks when administering, prescribing, or dispensing in situations where increased risk of misuse, abuse, or diversion is a concern. Has the highest potential for abuse and risk of producing fatal overdose due to respiratory depression. Ethanol, other opioids, and other CNS depressants (eg, sedative-hypnotics, skeletal muscle relaxants) can potentiate the respiratory-depressant effects and increase the risk of adverse outcomes, including death. (HP) A more concentrated sol and is for use in opioid-tolerant patients only; do not confuse with standard parenteral formulations of hydromorphone or other opioids, as overdose and death may result.

OTHER BRAND NAMES

Dilaudid-HP

ADULT DOSAGE

Pain

Opioid-Naive:

SQ/IM:

Initial: 1-2mg q2-3h as necessary

Titrate: Adjust dose according to severity of pain and adverse events, as well as patient's underlying disease and age

IV:

Initial: 0.2-1mg q2-3h, given slowly, over at least 2-3 min, depending on the dose

Titrate: Adjust dose to achieve acceptable analgesia and tolerable adverse events

Moderate to Severe Pain

HP:

Opioid-Tolerant Patients Requiring Higher Doses of Opioids:

Base starting dose on the prior dose of hydromorphone inj or on the prior dose of an alternate opioid; periodically reassess after the initial dosing

Conversions

From Morphine Sulfate: 10mg parenteral or 40-60mg oral

From Hydromorphone HCl: 1.3-2mg parenteral or 6.5-7.5mg oral

From Oxymorphone HCl: 1-1.1mg parenteral or 6.6mg oral

From Levorphanol Tartrate: 2-2.3mg parenteral or 4mg oral

From Meperidine HCl: 75-100mg parenteral or 300-400mg oral

From Methadone HCl: 10mg parenteral or 10-20mg oral

From Nalbuphine HCl: 10-12mg parenteral

From Butorphanol Tartrate: 1.5-2.5mg parenteral

PEDIATRIC DOSAGE

Pediatric use may not have been established

DOSE MODIFICATION

Renal Impairment

Initial: 1/4 to 1/2 the usual starting dose depending on the degree of impairment

Hepatic Impairment

Initial: 1/4 to 1/2 the usual starting dose depending on the extent of impairment

Elderly

Start at lower end of dosing range

ADMINISTRATION

SQ/IM/IV route

Dilaudid Inj and HP Inj are physically compatible/chemically stable for at least 24 hours at 25°C, protected from light in most large-volume parenteral sol

500mg/50mL Vial

Do not penetrate stopper with syringe; remove both flipseal and rubber stopper

Discard any unused portion

Reconstitution of Sterile Lyophilized HP Inj 250mg

Reconstitute immediately prior to use with 25mL of SWFI to provide a sol containing 10mg/mL of hydromorphone hydrochloride

HOW SUPPLIED

Inj: 1mg/mL, 2mg/mL, 4mg/mL, (HP) 10mg/mL [1mL, 5mL, ampule; 50mL, vial], 250mg

CONTRAINDICATIONS

Respiratory depression in the absence of resuscitative equipment or in unmonitored settings, acute or severe bronchial asthma, patients with, or at risk of developing, GI obstruction, especially paralytic ileus. (HP) Patients who are not opioid-tolerant.

WARNINGS/PRECAUTIONS

Respiratory depression occurs most frequently in elderly, debilitated, and those suffering from upper airway obstruction or conditions accompanied by hypoxia or hypercapnia; extreme caution with chronic obstructive pulmonary disease (COPD) or cor pulmonale, substantially decreased respiratory reserve, hypoxia, hypercapnia, or preexisting respiratory depression. May cause neonatal withdrawal syndrome. Respiratory depressant effects with carbon dioxide retention and secondary elevation of CSF pressure may be markedly exaggerated in the presence of head injury, other intracranial lesions, or preexisting increase in intracranial pressure (ICP). May produce effects on pupillary response and consciousness, which can obscure the clinical course and neurologic signs of further increase ICP in patients with head injuries. May cause severe hypotension, and may produce orthostatic hypotension in ambulatory patients; caution with circulatory shock. Contains sodium metabisulfite, which may cause allergic-type reactions, including anaphylactic symptoms and life-threatening or less severe asthmatic episodes in certain susceptible people. May obscure the diagnosis or clinical course in patients with acute abdominal conditions. May cause spasm of the sphincter of Oddi and diminish biliary and pancreatic secretions; caution with biliary tract disease, including acute pancreatitis. Caution in elderly/debilitated and those with severe pulmonary/hepatic/renal impairment, myxedema/hypothyroidism, adrenocortical insufficiency (eg, Addison's disease), CNS depression or coma, toxic psychoses, prostatic hypertrophy, urethral stricture, acute alcoholism, delirium tremens, or kyphoscoliosis associated with respiratory depression; reduce initial dose. May aggravate preexisting convulsions in patients with convulsive disorders, and may induce or aggravate seizures in some clinical settings. Mild to severe seizures and myoclonus reported in severely compromised patients administered high doses of parenteral hydromorphone. Caution with alcoholism and other drug dependencies. May impair mental/physical abilities. Physical dependence and tolerance may occur. Do not abruptly d/c.

ADVERSE REACTIONS

Respiratory depression, apnea, lightheadedness, dizziness, sedation, N/V, sweating, flushing, dysphoria, euphoria, dry mouth, pruritus.

DRUG INTERACTIONS

See Boxed Warning. Concomitant use with other CNS depressants (eg, general anesthetics, phenothiazines, centrally-acting antiemetics, tranquilizers) increases the risk of hypotension and profound sedation, potentially resulting in coma or death; use with caution and in reduced dosages. May enhance action of neuromuscular blocking agents and produce an increased degree of respiratory depression. May cause severe hypotension with phenothiazines, general anesthetics, or other agents that compromise vasomotor tone. Mixed agonist/antagonist analgesics (pentazocine, nalbuphine, butorphanol, buprenorphine) may reduce the analgesic effect and/or may precipitate withdrawal symptoms; use with caution. MAOIs may potentiate action; allow at least 14 days after discontinuing treatment with MAOIs before starting therapy. Concomitant use with anticholinergics or other medications with anticholinergic activity may increase risk of urinary retention and severe constipation, which may lead to paralytic ileus.

NURSING CONSIDERATIONS

Assessment: Assess for risk factors for drug abuse or addiction, pain type/severity, prior opioid therapy, opioid tolerance, respiratory depression, COPD, cor pulmonale, decreased respiratory reserve, hypoxia, hypercapnia, asthma, GI obstruction, renal/hepatic impairment, pregnancy/nursing status, possible drug interactions, or any other conditions where treatment is contraindicated or cautioned.

Monitoring: Monitor for respiratory depression, increase in ICP, hypotension, spasm of the sphincter of Oddi, aggravation/induction of convulsions/seizures, physical dependence, tolerance, and other adverse reactions. Monitor for signs of misuse, abuse, and addiction.

Patient Counseling: Discuss the risk of respiratory depression. Instruct to report adverse events experienced during therapy. Advise not to adjust dose or combine with alcohol or other CNS depressants without prescriber's consent. Inform that drug may impair mental/physical abilities; instruct to use caution when performing hazardous tasks (eg, operating machinery/driving). Advise to consult physician if pregnant or planning to become pregnant. Inform that drug has potential for abuse; instruct to protect it from theft and never to share with others. Instruct to avoid abrupt withdrawal.

Storage: 20-25°C (68-77°F); excursions permitted to 15-30°C (59-86°F). Protect from light. Diluted Sol: Stable for at least 24 hrs at 25°C (77°F), protected from light in most common large-volume parenteral sol.

DILAUDID ORAL – hydromorphone hydrochloride CII

Class: Opioid analgesic

Contains hydromorphone, a Schedule II controlled opioid agonist with the highest potential for abuse and risk of respiratory depression. Alcohol, other opioids, and CNS depressants (eg, sedative-hypnotics) potentiate respiratory depressant effects, increasing the risk of respiratory depression that may result in death.

ADULT DOSAGE

Pain

Periodically reassess after the initial dosing

Sol:

Usual: 2.5-10mg q3-6h ud by clinical situation

Tab:

Initial: 2-4mg q4-6h

Titrate: May increase gradually if analgesia is inadequate, as tolerance develops, or if pain severity increases

Sol/Tab:

Nonopioid-Tolerant:

Initial: 2-4mg q4h

Taking Opioids:

Base starting dose on prior opioid usage

Give only 1/2 to 2/3 of the estimated dose for the 1st few doses, then increase prn according to response

Chronic Pain:

Administer dose around-the-clock

May give a supplemental dose of 5-15% of the total daily usage q2h prn

Conversions

From Morphine Sulfate: 10mg parenteral or 40-60mg oral

From Hydromorphone HCl: 1.3-2mg parenteral or 6.5-7.5mg oral

From Oxymorphone HCl: 1-1.1mg parenteral or 6.6mg oral

From Levorphanol Tartrate: 2-2.3mg parenteral or 4mg oral

From Meperidine HCl: 75-100mg parenteral or 300-400mg oral

From Methadone HCl: 10mg parenteral or 10-20mg oral

PEDIATRIC DOSAGE

Pediatric use may not have been established

DOSE MODIFICATION

Renal Impairment

Moderate-Severe:

Start on a lower dose and closely monitor during titration

Use oral liquid to adjust the dose

Hepatic Impairment

Moderate:

Start on a lower dose and closely monitor during titration

Use oral liquid to adjust the dose

Elderly

Start at lower end of dosing range

ADMINISTRATION

Oral route

HOW SUPPLIED

Sol: 1mg/mL [473mL]; Tab: 2mg, 4mg, 8mg* *scored

CONTRAINDICATIONS

Respiratory depression in the absence of resuscitative equipment, status asthmaticus, obstetrical analgesia.

WARNINGS/PRECAUTIONS

Respiratory depression is more likely to occur in elderly, debilitated, and those suffering from conditions accompanied by hypoxia or hypercapnia; extreme caution with chronic obstructive pulmonary disease (COPD) or cor pulmonale, substantially decreased respiratory reserve, hypoxia, hypercapnia, or preexisting respiratory depression. May cause neonatal withdrawal syndrome. Respiratory depressant effects with carbon dioxide retention and secondary elevation of CSF pressure may be markedly exaggerated in the presence of head injury, other intracranial lesions, or preexisting increase in intracranial pressure (ICP). May produce effects on pupillary response and consciousness, which can obscure the clinical course and neurologic signs of further increase in ICP in patients with head injuries. May cause severe hypotension; caution with circulatory shock. Contains sodium metabisulfite; may cause allergic-type reactions, including anaphylactic symptoms and life-threatening or less severe asthmatic episodes in certain susceptible people. Caution in elderly/debilitated and those with severe pulmonary/hepatic/renal impairment, myxedema/hypothyroidism, adrenocortical insufficiency (eg, Addison's disease), CNS depression or coma, toxic psychoses, prostatic hypertrophy, urethral stricture, gallbladder disease, acute alcoholism, delirium tremens, kyphoscoliosis, or following GI surgery; reduce initial dose. May obscure the diagnosis or clinical course in patients with acute abdominal conditions. May aggravate preexisting convulsions in patients with convulsive disorders. Mild to severe seizures and myoclonus reported in severely compromised patients administered high doses of parenteral hydromorphone. Caution with alcoholism and other drug dependencies. May impair mental/physical abilities. May produce orthostatic hypotension in ambulatory patients. May cause spasm of the sphincter of Oddi; caution in patients about to undergo biliary tract surgery. Physical dependence and tolerance may occur. Do not abruptly d/c.

ADVERSE REACTIONS

Respiratory depression, apnea, lightheadedness, dizziness, sedation, N/V, sweating, flushing, dysphoria, euphoria, dry mouth, pruritus.

DRUG INTERACTIONS

See Boxed Warning. Concomitant use with other CNS depressants (eg, general anesthetics, phenothiazines, tranquilizers) may produce additive depressant effects; use with caution and in reduced dosages. Do not give with alcohol. May enhance action of neuromuscular blocking agents and produce an excessive degree of respiratory depression. May cause severe hypotension with phenothiazines or general anesthetics. Mixed agonist/antagonist analgesics (pentazocine, nalbuphine, butorphanol, buprenorphine) may reduce the analgesic effect and/or may precipitate withdrawal symptoms; use with caution.

NURSING CONSIDERATIONS

Assessment: Assess for risk factors for drug abuse or addiction, pain type/severity, prior opioid therapy, opioid tolerance, respiratory depression, COPD, cor pulmonale, decreased respiratory reserve, hypoxia, hypercapnia, asthma, renal/hepatic impairment, pregnancy/nursing status, possible drug interactions, or any other conditions where treatment is contraindicated or cautioned.

Monitoring: Monitor for respiratory depression, sedation, CNS depression, aggravation/induction of seizures/convulsions, increase in ICP, hypotension, tolerance, physical dependence, and other adverse reactions. Routinely monitor for signs of misuse, abuse, and addiction.

Patient Counseling: Inform that medication may cause severe adverse effects (eg, respiratory depression) if not taken ud. Instruct to report pain and adverse experiences occurring during therapy. Advise not to adjust dose or combine with alcohol or other CNS depressants without prescriber's consent. Inform that drug may impair mental/physical abilities; instruct to use caution when performing hazardous tasks (eg, operating machinery/driving). Advise to consult physician if pregnant or planning to become pregnant. Inform that drug has potential for abuse; instruct to protect it from theft and never to share with others. Advise to avoid abrupt withdrawal if taking medication for more than a few weeks and cessation of therapy is indicated. Instruct to keep drug in a secure place, and to destroy unused tabs by flushing down toilet.

Storage: 25°C (77°F); excursions permitted to 15-30°C (59-86°F). Protect from light.

DILTIAZEM INJECTION – diltiazem hydrochloride

RX

Class: Calcium channel blocker (nondihydropyridine)

ADULT DOSAGE

Atrial Fibrillation/Flutter

Bolus: 0.25mg/kg IV over 2 min
If no response after 15 min, may give 2nd dose of 0.35mg/kg over 2 min

Continuous Infusion: 0.25-0.35mg/kg IV bolus, then 10mg/hr
Titrate: Increase by 5mg/hr
Max: 15mg/hr and duration up to 24 hrs

PEDIATRIC DOSAGE

Pediatric use may not have been established

DOSE MODIFICATION

Elderly

Start at lower end of dosing range

ADMINISTRATION

IV route

Dilute in normal saline, D5W, or D5W/0.45% NaCl. Refer to PI for more details

Incompatibilities

Do not mix w/ any other drugs in the same container and is recommended not to be coinfused in the same IV line
Physical incompatibilities (precipitate formation or cloudiness) were observed when diltiazem was infused in the same IV line w/ the following: acetazolamide, acyclovir, aminophylline, ampicillin, ampicillin sodium/sulbactam sodium, cefamandole, cefoperazone, diazepam, furosemide, hydrocortisone sodium succinate, insulin (regular: 100 U/mL), methylprednisolone sodium succinate, mezlocillin, nafcillin, phenytoin, rifampin, and sodium bicarbonate

HOW SUPPLIED

Inj: 5mg/mL

CONTRAINDICATIONS

Sick sinus syndrome and 2nd- or 3rd-degree atrioventricular (AV) block (except with functioning pacemaker), severe hypotension, cardiogenic shock, concomitant IV β-blockers or within a few hrs of use, A-fib/flutter associated with accessory bypass tract (eg, Wolff-Parkinson-White [WPW] syndrome, short PR syndrome), ventricular tachycardia.

WARNINGS/PRECAUTIONS

Initiate in setting with resuscitation capabilities. Caution if hemodynamically compromised, and with renal, hepatic, or ventricular dysfunction. Monitor ECG continuously and BP frequently. Symptomatic hypotension, acute hepatic injury reported. D/C if high-degree AV block occurs in sinus rhythm or if persistent rash occurs. Ventricular premature beats may be present on conversion of PSVT to sinus rhythm.

ADVERSE REACTIONS

Hypotension, inj-site reactions (eg, itching, burning), vasodilation (flushing), arrhythmias.

DRUG INTERACTIONS

See Contraindications. Caution with drugs that decrease peripheral resistance, intravascular volume, myocardial contractility or conduction. Increased AUC of midazolam, triazolam, buspirone, quinidine, and lovastatin, which may require a dose adjustment due to increased clinical effects or increased adverse events. Elevates carbamazepine levels, which may result in toxicity. Cyclosporine may need dose adjustment. Potentiates the depression of cardiac contractility, conductivity, automaticity, and vascular dilation with anesthetics. Possible bradycardia, AV block, and contractility depression with oral β-blockers. Possible competitive inhibition of metabolism with drugs metabolized by CYP450. Avoid rifampin. Monitor for excessive slowing of HR and/or AV block with digoxin. Cimetidine increases peak diltiazem plasma levels and AUC.

NURSING CONSIDERATIONS

Assessment: Assess for sick sinus syndrome and 2nd- or 3rd-degree AV block, presence of functioning pacemaker, severe hypotension, cardiogenic shock, A-fib/flutter associated with accessory bypass tract (eg, WPW syndrome, short PR syndrome), ventricular tachycardia, wide complex tachycardia, acute myocardial infarction, congestive heart failure, pulmonary congestion documented by x-ray, hypertrophic cardiomyopathy, renal/hepatic impairment, pregnancy/nursing status, and possible drug interactions.

Monitoring: Initiation of therapy should be done in setting with monitoring and resuscitation capabilities, including DC cardioversion/defibrillation. Monitor BP, HR, LFTs, and ECG. Monitor for hemodynamic deterioration, ventricular fibrillation, cardiac conduction abnormalities (eg, 2nd- or

3rd-degree AV block), ventricular premature beats, dermatologic events (erythema multiforme/exfoliative dermatitis), and acute hepatic injury.

Patient Counseling: Inform that initiation of therapy should be done in a setting with monitoring and resuscitation capabilities, including DC cardioversion/defibrillation. Inform of risks/benefits and instruct to report adverse reactions. Advise to notify physician if pregnant/nursing.

Storage: 2-8°C (36-46°F). Do not freeze. Room temperature for up to 1 month. Destroy after 1 month. Diluted Sol: D5W, 0.9% NaCl, or D5W & 0.45% NaCl: Stable at 20-25°C (68-77°F) or 2-8°C (36-46°F) for at least 24 hrs when stored in a glass or polyvinyl chloride bag.

DIOVAN — valsartan RX

Class: Angiotensin II receptor antagonist

D/C when pregnancy is detected. Drugs that act directly on the renin-angiotensin system (RAS) can cause injury/death to the developing fetus.

ADULT DOSAGE

Hypertension

Initial: 80mg or 160mg qd
Titrate: May increase to a max of 320mg qd
May add diuretic if BP not controlled

Heart Failure

NYHA Class II-IV
Initial: 40mg bid
Titrate: May increase to 80mg and 160mg bid (use highest dose tolerated)
Max: 320mg/day in divided doses

Post-Myocardial Infarction

Initial: 20mg bid as early as 12 hrs after MI
Titrate: May increase to 40mg bid w/in 7 days, w/ subsequent titrations to 160mg bid as tolerated
Maint: 160mg bid
Consider reducing dose if symptomatic hypotension or renal dysfunction occurs

PEDIATRIC DOSAGE

Hypertension

6-16 Years:
Initial: 1.3mg/kg qd (up to 40mg total)
Titrate: Adjust dose according to BP response
Max: 2.7mg/kg (up to 160mg) qd

DOSE MODIFICATION

Concomitant Medications
Heart Failure:
Concomitant Diuretics: Consider reducing diuretic dose

ADMINISTRATION

Oral route

Take w/ or w/o food
Use of a sus is recommended for children who cannot swallow tabs, or if calculated dosage does not correspond to available tab strength
Adjust dose accordingly when switching dosage forms; exposure w/ sus is 1.6X greater than w/ tab

Preparation of Sus (for 160mL of a 4mg/mL Sus)

1. Add 80mL of Ora-Plus oral suspending vehicle to an amber glass bottle containing 8 Diovan 80mg tabs, and shake for a minimum of 2 min
2. Allow the sus to stand for a minimum of 1 hr
3. After the standing time, shake the sus for a minimum of 1 additional min
4. Add 80mL of Ora-Sweet SF oral sweetening vehicle to the bottle and shake the sus for at least 10 sec to disperse the ingredients
5. The sus is homogenous and can be stored for either up to 30 days at room temperature (below 30°C/86°F) or up to 75 days at refrigerated conditions (2-8°C/35-46°F) in the glass bottle
6. Shake the bottle well (at least 10 sec) prior to dispensing the sus

HOW SUPPLIED

Tab: 40mg*, 80mg, 160mg, 320mg *scored

CONTRAINDICATIONS

Coadministration with aliskiren in patients with diabetes.

WARNINGS/PRECAUTIONS

Symptomatic hypotension may occur in patients with an activated RAS (eg, volume- and/or salt-depleted patients receiving high doses of diuretics); correct this condition prior to therapy. Caution when initiating therapy in patients with HF or post-MI. Renal function changes may occur; caution in patients whose renal function depend in part on the activity of the RAS (eg, renal artery stenosis, chronic kidney disease, severe CHF, volume depletion). Consider withholding or discontinuing therapy if clinically significant decrease in renal function develops. Increased K^+ in some patients with HF reported, and more likely to occur in patients with preexisting renal impairment; dose reduction and/or discontinuation of therapy may be required. Do not readminister to patients who have had angioedema. Caution with dosing in patients with hepatic or severe renal impairment.

ADVERSE REACTIONS

Headache, abdominal pain, cough, increased BUN, hyperkalemia, dizziness, hypotension, SrCr elevation, viral infection, fatigue, diarrhea, arthralgia, back pain.

DRUG INTERACTIONS

See Contraindications. Dual blockade of the RAS is associated with increased risk of hypotension, hyperkalemia, and changes in renal function (including acute renal failure); avoid combined use of RAS inhibitors, or closely monitor BP, renal function, and electrolytes with concomitant agents that also affect the RAS. Avoid with aliskiren in patients with renal impairment (GFR <60mL/min). Inhibitors of the hepatic uptake transporter OATP1B1 (rifampin, cyclosporine) and the hepatic efflux transporter MRP2 (ritonavir) may increase exposure. Other agents that block the RAS, K^+-sparing diuretics, K^+ supplements, or salt substitutes containing K^+ may increase serum K^+ levels, and in HF patients may increase SrCr; monitor serum K^+ levels. Greater antihypertensive effect with atenolol. NSAIDs, including selective COX-2 inhibitors, may result in deterioration of renal function, including possible acute renal failure, and may attenuate antihypertensive effect. Increased lithium levels and lithium toxicity reported; monitor serum lithium levels during concomitant use.

NURSING CONSIDERATIONS

Assessment: Assess for hypersensitivity to the drug and its components, hepatic/renal impairment, volume/salt depletion, renal artery stenosis, HF, pregnancy/nursing status, and possible drug interactions.

Monitoring: Monitor for signs/symptoms of hypotension and other adverse reactions. Monitor electrolytes, BP, and renal function.

Patient Counseling: Counsel about the risk/benefits of therapy and possible adverse effects. Inform of consequences of exposure during pregnancy and discuss treatment options with women planning to become pregnant. Instruct to report pregnancies to physician as soon as possible.

Storage: (Tab) 25°C (77°F); excursions permitted to 15-30°C (59-86°F). Protect from moisture. (Sus) <30°C (86°F) for up to 30 days or at 2-8°C (35-46°F) for up to 75 days.

DIOVAN HCT – hydrochlorothiazide/valsartan RX

Class: Angiotensin II receptor antagonist/thiazide diuretic

D/C when pregnancy is detected. Drugs that act directly on the renin-angiotensin system (RAS) can cause injury/death to the developing fetus.

ADULT DOSAGE

Hypertension

Initial: 160mg-12.5mg qd
Titrate: May increase after 1-2 weeks of therapy
Max: 320mg-25mg qd

Add-On Therapy:

Use if not adequately controlled with valsartan (or another ARB) alone or HCTZ alone
With dose-limiting adverse reactions to either component alone, may switch to therapy containing a lower dose of that component
Titrate: May increase after 3-4 weeks of therapy if BP uncontrolled
Max: 320mg-25mg

Replacement Therapy:

May substitute for titrated components

PEDIATRIC DOSAGE

Pediatric use may not have been established

ADMINISTRATION

Oral route

Take with or without food

HOW SUPPLIED

Tab: (Valsartan-HCTZ) 80mg-12.5mg, 160mg-12.5mg, 160mg-25mg, 320mg-12.5mg, 320mg-25mg

CONTRAINDICATIONS

Anuria, sulfonamide-derived drug hypersensitivity. Coadministration with aliskiren in patients with diabetes.

WARNINGS/PRECAUTIONS

Not for initial therapy with intravascular volume depletion. Symptomatic hypotension may occur in patients with activated RAS (eg, volume- and/or salt-depleted patients receiving high doses of diuretics); correct this condition prior to therapy. Renal function changes may occur including acute renal failure; caution in patients whose renal function depends in part on the activity of the RAS (eg, renal artery stenosis, chronic kidney disease, severe congestive heart failure, volume depletion). Consider withholding or discontinuing therapy if clinically significant decrease in renal function develops. May cause serum electrolyte abnormalities (eg, hyperkalemia, hypokalemia, hyponatremia, hypomagnesemia); correct hypokalemia and any coexisting hypomagnesemia prior to initiation of therapy and monitor periodically. D/C if hypokalemia is accompanied by clinical signs (eg, muscular weakness, paresis, ECG alterations). Increased K^+ in patients with heart failure (HF) reported; dose reduction or discontinuation of therapy may be required. Do not readminister to patients with angioedema. HCTZ: May cause hypersensitivity reactions and exacerbation or activation of systemic lupus erythematosus (SLE). May precipitate hepatic coma with hepatic impairment or progressive liver disease. May cause idiosyncratic reaction, resulting in acute transient myopia and acute angle-closure glaucoma; d/c as rapidly as possible. May alter glucose tolerance and increase serum cholesterol and TG levels. May cause or exacerbate hyperuricemia and precipitate gout in susceptible patients. May cause hypercalcemia.

ADVERSE REACTIONS

Dizziness, BUN elevations, hypokalemia, angioedema, dry cough, nasopharyngitis.

DRUG INTERACTIONS

See Contraindications. Increased lithium levels and lithium toxicity reported; monitor lithium levels during concomitant use. Valsartan: Dual blockade of the RAS is associated with increased risk of hypotension, hyperkalemia, and changes in renal function (including acute renal failure); avoid combined use of RAS inhibitors, or closely monitor BP, renal function, and electrolytes with concomitant agents that also affect the RAS. Avoid with aliskiren in patients with renal impairment (GFR <60mL/min). Greater antihypertensive effect with atenolol. Inhibitors of the hepatic uptake transporter OATP1B1 (rifampin, cyclosporine) or the hepatic efflux transporter MRP2 (ritonavir) may increase exposure. NSAIDs, including selective COX-2 inhibitors, may result in deterioration of renal function, including possible acute renal failure, and may attenuate antihypertensive effect. Other agents that block the RAS, K^+-sparing diuretics, K^+ supplements, or salt substitutes containing K^+ may increase serum K^+ levels, and in HF patients may increase SrCr; monitor serum K^+ levels. HCTZ: Dosage adjustment of antidiabetic drugs (eg, oral agents, insulin) may be required. May lead to symptomatic hyponatremia with carbamazepine. Ion exchange resins (eg, cholestyramine, colestipol) may reduce exposure; space dosing at least 4 hrs before or 4-6 hrs after the administration of ion exchange resins. Cyclosporine may increase risk of hyperuricemia and gout-type complications.

NURSING CONSIDERATIONS

Assessment: Assess for hypersensitivity to the drug and its components, anuria, history of sulfonamide-derived hypersensitivity or penicillin allergy, renal/hepatic impairment, volume/salt depletion, risk for acute renal failure, SLE, electrolyte imbalances, pregnancy/nursing status, and possible drug interactions.

Monitoring: Monitor for signs/symptoms of hypotension, hypersensitivity/idiosyncratic reactions, exacerbation or activation of SLE, myopia, angle-closure glaucoma, precipitation of gout or hyperuricemia, and other adverse reactions. Monitor BP, serum electrolytes, cholesterol, TG levels, and renal function periodically.

Patient Counseling: Inform about the consequences of exposure during pregnancy and discuss treatment options in women planning to become pregnant. Instruct to report pregnancies to physician as soon as possible. Caution about lightheadedness, especially during the 1st days of therapy; instruct to d/c and consult physician if syncope occurs. Caution that inadequate fluid intake, excessive perspiration, diarrhea, and vomiting may lead to an excessive fall in BP, with the same consequences of lightheadedness and possible syncope. Instruct to avoid use of K^+ supplements or salt substitutes containing K^+ without consulting a physician.

Storage: 25°C (77°F); excursions permitted to 15-30°C (59-86°F). Protect from moisture.

DITROPAN XL – oxybutynin chloride

Class: Anticholinergic

RX

ADULT DOSAGE
Overactive Bladder
Initial: 5 or 10mg qd at the same time each day
Titrate: May adjust dose in 5mg increments weekly
Max: 30mg/day

PEDIATRIC DOSAGE
Detrusor Overactivity
Associated w/ a Neurological Condition (eg, Spina Bifida):
≥6 Years:
Initial: 5mg qd at the same time each day
Titrate: May adjust dose in 5mg increments
Max: 20mg/day

ADMINISTRATION
Oral route
May be taken w/ or w/o food
Swallow tab whole w/ aid of liquids; do not chew, divide, or crush

HOW SUPPLIED
Tab, Extended-Release: 5mg, 10mg, 15mg

CONTRAINDICATIONS
Urinary retention, gastric retention and other severe decreased GI motility conditions, uncontrolled narrow-angle glaucoma.

WARNINGS/PRECAUTIONS
Angioedema of the face, lips, tongue, and/or larynx reported; d/c promptly and provide appropriate therapy if angioedema occurs. Associated w/ anticholinergic CNS effects; consider dose reduction or discontinuation if any occur. Caution w/ preexisting dementia treated w/ cholinesterase inhibitors, Parkinson's disease, myasthenia gravis, autonomic neuropathy, clinically significant bladder outflow obstruction, GI obstructive disorders, ulcerative colitis, intestinal atony, GERD, and preexisting severe GI narrowing (pathologic or iatrogenic). May decrease GI motility. May impair mental/physical abilities. Not recommended in pediatric patients who cannot swallow tab whole w/o chewing, dividing, or crushing.

ADVERSE REACTIONS
Dry mouth, constipation, diarrhea, headache, somnolence, dizziness, dyspepsia, nausea, blurred vision, dry eyes, insomnia.

DRUG INTERACTIONS
Concomitant use w/ other anticholinergic drugs may increase the frequency and/or severity of anticholinergic-like effects. May alter GI absorption of other drugs due to GI motility effects; caution w/ drugs w/ narrow therapeutic index. May antagonize effects of prokinetic agents (eg, metoclopramide). Increased levels w/ ketoconazole. Caution w/ CYP3A4 inhibitors (eg, antimycotics, macrolides); may alter mean pharmacokinetic parameters. Caution w/ drugs that may cause/exacerbate esophagitis (eg, bisphosphonates).

NURSING CONSIDERATIONS

Assessment: Assess for urinary/gastric retention, bladder outflow obstruction, GI narrowing/obstructive disorder, GERD, ulcerative colitis, uncontrolled narrow-angle glaucoma, Parkinson's disease, myasthenia gravis, autonomic neuropathy, dementia, hypersensitivity to the drug substance or other components of the product, any other conditions where treatment is contraindicated or cautioned, pregnancy/nursing status, and possible drug interactions.

Monitoring: Monitor for aggravation of myasthenia gravis or autonomic neuropathy, angioedema, hypersensitivity reactions, anticholinergic CNS effects, GI adverse reactions (eg, urinary retention, esophagitis, gastric retention), and other adverse reactions.

Patient Counseling: Inform that angioedema may occur and could result in life-threatening airway obstruction; advise to promptly d/c therapy and seek medical attention if experiencing swelling of the tongue, edema of the laryngopharynx, or difficulty breathing. Inform that heat prostration may occur when administered in high environmental temperature. Inform that drug may produce drowsiness, dizziness, or blurred vision; advise to exercise caution. Inform that alcohol may enhance drowsiness. Advise not to drive or operate heavy machinery until effects have been determined.

Storage: 25°C (77°F); excursions permitted to 15-30°C (59-86°F). Protect from moisture and humidity.

DOCETAXEL – docetaxel

RX

Class: Antimicrotubule agent

Increased treatment-related mortality reported with hepatic dysfunction, high-dose therapy, and in patients with non-small cell lung carcinoma (NSCLC) who had prior platinum-based chemotherapy with docetaxel at 100mg/m^2. Avoid if neutrophils <1500 cells/mm^3, bilirubin >ULN, or AST/ALT >1.5X ULN with alkaline phosphatase >2.5X ULN; may increase risk for the development of Grade 4 neutropenia, febrile neutropenia, infections, severe thrombocytopenia, severe stomatitis, severe skin toxicity, and toxic death. Obtain LFTs before each treatment cycle and frequent blood counts to monitor for neutropenia. Severe hypersensitivity reactions reported with dexamethasone premedication; d/c immediately if symptoms occur. Contraindicated with history of severe hypersensitivity reactions to other drugs formulated with polysorbate 80. Severe fluid retention may occur despite dexamethasone premedication.

OTHER BRAND NAMES

Taxotere

ADULT DOSAGE

Breast Cancer

Single Agent:

Locally advanced or metastatic breast cancer after failure of prior chemotherapy

60-100mg/m^2 IV over 1 hr every 3 weeks

Combination w/ Doxorubicin and Cyclophosphamide:

Adjuvant treatment of operable node-positive breast cancer

75mg/m^2 1 hr after doxorubicin 50mg/m^2 and cyclophosphamide 500mg/m^2 every 3 weeks for 6 courses

Prophylactic G-CSF may be used to mitigate risk of hematological toxicities

Non-Small Cell Lung Cancer

Single Agent:

Locally advanced or metastatic non-small cell lung cancer after failure of prior platinum-based chemotherapy

75mg/m^2 IV over 1 hr every 3 weeks

Combination w/ Cisplatin:

Unresectable, locally advanced or metastatic non-small cell lung cancer in chemotherapy-naive patients

75mg/m^2 IV over 1 hr immediately followed by cisplatin 75mg/m^2 over 30-60 min every 3 weeks

Metastatic Prostate Cancer

Combination w/ prednisone for androgen-independent (hormone refractory) metastatic prostate cancer

75mg/m^2 IV over 1 hr every 3 weeks + prednisone 5mg PO bid

Gastric Adenocarcinoma

Combination w/ cisplatin and fluorouracil for advanced gastric adenocarcinoma, including adenocarcinoma of the gastroesophageal junction, in chemotherapy-naive patients

75mg/m^2 IV over 1 hr, followed by cisplatin 75mg/m^2 IV over 1-3 hrs (both on Day 1 only), followed by fluorouracil 750mg/m^2/day IV over 24 hrs x 5 days, starting at end of cisplatin infusion

Repeat treatment every 3 weeks

Squamous Cell Carcinoma of the Head and Neck

Combination w/ cisplatin and fluorouracil for induction treatment of locally advanced

PEDIATRIC DOSAGE

Pediatric use may not have been established

squamous cell carcinoma of the head and neck (SCCHN)

Administer prophylaxis for neutropenic infections

Induction Followed by Radiotherapy:
Locally advanced inoperable SCCHN

75mg/m^2 IV over 1 hr, followed by cisplatin 75mg/m^2 IV over 1 hr, on Day 1, followed by fluorouracil as a continuous IV infusion at 750mg/m^2/day x 5 days

Administer every 3 weeks for 4 cycles; following chemotherapy, patients should receive radiotherapy

Induction Followed by Chemoradiotherapy:
Locally advanced (unresectable, low surgical cure, or organ preservation) SCCHN

75mg/m^2 IV over 1 hr on Day 1, followed by cisplatin 100mg/m^2 IV over 30 min to 3 hrs, followed by fluorouracil 1000mg/m^2/day as a continuous IV infusion from Day 1 to Day 4

Administer every 3 weeks for 3 cycles; following chemotherapy, patients should receive chemoradiotherapy

Premedication

All Patients:
Oral corticosteroids (see below for prostate cancer) such as dexamethasone 16mg/day (8mg bid) for 3 days starting 1 day prior to docetaxel administration

Prostate Cancer:
Given the concurrent use of prednisone, the recommended regimen is dexamethasone 8mg PO, at 12 hrs, 3 hrs, and 1 hr before docetaxel infusion

Gastric Adenocarcinoma/Head and Neck Cancer:
Patients must receive antiemetics and appropriate hydration for cisplatin administration

DOSE MODIFICATION

Hepatic Impairment

AST/ALT >2.5-≤5X ULN and Alkaline Phosphatase ≤2.5X ULN, or AST/ALT >1.5-≤5X ULN and Alkaline Phosphatase >2.5-≤5X ULN: Reduce docetaxel dose by 20%
AST/ALT >5X ULN and/or Alkaline Phosphatase >5X ULN: D/C treatment

Adverse Reactions

Breast Cancer:
Initial Dose 100mg/m^2:
Experience Febrile Neutropenia, Neutrophils <500 cells/mm^3 for >1 Week, or Severe/Cumulative Cutaneous Reactions: Reduce dose to 75mg/m^2; if reactions continue, either reduce dose to 55mg/m^2 or d/c treatment
Initial Dose 60mg/m^2:
Do Not Experience Febrile Neutropenia, Neutrophils <500 cells/mm^3 for >1 Week, Severe/Cumulative Cutaneous Reactions, or Severe Peripheral Neuropathy: May tolerate higher doses
≥Grade 3 Peripheral Neuropathy: D/C treatment

Combination Therapy in Adjuvant Treatment of Breast Cancer:
Febrile Neutropenia: Administer G-CSF in all subsequent cycles; if reaction continues, continue G-CSF and reduce docetaxel dose to 60mg/m^2
Grade 3 or 4 Stomatitis: Reduce docetaxel dose to 60mg/m^2
Severe/Cumulative Cutaneous Reactions or Moderate Neurosensory Signs and/or Symptoms: Reduce docetaxel dose to 60mg/m^2; if reactions continue at 60mg/m^2, d/c treatment

Non-Small Cell Lung Cancer:
Monotherapy:
Experience Febrile Neutropenia, Neutrophils <500 cells/mm^3 for >1 Week, or Severe/Cumulative Cutaneous Reactions, or Other Grade 3-4 Nonhematological Toxicities: Withhold treatment until toxicity resolves, then resume at 55mg/m^2
≥Grade 3 Peripheral Neuropathy: D/C treatment

Combination Therapy:
Nadir of Platelet Count During Previous Course of Therapy is <25000 cells/mm^3 w/ Febrile Neutropenia/Serious Nonhematologic Toxicities: Reduce docetaxel dose in subsequent cycles to 65mg/m^2; if further dose reduction is required, 50mg/m^2 is recommended

Prostate Cancer:
Experience Febrile Neutropenia, Neutrophils <500 cells/mm^3 for >1 Week, Severe/Cumulative Cutaneous Reactions, or Moderate Neurosensory Signs and/or Symptoms: Reduce docetaxel dose to 60mg/m^2; if reactions continue at 60mg/m^2, d/c treatment

Gastric Adenocarcinoma/Head and Neck Cancer:
Experience Episode of Febrile Neutropenia or Prolonged Neutropenia/Neutropenic Infection Occurs Despite G-CSF Use: Reduce docetaxel dose to 60mg/m^2; if subsequent episodes of complicated neutropenia occur, reduce docetaxel dose to 45mg/m^2. D/C if toxicities persist
Grade 4 Thrombocytopenia: Reduce docetaxel dose to 60mg/m^2; do not retreat w/ subsequent cycles until neutrophils recover to >1500 cells/mm^3 and platelets recover to >100,000 cells/mm^3. D/C if toxicities persist

Toxicities w/ Docetaxel in Combination w/ Cisplatin and Fluorouracil:
Grade 3 Diarrhea:
1st Episode: Reduce fluorouracil dose by 20%
2nd Episode: Reduce docetaxel dose by 20%

Grade 4 Diarrhea:
1st Episode: Reduce docetaxel and fluorouracil doses by 20%
2nd Episode: D/C treatment

Grade 3 Stomatitis/Mucositis:
1st Episode: Reduce fluorouracil dose by 20%
2nd Episode: Stop fluorouracil only, at all subsequent cycles
3rd Episode: Reduce docetaxel dose by 20%

Grade 4 Stomatitis/Mucositis:
1st Episode: Stop fluorouracil only, at all subsequent cycles
2nd Episode: Reduce docetaxel dose by 20%

Refer to PI for cisplatin and fluorouracil dose modifications

ADMINISTRATION
IV route

Administration Precautions
Contact of the docetaxel inj w/ plasticized PVC equipment or devices used to prepare sol for infusion is not recommended; store the final docetaxel dilution for infusion in bottles (glass, polypropylene) or plastic bags (polypropylene, polyolefin) and administer through polyethylene-lined administration sets

Preparation
Requires no prior dilution w/ a diluent and is ready to add to the infusion sol

Docetaxel Inj Concentrate (20mg/mL):
Do not use the two-vial formulation (inj concentrate and diluent) w/ the one-vial formulation

HOW SUPPLIED
Inj: 10mg/mL [2mL, 8mL, 16mL], (Taxotere) 20mg/mL [1mL, 4mL]

CONTRAINDICATIONS
Neutrophils <1500 cells/mm^3.

WARNINGS/PRECAUTIONS
Avoid subsequent cycles until neutrophils recover to level >1500 cells/mm^3 and platelets to >100,000 cells/mm^3. Severe fluid retention reported; monitor from the 1st dose for possible exacerbation of preexisting effusions. Acute myeloid leukemia or myelodysplasia may occur in adjuvant therapy (eg, adjuvant therapy in BC). Localized erythema of extremities with edema and desquamation reported; adjust dose if severe skin toxicity occurs. Severe neurosensory symptoms (eg, paresthesia, dysesthesia, pain) may develop; adjust dose if symptoms occur and d/c treatment if symptoms persist. Cystoid macular edema (CME) reported; d/c and initiate appropriate treatment if CME is diagnosed, and/or consider alternative non-taxane cancer treatment. Severe asthenia reported. May cause fetal harm. Caution in elderly. Intoxication reported due to alcohol content. Alcohol content of the drug may affect CNS; caution in whom alcohol intake should be avoided or minimized. Alcohol content of the drug may impair physical/mental abilities.

ADVERSE REACTIONS
Myalgia, alopecia, N/V, diarrhea, nail disorders, skin reactions, fluid retention, thrombocytopenia, anemia, neutropenia, infections, hypersensitivity, neuropathy, dysgeusia, constipation.

DRUG INTERACTIONS
Avoid with CYP3A4 inhibitors; reduce dose by 50% if coadministered with strong CYP3A4 inhibitors (eg, ketoconazole, clarithromycin, atazanavir). CYP3A4 inducers and substrates may alter metabolism. Protease inhibitors (eg, ritonavir) may increase exposure. Renal insufficiency and renal

failure reported with concomitant nephrotoxic drugs. Radiation pneumonitis may occur in patients receiving concomitant radiotherapy (rare).

NURSING CONSIDERATIONS

Assessment: Assess for history of severe hypersensitivity reactions to the drug or other drugs with polysorbate 80, preexisting effusion, hepatic impairment, pregnancy/nursing status, and possible drug interactions. Obtain baseline weight, CBC with platelets and differential count, and LFTs. Perform a comprehensive ophthalmologic examination in patients with impaired vision.

Monitoring: Monitor for fluid retention, acute myeloid leukemia, hematologic effects, skin toxicities, exacerbation of effusions, neurosensory symptoms, hepatic impairment, hypersensitivity reactions, asthenia, CME, and other adverse reactions. Monitor weight, CBC with platelets and differential count, and LFTs.

Patient Counseling: Inform about risks and benefits of therapy. Inform that drug may cause fetal harm; advise to avoid pregnancy and to use effective contraceptives. Explain the significance of oral corticosteroid administration to help facilitate compliance; instruct to report if not compliant. Instruct to report signs of hypersensitivity reactions, fluid retention, myalgia, or cutaneous/ neurologic reactions. Counsel about side effects that are associated with the drug. Explain the significance of routine blood cell counts. Instruct to monitor temperature frequently and immediately report any occurrence of fever. Explain about the possible side effects of the alcohol content in the drug, including possible side effects on the CNS. Advise patients in whom alcohol should be avoided or minimized to consider the alcohol content of the drug; inform that alcohol could impair their ability to drive or use machines immediately after infusion.

Storage: 20-25°C (68-77°F), (Taxotere) 2-25°C (36-77°F). Multi-use vials are stable for up to 28 days when stored at 2-8°C (36-46°F) after use. Protect from light. Reconstituted Sol: 0.9% NaCl or D5W: Stable at 2-25°C (36-77°F) for 4 hrs or (Taxotere) 6 hrs. (Taxotere) Infusion sol is stable in non-PVC bags up to 48 hrs at 2-8°C (36-46°F).

DOLOPHINE – methadone hydrochloride CII

Class: Opioid analgesic

Exposes patients and other users to the risk of opioid addiction, abuse, and misuse, leading to overdose and death; assess each patient's risk prior to prescribing, and monitor regularly for development of these behaviors/conditions. Serious, life-threatening, or fatal respiratory depression may occur; monitor for respiratory depression, especially during initiation or following a dose increase. Accidental ingestion, especially in children, can result in fatal overdose. QT interval prolongation and serious arrhythmia (torsades de pointes) occurred; closely monitor for changes in cardiac rhythm during initiation and titration. Prolonged use during pregnancy can result in neonatal opioid withdrawal syndrome; advise pregnant women of the risk and ensure availability of appropriate treatment. For detoxification and maintenance of opioid dependence, methadone should be administered in accordance with treatment standards, including limitations on unsupervised administration.

ADULT DOSAGE

Pain

Management of Pain Severe Enough to Require Daily, Around-The-Clock, Long-Term Opioid Treatment and for Which Alternative Treatment Options are Inadequate:
1st Opioid Analgesic: 2.5mg q8-12h
Titrate/Maint: Titrate to a dose that provides adequate analgesia and minimizes adverse reactions; may adjust dose every 1-2 days

Detoxification/Maintenance Treatment of Opioid Addiction

Initial: 20-30mg single dose; do not exceed 30mg
Evaluate after 2-4 hrs for same-day dosing adjustment; give additional 5-10mg (max 40mg/1st day) if withdrawal symptoms are not suppressed or if symptoms reappear
Use lower initial doses for expected low tolerance at treatment entry

Short-term Detoxification:
Titrate to 40mg/day in divided doses; after 2-3 days of stabilization, gradually decrease dose on a daily basis or at 2-day intervals depending on toleration of withdrawal symptoms

PEDIATRIC DOSAGE

Pediatric use may not have been established

Hospitalized patients may tolerate a daily reduction of 20% of the total daily dose; ambulatory patients may need a slower schedule

Titrate and Maint of Detoxification:
Usual: 80-120mg/day; titrate to a dose at which opioid withdrawal symptoms are prevented for 24 hrs

Medically Supervised Withdrawal After Maint Treatment:
Reduce dose by <10% of the established tolerance or maint dose; 10- to 14-day intervals should elapse between dose reductions

Acute Pain During Methadone Maint Treatment:
May require somewhat higher and/or more frequent doses than in nontolerant patients

Conversions

D/C all other around-the-clock opioid drugs when therapy is initiated

From Parenteral to Oral Methadone: Use conversion ratio of 1:2mg

From Other Oral Opioids: Refer to PI for calculations

DOSE MODIFICATION

Elderly

Start at lower end of dosing range

Other Important Modifications

Pregnancy: May need to increase dose or decrease dosing interval

ADMINISTRATION

Oral route

HOW SUPPLIED

Tab: 5mg*, 10mg* *scored

CONTRAINDICATIONS

Significant respiratory depression, acute or severe bronchial asthma in an unmonitored setting or in the absence of resuscitative equipment, known or suspected paralytic ileus.

WARNINGS/PRECAUTIONS

Reserve for use in patients for whom alternative analgesic treatment options (eg, nonopioid or IR opioid analgesics) are ineffective, not tolerated, or would be otherwise inadequate to provide sufficient management of pain. Not indicated as a prn analgesic. Deaths reported during conversion from chronic, high-dose treatment with other opioid agonists and during initiation of treatment of addiction in subjects previously abusing high doses of other agonists. Retained in the liver and then slowly released, prolonging the duration of potential toxicity, with repeated dosing. Life-threatening respiratory depression is more likely to occur in elderly, cachectic, or debilitated patients; monitor closely when initiating and titrating, and when given with drugs that depress respiration. Consider alternative nonopioid analgesics in patients with significant COPD or cor pulmonale, and in patients having a substantially decreased respiratory reserve, hypoxia, hypercapnia, or preexisting respiratory depression. May cause severe hypotension including orthostatic hypotension and syncope in ambulatory patients; increased risk in patients with compromised ability to maintain BP. Monitor for signs of sedation and respiratory depression in patients susceptible to the intracranial effects of carbon dioxide retention (eg, those with increased intracranial pressure or brain tumors). May obscure the clinical course in patients with head injury. Avoid with GI obstruction and impaired consciousness or coma. May cause spasm of sphincter of Oddi or increase serum amylase. May aggravate convulsions in patients with convulsive disorders and may induce or aggravate seizures. May impair mental/physical abilities. Abrupt discontinuation may lead to opioid withdrawal symptoms. Infants born to opioid-dependent mothers may be physically dependent and may exhibit respiratory difficulties and withdrawal symptoms. Caution in elderly.

ADVERSE REACTIONS

Respiratory depression, QT prolongation, arrhythmia, systemic hypotension, lightheadedness, dizziness, sedation, sweating, N/V.

DRUG INTERACTIONS

Concomitant use with other CNS depressants (eg, sedatives, tranquilizers, phenothiazines) may result in hypotension, profound sedation, coma, respiratory depression, and death; reduce dose of one or both drugs when combined therapy is considered. CYP3A4 inhibitors may cause decreased clearance leading to an increase in plasma levels and increased or prolonged opioid effects; these effects could be more pronounced with concomitant use of CYP2C9 and 3A4 inhibitors. CYP3A4 inducers may induce metabolism and, therefore, may increase clearance, leading to a decrease in plasma concentrations, lack of efficacy, or (possibly) development of a withdrawal syndrome in a patient who had developed physical dependence to therapy. Antiretroviral drugs (eg, abacavir, darunavir + ritonavir, efavirenz, lopinavir + ritonavir) may increase clearance or decrease plasma levels. May decrease levels of didanosine and stavudine. May increase area under the curve of zidovudine. Monitor for cardiac conduction changes with drugs known to have potential to prolong QT interval. Pharmacodynamic interactions may occur with potentially arrhythmogenic agents (eg, Class I and III antiarrhythmics, neuroleptics, TCAs, calcium channel blockers). Monitor closely with drugs capable of inducing electrolyte disturbances that may prolong QT interval, including diuretics, laxatives, and mineralocorticoid hormones. Mixed agonist/antagonist (eg, pentazocine, nalbuphine, butorphanol), and partial agonist (buprenorphine) analgesics may reduce the analgesic effect or precipitate withdrawal symptoms; avoid use. Severe reactions may occur with concurrent use or within 14 days of MAOI use. May increase levels of desipramine. Anticholinergics may increase risk of urinary retention and/or severe constipation, which may lead to paralytic ileus.

NURSING CONSIDERATIONS

Assessment: Assess for personal/family history or risk factors for drug abuse or addiction, general condition and medical status, opioid experience/tolerance, pain type/severity, previous opioid daily dose, type of prior analgesics used, respiratory depression, cardiac conduction abnormalities, COPD or other respiratory complications, GI obstruction, paralytic ileus, hepatic/renal impairment, previous hypersensitivity to drug, pregnancy/nursing status, possible drug interactions, and any other conditions where treatment is contraindicated or cautioned.

Monitoring: Monitor for signs/symptoms of respiratory depression, QT prolongation and arrhythmias, orthostatic hypotension, syncope, symptoms of worsening biliary tract disease, aggravation/induction of seizures, tolerance, physical dependence, mental/physical impairment, withdrawal syndrome, hypersensitivity reactions, and other adverse reactions. Monitor for signs of increased intracranial pressure with head injuries. Routinely monitor for signs of misuse, abuse, and addiction.

Patient Counseling: Inform that use of medication, even when taken as recommended, may result in addiction, abuse, and misuse. Instruct not to share with others and to take steps to protect from theft or misuse. Inform of the risks of life-threatening respiratory depression; advise how to recognize respiratory depression and to seek medical attention if breathing difficulties develop. Inform that accidental ingestion, especially in children, may result in respiratory depression or death. Instruct to dispose of unused tab by flushing down the toilet. Instruct to seek medical attention immediately if patient experiences symptoms suggestive of an arrhythmia. Inform female patients of reproductive potential that prolonged use of drug during pregnancy may result in neonatal opioid withdrawal syndrome, which may be life threatening if not recognized and treated. Inform that potentially serious additive effects may occur if drug is used with alcohol or other CNS depressants, and instruct not to use such drugs unless supervised by a healthcare provider. Advise to use drug exactly ud and not to d/c without 1st discussing the need for a tapering regimen with prescriber. Inform that drug may impair ability to perform potentially hazardous activities (eg, driving a car, operating heavy machinery). Advise about potential for severe constipation, including management instructions and when to seek medical attention. Inform that anaphylaxis may occur; advise how to recognize such a reaction and when to seek medical attention. Instruct nursing mothers to watch for signs of methadone toxicity in their infants (eg, increased sleepiness [more than usual], difficulty breastfeeding, breathing difficulties, limpness); instruct to inform physician immediately if these signs occur.

Storage: 25°C (77°F); excursions permitted to 15-30°C (59-86°F).

DORIBAX – doripenem RX

Class: Carbapenem

ADULT DOSAGE

Intra-Abdominal Infections

Complicated Infections:

500mg q8h by IV infusion over 1 hr for 5-14 days

Duration includes a possible switch to an appropriate PO therapy, after at least 3 days of parenteral therapy, once clinical improvement has been demonstrated

PEDIATRIC DOSAGE

Pediatric use may not have been established

Urinary Tract Infections

Complicated UTIs, Including Pyelonephritis: 500mg q8h by IV infusion over 1 hr for 10 days; may extend up to 14 days w/ concurrent bacteremia

Duration includes a possible switch to an appropriate PO therapy, after at least 3 days of parenteral therapy, once clinical improvement has been demonstrated

DOSE MODIFICATION

Renal Impairment

CrCl 30-50mL/min: 250mg IV (over 1 hr) q8h

CrCl >10 to <30mL/min: 250mg IV (over 1 hr) q12h

ADMINISTRATION

IV route

Do not mix w/ or physically add to sol containing other drugs

Preparation

500mg Dose:

Constitute 500mg vial w/ 10mL of sterile water for inj (SWFI) or 0.9% NaCl inj; gently shake to form a sus. Withdraw sus using a syringe (21-gauge needle) and add to infusion bag containing 100mL of normal saline or D5; gently shake until clear

250mg Dose:

Using 250mg Vial: Constitute 250mg vial w/ 10mL of SWFI or 0.9% NaCl inj; gently shake to form a sus. Withdraw sus using a syringe (21-gauge needle) and add to infusion bag containing 50mL or 100mL of normal saline or D5; gently shake until clear

Using 500mg Vial: Constitute 500mg vial w/ 10mL of SWFI or 0.9% NaCl inj; gently shake to form a sus. Withdraw sus using a syringe (21-gauge needle) and add to infusion bag containing 100mL of normal saline or D5. Remove 55mL of this sol from the bag and discard and infuse remaining sol

HOW SUPPLIED

Inj: 250mg, 500mg

WARNINGS/PRECAUTIONS

Not approved for the treatment of ventilator-associated bacterial pneumonia. Serious and occasionally fatal hypersensitivity (anaphylactic) and serious skin reactions reported; d/c if an allergic reaction occurs. Seizures reported; higher risk in patients with preexisting CNS disorders (eg, stroke, history of seizures), patients with compromised renal function, and patients given doses >500mg q8h. *Clostridium difficile*-associated diarrhea (CDAD) reported; d/c if CDAD is suspected or confirmed. May result in bacterial resistance with use in the absence of a proven/strongly suspected bacterial infection. Do not administer via inhalation route; pneumonitis reported. Caution in elderly.

ADVERSE REACTIONS

Headache, nausea, diarrhea, rash, phlebitis, anemia, pruritus, hepatic enzyme elevation, oral candidiasis.

DRUG INTERACTIONS

May reduce serum valproic acid levels to below the therapeutic concentration range, which may increase risk for breakthrough seizures; consider alternative antibacterial therapies for patients receiving valproic acid or sodium valproate, or if treatment with the drug is necessary, consider supplemental anticonvulsant therapy. Probenecid may increase levels; coadministration is not recommended.

NURSING CONSIDERATIONS

Assessment: Assess for ventilator-associated bacterial pneumonia, CNS disorders, renal impairment, pregnancy/nursing status, and possible drug interactions. Carefully assess for previous hypersensitivity reactions to drug, penicillin, cephalosporins, other β-lactams, or other allergens.

Monitoring: Monitor for hypersensitivity reactions, CDAD, seizures, development of drug-resistant bacteria, and other adverse reactions. Monitor renal function in patients with moderate or severe renal impairment and in elderly.

Patient Counseling: Advise that allergic reactions could occur and that serious reactions may require immediate treatment. Advise to report any previous hypersensitivity reactions to medications or allergens. Counsel that therapy should only be used to treat bacterial, not viral, infections. Instruct to take exactly ud; inform that skipping doses or not completing the full course of therapy may decrease effectiveness of treatment and increase bacterial resistance. Counsel to inform physician if patient has CNS disorders and if taking valproic acid or sodium valproate.

Storage: 25°C (77°F); excursions permitted to 15-30°C (59-86°F). Refer to PI for storage of constituted sol.

DORYX – doxycycline hyclate

Class: Tetracyclines

RX

OTHER BRAND NAMES

Doxycycline Hyclate

ADULT DOSAGE

General Dosing

Treatment of the following infections caused by susceptible microorganisms: Rocky Mountain spotted fever, typhus fever and the typhus group, Q fever, rickettsialpox, tick fevers, lymphogranuloma venereum, granuloma inguinale, chancroid, respiratory tract infections, psittacosis (ornithosis), relapsing fever, plague, tularemia, cholera, *Campylobacter fetus* infections, brucellosis (in conjunction w/ streptomycin), bartonellosis, UTIs, trachoma, and inclusion conjunctivitis. Treatment of infections caused by susceptible strains of *Escherichia coli*, *Enterobacter aerogenes*, Shigella species, and Acinetobacter species. When penicillin (PCN) is contraindicated, treatment of the following infections caused by susceptible microorganisms: yaws, Vincent's infection, actinomycosis, and infections caused by Clostridium species. Adjunctive therapy in acute intestinal amebiasis and severe acne.

Initial: 100mg q12h on 1st day

Maint: 100mg qd or 50mg q12h

More Severe Infections (eg, Chronic UTIs):

100mg q12h

Streptococcal Infections:

Continue therapy for 10 days

Acute Epididymo-Orchitis

Caused by *Chlamydia trachomatis*:

100mg bid for at least 10 days

Malaria

Prophylaxis:

100mg qd, beginning 1 or 2 days before travel, continuing daily during travel, and for 4 weeks after departure from malarious area

Inhalational Anthrax (Postexposure)

100mg bid for 60 days

Urethral Infections

Uncomplicated Infections Caused by *Chlamydia trachomatis*:

100mg bid for 7 days

Alternate Dosing:

200mg qd for 7 days (Doryx)

Endocervical Infections

Uncomplicated Infections Caused by *Chlamydia trachomatis*:

100mg bid for 7 days

Alternate Dosing:

200mg qd for 7 days (Doryx)

Rectal Infections

Uncomplicated Infections Caused by *Chlamydia trachomatis*:

100mg bid for 7 days

PEDIATRIC DOSAGE

General Dosing

>8 Years:

≤45kg:

4.4mg/kg divided into 2 doses on 1st day, followed by 2.2mg/kg qd or as 2 divided doses, on subsequent days

More Severe Infections (eg, Chronic UTIs):

May use up to 4.4mg/kg

>45kg:

Initial: 100mg q12h on 1st day

Maint: 100mg qd or 50mg q12h

More Severe Infections (eg, Chronic UTIs):

100mg q12h

Streptococcal Infections:

Continue therapy for 10 days

Malaria

Prophylaxis:

>8 Years:

2mg/kg qd up to 100mg qd, beginning 1 or 2 days before travel, continuing daily during travel and for 4 weeks after departure from malarious area

Inhalational Anthrax (Postexposure)

<45kg:

2.2mg/kg bid for 60 days

>45kg:

100mg bid for 60 days

Gonococcal Infections

Uncomplicated Infections (Except Anorectal Infections in Men):
100mg bid for 7 days
Alternate Dosing:
Single visit dose of 300mg stat followed in 1 hr by a second 300mg dose

Nongonococcal Urethritis

Caused by *Ureaplasma urealyticum*:
100mg bid for 7 days

Syphilis

Early (<1-Year Duration):
100mg bid for 2 weeks
>1-Year Duration:
100mg bid for 4 weeks

ADMINISTRATION

Oral route

Administer w/ adequate amounts of fluid
May be given w/ food or milk if gastric irritation occurs
May administer 200mg tab w/o regard to meals

Administering w/ Applesauce
May break up tab and sprinkle contents (delayed-release pellets) over a spoonful of applesauce
Do not crush or damage the pellets when breaking up the tab
Swallow applesauce/pellet mixture immediately w/o chewing; may follow w/ a glass of water

HOW SUPPLIED

Tab, Delayed-Release: 100mg*, 150mg*, 200mg*; (Generic) 75mg* *scored

WARNINGS/PRECAUTIONS

May cause permanent discoloration of the teeth (yellow-gray-brown) if used during tooth development (last 1/2 of pregnancy, infancy, and childhood to 8 yrs of age); do not use in this age group, except for anthrax. Enamel hypoplasia reported. *Clostridium difficile*-associated diarrhea (CDAD) reported; d/c if CDAD is suspected or confirmed. Photosensitivity, manifested by an exaggerated sunburn reaction, reported; d/c at the 1st evidence of skin erythema. May result in bacterial resistance if used in the absence of proven or suspected bacterial infection, or a prophylactic indication; take appropriate measures if superinfection develops. Bulging fontanels in infants and benign intracranial HTN in adults reported. May decrease fibula growth rate in prematures. May cause an increase in BUN. When used for malaria prophylaxis, patient may still transmit the infection to mosquitoes outside endemic areas. False elevations of urinary catecholamines may occur due to interference w/ the fluorescence test.

ADVERSE REACTIONS

N/V, diarrhea, bacterial vaginitis.

DRUG INTERACTIONS

Depresses plasma prothrombin activity; may require downward adjustment of anticoagulant dose. May interfere w/ bactericidal action of PCN; avoid concurrent use. Impaired absorption w/ bismuth subsalicylate, antacids containing aluminum, Ca^{2+}, or Mg^{2+}, and iron-containing preparations. May render oral contraceptives less effective. Decreased $T_{1/2}$ w/ barbiturates, carbamazepine, and phenytoin. Fatal renal toxicity reported w/ methoxyflurane.

NURSING CONSIDERATIONS

Assessment: Assess for hypersensitivity to drug or any tetracyclines, pregnancy/nursing status, and possible drug interactions. Perform culture and susceptibility testing.

Monitoring: Monitor for CDAD, photosensitivity, skin erythema, superinfection, benign intracranial HTN in adults, and other adverse reactions. In long-term therapy, perform periodic lab evaluation of organ systems, including hematopoietic, renal, and hepatic studies.

Patient Counseling: Apprise of the potential hazard to fetus if used during pregnancy. Inform that therapy does not guarantee protection against malaria; advise to use measures that help avoid contact w/ mosquitoes. Advise to avoid excessive sunlight or artificial UV light and to d/c therapy if phototoxicity (eg, skin eruptions) occurs; advise to consider use of sunscreen or sunblock. Inform that absorption of drug is reduced when taken w/ bismuth subsalicylate, antacids containing aluminum, Ca^{2+}, or Mg^{2+}, iron-containing preparations, and w/ foods, especially those that contain Ca^{2+}. Inform that drug may increase the incidence of vaginal candidiasis. Inform that diarrhea may be experienced and instruct to immediately contact physician if watery and bloody stools (w/ or w/o stomach cramps and fever) occur, even as late as ≥2 months after the last dose. Counsel that therapy should only be used to treat bacterial, not viral, infections. Instruct to take exactly ud even if the patient feels better early in the course of therapy. Inform that skipping doses or not completing the full course of therapy may decrease effectiveness of treatment and increase bacterial resistance.

Storage: 20-25°C (68-77°F); excursions permitted to 15-30°C (59-86°F). (Generic) 25°C (77°F); excursions permitted to 15-30°C (59-86°F). Protect from light.

DOXIL – doxorubicin hydrochloride liposome RX

Class: Anthracycline

May cause myocardial damage, including CHF, as the total cumulative dose approaches 550mg/m^2; include prior use of other anthracyclines or anthracenediones in total cumulative dose calculations. Risk of cardiomyopathy may be increased at lower cumulative doses w/ prior mediastinal irradiation. Acute infusion-related reactions occurred in patients w/ solid tumors. Serious, life-threatening, and fatal infusion reactions reported.

ADULT DOSAGE

Ovarian Carcinoma

Progressed/Recurred After Platinum-Based Therapy:
50mg/m^2 IV over 60 min every 28 days until disease progression or unacceptable toxicity

AIDS-Related Kaposi's Sarcoma

After Failure of/Intolerance to Prior Systemic Chemotherapy:
20mg/m^2 IV over 60 min every 21 days until disease progression or unacceptable toxicity

Multiple Myeloma

In patients who have not previously received bortezomib and have received at least 1 prior therapy

30mg/m^2 IV over 60 min on Day 4 of each 21-day cycle for 8 cycles or until disease progression or unacceptable toxicity

Administer therapy after bortezomib on Day 4 of each cycle

PEDIATRIC DOSAGE

Pediatric use may not have been established

DOSE MODIFICATION

Hepatic Impairment
Serum bilirubin >1.2mg/dL: Reduce dose
Adverse Reactions
Hand-Foot Syndrome:
Grade 1:
If previous Grade 3 or 4, delay dose up to 2 weeks, then decrease by 25%
Grade 2:
Delay dosing up to 2 weeks or until resolved to Grade 0-1
If resolved to Grade 0-1 w/in 2 weeks, continue treatment at previous dose if no previous Grade 3 or 4 toxicity, or decrease dose by 25% if previous Grade 3 or 4 toxicity
D/C if no resolution after 2 weeks
Grade 3 or 4:
Delay dosing up to 2 weeks or until resolved to Grade 0-1, then decrease dose by 25%
D/C if no resolution after 2 weeks

Stomatitis:
Grade 1:
If previous Grade 3 or 4, delay dose up to 2 weeks, then decrease by 25%
Grade 2:
Delay dosing up to 2 weeks or until resolved to Grade 0-1
If resolved to Grade 0-1 w/in 2 weeks, continue treatment at previous dose if no previous Grade 3 or 4 toxicity, or decrease dose by 25% if previous Grade 3 or 4 toxicity
D/C if no resolution after 2 weeks
Grade 3 or 4:
Delay dosing up to 2 weeks or until resolved to Grade 0-1; decrease dose by 25% and return to original dose interval
D/C if no resolution after 2 weeks

Neutropenia/Thrombocytopenia:
Grade 2 or 3:
Delay until ANC ≥1500 and platelet count ≥75,000; resume treatment at previous dose
Grade 4:
Delay until ANC ≥1500 and platelet count ≥75,000; resume at 25% dose reduction or continue previous dose w/ prophylactic granulocyte growth factor

Toxicities w/ Bortezomib:
Fever >38°C and ANC <1000:
Withhold dose for this cycle if before Day 4; decrease dose by 25% if after Day 4 of previous cycle
On any Day of Administration After Day 1 of Each Cycle:
Platelet Count <25,000 or Hgb <8g/dL or ANC <500: Withhold dose for this cycle if before Day 4; decrease dose by 25% if after Day 4 of previous cycle and if bortezomib is reduced for hematologic toxicity
Grade 3 or 4 Nonhematologic Toxicity: Do not dose until Grade <2, then reduce dose by 25%
Suspected Extravasation:
D/C for burning or stinging sensation or other evidence indicating perivenous infiltration or extravasation
Do not remove the needle until attempts are made to aspirate extravasated fluid
Do not flush the line; avoid applying pressure to the site
Apply ice to site intermittently for 15 min qid for 3 days
Elevate extremity if extravasation is in an extremity

ADMINISTRATION

IV route

Administer 1st dose at an initial rate of 1mg/min; if no infusion-related adverse reactions are observed, increase infusion rate to complete the administration of therapy over 1 hr
Do not administer as an undiluted sus or IV bolus
Do not use w/ in-line filters
Do not rapidly flush the IV line
Do not mix w/ other drugs

Preparation
Dilute doses up to 90mg in 250mL of D5 inj prior to administration
Dilute doses >90mg in 500mL of D5 inj prior to administration
Administer w/in 24 hrs

HOW SUPPLIED

Inj: 2mg/mL [10mL, 25mL]

WARNINGS/PRECAUTIONS

Do not substitute for doxorubicin HCl inj. Administer only when potential benefits outweigh the risk in patients w/ a history of cardiovascular disease (CVD). Temporarily stop therapy in the event of an infusion-related reaction until resolution then resume at a reduced infusion rate; d/c infusion for serious or life-threatening infusion-related reactions. Hand-foot syndrome (HFS) reported; d/c if HFS is severe and debilitating. Secondary oral cancers, primarily squamous cell carcinoma, reported w/ long-term (>1 yr) exposure; examine at regular intervals for the presence of oral ulceration/ discomfort. May cause fetal harm.

ADVERSE REACTIONS

Myocardial damage, acute infusion-related reactions, neutropenia, anemia, thrombocytopenia, stomatitis, fever, fatigue, N/V, asthenia, diarrhea, constipation, HFS, rash, anorexia.

NURSING CONSIDERATIONS

Assessment: Assess for drug hypersensitivity, history of CVD, hepatic dysfunction, pregnancy/ nursing status. Assess left ventricular cardiac function (eg, multigated acquisition, echocardiogram).

Monitoring: Monitor for signs/symptoms of myocardial damage, infusion-related reactions, HFS, secondary oral cancers, and other adverse reactions. Monitor cardiac function.

Patient Counseling: Advise to contact physician if a new onset of fever, symptoms of an infection, or symptoms of HF develop. Advise about the symptoms of infusion-related reactions and instruct to seek immediate medical attention if any of these symptoms develop. Advise to notify physician if symptoms of HFS or stomatitis develops. Advise females of reproductive potential of the potential risk to a fetus and to inform physician w/ a known or suspected pregnancy. Advise females and males of reproductive potential to use effective contraception during and for 6 months following treatment, and that therapy may cause temporary or permanent infertility. Advise females not to breastfeed during treatment. Inform that a reddish-orange color may appear in urine and other body fluids.

Storage: 2-8°C (36-46°F). Do not freeze.

Doxy 100 – doxycycline

RX

Class: Tetracyclines

ADULT DOSAGE

General Dosing

Initial: 200mg IV administered in 1 or 2 infusions on 1st day
Maint: 100-200mg/day IV depending on severity of infection, w/ 200mg administered in 1 or 2 infusions
Group A β-Hemolytic Streptococci Infections: Treat for at least 10 days

Syphilis

Primary and Secondary: 300mg/day IV for at least 10 days

Inhalational Anthrax (Postexposure)

100mg IV bid; institute oral therapy as soon as possible and continue therapy for a total of 60 days

PEDIATRIC DOSAGE

General Dosing

>8 Years:
≤100 lbs:
Initial: 2mg/lb IV administered in 1 or 2 infusions on 1st day
Maint: 1-2mg/lb/day IV given as 1 or 2 infusions, depending on severity of infection
>100 lbs:
Initial: 200mg IV administered in 1 or 2 infusions on 1st day
Maint: 100-200mg/day IV depending on severity of infection, w/ 200mg administered in 1 or 2 infusions
Group A β-Hemolytic Streptococci Infections: Treat for at least 10 days

Inhalational Anthrax (Postexposure)

<100 lbs: 1mg/lb IV bid; institute oral therapy as soon as possible and continue therapy for a total of 60 days

ADMINISTRATION

IV route
Avoid rapid administration
Do not inject IM or SQ

Preparation

Reconstitute w/ 10mL of SWFI or any compatible IV sol
Withdraw entire reconstituted sol from vial and further dilute w/ 100-1000mL of compatible IV sol to achieve desired concentrations of 0.1-1mg/mL
Concentrations <0.1mg/mL or >1mg/mL not recommended

Infusion Duration

May vary w/ dose, but is usually 1-4 hrs
Recommended infusion time for 100mg of a 0.5mg/mL sol is 1hr

Compatible IV Solutions

NaCl Inj
D5 Inj
Ringer's Inj
Invert Sugar, 10% in water
Lactated Ringer's Inj
D5 in Lactated Ringer's
Normosol-M in D5W
Normosol-R in D5W
Plasma-Lyte 56 in D5
Plasma-Lyte 148 in D5
Refer to PI for further stability information

HOW SUPPLIED

Inj: 100mg

WARNINGS/PRECAUTIONS

May cause permanent discoloration of the teeth (yellow-gray-brown) if used during tooth development (last 1/2 of pregnancy, infancy, and childhood to 8 yrs of age); do not use in this age group, except for anthrax. Enamel hypoplasia reported. Mild to life-threatening pseudomembranous colitis reported. Photosensitivity manifested by an exaggerated sunburn reaction reported; d/c at the 1st evidence of skin erythema. May cause an increase in BUN. May result in bacterial resistance if used in the absence of proven or suspected bacterial infection, or a prophylactic indication; take appropriate measures if superinfection develops.

ADVERSE REACTIONS

Anorexia, N/V, diarrhea, glossitis, dysphagia, maculopapular/erythematous rash, urticaria, angioneurotic edema, anaphylaxis, pericarditis, hemolytic anemia, thrombocytopenia, neutropenia, eosinophilia.

DRUG INTERACTIONS

Depresses plasma prothrombin activity; may require downward adjustment of anticoagulant dose. May interfere with bactericidal action of PCN; avoid concurrent use.

NURSING CONSIDERATIONS

Assessment: Assess for hypersensitivity to drug or any tetracyclines, pregnancy/nursing status, and possible drug interactions. Perform culture and susceptibility testing. In venereal diseases when coexistent syphilis is suspected, perform a dark-field exam and blood serology.

Monitoring: Monitor for pseudomembranous colitis, photosensitivity, skin erythema, superinfection, discoloration of the teeth, and other adverse reactions. In venereal diseases when coexistent syphilis is suspected, repeat blood serology monthly for at least 4 months. In long-term therapy, perform periodic lab evaluation of organ systems, including hematopoietic, renal, and hepatic studies.

Patient Counseling: Advise patients apt to be exposed to direct sunlight or UV light that photosensitivity manifested by an exaggerated sunburn reaction may occur; instruct to d/c treatment at the 1st evidence of skin erythema. Instruct to notify physician if pregnant/breastfeeding. Counsel that therapy should only be used to treat bacterial, not viral, infections. Instruct to take exactly ud even if the patient feels better early in the course of therapy. Inform that skipping doses or not completing the full course of therapy may decrease effectiveness of treatment and increase bacterial resistance.

Storage: 20-25°C (68-77°F). Protect from light. Refer to PI for stability information of reconstituted/diluted sol.

DRISDOL — ergocalciferol **RX**

Class: Vitamin D analogue

ADULT DOSAGE

Hypoparathyroidism

50,000-200,000 IU daily given concomitantly w/ calcium lactate 4g six times/day

Vitamin D Resistant Rickets

12,000-500,000 IU daily

Other Indications

Familial Hypophosphatemia

PEDIATRIC DOSAGE

Hypoparathyroidism

50,000-200,000 IU daily given concomitantly w/ calcium lactate 4g six times/day

Vitamin D Resistant Rickets

12,000-500,000 IU daily

Other Indications

Familial Hypophosphatemia

DOSE MODIFICATION

Elderly

Start at low end of dosing range

ADMINISTRATION

Oral route

HOW SUPPLIED

Cap: 1.25mg (50,000 IU vitamin D)

CONTRAINDICATIONS

Hypercalcemia, malabsorption syndrome, abnormal sensitivity to the toxic effects of vitamin D, hypervitaminosis D.

WARNINGS/PRECAUTIONS

Avoid in infants with idiopathic hypercalcemia. Exercise great care in dose adjustment to prevent serious toxic effects; the range between therapeutic and toxic doses is narrow in vitamin D resistant rickets. Monitor serum calcium levels frequently with high doses. Perform monthly bone x-ray until condition is corrected and stabilized. IV calcium, parathyroid hormone, and/or dihydrotachysterol may be needed when treating hypoparathyroidism. Maintain normal serum phosphorus levels (eg, dietary phosphate restriction and/or administration of aluminum gels) when treating hyperphosphatemia to prevent metastatic calcification. Maintain adequate dietary calcium. Contains FD&C Yellow No. 5 (tartrazine), which can cause allergic reactions (including bronchial asthma). Avoid excess use of vitamin D during normal pregnancy, unless unique case outweighs the significant hazards. Caution in elderly.

ADVERSE REACTIONS

Anemia, anorexia, constipation, nausea, stiffness, weakness, calcification of soft tissues, impaired renal function, HTN.

DRUG INTERACTIONS

Impaired absorption with mineral oil. Thiazide diuretics may cause hypercalcemia in hypoparathyroid patients.

NURSING CONSIDERATIONS

Assessment: Assess for hypercalcemia, malabsorption syndrome, and hypervitaminosis D prior to treatment. Assess for hypersensitivity to vitamin D in infants with idiopathic hypercalcemia.

Evaluate vitamin D consumption patient is receiving from other sources (eg, fortified foods, dietary supplements, self administered and prescription drugs) prior to therapy. Assess use in patients with decreased hepatic/renal or cardiac function. Assess for pregnancy/nursing status and possible drug interactions.

Monitoring: Monitor vitamin D intake from other sources during therapy. Monitor for clinical response to therapy and adjust dosing accordingly. Monitor for adverse reactions. Perform frequent monitoring of blood calcium levels in patients on high doses. In patients treated for hypoparathyroidism, monitor need for IV calcium, parathyroid hormone, and/or dihydrotachysterol, have blood calcium levels and blood phosphorus levels checked every 2 weeks, and perform x-rays once a month. Monitor serum calcium in infants with nursing mother given large doses of vitamin D.

Patient Counseling: Counsel about signs/symptoms of hypervitaminosis D (hypercalcemia, impaired renal function, calcification of soft tissues, and decline in growth rate in infants and children). Inform that effects of vitamin D can persist for more than 2 months.

Storage: 25°C (77°F); excursions permitted to 15-30°C (59-86°F). Protect from light.

DUAC — benzoyl peroxide/clindamycin phosphate RX

Class: Antibacterial/keratolytic

ADULT DOSAGE

Inflammatory Acne Vulgaris

Apply a thin layer to the face qd (pm or ud)

PEDIATRIC DOSAGE

Inflammatory Acne Vulgaris

≥12 Years:

Apply a thin layer to the face qd (pm or ud)

ADMINISTRATION

Topical route

Wash skin gently, rinse w/ warm water, and pat dry before application

HOW SUPPLIED

Gel: (Clindamycin/Benzoyl Peroxide) 1.2%/5% [45g]

CONTRAINDICATIONS

History of regional enteritis, ulcerative colitis (UC), pseudomembranous colitis, or antibiotic-associated colitis.

WARNINGS/PRECAUTIONS

Avoid contact w/ the eyes, mouth, lips, mucous membranes, or broken skin areas. Diarrhea, bloody diarrhea, and colitis (including pseudomembranous colitis) reported; d/c if significant diarrhea occurs. Severe colitis, which may result in death, reported following oral or parenteral administration w/ an onset of up to several weeks following cessation of therapy. May cause increased sensitivity to sunlight; minimize sun exposure (including use of tanning beds or sun lamps) following application. Caution in patients who may be required to have considerable sun exposure due to occupation and those w/ inherent sensitivity to sun.

ADVERSE REACTIONS

Facial local skin reactions (eg, erythema, peeling, burning, dryness).

DRUG INTERACTIONS

Avoid w/ erythromycin-containing products. Antiperistaltic agents (eg, opiates, diphenoxylate w/ atropine) may prolong and/or worsen severe colitis. Caution w/ concomitant topical acne therapies (eg, peeling, desquamating, or abrasive agents) because of possible cumulative irritancy effect; if irritancy or dermatitis occurs, reduce frequency of application or temporarily interrupt treatment and resume once the irritation subsides, or d/c treatment if irritation persists. May enhance action of other neuromuscular blocking agents; use w/ caution. May cause skin and facial hair to temporarily change color (yellow/orange) w/ topical sulfone products.

NURSING CONSIDERATIONS

Assessment: Assess for hypersensitivity to drug or lincomycin; history of regional enteritis, UC, pseudomembranous colitis, or antibiotic-associated colitis; pregnancy/nursing status; and possible drug interactions. Assess use in patients who may be required to have considerable sun exposure due to occupation and those w/ inherent sensitivity to the sun.

Monitoring: Monitor for signs/symptoms of diarrhea, colitis, local skin reactions, and other adverse reactions. For colitis, perform stool culture and assay for *Clostridium difficile* toxin.

Patient Counseling: Counsel to d/c use and contact physician immediately if an allergic reaction (eg, severe swelling, SOB) develops. Inform that drug may cause irritation (eg, erythema, scaling, itching, or burning), especially when used in combination w/ other topical acne therapies. Advise to limit exposure to sunlight, wear protective clothing (eg, hat), and use sunscreen. Inform that drug may bleach hair or colored fabric. Inform that drug may cause skin and facial hair to temporarily change color (yellow/orange) when used w/ topical sulfone products.

Storage: Do not freeze. Prior to Dispensing: 2-8°C (36-46°F). After Dispensing: Room temperature up to 25°C (77°F). Keep tube tightly closed.

DUAVEE – bazedoxifene/conjugated estrogens **RX**

Class: Estrogen/estrogen agonist and antagonist

Do not take additional estrogens. Increased risk of endometrial cancer in a woman with a uterus who uses unopposed estrogens. Perform adequate diagnostic measures to rule out malignancy in postmenopausal women with undiagnosed persistent or recurring abnormal genital bleeding. Should not be used for the prevention of cardiovascular disease (CVD) or dementia. Increased risk of stroke and deep vein thrombosis (DVT) reported in postmenopausal women (50-79 yrs of age) treated with daily oral conjugated estrogens alone. Increased risk of probable dementia reported in postmenopausal women ≥65 yrs of age treated with daily conjugated estrogens alone. Estrogens should be prescribed at the lowest effective dose and for the shortest duration consistent with treatment goals and risks.

ADULT DOSAGE

Menopausal Vasomotor Symptoms

Moderate to Severe:
Usual: 1 tab daily

Postmenopausal Osteoporosis

Prevention:
Usual: 1 tab daily
Add supplemental Ca^{2+}/vitamin D if patient has inadequate dietary intake

PEDIATRIC DOSAGE

Pediatric use may not have been established

ADMINISTRATION

Oral route

Swallow tab whole; take w/o regard to meals

HOW SUPPLIED

Tab: (Conjugated Estrogens [CE]/Bazedoxifene) 0.45mg/20mg

CONTRAINDICATIONS

Undiagnosed abnormal uterine bleeding, known/suspected/history of breast cancer, known/suspected estrogen-dependent neoplasia, active/history of DVT/pulmonary embolism (PE), active/history of arterial thromboembolic disease (eg, stroke, myocardial infarction), known hepatic impairment or disease, known protein C/protein S/antithrombin deficiency or other known thrombophilic disorders, pregnancy, women who may become pregnant, and nursing mothers.

WARNINGS/PRECAUTIONS

D/C immediately if stroke or DVT occurs or is suspected. Caution in patients with risk factors for arterial vascular disease and/or venous thromboembolism. If feasible, d/c at least 4-6 weeks before surgery of the type associated with an increased risk of thromboembolism, or during periods of prolonged immobilization. May increase risk of ovarian cancer and gallbladder disease requiring surgery. Retinal vascular thrombosis reported; d/c pending exam if sudden partial/complete loss of vision, or sudden onset of proptosis, diplopia, or migraine occurs. D/C permanently if exam reveals papilledema or retinal vascular lesions. May elevate BP and thyroid-binding globulin levels. May elevate plasma TGs, leading to pancreatitis in patients with preexisting hypertriglyceridemia. Caution with history of cholestatic jaundice associated with past estrogen use or with pregnancy; d/c in case of recurrence. May cause fluid retention. Caution with hypoparathyroidism; hypocalcemia may occur. May exacerbate symptoms of angioedema in women with hereditary angioedema. May exacerbate asthma, diabetes mellitus (DM), epilepsy, migraine, porphyria, systemic lupus erythematosus (SLE), and hepatic hemangiomas. Not recommended for use in patients >75 yrs of age and in patients with renal impairment. May affect certain endocrine and blood components in lab tests.

ADVERSE REACTIONS

Muscle spasms, nausea, diarrhea, dyspepsia, upper abdominal pain, oropharyngeal pain, dizziness, neck pain.

DRUG INTERACTIONS

Do not take progestins. CE: CYP3A4 inducers (eg, St. John's wort preparations, phenobarbital, carbamazepine) may decrease levels and may decrease therapeutic effects and/or result in changes in the uterine bleeding profile. CYP3A4 inhibitors (eg, erythromycin, clarithromycin, ketoconazole) may increase levels and may increase the risk of endometrial hyperplasia; monitor if CYP3A4 inhibitor is chronically administered (>30 days). Women dependent on thyroid hormone replacement therapy who are also receiving estrogens may require increased doses of their thyroid replacement therapy; monitor thyroid function. Bazedoxifene: Substances known to induce uridine diphosphate glucuronosyltransferase (eg, rifampin, phenobarbital, carbamazepine) may increase metabolism, decrease exposure, and may be associated with an increase in risk of endometrial hyperplasia.

NURSING CONSIDERATIONS

Assessment: Assess for undiagnosed abnormal uterine bleeding, presence/history of breast cancer, estrogen-dependent neoplasia, active/history of DVT/PE/arterial thromboembolic disease, hepatic impairment/disease, history of cholestatic jaundice, drug hypersensitivity, renal impairment, pregnancy/nursing status, any other conditions where treatment may be contraindicated or cautioned, and possible drug interactions.

Monitoring: Monitor for signs/symptoms of CVD; malignant neoplasms; gallbladder disease; dementia; visual abnormalities; BP and plasma TG elevations; pancreatitis; cholestatic jaundice; hypothyroidism; fluid retention; exacerbation of asthma, DM, epilepsy, migraine, porphyria, SLE, and hepatic hemangiomas; and other adverse reactions. Perform annual breast exam; schedule mammography based on age, risk factors, and prior mammogram results. Perform adequate diagnostic measures in patients with undiagnosed persistent or recurring genital bleeding. Perform periodic evaluation to determine treatment need.

Patient Counseling: Advise to immediately report to physician any signs/symptoms related to venous thrombosis and thromboembolic events. Inform postmenopausal women of the importance of reporting vaginal bleeding to physician as soon as possible. Inform postmenopausal women of possible serious reactions of therapy (eg, cardiovascular disorders, malignant neoplasms, probable dementia), and possible less serious but common adverse reactions (eg, muscle spasms, nausea, diarrhea). Advise to add supplemental Ca^{+2} and/or vitamin D to the diet if daily intake is inadequate. Instruct to remove only 1 tab from the blister package at the time of use.

Storage: 20-25°C (68-77°F); excursions permitted to 15-30°C (59-86°F). Keep in original container to protect from moisture; do not place in pill boxes or pill organizers. After opening foil pouch, use within 60 days.

DUEXIS – famotidine/ibuprofen

Class: H_2-blocker/NSAID

RX

NSAIDs may increase risk of serious cardiovascular (CV) thrombotic events, myocardial infarction (MI), and stroke; increased risk with duration of use and with CV disease (CVD) or risk factors for CVD. Increased risk of serious GI adverse reactions (eg, bleeding, ulceration, and perforation of stomach/intestines) that can be fatal and occur anytime during use and without warning symptoms; elderly patients are at greater risk. Contraindicated for the treatment of perioperative pain in the setting of coronary artery bypass graft (CABG) surgery.

ADULT DOSAGE

Rheumatoid Arthritis

Relief of signs/symptoms of rheumatoid arthritis and to decrease the risk of developing upper GI ulcers in patients taking ibuprofen for this indication

1 tab tid

Osteoarthritis

Relief of signs/symptoms of osteoarthritis and to decrease the risk of developing upper GI ulcers in patients taking ibuprofen for this indication

1 tab tid

PEDIATRIC DOSAGE

Pediatric use may not have been established

ADMINISTRATION

Oral route

Swallow whole; do not cut, chew, divide, or crush

HOW SUPPLIED

Tab: (Ibuprofen/Famotidine) 800mg/26.6mg

CONTRAINDICATIONS

Patients who have experienced asthma, urticaria, or allergic reactions after taking aspirin (ASA) or other NSAIDs. Patients in the late stages of pregnancy. Treatment of perioperative pain in the setting of CABG surgery.

WARNINGS/PRECAUTIONS

Use for the shortest possible duration. Symptomatic response does not preclude the presence of gastric malignancy. D/C with active and clinically significant bleeding. Periodically monitor Hgb if initial Hgb ≤10g and long-term therapy is going to be received. D/C if visual disturbances occur and perform ophthalmologic exam. May mask signs of inflammation and fever. Ibuprofen: May cause HTN or worsen preexisting HTN; caution with HTN, and monitor BP closely. Fluid retention and edema reported; caution with fluid retention or heart failure (HF). Caution with history of ulcer disease or GI bleeding, or risk factors for GI bleeding (eg, prolonged NSAID therapy, older age, poor general health status); monitor for GI ulceration/bleeding, and d/c if serious GI adverse reaction occurs. May exacerbate inflammatory bowel disease (IBD). Renal injury reported with long-term use; increased risk with renal/hepatic impairment, HF, and in elderly. D/C if clinical signs and symptoms consistent with renal disease develop. Anaphylaxis may occur; avoid with ASA triad. May cause serious skin adverse reactions; d/c at 1st appearance of skin rash or any sign of hypersensitivity. May cause elevated LFTs or severe hepatic reactions; d/c if liver disease or systemic manifestations occur. Anemia may occur; monitor Hgb/Hct if signs/symptoms of anemia develop with long-term use. May inhibit platelet aggregation and prolong bleeding time; monitor patients with coagulation disorders. Caution with preexisting asthma and avoid with ASA-sensitive asthma. Aseptic meningitis with fever and coma observed on rare occasions. Not a substitute for corticosteroids or for the treatment of corticosteroid insufficiency. Caution in elderly and debilitated. Famotidine: CNS adverse effects reported with moderate (CrCl <50mL/min) and severe renal insufficiency (CrCl <10mL/min); not recommended with CrCl <50mL/min.

ADVERSE REACTIONS

CV thrombotic events, MI, stroke, GI bleeding/ulceration/perforation, nausea, diarrhea, constipation, upper abdominal pain, headache, dyspepsia, upper respiratory tract infection, HTN.

DRUG INTERACTIONS

Increased risk of GI bleeding with oral corticosteroids, anticoagulants (eg, warfarin), antiplatelet drugs (including low-dose ASA), smoking, alcohol, and SSRIs. Risk of renal toxicity when coadministered with diuretics and ACE inhibitors. Avoid with other ibuprofen-containing products. Bleeding reported with coumarin-type anticoagulants. Increased risk of adverse events with ASA. May diminish effects of ACE inhibitors, thiazides, and loop (eg, furosemide) diuretics. May increase lithium levels; monitor for lithium toxicity. May enhance methotrexate toxicity; use with caution. Delayed absorption with cholestyramine.

NURSING CONSIDERATIONS

Assessment: Assess for CABG surgery, CVD, a history of hypersensitivity to ASA or other NSAIDs, or any other conditions where treatment is contraindicated or cautioned. Assess for pregnancy/nursing status and for possible drug interactions. Obtain baseline BP, LFTs, CBC, and renal function.

Monitoring: Monitor for CV thrombotic events, GI events, active bleeding, anemia, anaphylaxis, skin reactions, visual disturbances, and other adverse reactions. Monitor BP, LFTs, renal function, CBC, and chemistry profiles.

Patient Counseling: Inform of possible serious CV and GI side effects. Advise to d/c drug immediately and contact physician if any type of rash develops. Instruct to d/c therapy and seek immediate medical therapy if nephrotoxicity, hepatotoxicity, or anaphylaxis occurs. Advise to report signs/symptoms of unexplained weight gain or edema to physician. Inform that medication should be avoided in late pregnancy. Instruct on what to do if a dose is missed.

Storage: 25°C (77°F); excursions permitted to 15-30°C (59-86°F).

DULERA – formoterol fumarate dihydrate/mometasone furoate RX

Class: Beta$_2$-agonist/corticosteroid

Long-acting β_2-adrenergic agonists (LABAs), such as formoterol, increase the risk of asthma-related death. LABAs may increase the risk of asthma-related hospitalization in pediatric patients and adolescents. Use only for patients not adequately controlled on a long-term asthma control medication (eg, inhaled corticosteroid) or whose disease severity clearly warrants initiation of treatment with both an inhaled corticosteroid and LABA. Do not use if asthma is adequately controlled on low- or medium-dose inhaled corticosteroids.

ADULT DOSAGE

Asthma

Previously on Inhaled Medium Dose Corticosteroids:
2 inh of 100mcg-5mcg bid (am and pm)
Max: 400mcg-20mcg daily

Previously on Inhaled High Dose Corticosteroids:
2 inh of 200mcg-5mcg bid (am and pm)

PEDIATRIC DOSAGE

Asthma

≥12 Years:
Previously on Inhaled Medium Dose Corticosteroids:
2 inh of 100mcg-5mcg bid (am and pm)
Max: 400mcg-20mcg daily

Max: 800mcg-20mcg daily
Do not use >2 inh bid of the prescribed strength. If inadequate response after 2 weeks of therapy, higher strength may provide additional asthma control

Previously on Inhaled High Dose Corticosteroids:
2 inh of 200mcg-5mcg bid (am and pm)
Max: 800mcg-20mcg daily
Do not use >2 inh bid of the prescribed strength. If inadequate response after 2 weeks of therapy, higher strength may provide additional asthma control

ADMINISTRATION

Oral inh route

After inh, rinse mouth with water without swallowing
Shake well before use
Refer to PI for proper administration

Priming

Hold in the upright position and release 4 actuations (puffs) into the air, away from your face
After priming 4 times, the dose counter should read either "60" or "120"
If Dulera is not used for more than 5 days, prime again before use

HOW SUPPLIED

MDI: (Mometasone-Formoterol) 100mcg-5mcg/inh, 200mcg-5mcg/inh [60, 120 inh]

CONTRAINDICATIONS

Primary treatment of status asthmaticus or other acute episodes of asthma where intensive measures are required.

WARNINGS/PRECAUTIONS

Not indicated for the relief of acute bronchospasm. Do not initiate during rapidly deteriorating/potentially life-threatening episodes of asthma. D/C regular use of oral/inhaled short-acting β_2-agonists (SABAs) prior to treatment. Cardiovascular (CV) effects and fatalities reported with excessive use; do not use an additional LABA. *Candida albicans* infections of mouth and pharynx reported; treat and, if needed, interrupt therapy. Increased susceptibility to infections. May lead to serious/fatal course of chickenpox or measles; avoid exposure and, if exposed, consider prophylaxis/treatment. Caution with active/quiescent tuberculosis (TB), untreated systemic fungal, bacterial, viral, or parasitic infections, or ocular herpes simplex. Deaths due to adrenal insufficiency reported with transfer from systemic to inhaled corticosteroids; wean slowly from systemic corticosteroid use after transferring to therapy. Resume oral corticosteroids during periods of stress or a severe asthma attack if patient previously withdrawn from systemic corticosteroid. Transferring from systemic to inhalation therapy may unmask previously suppressed allergic conditions (eg, rhinitis, conjunctivitis, eczema). Observe for systemic corticosteroid withdrawal effects. Reduce dose slowly if hypercorticism and adrenal suppression appear. Inhalation induced bronchospasm with immediate increase in wheezing may occur; d/c immediately and institute alternative therapy. Immediate hypersensitivity reactions, and CV and CNS effects may occur. Decreases in bone mineral density (BMD) reported; caution with major risk factors for decreased bone mineral content, including chronic use of drugs that can reduce bone mass (eg, anticonvulsants, corticosteroids). May reduce growth velocity in pediatric patients. Glaucoma, increased intraocular pressure (IOP), and cataracts reported. Caution in elderly and patients with CV disorders, aneurysm, pheochromocytoma, convulsive disorders, thyrotoxicosis, and in patients unusually responsive to sympathomimetic amines. May cause changes in blood glucose and serum K^+ levels.

ADVERSE REACTIONS

Nasopharyngitis, sinusitis, headache, dysphonia.

DRUG INTERACTIONS

Do not use with other medications containing LABA; increased risk of CV effects. Caution with ketoconazole, other known strong CYP3A4 inhibitors (eg, ritonavir, clarithromycin, itraconazole), and non-K^+-sparing diuretics (eg, loop or thiazide diuretics). Elevated risk of arrhythmias with concomitant anesthesia with halogenated hydrocarbons. Mometasone: Increased plasma concentration with oral ketoconazole and increased systemic exposure with CYP3A4 inhibitors. Formoterol: Potentiation of sympathetic effects with additional adrenergic drugs; use with caution. Potentiation of hypokalemic effect with xanthine derivatives and diuretics. Caution with MAOIs, TCAs, macrolides, drugs known to prolong QTc interval or within 2 weeks of discontinuing such agents; effect on CV system may be potentiated. Use with β-blockers may block effects and produce severe bronchospasm in asthma patients; if needed, consider cardioselective β-blocker with caution.

NURSING CONSIDERATIONS

Assessment: Assess for status asthmaticus, acute asthma episodes, rapidly deteriorating asthma, known hypersensitivity to any drug component, risk factors for decreased bone mineral content, CV or convulsive disorders, thyrotoxicosis, other conditions where treatment is contraindicated or cautioned, pregnancy/nursing status, and possible drug interactions. Obtain baseline BMD and lung function.

Monitoring: Monitor for localized oral *C. albicans* infections, glaucoma, increased IOP, cataracts, CV/CNS effects, hypercorticism, adrenal suppression, inhalation induced bronchospasm, hypokalemia, hyperglycemia, hypersensitivity reactions, signs of increased drug exposure with hepatic impairment, and other adverse reactions. Monitor BMD and lung function. Perform regular eye examinations. Monitor growth in pediatric patients routinely.

Patient Counseling: Inform about increased risk of asthma-related hospitalization in pediatric patients/adolescents and asthma-related death. Instruct not to use to relieve acute asthma symptoms, if symptoms arise between doses, use an inhaled SABA for immediate relief. Instruct to seek medical attention if symptoms worsen, if lung function decreases, or if more inhalations than usual of a SABA are needed. If a dose is missed, instruct to take next dose at the same time patients normally do. Instruct not to d/c or reduce therapy without physician's guidance. Instruct not to use with other LABAs. Advise to avoid exposure to chickenpox or measles and, if exposed, consult physician without delay. Inform of potential worsening of existing TB, fungal, bacterial, viral, or parasitic infections, or ocular herpes simplex. Inform about risks of hypercorticism and adrenal suppression, decreased BMD, cataracts or glaucoma, oropharyngeal candidiasis, and reduced growth velocity in pediatric patients. Inform of adverse events associated with β_2-agonists. Instruct regarding use of therapy.

Storage: 20-25°C (68-77°F); excursions permitted to 15-30°C (59-86°F). Do not puncture. Do not use or store near heat or open flame. 60-inhalation inhaler: Store with the mouthpiece down or in a horizontal position after priming.

DUONEB – albuterol sulfate/ipratropium bromide — RX

Class: Anticholinergic/beta$_2$-agonist

ADULT DOSAGE

Bronchospasm

Associated w/ COPD:
3mL qid via nebulizer
May give up to 2 additional 3mL doses/day, prn

PEDIATRIC DOSAGE

Pediatric use may not have been established

ADMINISTRATION

Inh route

Administer via jet nebulizer connected to an air compressor w/ an adequate air flow, equipped w/ a mouthpiece or suitable face mask

HOW SUPPLIED

Sol, Inhalation: (Ipratropium Bromide-Albuterol Sulfate) 0.5mg-3mg/3mL

CONTRAINDICATIONS

History of hypersensitivity to atropine and its derivatives.

WARNINGS/PRECAUTIONS

Paradoxical bronchospasm may occur; d/c immediately and institute alternative therapy if occurs. Fatalities reported with excessive use of inhaled products containing sympathomimetic amines and with home use of nebulizers. May produce significant cardiovascular (CV) effects (eg, ECG changes). Immediate hypersensitivity reactions reported. Caution with CV disorders (eg, coronary insufficiency, cardiac arrhythmias, HTN), convulsive disorders, hyperthyroidism, diabetes mellitus (DM), narrow-angle glaucoma, prostatic hypertrophy, bladder neck obstruction, hepatic/renal insufficiency, and in patients unusually responsive to sympathomimetic amines. Aggravation of preexisting DM and ketoacidosis reported with large doses of IV albuterol. May decrease serum K^+.

ADVERSE REACTIONS

Lung disease, pharyngitis, pain, chest pain, diarrhea, dyspepsia, nausea, leg cramps, bronchitis, pneumonia, UTI, constipation, voice alterations.

DRUG INTERACTIONS

Additive effects with other anticholinergic drugs; use with caution. Other sympathomimetic agents may increase risk of adverse CV effects; use with caution. β-blockers and albuterol inhibit the effect of each other; use β-blockers with caution in patients with hyperreactive airways. ECG changes and/or hypokalemia that may result from non-K^+-sparing diuretics (eg, loop or thiazide diuretics) may be worsened by β-agonists; use with caution. Administration with MAOIs or TCAs, or within 2 weeks of discontinuation of such agents may potentiate the action of albuterol on CV system; use with extreme caution.

NURSING CONSIDERATIONS

Assessment: Assess for history of hypersensitivity to atropine and its derivatives, CV disorders, convulsive disorders, hyperthyroidism, DM, narrow-angle glaucoma, prostatic hypertrophy, bladder neck obstruction, hepatic/renal insufficiency, pregnancy/nursing status, and possible drug interactions. Assess use in patients unusually responsive to sympathomimetic amines.

Monitoring: Monitor for signs/symptoms of hypersensitivity reactions, paradoxical bronchospasm, CV effects, and other adverse reactions. Monitor pulse rate and BP. Reassess therapy if signs of worsening COPD occur.

Patient Counseling: Advise not to exceed recommended dose or frequency without consulting physician. Instruct to contact physician if symptoms worsen. Instruct to avoid exposing eyes to this product as temporary pupillary dilation, blurred vision, eye pain, or precipitation/worsening of narrow-angle glaucoma may occur. Inform that proper nebulizer technique should be assured, particularly if a mask is used. Instruct to contact physician if pregnancy occurs or nursing is started while on therapy.

Storage: 2-25°C (36-77°F). Store in pouch until time of use. Protect from light.

DURAGESIC — fentanyl

Class: Opioid analgesic

CII

Exposes patients and other users to the risk of opioid addiction/abuse/misuse, which may lead to overdose and death; assess risk prior to therapy and monitor all patients regularly for development of these behaviors or conditions. Serious, life-threatening, or fatal respiratory depression may occur; monitor especially during initiation or following a dose increase. Contraindicated for use as a prn analgesic, in nonopioid tolerant patients, in acute pain, and in postoperative pain. Deaths due to fatal overdose have occurred from accidental exposure; strict adherence to handling/disposal instructions is of utmost importance to prevent accidental exposure. Prolonged use during pregnancy may result in neonatal opioid withdrawal syndrome. Concomitant use with all CYP3A4 inhibitors and discontinuation of a concomitantly administered CYP3A4 inducer may increase plasma concentrations and potentially cause fatal respiratory depression; monitor patients during concomitant therapy. Exposure of application site and surrounding area to direct external heat sources may increase absorption and result in fatal overdose and death; patients who develop fever or increased core body temperature due to strenuous exertion are at increased risk and may require dose adjustment.

ADULT DOSAGE

Severe Pain (Daily, Around-the-Clock Management)

Opioid-Tolerant Patients:

D/C or taper all other ER and around-the-clock opioids when beginning therapy

25-300mcg/hr reapplied q72hr; initiate dosing regimen for each patient individually, taking into account the patient's prior analgesic treatment (refer to PI for dose conversions)

Titrate dose based on daily dose of supplemental opioid analgesics required on the 2nd or 3rd day of initial application; use the ratio of 45mg/24 hrs of oral morphine to a 12mcg/hr increase in fentanyl dose

Evaluate for further titration after no less than two 3-day applications before any further increase in dose

A small portion of patients may require systems to be applied q48h; an increase in dose should be evaluated before changing dosing interval

PEDIATRIC DOSAGE

Severe Pain (Daily, Around-the-Clock Management)

Opioid-Tolerant Patients:

≥2 Years:

D/C or taper all other ER and around-the-clock opioids when beginning therapy

25-300mcg/hr reapplied q72hr; initiate dosing regimen for each patient individually, taking into account the patient's prior analgesic treatment (refer to PI for dose conversions)

Titrate dose based on daily dose of supplemental opioid analgesics required on the 2nd or 3rd day of initial application; use the ratio of 45mg/24 hrs of oral morphine to a 12mcg/hr increase in fentanyl dose

Evaluate for further titration after no less than two 3-day applications before any further increase in dose

A small portion of patients may require systems to be applied q48h; an increase in dose should be evaluated before changing dosing interval

DOSE MODIFICATION

Renal Impairment

Mild to Moderate: Start w/ one half of the usual dosage

Severe: Avoid use

Hepatic Impairment

Mild to Moderate: Start w/ one half of the usual dosage

Severe: Avoid use

Discontinuation

Significant amounts of fentanyl continue to be absorbed from the skin for ≥24 hrs after the patch is removed

Converting to Another Opioid:

1. Remove patch and titrate the dose of the new analgesic based upon the patient's report of pain until adequate analgesia has been attained
2. Upon system removal, ≥17 hrs are required for a 50% decrease in serum fentanyl concentrations

Not Converting to Another Opioid:
Use a gradual downward titration (eg, having the dose every 6 days), in order to reduce the possibility of withdrawal symptoms; it is not known at what dose level fentanyl may be discontinued w/o producing the signs and symptoms of opioid withdrawal

Elderly
Start at lower end of the dosing range

ADMINISTRATION

Transdermal route

Application and Handling Instructions
1. Apply to intact, non-irritated, and non-irradiated skin on a flat surface such as the chest, back, flank, or upper arm; in young children and persons w/ cognitive impairment, adhesion should be monitored and the upper back is the preferred location to minimize the potential of inappropriate patch removal
2. Hair at the application site may be clipped (not shaved) prior to system application
3. If the application site must be cleansed prior to application of the patch, do so w/ clear water; do not use soaps, oils, lotions, alcohol, or any other agents that might irritate the skin or alter its characteristics. Allow the skin to dry completely prior to patch application
4. Apply immediately upon removal from the sealed package; the patch must not be altered (eg, cut) in any way prior to application. Do not use if the pouch seal is broken or if the patch is cut or damaged
5. Press the transdermal system firmly in place w/ the palm of the hand for 30 sec, making sure the contact is complete, especially around the edges
6. Each patch may be worn continuously for 72 hrs; the next patch is applied to a different skin site after removal of the previous transdermal system
7. If problems w/ adhesion of the patch occur, the edges of the patch may be taped w/ first aid tape; if adhesion problems persist, the patch may be overlayed w/ a transparent adhesive film dressing
8. If the patch falls off before 72 hrs, dispose of it by folding in 1/2 and flushing down the toilet; a new patch may be applied to a different skin site
9. Patients (or caregivers) should wash their hands immediately w/ soap and water after applying patch
10. Contact w/ unwashed or unclothed application sites can result in secondary exposure and should be avoided

Disposal Instructions
1. Patients should dispose of used patches immediately upon removal by folding the adhesive side of the patch to itself, then flushing down the toilet
2. Unused patches should be removed from their pouches, the protective liners removed, the patches folded so that the adhesive side of the patch adheres to itself, and immediately flushed down the toilet
3. Patients should dispose of any patches remaining from a prescription as soon as they are no longer needed

HOW SUPPLIED

Patch: 12mcg/hr, 25mcg/hr, 50mcg/hr, 75mcg/hr, 100mcg/hr [5[s]]

CONTRAINDICATIONS

Opioid-intolerant patients; management of acute/intermittent pain, or in patients who require opioid analgesia for a short period; management of postoperative pain, including use after outpatient/day surgeries (eg, tonsillectomies); management of mild pain; significant respiratory compromise, especially if adequate monitoring and resuscitative equipment are not readily available; acute or severe bronchial asthma; diagnosis or suspicion of paralytic ileus.

WARNINGS/PRECAUTIONS

Should be prescribed only by healthcare professionals knowledgeable in the use of potent opioids for the management of chronic pain. Reserve for use in patients for whom alternative treatment options (eg, nonopioid analgesics, immediate-release opioids) are ineffective, not tolerated, or would be otherwise inadequate to provide sufficient management of pain. Do not use as the 1st opioid. Risk of addiction is increased with personal/family history of substance abuse or mental illness. Prescribe smallest appropriate quantity. Closely monitor elderly, cachectic, or debilitated patients for respiratory depression. May decrease respiratory drive to the point of apnea in patients with chronic pulmonary disease; consider use of other nonopioid analgesic alternatives if possible. Avoid in patients who may be susceptible to the intracranial effects of CO_2 retention. May obscure clinical course of head injury and may increase intracranial pressure (ICP); monitor patients with brain tumors. May cause severe hypotension, including orthostatic hypotension and syncope, in ambulatory patients; increased risk with reduced blood volume. May produce bradycardia. Avoid use with severe hepatic/renal impairment. May cause spasm of the sphincter of Oddi; monitor patients with biliary tract disease (eg, acute pancreatitis). May cause increases in serum amylase concentration. Tolerance and physical dependence may develop during chronic therapy. May impair mental/physical abilities. Significant absorption from the skin continues for ≥24 hrs after patch removal. Avoid abrupt discontinuation; use a gradual downward dose titration. Not for use in women during and immediately prior to labor.

ADVERSE REACTIONS

Respiratory depression, N/V, constipation, diarrhea, headache, muscle spasms, malaise, palpitations, dizziness, insomnia, somnolence, fatigue, feeling cold, hyperhidrosis, anorexia.

DRUG INTERACTIONS

See Boxed Warning. Monitor respiratory depression when given with other drugs that depress respiration. Concomitant use with CNS depressants (eg, other opioids, sedatives, alcohol) may cause respiratory depression, hypotension, profound sedation, coma, or death; closely monitor and reduce dose of 1 or both agents. Coadministration with CYP3A4 inducers may lead to lack of efficacy of fentanyl or development of withdrawal; monitor for signs of opioid withdrawal and consider dose adjustments until stable drug effects are achieved. Avoid concomitant use with MAOIs or within 14 days of stopping such treatment. Mixed agonist/antagonist (eg, pentazocine, nalbuphine, butorphanol) or partial agonist (buprenorphine) analgesics may reduce analgesic effect or may precipitate withdrawal symptoms; avoid concomitant use. Monitor for signs of urinary retention or reduced GI motility with anticholinergics or other medications with anticholinergic activity.

NURSING CONSIDERATIONS

Assessment: Assess for degree of opioid tolerance, type and severity of pain, risks for opioid abuse, addiction, or misuse, paralytic ileus, acute/severe bronchial asthma, history of hypersensitivity to drug or any component of patch, debilitation, seizures, biliary tract disease, any other conditions where treatment is contraindicated or cautioned, pregnancy/nursing status, and possible drug interactions.

Monitoring: Monitor for signs/symptoms of respiratory depression, bradycardia, worsening of biliary tract disease, increased ICP, increased serum amylase levels, increased body temperature/fever, abuse, misuse, addiction, tolerance/physical dependence, opioid withdrawal syndrome in neonates born to mothers on prolonged therapy during pregnancy, and other adverse reactions.

Patient Counseling: Inform that use of patch may result in addiction, abuse, and misuse, which may lead to overdose or death; instruct not to share with others and protect from theft, misuse, and from children. Inform of the risk of life-threatening respiratory depression; advise on how to recognize respiratory depression and to seek medical attention. Instruct to avoid accidental contact when holding or caring for children. Instruct to immediately take patch off if it dislodges and accidentally sticks to the skin of another person, wash exposed area with water, and seek medical attention. Advise to never change the dose/number of patches unless instructed. Advise how to safely taper medication and not to stop abruptly. Warn of the potential for temperature-dependent increases in drug release from patch; instruct to avoid strenuous exertion that may increase body temperature and avoid exposing application site and surrounding area to direct external heat sources. Counsel that medication may impair mental and/or physical ability; instruct patients to refrain from potentially hazardous tasks until therapy is established that they have not been adversely affected. Inform of pregnancy risks and advise women of childbearing potential who become/are planning to become pregnant to consult physician prior to initiating or continuing therapy. Advise to notify physician of all medications currently being taken and avoid using other CNS depressants and alcohol. Inform that severe constipation may develop. Instruct to refer to the instructions for use for proper disposal of patch.

Storage: Up to 25°C (77°F); excursions permitted to 15-30°C (59-86°F). Store in original unopened pouch.

DURAMORPH — morphine sulfate CII

Class: Opioid analgesic

Risk of severe adverse effects with epidural or intrathecal route; observe patients in a fully equipped and staffed environment for at least 24 hrs after initial dose. Naloxone inj and resuscitative equipment should be immediately available in case of life-threatening or intolerable side effects and whenever therapy is initiated. Intrathecal dosage is usually 1/10 that of epidural dosage. Remove any contaminated clothing and rinse affected area with water if accidental dermal exposure occurs. Associated with risk of overdosage, diversion, and abuse; special measures must be taken to control this product within the hospital/clinic. Do not use if color is darker than pale yellow, if it is discolored in any other way, or if it contains a precipitate.

ADULT DOSAGE

Pain

Unresponsive to Non-Narcotic Analgesics:

IV:

Initial: 2-10mg/70kg

Epidural:

Initial: 5mg in the lumbar region

If adequate pain relief is not achieved w/in 1 hr, may give incremental doses of 1-2mg at intervals sufficient to assess effectiveness

PEDIATRIC DOSAGE

Pediatric use may not have been established

Max: 10mg/24 hrs
Intrathecal:
Usual: Single 0.2-1mg dose in the lumbar area; usually 1/10 of the epidural dose
Do not inject more than 2mL of the 5mg/10mL ampul or 1mL of the 10mg/10mL ampul
Repeated inj not recommended; consider alternate routes if pain recurs

ADMINISTRATION
IV/Epidural/Intrathecal route

Proper placement of a needle or catheter in the epidural space should be verified before inj
Limit administration by epidural/intrathecal routes to lumbar area

Intrathecal
May administer a constant IV infusion of 0.6mg/hr naloxone for 24 hrs after intrathecal inj to reduce incidence of potential side effects

HOW SUPPLIED
Inj: 0.5mg/mL, 1mg/mL [10mL]

CONTRAINDICATIONS
Medical conditions that would preclude the administration of opioids by the IV route (acute bronchial asthma, upper airway obstruction).

WARNINGS/PRECAUTIONS
Not for use in continuous microinfusion devices. May be habit forming. Administration should be limited to use by those familiar with respiratory depression management. Rapid IV administration may result in chest-wall rigidity. Prior to any epidural or intrathecal administration, assess for patient conditions (eg, infection at the inj site, bleeding diathesis, anticoagulant therapy) which call for special evaluation of the benefit versus risk potential. Should be administered by or under the direction of a physician experienced in the techniques and familiar with the patient management problems associated with epidural or intrathecal administration. Severe respiratory depression up to 24 hrs following epidural/intrathecal administration reported. Unusual acceleration of neuraxial morphine requirements may occur, which may cause concern regarding systemic absorption and the hazards of large doses; patients may benefit from hospitalization and detoxification. Myoclonic-like spasm of the lower extremities reported with intrathecal doses of >20mg/day; after detoxification, may resume treatment at lower doses. Higher incidence of respiratory depression with intrathecal than epidural use. Seizures may result from high doses; caution with known seizure disorders. Extreme caution with head injury or increased intracranial pressure; pupillary changes (miosis) may obscure the existence, extent, and course of intracranial pathology. High neuraxial doses may produce myoclonic events. Maintain a high index of suspicion for adverse drug reactions when evaluating altered mental status or movement abnormalities. Caution with decreased respiratory reserve (eg, emphysema, severe obesity, kyphoscoliosis, paralysis of the phrenic nerve). Avoid with chronic asthma, upper airway obstruction, or in any other chronic pulmonary disorder. Use caution when administering epidurally to patients with reduced metabolic rates and with hepatic and/or renal dysfunction. Smooth muscle hypertonicity may result in biliary colic. Initiation of neuraxial opiate analgesia is frequently associated with micturition disturbances, especially in males with prostatic enlargement. Monitor patients with reduced circulating blood volume or impaired myocardial function for possible occurrence of orthostatic hypotension. May cause severe hypotension when ability to maintain BP has already been compromised by a depleted blood volume. Avoid abrupt withdrawal. Caution in elderly.

ADVERSE REACTIONS
Respiratory depression/arrest, convulsions, dysphoric reactions, toxic psychoses, pruritus, urinary retention, constipation, lumbar puncture-type headache.

DRUG INTERACTIONS
CNS depressants (eg, alcohol, sedatives, antihistaminics, psychotropic drugs) potentiate depressant effects. Neuroleptics may increase risk of respiratory depression. Monitor for possible occurrence of orthostatic hypotension in patients on sympatholytic drugs. May cause severe hypotension with concurrent administration of drugs such as phenothiazines or general anesthetics.

NURSING CONSIDERATIONS

Assessment: Assess for patient's general condition and medical status, renal/hepatic impairment, hypersensitivity to drug, any other conditions where treatment is contraindicated or cautioned, pregnancy/nursing status, and possible drug interactions.

Monitoring: Monitor for signs/symptoms of respiratory depression, seizures, myoclonic events, biliary colic, urinary retention, orthostatic hypotension, drug abuse/dependence, and other adverse reactions.

Patient Counseling: Inform about risks and benefits of therapy. Inform of adverse reactions that may occur. Instruct to inform physician of other medications being taken. Inform that medication has potential for abuse and dependence.

Storage: 20-25°C (68-77°F); excursions permitted to 15-30°C (59-86°F). Protect from light. Do not freeze. Do not heat-sterilize.

DYAZIDE – hydrochlorothiazide/triamterene RX

Class: K^+-sparing diuretic/thiazide diuretic

Abnormal elevation of serum K^+ levels (≥5.5mEq/L) may occur w/ all K^+-sparing diuretic combinations. Hyperkalemia is more likely to occur w/ renal impairment and diabetes (even w/o evidence of renal impairment), and in elderly or severely ill; monitor serum K^+ levels at frequent intervals.

ADULT DOSAGE

Edema

1-2 caps PO qd

Hypertension

1-2 caps PO qd

PEDIATRIC DOSAGE

Pediatric use may not have been established

ADMINISTRATION

Oral route

HOW SUPPLIED

Cap: (HCTZ-Triamterene) 25mg-37.5mg

CONTRAINDICATIONS

Anuria, acute and chronic renal insufficiency or significant renal impairment, sulfonamide hypersensitivity, preexisting elevated serum K^+ (hyperkalemia), K^+-sparing agents (eg, spironolactone, amiloride, or other formulations containing triamterene), K^+ salt substitutes, K^+ supplements (except w/ severe hypokalemia).

WARNINGS/PRECAUTIONS

Avoid in severely ill in whom respiratory or metabolic acidosis may occur; if used, frequent evaluations of acid/base balance and serum electrolytes are necessary. May cause idiosyncratic reaction, resulting in acute transient myopia and acute angle-closure glaucoma; d/c as rapidly as possible. Caution w/ diabetes; may cause hyperglycemia and glycosuria. Diabetes mellitus (DM) may become manifest. Caution w/ hepatic impairment; may precipitate hepatic coma w/ severe liver disease. Corrective measures must be taken if hypokalemia develops; d/c and initiate potassium chloride (KCl) supplementation if serious hypokalemia develops (serum K^+ <3.0mEq/L). May potentiate electrolyte imbalance w/ heart failure, renal disease, or cirrhosis of the liver. May cause hypochloremia. Dilutional hyponatremia may occur in edematous patients in hot weather. Caution w/ history of renal stones. May increase BUN and SrCr. May decrease serum PBI levels. Decreased Ca^{2+} excretion reported. Changes in parathyroid glands w/ hypercalcemia and hypophosphatemia reported during prolonged therapy. May interfere w/ the fluorescent measurement of quinidine.

ADVERSE REACTIONS

Muscle cramps, N/V, pancreatitis, weakness, arrhythmia, impotence, dry mouth, jaundice, paresthesia, renal stones, anaphylaxis, acute renal failure, hyperkalemia, hyponatremia.

DRUG INTERACTIONS

See Contraindications. Increased risk of hyperkalemia w/ ACE inhibitors, blood from blood bank, and low-salt milk. Increased risk of severe hyponatremia w/ chlorpropamide. Possible interaction resulting in acute renal failure w/ indomethacin; caution w/ NSAIDs. Avoid w/ lithium due to risk of lithium toxicity. Decreased arterial responsiveness to norepinephrine. Amphotericin B, corticosteroids, and corticotropin may intensify electrolyte imbalance, particularly hypokalemia. Adjust dose of antigout drugs to control hyperuricemia and gout. May decrease effect of oral anticoagulants. May alter insulin requirements. Increased paralyzing effects of nondepolarizing muscle relaxants (eg, tubocurarine). Reduced K^+ levels w/ chronic or overuse of laxatives or use of exchange resins (eg, sodium polystyrene sulfonate). May reduce effectiveness of methenamine. May potentiate action of other antihypertensive drugs (eg, β-blockers).

NURSING CONSIDERATIONS

Assessment: Assess for anuria, renal/hepatic impairment, sulfonamide hypersensitivity, hyperkalemia, diabetes, history of renal stones, pregnancy/nursing status, and for possible drug interactions. Obtain baseline BUN, SrCr, and serum electrolytes.

Monitoring: Monitor for signs/symptoms of hype/hypokalemia, hyperglycemia, hypochloremia, renal stones, and for electrolyte imbalance. Monitor for hepatic coma in patients w/ severe liver disease. Monitor serum K^+ levels, BUN, SrCr, and serum electrolytes.

Patient Counseling: Inform about risks/benefits of therapy. Advise to seek medical attention if symptoms of hyperkalemia (eg, paresthesias, muscular weakness, fatigue), hypokalemia, hyperglycemia, renal stones, electrolyte imbalance (eg, dry mouth, thirst, weakness), or hypersensitivity reactions occur.

Storage: 20-25°C (68-77°F); excursions permitted to 15-30°C (59-86°F). Protect from light. Dispense in a tight, light-resistant container.

DYMISTA – azelastine hydrochloride/fluticasone propionate RX

Class: Corticosteroid/H_1-antagonist

ADULT DOSAGE

Seasonal Allergic Rhinitis

1 spray in each nostril bid

PEDIATRIC DOSAGE

Seasonal Allergic Rhinitis

≥6 Years:
1 spray in each nostril bid

DOSE MODIFICATION

Elderly

Dose cautiously; start at lower end of dosing range

ADMINISTRATION

Intranasal route

Shake the bottle gently before each use

Priming

Prime pump before initial use by releasing 6 sprays or until a fine mist appears
Reprime w/ 1 spray or until a fine mist appears if not used for ≥14 days

HOW SUPPLIED

Spray: (Azelastine/Fluticasone) (137mcg/50mcg)/spray [23g]

WARNINGS/PRECAUTIONS

Somnolence reported; may impair mental/physical abilities. Epistaxis reported. Nasal ulceration and septal perforation reported; avoid w/ recent nasal ulcers, nasal surgery, or nasal trauma. Development of localized infections of the nose and pharynx w/ *Candida albicans* may occur; may require discontinuation and treatment w/ appropriate local therapy if infection develops. Examine periodically for evidence of *Candida* infection or other signs of adverse effects on nasal mucosa if used over several months or longer. D/C slowly if hypercorticism and adrenal suppression occur. Fluticasone: May result in development of glaucoma and/or cataracts; closely monitor patients w/ change in vision or w/ history of increased IOP, glaucoma, and/or cataracts. May increase susceptibility to infections; caution w/ active or quiescent tuberculosis (TB) of the respiratory tract; untreated local or systemic fungal or bacterial infections; systemic viral or parasitic infections; or ocular herpes simplex. Avoid exposure to chickenpox and measles. Risk of adrenal insufficiency and withdrawal symptoms when replacing systemic corticosteroids w/ topical corticosteroids. May cause growth velocity reduction in pediatric patients.

ADVERSE REACTIONS

Dysgeusia, headache, epistaxis, pyrexia, cough, nasal congestion, rhinitis, viral infection, URTI, pharyngitis, pain, diarrhea, N/V, otitis media/externa.

DRUG INTERACTIONS

Avoid w/ alcohol or other CNS depressants. Fluticasone: Ritonavir and other strong CYP3A4 inhibitors may increase exposure; not recommended w/ ritonavir and caution w/ other potent CYP3A4 inhibitors (eg, ketoconazole). Concomitant use of intranasal corticosteroids w/ other inhaled corticosteroids could increase the risk of signs/symptoms of hypercorticism and/or hypothalamic-pituitary-adrenal axis suppression.

NURSING CONSIDERATIONS

Assessment: Assess for recent nasal ulcers/surgery/trauma, active or quiescent TB, systemic viral/parasitic infections, ocular herpes simplex, untreated fungal/bacterial infections, history of IOP, glaucoma, cataracts, pregnancy/nursing status, and possible drug interactions.

Monitoring: Monitor for somnolence, epistaxis, nasal ulceration, nasal septal perforation, changes in vision, glaucoma, cataracts, hypercorticism, adrenal suppression, and for the development/exacerbation of infections. Routinely monitor growth of pediatric patients.

Patient Counseling: Caution against engaging in hazardous occupations requiring complete mental alertness and motor coordination (eg, driving, operating machinery). Advise to avoid w/ alcohol and other CNS depressants. Instruct to inform physician if a change in vision is noted. Instruct to avoid exposure to chickenpox or measles and, if exposed, to consult physician w/o delay. Inform of potential worsening of existing TB, fungal, bacterial, viral or parasitic infections, or ocular herpes simplex. Counsel that corticosteroids may cause reduction in growth velocity in pediatric patients. Instruct to avoid spraying into eyes; if sprayed in the eyes, instruct to flush eyes w/ water for at least 10 min. Discard the bottle after 120 medicated sprays have been used. Instruct to notify physician of all medications currently taking.

Storage: 20-25°C (68-77°F). Store upright w/ dust cap in place. Protect from light. Do not store in the freezer or refrigerator.

EDARBI – azilsartan medoxomil RX

Class: Angiotensin II receptor antagonist

D/C when pregnancy is detected. Drugs that act directly on the renin-angiotensin system (RAS) can cause injury/death to the developing fetus.

ADULT DOSAGE

Hypertension

Usual: 80mg qd

W/ High Dose Diuretics:

Initial: 40mg qd

PEDIATRIC DOSAGE

Pediatric use may not have been established

ADMINISTRATION

Oral route

Take w/ or w/o food

HOW SUPPLIED

Tab: 40mg, 80mg

CONTRAINDICATIONS

Coadministration with aliskiren in patients with diabetes.

WARNINGS/PRECAUTIONS

Symptomatic hypotension may occur in patients with an activated RAS (eg, volume- and/or salt-depleted patients receiving high doses of diuretics); correct this condition prior to therapy or start treatment at 40mg. Changes in renal function may occur. Oliguria and/or progressive azotemia and (rarely) acute renal failure and/or death may occur in patients whose renal function is dependent on the RAS (eg, severe CHF, renal artery stenosis, volume depletion). Increases in SrCr or BUN in patients with renal artery stenosis reported.

ADVERSE REACTIONS

Dizziness, postural dizziness, nausea, asthenia, fatigue, muscle spasm, cough, diarrhea.

DRUG INTERACTIONS

See Contraindications. NSAIDs, including selective COX-2 inhibitors, may deteriorate renal function and attenuate the antihypertensive effect. Dual blockade of the RAS is associated with increased risks of hypotension, hyperkalemia, and changes in renal function (including acute renal failure); avoid combined use of RAS inhibitors. Closely monitor BP, renal function, and electrolytes with concomitant agents that also affect the RAS. Avoid with aliskiren in patients with renal impairment (GFR <60mL/min). Increases in lithium levels and lithium toxicity reported; monitor lithium levels. Increases in SrCr may be larger with chlorthalidone or HCTZ.

NURSING CONSIDERATIONS

Assessment: Assess for volume/salt depletion, renal impairment, CHF, renal artery stenosis, diabetes, pregnancy/nursing status, and possible drug interactions.

Monitoring: Monitor for signs/symptoms of hypotension and other adverse reactions. Monitor BP and renal function.

Patient Counseling: Inform of pregnancy risks; instruct to notify physician as soon as possible if pregnant/planning to become pregnant. Advise to seek medical attention if symptoms of hypotension or other adverse events occur.

Storage: 25°C (77°F); excursions permitted to 15-30°C (59-86°F). Protect from moisture and light.

EDARBYCLOR – azilsartan medoxomil/chlorthalidone RX

Class: Angiotensin II receptor antagonist/thiazide diuretic

D/C when pregnancy is detected. Drugs that act directly on the renin-angiotensin system (RAS) can cause injury/death to the developing fetus.

ADULT DOSAGE

Hypertension

Initial: 40mg-12.5mg qd
Titrate: May increase to 40mg-25mg after 2-4 weeks prn to achieve BP goals
Max: 40mg-25mg

Add-On Therapy:
Use if not adequately controlled on ARBs or diuretic monotherapy
Replacement Therapy:
May receive the corresponding dose of the titrated individual components

PEDIATRIC DOSAGE

Pediatric use may not have been established

DOSE MODIFICATION

Adverse Reactions

Dose-Limiting Adverse Reaction on Chlorthalidone: Initially give w/ a lower dose of chlorthalidone

ADMINISTRATION

Oral route

Take w/ or w/o food

HOW SUPPLIED

Tab: (Azilsartan-Chlorthalidone) 40mg-12.5mg, 40mg-25mg

CONTRAINDICATIONS

Anuria. Coadministration with aliskiren in patients with diabetes.

WARNINGS/PRECAUTIONS

Symptomatic hypotension may occur in patients with activated RAS (eg, volume- and/or salt-depleted patients receiving high doses of diuretics); correct this condition prior to therapy. Consider withholding or discontinuing therapy if progressive renal impairment becomes evident. Azilsartan: Changes in renal function may occur. Oliguria and/or progressive azotemia and (rarely) acute renal failure and/or death may occur in patients whose renal function is dependent on the RAS (eg, severe CHF). Increases in BUN or SrCr in patients with renal artery stenosis reported. Chlorthalidone: May cause fetal/neonatal jaundice and thrombocytopenia. May precipitate azotemia with renal disease. May cause hypokalemia, hyperuricemia, and/or precipitate frank gout. May precipitate hepatic coma in patients with hepatic dysfunction or progressive liver disease.

ADVERSE REACTIONS

Dizziness, syncope, hypotension, diarrhea, nausea, asthenia, fatigue, muscle spasm, cough, rash, headache, GI upset, elevation of uric acid and cholesterol.

DRUG INTERACTIONS

See Contraindications. May increase risk of symptomatic hypotension with high-dose diuretics. May increase risk of lithium toxicity; monitor lithium levels. Azilsartan: NSAIDs, including selective COX-2 inhibitors, may deteriorate renal function and attenuate the antihypertensive effect. Dual blockade of the RAS is associated with increased risks of hypotension, hyperkalemia, and changes in renal function (including acute renal failure); avoid combined use of RAS inhibitors. Closely monitor BP, renal function, and electrolytes with concomitant agents that affect the RAS. Avoid with aliskiren in patients with renal impairment (GFR <60mL/min). Chlorthalidone: Coadministration with digitalis may exacerbate the adverse effect of hypokalemia.

NURSING CONSIDERATIONS

Assessment: Assess for anuria, volume/salt depletion, CHF, renal/hepatic function, renal artery stenosis, pregnancy/nursing status, and possible drug interactions. Obtain baseline BP.

Monitoring: Monitor for signs/symptoms of hypotension, hypokalemia, hyperuricemia, precipitation of frank gout, and other adverse reactions. Monitor BP, serum electrolytes, and hepatic/renal function.

Patient Counseling: Inform about the consequences of exposure during pregnancy and discuss treatment options in women planning to become pregnant. Instruct to report pregnancy to the physician as soon as possible. If a dose is missed, instruct to take it later in the same day; advise not to double the dose on the following day. Instruct to report gout symptoms and lightheadedness; advise to d/c and consult physician if syncope occurs. Inform that dehydration from excessive perspiration, vomiting, and diarrhea may lead to an excessive fall in BP; advise to consult physician if these occur. Advise patients with renal impairment to receive periodic blood tests while on therapy.

Storage: 25°C (77°F); excursions permitted to 15-30°C (59-86°F). Protect from moisture and light.

EDLUAR – zolpidem tartrate **CIV**

Class: Imidazopyridine hypnotic

ADULT DOSAGE

Insomnia

Short-Term Treatment of Insomnia Characterized by Difficulties w/ Sleep Initiation:
Initial: 5mg (women), and either 5mg or 10mg (men), taken qhs
Titrate: May increase to 10mg if the 5mg dose is not effective
Max: 10mg qhs

PEDIATRIC DOSAGE

Pediatric use may not have been established

DOSE MODIFICATION

Concomitant Medications
Use w/ CNS Depressants: May need to adjust dose of zolpidem

Hepatic Impairment
Hepatic Insufficiency:
Usual: 5mg qhs

Elderly
Elderly/Debilitated:
Usual: 5mg qhs

ADMINISTRATION

SL route

Take immediately before hs w/ at least 7-8 hrs remaining before the planned time of awakening
Do not take w/ or immediately after a meal
Place tab under tongue; do not swallow tab or take w/ water

HOW SUPPLIED

Tab, SL: 5mg, 10mg

WARNINGS/PRECAUTIONS

Increased risk of next-day psychomotor impairment if taken with less than a full night of sleep remaining (7-8 hrs). May impair mental/physical abilities. Initiate only after careful evaluation; failure of insomnia to remit after 7-10 days of treatment may indicate presence of a primary psychiatric and/or medical illness. Angioedema and anaphylaxis reported; do not rechallenge if such reactions develop. Abnormal thinking, behavior changes, and visual/auditory hallucinations reported. Complex behaviors (eg, sleep-driving) while not fully awake reported; consider discontinuation if a sleep-driving episode occurs. Amnesia, anxiety, and other neuropsychiatric symptoms may occur. Worsening of depression, and suicidal thoughts and actions (including completed suicides) reported primarily in depressed patients; prescribe the least amount of drug that is feasible at a time. Caution with compromised respiratory function; prior to prescribing, consider the risks of respiratory depression in patients with respiratory impairment (eg, sleep apnea, myasthenia gravis). Withdrawal signs and symptoms reported following rapid dose decrease or abrupt discontinuation; monitor for tolerance, abuse, and dependence.

ADVERSE REACTIONS

Drowsiness, dizziness, headache, diarrhea, drugged feeling, lethargy, dry mouth, back pain, pharyngitis, sinusitis, allergy.

DRUG INTERACTIONS

See Dosage. Increased risk of CNS depression and complex behaviors with other CNS depressants (eg, benzodiazepines, opioids, TCAs, alcohol). Use with other sedative-hypnotics (eg, other zolpidem products) at hs or the middle of the night is not recommended. Increased risk of next-day psychomotor impairment with other CNS depressants or drugs that increase zolpidem levels. May decrease peak levels of imipramine. Additive effect of decreased alertness with imipramine or chlorpromazine. Additive adverse effect on psychomotor performance with chlorpromazine or alcohol. Sertraline and CYP3A inhibitors may increase exposure. Fluoxetine may increase $T_{1/2}$. Rifampin (a CYP3A4 inducer) may reduce exposure, pharmacodynamic effects, and efficacy. Ketoconazole (a potent CYP3A4 inhibitor) may increase pharmacodynamic effects; consider lower dose of zolpidem.

NURSING CONSIDERATIONS

Assessment: Assess for physical and/or psychiatric disorder, depression, compromised respiratory function, sleep apnea, myasthenia gravis, hepatic impairment, history of drug/alcohol addiction or abuse, hypersensitivity to the drug, pregnancy/nursing status, and possible drug interactions.

Monitoring: Monitor for angioedema, anaphylaxis, emergence of any new behavioral signs/symptoms of concern, respiratory depression, withdrawal signs/symptoms, tolerance, abuse, dependence, and other adverse reactions.

Patient Counseling: Inform about the benefits and risks of treatment. Instruct to take only as prescribed; advise to wait at least 8 hrs after dosing before driving or engaging in other activities requiring full mental alertness. Instruct to contact physician immediately if any adverse reactions (eg, severe anaphylactic/anaphylactoid reactions, sleep-driving or other complex behaviors, suicidal thoughts) develop. Advise not to use the drug if patient drank alcohol that pm or before bed. Instruct not to increase the dose and to inform physician if it is believed that the drug does not work.

Storage: 20-25°C (68-77°F). Protect from light and moisture.

EDURANT – rilpivirine **RX**

Class: Non-nucleoside reverse transcriptase inhibitor

ADULT DOSAGE

HIV-1 Infection

Combination with Other Antiretrovirals
Treatment-Naive and HIV-RNA ≤1000,000 copies/mL at Initiation:
25mg qd

PEDIATRIC DOSAGE

Pediatric use may not have been established

DOSE MODIFICATION

Concomitant Medications

Rifabutin: Increase dose to 50mg qd
Decrease dose to 25mg qd when coadministration is stopped

ADMINISTRATION

Oral route

Take with a meal

HOW SUPPLIED

Tab: 25mg

CONTRAINDICATIONS

Concomitant use with carbamazepine, oxcarbazepine, phenobarbital, phenytoin, rifampin, rifapentine, proton pump inhibitors (eg, esomeprazole, lansoprazole, omeprazole, pantoprazole, rabeprazole), systemic dexamethasone (more than a single dose), and St. John's wort.

WARNINGS/PRECAUTIONS

Depressive disorders reported; immediate medical evaluation is recommended if severe depressive symptoms occur. Hepatotoxicity reported; monitor LFTs before and during treatment in patients with underlying hepatic disease or marked transaminase elevations; consider monitoring in patients without preexisting hepatic dysfunction or other risk factors. Immune reconstitution syndrome, redistribution/accumulation of body fat, and autoimmune disorders (eg, Graves' disease, polymyositis, Guillain-Barre syndrome) in the setting of immune reconstitution reported. Caution with severe renal impairment or end-stage renal disease (ESRD); monitor for adverse effects. Caution in elderly.

ADVERSE REACTIONS

Lab abnormalities (increased SrCr, AST/ALT, total bilirubin, total cholesterol, LDL), depressive disorders, insomnia, headache, rash.

DRUG INTERACTIONS

See Contraindications and Dosage. Coadministration with CYP3A inducers or drugs that increase gastric pH may result in decreased levels and loss of virologic response and possible resistance to rilpivirine. CYP3A inhibitors may increase levels. Not recommended with delavirdine and other non-nucleoside reverse transcriptase inhibitors (NNRTIs). Concomitant didanosine should be given on an empty stomach and at least 2 hrs before or at least 4 hrs after therapy. Darunavir/ritonavir (RTV), lopinavir/RTV, unboosted protease inhibitors (PIs) or other boosted PIs (with RTV), may increase levels. Monitor for breakthrough fungal infections with azole antifungals. Clarithromycin, erythromycin, or telithromycin may increase levels; consider alternatives (eg, azithromycin) when possible. Rifabutin may decrease levels. Administer antacids either at least 2 hrs before or at least 4 hrs after therapy. Administer H_2-receptor antagonists at least 12 hrs before or at least 4 hrs after therapy. Clinical monitoring recommended with methadone as methadone maintenance therapy may need to be adjusted in some patients. Caution with drugs that have a known risk of torsades de pointes.

NURSING CONSIDERATIONS

Assessment: Assess for severe renal impairment or ESRD, underlying hepatic disease, marked transaminase elevations, pregnancy/nursing status, and possible drug interactions.

Monitoring: Monitor for depressive disorders, immune reconstitution syndrome, autoimmune disorders, fat redistribution/accumulation, hepatotoxicity, and other adverse reactions.

Patient Counseling: Inform that product is not a cure for HIV infection; advise that continuous therapy is necessary to control HIV infection and decrease HIV-related illnesses. Advise to continue to practice safer sex and to use latex or polyurethane condoms. Instruct never to reuse or share needles. Inform mothers to avoid nursing to reduce risk of transmission of HIV to their baby. Advise to take medication ud. Advise not to alter the dose or d/c therapy without consulting physician. If a dose is missed within 12 hrs of the time it is usually taken, instruct to take as soon as possible with a meal and then to take the next dose at the regular scheduled time. If dose is missed by >12 hrs of the time it is usually taken, instruct not to take the missed dose, but resume the usual dosing schedule. Advise to report to physician the use of any other prescription/nonprescription or herbal products (eg, St. John's wort). Instruct to seek medical evaluation if depressive symptoms are experienced. Inform that hepatotoxicity has been reported and redistribution/accumulation of body fat may occur.

Storage: 25°C (77°F); excursions permitted to 15-30°C (59-86°F). Protect from light.

EFFEXOR XR – venlafaxine

RX

Class: Serotonin and norepinephrine reuptake inhibitor

Antidepressants increased the risk of suicidal thoughts and behavior in children, adolescents, and young adults in short-term studies. Monitor closely for clinical worsening and emergence of suicidal thoughts and behaviors.

ADULT DOSAGE

Major Depressive Disorder

Initial: 75mg/day as a single dose, or 37.5mg/day for 4-7 days and then increase to 75mg/day
Titrate: May increase by increments of up to 75mg/day at ≥4-day intervals
Max: 225mg/day

Anxiety Disorders

Generalized Anxiety Disorder:
Initial: 75mg/day as a single dose, or 37.5mg/day for 4-7 days and then increase to 75mg/day
Titrate: May increase by increments of up to 75mg/day at ≥4-day intervals
Max: 225mg/day
Social Anxiety Disorder:
75mg/day as a single dose

Panic Disorder

W/ or w/o Agoraphobia:
Initial: 37.5mg/day for 7 days
Titrate: May increase by increments of up to 75mg/day at ≥7-day intervals
Max: 225mg/day

Dosing Considerations with MAOIs

Switching to/from an MAOI for Psychiatric Disorders:
Allow at least 14 days between discontinuation of an MAOI and initiation of treatment, and allow at least 7 days between discontinuation of treatment and initiation of an MAOI

W/ Other MAOIs (eg, Linezolid, IV Methylene Blue):
Do not start venlafaxine in patient being treated w/ linezolid or IV methylene blue. Consider other interventions (eg, hospitalization) in patients who require more urgent treatment of a psychiatric condition
If acceptable alternatives are not available,

PEDIATRIC DOSAGE

Pediatric use may not have been established

d/c venlafaxine and administer linezolid or IV methylene blue. Monitor for serotonin syndrome for 7 days or until 24 hrs after the last dose of linezolid or IV methylene blue, whichever comes 1st. May resume venlafaxine therapy 24 hrs after last dose of linezolid or IV methylene blue

DOSE MODIFICATION

Renal Impairment

Mild (CrCl 60-89mL/min) or Moderate (CrCl 30-59mL/min): Reduce total daily dose by 25-50%
Severe (CrCl <30mL/min) or Hemodialysis: Reduce total daily dose by ≥50%

Hepatic Impairment

Mild to Moderate (Child-Pugh 5-9): Reduce total daily dose by 50%
Severe (Child-Pugh 10-15) or Hepatic Cirrhosis: May need to reduce by ≥50%

Discontinuation

Gradually reduce (eg, reducing daily dose by 75mg at 1-week intervals)

Other Important Modifications

Switching from Effexor Immediate-Release Tab:
Give the nearest equivalent dose (mg/day); individual dose adjustments may be necessary

ADMINISTRATION

Oral route
Take w/ food at same time each day, either in am or pm
Swallow whole w/ fluid and do not divide, crush, chew, or place in water
May administer by carefully opening the cap and sprinkling the entire contents on a spoonful of applesauce; swallow immediately w/o chewing and follow w/ glass of water

HOW SUPPLIED

Cap, Extended-Release: 37.5mg, 75mg, 150mg

CONTRAINDICATIONS

Use of an MAOI for psychiatric disorders either concomitantly or w/in 7 days of discontinuing treatment. Treatment w/in 14 days of discontinuing an MAOI for psychiatric disorders. Starting treatment in patients being treated w/ other MAOIs (eg, linezolid, IV methylene blue).

WARNINGS/PRECAUTIONS

Not approved for the treatment of bipolar depression. Serotonin syndrome reported; d/c immediately and initiate supportive symptomatic treatment. Dose-related increases in systolic and diastolic BP, as well as sustained HTN, reported; control preexisting HTN before initiating treatment and consider dose reduction or discontinuation for patients who experience a sustained increase in BP. May increase the risk of bleeding events. Pupillary dilation that occurs following use may trigger an angle-closure attack in a patient w/ anatomically narrow angles who does not have a patent iridectomy. Mania/hypomania reported. Avoid abrupt discontinuation; gradually reduce dose. Seizures reported; d/c if seizures develop. Hyponatremia may occur; consider discontinuation in patients w/ symptomatic hyponatremia. Interstitial lung disease (ILD) and eosinophilic pneumonia rarely reported; consider discontinuation if symptoms occur. Caution w/ preexisting HTN or cardiovascular (CV) or cerebrovascular conditions that might be compromised by increases in BP, history of mania/hypomania, history of seizures, renal/hepatic impairment, and in the elderly. False (+) urine immunoassay screening tests for phencyclidine and amphetamines reported.

ADVERSE REACTIONS

Asthenia, sweating, N/V, constipation, anorexia, dry mouth, dizziness, insomnia, nervousness, somnolence, abnormal ejaculation/orgasm, impotence, decreased libido.

DRUG INTERACTIONS

See Contraindications. May cause serotonin syndrome w/ other serotonergic drugs (eg, triptans, TCAs, fentanyl) and w/ drugs that impair metabolism of serotonin; d/c immediately if this occurs. Not recommended w/ weight-loss agents or tryptophan supplements. Increased risk of hyponatremia w/ diuretics. Increased risk of bleeding w/ aspirin (ASA), NSAIDs, warfarin, and other anticoagulants or other drugs known to affect platelet function. Avoid w/ ethanol. Increased levels w/ cimetidine; caution in patients w/ HTN, hepatic dysfunction, or in the elderly. Increased levels w/ ketoconazole; use w/ caution. May increase metoprolol levels; use w/ caution and monitor BP. Caution w/ other CNS-active drugs.

NURSING CONSIDERATIONS

Assessment: Assess for history of mania/hypomania, seizures, HTN, susceptibility to angle-closure glaucoma, drug abuse, CV/cerebrovascular conditions, volume depletion, hepatic/renal impairment, hypersensitivity to the drug, pregnancy/nursing status, and possible drug interactions. Perform adequate screening to determine if patient is at risk for bipolar disorder; such screening should include a detailed psychiatric history, including a family history of suicide, bipolar disorder, and depression.

Monitoring: Monitor for signs/symptoms of clinical worsening, suicidality, unusual behavior, serotonin syndrome, sustained HTN, abnormal bleeding, angle-closure glaucoma, activation of mania/hypomania, hyponatremia, seizures, ILD, eosinophilic pneumonia, and other adverse reactions. Monitor BP. If discontinued abruptly, monitor for discontinuation symptoms (eg, dysphoric mood, confusion, agitation). Carefully monitor patients receiving concomitant warfarin therapy when treatment is initiated or discontinued. Periodically reassess to determine the need for maintenance or continued treatment.

Patient Counseling: Inform about the risks and benefits of therapy. Advise to look for emergence of suicidality, worsening of depression, and unusual changes in behavior, especially early during treatment and when the dose is adjusted up or down. Advise not to use concomitantly w/ other venlafaxine- or desvenlafaxine-containing products. Instruct not to take w/ an MAOI or w/in 14 days of stopping an MAOI and to allow 7 days after stopping treatment before starting an MAOI. Caution about the risk of serotonin syndrome. Advise that they should have regular BP monitoring during therapy. Caution that concomitant use w/ ASA, NSAIDs, warfarin, or other drugs that affect coagulation may increase the risk of bleeding. Inform about the risk of angle-closure glaucoma in susceptible individuals. Advise patients, families, and caregivers to observe for signs of activation of mania/hypomania. Advise that elevations in total cholesterol, LDL, and TGs may occur and that measurement of serum lipids may be considered. Advise not to stop taking medication w/o first talking w/ healthcare professional; inform that discontinuation effects may occur when stopping treatment. Caution against operating hazardous machinery (including automobiles) until reasonably certain that therapy does not adversely affect ability to engage in such activities. Advise to avoid alcohol while on therapy. Advise to notify physician if allergic phenomena develops, or if pregnant, intending to become pregnant, or if breastfeeding. Inform that spheroids may be passed in the stool or via colostomy.

Storage: 20-25°C (68-77°F).

EFFIENT — prasugrel

RX

Class: Platelet aggregation inhibitor

May cause significant, sometimes fatal, bleeding; risk factors include <60kg body weight, propensity to bleed, and concomitant use of medications that increase risk of bleeding (eg, warfarin, heparin, fibrinolytic therapy, chronic use of NSAIDs). Do not use in patients with active pathological bleeding or a history of transient ischemic attack (TIA) or stroke. Not recommended in patients ≥75 yrs of age, due to increased risk of fatal and intracranial bleeding and uncertain benefit, except in high-risk situations (diabetes or history of prior MI) where the effect appears to be greater and use may be considered. Do not start in patients likely to undergo urgent CABG; d/c at least 7 days prior to any surgery, when possible. Suspect bleeding in any patient who is hypotensive and has recently undergone coronary angiography, percutaneous coronary intervention (PCI), CABG, or other surgical procedures. If possible, manage bleeding without discontinuing the drug. Discontinuing, particularly in the 1st few weeks after acute coronary syndrome (ACS), increases the risk of subsequent cardiovascular (CV) events.

ADULT DOSAGE

Acute Coronary Syndrome

To reduce the rate of cardiovascular thrombotic events (including stent thrombosis) in patients who are to be managed w/ percutaneous coronary intervention as follows: patients w/ unstable angina or non-ST-elevation MI or patients with ST-elevation MI when managed w/ primary or delayed percutaneous coronary intervention

LD: 60mg as a single dose
Maint: 10mg qd
Take w/ aspirin (75-325mg/day)

PEDIATRIC DOSAGE

Pediatric use may not have been established

DOSE MODIFICATION

Dose Reductions

Low Body Weight:

<60kg: Consider lowering the maint dose to 5mg qd

ADMINISTRATION

Oral route

Take PO w/ or w/o food
Do not break the tab

HOW SUPPLIED

Tab: 5mg, 10mg

CONTRAINDICATIONS
Active pathological bleeding (eg, peptic ulcer, intracranial hemorrhage), history of prior TIA or stroke.

WARNINGS/PRECAUTIONS
Withholding a dose will not be useful in managing a bleeding event or the risk of bleeding associated with an invasive procedure. D/C for active bleeding, elective surgery, stroke, or TIA. Avoid therapy lapses; if temporary discontinuation is needed because of an adverse event(s), restart as soon as possible. Thrombotic thrombocytopenic purpura (TTP) reported; may occur after a brief exposure (<2 weeks) and requires urgent treatment (eg, plasmapheresis). Hypersensitivity including angioedema reported. Risk for bleeding with severe hepatic impairment or moderate to severe renal impairment.

ADVERSE REACTIONS
Bleeding, HTN, hypercholesterolemia/hyperlipidemia, headache, back pain, dyspnea, nausea, dizziness, cough, hypotension, fatigue, noncardiac chest pain.

DRUG INTERACTIONS
See Boxed Warning.

NURSING CONSIDERATIONS

Assessment: Assess for active pathological bleeding, history of prior TIA or stroke, other risk factors for bleeding, hypersensitivity, pregnancy/nursing status, and possible drug interactions. Assess likelihood of undergoing urgent CABG.

Monitoring: Monitor for signs/symptoms of bleeding, TTP, hypersensitivity, stroke, TIA, and other adverse reactions.

Patient Counseling: Inform about the benefits and risks of treatment. Instruct to take exactly as prescribed and not to d/c without consulting the prescribing physician. Inform that patient may bruise and bleed more easily and that bleeding will take longer than usual to stop. Advise to report to physician any unanticipated, prolonged, or excessive bleeding, or blood in stool/urine. Inform that TTP, a rare but serious condition, has been reported; instruct to seek prompt medical attention if experiencing unexplained fever, weakness, extreme skin paleness, purple skin patches, yellowing of skin/eyes, or neurological changes. Inform that hypersensitivity reactions may occur. Instruct to notify physicians and dentists about therapy before scheduling any invasive procedure.

Storage: 25°C (77°F); excursions permitted to 15-30°C (59-86°F).

EFUDEX – fluorouracil RX

Class: Antimetabolite

ADULT DOSAGE

Multiple Actinic or Solar Keratoses

Apply sufficient amount to cover the lesions bid. Continue use until inflammatory response reaches the erosion stage

Usual Duration: 2-4 weeks

Superficial Basal Cell Carcinomas

5%:
Apply sufficient amount to cover the lesions bid. Continue use for at least 3-6 weeks

May be required for as long as 10-12 weeks before lesions are obliterated

Use when conventional methods are impractical (eg, w/ multiple lesions or difficult treatment sites)

PEDIATRIC DOSAGE

Pediatric use may not have been established

ADMINISTRATION
Topical route

Apply preferably w/ a nonmetal applicator or suitable glove
If applied w/ the fingers, wash the hands immediately afterward

HOW SUPPLIED
Cre: 5% [40g]; Sol: 2%, 5% [10mL, 25mL]

CONTRAINDICATIONS
Women who are or may become pregnant. Dihydropyrimidine dehydrogenase (DPD) enzyme deficiency.

WARNINGS/PRECAUTIONS

Avoid application to mucous membranes; local inflammation and ulceration may occur. If any occlusive dressing is used in treatment of basal cell carcinoma, there may be an increase in the severity of inflammatory reactions in the adjacent normal skin; a porous gauze dressing may be applied for cosmetic reasons without increase in reaction. Minimize exposure to UV rays during and immediately following treatment; intensity of the reaction may be increased. D/C if symptoms of DPD enzyme deficiency develop. Increased absorption through ulcerated or inflamed skin may occur. Not for ophthalmic, oral, or intravaginal use.

ADVERSE REACTIONS

Burning, crusting, allergic contact dermatitis, pruritus, scarring, rash, soreness, ulceration, leukocytosis.

NURSING CONSIDERATIONS

Assessment: Assess for drug hypersensitivity, DPD enzyme deficiency, skin ulceration/inflammation, and pregnancy/nursing status.

Monitoring: Monitor for local reactions, and other adverse effects. Biopsy solar keratoses that do not respond to confirm the diagnosis. Perform follow-up biopsies as indicated in the management of superficial basal cell carcinoma.

Patient Counseling: Inform that the reaction in the treated areas may be unsightly during therapy and, usually, for several weeks following cessation of therapy. Instruct to avoid exposure to UV rays during and immediately following treatment. Advise not to apply on the eyelids or directly into the eyes, nose, or mouth.

Storage: 25°C (77°F); excursions permitted to 15-30°C (59-86°F).

EGRIFTA – tesamorelin RX

Class: Growth hormone-releasing factor

ADULT DOSAGE

Lipodystrophy

Reduction of Excess Abdominal Fat in HIV-Infected Patients:
2mg SQ in the abdomen qd

PEDIATRIC DOSAGE

Pediatric use may not have been established

ADMINISTRATION

SQ route
Rotate inj sites to different areas of the abdomen
Do not inject into scar tissue, bruises, or the navel
Administer immediately following reconstitution

Reconstitution

Two vials of tesamorelin must be reconstituted w/ the diluent provided
1. Reconstitute the first vial w/ 2.2mL of diluent
2. Mix by rolling the vial gently in hands for 30 sec; do not shake
3. Reconstitute the second vial w/ the entire sol from the first vial
4. Mix by rolling the vial gently in hands for 30 sec; do not shake

HOW SUPPLIED

Inj: 1mg

CONTRAINDICATIONS

Pregnancy, newly diagnosed or recurrent active malignancy, disruption of hypothalamic-pituitary axis due to hypophysectomy, hypopituitarism, pituitary tumor/surgery, head irradiation or head trauma, hypersensitivity to mannitol.

WARNINGS/PRECAUTIONS

Carefully consider whether to continue treatment in patients who do not show clear efficacy response. Not indicated for weight loss management (weight neutral effect). Initiate therapy after careful evaluation of the potential benefit of treatment for patients with history of nonmalignant neoplasms or history of treated and stable malignancies. Carefully consider the increased background risk of malignancies in HIV-positive patients before initiation of therapy. Stimulates growth hormone (GH) production and increases serum insulin growth factor-1 (IGF-1); monitor IGF-1 levels closely and consider discontinuation of therapy in patients with persistent elevations of IGF-1 levels (eg, >3 standard deviation scores), particularly if the efficacy response is not robust. Fluid retention may occur. May cause glucose intolerance and increase the risk for developing diabetes. Hypersensitivity reactions may occur; d/c treatment immediately when suspected. May cause inj-site reactions. Consider discontinuation in critically ill patients; increased mortality in patients with acute critical illness due to complications following open heart surgery, abdominal surgery, or multiple accidental trauma, or those with acute respiratory failure.

ADVERSE REACTIONS

Arthralgia, pain in extremity, peripheral edema, inj-site reactions (eg, erythema, pruritus, pain), myalgia, paresthesia, hypoesthesia, nausea, rash.

DRUG INTERACTIONS

May modulate CYP450 mediated antipyrine clearance; monitor carefully in combination with other drugs known to be metabolized by CYP450 liver enzymes. May require an increase in maintenance or stress doses of glucocorticoids following initiation of therapy, particularly in patients treated with cortisone acetate and prednisone.

NURSING CONSIDERATIONS

Assessment: Assess for hypersensitivity to the drug and/or mannitol, hypothalamic-pituitary axis disruption due to hypophysectomy, hypopituitarism, pituitary tumor/surgery, head irradiation or head trauma, active malignancy, history of nonmalignant neoplasms or treated and stable malignancies, diabetes, acute critical illness, pregnancy/nursing status, and possible drug interactions. Evaluate glucose status.

Monitoring: Monitor for fluid retention, hypersensitivity/inj-site reactions, and other adverse reactions. Monitor for response and IGF-1 levels. Monitor for changes in glucose metabolism periodically in patients who develop impaired glucose tolerance or diabetes and for potential development or worsening of retinopathy in patients with diabetes.

Patient Counseling: Advise that treatment may cause symptoms consistent with fluid retention. Instruct to seek prompt medical attention and to d/c therapy immediately when hypersensitivity reactions occur. Advise to rotate inj site to reduce incidence of inj-site reactions. Counsel not to share syringe with another person, even if the needle is changed. Instruct women to d/c treatment if pregnant and not to breastfeed.

Storage: Unreconstituted: 2-8°C (36-46°F). Reconstituted: Do not freeze or refrigerate. Diluent/Syringes/Needles: 20-25°C (68-77°F). Protect from light. Keep in the original box until use.

ELIDEL – pimecrolimus RX

Class: Macrolactam ascomycin derivative

Rare cases of malignancy (eg, skin and lymphoma) reported with topical calcineurin inhibitors, including pimecrolimus, although causal relationship is not established. Avoid long-term use, and application should be limited to areas of involvement with atopic dermatitis. Not indicated for children <2 yrs or age.

ADULT DOSAGE

Atopic Dermatitis

Short-term/noncontinuous chronic treatment (2nd line) of mild to moderate atopic dermatitis in patients who have failed to respond adequately to other topical treatments, or when those treatments are not advisable

Apply thin layer to the affected skin bid until signs and symptoms resolve

Reexamine if signs and symptoms persist beyond 6 weeks

PEDIATRIC DOSAGE

Atopic Dermatitis

Short-term/noncontinuous chronic treatment (2nd line) of mild to moderate atopic dermatitis in patients who have failed to respond adequately to other topical treatments, or when those treatments are not advisable

≥2 Years:

Apply thin layer to the affected skin bid until signs and symptoms resolve

Reexamine if signs and symptoms persist beyond 6 weeks

ADMINISTRATION

Topical route

HOW SUPPLIED

Cre: 1% [30g, 60g, 100g]

WARNINGS/PRECAUTIONS

Avoid with malignant or premalignant skin conditions, Netherton's syndrome, or other skin diseases that may increase the potential for systemic absorption. Avoid in immunocompromised patients. May cause local symptoms, such as skin burning or pruritus, and may improve as the lesions of atopic dermatitis resolve. Resolve bacterial or viral infections at treatment sites before starting treatment. Increased risk of varicella zoster and herpes simplex virus infection, or eczema herpeticum. Skin papilloma/warts reported; consider discontinuation until complete resolution is achieved if skin papillomas worsen or do not respond to conventional therapy.

Lymphadenopathy reported; d/c if lymphadenopathy of uncertain etiology or in the presence of acute infectious mononucleosis. Minimize or avoid natural or artificial sunlight exposure during treatment.

ADVERSE REACTIONS
Application-site burning, application-site reaction, influenza, nasopharyngitis, headache, URTI, sore throat, hypersensitivity, cough, pyrexia, N/V, skin infection, abdominal pain.

DRUG INTERACTIONS
Caution with CYP3A4 inhibitors (eg, erythromycin, ketoconazole, calcium channel blockers) in patients with widespread and/or erythrodermic disease.

NURSING CONSIDERATIONS

Assessment: Assess for malignant or premalignant skin conditions, Netherton's syndrome, or other skin diseases that may increase the potential for systemic absorption, immunocompromised state, viral/bacterial skin infections, pregnancy/nursing status, and possible drug interactions.

Monitoring: Monitor for varicella virus infection, herpes simplex virus infection, eczema herpeticum, skin papilloma/warts, lymphomas, lymphadenopathy, skin malignancies, local symptoms, and other adverse reactions.

Patient Counseling: Instruct to use ud. Inform not to use continuously for a long time and to use only on areas of skin with eczema. Instruct not to use sun lamps, tanning beds, or get treatment with UV light therapy. Advise to limit sun exposure, wear loose fitting clothing that protects the treated area from the sun, and not to cover treated skin area with bandages, dressings, or wraps. Inform that the medication is for use on the skin only; instruct to avoid contact with eyes, nose, mouth, vagina, or rectum (mucous membranes). Instruct to wash hands and dry skin before applying cre and not to bathe, shower, or swim after application.

Storage: 25°C (77°F); excursions permitted to 15-30°C (59-86°F). Do not freeze.

ELIGARD — leuprolide acetate RX

Class: Synthetic gonadotropin-releasing hormone analogue

ADULT DOSAGE

Advanced Prostate Cancer

Palliative Treatment:
7.5mg: 1 inj every month
22.5mg: 1 inj every 3 months
30mg: 1 inj every 4 months
45mg: 1 inj every 6 months

PEDIATRIC DOSAGE

Pediatric use may not have been established

ADMINISTRATION
SQ route

Inj site should vary periodically; avoid areas w/ brawny or fibrous SQ tissue or locations that could be rubbed or compressed (eg, w/ a belt or clothing waistband)
Use gloves during mixing and administration

Administration Procedure
Important: Allow the product to reach room temperature before using. Once mixed, administer w/ in 30 min; refer to PI for mixing procedure
Choose an inj site on the abdomen, upper buttocks, or anywhere w/ adequate amounts of SQ tissue that does not have excessive pigment, nodules, lesions, or hair; choose an area that has not recently been used

HOW SUPPLIED
Inj: 7.5mg, 22.5mg, 30mg, 45mg

CONTRAINDICATIONS
Women who are or may become pregnant.

WARNINGS/PRECAUTIONS
Transient increase in serum concentrations of testosterone and worsening of symptoms or onset of new signs/symptoms (eg, bone pain, neuropathy, hematuria) during the 1st few weeks of therapy may occur. Cases of ureteral obstruction and/or spinal cord compression reported; institute standard treatment if these complications occur. Closely monitor patients w/ metastatic vertebral lesions and/or urinary tract obstruction during 1st few weeks of therapy. Suppresses pituitary-gonadal system; may affect results of diagnostic tests of pituitary gonadotropic and gonadal functions conducted during and after therapy. Hyperglycemia and increased risk of developing diabetes, MI, sudden cardiac death, and stroke reported. May prolong QT/QTc interval; consider whether the benefits outweigh the potential risks in patients w/ congenital long

QT syndrome, CHF, frequent electrolyte abnormalities, and in patients taking drugs known to prolong the QT interval.

ADVERSE REACTIONS

Hot flashes/sweats, inj-site reactions (eg, transient burning/stinging, pain, erythema, bruising, pruritus), malaise/fatigue, testicular atrophy, weakness, gynecomastia, myalgia, arthralgia, dizziness, decreased libido, clamminess, night sweats, nausea.

NURSING CONSIDERATIONS

Assessment: Assess for hypersensitivity to drug, metastatic vertebral lesions, urinary tract obstructions, congenital long QT syndrome, CHF, electrolyte abnormalities and diabetes mellitus. Obtain baseline serum testosterone levels and prostate specific antigen (PSA) levels. Obtain baseline blood glucose and/or HbA1c levels. Correct electrolyte abnormalities.

Monitoring: Monitor for worsening/occurrence of signs/symptoms of prostate cancer, spinal cord compression, ureteral obstruction, signs/symptoms suggestive of cardiovascular disease development, and other adverse reactions. Periodically monitor blood glucose, HbA1c, testosterone, and PSA levels. Consider periodic monitoring of ECG and electrolytes.

Patient Counseling: Inform that hot flashes may be experienced. Advise that increased bone pain, difficulty in urinating, and onset or aggravation of weakness or paralysis may be experienced during the 1st few weeks of therapy. Instruct to notify physician if new or worsened symptoms develop after beginning treatment. Inform about inj-site related adverse reactions (eg, transient burning/stinging, pain, bruising, redness); instruct to notify physician if such reactions do not resolve. Advise to contact physician immediately if an allergic reaction develops.

Storage: 2-8°C (35.6-46.4°F).

ELIMITE — permethrin

RX

Class: Pyrethroid scabicidal agent

ADULT DOSAGE

Scabies Infestations

Infestation w/ *Sarcoptes scabiei*:
Thoroughly massage into skin from head to soles of feet; remove by washing after 8-14 hrs
One application is generally curative; retreat if living mites present after 14 days
Usually 30g is sufficient for an average adult

PEDIATRIC DOSAGE

Scabies Infestations

Infestation w/ *Sarcoptes scabiei*:

≥2 Months of Age:
Thoroughly massage into skin from head to soles of feet (scalp, temple and forehead on infants); remove by washing after 8-14 hrs
One application is generally curative; retreat if living mites present after 14 days

ADMINISTRATION

Topical route

HOW SUPPLIED

Cre: 5% [60g]

WARNINGS/PRECAUTIONS

D/C if hypersensitivity occurs. Scabies infestation is often accompanied by pruritus, edema, and erythema; treatment may temporarily exacerbate these conditions.

ADVERSE REACTIONS

Burning, stinging, pruritus.

NURSING CONSIDERATIONS

Assessment: Assess for previous hypersensitivity to the drug or any synthetic pyrethroid or pyrethrin, and pregnancy/nursing status.

Monitoring: Monitor for hypersensitivity, exacerbation of pruritus, edema, or erythema, and other adverse reactions.

Patient Counseling: Inform that itching, mild burning, and/or stinging may occur after application; instruct to consult physician if irritation persists. Advise to avoid contact with eyes during application and to flush with water immediately if medication gets in the eyes.

Storage: 20-25°C (68-77°F).

ELIQUIS – apixaban

RX

Class: Selective factor Xa inhibitor

Premature discontinuation increases the risk of thrombotic events. If therapy must be discontinued for a reason other than pathological bleeding or completion of a course of therapy, consider coverage with another anticoagulant. Epidural or spinal hematomas may occur in patients treated with apixaban who are receiving neuraxial anesthesia or undergoing spinal puncture; long-term or permanent paralysis may result. Increased risk of developing epidural/spinal hematomas by the use of indwelling epidural catheters, concomitant use of other drugs that affect hemostasis, (eg, NSAIDs, platelet inhibitors, other anticoagulants), history of traumatic or repeated epidural or spinal punctures, history of spinal deformity or spinal surgery, and when optimal timing between the administration of therapy and neuraxial procedure is not known. Monitor frequently for signs/symptoms of neurologic impairment; urgent treatment is necessary if neurologic compromise is noted. Consider benefits and risks before neuraxial intervention in patients anticoagulated or to be anticoagulated.

ADULT DOSAGE

Reduce Risk of Stroke and Systemic Embolism in Nonvalvular Atrial Fibrillation

Usual: 5mg bid

Deep Vein Thrombosis/Pulmonary Embolism

DVT:

Following Hip or Knee Replacement Surgery:

Usual: 2.5mg bid

Give initial dose 12-24 hrs after surgery

Treatment Duration:

Hip Replacement Surgery: 35 days

Knee Replacement Surgery: 12 days

DVT/PE Treatment:

Usual: 10mg bid for 7 days, followed by 5mg bid

Risk Reduction of Recurrent DVT/PE:

Usual: 2.5mg bid after at least 6 months of treatment for DVT or pulmonary embolism

Conversions

Switching from Warfarin to Apixaban:

D/C warfarin and start apixaban when INR < 2.0

Switching to Warfarin:

D/C therapy and begin both a parenteral anticoagulant and warfarin at the time the next dose of apixaban would have been taken, d/c parenteral anticoagulant when INR reaches an acceptable range

Conversion to/from Anticoagulants Other Than Warfarin:

D/C agent being taken and begin the other at the next scheduled dose

PEDIATRIC DOSAGE

Pediatric use may not have been established

DOSE MODIFICATION

Concomitant Medications

Strong Dual CYP3A4 and P-gp Inhibitors (eg, Ketoconazole, Itraconazole, Ritonavir):

Usual: For patients receiving apixaban doses >2.5mg bid, reduce apixaban dose by 50%; if already taking 2.5mg bid, avoid coadministration w/ strong dual inhibitors of CYP3A4 and P-gp

Renal Impairment

Nonvalvular A-Fib Patients w/ ESRD Maintained on Hemodialysis:

Usual: 5mg bid; reduce dose to 2.5mg bid (if patient is ≥80 yrs of age or ≤60kg)

Hepatic Impairment

Severe: Not recommended

Other Important Modifications

Dosage Adjustments in Nonvalvular A-Fib Patients w/ Any Two of the Following: ≥80 Years, ≤60kg, or SrCr ≥1.5mg/dL:

Usual: 2.5mg bid

Elective Surgery/Invasive Procedures:

D/C at least 48 hrs prior to elective surgery or invasive procedures w/ moderate/high risk of unacceptable/clinically significant bleeding, or at least 24 hrs w/ a low risk of bleeding or where bleeding would be noncritical in location and easily controlled

Bridging anticoagulation during the 24-48 hrs after discontinuing therapy and prior to the intervention is not generally required

Restart therapy after the surgical or other procedures as soon as adequate hemostasis has been established

ADMINISTRATION

Oral route

May crush and suspend tab in 60mL D5W and immediately deliver through a NG tube if unable to swallow tabs whole

HOW SUPPLIED

Tab: 2.5mg, 5mg

CONTRAINDICATIONS

Active pathological bleeding.

WARNINGS/PRECAUTIONS

Not recommended in patients with severe hepatic impairment or with prosthetic heart valves. May increase the risk of bleeding and cause serious, potentially fatal bleeding; d/c in patients with active pathological hemorrhage. Specific antidote for apixaban is not available; activated oral charcoal reduces apixaban absorption. In patients who receive both apixaban and neuraxial anesthesia, removal of indwelling epidural or intrathecal catheters should not be earlier than 24 hrs after the last administration of apixaban; next dose of apixaban should not be administered earlier than 5 hrs after the removal of the catheter. If traumatic spinal/epidural puncture occurs, delay administration of apixaban for 48 hrs. Initiation of treatment is not recommended as an alternative to unfractionated heparin for the initial treatment of patients with pulmonary embolism who present with hemodynamic instability or who may receive thrombolysis or pulmonary embolectomy.

ADVERSE REACTIONS

Bleeding.

DRUG INTERACTIONS

See Boxed Warning and Dosage. CYP3A4 and P-gp inhibitors may increase exposure and increase the risk of bleeding. CYP3A4 and P-gp inducers may decrease exposure and increase the risk of stroke and other thromboembolic events. Avoid with strong dual inducers of CYP3A4 and P-gp (eg, rifampin, carbamazepine, phenytoin, St. John's wort). Increased risk of bleeding with drugs affecting hemostasis, including aspirin (ASA) and other antiplatelet agents, other anticoagulants, heparin, thrombolytics, SSRIs, SNRIs, NSAIDs, and fibrinolytics.

NURSING CONSIDERATIONS

Assessment: Assess for drug hypersensitivity, active pathological bleeding, prosthetic heart valves, PE with hemodynamic instability or patients who may receive thrombolysis or pulmonary embolectomy, hepatic/renal impairment, pregnancy/nursing status, and possible drug interactions.

Monitoring: Monitor for active pathological hemorrhage and other adverse reactions. Monitor for thrombotic events in patients discontinuing therapy. In patients undergoing neuraxial anesthesia or spinal puncture, monitor for epidural or spinal hematomas and neurological impairment.

Patient Counseling: Instruct not to d/c without consulting physician. Inform that it may take longer than usual for bleeding to stop, and that patient may bruise/bleed more easily. Advise on how to recognize bleeding/symptoms of hypovolemia and of the urgent need to report any unusual bleeding to physician. Instruct to inform physicians and dentists if taking apixaban, and/or any other product known to affect bleeding (eg, nonprescription drugs such as ASA or NSAIDs), before any surgery/medical/dental procedure is scheduled and before any new drug is taken. Advise patients having neuraxial anesthesia or spinal puncture to watch for signs/symptoms of spinal/epidural hematomas (eg, numbness, weakness of legs, bowel/bladder dysfunction); instruct to contact physician immediately if symptoms occur. Advise to inform physician if pregnant or planning to become pregnant, or if breastfeeding or intending to breastfeed during treatment. If a dose is missed, instruct to take as soon as possible on the same day and that bid administration should be resumed; instruct not to double the dose to make up for a missed dose.

Storage: 20-25°C (68-77°F); excursions permitted to 15-30°C (59-86°F).

ELOCON – mometasone furoate RX

Class: Corticosteroid

ADULT DOSAGE

Inflammatory and Pruritic Manifestations of Corticosteroid-Responsive Dermatoses

Cre/Oint:

Apply a thin film to affected skin areas qd

Lot:

Apply a few drops to affected skin areas qd and massage lightly until it disappears

PEDIATRIC DOSAGE

Inflammatory and Pruritic Manifestations of Corticosteroid-Responsive Dermatoses

≥2 Years:

Cre/Oint:

Apply a thin film to affected skin areas qd; safety and efficacy for >3 weeks have not been established

Cre/Lot/Oint:
D/C therapy when control is achieved; reassess diagnosis if no improvement seen within 2 weeks

≥12 Years:
Lot:
Apply a few drops to affected skin areas qd and massage lightly until it disappears
Cre/Lot/Oint:
D/C therapy when control is achieved; reassess diagnosis if no improvement seen within 2 weeks

ADMINISTRATION
Topical route

Avoid use with occlusive dressings unless directed by physician
Should not be applied in the diaper area if the child still requires diapers or plastic pants, as these garments may constitute occlusive dressing

HOW SUPPLIED
Cre: 0.1% [15g, 50g]; Lot: 0.1% [30mL, 60mL]; Oint: 0.1% [15g, 45g]

WARNINGS/PRECAUTIONS
Not for oral, ophthalmic, or intravaginal use. Avoid use on the face, groin, or axillae. Avoid use with occlusive dressings. Systemic absorption may produce reversible hypothalamic pituitary adrenal (HPA) axis suppression with the potential for glucocorticosteroid insufficiency, manifestations of Cushing's syndrome, hyperglycemia, and glucosuria. Periodically evaluate for HPA-axis suppression and, if noted, gradually withdraw drug, reduce frequency of application, or substitute a less potent corticosteroid. Factors predisposing to HPA-axis suppression include use of high-potency steroids, large treatment surface areas, prolonged use, use of occlusive dressings, altered skin barrier, liver failure, and young age. Glucocorticosteroid insufficiency may occur, requiring supplemental systemic corticosteroids. Pediatric patients may be more susceptible to systemic toxicity. D/C and institute appropriate therapy if irritation develops. Use appropriate antifungal or antibacterial agent if concomitant skin infections are present or develop; if favorable response does not occur promptly, d/c until infection is controlled. Caution in elderly. (Cre/Oint) Safety and efficacy of use in pediatric patients for >3 weeks have not been established.

ADVERSE REACTIONS
Burning, irritation, dryness, secondary infection, acneiform reaction, folliculitis, hypertrichosis, hypopigmentation, perioral dermatitis, allergic contact dermatitis, striae, miliaria, skin atrophy.

NURSING CONSIDERATIONS

Assessment: Assess for presence of concomitant skin infections, severity of dermatoses, factors that predispose to HPA-axis suppression, and pregnancy/nursing status.

Monitoring: Monitor for signs/symptoms of HPA-axis suppression, Cushing's syndrome, hyperglycemia, glucosuria, irritation, allergic contact dermatitis (eg, failure to heal), skin infections, and other adverse reactions. Perform periodic monitoring of HPA-axis suppression using adrenocorticotropic hormone stimulation test. Monitor for systemic toxicity (eg, adrenal suppression, intracranial HTN) in pediatric patients. Monitor response to therapy.

Patient Counseling: Instruct to use externally ud. Advise not to use on face, underarms, or groin areas. Instruct to avoid contact with eyes. Advise not to use for any disorder other than that for which it was prescribed. Inform not to bandage, cover, or wrap treated skin area unless directed by a physician. Instruct to report any signs of local adverse reactions to physician. Advise not to use medication for treatment of diaper dermatitis and not to apply to diaper area. Instruct to d/c use when control is achieved and to notify physician if no improvement seen within 2 weeks. Advise that other corticosteroid-containing products should not be used without first consulting with the physician.

Storage: 25°C (77°F); excursions permitted to 15-30°C (59-86°F). (Cre) Avoid excessive heat.

EMEND CAPSULES – aprepitant **RX**

Class: Substance P/neurokinin 1 receptor antagonist

ADULT DOSAGE
Chemotherapy-Associated Nausea/Vomiting
Prevention:
Day 1: 125mg 1 hr prior to chemotherapy
Days 2 and 3: 80mg qam

Administer as part of a regimen that includes a corticosteroid and a 5-HT_3 antagonist; refer to PI

Postoperative Nausea/Vomiting
Prevention:
40mg within 3 hrs prior to induction of anesthesia

PEDIATRIC DOSAGE
Pediatric use may not have been established

ADMINISTRATION

Oral route

Take w/ or w/o food

HOW SUPPLIED

Cap: 40mg, 80mg, 125mg

CONTRAINDICATIONS

Concomitant use with pimozide, terfenadine, astemizole, or cisapride.

WARNINGS/PRECAUTIONS

Not recommended for chronic continuous use for prevention of N/V. Caution with severe hepatic impairment (Child-Pugh score >9).

ADVERSE REACTIONS

Asthenia/fatigue, N/V, constipation, diarrhea, hiccups, anorexia, headache, dehydration, pruritus, dizziness, alopecia, hypotension, pyrexia.

DRUG INTERACTIONS

See Contraindications. May increase concentrations of CYP3A4 substrates (eg, vinblastine, vincristine, ifosfamide, midazolam); use with caution; refer to PI for dose adjustment recommendations for methylprednisolone and oral dexamethasone. May decrease concentrations of CYP2C9 substrates (eg, warfarin, tolbutamide, phenytoin). Coadministration with warfarin may decrease PT/INR; in patients on chronic warfarin therapy, closely monitor INR in the 2-week period, particularly at 7-10 days, following initiation of aprepitant with each chemotherapy cycle, or following administration of aprepitant for the prevention of postoperative N/V. May reduce efficacy of hormonal contraceptives; use alternative or backup methods of contraception during treatment and for 1 month after the last dose. CYP3A4 inhibitors may increase concentrations; caution with strong inhibitors (eg, ketoconazole, itraconazole, nefazodone) and moderate inhibitors (eg, diltiazem) of CYP3A4. CYP3A4 inducers (eg, rifampin, carbamazepine, phenytoin) may decrease concentrations and efficacy. May increase concentrations of diltiazem. Coadministration with paroxetine may decrease levels of both drugs.

NURSING CONSIDERATIONS

Assessment: Assess for hypersensitivity to drug, severe hepatic impairment, pregnancy/nursing status, and possible drug interactions.

Monitoring: Monitor for hypersensitivity reactions and other adverse reactions. Monitor INR closely with warfarin.

Patient Counseling: Instruct to take drug only as prescribed. Instruct to d/c medication and contact physician immediately if patient experiences an allergic reaction. Advise to inform physician if using any other prescription, nonprescription medication, or herbal products. Inform that drug may reduce efficacy of hormonal contraceptives; advise to use alternative or backup methods of contraception during therapy and for 1 month after the last dose.

Storage: 20-25°C (68-77°F).

EMEND FOR INJECTION – fosaprepitant dimeglumine RX

Class: Substance P/neurokinin 1 receptor antagonist

ADULT DOSAGE

Chemotherapy-Associated Nausea/Vomiting

Prevention:
Highly Emetogenic Chemotherapy:
Single-Dose Regimen:
150mg on Day 1 only as an infusion over 20-30 min initiated approx 30 min prior to chemotherapy

Highly and Moderately Emetogenic Chemotherapy:
3-Day Dosing Regimen:
Day 1: 115mg as an infusion over 15 min initiated 30 min prior to chemotherapy; 125mg aprepitant caps may be substituted for inj
Days 2 and 3: 80mg aprepitant caps

Both regimens should be administered in conjunction w/ a corticosteroid and a 5-HT_3 antagonist; refer to PI

PEDIATRIC DOSAGE

Pediatric use may not have been established

ADMINISTRATION
IV route

Preparation of 115mg Inj
1. Inject 5mL 0.9% NaCl for Inj (normal saline [NS]) into the vial. Assure that NS is added to the vial along the vial wall in order to prevent foaming. Swirl the vial gently; avoid shaking and jetting saline into the vial
2. Prepare an infusion bag filled w/ 110mL of NS
3. Withdraw entire volume from the vial and transfer into infusion bag containing 110mL of NS to yield a total volume of 115mL and a final concentration of 1mg/1mL
4. Gently invert the bag 2-3 times

Preparation of 150mg Inj
1. Inject 5mL NS into the vial. Assure that NS is added to the vial along the vial wall in order to prevent foaming. Swirl the vial gently; avoid shaking and jetting saline into the vial
2. Prepare an infusion bag filled w/ 145mL of NS
3. Withdraw entire volume from the vial and transfer into infusion bag containing 145mL of NS to yield a total volume of 150mL and a final concentration of 1mg/1mL
4. Gently invert the bag 2-3X

HOW SUPPLIED
Inj: 115mg, 150mg

CONTRAINDICATIONS
Hypersensitivity to polysorbate 80. Concomitant use with pimozide or cisapride.

WARNINGS/PRECAUTIONS
Immediate hypersensitivity reactions reported; avoid reinitiating infusion if hypersensitivity occurs during 1st-time use. Not recommended for chronic continuous use for prevention of N/V. Caution with severe hepatic impairment (Child-Pugh score >9).

ADVERSE REACTIONS
Infusion-site reactions (erythema, pruritus, pain, induration), BP increased, thrombophlebitis.

DRUG INTERACTIONS
See Contraindications. May increase concentrations of CYP3A4 substrates (eg, vinblastine, vincristine, ifosfamide, midazolam); use with caution; refer to PI for dose adjustment recommendations for methylprednisolone and oral dexamethasone. May reduce efficacy of hormonal contraceptives; use alternative or backup methods of contraception during treatment and for 1 month after the last dose. May decrease concentrations of CYP2C9 substrates (eg, warfarin, tolbutamide). Coadministration with warfarin may decrease PT/INR; in patients on chronic warfarin therapy, closely monitor INR in the 2-week period, particularly at 7-10 days, following initiation of fosaprepitant with each chemotherapy cycle. CYP3A4 inhibitors may increase concentrations; caution with strong inhibitors (eg, ketoconazole, itraconazole, nefazodone) and moderate inhibitors (eg, diltiazem) of CYP3A4. CYP3A4 inducers (eg, rifampin, carbamazepine, phenytoin) may decrease concentrations and efficacy. May increase concentrations of diltiazem. Coadministration with paroxetine may decrease levels of both drugs.

NURSING CONSIDERATIONS

Assessment: Assess for hypersensitivity to drug or its components, severe hepatic impairment, pregnancy/nursing status, and possible drug interactions.

Monitoring: Monitor for hypersensitivity reactions and other adverse reactions. Monitor INR closely with warfarin.

Patient Counseling: Instruct to d/c medication and inform physician immediately if patient experiences an allergic reaction. Counsel patients who develop an infusion-site reaction on how to care for the local reaction and when to seek further evaluation. Advise to inform physician if using any other prescription, nonprescription medication, or herbal products. Inform that drug may reduce efficacy of hormonal contraceptives; advise to use alternative or backup methods of contraception during therapy and for 1 month after the last dose.

Storage: 2-8°C (36-46°F). Reconstituted Sol: Stable for 24 hrs at ≤25°C (77°F).

EMLA – lidocaine/prilocaine RX

Class: Acetamide local anesthetic

ADULT DOSAGE
Topical Anesthetic
Apply thick layer of cre to intact skin and cover w/ occlusive dressing
Minor Dermal Procedure:
Apply 2.5g over 20-25cm^2 of skin surface for at least 1 hr

PEDIATRIC DOSAGE
Topical Anesthetic
Intact Skin:
0-3 Months of Age:
<5kg:
Max: 1g/10cm^2 for up to 1 hr
3-12 Months of Age:

Major Dermal Procedure:
Apply 2g/10cm² of skin for 2 hrs

As an Adjunct Prior to Local Anesthetic Infiltration on Adult Male Genital Skin:
Apply 1g/10cm² of skin surface for 15 min

Minor Procedures on the Female External Genitalia (eg, Removal of Condylomata Acuminata) and Pretreatment for Anesthetic Infiltration:
Apply 5-10g for 5-10 min

>5kg:
Max: 2g/20cm² for up to 4 hrs

1-6 Years:
>10kg:
Max: 10g/100cm² for up to 4 hrs

7-12 Years:
>20kg:
Max: 20g/200cm² for up to 4 hrs
If >3 months and does not meet minimum weight requirement, max dose restricted to corresponding weight

ADMINISTRATION
Topical route
Not for ophthalmic use

HOW SUPPLIED
Cre: (Lidocaine-Prilocaine) 2.5%-2.5%

WARNINGS/PRECAUTIONS
Application to larger areas or for longer than recommended times may result in serious adverse effects. Should not be used where penetration or migration beyond the tympanic membrane into the middle ear is possible. Avoid w/ congenital or idiopathic methemoglobinemia and in infants <12 months of age receiving treatment w/ methemoglobin-inducing agents. Very young or patients w/ G6PD deficiency are more susceptible to methemoglobinemia. Reports of methemoglobinemia in infants and children following excessive applications. Monitor neonates and infants up to 3 months of age for Met-Hb levels before, during, and after application. Repeated doses may increase blood levels; caution in patients who may be more susceptible to systemic effects (eg, acutely ill, debilitated, elderly). Avoid eye contact and application to open wounds. Has been shown to inhibit viral and bacterial growth. Caution w/ severe hepatic disease and in patients w/ drug sensitivities.

ADVERSE REACTIONS
Erythema, edema, abnormal sensations, paleness (pallor or blanching), altered temperature sensations, burning sensation, itching, rash.

DRUG INTERACTIONS
Additive and potentially synergistic toxic effects w/ Class I antiarrhythmic drugs (eg, tocainide, mexiletine). May have additive cardiac effects w/ Class III antiarrhythmic drugs (eg, amiodarone, bretylium, sotalol, dofetilide). Avoid drugs associated w/ drug-induced methemoglobinemia (eg, sulfonamides, acetaminophen, acetanilid, aniline dyes, benzocaine, chloroquine, dapsone, naphthalene, nitrates/nitrites, nitrofurantoin, nitroglycerin, nitroprusside, phenobarbital, phenytoin, primaquine, pamaquine, para-aminosalicylic acid, phenacetin, quinine). Caution w/ other products containing lidocaine/prilocaine; consider the amount absorbed from all formulations.

NURSING CONSIDERATIONS

Assessment: Assess for congenital or idiopathic methemoglobinemia, G6PD deficiency, hepatic disease, open wounds, presence of acute illness, presence of debilitation, history of drug sensitivities, pregnancy/nursing status, and for possible drug interactions. In neonates and infants ≤3 months of age, obtain Met-Hb levels prior to application.

Monitoring: Monitor for signs/symptoms of methemoglobinemia, ototoxicity, local skin reactions and for allergic/anaphylactoid reactions. Monitor Met-Hb levels in neonates and infants ≤3 months of age during and after application.

Patient Counseling: Inform about potential risks/benefits of drug. Advise to avoid inadvertent trauma to treated area. Instruct not to apply near eyes or on open wounds. Apply ud by physician. Advise to notify physician if pregnant/nursing or planning to become pregnant. Instruct to remove cre and consult physician if child becomes very dizzy, excessively sleepy, or develops duskiness on the face or lips after application.

Storage: 20-25°C (68-77°F). Keep tightly closed.

EMTRIVA – emtricitabine RX

Class: Nucleoside reverse transcriptase inhibitor

Lactic acidosis and severe hepatomegaly with steatosis, including fatal cases, reported with the use of nucleoside analogues alone or in combination with other antiretrovirals. Not approved for the treatment of chronic hepatitis B virus (HBV) infection. Severe acute exacerbations of hepatitis B reported in patients who have discontinued therapy. Closely monitor hepatic function with both clinical and lab follow-up for at least several months in patients who are coinfected with HIV-1 and HBV and d/c therapy. If appropriate, initiation of antihepatitis B therapy may be warranted.

ADULT DOSAGE
HIV-1 Infection
Combination with Other Antiretrovirals:
Cap:
200mg qd
Sol:
240mg (24mL) qd

PEDIATRIC DOSAGE
HIV-1 Infection
Combination with Other Antiretrovirals
0-3 Months of Age:
Sol:
3mg/kg qd
3 Months-17 Years:
Cap:
>33kg: 200mg qd
Sol:
6mg/kg qd
Max: 240mg (24mL) qd

DOSE MODIFICATION
Renal Impairment
CrCl 30-49mL/min:
Cap: 200mg q48h
Sol: 120mg (12mL) q24h
CrCl 15-29mL/min:
Cap: 200mg q72h
Sol: 80mg (8mL) q24h
CrCl <15mL/min or on Hemodialysis:
Cap: 200mg q96h; give dose after dialysis, if dosing on day of dialysis
Sol: 60mg (6mL) q24h; give dose after dialysis, if dosing on day of dialysis

ADMINISTRATION
Oral route
Take without regard to food

HOW SUPPLIED
Cap: 200mg; Sol: 10mg/mL [170mL]

WARNINGS/PRECAUTIONS
Obesity and prolonged nucleoside exposure may be risk factors for lactic acidosis and severe hepatomegaly with steatosis. Caution with known risk factors for liver disease. D/C if lactic acidosis or pronounced hepatotoxicity develops. Test for chronic HBV before initiating therapy. Reduce dose and closely monitor clinical response and renal function with renal impairment. Redistribution/accumulation of body fat and immune reconstitution syndrome reported. Autoimmune disorders (eg, Graves' disease, polymyositis, Guillain-Barre syndrome) in the setting of immune reconstitution reported. Caution in elderly.

ADVERSE REACTIONS
Lactic acidosis, severe hepatomegaly with steatosis, headache, diarrhea, nausea, fatigue, dizziness, depression, insomnia, abnormal dreams, rash, abdominal pain, asthenia, increased cough, rhinitis.

DRUG INTERACTIONS
Do not coadminister with emtricitabine- or lamivudine-containing products.

NURSING CONSIDERATIONS

Assessment: Assess for previous hypersensitivity, risk factors for lactic acidosis and liver disease, HBV infection, renal impairment, pregnancy/nursing status, and possible drug interactions.

Monitoring: Monitor for signs/symptoms of lactic acidosis, severe hepatomegaly with steatosis, hepatotoxicity, redistribution/accumulation of body fat, immune reconstitution syndrome, autoimmune disorders, and other adverse reactions. Closely monitor hepatic function with both clinical and lab follow-up for at least several months in patients who are coinfected with HIV-1 and HBV and d/c therapy. Closely monitor clinical response and renal function with renal impairment.

Patient Counseling: Inform that therapy is not a cure for HIV-1 infection and illnesses associated with HIV-1 infection, including opportunistic infections, may continue. Instruct not to breastfeed, and not to share needles or other injection equipment and personal items that can have blood or body fluids on them (eg, toothbrushes, razor blades). Advise to always practice safer sex by using a latex or polyurethane condom to lower the chance of sexual contact with semen, vaginal secretions, or blood. Inform that it is important to take drug with combination therapy on a regular dosing schedule to avoid missing doses. Instruct to notify physician if symptoms suggestive of lactic acidosis or pronounced hepatotoxicity (eg, N/V, unusual or unexpected stomach discomfort, weakness) develop.

Storage: (Cap) 25°C (77°F); excursions permitted to 15-30°C (59-86°F). (Sol) 2-8°C (36-46°F). Use within 3 months if stored at 25°C (77°F).

ENABLEX – darifenacin RX

Class: Muscarinic antagonist

ADULT DOSAGE

Overactive Bladder

Initial: 7.5mg qd w/ water
Titrate: May increase to 15mg qd as early as 2 weeks after starting therapy based on individual response

PEDIATRIC DOSAGE

Pediatric use may not have been established

DOSE MODIFICATION

Concomitant Medications
Potent CYP3A4 Inhibitors:
Max: 7.5mg/day

Hepatic Impairment
Moderate (Child-Pugh B):
Max: 7.5mg/day
Severe (Child-Pugh C): Not recommended

ADMINISTRATION

Oral route

Take w/ or w/o food

HOW SUPPLIED

Tab, Extended-Release: 7.5mg, 15mg

CONTRAINDICATIONS

Urinary retention, gastric retention, uncontrolled narrow-angle glaucoma, and in patients at risk for these conditions.

WARNINGS/PRECAUTIONS

Risk of urinary retention; caution with significant bladder outflow obstruction. Risk of gastric retention; caution with GI obstructive disorders. May decrease GI motility; caution with severe constipation, ulcerative colitis, and myasthenia gravis. Caution with moderate hepatic impairment and in patients being treated for narrow-angle glaucoma. Angioedema reported; d/c and institute appropriate therapy if involvement of the tongue, hypopharynx, or larynx occurs. CNS anticholinergic effects (eg, headache, confusion, hallucinations, somnolence) reported; monitor for signs of anticholinergic CNS effects (particularly after beginning treatment or increasing the dose) and d/c or reduce dose if this occurs.

ADVERSE REACTIONS

Dry mouth, constipation, dyspepsia, abdominal pain, nausea, UTI, headache, flu syndrome.

DRUG INTERACTIONS

Pharmacokinetics may be altered by CYP3A4 inducers and CYP2D6/CYP3A4 inhibitors. Caution with medications metabolized by CYP2D6 and which have a narrow therapeutic window (eg, flecainide, thioridazine, TCAs). May increase the frequency and/or severity of dry mouth, constipation, blurred vision, and other anticholinergic pharmacologic effects with other anticholinergic agents. May alter the absorption of some concomitantly administered drugs due to effects on GI motility. Increased concentration with cimetidine, erythromycin, fluconazole, or ketoconazole. May increase imipramine and desipramine (imipramine active metabolite) concentrations.

NURSING CONSIDERATIONS

Assessment: Assess for urinary retention, gastric retention, narrow-angle glaucoma and risk for these conditions, bladder outflow obstruction, GI obstructive disorders, severe constipation, ulcerative colitis, myasthenia gravis, hepatic impairment, pregnancy/nursing status, and possible drug interactions.

Monitoring: Monitor for symptoms of urinary retention, gastric retention, decreased GI motility, and for angioedema (face, lips, tongue, hypopharynx, larynx). Monitor for signs of anticholinergic CNS effects (particularly after beginning treatment or increasing the dose).

Patient Counseling: Advise that dizziness or blurred vision may occur; instruct to exercise caution when engaging in potentially dangerous activities. Instruct to take qd with liquid. Instruct to swallow whole; advise to not chew, divide, or crush. Inform that symptoms of constipation, urinary retention, heat prostration when used in a hot environment, or angioedema may occur. Advise to d/c therapy and seek medical attention if edema of the tongue or laryngopharynx, or difficulty breathing occurs. Advise to read the patient information leaflet before starting therapy.

Storage: 25°C (77°F); excursions permitted to 15-30°C (59-86°F). Protect from light.

ENALAPRIL/HCTZ – enalapril maleate/hydrochlorothiazide RX

Class: ACE inhibitor/thiazide diuretic

D/C when pregnancy is detected. Drugs that act directly on the renin-angiotensin system (RAS) can cause injury/death to developing fetus.

OTHER BRAND NAMES
Vaseretic

ADULT DOSAGE
Hypertension

Uncontrolled BP on Enalapril/HCTZ Monotherapy:
Initial: 5mg/12.5mg or 10mg/25mg qd
Titrate: Increase dose based on clinical response. May increase HCTZ dose after 2-3 weeks
Max: 20mg/50mg qd

Replacement Therapy: May substitute for titrated components

PEDIATRIC DOSAGE
Pediatric use may not have been established

DOSE MODIFICATION
Elderly
Start at lower end of dosing range

ADMINISTRATION
Oral route

HOW SUPPLIED
Tab: (Enalapril/HCTZ) 5mg/12.5mg; (Vaseretic) 10mg/25mg* *scored

CONTRAINDICATIONS
Hereditary/idiopathic angioedema, anuria, hypersensitivity to other sulfonamide-derived drugs, history of ACE inhibitor-associated angioedema. Coadministration with aliskiren in patients with diabetes mellitus (DM).

WARNINGS/PRECAUTIONS
Not for initial therapy. Avoid if CrCl ≤30mL/min. Caution in elderly. Enalapril: Excessive hypotension may occur in salt/volume-depleted patients (eg, patients treated vigorously with diuretics or dialysis). Excessive hypotension associated with oliguria and/or progressive azotemia, and with acute renal failure (rare) and/or death has been observed in CHF patients; monitor closely upon initiation and during first 2 weeks of therapy and when dose is increased. Head/neck angioedema reported; d/c and administer appropriate therapy. Intestinal angioedema reported. More reports of angioedema in blacks than nonblacks. Anaphylactoid reactions reported during desensitization with hymenoptera venom, dialysis with high-flux membranes, and LDL apheresis with dextran sulfate absorption. Neutropenia/agranulocytosis reported; monitor WBCs in patients with collagen vascular disease and renal disease. Associated with syndrome that starts with cholestatic jaundice and progresses to fulminant hepatic necrosis and sometimes death (rare); d/c if jaundice or marked elevations of hepatic enzymes occur. Caution with left ventricular outflow obstruction. May cause changes in renal function; may be associated with oliguria and/or progressive azotemia and rarely with acute renal failure or death in severe heart failure patients whose renal function depends on the renin-angiotensin-aldosterone system. May increase BUN/SrCr in patients with renal artery stenosis or with no preexisting renal vascular disease; monitor renal function during the 1st few weeks of therapy in patients with renal artery stenosis. Hyperkalemia and persistent nonproductive cough reported. Hypotension may occur with major surgery or during anesthesia. HCTZ: May precipitate azotemia in patients with renal disease; caution with severe renal disease. Consider withholding or discontinuing therapy if progressive renal impairment occurs. Caution with hepatic impairment or progressive liver disease; may precipitate hepatic coma. Sensitivity reactions may occur. May exacerbate/activate systemic lupus erythematosus (SLE). May cause idiosyncratic reaction, resulting in acute transient myopia and acute angle-closure glaucoma; d/c as rapidly as possible. Observe for signs of fluid or electrolyte imbalance (eg, hyponatremia, hypochloremic alkalosis, hypokalemia). Hyperuricemia, gout precipitation, manifestations of latent DM, hypomagnesemia, hypercalcemia, and increased cholesterol and TG levels may occur. D/C before testing for parathyroid function. Enhanced effects in postsympathectomy patients. Hypokalemia may sensitize or exaggerate the response of the heart to toxic effects of digitalis.

ADVERSE REACTIONS
Dizziness, cough, fatigue, headache.

DRUG INTERACTIONS
See Contraindications. Dual blockade of the RAS is associated with increased risks of hypotension, hyperkalemia, and changes in renal function (including acute renal failure); avoid combined use of RAS inhibitors, or closely monitor BP, renal function, and electrolytes with concomitant agents that

affect the RAS. Avoid with aliskiren in patients with renal impairment (GFR <60mL/min). NSAIDs, including selective COX-2 inhibitors, may diminish effects of diuretics and ACE inhibitors, and may cause deterioration of renal function. Increased risk of lithium toxicity; avoid with lithium. Enalapril: Hypotension risk, and increased BUN/SrCr with diuretics. Antihypertensive agents that cause renin release (eg, diuretics) may augment effect. Increased risk of hyperkalemia with K^+-sparing diuretics, K^+ supplements, and/or K^+-containing salt substitutes. Nitritoid reactions reported with injectable gold. HCTZ: Potentiation of orthostatic hypotension may occur with alcohol, barbiturates, and narcotics. Dose adjustment of the antidiabetic drug (oral agents and insulin) may be required. Potentiation may occur with other antihypertensives. Cholestyramine and colestipol resins impair absorption. Corticosteroids and adrenocorticotropic hormone may intensify electrolyte depletion, particularly hypokalemia. May decrease response to pressor amines (eg, norepinephrine). May increase responsiveness to nondepolarizing skeletal muscle relaxants (eg, tubocurarine).

NURSING CONSIDERATIONS

Assessment: Assess for hereditary/idiopathic or history of ACE inhibitor-associated angioedema, anuria, DM, volume/salt depletion, hypersensitivity to the drug or sulfonamide-derived drugs, CHF, left ventricular outflow obstruction, collagen vascular disease, SLE, risk factors for hyperkalemia, renal/hepatic function, pregnancy/nursing status, and possible drug interactions.

Monitoring: Monitor for signs/symptoms of angioedema, exacerbation/activation of SLE, idiosyncratic reaction, latent DM, fluid/electrolyte imbalance, hypercalcemia, hypomagnesemia, hyperuricemia or precipitation of gout, sensitivity reactions, and other adverse reactions. Periodically monitor WBCs in patients with collagen vascular disease and renal disease. Monitor BP, serum electrolytes, renal/hepatic function, and cholesterol/TG levels.

Patient Counseling: Inform about fetal risks if taken during pregnancy and discuss treatment options in women planning to become pregnant; instruct to report pregnancy to physician as soon as possible. Instruct to d/c therapy and immediately report any signs/symptoms of angioedema. Instruct to report lightheadedness and to d/c therapy if actual syncope occurs. Inform that excessive perspiration, dehydration, and other causes of volume depletion may lead to an excessive fall in BP. Instruct not to use salt substitutes containing K^+ without consulting physician, and to report promptly any signs/symptoms of infection.

Storage: Protect from moisture. (Enalapril-HCTZ) 20-25°C (68-77°F). (Vaseretic) 25°C (77°F); excursions permitted to 15-30°C (59-86°F).

ENBREL – etanercept RX

Class: TNF-blocker

Increased risk for developing serious infections (eg, active TB, latent TB reactivation, invasive fungal infections, bacterial/viral infections, opportunistic infections) leading to hospitalization or death, mostly w/ concomitant use w/ immunosuppressants (eg, methotrexate [MTX], corticosteroids). D/C if serious infection or sepsis develops. Active/latent reactivation of TB may present w/ disseminated or extrapulmonary disease; test for latent TB before and during therapy and initiate treatment for latent TB prior to therapy. Consider empiric antifungal therapy in patients at risk for invasive fungal infections who develop severe systemic illness. Monitor for development of infection during and after treatment, including development of TB in patients who tested (-) for latent TB infection prior to therapy. Lymphoma and other malignancies, some fatal, reported in children and adolescents.

ADULT DOSAGE

Plaque Psoriasis

Initial: 50mg twice weekly for 3 months
Maint: 50mg once weekly

Rheumatoid Arthritis

50mg weekly
Max: 50mg/week

May continue MTX, glucocorticoids, salicylates, NSAIDs, or analgesics during treatment

Psoriatic Arthritis

50mg weekly
Max: 50mg/week

May continue MTX, glucocorticoids, salicylates, NSAIDs, or analgesics during treatment

Ankylosing Spondylitis

50mg weekly
Max: 50mg/week

May continue MTX, glucocorticoids, salicylates, NSAIDs, or analgesics during treatment

PEDIATRIC DOSAGE

Juvenile Idiopathic Arthritis

Moderately to Severely Active:
≥2 Years:
<63kg: 0.8mg/kg weekly
≥63kg: 50mg weekly

May continue glucocorticoids, NSAIDs, or analgesics during treatment

ADMINISTRATION

SQ route

Leave at room temperature for about 15-30 min before injecting
Do not mix contents of one vial of Enbrel sol w/ the contents of another vial of Enbrel
Do not add any other medications to sol containing Enbrel
Do not reconstitute Enbrel w/ other diluents
Do not filter reconstituted solution during preparation or administration

Preparation Using the Single-use Prefilled Syringe/SureClick Autoinjector

Check to see if the amount of liquid in the prefilled syringe falls between the 2 purple fill level indicator lines; do not use if the syringe does not have the right amount of liquid

Preparation Using the Multiple-Use Vial

Reconstitute w/ 1mL of Sterile Bacteriostatic Water for Inj (0.9% benzyl alcohol)
Do not use vial adaptor if multiple doses are to be withdrawn from the vial; use a 25-gauge needle if the vial will be used for multiple doses

If Using Vial Adapter:

1. Twist adapter onto the diluents syringe
2. Place vial adapter over Enbrel vial and inter vial adapter into vial stopper
3. Push down on plunger to inject diluents into Enbrel vial
4. Keeping the diluent syringe in place, gently swirl the contents of the Enbrel vial during dissolution
5. Withdraw the correct dose of reconstituted sol into the syringe
6. Remove the syringe from the vial adapter or remove the 25-gauge needle from the syringe
7. Attach a 27-gauge needle to inject Enbrel

HOW SUPPLIED

Inj: 25mg [multiple-use vial, single-use prefilled syringe], 50mg [single-use prefilled syringe, single-use prefilled SureClick autoinjector]

CONTRAINDICATIONS

Sepsis.

WARNINGS/PRECAUTIONS

Do not initiate in patients w/ an active infection. Increased risk of infection in patients >65 yrs of age and in patients w/ comorbid conditions. New onset or exacerbation of CNS and peripheral nervous system demyelinating disorders, acute and chronic leukemia, new onset and worsening of CHF, melanoma and non-melanoma skin cancer, and Merkel cell carcinoma reported; consider periodic skin examinations for all patients at increased risk for skin cancer. Pancytopenia, including aplastic anemia, reported. Reactivation of hepatitis B in patients who were previously infected w/ hepatitis B virus (HBV) reported; closely monitor for signs of active HBV infection during and for several months after therapy. Consider discontinuing therapy and initiating antiviral therapy w/ appropriate supportive treatment if HBV reactivation develops. Allergic reactions reported; d/c immediately and initiate appropriate therapy if an anaphylactic or other serious allergic reaction occurs. Needle cover of prefilled syringe and needle cover w/in the needle cap of autoinjector contain dry natural rubber, which may cause allergic reactions in latex-sensitive individuals. If possible, pediatric patients should be brought up to date w/ all immunizations in agreement w/ current immunization guidelines prior to initiating therapy. May result in the formation of autoantibodies and in the development of a lupus-like syndrome or autoimmune hepatitis; d/c and evaluate patient if a lupus-like syndrome or autoimmune hepatitis develops. Caution w/ moderate to severe alcoholic hepatitis and in the elderly. Patients w/ a significant exposure to varicella virus should temporarily d/c therapy and be considered for prophylactic treatment w/ varicella zoster immune globulin.

ADVERSE REACTIONS

Infections, sepsis, malignancies, inj-site reactions, diarrhea, rash, pyrexia, pruritus.

DRUG INTERACTIONS

See Boxed Warning. Avoid w/ live vaccines; pediatric patients should be brought up-to-date w/ all immunizations in agreement w/ current immunization guidelines prior to initiating therapy. Not recommended w/ anakinra or abatacept; may increase risk of serious infections. Not recommended in patients w/ Wegener's granulomatosis receiving immunosuppressive agents; increased incidence of noncutaneous solid malignancies when added to standard therapy (eg, cyclophosphamide). Not recommended w/ cyclophosphamide. Mild decrease in mean neutrophil counts reported w/ sulfasalazine. Hypoglycemia reported following initiation of therapy in patients receiving antidiabetic medication; reduction in antidiabetic medication may be necessary.

NURSING CONSIDERATIONS

Assessment: Assess for sepsis, active/chronic/recurrent infection, history of an opportunistic infection, recent travel in areas of endemic TB or endemic mycoses, underlying conditions that may predispose to infection, central or peripheral nervous system demyelinating disorders, CHF, history of significant hematologic abnormalities, latex sensitivity, alcoholic hepatitis, risk for skin cancer, pregnancy/nursing status, and possible drug interactions. Test for latent TB infection and for HBV infection. Assess immunization history in pediatric patients.

Monitoring: Monitor for development of infection during and after treatment. Monitor for sepsis, central or peripheral nervous system demyelinating disorders, malignancies, new or worsening

CHF, hematologic abnormalities, allergic reactions, lupus-like syndrome, autoimmune hepatitis, and other adverse reactions. Monitor for active TB and periodically test for latent TB. Monitor for HBV reactivation during therapy and for several months following termination of therapy. Consider periodic skin examinations for all patients at increased risk for skin cancer.

Patient Counseling: Advise of the potential risks and benefits of therapy. Inform that therapy may lower the ability of immune system to fight infections; instruct to contact physician if any symptoms of infection, TB, or HBV develop. Advise to report any signs of new/worsening medical conditions (eg, CNS demyelinating disorders, CHF, autoimmune disorders) or any symptoms suggestive of pancytopenia. Counsel about the risk of lymphoma and other malignancies. Instruct to seek immediate medical attention if any symptoms of a severe allergic reaction develop. Advise that the needle cover of prefilled syringe and the needle cover w/in the needle cap of the autoinjector contain dry natural rubber (a derivative of latex), which may cause allergic reactions in individuals sensitive to latex. Instruct in inj technique, as well as proper syringe and needle disposal, and caution against reuse of needles and syringes. Advise to inform physician if pregnant/breastfeeding.

Storage: 2-8°C (36-46°F). Do not shake. Protect from light or physical damage. Storage at room temperature for a max single period of 14 days is permissible, w/ protection from light, sources of heat, and (vial) humidity; once the product has been stored at room temperature, do not place back into the refrigerator. Discard if not used w/in 14 days at room temperature. Do not store in extreme heat or cold. Do not freeze. (Vial) Reconstituted Sol: Use immediately or may refrigerate for up to 14 days.

ENJUVIA – synthetic conjugated estrogens, B RX

Class: Estrogen

Estrogens increase the risk of endometrial cancer. Perform adequate diagnostic measures, including endometrial sampling, to rule out malignancy with undiagnosed persistent or recurrent abnormal vaginal bleeding. Should not be used for the prevention of cardiovascular (CV) disease or dementia. Increased risks of MI, stroke, invasive breast cancer, pulmonary embolism (PE), and deep vein thrombosis (DVT) in postmenopausal women (50-79 yrs) reported. Increased risk of developing probable dementia in postmenopausal women ≥65 yrs reported. Should be prescribed at the lowest effective dose and for the shortest duration consistent with treatment goals and risks.

ADULT DOSAGE

Menopause

Moderate to Severe Vasomotor Symptoms:
Initial: 0.3mg qd
Titrate: Dose adjust based on individual response
Maint: 0.3-1.25mg qd

Vaginal Dryness and Pain w/ Intercourse/ Vulvar and Vaginal Atrophy:
Initial/Maint: 0.3mg qd

Reevaluate treatment need periodically (eg, 3- to 6-month intervals)

PEDIATRIC DOSAGE

Pediatric use may not have been established

ADMINISTRATION

Oral route

HOW SUPPLIED

Tab: 0.3mg, 0.45mg, 0.625mg, 0.9mg, 1.25mg

CONTRAINDICATIONS

Undiagnosed abnormal genital bleeding, known/suspected/history of breast cancer, known/ suspected estrogen-dependent neoplasia, active or history of DVT/PE, active or recent arterial thromboembolic disease (eg, stroke, MI), liver dysfunction or disease, known/suspected pregnancy.

WARNINGS/PRECAUTIONS

Increased risk of CV events; d/c immediately if these occur or are suspected. Caution in patients with risk factors for arterial vascular disease and/or venous thromboembolism. If feasible, d/c at least 4-6 weeks before surgery of the type associated with an increased risk of thromboembolism, or during prolonged immobilization. May increase the risk of breast/endometrial/ovarian cancer and gallbladder disease. Consider addition of progestin for women with a uterus or with residual endometriosis posthysterectomy. May lead to severe hypercalcemia in patients with breast cancer and bone metastases; d/c and take appropriate measures if hypercalcemia occurs. Retinal vascular thrombosis reported; d/c pending examination if sudden partial/complete loss of vision or sudden onset of proptosis, diplopia, or migraine occurs. If examination reveals papilledema or retinal vascular lesions, d/c therapy permanently. May elevate BP, thyroid-binding globulin levels, or plasma TGs, leading to pancreatitis and other complications. Caution in patients with history of cholestatic jaundice; d/c in case of recurrence. May cause fluid retention; caution with cardiac/renal dysfunction. Caution with severe hypocalcemia. May exacerbate endometriosis, asthma, diabetes mellitus (DM), epilepsy, migraine or porphyria, systemic lupus erythematosus (SLE), and hepatic hemangiomas; use with caution. May affect certain endocrine function tests, HDL, LDL, TG levels, and blood components in lab tests.

ADVERSE REACTIONS

Abdominal pain, flu syndrome, headache, pain, flatulence, nausea, dizziness, paresthesia, bronchitis, rhinitis, sinusitis, breast pain, dysmenorrhea, vaginitis.

DRUG INTERACTIONS

CYP3A4 inducers (eg, St. John's wort, phenobarbital, carbamazepine, rifampin) may decrease levels, which may decrease therapeutic effects and/or change uterine bleeding profile. CYP3A4 inhibitors (eg, erythromycin, clarithromycin, ketoconazole, itraconazole, ritonavir, grapefruit juice) may increase levels, which may result in side effects. Patients concomitantly receiving thyroid replacement therapy and estrogens may require increased doses of thyroid hormone.

NURSING CONSIDERATIONS

Assessment: Assess for undiagnosed abnormal genital bleeding, presence/history of breast cancer estrogen-dependent neoplasia, active/history of DVT/PE, active or recent (eg, within past yr) arterial thromboembolic disease (eg, stroke, MI), liver dysfunction/disease, pregnancy/nursing status, any other conditions where treatment is contraindicated or cautioned, need for progestin therapy, and possible drug interactions. Assess use in patient ≥65 yrs and in those with preexisting hypertriglyceridemia, history of cholestatic jaundice, or presence of hypothyroidism, hypocalcemia, asthma, DM, epilepsy, migraine, porphyria, SLE, and hepatic hemangiomas.

Monitoring: Monitor for signs/symptoms of CV disorders (eg, stroke, MI), malignant neoplasms (eg, endometrial, breast/ovarian cancer), dementia, gallbladder disease, hypercalcemia, visual abnormalities, elevations in BP, fluid retention, elevations in serum TGs, pancreatitis, hypothyroidism, hypocalcemia, exacerbation of endometriosis, and for other conditions (eg, asthma, DM, epilepsy, migraine, SLE). Perform annual breast exam; schedule mammography based on age, risk factors, and prior mammogram results. Monitor thyroid function in patients on thyroid replacement therapy, and monitor BP. Periodically evaluate (every 3-6 months) to determine need for therapy. If undiagnosed, persistent, or recurring abnormal vaginal bleeding occurs, perform proper diagnostic testing (eg, endometrial sampling) to rule out malignancy.

Patient Counseling: Inform that therapy increases the risk for uterine cancer and may increase the chances of getting a heart attack, stroke, breast cancer, and blood clots. Advise to report breast lumps, unusual vaginal bleeding, dizziness or faintness, changes in speech, severe headaches, chest pain, SOB, leg pains, vision changes, or vomiting. Instruct to notify physician if taking other medications or if planning surgery or prolonged immobilization. Advise to have yearly breast examinations by a physician and to perform monthly breast self-examinations. Instruct to take exactly ud.

Storage: 20-25°C (68-77°F).

ENTEREG – alvimopan **RX**

Class: Opioid antagonist

Potential risk of myocardial infarction with long-term use; for short-term hospital use only. Available only through a restricted program for short-term use (15 doses) under a Risk Evaluation and Mitigation Strategy called the Entereg Access Support and Education (E.A.S.E.) Program.

ADULT DOSAGE

Postoperative Gastrointestinal Recovery

To Accelerate the Time to Upper and Lower GI Recovery Following Surgeries that Include Partial Bowel Resection w/ Primary Anastomosis:

Usual: 12mg given 30 min to 5 hrs prior to surgery followed by 12mg bid beginning the day after surgery until discharge for a max of 7 days

Max: 15 doses

PEDIATRIC DOSAGE

Pediatric use may not have been established

DOSE MODIFICATION

Renal Impairment

ESRD: Not recommended

Hepatic Impairment

Severe: Not recommended

ADMINISTRATION

Oral route

HOW SUPPLIED
Cap: 12mg

CONTRAINDICATIONS
Patients who have taken therapeutic doses of opioids for >7 consecutive days immediately prior to therapy.

WARNINGS/PRECAUTIONS
Increased sensitivity to therapy and occurrence of GI adverse reactions (eg, abdominal pain, N/V, diarrhea) are expected with patients recently exposed to opioids; monitor patients receiving >3 doses of an opioid within the week prior to surgery for GI adverse reactions. Not recommended with severe hepatic impairment, end-stage renal disease, complete GI obstruction/surgery for correction of complete bowel obstruction, or pancreatic/gastric anastomosis. Closely monitor patients with mild-to-moderate hepatic impairment/mild-to-severe renal impairment and Japanese patients for possible adverse effects (eg, diarrhea, GI pain, cramping); d/c if adverse events occur.

ADVERSE REACTIONS
Dyspepsia.

DRUG INTERACTIONS
See Contraindications.

NURSING CONSIDERATIONS

Assessment: Assess for hepatic/renal impairment, complete GI obstruction/surgery for correction of complete bowel obstruction, pancreatic/gastric anastomosis, history of opioid use, and pregnancy/nursing status.

Monitoring: Monitor for GI adverse reactions, and other adverse effects.

Patient Counseling: Instruct to disclose long-term or intermittent opioid pain therapy, including any use of opioids in the week prior to receiving therapy; inform that recent use of opioids may increase susceptibility to adverse reactions, primarily those limited to the GI tract (eg, abdominal pain, N/V, diarrhea). Advise that therapy is for hospital use only for no more than 7 days after bowel resection surgery. Inform that dyspepsia may occur.

Storage: 25°C (77°F); excursions permitted to 15-30°C (59-86°F).

ENTOCORT EC – budesonide RX

Class: Corticosteroid

ADULT DOSAGE

Crohn's Disease

Mild to Moderate Active Crohn's Disease of the Ileum and/or Ascending Colon:
Usual: 9mg qd, in the am for up to 8 weeks; repeated 8-week courses may be given for recurring episodes of active disease
Maint of Clinical Remission:
6mg qd for up to 3 months; if symptom control is still maintained at 3 months, attempt to taper to complete cessation

PEDIATRIC DOSAGE
Pediatric use may not have been established

DOSE MODIFICATION

Concomitant Medications
CYP3A4 Inhibitors: Monitor for increased signs and/or symptoms of hypercorticism if concomitant administration w/ ketoconazole or any other CYP3A4 inhibitor is indicated; consider reducing dose

Hepatic Impairment
Moderate to Severe: Monitor for increased signs and/or symptoms of hypercorticism; consider reducing dose

Elderly
Start at lower end of dosing range

ADMINISTRATION
Oral route

Swallow caps whole; do not chew or break

HOW SUPPLIED
Cap: 3mg

WARNINGS/PRECAUTIONS
May reduce response of hypothalamic-pituitary-adrenal axis to stress. Supplement with systemic glucocorticosteroids if undergoing surgery or other stressful situations. Increased risk of infection;

avoid exposure to varicella/varicella zoster and measles. Caution with tuberculosis (TB), HTN, diabetes mellitus (DM), osteoporosis, peptic ulcer, glaucoma, cirrhosis, cataracts, or family history of DM or glaucoma. Replacement of systemic glucocorticosteroids may unmask allergies. Chronic use may cause hypercorticism and adrenal suppression.

ADVERSE REACTIONS

Headache, respiratory infection, N/V, back pain, dyspepsia, dizziness, abdominal pain, diarrhea, flatulence, sinusitis, viral infection, arthralgia, benign intracranial HTN, signs/symptoms of hypercorticism.

DRUG INTERACTIONS

Ketoconazole caused an eight-fold increase of systemic exposure to oral budesonide. Increased levels with CYP3A4 inhibitors (eg, ketoconazole, saquinavir, erythromycin, grapefruit); monitor for increased signs and symptoms of hypercorticism and reduce budesonide dose if coadministered.

NURSING CONSIDERATIONS

Assessment: Assess for liver disease, history of chickenpox or measles, TB, HTN, osteoporosis, peptic ulcers, cataracts, history and/or family history of DM or glaucoma, and possible drug interactions. Obtain baseline LFTs.

Monitoring: Monitor LFTs periodically and for signs/symptoms of hypercorticism and hypersensitivity reactions.

Patient Counseling: Advise to swallow whole; do not chew or break. Instruct to avoid consumption of grapefruit and grapefruit juice during therapy. Caution to take particular care to avoid exposure to chickenpox or measles.

Storage: 25° (77°F); excursions permitted to 15-30°C (59-86°F). Keep container tightly closed.

ENTYVIO — vedolizumab

RX

Class: Monoclonal antibody/integrin receptor antagonist

ADULT DOSAGE

Ulcerative Colitis

Moderately to Severely Active:

For inducing/maintaining clinical response and remission, improving endoscopic appearance of the mucosa, and achieving corticosteroid-free remission in patients who have had an inadequate response w/, lost response to, or were intolerant to a TNF blocker or immunomodulator; or had an inadequate response w/, were intolerant to, or demonstrated dependence on corticosteroids

Usual: 300mg IV infusion over 30 min at 0, 2, and 6 weeks and then every 8 weeks thereafter

D/C if no evidence of therapeutic benefit seen by Week 14

Crohn's Disease

Moderately to Severely Active:

For achieving clinical response and remission, and achieving corticosteroid-free remission in patients who have had an inadequate response w/, lost response to, or were intolerant to a TNF blocker or immunomodulator; or had an inadequate response w/, were intolerant to, or demonstrated dependence on corticosteroids

Usual: 300mg IV infusion over 30 min at 0, 2, and 6 weeks and then every 8 weeks thereafter

D/C if no evidence of therapeutic benefit seen by Week 14

PEDIATRIC DOSAGE

Pediatric use may not have been established

ADMINISTRATION

IV route

Do not administer as an IV push or bolus

Lyophilized powder must be reconstituted w/ sterile water for inj (SWFI) and diluted in 250mL of sterile 0.9% NaCl inj prior to administration

After infusion is complete, flush w/ 30mL of sterile 0.9% NaCl inj

Reconstitution
1. Reconstitute vial containing lyophilized powder w/ 4.8mL of SWFI using a syringe w/ a 21- to 25-gauge needle
2. Insert the syringe needle into the vial through the center of the stopper and direct the stream of SWFI to the glass wall of the vial to avoid excessive foaming
3. Gently swirl vial for at least 15 sec; do not vigorously shake or invert
4. Allow sol to sit for up to 20 min at room temperature to allow for reconstitution and for any foam to settle; may swirl and inspect for dissolution during this time. If not fully dissolved after 20 min, allow another 10 min for dissolution; do not use vial if the drug product is not dissolved w/in 30 min
5. Prior to withdrawing the reconstituted sol from vial, gently invert vial 3X
6. Withdraw 5mL (300mg) of reconstituted sol using a syringe w/ a 21- to 25- gauge needle

Dilution
Add the 5mL (300mg) of reconstituted sol to 250mL of 0.9% NaCl and gently mix infusion bag; once reconstituted and diluted, use infusion sol as soon as possible
Do not add other medicinal products to the prepared infusion sol or IV infusion set
May store infusion sol for up to 4 hrs at 2°-8°C (36°-46°F), if necessary; do not freeze

HOW SUPPLIED
Inj: 300mg

WARNINGS/PRECAUTIONS
Hypersensitivity reactions reported; d/c immediately and initiate appropriate treatment if anaphylaxis or other serious allergic reactions occur. Increased risk for developing infections; not recommended in patients with active, severe infections until the infections are controlled. Consider withholding treatment if a severe infection develops. Consider screening for tuberculosis according to the local practice. Progressive multifocal leukoencephalopathy (PML) may occur; monitor for any new onset, or worsening, of neurological signs and symptoms. If PML is suspected, withhold dosing and refer to a neurologist; if confirmed, d/c dosing permanently. Elevations of transaminase and/or bilirubin reported; d/c if jaundice or other evidence of significant liver injury develops. Prior to initiating treatment, all patients should be brought up to date with all immunizations according to current immunization guidelines.

ADVERSE REACTIONS
Nasopharyngitis, headache, arthralgia, nausea, pyrexia, upper respiratory tract infection, fatigue, cough, bronchitis, influenza, back pain, rash, pruritus, sinusitis, oropharyngeal pain, pain in extremities.

DRUG INTERACTIONS
Avoid with natalizumab; potential for increased risk of PML and other infections. Avoid with TNF blockers; potential for increased risk of infections. Live vaccines may be administered concurrently with therapy only if the benefits outweigh the risks.

NURSING CONSIDERATIONS

Assessment: Assess for hypersensitivity to drug, infections, history of recurring severe infections, pregnancy/nursing status, and possible drug interactions. Assess immunization history.

Monitoring: Monitor for infusion/hypersensitivity reactions, infections, PML, liver injury, and other adverse reactions.

Patient Counseling: Instruct to report immediately if symptoms consistent with a hypersensitivity reaction occur during or following infusion. Advise to notify physician if any signs/symptoms of infection develop. Instruct to report immediately any symptoms that may indicate PML (new onset or worsening of neurological signs/symptoms) and/or liver injury (eg, fatigue, anorexia, right upper abdominal discomfort, dark urine, jaundice).

Storage: 2-8°C (36-46°F). Protect from light. Infusion Sol: 2-8°C (36-46°F) for up to 4 hrs. Do not freeze.

EPIDUO – adapalene/benzoyl peroxide RX

Class: Antibacterial/keratolytic

ADULT DOSAGE
Acne Vulgaris
Apply a thin film to affected areas of the face and/or trunk qd after washing. Use a pea-sized amount for each area of the face (eg, forehead, chin, each cheek)

PEDIATRIC DOSAGE
Acne Vulgaris
≥9 Years:
Apply a thin film to affected areas of the face and/or trunk qd after washing. Use a pea-sized amount for each area of the face (eg, forehead, chin, each cheek)

ADMINISTRATION
Topical route

Apply after washing

HOW SUPPLIED
Gel: (Adapalene-Benzoyl Peroxide) 0.1%-2.5% [45g]

WARNINGS/PRECAUTIONS
Not for oral, ophthalmic, or intravaginal use. Minimize exposure to sunlight and sunlamps; use sunscreen and protective apparel if exposure cannot be avoided. Exercise caution in patients with high levels of sun exposure and those with inherent sensitivity to sun. Extreme weather may cause irritation. Avoid contact with the eyes, lips, and mucous membranes. Avoid application to cuts, abrasions, eczematous, or sunburned skin. Erythema, scaling, dryness, stinging/burning, and irritant and allergic contact dermatitis may occur; depending on severity, may apply moisturizer, reduce frequency of application, or d/c use. Avoid waxing as a depilatory method on the treated skin.

ADVERSE REACTIONS
Local cutaneous reactions (eg, erythema, scaling, stinging/burning, dryness), contact dermatitis.

DRUG INTERACTIONS
Caution with concomitant topical acne therapy, especially with peeling, desquamating, or abrasive agents. Avoid with other potentially irritating topical products (medicated or abrasive soaps and cleansers, soaps and cosmetics that have strong skin-drying effect, and products with high concentrations of alcohol, astringents, spices, or limes).

NURSING CONSIDERATIONS

Assessment: Assess for presence of cuts, abrasions, eczematous, or sunburned skin at the treatment site. Assess for pregnancy/nursing status and possible drug interactions. Assess if patient has high levels of sun exposure or inherent sensitivity to the sun.

Monitoring: Monitor for irritation, erythema, scaling, dryness, stinging/burning, and other adverse reactions.

Patient Counseling: Advise to cleanse area with mild or soapless cleanser and to pat dry. Advise to avoid contact with the eyes, lips, and mucous membranes. Instruct not to use more than the recommended amount. Inform that drug may cause irritation and may bleach hair and colored fabric. Instruct to minimize exposure to sunlight and sunlamps. Recommend to use sunscreen products and protective apparel when exposure to sunlight cannot be avoided.

Storage: 25°C (77°F); excursions permitted to 15-30°C (59-86°F). Keep tube tightly closed. Protect from light. Keep away from heat.

EPIFOAM – hydrocortisone acetate/pramoxine hydrochloride RX

Class: Anesthetic/corticosteroid

ADULT DOSAGE

Inflammatory and Pruritic Manifestations of Corticosteroid-Responsive Dermatoses

Apply a small amount to the affected area tid-qid depending on severity of condition

PEDIATRIC DOSAGE

Inflammatory and Pruritic Manifestations of Corticosteroid-Responsive Dermatoses

Apply a small amount to the affected area tid-qid depending on severity of condition

ADMINISTRATION
Topical route

May use occlusive dressings for management of psoriasis or recalcitrant conditions; d/c occlusive dressing if infection develops

Shake container vigorously for 5-10 sec before each use
May also dispense a small amount to a pad and apply to affected areas
Rinse container and cap w/ warm water after use
Do not insert container into vagina or anus

HOW SUPPLIED
Foam: (Hydrocortisone-Pramoxine) 1%-1% [10g]

WARNINGS/PRECAUTIONS
Not for prolonged use. D/C if redness, pain, irritation, or swelling persists. Systemic absorption may produce reversible hypothalamic-pituitary-adrenal (HPA) axis suppression, manifestations of Cushing's syndrome, hyperglycemia, and glucosuria; evaluate periodically for evidence of HPA-axis suppression when large dose is applied to large surface areas or under an occlusive dressing. Withdraw treatment, reduce frequency of application, or substitute with a less potent steroid if HPA-axis suppression is noted. Application of more potent steroids, use over large

surface areas, prolonged use, and the addition of occlusive dressings may augment systemic absorption. Signs and symptoms of steroid withdrawal may occur requiring supplemental systemic corticosteroids. D/C and institute appropriate therapy if irritation occurs. Use appropriate antifungal or antibacterial agent in the presence of dermatological infections; if favorable response does not occur promptly, d/c until infection is controlled. Pediatrics may be more susceptible to systemic toxicity. Chronic therapy may interfere with growth and development of pediatrics.

ADVERSE REACTIONS

Burning, itching, irritation, dryness, folliculitis, hypertrichosis, acneiform eruptions, hypopigmentation, perioral dermatitis, allergic contact dermatitis, maceration, secondary infection, skin atrophy, striae, miliaria.

NURSING CONSIDERATIONS

Assessment: Assess for previous hypersensitivity to any components of the drug, dermatological infections, and pregnancy/nursing status.

Monitoring: Monitor for signs/symptoms of reversible HPA-axis suppression, Cushing's syndrome, hyperglycemia, glucosuria, skin irritation, skin infections, systemic toxicity in pediatrics, hypersensitivity reactions, and other adverse reactions. When large dose is applied to large surface area or under occlusive dressings, monitor for HPA-axis suppression by using urinary free cortisol and adrenocorticotropic hormone stimulation tests. Monitor for signs/symptoms of steroid withdrawal following discontinuation.

Patient Counseling: Instruct to use externally and ud; instruct to avoid contact with eyes. Advise not to use for any disorder other than for which it was prescribed. Instruct not to bandage, cover, or wrap treated skin, unless directed by physician. Advise to report any signs of local adverse reactions, especially under occlusive dressing. Instruct not to use tight-fitting diapers or plastic pants on a child being treated in the diaper area, as these garments may constitute occlusive dressings.

Storage: 20-25°C (68-77°F). Store upright. Do not store at temperatures >120°F (49°C). Do not burn or puncture the aerosol container. Do not refrigerate.

EpiPen – epinephrine RX

Class: Sympathomimetic catecholamine

OTHER BRAND NAMES

EpiPen Jr.

ADULT DOSAGE

Emergency Treatment of Type I Allergic Reactions

Including anaphylaxis to stinging and biting insects, allergen immunotherapy, foods, drugs, diagnostic testing substances, and other allergens, as well as idiopathic or exercise-induced anaphylaxis

15-30kg:
EpiPen Jr: 0.15mg

≥30kg:
EpiPen: 0.3mg

Severe Persistent Anaphylaxis:
Repeat inj may be necessary

PEDIATRIC DOSAGE

Emergency Treatment of Type I Allergic Reactions

Including anaphylaxis to stinging and biting insects, allergen immunotherapy, foods, drugs, diagnostic testing substances, and other allergens, as well as idiopathic or exercise-induced anaphylaxis

15-30kg:
EpiPen Jr: 0.15mg

≥30kg:
EpiPen: 0.3mg

Severe Persistent Anaphylaxis:
Repeat inj may be necessary

ADMINISTRATION

IM/SQ route
Inject into the anterolateral aspect of the thigh, through clothing if necessary
Consider using other forms of injectable epinephrine if doses <0.15mg are deemed necessary

HOW SUPPLIED

Inj: (EpiPen Jr) 0.15mg/0.3mL; (EpiPen) 0.3mg/0.3mL

WARNINGS/PRECAUTIONS

Intended for immediate administration in patients who are determined to be at increased risk for anaphylaxis, including those with a history of anaphylactic reactions. Intended for immediate administration as emergency supportive therapy only and is not a substitute for immediate medical care. More than 2 sequential doses should only be administered under direct medical supervision. Do not inject IV. Large doses or accidental IV inj use may result in cerebral hemorrhage due to sharp rise in BP; rapidly acting vasodilators can counteract the marked pressor effects of epinephrine. Do not inject into buttock; may not provide effective treatment of anaphylaxis. Do not inject into digits, hands, or feet; may result in loss of blood flow to the affected area. Contains sodium metabisulfite; may cause allergic-type reactions, including anaphylactic symptoms or life-threatening or less severe asthmatic episodes in certain susceptible persons. Caution in patients with heart disease, hyperthyroidism, diabetes mellitus (DM), elderly, pregnant women. May temporarily worsen symptoms of Parkinson's disease.

ADVERSE REACTIONS

Anxiety, apprehensiveness, restlessness, tremor, weakness, dizziness, sweating, palpitations, pallor, N/V, headache, respiratory difficulties.

DRUG INTERACTIONS

May precipitate/aggravate angina pectoris as well as produce ventricular arrhythmias with drugs that may sensitize the heart to arrhythmias; use with caution. Monitor for cardiac arrhythmias with antiarrhythmics, cardiac glycosides, and diuretics. Effects may be potentiated by TCAs, MAOIs, levothyroxine sodium, and certain antihistamines (notably, chlorpheniramine, tripelennamine, diphenhydramine). Cardiostimulating and bronchodilating effects are antagonized by β-adrenergic blockers (eg, propranolol). Vasoconstricting and hypertensive effects are antagonized by α-adrenergic blockers (eg, phentolamine). Ergot alkaloids may reverse pressor effects.

NURSING CONSIDERATIONS

Assessment: Assess for risk of anaphylaxis, heart disease, hyperthyroidism, DM, Parkinson's disease, pregnancy/nursing status, and for possible drug interactions.

Monitoring: Monitor for allergic-type reactions, angina pectoris, ventricular arrhythmias, cerebral hemorrhage, and other adverse reactions. Monitor HR and BP.

Patient Counseling: Advise that therapy may produce signs and symptoms that include increased HR, sensation of more forceful heartbeat, palpitations, sweating, N/V, difficulty breathing, pallor, dizziness, weakness or shakiness, headache, apprehension, nervousness, or anxiety; advise that these signs and symptoms usually subside rapidly, especially with rest, quiet, and recumbency. Inform that patients may develop more severe or persistent effects if they have HTN or hyperthyroidism. Inform that patients may experience angina if they have coronary artery disease. Advise that patients may develop increased blood glucose levels following administration if they have DM. Advise that a temporary worsening of symptoms may be noticed if patient has Parkinson's disease. Instruct to seek immediate medical care in case of accidental inj.

Storage: 20-25°C (68-77°F); excursions permitted to 15-30°C (59-86°F). Store in the carrier tube provided. Protect from light. Do not refrigerate.

EPIVIR – lamivudine

RX

Class: Nucleoside reverse transcriptase inhibitor

Lactic acidosis and severe hepatomegaly w/ steatosis, including fatal cases, reported w/ nucleoside analogues; suspend treatment if lactic acidosis or pronounced hepatotoxicity occurs. Severe acute exacerbations of hepatitis B reported in patients coinfected w/ hepatitis B virus (HBV) upon discontinuation of therapy; closely monitor hepatic function for at least several months. If appropriate, initiation of antihepatitis B therapy may be warranted. Epivir tabs and sol, used to treat HIV-1 infection, contain higher dose of lamivudine than Epivir-HBV tabs and sol, used to treat chronic HBV infection; only use appropriate dosing forms for HIV-1 treatment.

ADULT DOSAGE

HIV-1 Infection

Combination w/ Other Antiretrovirals:
150mg bid or 300mg qd

PEDIATRIC DOSAGE

HIV-1 Infection

Combination w/ Other Antiretrovirals:
≥3 Months:
Sol:
4mg/kg bid or 8mg/kg qd
Max: 300mg/day

Tab:
QD Dosing Regimen:
14-<20kg: 150mg
≥20-<25kg: 225mg
≥25kg: 300mg

BID Dosing Regimen (Using Scored 150mg Tab):
14-<20kg:
AM Dose: 75mg
PM Dose: 75mg
≥20-<25kg:
AM Dose: 75mg
PM Dose: 150mg
≥25kg:
AM Dose: 150mg
PM Dose: 150mg

DOSE MODIFICATION
Renal Impairment
CrCl 30-49mL/min: 150mg qd
CrCl 15-29mL/min: 150mg 1st dose, then 100mg qd
CrCl 5-14mL/min: 150mg 1st dose, then 50mg qd
CrCl <5mL/min: 50mg 1st dose, then 25mg qd
Consider dose reduction and/or increase in dosing interval in pediatric patients w/ renal impairment

ADMINISTRATION
Oral route

Take w/ or w/o food

HOW SUPPLIED
Sol: 10mg/mL [240mL]; Tab: 150mg*, 300mg *scored

WARNINGS/PRECAUTIONS
Obesity and prolonged nucleoside exposure may be risk factors for lactic acidosis and severe hepatomegaly w/ steatosis. Caution w/ known risk factors for liver disease. Emergence of lamivudine-resistant HBV reported. Caution in pediatric patients w/ history of prior antiretroviral nucleoside exposure, history of pancreatitis, or other significant risk factors for development of pancreatitis; d/c if pancreatitis develops. Immune reconstitution syndrome reported. Autoimmune disorders (eg, Graves' disease, polymyositis, Guillain-Barre syndrome) reported to occur in the setting of immune reconstitution and can occur many months after initiation of treatment. Redistribution/accumulation of body fat may occur. Caution in elderly.

ADVERSE REACTIONS
Lactic acidosis, severe hepatomegaly w/ steatosis, headache, malaise, fatigue, N/V, diarrhea, nasal signs/symptoms, neuropathy, insomnia, musculoskeletal pain, cough, fever, dizziness.

DRUG INTERACTIONS
Not recommended w/ other lamivudine-containing products, emtricitabine-containing products, and zalcitabine. Hepatic decompensation reported in HIV-1/hepatitis C virus coinfected patients receiving interferon-alfa w/ or w/o ribavirin; closely monitor for treatment-associated toxicities. Possible interaction w/ drugs whose main route of elimination is active renal secretion via the organic cationic transport system (eg, trimethoprim).

NURSING CONSIDERATIONS

Assessment: Assess for hepatic/renal impairment, risk factors for lactic acidosis, HIV-1 and HBV coinfection, previous hypersensitivity, pregnancy/nursing status, and possible drug interactions. In pediatric patients, assess for a history of prior antiretroviral nucleoside exposure, a history of pancreatitis, or risk factors for pancreatitis. Consider HIV-1 viral load and CD4+ cell count/percentage when selecting the dosing interval for patients initiating treatment w/ oral sol.

Monitoring: Monitor for signs/symptoms of pancreatitis, immune reconstitution syndrome (eg, opportunistic infections), autoimmune disorders, fat redistribution/accumulation, lactic acidosis, hepatomegaly w/ steatosis, hepatitis B exacerbation, hepatic/renal dysfunction, and hypersensitivity reactions. Monitor hepatic function closely for several months in patients w/ HIV/HBV coinfection who d/c therapy. Monitor CBC.

Patient Counseling: Inform that drug may rarely cause a serious condition called lactic acidosis w/ liver enlargement. Instruct to discuss any changes in regimen w/ physician. Instruct not to take concomitantly w/ emtricitabine- or other lamivudine-containing products. Advise parents or guardians of pediatric patients to monitor for signs and symptoms of pancreatitis. Advise that drug is not a cure for HIV-1 infection and continuous therapy is necessary to control HIV-1 infection and decrease HIV-related illness. Inform that redistribution/accumulation of body fat may occur. Advise diabetic patients that each 15mL dose of sol contains 3g of sucrose. Advise to avoid doing things that can spread HIV-1 to others. Inform to take all HIV medications exactly as prescribed.

Storage: (Tab) 25°C (77°F); excursions permitted to 15-30°C (59-86°F). (Sol) 25°C (77°F).

EPIVIR-HBV – lamivudine

RX

Class: Nucleoside reverse transcriptase inhibitor

Lactic acidosis and severe hepatomegaly with steatosis, including fatal cases, reported with nucleoside analogues. Suspend treatment if lactic acidosis or pronounced hepatotoxicity occurs. Severe acute exacerbations of hepatitis B reported upon discontinuation of therapy; closely monitor hepatic function for at least several months. If appropriate, initiation of antihepatitis B therapy may be warranted. Not approved for treatment of HIV infection. Lamivudine dosage in Epivir-HBV is subtherapeutic and monotherapy is inappropriate for treatment of HIV infection. HIV-1 resistance may emerge in chronic hepatitis B-infected patients with unrecognized/untreated HIV infection. Offer HIV counseling and testing to all patients prior to therapy and periodically thereafter.

ADULT DOSAGE

Chronic Hepatitis B

100mg qd

PEDIATRIC DOSAGE

Chronic Hepatitis B

2-17 Years:
3mg/kg qd
Max: 100mg/day

DOSE MODIFICATION

Renal Impairment

CrCl 30-49mL/min: 100mg 1st dose, then 50mg qd
CrCl 15-29mL/min: 100mg 1st dose, then 25mg qd
CrCl 5-14mL/min: 35mg 1st dose, then 15mg qd
CrCl <5mL/min: 35mg 1st dose, then 10mg qd

ADMINISTRATION

Oral route

Take with or without food
Tabs and oral sol are interchangeable
Use oral sol for doses <100mg
Do not use with other medications that contain lamivudine or emtricitabine
Refer to PI for assessing patients during treatment

HOW SUPPLIED

Sol: 5mg/mL [240mL]; Tab: 100mg

WARNINGS/PRECAUTIONS

Consider initiation of treatment only when use of an alternative antiviral agent with a higher genetic barrier to resistance is not available/appropriate. Obesity and prolonged nucleoside exposure may be risk factors for lactic acidosis and severe hepatomegaly with steatosis. Caution with known risk factors for liver disease. Emergence of resistance-associated HBV substitutions reported; monitor ALT and HBV DNA levels if suspected. Not approved for patients dually infected with HBV and HIV. Epivir HBV contains a lower lamivudine dose than Epivir, Combivir, Epzicom, and Trizivir. If a decision is made to administer lamivudine to such coinfected patients, use the higher dosage indicated for HIV therapy as part of an appropriate combination regimen and refer to PI of such drugs. Caution in elderly patients.

ADVERSE REACTIONS

Lactic acidosis, severe hepatomegaly with steatosis, exacerbations of hepatitis B, ear/nose/throat infections, sore throat, diarrhea, serum lipase increase, CPK increase, ALT increase, thrombocytopenia.

DRUG INTERACTIONS

Avoid with other lamivudine- and emtricitabine-containing products. Possible interaction with other drugs whose main route of elimination is active renal secretion via the organic cationic transport system (eg, trimethoprim).

NURSING CONSIDERATIONS

Assessment: Assess for hepatic/renal impairment, previous nucleoside exposure, risk factors for liver disease, HIV infection, hypersensitivity to drug, pregnancy/nursing status, and possible drug interactions. Perform HIV counseling and testing. Obtain baseline ALT and HBV DNA levels.

Monitoring: Monitor for renal/hepatic dysfunction, loss of therapeutic response (eg, persistent ALT elevation, increasing HBV DNA levels after an initial decline below assay limit, progression of clinical signs/symptoms of hepatic disease, worsening of hepatic necroinflammatory findings), signs/symptoms of lactic acidosis, hepatomegaly with steatosis, emergence of resistant HIV, hepatitis B exacerbation, and hypersensitivity reactions. Monitor hepatic function closely for several months in patients who d/c therapy.

Patient Counseling: Advise to remain under the care of a physician during therapy and to report any new symptoms or concurrent medications. Inform that drug is not a cure for hepatitis B and that long-term benefits and relationship of initial treatment response to outcomes (eg, hepatocellular carcinoma, decompensated cirrhosis) are unknown. Inform that liver disease deterioration may occur upon discontinuation. Instruct to discuss any changes in regimen with physician. Inform that emergence of resistant HBV and worsening of disease can occur; advise to report any new symptoms to physician. Counsel on importance of HIV testing to avoid inappropriate therapy and development of resistant HIV. Inform that drug contains a lower dose of lamivudine than Epivir, Combivir, Epzicom, and Trizivir; instruct not to take concurrently with these products. Instruct not to take concurrently with emtricitabine-containing products (eg, Atripla, Complera, Emtriva, Stribild, Truvada). Inform that therapy has not been shown to reduce the risk of HBV transmission through sexual contact/blood contamination. Instruct to avoid doing things that can spread HBV infection to others. Inform diabetics that each 20mL dose of oral sol contains 4g of sucrose.

Storage: Tab: 25°C (77°F); excursions permitted to 15-30°C (59-86°F). Sol: 20-25°C (68-77°F); store in tightly closed bottles.

EPOGEN – epoetin alfa RX

Class: Erythropoiesis stimulator

Increased risk of death, MI, stroke, venous thromboembolism (VTE), thrombosis of vascular access, and tumor progression or recurrence. Use the lowest dose sufficient to reduce/avoid the need for RBC transfusions. Chronic Kidney Disease (CKD): Greater risks for death, serious adverse cardiovascular (CV) reactions, and stroke when administered to target Hgb level >11g/dL. Cancer: Shortened overall survival and/or increased risk of tumor progression or recurrence in patients with breast, non-small cell lung, head and neck, lymphoid, and cervical cancers. Must enroll in and comply with the ESA APPRISE Oncology Program to prescribe and/or dispense drug to patients. Use only for anemia from myelosuppressive chemotherapy. Not indicated for patients receiving myelosuppressive chemotherapy when anticipated outcome is cure. D/C following completion of a chemotherapy course. Perisurgery: Due to increased risk of deep venous thrombosis (DVT), DVT prophylaxis is recommended.

ADULT DOSAGE

Anemia

Chronic Kidney Disease Associated Anemia:
Initiate When:
On Dialysis: Hgb <10g/dL
Not On Dialysis: Hgb <10g/dL, the rate of Hgb decline indicates likelihood of requiring a RBC transfusion, and reducing the risk of alloimmunization and/or other RBC transfusion-related risks is a goal
Initial: 50-100 U/kg IV/SQ 3X/week
Titrate:
On Dialysis: When Hgb approaches/exceeds 11g/dL, reduce or interrupt dose
Not On Dialysis: When Hgb approaches/exceeds 10g/dL, reduce or interrupt dose
All Chronic Kidney Disease Patients:
Do not increase dose more frequently than once every 4 weeks; decreases in dose may occur more frequently
If Hgb rises rapidly (eg, >1g/dL in any 2-week period), decrease dose by 25% or more prn to reduce rapid responses
If Hgb has not increased by >1g/dL after 4 weeks, increase dose by 25%
If no response after 12-week escalation period, use lowest dose to maintain sufficient Hgb level to reduce need for RBC transfusions and evaluate other causes of anemia

Zidovudine (≤4200mg) Associated Anemia in HIV-Infected Patients w/ Endogenous Serum Erythropoietin Levels of ≤500 mU/mL:
Initial: 100 U/kg IV/SQ 3X/week
Titrate:
Hgb Does Not Increase After 8 Weeks of Therapy: Increase by 50-100 U/kg at 4- to 8- week intervals until Hgb reaches a level needed to avoid RBC transfusions or 300 U/kg
Hgb >12g/dL: Withhold dose. When Hgb <11g/dL, resume at 25% below the previous dose

PEDIATRIC DOSAGE

Anemia

Chronic Kidney Disease Associated Anemia:
1 Month-16 Years:
On Dialysis:
Initial: 50 U/kg IV/SQ 3X weekly
Titrate: When Hgb approaches/exceeds 11g/dL, reduce or interrupt dose
Do not increase dose more frequently than once every 4 weeks; decreases in dose may occur more frequently
If Hgb rises rapidly (eg, >1g/dL in any 2-week period), decrease dose by 25% or more prn to reduce rapid responses
If Hgb has not increased by >1g/dL after 4 weeks, increase dose by 25%
If no response after 12-week escalation period, use lowest dose to maintain sufficient Hgb level to reduce need for RBC transfusions and evaluate other causes of anemia

Chemotherapy Associated Anemia:
5-18 Years:
Initial: 600 U/kg IV weekly until completion of a chemotherapy course
Titrate:
Dose Reduction: Reduce by 25% if Hgb increases >1g/dL in any 2-week period or Hgb reaches a level needed to avoid RBC transfusions. Withhold if Hgb exceeds level needed to avoid RBC transfusions; reinitiate at 25% below previous dose when Hgb approaches a level where RBC transfusions may be required
Dose Increase: If Hgb increases by <1g/dL and remains below 10g/dL after initial 4 weeks, increase dose to 900 U/kg weekly
D/C therapy if there is no response in Hgb levels or if RBC transfusions are still required after 8 weeks
Max: 60,000 U/week

D/C if increase in Hgb is not achieved at a dose of 300 U/kg for 8 weeks

Chemotherapy Associated Anemia:
Initiate when Hgb <10g/dL and if there is a minimum of 2 additional months of planned chemotherapy
Initial: 150 U/kg SQ 3X/week or 40,000 U SQ weekly until completion of a chemotherapy course
Titrate:
Dose Reduction: Reduce by 25% if Hgb increases >1g/dL in any 2-week period or reaches a level needed to avoid RBC transfusions. Withhold if Hgb exceeds level needed to avoid RBC transfusions; reinitiate at 25% below previous dose when Hgb approaches a level where RBC transfusions may be required
Dose Increase: If Hgb increases by <1g/dL and remains below 10g/dL after initial 4 weeks, increase dose to 300 U/kg 3X/week or 60,000 U/week
D/C therapy if there is no response in Hgb levels or if RBC transfusions are still required after 8 weeks

Surgery Patients:
Used to reduce the need for allogeneic RBC transfusions among patients w/ perioperative Hgb >10-≤13g/dL who are at high risk for perioperative blood loss from elective, noncardiac, nonvascular surgery
Usual: 300 U/kg/day SQ qd for 10 days before, on the day of, and for 4 days after surgery; or 600 U/kg SQ in 4 doses administered 21, 14, and 7 days before surgery and on the day of surgery. Deep vein thrombosis prophylaxis is recommended

DOSE MODIFICATION
Elderly
Individualize dose selection and adjustment to achieve and maintain target Hgb

ADMINISTRATION
IV/SQ route

IV route is recommended for chronic kidney disease patients on hemodialysis

Preparation/Administration
Do not shake; do not use if shaken or frozen
Preservative-free single-use vials may be admixed in a syringe w/ bacteriostatic 0.9% NaCl inj, w/ benzyl alcohol 0.9% in a 1:1 ratio
Do not dilute or mix w/ other drug sol
Do not re-enter preservative-free vials; discard unused portions
Store unused portions of multidose vials at 36-46°F (2-8°C); discard after 21 days after initial entry

HOW SUPPLIED
Inj: 2000 U/mL, 3000 U/mL, 4000 U/mL, 10,000 U/mL [single-dose vial]; 10,000 U/mL [2mL], 20,000 U/mL [1mL] [multidose vial]

CONTRAINDICATIONS
Uncontrolled HTN, pure red cell aplasia (PRCA) that begins after treatment with epoetin alfa or other erythropoietin protein drugs. (Multidose Vials) Neonates, infants, pregnant women, and nursing mothers.

WARNINGS/PRECAUTIONS
Not indicated for use in patients with cancer receiving hormonal agents, biologic products, or radiotherapy, unless also receiving concomitant myelosuppressive chemotherapy; in patients scheduled for surgery who are willing to donate autologous blood; in patients undergoing cardiac/vascular surgery; or as a substitute for RBC transfusions in patients requiring immediate correction of anemia. Evaluate transferrin saturation and serum ferritin prior to and during treatment; administer supplemental iron when serum ferritin is <100mcg/L or serum transferrin saturation is <20%. Correct/exclude other causes of anemia (eg, vitamin deficiency, metabolic/chronic

inflammatory conditions, bleeding) before initiating therapy. Hypertensive encephalopathy and seizures reported in patients with CKD; increases risk of seizures in CKD patients. Appropriately control HTN prior to initiation of and during treatment; reduce/withhold therapy if BP becomes difficult to control. PRCA and severe anemia, with or without other cytopenias that arise following the development of neutralizing antibodies to erythropoietin, reported. Withhold and evaluate for neutralizing antibodies to erythropoietin if severe anemia and low reticulocyte count develop; d/c permanently if PRCA develops, and do not switch to other erythropoiesis-stimulating agents. Serious allergic reactions may occur; immediately and permanently d/c therapy. Contains albumin; may carry an extremely remote risk for transmission of viral diseases or Creutzfeldt-Jakob disease. Patients may require adjustments in their dialysis prescriptions after initiation of therapy, or require increased anticoagulation with heparin to prevent clotting of extracorporeal circuit during hemodialysis. Multidose vial contains benzyl alcohol; benzyl alcohol is associated with serious adverse events and death, particularly in pediatric patients.

ADVERSE REACTIONS

MI, stroke, VTE, thrombosis of vascular access, tumor progression/recurrence, pyrexia, N/V, HTN, cough, arthralgia, dizziness, pruritus, rash, headache.

NURSING CONSIDERATIONS

Assessment: Assess for uncontrolled HTN, previous hypersensitivity to the drug, causes of anemia, pregnancy/nursing status, and other conditions where treatment is contraindicated or cautioned. Obtain baseline Hgb levels, transferrin saturation, and serum ferritin.

Monitoring: Monitor for signs/symptoms of an allergic reaction, CV/thromboembolic events, stroke, premonitory neurologic symptoms, PRCA, severe anemia, progression/recurrence of tumor, and other adverse reactions. Monitor BP, transferrin saturation, and serum ferritin. Following initiation of therapy and after each dose adjustment, monitor Hgb weekly until Hgb is stable, then at least monthly, and to maintain Hgb sufficient to minimize need for RBC transfusions.

Patient Counseling: Inform of the risks and benefits of therapy, and of the increased risks of mortality, serious CV reactions, thromboembolic reactions, stroke, and tumor progression. Advise of the need to have regular lab tests for Hgb. Inform cancer patients that they must sign the patient-physician acknowledgment form prior to therapy. Instruct to undergo regular BP monitoring, adhere to prescribed antihypertensive regimen, and follow recommended dietary restrictions. Advise to contact physician for new-onset neurologic symptoms or change in seizure frequency. Instruct regarding proper disposal and caution against reuse of needles, syringes, or unused portions of single-dose vials.

Storage: 2-8°C (36-46°F). Do not freeze; do not use if it has been frozen. Protect from light. Discard unused portions of multidose vials 21 days after initial entry.

EPZICOM – abacavir sulfate/lamivudine — RX

Class: Nucleoside reverse transcriptase inhibitor

Lactic acidosis and severe hepatomegaly w/ steatosis, including fatal cases, reported w/ nucleoside analogues. Abacavir: Serious and sometimes fatal hypersensitivity reactions (multiorgan clinical syndrome) reported; d/c as soon as suspected and never restart therapy w/ any abacavir-containing product. Patients w/ HLA-B*5701 allele are at high risk for hypersensitivity; screen for HLA-B*5701 allele prior to therapy. Lamivudine: Severe acute exacerbations of hepatitis B reported in patients coinfected w/ hepatitis B virus (HBV) upon discontinuation of therapy; closely monitor hepatic function for at least several months. If appropriate, initiation of antihepatitis B therapy may be warranted.

ADULT DOSAGE

HIV-1 Infection

Combination w/ Other Antiretrovirals:
1 tab qd

PEDIATRIC DOSAGE

Pediatric use may not have been established

DOSE MODIFICATION

Renal Impairment

CrCl <50mL/min: Not recommended

Hepatic Impairment

No recommended

ADMINISTRATION

Oral route

HOW SUPPLIED

Tab: (Abacavir/Lamivudine) 600mg/300mg

CONTRAINDICATIONS

Hepatic impairment.

WARNINGS/PRECAUTIONS

Obesity and prolonged nucleoside exposure may be risk factors for lactic acidosis and severe hepatomegaly w/ steatosis. Caution w/ known risk factors for liver disease; suspend therapy if clinical or lab findings suggestive of lactic acidosis or pronounced hepatotoxicity develop. Immune reconstitution syndrome reported. Autoimmune disorders (eg, Graves' disease, polymyositis, Guillain-Barre syndrome) reported to occur in the setting of immune reconstitution and can occur many months after initiation of treatment. Redistribution/accumulation of body fat may occur. Cross-resistance potential w/ nucleoside reverse transcriptase inhibitors reported. Caution in elderly. Abacavir: Increased risk of MI reported; consider the underlying risk of coronary heart disease when prescribing therapy. Lamivudine: Emergence of lamivudine-resistant HBV reported.

ADVERSE REACTIONS

Lactic acidosis, severe hepatomegaly w/ steatosis, hypersensitivity, insomnia, depression/depressed mood, headache/migraine, fatigue/malaise, dizziness/vertigo, nausea, diarrhea, rash, pyrexia.

DRUG INTERACTIONS

Avoid w/ other abacavir-, lamivudine-, and/or emtricitabine-containing products. Abacavir: Ethanol may decrease elimination causing an increase in overall exposure. May increase oral methadone clearance. Lamivudine: Hepatic decompensation may occur in HIV-1/hepatitis C virus (HCV) coinfected patients receiving interferon-alfa w/ or w/o ribavirin; closely monitor for treatment-associated toxicities.

NURSING CONSIDERATIONS

Assessment: Assess medical history for prior exposure to any abacavir-containing product. Assess for HBV infection, history of hypersensitivity reactions, HLA-B*5701 status, hepatic/renal impairment, risk factors for coronary heart disease and lactic acidosis, pregnancy/nursing status, and possible drug interactions.

Monitoring: Monitor for signs/symptoms of hypersensitivity reactions, lactic acidosis, hepatomegaly w/ steatosis, immune reconstitution syndrome (eg, opportunistic infections), autoimmune disorders, fat redistribution/accumulation, MI, and other adverse reactions. Monitor hepatic/renal function. Closely monitor hepatic function for several months after discontinuing therapy.

Patient Counseling: Inform patients regarding hypersensitivity reactions w/ abacavir; instruct to contact physician immediately if symptoms develop and not to restart or replace w/ any other abacavir-containing products w/o medical consultation. Inform that the drug may cause lactic acidosis w/ hepatomegaly. Inform patients coinfected w/ HIV-1 and HBV that deterioration of liver disease has occurred in some cases when treatment w/ lamivudine was discontinued; instruct to discuss any changes of regimen w/ the physician. Inform that hepatic decompensation has occurred in HIV-1/HCV coinfected patients w/ interferon alfa w/ or w/o ribavirin. Inform that redistribution/accumulation of body fat may occur. Advise that drug is not a cure for HIV-1 infection and continuous therapy is necessary to control HIV-1 infection and decrease HIV-related illness. Inform patients to take all HIV medications exactly as prescribed. Advise not to re-use/share needles/other inj equipment/personal items (eg, toothbrush, razor blades), to continue to practice safer by using latex or polyurethane condoms, and not to breastfeed.

Storage: 25°C (77°F); excursions permitted to 15-30°C (59-86°F).

ERBITUX – cetuximab

RX

Class: Epidermal growth factor receptor (EGFR) antagonist

Serious infusion reactions, some fatal, reported; immediately interrupt and permanently d/c infusion if these reactions occur. Cardiopulmonary arrest and/or sudden death occurred in patients w/ squamous cell carcinoma of the head and neck (SCCHN) treated w/ cetuximab in combination w/ radiation therapy or w/ European Union-approved cetuximab in combination w/ platinum-based therapy w/ 5-fluorouracil (5-FU); closely monitor serum electrolytes during and after therapy.

ADULT DOSAGE

Squamous Cell Carcinoma of the Head and Neck

W/ Radiation Therapy for the Initial Treatment of Locally or Regionally Advanced Squamous Cell Carcinoma of the Head and Neck (SCCHN):

Initial: 400mg/m^2 administered 1 week prior to initiation of a course of radiation therapy as a 120-min IV infusion

Maint: 250mg/m^2 infused over 60 min weekly for the duration of radiation therapy (6-7 weeks)

PEDIATRIC DOSAGE

Pediatric use may not have been established

Max Infusion Rate: 10mg/min

Complete administration 60 min prior to radiation therapy

W/ Platinum-Based Therapy w/ 5-FU for the 1st-Line Treatment of Patients w/ Recurrent Locoregional Disease or Metastatic SCCHN:
Initial: 400mg/m^2 administered on the day of initiation of platinum-based therapy w/ 5-FU as a 120-min IV infusion
Maint: 250mg/m^2 infused over 60 min weekly until disease progression or unacceptable toxicity
Max Infusion Rate: 10mg/min
Complete administration 60 min prior to platinum-based therapy w/ 5-FU

As Monotherapy in Patients w/ Recurrent/ Metastatic SCCHN for Whom Prior Platinum-Based Therapy Failed:
Initial: 400mg/m^2 administered as a 120-min IV infusion
Maint: 250mg/m^2 infused over 60 min weekly until disease progression or unacceptable toxicity
Max Infusion Rate: 10mg/min

Metastatic Colorectal Cancer

Treatment of K-Ras mutation negative (wild-type), epidermal growth factor receptor (EGFR)-expressing, metastatic colorectal cancer in combination w/ FOLFIRI (irinotecan, 5-FU, leucovorin) for 1st-line treatment, in combination w/ irinotecan in patients who are refractory to irinotecan-based chemotherapy, and as monotherapy in patients who have failed oxaliplatin- and irinotecan-based chemotherapy or are intolerant to irinotecan
Initial: 400mg/m^2 administered as a 120-min IV infusion; complete administration 60 min prior to FOLFIRI
Maint: 250mg/m^2 infused over 60 min weekly until disease progression or unacceptable toxicity; complete administration 60 min prior to FOLFIRI
Max Infusion Rate: 10mg/min

Premedication

H_1-antagonist (eg, 50mg diphenhydramine) IV 30-60 min prior to 1st dose; premedication for subsequent doses should be based on clinical judgment and presence/severity of prior infusion reactions

DOSE MODIFICATION

Adverse Reactions

NCI CTC Grade 1 or 2 and Non-Serious NCI CTC Grade 3 Infusion Reaction:
Reduce infusion rate by 50%; immediately and permanently d/c for serious infusion reactions, requiring medical intervention and/or hospitalization

Severe Acneiform Rash (NCI CTC Grade 3 or 4):
1st Occurrence: Delay infusion 1-2 weeks
W/ Improvement: Continue at 250mg/m^2
No Improvement: D/C treatment

2nd Occurrence: Delay infusion 1-2 weeks
W/ Improvement: Reduce to 200mg/m^2
No Improvement: D/C treatment

3rd Occurrence: Delay infusion 1-2 weeks
W/ Improvement: Reduce to 150mg/m^2
No Improvement: D/C treatment

4th Occurrence: D/C treatment

ADMINISTRATION
IV route

Do not administer as IV push or bolus
Administer via infusion pump or syringe pump
Administer through low protein binding 0.22-µm in-line filter
Do not shake or dilute

HOW SUPPLIED
Inj: 2mg/mL [50mL, 100mL]

WARNINGS/PRECAUTIONS
Caution when used in combination w/ radiation therapy or platinum-based therapy w/ 5-FU in head and neck cancer patients w/ history of coronary artery disease (CAD), CHF, or arrhythmias. Interstitial lung disease (ILD) reported; interrupt for acute onset or worsening of pulmonary symptoms and permanently d/c if ILD is confirmed. Dermatologic toxicities (eg, acneiform rash, skin drying/fissuring, paronychial inflammation, infectious sequelae, hypertrichosis) reported. Life-threatening and fatal bullous mucocutaneous disease w/ blisters, erosions, and skin sloughing has also been observed; limit sun exposure during therapy. Addition of cetuximab to radiation and cisplatin in patients reported to increase incidence of Grade 3-4 mucositis, radiation recall syndrome, acneiform rash, cardiac events, and electrolyte disturbances compared to radiation and cisplatin alone; addition of cetuximab did not improve progression-free survival. Hypomagnesemia and electrolyte abnormalities reported; replete electrolytes as necessary. Do not resume nursing earlier than 60 days following the last dose of therapy if nursing is interrupted. Not indicated for the treatment of K-ras mutation-positive colorectal cancer.

ADVERSE REACTIONS
Cardiopulmonary arrest, infusion reactions, cutaneous reactions (eg, rash, pruritus, nail changes), headache, diarrhea, infection, dermatologic toxicity, radiation dermatitis, sepsis, renal failure, ILD, pulmonary embolus.

NURSING CONSIDERATIONS

Assessment: Assess for history of CAD, CHF, arrhythmias, pulmonary disorders, pregnancy/nursing status, and possible drug interactions. Obtain serum electrolyte levels (Mg^{2+}, K^{+}, Ca^{2+}). Determine K-ras mutation and EGFR-expression status in colorectal tumors using FDA-approved tests.

Monitoring: Monitor for signs/symptoms of infusion reactions, cardiopulmonary arrest, acute onset or worsening of pulmonary symptoms, dermatologic toxicities and infectious sequelae, and for other adverse reactions. Monitor patients for 1 hr after infusion in a setting w/ resuscitation equipment and other agents necessary to treat anaphylaxis, and for a longer period to confirm resolution of the event in patients requiring treatment for infusion reactions. Periodically monitor for hypomagnesemia, hypocalcemia, and hypokalemia during and for at least 8 weeks after therapy.

Patient Counseling: Advise to report to physician signs/symptoms of infusion reactions. Inform of pregnancy/nursing risks; advise to use adequate contraception during and for 6 months after last dose for both males and females. Inform that nursing is not recommended during and for 2 months following last dose of therapy. Instruct to limit sun exposure (eg, use of sunscreen, wear hats) during and for 2 months after last dose of therapy.

Storage: Vials: 2-8°C (36-46°F). Do not freeze. Infusion Containers: Stable for up to 12 hrs at 2-8°C (36-46°F) and up to 8 hrs at 20-25°C (68-77°F).

ERIVEDGE – vismodegib

RX

Class: Hedgehog pathway inhibitor

May result in embryo-fetal death or severe birth defects. Verify pregnancy status prior to initiation of therapy. Advise male and female patients of these risks. Advise female patients of the need for contraception and advise male patients of the potential risk of exposure through semen.

ADULT DOSAGE

Basal Cell Carcinoma

Metastatic basal cell carcinoma, or locally advanced basal cell carcinoma that has recurred following surgery or in patients who are not candidates for surgery, and who are not candidates for radiation

Usual: 150mg qd until disease progression or until unacceptable toxicity

PEDIATRIC DOSAGE

Pediatric use may not have been established

ADMINISTRATION
Oral route
Take w/ or w/o food
Swallow caps whole; do not open or crush caps

HOW SUPPLIED
Cap: 150mg

WARNINGS/PRECAUTIONS
Do not donate blood or blood products while on therapy and for at least 7 months after the last dose.

ADVERSE REACTIONS
Muscle spasm, alopecia, dysgeusia, weight loss, fatigue, N/V, diarrhea, decreased appetite, constipation, arthralgia, ageusia.

DRUG INTERACTIONS
P-glycoprotein inhibitors (eg, clarithromycin, erythromycin, azithromycin) may increase systemic exposure and incidence of adverse events. Drugs that alter upper GI tract pH (eg, proton pump inhibitors, H_2-receptor antagonists, antacids) may alter solubility and reduce bioavailability.

NURSING CONSIDERATIONS

Assessment: Assess pregnancy/nursing status, and for possible drug interactions.

Monitoring: Monitor for disease progression, toxicities, and other adverse reactions.

Patient Counseling: Inform that drug may cause embryo-fetal death or severe birth defects; instruct female patients of reproductive potential to use a highly effective form of contraception while on therapy and for at least 7 months after the last dose. Instruct male patients, even those with prior vasectomy, to use condoms with spermicide during sexual intercourse with female partners while on therapy and for at least 2 months after the last dose. Instruct to immediately contact physician if pregnancy occurs or is suspected following exposure to drug. Instruct to immediately report any pregnancy exposure to drug and encourage participation in the Erivedge pregnancy pharmacovigilance program. Inform female patients of the potential for serious adverse reactions in nursing infants. Advise not to donate blood or blood products while on therapy and for at least 7 months after the last dose.

Storage: 20-25°C (68-77°F); excursions permitted between 15-30°C (59-86°F).

ERTACZO – sertaconazole nitrate RX

Class: Azole antifungal

ADULT DOSAGE

Fungal Infections

Interdigital Tinea Pedis Caused by *Trichophyton rubrum*, *Trichophyton mentagrophytes*, and *Epidermophyton floccosum*:
Apply sufficient amount to cover both the affected areas between the toes and the immediately surrounding healthy skin bid for 4 weeks

PEDIATRIC DOSAGE

Fungal Infections

Interdigital Tinea Pedis Caused by *Trichophyton rubrum*, *Trichophyton mentagrophytes*, and *Epidermophyton floccosum*:

≥12 Years:
Apply sufficient amount to cover both the affected areas between the toes and the immediately surrounding healthy skin bid for 4 weeks

ADMINISTRATION
Topical route
Wash hands after applying medication
Dry affected area(s) thoroughly before application if used after bathing

HOW SUPPLIED
Cre: 2% [60g]

WARNINGS/PRECAUTIONS
D/C and institute appropriate therapy if irritation occurs. Caution in patients sensitive to imidazole antifungals; cross-reactivity may occur.

ADVERSE REACTIONS
Contact dermatitis, dry skin, burning skin, application site skin tenderness.

NURSING CONSIDERATIONS

Assessment: Assess for hypersensitivity to imidazole antifungals and pregnancy/nursing status.

Monitoring: Monitor for irritation and other adverse reactions.

Patient Counseling: Instruct to use externally and ud. Instruct to use medication for the full treatment time, even though symptoms may have improved. Instruct to inform physician if area of application shows signs of increased irritation, redness, itching, burning, blistering, swelling, or oozing. Instruct to avoid the use of occlusive dressings unless directed by physician. Advise not to use for any disorder other than that for which it was prescribed.

Storage: 20-25°C (68-77°F); excursions permitted to 15-30°C (59-86°F).

ESTRACE – estradiol

Class: Estrogen

RX

Estrogens increase the risk of endometrial cancer. Perform adequate diagnostic measures, including endometrial sampling, to rule out malignancy w/ undiagnosed persistent or recurrent abnormal vaginal bleeding. Should not be used for the prevention of cardiovascular disease. Increased risk of MI, stroke, invasive breast cancer, pulmonary embolism (PE), and DVT in postmenopausal women (50-79 yrs of age) reported. Increased risk of developing probable dementia in postmenopausal women ≥65 yrs of age reported. Should be prescribed at the lowest effective dose and for the shortest duration consistent w/ treatment goals and risks.

ADULT DOSAGE

Menopause

Vulvar/Vaginal Atrophy:
Cre:
Initial: 2-4g/day for 1-2 weeks, then gradually decrease to 1/2 initial dose for 1-2 weeks
Maint: 1g 1-3X/week
Attempt to d/c or taper at 3- to 6-month intervals

Vasomotor Symptoms/Vulvar and Vaginal Atrophy:
Moderate to Severe:
Tab:
Initial: 1-2mg/day
Titrate: Adjust as necessary to control presenting symptoms
Maint: Minimal effective dose should be determined by titration
Administer cyclically (eg, 3 weeks on and 1 week off)
Attempt to d/c or taper at 3- to 6-month intervals

Hypoestrogenism

Due to Hypogonadism, Castration, or Primary Ovarian Failure:
Tab:
Initial: 1-2mg/day
Titrate: Adjust as necessary to control presenting symptoms
Maint: Minimal effective dose should be determined by titration

Breast Cancer

Palliative Treatment in Appropriately Selected Women and Men w/ Metastatic Disease:
Tab:
Usual: 10mg tid for at least 3 months

Prostate Carcinoma

Palliative Treatment of Advanced Androgen-Dependent Carcinoma:
Tab:
Usual: 1-2mg tid

Osteoporosis

Prevention:
Tab:
Consider therapy for women at risk of osteoporosis and for whom non-estrogen medications are not appropriate, when used solely for prevention of postmenopausal osteoporosis

PEDIATRIC DOSAGE

Pediatric use may not have been established

ADMINISTRATION

Cre

Intravaginal route

Tab

Oral route

HOW SUPPLIED

Cre: 0.01% [42.5g]; Tab: 0.5mg*, 1mg*, 2mg* *scored

CONTRAINDICATIONS

Undiagnosed abnormal genital bleeding, known/suspected/history of breast cancer, known/suspected estrogen-dependent neoplasia, active/history of DVT/PE, active or recent arterial thromboembolic disease (eg, stroke, MI), liver dysfunction or disease, known/suspected pregnancy.

WARNINGS/PRECAUTIONS

D/C immediately if stroke, DVT, PE, or MI occur or is suspected. Caution in patients w/ risk factors for arterial vascular disease and/or venous thromboembolism. If feasible, d/c at least 4-6 weeks before surgery of the type associated w/ an increased risk of thromboembolism, or during periods of prolonged immobilization. May increase the risk of gallbladder disease and ovarian cancer. May lead to severe hypercalcemia in patients w/ breast cancer and bone metastases; d/c and take appropriate measures if hypercalcemia occurs. Retinal vascular thrombosis reported; d/c pending exam if sudden partial/complete loss of vision, or sudden onset of proptosis, diplopia, or migraine occurs. D/C permanently if exam reveals papilledema or retinal vascular lesions. Consider addition of progestin for women w/ a uterus or w/ residual endometriosis post-hysterectomy. May elevate BP and thyroid-binding globulin levels. May elevate plasma TGs leading to pancreatitis in patients w/ preexisting hypertriglyceridemia. Caution w/ impaired liver function, and history of cholestatic jaundice associated w/ past estrogen use or w/ pregnancy; d/c in case of recurrence. May cause fluid retention; caution w/ cardiac/renal impairment. Caution w/ severe hypocalcemia. May exacerbate endometriosis, asthma, diabetes mellitus, epilepsy, migraine, porphyria, systemic lupus erythematosus, and hepatic hemangiomas; use w/ caution. May affect certain endocrine and blood components in lab tests. (Tab) 2mg tab contains tartrazine, which may cause allergic-type reactions (eg, bronchial asthma) in certain susceptible individuals.

ADVERSE REACTIONS

Vaginal bleeding pattern changes, vaginitis, breast tenderness, galactorrhea, N/V, thrombophlebitis, melasma, abdominal cramps, headache, mental depression, weight changes, edema, libido changes, MI, PE.

DRUG INTERACTIONS

CYP3A4 inducers (eg, St. John's wort preparations, phenobarbital, carbamazepine, rifampin) may decrease levels, which may decrease therapeutic effects and/or change uterine bleeding profile. CYP3A4 inhibitors (eg, erythromycin, ketoconazole, ritonavir, grapefruit juice) may increase levels, which may result in side effects. Patients concomitantly receiving thyroid replacement therapy and estrogens may require increased doses of thyroid replacement therapy; monitor thyroid function.

NURSING CONSIDERATIONS

Assessment: Assess for undiagnosed abnormal genital bleeding, presence/history of breast cancer, estrogen-dependent neoplasia, active/history of DVT/PE/arterial thromboembolic disease, liver impairment/disease, history of cholestatic jaundice, drug hypersensitivity, pregnancy/nursing status, any other conditions where treatment is contraindicated or cautioned, need for progestin therapy, and possible drug interactions.

Monitoring: Monitor for signs/symptoms of CV events, malignant neoplasms, dementia, gallbladder disease, hypercalcemia, visual abnormalities, BP and serum TG elevations, pancreatitis, fluid retention, cholestatic jaundice, exacerbation of endometriosis and other conditions, and other adverse reactions. Perform annual breast exam; schedule mammography based on age, risk factors, and prior mammogram results. Monitor thyroid function in patients on thyroid hormone replacement therapy. Periodically evaluate (every 3-6 months) to determine need for therapy. In cases of undiagnosed, persistent, or recurrent abnormal vaginal bleeding, perform adequate diagnostic measures (eg, endometrial sampling) to rule out malignancy.

Patient Counseling: Inform of the risks/benefits of therapy. Inform that medication increases risk for breast/uterine cancer. Advise to contact physician if breast lumps, unusual vaginal bleeding, dizziness or faintness, changes in speech, severe headaches, chest pain, SOB, leg pain, visual changes, or vomiting occur. Advise to have yearly breast exams by a physician and perform monthly breast self-exams. Advise to notify physician if pregnant/nursing.

Storage: (Cre) Room temperature. Protect from temperatures in excess of 40°C (104°F). (Tab) 20-25°C (68-77°F).

ESTRADERM – estradiol

Class: Estrogen

RX

Estrogens increase the risk of endometrial cancer. Perform adequate diagnostic measures, including endometrial sampling, to rule out malignancy w/ undiagnosed persistent or recurrent abnormal vaginal bleeding. Should not be used for the prevention of cardiovascular disease (CVD) or dementia. Increased risk of MI, stroke, invasive breast cancer, pulmonary emboli (PE), and deep vein thrombosis (DVT) in postmenopausal women (50-79 yrs of age) reported. Increased risk of developing probable dementia in postmenopausal women ≥65 yrs of age reported. Should be prescribed at the lowest effective dose and for the shortest duration consistent w/ treatment goals and risks.

ADULT DOSAGE

Postmenopausal Osteoporosis

Prevention:
Initial: 0.05mg/day as soon as possible after menopause

Reevaluate treatment need periodically (eg, 3- to 6-month intervals)

Hypoestrogenism

Due to Hypogonadism/Castration/Primary Ovarian Failure:
0.05mg ud

Reevaluate treatment need periodically (eg, 3- to 6-month intervals)

Menopause

Vasomotor Symptoms/Vulvar and Vaginal Atrophy:
Initial: 0.05mg twice weekly

Reevaluate treatment need periodically (eg, 3- to 6-month intervals)

PEDIATRIC DOSAGE

Pediatric use may not have been established

DOSE MODIFICATION

Concomitant Medications

Women Currently on Oral Estrogens: Initiate 1 week after withdrawal of oral hormonal therapy, or sooner if menopausal symptoms reappear in <1 week

Other Important Modifications

Patients w/o Intact Uterus: Administer therapy continuously
Patients w/ Intact Uterus: Administer on a cyclic schedule (eg, 3 weeks on, followed by 1 week off)

ADMINISTRATION

Transdermal route

Place adhesive side on a clean, dry area of skin on trunk of body (including buttocks and abdomen); area selected should not be oily, damaged, or irritated
Site selected should be one that is not exposed to sunlight
Do not apply to breasts and/or waistline
Replace system twice weekly; rotate application sites w/ an interval of at least 1 week allowed between applications to a particular site
Apply immediately after opening pouch and removing the protective liner
Press system firmly in place w/ palm of the hand for about 10 sec
If the system falls off, reapply the same one. If necessary, a new system may be applied; in either case, continue original treatment schedule

HOW SUPPLIED

Patch: 0.05mg/day, 0.1mg/day [8[s]]

CONTRAINDICATIONS

Undiagnosed abnormal genital bleeding, known/suspected/history of breast cancer, known/suspected estrogen-dependent neoplasia, active or history of DVT/PE, active or recent arterial thromboembolic disease (eg, stroke, MI), liver dysfunction or disease, known/suspected pregnancy.

WARNINGS/PRECAUTIONS

D/C immediately if stroke, DVT, PE, or MI occurs or is suspected. Caution in patients w/ risk factors for arterial vascular disease and/or venous thromboembolism (VTE). If feasible, d/c at least 4-6 weeks before surgery of the type associated w/ an increased risk of thromboembolism, or during periods of prolonged immobilization. May increase risk of breast/ovarian/endometrial cancer and gallbladder disease. Consider addition of progestin for women w/ a uterus or w/ residual endometriosis posthysterectomy. May lead to severe hypercalcemia in patients w/ breast cancer and bone metastases; d/c and take appropriate measures if hypercalcemia occurs. Retinal vascular thrombosis reported; if sudden partial or complete loss of vision, sudden onset of proptosis, diplopia, or migraine occurs, d/c pending examination. If examinations reveal papilledema or retinal vascular lesions, d/c permanently. May elevate BP, thyroid-binding globulin levels, and plasma TG levels leading to pancreatitis and other complications. Caution w/ history of cholestatic jaundice; d/c in case of recurrence. May cause fluid retention; caution w/ cardiac/renal dysfunction. Caution w/ impaired liver function and severe hypocalcemia. May exacerbate endometriosis, asthma, diabetes mellitus (DM), epilepsy, migraine, porphyria, systemic lupus erythematosus (SLE), and hepatic hemangiomas; use w/ caution. May affect certain endocrine and blood components in lab tests.

ADVERSE REACTIONS

Altered vaginal bleeding, vaginal candidiasis, breast tenderness/enlargement, N/V, chloasma, melasma, weight changes, VTE, pulmonary embolism, MI, stroke, application-site redness/ irritation.

DRUG INTERACTIONS

CYP3A4 inducers (eg, St. John's wort, phenobarbital, carbamazepine, rifampin) may decrease levels, which may decrease therapeutic effects and/or change uterine bleeding profile. CYP3A4 inhibitors (eg, erythromycin, ketoconazole, ritonavir, grapefruit juice) may increase levels, which may result in side effects. Patients concomitantly receiving thyroid hormone replacement therapy and estrogens may require increased doses of their thyroid replacement therapy.

NURSING CONSIDERATIONS

Assessment: Assess for undiagnosed abnormal genital bleeding, presence/history of breast cancer, estrogen-dependent neoplasia, active or history of DVT/PE, active or recent (w/in past yr) arterial thromboembolic disease, liver dysfunction/disease, known/suspected pregnancy, any other conditions where treatment is contraindicated or cautioned, need for progestin therapy, and possible drug interactions. Assess use in women ≥65 yrs, nursing patients, and those w/ hypertriglyceridemia, hypothyroidism, DM, asthma, epilepsy, migraine or porphyria, SLE, and hepatic hemangiomas.

Monitoring: Monitor for signs/symptoms of CVD, malignant neoplasms, dementia, gallbladder disease, hypercalcemia, visual abnormalities, hypertriglyceridemia, pancreatitis, hypothyroidism, fluid retention, cholestatic jaundice, exacerbation of endometriosis and other conditions. Perform annual breast exam; schedule mammography based on age, risk factors, and prior mammogram results. Regularly monitor BP, thyroid function in patients on thyroid replacement therapy, and periodically evaluate (every 3-6 months) to determine need for therapy. In case of undiagnosed, persistent, or recurrent vaginal bleeding in women w/ uterus, perform adequate diagnostic testing measures (eg, endometrial sampling) to rule out malignancy.

Patient Counseling: Inform that therapy may increase the risk for uterine cancer and may increase chances of getting a heart attack, stroke, breast cancer, blood clots, and dementia. Instruct to report to physician any breast lumps, unusual vaginal bleeding, dizziness and faintness, changes in speech, severe headaches, chest pain, SOB, leg pains, changes in vision, or vomiting. Advise to notify physician if pregnant or nursing. Instruct to have annual breast examination by a physician and perform monthly breast self-examination. Instruct to place medication system on clean, dry skin on the trunk (including buttocks and abdomen); site should not be exposed to sunlight; area should not be oily, damaged, or irritated; and should not be applied on breasts or waistline. Counsel to rotate application sites w/ an interval of 1 week, and to apply immediately after opening pouch. Inform that if medication system falls off, reapply same system or apply new system prn and continue w/ original treatment schedule.

Storage: Do not store above 30°C (86°F). Do not store unpouched.

ESTRING – estradiol RX

Class: Estrogen

Increased risk of endometrial cancer in a woman w/ a uterus who uses unopposed estrogens. Adding a progestin to estrogen therapy reduces the risk of endometrial hyperplasia. Adequate diagnostic measures should be undertaken to rule out malignancy in all cases of undiagnosed, persistent or recurring abnormal genital bleeding. Should not be used for the prevention of cardiovascular (CV) disease or dementia. Increased risk of stroke and DVT reported in postmenopausal women (50-79 yrs of age) treated w/ daily oral conjugated estrogens (CE) alone and when combined w/ medroxyprogesterone acetate (MPA). Increased risk of developing probable dementia reported in postmenopausal women ≥65 yrs of age treated w/ daily CE alone and when combined w/ MPA. Increased risks of pulmonary embolism (PE), MI, and invasive breast cancer reported in postmenopausal women (50-79 yrs of age) treated w/ daily oral CE combined w/ MPA. Should be prescribed at the lowest effective dose and for the shortest duration consistent w/ treatment goals and risks.

ADULT DOSAGE

Menopause

Moderate to Severe Vulvar and Vaginal Atrophy:

Insert 1 ring as deeply as possible into the upper 1/3 of the vaginal vault; ring should remain in place for 3 months

Reassess need to continue treatment at 3- or 6-month intervals

PEDIATRIC DOSAGE

Pediatric use may not have been established

ADMINISTRATION

Intravaginal route

Retention of the ring for >90 days does not represent overdosage, but will result in progressively greater underdosage w/ the risk of loss of efficacy and increasing risk of vaginal infections and/or erosions

Insertion

1. Press ring into an oval and insert into upper 3rd of vaginal vault; exact position is not critical
2. If patient feels discomfort, the ring is probably not far enough inside
3. Gently push ring further into vagina

Use

The ring should be left in place continuously for 90 days and then, if continuation of therapy is deemed appropriate, replaced by a new ring

The ring should not interfere w/ sexual intercourse

Straining at defecation may make the ring move down in the lower part of the vagina; it may be pushed up again w/ a finger

If the ring is expelled totally from the vagina during the 90-day treatment period, rinse in lukewarm water and reinsert

Removal

Remove by hooking a finger through the ring and pulling it out

HOW SUPPLIED

Vaginal Ring: 2mg

CONTRAINDICATIONS

Undiagnosed abnormal genital bleeding, known/suspected/history of breast cancer, known/suspected estrogen-dependent neoplasia, active/history of DVT/PE/arterial thromboembolic disease (eg, stroke, MI), known liver impairment/disease, known protein C/protein S/antithrombin deficiency or other known thrombophilic disorders, known/suspected pregnancy.

WARNINGS/PRECAUTIONS

D/C immediately if stroke, DVT, PE, or MI occurs or is suspected. If feasible, d/c at least 4-6 weeks before surgery of the type associated w/ an increased risk of thromboembolism, or during periods of prolonged immobilization. May increase risk of gallbladder disease requiring surgery and risk of ovarian cancer. May lead to severe hypercalcemia in patients w/ breast cancer and bone metastases; d/c and take appropriate measures if hypercalcemia occurs. Retinal vascular thrombosis reported; d/c therapy pending exam if sudden partial/complete loss of vision, or sudden onset of proptosis, diplopia, or migraine occurs. D/C if exam reveals papilledema or retinal vascular lesions. May exacerbate symptoms of angioedema in women w/ hereditary angioedema. May increase BP and thyroid-binding globulin levels. May be associated w/ elevations of plasma TGs, leading to pancreatitis in patients w/ preexisting hypertriglyceridemia; consider discontinuation if pancreatitis occurs. Caution w/ history of cholestatic jaundice associated w/ past estrogen use or w/ pregnancy; d/c in case of recurrence. Caution w/ hypoparathyroidism; hypocalcemia may occur. May cause fluid retention. Cases of malignant transformation of residual endometrial implants reported in women treated posthysterectomy w/ estrogen therapy alone; consider addition of progestin for these patients. May exacerbate asthma, diabetes mellitus, epilepsy, migraine, porphyria, systemic lupus erythematosus, and hepatic hemangiomas. A narrow vagina, vaginal stenosis, prolapse, or a vaginal infection may make the vagina more susceptible to irritation/ulceration. If a vaginal infection develops, remove and reinsert only after the infection is appropriately treated. May affect certain endocrine and blood components in lab tests.

ADVERSE REACTIONS

Headache, leukorrhea, back pain, genital moniliasis, sinusitis, vaginitis, vaginal discomfort/pain, vaginal hemorrhage, arthritis, insomnia, abdominal pain, upper respiratory tract infection, asymptomatic genital bacterial growth, arthralgia.

DRUG INTERACTIONS

CYP3A4 inducers (eg, St. John's wort preparations, phenobarbital, carbamazepine) may decrease levels, possibly resulting in a decrease in systemic effects and/or changes in the uterine bleeding profile. CYP3A4 inhibitors (eg, erythromycin, ketoconazole, grapefruit juice) may increase levels, and may result in side effects. Patients concomitantly receiving thyroid hormone replacement therapy and estrogens may require increased doses of thyroid replacement therapy; monitor thyroid function.

NURSING CONSIDERATIONS

Assessment: Assess for abnormal genital bleeding, presence/history of breast cancer, estrogen-dependent neoplasia, active/history of DVT/PE/arterial thromboembolic disease, liver impairment/disease, thrombophilic disorders, known anaphylactic reaction or angioedema/hypersensitivity to the drug, pregnancy/nursing status, and any other conditions where treatment is contraindicated or cautioned, need for progestin therapy, and possible drug interactions.

Monitoring: Monitor for signs/symptoms of CV disorders, malignant neoplasms, dementia, gallbladder disease, hypercalcemia, visual abnormalities, BP and plasma TG elevations, pancreatitis, cholestatic jaundice, hypothyroidism, fluid retention, exacerbation of endometriosis or other conditions, vaginal irritation/infection, and other adverse reactions. Perform adequate diagnostic measures (eg, endometrial sampling) in patients w/ undiagnosed, persistent or recurring abnormal genital bleeding. Perform annual breast exam; schedule mammography based on age, risk factors, and prior mammogram results. Monitor thyroid function if on thyroid hormone replacement therapy. Reassess need to continue treatment at 3- or 6-month intervals.

Patient Counseling: Inform of risks and benefits of therapy. Instruct to use ud. Advise of possible serious adverse reactions of therapy (eg, CV disorders, malignant neoplasms, probable dementia). Instruct to notify physician if signs/symptoms of vaginal irritation, abnormal vaginal bleeding, or any adverse reactions occur. Advise to have yearly breast exams by a physician and to perform monthly breast self-exams. Inform that the ring may be expelled from the vagina during bowel movement, straining or w/ constipation; if this occurs, rinse in lukewarm water and reinsert.

Storage: 15-30°C (59-86°F).

ETODOLAC – etodolac **RX**

Class: NSAID

NSAIDs may increase risk of serious cardiovascular (CV) thrombotic events, MI, and stroke, which can be fatal; increased risk with duration of use and with cardiovascular disease (CVD) or risk factors for CVD. Increased risk of serious GI adverse events (eg, bleeding, ulceration, stomach/intestinal perforation) that can be fatal and occur anytime during use without warning symptoms; elderly patients are at a greater risk. Contraindicated for the treatment of perioperative pain in the setting of CABG surgery.

ADULT DOSAGE

Acute Pain

Usual: 200-400mg q6-8h
Max: 1000mg/day

Use lowest effective dose for the shortest duration; after observing response to initial therapy, adjust dose and frequency

Osteoarthritis

Acute and Long-Term Management of Signs/Symptoms:
Initial: 300mg bid-tid, or 400mg bid, or 500mg bid
May give a lower dose of 600mg/day for long-term use
Max: 1000mg/day
Use lowest effective dose for the shortest duration; after observing response to initial therapy, adjust dose and frequency

Rheumatoid Arthritis

Acute and Long-Term Management of Signs/Symptoms:

Initial: 300mg bid-tid, or 400mg bid, or 500mg bid
May give a lower dose of 600mg/day for long-term use
Max: 1000mg/day

Use lowest effective dose for the shortest duration; after observing response to initial therapy, adjust dose and frequency

PEDIATRIC DOSAGE

Pediatric use may not have been established

DOSE MODIFICATION

Hepatic Impairment

Severe: Consider reducing dose

Elderly

Caution w/ dose selection

ADMINISTRATION

Oral route

HOW SUPPLIED

Cap: 200mg, 300mg; Tab: 400mg, 500mg

CONTRAINDICATIONS

History of asthma, urticaria, or other allergic-type reactions with aspirin (ASA) or other NSAIDs. Treatment of perioperative pain in the setting of CABG surgery.

WARNINGS/PRECAUTIONS

May cause HTN or worsen preexisting HTN. Fluid retention and edema reported; caution with fluid retention or heart failure (HF). Extreme caution with prior history of ulcer disease, GI bleeding, or risk factors for GI bleeding (eg, prolonged NSAID therapy, older age, poor general health status); d/c if serious GI event occurs. Renal papillary necrosis and other renal injury reported after long-term use; increased risk with renal/hepatic impairment, HF, and elderly. Caution with preexisting kidney disease. Not recommended for use with advanced renal disease. Caution with mild to moderate renal impairment. Anaphylactoid reactions may occur. Avoid with ASA triad. Caution with asthma and avoid with ASA-sensitive asthma. May cause serious skin adverse events (eg, exfoliative dermatitis, Stevens-Johnson syndrome, toxic epidermal necrolysis); d/c at 1st appearance of skin rash or any other signs of hypersensitivity. Avoid in late pregnancy; may cause premature closure of ductus arteriosus. Not a substitute for corticosteroids or for the treatment of corticosteroid insufficiency; may mask signs of inflammation and fever. May cause elevations of LFTs or severe hepatic reactions (eg, jaundice, fulminant hepatitis, liver necrosis, hepatic failure); d/c if liver disease or systemic manifestations occur, or if abnormal LFTs persist/worsen. Anemia reported; monitor Hgb/Hct if signs or symptoms of anemia develop. May inhibit platelet aggregation and prolong bleeding time; monitor patients with coagulation disorders. Caution in debilitated and elderly. Lab test interactions may occur.

ADVERSE REACTIONS

Abdominal pain, constipation, diarrhea, dyspepsia, flatulence, heartburn, N/V, GI ulcers, abnormal renal function, anemia, dizziness, headaches, increased bleeding time, pruritus, rashes.

DRUG INTERACTIONS

May impair response with thiazides or loop diuretics. Increased risk of GI bleeding with oral corticosteroids, anticoagulants, alcohol use, and smoking. Risk of renal toxicity with diuretics and ACE inhibitors. May diminish antihypertensive effect of ACE inhibitors. May decrease peak concentration with antacids. Not recommended with ASA; may increase adverse effects. May elevate cyclosporine, digoxin, and methotrexate (MTX) levels. May enhance nephrotoxicity associated with cyclosporine. Avoid use prior to or concomitantly with high doses of MTX. May enhance MTX toxicity; caution with concomitant use. May reduce natriuretic effect of furosemide and thiazides in some patients, with possible loss of BP control; monitor for signs of renal insufficiency/failure and diuretic efficacy. May increase lithium levels and reduce lithium clearance; monitor for signs of lithium toxicity, and assess lithium levels when NSAID dosage adjustments are required. Phenylbutazone may increase free fraction of etodolac; not recommended concomitantly. Caution with warfarin; prolonged PT, with or without bleeding, may occur with warfarin; monitor patients carefully.

NURSING CONSIDERATIONS

Assessment: Assess for previous hypersensitivity to the drug or any of its components; history of asthma, urticaria, or allergic-type reactions with ASA or other NSAIDs; ASA triad; CVD; risk factors for CVD; HTN; fluid retention; HF; history of ulcer disease; history of/risk factors for GI bleeding; general health status; renal/hepatic impairment; coagulation disorders; pregnancy/nursing status; and possible drug interactions. Obtain baseline CBC and BP.

Monitoring: Monitor for bleeding time, GI bleeding/ulceration/perforation, CV thrombotic events, MI, HTN, stroke, fluid retention, edema, asthma, hypersensitivity, and other adverse reactions. Monitor for BP, LFTs, and renal function. Monitor for CBC and chemistry profile periodically with long-term use.

Patient Counseling: Inform to seek medical advice if symptoms of CV events, GI ulceration/ bleeding, skin/hypersensitivity reactions, unexplained weight gain or edema, hepatotoxicity, or anaphylactoid reactions occur. Instruct to avoid use in late pregnancy.

Storage: 20-25°C (68-77°F). (Cap) Protect from moisture. (Tab) Store in original container until ready to use.

EVISTA – raloxifene hydrochloride

RX

Class: Selective estrogen receptor modulator

Increased risk of deep vein thrombosis (DVT) and pulmonary embolism (PE) reported. Avoid use in women with active or past history of venous thromboembolism (VTE). Increased risk of death due to stroke in postmenopausal women with documented coronary heart disease or at increased risk for major coronary events; consider risk-benefit balance in women at risk for stroke.

ADULT DOSAGE

Osteoporosis

Treatment and Prevention in Postmenopausal Women:
60mg qd

Ca^{2+} and Vitamin D Supplementation:
Total Daily Ca^{2+} Requirement: 1500mg/day
Vitamin D: 400-800 IU/day

Reduction in Risk of Invasive Breast Cancer

Postmenopausal Women w/ Osteoporosis/ Postmenopausal Women at High Risk for Invasive Breast Cancer:
60mg qd

Ca^{2+} and Vitamin D Supplementation:
Total Daily Ca^{2+} Requirement: 1500mg/day
Vitamin D: 400-800 IU/day

PEDIATRIC DOSAGE

Pediatric use may not have been established

ADMINISTRATION

Oral route

May be given at any time of day w/o regard to meals

HOW SUPPLIED

Tab: 60mg

CONTRAINDICATIONS

Active/past history of VTE (eg, DVT, PE, retinal vein thrombosis), pregnancy, women who may become pregnant, nursing mothers.

WARNINGS/PRECAUTIONS

VTE events, including superficial venous thrombophlebitis, reported. D/C at least 72 hrs prior to and during prolonged immobilization (eg, postsurgical recovery, prolonged bed rest); resume therapy only after patient is fully ambulatory. Caution in women at risk of thromboembolic disease for other reasons (eg, CHF, superficial thrombophlebitis, active malignancy). Should not be used for primary or secondary prevention of cardiovascular disease (CVD). Avoid use in premenopausal women. Monitor serum TG levels in women with history of hypertriglyceridemia in response to treatment with estrogen or estrogen plus progestin. Use in women with history of breast cancer has not been adequately studied. Caution with hepatic impairment or with moderate or severe renal impairment. Not recommended for use in men. Monitor for unexplained uterine bleeding and breast abnormalities.

ADVERSE REACTIONS

DVT, PE, hot flashes, leg cramps, infection, flu syndrome, headache, N/V, diarrhea, peripheral edema, arthralgia, vaginal bleeding, pharyngitis, sinusitis, cough increased.

DRUG INTERACTIONS

Avoid concomitant administration with cholestyramine, other anion exchange resins, and systemic estrogens. Monitor PT with warfarin and other warfarin derivatives. Caution with certain other highly protein-bound drugs (eg, diazepam, diazoxide, lidocaine).

NURSING CONSIDERATIONS

Assessment: Assess for active or history of VTE (eg, DVT, PE, retinal vein thrombosis), CVD, risk factors for stroke, history of breast cancer, history of hypertriglyceridemia, prolonged immobilization, renal/hepatic impairment, pregnancy/nursing status, and for possible drug interactions. Perform breast exams and mammograms prior to treatment.

Monitoring: Monitor for VTE (eg, DVT, PE, retinal vein thrombosis), stroke, unexplained uterine bleeding, breast abnormalities, and other adverse reactions. Monitor serum TG levels with history of hypertriglyceridemia. Monitor PT with warfarin and other warfarin derivatives. Perform regular breast exams and mammograms after initial treatment.

Patient Counseling: For osteoporosis treatment/prevention, instruct to take supplemental Ca^{2+} and/or vitamin D if intake is inadequate. Counsel on weight-bearing exercise and modification of certain behavioral factors (eg, smoking, excessive alcohol consumption) for osteoporosis treatment/prevention. Advise to d/c therapy at least 72 hrs prior to and during prolonged immobilization. Instruct to avoid prolonged restrictions of movement during travel. Counsel that therapy may increase incidence of hot flashes or hot flashes may occur upon initiation of therapy. Inform that regular breast exams and mammography should be done before initiation of therapy and should continue during therapy.

Storage: 20-25°C (68-77°F); excursions permitted to 15-30°C (59-86°F).

EVOCLIN – clindamycin phosphate — RX

Class: Lincomycin derivative

ADULT DOSAGE

Acne Vulgaris

Apply enough to cover entire affected area(s) qd

D/C if no improvement after 6-8 weeks or if condition worsens

PEDIATRIC DOSAGE

Acne Vulgaris

≥12 Years:

Apply enough to cover entire affected area(s) qd

D/C if no improvement after 6-8 weeks or if condition worsens

ADMINISTRATION

Topical route

Not for oral, ophthalmic, or intravaginal use

Wash skin with mild soap and allow to fully dry before application

HOW SUPPLIED

Foam: 1% [50g, 100g]

CONTRAINDICATIONS

History of regional enteritis, ulcerative colitis, or antibiotic-associated colitis (including pseudomembranous colitis).

WARNINGS/PRECAUTIONS

Diarrhea, bloody diarrhea, and colitis (including pseudomembranous colitis) reported; d/c if significant diarrhea occurs. May cause irritation; d/c if irritation or dermatitis occurs. Avoid contact with eyes, mouth, lips, other mucous membranes, or areas of broken skin; rinse thoroughly with water if contact occurs. Caution in atopic individuals.

ADVERSE REACTIONS

Diarrhea, bloody diarrhea, colitis, headache, application-site burning.

DRUG INTERACTIONS

Antiperistaltic agents (eg, opiates, diphenoxylate with atropine) may prolong and/or worsen severe colitis. Avoid with topical/oral erythromycin-containing products due to possible antagonism to clindamycin. May enhance the action of other neuromuscular blockers; use with caution. Caution with concomitant topical acne therapy (eg, peeling, desquamating, abrasive agents) due to possible cumulative irritancy effect.

NURSING CONSIDERATIONS

Assessment: Assess for history of regional enteritis/ulcerative colitis or antibiotic-associated colitis (including pseudomembranous colitis), pregnancy/nursing status, and possible drug interactions. Assess use in atopic individuals.

Monitoring: Monitor for significant diarrhea, colitis, and irritation/dermatitis. For colitis, perform stool culture and assay for *Clostridium difficile* toxin.

Patient Counseling: Instruct to dispense foam directly into cap or onto cool surface, then apply enough to cover the face. Instruct to wash hands after application, and to avoid contact with eyes, mouth, lips, other mucous membranes, or areas of broken skin; instruct to rinse thoroughly with water if contact occurs. Inform that irritation (eg, erythema, scaling, itching, burning, stinging) may occur; advise to d/c if excessive irritancy or dermatitis occurs. Instruct to d/c and contact physician if experiencing severe diarrhea or GI discomfort. Inform that medication is flammable; avoid fire, flame, and/or smoking during and immediately following application.

Storage: 20-25°C (68-77°F). Do not expose to heat or store at >49°C (120°F). Contents under pressure; do not puncture or incinerate.

Evzio – naloxone hydrochloride

RX

Class: Opioid antagonist

ADULT DOSAGE

Opioid Overdose

Emergency treatment of known or suspected opioid overdose, as manifested by respiratory and/or CNS depression

Usual: Administer initial dose (0.4mg) IM/SQ into the anterolateral aspect of the thigh, through clothing if necessary, and seek emergency medical assistance

If desired response is not obtained after 2 or 3 min, may administer another dose; if there is still no response and additional doses are available, may administer additional doses every 2-3 min until emergency medical assistance arrives

Reversal of respiratory depression by partial agonists or mixed agonists/antagonists (eg, buprenorphine, pentazocine) may be incomplete or require higher doses of naloxone

PEDIATRIC DOSAGE

Opioid Overdose

Emergency treatment of known or suspected opioid overdose, as manifested by respiratory and/or CNS depression

Usual: Administer initial dose (0.4mg) IM/SQ into the anterolateral aspect of the thigh, through clothing if necessary, and seek emergency medical assistance

If desired response is not obtained after 2 or 3 min, may administer another dose; if there is still no response and additional doses are available, may administer additional doses every 2-3 min until emergency medical assistance arrives

Reversal of respiratory depression by partial agonists or mixed agonists/antagonists (eg, buprenorphine, pentazocine) may be incomplete or require higher doses of naloxone

ADMINISTRATION

IM/SQ route

For single use only; do not attempt to reuse
If voice instruction system does not operate properly, device will still deliver intended dose when properly administered
Once the red safety guard is removed, use immediately or dispose properly; do not attempt to replace the red safety guard once it is removed
Upon actuation, the needle is automatically inserted and delivers 0.4mg naloxone inj, then retracts the needle fully into its housing

Pediatrics

<1 Year: Caregiver should pinch the thigh muscle while administering the treatment

HOW SUPPLIED

Inj: 0.4mg/0.4mL

WARNINGS/PRECAUTIONS

Not a substitute for emergency medical care. May precipitate an acute abstinence syndrome in patients who are opioid dependent. In neonates, opioid withdrawal may be life-threatening if not recognized and properly treated; signs and symptoms may include convulsions, excessive crying, and hyperactive reflexes. Abrupt postoperative reversal of opioid depression may result in N/V, sweating, tremulousness, tachycardia, hypotension, HTN, seizures, ventricular tachycardia and fibrillation, pulmonary edema, and cardiac arrest; caution in patients with preexisting cardiac disease or who have received medications with potential adverse cardiovascular effects.

ADVERSE REACTIONS

Hypotension, HTN, ventricular tachycardia and fibrillation, dyspnea, pulmonary edema, cardiac arrest.

NURSING CONSIDERATIONS

Assessment: Assess for hypersensitivity to drug, opioid dependence, cardiac disease, and pregnancy/nursing status.

Monitoring: Monitor for precipitation of opioid withdrawal and for other adverse reactions.

Patient Counseling: Instruct patients, family members, and caregivers on how to recognize the signs/symptoms of an opioid overdose requiring the use of drug, and how to properly use it. Instruct to seek emergency medical assistance after administering the 1st dose. Advise that the reversal of respiratory depression by partial agonists or mixed agonist/antagonists may be incomplete. Inform that use in patients who are opioid dependent may precipitate an acute abstinence syndrome.

Storage: 15-25°C (59-77°F); excursions permitted between 4-40°C (39-104°F).

EXELON – rivastigmine

RX

Class: Acetylcholinesterase inhibitor

ADULT DOSAGE

Alzheimer's Disease

Cap/Sol:
Mild to Moderate Dementia:
Initial: 1.5mg bid
Titrate: May increase to 3mg bid after at least 2 weeks; subsequent increases to 4.5mg bid and 6mg bid should be attempted after a minimum of 2 weeks at the previous dose
Usual: 6-12mg/day (3-6mg bid)
Max: 12mg/day (6mg bid)

Patch:
Mild to Moderate Dementia:
Initial: Apply one 4.6mg/24 hrs patch qd
Titrate: Increase dose only after a minimum of 4 weeks at the previous dose
Maint: 9.5mg/24 hrs qd or 13.3mg/24 hrs qd
Max: 13.3mg/24 hrs

Severe Dementia:
Initial: Apply one 4.6mg/24 hrs patch qd
Titrate: Increase dose only after a minimum of 4 weeks at the previous dose
Maint: 13.3mg/24 hrs qd
Max: 13.3mg/24 hrs

Parkinson's Disease

Mild to Moderate Dementia:
Cap/Sol:
Initial: 1.5mg bid
Titrate: May increase to 3mg bid after at least 4 weeks; subsequent increases to 4.5mg bid and 6mg bid should be attempted after a minimum of 4 weeks at the previous dose
Max: 12mg/day (6mg bid)

Patch:
Initial: Apply one 4.6mg/24 hrs patch qd
Titrate: Increase dose only after a minimum of 4 weeks at the previous dose
Maint: 9.5mg/24 hrs qd or 13.3mg/24 hrs qd
Max: 13.3mg/24 hrs

Conversions

Switching to Patch from Cap/Sol:
Total Daily PO Dose <6mg: 4.6mg/24 hrs patch
Total Daily PO Dose 6-12mg: 9.5mg/24 hrs patch

Apply first patch on the day following the last oral dose

PEDIATRIC DOSAGE

Pediatric use may not have been established

DOSE MODIFICATION

Renal Impairment

Moderate to Severe:
Cap/Sol: May only be able to tolerate lower doses

Hepatic Impairment

Mild to Moderate (Child-Pugh 5-9):
Cap/Sol: May only be able to tolerate lower doses
Patch: Consider using the 4.6mg/24 hrs patch as both initial and maint dose

Adverse Reactions

Treatment Interruption:
Cap/Sol:
≤3-Day Interruption: Restart treatment w/ same or lower dose
>3-Day Interruption: Restart treatment w/ 1.5mg bid and titrate

Patch:
≤3-Day Interruption: Restart w/ same or lower strength patch
>3-Day Interruption: Restart w/ 4.6mg/24 hrs patch and titrate

Other Important Modifications
Low Body Weight (<50kg):
Cap/Sol: Consider reducing dose if toxicities develop
Patch: Consider reducing maint dose to the 4.6mg/24 hrs patch if toxicities develop

ADMINISTRATION

Oral/Transdermal route

Cap/Sol
Take w/ meals in divided doses in am and pm
Cap and sol may be interchanged at equal doses
Sol Administration Instructions:
Remove the oral dosing syringe provided in its protective case, and using the provided syringe, withdraw the prescribed amount of sol from container
Each dose of sol may be swallowed directly from the syringe or 1st mixed w/ a small glass of water, cold fruit juice, or soda

Patch
Do not use the patch if the pouch seal is broken or the patch is cut, damaged, or changed in any way
Apply once a day; press down firmly for 30 sec until the edges stick well when applying to clean, dry, hairless, intact, healthy skin in a place that will not be rubbed against by tight clothing
Use the upper or lower back as the site of application. If sites on the back are not accessible, apply the patch to the upper arm or chest; do not apply to a skin area where cre, lot, or powder has recently been applied
Do not apply to skin that is red, irritated, or cut
Replace w/ a new patch every 24 hrs. Instruct patients to only wear 1 patch at a time. If a patch falls off or if a dose is missed, apply a new patch immediately and then replace this patch the following day at the usual application time
Change the site of patch application daily, although a new patch can be applied to the same general area (eg, another spot on the upper back) on consecutive days. Do not apply a new patch to the same location for at least 14 days
Patch may be worn during bathing and in hot weather; avoid long exposure to external heat sources (excessive sunlight, saunas, solariums)
Place used patches in the previously saved pouch and discard in the trash, away from pets or children

HOW SUPPLIED

Cap: 1.5mg, 3mg, 4.5mg, 6mg; Sol: 2mg/mL [120mL]; Patch: 4.6mg/24 hrs, 9.5mg/24 hrs, 13.3mg/24 hrs [30[s]]

CONTRAINDICATIONS

Previous history of application-site reactions w/ rivastigmine transdermal patch suggestive of allergic contact dermatitis, (Oral) in the absence of negative allergy testing.

WARNINGS/PRECAUTIONS

May cause dose-related GI adverse reactions (eg, significant N/V, diarrhea, anorexia/decreased appetite, and weight loss). Disseminated allergic dermatitis irrespective of route of administration reported; d/c if these occur. In patients who develop application-site reactions to patch suggestive of allergic contact dermatitis and who still require therapy, switch to oral therapy only after negative allergy testing and under close medical supervision. May increase gastric acid secretion; monitor for symptoms of active/occult bleeding. Caution in those at increased risk of developing ulcers. May have vagotonic effects on HR (eg, bradycardia), which may be particularly important in sick sinus syndrome or supraventricular cardiac conduction conditions. May cause urinary obstruction and seizures. Caution in patients w/ asthma and obstructive pulmonary disease. May exacerbate or induce extrapyramidal symptoms and impair mental/physical abilities. Caution in patients w/ low or high body weights. (Oral) Syncopal episodes reported. Worsening of parkinsonian symptoms, particularly tremor, observed in patients treated w/ cap. (Patch) Skin application-site reactions may occur. Allergic contact dermatitis should be suspected if application-site reactions spread beyond the patch size; d/c treatment if there is evidence of more intense local reaction (eg, increasing erythema, edema, papules), and if symptoms do not significantly improve w/in 48 hrs after patch removal.

ADVERSE REACTIONS

N/V, anxiety, decreased weight, anorexia, headache, dizziness, fatigue, diarrhea, depression, asthenia, tremor, dyspepsia. (Oral) Abdominal pain.

DRUG INTERACTIONS

Increased risk of additive extrapyramidal adverse reactions w/ metoclopramide; avoid concomitant use. May increase cholinergic effects of other cholinomimetics and may interfere w/ the activity of anticholinergics (eg, oxybutynin, tolterodine); avoid concomitant use unless clinically necessary. Additive bradycardic effects resulting in syncope may occur w/ β-blockers, especially cardioselective β-blockers (eg, atenolol); avoid concomitant use. May exaggerate succinylcholine-type muscle relaxation during anesthesia. Caution w/ NSAIDs; monitor for symptoms of active/occult bleeding.

NURSING CONSIDERATIONS

Assessment: Assess for hypersensitivity to drug, history of GI ulcer disease, sick sinus syndrome, supraventricular cardiac conduction conditions, asthma or obstructive pulmonary disease, pregnancy/nursing status, and possible drug interactions. Assess body weight, for history of application-site reactions w/ rivastigmine patch suggestive of allergic contact dermatitis, and hepatic impairment. (Oral) Assess for renal impairment.

Monitoring: Monitor for signs/symptoms of active or occult GI bleeding, hypersensitivity reactions, extrapyramidal symptoms, urinary obstruction, seizures, GI adverse events, cardiac conduction effects, and other adverse reactions. Closely monitor patients w/ high or low body weight. Monitor for toxicities (eg, excessive N/V) in patients w/ low body weight. (Patch) Monitor for skin reactions (allergic contact dermatitis).

Patient Counseling: Instruct caregivers to monitor for GI adverse reactions and to inform physician if these occur. Inform that allergic skin reactions have been reported regardless of formulation; instruct to consult physician immediately in case of skin reaction while on therapy. Instruct to d/c if disseminated skin hypersensitivity reaction occurs. Advise that therapy may exacerbate or induce extrapyramidal symptoms. (Patch) Instruct to rotate application site, not to use the same site w/in 14 days, to replace patch q24h at consistent time of day, and to wear only 1 patch at a time. Instruct to avoid exposure to external heat for long periods. Instruct on proper usage and discarding of patch. In case of accidental contact w/ eyes or if eyes become red after handling the patch, instruct to rinse immediately w/ plenty of water and seek medical advice if symptoms do not resolve. Advise not to take rivastigmine cap or oral sol, or other drugs w/ cholinergic effects while wearing patch. Instruct to inform physician if application-site reactions spread beyond the patch size, if there is evidence of more intense local reaction, and if symptoms do not significantly improve w/in 48 hrs after patch removal.

Storage: 25°C (77°F); excursions permitted to 15-30°C (59-86°F). (Sol) Store in upright position and protect from freezing. Stable for up to 4 hrs at room temperature if combined w/ cold fruit juice or soda. (Patch) Keep in sealed pouch until use.

EXFORGE – amlodipine/valsartan — RX

Class: ARB/calcium channel blocker (dihydropyridine)

D/C when pregnancy is detected. Drugs that act directly on the renin-angiotensin system (RAS) can cause injury/death to the developing fetus.

ADULT DOSAGE

Hypertension

Initial: 5mg-160mg qd
Titrate: May increase after 1-2 weeks of therapy to control BP
Max: 10mg-320mg qd

Add-On Therapy:
May be used if BP is not adequately controlled w/ amlodipine (or another dihydropyridine calcium channel blocker) or valsartan (or another ARB) alone
Patients w/ dose-limiting adverse reactions to either component alone may be switched to therapy containing a lower dose of that component
Titrate: May increase dose if BP remains uncontrolled after 3-4 weeks of therapy
Max: 10mg-320mg qd

Replacement Therapy:
May substitute for individually titrated components

May be administered w/ other antihypertensive agents

PEDIATRIC DOSAGE

Pediatric use may not have been established

DOSE MODIFICATION

Hepatic Impairment
Consider lower doses

Elderly
Start at lower end of dosing range

ADMINISTRATION
Oral route
Take w/ or w/o food

HOW SUPPLIED
Tab: (Amlodipine-Valsartan) 5mg-160mg, 10mg-160mg, 5mg-320mg, 10mg-320mg

CONTRAINDICATIONS
Coadministration with aliskiren in patients with diabetes.

WARNINGS/PRECAUTIONS
Symptomatic hypotension may occur in patients with an activated RAS (eg, volume- and/or salt-depleted patients receiving high doses of diuretics); correct volume depletion prior to therapy. Caution when initiating therapy in patients with HF or recent MI, and in patients undergoing surgery/dialysis. Renal function changes may occur; caution in patients whose renal function may depend in part on the activity of the RAS (eg, renal artery stenosis, severe HF, post-MI, volume depletion). Consider withholding or discontinuing if clinically significant decrease in renal function develops. Amlodipine: Caution with severe aortic stenosis. Worsening angina and acute MI may develop after starting or increasing dose, particularly with severe obstructive CAD. Valsartan: Increased K^+ in some patients with HF reported, and more likely to occur in patients with preexisting renal impairment; dose reduction and/or discontinuation of therapy may be required. Do not readminister to patients who have had angioedema. Caution in elderly and with liver disease.

ADVERSE REACTIONS
Increased BUN, peripheral edema, nasopharyngitis, hyperkalemia.

DRUG INTERACTIONS
See Contraindications. Amlodipine: May increase simvastatin exposure; limit simvastatin dose to 20mg/day. Increased systemic exposure with CYP3A4 inhibitors (moderate and strong) warranting dose reduction; monitor for symptoms of hypotension and edema to determine the need for dose adjustment. Monitor BP when coadministered with CYP3A4 inducers. Valsartan: Dual blockade of the RAS is associated with increased risks of hypotension, hyperkalemia, and changes in renal function (including acute renal failure); avoid combined use of RAS inhibitors, or closely monitor BP, renal function, and electrolytes with concomitant agents that also affect the RAS. Avoid with aliskiren in patients with renal impairment (GFR <60mL/min). Greater antihypertensive effect with atenolol. Other agents that block the RAS, K^+-sparing diuretics, K^+ supplements, or salt substitutes containing K^+ may increase serum K^+ levels, and in HF patients may increase SrCr; monitor serum K^+ levels. NSAIDs, including selective COX-2 inhibitors, may result in deterioration of renal function, including possible acute renal failure, and may attenuate antihypertensive effect. Inhibitors of the hepatic uptake transporter OATP1B1 (rifampin, cyclosporine) and the hepatic efflux transporter MRP2 (ritonavir) may increase exposure. Increases in lithium levels and lithium toxicity reported; monitor serum lithium levels during concomitant use.

NURSING CONSIDERATIONS

Assessment: Assess for hypersensitivity to any component of the drug, volume/salt depletion, HF, recent MI, renal artery stenosis, severe aortic stenosis, severe obstructive CAD, renal/hepatic impairment, pregnancy/nursing status, and possible drug interactions.

Monitoring: Monitor for signs/symptoms of hypotension, hyperkalemia, hypersensitivity reactions, and other adverse reactions. Monitor for symptoms of angina or MI, particularly in patients with severe obstructive CAD, after dosage initiation or increase. Monitor BP, serum electrolytes, and renal function.

Patient Counseling: Counsel about risks/benefits of therapy. Inform of the consequences of exposure during pregnancy and the treatment options in women planning to become pregnant; instruct to report pregnancy to physician as soon as possible.

Storage: 25°C (77°F); excursions permitted to 15-30°C (59-86°F). Protect from moisture.

Exforge HCT – amlodipine/hydrochlorothiazide/valsartan RX

Class: ARB/calcium channel blocker (dihydropyridine)/thiazide diuretic

D/C when pregnancy is detected. Drugs that act directly on the renin-angiotensin system (RAS) can cause injury/death to the developing fetus.

ADULT DOSAGE

Hypertension

Usual: Dose qd
Titrate: May increase dose after 2 weeks
Max: 10mg-320mg-25mg qd

Add-On/Switch Therapy:
May use for patients not adequately controlled

PEDIATRIC DOSAGE
Pediatric use may not have been established

on any 2 of the following: calcium channel blockers (CCBs), ARBs, and diuretics

Patients w/ dose-limiting adverse reactions to an individual component while on any dual combination of the components of therapy may be switched to a lower dose of that component

Replacement Therapy:

May substitute for individually titrated components

May be administered w/ other antihypertensive agents

DOSE MODIFICATION

Hepatic Impairment

Consider lower doses

Elderly

Consider lower initial doses

ADMINISTRATION

Oral route

Take w/ or w/o food

HOW SUPPLIED

Tab: (Amlodipine-Valsartan-HCTZ) 5mg-160mg-12.5mg, 5mg-160mg-25mg, 10mg-160mg-12.5mg, 10mg-160mg-25mg, 10mg-320mg-25mg

CONTRAINDICATIONS

Anuria, sulfonamide-derived drug hypersensitivity. Coadministration with aliskiren in patients with diabetes.

WARNINGS/PRECAUTIONS

Not for initial therapy of HTN. Symptomatic hypotension may occur in patients with activated RAS (eg, volume- and/or salt-depleted patients receiving high doses of diuretics); correct this condition prior to therapy. Avoid with aortic or mitral stenosis or obstructive hypertrophic cardiomyopathy. Renal function changes, including acute renal failure, may occur; caution in patients whose renal function depend in part on the activity of the RAS (eg, renal artery stenosis, severe heart failure [HF], post-MI, volume depletion). Consider withholding or discontinuing therapy if clinically significant decrease in renal function develops. May cause serum electrolyte abnormalities (eg, hyper/hypokalemia, hyponatremia, hypomagnesemia); correct hypokalemia and any coexisting hypomagnesemia prior to initiation of therapy. D/C if hypokalemia is accompanied by clinical signs (eg, muscular weakness, paresis, ECG alterations). Do not readminister to patients who have had angioedema. Amlodipine: Worsening angina and acute MI may develop after starting or increasing dose, particularly in patients with severe obstructive coronary artery disease (CAD). Valsartan: Increased K^+ in some patients with HF reported, and more likely to occur in patients with preexisting renal impairment; dose reduction and/or discontinuation of diuretic and/or valsartan may be required. HCTZ: May cause hypersensitivity reactions and exacerbation or activation of systemic lupus erythematosus (SLE). Minor alterations of fluid and electrolyte balance may precipitate hepatic coma in patients with hepatic dysfunction or progressive liver disease. May cause idiosyncratic reaction, resulting in acute transient myopia and acute angle-closure glaucoma; d/c as rapidly as possible. May alter glucose tolerance and increase serum cholesterol and TG levels. May cause or exacerbate hyperuricemia and precipitate gout in susceptible patients. May cause hypercalcemia.

ADVERSE REACTIONS

Increased BUN, hypokalemia, dizziness, edema, headache.

DRUG INTERACTIONS

See Contraindications. Amlodipine: May increase simvastatin exposure; limit simvastatin dose to 20mg/day. Increased systemic exposure with CYP3A inhibitors (moderate and strong) warranting dose reduction; monitor for symptoms of hypotension and edema to determine the need for dose adjustment. Monitor BP when coadministered with CYP3A4 inducers. Valsartan: Dual blockade of the RAS is associated with increased risk of hypotension, hyperkalemia, and changes in renal function (including acute renal failure); avoid combined use of RAS inhibitors, or closely monitor BP, renal function, and electrolytes with concomitant agents that also affect the RAS. Avoid with aliskiren in patients with renal impairment (GFR <60mL/min). Greater antihypertensive effect with atenolol. Other agents that block the RAS, K^+-sparing diuretics, K^+ supplements, or salt substitutes containing K^+ may lead to increases in serum K^+, and in HF patients to increases in SrCr; monitor serum K^+ levels. NSAIDs, including selective COX-2 inhibitors, may deteriorate renal function and attenuate antihypertensive effect. HCTZ: Dosage adjustment of antidiabetic drugs (eg, oral agents, insulin) may be required. May lead to symptomatic hyponatremia with carbamazepine. Ion exchange resins (eg, cholestyramine, colestipol) may reduce exposure; space dosing at least 4 hrs before or 4-6 hrs after the administration of resins. Cyclosporine may increase risk of hyperuricemia and gout-type complications. Valsartan-HCTZ: Increases in lithium levels and lithium toxicity reported; monitor serum lithium levels during concomitant use.

NURSING CONSIDERATIONS

Assessment: Assess for hypersensitivity to the drug and its components, anuria, sulfonamide-derived drug or PCN hypersensitivity, history of allergy or bronchial asthma, renal/hepatic impairment, HF, aortic or mitral stenosis, renal artery stenosis, obstructive hypertrophic cardiomyopathy, SLE, volume/salt depletion, electrolyte imbalances, CAD, pregnancy/nursing status, and possible drug interactions.

Monitoring: Monitor for signs/symptoms of hypotension, hypersensitivity/idiosyncratic reactions, metabolic disturbances, myopia and angle-closure glaucoma, worsening angina or acute MI, fluid imbalance, exacerbation or activation of SLE, hyperglycemia, hyperuricemia or precipitation of gout, increases in cholesterol and TG levels, and other adverse reactions. Monitor BP, serum electrolytes, BUN, and renal function.

Patient Counseling: Inform of the consequences of exposure during pregnancy and the treatment options in women planning to become pregnant; instruct to report pregnancy to physician as soon as possible. Inform that lightheadedness may occur, especially during the 1st days of therapy; if syncope occurs, instruct to d/c therapy until physician has been consulted. Caution that inadequate fluid intake, excessive perspiration, diarrhea, or vomiting may lead to an excessive fall in BP, which may result in lightheadedness and possible syncope. Instruct to avoid K^+ supplements or salt substitutes containing K^+ without consulting prescribing physician.

Storage: 25°C (77°F); excursions permitted to 15-30°C (59-86°F). Protect from moisture.

EXTAVIA – interferon beta-1b

RX

Class: Biological response modifier

ADULT DOSAGE

Multiple Sclerosis

Relapsing Forms:
Initial: 0.0625mg SQ qod
Titrate: Increase over 6 weeks to 0.25mg qod SQ

Titration Schedule:
Week 1-2: 0.0625mg (0.25mL)
Week 3-4: 0.125mg (0.5mL)
Week 5-6: 0.1875mg (0.75mL)
Week 7 and After: 0.25mg (1mL)

Premedication for Flu-Like Symptoms:
Concurrent use of analgesics and/or antipyretics may help ameliorate flu-like symptoms on treatment days

PEDIATRIC DOSAGE

Pediatric use may not have been established

ADMINISTRATION

SQ route

Rotate inj sites

Reconstitution

Attach prefilled syringe containing diluent (NaCl, 0.54% Sol) to Extavia vial using vial adapter
Slowly inject 1.2mL of diluent into Extavia vial
Gently swirl vial to dissolve drug completely; do not shake
Foaming may occur during reconstitution or if vial is swirled or shaken too vigorously; if foaming occurs, allow vial to sit undisturbed until foam settles
Keeping syringe and vial adapter in place, turn assembly over so that vial is on top; withdraw appropriate dose of Extavia sol
Remove vial from vial adapter before injecting Extavia

HOW SUPPLIED

Inj: 0.3mg

CONTRAINDICATIONS

Hypersensitivity to albumin (human), mannitol.

WARNINGS/PRECAUTIONS

Severe hepatic injury including hepatic failure (rare) and asymptomatic elevation of serum transaminases reported; consider discontinuing therapy if serum transaminase levels significantly increase, or if associated with clinical symptoms (eg, jaundice). Anaphylaxis (rare) and other allergic reactions reported; d/c if anaphylaxis occurs. Depression and suicide reported; consider discontinuation of therapy if depression develops. Congestive heart failure (CHF), cardiomyopathy, and cardiomyopathy with CHF reported; monitor for worsening of cardiac condition during initiation of and continued treatment in patients with preexisting CHF. Consider discontinuation of therapy if worsening of CHF occurs with no other etiology. Inj-site necrosis/reactions reported; avoid administration into affected area until fully healed in patients who continue therapy after inj-site necrosis has occurred. If multiple lesions occur, d/c until healed. Leukopenia and seizures reported. May require more intensive monitoring of CBC, with differential and platelet counts in patients with myelosuppression.

ADVERSE REACTIONS

Inj-site reaction, lymphopenia, flu-like symptoms, myalgia, leukopenia, neutropenia, increased liver enzymes, headache, hypertonia, pain, rash, insomnia, abdominal pain, asthenia.

DRUG INTERACTIONS

Potential risk for hepatic injury with hepatotoxic drugs and alcohol.

NURSING CONSIDERATIONS

Assessment: Assess for hypersensitivity to the drug or human albumin, preexisting CHF, myelosuppression, pregnancy/nursing status, and possible drug interactions.

Monitoring: Monitor for hepatic injury, anaphylaxis, depression, suicidal ideation, worsening of CHF, inj-site necrosis/reactions, leukopenia, flu-like symptom complex, and other adverse reactions. Monitor CBC and differential WBC count, platelet counts and blood chemistries, including LFTs at regular intervals (1, 3, and 6 months) following introduction, and then periodically thereafter in the absence of clinical symptoms.

Patient Counseling: Instruct on proper aseptic technique and procedures. Advise not to reuse needles/syringes and instruct on safe disposal procedures. Inform of the importance of rotating inj sites with each dose. Instruct to notify physician if pregnant, planning to become pregnant, or if any adverse reactions (eg, hepatic dysfunction, allergic reactions, anaphylaxis, worsening of cardiac condition, inj-site necrosis, seizures) occur. Inform that symptoms of depression or suicidal ideation may occur and instruct to notify physician immediately if these occur. Inform that flu-like symptoms are common following initiation of therapy. Instruct to take missed dose as soon as patient remembers or is able to, but not to take on 2 consecutive days.

Storage: 20-25°C (68-77°F); excursions of 15-30°C (59-86°F) are permitted for up to 3 months. After reconstitution, if not used immediately, refrigerate and use within 3 hrs. Do not freeze.

EXTINA – ketoconazole RX

Class: Azole antifungal

ADULT DOSAGE

Seborrheic Dermatitis

Apply to affected area(s) bid for 4 weeks

PEDIATRIC DOSAGE

Seborrheic Dermatitis

≥12 Years:

Apply to affected area(s) bid for 4 weeks

ADMINISTRATION

Topical route

1. Hold the container upright, and dispense foam into the cap of the can or other cool surface in an amount sufficient to cover the affected area(s)
2. Dispensing directly onto hands is not recommended, as the foam will begin to melt immediately upon contact with warm skin
3. Pick up small amounts of foam with the fingertips, and gently massage into the affected area(s) until the foam disappears
4. For hair-bearing areas, part the hair, so that foam may be applied directly to the skin (rather than on the hair)

HOW SUPPLIED

Foam: 2% [50g, 100g]

WARNINGS/PRECAUTIONS

Not for ophthalmic, oral, or intravaginal use. Safety and efficacy for the treatment of fungal infections not established. May cause contact sensitization, including photoallergenicity. Contents are flammable; avoid fire, flame, and/or smoking during and immediately following application. Hepatitis, lowered testosterone, and adrenocorticotropic hormone-induced corticosteroid serum levels reported with orally administered ketoconazole; not seen with topical ketoconazole.

ADVERSE REACTIONS

Application-site burning, application-site reactions (eg, dryness, erythema, irritation, paresthesia, pruritus, rash, warmth), photoallergenicity, contact sensitization.

NURSING CONSIDERATIONS

Assessment: Assess pregnancy/nursing status.

Monitoring: Monitor for contact sensitization and application-site reactions.

Patient Counseling: Instruct to use ud. Instruct to avoid fire, flame, and/or smoking during and immediately following application. Instruct not to apply directly to hands; apply to affected areas using the fingertips. Inform that skin irritation and contact sensitization may occur; instruct to inform a physician if the area shows signs of increased irritation, and to report any signs of adverse reactions. Instruct to wash hands after application.

Storage: 20-25°C (68-77°F). Do not store under refrigerated conditions or in direct sunlight. Do not expose containers to heat or store at temperatures above 49°C (120°F). Do not puncture and/or incinerate container.

EYLEA – aflibercept

RX

Class: Vascular endothelial growth factor (VEGF) inhibitor

ADULT DOSAGE

Neovascular (Wet) Age-Related Macular Degeneration

Usual: 2mg (0.05mL) every 4 weeks for first 12 weeks, followed by 2mg once every 8 weeks

Macular Edema

Following Retinal Vein Occlusion:
Usual: 2mg (0.05mL) once every 4 weeks

Diabetic Macular Edema

Usual: 2mg (0.05mL) every 4 weeks for first 5 inj, followed by 2mg once every 8 weeks

Diabetic Retinopathy

W/ Diabetic Macular Edema:
Usual: 2mg (0.05mL) every 4 weeks for first 5 inj, followed by 2mg once every 8 weeks

PEDIATRIC DOSAGE

Pediatric use may not have been established

ADMINISTRATION

Intravitreal route

Procedure should be carried out under controlled aseptic conditions
Adequate anesthesia and a topical broad-spectrum microbicide should be given prior to inj
Each vial should only be used for the treatment of a single eye; if the contralateral eye requires treatment, use a new vial and change sterile field, syringe, gloves, drapes, eyelid speculum, filter, and inj needles before administering to other eye
After inj, any unused product must be discarded

Preparation

1. Perform inj w/ a 30-gauge x 1/2-inch inj needle
2. Remove protective plastic cap from vial and clean top of vial w/ alcohol wipe
3. Remove 19-gauge x 1.5-inch, 5-micron filter needle and 1-mL syringe supplied in carton from pouches; attach filter needle to syringe by twisting it onto Luer lock syringe tip
4. Push filter needle into center of vial stopper until needle is completely inserted into vial and tip touches the bottom or bottom edge of vial
5. Withdraw all of vial contents into syringe, keeping vial in an upright position, slightly inclined to ease complete withdrawal; to deter introduction of air, ensure bevel of filter needle is submerged into liquid. Continue to tilt vial during withdrawal keeping bevel of filter needle submerged in liquid
6. Ensure that plunger rod is drawn sufficiently back when emptying vial in order to completely empty filter needle
7. Remove filter needle from syringe and properly dispose of filter needle; do not use filter needle for intravitreal inj
8. Remove 30-gauge x 1/2-inch inj needle from plastic pouch and attach inj needle to syringe by firmly twisting inj needle onto Luer lock syringe tip
9. When ready to administer, remove plastic needle shield from needle
10. Holding syringe w/ needle pointing up, check for bubbles; if there are bubbles, gently tap syringe w/ finger until bubbles rise to top
11. To eliminate all bubbles and to expel excess drug, slowly depress plunger so that plunger tip aligns w/ line that marks 0.05mL on syringe

HOW SUPPLIED

Inj: 40mg/mL [0.05mL]

CONTRAINDICATIONS

Ocular/periocular infections, active intraocular inflammation.

WARNINGS/PRECAUTIONS
Endophthalmitis and retinal detachments may occur. Acute increases in IOP noted w/in 60 min of inj. Sustained increases in IOP reported after repeated dosing. Monitor IOP and perfusion of the optic nerve head and manage appropriately. Potential risk of arterial thromboembolic events (ATEs) (eg, nonfatal stroke, nonfatal MI, vascular death).

ADVERSE REACTIONS
Conjunctival hemorrhage, ocular hyperemia, eye pain, cataract, vitreous detachment/floaters, IOP increased, corneal epithelium defect, retinal pigment epithelium detachment, inj-site pain, foreign body sensation in eyes, lacrimation increased.

NURSING CONSIDERATIONS

Assessment: Assess for hypersensitivity to the drug, ocular/periocular infections, active intraocular inflammation, and pregnancy/nursing status.

Monitoring: Monitor for signs/symptoms of endophthalmitis, retinal detachment, ATEs, and other adverse reactions. Monitor IOP and perfusion of the optic nerve head.

Patient Counseling: Advise to seek immediate care from an ophthalmologist if eye becomes red, sensitive to light, painful, or develops a change in vision in the days following administration. Inform that temporary visual disturbances may be experienced after inj and the associated eye examinations; advise not to drive or use machinery until visual function has recovered sufficiently.

Storage: 2-8°C (36-46°F). Do not freeze. Protect from light.

FABIOR – tazarotene RX

Class: Retinoid

ADULT DOSAGE

Acne Vulgaris

Lightly cover affected area with thin layer qpm

PEDIATRIC DOSAGE

Acne Vulgaris

≥12 Years:
Lightly cover affected area with thin layer qpm

ADMINISTRATION
Topical route

1. Shake can before use
2. Clean and dry affected area
3. Dispense a small amount of foam into the palm of hand
4. Gently massage the foam into skin until foam disappears
5. Wash hands after application

HOW SUPPLIED
Foam: 0.1% [50g, 100g]

CONTRAINDICATIONS
Pregnancy.

WARNINGS/PRECAUTIONS
Not for oral, ophthalmic, or intravaginal use; avoid contact with any of these areas. Females of childbearing potential should use adequate birth-control measures during treatment. Obtain negative pregnancy test result (sensitivity down to at least 25 mIU/mL for human chorionic gonadotropin [hCG]) within 2 weeks prior to therapy; initiate therapy during normal menstrual period. Caution with history of local tolerability reactions or local hypersensitivity. May cause severe irritation; do not use on abraded or eczematous skin. Avoid contact with mouth, eyes, and mucous membranes; rinse well with water in case of accidental contact. May cause skin redness, peeling, burning or excessive pruritus; d/c therapy until integrity of skin is restored or reduce dosing interval if these occur. D/C treatment if irritation persists. Weather extremes (eg, wind, cold) may be more irritating. Avoid exposure to sunlight (including sunlamps); if exposure is necessary, use sunscreens and protective clothing. Avoid with sunburn. Caution with personal or family history of skin cancer. Propellant in drug is flammable; avoid fire, flame, and/or smoking during and immediately following application.

ADVERSE REACTIONS
Application-site irritation/dryness/erythema/exfoliation.

DRUG INTERACTIONS
Avoid with dermatologic medications and cosmetics that have a strong drying effect. Oxidizing agents (eg, benzoyl peroxide) may cause degradation and may reduce clinical efficacy; if combination is required, apply at different times of the day. Cumulative irritant effect may occur with topical acne therapy; use with caution. Possibility of augmented photosensitivity increased with photosensitizers (eg, thiazides, tetracyclines, fluoroquinolones, phenothiazines, sulfonamides); use with caution.

NURSING CONSIDERATIONS

Assessment: Assess for hypersensitivity, eczematous skin, sunburn, considerable sun exposure due to occupation, sunlight sensitivity, personal or family history of skin cancer, pregnancy/nursing status, and possible drug interactions. Obtain negative pregnancy test result (sensitivity down to at least 25 mIU/mL for hCG) within 2 weeks prior to therapy.

Monitoring: Monitor for local irritation (skin redness, peeling, burning or excessive pruritus) and other adverse reactions.

Patient Counseling: Advise to use effective method of contraception during treatment to avoid pregnancy; advise to d/c medication and contact physician if pregnancy occurs. Instruct to reduce application frequency or temporarily interrupt treatment if undue irritation (redness, peeling, discomfort) occurs; inform that treatment may be resumed once irritation subsides. Instruct to avoid exposure of treated areas to either natural or artificial sunlight (eg, tanning beds, sunlamps). Instruct to avoid contact with mouth, eyes, and mucous membranes; rinse well with water in case of accidental contact. Instruct to avoid fire, flame, or smoking during and immediately following application since foam is flammable. Instruct to wash hands after application.

Storage: 20-25°C (68-77°F); excursions permitted to 15-30°C (59-86°F). Protect from freezing. Do not expose to heat or store at >49°C (120°F).

FACTIVE – gemifloxacin mesylate RX

Class: Fluoroquinolone

Fluoroquinolones are associated with an increased risk of tendinitis and tendon rupture in all ages. Risk is further increased in patients >60 yrs, patients taking corticosteroids, and with kidney, heart, or lung transplants. May exacerbate muscle weakness with myasthenia gravis; avoid in patients with known history of myasthenia gravis.

ADULT DOSAGE

Acute Bacterial Exacerbation of Chronic Bronchitis

320mg qd for 5 days

Community-Acquired Pneumonia

Mild to Moderate Severity:

Due to *Streptococcus pneumoniae*, *Haemophilus influenzae*, *Mycoplasma pneumoniae*, or *Chlamydia pneumoniae*:
320mg qd for 5 days

Due to Multidrug Resistant *S. pneumoniae*, *Klebsiella pneumoniae*, or *Moraxella catarrhalis*:
320mg qd for 7 days

PEDIATRIC DOSAGE

Pediatric use may not have been established

DOSE MODIFICATION

Renal Impairment

CrCl ≤40mL/min or Dialysis: 160mg q24h

ADMINISTRATION

Oral route

Take w/ or w/o food; swallow whole w/ fluids

HOW SUPPLIED

Tab: 320mg* *scored

WARNINGS/PRECAUTIONS

D/C if pain, swelling, inflammation, or rupture of a tendon occurs. May prolong QT interval; avoid with history of QTc interval prolongation or uncontrolled electrolyte disorders, and caution with proarrhythmic conditions. Serious and sometimes fatal hypersensitivity reactions reported; d/c if skin rash, jaundice, or any other sign of hypersensitivity appears and institute appropriate therapy. Rare cases of sensory or sensorimotor axonal polyneuropathy, resulting in paresthesias, hypoesthesias, dysesthesias, and weakness reported. CNS effects (infrequent) reported; caution with CNS diseases (eg, epilepsy or patients predisposed to convulsions), and d/c if CNS stimulation occurs. Convulsions, toxic psychoses, and increased intracranial pressure (including pseudotumor cerebri) reported. *Clostridium difficile*-associated diarrhea (CDAD) reported. May cause photosensitivity/phototoxicity reactions; d/c if photosensitivity/phototoxicity occurs. Avoid excessive exposure to source of light. Liver enzyme elevations reported. Caution in elderly and with renal impairment. Maintain adequate hydration. May result in bacterial resistance with prolonged use or use in the absence of a proven/suspected bacterial infection or a prophylactic indication; take appropriate measures if superinfection develops.

ADVERSE REACTIONS
Diarrhea, rash, N/V, headache, abdominal pain, dizziness.

DRUG INTERACTIONS
See Boxed Warning. Avoid Mg^{2+}- or aluminum-containing antacids, ferrous sulfate (iron), Videx (didanosine) chewable/buffered tab or pediatric powder for oral sol, and multivitamin preparations containing zinc or other metal cations, within 3 hrs before or 2 hrs after therapy and sucralfate within 2 hrs of therapy. Calcium carbonate may decrease levels. Reduced levels with oral estrogen/progesterone contraceptive product. Increased levels with cimetidine, omeprazole, probenecid. Avoid Class IA (eg, quinidine, procainamide) or Class III (eg, amiodarone, sotalol) antiarrhythmics. Caution with drugs that prolong the QTc interval (eg, erythromycin, antipsychotics, TCAs). Increased INR or PT and/or clinical episodes of bleeding reported with warfarin or its derivatives.

NURSING CONSIDERATIONS

Assessment: Assess for hypersensitivity to drug, factors that increase the risk of tendon rupture, history of myasthenia gravis and QTc interval prolongation, uncontrolled electrolyte disorders, proarrhythmic conditions, CNS disease, pregnancy/nursing status, and possible drug interactions. Obtain baseline renal function and LFTs.

Monitoring: Monitor for signs/symptoms of tendinitis or tendon rupture, muscle weakness exacerbation, hypersensitivity and photosensitivity/phototoxicity reactions, peripheral neuropathy, CNS effects, and CDAD. Monitor renal function and LFTs.

Patient Counseling: Instruct to contact physician and advise to rest, refrain from exercise, and d/c therapy if pain, swelling, or inflammation of a tendon, or weakness or inability to move joints occur. Inform that drug may worsen myasthenia gravis symptoms; immediately contact physician if muscle weakness worsens or breathing problems occur. Inform that drug treats bacterial, not viral, infections. Instruct to take drug exactly ud, swallow whole, drink fluids liberally, and not to skip doses. Instruct to d/c therapy and notify physician if rash or other allergic reaction develops. Counsel to notify physician if watery and bloody stools, palpitations, sunburn-like reaction, or skin eruption occurs, and about medications taken concurrently. Instruct not to engage in activities requiring mental alertness and coordination if dizziness occurs, and to minimize or avoid sun/UV light exposure.

Storage: 25°C (77°F); excursions permitted to 15-30°C (59-86°F). Protect from light.

FAMOTIDINE – famotidine **RX**

Class: H_2-blocker

OTHER BRAND NAMES
Pepcid

ADULT DOSAGE

Active Duodenal Ulcer

IV:
20mg q12h

PO:
Acute Therapy:
20mg bid or 40mg qhs for 4-8 weeks
Maint Therapy:
20mg qhs

Gastroesophageal Reflux Disease

Short-term Treatment of GERD:
20mg bid for up to 6 weeks

Short-term Treatment of GERD w/ Esophagitis:
20 or 40mg bid for up to 12 weeks

Pathological Hypersecretory Conditions

Treatment of Pathological Hypersecretory Conditions (eg, Zollinger-Ellison Syndrome, Multiple Endocrine Adenomas):
PO:
Initial: 20mg q6h
Titrate: Adjust dose to individual patient needs and continue as long as clinically indicated
Oral doses up to 160mg q6h have been administered to some patients w/ severe Zollinger-Ellison syndrome

PEDIATRIC DOSAGE

Peptic Ulcer

1-16 Years:
PO:
Initial: 0.5mg/kg/day qhs or divided bid
Max: 40mg/day
IV:
0.25mg/kg over ≥2 min or as 15-min infusion q12h
Max: 40mg/day

Individualize dose based on response and/or gastric/esophageal pH determination and endoscopy

Gastroesophageal Reflux Disease

Sus:
<3 Months of Age:
0.5mg/kg/dose qd for up to 8 weeks

3 Months of Age-<1 Year:
0.5mg/kg/dose bid

GERD w/ or w/o Esophagitis:
1-16 Years:
PO:
Initial: 1mg/kg/day divided bid
Max: 40mg bid

Individualize dose based on response and/or gastric/esophageal pH determination and endoscopy

IV:
Initial: 20mg q12h
Titrate: Adjust dose to individual patient needs and continue as long as clinically indicated

Gastric Ulcers

Acute Therapy for Active Benign Gastric Ulcer:
PO:
40mg qhs

IV:
20mg q12h

DOSE MODIFICATION

Renal Impairment
Moderate (CrCl <50mL/min) or Severe (CrCl <10mL/min): May reduce to 1/2 dose, or prolong dosing interval to 36-48 hrs

ADMINISTRATION

IV/Oral route

May take w/ antacids if needed

Preparation
IV Sol:
Dilute 2mL of famotidine inj w/ 0.9% NaCl or other compatible IV sol to a total volume of either 5mL or 10mL and inject over a period of not less than 2 min
IV Infusion Sol:
Dilute 2mL of famotidine inj w/ 100mL of D5W or other compatible sol, and infuse over 15-30 min
Oral Sus preparation:
Slowly add 46mL of purified water and shake vigorously for 5-10 sec immediately after adding the water and immediately before use
Stability:
When added to or diluted w/ Water for Inj, 0.9% NaCl, D5W and D10W, or Lactated Ringer's Inj, diluted famotidine inj is physically and chemically stable for 7 days at room temperature
When added to or diluted w/ sodium bicarbonate Inj 5%, famotidine inj at a concentration of 0.2mg/mL is physically and chemically stable for 7 days at room temperature

HOW SUPPLIED

Inj: 10mg/mL [2mL, 4mL, 20mL]; 20mg/50mL [50mL]; Sus: (Pepcid) 40mg/5mL [50mL]; Tab: (Pepcid) 20mg, 40mg

WARNINGS/PRECAUTIONS

Symptomatic response to therapy does not preclude presence of gastric malignancy. CNS adverse effects reported with moderate and severe renal insufficiency; may need to prolong dosing intervals or lower dose. Caution in elderly. (Inj) For IV use only. (Tab) Very rarely, prolonged QT interval reported in patients with impaired renal function whose dose/dosing interval may not have been adjusted appropriately.

ADVERSE REACTIONS

Headache, agitation.

NURSING CONSIDERATIONS

Assessment: Assess for hypersensitivity to the drug or to other H_2-receptor antagonists, renal insufficiency, gastric malignancy, pregnancy/nursing status, and possible drug interactions.

Monitoring: Monitor for hypersensitivity reactions and other adverse reactions. Monitor renal function in the elderly.

Patient Counseling: Inform of risks/benefits of therapy. Instruct to contact physician if hypersensitivity or other adverse reactions develop. Advise to avoid nursing while on medication.

Storage: (Inj) 2-8°C (36-46°F). Bring to room temperature if sol freezes. Diluted Sol: Stable at room temperature for 7 days. Refrigeration and use within 48 hrs is recommended if not used immediately after preparation. (Premixed Inj) 25°C (77°F); avoid exposure to excessive heat; brief exposure to temperatures ≤35°C (95°F) does not adversely affect product. (Sus) 25°C (77°F); excursions permitted to 15-30°C (59-86°F). Protect from freezing. Discard unused suspension after 30 days. (Tab) Controlled room temperature.

FAMVIR – famciclovir

RX

Class: Nucleoside analogue

ADULT DOSAGE

Herpes Zoster

500mg q8h for 7 days
Initiate as soon as diagnosed

Herpes

Orolabial/Genital:

Recurrent in HIV-Infected Patients:

500mg bid for 7 days
Initiate at 1st sign/symptom

Herpes Labialis (Cold Sores)

Recurrent:

1500mg single dose
Initiate at 1st sign/symptom

Genital Herpes

Recurrent Episodes:

1000mg bid for 1 day
Initiate at 1st sign/symptom

Suppressive Therapy:

250mg bid

PEDIATRIC DOSAGE

Pediatric use may not have been established

DOSE MODIFICATION

Renal Impairment

Recurrent Herpes Labialis:

CrCl 40-59mL/min: 750mg single dose
CrCl 20-39mL/min: 500mg single dose
CrCl <20mL/min: 250mg single dose
Hemodialysis: 250mg single dose following dialysis

Recurrent Genital Herpes:

CrCl 40-59mL/min: 500mg q12h for 1 day
CrCl 20-39mL/min: 500mg single dose
CrCl <20mL/min: 250mg single dose
Hemodialysis: 250mg single dose following dialysis

Suppression of Recurrent Genital Herpes:

CrCl 20-39mL/min: 125mg q12h
CrCl <20mL/min: 125mg q24h
Hemodialysis: 125mg following each dialysis

Herpes Zoster:

CrCl 40-59mL/min: 500mg q12h
CrCl 20-39mL/min: 500mg q24h
CrCl <20mL/min: 250mg q24h
Hemodialysis: 250mg following each dialysis

Recurrent Orolabial/Genital Herpes in HIV-Infected Patients:

CrCl 20-39mL/min: 500mg q24h
CrCl <20mL/min: 250mg q24h
Hemodialysis: 250mg following each dialysis

ADMINISTRATION

Oral route
Take with or without food

HOW SUPPLIED

Tab: 125mg, 250mg, 500mg

WARNINGS/PRECAUTIONS

Acute renal failure reported in patients with underlying renal disease who have received inappropriately high doses. Caution in elderly and with renal impairment.

ADVERSE REACTIONS

Headache, N/V, diarrhea, elevated lipase, ALT elevation, fatigue, flatulence, pruritus, rash, neutropenia, abdominal pain, dysmenorrhea, migraine.

DRUG INTERACTIONS

Probenecid or other drugs significantly eliminated by active renal tubular secretion may increase levels of penciclovir. Potential interaction with drugs metabolized by and/or inhibiting aldehyde oxidase. Raloxifene may decrease formation of penciclovir.

NURSING CONSIDERATIONS

Assessment: Assess for hypersensitivity to the drug, renal impairment, pregnancy/nursing status, and possible drug interactions.

Monitoring: Monitor renal function and for adverse reactions.

Patient Counseling: Inform to take exactly ud. Advise to initiate treatment at earliest signs/symptoms of recurrence of cold sores, at the 1st sign/symptom of recurrent genital herpes if episodic therapy is indicated, and as soon as possible after a diagnosis of herpes zoster. Inform that drug is not a cure for cold sores or genital herpes. Advise to avoid contact with lesions or intercourse when lesions and/or symptoms are present to avoid infecting partners. Counsel to use safer sex practices. Instruct to refrain from driving or operating machinery if dizziness, somnolence, confusion, or other CNS disturbances occur. Inform that drug contains lactose; instruct to notify physician if with rare hereditary problems of galactose intolerance, a severe lactase deficiency, or glucose-galactose malabsorption.

Storage: 25°C (77°F); excursions permitted to 15-30°C (59-86°F).

FARXIGA – dapagliflozin RX

Class: Sodium-glucose cotransporter 2 (SGLT2) inhibitor

ADULT DOSAGE

Type 2 Diabetes Mellitus

Initial: 5mg qam

Titrate: May increase to 10mg qd

PEDIATRIC DOSAGE

Pediatric use may not have been established

DOSE MODIFICATION

Renal Impairment

eGFR <60mL/min: Do not initiate treatment

D/C therapy when eGFR is persistently <60mL/min

ADMINISTRATION

Oral route

Take w/ or w/o food

HOW SUPPLIED

Tab: 5mg, 10mg

CONTRAINDICATIONS

Severe renal impairment, ESRD, patients on dialysis.

WARNINGS/PRECAUTIONS

Not recommended for type 1 diabetes mellitus (DM) or for treatment of diabetic ketoacidosis. Do not initiate in patients with an eGFR <60mL/min. Causes intravascular volume contraction. Symptomatic hypotension may occur, particularly in patients with renal impairment (eGFR <60mL/min), elderly patients, or patients on loop diuretics; correct volume status before initiating treatment in patients with ≥1 of these characteristics. Increases SrCr and decreases eGFR; caution in elderly patients and patients with renal impairment. Adverse reactions related to renal function may occur. D/C when eGFR is persistently <60mL/min. Increases risk of genital mycotic infections. Increases in LDL levels reported. Newly diagnosed cases of bladder cancer reported; do not use in patients with active bladder cancer and caution in patients with prior history of bladder cancer. Hypersensitivity reactions (eg, angioedema, urticaria, hypersensitivity) reported; d/c and treat if this occurs and monitor until signs/symptoms resolve. Caution in patients with severe hepatic impairment. Monitoring glycemic control with urine glucose tests or 1,5-anhydroglucitol assay is not recommended.

ADVERSE REACTIONS

Genital mycotic infections, nasopharyngitis, UTIs, back pain, increased urination.

DRUG INTERACTIONS

May increase risk of hypoglycemia when combined with insulin or an insulin secretagogue; a lower dose of insulin or insulin secretagogue may be required.

NURSING CONSIDERATIONS

Assessment: Assess for diabetic ketoacidosis, type of DM, volume status, risk for genital mycotic infections, active/history of bladder cancer, drug hypersensitivity, pregnancy/nursing status, and possible drug interactions. Assess baseline renal/hepatic function, LDL levels, and BP.

Monitoring: Monitor for signs/symptoms of hypotension, genital mycotic infections, hypersensitivity reactions, and other adverse reactions. Monitor renal function and LDL levels.

Patient Counseling: Inform of the risks, benefits, and alternative modes of therapy. Advise about the importance of adherence to dietary instructions, regular physical activity, periodic blood glucose monitoring and HbA1c testing, recognition and management of hypo/hyperglycemia, and assessment of diabetes complications. Instruct to seek medical advice promptly during periods of stress (eg, fever, trauma, infection, surgery) as medication requirements may change. Instruct to immediately inform physician if pregnant, breastfeeding, planning to become pregnant or to breastfeed, or if experiencing signs/symptoms of hypotension or bladder cancer. Instruct to have adequate fluid intake. Counsel on the signs/symptoms of vaginal yeast infection, balanitis, balanoposthitis, and UTI; inform of treatment options and when to seek medical advice. Instruct to d/c therapy and consult physician if any signs/symptoms suggesting an allergic reaction or angioedema develop.

Storage: 20-25°C (68-77°F); excursions permitted between 15-30°C (59-86°F).

FELODIPINE ER – felodipine

RX

Class: Calcium channel blocker (dihydropyridine)

ADULT DOSAGE

Hypertension

Initial: 5mg qd
Titrate: May decrease to 2.5mg qd or increase to 10mg qd at intervals of not <2 weeks, depending on the patient's response
Range: 2.5-10mg qd

PEDIATRIC DOSAGE

Pediatric use may not have been established

DOSE MODIFICATION

Hepatic Impairment
Initial: 2.5mg qd

Elderly
Initial: 2.5mg qd

ADMINISTRATION

Oral route
Take regularly either w/o food or w/ a light meal
Swallow whole; do not crush or chew

HOW SUPPLIED

Tab, Extended-Release: 2.5mg, 5mg, 10mg

WARNINGS/PRECAUTIONS

May occasionally precipitate significant hypotension and, rarely, syncope. May lead to reflex tachycardia, which may precipitate angina pectoris. Caution with heart failure (HF) or compromised ventricular function, particularly in combination with a β-blocker. Closely monitor BP during dose adjustment in patients with hepatic impairment and in elderly. Peripheral edema reported. Caution in elderly.

ADVERSE REACTIONS

Peripheral edema, headache, asthenia, dyspepsia, dizziness, upper respiratory infection, flushing.

DRUG INTERACTIONS

CYP3A4 inhibitors (eg, ketoconazole, erythromycin, grapefruit juice, cimetidine) may increase plasma levels by several-fold. Decreased levels with long-term anticonvulsant therapy (eg, phenytoin, carbamazepine, phenobarbital); consider alternative antihypertensive therapy. May increase metoprolol and tacrolimus levels; monitor tacrolimus blood concentration and adjust tacrolimus dose if needed.

NURSING CONSIDERATIONS

Assessment: Assess for hypersensitivity to the drug, HF, compromised ventricular function, hepatic impairment, pregnancy/nursing status, and possible drug interactions.

Monitoring: Monitor for syncope, angina pectoris, peripheral edema, and other adverse reactions. Monitor BP.

Patient Counseling: Inform that mild gingival hyperplasia (gum swelling) has been reported and that good dental hygiene decreases its incidence and severity.

Storage: 20-25°C (68-77°F). Protect from light.

Femara – letrozole

RX

Class: Nonsteroidal aromatase inhibitor

ADULT DOSAGE

Breast Cancer

Adjuvant Treatment of Postmenopausal Women w/ Hormone Receptor Positive Early Breast Cancer:
2.5mg qd; d/c at relapse

Extended Adjuvant Treatment of Early Breast Cancer in Postmenopausal Women, Who Have Received 5 Years of Adjuvant Tamoxifen Therapy:
2.5mg qd; d/c at tumor relapse

1st-Line Treatment of Postmenopausal Women w/ Hormone Receptor Positive or Unknown, Locally Advanced or Metastatic Breast Cancer; Treatment of Advanced Breast Cancer in Postmenopausal Women w/ Disease Progression Following Antiestrogen Therapy:
2.5mg qd; continue until tumor progression is evident

PEDIATRIC DOSAGE

Pediatric use may not have been established

DOSE MODIFICATION

Hepatic Impairment

Cirrhosis/Severe Hepatic Dysfunction: 2.5mg qod

ADMINISTRATION

Oral route

Take w/o regard to meals

HOW SUPPLIED

Tab: 2.5mg

CONTRAINDICATIONS

Women who are or may become pregnant.

WARNINGS/PRECAUTIONS

May decrease bone mineral density (BMD); consider monitoring BMD. Bone fractures and osteoporosis reported. Hypercholesterolemia reported; consider monitoring serum cholesterol levels. Reduce dose by 50% with cirrhosis and severe hepatic impairment. May impair physical/mental abilities. Moderate decreases in lymphocyte counts and thrombocytopenia reported.

ADVERSE REACTIONS

Hypercholesterolemia, hot flushes, fatigue, edema, arthralgia/arthritis, myalgia, headache, dizziness, night sweats, nausea, back pain, bone fractures, weight increase, depression, osteopenia.

DRUG INTERACTIONS

Reduced plasma levels with coadministered tamoxifen.

NURSING CONSIDERATIONS

Assessment: Assess for premenopausal endocrine status, cirrhosis or hepatic impairment, pregnancy/nursing status, and possible drug interactions.

Monitoring: Monitor for bone fractures, osteoporosis, fatigue, dizziness, somnolence, and other adverse reactions. Monitor BMD and serum cholesterol levels.

Patient Counseling: Inform that the drug is contraindicated in pregnant women and women of premenopausal endocrine status. Counsel perimenopausal and recently postmenopausal women to use contraception until postmenopausal status is fully established. Advise about possible fatigue, dizziness, and somnolence; caution against operating machinery/driving. Advise that BMD may be monitored while on therapy.

Storage: 25°C (77°F); excursions permitted to 15-30°C (59-86°F).

FENTANYL INJECTION – fentanyl citrate CII

Class: Opioid analgesic

ADULT DOSAGE

Anesthesia

Premedication:
50-100mcg (1-2mL) IM 30-60 min prior to surgery

General Anesthesia:
50-100mcg/kg (1-2mL/kg) w/ oxygen and a muscle relaxant
Max: 150mcg/kg (3mL/kg)

Adjunct to General Anesthesia:
Low Dose: 2mcg/kg (0.04mL/kg)
Moderate Dose: 2-20mcg/kg (0.04-0.4mL/kg)
High-Dose: 20-50mcg/kg (0.4-1mL/kg)

Adjunct to Regional Anesthesia:
50-100mcg (1-2mL) IM or slow IV over 1-2 min

Postoperatively (Recovery Room):
50-100mcg (1-2mL); repeat dose in 1-2 hrs prn

Administer w/ a neuroleptic (eg, droperidol inj) for the induction of anesthesia and as an adjunct in the maint of general and regional anesthesia

Use w/ oxygen in selected high-risk patients (eg, those undergoing open-heart surgery or certain complicated neurological or orthopedic procedures)

PEDIATRIC DOSAGE

Anesthesia

2-12 Years:
Induction/Maint: 2-3mcg/kg

DOSE MODIFICATION

Elderly
Reduce initial dose

Other Important Modifications
Debilitated Patients: Reduce initial dose

ADMINISTRATION

IM/IV route

HOW SUPPLIED

Inj: 50mcg/mL [5mL]

WARNINGS/PRECAUTIONS

Administer only if specifically trained in the use of IV anesthetics and management of the respiratory effects of potent opioids. An opioid antagonist, resuscitative and intubation equipment, and oxygen should be readily available. Fluids and other countermeasures to manage hypotension should be available when used w/ tranquilizers. Initial dose reduction recommended w/ narcotic analgesia for recovery. May cause muscle rigidity, particularly w/ muscles used for respiration. Adequate facilities should be available for postoperative monitoring and ventilation. May cause euphoria, miosis, bradycardia, and bronchoconstriction. Caution in respiratory depression-susceptible patients (eg, comatose patients w/ head injury or brain tumor); may obscure the clinical course of patients w/ head injury. Caution w/ COPD, decreased respiratory reserve, potentially compromised respiration, liver/kidney dysfunction, and cardiac bradyarrhythmias. Monitor vital signs routinely.

ADVERSE REACTIONS

Respiratory depression, apnea, rigidity, bradycardia.

DRUG INTERACTIONS

Severe and unpredictable potentiation w/ MAOIs; appropriate monitoring and availability of vasodilators and β-blockers for HTN treatment is indicated. Additive or potentiating effects w/ other CNS depressants (eg, barbiturates, tranquilizers, narcotics, general anesthetics); reduce dose of other CNS depressants. Reports of cardiovascular (CV) depression w/ nitrous oxide. Alteration of respiration w/ certain forms of conduction anesthesia (eg, spinal anesthesia, some peridural anesthetics). Decreased pulmonary arterial pressure and hypotension w/ tranquilizers (eg, droperidol). May increase BP in patients w/ or w/o HTN w/ droperidol. May cause CV depression w/ diazepam.

NURSING CONSIDERATIONS

Assessment: Assess level of pain intensity, patient's general condition and medical status, or any other conditions where treatment is contraindicated or cautioned. Assess for history of hypersensitivity, pregnancy/nursing status, renal/hepatic function, and possible drug interactions. Assess use in elderly and debilitated patients.

Monitoring: Monitor for signs/symptoms of respiratory depression, muscle rigidity, medication abuse, and drug dependence. If given w/ nitrous oxide, monitor for CV depression. If administered w/ a tranquilizer, monitor for hypotension and hypovolemia. If combined w/ droperidol, monitor for increases in BP; perform ECG monitoring. Perform routine monitoring of vital signs.

Patient Counseling: Advise patient about the benefits and risks of the medication. Instruct to notify physician if any adverse reactions occur.

Storage: 20-25°C (68-77°F); excursions permitted to 15-30°C (59-86°F). Protect from light.

FENTORA – fentanyl CII

Class: Opioid analgesic

Fatal respiratory depression may occur. Contraindicated in the management of acute or postoperative pain (eg, headache/migraine) and in opioid-nontolerant patients. Keep out of reach of children. Concomitant use with CYP3A4 inhibitors may increase plasma levels, and may cause fatal respiratory depression. Do not convert patients on a mcg-per-mcg basis from any other fentanyl products to Fentora. Do not substitute for any other fentanyl products; may result in fatal overdose. Contains fentanyl with abuse liability similar to other opioid analgesics. Available only through a restricted program called Transmucosal Immediate Release Fentanyl Risk Evaluation Mitigation Strategy (TIRF REMS) Access program due to risk of misuse, abuse, addiction, and overdose. Outpatients, healthcare professionals who prescribe to outpatients, pharmacies, and distributors must enroll in this program.

ADULT DOSAGE

Cancer Pain

Breakthrough Pain:
Initial: 100mcg
Max: 2 doses/episode of breakthrough pain
Titrate:
If higher dose is needed, may give two 100mcg tabs (1 on each side of the mouth) w/their next breakthrough pain episode
May titrate to two 100mcg tabs on each side of mouth (total of four 100mcg tabs), if pain is not adequately controlled
For doses >400mcg, titrate using multiples of 200mcg tabs
Do not use >4 tabs simultaneously
Maint:
Once titrated to effective dose, use only 1 tab of the appropriate strength per breakthrough pain episode
If breakthrough pain is not relieved after 30 min, may give only 1 additional dose of the same strength for that episode; wait at least 4 hrs before treating another breakthrough pain episode
If >4 episodes/day are experienced, dose of the around-the-clock opioid should be reevaluated

Conversions

Initial Fentora Dose Based on Current Actiq Dose:
200mcg of Actiq: 100mcg
400mcg of Actiq: 100mcg
600mcg of Actiq: 200mcg
800mcg of Actiq: 200mcg
1200mcg of Actiq: 2 x 200mcg tabs
1600mcg of Actiq: 2 x 200mcg tabs
Titrate to effective dose

PEDIATRIC DOSAGE

Pediatric use may not have been established

DOSE MODIFICATION

Discontinuation
Gradual downward titration is recommended

ADMINISTRATION

Buccal/SL route

Do not split, crush, suck, chew, or swallow whole
Do not attempt to push tab through the blister as this may cause damage to the tab
Immediately place entire tab in the buccal cavity (above a rear molar, between the upper cheek and gum)
Once effective dose is determined during titration, an alternate route is SL
Leave tab in place until it has disintegrated (usually about 14-25 min)
If remnants from the tab remain after 30 min, may swallow w/ a glass of water
Alternate sides of the mouth when administering subsequent doses in the buccal cavity

HOW SUPPLIED

Tab, Buccal: 100mcg, 200mcg, 400mcg, 600mcg, 800mcg

CONTRAINDICATIONS

Opioid-nontolerant patients, management of acute or postoperative pain, including headache/migraine and dental pain.

WARNINGS/PRECAUTIONS

Increased risk of respiratory depression in patients with underlying respiratory disorders and in elderly/debilitated. May impair mental and/or physical abilities. Caution with chronic obstructive pulmonary disease or preexisting medical conditions predisposing to respiratory depression; may further decrease respiratory drive to the point of respiratory failure. May obscure clinical course of head injuries; use extreme caution in patients who may be susceptible to the intracranial effects of carbon dioxide retention (eg, with evidence of increased intracranial pressure or impaired consciousness). Application-site reactions (paresthesia, ulceration, bleeding) reported. Avoid use during labor and delivery. Caution with renal/hepatic impairment, bradyarrhythmias, and in elderly.

ADVERSE REACTIONS

Respiratory depression, headache, N/V, constipation, dizziness, dyspnea, somnolence, fatigue, anemia, asthenia, abdominal pain, dehydration, peripheral edema, diarrhea, anorexia.

DRUG INTERACTIONS

See Boxed Warning. CYP3A4 inducers (eg, carbamazepine, efavirenz, modafinil, phenobarbital, pioglitazone, rifampin, St. John's wort) may decrease levels. Respiratory depression is more likely to occur when given with other drugs that depress respiration. Increased depressant effects with other CNS depressants (eg, sedatives, hypnotics, tranquilizers, skeletal muscle relaxants, sedating antihistamines, alcohol); consider adjusting fentanyl dose if warranted. Not recommended for use in patients who have received MAOIs within 14 days.

NURSING CONSIDERATIONS

Assessment: Assess for degree of opioid tolerance, previous opioid dose, type and severity of pain, general condition and medical status, and any other conditions where treatment is contraindicated or cautioned. Assess for hypersensitivity to the drug, renal/hepatic impairment, pregnancy/nursing status, and possible drug interactions.

Monitoring: Monitor for signs/symptoms of respiratory depression, impairment of mental/physical abilities, application-site reactions, bradycardia, drug abuse/addiction, and other adverse reactions.

Patient Counseling: Instruct outpatients to enroll in the TIRF REMS Access program. Instruct to keep drug out of reach of children. Advise to take ud and to not share it with anyone else. Instruct to notify physician if breakthrough pain is not alleviated or worsens after taking the drug. Inform that drug may impair mental/physical abilities; caution against performing activities that require high level of attention (eg, operating machinery/driving). Advise not to combine with alcohol, sleep aids, or tranquilizers except by order of prescribing physician. Instruct to notify physician if pregnant or planning to become pregnant. Inform of proper storage, administration, and disposal.

Storage: 20-25°C (68-77°F); excursions permitted to 15-30°C (59-86°F). Protect from freezing and moisture.

FETZIMA – levomilnacipran RX

Class: Serotonin and norepinephrine reuptake inhibitor

Antidepressants increased the risk of suicidal thoughts and behavior in children, adolescents, and young adults in short-term studies. Monitor and observe closely for worsening, and for emergence of suicidal thoughts and behaviors. Not approved for use in pediatric patients.

ADULT DOSAGE

Major Depressive Disorder

Initial: 20mg qd for 2 days
Titrate: Increase to 40mg qd. Based on efficacy and tolerability, may then be increased in increments of 40mg at intervals of ≥2 days
Range: 40-120mg qd

PEDIATRIC DOSAGE

Pediatric use may not have been established

Max: 120mg qd
Periodically reassess need for maint treatment and the appropriate dose

Dosing Considerations with MAOIs

Switching to/from an MAOI for Psychiatric Disorders:
Allow at least 14 days between discontinuation of an MAOI and initiation of treatment, and allow at least 7 days between discontinuation of treatment and initiation of an MAOI

W/ Other MAOIs (eg, Linezolid, IV Methylene Blue):
Do not start levomilnacipran in patients being treated w/ linezolid or IV methylene blue
In patients already receiving levomilnacipran, if acceptable alternatives are not available and benefits outweigh risks, d/c levomilnacipran and administer linezolid or IV methylene blue; monitor for serotonin syndrome for 2 weeks or until 24 hrs after the last dose of linezolid or IV methylene blue, whichever comes 1st. May resume levomilnacipran therapy 24 hrs after the last dose of linezolid or IV methylene blue

---

DOSE MODIFICATION

Concomitant Medications
Use w/ Strong CYP3A4 Inhibitors:
Max: 80mg qd

Renal Impairment
Moderate (CrCl 30-59mL/min):
Max Maint: 80mg qd
Severe (CrCl 15-29mL/min):
Max Maint: 40mg qd
ESRD: Not recommended

Discontinuation
Gradually reduce dose, whenever possible; if intolerable symptoms occur following a dose decrease or upon discontinuation of treatment, consider resuming previously prescribed dose and decreasing the dose at a more gradual rate

ADMINISTRATION
Oral route
Take at the same time each day, w/ or w/o food
Swallow cap whole; do not open, chew, or crush

HOW SUPPLIED
Cap, Extended-Release: 20mg, 40mg, 80mg, 120mg; (Titration Pack) 20mg [2^s], 40mg [26^s]

CONTRAINDICATIONS
Use of an MAOI for psychiatric disorders either concomitantly or within 7 days of stopping treatment. Treatment within 14 days of stopping an MAOI for psychiatric disorders. Starting treatment in patients being treated with other MAOIs (eg, linezolid, IV methylene blue).

WARNINGS/PRECAUTIONS
Not recommended for patients with end-stage renal disease. Not approved for the treatment of bipolar depression. Serotonin syndrome reported; d/c immediately if symptoms occur and initiate supportive symptomatic treatment. Associated with increases in BP and HR; control preexisting HTN or treat preexisting tachyarrhythmias and other cardiac disease before initiating treatment. Caution with preexisting HTN, cardiovascular (CV) or cerebrovascular conditions that might be compromised by increases in BP. Consider discontinuation or other appropriate medical intervention if sustained increase in BP or HR occurs. May increase risk of bleeding events. Pupillary dilation that occurs following therapy may trigger an angle-closure attack in a patient with anatomically narrow angles who does not have a patent iridectomy. May affect urethral resistance; caution in patients prone to obstructive urinary disorders. If symptoms of urinary hesitation, urinary retention, or dysuria develop, consider discontinuation or other appropriate medical intervention. Activation of mania/hypomania reported; caution with history or family history of bipolar disorder, mania, or hypomania. Seizures reported; caution in patients with a seizure disorder. Discontinuation symptoms may occur. Avoid abrupt discontinuation; reduce dose gradually whenever possible. Hyponatremia may occur; elderly and volume-depleted patients may be at greater risk. D/C in patients with symptomatic hyponatremia and institute appropriate medical intervention.

ADVERSE REACTIONS

N/V, constipation, hyperhidrosis, HR/BP increased, erectile dysfunction, tachycardia, palpitations, testicular pain, ejaculation disorder, urinary hesitation, hot flush, hypotension, HTN, decreased appetite.

DRUG INTERACTIONS

See Contraindications and Dosage. May cause serotonin syndrome with other serotonergic drugs (eg, triptans, TCAs, fentanyl, lithium, St. John's wort) and with drugs that impair metabolism of serotonin; d/c immediately if serotonin syndrome occurs. Caution with NSAIDs, aspirin (ASA), warfarin, and other drugs that affect coagulation or bleeding due to potential increased risk of bleeding. Increased exposure with CYP3A4 inhibitor ketoconazole. Caution with other CNS-active drugs, including those with a similar mechanism of action. Do not give with alcohol; pronounced accelerated drug release may occur. Caution with drugs that increase BP and HR. Increased risk of hyponatremia with diuretics.

NURSING CONSIDERATIONS

Assessment: Assess for risk for bipolar disorder, HTN, CV/cerebrovascular conditions, tachyarrhythmias, susceptibility to angle-closure glaucoma/obstructive urinary disorders, history of mania/hypomania, seizure disorder, volume depletion, hypersensitivity to the drug, renal impairment, pregnancy/nursing status, and possible drug interactions.

Monitoring: Monitor for signs/symptoms of clinical worsening, suicidality, unusual changes in behavior, serotonin syndrome, bleeding events, angle-closure glaucoma, urinary hesitation/retention, dysuria, activation of mania/hypomania, seizures, discontinuation symptoms, hyponatremia, and other adverse reactions. Monitor BP and HR periodically. Periodically reassess the need for maintenance treatment and the appropriate dose.

Patient Counseling: Advise about the benefits and risks of therapy and counsel on its appropriate use. Counsel to look for the emergence of suicidality, especially early during treatment and when the dose is adjusted up or down. Caution about the risk of serotonin syndrome, particularly with the concomitant use with other serotonergic agents. Inform that concomitant use with ASA, NSAIDs, warfarin, or other drugs that affect coagulation may increase the risk of abnormal bleeding. Inform that drug can cause mild pupillary dilation, which in susceptible individuals, can lead to an episode of angle-closure glaucoma. Advise to have BP and HR monitored regularly, to observe for signs of activation of mania/hypomania, to avoid alcohol consumption, and not to d/c therapy without notifying physician. Caution against operating hazardous machinery until reasonably certain that therapy does not adversely affect ability to engage in such activities. Advise to notify physician if allergic reactions develop, if pregnant/intending to become pregnant, or if breastfeeding.

Storage: 25°C (77°F); excursions permitted between 15-30°C (59-86°F).

FINACEA – azelaic acid RX

Class: Dicarboxylic acid antimicrobial

ADULT DOSAGE

Rosacea

Inflammatory Papules/Pustules of Mild to Moderate Rosacea:

Apply and gently massage thin layer into affected areas on the face bid (am and pm)

Reassess if no improvement observed upon completing 12 weeks of therapy

PEDIATRIC DOSAGE

Pediatric use may not have been established

ADMINISTRATION

Topical route

Cleanse affected area w/ very mild soaps or soapless cleansing lotion and pat dry w/ soft towel before application

Cosmetics may be applied after the application of gel has dried

Avoid the use of occlusive dressings or wrappings

Avoid spicy foods, thermally hot foods and drinks, and alcoholic beverages

HOW SUPPLIED

Gel: 15% [45g pump, 50g tube]

WARNINGS/PRECAUTIONS

Cases of adverse skin reactions due to hypersensitivity reported; d/c if hypersensitivity develops and institute appropriate therapy. Skin irritation (eg, pruritus, burning, stinging) may occur during 1st few weeks of treatment; d/c if sensitivity or severe irritation develops/persists and institute appropriate therapy. Hypopigmentation reported. Avoid contact w/ eyes, mouth, and other mucous membranes.

ADVERSE REACTIONS

Burning/stinging/tingling, pruritus, scaling/dry skin/xerosis, erythema/irritation.

NURSING CONSIDERATIONS

Assessment: Assess for pregnancy/nursing status.

Monitoring: Monitor for sensitivity reactions or skin irritation/reaction and other adverse reactions. Monitor for early signs of hypopigmentation in patients w/ dark complexion.

Patient Counseling: Inform that medication is for external use only. Instruct to avoid contact w/ eyes, mouth, and other mucous membranes; if contact w/ eyes occurs, instruct to wash eyes w/ large amounts of water and to consult physician if eye irritation persists. Advise to avoid alcoholic cleansers, tinctures and astringents, abrasives, and peeling agents. Instruct to wash hands immediately after application. Inform that cosmetics may be applied after application of gel has dried. Instruct to avoid using occlusive dressings or wrappings and to avoid eating spicy foods, alcoholic beverages, and thermally hot food and drinks. Inform that skin irritation may occur, usually during 1st few weeks of treatment; if irritation is excessive or persists, or allergic reactions occur, instruct to d/c therapy and consult a physician. Instruct to report abnormal changes in skin color. Instruct on how to properly use pump.

Storage: 25°C (77°F); excursions permitted to 15-30°C (59-86°F).

FIORICET – acetaminophen/butalbital/caffeine RX

Class: Analgesic/barbiturate

Associated w/ cases of acute liver failure, at times resulting in liver transplant and death. Most cases of liver injury are associated w/ acetaminophen (APAP) use at doses >4000mg/day, and often involve >1 APAP-containing product.

ADULT DOSAGE

Tension Headache

Relief of the Symptom Complex of Tension (or Muscle Contraction) Headache:
1-2 caps q4h prn
Max: 6 caps/day

PEDIATRIC DOSAGE

Tension Headache

Relief of the Symptom Complex of Tension (or Muscle Contraction) Headache:
≥12 Years:
1-2 caps q4h prn
Max: 6 caps/day

DOSE MODIFICATION

Elderly

Start at lower end of dosing range

ADMINISTRATION

Oral route

HOW SUPPLIED

Cap: (Butalbital-APAP-Caffeine) 50mg-300mg-40mg

CONTRAINDICATIONS

Porphyria.

WARNINGS/PRECAUTIONS

Not for extended and repeated use; may be habit-forming and potentially abusable. Increased risk of acute liver failure in patients w/ underlying liver disease. May cause serious skin reactions (eg, acute generalized exanthematous pustulosis, Stevens-Johnson syndrome, toxic epidermal necrolysis), which can be fatal; d/c at the 1st appearance of skin rash or any other sign of hypersensitivity. Hypersensitivity and anaphylaxis reported; d/c immediately if signs/symptoms occur. Caution w/ severe renal/hepatic impairment, acute abdominal conditions, and in elderly or debilitated patients. Lab test interactions may occur.

ADVERSE REACTIONS

Acute liver failure, drowsiness, lightheadedness, dizziness, sedation, SOB, N/V, abdominal pain, intoxicated feeling.

DRUG INTERACTIONS

CNS effects may be enhanced by MAOIs. May enhance CNS depressant effects of other narcotic analgesics, alcohol, general anesthetics, tranquilizers (eg, chlordiazepoxide), sedative hypnotics, or other CNS depressants. Increased risk of acute liver failure w/ alcohol ingestion.

NURSING CONSIDERATIONS

Assessment: Assess for hypersensitivity or intolerance to any component of the drug, porphyria, alcohol intake, renal/hepatic impairment, or any other conditions where treatment is contraindicated or cautioned, pregnancy/nursing status, and for possible drug interactions.

Monitoring: Monitor for signs/symptoms of hepatotoxicity, skin/hypersensitivity/anaphylactic reactions, drug abuse/dependence, and other adverse reactions. Monitor effects of therapy w/ serial LFTs and/or renal function tests in patients w/ severe hepatic or renal disease.

Patient Counseling: Instruct to look for APAP on package labels and not to use >1 APAP-containing product. Instruct to seek medical attention immediately upon ingestion of >4000mg/day of APAP, even if patient is feeling well. Inform that drug may impair mental/physical abilities; advise to avoid performing hazardous tasks (eg, driving/operating machinery). Instruct to avoid drinking alcohol or taking other CNS depressants. Inform that therapy may be habit-forming; advise to take ud. Instruct to d/c and contact physician immediately if signs of allergy (eg, rash or difficulty breathing) develop.

Storage: 20-25°C (68-77°F).

FLAGYL – metronidazole

Class: Nitroimidazole

RX

Shown to be carcinogenic in mice and rats. Avoid unnecessary use. Should be reserved for the conditions for which it is indicated.

ADULT DOSAGE

Anaerobic Bacterial Infections

IV metronidazole is usually administered initially in the treatment of most serious infections

Cap/Tab:

Usual: 7.5mg/kg q6h

Max: 4g/24 hrs

Duration: 7-10 days; bone/joint, lower respiratory tract, and endocardium infections may require longer treatment

Trichomoniasis

Female:

Seven-Day Course of Treatment:

Cap:

375mg bid for 7 consecutive days

Tab:

250mg tid for 7 consecutive days

One-Day Treatment:

Tab:

2g given as a single dose or in two divided doses of 1g each, given in the same day

When repeat courses are required, allow an interval of 4-6 weeks between courses, and reconfirm presence of the trichomonas

Male:

Cap/Tab:

Individualize treatment as it is for the female

Amebiasis

Acute Intestinal Amebiasis (Acute Amebic Dysentery):

Cap/Tab:

750mg tid for 5-10 days

Amebic Liver Abscess:

Cap/Tab:

750mg tid for 5-10 days

Tab:

500mg tid for 5-10 days

PEDIATRIC DOSAGE

Amebiasis

Cap/Tab:

35-50mg/kg/24 hrs, divided into 3 doses, for 10 days

DOSE MODIFICATION

Renal Impairment

Cap/Tab:

Hemodialysis: Consider supplementation of metronidazole dosage following hemodialysis session, if administration cannot be separated from hemodialysis session

Hepatic Impairment
Severe (Child-Pugh C):
Cap:
Amebiasis: 375mg q8h for 5-10 days
Trichomoniasis: 375mg q24h for 7 days
Tab:
Reduce dosage by 50%

ADMINISTRATION
Oral route

HOW SUPPLIED
Cap: 375mg; Tab: 250mg, 500mg

CONTRAINDICATIONS
Disulfiram use w/in the last 2 weeks. Consumption of alcohol or products containing propylene glycol during and for at least 3 days after therapy. Use during the 1st trimester of pregnancy in trichomoniasis patients.

WARNINGS/PRECAUTIONS
Cases of encephalopathy and peripheral neuropathy (including optic neuropathy), convulsive seizures, and aseptic meningitis reported; promptly evaluate benefit/risk ratio of the continuation of therapy if abnormal neurologic signs/symptoms appear. Known or previously unrecognized candidiasis may present more prominent symptoms during therapy and requires treatment w/ a candidacidal agent. Caution w/ hepatic/renal impairment, evidence of or history of blood dyscrasia, and in the elderly. Mild leukopenia reported; monitor total and differential leukocyte counts before and after therapy. May result in bacterial/parasitic resistance if used in the absence of proven or suspected bacterial/parasitic infection, or a prophylactic indication. Lab test interactions may occur. (Tab) In pregnant patients for whom alternative treatment has been inadequate, the one-day course of therapy should not be used.

ADVERSE REACTIONS
Headache, syncope, dizziness, vertigo, incoordination, nausea, diarrhea, epigastric distress, abdominal cramping, constipation, unpleasant metallic taste, erythematous rash, pruritus, urticaria, dysuria.

DRUG INTERACTIONS
See Contraindications. May potentiate anticoagulant effect of warfarin and other oral coumarin anticoagulants, resulting in PT prolongation; carefully monitor PT and INR. May increase serum lithium, and may cause lithium toxicity; obtain serum lithium and SrCr levels several days after beginning metronidazole. May increase busulfan concentrations, which can result in increased risk for serious busulfan toxicity; avoid concomitant use, or, if coadministration is medically needed, frequently monitor busulfan concentration and adjust busulfan dose accordingly. Simultaneous administration of drugs that decrease microsomal liver enzyme activity (eg, cimetidine) may prolong $T_{1/2}$ and decrease clearance. Simultaneous administration of drugs that induce microsomal liver enzymes (eg, phenytoin, phenobarbital) may accelerate elimination, resulting in reduced levels. Impaired clearance of phenytoin reported.

NURSING CONSIDERATIONS

Assessment: Assess for candidiasis, alcohol use, hepatic/renal impairment, evidence/history of blood dyscrasia, hypersensitivity to drug or other nitroimidazole derivatives, pregnancy/nursing status, and possible drug interactions. Obtain total and differential leukocyte counts.

Monitoring: Monitor for abnormal neurologic signs/symptoms, candidiasis, and other adverse reactions. Monitor total and differential leukocyte counts after therapy. Monitor PT and INR w/ oral coumarin anticoagulants (eg, warfarin).

Patient Counseling: Instruct to d/c consumption of alcoholic beverages or products containing propylene glycol while taking the drug and for at least 3 days afterward. Counsel that therapy should only be used to treat bacterial and parasitic, not viral, infections. Instruct to take exactly ud. Inform that skipping doses or not completing the full course of therapy may decrease effectiveness of treatment and increase bacterial resistance.

Storage: (Cap) 15-25°C (59-77°F). (Tab) <25°C (77°F). Protect from light.

FLAGYL ER – metronidazole RX

Class: Nitroimidazole

Shown to be carcinogenic in mice and rats. Avoid unnecessary use. Should be reserved for the conditions for which it is indicated.

ADULT DOSAGE
Bacterial Vaginosis
Nonpregnant Women:
750mg qd for 7 consecutive days

PEDIATRIC DOSAGE
Bacterial Vaginosis
Post-Menarche/Nonpregnant Females:
750mg qd for 7 consecutive days

DOSE MODIFICATION

Renal Impairment

Hemodialysis: If administration cannot be separated from hemodialysis session, consider supplementation of dosage following the session, depending on patient's clinical situation

Elderly

May need to adjust dose based on serum levels

ADMINISTRATION

Oral route

Take at least 1 hr ac or 2 hrs pc
Do not split, chew, or crush

HOW SUPPLIED

Tab, Extended-Release: 750mg

CONTRAINDICATIONS

Disulfiram use within the last 2 weeks. Consumption of alcohol or products containing propylene glycol during and for at least 3 days after therapy.

WARNINGS/PRECAUTIONS

Cases of encephalopathy and peripheral neuropathy (including optic neuropathy), convulsive seizures, and aseptic meningitis reported; promptly evaluate benefit/risk ratio of the continuation of therapy if abnormal neurologic signs/symptoms appear. Known or previously unrecognized candidiasis may present more prominent symptoms during therapy and requires treatment with a candidacidal agent. Do not administer to patients with severe (Child-Pugh C) hepatic impairment unless benefits outweigh risks. Caution with hepatic/renal impairment, evidence of or history of blood dyscrasia, and in the elderly. Mild leukopenia reported; monitor total and differential leukocyte counts before and after therapy. May result in bacterial resistance if used in the absence of proven or suspected bacterial infection, or a prophylactic indication. Lab test interactions may occur.

ADVERSE REACTIONS

Headache, vaginitis, nausea, metallic taste, bacterial infection, influenza-like symptoms, genital pruritus, abdominal pain, dizziness, diarrhea, upper respiratory tract infection, rhinitis, sinusitis, pharyngitis, dysmenorrhea.

DRUG INTERACTIONS

See Contraindications. May potentiate anticoagulant effect of warfarin and other oral coumarin anticoagulants, resulting in PT prolongation; carefully monitor PT and INR. May increase serum lithium, and may cause lithium toxicity; obtain serum lithium and SrCr levels several days after beginning metronidazole. May increase busulfan concentrations, which can result in increased risk for serious busulfan toxicity; avoid concomitant use, or, if coadministration is medically needed, frequently monitor busulfan concentration and adjust busulfan dose accordingly. Simultaneous administration of drugs that decrease microsomal liver enzyme activity (eg, cimetidine) may prolong $T_{1/2}$ and decrease clearance. Simultaneous administration of drugs that induce microsomal liver enzymes (eg, phenytoin, phenobarbital) may accelerate elimination, resulting in reduced levels. Impaired clearance of phenytoin reported.

NURSING CONSIDERATIONS

Assessment: Assess for candidiasis, alcohol use, hepatic/renal impairment, evidence/history of blood dyscrasia, hypersensitivity to drug or other nitroimidazole derivatives, pregnancy/nursing status, and possible drug interactions. Obtain total and differential leukocyte counts.

Monitoring: Monitor for abnormal neurologic signs/symptoms, candidiasis, and other adverse reactions. Monitor total and differential leukocyte counts after therapy. Monitor PT and INR with oral coumarin anticoagulants (eg, warfarin).

Patient Counseling: Instruct to d/c consumption of alcoholic beverages or products containing propylene glycol while taking the drug and for at least 3 days afterward. Counsel that therapy should only be used to treat bacterial, not viral (eg, common cold), infections. Instruct to take exactly ud. Inform that skipping doses or not completing full course of therapy may decrease effectiveness of treatment and increase bacterial resistance.

Storage: 25°C (77°F); excursions permitted to 15-30°C (59-86°F). Store in a dry place.

FLECAINIDE – flecainide acetate

RX

Class: Class IC antiarrhythmic

Excessive mortality or nonfatal cardiac arrest rate reported in patients with asymptomatic non-life-threatening ventricular arrhythmias who had MI >6 days but <2 yrs previously. It is prudent to consider the risks of Class IC agents, coupled with the lack of any evidence of improved survival, generally unacceptable in patients without life-threatening ventricular arrhythmias, even if patients are experiencing unpleasant, but not life-threatening, symptoms or signs. Ventricular tachycardia (VT) reported in patients treated for paroxysmal atrial fibrillation/flutter (PAF). Use not recommended in patients with chronic A-fib. Case reports of ventricular proarrhythmic effects in patients treated for A-fib/atrial flutter (A-flutter) have included increased premature ventricular contractions (PVCs), VT, ventricular fibrillation (VF), and death. Patients treated for A-flutter have been reported with 1:1 atrioventricular (AV) conduction due to slowing the atrial rate. A paradoxical increase in ventricular rate also may occur in patients with A-fib. Concomitant negative chronotropic therapy (eg, digoxin, β-blockers) may lower the risk of this complication.

ADULT DOSAGE

Paroxysmal Supraventricular Tachycardia

Prevention of paroxysmal supraventricular tachycardias, including atrioventricular nodal reentrant tachycardia, atrioventricular reentrant tachycardia, and other supraventricular tachycardias of unspecified mechanism associated w/ disabling symptoms in patients w/o structural heart disease

Initial: 50mg q12h
Titrate: May increase in increments of 50mg bid every 4 days until efficacy is achieved
Max: 300mg/day
Inadequately Controlled: May dose at 8h intervals

Paroxysmal Atrial Fibrillation/Flutter

Prevention of paroxysmal atrial fibrillation/flutter associated w/ disabling symptoms in patients w/o structural heart disease

Initial: 50mg q12h
Titrate: May increase in increments of 50mg bid every 4 days until efficacy is achieved
Inadequately Controlled: May dose at 8h intervals

May achieve substantial increase in efficacy w/o a substantial increase in discontinuations for adverse experiences by increasing the dose from 50-100mg bid

Ventricular Arrhythmias

Prevention of documented ventricular arrhythmias (life-threatening)

Sustained Ventricular Tachycardia:
Initial: 100mg q12h
Titrate: May increase in increments of 50mg bid every 4 days until efficacy is achieved
Max: 400mg/day

PEDIATRIC DOSAGE

Arrhythmias

<6 Months of Age:
Initial: 50mg/m²/day divided into 2 or 3 equally spaced doses

>6 Months of Age:
Initial: 100mg/m²/day divided into 2 or 3 equally spaced doses

Max: 200mg/m²/day

DOSE MODIFICATION

Concomitant Medications

Amiodarone: Reduce dose by 50%

Renal Impairment

Less Severe Renal Disease:
Initial: 100mg q12h
Severe (CrCl ≤35mL/min):
Initial: 100mg qd or 50mg bid

Other Important Modifications

Transferring from Another Antiarrhythmic: Allow at least 2-4 plasma half-lives to elapse for the drug being discontinued before starting therapy

Inadequately Controlled Patients: May dose at 8h intervals. Once adequate control is achieved, may be possible to reduce the dose as necessary in some patients. Evaluate efficacy at lower dose in these patients

ADMINISTRATION

Oral route

Initiate therapy in-hospital w/ rhythm monitoring for patients w/ sustained ventricular tachycardia

HOW SUPPLIED
Tab: 50mg, 100mg*, 150mg* *scored

CONTRAINDICATIONS
Preexisting 2nd- or 3rd-degree AV block, right bundle branch block associated with left hemiblock (without a pacemaker), presence of cardiogenic shock.

WARNINGS/PRECAUTIONS
May cause new or worsened supraventricular or ventricular arrhythmias. May cause or worsen CHF; caution with history of CHF or myocardial dysfunction. Close attention must be given to maintenance of cardiac function. Slows cardiac conduction, producing dose-related increases in PR, QRS, and QT intervals; may consider dose reduction. Rare cases of torsades de pointes-type arrhythmia reported. Conduction changes (eg, sinus pause, sinus arrest, symptomatic bradycardia, 2nd- or 3rd-degree AV block) reported; manage on the lowest effective dose. D/C therapy if 2nd- or 3rd-degree AV block, or right bundle branch block associated with a left hemiblock occurs, unless a temporary or implanted ventricular pacemaker is in place to ensure an adequate ventricular rate. Extreme caution with sick sinus syndrome. May increase endocardial pacing thresholds and suppress ventricular escape rhythms; caution in patients with permanent pacemakers or temporary pacing electrodes. Should not be administered with existing poor thresholds or nonprogrammable pacemakers unless suitable pacing rescue is available. Hypokalemia/hyperkalemia may alter effects. Should not be used in hepatic impairment unless benefits clearly outweigh the risks; if used, caution in dosage increases. Start therapy of patients with sustained VT and pediatric patients in the hospital with rhythm monitoring.

ADVERSE REACTIONS
Cardiac arrest, increased PVCs, VT, VF, arrhythmias, CHF, dizziness, visual disturbances, headache, fatigue, nausea, palpitation, dyspnea, chest pain, asthenia.

DRUG INTERACTIONS
Coadministration may increase digoxin levels. Additive negative inotropic effects with β-blockers (eg, propranolol). Concomitant enzyme inducers (phenytoin, phenobarbital, carbamazepine) may increase the rate of elimination. Cimetidine may increase levels and $T_{1/2}$. CYP2D6 inhibitors (eg, quinidine) may increase levels in patients that are on chronic flecainide therapy, especially if they are extensive metabolizers. Amiodarone may increase levels, if flecainide dosage is not reduced. Avoid with disopyramide, verapamil, nifedipine, or diltiazem. Milk may inhibit absorption in infants; consider a reduction in flecainide dosage when milk is removed from diet of infants.

NURSING CONSIDERATIONS

Assessment: Assess for preexisting 2nd- or 3rd-degree AV block, right bundle branch block associated with a left hemiblock, implanted pacemaker, asymptomatic non-life-threatening ventricular arrhythmia, A-fib/A-flutter, cardiogenic shock, MI, cardiomyopathy, preexisting CHF or low ejection fractions (<30%), sick sinus syndrome, hypersensitivity, pregnancy/nursing status, renal/hepatic impairment, and possible drug interactions. Correct preexisting hypokalemia or hyperkalemia prior to therapy. Determine pacing threshold in patients with pacemaker.

Monitoring: Monitor for paradoxical increase in ventricular rate, new or worsened supraventricular/ventricular arrhythmias, worsening of CHF, effects on cardiac conduction, bradycardia, hypersensitivity reactions, and other adverse reactions. Monitor for plasma trough levels and ECGs either after initiation or change in dose, whether the dose was increased for lack of effectiveness, or increased growth of pediatric patient. Periodically monitor plasma levels with renal/hepatic impairment, CHF, and/or if on concurrent amiodarone therapy. Determine pacing threshold in patients with pacemakers after 1 week and at regular intervals thereafter.

Patient Counseling: Inform about risks/benefits of therapy and instruct to report any adverse reactions to physician.

Storage: 20-25°C (68-77°F).

FLECTOR – diclofenac epolamine RX

Class: NSAID

NSAIDs may cause an increased risk of serious cardiovascular (CV) thrombotic events, MI, stroke, and serious GI adverse events including bleeding, ulceration, and perforation of the stomach or intestines that can be fatal. Patients with CV disease (CVD) or risk factors for CVD may be at greater risk. Elderly patients are at a greater risk for GI events. Contraindicated in the perioperative setting of coronary artery bypass graft (CABG) surgery.

ADULT DOSAGE

Acute Pain

Due to Minor Strains, Sprains, and Contusions:
Apply 1 patch to most painful area bid

PEDIATRIC DOSAGE

Pediatric use may not have been established

ADMINISTRATION
Transdermal route

HOW SUPPLIED
Patch: 180mg (1.3%) [5[s]]

CONTRAINDICATIONS
History of asthma, urticaria, or allergic-type reactions after taking aspirin (ASA) or other NSAIDs. Treatment of perioperative pain in the setting of CABG surgery. Use on non-intact or damaged skin.

WARNINGS/PRECAUTIONS
Use lowest effective dose for shortest duration possible. Extreme caution with history of ulcer disease/GI bleeding. Cases of severe hepatic reactions reported. May cause elevations of LFTs; d/c if abnormal LFTs persist or worsen, liver disease develops, or systemic manifestations occur. May lead to new onset or worsening of preexisting HTN; monitor BP closely. Fluid retention and edema reported; caution with fluid retention/heart failure (HF). Caution when initiating treatment in patients with considerable dehydration. Renal papillary necrosis and other renal injury reported after long-term use; increased risk with renal/hepatic impairment, HF, and elderly. Not recommended for use with advanced renal disease; if therapy must be initiated, monitor renal function. Anaphylactic reactions may occur; avoid in patients with aspirin (ASA) triad. May cause serious skin adverse events (eg, exfoliative dermatitis, Stevens-Johnson syndrome [SJS], toxic epidermal necrolysis [TEN]); d/c at 1st appearance of skin rash or any other signs of hypersensitivity. Avoid starting at 30 weeks gestation; may cause premature closure of ductus arteriosus. Cannot replace corticosteroids or treat corticosteroid insufficiency. May diminish the utility of diagnostic signs in detecting complications of presumed noninfectious, painful conditions. Anemia may occur; monitor Hgb/Hct if signs/symptoms of anemia develop with long-term use. May inhibit platelet aggregation and prolong bleeding time; monitor patients with coagulation disorders. Caution with preexisting asthma and avoid with ASA-sensitive asthma. Avoid contact with eyes and mucosa. D/C if abnormal renal tests persist or worsen. Caution in elderly and debilitated patients.

ADVERSE REACTIONS
CV thrombotic events, MI, stroke, GI adverse events, application-site reactions (eg, pruritus, dermatitis), headache, paresthesia, somnolence.

DRUG INTERACTIONS
Increased adverse effects with ASA; avoid use. May result in higher rate of hemorrhage, more frequent abnormal creatinine, urea, and Hgb with oral NSAIDs; avoid combination unless benefit outweighs risk. May diminish antihypertensive effect of ACE inhibitors. Patients taking thiazides or loop diuretics may have impaired response to these therapies. Increased risk of renal toxicity with diuretics and ACE inhibitors. May reduce natriuretic effect of furosemide and thiazides; monitor for signs of renal failure and diuretic efficacy. May increase lithium levels; monitor for toxicity. May enhance methotrexate toxicity and cyclosporine nephrotoxicity; caution with coadministration. Increased risk of GI bleeding with oral corticosteroids, anticoagulants (eg, warfarin), smoking, and alcohol. Synergistic effects on GI bleeding with anticoagulants (eg, warfarin). Caution with drugs known to be potentially hepatotoxic (eg, acetaminophen [APAP], certain antibiotics, antiepileptics).

NURSING CONSIDERATIONS

Assessment: Assess for history of asthma, urticaria, or allergic-type reactions with ASA or other NSAIDs, ASA triad, CVD, risk factors for CVD, HTN, fluid retention, HF, history of ulcer disease, history of/risk factors for GI bleeding, general health status, history of renal/hepatic impairment, coagulation disorders, dehydration, tobacco/alcohol use, pregnancy/nursing status, and for possible drug interactions. Assess that skin at application site is intact and not damaged. Obtain baseline CBC and BP.

Monitoring: Monitor BP, CBC, LFTs, renal function, and chemistry profile periodically. Monitor for GI bleeding/ulceration/perforation, CV thrombotic events, MI, stroke, HTN, fluid retention, edema, skin/allergic reactions, and other adverse reactions.

Patient Counseling: Instruct only to use on intact skin. Advise to wash hands after applying, handling, or removing the patch. Instruct not to wear patch during bathing or showering. Instruct to avoid contact with eyes and mucosa; advise that if eye contact occurs, to wash out the eye with water or saline immediately and consult physician if irritation persists for >1 hr. Counsel to seek medical attention if symptoms of hepatotoxicity, anaphylactic reactions, skin and hypersensitivity reactions, CV events, GI ulceration and bleeding, bronchospasm, weight gain, or edema occurs. Inform of pregnancy risks. Instruct to tape down edges of patch if it begins to peel-off; if problems with adhesion persist, recommend to overlay the patch with a mesh netting sleeve. Advise to avoid coadministration with unprescribed APAP.

Storage: 25°C (77°F); excursions permitted to 15-30°C (59-86°F). Keep sealed at all times when not in use.

FLOMAX – tamsulosin hydrochloride

RX

Class: Alpha$_1$-antagonist

ADULT DOSAGE

Benign Prostatic Hyperplasia

0.4mg qd 30 min after the same meal each day

Titrate: May increase to 0.8mg qd after 2-4 weeks if response is inadequate

If therapy is discontinued or interrupted for several days at either the 0.4mg or 0.8mg dose, restart w/ 0.4mg qd

PEDIATRIC DOSAGE

Pediatric use may not have been established

ADMINISTRATION

Oral route

Do not crush, chew, or open cap

HOW SUPPLIED

Cap: 0.4mg

WARNINGS/PRECAUTIONS

Orthostasis/syncope may occur; caution to avoid situations in which injury could result should syncope occur. May cause priapism. Prostate cancer and BPH frequently coexist. Intraoperative floppy iris syndrome (IFIS) observed during cataract and glaucoma surgery; initiation of therapy in patients who are scheduled for cataract or glaucoma surgery is not recommended. Allergic reaction reported (rare) in patients with sulfa allergy.

ADVERSE REACTIONS

Headache, dizziness, rhinitis, infection, abnormal ejaculation, asthenia, back pain, diarrhea, pharyngitis, chest pain, cough increased, somnolence, insomnia, sinusitis, nausea.

DRUG INTERACTIONS

Avoid with other α-adrenergic blockers. Caution with cimetidine, particularly at a dose >0.4mg, and warfarin. Avoid with strong inhibitors of CYP3A4 (eg, ketoconazole). Caution with moderate inhibitors of CYP3A4 (eg, erythromycin), with strong (eg, paroxetine) or moderate (eg, terbinafine) inhibitors of CYP2D6, and in patients known to be CYP2D6 poor metabolizers, particularly at a dose >0.4mg. Caution with PDE-5 inhibitors; may cause symptomatic hypotension.

NURSING CONSIDERATIONS

Assessment: Assess for BPH, known hypersensitivity, sulfa allergy, and possible drug interactions. Assess if patient is planning to undergo cataract/glaucoma surgery. Screen for the presence of prostate cancer.

Monitoring: Monitor for signs/symptoms of orthostasis, syncope, priapism, IFIS, allergic reactions, and other adverse reactions. Monitor for the presence of prostate cancer at regular intervals.

Patient Counseling: Advise patient about the possible occurrence of symptoms related to orthostatic hypotension; caution about driving, operating machinery, or performing hazardous tasks. Advise that therapy should not be used in combination with strong inhibitors of CYP3A4. Advise about the possibility of priapism and to seek immediate medical attention if it occurs. Inform of the importance of screening for prostate cancer prior to therapy and at regular intervals afterwards. Advise to inform ophthalmologist of drug use if considering cataract or glaucoma surgery.

Storage: 25°C (77°F); excursions permitted to 15-30°C (59-86°F).

FLONASE – fluticasone propionate

RX

Class: Corticosteroid

ADULT DOSAGE

Perennial Nonallergic Rhinitis

Initial: 2 sprays/nostril qd or 1 spray/nostril bid
Maint: 1 spray/nostril qd
Max: 2 sprays/nostril qd (200mcg/d)

PEDIATRIC DOSAGE

Perennial Nonallergic Rhinitis

≥4 Years:
Initial: 1 spray/nostril qd
Titrate: May increase to 2 sprays/nostril qd if response is inadequate, then return to 1 spray/nostril qd once adequate control is achieved
Max: 2 sprays/nostril qd (200mcg/d)

DOSE MODIFICATION

Elderly

Start at lower end of dosing range

ADMINISTRATION

Intranasal route

Shake gently before each use

Priming

Prime before using for the 1st time or after a period of non-use (≥1 week) by shaking the contents well and releasing 6 sprays into the air, away from the face

HOW SUPPLIED

Spray: 50mcg/spray [120 sprays]

WARNINGS/PRECAUTIONS

May cause local nasal effects (eg, epistaxis, nasal ulceration, *Candida* infections, nasal septum perforation, impaired wound healing). When localized infections of the nose and pharynx with *Candida albicans* develop, may need to treat and d/c therapy. Avoid with recent nasal ulcers, nasal surgery, or nasal trauma until healing has occurred. Glaucoma and/or cataracts may develop; closely monitor patients with a change in vision or with a history of increased IOP, glaucoma, and/or cataracts. Hypersensitivity reactions reported; d/c if such reactions occur. May increase susceptibility to infections, caution with active or quiescent TB, systemic fungal, bacterial, viral or parasitic infections; or ocular herpes simplex. Avoid exposure to chickenpox and measles. D/C slowly if hypercorticism and adrenal suppression occur. Risk of adrenal insufficiency and withdrawal symptoms when replacing systemic corticosteroids with topical corticosteroids. May reduce growth velocity in pediatric patients. Caution with hepatic disease.

ADVERSE REACTIONS

Headache, pharyngitis, epistaxis, nasal burning/irritation, N/V, asthma symptoms, cough.

DRUG INTERACTIONS

Not recommended with strong CYP3A4 inhibitors (eg, ritonavir, clarithromycin, ketoconazole); increased systemic corticosteroid adverse effects may occur.

NURSING CONSIDERATIONS

Assessment: Assess for drug hypersensitivity, active or quiescent TB, systemic fungal/bacterial/viral/parasitic infections, ocular herpes simplex, recent nasal ulcers/surgery/trauma, history of increased IOP, glaucoma, or cataracts, hepatic disease, pregnancy/nursing status, and possible drug interactions. Assess if patients have not been immunized or exposed to infections, such as measles or chickenpox.

Monitoring: Monitor for epistaxis, nasal ulceration, nasal septal perforation, impaired wound healing, changes in vision, glaucoma, cataracts, hypersensitivity reactions, infections (eg, chickenpox, measles), hypercorticism, adrenal suppression, hypoadrenalism (in infants born of mothers receiving corticosteroids during pregnancy), and other adverse reactions. Examine periodically for evidence of nasal *Candida* infections. Routinely monitor growth of pediatric patients. Monitor for adrenal insufficiency and withdrawal symptoms when replacing systemic corticosteroid with topical corticosteroid.

Patient Counseling: Inform of possible local nasal effects, glaucoma, cataracts, hypersensitivity reactions, immunosuppression, and reduced growth velocity (in pediatric patients). Advise patients who have experienced recent nasal ulcers, surgery, or trauma to not use therapy until healing has occurred. Instruct to notify physician if a change in vision develops, and to d/c therapy if hypersensitivity reactions occur. Instruct to avoid exposure to chickenpox or measles; if exposed, advise to consult physician without delay. Instruct to use spray on a regular basis, and not to increase prescribed dosage; advise to contact physician if symptoms do not improve or if condition worsens. Instruct to avoid spraying in eyes and mouth. Advise women to contact physician if they become pregnant.

Storage: 4-30°C (39-86°F).

FLOVENT HFA – fluticasone propionate RX

Class: Corticosteroid

ADULT DOSAGE

Asthma

Prophylactic Maint Treatment:

Previous Therapy:
Bronchodilators Alone:
Initial: 88mcg bid
Max: 440mcg bid

Inhaled Corticosteroids:
Initial: 88-220mcg bid
Max: 440mcg bid

PEDIATRIC DOSAGE

Asthma

Prophylactic Maint Treatment:
4-11 Years:
Initial/Max: 88mcg bid

≥12 Years:
Previous Therapy:
Bronchodilators Alone:
Initial: 88mcg bid
Max: 440mcg bid

Oral Corticosteroids:
Initial: 440mcg bid
Max: 880mcg bid

Reduce oral prednisone no faster than 2.5-5mg/day on a weekly basis beginning after at least 1 week of fluticasone therapy

Titrate:
Reduce to lowest effective dose once asthma stability is achieved. Higher dosages may provide additional asthma control if response to initial dose is inadequate after 2 weeks

Inhaled Corticosteroids:
Initial: 88-220mcg bid
Max: 440mcg bid

Oral Corticosteroids:
Initial: 440mcg bid
Max: 880mcg bid

Reduce oral prednisone no faster than 2.5-5mg/day on a weekly basis beginning after at least 1 week of fluticasone therapy

Titrate:
Reduce to lowest effective dose once asthma stability is achieved. Higher dosages may provide additional asthma control if response to initial dose is inadequate after 2 weeks

ADMINISTRATION

Oral inh route

Rinse mouth after inh
Shake well for 5 sec before each spray

Priming
Prime the inhaler before using for the first time by releasing 4 test sprays into the air, shaking well for 5 sec before each spray
If the inhaler has not been used for more than 7 days or has been dropped, prime inhaler by shaking well for 5 sec and releasing 1 spray into the air

HOW SUPPLIED

MDI: 44mcg/inh, 110mcg/inh, 220mcg/inh [120 inhalations]

CONTRAINDICATIONS

Primary treatment of status asthmaticus or other acute episodes of asthma where intensive measures are required.

WARNINGS/PRECAUTIONS

Not indicated for acute bronchospasm relief. *Candida albicans* infections of mouth and pharynx reported; treat and/or interrupt therapy if needed. Increased susceptibility to infections. May lead to serious/fatal course of chickenpox or measles in children; avoid exposure, and if exposed, consider prophylaxis/treatment. Caution with active/quiescent tuberculosis (TB), systemic fungal/bacterial/viral/parasitic infections, or ocular herpes simplex. Deaths due to adrenal insufficiency reported during and after transfer from systemic to inhaled corticosteroids; wean slowly from systemic corticosteroid use after transferring to therapy. Resume oral corticosteroids during periods of stress or a severe asthma attack in patients previously withdrawn from systemic corticosteroids. Transfer from systemic to inhaled corticosteroids may unmask allergic conditions previously suppressed by systemic therapy (eg, rhinitis, conjunctivitis, eczema). Monitor for systemic corticosteroid effects. Reduce dose slowly and consider other treatments if hypercorticism and adrenal suppression/crisis occur. Immediate hypersensitivity reactions may occur. Decreases in bone mineral density (BMD) reported with long-term use; caution with major risk factors for decreased bone mineral content, including chronic use of drugs that can reduce bone mass (eg, anticonvulsants, oral corticosteroids). May cause reduction in growth velocity in pediatric patients; routinely monitor growth. Glaucoma, increased intraocular pressure (IOP), and cataracts reported with long-term use. Systemic eosinophilic conditions, and vasculitis consistent with Churg-Strauss syndrome may occur. Paradoxical bronchospasm with immediate increase in wheezing may occur; treat immediately with an inhaled short-acting bronchodilator; d/c and institute alternative therapy. Closely monitor patients with hepatic disease.

ADVERSE REACTIONS

Upper respiratory tract infection/inflammation, throat irritation, sinusitis/sinus infection, hoarseness/dysphonia, candidiasis, cough, bronchitis, headache.

DRUG INTERACTIONS

Not recommended with strong CYP3A4 inhibitors (eg, ritonavir [RTV], atazanavir, clarithromycin, indinavir, itraconazole, nefazodone, nelfinavir, saquinavir, ketoconazole, telithromycin); increased systemic corticosteroid adverse effects may occur. RTV and ketoconazole may increase exposure and reduce cortisol levels.

NURSING CONSIDERATIONS

Assessment: Assess for hypersensitivity to drug, status asthmaticus, acute bronchospasm, active/quiescent TB, ocular herpes simplex, systemic infections, risk factors for decreased bone mineral content, history of increased IOP, glaucoma, cataracts, hepatic impairment, pregnancy/nursing status, and possible drug interactions.

Monitoring: Monitor for signs of infection, systemic corticosteroid effects (eg, hypercorticism, adrenal suppression), hypersensitivity reactions, decreased BMD, glaucoma, increased IOP, cataracts, paradoxical bronchospasm, eosinophilic conditions, asthma instability, hypoadrenalism (in infants born to a mother who received corticosteroids during pregnancy), and other adverse reactions. Monitor growth in pediatric patients routinely. Closely monitor patients with hepatic disease.

Patient Counseling: Advise to contact physician if oropharyngeal candidiasis develops. Advise to rinse the mouth with water without swallowing after inh to help reduce the risk of thrush. Inform that product is not a bronchodilator and not intended for use as rescue medicine for acute asthma exacerbations; instruct to contact physician immediately if deterioration of asthma occurs. Instruct to avoid exposure to chickenpox or measles and to consult physician without delay if exposed. Inform about risks of immunosuppression, hypercorticism, adrenal suppression, reduction in BMD, reduced growth velocity in pediatric patients, and ocular effects. Instruct to d/c therapy if immediate hypersensitivity reactions occur. Instruct to use at regular intervals ud and not to stop use abruptly; advise to contact physician immediately if use is discontinued. Instruct to avoid spraying in eyes. Advise women to contact physician if they become pregnant while on therapy.

Storage: 20-25°C (68-77°F); excursions permitted to 15-30°C (59-86°F). Store with mouthpiece down. Do not puncture, use/store near heat or open flame, or throw canister into fire/incinerator. Exposure to temperatures >49°C (120°F) may cause bursting. Discard when counter reads 000.

FLUDROCORTISONE – fludrocortisone acetate — RX

Class: Corticosteroid

ADULT DOSAGE

Addison's Disease

Primary and Secondary Adrenocortical Insufficiency:
Usual: 0.1mg/day
Range: 0.1mg 3X weekly to 0.2mg/day

Preferably administered w/ cortisone (10-37.5mg/day in divided doses) or hydrocortisone (10-30mg/day in divided doses)

Salt-Losing Adrenogenital Syndrome

0.1-0.2mg/day

PEDIATRIC DOSAGE

Pediatric use may not have been established

DOSE MODIFICATION

Adverse Reactions

Addison's Disease:
Transient HTN: Reduce dose to 0.05mg/day

ADMINISTRATION

Oral route

HOW SUPPLIED

Tab: 0.1mg* *scored

CONTRAINDICATIONS

Systemic fungal infections.

WARNINGS/PRECAUTIONS

May mask signs of infection, and new infections may appear during therapy. There may be decreased resistance and inability to localize infection; promptly control infection with suitable antimicrobial therapy. Prolonged use may produce posterior subcapsular cataracts, glaucoma with possible damage to optic nerves, and secondary ocular infections due to fungi or viruses. May cause elevation of BP, salt and water retention, and increased K^+ excretion; carefully monitor dosage and salt intake to avoid HTN, edema, or weight gain. Periodic serum electrolyte monitoring is advisable during prolonged therapy; dietary salt restriction and K^+ supplementation may be necessary. May increase Ca^{2+} excretion. Use in patients with active tuberculosis (TB) should be restricted to fulminating or disseminated cases in conjunction with an appropriate antituberculous regimen. Reactivation of TB may occur; caution in patients with latent TB or tuberculin reactivity; patients on prolonged therapy should receive chemoprophylaxis. Avoid exposure to chickenpox or measles. Adverse effects may occur by too rapid withdrawal or by continued use of large doses. Enhanced effects with hypothyroidism and cirrhosis. To avoid drug-induced adrenal insufficiency, supportive dosage may be required in times of stress (eg, trauma, surgery, severe illness) both during treatment and for a yr afterwards. Use lowest possible dose; gradually reduce dosage when possible. Caution with ocular herpes simplex, nonspecific ulcerative colitis, HTN, diverticulitis, fresh intestinal anastomoses, active/latent peptic ulcer, renal insufficiency, osteoporosis, and myasthenia gravis. Psychic derangements may appear and existing emotional instability or psychotic tendencies may be aggravated. Lab test interactions may occur.

ADVERSE REACTIONS

HTN, CHF, edema, cardiac enlargement, K^+ loss, hypokalemic alkalosis.

DRUG INTERACTIONS

Decreased pharmacologic effect and increased ulcerogenic effect of aspirin (ASA); monitor salicylate levels or therapeutic effect of ASA and adjust salicylate dosage accordingly if effect is altered. Caution with ASA in patients with hypoprothrombinemia. Enhanced hypokalemia with amphotericin B or K^+-depleting diuretics (eg, benzothiadiazines, furosemide, ethacrynic acid) and enhanced possibility of arrhythmias or digitalis toxicity associated with hypokalemia with digitalis glycosides; monitor serum K^+ levels and use K^+ supplements if necessary. Rifampin, barbiturates, or phenytoin may diminish steroid effect; increase steroid dosage accordingly. Decreased PT response with oral anticoagulants; monitor prothrombin levels and adjust anticoagulant dosage accordingly. Diminished effect of oral hypoglycemics and insulin; monitor for symptoms of hyperglycemia and adjust dosage of antidiabetic drug upward if necessary. Enhanced tendency toward edema with anabolic steroids (particularly C-17 alkylated androgens [eg, oxymetholone, methandrostenolone, norethandrolone]); use with caution especially in patients with hepatic/cardiac disease. May require a reduction of corticosteroid dose when estrogen therapy is initiated, and may require increased amounts when estrogen is terminated. Avoid smallpox vaccination and other immunizations; possible hazards of neurologic complications and a lack of antibody response.

NURSING CONSIDERATIONS

Assessment: Assess for hypersensitivity to drug, systemic fungal infections, active/latent TB, HTN, renal insufficiency, psychotic tendencies, hypothyroidism, osteoporosis, myasthenia gravis, peptic ulcer, fresh intestinal anastomoses, ocular herpes simplex, diverticulitis, ulcerative colitis, other conditions where treatment is cautioned, pregnancy/nursing status, and possible drug interactions.

Monitoring: Monitor for infections, edema, weight gain, psychic derangement, cataracts, latent TB reactivation, and other adverse reactions. Monitor dosage, salt intake, serum electrolytes, and BP. Monitor for remission or exacerbations of disease and stress (surgery, infection, trauma). Monitor prothrombin levels if used with oral anticoagulants.

Patient Counseling: Advise to report any medical history of heart disease, high BP, and kidney/liver disease, and to report current use of any medicines. Instruct to avoid exposure to chickenpox or measles and, if exposed, to obtain medical advice. Inform of steroid-dependent status and of increased dosage requirement with stress; advise to carry medical identification indicating this dependence and, if necessary, instruct to carry an adequate supply of medication for emergency use. Inform of the importance of regular follow-up visits and the need to promptly notify physician of dizziness, severe or continuing headaches, swelling of feet or lower legs, or unusual weight gain. Instruct to take only ud, to take a missed dose as soon as possible, unless it is almost time for next dose, and not to double next dose.

Storage: 15-30°C (59-86°F). Avoid excessive heat.

FOCALIN – dexmethylphenidate hydrochloride CII

Class: Sympathomimetic amine

Caution with history of drug dependence or alcoholism. Chronic, abusive use may lead to marked tolerance and psychological dependence with varying degrees of abnormal behavior may occur with chronic abusive use. Frank psychotic episodes may occur, especially with parenteral abuse. Careful supervision is required during withdrawal from abusive use, since severe depression may occur. Withdrawal following chronic use may unmask symptoms of underlying disorder that may require follow-up.

ADULT DOSAGE

Attention-Deficit Hyperactivity Disorder

Refer to pediatric dosing

PEDIATRIC DOSAGE

Attention-Deficit Hyperactivity Disorder

≥6 Years:

Methylphenidate-Naive:

Initial: 5mg/day (2.5mg bid)

Titrate: May adjust weekly in 2.5-5mg increments

Max: 20mg/day (10mg bid)

Currently on Methylphenidate:

Initial: 1/2 the dose of racemic methylphenidate

Max: 20mg/day (10mg bid)

Periodically reevaluate the long-term usefulness of the drug

DOSE MODIFICATION

Adverse Reactions

Reduce dose or d/c if paradoxical aggravation of symptoms or other adverse events occur
D/C if no improvement seen after appropriate dosage adjustment over 1 month

ADMINISTRATION

Oral route

Take w/ or w/o food
Administer bid, at least 4 hrs apart

HOW SUPPLIED

Tab: 2.5mg, 5mg, 10mg

CONTRAINDICATIONS

Marked anxiety, tension, agitation, glaucoma, motor tics, or family history or diagnosis of Tourette's syndrome. Treatment with MAOIs or within a minimum of 14 days following discontinuation of an MAOI.

WARNINGS/PRECAUTIONS

Avoid in patients with known serious structural cardiac abnormalities, cardiomyopathy, serious heart rhythm abnormalities, coronary artery disease, or other serious cardiac problems. Sudden death reported in children and adolescents with structural cardiac abnormalities or other serious heart problems. Sudden death, stroke, and myocardial infarction (MI) reported in adults. May cause modest increase in average BP and HR; caution in patients whose underlying medical conditions might be compromised by increases in BP or HR. Prior to treatment, perform medical history (including assessment for family history of sudden death or ventricular arrhythmia) and physical exam to assess for presence of cardiac disease. Promptly perform cardiac evaluation if symptoms of cardiac disease develop during treatment. May exacerbate symptoms of behavior disturbance and thought disorder in patients with a preexisting psychotic disorder. May induce mixed/manic episode in patients with comorbid bipolar disorder. May cause treatment-emergent psychotic or manic symptoms at usual doses in children and adolescents without a prior history of psychotic illness or mania; discontinuation may be appropriate if such symptoms occur. Aggressive behavior or hostility reported in children and adolescents. May cause long-term suppression of growth in children; may need to interrupt treatment in patients not growing or gaining height or weight as expected. May lower convulsive threshold; d/c in the presence of seizures. Priapism reported; immediate medical attention should be sought if abnormally sustained or frequent and painful erections develop. Associated with peripheral vasculopathy, including Raynaud's phenomenon; monitor for digital changes. Difficulties with accommodation and blurring of vision reported. Periodically monitor CBC, differential, and platelet counts during prolonged therapy.

ADVERSE REACTIONS

Abdominal pain, fever, anorexia, nausea.

DRUG INTERACTIONS

See Contraindications. May decrease the effectiveness of drugs used to treat HTN. Caution with pressor agents. May inhibit metabolism of coumarin anticoagulants, anticonvulsants (eg, phenobarbital, phenytoin, primidone) and some antidepressants (eg, TCAs, SSRIs); downward dose adjustments and monitoring of plasma drug concentration (or coagulation times for coumarin) of these drugs may be necessary when initiating or discontinuing dexmethylphenidate.

NURSING CONSIDERATIONS

Assessment: Assess for previous hypersensitivity to the drug, history of drug dependence or alcoholism, marked anxiety, agitation, tension, glaucoma, motor tics, family history or diagnosis of Tourette's syndrome, preexisting psychotic disorder, comorbid bipolar disorder, history of seizures, medical conditions that might be compromised by increases in BP or HR, any other conditions where treatment is contraindicated or cautioned, pregnancy/nursing status, and possible drug interactions. Perform a careful history (including assessment for a family history of sudden death or ventricular arrhythmia) and physical exam to assess for the presence of cardiac disease, and perform further cardiac evaluation if findings suggest such disease (eg, ECG, echocardiogram). Adequately screen patients with comorbid depressive symptoms to determine if they are at risk for bipolar disorder (eg, detailed psychiatric history, including a family history of suicide, bipolar disorder, and depression).

Monitoring: Monitor for signs/symptoms of cardiac disease, exacerbation of behavioral disturbance and thought disorder, psychosis, mania, appearance of or worsening of aggressive behavior or hostility, seizures, priapism, digital changes, visual disturbances, and other adverse reactions. Monitor BP and HR. During prolonged use, periodically evaluate usefulness of therapy and monitor CBC, differential, and platelet counts. In pediatric patients, monitor growth.

Patient Counseling: Inform about risks and benefits of treatment. Counsel on the appropriate use of the medication. Advise of the possibility of priapism; instruct to seek immediate medical attention in the event of priapism. Instruct to report to physician any new numbness, pain, skin color change, sensitivity to temperature in fingers or toes, or any signs of unexplained wounds appearing on the fingers or toes.

Storage: 25°C (77°F); excursions permitted to 15-30°C (59-86°F). Protect from light and moisture.

FOCALIN XR – dexmethylphenidate hydrochloride CII

Class: Sympathomimetic amine

Caution with history of drug dependence or alcoholism. Marked tolerance and psychological dependence with varying degrees of abnormal behavior may occur with chronic abusive use. Frank psychotic episodes may occur, especially with parenteral abuse. Careful supervision is required during withdrawal from abusive use, since severe depression may occur. Withdrawal following chronic therapeutic use may unmask symptoms of underlying disorder that may require follow-up.

ADULT DOSAGE

Attention-Deficit Hyperactivity Disorder

Methylphenidate-Naive:
Initial: 10mg qam
Titrate: May adjust weekly in 10mg increments
Max: 40mg/day

Currently on Methylphenidate:
Initial: 1/2 of methylphenidate total daily dose

Currently on Dexmethylphenidate Immediate-Release:
May switch to the same daily dose of the extended-release

Periodically reevaluate the long-term usefulness of the drug

PEDIATRIC DOSAGE

Attention-Deficit Hyperactivity Disorder

≥6 Years:
Methylphenidate-Naive:
Initial: 5mg qam
Titrate: May adjust weekly in 5mg increments
Max: 30mg/day

Currently on Methylphenidate:
Initial: 1/2 of methylphenidate total daily dose

Currently on Dexmethylphenidate Immediate-Release:
May switch to the same daily dose of the ER

Periodically reevaluate the long-term usefulness of the drug

DOSE MODIFICATION

Adverse Reactions

Reduce dose or d/c if paradoxical aggravation of symptoms or other adverse events occur
D/C if no improvement seen after appropriate dosage adjustment over 1 month

ADMINISTRATION

Oral route

Swallow caps whole or sprinkle contents on a spoonful of applesauce
Do not crush, chew, or divide
Consume drug and applesauce mixture immediately; do not store for future use

HOW SUPPLIED

Cap, Extended-Release (ER): 5mg, 10mg, 15mg, 20mg, 25mg, 30mg, 35mg, 40mg

CONTRAINDICATIONS

Marked anxiety, tension, agitation, glaucoma, motor tics or family history or diagnosis of Tourette's syndrome. Treatment with MAOIs or within a minimum of 14 days following discontinuation of an MAOI.

WARNINGS/PRECAUTIONS

Avoid in patients with known serious structural cardiac abnormalities, cardiomyopathy, serious heart rhythm abnormalities, coronary artery disease, or other serious cardiac problems. Sudden death reported in children and adolescents with structural cardiac abnormalities or other serious heart problems. Sudden death, stroke, MI reported in adults. May cause modest increase in average BP and HR; caution with HTN, heart failure, recent MI, or ventricular arrhythmia. Prior to treatment, perform a medical history (including assessment for family history of sudden death or ventricular arrhythmia) and physical exam to assess for the presence of cardiac disease. Promptly perform cardiac evaluation if symptoms of cardiac disease develop during treatment. May exacerbate symptoms of behavior disturbance and thought disorder in patients with preexisting psychotic disorder. Caution in patients with comorbid bipolar disorder; may induce mixed/manic episodes. May cause treatment-emergent psychotic or manic symptoms (eg, hallucinations, delusional thinking, mania) in children and adolescents without prior history of psychotic illness or mania; discontinuation may be appropriate if such symptoms occur. Aggressive behavior or hostility reported in children and adolescents. May cause long-term suppression of growth in children; monitor growth, and may need to interrupt treatment in patients not growing or gaining height or weight as expected. May lower convulsive threshold; d/c in the presence of seizures. Priapism reported; seek immediate medical attention if abnormally sustained or frequent and painful erections develop. Associated with peripheral vasculopathy, including Raynaud's phenomenon; monitor for digital changes. Difficulties with accommodation and blurring of vision reported. Periodically monitor CBC, differential, and platelet counts during prolonged therapy.

ADVERSE REACTIONS

Dyspepsia, headache, anxiety, insomnia, anorexia, dry mouth, pharyngolaryngeal pain, feeling jittery, dizziness, decreased appetite, vomiting.

DRUG INTERACTIONS

See Contraindications. May decrease the effectiveness of drugs used to treat HTN. Caution with pressor agents. May inhibit metabolism of coumarin anticoagulants, anticonvulsants (eg, phenobarbital, phenytoin, primidone), and tricyclic drugs (eg, imipramine, clomipramine, desipramine); downward dose adjustments and monitoring of plasma drug concentration (or coagulation times for coumarin) of these drugs may be necessary when initiating or discontinuing therapy. Antacids or acid suppressants could alter drug release.

NURSING CONSIDERATIONS

Assessment: Assess for previous hypersensitivity to the drug, history of drug dependence or alcoholism, marked anxiety, tension, agitation, glaucoma, motor tics, family history or diagnosis of Tourette's syndrome, preexisting psychotic disorder, comorbid bipolar disorder, cardiac disease, medical conditions that might be compromised by increases in BP and HR, any other conditions where treatment is cautioned, pregnancy/nursing status, and possible drug interactions.

Monitoring: Monitor BP, HR, and for signs/symptoms of cardiac disease (eg, exertional chest pain, unexplained syncope), exacerbation of behavioral disturbance and thought disorder, psychosis, mania, appearance of or worsening of aggressive behavior or hostility, seizures, priapism, digital changes, visual disturbances, and other adverse reactions. During prolonged use, periodically reevaluate usefulness of therapy and monitor CBC, differential, and platelet counts. In pediatric patients, monitor growth.

Patient Counseling: Inform about benefits and risks of treatment. Counsel on the appropriate use of the medication. Advise of the possibility of priapism; instruct to seek immediate medical attention in the event of priapism. Instruct to report to physician any new numbness, pain, skin color change, sensitivity to temperature in fingers or toes, or any signs of unexplained wounds appearing on fingers or toes.

Storage: 25°C (77°F); excursions permitted to 15-30°C (59-86°F).

Folic Acid – folic acid

RX

Class: Erythropoiesis agent

ADULT DOSAGE

Anemia

Megaloblastic Anemias (Due to Folic Acid Deficiency)/Anemias of Nutritional Origin, Pregnancy, Infancy, or Childhood:
Usual: Up to 1mg/day. Resistant cases may require larger doses
Maint: 0.4mg
Pregnant and Lactating Women: 0.8mg
Minimum: 0.1mg/day

May need to increase maint level in the presence of alcoholism, hemolytic anemia, anticonvulsant therapy, or chronic infection

PEDIATRIC DOSAGE

Anemia

Megaloblastic Anemias (Due to Folic Acid Deficiency)/Anemias of Nutritional Origin, Pregnancy, Infancy, or Childhood:
Usual: Up to 1mg/day. Resistant cases may require larger doses
Maint:
Infants: 0.1mg
<4 Years: Up to 0.3mg
>4 Years: 0.4mg
Minimum: 0.1mg/day

May need to increase maint level in the presence of alcoholism, hemolytic anemia, anticonvulsant therapy, or chronic infection

ADMINISTRATION

Oral route

HOW SUPPLIED

Tab: 1mg* *scored

WARNINGS/PRECAUTIONS

Folic acid alone is improper therapy for pernicious anemia and other megaloblastic anemias in which vitamin B12 is deficient. Folic acid >0.1mg/day may obscure pernicious anemia in that hematologic remission may occur while neurologic manifestations remain progressive; potential danger exists in administering folic acid to patients w/ undiagnosed anemia.

ADVERSE REACTIONS

Allergic sensitization.

DRUG INTERACTIONS

Antagonizes anticonvulsant action of phenytoin; increased doses may be required in a patient whose epilepsy is completely controlled by phenytoin. False low serum and red cell folate levels may occur w/ antibiotics (eg, tetracycline), which suppress the growth of Lactobacillus casei.

NURSING CONSIDERATIONS

Assessment: Assess for alcoholism, hemolytic anemia, chronic infection, pernicious anemia and other megaloblastic anemias, previous intolerance to the drug, pregnancy/nursing status, and possible drug interactions.

Monitoring: Monitor for allergic sensitization, and obtain CBC.

Patient Counseling: Inform of risks and benefits of therapy.

Storage: 20-25°C (68-77°F).

FORADIL – formoterol fumarate RX

Class: Beta$_2$-agonist

Long-acting β_2-adrenergic agonists (LABAs) may increase the risk of asthma-related death. Contraindicated in asthma without use of a long-term asthma control medication (eg, inhaled corticosteroid). Do not use if asthma is adequately controlled on low- or medium-dose inhaled corticosteroids. LABAs may increase risk of asthma-related hospitalization in pediatric patients and adolescents; ensure adherence with both long-term asthma control medication and LABAs.

ADULT DOSAGE

Asthma

Combination w/ Long-Term Asthma Control Medication:
One 12mcg cap q12h
Max: 24mcg/day

Exercise-Induced Bronchospasm

Acute Prevention:
One 12mcg cap at least 15 min before exercise prn; additional doses should not be used for 12 hrs after administration

Additional dose should not be used for prevention of exercise-induced bronchospasm if already receiving bid dosing for asthma

Chronic Obstructive Pulmonary Disease

Maint Treatment of Bronchoconstriction:
One 12mcg cap q12h
Max: 24mcg/day

PEDIATRIC DOSAGE

Asthma

Combination w/ Long-Term Asthma Control Medication:
≥5 Years:
One 12mcg cap q12h
Max: 24mcg/day

Exercise-Induced Bronchospasm

Acute Prevention:
≥5 Years:
One 12mcg cap at least 15 min before exercise prn; additional doses should not be used for 12 hrs after administration

Additional doses should not be used for prevention of exercise-induced bronchospasm if already receiving bid dosing for asthma

ADMINISTRATION

Oral inh route

Administer caps only using the Aerolizer Inhaler; caps should not be swallowed

Only remove caps from blister immediately before use

HOW SUPPLIED

Cap, Inh: 12mcg [12^s, 60^s]

CONTRAINDICATIONS

Treatment of asthma without concomitant use of long-term asthma control medication (eg, inhaled corticosteroid). Primary treatment of status asthmaticus or other acute episodes of asthma or COPD where intensive measures are required. History of hypersensitivity to milk proteins.

WARNINGS/PRECAUTIONS

Not indicated for the relief of acute bronchospasm. Should not be initiated with significantly worsening, acutely deteriorating, or potentially life-threatening episodes of asthma or COPD. D/C regular use of inhaled, short-acting β_2-agonists (SABAs) when beginning treatment; use only for relief of acute asthma symptoms. Not a substitute for oral/inhaled corticosteroids. Do not use more often or at doses higher than recommended or with other LABAs (eg, salmeterol xinafoate, arformoterol tartrate). D/C if paradoxical bronchospasm or clinically significant cardiovascular (CV) effects occur. Caution in patients with CV disorders (eg, coronary insufficiency, cardiac arrhythmias, HTN, aneurysm, pheochromocytoma), convulsive disorders, thyrotoxicosis, preexisting diabetes mellitus (DM), and ketoacidosis. Caution in patients who are unusually responsive to sympathomimetic amines. ECG changes, immediate hypersensitivity reactions, significant hypokalemia, and changes in blood glucose may occur. Contains lactose; may cause allergic reactions in patients with severe milk protein allergy.

ADVERSE REACTIONS

Viral infection, URTI, CV events, asthma exacerbations, bronchitis, back pain, pharyngitis, chest pain.

DRUG INTERACTIONS

Adrenergic drugs may potentiate sympathetic effects; use with caution. Xanthine derivatives or systemic corticosteroids may potentiate any hypokalemic effect. ECG changes or hypokalemia that may result from non-K^+-sparing diuretics (eg, loop/thiazide diuretics) can be acutely worsened; use with caution. MAOIs, TCAs, macrolides, and drugs known to prolong the QTc interval may potentiate effect on CV system; use with extreme caution. Drugs known to prolong the QTc interval have an increased risk of ventricular arrhythmias. Use with β-blockers may block effects and produce severe bronchospasm in asthmatic patients; if needed, consider cardioselective β-blocker with caution. Elevated risk of arrhythmias with concomitant anesthesia with halogenated hydrocarbons.

NURSING CONSIDERATIONS

Assessment: Assess for previous hypersensitivity to the drug or milk proteins, CV disorders, convulsive disorders, thyrotoxicosis, DM, ketoacidosis, pregnancy/nursing status, and possible drug interactions. Assess use in patients unusually responsive to sympathomimetic amines. Obtain baseline serum K^+ and blood glucose levels. In patients with asthma, assess for status asthmaticus or presence of an acute asthma episode and assess for use of long-term asthma control medication. In patients with COPD, assess for presence of an acute COPD episode.

Monitoring: Monitor for paradoxical bronchospasm, signs of worsening asthma, CV effects, hypersensitivity reactions, aggravation of DM, and ketoacidosis. Monitor pulse rate, BP, ECG changes, and serum K^+ and blood glucose levels.

Patient Counseling: Inform of the risks and benefits of therapy. Instruct not to use to relieve acute asthma symptoms or exacerbations of COPD. Advise to seek medical attention if symptoms worsen, if treatment becomes less effective, or if more than usual inhalations of SABA are needed. Instruct not to exceed prescribed dose, d/c, or reduce dose without 1st contacting physician. Inform that treatment may lead to palpitations, chest pain, rapid HR, tremor, or nervousness. Advise to administer only via the Aerolizer device, to always use the new device that comes with each refill, and not to use the device for other medications. Instruct not to use with a spacer and never to exhale into the device. Advise to avoid exposing caps to moisture and to handle with dry hands. Advise to strictly follow storage conditions, remove cap from blister only immediately before use, and pierce caps only once. Advise to contact physician if patient is pregnant/nursing or if patient has severe milk protein allergy.

Storage: Prior to Dispensing: 2-8°C (36-46°F). After Dispensing: 20-25°C (68-77°F). Protect from heat and moisture. Always store caps in blister and only remove from blister immediately before use.

Forfivo XL – bupropion hydrochloride

RX

Class: Aminoketone

Antidepressants increased the risk of suicidal thinking and behavior (suicidality) in children, adolescents, and young adults in short-term studies of major depressive disorder (MDD) and other psychiatric disorders. Monitor and observe closely for clinical worsening, suicidality, or unusual changes in behavior. Not approved for use in pediatric patients. Not approved for smoking cessation; serious neuropsychiatric events reported in patients taking bupropion for smoking cessation.

ADULT DOSAGE

Major Depressive Disorder

Usual: 1 tab (450mg) qd

Do not initiate treatment w/ Forfivo XL; use another bupropion formulation for initial dose titration

May be used in patients who are receiving 300mg/day of another bupropion formulation for at least 2 weeks, and require a dosage of 450mg/day

Patients currently being treated w/ other bupropion products at 450mg/day may be switched to equivalent dose of Forfivo XL qd

Periodically reevaluate long-term usefulness of the drug

PEDIATRIC DOSAGE

Pediatric use may not have been established

DOSE MODIFICATION

Renal Impairment

Not recommended

Hepatic Impairment
Not recommended

ADMINISTRATION
Oral route

Take w/o regard to meals
Swallow whole; do not crush, divide, or chew

HOW SUPPLIED
Tab, Extended-Release: 450mg

CONTRAINDICATIONS
Seizure disorder, treated currently with other bupropion products, current/prior diagnosis of bulimia or anorexia nervosa, undergoing abrupt discontinuation of alcohol or sedatives, and concurrent use of MAOIs or initiation of treatment within 14 days of discontinuation of an MAOI.

WARNINGS/PRECAUTIONS
Not recommended in patients with hepatic/renal impairment. May precipitate a mixed/manic episode in patients at risk for bipolar disorder. Screen for bipolar disorder; not approved for treatment of bipolar depression. Dose-related risk of seizures; d/c and do not restart treatment if seizure occurs. Increased risk of seizure in patients with history of head trauma or prior seizure, CNS tumor, or severe hepatic cirrhosis. Neuropsychiatric signs and symptoms (eg, delusions, hallucinations, psychosis, concentration disturbance, paranoia, confusion) reported; d/c if these reactions occur. Pupillary dilation that occurs following use may trigger an angle-closure attack in a patient with anatomically narrow angles who does not have a patent iridectomy. HTN reported; caution with recent myocardial infarction or unstable heart disease. Increased restlessness, agitation, anxiety, and insomnia reported, especially shortly after initiation of treatment. If weight loss is a major presenting sign of a patient's depressive illness, the anorectic and/or weight-reducing potential of the product should be considered. D/C treatment if allergic or anaphylactoid/anaphylactic reactions occur. Arthralgia, myalgia, fever with rash, and other symptoms suggestive of delayed hypersensitivity reported; these symptoms may resemble serum sickness. False (+) urine immunoassay screening tests for amphetamines reported. Caution in elderly.

ADVERSE REACTIONS
Dry mouth, nausea, insomnia, dizziness, pharyngitis, abdominal pain, agitation, anxiety, tremor, palpitation, sweating, tinnitus, myalgia, anorexia, urinary frequency.

DRUG INTERACTIONS
See Contraindications. Caution with drugs that lower seizure threshold (eg, other antidepressants, antipsychotics, theophylline, systemic steroids). Increased seizure risk with excessive alcohol or sedative use; opiate, cocaine, or stimulant addiction; and use of OTC stimulants or anorectics, oral hypoglycemics, or insulin. Avoid with alcohol. Monitor for HTN with nicotine replacement therapy. Potential interaction with CYP2B6 substrates, inhibitors, or inducers (eg, orphenadrine, thiotepa, cyclophosphamide). Decreased levels with ritonavir or ritonavir/lopinavir and efavirenz; may need to increase bupropion dose but max dose should not be exceeded. Not recommended with ticlopidine or clopidogrel. Paroxetine, sertraline, norfluoxetine, nelfinavir, and fluvoxamine may inhibit hydroxylation. Cimetidine may increase levels of some active metabolites. Carbamazepine, phenytoin, and phenobarbital may induce metabolism. Caution with drugs that are metabolized by CYP2D6 (eg, certain antidepressants, antipsychotics, β-blockers, type 1C antiarrhythmics); consider dose reduction of concomitant medication. May reduce efficacy of drugs that require metabolic activation by CYP2D6 to be effective (eg, tamoxifen). May increase citalopram levels. Caution with levodopa or amantadine.

NURSING CONSIDERATIONS

Assessment: Assess for bipolar disorder, hepatic/renal impairment, seizure disorders or conditions that may increase risk of seizure, susceptibility to angle-closure glaucoma, hypersensitivity to the drug, any other conditions where treatment is contraindicated or cautioned, pregnancy/nursing status, and possible drug interactions. Obtain baseline BP.

Monitoring: Monitor for clinical worsening, suicidality, unusual changes in behavior, seizures, increased restlessness, agitation, anxiety, insomnia, neuropsychiatric signs/symptoms, activation of mania/hypomania, HTN, changes in weight/appetite, angle-closure glaucoma, anaphylactoid/anaphylactic reactions, delayed hypersensitivity and other adverse reactions. Reassess periodically to determine need for maintenance treatment.

Patient Counseling: Inform of the benefits/risks of therapy. Advise patients and caregivers of need for close observation for clinical worsening, suicidality, or unusual changes in behavior. Inform that product contains same active ingredient found in Zyban. Instruct to d/c and not to restart if seizure occurs while on therapy. Inform that therapy may impair mental/physical abilities; advise to refrain from operating hazardous machinery/driving until effects of therapy are known. Inform that excessive use or abrupt discontinuation of alcohol or sedatives may alter seizure threshold; advise to minimize or avoid alcohol use. Caution about risk of angle-closure glaucoma. Instruct to notify physician if taking/planning to take any prescription or OTC medications. Advise to contact physician if pregnant or intending to become pregnant during therapy.

Storage: 20-25°C (68-77°F).

FORTAMET – metformin hydrochloride

RX

Class: Biguanide

Lactic acidosis reported (rare). May occur in association w/ other conditions such as diabetes mellitus (DM) w/ significant renal insufficiency, CHF, and conditions w/ risk of hypoperfusion and hypoxemia. Risk increases w/ the degree of renal dysfunction and age. Avoid in patients ≥80 yrs unless renal function is normal. Avoid w/ clinical/lab evidence of hepatic disease. Temporarily d/c prior to IV radiocontrast studies or surgical procedures. Caution against excessive alcohol intake; may potentiate effects of metformin on lactate metabolism. Withhold in the presence of any condition associated w/ hypoxemia, dehydration, or sepsis. Regularly monitor renal function and use minimum effective dose to decrease risk. If lactic acidosis is suspected, immediately d/c and institute general supportive measures.

ADULT DOSAGE

Type 2 Diabetes Mellitus

≥17 Years:
Initial: 500-1000mg qd
Titrate: May increase in increments of 500mg weekly
Max: 2500mg/day

Transfer From Other Antidiabetic Therapy:
From Standard Oral Hypoglycemic Agents Other Than Chlorpropamide: No transition period necessary
From Chlorpropamide: Exercise care during first 2 weeks for overlapping drug effects and possible hypoglycemia

PEDIATRIC DOSAGE

Pediatric use may not have been established

DOSE MODIFICATION

Concomitant Medications

Oral Sulfonylurea Therapy:
If unresponsive to 4 weeks of max dose of metformin HCl extended-release (ER) monotherapy, consider gradual addition of an oral sulfonylurea while continuing metformin HCl ER at max dose
If patients have not satisfactorily responded to 1-3 months of concomitant therapy (max dose of metformin HCl ER and max dose of an oral sulfonylurea), consider therapeutic alternatives (eg, switching to insulin w/ or w/o metformin HCl ER)

Insulin Therapy:
Initial: 500mg qd while continuing current insulin dose
Titrate: May increase by 500mg after approx 1 week and by 500mg every week thereafter
Max: 2500mg/day
Decrease insulin dose by 10-25% if FPG <120mg/dL

Hepatic Impairment

Avoid in patients w/ clinical or laboratory evidence of hepatic disease

Elderly

Initial/Maint: Use conservative dosing
Do not titrate to max dose

Other Important Modifications

Debilitated/Malnourished Patients:
Do not titrate to max dose

ADMINISTRATION

Oral route

Take w/ a full glass of water w/ pm meal

HOW SUPPLIED

Tab, Extended-Release: 500mg, 1000mg

CONTRAINDICATIONS

Renal disease/dysfunction (eg, SrCr ≥1.5mg/dL [males], ≥1.4mg/dL [females], or abnormal CrCl), acute or chronic metabolic acidosis, including diabetic ketoacidosis w/ or w/o coma.

WARNINGS/PRECAUTIONS

Lactic acidosis may be suspected in diabetic patients w/ metabolic acidosis lacking evidence of ketoacidosis (ketonuria and ketonemia). Caution w/ concomitant medications that may affect renal function, result in significant hemodynamic change, or interfere w/ the disposition of metformin. Temporarily d/c prior to surgical procedures associated w/ restricted oral intake. Temporarily withhold drug before, during, and 48 hrs after radiologic studies w/ IV iodinated contrast materials; reinstitute only when renal function is normal. D/C in hypoxic states (eg, shock, CHF, acute myocardial infarction [MI]), dehydration, and sepsis. Avoid w/ hepatic impairment. May decrease vitamin B12 levels. Increased risk of hypoglycemia in elderly, debilitated/malnourished, adrenal or pituitary insufficiency, or alcohol intoxication. Temporarily withhold metformin and administer insulin if loss of glycemic control occurs due to stress; reinstitute metformin after acute episode is resolved.

ADVERSE REACTIONS

Lactic acidosis, infection, diarrhea, nausea, headache, dyspepsia, rhinitis, flatulence, abdominal pain.

DRUG INTERACTIONS

Furosemide, nifedipine, cimetidine, and cationic drugs (eg, amiloride, digoxin, morphine) may increase metformin levels. Thiazides, other diuretics, corticosteroids, phenothiazines, thyroid products, estrogens, oral contraceptives, phenytoin, nicotinic acid, sympathomimetics, calcium channel blockers, and isoniazid may cause hyperglycemia and loss of glycemic control. May decrease furosemide levels.

NURSING CONSIDERATIONS

Assessment: Assess for hypoxic states (eg, acute CHF, acute MI, cardiovascular collapse), septicemia, acute/chronic metabolic acidosis, adrenal/pituitary insufficiency, alcoholism, pregnancy/nursing status, and possible drug interactions. Evaluate for other medical conditions, and for any IV radiocontrast study or surgical procedure. Assess FPG, HbA1c, renal function, LFTs, and hematologic parameters (eg, Hgb/Hct, RBC indices).

Monitoring: Monitor for lactic acidosis, hypoglycemia, prerenal azotemia, hypoxic states, hypersensitivity reactions, and other adverse reactions. Monitor FPG, HbA1c, renal function (eg, SrCr), LFTs, and hematologic parameters (eg, Hgb/Hct, RBC indices).

Patient Counseling: Inform of the potential risks, benefits, and alternative modes of therapy. Inform about the importance of adherence to dietary instructions, regular exercise programs, and regular testing of blood glucose, HbA1c, renal function, and hematologic parameters. Inform of the risk of lactic acidosis w/ therapy and to contact physician if unexplained hyperventilation, myalgia, malaise, unusual somnolence, or other nonspecific symptoms occur. Counsel against excessive alcohol intake. Explain risks, symptoms, and conditions that predispose to the development of hypoglycemia when initiating combination therapy. Instruct that drug must be taken w/ food, swallowed whole w/ a full glass of water and should not be chewed, cut, or crushed, and that inactive ingredients may be eliminated in the feces as a soft mass.

Storage: 20-25°C (68-77°F); excursions permitted to 15-30°C (59-86°F). Keep tightly closed. Protect from light and moisture. Avoid excessive heat and humidity.

FORTAZ – ceftazidime RX

Class: Cephalosporin (3rd generation)

ADULT DOSAGE

General Dosing

Usual: 1g IM/IV q8-12h

Continue therapy for 2 days after signs and symptoms of infection have disappeared; complicated infections may require longer duration of therapy

Serious Gynecological/Intra-Abdominal/Life-Threatening Infections:
Usual: 2g IV q8h

Urinary Tract Infections

Uncomplicated: 250mg IM/IV q12h
Complicated: 500mg IM/IV q8-12h

Bone/Joint Infections

Usual: 2g IV q12h

Pneumonia

Uncomplicated: 500mg-1g IM/IV q8h

Skin and Skin Structure Infections

Mild: 500mg-1g IM/IV q8h

Meningitis

Usual: 2g IV q8h

Lung Infection

Caused by *Pseudomonas* spp. in Cystic Fibrosis:

Usual: 30-50mg/kg IV q8h
Max: 6g/day

PEDIATRIC DOSAGE

General Dosing

Neonates (0-4 Weeks of Age): 30mg/kg IV q12h

1 Month-12 Years:
Usual: 30-50mg/kg IV q8h
Max: 6g/day

Use higher doses for immunocompromised patients with cystic fibrosis or meningitis

DOSE MODIFICATION

Renal Impairment

If normal recommended dose is lower than recommended dose for renal impairment, the lower dose should be used

CrCl 31-50mL/min: 1g q12h
CrCl 16-30mL/min: 1g q24h
CrCl 6-15mL/min: 500mg q24h
CrCl <5mL/min: 500mg q48h

Other Important Modifications

Hemodialysis: May receive 1g LD, followed by 1g after each hemodialysis period
Intraperitoneal/Continuous Peritoneal Dialysis: May receive 1g LD, followed by 500mg q24h
May include ceftazidime inj in dialysis fluid at a concentration of 250mg/2L dialysis fluid

ADMINISTRATION

IM/IV route

Avoid intra-arterial administration

IM

Administer into large muscle mass (eg, upper outer quadrant of gluteus maximus or lateral part of thigh)
Reconstitute 500mg vial or 1g vial with 1.5mL or 3mL (respectively) of appropriate diluent (eg, Sterile Water for Inj, Bacteriostatic Water for Inj, or 0.5% or 1% Lidocaine HCl Inj)

IV

Do not use plastic containers in series connections
Add 5.3mL of diluent to 500mg IV vial, 10mL of diluent to 1g or 2g IV vial, or 26mL of diluent to 6g pharmacy bulk package vial; constitute with Sterile Water for Inj
Direct Intermittent IV Administration: Slowly inject directly into the vein over 3-5 min, or give through tubing of administration set while patient is also receiving one of the compatible IV fluids
IV Infusion: Constitute 500mg, 1g, or 2g vial and withdraw 5mL, 10mL, or 11.5mL (respectively) to IV container with a compatible IV fluid
Intermittent IV Infusion with Y-Type Administration Set: Administer with compatible solutions; do not infuse with sol containing ceftazidime

Compatible IV Fluid for Solutions with Concentrations Between 1-40mg/mL

0.9% NaCl Inj
1/6 M Sodium Lactate Inj
5% Dextrose Inj
5% Dextrose and 0.225% NaCl Inj
5% Dextrose and 0.45% NaCl Inj
5% Dextrose and 0.9% NaCl Inj
10% Dextrose Inj
Ringer's Inj
Lactated Ringer's Inj
10% Invert Sugar in Water for Inj
Normosol-M in 5% Dextrose Inj
Refer to PI for additional administration instructions

HOW SUPPLIED

Inj: 500mg, 1g, 2g; 1g, 2g [ADD-Vantage]; 1g/50mL, 2g/50mL [Galaxy]. Also available as a Pharmacy Bulk Package.

WARNINGS/PRECAUTIONS

Cross hypersensitivity among β-lactam antibiotics reported; caution with penicillin (PCN) sensitivity. D/C if allergic reaction occurs. *Clostridium difficile*-associated diarrhea (CDAD) reported. May result in bacterial resistance with prolonged use or use in the absence of a proven/suspected bacterial infection or a prophylactic indication; take appropriate measures if superinfection develops. Elevated levels with renal insufficiency may lead to seizures, encephalopathy, coma, asterixis, myoclonia, and neuromuscular excitability. Associated with fall in prothrombin activity; caution with renal/hepatic impairment, poor nutritional state, and protracted course of antimicrobial therapy. Caution with colitis, history of GI disease, and elderly. Distal necrosis may occur after inadvertent intra-arterial administration. Lab test interactions may occur.

ADVERSE REACTIONS

Allergic reactions, increased ALT/AST/GGT/LDH, eosinophilia, local/GI reactions.

DRUG INTERACTIONS

Nephrotoxicity reported with aminoglycosides or potent diuretics (eg, furosemide). Avoid with chloramphenicol. May reduce efficacy of combined oral estrogen/progesterone contraceptives.

NURSING CONSIDERATIONS

Assessment: Assess for history of hypersensitivity to cephalosporins/PCNs, history of GI disease, colitis, renal/hepatic impairment, nursing status, and for possible drug interactions.

Monitoring: Monitor for signs and symptoms of hypersensitivity reactions, CDAD, LDH, LFTs, renal function, PT, hemolytic anemia, and for superinfection. Monitor for seizures, encephalopathy, coma, asterixis, neuromuscular excitability, and myoclonia with renal impairment. Perform periodic susceptibility testing.

Patient Counseling: Inform that therapy only treats bacterial, not viral, infections. Instruct to take exactly ud; explain that skipping doses or not completing full course may decrease effectiveness and increase resistance. Advise that patient may experience diarrhea; instruct to notify physician if watery/bloody stools (with/without stomach cramps and fever) occur.

Storage: 15-30°C (59-86°F), in dry state. Protect from light. Frozen as premixed sol should not be stored above -20°C.

FORTEO – teriparatide (rDNA origin) RX

Class: Recombinant human parathyroid hormone

Prescribe only when benefits outweigh risks; do not prescribe for patients who are at increased baseline risk for osteosarcoma (including those with Paget's disease of bone or unexplained alkaline phosphatase elevations, pediatric and young adult patients with open epiphyses, or prior external beam or implant radiation therapy involving the skeleton).

ADULT DOSAGE

Osteoporosis

High Risk for Fracture:

Postmenopausal Women w/ Osteoporosis:
20mcg qd

Primary or Hypogonadal Osteoporosis in Men:
20mcg qd

Glucocorticoid-Induced Osteoporosis:
20mcg qd

PEDIATRIC DOSAGE

Pediatric use may not have been established

ADMINISTRATION

SQ route

Inject into the thigh or abdominal wall
Administer initially under circumstances where the patient can sit or lie down if symptoms of orthostatic hypotension occur

HOW SUPPLIED

Inj: 250mcg/mL [2.4mL]

WARNINGS/PRECAUTIONS

Use for >2 yrs during a patient's lifetime is not recommended. Do not give in patients with bone metastases or history of skeletal malignancies, metabolic bone diseases other than osteoporosis, preexisting hypercalcemia, or underlying hypercalcemic disorder (eg, primary hyperparathyroidism). Transiently increases serum Ca^{2+}. Consider measurement of urinary Ca^{2+} excretion if active urolithiasis or preexisting hypercalciuria are suspected; caution in patients with active or recent urolithiasis. Transient episodes of symptomatic orthostatic hypotension reported with administration of initial doses; administer initially under circumstances where the patient can sit or lie down if symptoms of orthostatic hypotension occur.

ADVERSE REACTIONS

Pain, arthralgia, rhinitis, asthenia, N/V, dizziness, headache, HTN, increased cough, pharyngitis, constipation, dyspepsia, diarrhea, rash, insomnia.

DRUG INTERACTIONS

Hypercalcemia may predispose to digitalis toxicity; caution if taking digoxin concomitantly.

NURSING CONSIDERATIONS

Assessment: Assess for increased baseline risk for osteosarcoma, bone metastases or history of skeletal malignancies, metabolic bone disease other than osteoporosis, hypercalcemia, hypercalcemic disorder, hypercalciuria, active or recent urolithiasis, hypersensitivity to drug, pregnancy/nursing status, and possible drug interactions. Consider measurement of urinary Ca^{2+} excretion if active urolithiasis or preexisting hypercalciuria are suspected.

Monitoring: Monitor for signs/symptoms of osteosarcoma, orthostatic hypotension, and other adverse reactions.

Patient Counseling: Inform of potential risk of osteosarcoma and encourage to enroll in the voluntary Forteo Patient Registry. Instruct to sit or lie down if lightheadedness or palpitations following inj develop; if symptoms persist or worsen, advise to consult physician before continuing treatment. Instruct to contact physician if persistent symptoms of hypercalcemia (eg, N/V, constipation, lethargy, muscle weakness) develop. Counsel on roles of supplemental Ca^{2+} and/or vitamin D, weight-bearing exercise, and modification of certain behavioral factors (eg, smoking, alcohol consumption). Instruct on proper use of delivery device (pen) and proper disposal of needles; advise not to share pen with other patients and not to transfer contents to a syringe.

Storage: 2-8°C (36-46°F). Recap pen when not in use. Minimize time out of the refrigerator during the use period; may deliver dose immediately following removal from the refrigerator. Do not freeze; do not use if it has been frozen. Discard after the 28-day use period.

FORTESTA – testosterone CIII

Class: Androgen

Virilization reported in children secondarily exposed to testosterone gel. Children should avoid contact with unwashed or unclothed application sites in men using testosterone gel. Advise patients to strictly adhere to recommended instructions for use.

ADULT DOSAGE

Testosterone Replacement Therapy

Congenital/Acquired Primary Hypogonadism or Hypogonadotropic Hypogonadism in Males:

Initial: Apply 40mg qam
Titrate: May adjust between 10-70mg based on serum testosterone concentration from a single blood draw 2 hrs after application at 14 days, and 35 days after starting treatment or following dose adjustment
Titration Based on Total Serum Testosterone Concentration 2 Hrs Post Application:
<500ng/dL: Increase daily dose by 10mg
≥500-<1250ng/dL: Continue on current dose
≥1250-<2500ng/dL: Decrease daily dose by 10mg
≥2500ng/dL: Decrease daily dose by 20mg
Max: 70mg

PEDIATRIC DOSAGE

Pediatric use may not have been established

ADMINISTRATION

Topical route

Apply to intact skin of the thighs
Avoid swimming, showering, or washing the administration site for a minimum of 2 hrs after application
Prime canister pump in upright position, slowly and fully depress actuator 8X
Refer to PI for further administration instructions

HOW SUPPLIED

Gel: 10mg/actuation [120 actuations]

CONTRAINDICATIONS

Breast carcinoma or known/suspected prostate carcinoma in men; women who are or may become pregnant, or are breastfeeding.

WARNINGS/PRECAUTIONS

Application site and dose are not interchangeable with other topical testosterone products. Patients with BPH and geriatric patients may be at increased risk of worsening of signs/symptoms of BPH. May increase risk for prostate cancer. Risk of virilization in women due to secondary exposure; d/c until cause is identified. Not indicated for use in women. Increases in Hct/RBC mass may increase risk for thromboembolic events; may require dose reduction or discontinuation of therapy until Hct decreases to an acceptable concentration. Venous thromboembolic events (VTEs), including deep vein thrombosis and pulmonary embolism, reported; d/c treatment and initiate workup and management if venous thromboembolic event is suspected. Suppression of spermatogenesis may occur with large doses. Prolonged use of high doses of orally active 17-α-alkyl androgens may cause serious hepatic effects (eg, peliosis hepatis, hepatic neoplasms, cholestatic hepatitis, jaundice). Risk of edema with or without congestive heart failure (CHF) in patients with preexisting cardiac, renal, or hepatic disease. Gynecomastia may develop and persist. May potentiate sleep apnea. Changes in serum lipid profile may require dose adjustment or discontinuation of therapy. Caution in cancer patients at risk of hypercalcemia and associated hypercalciuria. May decrease levels of thyroxin-binding globulins, resulting in decreased total T4 serum levels and increased resin uptake of T3 and T4. Flammable; avoid fire, flame, or smoking until the gel has dried.

ADVERSE REACTIONS
Application-site reactions.

DRUG INTERACTIONS
Changes in insulin sensitivity or glycemic control may occur; may decrease blood glucose and, therefore, decrease insulin requirements in diabetic patients. Adrenocorticotropic hormone or corticosteroids may increase fluid retention; caution in patients with cardiac, renal, or hepatic disease. Changes in anticoagulant activity may occur; frequently monitor INR and PT in patients taking anticoagulants, especially at initiation and termination of androgen therapy.

NURSING CONSIDERATIONS

Assessment: Assess for BPH, prostate cancer, cardiac/renal/hepatic disease, obesity, chronic lung disease, conditions where treatment is contraindicated or cautioned, and for possible drug interactions. Check Hct prior to therapy.

Monitoring: Monitor for prostate carcinoma, edema with or without CHF, gynecomastia, worsening of signs/symptoms of BPH, sleep apnea, VTEs, and other adverse reactions. Perform periodic monitoring of Hgb, LFTs, prostate-specific antigen, and serum lipid profile. Obtain serum testosterone levels 14 days and 35 days after initiation of therapy or following dose adjustment. In cancer patients at risk for hypercalcemia, regularly monitor serum Ca^{2+} levels. Reevaluate Hct 3-6 months after start of therapy, then annually.

Patient Counseling: Inform that men with known or suspected prostate/breast cancer should not use androgen therapy. Advise to report signs/symptoms of secondary exposure in children and in women to the physician. Inform that children and women should avoid contact with unwashed or unclothed application sites of men using testosterone gel. Instruct to apply ud; instruct to cover application site with clothing after gel dries, and wash application site with soap and water prior to direct skin-to-skin contact with others. Inform about possible adverse reactions. Inform that drug is flammable; instruct to avoid fire, flame, or smoking until the gel has dried. Advise not to share the medication with anyone. Instruct to adhere to all the recommended monitoring, to wait 2 hrs before swimming or washing following application, and to report changes in their state of health.

Storage: 20-25°C (68-77°F); excursions permitted to 15-30°C (59-86°F). Do not freeze. Discard used canisters in household trash in a manner that prevents accidental application or ingestion by children or pets.

FOSAMAX PLUS D – alendronate sodium/cholecalciferol RX

Class: Bisphosphonate/vitamin D analogue

ADULT DOSAGE

Osteoporosis

Treatment of Osteoporosis in Postmenopausal Women/Treatment to Increase Bone Mass in Men w/ Osteoporosis:
Usual: 1 tab (70mg/2800 IU or 70mg/5600 IU) once weekly

For most osteoporotic women/men, appropriate dose is 70mg/5600 IU once weekly

Periodically reevaluate need for continued therapy

Missed Dose

If once-weekly dose is missed, administer 1 tab on am after patient remembers; do not take 2 tabs on same day, but return to taking 1 tab once a week, as originally scheduled on chosen day

PEDIATRIC DOSAGE

Pediatric use may not have been established

DOSE MODIFICATION

Renal Impairment
CrCl <35mL/min: Not recommended

ADMINISTRATION
Oral route

Take upon arising for the day
Swallow tabs w/ full glass of water (6-8 oz); do not chew or suck on the tab
Take at least 1/2 hr before the 1st food, beverage, or medication of the day w/ plain water only
Do not lie down for at least 30 min and until after 1st food of the day

Recommendations for Ca^{2+} and Vitamin D Supplementation

If dietary intake is inadequate, patients should take supplemental Ca^{2+}; patients at increased risk for vitamin D insufficiency may need additional vitamin D supplementation

Patients w/ GI malabsorption syndromes may require higher doses of vitamin D supplementation and measurement of 25-hydroxyvitamin D should be considered

HOW SUPPLIED

Tab: (Alendronate/Cholecalciferol) 70mg/2800 IU, 70mg/5600 IU

CONTRAINDICATIONS

Esophageal abnormalities that delay esophageal emptying (eg, stricture, achalasia), inability to stand or sit upright for at least 30 min, hypocalcemia.

WARNINGS/PRECAUTIONS

Do not use alone to treat vitamin D deficiency. Consider discontinuation after 3-5 yrs of use in patients at low-risk for fracture; periodically reevaluate risk for fracture in patients who d/c therapy. May cause local irritation of the upper GI mucosa; caution w/ active upper GI problems (eg, Barrett's esophagus, dysphagia, other esophageal diseases, gastritis, duodenitis, ulcers). Esophageal reactions (eg, esophagitis, esophageal ulcers/erosions) reported; d/c if dysphagia, odynophagia, retrosternal pain, or new/worsening heartburn develops. Use under appropriate supervision in patients who cannot comply w/ dosing instructions due to mental disability. Gastric and duodenal ulcers reported. Treat hypocalcemia or other disorders affecting mineral metabolism (eg, vitamin D deficiency) prior to therapy. Asymptomatic decreases in serum Ca^{2+} and phosphate may occur. Severe and occasionally incapacitating bone, joint, and/or muscle pain reported; d/c if severe symptoms develop. Osteonecrosis of the jaw (ONJ) reported; risk may increase w/ duration of exposure to drug. If invasive dental procedures are required, discontinuation of treatment may reduce risk for ONJ. Consider discontinuation if ONJ develops. Atypical, low-energy, or low trauma fractures of the femoral shaft reported; evaluate any patient w/ a history of bisphosphonate exposure who presents w/ thigh/groin pain to rule out incomplete femur fracture, and consider interruption of therapy. Vitamin D3 supplementation may worsen hypercalcemia and/or hypercalciuria in patients w/ diseases associated w/ unregulated overproduction of 1,25-dihydroxyvitamin D (eg, leukemia, lymphoma, sarcoidosis).

ADVERSE REACTIONS

Abdominal pain, musculoskeletal pain, nausea, dyspepsia, constipation, diarrhea.

DRUG INTERACTIONS

Ca^{2+} supplements, antacids, or oral medications containing multivalent cations will interfere w/ absorption of alendronate; wait at least 1/2 hr after dosing before taking any other oral medications. NSAID use is associated w/ GI irritation; use w/ caution. Alendronate: Increased incidence of upper GI adverse events in patients receiving concomitant therapy w/ daily doses of alendronate >10mg and aspirin-containing products. Cholecalciferol: Olestra, mineral oils, orlistat, and bile acid sequestrants (eg, cholestyramine, colestipol) may impair absorption; consider additional supplementation. Anticonvulsants, cimetidine, and thiazides may increase catabolism; consider additional supplementation.

NURSING CONSIDERATIONS

Assessment: Assess for esophageal abnormalities, ability to stand or sit upright for at least 30 min, hypocalcemia, risk for ONJ, active upper GI problems, mental disability, renal impairment, drug hypersensitivity, any other conditions where treatment is contraindicated or cautioned, pregnancy/nursing status, and possible drug interactions.

Monitoring: Monitor for signs/symptoms of ONJ, atypical fractures, esophageal reactions, musculoskeletal pain, hypocalcemia, and other adverse events. Monitor urine and serum Ca^{2+} in patients w/ diseases associated w/ unregulated overproduction of 1,25-dihydroxyvitamin D. Periodically reevaluate the need for continued therapy.

Patient Counseling: Instruct to take supplemental Ca^{2+} and vitamin D if dietary intake is inadequate. Counsel to consider weight-bearing exercise along w/ the modification of certain behavioral factors (eg, cigarette smoking, excessive alcohol consumption), if these factors exist. Instruct to take upon arising for the day and at least 1/2 hr before the 1st food, beverage, or other medication of the day w/ plain water only; advise to swallow tab w/ 6-8 oz of water. Advise to avoid lying down for at least 30 min after taking the drug and until after 1st food of the day. Instruct to follow all dosing instructions and inform that failure to follow them may increase risk of esophageal problems. Advise to d/c and consult physician if symptoms of esophageal disease develop. Instruct that if a once-weekly dose is missed, to take 1 dose on the am after patient remembers and to return to taking 1 dose once a week, as originally scheduled on patient's chosen day; instruct not to take 2 doses on the same day.

Storage: 20-25°C (68-77°F); excursions permitted to 15-30°C (59-86°F). Protect from moisture and light.

FOSINOPRIL – fosinopril sodium

RX

Class: ACE inhibitor

May cause injury and even death to the developing fetus during the 2nd and 3rd trimesters of pregnancy. D/C when pregnancy is detected.

ADULT DOSAGE

Hypertension

Initial: 10mg qd
Titrate: May adjust dosage based on BP response
Usual: 20-40mg qd

Divide daily dose if trough response is inadequate
Diuretic may be added if BP is not adequately controlled with therapy alone

Heart Failure

Adjunct to diuretics with or without digitalis
Initial: 10mg qd
Titrate: Increase over several weeks as tolerated
Usual: 20-40mg qd
Max: 40mg qd

PEDIATRIC DOSAGE

Hypertension

≥6 Years:
>50kg: 5-10mg qd

DOSE MODIFICATION

Concomitant Medications

HTN:

Currently Treated with Diuretic:
D/C diuretic 2-3 days prior to initiating therapy, if possible. May resume diuretic therapy if BP is not controlled with therapy alone
Initial: 10mg qd with careful monitoring until BP is stabilized

Renal Impairment

HF:

Moderate to Severe Renal Failure/Vigorous Diuresis:
Initial: 5mg

Elderly

Start at lower end of dosing range

ADMINISTRATION

Oral route.

HOW SUPPLIED

Tab: 10mg*, 20mg, 40mg *scored

CONTRAINDICATIONS

History of ACE inhibitor-associated angioedema.

WARNINGS/PRECAUTIONS

Head and neck angioedema reported; d/c and administer appropriate therapy if laryngeal stridor or angioedema of the face, lips, tongue, mucous membranes, glottis, or extremities occurs. More reports of angioedema in blacks than nonblacks. Intestinal angioedema reported; monitor for abdominal pain. Anaphylactoid reactions reported during desensitization with hymenoptera venom, dialysis with high-flux membranes, and LDL apheresis with dextran sulfate absorption. Symptomatic hypotension may occur, most likely in patients with volume and/or salt depletion; correct depletion prior to therapy. Excessive hypotension associated with oliguria, azotemia, and rarely acute renal failure and death may occur in patients with HF, with or without associated renal insufficiency; monitor closely during the first 2 weeks of treatment and whenever dose of therapy or diuretic is increased. May cause agranulocytosis and bone marrow depression; consider monitoring of WBC in patients with collagen-vascular disease, especially with renal impairment. Rarely, associated with syndrome that starts with cholestatic jaundice and progresses to fulminant hepatic necrosis and sometimes death; d/c if jaundice or marked elevation of hepatic enzymes occur. May cause renal function changes. May increase BUN and SrCr levels with renal artery stenosis or with no preexisting renal vascular disease; may need to reduce dose of therapy and/or d/c diuretic. Hyperkalemia reported; risk factors include diabetes mellitus (DM) and renal insufficiency. Hypotension may occur with surgery or during anesthesia. Persistent nonproductive cough reported. Caution in elderly.

ADVERSE REACTIONS

Dizziness, cough, hypotension, musculoskeletal pain.

DRUG INTERACTIONS
May increase lithium levels and symptoms of lithium toxicity; frequently monitor serum lithium levels. Hypotension risk with diuretics. Increased risk of hyperkalemia with K^+-sparing diuretics (eg, spironolactone, amiloride, triamterene), K^+-containing salt substitutes, or K^+ supplements; use with caution. Antacids may impair absorption; separate doses by 2 hrs. Nitritoid reactions reported rarely with injectable gold (sodium aurothiomalate).

NURSING CONSIDERATIONS

Assessment: Assess for history of angioedema, hypersensitivity to drug, volume/salt depletion, collagen vascular disease, DM, renal artery stenosis, HF, renal impairment, pregnancy/nursing status, and possible drug interactions.

Monitoring: Monitor for signs/symptoms of hypotension, anaphylactoid or hypersensitivity reactions, head/neck/intestinal angioedema, agranulocytosis, neutropenia, bone marrow depression, hyperkalemia, and other adverse reactions. Monitor BP and renal/hepatic function. Consider monitoring WBCs in patients with collagen vascular disease, especially if with renal impairment.

Patient Counseling: Instruct to d/c therapy and immediately report signs/symptoms of angioedema. Caution about lightheadedness, especially during the 1st few days of therapy; advise to d/c therapy and consult physician if syncope occurs. Caution that inadequate fluid intake or excessive perspiration, diarrhea, or vomiting may lead to an excessive fall in BP resulting in lightheadedness or syncope. Instruct to avoid using K^+ supplements or salt substitutes-containing K^+ without consulting physician. Advise to report any symptoms of infection. Inform of pregnancy risks during the 2nd or 3rd trimesters and instruct to report to physician as soon as possible if pregnant.

Storage: 20-25°C (68-77°F). Protect from moisture.

FOSINOPRIL/HCTZ – fosinopril sodium/hydrochlorothiazide RX

Class: ACE inhibitor/thiazide diuretic

D/C when pregnancy is detected. Drugs that act directly on the renin-angiotensin system (RAS) can cause injury/death to developing fetus.

ADULT DOSAGE

Hypertension

Not Controlled with Fosinopril/HCTZ Monotherapy:
10mg-12.5mg tab or 20mg-12.5mg tab qd
Titrate: Dosage must be guided by clinical response

PEDIATRIC DOSAGE

Pediatric use may not have been established

DOSE MODIFICATION

Elderly
Start at lower end of dosing range

ADMINISTRATION
Oral route

HOW SUPPLIED
Tab: (Fosinopril-HCTZ) 10mg-12.5mg, 20mg-12.5mg* *scored

CONTRAINDICATIONS
Anuria and hypersensitivity to other sulfonamide-derived drugs.

WARNINGS/PRECAUTIONS
Not indicated for initial therapy. Caution in elderly and with severe renal disease. Avoid if CrCl <30mL/min. Caution with impaired hepatic function or progressive liver disease; may precipitate hepatic coma. Fosinopril: Angioedema reported; d/c and administer appropriate therapy if laryngeal stridor or angioedema of the face, tongue, or glottis occurs. Higher rate of angioedema in blacks than nonblacks. Intestinal angioedema reported; monitor for abdominal pain. Anaphylactoid reactions reported during desensitization with hymenoptera venom, dialysis with high-flux membranes, and LDL apheresis with dextran sulfate absorption. Symptomatic hypotension may occur, most likely in patients with volume and/or salt depletion; correct volume and/or salt depletion prior to therapy. Excessive hypotension associated with oliguria, azotemia, and rarely acute renal failure and/or death may occur in patients with congestive heart failure (CHF); monitor closely during the first 2 weeks of treatment and when dose is increased. May cause changes in renal function. May increase BUN and SrCr levels with renal artery stenosis and with no preexisting renal vascular disease; monitor renal function during 1st few weeks of therapy in patients with renal

artery stenosis. May cause agranulocytosis and bone marrow depression; consider monitoring of WBCs in patients with collagen vascular disease and renal disease. Rarely, associated with syndrome that starts with cholestatic jaundice and progresses to fulminant necrosis and sometimes death; d/c if jaundice or marked hepatic enzyme elevations occur. Hyperkalemia and persistent nonproductive cough reported. Hypotension may occur with surgery or during anesthesia. HCTZ: May precipitate azotemia with severe renal disease. May exacerbate or activate systemic lupus erythematosus (SLE). Dilutional hyponatremia may occur in edematous patients; institute appropriate therapy of water restriction rather than salt administration, except for life-threatening hyponatremia. May increase cholesterol, TGs, uric acid levels, and decrease glucose tolerance. Hyponatremia, hypokalemia, and hypochloremic alkalosis reported. Hypokalemia may sensitize or exaggerate the response of the heart to toxic effects of digitalis. Pathological changes in the parathyroid glands, with hypercalcemia and hypophosphatemia observed with prolonged therapy. May enhance effects in postsympathectomy patients. Neutropenia/agranulocytosis reported. Lab test interactions may occur.

ADVERSE REACTIONS

Headache, cough, fatigue, dizziness.

DRUG INTERACTIONS

Dual blockade of the RAS is associated with increased risks of hypotension, hyperkalemia, and changes in renal function (including acute renal failure); closely monitor BP, renal function, and electrolytes with concomitant agents that also affect the RAS. Avoid concomitant use of aliskiren in patients with diabetes and with renal impairment (GFR <60mL/min). Increased risk of hyperkalemia with K^+-sparing diuretics, K^+ supplements, or K^+-containing salt substitutes; use with caution and monitor serum K+ frequently. Caution with other antihypertensives. May alter insulin requirements in diabetic patients. May increase lithium levels and risk of toxicity; use with caution and monitor serum lithium levels frequently. Nitritoid reactions reported rarely with injectable gold (eg, sodium aurothiomalate). Fosinopril: Antacids (aluminum hydroxide, magnesium hydroxide, simethicone) may impair absorption; separate doses by 2 hrs. HCTZ: May potentiate action of other antihypertensives, especially ganglionic or peripheral adrenergic-blocking drugs. May decrease effectiveness of methenamine. May increase responsiveness to tubocurarine. May decrease arterial responsiveness to norepinephrine. NSAIDs may decrease diuretic, natriuretic, and antihypertensive effects. Cholestyramine or colestipol resins reduce absorption. Increased risk of hypokalemia with corticosteroids and adrenocorticotropic hormone.

NURSING CONSIDERATIONS

Assessment: Assess for anuria, history of allergy or bronchial asthma, hypersensitivity to drug or to sulfonamides, volume/salt depletion, CHF, SLE, renal/hepatic function, collagen vascular disease, risk factors for hyperkalemia, pregnancy/nursing status, and possible drug interactions.

Monitoring: Monitor for signs/symptoms of angioedema, agranulocytosis, anaphylactoid/hypersensitivity reactions, hypotension, exacerbation/activation of SLE, and other adverse reactions. Monitor BP, serum electrolytes, serum uric acid levels, hepatic/renal function, cholesterol/TG levels, and glucose tolerance. Monitor WBCs in patients with collagen vascular disease and renal impairment.

Patient Counseling: Inform females of childbearing age of the consequences of exposure during pregnancy and of the treatment options for women planning to become pregnant; report pregnancy to physician as soon as possible. Instruct to d/c therapy and immediately report signs/symptoms of angioedema (eg, swelling of face, eyes, lips, tongue, difficulty breathing). Caution that lightheadedness can occur, especially during the 1st days of therapy and advise to report to physician; instruct to d/c therapy and consult physician if syncope occurs. Caution that inadequate fluid intake, excessive perspiration, diarrhea, or vomiting can lead to excessive fall in BP, resulting in lightheadedness or syncope. Instruct not to use salt substitutes containing K^+ or K^+ supplements without consulting physician. Instruct to promptly report any indication of infection (eg, sore throat, fever).

Storage: 20-25°C (68-77°F). Protect from moisture.

FRAGMIN — dalteparin sodium RX

Class: Low molecular weight heparin

Epidural or spinal hematomas may occur in patients anticoagulated w/ low molecular weight heparins (LMWHs) or heparinoids and are receiving neuraxial anesthesia or undergoing spinal puncture; may result in long-term or permanent paralysis. Increased risk of developing epidural or spinal hematomas in patients using indwelling epidural catheters, concomitant use of other drugs that affect hemostasis (eg, NSAIDs, platelet inhibitors, other anticoagulants), history of traumatic or repeated epidural or spinal punctures, history of spinal deformity or spinal surgery, or unknown optimal timing between administration of therapy and neuraxial procedures. Monitor frequently for signs/symptoms of neurologic impairment; if neurologic compromise is noted, urgent treatment is necessary. Consider benefits and risks before neuraxial intervention in patients anticoagulated or to be anticoagulated for thromboprophylaxis.

ADULT DOSAGE

Unstable Angina

Prophylaxis of Ischemic Complications:

Usual: 120 IU/kg q12h w/ PO aspirin therapy (75-165mg qd) until clinically stabilized
Usual Duration: 5-8 days
Max: 10,000 IU q12h

Non-Q-Wave Myocardial Infarction

Prophylaxis of Ischemic Complications:

Usual: 120 IU/kg q12h w/ PO aspirin therapy (75-165mg qd) until clinically stabilized
Usual Duration: 5-8 days
Max: 10,000 IU q12h

Deep Vein Thrombosis

Prophylaxis Following Hip Replacement Surgery:
1st Dose Preop PM Before Surgery:
Usual: 5000 IU 10-14 hrs preop, then 5000 IU 4-8 hrs postop, then 5000 IU qd for 5-10 days postop (up to 14 days)
1st Dose Preop Day of Surgery:
Usual: 2500 IU w/in 2 hrs preop, then 2500 IU 4-8 hrs postop, then 5000 IU qd for 5-10 days postop (up to 14 days)
1st Dose Postop:
Usual: 2500 IU 4-8 hrs postop then 5000 IU qd for 5-10 days postop (up to 14 days)
Prophylaxis in Patients Undergoing Abdominal Surgery:
Risk of Thromboembolic Complications: 2500 IU 1-2 hrs preop then qd for 5-10 days postop
High Risk of Thromboembolic Complications: 5000 IU pm preop then qd for 5-10 days postop
Abdominal Surgery w/ Malignancy: 2500 IU 1-2 hrs preop, followed by 2500 IU 12 hrs later, then 5000 IU qd for 5-10 days postop

Prophylaxis in Medical Patients at Risk Due to Severely Restricted Mobility During Acute Illness: 5000 IU qd for 12-14 days

Venous Thromboembolism

Extended Treatment of Symptomatic VTE in Patients w/ Cancer:

Usual: 200 IU/kg qd for first 30 days, then 150 IU/kg qd for months 2-6
Max: 18,000 IU/day

PEDIATRIC DOSAGE

Pediatric use may not have been established

DOSE MODIFICATION

Renal Impairment
Extended Treatment of Symptomatic VTE in Cancer Patients:
Severe (CrCl <30mL/min): Monitor anti-factor Xa levels to determine appropriate dose; target anti-Xa range is 0.5-1.5 IU/mL. When monitoring anti-Xa levels, perform sampling 4-6 hrs after dosing and only after the patient has received 3-4 doses

Adverse Reactions
Thrombocytopenia:
In Patients w/ Cancer and Acute Symptomatic VTE:
Platelet Count <50,000/mm^3: D/C therapy until platelet count recovers to >50,000/mm^3
Platelet Count 50,000-100,000/mm^3: Reduce daily dose by 2500 IU until platelet count recovers to ≥100,000/mm^3

ADMINISTRATION

SQ route

Do not inject IM
Do not mix w/ other inj or infusions unless compatible

SQ Injection Technique

May inject in the U-shape area around the navel, the upper outer side of the thigh, or the upper outer quadrangle of the buttock; vary inj site daily

Use thumb and forefinger to lift a fold of skin when injecting to the navel area or thigh; entire length of needle should be inserted at a 45-90° angle

Do not expel air bubble from fixed dose syringe prior to inj; air bubble may be expelled from graduated syringes

HOW SUPPLIED

Inj: 2500 IU, 5000 IU [0.2mL syringe], 7500 IU [0.3mL syringe], 10,000 IU [0.4mL, 1mL syringe], 12,500 IU [0.5mL syringe], 15,000 IU [0.6mL syringe], 18,000 IU [0.72mL syringe], 95,000 IU [3.8mL, 9.5mL vial]

CONTRAINDICATIONS

Active major bleeding, history of heparin-induced thrombocytopenia or heparin-induced thrombocytopenia w/ thrombosis, as treatment for unstable angina/non-Q wave MI and for prolonged VTE prophylaxis in patients undergoing epidural/neuraxial anesthesia, and hypersensitivity to heparin or to pork products.

WARNINGS/PRECAUTIONS

Not indicated for acute treatment of VTE. Consider pharmacokinetic profile of dalteparin to reduce the potential risk of bleeding associated w/ concurrent use w/ epidural or spinal anesthesia/analgesia or spinal puncture. Placement or removal of catheter should be delayed for at least 12 hrs after administration of 2500 IU qd, at least 15 hrs after administration of 5000 IU qd, and at least 24 hrs after administration of higher doses (200 IU/kg qd, 120 IU/kg bid) of therapy. For patients w/ CrCl <30mL/min, consider doubling the timing of removal of catheter, at least 24 hrs for the lower prescribed dose and at least 48 hrs for the higher dose. Extreme caution in patients w/ increased risk of hemorrhage (eg, severe uncontrolled HTN, bacterial endocarditis, hemorrhagic stroke, shortly after brain, spinal, or ophthalmological surgery). May enhance the risk of bleeding w/ thrombocytopenia or platelet defects, severe liver/kidney insufficiency, hypertensive or diabetic retinopathy, and recent GI bleeding. Bleeding may occur at any site during therapy. Heparin-induced thrombocytopenia may occur. Multidose vial contains benzyl alcohol as a preservative; associated w/ fatal "gasping syndrome" in premature infants. Caution in pregnant women; use preservative-free formulations, where possible. Caution in elderly, particularly w/ low body weight (<45kg) and those predisposed to decreased renal function.

ADVERSE REACTIONS

Inj-site hematoma, bleeding, inj-site pain, thrombocytopenia, elevation of serum transaminases (ALT/AST).

DRUG INTERACTIONS

See Boxed Warning and Contraindications. Caution w/ oral anticoagulants, platelet inhibitors, and thrombolytic agents due to increased risk of bleeding.

NURSING CONSIDERATIONS

Assessment: Assess for hypersensitivity reaction to drug/heparin or pork products, conditions that increase risk of hematomas/hemorrhage, renal/hepatic impairment, any other conditions where treatment is contraindicated or cautioned, pregnancy/nursing status, and possible drug interactions.

Monitoring: Monitor for bleeding, thrombocytopenia, hypersensitivity reactions, and other adverse reactions. Monitor for signs/symptoms of spinal or epidural hematomas and neurologic impairment in patients receiving neuraxial anesthesia or undergoing spinal puncture. Perform periodic CBCs w/ platelet count, blood chemistry, and stool occult blood tests. Monitor anti-factor Xa levels in patients w/ severe renal impairment or if abnormal coagulation parameters or bleeding occurs.

Patient Counseling: Inform patients who had neuraxial anesthesia/spinal puncture, particularly if taking concomitant NSAIDs, platelet inhibitors, or other anticoagulants to watch for signs/symptoms of spinal/epidural hematoma (eg, tingling, numbness [especially in the lower limbs], muscular weakness); instruct to notify physician immediately if any of these occur. Instruct to d/c use of ASA or other NSAIDs prior to therapy whenever possible. Inform about injecting instructions if therapy is to continue after discharge from hospital. Instruct to report to physician any unusual bleeding, bruising, or signs of thrombocytopenia (eg, rash of dark red spots under skin). Inform that it will take longer than usual to stop bleeding and may bruise and/or bleed more easily while on therapy. Advise to inform healthcare providers of intake of dalteparin and/or any other product known to affect bleeding before any surgery is scheduled, or before any new drug is taken. Instruct to inform physicians and dentists of all medications being taken, including those obtained w/o prescription.

Storage: 20-25°C (68-77°F). (Multiple Dose Vial): Room temperature for ≤2 weeks after 1st penetration of the rubber stopper. Discard any unused sol after 2 weeks.

FROVA – frovatriptan succinate RX

Class: $5\text{-}HT_{1B/1D}$ agonist

ADULT DOSAGE

Migraine

W/ or w/o Aura:

Usual: 2.5mg w/ fluids

May administer 2nd dose 2 hrs after 1st dose if migraine recurs after initial relief

Max: 7.5mg/day

Safety of treating >4 migraines/30 days not known

PEDIATRIC DOSAGE

Pediatric use may not have been established

ADMINISTRATION

Oral route

HOW SUPPLIED

Tab: 2.5mg

CONTRAINDICATIONS

Ischemic coronary artery disease (CAD) (eg, angina pectoris, history of MI, documented silent ischemia) or coronary artery vasospasm (eg, Prinzmetal's angina), Wolff-Parkinson-White syndrome or arrhythmias associated with other cardiac accessory conduction pathway disorders, history of stroke, transient ischemic attack, or history of hemiplegic or basilar migraine, peripheral vascular disease, ischemic bowel disease, uncontrolled HTN. Recent use (within 24 hrs) of another $5\text{-}HT_1$ agonist, an ergotamine-containing or ergot-type medication (eg, dihydroergotamine, methysergide).

WARNINGS/PRECAUTIONS

Use only if a clear diagnosis of migraine has been established. If no treatment response for the 1st migraine attack, reconsider diagnosis before treating any subsequent attacks. Not indicated for prevention of migraine attacks. Serious cardiac adverse reactions, including acute MI, reported. May cause coronary artery vasospasm (Prinzmetal's angina). Perform cardiovascular (CV) evaluation in triptan-naive patients who have multiple CV risk factors prior to therapy; consider administering 1st dose in a medically supervised setting and perform ECG immediately following administration in patients with a negative CV evaluation. Consider periodic CV evaluation in intermittent long-term users who have CV risk factors. Life-threatening cardiac rhythm disturbances (eg, ventricular tachycardia/fibrillation leading to death) reported; d/c if these occur. Sensations of pain, tightness, pressure, and heaviness reported in the chest, throat, neck, and jaw after treatment and are usually noncardiac in origin; perform a cardiac evaluation if at high cardiac risk. Cerebral/subarachnoid hemorrhage, stroke, and other cerebrovascular events reported. Care should be taken to exclude other potentially serious neurological conditions before treatment. May cause noncoronary vasospastic reactions (eg, peripheral vascular ischemia, GI vascular ischemia and infarction [presenting with abdominal pain and bloody diarrhea], splenic infarction, Raynaud's syndrome); rule out vasospastic reaction before using if experiencing signs/symptoms suggestive of noncoronary vasospasm reaction. Transient and permanent blindness and significant partial vision loss reported. Overuse of acute migraine drugs may lead to exacerbation of headache (medication overuse headache); detoxification, including withdrawal of the overused drugs, and treatment of withdrawal symptoms may be necessary. Serotonin syndrome may occur; d/c if serotonin syndrome is suspected. Significant elevation in BP, including hypertensive crisis with acute impairment of organ systems, reported; monitor BP. Anaphylaxis, anaphylactoid, and hypersensitivity reactions including angioedema reported; more likely to occur in patients with history of sensitivity to multiple allergens. Caution with severe hepatic impairment.

ADVERSE REACTIONS

Dizziness, fatigue, headache, paresthesia, flushing, dry mouth, hot or cold sensation, skeletal pain.

DRUG INTERACTIONS

See Contraindications. Serotonin syndrome reported with SSRIs, SNRIs, TCAs, and MAOIs.

NURSING CONSIDERATIONS

Assessment: Assess for ischemic CAD, coronary artery vasospasm, uncontrolled HTN, neurological conditions, hepatic impairment, history of sensitivity to multiple allergens, drug hypersensitivity, any conditions where treatment is cautioned or contraindicated, pregnancy/nursing status, and possible drug interactions. Perform CV evaluation in triptan-naive patients prior to therapy who have multiple CV risk factors.

Monitoring: Monitor for cardiac adverse reactions, coronary artery vasospasm, cardiac rhythm disturbances, cerebrovascular events, noncoronary vasospastic reactions, serotonin syndrome, BP elevation, exacerbation of headache, anaphylactic/hypersensitivity reactions, ophthalmic changes, and other adverse events. Consider periodic CV evaluation in intermittent long-term users who have CV risk factors. Perform ECG immediately following administration in patients with a negative CV evaluation.

Patient Counseling: Inform that drug may cause serious CV side effects, to be alert for the signs/symptoms of chest pain, SOB, weakness, and slurring of speech, and to ask for medical advice when observing any indicative signs/symptoms. Inform that anaphylactic/anaphylactoid reactions have occurred and that they are more likely to occur in patients with history of sensitivity to multiple allergens. Inform that overuse (≥10 days/month) may lead to exacerbation of headache; encourage to record headache frequency and drug use. Caution about the risk of serotonin syndrome. Advise to notify physician if pregnant/nursing or planning to become pregnant.

Storage: 25°C (77°F); excursions permitted to 15-30°C (59-86°F). Protect from moisture.

FULYZAQ – crofelemer RX

Class: Antidiarrheal

ADULT DOSAGE

Noninfectious Diarrhea

Symptomatic Relief in Patients w/ HIV/AIDS on Antiretroviral Therapy

125mg bid

PEDIATRIC DOSAGE

Pediatric use may not have been established

ADMINISTRATION

Oral route

Take w/ or w/o food
Swallow whole; do not crush or chew

HOW SUPPLIED

Tab, Delayed-Release: 125mg

WARNINGS/PRECAUTIONS

Not indicated for the treatment of infectious diarrhea; rule out infectious etiologies of diarrhea before initiating therapy.

ADVERSE REACTIONS

URTI, bronchitis, cough, flatulence, increased bilirubin.

NURSING CONSIDERATIONS

Assessment: Assess etiology of diarrhea and pregnancy/nursing status.

Monitoring: Monitor for adverse reactions.

Patient Counseling: Instruct to take ud.

Storage: 20-25°C (68-77°F); excursions permitted between 15-30°C (59-86°F).

FUROSEMIDE – furosemide RX

Class: Loop diuretic

OTHER BRAND NAMES

Lasix

ADULT DOSAGE

Edema

Associated w/ CHF, Liver Cirrhosis, and Renal Disease (Nephrotic Syndrome):

PO:

Initial: 20-80mg as a single dose
Titrate: May repeat the same dose if needed or increase dose by 20mg or 40mg; give dose no sooner than 6-8 hrs after the previous dose until desired diuretic effect has been obtained; give individually determined single dose qd or bid
Severe Edematous States: May carefully titrate dose up to 600mg/day

Consider giving on 2-4 consecutive days each week

PEDIATRIC DOSAGE

Edema

Associated w/ CHF, Liver Cirrhosis, and Renal Disease (Nephrotic Syndrome):

PO:

Initial: 2mg/kg as a single dose
Titrate: May increase by 1 or 2mg/kg no sooner than 6-8 hrs after the previous dose, if diuretic response is not satisfactory after the initial dose
Maint: Adjust to the minimum effective level
Max: 6mg/kg

Inj:

Initial: 1mg/kg IV/IM
Titrate: May increase by 1mg/kg no sooner

Closely monitor when exceeding 80mg/day for prolonged periods
Inj:
Initial: 20-40mg as a single dose IV/IM; give IV dose slowly (1-2 min)
Titrate: May repeat the same dose if needed or increase by 20mg no sooner than 2 hrs after the previous dose; give individually determined single dose qd or bid

Hypertension

PO:
Initial: 40mg bid
Titrate: Adjust dose according to response

Add other antihypertensive agents if response is not satisfactory

Acute Pulmonary Edema

Inj:
Initial: 40mg IV slowly (over 1-2 min)
Titrate: May increase to 80mg IV slowly (over 1-2 min), if satisfactory response does not occur within 1 hr

Additional therapy (eg, digitalis, oxygen) may be administered concomitantly if necessary

than 2 hrs after the previous dose, if response is not satisfactory
Max: 6mg/kg
Premature Infants: 1mg/kg/day

DOSE MODIFICATION
Elderly
PO/Inj:
Start at lower end of dosing range

Concomitant Medications
Antihypertensives:
PO:
Reduce dose of other agents by at least 50%
May further reduce dose or d/c therapy of other antihypertensive drugs as BP falls

ADMINISTRATION
Oral/IV/IM route

Inj

Add furosemide inj to NaCl inj, D5, lactated Ringer's inj after pH has been adjusted to above 5.5
Administer as a controlled IV infusion at a rate no greater than 4mg/min
Care must be taken to ensure that the pH of the prepared infusion sol is in the weakly alkaline to neutral range
Acid sol, including other parenteral medications (eg, labetalol, ciprofloxacin, amrinone, milrinone), must not be administered concurrently in the same infusion because they may cause precipitation of the furosemide
Furosemide inj should not be added to a running IV line containing any of these acidic products

HOW SUPPLIED
Inj: 10mg/mL [2mL, 4mL, 10mL]; Sol: 10mg/mL [60mL, 120mL], 40mg/5mL [500mL]; Tab: (Lasix) 20mg, 40mg*, 80mg *scored

CONTRAINDICATIONS
Anuria.

WARNINGS/PRECAUTIONS
May lead to profound diuresis with water and electrolyte depletion if given in excessive amounts; careful medical supervision required and dose and dose schedule must be adjusted to individual patient's needs. Initiate therapy in hospital with hepatic cirrhosis and ascites. Do not institute therapy until basic condition is improved in patients with hepatic coma and in states of electrolyte depletion. D/C if increasing azotemia and oliguria occur during treatment of severe progressive renal disease. Tinnitus, reversible or irreversible hearing impairment, and deafness reported. Ototoxicity is associated with rapid inj, severe renal impairment, use of higher than recommended doses, hypoproteinemia, or concomitant use with aminoglycoside antibiotics, ethacrynic acid, or other ototoxic drugs; control IV infusion rate if using high dose parenteral therapy. Excessive diuresis may cause dehydration, blood volume reduction with circulatory collapse, vascular thrombosis and embolism, particularly in elderly. Monitor for fluid/electrolyte imbalance (hyponatremia, hypochloremia alkalosis, hypokalemia, hypomagnesemia, or hypocalcemia), liver/kidney damage, blood dyscrasias, or other idiosyncratic reactions. Increased in blood glucose and alterations in glucose tolerance tests, and rarely, precipitation of diabetes mellitus (DM) reported. May cause

acute urinary retention in patients with severe symptoms of urinary retention; monitor carefully, especially during the initial stages of treatment. May lead to a higher incidence of deterioration in renal function after receiving radiocontrast in patients at high risk for radiocontrast nephropathy. May potentiate ototoxicity and effect of therapy may be weakened in patients with hypoproteinemia. Asymptomatic hyperuricemia may occur and gout may rarely be precipitated. Caution in patients with sulfonamide allergy. May activate/exacerbate systemic lupus erythematosus (SLE). May precipitate nephrocalcinosis/nephrolithiasis in premature infants and children <4 yrs of age with no history of prematurity; monitor renal function and consider renal ultrasonography. May increase risk of persistence of patent ductus arteriosus in premature infants during the 1st weeks of life. May interfere with certain lab tests. Caution in elderly. (Inj) Use only in patients unable to take PO medication or in emergency situations; replace with PO therapy as soon as practical. May develop plasma level with potential toxic effects in premature infants with post conceptual age (gestational plus postnatal) <31 weeks receiving doses exceeding 1mg/kg/24 hrs. May cause hearing loss in neonates.

ADVERSE REACTIONS

Pancreatitis, jaundice, anorexia, paresthesias, diarrhea, N/V, dizziness, rash, urticaria, photosensitivity, fever, thrombophlebitis, restlessness, aplastic anemia, eosinophilia.

DRUG INTERACTIONS

May increase ototoxic potential of aminoglycoside antibiotics; avoid this combination, except in life-threatening situations. Avoid with ethacrynic acid and lithium. May experience salicylate toxicity at lower doses with concomitant high doses of salicylates for rheumatic disease. May antagonize skeletal muscle relaxing effect of tubocurarine. May potentiate action of succinylcholine. Potentiation of therapeutic effect of other antihypertensive drugs. Potentiation occurs with ganglionic or peripheral adrenergic blockers. May decrease arterial responsiveness to norepinephrine. Reduced CrCl in patients with chronic renal insufficiency with acetylsalicylic acid. Increased BUN, SrCr, and K^+ levels, and weight gain reported with NSAIDs. Hypokalemia may develop with adrenocorticotropic hormone and corticosteroids. Reduced natriuretic and antihypertensive effects with indomethacin. Indomethacin may affect plasma renin levels, aldosterone excretion, and renin profile evaluation. Digitalis may exaggerate metabolic effects of hypokalemia. (Inj/Tab) Avoid with chloral hydrate. May enhance nephrotoxicity of nephrotoxic drugs (eg, cisplatin) if furosemide is not given in lower doses and with positive fluid balance. Severe hypotension and renal function deterioration including renal failure may occur; interruption or reduction in dose of furosemide, ACE inhibitors, or ARBs may be necessary. Phenytoin interferes with renal action. Methotrexate and other drugs that undergo significant renal tubular secretion may reduce the effect of furosemide. May increase the risk of cephalosporin-induced nephrotoxicity. Increased risk of gouty arthritis with cyclosporine. Hypokalemia may develop with licorice in large amounts, or prolonged use of laxatives. (Tab/Sol) Reduced natriuretic and antihypertensive effects with sucralfate; separate intake by at least 2 hrs.

NURSING CONSIDERATIONS

Assessment: Assess for anuria, sulfonamide/drug hypersensitivity, SLE, hepatic/renal impairment, hypoproteinemia, pregnancy/nursing status, and possible drug interactions.

Monitoring: Monitor for signs/symptoms of fluid/electrolyte imbalance, blood dyscrasias, hyperglycemia and alterations in glucose tolerance tests, hyperuricemia, precipitation of gout or DM, ototoxicity, dehydration, blood volume reduction with circulatory collapse, vascular thrombosis and embolism, acute urinary retention, and other adverse reactions. Monitor serum electrolytes, carbon dioxide, creatinine, and BUN frequently during 1st few months of therapy, then periodically thereafter. Monitor urine and blood glucose periodically in diabetics. Monitor renal function and perform renal ultrasonography in pediatric patients.

Patient Counseling: Advise that patient may experience symptoms from excessive fluid and/or electrolyte losses. Advise that postural hypotension can be managed by getting up slowly. Inform patients with DM that drug may increase blood glucose levels and affect urine glucose tests. Advise that skin may be more sensitive to sunlight during therapy. Advise hypertensive patients to avoid medications that may increase BP, including OTC products for appetite suppression and cold symptoms.

Storage: Protect from light. (Inj) 20-25°C (68-77°F). (Tab/Sol) 25°C (77°F); excursions permitted to 15-30°C (59-86°F).

FYCOMPA – perampanel **CIII**

Class: AMPA glutamate receptor antagonist (non-competitive)

Serious or life-threatening psychiatric and behavioral adverse reactions including aggression, hostility, irritability, anger, and homicidal ideation and threats reported; monitor these reactions as well as changes in mood, behavior, or personality that are not typical for the patient, particularly during the titration period and at higher doses. Reduce dose if these symptoms occur and d/c immediately if symptoms are severe or are worsening.

ADULT DOSAGE

Partial Onset Seizures

Adjunctive therapy in patients w/ or w/o secondarily generalized seizures w/ epilepsy

Absence of Enzyme-Inducing Anti-Epileptic Drugs:

Initial: 2mg qhs

Titrate: Increase by 2mg/day increments no more than every week to 4-8mg qhs

Usual: 8-12mg qd

Presence of Enzyme-Inducing Anti-Epileptic Drugs (eg, Phenytoin, Carbamazepine, Oxcarbazepine):

Initial: 4mg qd

PEDIATRIC DOSAGE

Partial Onset Seizures

Adjunctive therapy in patients w/ or w/o secondarily generalized seizures w/ epilepsy

≥12 Years:

Absence of Enzyme-Inducing Anti-Epileptic Drugs:

Initial: 2mg qhs

Titrate: Increase by 2mg/day increments no more than every week to 4-8mg qhs

Usual: 8-12mg qd

Presence of Enzyme-Inducing Anti-Epileptic Drugs (eg, Phenytoin, Carbamazepine, Oxcarbazepine:

Initial: 4mg qd

DOSE MODIFICATION

Renal Impairment

Moderate: Monitor closely and titrate slowly

Severe/Undergoing Hemodialysis: Not recommended for use

Hepatic Impairment

Mild and Moderate:

Initial: 2mg/day

Titrate: Increase by 2mg/day every 2 weeks

Max: 6mg/day (mild), 4mg/day (moderate)

Severe: Not recommended for use

Elderly

Dosage increases during titration are no more than every 2 weeks

ADMINISTRATION

Oral route

HOW SUPPLIED

Tab: 2mg, 4mg, 6mg, 8mg, 10mg, 12mg

WARNINGS/PRECAUTIONS

Not recommended with severe hepatic/renal impairment, or if undergoing hemodialysis. Increased risk of suicidal thoughts or behavior. May increase dose-related events related to dizziness, disturbance in gait/coordination, somnolence, and fatigue-related events. May impair mental and physical abilities. Increased risk of falls may occur. Potential of increased seizure frequency with abrupt withdrawal; gradual withdrawal generally recommended. Caution with moderate renal impairment and in elderly.

ADVERSE REACTIONS

Dizziness, somnolence, fatigue, irritability, falls, N/V, ataxia, balance disorder, gait disturbance, vertigo, weight gain, upper respiratory tract infection, headache.

DRUG INTERACTIONS

Concomitant use with oral or implant contraceptives containing levonorgestrel may render them less effective due to reduced exposure; additional non-hormonal forms of contraception recommended. CYP450 inducers (eg, carbamazepine, phenytoin, oxcarbazepine) may decrease levels; monitor for clinical response and tolerability. Avoid concomitant use with other strong CYP3A inducers (eg, rifampin, St. John's wort). CNS depressants (eg, benzodiazepines, narcotics, barbiturates, sedating antihistamines) including alcohol may increase CNS depression; use caution when administering with these agents.

NURSING CONSIDERATIONS

Assessment: Assess for psychiatric history, behavioral problems, hepatic/renal impairment, pregnancy/nursing status, and possible drug interactions.

Monitoring: Monitor for signs/symptoms of psychiatric and behavioral reactions, suicidal behavior and ideation, dizziness, gait disturbance, somnolence, worsening of depression, clinical response and tolerability, fatigue, falls, and other adverse reactions.

Patient Counseling: Inform about the risks and benefits of therapy. Explain the need to monitor for the emergence of anger, aggression, hostility, unusual changes in mood, personality/behavior, and other behavioral symptoms; advise to report any such symptoms immediately to physician. Counsel patients, caregivers, and families that therapy may increase risk of suicidal thinking and behavior. Inform that therapy may cause dizziness, gait disturbance, somnolence, and fatigue; advise not to drive, operate complex machinery, or engage in hazardous activities until accustomed to any such effects associated with therapy. Explain that therapy may cause falls and injuries. Inform that therapy may decrease efficacy of contraceptives containing levonorgestrel, and may enhance the impairment effects of alcohol and other CNS depressants. Explain that abrupt discontinuation of therapy may increase seizure frequency. Inform that therapy is a controlled substance that can be misused and abused. Encourage patient to enroll in the North American Antiepileptic Drug Pregnancy Registry if pregnant.

Storage: 25°C (77°F); excursions permitted to 15-30°C (59-86°F).

GARDASIL – human papillomavirus quadrivalent (types 6, 11, 16, and 18) vaccine, recombinant RX

Class: Vaccine

ADULT DOSAGE

Human Papillomavirus

Vaccination of girls and women 9-26 yrs of age for the prevention of cervical, vulvar, vaginal, and anal cancer caused by human papillomavirus (HPV) types 16 and 18; genital warts (condyloma acuminata) caused by HPV types 6 and 11; and cervical intraepithelial neoplasia (CIN) grade 2/3 and cervical adenocarcinoma in situ, CIN grade 1, vulvar intraepithelial neoplasia (VIN) grades 2 and 3, vaginal intraepithelial neoplasia (VaIN) grades 2 and 3, and anal intraepithelial neoplasia (AIN) grades 1, 2, and 3 caused by HPV types 6, 11, 16, and 18. Vaccination of boys and men 9-26 yrs of age for the prevention of anal cancer caused by HPV types 16 and 18; genital warts (condyloma acuminata) caused by HPV types 6 and 11; and AIN grades 1, 2, and 3 caused by HPV types 6, 11, 16, and 18

≤26 Years:

0.5mL dose at the following schedule: 0, 2, and 6 months

PEDIATRIC DOSAGE

Human Papillomavirus

Vaccination of girls and women 9-26 yrs of age for the prevention of cervical, vulvar, vaginal, and anal cancer caused by human papillomavirus (HPV) types 16 and 18; genital warts (condyloma acuminata) caused by HPV types 6 and 11; and cervical intraepithelial neoplasia (CIN) grade 2/3 and cervical adenocarcinoma in situ, CIN grade 1, vulvar intraepithelial neoplasia (VIN) grades 2 and 3, vaginal intraepithelial neoplasia (VaIN) grades 2 and 3, and anal intraepithelial neoplasia (AIN) grades 1, 2, and 3 caused by HPV types 6, 11, 16, and 18. Vaccination of boys and men 9-26 yrs of age for the prevention of anal cancer caused by HPV types 16 and 18; genital warts (condyloma acuminata) caused by HPV types 6 and 11; and AIN grades 1, 2, and 3 caused by HPV types 6, 11, 16, and 18

≥9 Years:

0.5mL dose at the following schedule: 0, 2, and 6 months

ADMINISTRATION

IM route

Shake well before use

Administer in the deltoid region of the upper arm or in the higher anterolateral area of the thigh

Do not dilute or mix w/ other vaccines

Single-Dose Vial

Withdraw the 0.5mL dose of vaccine using a sterile needle/syringe and use promptly

Prefilled Syringe

Attach needle by twisting in clockwise direction until needle fits securely on syringe; administer entire dose as per standard protocol

HOW SUPPLIED

Inj: 0.5mL

CONTRAINDICATIONS

Hypersensitivity, including severe allergic reactions to yeast.

WARNINGS/PRECAUTIONS

Syncope may occur; observe for 15 min after administration. Appropriate medical treatment and supervision must be readily available in case of anaphylactic reactions. Women should continue to undergo cervical cancer screening. Recipients should not d/c anal cancer screening if it has been recommended by healthcare provider. Does not protect against disease from vaccine and non-vaccine HPV types to which a person has previously been exposed through sexual activity. Not intended for treatment of active external genital lesions; cervical, vulvar, vaginal, and anal cancers; CIN; VIN; VaIN; or AIN. Vaccination may not result in protection in all vaccine recipients. Response to vaccine may be diminished in immunocompromised individuals.

ADVERSE REACTIONS

Inj-site pain/swelling/erythema/pruritus, pyrexia, nausea, dizziness, diarrhea, headache.

DRUG INTERACTIONS

Immunosuppressive therapies, including irradiation, antimetabolites, alkylating agents, cytotoxic drugs, and corticosteroids (used in greater than physiologic doses), may reduce the immune responses to vaccines.

NURSING CONSIDERATIONS

Assessment: Assess for hypersensitivity to yeast or the vaccine, immunocompromised conditions, pregnancy/nursing status, and possible drug interactions.

Monitoring: Monitor for syncope, anaphylactic reactions, and other adverse reactions.

Patient Counseling: Inform about benefits and risks associated w/ vaccine. Instruct women to continue to undergo cervical cancer screening per standard of care. Advise not to d/c anal cancer screening if recommended by physician. Inform that vaccine does not provide protection against disease from vaccine and non-vaccine HPV types to which a person has previously been exposed through sexual activity. Inform that syncope may occur following vaccination. Advise that vaccine is not recommended during pregnancy. Counsel about the importance of completing the immunization series unless contraindicated. Instruct to report any adverse reactions to physician.

Storage: 2-8°C (36-46°F). Do not freeze. Protect from light. Administer as soon as possible after being removed from refrigeration; can be out of refrigeration (≤25°C [77°F]) for a total time of not more than 72 hrs.

GELNIQUE – oxybutynin

RX

Class: Muscarinic antagonist

ADULT DOSAGE

Overactive Bladder

3% Gel:
Apply 3 pumps (84mg/day) qd

10% Gel:
Apply contents of 1 sachet qd

PEDIATRIC DOSAGE

Pediatric use may not have been established

ADMINISTRATION

Topical route

Apply to clean, dry, intact skin on the abdomen, upper arms/shoulders, or thighs
Apply immediately after actuating the dose (3% Gel), or after the sachets are opened and contents expelled (10% Gel)
Rotate application sites; avoid use of same site on consecutive days
Wash hands immediately after application

HOW SUPPLIED

Gel: 3% [92g], (Chloride) 10% [1g, 30^{s}]

CONTRAINDICATIONS

Urinary/gastric retention, uncontrolled narrow-angle glaucoma.

WARNINGS/PRECAUTIONS

For topical application only. Flammable; avoid open fire or smoking until gel has dried. Caution with bladder outflow obstruction, GI obstructive disorders, gastroesophageal reflux, and myasthenia gravis. May decrease GI motility; caution with conditions such as ulcerative colitis or intestinal atony. Angioedema may occur; d/c and provide appropriate therapy if this occurs. Skin transference may occur; cover application site with clothing after gel has dried. CNS anticholinergic effects (eg, headache, dizziness, somnolence) reported; consider discontinuation or (3% Gel) dose reduction if these occur. May impair mental/physical abilities. (3% Gel) Caution in patients being treated for narrow-angle glaucoma. (10% Gel) Skin hypersensitivity may occur; d/c if hypersensitivity develops.

ADVERSE REACTIONS

Dry mouth, application-site reactions (eg, erythema, rash), urinary tract infection, nasopharyngitis, (3% Gel) conjunctivitis, (10% Gel) upper respiratory tract infections.

DRUG INTERACTIONS

Caution with drugs (eg, bisphosphonates) that may cause or exacerbate esophagitis. Concomitant use with other anticholinergic (antimuscarinic) agents may increase the frequency and/or severity of dry mouth, constipation, blurred vision, somnolence, and other anticholinergic pharmacological effects.

NURSING CONSIDERATIONS

Assessment: Assess for urinary/gastric retention, uncontrolled narrow-angle glaucoma, bladder outflow obstruction, GI obstructive disorders, ulcerative colitis or intestinal atony, gastroesophageal reflux, myasthenia gravis, pregnancy/nursing status, and for possible drug interactions.

Monitoring: Monitor for signs/symptoms of urinary retention, gastric retention, esophagitis, angioedema, CNS effects, and other adverse reactions.

Patient Counseling: Advise that therapy is for topical application only and should not be ingested. Instruct not to apply to recently shaved skin surfaces. Advise to avoid showering or water immersion for 1 hr after application. Counsel to cover treated sites with clothing if close skin-to-skin contact is anticipated. Instruct to avoid open fire or smoking until gel has dried. Advise that adverse reactions related to anticholinergic pharmacological activity may occur. Inform that heat prostration may occur in hot environment. Advise to exercise caution in engaging in potentially dangerous activities until effects have been determined. Inform that alcohol may enhance drowsiness. Instruct to avoid skin with open sores, wounds, irritation, scars, and tattoos. Advise to thoroughly rinse eyes right away with warm, clean water if gel gets in the eyes and to seek medical attention if needed. (3% Gel) Instruct not to use any gel that comes out while priming. Advise not to apply to breasts/ genital area.

Storage: Protect from moisture and humidity. Discard used sachets/pump dispensers in a manner that prevents accidental application or ingestion by children, pets, or others. (3% Gel) 25°C (77°F); excursions permitted to 15-30°C (59-86°F). (10% Gel) 20-25°C (68-77°F).

GEMCITABINE – gemcitabine **RX**

Class: Nucleoside metabolic inhibitor

OTHER BRAND NAMES

Gemzar

ADULT DOSAGE

Ovarian Carcinoma

In combination w/ carboplatin for advanced ovarian cancer that has relapsed ≥6 months after completion of platinum-based therapy

Usual: 1000mg/m^2 IV infusion over 30 min on Days 1 and 8 of each 21-day cycle + carboplatin AUC 4 IV after gemcitabine administration on Day 1 of each 21-day cycle

Metastatic Breast Cancer

In combination w/ paclitaxel for 1st-line treatment of metastatic breast cancer after failure of prior anthracycline-containing adjuvant chemotherapy, unless anthracyclines were clinically contraindicated

Usual: 1250mg/m^2 IV over 30 min on Days 1 and 8 of each 21-day cycle; administer paclitaxel at 175mg/m^2 on Day 1 as a 3-hr IV infusion before gemcitabine administration

Non-Small Cell Lung Cancer

In combination w/ cisplatin for 1st-line treatment of patients w/ inoperable, locally advanced (Stage IIIA or IIIB), or metastatic (Stage IV) non-small cell lung cancer

Every 4-Week Schedule:
Usual: 1000mg/m^2 IV over 30 min on Days 1, 8, and 15; administer cisplatin IV at 100mg/m^2 on Day 1 after gemcitabine infusion

Every 3-Week Schedule:
Usual: 1250mg/m^2 IV over 30 min on Days 1 and 8; administer cisplatin IV at 100mg/m^2 on Day 1 after gemcitabine infusion

Pancreatic Adenocarcinoma

1st-line treatment for patients w/ locally advanced (nonresectable Stage II or Stage III) or metastatic (Stage IV) adenocarcinoma of the pancreas; for patients previously treated w/ 5-FU

Usual: 1000mg/m^2 IV over 30 min

Treatment Schedule:
Weeks 1-8: Weekly dosing for the first 7 weeks, followed by 1-week rest
After Week 8: Weekly dosing on Days 1, 8, and 15 of 28-day cycles

PEDIATRIC DOSAGE

Pediatric use may not have been established

DOSE MODIFICATION

Adverse Reactions

Ovarian Cancer:

Myelosuppression on Treatment Day 1:

Absolute Granulocyte Count (AGC) <1500 x 10^6/L or Platelet Count <100,000 x 10^6/L: Delay treatment cycle

Myelosuppression on Treatment Day 8:

AGC 1000-1499 x 10^6/L or Platelet Count 75,000-99,999 x 10^6/L: Administer 50% of full dose

AGC <1000 x 10^6/L or Platelet Count <75,000 x 10^6/L: Hold therapy

Myelosuppression in Previous Cycle:

Permanently reduce dose to 800mg/m^2 on Days 1 and 8 for initial occurrence of any of the following:

1. AGC <500 x 10^6/L for >5 days
2. AGC <100 x 10^6/L for >3 days
3. Febrile neutropenia
4. Platelets <25,000 x 10^6/L
5. Cycle delay of >1 week due to toxicity

If any of the above toxicities occur after initial dose reduction, permanently reduce dose to 800mg/m^2 on Day 1 only

Breast Cancer:

Myelosuppression on Treatment Day 1:

AGC <1500 x 10^6/L or Platelet Count <100,000 x 10^6/L: Hold therapy

Myelosuppression on Treatment Day 8:

AGC 1000-1199 x 10^6/L or Platelet Count 50,000-75,000 x 10^6/L: Administer 75% of full dose

AGC 700-999 x 10^6/L and Platelet Count ≥50,000 x 10^6/L: Administer 50% of full dose

AGC <700 x 10^6/L or Platelet Count <50,000 x 10^6/L: Hold therapy

Non-Small Cell Lung Cancer/Pancreatic Cancer:

Myelosuppression:

AGC 500-999 x 10^6/L or Platelet Count 50,000-99,999 x 10^6/L: Administer 75% of full dose

AGC <500 x 10^6/L or Platelet Count <50,000 x 10^6/L: Hold therapy

Nonhematologic Toxicities in Any Indication:

Permanently d/c gemcitabine for any of the following:

1. Unexplained dyspnea or other evidence of severe pulmonary toxicity
2. Severe hepatic toxicity
3. Hemolytic-uremic syndrome
4. Capillary leak syndrome
5. Posterior reversible encephalopathy syndrome

Other Severe (Grade 3 or 4) Nonhematologic Toxicities: Hold therapy or reduce dose by 50% until toxicity resolves; no dose modifications are recommended for alopecia, nausea, or vomiting

ADMINISTRATION

IV route

Preparation for IV Infusion

1. Reconstitute the vials w/ 0.9% NaCl inj w/o preservatives:

200mg Vial: Add 5mL

1g Vial: Add 25mL

2g Vial: Add 50mL

These dilutions yield a gemcitabine concentration of 38mg/mL

Prior to administration, dilute the appropriate amount of drug w/ 0.9% NaCl inj; final concentrations may be as low as 0.1mg/mL

Handling Precautions

Immediately wash the skin thoroughly or rinse the mucosa w/ copious amounts of water if gemcitabine for inj contacts the skin or mucus membranes

HOW SUPPLIED

Inj: 2g; (Gemzar) 200mg, 1g

WARNINGS/PRECAUTIONS

Prolongation of infusion time beyond 60 min or more frequent than weekly dosing resulted in an increased incidence of clinically significant hypotension, severe flu-like symptoms, myelosuppression, and asthenia. Myelosuppression manifested by neutropenia, thrombocytopenia, and anemia occurs w/ monotherapy; increased risk when combined w/ other cytotoxic drugs. Pulmonary toxicity (eg, interstitial pneumonitis, pulmonary fibrosis/edema, adult respiratory distress syndrome) reported; may lead to fatal respiratory failure despite discontinuation of therapy. D/C if unexplained dyspnea (w/ or w/o bronchospasm) or any evidence of pulmonary toxicity develops. Hemolytic-uremic syndrome (HUS), including fatalities from renal failure or the requirement for dialysis, may occur; consider the diagnosis of HUS if anemia (w/ evidence of microangiopathic hemolysis, elevation of bilirubin/lactate dehydrogenase, or reticulocytosis), severe thrombocytopenia, or evidence of renal failure (SrCr/BUN elevation) develops. Permanently d/c therapy in patients w/ HUS or severe renal impairment. Liver injury, including liver failure and death, reported alone or in combination w/ other potentially hepatotoxic drugs; administration in patients w/ concurrent liver metastases or a preexisting history of hepatitis, alcoholism, or liver cirrhosis may lead to exacerbation of the underlying hepatic insufficiency. D/C if severe liver injury develops. May cause fetal harm. Capillary leak syndrome (CLS) w/ severe consequences reported; d/c if CLS develops. Posterior reversible encephalopathy syndrome (PRES) reported; confirm the diagnosis of PRES w/ MRI and d/c if PRES develops.

ADVERSE REACTIONS

N/V, anemia, increased ALT/AST/alkaline phosphatase, neutropenia, proteinuria, fever, hematuria, rash, thrombocytopenia, dyspnea, edema, diarrhea, hemorrhage, infection.

DRUG INTERACTIONS

Not indicated for use in combination w/ radiation therapy; life-threatening mucositis, especially esophagitis and pneumonitis occurred w/ concurrent thoracic radiation (given together or ≤7 days apart). Radiation recall reported in patients who received gemcitabine after prior radiation (given >7 days apart).

NURSING CONSIDERATIONS

Assessment: Assess for hypersensitivity to drug, renal/hepatic dysfunction, pregnancy/nursing status, and possible drug interactions. Obtain CBC, including differential and platelet count, prior to each dose.

Monitoring: Monitor for signs/symptoms of myelosuppression, pulmonary toxicity, HUS, CLS, PRES, and other adverse reactions. Periodically monitor renal/hepatic function.

Patient Counseling: Inform of the risks and benefits of therapy. Advise of the potential need for blood transfusions and increased susceptibility to infections. Instruct to immediately contact physician if any signs/symptoms of infection, fever, prolonged/unexpected bleeding, bruising, SOB, wheezing, cough, changes in the color/volume of urine output, jaundice, or pain/tenderness in the right upper abdominal quadrant develops. Inform that drug may cause fetal harm; instruct to notify physician if pregnant or nursing.

Storage: 20-25°C (68-77°F); excursions permitted between 15-30°C (59-86°F). Reconstituted Sol: 20-25°C (68-77°F) for 24 hrs. Do not refrigerate.

GEODON – ziprasidone hydrochloride; ziprasidone mesylate RX

Class: Atypical antipsychotic

Elderly patients w/ dementia-related psychosis treated w/ antipsychotic drugs are at an increased risk of death; most deaths appeared to be cardiovascular (CV) (eg, HF, sudden death) or infectious (eg, pneumonia) in nature. Not approved for treatment of dementia-related psychosis.

ADULT DOSAGE

Schizophrenia

PO:

Initial: 20mg bid

Titrate: May adjust up to 80mg bid at intervals of not <2 days

Max: 80mg bid

Periodically reassess need for maintenance treatment

Acute Agitation in Schizophrenia:

IM:

Usual: 10mg (may give q2h) to 20mg (may give q4h)

Max: 40mg/day

If long-term therapy is indicated, replace w/ oral formulation as soon as possible

Bipolar I Disorder

Mixed or Manic Episodes:

PO:

Acute (Monotherapy):

Initial: 40mg bid

Titrate: May increase to 60mg or 80mg bid on 2nd day of treatment, and subsequently adjust based on tolerance and efficacy w/in the range 40-80mg bid

Maint (Adjunct to Lithium or Valproate):

Continue treatment at the same dose on which the patient was initially stabilized, w/in the range of 40-80mg bid. Periodically reassess need for maintenance treatment

PEDIATRIC DOSAGE

Pediatric use may not have been established

DOSE MODIFICATION

Elderly

Start at lower end of dosing range

ADMINISTRATION

Oral/IM route

Caps

Take w/ food

Inj

Add 1.2mL of Sterile Water for Inj to vial and shake vigorously until all the drug is dissolved

Draw up 0.5mL of reconstituted sol to administer a 10mg dose; draw up 1mL of reconstituted sol to administer a 20mg dose

Do not mix w/ other medicinal products or solvents other than Sterile Water for Inj

HOW SUPPLIED

Cap: 20mg, 40mg, 60mg, 80mg; Inj: 20mg/mL

CONTRAINDICATIONS

Recent acute MI, uncompensated HF, or known history of QT prolongation (including congenital long QT syndrome). Concomitant use w/ dofetilide, sotalol, quinidine, other class IA/III antiarrhythmics, mesoridazine, thioridazine, chlorpromazine, droperidol, pimozide, sparfloxacin, gatifloxacin, moxifloxacin, halofantrine, mefloquine, pentamidine, arsenic trioxide, levomethadyl acetate, dolasetron mesylate, probucol, tacrolimus, or other drugs that prolong QT interval.

WARNINGS/PRECAUTIONS

Avoid in patients w/ history of cardiac arrhythmias. D/C in patients w/ persistent QTc measurements >500 msec. Hypokalemia and/or hypomagnesemia may increase risk of QT prolongation and arrhythmia; replete those electrolytes before treatment. Initiate further evaluation if symptoms of torsades de pointes occur. Neuroleptic malignant syndrome (NMS) reported; d/c therapy and institute symptomatic treatment. Drug reaction w/ eosinophilia and systemic symptoms (DRESS) reported; d/c if suspected. May cause tardive dyskinesia (TD), especially in the elderly; consider discontinuation if this occurs. Associated w/ metabolic changes (eg, hyperglycemia and diabetes mellitus [DM] sometimes associated w/ ketoacidosis or hyperosmolar coma, dyslipidemia, weight gain) that may increase CV/cerebrovascular risk. Rash and/or urticaria reported; d/c upon appearance of rash. May induce orthostatic hypotension and syncope; caution w/ CV disease, cerebrovascular disease, or conditions that predispose to hypotension. Leukopenia, neutropenia, and agranulocytosis reported; d/c in patients w/ severe neutropenia (ANC <1000/ mm^3) or at 1st sign of decline in WBCs in patients w/ preexisting low WBC count or history of drug-induced leukopenia/neutropenia. Seizures reported. May cause esophageal dysmotility and aspiration; caution in patients at risk for aspiration pneumonia. May elevate prolactin levels. May impair physical/mental abilities. Somnolence and priapism reported. May disrupt the body's ability to reduce core body temperature. Caution in those at risk for suicide and in elderly patients. Caution w/ renal impairment when administered IM. Concomitant use of IM and oral preparations in schizophrenic patients is not recommended.

ADVERSE REACTIONS

N/V, rash, diarrhea, somnolence, dizziness, headache, extrapyramidal symptoms, respiratory tract infection, akathisia, abnormal vision, asthenia, constipation, dry mouth, anxiety. (Inj) Inj-site pain.

DRUG INTERACTIONS

See Contraindications. Caution w/ centrally acting drugs and medications w/ anticholinergic activity. May enhance effects of certain antihypertensives. May antagonize effects of levodopa and dopamine agonists. Decreased levels w/ carbamazepine. Increased levels w/ CYP3A4 inhibitors (eg, ketoconazole). Periodically monitor serum electrolytes w/ diuretics.

NURSING CONSIDERATIONS

Assessment: Assess for drug hypersensitivity, history of QT prolongation, recent acute MI, uncompensated HF, dementia-related psychosis, history of seizures/conditions that lower seizure threshold, other conditions where treatment is contraindicated or cautioned, pregnancy/nursing status, and possible drug interactions. Obtain baseline serum electrolytes (K^+, Mg^{2+}) in patients at risk for significant electrolyte disturbances. Obtain baseline FPG in patients w/ DM or at risk for DM. Obtain baseline CBC if at risk for leukopenia/neutropenia.

Monitoring: Monitor for QT prolongation, torsades de pointes, NMS, DRESS, TD, metabolic changes, rash, orthostatic hypotension, seizures, esophageal dysmotility, aspiration, suicidal ideation, hypokalemia, hypomagnesemia, and other adverse reactions. Monitor CBC frequently during the 1st few months of therapy in patients w/ preexisting low WBCs or history of drug-induced leukopenia/ neutropenia. Monitor for fever or other signs/symptoms of infection in patients w/ neutropenia. Monitor for worsening of glucose control in patients w/ DM and monitor FPG in patients at risk for DM. Reassess periodically to determine need for maintenance treatment.

Patient Counseling: Inform of the risks and benefits of therapy. Advise to inform physician of any history of QT prolongation, recent acute MI, uncompensated HF, risk for electrolyte abnormalities, history of cardiac arrhythmia, or if taking other QT-prolonging drugs. Instruct to report conditions that increase risk for electrolyte disturbances (eg, hypokalemia, taking diuretics, prolonged diarrhea) and if dizziness, palpitations, or syncope occurs. Instruct to report to physician at the earliest onset any signs/symptoms that may be associated w/ DRESS.

Storage: 25°C (77°F); excursions permitted to 15-30°C (59-86°F). (Inj) Protect from light. Reconstituted Sol: 15-30°C (59-86°F) for up to 24 hrs when protected from light, or refrigerate at 2-8°C (36-46°F) for up to 7 days.

GIAZO – balsalazide disodium

RX

Class: 5-aminosalicylic acid derivative

ADULT DOSAGE

Ulcerative Colitis

Mildly to Moderately Active:
Males: 3 tabs bid (6.6g/day) for up to 8 weeks

PEDIATRIC DOSAGE

Pediatric use may not have been established

ADMINISTRATION

Oral route

Take w/ or w/o food

HOW SUPPLIED

Tab: 1.1g

WARNINGS/PRECAUTIONS

Associated with acute intolerance syndrome (eg, cramping, acute abdominal pain and bloody diarrhea, fever, headache, and rash) that may be difficult to distinguish from exacerbation of ulcerative colitis; observe closely for worsening of symptoms and d/c therapy if acute intolerance syndrome is suspected. Renal impairment, including minimal change nephropathy, acute/chronic interstitial nephritis, and renal failure, reported; evaluate renal function prior to initiation and periodically while on therapy. Caution with known renal dysfunction or history of renal disease. Hepatic failure reported in patients with preexisting liver disease; use caution and consider LFTs in patients with liver disease. Caution in elderly; closely monitor blood cell counts during therapy.

ADVERSE REACTIONS

Headache, nasopharyngitis, anemia, diarrhea, fatigue, pharyngolaryngeal pain, urinary tract infection, GI disorders.

NURSING CONSIDERATIONS

Assessment: Assess for hypersensitivity to salicylates, aminosalicylates, or their metabolites, and renal/hepatic function.

Monitoring: Monitor for signs/symptoms of acute intolerance syndrome, renal/hepatic impairment, and other adverse reactions. Monitor blood cell counts in elderly.

Patient Counseling: Instruct not to take drug if hypersensitive to salicylates (eg, aspirin). Advise patients who need to control Na^+ intake that the recommended dosing of 6.6g/day provides about 756mg of Na^+/day. Instruct to contact physician if worsening of ulcerative colitis symptoms is experienced. Instruct to inform physician if they have or are later diagnosed with renal dysfunction and/or liver disease.

Storage: 20-25°C (68-77°F); excursions permitted between 15-30°C (59-86°F).

GLEEVEC – imatinib mesylate

RX

Class: Kinase inhibitors

ADULT DOSAGE

Hypereosinophilic Syndrome/Chronic Eosinophilic Leukemia

FIP1L1-PDGFRα Fusion Kinase-Negative/ Unknown:
400mg qd

Demonstrated FIP1L1-PDGFRα Fusion Kinase:
Initial: 100mg qd
Titrate: May increase to 400mg qd

Dermatofibrosarcoma Protuberans

Unresectable, Recurrent, and/or Metastatic:
800mg/day (as 400mg bid)

PEDIATRIC DOSAGE

Ph+ Chronic Myeloid Leukemia

Newly Diagnosed Patients in Chronic Phase:
≥1 Year:
340mg/m^2/day
Max: 600mg/day

Dose can be given qd or split in 2 (am and pm)

Ph+ Acute Lymphoblastic Leukemia

In Combination w/ Chemotherapy for Newly Diagnosed Patients:
≥1 Year:
340mg/m^2 qd
Max: 600mg qd

Kit (CD117)-Positive Gastrointestinal Stromal Tumors

Unresectable and/or Metastatic Malignant:
400mg qd
Titrate: May increase up to 800mg/day (as 400mg bid)

Adjuvant Treatment Following Complete Gross Resection:
400mg qd; optimal treatment duration unknown

Ph+ Chronic Myeloid Leukemia

Chronic Phase:
400mg qd
Titrate: May increase to 600mg qd

Accelerated Phase/Blast Crisis:
600mg qd
Titrate: May increase to 800mg/day (as 400mg bid)

Ph+ Acute Lymphoblastic Leukemia

Relapsed/Refractory:
600mg qd

Myelodysplastic/Myeloproliferative Diseases

Associated w/ PDGFR Gene Re-Arrangements:
400mg qd

Aggressive Systemic Mastocytosis

W/O D816V c-Kit Mutation:
400mg qd

c-Kit Mutational Status Unknown/Unavailable:
400mg qd may be considered for patients not responding satisfactorily to other therapies

Associated w/ Eosinophilia:
Initial: 100mg qd
Titrate: May increase to 400mg qd

DOSE MODIFICATION

Concomitant Medications
Strong CYP3A4 Inducers: Avoid use; if necessary, increase imatinib dose by at least 50%

Renal Impairment
Mild (CrCl 40-59mL/min):
Max: 600mg

Moderate (CrCl 20-39mL/min):
Initial: Reduce dose by 50%
Max: 400mg

Hepatic Impairment
Severe: Reduce dose by 25%

Adverse Reactions
Bilirubin >3X IULN/Liver Transaminases >5X IULN:
1. Withhold therapy until bilirubin levels return to <1.5X IULN and transaminase levels to <2.5X IULN
2. Continue treatment at a reduced daily dose:
Adults: 400mg to 300mg, 600mg to 400mg, or 800mg to 600mg
Pediatrics: 340mg/m^2/day to 260mg/m^2/day

Severe Nonhematologic (eg, Severe Hepatotoxicity, Severe Fluid Retention):
Withhold therapy until the event has resolved; resume treatment as appropriate depending on initial severity of event
Neutropenia/Thrombocytopenia:
ANC <1.0 x 10^9/L and/or Platelets <50 x 10^9/L:
Adults:
Initial Dose 100mg:
1. Withhold treatment until ANC ≥1.5 x 10^9/L and platelets ≥75 x 10^9/L
2. Resume treatment at previous dose (dose before severe adverse reaction)

Initial Dose 400mg:
1. Withhold treatment until ANC ≥1.5 x 10^9/L and platelets ≥75 x 10^9/L

2. Resume treatment at the original starting dose of 400mg
3. If recurrence of ANC <1.0 x 10^9/L and/or platelets <50 x 10^9/L, repeat step 1 and resume at a reduced dose of 300mg

Initial Dose 800mg:
1. Withhold treatment until ANC ≥1.5 x 10^9/L and platelets ≥75 x 10^9/L
2. Resume treatment at 600mg
3. In the event of recurrence of ANC <1.0 x 10^9/L and/or platelets <50 x 10^9/L, repeat step 1 and resume at reduced dose of 400mg

Pediatrics:
Initial Dose 340mg/m²:
1. Withhold treatment until ANC ≥1.5 x 10^9/L and platelets ≥75 x 10^9/L
2. Resume treatment at previous dose (dose before severe adverse reaction)
3. In the event of recurrence of ANC <1.0 x 10^9/L and/or platelets <50 x 10^9/L, repeat step 1 and resume at reduced dose of 260mg/m²

ANC <0.5 x 10^9/L and/or Platelets <10 x 10^9/L:
Adults:
Initial Dose 600mg:
1. Check if cytopenia is related to leukemia (marrow aspirate or biopsy)
2. If cytopenia is unrelated to leukemia, reduce dose to 400mg
3. If cytopenia persists 2 weeks, reduce further to 300mg
4. If cytopenia persists 4 weeks and is still unrelated to leukemia, withhold treatment until ANC ≥1 x 10^9/L and platelets ≥20 x 10^9/L and then resume treatment at 300mg

ADMINISTRATION

Oral route

Take w/ a meal and a large glass of water
Do not crush tab

Patients Unable to Swallow Tabs
1. Disperse tabs in a glass of water or apple juice
2. Required number of tabs should be placed in the appropriate volume of beverage (approx 50mL for a 100mg tab and 200mL for a 400mg tab)
3. Stir w/ a spoon and administer immediately after complete disintegration of tab

HOW SUPPLIED

Tab: 100mg*, 400mg* *scored

WARNINGS/PRECAUTIONS

Edema and serious fluid retention reported. Hematologic toxicity (eg, anemia/neutropenia/thrombocytopenia) reported. CHF and left ventricular dysfunction reported; carefully monitor patients w/ cardiac disease or risk factors for cardiac failure or history of renal failure, and evaluate/treat any patient w/ cardiac or renal failure. Hepatotoxicity may occur. Grade 3/4 hemorrhages in clinical studies in patients w/ newly diagnosed CML and w/ GIST reported. GI tumor sites may be the source of GI hemorrhages; GI hemorrhage in patients w/ newly diagnosed Ph+ CML, and gastric antral vascular ectasia reported. GI irritation/perforation reported. In patients w/ HES w/ occult infiltration of HES cells w/in the myocardium, cases of cardiogenic shock/left ventricular dysfunction have been associated w/ HES cell degranulation upon initiation of therapy; reversible w/ administration of systemic steroids, circulatory support measures, and temporarily withholding treatment. Consider echocardiogram and determination of serum troponin in patients w/ HES/CEL, MDS/MPD, or ASM associated w/ high eosinophil levels; if either is abnormal, consider prophylactic use of systemic steroids (1-2mg/kg) for 1-2 weeks concomitantly at initiation of therapy. Bullous dermatologic reactions, including erythema multiforme and Stevens-Johnson syndrome, reported. May cause fetal harm; sexually active female patients of reproductive potential should use highly effective contraception. Growth retardation reported in children and preadolescents; closely monitor growth. Tumor lysis syndrome (TLS) reported in patients w/ CML, GIST, ALL, and eosinophilic leukemia; caution in patients at risk of TLS (those w/ tumors w/ high proliferative rate or high tumor burden prior to treatment), and correct dehydration and treat high uric acid levels prior to initiation of treatment. May impair mental/physical abilities.

ADVERSE REACTIONS

N/V, edema, muscle cramps, musculoskeletal pain, diarrhea, rash, fatigue, headache, asthenia, abdominal pain, hemorrhage, malaise, neutropenia, anemia, anorexia.

DRUG INTERACTIONS

See Dose Modification. Increased levels w/ CYP3A4 inhibitors; caution w/ strong CYP3A4 inhibitors (eg, ketoconazole, nefazodone, clarithromycin); avoid w/ grapefruit juice. Decreased levels w/ CYP3A4 inducers (eg, rifampin, St. John's wort, enzyme-inducing antiepileptic drugs); consider alternative therapeutic agents w/ less enzyme induction potential when CYP3A4 inducers are indicated. Increases levels of simvastatin, metoprolol, and CYP3A4 metabolized drugs (eg, dihydropyridine calcium channel blockers, triazolo-benzodiazepines, certain HMG-CoA reductase inhibitors); caution w/ CYP3A4/CYP2D6 substrates that have a narrow therapeutic window (eg, alfentanil, cyclosporine, ergotamine). Switch from warfarin to low molecular weight or standard heparin if anticoagulation is required during therapy. When concomitantly used w/ chemotherapy, liver toxicity reported; monitor hepatic function. Hypothyroidism reported in thyroidectomy patients undergoing levothyroxine replacement; closely monitor TSH levels.

NURSING CONSIDERATIONS

Assessment: Assess for cardiac disease, renal impairment, dehydration, high uric acid levels, pregnancy/nursing status, and possible drug interactions. Perform echocardiogram and determine troponin levels in patients w/ HES/CEL and w/ MDS/MPD or ASM associated w/ high eosinophil levels. Obtain baseline CBC and LFTs.

Monitoring: Monitor for signs and symptoms of fluid retention, CHF, left ventricular dysfunction, hemorrhage, GI disorders, TLS, bullous dermatologic reactions, and other adverse events. Perform CBCs weekly for the 1st month, biweekly for the 2nd month, and periodically thereafter. Monitor LFTs monthly or as clinically indicated. Monitor growth in children, and TSH levels in thyroidectomy patients undergoing levothyroxine replacement.

Patient Counseling: Instruct to take drug exactly as prescribed and not to change the dose or to stop taking the medication unless told to do so by physician. Advise women of reproductive potential to avoid becoming pregnant and instruct to notify physician if pregnant. Instruct sexually active females to use highly effective contraception. Instruct to avoid breastfeeding while on therapy. Advise to contact physician if patient is experiencing any side effects during therapy or has a history of cardiac disease or risk factors for cardiac failure. Inform that the drug and certain other medicines can interact w/ each other; advise to inform physician if taking/planning to take iron supplements. Inform to avoid grapefruit juice and other foods known to inhibit CYP3A4 while on therapy. Advise that growth retardation has been reported in children and preadolescents, and that growth should be monitored. Caution about driving a car or operating machinery.

Storage: 25°C (77°F); excursions permitted to 15-30°C (59-86°F). Protect from moisture.

GLIMEPIRIDE – glimepiride RX

Class: Sulfonylurea (2nd generation)

OTHER BRAND NAMES

Amaryl

ADULT DOSAGE

Type 2 Diabetes Mellitus

Initial: 1mg or 2mg qd

Titrate: After reaching 2mg/day, may further increase dose in increments of 1mg or 2mg based on glycemic response, not more frequently than every 1-2 weeks

Max: 8mg qd

PEDIATRIC DOSAGE

Pediatric use may not have been established

DOSE MODIFICATION

Concomitant Medications

Colesevelam: Administer at least 4 hrs prior to colesevelam

Renal Impairment

Initial: 1mg qd

Titrate: Adjust conservatively

Max: 8mg qd

Elderly

Initial: 1mg qd

Titrate: Adjust conservatively

Max: 8mg qd

ADMINISTRATION

Oral route

Administer w/ breakfast or the 1st main meal of the day

HOW SUPPLIED

Tab: 3mg*, 6mg*, 8mg*; (Amaryl) 1mg*, 2mg*, 4mg* *scored

WARNINGS/PRECAUTIONS

Not for treatment of type 1 DM or diabetic ketoacidosis. Patients being transferred from longer $T_{1/2}$ sulfonylureas (eg, chlorpropamide) may have overlapping drug effect for 1-2 weeks; monitor for hypoglycemia. May cause severe hypoglycemia, which may impair mental/physical abilities; caution in patients predisposed to hypoglycemia. Early warning symptoms of hypoglycemia may be different/less pronounced in patients with autonomic neuropathy and in the elderly.

Hypersensitivity reactions (eg, anaphylaxis, angioedema, Stevens-Johnson syndrome) reported; if suspected, promptly d/c therapy, assess for other potential causes for the reaction, and institute alternative treatment. May cause hemolytic anemia; caution with G6PD deficiency and consider the use of a non-sulfonylurea alternative. Increased risk of cardiovascular mortality. Caution in elderly.

ADVERSE REACTIONS

Dizziness, nausea, asthenia, headache, hypoglycemia, flu syndrome.

DRUG INTERACTIONS

See Dosage. Oral antidiabetic medications, pramlintide acetate, insulin, ACE inhibitors, H_2-receptor antagonists, fibrates, propoxyphene, pentoxifylline, somatostatin analogues, anabolic steroids and androgens, cyclophosphamide, phenyramidol, guanethidine, fluconazole, sulfinpyrazone, tetracyclines, clarithromycin, disopyramide, quinolones, and drugs that are highly protein-bound (eg, fluoxetine, NSAIDs, salicylates, sulfonamides, chloramphenicol, coumarins, probenecid, MAOIs) may increase glucose-lowering effect; monitor for hypoglycemia during coadministration and for worsening glycemic control during withdrawal of these drugs. Danazol, glucagon, somatropin, protease inhibitors, atypical antipsychotics (eg, olanzapine, clozapine), barbiturates, diazoxide, laxatives, rifampin, thiazides and other diuretics, corticosteroids, phenothiazines, thyroid hormones, estrogens, oral contraceptives, phenytoin, nicotinic acid, sympathomimetics (eg, epinephrine, albuterol, terbutaline), and isoniazid may reduce glucose-lowering effect; monitor for worsening glycemic control during coadministration and for hypoglycemia during withdrawal of these drugs. β-blockers, clonidine, reserpine, and alcohol intake may potentiate or weaken glucose-lowering effect. Signs of hypoglycemia may be reduced or absent with sympatholytic drugs (eg, β-blockers, clonidine, guanethidine, reserpine). Potential interaction leading to severe hypoglycemia reported with oral miconazole. May interact with inhibitors (eg, fluconazole) and inducers (eg, rifampin) of CYP2C9. Colesevelam may reduce levels.

NURSING CONSIDERATIONS

Assessment: Assess for hypersensitivity to drug or sulfonamide derivatives, predisposition to hypoglycemia, autonomic neuropathy, G6PD deficiency, pregnancy/nursing status, and possible drug interactions.

Monitoring: Monitor for hypoglycemia, hypersensitivity reactions, hemolytic anemia, and other adverse reactions.

Patient Counseling: Inform about importance of adherence to dietary instructions, a regular exercise program, and regular testing of blood glucose. Advise about potential side effects (eg, hypoglycemia, weight gain). Inform about the symptoms and treatment of hypoglycemia, and the conditions that predispose to it. Inform that ability to concentrate and react may be impaired as a result of hypoglycemia; caution when driving/operating machinery. Advise to inform physician if pregnant/breastfeeding or contemplating pregnancy/breastfeeding.

Storage: 20-25°C (68-77°F). (Amaryl) 25°C (77°F); excursions permitted to 20-25°C (68-77°F).

GLUCAGON — glucagon (rDNA origin)

RX

Class: Glucagon

ADULT DOSAGE

Hypoglycemia

Severe:

>20kg:

1mg (1 U) SQ/IM/IV

Diagnostic Aid

Relaxation of the Stomach:

IV:

0.5mg (0.5 U)

IM:

2mg (2 U)

Relaxation of Duodenum/Small Bowel:

IV:

0.25-0.5mg (0.25-0.5 U) or 2mg (2 U)

IM:

1mg (1 U) or 2mg (2 U)

Relaxation of the Colon:

IM:

2mg (2 U) 10 min prior to procedure

PEDIATRIC DOSAGE

Hypoglycemia

Severe:

<20kg:

0.5mg (0.5 U) or a dose equivalent to 20-30mcg/kg

>20kg:

1mg (1 U) SQ/IM/IV

DOSE MODIFICATION

Elderly

Start at lower end of dosing range

ADMINISTRATION

IM/IV/SQ routes

The diluent is provided for use only in the preparation of glucagon for parenteral inj
Do not use at concentrations >1mg/mL (1 U/mL)
Use reconstituted glucagon immediately; discard any unused portion

Severe Hypoglycemia

1. Treat initially w/ IV glucose if possible; if parenteral glucose cannot be used, dissolve the lyophilized glucagon using the accompanying diluting sol and use immediately
2. An unconscious patient will usually awaken w/in 15 min following the glucagon inj. If the response is delayed, there is no contraindication to the administration of an additional dose of glucagon; however, emergency aid should be sought so that parenteral glucose can be given
3. After the patient responds, supplemental carbohydrate should be given to restore liver glycogen and to prevent secondary hypoglycemia

Diagnostic Aid

1. Dissolve the lyophilized glucagon using the accompanying diluting sol and use immediately
2. Select dose depending on the onset and duration of effect required for the examination; refer to PI

HOW SUPPLIED

Inj: 1mg/mL (1 U/mL)

CONTRAINDICATIONS

Pheochromocytoma.

WARNINGS/PRECAUTIONS

Caution with a history suggestive of insulinoma and/or pheochromocytoma. In patients with insulinoma, IV glucagon may produce an initial increase in blood glucose and then subsequently cause hypoglycemia. In the presence of pheochromocytoma, may cause the tumor to release catecholamines, which may result in a sudden and marked increase in BP. Generalized allergic reactions (eg, urticaria, respiratory distress, and hypotension) reported. Effective in treating hypoglycemia only if sufficient liver glycogen is present. Little or no help in states of starvation, adrenal insufficiency, or chronic hypoglycemia; treat with glucose.

ADVERSE REACTIONS

N/V, allergic reactions, urticaria, respiratory distress, hypotension.

DRUG INTERACTIONS

Addition of an anticholinergic during diagnostic examination may increase side effects.

NURSING CONSIDERATIONS

Assessment: Assess if patient is in state of starvation, has adrenal insufficiency or chronic hypoglycemia. Assess for history suggestive of insulinoma and/or pheochromocytoma, pregnancy/nursing status, and possible drug interactions.

Monitoring: Monitor for signs/symptoms of an allergic reaction, HTN, and hypoglycemia. Monitor blood glucose levels in patients with hypoglycemia until asymptomatic.

Patient Counseling: Instruct patient and family members in event of emergency how to properly prepare and administer glucagon. Inform about measures to prevent hypoglycemia, including following a uniform regimen on a regular basis, careful adjustment of the insulin program, frequent testing of blood or urine for glucose, and routinely carrying hyperglycemic agents to quickly elevate blood glucose levels (eg, sugar, candy, readily absorbed carbohydrates). Inform about symptoms of hypoglycemia and how to treat it appropriately. Inform caregivers that if patient is hypoglycemic, they should be kept alert and hypoglycemia should be treated as quickly as possible to prevent CNS damage. Advise to inform physician when hypoglycemia occurs.

Storage: Before reconstitution: 20-25°C (68-77°F); excursions allowed between 15-30°C (59-86°F).

GLUCOPHAGE XR – metformin hydrochloride RX

Class: Biguanide

Lactic acidosis reported (rare); increased risk with increased age, diabetes mellitus (DM), renal dysfunction, CHF, and conditions with risk of hypoperfusion and hypoxemia. Avoid use in patients ≥80 yrs of age unless renal function is normal. Withhold therapy in the presence of any condition associated with hypoxemia, dehydration, or sepsis. Avoid with clinical or lab evidence of hepatic disease. Caution against excessive alcohol intake; may potentiate the effects of metformin on lactate metabolism. Temporarily d/c prior to any IV radiocontrast study or surgical procedures. D/C use and institute appropriate therapy if lactic acidosis occurs.

OTHER BRAND NAMES
Glucophage

ADULT DOSAGE
Type 2 Diabetes Mellitus
Tab:
Initial: 500mg bid or 850mg qd w/ meals
Titrate: Increase by 500mg/week or 850mg every 2 weeks, up to a total of 2000mg/day given in divided doses; may also titrate from 500mg bid to 850mg bid after 2 weeks
Max: 2550mg/day; doses >2000mg/day may be better tolerated given tid
Tab, ER:
Initial: 500mg qd w/ pm meal
Titrate: Increase by 500mg/week
Max: 2000mg/day; consider 1000mg bid if unable to achieve glycemic control on 2000mg qd

PEDIATRIC DOSAGE
Type 2 Diabetes Mellitus
10-16 Years:
Tab:
Initial: 500mg bid w/ meals
Titrate: Increase by 500mg/week
Max: 2000mg/day

DOSE MODIFICATION
Concomitant Medications
Insulin Therapy in Adults:
Initial: 500mg qd while continuing current insulin dose
Titrate: Increase by 500mg/week; decrease insulin dose by 10-25% when FPG <120mg/dL
Max: 2500mg/day (tab) and 2000mg/day (tab, ER)
Oral Sulfonylurea Therapy in Adults:
Consider gradual addition of an oral sulfonylurea if unresponsive to 4 weeks of max dose of Glucophage or Glucophage XR monotherapy; if patients have not satisfactorily responded to 1-3 months of concomitant therapy, consider therapeutic alternatives (eg, switching to insulin w/ or w/o Glucophage or Glucophage XR)
Elderly
Dose conservatively; do not titrate to max dose
Other Important Modifications
Transferring Patients from Chlorpropamide: Exercise care during the first 2 weeks because of the prolonged retention of chlorpropamide in the body
Debilitated/Malnourished: Do not titrate to max dose

ADMINISTRATION
Oral route
Tab
Give in divided doses w/ meals
Tab, ER
Give qd w/ the pm meal
Must be swallowed whole; do not crush or chew

HOW SUPPLIED
Tab: (Glucophage) 500mg, 850mg, 1000mg; Tab, ER: (Glucophage XR) 500mg, 750mg

CONTRAINDICATIONS
Renal disease/dysfunction (eg, SrCr ≥1.5mg/dL [males], ≥1.4mg/dL [females], or abnormal CrCl), acute or chronic metabolic acidosis, diabetic ketoacidosis with or without coma. D/C temporarily (48 hrs) for radiologic studies with intravascular iodinated contrast materials.

WARNINGS/PRECAUTIONS
D/C therapy if conditions associated with lactic acidosis and characterized by hypoxemia states (eg, acute CHF, cardiovascular [CV] collapse, acute MI), or prerenal azotemia develop. D/C therapy if temporary loss of glycemic control occurs due to stress; temporarily give insulin and reinstitute after acute episode is resolved. May decrease serum vitamin B12 levels. Increased risk of hypoglycemia in elderly, debilitated/malnourished or with adrenal or pituitary insufficiency or alcohol intoxication. Consider therapeutic alternatives, including initiation of insulin, if secondary failure occurs. Caution in elderly.

ADVERSE REACTIONS
Lactic acidosis, diarrhea, N/V, flatulence, asthenia, abdominal discomfort, hypoglycemia, dizziness, dyspnea, taste disorder, chest discomfort, flu syndrome, palpitations, indigestion.

DRUG INTERACTIONS
See Boxed Warning and Contraindications. May increase levels with furosemide, nifedipine, cimetidine, cationic drugs (eg, digoxin, amiloride, procainamide, quinidine, quinine, ranitidine, trimethoprim, vancomycin, triamterene, morphine). Observe for loss of glycemic control

with thiazides, other diuretics, corticosteroids, phenothiazines, thyroid products, estrogens, oral contraceptives, phenytoin, nicotinic acid, sympathomimetics, calcium channel blockers, and isoniazid. May interact with highly protein-bound drugs (eg, salicylates, sulfonamides, chloramphenicol, probenecid). May decrease furosemide or glyburide levels. Caution with drugs that may affect renal function or result in significant hemodynamic change or may interfere with the disposition of metformin. Hypoglycemia may occur with concomitant use of other glucose-lowering agents (eg, sulfonylureas, insulin). May overlap drug effects when transferred from chlorpropamide. Hypoglycemia may be difficult to recognize with β-adrenergic blocking drugs.

NURSING CONSIDERATIONS

Assessment: Assess for renal/hepatic impairment, acute/chronic metabolic acidosis, presence of a hypoxic state (eg, acute CHF, acute MI, CV collapse), dehydration, sepsis, alcoholism, nutritional status, adrenal/pituitary insufficiency, pregnancy/nursing status, and for possible drug interactions. Assess baseline renal function, FPG, HbA1c, and hematological parameters (Hct, Hgb, RBC indices).

Monitoring: Monitor for lactic/metabolic acidosis, ketoacidosis, hypoglycemia, hypoxemia (eg, CV collapse, acute CHF, acute MI), prerenal azotemia, and for decreases in vitamin B12 levels. Monitor FPG, HbA1c, renal function (eg, SrCr, CrCl), and hematological parameters (eg, Hgb, Hct, RBC indices).

Patient Counseling: Inform of the potential risks and benefits of therapy. Inform about the importance of adherence to dietary instructions and a regular exercise program. Inform of the risk of developing lactic acidosis during therapy; advise to d/c therapy immediately and contact physician if unexplained hyperventilation, myalgia, malaise, unusual somnolence, or other nonspecific symptoms occur. Instruct to avoid excessive alcohol intake. Counsel to take tab with meals and ER tab with pm meal. Instruct that ER tab must be swallowed whole and not crushed or chewed.

Storage: 20-25°C (68-77°F); excursions permitted to 15-30°C (59-86°F).

GLUCOTROL – glipizide RX

Class: Sulfonylurea (2nd generation)

ADULT DOSAGE

Type 2 Diabetes Mellitus

Initial: 5mg qd
Titrate: Increase by 2.5-5mg every several days; may divide dose if response to single dose is not satisfactory
Max qd Dose: 15mg
Max Total Daily Dose: 40mg

Doses >15mg/day should be divided

Switching from Insulin:
Daily Insulin Requirement:
≤20 U/day: D/C insulin and begin glipizide at usual dose
>20 U/day: Reduce insulin dose by 50% and begin glipizide at usual dose; subsequent insulin reductions should depend on individual patient response

Switching from Longer Half-Life Sulfonylureas (eg, Chlorpropamide):
Observe patient carefully for 1-2 weeks

PEDIATRIC DOSAGE

Pediatric use may not have been established

DOSE MODIFICATION

Concomitant Medications
Colesevelam: Administer glipizide at least 4 hrs prior to colesevelam

Renal Impairment
Initial/Maint: Dose conservatively

Hepatic Impairment
Initial: 2.5mg qd
Maint: Dose conservatively

Elderly
Initial: 2.5mg qd
Maint: Dose conservatively

Other Important Modifications
Debilitated/Malnourished Patients:
Initial/Maint: Dose conservatively

ADMINISTRATION

Oral route

Administer approx 30 min ac

HOW SUPPLIED

Tab: 5mg*, 10mg* *scored

CONTRAINDICATIONS

Type 1 diabetes mellitus (DM) or diabetic ketoacidosis, with or without coma.

WARNINGS/PRECAUTIONS

Caution during first 1-2 weeks of therapy if transferring from longer $T_{1/2}$ sulfonylureas (eg, chlorpropamide). Consider hospitalization during the insulin withdrawal period if patient has been receiving >40 U/day of insulin. May be associated with increased risk of cardiovascular mortality. May produce severe hypoglycemia; increased risk in elderly, debilitated, or malnourished patients; with renal/hepatic impairment, or adrenal/pituitary insufficiency; when caloric intake is deficient; or after severe/prolonged exercise. Loss of glycemic control may occur when exposed to stress (eg, fever, trauma, infection, surgery); may be necessary to d/c therapy and administer insulin. Secondary failure may occur over time. May cause hemolytic anemia; caution with G6PD deficiency and consider a non-sulfonylurea alternative. Caution in elderly.

ADVERSE REACTIONS

Hypoglycemia, GI disturbances, dizziness, drowsiness, headache, porphyria cutanea tarda, photosensitivity reactions, leukopenia, agranulocytosis, thrombocytopenia, hemolytic anemia.

DRUG INTERACTIONS

See Dosage. Hypoglycemic effects may be potentiated by NSAIDs, some azoles, other highly protein-bound drugs, salicylates, sulfonamides, chloramphenicol, probenecid, coumarins, MAOIs, and β-blockers; monitor closely for hypoglycemia during coadministration and for loss of glycemic control when such drugs are withdrawn. Potential interaction leading to severe hypoglycemia reported with oral miconazole. Fluconazole may increase levels. Thiazides and other diuretics, corticosteroids, phenothiazines, thyroid products, estrogens, oral contraceptives, phenytoin, nicotinic acid, sympathomimetics, calcium channel blockers, and isoniazid may produce hyperglycemia and may lead to loss of glycemic control; monitor closely for loss of control during coadministration and for hypoglycemia when such drugs are withdrawn. Increased likelihood of hypoglycemia with alcohol and use of >1 glucose-lowering drug. May be difficult to recognize hypoglycemia with β-blockers. Caution with salicylate or dicumarol. Colesevelam may reduce levels.

NURSING CONSIDERATIONS

Assessment: Assess for previous hypersensitivity to drug, renal/hepatic impairment, type of DM, diabetic ketoacidosis, risk factors for hypoglycemia, G6PD deficiency, pregnancy/nursing status, and possible drug interactions. Obtain baseline FPG and HbA1c levels.

Monitoring: Monitor for hypoglycemia, loss of glycemic control when exposed to stress, hypersensitivity reactions, secondary failure, hemolytic anemia, and other adverse reactions. Monitor blood/urine glucose and HbA1c levels periodically.

Patient Counseling: Inform of the risks, benefits, and alternative modes of therapy. Counsel about the importance of adherence to dietary instructions, regular exercise program, and regular testing of urine and/or blood glucose. Inform about the symptoms, treatment, and predisposing conditions of hypoglycemia, as well as primary and secondary failure. During the insulin withdrawal period, instruct to test for sugar and ketone bodies in urine at least tid and to contact physician immediately if these tests are abnormal.

Storage: <30°C (86°F).

Glucotrol XL – glipizide RX

Class: Sulfonylurea (2nd generation)

ADULT DOSAGE

Type 2 Diabetes Mellitus

Initial: 5mg qd; may start at lower dose if sensitive to hypoglycemic drugs
Usual: 5-10mg qd
Max: 20mg/day

PEDIATRIC DOSAGE

Pediatric use may not have been established

Switching from IR Glipizide:
May give qd dose at the nearest equivalent total daily dose, or may titrate to the appropriate dose starting w/ 5mg qd

Switching from Insulin:
Daily Insulin Requirement:
≤20 U/day: D/C insulin and begin Glucotrol XL at usual dose
>20 U/day: Reduce insulin dose by 50% and begin Glucotrol XL at usual dose; subsequent insulin reductions should depend on individual patient response

Switching from Longer Half-Life Sulfonylureas (eg, Chlorpropamide):
Observe patient carefully for 1-2 weeks

DOSE MODIFICATION

Concomitant Medications
Other Blood-Glucose-Lowering Agents: Initiate at lowest recommended dose
When adding Glucotrol XL to other blood-glucose-lowering agents, initiate Glucotrol XL at 5mg; may start at lower dose if sensitive to hypoglycemic drugs
Colesevelam: Administer Glucotrol XL at least 4 hrs prior to colesevelam

Renal Impairment
Initial/Maint: Dose conservatively

Hepatic Impairment
Initial/Maint: Dose conservatively

Elderly
Initial/Maint: Dose conservatively

Other Important Modifications
Debilitated/Malnourished Patients:
Initial/Maint: Dose conservatively

ADMINISTRATION

Oral route

Administer w/ breakfast
Swallow tab whole; do not chew, divide, or crush

HOW SUPPLIED

Tab, ER: 2.5mg, 5mg, 10mg

CONTRAINDICATIONS

Type 1 DM, diabetic ketoacidosis, with or without coma.

WARNINGS/PRECAUTIONS

Patients being transferred from longer $T_{1/2}$ sulfonylureas (eg, chlorpropamide) may have overlapping drug effect; observe carefully (1-2 weeks) for hypoglycemia. Consider hospitalization during the insulin withdrawal period if patient has been receiving >40 U/day. May be associated with increased risk of cardiovascular mortality. Obstructive symptoms (rare) reported in patients with known strictures in association with ingestion of another non-deformable sustained release formulation; caution with preexisting severe GI narrowing (pathologic or iatrogenic). Markedly reduced GI retention times of the drug may influence clinical efficacy. May produce severe hypoglycemia; increased risk in elderly, debilitated, or malnourished patients; with renal/hepatic impairment or adrenal/pituitary insufficiency; when caloric intake is deficient; or after severe/prolonged exercise. Loss of glycemic control may occur when exposed to stress (eg, fever, trauma, infection, surgery); may be necessary to d/c therapy and administer insulin. Secondary failure may occur over time; assess adequacy of dose adjustment and adherence to diet. May cause hemolytic anemia; caution with G6PD deficiency and consider a non-sulfonylurea alternative.

ADVERSE REACTIONS

Hypoglycemia, asthenia, headache, dizziness, diarrhea, nervousness, tremor, flatulence.

DRUG INTERACTIONS

See Dosage. Hypoglycemic effects may be potentiated by NSAIDs and other highly protein-bound drugs, salicylates, sulfonamides, chloramphenicol, probenecid, coumarins, MAOIs, and β-blockers; monitor closely for hypoglycemia during coadministration and for loss of glycemic control during withdrawal of these drugs. Potential interaction leading to severe hypoglycemia reported with oral miconazole. Thiazides and other diuretics, corticosteroids, phenothiazines, thyroid products, estrogens, oral contraceptives, phenytoin, nicotinic acid, sympathomimetics, calcium channel blockers, and isoniazid may produce hyperglycemia and may lead to loss of glycemic control; monitor closely for loss of control during coadministration and for hypoglycemia during withdrawal of these drugs. Increased likelihood of hypoglycemia with alcohol and use of >1 glucose-lowering drug. May be difficult to recognize hypoglycemia with β-blockers. Caution with salicylate or dicumarol. Fluconazole may increase levels. Colesevelam may reduce levels.

NURSING CONSIDERATIONS

Assessment: Assess for previous hypersensitivity to drug, renal/hepatic impairment, type of DM, diabetic ketoacidosis, risk factors for hypoglycemia, severe GI narrowing, G6PD deficiency, pregnancy/nursing status, and for possible drug interactions. Obtain baseline FPG and HbA1c levels.

Monitoring: Monitor for hypoglycemia, loss of glycemic control when exposed to stress, hypersensitivity reactions, secondary failure, hemolytic anemia, and other adverse reactions. Monitor blood and urine glucose periodically and HbA1c levels every 3 months.

Patient Counseling: Inform of the risks, benefits, and alternative modes of therapy. Counsel not to be concerned if tab-like material is noticed in the stool. Inform about the importance of adherence to dietary instructions, of a regular exercise program, and of regular testing of urine and/or blood glucose. Inform about the symptoms and treatment of hypoglycemia, the conditions that predispose to its development, as well as primary and secondary failure. During the insulin withdrawal period, instruct to test for sugar and ketone bodies in urine at least tid and to contact physician immediately if these tests are abnormal.

Storage: 15-30°C (59-86°F). Protect from moisture and humidity.

GLUCOVANCE – glyburide/metformin hydrochloride RX

Class: Biguanide/sulfonylurea

Lactic acidosis may occur due to metformin accumulation; risk increases with CHF, degree of renal dysfunction, and patient's age. Regularly monitor renal function and use the minimum effective dose of metformin. Do not initiate in patients ≥80 yrs of age unless measurement of CrCl demonstrates that renal function is not reduced. Promptly withhold therapy in the presence of any condition associated with hypoxemia, dehydration, or sepsis. Avoid with clinical or lab evidence of hepatic disease. Caution against excessive alcohol intake; alcohol potentiates the effects of metformin on lactate metabolism. Temporarily d/c therapy prior to any intravascular radiocontrast study and for any surgical procedure. D/C use immediately and promptly institute general supportive measures if lactic acidosis occurs. Prompt hemodialysis is recommended to correct the acidosis and remove the accumulated metformin.

ADULT DOSAGE

Type 2 Diabetes Mellitus

Currently on Diet and Exercise:
Initial: 1.25mg/250mg qd w/ a meal; may use 1.25mg/250mg bid w/ the am and pm meals if baseline HbA1c >9% or FPG >200mg/dL
Titrate: Increase by 1.25mg/250mg/day every 2 weeks
Max: 20mg/2000mg/day

Currently on a Sulfonylurea and/or Metformin:
Initial: 2.5mg/500mg or 5mg/500mg bid w/ the am and pm meals; starting dose should not exceed daily doses of the sulfonylurea or metformin already being taken
Titrate: Increase by no more than 5mg/500mg/day
Max: 20mg/2000mg/day

Addition of Thiazolidinediones:
Continue current dose of Glucovance and initiate thiazolidinedione at its recommended starting dose

PEDIATRIC DOSAGE

Pediatric use may not have been established

DOSE MODIFICATION

Concomitant Medications

Colesevelam: Administer Glucovance at least 4 hrs prior to colesevelam

Elderly

Initial/Maint: Dose conservatively; do not titrate to max dose

Adverse Reactions

Hypoglycemia w/ Glucovance/Thiazolidinedione Combination: Consider reducing the dose of the glyburide component; consider adjusting the dosages of the other components of the regimen as clinically warranted

Other Important Modifications

Debilitated/Malnourished Patients: Do not titrate to max dose

ADMINISTRATION

Oral route

HOW SUPPLIED

Tab: (Glyburide/Metformin) 1.25mg/250mg, 2.5mg/500mg, 5mg/500mg

CONTRAINDICATIONS

Renal disease or dysfunction (eg, SrCr ≥1.5mg/dL [males], ≥1.4mg/dL [females], or abnormal CrCl), acute or chronic metabolic acidosis, including diabetic ketoacidosis, with or without coma. Coadministration with bosentan. Temporarily d/c in patients undergoing radiologic studies involving intravascular administration of iodinated contrast materials.

WARNINGS/PRECAUTIONS

May be associated with increased cardiovascular (CV) mortality. May cause hypoglycemia; increased risk when caloric intake is deficient; when strenuous exercise is not compensated by caloric supplementation; with renal/hepatic insufficiency, adrenal/pituitary insufficiency, alcohol intoxication; or in elderly, debilitated, or malnourished patients. Not recommended during pregnancy. Caution in elderly. Glyburide: May cause hemolytic anemia; caution with G6PD deficiency. Metformin: Assess renal function before initiation of therapy and at least annually thereafter; d/c with evidence of renal impairment. Temporarily d/c at the time of or prior to radiologic studies involving the use of intravascular iodinated contrast materials, withhold for 48 hrs subsequent to the procedure, and reinstitute only if renal function is normal. D/C promptly if CV collapse (shock), acute CHF, acute MI and other conditions characterized by hypoxemia occur. Temporarily suspend for any surgical procedure (except minor procedures not associated with restricted intake of food and fluids); restart when oral intake is resumed and renal function is normal. May decrease serum vitamin B12 levels; monitor hematologic parameters annually. Caution in patients predisposed to developing subnormal vitamin B12 levels (eg, those with inadequate vitamin B12 or Ca^{2+} intake or absorption). Evaluate patients previously well controlled on therapy who develop lab abnormalities or clinical illness for evidence of ketoacidosis or lactic acidosis; d/c if acidosis occurs.

ADVERSE REACTIONS

Lactic acidosis, upper respiratory infection, N/V, abdominal pain, headache, dizziness, diarrhea.

DRUG INTERACTIONS

See Boxed Warning, Contraindications, and Dosage. Increased risk of hypoglycemia with other glucose-lowering agents or ethanol. May be difficult to recognize hypoglycemia with β-blockers. Thiazides and other diuretics, corticosteroids, phenothiazines, thyroid products, estrogens, oral contraceptives, phenytoin, nicotinic acid, sympathomimetics, calcium channel blockers, and isoniazid may produce hyperglycemia and may lead to loss of glycemic control; monitor closely for loss of control during coadministration and for hypoglycemia during withdrawal of these drugs. Weight gain observed with the addition of rosiglitazone to therapy. Monitor LFTs during coadministration with a thiazolidinedione. Metformin: Caution with drugs that may affect renal function or result in significant hemodynamic change or may interfere with the disposition of metformin (eg, cationic drugs eliminated by renal tubular secretion). Furosemide, nifedipine, and cimetidine may increase levels. May decrease furosemide levels. Cationic drugs that are eliminated by renal tubular secretion (eg, cimetidine, amiloride, digoxin, morphine, quinidine, vancomycin) may potentially produce an interaction; monitor and adjust dose of therapy and/or the interfering drug. Glyburide: Hypoglycemic effects may be potentiated by NSAIDs and other highly protein-bound drugs, salicylates, sulfonamides, chloramphenicol, probenecid, coumarins, MAOIs, and β-blockers; monitor closely for hypoglycemia during coadministration and for loss of glycemic control during withdrawal of these drugs. Possible interaction with ciprofloxacin (a fluoroquinolone antibiotic), resulting in potentiation of hypoglycemic action. Potential interaction leading to severe hypoglycemia reported with oral miconazole. Colesevelam may reduce levels.

NURSING CONSIDERATIONS

Assessment: Assess for metabolic acidosis, diabetic ketoacidosis, risk factors for lactic acidosis, renal/hepatic impairment, presence of malnourishment or debilitation, adrenal/pituitary insufficiency, alcoholism, G6PD deficiency, hypoxemia, inadequate vitamin B12 or Ca^{2+} intake/absorption, previous hypersensitivity to the drug, pregnancy/nursing status, and possible drug interactions. Assess if patient is planning to undergo any surgical procedure, or radiologic studies involving the use of intravascular iodinated contrast materials. Obtain baseline FPG and HbA1c levels, and hematologic parameters.

Monitoring: Monitor for signs/symptoms of lactic acidosis, CV effects, hypoglycemia, hemolytic anemia, and other adverse reactions. Monitor for changes in clinical status. Monitor renal function, especially in elderly, at least annually. Monitor hematologic parameters annually. Perform routine serum vitamin B12 measurements at 2- to 3-yr intervals in patients predisposed to developing subnormal vitamin B12 levels. Monitor FPG and HbA1c levels periodically.

Patient Counseling: Inform of the risks, benefits, and alternative modes of therapy. Advise on the importance of adherence to dietary instructions, regular exercise program, and regular testing of blood glucose, HbA1c, renal function, and hematologic parameters. Inform of the risk of lactic acidosis; instruct to d/c therapy immediately and notify physician if unexplained hyperventilation, myalgia, malaise, unusual somnolence, or other nonspecific symptoms occur. Inform of the risk of hypoglycemia. Counsel against excessive alcohol intake.

Storage: Up to 25°C (77°F).

GLUMETZA – metformin hydrochloride — RX

Class: Biguanide

Lactic acidosis may occur due to metformin accumulation; increased risk with conditions such as sepsis, dehydration, excess alcohol intake, hepatic/renal impairment, and acute CHF. If acidosis is suspected, d/c and hospitalize patient immediately.

ADULT DOSAGE

Type 2 Diabetes Mellitus

Initial: 500mg qd
Titrate: May increase by 500mg no sooner than every 1-2 weeks if higher dose is needed and there are no GI adverse reactions
Max: 2000mg/day

Already Receiving Immediate-Release Metformin:
May switch to metformin (tab, extended release) qd at the same total daily dose, up to 2000mg/day

PEDIATRIC DOSAGE

Pediatric use may not have been established

DOSE MODIFICATION

Concomitant Medications

Insulin Secretagogue (Eg, Sulfonylurea)/Insulin:
May require lower doses of insulin secretagogue/insulin

Hepatic Impairment
Avoid use

Elderly
Start at lower end of dosing range

ADMINISTRATION

Oral route

Take w/ pm meal
Swallow whole; do not split, crush, or chew

HOW SUPPLIED

Tab, Extended-Release: 500mg, 1000mg

CONTRAINDICATIONS

Renal impairment (SrCr ≥1.5mg/dL [males], ≥1.4mg/dL [females], or abnormal CrCl), acute or chronic metabolic acidosis, including diabetic ketoacidosis.

WARNINGS/PRECAUTIONS

Not for treatment of type 1 diabetes or diabetic ketoacidosis. Verify renal function is normal prior to starting therapy and at least annually thereafter. Avoid use in patients ≥80 yrs unless renal function is not reduced. D/C if conditions associated with hypoxemia, cardiovascular (CV) collapse, acute MI, acute CHF, or prerenal azotemia develop. Acute alteration of renal function and lactic acidosis reported with intravascular iodinated contrast materials (eg, IV urogram, IV cholangiography, angiography, computed tomography); temporarily d/c at time of or prior to procedure, withhold for 48 hrs subsequent to procedure, and reinstitute only after renal function is normal. D/C prior to any surgical procedure necessitating restricted food/fluid intake; restart after oral intake resumed and renal function found to be normal. May decrease serum vitamin B12levels; measure hematologic parameters annually. Increased risk of hypoglycemia in elderly, debilitated/malnourished, adrenal/ pituitary insufficiency, and alcohol intoxication. Caution in elderly.

ADVERSE REACTIONS

Lactic acidosis (signs may include malaise, myalgia, respiratory distress, increasing somnolence, abdominal distress), hypoglycemia, diarrhea, nausea.

DRUG INTERACTIONS

Hypoglycemia may occur with other glucose-lowering agents (eg, sulfonylureas, insulin) or ethanol; may require lower doses of insulin secretagogues (eg, sulfonylurea) or insulin. Alcohol may potentiate effect on lactate metabolism; caution against excessive alcohol intake. Caution with medications that may affect renal function or result in significant hemodynamic change or may interfere with the disposition of metformin, such as cationic drugs (eg, amiloride, cimetidine, digoxin, morphine, procainamide, quinidine, quinine, ranitidine, triamterene, trimethoprim, vancomycin) that are eliminated by renal tubular secretion; dosage adjustment recommended. Caution with topiramate or other carbonic anhydrase inhibitors (eg, zonisamide, acetazolamide, dichlorphenamide); may increase risk of lactic acidosis. Risk of hyperglycemia and loss of blood glucose control with thiazides and other diuretics, corticosteroids, phenothiazines, thyroid products, estrogens, oral contraceptives, phenytoin, nicotinic acid, sympathomimetics, calcium channel blockers, and isoniazid.

NURSING CONSIDERATIONS

Assessment: Assess for DM type, diabetic ketoacidosis, metabolic acidosis, sepsis, dehydration, excess alcohol intake, hepatic/renal impairment, CHF, hypoperfusion, hypoxemia, adequate vitamin B12or Ca^{2+} intake/absorption, adrenal/pituitary insufficiency, caloric intake, general health status, pregnancy/nursing status, and possible drug interactions. Obtain baseline FPG, HbA1c, SrCr, CrCl, and LFTs. Evaluate for other medical/surgical conditions.

Monitoring: Monitor for hypoglycemia, lactic acidosis, malaise, myalgia, respiratory distress, somnolence, abdominal distress, hypoxemia, dehydration, sepsis, hypothermia, hypotension, resistant bradyarrhythmias, CV collapse, acute CHF, acute MI, or prerenal azotemia. Monitor renal/hepatic function, HbA1c, FPG, and hematologic parameters. Monitor serum vitamin B12 measurements at 2- to 3-yr intervals if inadequate B12or Ca^{2+} intake/absorption.

Patient Counseling: Inform of the potential risks and benefits of the drug and of alternative modes of therapy. Counsel about the importance of adherence to dietary instructions, regular exercise program, regular testing of blood glucose, and HbA1c. Advise to seek medical advice during periods of stress (eg, fever, trauma, infection, surgery). Counsel about the risks/symptoms of, and conditions that predispose to the development of lactic acidosis. D/C and promptly seek medical attention if symptoms of unexplained hyperventilation, myalgia, malaise, unusual somnolence, or other nonspecific symptoms occur. Inform about the importance of regular testing of renal function and hematological parameters. Counsel against excessive alcohol intake, either acute or chronic, while on therapy. Inform that hypoglycemia may occur when used in conjunction with insulin secretagogues (eg, sulfonylureas, insulin). Instruct to swallow tab whole and to not crush or chew. Instruct that if a dose is missed, to not take 2 doses of 2000mg the same day. Inform that inactive ingredients may occasionally be eliminated in the feces as soft mass resembling the tab.

Storage: 20-25°C (68-77°F); excursions permitted to 15-30°C (59-86°F).

GRALISE – gabapentin

Class: GABA analogue

RX

ADULT DOSAGE

Postherpetic Neuralgia

Initial:
Day 1: 300mg qd
Titrate:
Day 2: 600mg qd
Days 3-6: 900mg qd
Days 7-10: 1200mg qd
Days 11-14: 1500mg qd
Day 15: 1800mg qd

If dose is reduced or substituted w/ an alternative medication, this should be done gradually over ≥1 week

PEDIATRIC DOSAGE

Pediatric use may not have been established

DOSE MODIFICATION

Renal Impairment

Initial: 300mg qd
Titrate: Follow the schedule listed above; individualize dose
CrCl ≥60mL/min: 1800mg qd
CrCl 30-60mL/min: 600-1800mg qd
CrCl <30mL/min/Hemodialysis: Do not administer

Discontinuation

D/C gradually over ≥1 week

ADMINISTRATION

Oral route

Take w/ pm meal
Swallow tabs whole; do not split, crush, or chew

HOW SUPPLIED

Tab: 300mg, 600mg

WARNINGS/PRECAUTIONS

Not interchangeable with other gabapentin products. Increased risk of suicidal thoughts or behavior; monitor for the emergence or worsening of depression, suicidal thoughts or behavior, and/or any unusual changes in mood or behavior. May have tumorigenic potential. Drug reaction with eosinophilia and systemic symptoms (DRESS)/multiorgan hypersensitivity reported; evaluate immediately if signs/symptoms are present, and d/c therapy if an alternative etiology cannot be established. Lab test interactions may occur.

ADVERSE REACTIONS

Dizziness, somnolence, headache, peripheral edema, diarrhea.

DRUG INTERACTIONS

Naproxen may increase absorption. May reduce levels of hydrocodone. Hydrocodone and morphine may increase area under the curve. Cimetidine may decrease oral clearance and CrCl. May increase C_{max} of norethindrone. Reduced bioavailability with an antacid containing aluminum hydroxide and magnesium hydroxide; take at least 2 hrs following the antacid.

NURSING CONSIDERATIONS

Assessment: Assess for preexisting tumors, depression, hypersensitivity to drug, renal function, pregnancy/nursing status, and possible drug interactions.

Monitoring: Monitor for emergence or worsening of depression, suicidal thoughts/behavior, and/or any unusual changes in mood/behavior, new or worsening tumors, DRESS, and other adverse reactions.

Patient Counseling: Advise that drug is not interchangeable with other formulations of gabapentin, and to take only as prescribed. Inform that drug may cause dizziness, somnolence, and other signs and symptoms of CNS depression; advise not to drive or operate machinery until sufficient experience on therapy is gained. Advise that if a dose is missed, to take drug with food as soon as remembered, or, if it is almost time for the next dose, to just skip the missed dose and take the next dose at the regular time; instruct not to take 2 doses at the same time. Inform that drug may increase the risk of suicidal thoughts and behavior; advise to report to physician any behaviors of concern.

Storage: 25°C (77°F); excursions permitted to 15-30°C (59-86°F).

HALCION – triazolam **CIV**

Class: Benzodiazepine

ADULT DOSAGE

Insomnia

Short-Term Treatment (Generally 7-10 Days): 0.25mg qhs; 0.125mg may be sufficient for some patients (eg, low body weight)
Max: 0.5mg

PEDIATRIC DOSAGE

Pediatric use may not have been established

DOSE MODIFICATION

Elderly

Initial: 0.125mg
Max: 0.25mg

Other Important Dose Modifications

Debilitated Patients:

Initial: 0.125mg
Max: 0.25mg

ADMINISTRATION

Oral route

HOW SUPPLIED

Tab: 0.25mg* *scored

CONTRAINDICATIONS

Pregnancy. Coadministration with medications that significantly impair the oxidative metabolism mediated by CYP3A (eg, ketoconazole, itraconazole, nefazodone, HIV protease inhibitors).

WARNINGS/PRECAUTIONS

Initiate only after careful evaluation; failure of insomnia to remit after 7-10 days of treatment may indicate presence of a primary psychiatric and/or medical illness. Use lowest effective dose, especially in elderly. Complex behaviors (eg, sleep-driving, preparing/eating food, making phone calls, having sex) reported; consider discontinuation if sleep-driving occurs. Severe anaphylactic and anaphylactoid reactions reported; do not rechallenge if angioedema develops. Increased daytime anxiety reported; may d/c if observed. Abnormal thinking, behavior changes, anterograde amnesia, paradoxical reactions, traveler's amnesia, and dose-related side effects (eg, drowsiness, dizziness, lightheadedness, amnesia) reported. Worsening of depression, including suicidal thinking, reported in primarily depressed patients. May impair mental/physical abilities. Respiratory depression and apnea reported in patients with compromised respiratory function. Caution in patients with signs or symptoms of depression that could be intensified by hypnotic drugs, renal/hepatic impairment, chronic pulmonary insufficiency, and sleep apnea. Dependence and tolerance to drug may develop; caution with history of alcoholism, drug abuse, or with marked personality disorders, due to increased risk of dependence. Withdrawal symptoms reported following abrupt discontinuation; avoid abrupt discontinuation, and taper dose gradually in any patient taking more than the lowest dose for more than a few weeks or with history of seizure.

ADVERSE REACTIONS

Drowsiness, dizziness, lightheadedness, headache, nervousness, coordination disorders/ataxia, N/V.

DRUG INTERACTIONS

See Contraindications. Avoid with very potent CYP3A inhibitors (eg, azole-type antifungals). Caution and consider triazolam dose reduction with drugs inhibiting CYP3A to a lesser but significant degree. Macrolide antibiotics (eg, erythromycin, clarithromycin) and cimetidine may increase levels; use with caution and consider triazolam dose reduction. Isoniazid, oral contraceptives, grapefruit juice, and ranitidine may increase levels; use with caution. Additive CNS depressant effects with psychotropic medications, anticonvulsants, antihistamines, ethanol, and other CNS depressants. Increased risk of complex behaviors with alcohol and other CNS depressants. Caution with fluvoxamine, diltiazem, verapamil, sertraline, paroxetine, ergotamine, cyclosporine, amiodarone, nicardipine, and nifedipine.

NURSING CONSIDERATIONS

Assessment: Assess for physical and/or psychiatric disorder, depression, compromised respiratory function, renal/hepatic impairment, chronic pulmonary insufficiency, sleep apnea, history of seizures, alcoholism or drug abuse, marked personality disorders, hypersensitivity to the drug, pregnancy/nursing status, and possible drug interactions.

Monitoring: Monitor for complex behaviors, anaphylactic/anaphylactoid reactions, increased daytime anxiety, emergence of any new behavioral signs/symptoms of concern, tolerance, dependence, withdrawal symptoms, and other adverse reactions.

Patient Counseling: Inform of the risks and benefits of therapy. Caution against engaging in hazardous activities requiring complete mental alertness (eg, operating machinery, driving). Instruct to immediately report to physician if any adverse reactions (eg, sleep-driving, other complex behaviors) develop. Caution about the concomitant ingestion of alcohol and other CNS depressant drugs during treatment. Instruct to notify physician if pregnant, planning to become pregnant, or if nursing.

Storage: 20-25°C (68-77°F).

HARVONI – ledipasvir/sofosbuvir RX

Class: HCV NS5A inhibitor/HCV nucleotide analogue NS5B polymerase inhibitor

ADULT DOSAGE

Chronic Hepatitis C (Genotype 1)

Treatment Naive w/ or w/o Cirrhosis:
1 tab qd for 12 weeks

Treatment for 8 weeks may be considered in patients w/o cirrhosis who have pretreatment HCV RNA <6 million IU/mL

Treatment Experienced w/o Cirrhosis:
1 tab qd for 12 weeks

Treatment Experienced w/ Cirrhosis:
1 tab qd for 24 weeks

PEDIATRIC DOSAGE

Pediatric use may not have been established

ADMINISTRATION

Oral route

Take w/ or w/o food

HOW SUPPLIED

Tab: (Ledipasvir/Sofosbuvir) 90mg/400mg

ADVERSE REACTIONS

Fatigue, headache, nausea, diarrhea, insomnia.

DRUG INTERACTIONS

P-gp inducers (eg, rifampin, St. John's wort) may decrease levels and may lead to a reduced therapeutic effect; concomitant use is not recommended. Not recommended w/ other products containing sofosbuvir. Coadministration w/ carbamazepine, phenytoin, phenobarbital, oxcarbazepine, rifabutin, rifapentine, or tipranavir/ritonavir (RTV) is not recommended; may decrease levels. Coadministration w/ simeprevir is not recommended; may increase levels of ledipasvir and simeprevir. Coadministration w/ rosuvastatin is not recommended; may increase levels of rosuvastatin, which is associated w/ increased risk of myopathy, including rhabdomyolysis. Coadministration w/ amiodarone is not recommended; may result in serious symptomatic bradycardia, as well as fatal cardiac arrest. If coadministration is required, cardiac monitoring in an in-patient setting for the first 48 hrs of coadministration is recommended, after which outpatient or self-monitoring of HR should occur on a daily basis through at least the first 2 weeks. Patients also taking β-blockers, or those w/ underlying cardiac comorbidities and/or advanced liver disease may be at increased risk for symptomatic bradycardia w/ coadministration of amiodarone. May increase digoxin levels; therapeutic concentration monitoring of digoxin is recommended. Separate administration w/ antacids by 4 hrs. H_2-receptor antagonists (eg, famotidine) may be administered simultaneously or 12 hrs apart from ledipasvir/sofosbuvir at a dose that does not exceed doses comparable to famotidine 40mg bid. Proton-pump inhibitor doses comparable to omeprazole ≤20mg can be administered simultaneously under fasted conditions. Monitor for tenofovir-associated adverse reactions in patients receiving concomitant therapy w/ the combination of efavirenz, emtricitabine, and tenofovir disoproxil fumarate (TDF). Coadministration w/ regimens containing TDF and an HIV protease inhibitor/RTV may increase tenofovir levels; consider alternative hepatitis C virus (HCV) or antiretroviral therapy to avoid increases in tenofovir exposures; if coadministration is necessary, monitor for tenofovir-associated adverse reactions. Coadministration w/ combination of elvitegravir, cobicistat, emtricitabine, and TDF is not recommended; may increase tenofovir levels. (Ledipasvir) May increase intestinal absorption of coadministered substrates of P-gp or breast cancer resistance protein. Drugs that increase gastric pH may decrease levels. Refer to PI for further information on drug interactions.

NURSING CONSIDERATIONS

Assessment: Assess for pregnancy/nursing status and possible drug interactions.

Monitoring: Monitor for adverse reactions.

Patient Counseling: Inform that therapy may interact w/ other drugs; advise to report to physician the use of any other medication or herbal products. Counsel that the effect of treatment of hepatitis C infection on transmission is not known, and that appropriate precautions to prevent transmission of HCV during treatment or in the event of treatment failure should be taken. Advise to take ud, on a regular dosing schedule.

Storage: Room temperature <30°C (86°F).

HAVRIX – hepatitis A vaccine

RX

Class: Vaccine

ADULT DOSAGE

Hepatitis A Vaccine

Active Immunization:

Single 1mL dose, then 1mL booster dose anytime between 6-12 months later

PEDIATRIC DOSAGE

Hepatitis A Vaccine

Active Immunization:

≥12 Months of Age:

Single 0.5mL dose, then 0.5mL booster dose anytime between 6-12 months later

ADMINISTRATION

IM route

Administer primary immunization at least 2 weeks prior to expected exposure to hepatitis A virus

Preparation

1. Shake well before use
2. For the prefilled syringes, attach a sterile needle and administer IM
3. For the vials, use a sterile needle and sterile syringe to withdraw the vaccine dose and administer IM
4. Changing needles between drawing vaccine from a vial and injecting it into a recipient is not necessary unless the needle has been damaged or contaminated
5. Use a separate sterile needle and syringe for each individual
6. Do not dilute to administer

Administration

1. Administer in the anterolateral aspect of the thigh in young children or in deltoid muscle of the upper arm in older children and adults; do not administer in the gluteal region
2. When concomitant administration of other vaccines or immune globulin is required, administer w/ different syringes and at different inj sites
3. Do not mix w/ any other vaccine or product in the same syringe or vial

HOW SUPPLIED

Inj: 720 EL.U./0.5mL, 1440 EL.U./mL [vial, prefilled syringe]

CONTRAINDICATIONS

History of severe allergic reaction to neomycin.

WARNINGS/PRECAUTIONS

Tip caps of prefilled syringes may contain natural rubber latex; may cause allergic reactions in latex-sensitive individuals. Syncope may occur and can be accompanied by transient neurological signs (eg, visual disturbance, paresthesia, tonic-clonic limb movements); procedures should be in place to avoid falling injury and to restore cerebral perfusion following syncope. Appropriate treatment and supervision must be available for possible anaphylactic reactions. Immunocompromised persons may have a diminished immune response to vaccine. May not prevent hepatitis A infection in individuals who have an unrecognized hepatitis A infection at the time of vaccination. May not protect all individuals. Lower antibody response reported in patients with chronic liver disease.

ADVERSE REACTIONS

Inj-site reactions (eg, soreness, pain, redness, swelling, induration), headache, irritability, drowsiness, loss of appetite, fever, fatigue, malaise, anorexia, nausea.

DRUG INTERACTIONS

Immunosuppressive therapies, including irradiation, antimetabolites, alkylating agents, cytotoxic drugs, and corticosteroids (used in greater than physiologic doses), may reduce the immune response to vaccine.

NURSING CONSIDERATIONS

Assessment: Assess for history of severe allergic reaction to hepatitis A vaccine or neomycin. Assess for latex sensitivity, immunosuppression, chronic liver disease, unrecognized hepatitis A infection, immunization status/vaccination history, pregnancy/nursing status, and possible drug interactions.

Monitoring: Monitor for allergic reactions, syncope, neurological signs, and other adverse reactions. Monitor immune response to vaccine.

Patient Counseling: Inform of the potential benefits and risks of immunization. Counsel about potential side effects and emphasize that the vaccine contains noninfectious killed viruses and cannot cause hepatitis A infection. Instruct to report any adverse events to physician.

Storage: 2-8°C (36-46°F). Do not freeze; discard if vaccine has been frozen.

HEPSERA – adefovir dipivoxil RX

Class: Nucleotide analogue reverse transcriptase inhibitor

Lactic acidosis and severe hepatomegaly with steatosis, including fatal cases, reported with the use of nucleoside analogues alone or in combination with other antiretrovirals. Severe acute exacerbations of hepatitis reported in patients who have discontinued therapy. Closely monitor hepatic function with both clinical and lab follow-up for at least several months in patients who d/c therapy. If appropriate, resumption of antihepatitis B therapy may be warranted. Chronic use may result in nephrotoxicity in patients at risk of or having underlying renal dysfunction; monitor renal function and adjust dose if required. HIV resistance may occur in patients with unrecognized or untreated HIV infection.

ADULT DOSAGE

Chronic Hepatitis B

10mg qd

PEDIATRIC DOSAGE

Chronic Hepatitis B

≥12 Years:

10mg qd

DOSE MODIFICATION

Renal Impairment

CrCl 30-49mL/min: 10mg q48h

CrCl 10-29mL/min: 10mg q72h

Hemodialysis: 10mg q7d following dialysis

ADMINISTRATION

Oral route

Take without regard to food

HOW SUPPLIED

Tab: 10mg

WARNINGS/PRECAUTIONS

Caution in adolescents with underlying renal dysfunction; monitor renal function closely. Offer HIV antibody testing before initiating therapy. Obesity and prolonged nucleoside exposure may be risk factors for lactic acidosis and severe hepatomegaly with steatosis. Caution with known risk factors for liver disease. D/C if findings suggestive of lactic acidosis or pronounced hepatotoxicity develop. Resistance to the drug can result in viral load rebound, which may result in exacerbation of hepatitis B, and in the setting of diminished hepatic function, lead to liver decompensation and possible fatal outcome. To reduce risk of resistance in patients with lamivudine-resistant hepatitis B virus (HBV), use adefovir dipivoxil in combination with lamivudine and not as monotherapy. To reduce risk of resistance in patients receiving monotherapy, consider modification of treatment if serum HBV DNA remains >1000 copies/mL with continued treatment. Caution in elderly.

ADVERSE REACTIONS

Nephrotoxicity, lactic acidosis, severe hepatomegaly with steatosis, asthenia, headache, abdominal pain, nausea, flatulence, diarrhea, dyspepsia.

DRUG INTERACTIONS

Avoid with tenofovir disoproxil fumarate (TDF) or TDF-containing products. Coadministration with drugs that reduce renal function or compete for active tubular secretion may increase levels of either adefovir and/or these coadministered drugs. Caution with nephrotoxic agents (eg, cyclosporine, tacrolimus, aminoglycosides, vancomycin, NSAIDs).

NURSING CONSIDERATIONS

Assessment: Assess for renal dysfunction, risk factors for lactic acidosis and liver disease, hypersensitivity, pregnancy/nursing status, and possible drug interactions. Perform HIV antibody testing and assess CrCl.

Monitoring: Monitor for signs/symptoms of lactic acidosis, hepatotoxicity, nephrotoxicity, clinical resistance, and other adverse reactions. Monitor hepatic function (in patients who d/c therapy) and renal function.

Patient Counseling: Inform of risks, benefits, and alternative modes of therapy. Instruct to follow a regular dosing schedule to avoid missing doses. Advise to immediately report any severe abdominal pain, muscle pain, yellowing of the eyes, dark urine, pale stools, and/or loss of appetite. Instruct to notify physician if any unusual/known symptom develops, persists, or worsens. Advise not to d/c therapy without informing physician. Advise that routine lab monitoring and follow-up is important during therapy. Inform of importance of obtaining HIV antibody testing prior to starting therapy. Counsel women of childbearing age about risks of drug exposure during pregnancy, and to notify physician if the patient becomes pregnant while on therapy. Inform pregnant patients about the pregnancy registry.

Storage: 25°C (77°F); excursions permitted to 15-30°C (59-86°F).

HERCEPTIN – trastuzumab RX

Class: Monoclonal antibody/HER2-blocker

May result in cardiac failure; incidence and severity were highest with anthracycline-containing chemotherapy regimens. Evaluate left ventricular function prior to and during treatment; d/c in patients receiving adjuvant therapy and withhold in patients with metastatic disease for clinically significant decrease in left ventricular function. May result in serious and fatal infusion reactions and pulmonary toxicity; interrupt infusion for dyspnea or clinically significant hypotension, and monitor until symptoms completely resolve. D/C for anaphylaxis, angioedema, interstitial pneumonitis, or acute respiratory distress syndrome. Exposure during pregnancy may result in oligohydramnios and oligohydramnios sequence manifesting as pulmonary hypoplasia, skeletal abnormalities, and neonatal death.

ADULT DOSAGE

HER2 Overexpressing Node Positive or Node Negative Breast Cancer

Adjuvant Treatment:
During and Following Paclitaxel, Docetaxel, or Docetaxel/Carboplatin:
Initial: 4mg/kg IV infusion over 90 min, then at 2mg/kg IV infusion over 30 min weekly during chemo for the first 12 weeks (paclitaxel or docetaxel) or 18 weeks (docetaxel/carboplatin)
Subsequent Doses: One week following the last weekly dose, give 6mg/kg IV infusion over 30-90 min every 3 weeks

Single Agent w/in 3 Weeks Following Completion of Multimodality Anthracycline-Based Chemotherapy Regimens:
Initial: 8mg/kg IV infusion over 90 min
Subsequent Doses: 6mg/kg IV infusion over 30-90 min every 3 weeks

Extending adjuvant treatment >1 year is not recommended

HER2 Overexpressing Metastatic Breast Cancer

Alone or in Combination w/ Paclitaxel:
Initial: 4mg/kg IV infusion over 90 min
Subsequent Doses: 2mg/kg IV infusion over 30 min once a week until disease progression

HER2 Overexpressing Metastatic Gastric or Gastroesophageal Junction Adenocarcinoma

Patients Who Have Not Received Prior Treatment for Metastatic Disease:
Combination w/ Cisplatin and Capecitabine or 5-Fluorouracil:
Initial: 8mg/kg IV infusion over 90 min
Subsequent Doses: 6mg/kg IV infusion over 30-90 min every 3 weeks until disease progression

PEDIATRIC DOSAGE

Pediatric use may not have been established

DOSE MODIFICATION

Adverse Reactions
Infusion Reactions:
Mild or Moderate: Decrease rate of infusion
Dyspnea/Clinical Significant Hypotension: Interrupt infusion
Severe/Life-threatening: D/C therapy

Cardiomyopathy:
Withhold Therapy for at Least 4 Weeks for Either of the Following:
1. ≥16% absolute decrease in LVEF from pretreatment values
2. LVEF below institutional limits of normal and ≥10% absolute decrease in LVEF from pretreatment values

May Resume Therapy if:
LVEF returns to normal limits and absolute decrease from baseline is ≤15% w/in 4-8 weeks

Permanently D/C Therapy if:
Persistent (>8 weeks) LVEF decline or for suspension of dosing on more than 3 occasions for cardiomyopathy

ADMINISTRATION
IV route

Do not administer as IV push or bolus
Do not mix w/ other drugs
Do not substitute for or w/ ado-trastuzumab emtansine

Reconstitution
1. Reconstitute each 440mg vial w/ 20mL of Bacteriostatic Water for Injection, USP containing 1.1% benzyl alcohol as a preservative to yield a multidose sol containing 21mg/mL
2. In patients w/ known hypersensitivity to benzyl alcohol, reconstitute w/ 20mL of SWFI w/o preservative to yield a single use sol

Dilution
1. Determine the dose (mg) and calculate the volume of the 21mg/mL reconstituted sol needed
2. Withdraw this amount from the vial and add it to an infusion bag containing 250mL of 0.9% NaCl Inj, USP
3. Gently invert the bag to mix the sol

HOW SUPPLIED
Inj: 440mg

WARNINGS/PRECAUTIONS
Do not substitute for or with ado-trastuzumab emtansine. Patients with symptomatic intrinsic lung disease or extensive tumor involvement of the lungs, resulting in dyspnea at rest, may have more severe pulmonary toxicity. Detection of HER2 protein overexpression is necessary for appropriate patient selection; use FDA-approved tests for the specific tumor type to assess HER2 protein overexpression and HER2 gene amplification.

ADVERSE REACTIONS
Cardiac failure, infusion reactions, pulmonary toxicity, fever, N/V, headache, nasopharyngitis, diarrhea, infections, fatigue, anemia, neutropenia, rash, weight loss, increased cough.

DRUG INTERACTIONS
See Boxed Warning. Higher incidence of neutropenia with myelosuppressive chemotherapy. Paclitaxel may increase trough concentrations.

NURSING CONSIDERATIONS

Assessment: Assess cardiac function, including baseline left ventricular ejection fraction (LVEF). Assess HER2 protein overexpression and HER2 gene amplification. Assess for symptomatic intrinsic lung disease or extensive tumor involvement of lungs, pregnancy/nursing status, and possible drug interactions.

Monitoring: Monitor for infusion reactions, pulmonary toxicity, neutropenia, and other adverse reactions. Monitor LVEF every 3 months during and upon completion of therapy, and every 6 months for at least 2 yrs following completion as a component of adjuvant therapy. Repeat LVEF measurement at 4-week intervals if therapy is withheld for significant left ventricular cardiac dysfunction.

Patient Counseling: Advise to contact physician immediately for new onset or worsening SOB, cough, swelling of ankles/legs/face, palpitations, weight gain of >5 lbs in 24 hrs, dizziness, or loss of consciousness. Inform that drug may cause fetal harm. Advise women of childbearing potential to use effective contraceptive methods during treatment and for a minimum of 6 months following therapy. Instruct not to breastfeed during treatment. Encourage women exposed to therapy during pregnancy to enroll in MotHER - the Herceptin Pregnancy Registry.

Storage: 2-8°C (36-46°F). Reconstituted with Bacteriostatic Water for Inj: 2-8°C (36-46°F) for 28 days. Reconstituted with Unpreserved Sterile Water for Inj: Use immediately. Diluted in Polyvinylchloride or Polyethylene Bags Containing 0.9% NaCl Inj: 2-8°C (36-46°F) for no more than 24 hrs prior to use. Do not freeze following reconstitution/dilution.

HORIZANT – gabapentin enacarbil

Class: GABA analogue

RX

ADULT DOSAGE

Restless Legs Syndrome

Moderate-Severe Primary Restless Legs Syndrome:
Usual: 600mg qd at about 5 pm

If dose is not taken at the recommended time, the next dose should be taken the following day as prescribed

Postherpetic Neuralgia

Initial: 600mg qam for 3 days
Titrate: Increase to 600mg bid (1200mg/day) on Day 4
Usual: 600mg bid

PEDIATRIC DOSAGE

Pediatric use may not have been established

DOSE MODIFICATION

Renal Impairment
Restless Leg Syndrome:
CrCl ≥60mL/min:
600mg/day
CrCl 30-59mL/min:
Initial: 300mg/day
Titrate: Increase to 600mg prn
CrCl 15-29mL/min:
300mg/day
CrCl <15mL/min:
300mg qod
CrCl <15mL/min on Hemodialysis:
Not recommended

Postherpetic Neuralgia:
CrCl ≥60mL/min:
Titration: 600mg qam for 3 days
Maint: 600mg bid
Tapering: 600mg qam for 1 week

CrCl 30-59mL/min:
Titration: 300mg qam for 3 days
Maint: 300mg bid; increase to 600mg bid if needed based on tolerability and efficacy
Tapering: Reduce current maint dose to qd in am for 1 week

CrCl 15-29mL/min:
Titration: 300mg qam on Day 1 and Day 3
Maint: 300mg qam; increase to 300mg bid if needed based on tolerability and efficacy
Tapering: If taking 300mg bid, reduce to 300mg qd in am for 1 week. If taking 300mg qd, no taper needed

CrCl <15mL/min:
Maint: 300mg qod in am; increase to 300mg qd in am if needed based on tolerability and efficacy

CrCl <15mL/min on Hemodialysis:
Maint: 300mg following every dialysis; increase to 600mg following every dialysis if needed based on tolerability and efficacy

ADMINISTRATION

Oral route

Take w/ food
Swallow tab whole; do not cut, crush, or chew

HOW SUPPLIED

Tab, Extended Release: 300mg, 600mg

WARNINGS/PRECAUTIONS

Not recommended for patients who are required to sleep during the day and remain awake at night or in RLS patients with CrCl <15mL/min on hemodialysis. May cause significant driving impairment, somnolence/sedation, and dizziness. Not interchangeable with other gabapentin products. Increases the risk of suicidal thoughts or behavior; monitor for the emergence or worsening of depression, suicidal thoughts/behavior, and/or any unusual changes in mood or behavior. Drug reaction with eosinophilia and systemic symptoms (DRESS)/multiorgan hypersensitivity reported;

evaluate immediately if signs/symptoms (eg, hypersensitivity, fever, lymphadenopathy) are present and d/c if alternative etiology cannot be established. For RLS patients, if recommended daily dose is exceeded, reduce dose to 600mg daily for 1 week prior to discontinuation to minimize potential for withdrawal seizure. For PHN patients receiving bid dose, reduce dose to qd for 1 week prior to discontinuation to minimize potential for withdrawal seizure. May have tumorigenic potential. Caution in elderly and with renal impairment.

ADVERSE REACTIONS

Somnolence/sedation, dizziness, headache, nausea, dry mouth, flatulence, fatigue, insomnia, irritability, feeling drunk/abnormal, peripheral edema, weight increase, vertigo.

DRUG INTERACTIONS

Drug is released faster from extended-release tab in the presence of alcohol; avoid alcohol consumption. Increased somnolence/sedation, dizziness, and nausea when taken in conjunction with morphine.

NURSING CONSIDERATIONS

Assessment: Assess for preexisting tumors, history of depression, pregnancy/nursing status, renal function (CrCl), and possible drug interactions.

Monitoring: Monitor for withdrawal seizures with discontinuation, somnolence/sedation, dizziness, emergence or worsening of depression, suicidal thoughts/behavior, and/or any unusual changes in mood/behavior, DRESS, development or worsening of tumors, renal function, and hypersensitivity reactions.

Patient Counseling: Inform that therapy may cause significant driving impairment, somnolence, and dizziness; advise not to drive or operate dangerous machinery until sufficient experience on therapy is gained. Counsel that treatment may increase the risk of suicidal thoughts and behavior; advise to report to physician any behaviors of concern. Advise that multiorgan hypersensitivity reactions may occur; instruct to contact physician if experiencing any signs or symptoms of this condition. Advise not to interchange with other gabapentin products. If the dose is missed, instruct to take the next dose at the time of the next scheduled dose. Instruct about how to d/c therapy. Advise to avoid alcohol when taking the drug.

Storage: 25°C (77°F); excursions permitted to 15-30°C (59-86°F). Protect from moisture.

HUMALOG — insulin lispro (rDNA origin) RX

Class: Insulin

ADULT DOSAGE

Diabetes Mellitus

IV/SQ:

Total Daily Insulin Requirement:

Usual: 0.5-1 U/kg/day

PEDIATRIC DOSAGE

Type 1 Diabetes Mellitus

≥3 Years:

SQ:

Total Daily Insulin Requirement:

Usual: 0.5-1 U/kg/day

DOSE MODIFICATION

Renal Impairment

Frequent glucose monitoring and insulin dose reduction may be required

Hepatic Impairment

Frequent glucose monitoring and insulin dose reduction may be required

ADMINISTRATION

IV/SQ route

SQ

Administer w/in 15 min ac or immediately pc

Generally used w/ an intermediate- or long-acting insulin

Inject in the abdominal wall, thigh, upper arm, or buttocks; rotate inj sites w/in the same region

If mixed w/ NPH insulin, draw insulin lispro into syringe 1st and inject immediately after mixing

Continuous SQ Infusion (Insulin Pump)

Do not use diluted or mixed insulins in external insulin pumps

Rotate infusion sites w/in the same region

Initial Programming of Pump:

Should be based on the total daily insulin dose of the previous regimen

Approx 50% of total dose is usually given as meal-related boluses, and remainder given as basal infusion

Change insulin in the reservoir at least every 7 days; change infusion sets and infusion set insertion site at least every 3 days

IV

Not approved for use in pediatrics

Use at concentrations from 0.1 U/mL to 1.0 U/mL in infusion systems containing 0.9% NaCl

HOW SUPPLIED

Inj: 100 U/mL [3mL, cartridge, KwikPen, vial; 10mL, vial]

CONTRAINDICATIONS

During episodes of hypoglycemia.

WARNINGS/PRECAUTIONS

KwikPen, cartridges, reusable pens, and syringes must never be shared between patients, even if needle is changed; may carry a risk for transmission of blood-borne pathogens. Any change in insulin regimen should be made cautiously and under medical supervision. Changes in strength, manufacturer, type, or method of administration may result in the need for a change in dosage. Stress, major illness, or changes in exercise or meal patterns may alter insulin requirements. Hypoglycemia may occur and may impair ability to concentrate and react. Severe, life-threatening, generalized allergy, including anaphylaxis, may occur. Hypokalemia may occur. Frequent glucose monitoring and insulin dose reduction may be necessary w/ renal/hepatic impairment. Malfunction of the insulin pump or infusion set or insulin degradation can rapidly lead to hyperglycemia or ketosis; prompt identification and correction of the cause is necessary. Train patients using continuous SQ infusion pump therapy to administer by inj and have alternate insulin therapy available in case of pump failure. IV administration should be under medical supervision w/ close monitoring of blood glucose and K^+ levels.

ADVERSE REACTIONS

Flu syndrome, pharyngitis, rhinitis, headache, pain, cough increased, infection, diarrhea, nausea, fever, abdominal pain, asthenia, bronchitis, myalgia, UTI.

DRUG INTERACTIONS

May require insulin dose adjustment and close monitoring w/ drugs that may increase blood glucose-lowering effect and susceptibility to hypoglycemia (eg, salicylates, sulfonamide antibiotics, MAOIs, ACE inhibitors, somatostatin analogues [eg, octreotide]), drugs that may reduce blood glucose-lowering effect (eg, corticosteroids, oral contraceptives, sympathomimetic agents [eg, epinephrine, albuterol, terbutaline], atypical antipsychotics, protease inhibitors), or drugs that may increase or reduce blood glucose-lowering effect (eg, β-blockers, clonidine, lithium salts, alcohol). Pentamidine may cause hypoglycemia, sometimes followed by hyperglycemia. Signs of hypoglycemia may be reduced w/ β-blockers, clonidine, guanethidine, and reserpine. Caution w/ K^+-lowering drugs or drugs sensitive to serum K^+ concentrations. Observe for signs/symptoms of heart failure (HF) if treated concomitantly w/ a peroxisome proliferator-activated receptor (PPAR)-gamma agonist (eg, thiazolidinedione); consider discontinuation or dose reduction of the PPAR-gamma agonist if HF develops.

NURSING CONSIDERATIONS

Assessment: Assess for predisposition to hypoglycemia, risk for hypokalemia, hypersensitivity, renal/hepatic impairment, pregnancy/nursing status, and possible drug interactions. Obtain baseline blood glucose and HbA1c levels.

Monitoring: Monitor for signs/symptoms of hypoglycemia, hypokalemia, allergic reactions, and other adverse effects. Monitor blood glucose, HbA1c, K^+ levels, and renal/hepatic function.

Patient Counseling: Advise to never share KwikPen, cartridge, reusable pen, or syringe w/ another person, even if needle is changed. Instruct on self-management procedures (eg, glucose monitoring, proper inj technique, management of hypo/hyperglycemia). Advise on handling of special situations, such as intercurrent conditions (eg, illness, stress, emotional disturbances), inadequate or skipped doses, inadvertent administration of an increased dose, inadequate food intake, and skipped meals. Instruct diabetic women to inform physician if pregnant or contemplating pregnancy. Counsel to always check label before each inj to avoid medication errors, such as accidental mix-ups. Instruct on how to use external infusion pump.

Storage: Unused: 2-8°C (36-46°F) until expiration date. Do not freeze; do not use if it has been frozen. Opened: <30°C (86°F) for up to 28 days. Protect from direct heat and light. (Vials) May refrigerate. (Cartridge/KwikPen) Do not refrigerate. Discard cartridge used in the D-Tron pumps after 7 days even if it still contains the drug. Diluted Humalog for SQ Inj: 5°C (41°F) for 28 days or 30°C (86°F) for 14 days. Do not dilute drug contained in a cartridge or drug used in an external insulin pump. IV Admixture: 2-8°C (36-46°F) for 48 hrs; may be used at room temperature for up to an additional 48 hrs.

HUMALOG MIX 50/50 – insulin lispro protamine (rDNA origin)/ insulin lispro (rDNA origin) RX

Class: Insulin

ADULT DOSAGE

Diabetes Mellitus

Individualize dose

PEDIATRIC DOSAGE

Pediatric use may not have been established

DOSE MODIFICATION

Renal Impairment

Careful glucose monitoring and dose adjustments may be necessary

Hepatic Impairment

Careful glucose monitoring and dose adjustments may be necessary

ADMINISTRATION

SQ route

Inject w/in 15 min ac

HOW SUPPLIED

Inj: (Insulin Lispro Protamine/Insulin Lispro) (50 U/50 U)/mL [3mL, KwikPen; 10mL, vial]

CONTRAINDICATIONS

During episodes of hypoglycemia.

WARNINGS/PRECAUTIONS

KwikPens and syringes must never be shared between patients, even if needle is changed; may carry a risk for transmission of blood-borne pathogens. Any change of insulin should be made cautiously and only under medical supervision. Changes in strength, manufacturer, type, species, or method of manufacture may result in the need for a change in dosage. Hypoglycemia and hypokalemia may occur; caution in patients in whom such potential side effects may be clinically relevant (eg, patients w/ autonomic neuropathy). Lipodystrophy and hypersensitivity may occur. Dosage adjustment may be necessary if patient changes physical activity or usual meal plan. Illness, emotional disturbances, or other stress may alter insulin requirements. Careful glucose monitoring and insulin dose adjustment may be necessary w/ hepatic/renal impairment. Inj-site redness/ swelling/itching and severe, life-threatening, generalized allergy may occur. Contains cresol as excipient; localized reactions and generalized myalgias reported. Antibody production reported. Caution in elderly.

ADVERSE REACTIONS

Hypoglycemia, allergic reactions, inj-site reactions, lipodystrophy, pruritus, rash.

DRUG INTERACTIONS

Drugs w/ hyperglycemic activity (eg, corticosteroids, certain lipid-lowering drugs [eg, niacin], oral contraceptives, phenothiazines, thyroid replacement therapy) may increase insulin requirements. Drugs that increase insulin sensitivity or have hypoglycemic activity (eg, salicylates, sulfa antibiotics, MAOIs, ACE inhibitors, inhibitors of pancreatic function [eg, octreotide]) may decrease insulin requirements. β-blockers may mask symptoms of hypoglycemia. Caution w/ K^+-lowering drugs or drugs sensitive to serum K^+ levels. Observe for signs/symptoms of heart failure (HF) if treated concomitantly w/ a peroxisome proliferator-activated receptor (PPAR)-gamma agonist (eg, thiazolidinedione); consider discontinuation or dose reduction of the PPAR-gamma agonist if HF develops.

NURSING CONSIDERATIONS

Assessment: Assess for presence of hypoglycemia or hypokalemia and for conditions where such potential side effects might be clinically relevant. Assess for hypersensitivity, renal/hepatic impairment, pregnancy/nursing status, and possible drug interactions. Obtain baseline blood glucose and HbA1c levels.

Monitoring: Monitor for signs/symptoms of hypoglycemia, hypokalemia, lipodystrophy, allergic reactions, antibody production, and other adverse effects. Monitor blood glucose, HbA1c, K^+ levels, and renal/hepatic function.

Patient Counseling: Inform of the potential risks and advantages of therapy and alternative therapies. Instruct not to mix drug w/ any other insulin. Inform of the importance of proper insulin storage, inj technique, timing of dosage, adherence to meal planning, regular physical activity, regular blood glucose monitoring, periodic HbA1c testing, recognition and management of hypo/ hyperglycemia, and periodic assessment for diabetes complications. Advise to inform physician if pregnant or planning to become pregnant. Instruct patients using insulin pen delivery device on how to properly use the delivery device, prime the pen to a stream of insulin, and properly dispose of needles. Advise not to share insulin pen w/ others.

Storage: Unopened: 2-8°C (36-46°F) until expiration date, or at room temperature (<30°C [86°F]) for 28 days (vial) or 10 days (KwikPen). Do not freeze; do not use if it has been frozen. Opened: <30°C (86°F) for 28 days (vial) or 10 days (KwikPen). Do not refrigerate KwikPen. Protect from direct heat and light.

HUMALOG MIX 75/25 – insulin lispro protamine (rDNA origin)/ insulin lispro (rDNA origin) RX

Class: Insulin

ADULT DOSAGE

Diabetes Mellitus

Individualize dose

PEDIATRIC DOSAGE

Pediatric use may not have been established

DOSE MODIFICATION

Renal Impairment

Frequent glucose monitoring and insulin dose reduction may be necessary

Hepatic Impairment

Frequent glucose monitoring and insulin dose reduction may be necessary

ADMINISTRATION

SQ route

Inject w/in 15 min ac

HOW SUPPLIED

Inj: (Insulin Lispro Protamine/Insulin Lispro) (75 U/25 U)/mL [3mL, KwikPen; 10mL, vial]

CONTRAINDICATIONS

During episodes of hypoglycemia.

WARNINGS/PRECAUTIONS

KwikPens and syringes must never be shared between patients, even if needle is changed; may carry a risk for transmission of blood-borne pathogens. Any change of insulin should be made cautiously and only under medical supervision. Changes in strength, manufacturer, type, species, or method of manufacture may result in the need for a change in dosage. Hypoglycemia and hypokalemia may occur; caution in patients in whom such potential side effects might be clinically relevant (eg, patients w/ autonomic neuropathy). Lipodystrophy and hypersensitivity may occur. Dosage adjustment may be necessary if patient changes physical activity or usual meal plan. Illness, emotional disturbances, or other stress may alter insulin requirements. Careful glucose monitoring and insulin dose adjustment may be necessary w/ hepatic/renal impairment. Inj-site redness/ swelling/itching, and severe, life-threatening, generalized allergy may occur. Contains cresol as excipient; localized reactions and generalized myalgias reported. Antibody production reported. Caution in elderly.

ADVERSE REACTIONS

Hypoglycemia, allergic reactions, inj-site reactions, lipodystrophy, pruritus, rash.

DRUG INTERACTIONS

Drugs w/ hyperglycemic activity (eg, corticosteroids, certain lipid-lowering drugs [eg, niacin], oral contraceptives, phenothiazines, thyroid replacement therapy) may increase insulin requirements. Drugs that increase insulin sensitivity or have hypoglycemic activity (eg, salicylates, sulfa antibiotics, MAOIs, ACE inhibitors, inhibitors of pancreatic function [eg, octreotide]) may decrease insulin requirements. β-blockers may mask symptoms of hypoglycemia. Caution w/ K^+-lowering drugs or drugs sensitive to serum K^+ levels. Observe for signs/symptoms of heart failure (HF) if treated concomitantly w/ a peroxisome proliferator-activated receptor (PPAR)-gamma agonist (eg, thiazolidinedione); consider discontinuation or dose reduction of the PPAR-gamma agonist if HF develops.

NURSING CONSIDERATIONS

Assessment: Assess for presence of hypoglycemia or hypokalemia and for conditions where such potential side effects might be clinically relevant. Assess for hypersensitivity, renal/hepatic impairment, pregnancy/nursing status, and possible drug interactions. Obtain baseline blood glucose and HbA1c levels.

Monitoring: Monitor for signs/symptoms of hypoglycemia, hypokalemia, lipodystrophy, allergic reactions, antibody production, and other adverse effects. Monitor blood glucose, HbA1c, K^+ levels, and renal/hepatic function.

Patient Counseling: Inform of the potential risks and advantages of therapy and alternative therapies. Instruct not to mix drug w/ any other insulin. Inform of the importance of proper insulin storage, inj technique, timing of dosage, adherence to meal planning, regular physical activity, regular blood glucose monitoring, periodic HbA1c testing, recognition and management of hypo/hyperglycemia, and periodic assessment for diabetes complications. Advise to inform physician if pregnant/planning to become pregnant. Instruct patients using insulin pen delivery device on how to properly use delivery device, prime the pen to a stream of insulin, and properly dispose of needles. Advise not to share insulin pen w/ others.

Storage: Unopened: 2-8°C (36-46°F) until expiration date, or room temperature (<30°C [86°F]) for 28 days (vial) or 10 days (KwikPen). Do not freeze; do not use if it has been frozen. Opened: <30°C (86°F) for 28 days (vial) or 10 days (KwikPen). Do not refrigerate KwikPen. Protect from direct heat and light.

HUMIRA – adalimumab

RX

Class: Monoclonal antibody/TNF-blocker

Increased risk of serious infections (eg, active tuberculosis [TB] including latent TB reactivation, invasive fungal, bacterial, viral, and other infections due to opportunistic pathogens) leading to hospitalization or death, mostly with concomitant use of immunosuppressants (eg, methotrexate [MTX], corticosteroids). D/C if serious infection or sepsis develops. Active/latent reactivation TB patients have frequently presented with disseminated or extrapulmonary disease; test for latent TB before and during therapy and initiate treatment for latent TB prior to adalimumab use. Invasive fungal infections reported; consider empiric antifungal therapy in patients at risk who develop severe systemic illness. Monitor patients closely for development of infection during and after treatment, including development of TB in patients who tested negative for latent TB infection prior to therapy. Lymphoma and other malignancies, some fatal, reported in children and adolescents. Postmarketing cases of aggressive and fatal hepatosplenic T-cell lymphoma (HSTCL) reported in patients with Crohn's disease (CD) or ulcerative colitis (UC) and the majority were in adolescent and young adult males; all of these patients were treated concomitantly with azathioprine or 6-mercaptopurine.

ADULT DOSAGE

Rheumatoid Arthritis

Moderately to Severely Active:
40mg every other week; may increase to 40mg every week in patients not taking concomitant methotrexate (MTX)

May be used alone or in combination w/ MTX or other non-biologic disease-modifying anti-rheumatic drugs

Psoriatic Arthritis

Active:
40mg every other week

May be used alone or in combination w/ other non-biologic disease-modifying anti-rheumatic drugs

Ankylosing Spondylitis

Active:
40mg every other week

Crohn's Disease

Moderately to severely active Crohn's disease in patients who have had an inadequate response to conventional therapy and have also lost response to or are intolerant to infliximab

Day 1: 160mg (given as four 40mg inj in 1 day or as two 40mg inj/day for 2 consecutive days)
Day 15: 80mg
Day 29 Onward: 40mg every other week

Plaque Psoriasis

Moderate to severe chronic plaque psoriasis in patients who are candidates for systemic therapy or phototherapy, and when other systemic therapies are medically less appropriate

Initial: 80mg
Maint: 40mg every other week starting 1 week after initial dose

PEDIATRIC DOSAGE

Juvenile Idiopathic Arthritis

Moderately to Severely Active Polyarticular Juvenile Idiopathic Arthritis:
≥4 Years:
15-<30kg: 20mg every other week
≥30kg: 40mg every other week

May be used alone or in combination w/ methotrexate

Ulcerative Colitis

Moderately to severely active ulcerative colitis in patients who have had an inadequate response to immunosuppressants

Day 1: 160mg (given as four 40mg inj in 1 day or as two 40mg inj/day for 2 consecutive days)
Day 15: 80mg
Day 29 Onward: 40mg every other week

Only continue if clinical remission is evident by 8 weeks (Day 57) of therapy

ADMINISTRATION
SQ route

Rotate inj sites; avoid areas where skin is tender, bruised, red, or hard

HOW SUPPLIED
Inj: 20mg/0.4mL [prefilled syringe], 40mg/0.8mL [prefilled syringe, prefilled pen, vial]

WARNINGS/PRECAUTIONS
Do not initiate in patients with an active infection. Increased risk of infection in patients >65 yrs of age and in patients with comorbid conditions. Malignancies, including acute and chronic leukemia, lymphoma, and nonmelanoma skin cancer (NMSC), reported in adults. Anaphylaxis and angioneurotic edema reported; d/c immediately and institute appropriate therapy if anaphylactic or other serious allergic reaction occurs. May increase risk of hepatitis B virus (HBV) reactivation in chronic carriers; closely monitor for signs of active HBV infection during and for several months after therapy termination. D/C if HBV reactivation develops and start effective antiviral therapy with appropriate supportive treatment. New onset or exacerbation of CNS and peripheral demyelinating diseases, new or worsening congestive heart failure (CHF), and hematologic system adverse reactions, including significant cytopenia (eg, thrombocytopenia, leukopenia) reported. May result in formation of autoantibodies and development of a lupus-like syndrome; d/c if symptoms suggestive of a lupus-like syndrome develop. If possible, JIA patients should be brought up to date with all immunizations in agreement with current immunizations guidelines prior to initiating therapy. Avoid latex sensitive patients handling the needle cover of the prefilled syringe because it contains dry rubber (latex). Caution in elderly.

ADVERSE REACTIONS
Infections, malignancies, inj-site reactions, headache, rash, nausea, flu syndrome, abdominal pain, hyperlipidemia, hypercholesterolemia, back pain, hematuria, increased alkaline phosphatase, HTN.

DRUG INTERACTIONS
See Boxed Warning. Reduced clearance with MTX. Concomitant administration with other biologic DMARDs (eg, anakinra, abatacept) or other TNF blockers is not recommended due to possible increased risk for infections and other potential pharmacological interactions. Avoid with live vaccines. Upon initiation or discontinuation of adalimumab in patients being treated with CYP450 substrates with a narrow therapeutic index, monitor therapeutic effect (eg, warfarin) or drug concentration (eg, cyclosporine, theophylline) and adjust individual dose of the drug product prn.

NURSING CONSIDERATIONS

Assessment: Assess for sepsis, active/chronic/recurrent infection, history of an opportunistic infection, recent travel in areas of endemic TB or endemic mycoses, underlying conditions that may predispose to infection, central or peripheral nervous system demyelinating disorders, CHF, latex sensitivity, drug hypersensitivity, pregnancy/nursing status, and for possible drug interactions. Test for latent TB infection and for HBV infection. Assess immunization history in pediatric patients. Perform a skin examination, particularly in patients with a medical history of prior prolonged immunosuppressant therapy or psoriasis patients with a history of psoralen plus ultraviolet light (PUVA) treatment for the presence of NMSC.

Monitoring: Monitor for development of infection during and after treatment. Monitor for malignancies, hypersensitivity reactions, neurological reactions, hematological reactions, worsening/new-onset CHF, lupus-like syndrome, and other adverse reactions. Monitor for active TB and periodically test for latent TB. Monitor for HBV reactivation during therapy and for several months following termination of therapy. Perform periodic skin examinations, particularly in patients with a medical history of prior prolonged immunosuppressant therapy or psoriasis patients with a history of PUVA treatment for the presence of NMSC.

Patient Counseling: Inform about the potential benefits/risks of therapy. Inform that therapy may lower the ability of immune system to fight infections; instruct to contact physician if any symptoms of infection, including TB, invasive fungal infections, or reactivation of HBV infections develop. Counsel about the risk of malignancies. Advise to seek immediate medical attention if any symptoms of a severe allergic reaction develops. Advise latex-sensitive patients that the needle cap of prefilled syringe contains latex. Advise to report to physician any signs of new/worsening medical conditions (eg, CHF, neurological disease, autoimmune disorders) or any symptoms suggestive of a cytopenia (eg, bleeding, bruising, persistent fever). Instruct on proper inj technique, as well as proper syringe and needle disposal.

Storage: 2-8°C (36-46°F). Do not freeze; do not use if frozen even if it has been thawed. Store in a cool carrier with an ice pack when traveling. Protect prefilled syringe from exposure to light. Store in original carton until time of administration.

HUMULIN 70/30 – NPH, human insulin isophane (rDNA origin)/ regular, human insulin (rDNA origin) OTC

Class: Insulin

ADULT DOSAGE

Diabetes Mellitus

Individualize dose

May need to adjust dosage based on metabolic needs, blood glucose monitoring results, and glycemic control goal
Administer SQ approx 30-45 min ac

PEDIATRIC DOSAGE

Pediatric use may not have been established

DOSE MODIFICATION

Renal Impairment

May require more frequent dose adjustment and blood glucose monitoring

Hepatic Impairment

May require more frequent dose adjustment and blood glucose monitoring

Other Important Modifications

May require dose adjustments w/ changes in physical activity/meal patterns, or during acute illness

ADMINISTRATION

SQ route

Should appear uniformly cloudy after mixing; do not use if particulate matter is seen
Do not mix w/ any other insulins/diluents
Administer in the abdominal wall, thigh, upper arm, or buttocks; rotate the inj site w/in the same region from 1 inj to the next
Do not administer IV/IM and do not use in an insulin infusion pump
Is a premixed insulin; independent adjustment of the basal or prandial dose is not possible
Refer to PI for further dosage information

HOW SUPPLIED

Inj: (Insulin Isophane/Regular) (70 U/30 U)/mL [3mL, vial, pen, KwikPen; 10mL, vial]

CONTRAINDICATIONS

During episodes of hypoglycemia.

WARNINGS/PRECAUTIONS

Pens and KwikPens must never be shared between patients, even if the needle is changed; may carry a risk for transmission of blood-borne pathogens. Changes in strength, manufacturer, type, or method of administration may affect glycemic control and predispose to hypo/hyperglycemia; these changes should be made cautiously and under close medical supervision and the frequency of blood glucose monitoring should be increased. Hypoglycemia may occur; increase frequency of blood glucose monitoring in patients at higher risk for hypoglycemia and patients who have reduced symptomatic awareness of hypoglycemia. Hypoglycemia may impair concentration ability and reaction time. Severe, life-threatening, generalized allergy, including anaphylaxis, may occur; if hypersensitivity reactions occur, d/c therapy, treat per standard of care, and monitor until symptoms and signs resolve. May cause hypokalemia.

ADVERSE REACTIONS

Hypoglycemia, allergic reactions, peripheral edema, lipodystrophy, weight gain, immunogenicity.

DRUG INTERACTIONS

May require dose adjustment and increased frequency of glucose monitoring w/ drugs that may increase the risk of hypoglycemia (eg, antidiabetic agents, salicylates, sulfonamide antibiotics), drugs that may decrease the glucose-lowering effect (eg, corticosteroids, isoniazid, niacin), or drugs that may increase or decrease glucose-lowering effect (eg, β-blockers, clonidine, lithium salts, alcohol). Pentamidine may cause hypoglycemia, sometimes followed by hyperglycemia. Signs and symptoms of hypoglycemia may be blunted w/ β-blockers, clonidine, guanethidine, and reserpine. Monitor K^+ levels w/ K^+-lowering medications or medications sensitive to serum K^+ concentrations. Observe for signs/symptoms of heart failure (HF) if treated concomitantly w/ a peroxisome proliferator-activated receptor (PPAR)-gamma agonist (eg, thiazolidinedione); consider discontinuation or dose reduction of the PPAR-gamma agonist if HF develops.

NURSING CONSIDERATIONS

Assessment: Assess for risk of hypoglycemia or hypokalemia, hypersensitivity, renal/hepatic impairment, pregnancy/nursing status, and possible drug interactions. Obtain baseline FPG and HbA1c.

Monitoring: Monitor for signs and symptoms of hypoglycemia, hypokalemia, hypersensitivity reactions, and other adverse reactions. Monitor FPG, HbA1c, and renal/hepatic function.

Patient Counseling: Advise never to share a pen or KwikPen w/ another person, even if the needle is changed. Instruct on self-management procedures, including glucose monitoring, proper inj technique, and management of hypo/hyperglycemia, and on handling of special situations, such as intercurrent conditions, inadequate or skipped insulin dose, inadvertent administration of an increased insulin dose, inadequate food intake, and skipped meals. Inform that hypoglycemia may impair ability to concentrate and react; advise to use caution when driving or operating machinery. Instruct to always check the label before each inj to avoid medication errors/accidental mix-ups. Inform on the symptoms of hypersensitivity reactions. Advise to inform physician if pregnant/contemplating pregnancy. Advise to use only if product contains no particulate matter and appears uniformly cloudy after mixing.

Storage: Protect from heat and light. Do not freeze; do not use if it has been frozen. (Vial) Unopened: 2-8°C (36-46°F) until expiration date, or room temperature <30°C (86°F) for 31 days. Opened: 2-8°C (36-46°F) or room temperature <30°C (86°F) for 31 days. (Pen/KwikPen) Unopened: 2-8°C (36-46°F) until expiration date, or room temperature <30°C (86°F) for 10 days. Opened: Room temperature <30°C (86°F) for 10 days. Do not refrigerate.

HUMULIN N – NPH, human insulin isophane (rDNA origin) OTC

Class: Insulin

ADULT DOSAGE

Diabetes Mellitus

Individualize dose

May need to adjust dosage based on metabolic needs, blood glucose monitoring results, and glycemic control goal

PEDIATRIC DOSAGE

Diabetes Mellitus

Individualize dose

May need to adjust dosage based on metabolic needs, blood glucose monitoring results, and glycemic control goal

DOSE MODIFICATION

Renal Impairment

May require frequent glucose monitoring and insulin dose adjustments

Hepatic Impairment

May require frequent glucose monitoring and insulin dose adjustments

Other Important Modifications

May require dose adjustments w/ changes in physical activity/meal patterns, or during acute illness

ADMINISTRATION

SQ route

Should appear uniformly cloudy after mixing; do not use if particulate matter is seen
Administer in the abdominal wall, thigh, upper arm, or buttocks; rotate the inj site w/in the same region from 1 inj to the next
Do not administer IV/IM and do not use in an insulin infusion pump

Mixing w/ Other Insulins

If Humulin N is mixed w/ Humulin R or Humalog, draw Humulin R or Humalog into syringe 1st; inject immediately after mixing

HOW SUPPLIED

Inj: 100 U/mL [3mL, vial, pen, KwikPen; 10mL, vial]

CONTRAINDICATIONS

During episodes of hypoglycemia.

WARNINGS/PRECAUTIONS

Pens and KwikPens must never be shared between patients, even if needle is changed; may carry a risk for transmission of blood-borne pathogens. Changes in strength, manufacturer, type, or method of administration may affect glycemic control and predispose to hypo/hyperglycemia; these changes should be made cautiously and under close medical supervision and the frequency of blood glucose monitoring should be increased. Hypoglycemia may occur; increase frequency of blood glucose monitoring in patients at higher risk for hypoglycemia and in patients who have reduced symptomatic awareness of hypoglycemia. Hypoglycemia may impair concentration ability and reaction time. Severe, life-threatening, generalized allergy, including anaphylaxis, may occur; if hypersensitivity reactions occur, d/c therapy, treat per standard of care, and monitor until symptoms and signs resolve. May cause hypokalemia.

ADVERSE REACTIONS

Hypoglycemia, allergic reactions, peripheral edema, lipodystrophy, weight gain, immunogenicity.

DRUG INTERACTIONS

May require dose adjustment and increased frequency of glucose monitoring w/ drugs that may increase the risk of hypoglycemia (eg, antidiabetic agents, salicylates, sulfonamide antibiotics), drugs that may decrease the glucose-lowering effect (eg, corticosteroids, isoniazid, niacin), or drugs that may increase or decrease glucose-lowering effect (eg, β-blockers, clonidine, lithium salts, alcohol). Pentamidine may cause hypoglycemia, sometimes followed by hyperglycemia. Signs and symptoms of hypoglycemia may be blunted w/ β-blockers, clonidine, guanethidine, and reserpine. Monitor K^+ levels w/ K^+-lowering medications or medications sensitive to serum K^+ concentrations. Observe for signs/symptoms of heart failure (HF) if treated concomitantly w/ a peroxisome proliferator-activated receptor (PPAR)-gamma agonist (eg, thiazolidinedione); consider discontinuation or dose reduction of the PPAR-gamma agonist if HF develops.

NURSING CONSIDERATIONS

Assessment: Assess for risk of hypoglycemia or hypokalemia, hypersensitivity, renal/hepatic impairment, pregnancy/nursing status, and possible drug interactions. Obtain baseline FPG and HbA1c.

Monitoring: Monitor for signs and symptoms of hypoglycemia, hypokalemia, hypersensitivity reactions, and other adverse reactions. Monitor FPG, HbA1c, and renal/hepatic function.

Patient Counseling: Advise never to share a pen or KwikPen w/ another person even if needle is changed. Instruct on self-management procedures, including glucose monitoring, proper inj technique, management of hypo/hyperglycemia, and on handling of special situations such as intercurrent conditions, inadequate or skipped insulin dose, inadvertent administration of an increased insulin dose, inadequate food intake, and skipped meals. Inform that hypoglycemia may impair ability to concentrate and react; advise to use caution when driving or operating machinery. Instruct to always check the label before each inj to avoid medication errors/accidental mix-ups. Educate on the symptoms of hypersensitivity reactions. Advise to inform physician if pregnant/contemplating pregnancy. Advise to use only if product contains no particulate matter and appears uniformly cloudy after mixing.

Storage: Protect from heat and light. Do not freeze; do not use if it has been frozen. (Vial) Unopened: 2-8°C (36-46°F) until expiration date, or room temperature <30°C (86°F) for 31 days. Opened: 2-8°C (36-46°F) or room temperature <30°C (86°F) for 31 days. (Pen/KwikPen) Unopened: 2-8°C (36-46°F) until expiration date, or room temperature <30°C (86°F) for 14 days. Opened: Room temperature <30°C (86°F) for 14 days. Do not refrigerate.

HUMULIN R – regular, human insulin (rDNA origin) OTC

Class: Insulin

ADULT DOSAGE

Diabetes Mellitus

Initial: 0.2-0.4 U/kg/day

Maint:

Total Daily Insulin Requirement: 0.5-1 U/kg/day; requirement may be substantially higher in insulin-resistant patients

PEDIATRIC DOSAGE

Diabetes Mellitus

Initial: 0.2-0.4 U/kg/day

Maint:

Total Daily Insulin Requirement: 0.5-1 U/kg/day; requirement may be substantially higher in insulin-resistant patients

Prepubertal Children: Average total daily insulin requirement varies from 0.7-1 U/kg/day, but may be much lower during the period of partial remission

DOSE MODIFICATION

Renal Impairment

May require frequent glucose monitoring and insulin dose reduction

Hepatic Impairment

May require frequent glucose monitoring and insulin dose reduction

ADMINISTRATION

SQ/IV route

May be used in combination w/ oral antihyperglycemics or longer-acting insulin products

SQ

Usually given ≥3X daily ac

Inj should be followed by a meal w/in approx 30 min

Inject in the abdominal wall, thigh, gluteal region, or upper arm; rotate inj sites w/in the same region

IV

Use at concentrations from 0.1-1 U/mL in infusion systems w/ the infusion fluids 0.9% NaCl using polyvinyl chloride infusion bags

Mixing of Insulins

Humulin R is often used in combination w/ intermediate- or long-acting insulins; when mixed w/ an intermediate-acting insulin (eg, NPH insulin isophane sus), draw Humulin R into the syringe first

A U-100 insulin syringe should always be used

HOW SUPPLIED

Inj: 100 U/mL [3mL, 10mL]

CONTRAINDICATIONS

Episodes of hypoglycemia.

WARNINGS/PRECAUTIONS

Needles or syringes must never be reused or shared between patients; may carry a risk for transmission of blood-borne pathogens. Any change in insulin should be made cautiously and only under medical supervision. Changes in strength, manufacturer, type, species, or method of administration may result in the need for a change in dosage. May require dosage adjustments w/ change in physical activity or usual meal plan. Stress, illness, or emotional disturbances may alter insulin requirements. Hypoglycemia may occur and may impair ability to concentrate and react; caution in patients w/ hypoglycemia unawareness and those predisposed to hypoglycemia (eg, pediatric population, those who fast or have erratic food intake). Hyperglycemia, diabetic ketoacidosis, or hyperosmolar coma may develop if taken less than needed. Hypokalemia may occur. Severe, life-threatening, generalized allergy, including anaphylaxis, may occur. Contains metacresol as excipient; localized reactions and generalized myalgias reported. May be administered IV under medical supervision; close monitoring of blood glucose and K^+ is required.

ADVERSE REACTIONS

Hypoglycemia, lipodystrophy, weight gain, peripheral edema.

DRUG INTERACTIONS

May require dose adjustment and close monitoring w/ drugs that may increase blood-glucose-lowering effect and susceptibility to hypoglycemia (eg, oral antihyperglycemics, salicylates, sulfa antibiotics), drugs that may reduce blood-glucose-lowering effect (eg, corticosteroids, isoniazid, certain lipid-lowering drugs [eg, niacin]), or drugs that may increase or decrease blood-glucose-lowering effect (eg, β-blockers, clonidine, lithium salts, alcohol). Pentamidine may cause hypoglycemia, which may sometimes be followed by hyperglycemia. β-blockers, clonidine, guanethidine, and reserpine may mask the signs of hypoglycemia. Caution w/ K^+-lowering medications or medications sensitive to serum K^+ concentrations. Observe for signs/symptoms of heart failure (HF) if treated concomitantly w/ a peroxisome proliferator-activated receptor (PPAR)-gamma agonist (eg, thiazolidinedione); consider discontinuation or dose reduction of the PPAR-gamma agonist if HF develops.

NURSING CONSIDERATIONS

Assessment: Assess for risk of hypoglycemia or hypokalemia, hypersensitivity, renal/hepatic impairment, pregnancy/nursing status, and possible drug interactions. Obtain baseline FPG and HbA1c.

Monitoring: Monitor for signs and symptoms of hypoglycemia, hypokalemia, allergic reactions, and other adverse reactions. Monitor FPG, HbA1c, and renal/hepatic function.

Patient Counseling: Instruct not to share syringes w/ other people, even if the needle has been changed. Instruct to always carry a quick source of sugar (eg, hard candy or glucose tabs). Counsel about proper dose preparation, administration technique, signs/symptoms of hypoglycemia, importance of frequent monitoring of blood glucose levels, and need for a balanced diet and regular exercise. Advise to always keep an extra supply of insulin as well as a spare syringe and needle on hand, and to always wear diabetic identification. Instruct to exercise caution when driving or operating machinery. Instruct to notify physician if pregnant/nursing, planning to become pregnant, or taking any other medications.

Storage: Do not use if it has been frozen. Unopened: 2-8°C (36-46°F). Do not freeze. Opened: <30°C (86°F). Protect from heat and light. Use w/in 31 days. Admixture: 2-8°C (36-46°F) for 48 hrs, then may use at room temperature for up to an additional 48 hrs.

HYDRALAZINE – hydralazine hydrochloride

RX

Class: Vasodilator

ADULT DOSAGE

Hypertension

Tab:

Initial: 10mg qid for the first 2-4 days

Titrate: Increase to 25mg qid for the balance of the 1st week, then increase to 50mg qid for the 2nd and subsequent weeks

Maint: Adjust to lowest effective levels

Resistant Patients: Up to 300mg/day

Individually titrate to the lowest effective dose when combined w/ thiazide and/or reserpine, or β-blocker

Severe Hypertension

Inj:

Usual: 20-40mg, repeated prn

PEDIATRIC DOSAGE

Hypertension

Tab:

Initial: 0.75mg/kg/day given qid

Titrate: May increase gradually over 3-4 weeks

Max: 7.5mg/kg/day or 200mg/day

Severe Hypertension

Inj:

Usual: 1.7-3.5mg/kg divided in 4-6 doses

DOSE MODIFICATION

Renal Impairment

Inj:

May require a lower dose, especially those w/ marked renal damage

ADMINISTRATION

Oral/IV/IM route

Inj

Use only when drug cannot be given PO

Do not add to infusion sol

HOW SUPPLIED

Inj: 20mg/mL [1mL]; Tab: 10mg, 25mg, 50mg, 100mg

CONTRAINDICATIONS

Coronary artery disease (CAD), mitral valvular rheumatic heart disease.

WARNINGS/PRECAUTIONS

D/C if systemic lupus erythematosus (SLE) symptoms (eg, glomerulonephritis) occur. May cause anginal attacks, ECG changes of myocardial ischemia, MI. Caution with suspected CAD, cerebrovascular accidents (CVA), and advanced renal damage. Postural hypotension reported. Peripheral neuritis reported; add pyridoxine if symptoms develop. Perform CBCs and antinuclear antibody (ANA) titer determinations before and periodically during prolonged therapy or if arthralgia, fever, chest pain, continued malaise, or unexplained signs/symptoms occur. Blood dyscrasias reported; d/c if such abnormalities develop.

ADVERSE REACTIONS

Headache, anorexia, N/V, diarrhea, palpitations, tachycardia, angina pectoris.

DRUG INTERACTIONS

Caution with MAOIs. Profound hypotension may occur with other potent parenteral antihypertensives (eg, diazoxide). May reduce pressor responses to epinephrine.

NURSING CONSIDERATIONS

Assessment: Assess for CAD, mitral valvular rheumatic heart disease, drug hypersensitivity, CVA, renal impairment, pregnancy/nursing status, and possible drug interactions. Obtain baseline CBCs and ANA titers.

Monitoring: Monitor for SLE symptoms, anginal attacks, ECG changes, MI, peripheral neuritis, hypotension, blood dyscrasias, and other adverse reactions. Monitor CBCs and ANA titers periodically during prolonged therapy. (Inj) Monitor BP frequently.

Patient Counseling: Inform of potential side effects and advise to take medication regularly and continuously ud.

Storage: 20-25°C (68-77°F).

HYDROCHLOROTHIAZIDE TABLETS – hydrochlorothiazide RX

Class: Thiazide diuretic

ADULT DOSAGE

Edema

For edema due to renal dysfunction (eg, nephrotic syndrome, acute glomerulonephritis, chronic renal failure), edema in pregnancy due to pathologic causes and adjunctive therapy for edema associated w/ congestive heart failure, hepatic cirrhosis, and corticosteroid and estrogen therapy
Usual: 25-100mg/day as a single or divided dose. May give qod or 3-5 days/week

Hypertension

Initial: 25mg qd
Titrate: May increase to 50mg/day as a single or 2 divided doses

PEDIATRIC DOSAGE

Diuresis

Usual: 1-2mg/kg/day in single or 2 divided doses
Max:
<6 Months: 3mg/kg/day in 2 divided doses
Infants up to 2 Years: 37.5mg/day
2-12 Years: 100mg/day

Hypertension

Usual: 1-2mg/kg/day in single or 2 divided doses
Max:
<6 Months: 3mg/kg/day in 2 divided doses
Infants up to 2 Years: 37.5mg/day
2-12 Years: 100mg/day

ADMINISTRATION
Oral route

HOW SUPPLIED
Tab: 12.5mg, 25mg*, 50mg* *scored

CONTRAINDICATIONS
Anuria, hypersensitivity to sulfonamide-derived drugs.

WARNINGS/PRECAUTIONS
Caution with severe renal disease; may precipitate azotemia. Caution with hepatic impairment or progressive liver disease; may precipitate hepatic coma. Sensitivity reactions may occur in patients with or without a history of allergy or bronchial asthma. Possibility of exacerbation/activation of systemic lupus erythematosus (SLE) reported. May cause idiosyncratic reaction, resulting in acute transient myopia and acute angle-closure glaucoma; d/c as rapidly as possible. Observe for evidence of fluid/electrolyte imbalance (eg, hyponatremia, hypochloremic alkalosis, hypokalemia). Hypokalemia may sensitize or exaggerate the response of the heart to toxic effects of digitalis. Hyperuricemia or precipitation of acute gout, hyperglycemia, manifestations of latent diabetes mellitus (DM), hypomagnesemia, hypercalcemia, and increases in cholesterol and TG levels may occur. Enhanced antihypertensive effects in postsympathectomy patients. Consider withholding or discontinuing therapy if progressive renal impairment becomes evident. D/C before testing for parathyroid function.

ADVERSE REACTIONS
Weakness, hypotension, pancreatitis, jaundice, diarrhea, aplastic anemia, agranulocytosis, anaphylactic reactions, muscle spasm, vertigo, paresthesia, renal failure, erythema multiforme, transient blurred vision, impotence.

DRUG INTERACTIONS
Potentiation of orthostatic hypotension may occur with alcohol, barbiturates, or narcotics. Dosage adjustment of antidiabetic drugs (oral agents and insulin) may be required. Additive effect or potentiation with other antihypertensives. Anionic exchange resins (eg, cholestyramine, colestipol) may impair absorption. Corticosteroids and adrenocorticotropic hormone may intensify electrolyte depletion, particularly hypokalemia. May decrease response to pressor amines (eg, norepinephrine). May increase responsiveness to nondepolarizing skeletal muscle relaxants (eg, tubocurarine). May increase risk of lithium toxicity; avoid concomitant use. NSAIDs may reduce diuretic, natriuretic, and antihypertensive effects.

NURSING CONSIDERATIONS

Assessment: Assess for anuria, hypersensitivity to drug or sulfonamide-derived drugs, renal/hepatic impairment, history of allergy or bronchial asthma, SLE, DM, postsympathectomy status, pregnancy/nursing status, and possible drug interactions.

Monitoring: Monitor for signs/symptoms of fluid/electrolyte imbalance, sensitivity reactions, exacerbation/activation of SLE, idiosyncratic reaction, hyperuricemia or precipitation of acute gout, hyperglycemia, latent DM, increases in cholesterol and TG levels, and other adverse reactions. Monitor serum electrolytes.

Patient Counseling: Inform of the risks and benefits of therapy. Advise to report to physician any adverse reactions.

Storage: 20-25°C (68-77°F).

HYDROXYZINE HCL – hydroxyzine hydrochloride

RX

Class: Piperazine antihistamine

ADULT DOSAGE

Pruritus

Management of pruritus due to allergic conditions (eg, chronic urticaria, atopic/contact dermatoses) and histamine-mediated pruritus

PO:

25mg tid or qid

Sedation

As premedication and following general anesthesia

PO:

50-100mg

Nausea/Vomiting

IM:

25-100mg; not for use in N/V of pregnancy

Surgery

As pre- and postoperative adjunctive medication to permit reduction in narcotic dosage, allay anxiety, and control emesis

IM:

25-100mg

Anxiety

PO:

Symptomatic relief of anxiety and tension associated w/ psychoneurosis and as an adjunct in organic disease states

50-100mg qid

IM:

Management of anxiety, tension, and psychomotor agitation in conditions of emotional stress. Useful in alleviating manifestations of anxiety/tension as in the preparation for dental procedures and in acute emotional problems. Management of anxiety associated w/ organic disturbances and as adjunctive therapy in alcoholism and allergic conditions w/ strong emotional overlay (eg, asthma, chronic urticaria, pruritus). Treatment of acutely disturbed or hysterical patient and acute/chronic alcoholic w/ anxiety withdrawal symptoms or delirium tremens

50-100mg immediately, and q4-6h prn

Pregnancy

As pre- and postpartum adjunctive medication to permit reduction in narcotic dosage, allay anxiety, and control emesis

IM:

25-100mg

PEDIATRIC DOSAGE

Pruritus

Management of pruritus due to allergic conditions (eg, chronic urticaria, atopic/contact dermatoses) and histamine-mediated pruritus

PO:

<6 Years:

50mg/day in divided doses

>6 Years:

50-100mg/day in divided doses

Sedation

As premedication and following general anesthesia

PO:

0.6mg/kg

Nausea/Vomiting

Excluding N/V of pregnancy

IM:

0.5mg/lb

Surgery

As pre- and postoperative adjunctive medication to permit reduction in narcotic dosage, allay anxiety, and control emesis

IM:

0.5mg/lb

Anxiety

Symptomatic relief of anxiety and tension associated w/ psychoneurosis and as an adjunct in organic disease states

PO:

<6 Years:

50mg/day in divided doses

>6 Years:

50-100mg/day in divided doses

DOSE MODIFICATION

Elderly

Start at lower end of dosing range

ADMINISTRATION

Oral/IM route

Adjust dose according to response

When treatment is initiated by IM route, subsequent doses may be administered orally

Inj

May be administered w/o further dilution

Inject well w/in the body of a relatively large muscle; preferred site in adults is the upper outer quadrant of the buttock or midlateral thigh and in children is the midlateral thigh

HOW SUPPLIED

Inj: 25mg/mL [1mL], 50mg/mL [1mL, 2mL, 10mL]; Syrup: 10mg/5mL [118mL, 473mL]; Tab: 10mg, 25mg, 50mg

CONTRAINDICATIONS

Early pregnancy. (Inj) SQ, intra-arterial, or IV administration. (PO) Known hypersensitivity to cetirizine or levocetirizine.

WARNINGS/PRECAUTIONS

Patients may be started on IM therapy when indicated and should be maintained on oral therapy whenever this route is practicable. Drowsiness may occur. May impair mental/physical abilities. Caution in elderly. (Inj) Should not be used as sole treatment of psychosis or of clearly demonstrated cases of depression. Inadvertent SQ inj may result in significant tissue damage. IM inj may result in severe inj-site reactions requiring surgical intervention. Inj into the deltoid area should be used only if well developed (eg, certain adults and older children), and then only with caution to avoid radial nerve injury. In infants and small children, inj into the periphery of the upper outer quadrant of the gluteal region should be used only when necessary, in order to minimize the possibility of damage to the sciatic nerve.

ADVERSE REACTIONS

Dry mouth, drowsiness, involuntary motor activity. (Tab, Syrup) Fixed drug eruptions.

DRUG INTERACTIONS

May potentiate CNS depressants (eg, narcotics, non-narcotic analgesics and barbiturates, alcohol); reduce dose of CNS depressants when administered concomitantly. Modify use of meperidine and barbiturates, on an individual basis, when used in preanesthetic adjunctive therapy. (Inj) Cardiac arrests and death reported when combined with other CNS depressants. Administration of meperidine may result in severe hypotension in the postoperative patient or any individual whose ability to maintain BP has been compromised by a depleted blood volume. Use meperidine with great caution and in reduced dosage in patients who are receiving other pre- and/or postoperative medications and in whom there is a risk of respiratory depression, hypotension, and profound sedation or coma occurring.

NURSING CONSIDERATIONS

Assessment: Assess for hypersensitivity to drug, (PO) cetirizine, or levocetirizine; pregnancy/nursing status; and for possible drug interactions.

Monitoring: Monitor for hypersensitivity reactions, drowsiness, and other adverse reactions. Periodically reassess the usefulness of therapy.

Patient Counseling: Inform about risks/benefits of therapy. Inform that drowsiness may occur; instruct to use caution when driving or operating heavy machinery. Instruct to notify physician if pregnant, nursing, or taking any other concomitant therapy.

Storage: 20-25°C (68-77°F). (Syrup) Protect from freezing. (Inj) Excursions permitted to 15-30°C (59-86°F). (Inj/Syrup) Protect from light.

HYZAAR – hydrochlorothiazide/losartan potassium RX

Class: Angiotensin II receptor antagonist/thiazide diuretic

D/C when pregnancy is detected. Drugs that act directly on the renin-angiotensin system (RAS) can cause injury/death to the developing fetus.

ADULT DOSAGE

Hypertension

Usual: 50mg-12.5mg qd
Max: 100mg-25mg qd

Replacement Therapy:
Combination may be substituted for titrated components

Severe Hypertension

Initial: 50mg-12.5mg qd
Titrate: If inadequate response after 2-4 weeks, increase to 100mg-25mg qd
Max: 100mg-25mg qd

PEDIATRIC DOSAGE

Pediatric use may not have been established

Hypertension with Left Ventricular Hypertrophy

Reduction in Risk of Stroke:
Initial: Losartan 50mg qd
Titrate: If inadequate BP reduction, add 12.5mg HCTZ or substitute w/ losartan-HCTZ 50mg-12.5mg
If additional BP reduction needed, substitute w/ losartan 100mg and HCTZ 12.5mg or losartan-HCTZ 100mg-12.5mg, followed by losartan 100mg and HCTZ 25mg or losartan-HCTZ 100mg-25mg
This may not apply to black patients

ADMINISTRATION

Oral route
Take w/ or w/o food

HOW SUPPLIED

Tab: (Losartan/HCTZ) 50mg/12.5mg, 100mg/12.5mg, 100mg/25mg

CONTRAINDICATIONS

Anuria, sulfonamide-derived drug hypersensitivity. Coadministration with aliskiren in patients with diabetes.

WARNINGS/PRECAUTIONS

Not indicated for initial therapy of HTN. Symptomatic hypotension may occur in intravascularly volume-depleted patients (eg, treated with diuretics); correct volume depletion before therapy. Not recommended with hepatic impairment requiring losartan titration. Not recommended with severe renal impairment (CrCl ≤30mL/min). Angioedema reported (rare). HCTZ: Caution with impaired hepatic function or progressive liver disease; may precipitate hepatic coma. Hypersensitivity reactions may occur. May cause exacerbation or activation of systemic lupus erythematosus (SLE). May cause idiosyncratic reaction, resulting in acute transient myopia and acute angle-closure glaucoma; d/c as rapidly as possible. Observe for clinical signs of fluid or electrolyte imbalance (hyponatremia, hypochloremic alkalosis, and hypokalemia). Hypokalemia may develop, especially with brisk diuresis, severe cirrhosis, or after prolonged therapy. Hypokalemia may cause cardiac arrhythmia and may sensitize/exaggerate the response of the heart to the toxic effects of digitalis. Hyperuricemia may occur or frank gout may be precipitated. May cause hyperglycemia, hypomagnesemia, hypercalcemia, and manifestations of latent diabetes mellitus (DM). D/C prior to parathyroid function tests. Enhanced effects in postsympathectomy patients. Consider withholding or discontinuing therapy if progressive renal impairment becomes evident. Increased cholesterol and TG levels reported. May precipitate azotemia in patients with renal disease. Losartan: Oliguria and/or progressive azotemia and acute renal failure and/or death (rare) may occur in patients whose renal function is dependent on the activity of the RAS (eg, severe congestive heart failure [CHF]). May increase SrCr and BUN levels in patients with renal artery stenosis.

ADVERSE REACTIONS

Hypokalemia, dizziness, URI.

DRUG INTERACTIONS

See Contraindications. NSAIDs, including selective COX-2 inhibitors, may decrease effects of diuretics and angiotensin II receptor antagonists and may deteriorate renal function. May reduce lithium clearance and increase risk of lithium toxicity; avoid concurrent use. Monitor serum lithium levels during concomitant use. HCTZ: Potentiation of orthostatic hypotension may occur with alcohol, barbiturates, or narcotics. Dose adjustment of antidiabetic drugs (oral agents, insulin) may be required. May cause additive effect or potentiation with other antihypertensives. Anionic exchange resins (eg, cholestyramine, colestipol) may impair absorption. Corticosteroids, adrenocorticotropic hormone, or glycyrrhizin (found in liquorice) may intensify electrolyte depletion, particularly hypokalemia. May decrease response to pressor amines (eg, norepinephrine). May increase response to nondepolarizing skeletal muscle relaxants (eg, tubocurarine). Losartan: Dual blockade of the RAS is associated with increased risks of hypotension, syncope, hyperkalemia, and changes in renal function (including acute renal failure); closely monitor BP, renal function, and electrolytes with concomitant agents that affect the RAS. Avoid with aliskiren in patients with renal impairment (GFR <60mL/min). Rifampin may reduce levels. Fluconazole may decrease levels of the active metabolite and increase levels of losartan. May increase serum K^+ with K^+-sparing diuretics (eg, spironolactone, triamterene, amiloride), K^+ supplements, or salt substitutes containing K^+.

NURSING CONSIDERATIONS

Assessment: Assess for hypersensitivity to the drug and its components, anuria, sulfonamide-derived drug hypersensitivity, history of penicillin allergy, volume/salt depletion, SLE, DM, CHF, hepatic/renal function, postsympathectomy status, cirrhosis, renal artery stenosis, pregnancy/nursing status, and possible drug interactions. Obtain baseline BP.

Monitoring: Monitor for signs/symptoms of fluid/electrolyte imbalance, exacerbation/activation of SLE, idiosyncratic reaction, latent DM, precipitation of gout, hypersensitivity reactions, and other adverse reactions. Monitor BP, serum electrolytes, renal/hepatic function, cholesterol, and TG levels periodically.

Patient Counseling: Inform females of childbearing potential of the consequences of exposure during pregnancy and of the treatment options for women planning to become pregnant. Instruct to report pregnancy to the physician as soon as possible. Counsel that lightheadedness may occur, especially during the 1st days of therapy; instruct to report to physician. Instruct to d/c therapy and consult physician if syncope occurs. Caution that inadequate fluid intake, excessive perspiration, diarrhea, or vomiting may lead to an excessive fall in BP, with the same consequences of lightheadedness and possible syncope. Instruct not to use K^+ supplements or salt substitutes containing K^+ without consulting physician.

Storage: 25°C (77°F); excursions permitted to 15-30°C (59-86°F). Protect from light.

ILEVRO – nepafenac RX

Class: NSAID

ADULT DOSAGE

Postoperative Inflammation/Ocular Pain

1 drop to the affected eye qd, beginning 1 day prior to cataract surgery, continued on the day of surgery, and through the first 2 weeks of postoperative period

Administer additional drop 30-120 min prior to surgery

PEDIATRIC DOSAGE

Postoperative Inflammation/Ocular Pain

≥10 Years:

1 drop to the affected eye qd, beginning 1 day prior to cataract surgery, continued on the day of surgery, and through the first 2 weeks of postoperative period

Administer additional drop 30-120 min prior to surgery

DOSE MODIFICATION

Concomitant Medications

Space dosing ≥5 min apart w/ other topical ophthalmic medications

ADMINISTRATION

Ocular route

Shake well before use

HOW SUPPLIED

Sus: 0.3% [1.7mL]

WARNINGS/PRECAUTIONS

Potential for increased bleeding time due to interference with thrombocyte aggregation. Increased bleeding of ocular tissues (eg, hyphemas) reported in conjunction with ocular surgery; caution with known bleeding tendencies. May slow or delay healing, or result in keratitis. Continued use may result in sight threatening epithelial breakdown, corneal thinning/erosion/ulceration/perforation; d/c if evidence of corneal epithelial breakdown occurs and monitor for corneal health. Caution with complicated ocular surgeries, corneal denervation, corneal epithelial defects, diabetes mellitus (DM), ocular surface diseases (eg, dry eye syndrome), rheumatoid arthritis (RA), or repeat ocular surgeries within a short period of time. Use >1 day prior to surgery or beyond 14 days post-surgery may increase risk and severity of corneal adverse events. Avoid use with contact lenses and during late pregnancy.

ADVERSE REACTIONS

Capsular opacity, decreased visual acuity, foreign body sensation, IOP, sticky sensation, conjunctival edema, corneal edema, dry eye, lid margin crusting, ocular discomfort, ocular hyperemia/pain/pruritus, photophobia, tearing, vitreous detachment.

DRUG INTERACTIONS

May increase potential for healing problems with topical steroids. Caution with agents that may prolong bleeding time.

NURSING CONSIDERATIONS

Assessment: Assess for previous hypersensitivity to the drug, bleeding tendencies, complicated or repeated ocular surgeries, corneal denervation, corneal epithelial defects, DM, ocular surface diseases, RA, contact lens use, pregnancy/nursing status, and possible drug interactions.

Monitoring: Monitor for hypersensitivity reactions, wound healing problems, keratitis, increased bleeding time, bleeding of ocular tissues in conjunction with ocular surgery, epithelial breakdown, corneal thinning/erosion/ulceration/perforation, and other adverse reactions.

Patient Counseling: Inform of possibility that slow or delayed healing may occur. Instruct to avoid allowing the tip of the container to contact the eye or surrounding structures. Advise that use of the same bottle for both eyes is not recommended. Instruct not to use while wearing contact lens. Advise to notify physician if an intercurrent ocular condition (eg, trauma or infection) develops or if undergoing ocular surgery to assess continuation of therapy.

Storage: 2-25°C (36-77°F). Protect from light.

IMDUR – isosorbide mononitrate RX

Class: Nitrate vasodilator

ADULT DOSAGE

Angina Pectoris

Prevention:

Initial: 30mg or 60mg qam

Titrate: Increase to 120mg qam after several days; rarely, 240mg qam may be required

PEDIATRIC DOSAGE

Pediatric use may not have been established

DOSE MODIFICATION

Elderly

Start at lower end of dosing range

ADMINISTRATION

Oral route

Take qam on arising

Swallow tab whole w/ a half-glassful of fluid; do not crush or chew

Do not break 30mg tab

HOW SUPPLIED

Tab, Extended-Release: 30mg*, 60mg*, 120mg *scored

WARNINGS/PRECAUTIONS

Not useful in aborting acute anginal episode. Not recommended for use in patients w/ acute MI or congestive heart failure; perform careful clinical or hemodynamic monitoring if used in these conditions. Severe hypotension, particularly w/ upright posture, may occur; caution in volume depleted, hypotensive, or elderly patients. Nitrate-induced hypotension may be accompanied by paradoxical bradycardia and increased angina pectoris. May aggravate angina caused by hypertrophic cardiomyopathy. May develop tolerance. Chest pain, acute MI, and sudden death reported during temporary withdrawal.

ADVERSE REACTIONS

Headache, dizziness, dry mouth, asthenia, cardiac failure, abdominal pain, earache, arrhythmia, hyperuricemia, arthralgia, purpura, anxiety, hypochromic anemia, atrophic vaginitis, bacterial infection.

DRUG INTERACTIONS

Sildenafil amplifies vasodilatory effects that can result in severe hypotension. Additive vasodilating effects w/ other vasodilators (eg, alcohol). Marked symptomatic orthostatic hypotension reported w/ calcium channel blockers; dose adjustments of either class of agents may be necessary.

NURSING CONSIDERATIONS

Assessment: Assess for drug hypersensitivity, hypotension, volume depletion, angina caused by hypertrophic cardiomyopathy, pregnancy/nursing status, possible drug interactions, and any other conditions where treatment is cautioned or contraindicated.

Monitoring: Monitor for hypotension w/ paradoxical bradycardia and increased angina pectoris, tachycardia, aggravation of angina caused by hypertrophic cardiomyopathy, tolerance, manifestations of true physical dependence (eg, chest pain, acute MI), and other adverse reactions.

Patient Counseling: Inform about the risks and benefits of therapy. Counsel to carefully follow the prescribed schedule of dosing. Advise that daily headaches may accompany treatment and instruct to avoid altering schedule of treatment as the headaches are a marker of the activity of the medication and loss of headache may be associated w/ loss of antianginal efficacy. Inform that treatment may be associated w/ lightheadedness on standing, especially just after rising from a recumbent/seated position and may be more frequent w/ alcohol consumption.

Storage: 20-25°C (68-77°F).

IMITREX – sumatriptan

RX

Class: 5-$HT_{1B/1D}$ agonist

ADULT DOSAGE

Cluster Headache

Inj:
Max Single Dose: 6mg SQ
Max Dose/24 hrs: Two 6mg inj separated by at least 1 hr; consider a 2nd dose only if some response to 1st inj was observed

Migraine

W/ or w/o Aura:
May use lower doses (1-5mg) if side effects are dose limiting

Inj:
Max Single Dose: 6mg SQ
Max Dose/24 hrs: Two 6mg inj separated by at least 1 hr; consider a 2nd dose only if some response to 1st inj was observed

Spray:
Usual: 5mg, 10mg, or 20mg
May administer 1 additional dose at least 2 hrs after 1st dose if migraine has not resolved or returns after transient improvement
5mg and 20mg doses are given as a single spray in 1 nostril; 10mg dose may be achieved by administering a single 5mg dose in each nostril
Max: 40mg/24 hrs

Tab:
Usual: 25mg, 50mg, or 100mg
May administer a 2nd dose at least 2 hrs after 1st dose if migraine has not resolved or returns after transient improvement
Max: 200mg/24 hrs

PEDIATRIC DOSAGE

Pediatric use may not have been established

DOSE MODIFICATION

Hepatic Impairment
Mild to Moderate:
Max Tab Single Dose: 50mg

Elderly
Start at lower end of dosing range

ADMINISTRATION

Oral/SQ/Nasal route

Inj
Use the 6mg single dose vial for patients receiving doses other than 4mg or 6mg; do not use autoinjector
Avoid IM or intravascular delivery

HOW SUPPLIED

Inj: 4mg/0.5mL, 6mg/0.5mL [syringe], 6mg/0.5mL [vial]; Spray: 5mg, 20mg [6^{s}]; Tab: 25mg, 50mg, 100mg

CONTRAINDICATIONS

Ischemic coronary artery disease (CAD) (eg, angina pectoris, history of MI, documented silent ischemia), coronary artery vasospasm (eg, Prinzmetal's angina), Wolff-Parkinson-White syndrome or arrhythmias associated with other cardiac accessory conduction pathway disorders, history of stroke or transient ischemic attack, history of hemiplegic/basilar migraine, peripheral vascular disease, ischemic bowel disease, uncontrolled HTN, and severe hepatic impairment. Recent use (within 24 hrs) of another 5-HT_1 agonist, or of an ergotamine-containing or ergot-type medication (eg, dihydroergotamine, methysergide). Concurrent administration or recent use (within 2 weeks) of an MAO-A inhibitor.

WARNINGS/PRECAUTIONS

Safety of treating >4 headaches/30 days not known. Use only where a clear diagnosis of migraine headache or (Inj) cluster headache has been established. Reconsider diagnosis of migraine or cluster headache before treating any subsequent attacks if patient does not respond to the 1st dose of therapy. Serious cardiac adverse reactions (eg, acute MI) reported. May cause coronary artery vasospasm and sensations of tightness, pain, pressure, and heaviness in the precordium, throat, neck, and jaw, usually noncardiac in origin. Perform cardiovascular (CV) evaluation in triptan-naive patients with multiple CV risk factors (eg, increased age, diabetes, HTN, smoking, obesity, strong family history of CAD) prior to therapy; if negative, consider administering 1st dose under medical supervision and perform an ECG immediately following administration. Consider periodic CV evaluation in intermittent long-term users with risk factors for CAD. Evaluate patients with signs/symptoms suggestive of angina following inj for the presence of CAD or Prinzmetal's angina before giving additional doses. Life-threatening cardiac rhythm disturbances (eg, ventricular tachycardia, ventricular fibrillation leading to death) reported; d/c if these occur. Cerebral/subarachnoid hemorrhage and stroke reported; d/c therapy if a cerebrovascular event occurs. Exclude other potentially serious neurological conditions prior to therapy in patients not previously diagnosed as migraineurs, and in migraineurs who present with atypical symptoms. May cause noncoronary vasospastic reactions (eg, peripheral vascular ischemia, GI vascular ischemia/infarction, splenic infarction, Raynaud's syndrome). May cause transient/permanent blindness and significant partial vision loss. Overuse of acute migraine drugs may lead to exacerbation of headache; detoxification, including drug withdrawal, and treatment of withdrawal symptoms may be necessary. Serotonin syndrome may occur; d/c if suspected. Significant elevation in BP, including hypertensive crisis with acute impairment of organ systems, reported. Anaphylactic/anaphylactoid reactions may occur. Seizures reported; caution with history of epilepsy or conditions associated with a lowered seizure threshold. Caution in elderly. (Spray) Local irritative symptoms reported.

ADVERSE REACTIONS

Atypical sensations, paresthesia, N/V, chest discomfort, neck pain/stiffness, throat discomfort, pressure sensation, dizziness, vertigo. (Inj) Feeling of tightness, flushing, inj-site reaction. (Spray) Bad/unusual taste.

DRUG INTERACTIONS

See Contraindications. Serotonin syndrome reported with SSRIs, SNRIs, TCAs, or MAOIs.

NURSING CONSIDERATIONS

Assessment: Confirm diagnosis of migraine or (Inj) cluster headache and exclude other potentially serious neurologic conditions and noncoronary vasospastic reactions prior to therapy. Assess for CV disease, HTN, hemiplegic/basilar migraine, hypersensitivity to drug, and any other conditions where treatment is cautioned or contraindicated. Assess hepatic function, pregnancy/nursing status, and for possible drug interactions.

Monitoring: Monitor for signs/symptoms of cardiac events, cerebrovascular events, peripheral vascular ischemia, GI vascular ischemia/infarction, serotonin syndrome, hypersensitivity reactions, HTN, and other adverse reactions. Perform periodic CV evaluation in intermittent long-term users with risk factors for CAD.

Patient Counseling: Inform that therapy may cause CV side effects and anaphylactic/anaphylactoid reactions. Instruct to seek medical attention if signs/symptoms of chest pain, SOB, irregular heartbeat, significant rise in BP, weakness, or slurring of speech occur. Inform that use of acute migraine drugs for ≥10 days/month may lead to an exacerbation of headache; encourage to record headache frequency and drug use (eg, by keeping a headache diary). Inform about the risk of serotonin syndrome. Inform that drug may cause somnolence and dizziness; instruct to evaluate ability to perform complex tasks during migraine attacks and after administration of drug. Inform that medication should not be used during pregnancy unless the potential benefit justifies the potential risk to the fetus; instruct to notify physician if breastfeeding or planning to breastfeed. (Inj) Instruct on proper use of inj, to avoid IM or intravascular delivery, and to use inj sites with adequate skin and SQ thickness to accommodate length of needle. (Spray) Inform that local irritation of the nose and throat may be experienced and that symptoms will generally resolve in <2 hrs. Instruct on proper use of spray and caution to avoid spraying in eyes.

Storage: 2-30°C (36-86°F). (Spray/Inj) Protect from light.

IMPAVIDO – miltefosine

RX

Class: Antileishmanial agent

May cause fetal harm; do not administer to pregnant women. Obtain a serum or urine pregnancy test in females of reproductive potential prior to prescribing therapy; advise to use effective contraception during therapy and for 5 months after therapy.

ADULT DOSAGE

Leishmaniasis

Treatment of visceral, cutaneous, and mucosal leishmaniasis caused by susceptible *Leishmania* species

30-44kg:
50mg bid w/ food (breakfast and dinner)

≥45kg:
50mg tid w/ food (breakfast, lunch, and dinner)

Treat for 28 consecutive days

PEDIATRIC DOSAGE

Leishmaniasis

Treatment of visceral, cutaneous, and mucosal leishmaniasis caused by susceptible *Leishmania* species

≥12 Yrs:

30-44kg:
50mg bid w/ food (breakfast and dinner)

≥45kg:
50mg tid w/ food (breakfast, lunch, and dinner)

Treat for 28 consecutive days

ADMINISTRATION

Oral route

Take w/ food to ameliorate GI adverse reactions
Swallow caps whole; do not chew or break

HOW SUPPLIED

Cap: 50mg

CONTRAINDICATIONS

Pregnancy, Sjogren-Larsson syndrome.

WARNINGS/PRECAUTIONS

Leishmania species studied in clinical trials were based on epidemiologic data. There may be geographic variation in clinical response of the same *Leishmania* species to therapy. May cause reproductive effects (eg, impaired fertility). Scrotal pain and decreased/absent ejaculation during therapy reported. Elevations of SrCr reported. Elevations in liver transaminases (ALT, AST) and bilirubin reported in the treatment of visceral leishmaniasis. Vomiting and/or diarrhea commonly occur during administration and may result in volume depletion; encourage fluid intake. Vomiting and/or diarrhea occurring during therapy may affect absorption of oral contraceptives, and therefore compromise their efficacy; additional nonhormonal or alternative method(s) of effective contraception should be used if vomiting and/or diarrhea occur. Thrombocytopenia reported in patients treated for visceral leishmaniasis. Stevens-Johnson syndrome (SJS) reported; d/c if an exfoliative or bullous rash is noted. Avoid breastfeeding for 5 months after therapy.

ADVERSE REACTIONS

N/V, decreased appetite, diarrhea, asthenia, motion sickness, headache, dizziness, abdominal pain, lymphangitis, pruritus, malaise, pyrexia, somnolence.

NURSING CONSIDERATIONS

Assessment: Assess for drug hypersensitivity, Sjogren-Larsson syndrome, pregnancy/nursing status, and possible drug interactions. Obtain a serum or urine pregnancy test in females of reproductive potential.

Monitoring: Monitor for reproductive effects, vomiting/diarrhea, volume depletion, SJS, and other adverse reactions. Monitor renal function weekly during therapy and for 4 weeks after end of therapy. Monitor liver transaminases and bilirubin. Monitor platelet count during therapy for visceral leishmaniasis.

Patient Counseling: Instruct to complete the full course of therapy. Inform that abdominal pain, N/V, and diarrhea are common side effects of therapy and instruct to inform physician if these GI side effects are severe or persistent. Instruct to consume sufficient fluids to avoid dehydration and, consequently, the risk of kidney injury. Advise women of reproductive potential to use effective contraception during therapy and for 5 months after therapy ends. Advise women who use oral contraceptives to use additional nonhormonal or alternative method(s) of effective contraception during therapy if vomiting and/or diarrhea occurs. Advise nursing mothers not to breastfeed during therapy and for 5 months after therapy is completed. Inform that drug may cause reproductive effects (eg, impaired fertility).

Storage: 20-25 °C (68-77 °F); excursions permitted to 15-30 °C (59-86 °F). Protect from light.

IMURAN – azathioprine RX

Class: Purine antagonist antimetabolite

Increased risk of malignancy with chronic immunosuppression. Malignancy (eg, post-transplant lymphoma, hepatosplenic T-cell lymphoma) reported in patients with inflammatory bowel disease. Physician should be familiar with this risk as well as mutagenic potential and possible hematologic toxicities.

OTHER BRAND NAMES

Azasan

ADULT DOSAGE

Renal Transplant

Adjunct Therapy for Prevention of Rejection in Renal Homotransplantation:
Initial: 3-5mg/kg/day, beginning at the time of transplant
Usually given as a single daily dose on the day of, and in a minority of cases 1-3 days before, transplantation
Maint: 1-3mg/kg/day

Rheumatoid Arthritis

Reduces Signs/Symptoms:
Initial: 1mg/kg/day (50-100mg) given qd or bid
Titrate: May increase dose by 0.5mg/kg/day increments beginning at 6-8 weeks and thereafter by steps at 4-week intervals
Max: 2.5mg/kg/day

May be considered refractory if no improvement after 12 weeks

Maint Therapy:
Use lowest effective dose; decrease by 0.5mg/kg/day or 25mg/day every 4 weeks to lowest effective dose while other therapy is kept constant

PEDIATRIC DOSAGE

Pediatric use may not have been established

DOSE MODIFICATION

Renal Impairment

Relatively oliguric patients, especially those with tubular necrosis in the immediate postcadaveric transplant period, may have delayed clearance, and are usually given lower doses

ADMINISTRATION

Oral route

HOW SUPPLIED

Tab: 50mg*, (Azasan) 75mg*, 100mg* *scored

CONTRAINDICATIONS

(RA) Pregnancy, patients previously treated with alkylating agents (eg, cyclophosphamide, chlorambucil, melphalan).

WARNINGS/PRECAUTIONS

Renal transplant patients are known to have an increased risk of malignancy. Risk of post-transplant lymphomas may be increased with aggressive immunosuppressive treatment; maintain therapy at the lowest effective levels. Acute myelogenous leukemia as well as solid tumors reported in patients with RA. Severe leukopenia, thrombocytopenia, anemias (eg, macrocytic anemia, pancytopenia), and severe bone marrow suppression may occur. Myelotoxicity risk may be increased in patients with intermediate thiopurine S-methyl transferase (TPMT) activity. Increased risk of severe, life-threatening myelotoxicity in patients with low or absent TPMT activity; consider alternative therapies. Caution in patients having one non-functional allele who are at risk for reduced TPMT activity; dose reduction is recommended in patients with reduced TPMT activity. Reduce dose or d/c temporarily if rapid fall in or persistently low leukocyte count, or other evidence of bone marrow depression occurs. Delayed hematologic suppression may occur. TPMT testing cannot be a substitute for CBC monitoring. Consider early drug discontinuation in patients with abnormal CBC results that do not respond to dose reduction. May cause fetal harm. GI hypersensitivity reaction characterized by severe N/V reported. Increased risk for bacterial, viral, fungal, protozoal, and opportunistic infections, including reactivation of latent infections that may lead to serious, including fatal, outcomes. JC virus-associated infection resulting in progressive multifocal leukoencephalopathy (PML) reported; consider reducing the amount of immunosuppression in patients who develop PML.

ADVERSE REACTIONS

Malignancy, hematologic toxicities, infections, N/V.

DRUG INTERACTIONS

See Contraindications. Combined use with disease-modifying antirheumatic drugs cannot be recommended. Caution with concomitant aminosalicylate derivatives (eg, sulfasalazine, mesalazine, olsalazine); may inhibit TPMT enzyme. Allopurinol inhibits one of the inactivation pathways; reduce azathioprine dose to approximately 1/3-1/4 of the usual dose and consider further dose reduction or alternative therapies for patients with low or absent TPMT activity. Drugs that may affect leukocyte production (eg, co-trimoxazole) may lead to exaggerated leukopenia, especially in renal transplant recipients. ACE inhibitors may induce anemia and severe leukopenia. May inhibit anticoagulant effect of warfarin. Use of ribavirin for hepatitis C has been reported to induce severe pancytopenia and may increase the risk of azathioprine-related myelotoxicity.

NURSING CONSIDERATIONS

Assessment: Assess for drug hypersensitivity, renal/hepatic dysfunction, previous treatment of RA with alkylating agents, pregnancy/nursing status, and for possible drug interactions. Conduct TPMT genotyping/phenotyping to identify absent or reduced TPMT activity.

Monitoring: Monitor for signs/symptoms of cytopenias, malignancies, infections, GI hypersensitivity reactions, and other adverse reactions. Monitor CBCs, including platelet counts, weekly during the 1st month, twice monthly for the 2nd and 3rd months of therapy, then monthly or more frequently if dose/therapy changes are necessary. Periodically monitor serum transaminases, alkaline phosphatase, and bilirubin levels. Consider TPMT testing in patients with abnormal CBC results unresponsive to dose reduction.

Patient Counseling: Inform about necessity of periodic blood counts while on therapy and risks of malignancy and infection. Instruct to report to physician any unusual bleeding/bruising or signs/symptoms of infections. Educate about proper dosage instructions, especially with impaired renal function or concomitant use with allopurinol. Inform of the potential risks during pregnancy and nursing; advise to notify physician if pregnant or nursing. Instruct patients with increased risk for skin cancer to limit exposure to sunlight and UV light (eg, wearing protective clothing, using a sunscreen).

Storage: 20-25°C (68-77°F). Protect from light.

INCIVEK – telaprevir RX

Class: HCV NS3/4A protease inhibitor

Fatal and nonfatal serious skin reactions, including Stevens-Johnson syndrome (SJS), drug reaction with eosinophilia and systemic symptoms (DRESS), and toxic epidermal necrolysis (TEN) reported. D/C combination therapy immediately if serious skin rash reactions, including rash with systemic symptoms or a progressive severe rash develop. Consider discontinuing other medications known to be associated with serious skin reactions. Promptly refer patients for urgent medical care.

ADULT DOSAGE

Chronic Hepatitis C (Genotype 1)

In Combination w/ Peginterferon Alfa and Ribavirin in Patients w/ Compensated Liver Disease, Including Cirrhosis:
1125mg bid (10-14 hrs apart)

Treatment Duration:

Treatment-Naive and Prior Relapse Patients
HCV RNA Not Detected at Weeks 4 and 12:
Triple therapy (telaprevir/peginterferon alfa/ribavirin) x 12 weeks; then dual therapy (peginterferon alfa/ribavirin) x 12 weeks
HCV RNA Detected at Weeks 4 and/or 12 (1000 IU/mL or less):
Triple therapy x 12 weeks; then dual therapy x 36 weeks

Prior Partial and Null Responder Patients
All Patients:
Triple therapy x 12 weeks; then dual therapy x 36 weeks

PEDIATRIC DOSAGE

Pediatric use may not have been established

DOSE MODIFICATION

Hepatic Impairment

Moderate to Severe (Child-Pugh Score B or C; score ≥7):
Not recommended for use

Discontinuation

HCV RNA >1000 IU/mL at Weeks 4 or 12:
D/C triple therapy (treatment complete at 12 weeks)

HCV RNA Detectable at Week 24:
D/C dual therapy

ADMINISTRATION

Oral route

Take w/ food (not low fat)
D/C telaprevir if peginterferon alfa or ribavirin is discontinued for any reason
Swallow whole; do not chew, crush, break, cut, or dissolve

HOW SUPPLIED

Tab: 375mg

CONTRAINDICATIONS

Women who are or may become pregnant and men whose female partners are pregnant. Concomitant use with drugs that are highly dependent on CYP3A for clearance and for which elevated plasma concentrations are associated with serious and/or life-threatening reactions and with strong CYP3A inducers (eg, alfuzosin, carbamazepine, phenobarbital, phenytoin, rifampin, dihydroergotamine, ergonovine, ergotamine, methylergonovine, cisapride, St. John's wort, lovastatin, simvastatin, pimozide, sildenafil, or tadalafil when used for treatment of pulmonary arterial HTN, oral midazolam, triazolam). Refer to the individual monographs for peginterferon alfa and ribavirin.

WARNINGS/PRECAUTIONS

Monitor patients with mild to moderate rashes for progression of rash or development of systemic symptoms; d/c if rash becomes severe; peginterferon alfa and ribavirin may be continued; if improvement is not observed within 7 days of discontinuing telaprevir, consider sequential or simultaneous interruption or discontinuation of ribavirin and/or peginterferon alfa. Female patients of childbearing potential and their male partners as well as male patients and their female partners must use 2 forms of effective nonhormonal contraception during treatment and for 6 months after all treatment has ended; female patients should have monthly pregnancy tests during this time. Anemia reported with peginterferon alfa and ribavirin therapy; addition of telaprevir to peginterferon alfa and ribavirin associated with an additional decrease in Hgb concentrations; monitor Hgb prior to and at least at Weeks 2, 4, 8, and 12 during combination treatment and as clinically appropriate. Reduce ribavirin dose for the management of anemia. Do not reduce dose or restart telaprevir after discontinuing from either rash or anemia. Hematology evaluations (including Hgb, white cell differential, and platelet count) are recommended prior to and at Weeks 2, 4, 8, and 12 and as clinically appropriate. Chemistry evaluations (including electrolytes, SrCr, uric acid, hepatic enzymes, bilirubin, and TSH) are recommended as frequently as hematology evaluations or as clinically appropriate. Caution in elderly. Must not be administered as monotherapy and must only be prescribed with both peginterferon alfa and ribavirin. Not recommended with moderate/severe hepatic impairment (Child-Pugh B or C, score ≥7) or with decompensated liver disease.

ADVERSE REACTIONS

Serious skin reactions, pruritus, anemia, N/V, hemorrhoids, diarrhea, anorectal discomfort, dysgeusia, fatigue, anal pruritus.

DRUG INTERACTIONS

See Contraindications. Dose adjustments of concomitant drugs made during treatment should be readjusted after completion of therapy. Avoid with colchicine in patients with renal/hepatic impairment; risk of toxicity. Not recommended with voriconazole; high doses of itraconazole or ketoconazole; rifabutin; systemic corticosteroids; salmeterol; darunavir, fosamprenavir, or lopinavir (all with ritonavir); and inhaled/nasal fluticasone or budesonide. Avoid use with atorvastatin. May increase levels of alfentanil, fentanyl, antiarrhythmics, statins, digoxin, clarithromycin, erythromycin, telithromycin, trazodone, azole antifungals, rifabutin, alprazolam, IV midazolam, amlodipine and other calcium channel blockers, corticosteroids, bosentan, atazanavir, tenofovir, colchicine, cyclosporine, sirolimus, tacrolimus, salmeterol, repaglinide, PDE-5 inhibitors, CYP3A substrates, inhaled/nasal fluticasone or budesonide, and drugs that are substrates for P-glycoprotein (P-gp), OATP1B1, and OATP2B1 transport. May decrease levels of escitalopram, zolpidem, efavirenz, ethinyl estradiol, darunavir, fosamprenavir, and methadone. Use lowest digoxin dose initially with careful titration and monitoring of serum digoxin concentrations. May alter concentrations of warfarin; monitor INR. Clarithromycin, erythromycin, telithromycin, azoles, and CYP3A/P-gp inhibitors may increase levels. Rifabutin, systemic dexamethasone, HIV protease inhibitors, efavirenz, and CYP3A/P-gp inducers may decrease levels. Refer to PI for dosing modifications when used with certain concomitant therapies.

NURSING CONSIDERATIONS

Assessment: Assess for hepatic impairment or decompensated liver disease, pregnancy/nursing status, men whose female partners are of childbearing potential, and for possible drug interactions. Perform baseline hematology evaluations (including Hgb, white cell differential, and platelet count) and chemistry evaluations (including electrolytes, SrCr, uric acid, hepatic enzymes, bilirubin, and TSH).

Monitoring: Monitor for SJS, DRESS, TEN, and other adverse reactions. Monitor HCV-RNA levels at Weeks 4, 12, and as clinically indicated. Perform hematology evaluations (including Hgb, white cell differential, and platelet count) at Weeks 2, 4, 8, and 12 and as clinically appropriate, and chemistry evaluations (including electrolytes, SrCr, uric acid, hepatic enzymes, bilirubin, and TSH) as frequently as hematology evaluations or as clinically appropriate. Perform a routine monthly pregnancy test in females during therapy and for 6 months after stopping treatment. Monitor INR when warfarin is coadministered.

Patient Counseling: Inform that drug must be used in combination with peginterferon alfa and ribavirin. Instruct female patients to notify physician immediately if pregnant and male patients if female partner is pregnant. Advise female patients of childbearing potential and their male partners as well as male patients and their female partners to use 2 nonhormonal methods of effective contraception during treatment and for 6 months after all treatment has ended. Inform that combination treatment may cause rash; advise to promptly report any skin changes or itching. Advise not to stop treatment due to rash unless instructed. Inform that the effect of treatment of hepatitis C on transmission is unknown and that appropriate precautions to prevent transmission should be taken. Inform about the importance of hydration and fluid intake. Instruct to recognize signs/symptoms of dehydration (eg, increased thirst, dry mouth, decreased urine output, and more concentrated urine); advise to notify physician if oral fluid intake is poor or if severe vomiting and/or diarrhea is experienced. If a dose is missed within 6 hrs of the time it is usually taken, instruct to take the prescribed dose with food as soon as possible and if >6 hrs has passed, instruct to not take the missed dose and to resume the usual dosing schedule. Counsel to ingest food containing around 20g of fat within 30 min prior to dose.

Storage: 25°C (77°F); excursions permitted to 15-30°C (59-86°F).

INDERAL LA – propranolol hydrochloride RX

Class: Nonselective beta-blocker

ADULT DOSAGE

Hypertension

Initial: 80mg qd
Titrate: May increase to 120mg qd or higher until adequate BP control is achieved
Maint: 120-160mg qd; 640mg/day may be required

Angina Pectoris

Initial: 80mg qd
Titrate: Increase gradually at 3- to 7-day intervals until optimal response is obtained
Maint: 160mg qd
Max: 320mg qd

Reduce dose gradually over a period of a few weeks if therapy is to be discontinued

Migraine

Initial: 80mg qd
Usual: 160-240mg qd

D/C gradually if a satisfactory response is not obtained w/in 4-6 weeks after reaching maximal dose

Hypertrophic Subaortic Stenosis

Usual: 80-160mg qd

PEDIATRIC DOSAGE

Pediatric use may not have been established

DOSE MODIFICATION

Elderly

Start at lower end of dosing range

ADMINISTRATION

Oral route

HOW SUPPLIED

Cap, Extended-Release: 60mg, 80mg, 120mg, 160mg

CONTRAINDICATIONS

Cardiogenic shock, sinus bradycardia and >1st-degree block, bronchial asthma.

WARNINGS/PRECAUTIONS

Exacerbation of angina and myocardial infarction (MI) following abrupt discontinuation reported; when discontinuation is planned, reduce dose gradually over at least a few weeks. Reinstitute therapy if exacerbation of angina occurs upon interruption and take other measures for management of angina pectoris; follow same procedure in patients at risk of occult atherosclerotic heart disease who are given propranolol for other indication since coronary artery disease may be unrecognized. Hypersensitivity reactions (eg, anaphylactic/anaphylactoid reactions) and cutaneous reactions (eg, Stevens-Johnson syndrome, toxic epidermal necrolysis, exfoliative dermatitis, erythema multiforme, and urticaria) reported. May precipitate more severe failure in patients with CHF; avoid with overt CHF and caution in patients with history of heart failure (HF) who are well-compensated and are receiving diuretics prn. Continued use in patients without history of HF may cause cardiac failure. Caution with bronchospastic lung disease, Wolff-Parkinson-White (WPW) syndrome, tachycardia, and hepatic/renal impairment. Chronically administered therapy should not be routinely withdrawn prior to major surgery; however, may augment risks of general anesthesia and surgical procedures. May prevent appearance of signs/symptoms of acute hypoglycemia. Caution with labile insulin-dependent diabetics; may be more difficult to adjust insulin dose. May mask certain clinical signs of hyperthyroidism; abrupt withdrawal may be followed by an exacerbation of symptoms of hyperthyroidism, including thyroid storm. May reduce IOP. Patients with history of severe anaphylactic reaction to a variety of allergens may be more reactive to repeated accidental/diagnostic/therapeutic challenge; may be unresponsive to usual doses of epinephrine. Lab test interactions may occur (eg, changes to thyroid function tests), including in patients with HTN/severe HF. Not for treatment of hypertensive emergencies. Caution in elderly.

ADVERSE REACTIONS

Bradycardia, CHF, hypotension, lightheadedness, mental depression, N/V, agranulocytosis, systemic lupus erythematosus, urticaria, alopecia.

DRUG INTERACTIONS

Administration with drugs that have an effect on CY2D6, 1A2, or C19 metabolic pathways may lead to clinically relevant drug interactions and changes on its efficacy and/or toxicity; use with caution. Alcohol may increase levels. Propafenone and amiodarone may cause additive effects. Quinidine may increase levels and may cause postural hypotension. Reduced clearance of lidocaine and lidocaine toxicity reported following coadministration. Caution with drugs that slow atrioventricular (AV) nodal conduction (eg, digitalis, lidocaine, calcium channel blocker); increased risk of bradycardia with digitalis. Bradycardia, HF, and cardiovascular collapse reported with verapamil. Bradycardia, hypotension, high-degree heart block, and HF reported with diltiazem. ACE inhibitors may cause hypotension, particularly in the setting of acute MI. May antagonize effects of clonidine; administer cautiously to patients withdrawing from clonidine. May prolong 1st dose hypotension with prazosin. Postural hypotension reported with terazosin or doxazosin. May cause excessive reduction of resting sympathetic nervous activity with catecholamine-depleting drugs (eg, reserpine). May experience uncontrolled HTN with epinephrine. Effects can be reversed by β-receptor agonists (eg, dobutamine or isoproterenol). May reduce sensitivity to dobutamine stress echocardiography in patients undergoing evaluation for MI. May reduce efficacy with indomethacin and NSAIDs. May exacerbate hypotensive effects of MAOIs or TCAs. May depress myocardial contractility with methoxyflurane and trichloroethylene. May increase levels of warfarin; monitor PT. Hypotension and cardiac arrest reported with haloperidol. May lower T3 concentration with thyroxine.

NURSING CONSIDERATIONS

Assessment: Assess for cardiogenic shock, sinus bradycardia, AV heart block, bronchial asthma, CHF, bronchospastic lung disease, hyperthyroidism, diabetes, WPW syndrome, tachycardia, hepatic/renal impairment, history of HF, risk for occult atherosclerotic heart disease, hypersensitivity to drug, pregnancy/nursing status, and possible drug interactions.

Monitoring: Monitor for signs/symptoms of cardiac failure, hypoglycemia, decreased IOP, hyperthyroidism, withdrawal symptoms, hypersensitivity reactions, and other adverse reactions. Monitor PT with warfarin.

Patient Counseling: Inform of the risks/benefits of therapy. Instruct not to interrupt or d/c therapy without consulting physician. Inform that therapy may interfere with glaucoma screening test.

Storage: 20-25°C (68-77°F); excursions permitted to 15-30°C (59-86°F). Protect from light, moisture, freezing, and excessive heat.

INDOMETHACIN – indomethacin

RX

Class: NSAID

NSAIDs may cause an increased risk of serious cardiovascular (CV) thrombotic events, MI, stroke, and serious GI adverse events, including bleeding, ulceration, and perforation of the stomach or intestines. Contraindicated for the treatment of perioperative pain in the setting of CABG surgery.

OTHER BRAND NAMES

Indocin

ADULT DOSAGE

Ankylosing Spondylitis

Moderate to Severe Active Stages:
Initial: 25mg (5mL) bid-tid
Titrate: May increase by 25mg (5mL) or 50mg (10mL) at weekly intervals
Max: 150-200mg (30-40mL)/day

May give a large portion (up to a max of 100mg [20mL]) of the total daily dose hs in patients who have persistent night pain and/or morning stiffness

Rheumatoid Arthritis

Moderate to Severe Active Stages (Including Acute Flares of Chronic Disease):
Initial: 25mg (5mL) bid-tid
Titrate: May increase by 25mg (5mL) or 50mg (10mL) at weekly intervals
Max: 150-200mg (30-40mL)/day

May give a large portion (up to a max of 100mg [20mL]) of the total daily dose hs in patients who have persistent night pain and/or morning stiffness

Osteoarthritis

Moderate to Severe Active Stages:
Initial: 25mg (5mL) bid-tid
Titrate: May increase by 25mg (5mL) or 50mg (10mL) at weekly intervals
Max: 150-200mg (30-40mL)/day

May give a large portion (up to a max of 100mg [20mL]) of the total daily dose hs in patients who have persistent night pain and/or morning stiffness

Bursitis/Tendinitis

Acute Painful Shoulder:
Active Stages:
75-150mg (15-30mL)/day given in 3 or 4 divided doses; d/c after signs/symptoms of inflammation have been controlled for several days; usual course of therapy is 7-14 days

Acute Gouty Arthritis

Active Stages:
50mg (10mL) tid until pain is tolerable, then reduce dose to d/c

PEDIATRIC DOSAGE

Osteoarthritis

Moderate to Severe Active Stages:
≥2 Years:
Should not be prescribed for patients ≤14 yrs of age unless necessary
Initial: 1-2mg/kg/day given in divided doses
Max: 4mg/kg/day or 150-200mg/day, whichever is less
>14 Years:
Initial: 25mg (5mL) bid-tid
Titrate: May increase by 25mg (5mL) or 50mg (10mL) at weekly intervals
Max: 150-200mg (30-40mL)/day

May give a large portion (up to a max of 100mg [20mL]) of the total daily dose hs in patients who have persistent night pain and/or morning stiffness

Bursitis/Tendinitis

Acute Painful Shoulder:
Active Stages:
≥2 Years:
Should not be prescribed for patients ≤14 yrs of age unless necessary
Initial: 1-2mg/kg/day given in divided doses
Max: 4mg/kg/day or 150-200mg/day, whichever is less
>14 Years:
75-150mg (15-30mL)/day given in 3 or 4 divided doses; d/c after signs/symptoms of inflammation have been controlled for several days; usual course of therapy is 7-14 days

Acute Gouty Arthritis

Active Stages:
≥2 Years:
Should not be prescribed for patients ≤14 yrs of age unless necessary
Initial: 1-2mg/kg/day given in divided doses
Max: 4mg/kg/day or 150-200mg/day, whichever is less
>14 Years:
50mg (10mL) tid until pain is tolerable, then reduce dose to d/c

Rheumatoid Arthritis

Moderate to Severe Active Stages (Including Acute Flares of Chronic Disease):
≥2 Years:
Should not be prescribed for patients ≤14 yrs of age unless necessary
Initial: 1-2mg/kg/day given in divided doses
Max: 4mg/kg/day or 150-200mg/day, whichever is less

>14 Years:
Initial: 25mg (5mL) bid-tid

Titrate: May increase by 25mg (5mL) or 50mg (10mL) at weekly intervals
Max: 150-200mg (30-40mL)/day

May give a large portion (up to a max of 100mg [20mL]) of the total daily dose hs in patients who have persistent night pain and/or morning stiffness

Ankylosing Spondylitis

Moderate to Severe Active Stages:
≥2 Years:
Should not be prescribed for patients ≤14 yrs of age unless necessary
Initial: 1-2mg/kg/day given in divided doses
Max: 4mg/kg/day or 150-200mg/day, whichever is less
>14 Years:
Initial: 25mg (5mL) bid-tid
Titrate: May increase by 25mg (5mL) or 50mg (10mL) at weekly intervals
Max: 150-200mg (30-40mL)/day

May give a large portion (up to a max of 100mg [20mL]) of the total daily dose hs in patients who have persistent night pain and/or morning stiffness

ADMINISTRATION
Oral route

Take w/ food

HOW SUPPLIED
Cap: 25mg, 50mg; Sus: (Indocin) 25mg/5mL [237mL]

CONTRAINDICATIONS
Aspirin (ASA) or other NSAID allergy that precipitates acute asthmatic attack, urticaria, or rhinitis. Treatment of perioperative pain in the setting of CABG surgery.

WARNINGS/PRECAUTIONS
Use the lowest effective dose for the shortest duration consistent with individual treatment goals. Not a substitute for corticosteroids or to treat corticosteroid insufficiency. May lead to onset of new HTN or worsening of preexisting HTN; monitor BP closely. Fluid retention and edema reported; caution with fluid retention or HF. Renal papillary necrosis and other renal injury reported after long-term use. Not recommended for use with advanced renal disease; if therapy must be initiated, monitor renal function. Anaphylactoid reactions may occur; avoid in patient with ASA triad. May cause serious skin adverse events (eg, exfoliative dermatitis, Stevens-Johnson syndrome [SJS], and toxic epidermal necrolysis [TEN]); d/c at the first appearance of skin rash or any other signs of hypersensitivity. Avoid in late pregnancy; may cause premature closure of ductus arteriosus. May cause elevations of LFTs; d/c if liver disease develops or systemic manifestations occur. Anemia may occur; with long-term use, monitor Hgb/Hct if signs or symptoms of anemia develop. May inhibit platelet aggregation and prolong bleeding time; monitor with coagulation disorders. Caution with preexisting asthma and avoid with ASA-sensitive asthma. Corneal deposits and retinal disturbances reported with prolonged therapy; d/c if such changes are observed. Blurred vision may be significant; perform eye exams at periodic intervals during prolonged therapy. May aggravate depression or other psychiatric disturbances, epilepsy, and parkinsonism; use with caution. D/C if severe CNS adverse reactions develop. May impair mental/physical abilities. Caution in elderly.

ADVERSE REACTIONS
Headache, dizziness, upper GI ulcers, GI bleeding, GI perforation, N/V, dyspepsia, heartburn, epigastric pain, indigestion.

DRUG INTERACTIONS
May diminish antihypertensive effect of ACE inhibitors (eg, captopril) and angiotensin II antagonists (eg, losartan). Avoid with ASA, salicylates, diflunisal, triamterene, and other NSAIDs. May reduce the diuretic, natriuretic, and antihypertensive effects of loop, K^+-sparing, and thiazide diuretics. Increased levels of digoxin reported. Reduced basal plasma renin activity (PRA), as well as those elevations of PRA induced by furosemide reported. May decrease lithium clearance; monitor for toxicity. Caution with methotrexate; may enhance methotrexate toxicity. May increase levels with probenecid. Caution with cyclosporine and anticoagulants. Blunting of the antihypertensive effects of β-blockers reported. May increase risk of serious GI bleeding when used concomitantly with oral corticosteroids or anticoagulants, alcohol, or smoking.

NURSING CONSIDERATIONS

Assessment: Assess for history of asthma, urticaria or allergic-type reaction after previous use of NSAIDs, history of ulcer disease or GI bleeding, coagulation disorders or anticoagulant therapy, concomitant use of corticosteroids, smoking, alcohol use, age, health status, anemia, renal/hepatic impairment, pregnancy/nursing status, any other conditions where treatment is cautioned or contraindicated, and possible drug interactions.

Monitoring: Monitor BP during initiation of therapy and thereafter. Monitor platelet function, CBCs, LFTs, dexamethasone suppression tests, renal function, and chemistry profile. Monitor for signs/symptoms of anaphylactic/anaphylactoid reactions, adverse skin events (eg, exfoliative dermatitis, SJS, TEN), eosinophilia, rash, corneal deposits and retinal disturbances with periodic ophthalmic exam, CNS effects, aggravation of depression or other psychiatric disturbances, GI bleeding/ulceration and perforation, anemia, CV thrombotic events, MI, stroke, new or worsening HTN, renal toxicity, and hyperkalemia.

Patient Counseling: Inform about potential serious side effects (eg, CV side effects such as MI or stroke); instruct to seek medical attention if signs/symptoms of chest pain, SOB, weakness, slurred speech, skin rash, blisters or fever, GI effects, bleeding, ulceration and perforation, signs of anaphylactic/anaphylactoid reaction, or hepatic toxicity occurs. Advise to notify physician if weight gain/edema occurs. Inform of risks if used during pregnancy and to use caution while performing hazardous tasks (eg, operating machinery/driving).

Storage: (Cap) 20-25°C (68-77°F). Protect from light. Dispense in a tight, light-resistant container. (Sus) Below 30°C (86°F); avoid >50°C (122°F). Protect from freezing.

INFUMORPH – morphine sulfate CII

Class: Opioid analgesic

Not recommended for single-dose IV, IM or SQ administration. Risk of severe adverse effects; observe patients in a fully equipped and staffed environment for at least 24 hrs after the initial (single) test dose, and as appropriate, for the 1st several days after catheter implantation. Improper or erroneous substitution of Infumorph 200 or 500 (10 or 25mg/mL, respectively) for regular Duramorph (0.5 or 1mg/mL) is likely to result in serious overdosage, leading to seizures, respiratory depression, and possibly, fatal outcome. Naloxone inj and resuscitative equipment should be immediately available for use in case of life-threatening or intolerable side effects and whenever therapy is initiated or manipulation/refilling of the reservoir system takes place. Remove any contaminated clothing and rinse affected area with water if accidental dermal exposure occurs. Associated with risk of overdosage, diversion and abuse; special measures must be taken to control this product within the hospital/clinic. Do not use if the sol in the unopened ampul contains a precipitate that does not disappear upon shaking. After removal, do not use unless the sol is colorless or pale yellow.

ADULT DOSAGE

Chronic Intractable Pain

Individualize dose based on in-hospital evaluation of the response to a serial single-dose intrathecal or epidural bolus inj of regular Duramorph 0.5mg/mL or 1mg/mL, w/ close observation of the analgesic efficacy and adverse effects prior to surgery involving the continuous microinfusion device

Intrathecal:
Opioid Intolerant:
Initial: 0.2-1mg/day in the lumbar region
Opioid Tolerant:
Usual Range: 1-10mg/day
Individualize upper daily dose limit for each patient

Doses >20mg/day associated w/ higher risk of serious side effects; use w/ caution

Epidural:
Opioid Intolerant:
Initial: 3.5-7.5mg/day
Continuous Epidural Infusion:
Opioid Tolerant:
Initial: 4.5-10mg/day
Dose requirements may increase to 20-30mg/day; individualize upper daily limit for each patient

PEDIATRIC DOSAGE

Pediatric use may not have been established

ADMINISTRATION
Epidural/Intrathecal route

Withdraw desired amount of morphine from the ampul through a microfilter
Filter through a microfilter ≤5mcg before injecting into the microinfusion device
If dilution is required, 0.9%NaCl is recommended

HOW SUPPLIED
Inj: 10mg/mL, 25mg/mL [20mL]

CONTRAINDICATIONS
(For neuraxial analgesia use) Infection at inj microinfusion site, concomitant anticoagulant therapy, uncontrolled bleeding diathesis, any other concomitant therapy or medical condition that would render epidural or intrathecal administration of medication especially hazardous.

WARNINGS/PRECAUTIONS
May be habit-forming. Developed for use in continuous microinfusion devices; not for single-dose neuraxial inj. Chronic neuraxial opioid analgesia is appropriate only when less invasive means of controlling pain failed and should only be undertaken by those experienced in applying this treatment in a setting where its complications can be managed adequately. Inflammatory masses (eg, granulomas) reported; monitor for new neurologic signs/symptoms in patients receiving continuous infusion via indwelling intrathecal catheter and further assessment or intervention should be based on the clinical condition of the patient. Unusual acceleration of neuraxial morphine requirement may occur, causing concern regarding systemic absorption and the hazards of large doses; may benefit from hospitalization/detoxification. Myoclonic-like spasm of the lower extremities reported with intrathecal doses of >20mg/day; may need detoxification. May resume treatment at lower doses after detoxification. High neuraxial doses may produce myoclonic events. Limit intrathecal route to lumbar area. Caution with head injury or increased intracranial pressure; pupillary changes (miosis) may obscure the existence, extent, and course of intracranial pathology. Caution with decreased respiratory reserve (eg, emphysema, severe obesity, kyphoscoliosis, paralysis of the phrenic nerve), hepatic/renal dysfunction, and in elderly. Avoid with chronic asthma, upper airway obstruction, or any other chronic pulmonary disorder. Smooth muscle hypertonicity may result in biliary colic. Initiation of neuraxial opiate analgesia is associated with micturition disturbances, especially in males with prostatic enlargement. Orthostatic hypotension may occur with reduced circulating blood volume and myocardial dysfunction. Avoid abrupt withdrawal.

ADVERSE REACTIONS
Respiratory depression, myoclonus, inflammatory mass formation, dysphoric reactions, pruritus, urinary retention, constipation, lumbar puncture-type headache, peripheral edema.

DRUG INTERACTIONS
See Contraindications. CNS depressants (eg, alcohol, sedatives, antihistamines, psychotropics) may potentiate depressant effects. Neuroleptics may increase risk of respiratory depression. Withdrawal symptoms may occur upon administration of a narcotic antagonist. Monitor for orthostatic hypotension in patients on sympatholytic drugs.

NURSING CONSIDERATIONS

Assessment: Assess for patient's general condition and medical status, any other conditions where treatment is contraindicated or cautioned, renal/hepatic impairment, pregnancy/nursing status, and possible drug interactions.

Monitoring: Monitor for signs/symptoms of respiratory depression, myoclonic events, biliary colic, urinary retention, orthostatic hypotension, drug abuse/dependence, and other adverse reactions.

Patient Counseling: Inform about risks and benefits of therapy. Inform of adverse reactions that may occur. Instruct to inform physician of other medications taken.

Storage: 20-25°C (68-77°F); excursions permitted to 15-30°C (59-86°F). Protect from light. Do not freeze. Discard any unused portion. Do not heat-sterilize.

INLYTA – axitinib

RX

Class: Kinase inhibitors

ADULT DOSAGE
Advanced Renal Cell Carcinoma
Initial: 5mg bid (q12h)

PEDIATRIC DOSAGE
Pediatric use may not have been established

DOSE MODIFICATION

Hepatic Impairment

Moderate (Child-Pugh Class B): Reduce dose by half

Titrate: Increase or decrease dose based on individual safety and tolerability

Adverse Reactions

May require temporary interruption or permanent discontinuation, and/or dose reduction to 3mg bid

May further reduce to 2mg bid if needed

Concomitant Medications

Strong CYP3A4/5 Inhibitors:

Avoid coadministration, but if needed, decrease dose by half and increase or decrease subsequent doses based on individual safety and tolerability

Strong CYP3A4/5 Inhibitors Discontinuation:

Allow 3-5 half-lives of CYP3A4/5 inhibitor to elapse after discontinuation before returning to dose used prior to coadministration

Other Important Modifications

Normotensive/No Concomitant Antihypertensive/Tolerated for ≥2 Consecutive Weeks with No Adverse Reaction >Grade 2:

May increase to 7mg bid, and further to 10mg bid (using the same criteria)

ADMINISTRATION

Oral route

Take with or without food

Swallow whole with a glass of water

HOW SUPPLIED

Tab: 1mg, 5mg

WARNINGS/PRECAUTIONS

HTN/Hypertensive crisis reported; treat prn with standard antihypertensive therapy. Reduce dose if persistent HTN occurs despite antihypertensive therapy; d/c if HTN is severe and persistent or if hypertensive crisis develops. Arterial/venous thromboembolic events reported; caution with history of or risk for arterial/venous thromboembolic events. Hemorrhagic events reported; do not use in patients with evidence of untreated brain metastasis or recent active GI bleeding. Temporarily interrupt treatment if any bleeding requiring medical intervention occurs. Cardiac failure reported; management may require permanent discontinuation of therapy. GI perforation/fistulas, hypothyroidism, and hyperthyroidism reported. Treat thyroid dysfunction according to standard medical practice to maintain euthyroid state. D/C treatment at least 24 hrs prior to surgery; resume therapy after surgery based on clinical judgment of adequate wound healing. D/C if reversible posterior leukoencephalopathy (RPLS) occurs. Proteinuria reported; reduce dose or interrupt temporarily if moderate to severe proteinuria develops. Increased ALT reported. Caution with moderate hepatic impairment and with end-stage renal disease (CrCl <15mL/min). May cause fetal harm.

ADVERSE REACTIONS

Diarrhea, HTN, fatigue, decreased appetite, N/V, dysphonia, palmar-plantar erythrodysesthesia syndrome, weight decrease, asthenia, constipation, hypothyroidism, cough, mucosal inflammation, arthralgia, stomatitis.

DRUG INTERACTIONS

See Dosage. Avoid with grapefruit, grapefruit juice, and strong CYP3A4/5 inducers (eg, rifampin, dexamethasone, phenytoin, St. John's wort). Moderate CYP3A4/5 inducers (eg, bosentan, efavirenz, etravirine) may reduce exposure; avoid use if possible.

NURSING CONSIDERATIONS

Assessment: Assess for HTN, risk for/history of arterial/venous thromboembolic events, untreated brain metastasis, recent active GI bleeding, thyroid dysfunction, proteinuria, renal/hepatic impairment, pregnancy/nursing status, and possible drug interactions. Obtain baseline AST, ALT, and bilirubin levels. Control BP prior to initiation of treatment.

Monitoring: Monitor for HTN/hypertensive crisis, thromboembolic events, hemorrhage, symptoms of GI perforation/fistula, thyroid dysfunction, RPLS, proteinuria, signs/symptoms of cardiac failure, and other adverse events. Monitor AST, ALT, and bilirubin levels periodically.

Patient Counseling: Inform about benefits/risks of therapy. Inform that HTN may develop; instruct to have BP monitored regularly during treatment. Instruct to inform physician if experiencing symptoms suggestive of thromboembolic events, abnormal thyroid function, any bleeding episodes, or persistent/severe abdominal pain. Advise that cardiac failure may develop during therapy and that signs/symptoms should be monitored regularly during treatment. Advise to inform physician if patient has an unhealed wound or has surgery scheduled. Advise to inform physician if patient has worsening of neurological function consistent with RPLS (eg, headache, seizure, lethargy, confusion, blindness, other visual and neurologic disturbances). Advise to avoid becoming pregnant while on therapy and counsel both male and female patients to use effective birth control. Instruct female patients not to breastfeed while receiving treatment. Advise to inform physician about all concomitant medications, vitamins, or dietary and herbal supplements. Instruct not to take additional dose if the patient vomits or misses a dose and to take the next dose at the usual time.

Storage: 20-25°C (68-77°F); excursions permitted to 15-30°C (59-86°F).

InnoPran XL – propranolol hydrochloride RX

Class: Nonselective beta-blocker

Exacerbation of angina pectoris and myocardial infarction (MI) reported following abrupt discontinuation. When discontinuing chronically administered drug, particularly in ischemic heart disease, gradually reduce dose over a period of 1-2 weeks and monitor patients. Promptly resume therapy at least temporarily and take other measures appropriate for the management of unstable angina if angina markedly worsens or acute coronary insufficiency develops. Caution against interruption or discontinuation of therapy without a physician's advice. Coronary artery disease (CAD) may be unrecognized; avoid abrupt discontinuation of therapy even in patient treated only for HTN.

ADULT DOSAGE

Hypertension

Initial: 80mg qhs taken consistently, either on empty stomach or with food

Titrate: May titrate to 120mg qhs PRN for BP control

Max: 120mg qhs

PEDIATRIC DOSAGE

Pediatric use may not have been established

DOSE MODIFICATION

Elderly

Start at lower end of dosing range

ADMINISTRATION

Oral route

HOW SUPPLIED

Cap, Extended-Release: 80mg, 120mg

CONTRAINDICATIONS

Cardiogenic shock or decompensated heart failure (HF), sinus bradycardia, sick sinus syndrome and >1st-degree heart block (unless a permanent pacemaker is in place), bronchial asthma.

WARNINGS/PRECAUTIONS

May cause depression of myocardial contractility and precipitate HF and cardiogenic shock; may be necessary to lower dose or d/c therapy. Avoid routine withdrawal prior to surgery. May mask tachycardia occurring with hypoglycemia and hyperthyroidism. Abrupt withdrawal may precipitate thyroid storm. Bradycardia including sinus pause, heart block, and cardiac arrest reported. Increased risk in patients with 1st-degree AV block, sinus node dysfunction, and conduction disorders (eg, Wolff-Parkinson-White). D/C or reduce dose if severe bradycardia occurs. Patients treated for severe anaphylactic reaction may be unresponsive to usual doses of epinephrine; consider other medications (eg, IV fluids, glucagon). Caution in elderly.

ADVERSE REACTIONS

Fatigue, dizziness, constipation.

DRUG INTERACTIONS

Increased concentrations with warfarin; monitor PT. Increased concentrations with propafenone. Increase levels with CYP2D6 inhibitors (eg, bupropion, fluoxetine, paroxetine, quinidine), CYP1A2 inhibitors (eg, ciprofloxacin, enoxamine, fluvoxamine), and CYP2C19 inhibitors (eg, fluconazole, fluvoxamine, ticlopidine). Decreased levels with CYP1A2 inducers (eg, phenytoin, montelukast, smoking) and CYP2C19 inducers (eg, rifampin), and cholestyramine and colestipol, leading to loss of efficacy. May antagonize antihypertensive effects of clonidine; may result to rebound HTN if withdrawn abruptly. May prolong 1st dose hypotension and syncope with prazosin. May reduce sensitivity to dobutamine stress echocardiography in patients undergoing evaluation for myocardial ischemia. May exacerbate hypotensive effects of MAOIs or TCAs. NSAIDs may attenuate the antihypertensive effect of β-adrenoreceptor blocking agents. Increased risk of significant bradycardia with non-dihydropyridine calcium-channel blockers (eg, verapamil, diltiazem), digoxin, or clonidine.

NURSING CONSIDERATIONS

Assessment: Assess for cardiogenic shock, decompensated HF, sinus bradycardia, sick sinus syndrome, AV heart block, presence of pacemaker, bronchial asthma, hepatic or renal impairment, hyperthyroidism, hypoglycemia, history of anaphylactic reactions, possible drug interactions, and pregnancy/nursing status.

Monitoring: Monitor for signs/symptoms of HF, hyperthyroidism, hypoglycemia, anaphylactic reactions, and other adverse reactions. Monitor HR and PT.

Patient Counseling: Inform about risks and benefits of therapy. Instruct not to interrupt or d/c therapy without a physician's advice. Advise to contact physician if signs/symptoms of HF worsens (eg, weight gain or increasing SOB).

Storage: 25°C (77°F); excursions permitted to 15-30°C (59-86°F).

INSPRA – eplerenone RX

Class: Aldosterone blocker

ADULT DOSAGE

Congestive Heart Failure Post-Myocardial Infarction

Initial: 25mg qd
Titrate: Increase to 50mg qd, preferably w/in 4 weeks as tolerated
Dose Adjustment in CHF Post-MI Once Treatment Has Begun:
Serum K^+ <5.0mEq/L:
Increase from 25mg qod to 25mg qd
Increase from 25mg qd to 50mg qd
Serum K^+ 5.0-5.4mEq/L:
No adjustment
Serum K^+ 5.5-5.9mEq/L:
Decrease from 50mg qd to 25mg qd
Decrease from 25mg qd to 25mg qod
Decrease from 25mg qod to withhold
Serum K^+ ≥6mEq/L:
Withhold and restart at 25mg qod when serum K^+ <5.5mEq/L

Hypertension

Initial: 50mg qd
Titrate: Increase to 50mg bid if BP response is inadequate
Max: 100mg/day

PEDIATRIC DOSAGE

Pediatric use may not have been established

DOSE MODIFICATION

Concomitant Medications

Hypertensive Patients Receiving Moderate CYP3A4 Inhibitors:
Initial: 25mg qd

ADMINISTRATION

Oral route

May be administered w/ or w/o food

HOW SUPPLIED

Tab: 25mg, 50mg

CONTRAINDICATIONS

All Patients: Serum K^+ >5.5mEq/L at initiation, CrCl ≤30mL/min, concomitant administration of strong CYP3A4 inhibitors (eg, ketoconazole, itraconazole, nefazodone, troleandomycin, clarithromycin, ritonavir, nelfinavir). Patients Treated for HTN: Type 2 diabetes w/ microalbuminuria, SrCr >2mg/dL (males) or >1.8mg/dL (females), CrCl <50mL/min, concomitant administration of K^+ supplements or K^+-sparing diuretics (eg, amiloride, spironolactone, triamterene).

WARNINGS/PRECAUTIONS

Minimize the risk of hyperkalemia w/ proper patient selection and monitoring. Caution in patients w/ CHF post-MI who have SrCr >2mg/dL (males) or >1.8mg/dL (females), or CrCl ≤50mL/min, or who are diabetic (especially those w/ proteinuria). Increased risk of hyperkalemia in patients w/ decreased renal function.

ADVERSE REACTIONS

Hyperkalemia, dizziness, increased SrCr/TGs.

DRUG INTERACTIONS

See Contraindications and Dose Modification. Monitor serum K^+ and SrCr in 3-7 days in patients who start taking a moderate CYP3A4 inhibitor. Increased risk of hyperkalemia w/ an ACE inhibitor and/or an ARB; closely monitor serum K^+ and renal function, especially in patients at risk for impaired renal function (eg, elderly). Monitor serum lithium levels frequently if coadministered w/ lithium. When used w/ NSAIDs, observe to determine whether the desired effect on BP is obtained and monitor for changes in serum K^+ levels.

NURSING CONSIDERATIONS

Assessment: Assess for type 2 diabetes w/ microalbuminuria/proteinuria, pregnancy/nursing status, and possible drug interactions. Assess serum K^+ levels and renal function (eg, CrCl, SrCr).

Monitoring: Monitor for signs/symptoms of hyperkalemia and other adverse reactions. Monitor serum K^+ w/in the 1st week, at 1 month after start of treatment or dose adjustment, and periodically thereafter. Monitor BP and renal function.

Patient Counseling: Advise not to use K^+ supplements or salt substitutes containing K^+ w/o consulting the prescribing physician. Instruct to contact physician if dizziness, diarrhea, vomiting, rapid or irregular heartbeat, lower extremity edema, or difficulty breathing occurs. Inform that periodic monitoring of BP and serum K^+ is important.

Storage: 25°C (77°F); excursions permitted to 15-30°C (59-86°F).

INTELENCE — etravirine RX

Class: Non-nucleoside reverse transcriptase inhibitor

ADULT DOSAGE

HIV-1 Infection

Combination with Other Antiretrovirals
Treatment-Experienced:
Evidence of Viral Replication and HIV-1 Strains Resistant to an NNRTI and Other Antiretroviral:
200mg bid

PEDIATRIC DOSAGE

HIV-1 Infection

Combination with Other Antiretrovirals
Treatment-Experienced:
Evidence of Viral Replication and HIV-1 Strains Resistant to an NNRTI and Other Antiretroviral:
6-<18 Years:
≥16-<20kg: 100mg bid
≥20-<25kg: 125mg bid
≥25-<30kg: 150mg bid
≥30kg: 200mg bid

ADMINISTRATION
Oral route

Take after a meal
Swallow whole with liquid
May be dispersed in glass of water if unable to swallow whole
Refer to PI for further instructions

HOW SUPPLIED
Tab: 25mg*, 100mg, 200mg *scored

WARNINGS/PRECAUTIONS
Severe, potentially life-threatening, and fatal skin reactions (eg, erythema multiforme, toxic epidermal necrolysis, Stevens-Johnson syndrome), and hypersensitivity reactions including drug rash with eosinophilia and systemic symptoms reported; d/c immediately if these occur and initiate appropriate therapy. Immune reconstitution syndrome, autoimmune disorders (eg, Graves' disease, polymyositis, Guillain-Barre syndrome) in the setting of immune reconstitution, and redistribution/accumulation of body fat reported. Caution in elderly.

ADVERSE REACTIONS
Rash, peripheral neuropathy.

DRUG INTERACTIONS
May alter therapeutic effect and adverse reaction profile with drugs that induce, inhibit, or are substrates of CYP3A, CYP2C9, and CYP2C19, or are transported by P-glycoprotein. Avoid with other NNRTIs, delavirdine, rilpivirine, atazanavir (ATV) without low-dose ritonavir (RTV), fosamprenavir (FPV) without low-dose RTV, FPV/RTV, tipranavir/RTV, indinavir without low-dose RTV, nelfinavir without low-dose RTV, RTV (600mg bid), carbamazepine, phenobarbital, phenytoin, rifampin, rifapentine, and St. John's wort. Coadministration with boceprevir is not recommended in the presence of other drugs which may further decrease etravirine exposure (eg, darunavir/RTV, lopinavir/RTV, saquinavir/RTV, tenofovir disoproxil fumarate, or rifabutin). Caution with digoxin; use lowest dose initially. May increase levels of nelfinavir without RTV, digoxin, warfarin (monitor INR), anticoagulants, 14-OH-clarithromycin, voriconazole, diazepam, boceprevir, fluvastatin, and pitavastatin. May increase maraviroc levels in the presence of a potent CYP3A inhibitor (eg, RTV boosted protease inhibitor). May decrease levels of maraviroc, antiarrhythmics, itraconazole, ketoconazole, rifabutin, telaprevir, atorvastatin, lovastatin, simvastatin, immunosuppressant,

and clopidogrel (active) metabolite. May decrease dolutegravir levels; should only be used with dolutegravir when coadministered with ATV/RTV, darunavir/RTV, or lopinavir/RTV. Fluconazole and voriconazole may increase exposure. Posaconazole, itraconazole, or ketoconazole may increase levels. May decrease clarithromycin exposure. Caution with artemether/lumefantrine. Efavirenz, nevirapine, rifabutin, systemic dexamethasone, and boceprevir may decrease levels. Darunavir/RTV, lopinavir/RTV, and saquinavir/RTV may decrease exposure. Consider alternatives to clarithromycin, such as azithromycin, for treatment of Mycobacterium avium complex. Monitor for withdrawal symptoms when coadministered with methadone, buprenorphine, buprenorphine/naloxone. May need to alter sildenafil dose. Refer to PI for additional drug interaction information.

NURSING CONSIDERATIONS

Assessment: Assess treatment history, pregnancy/nursing status, and for possible drug interactions. Perform resistance testing where possible.

Monitoring: Monitor for signs/symptoms of severe skin/hypersensitivity reactions, body fat redistribution/accumulation, immune reconstitution syndrome (eg, opportunistic infections), autoimmune disorders, and other adverse reactions. Monitor clinical status, including liver transaminases. Monitor INR when combined with warfarin.

Patient Counseling: Inform that product is not a cure for HIV infection and patients may continue to develop opportunistic infections and other complications associated with HIV disease. Advise to avoid doing things that can spread HIV-1 infection to others. Advise to take medication ud. Instruct to always use in combination with other antiretrovirals. Advise not to alter dose or d/c therapy without consulting physician. If a dose is missed within 6 hrs of time usually taken, instruct to take as soon as possible following a meal. If scheduled time exceeds 6 hrs, instruct not to take the missed dose and resume the usual dosing schedule. Advise to report to physician the use of any other prescription/nonprescription or herbal products (eg, St. John's wort). Counsel to d/c and notify physician if severe rash develops. Advise that redistribution or accumulation of body fat may occur.

Storage: 25°C (77°F); excursions permitted to 15-30°C (59-86°F). Store in the original bottle. Protect from moisture.

INTERMEZZO – zolpidem tartrate CIV

Class: Imidazopyridine hypnotic

ADULT DOSAGE

Insomnia

As needed treatment when a middle-of-the-night awakening is followed by difficulty returning to sleep

Usual/Max: 1.75mg (women), 3.5mg (men) once per night prn

PEDIATRIC DOSAGE

Pediatric use may not have been established

DOSE MODIFICATION

Concomitant Medications

CNS Depressants: 1.75mg, once per night

Other Sedative-Hypnotics (eg, Other Zolpidem Products): Not recommended

Hepatic Impairment

Usual: 1.75mg, once per night if needed

Elderly

>65 Years: 1.75mg, once per night if needed

ADMINISTRATION

SL route

Take in bed only if patient has ≥4 hrs of bedtime remaining before planned time of waking

Place under tongue and allow to disintegrate completely before swallowing; do not swallow whole

Do not administer w/ or immediately after a meal

Remove tab from pouch just prior to dosing

HOW SUPPLIED

Tab, SL: 1.75mg, 3.5mg

WARNINGS/PRECAUTIONS

Not indicated for treatment of middle-of-the-night insomnia when patient has fewer than 4 hrs of bedtime remaining before planned time of waking. Has CNS depressant effects; may be at risk for next-day driving and psychomotor impairment if taken with <4 hrs of bedtime remaining or if higher than recommended dose is taken. Initiate only after careful evaluation; failure of insomnia to remit after 7-10 days of treatment may indicate presence of a primary psychiatric and/or medical illness. Severe anaphylactic/anaphylactoid reactions reported; do not rechallenge if angioedema or anaphylaxis develops. Abnormal thinking, behavior changes, and visual/auditory hallucinations reported. Complex behaviors (eg, sleep-driving) reported; consider discontinuation if a "sleep-driving" episode occurs. Amnesia, anxiety, and other neuropsychiatric symptoms may occur. Worsening of depression, and suicidal thoughts and actions (including complete suicide) reported in primarily depressed patients; prescribe the lowest number of tabs feasible at any one time. Caution with compromised respiratory function, including sleep apnea and myasthenia gravis. Withdrawal signs/symptoms reported following rapid dose decrease or abrupt discontinuation; monitor for tolerance, abuse, and dependence. Caution in elderly.

ADVERSE REACTIONS

Nausea, fatigue, headache.

DRUG INTERACTIONS

Use with other sedative-hypnotics (including other zolpidem products) at bedtime or the middle of the night is not recommended. May increase risk of CNS depression with other CNS depressants (eg, benzodiazepines, opioids, TCAs, alcohol); dose adjustments of zolpidem and of other concomitant CNS depressants may be necessary. Increased risk of next-day driving impairment and psychomotor impairment with other CNS depressants or other drugs that increase blood levels of zolpidem. Increased risk of complex behaviors with alcohol and other CNS depressants. May have additive effects of decreased alertness and psychomotor performance with imipramine, chlorpromazine, and alcohol. Caution with chronic haloperidol administration. Sertraline may increase exposure and increase pharmacodynamic effect. CYP3A inhibitors may increase exposure. May increase $T_{1/2}$ with multiple doses of fluoxetine. Rifampin may reduce exposure and decrease efficacy. Increased pharmacodynamic effects with ketoconazole; consider using a lower dose of zolpidem.

NURSING CONSIDERATIONS

Assessment: Assess for psychiatric and/or medical illness, respiratory impairment, myasthenia gravis, hepatic impairment, hypersensitivity to the drug, pregnancy/nursing status, and possible drug interactions.

Monitoring: Monitor for signs/symptoms CNS depression, respiratory depression, abnormal thinking, behavioral changes, visual/auditory hallucinations, complex behaviors, worsening of depression, suicidal thoughts/actions, angioedema/anaphylaxis, and other adverse reactions. Monitor for withdrawal signs/symptoms following rapid dose decrease or abrupt discontinuation.

Patient Counseling: Inform about the benefits and risks of treatment. Instruct patient to take as prescribed. Counsel that medication has the potential to cause next-day impairment, and the risk is increased if dosing instructions are not carefully followed. Advise to wait at least 4 hrs after dosing and until they feel fully awake before driving or engaging in other activities requiring mental alertness. Inform that severe anaphylactic and anaphylactoid reactions may occur; instruct to notify physician immediately if signs/symptoms occur. Instruct to inform families that therapy has been associated with "sleep-driving" and other complex behaviors while not being fully awake; instruct to call healthcare providers immediately if symptoms develop. Instruct to report immediately any suicidal thoughts. Advise not to take medication if alcohol has been consumed on that day or before going to bed.

Storage: 20-25°C (68-77°F); excursion permitted between 15-30°C (59-86°F). Protect from moisture. Do not remove tab from unit-dose pouch until time of use.

INTRON A – interferon alfa-2b, recombinant RX

Class: Biological response modifier

May cause or aggravate fatal or life-threatening neuropsychiatric, autoimmune, ischemic, and infectious disorders. Monitor closely with periodic clinical and lab evaluations. D/C in patients with persistently severe or worsening signs/symptoms of these conditions.

ADULT DOSAGE

Malignant Melanoma

≥18 Years:

Induction: 20 MIU/m^2 IV, over 20 min, 5 consecutive days/week for 4 weeks

Maint: 10 MIU/m^2 SQ 3X/week for 48 weeks

Follicular Lymphoma

≥18 Years:

5 MIU SQ 3X/week for up to 18 months

Chronic Hepatitis B

≥18 Years:

5 MIU IM/SQ qd or 10 MIU IM/SQ 3X/week for 16 weeks

PEDIATRIC DOSAGE

Chronic Hepatitis C

≥3 Years:

3 MIU IM/SQ 3X/week

In patients tolerating therapy with normalization of ALT at 16 weeks of treatment, extend therapy for 18-24 months

In patients who do not normalize their ALTs or have persistently high levels of HCV RNA after 16 weeks of therapy, consider discontinuing therapy

AIDS-Related Kaposi's Sarcoma

≥18 Years:
30 MIU/m²/dose IM/SQ 3X/week until disease progression or maximal response has been achieved after 16 weeks of treatment

Condylomata Acuminata

≥18 Years:
1 MIU/lesion 3X/week alternating days for 3 weeks
Max: 5 lesions/course
An additional course may be administered at 12-16 weeks

Chronic Hepatitis C

≥18 Years:
3 MIU IM/SQ 3X/week

In patients tolerating therapy with normalization of ALT at 16 weeks of treatment, extend therapy for 18-24 months
In patients who do not normalize their ALTs or have persistently high levels of HCV RNA after 16 weeks of therapy, consider discontinuing therapy

Hairy Cell Leukemia

≥18 Years:
2 MIU/m² IM/SQ 3X/week for up to 6 months

Chronic Hepatitis B

≥1 Year:
3 MIU/m² SQ 3X/week for 1 week, then 6 MIU/m² SQ 3X/week for total therapy of 16-24 weeks
Max: 10 MIU/m² 3X/week

DOSE MODIFICATION

Adverse Reactions

Hairy Cell Leukemia:
Severe: Reduce dose by 50% or temporarily withhold therapy until ADRs abate, then resume at 50%; permanently d/c if ADRs persist or recur following dose adjustment. D/C for progressive disease or failure to respond after 6 months of treatment

Malignant Melanoma:
Severe (Including Granulocytes >250/mm³ but <500/mm³ or SGPT/SGOT >5-10X ULN): Withhold until ADRs abate, then restart at 50% of the previous dose
Permanently D/C for:
Toxicity that does not abate after withholding treatment
Severe adverse reactions that recur in patients receiving reduced doses
Granulocytes <250/mm³ or SGPT/SGOT >10X ULN

Follicular Lymphoma:
Neutrophils >1000/mm³, but <1500/mm³: Reduce dose by 50%; may re-escalate to starting dose when ANC >1500/mm³
Neutrophils <1500/mm³ or Platelets <75,000/mm³: Delay chemotherapy cycle
Neutrophils <1000/mm³ or Platelets <50,000/mm³: Withhold therapy
SGOT >5X ULN or SCr >2.0 mg/dL: Permanently d/c

AIDS-Related Kaposi's Sarcoma:
Severe: Reduce dose by 50% or withhold; resume at reduced dose if ADRs abate with interruption of dosing. Permanently d/c if ADRs persist or recur following dose adjustment

Chronic Hepatitis C:
Severe: Reduce dose by 50% or temporarily d/c until ADRs abate; d/c therapy if intolerance persists after dose adjustment

Chronic Hepatitis B:
Severe ADRs or Lab Abnormalities: Reduce dose by 50% or d/c if appropriate, until the adverse reactions abate; d/c therapy if intolerance persists after dose adjustment
WBCs <1.5 x 10⁹/L or Granulocytes <0.75 x 10⁹/L or Platelets <50 x 10⁹/L: Reduce dose by 50%
WBCs <1.0 x 10⁹/L or Granulocytes <0.5 x 10⁹/L or Platelets <25 x 10⁹/L: Permanently d/c

ADMINISTRATION

IM/SQ/IV/Intralesional route

Administer in the pm when possible
Refer to PI for preparation and further administration instructions

Hairy Cell Leukemia
Platelets <50,000/mm³: Administer by SQ route

HOW SUPPLIED

Inj: 10 MIU, 18 MIU, 50 MIU [powder]; 18 MIU, 25 MIU [sol]

CONTRAINDICATIONS
Autoimmune hepatitis, decompensated liver disease. When used with Rebetol, refer to the individual monograph.

WARNINGS/PRECAUTIONS
Caution with coagulation disorders (eg, thrombophlebitis, pulmonary embolism), severe myelosuppression, debilitating medical conditions (eg, history of pulmonary disease, diabetes mellitus [DM] prone to ketoacidosis). Cardiovascular (CV) adverse experiences (eg, arrhythmia, cardiomyopathy, myocardial infarction [MI]), and ischemic and hemorrhagic cerebrovascular events reported; caution with history of CV disease (CVD). Depression and suicidal behavior reported; d/c if psychiatric problems are severe, or if symptoms persist or worsen. Obtundation, coma, and encephalopathy may occur in some patients, usually in elderly, treated with higher doses. May suppress bone marrow function and may result in severe cytopenias; d/c if severe decreases in neutrophil ($<0.5 \times 10^9$/L) or platelet counts ($<25 \times 10^9$/L) occur. Ophthalmologic disorders may be induced or aggravated; conduct baseline eye exam and monitor periodically with preexisting ophthalmologic disorders. D/C if new or worsening ophthalmologic disorders develop. Thyroid abnormalities and DM reported; d/c if these conditions develop and cannot be normalized by medication. Hepatotoxicity and autoimmune disorders reported; monitor or d/c if appropriate. D/C if signs/symptoms of liver failure develop. Avoid in patients with a history of autoimmune disease and in patients who are immunosuppressed transplant recipients. Pulmonary disorders may be induced or aggravated. Closely monitor if the chest x-ray shows pulmonary infiltrates or there is evidence of pulmonary function impairment and d/c if appropriate. Powder formulation contains albumin; carries an extremely remote risk for transmission of viral diseases and Creutzfeldt-Jakob disease. Should not be used with rapidly progressive visceral disease. Acute serious hypersensitivity reactions reported; d/c immediately if an acute reaction develops. New or exacerbated sarcoidosis, exacerbated psoriasis, and hypertriglyceridemia reported. D/C if persistently elevated TG levels associated with symptoms of potential pancreatitis occur. Do not interchange brands. Caution in elderly.

ADVERSE REACTIONS
Neuropsychiatric/autoimmune/ischemic/infectious disorders, flu-like symptoms, fatigue, fever, chills, neutropenia, myalgia, anorexia, N/V, rigors, headache, GI disorders.

DRUG INTERACTIONS
May increase theophylline levels. Caution with other potentially myelosuppressive agents (eg, zidovudine). Higher incidence of neutropenia with zidovudine. Peripheral neuropathy reported when used in combination with telbivudine. Hemolytic anemia, dental, and periodontal disorders reported when used in combination with ribavirin.

NURSING CONSIDERATIONS

Assessment: Assess for history of psychiatric disorders, CVD, autoimmune, and ophthalmologic disorders, hepatic/renal impairment, hypersensitivity reactions, or any other condition where treatment is contraindicated or cautioned. Assess pregnancy/nursing status and for possible drug interactions. Obtain baseline chest x-ray, standard hematologic tests (including Hgb, complete and differential WBC counts, and platelet count), blood chemistries (electrolytes, LFTs, and TSH), and eye exam. Perform ECG in patients with preexisting cardiac abnormalities and/or in advanced stages of cancer. Perform liver biopsy in patients with chronic hepatitis B and chronic hepatitis C. Test for presence of HCV antibody in patients with chronic hepatitis C.

Monitoring: Monitor for occurrence or aggravation of neuropsychiatric, autoimmune, ischemic, and infectious disorders; hypersensitivity reactions; exacerbation of preexisting psoriasis or sarcoidosis, development of new sarcoidosis; renal/hepatic dysfunction; and other adverse reactions. Closely monitor patients with a history of MI or arrhythmic disorder, liver/pulmonary function abnormalities, and WBC counts in myelosuppressed patients and in those receiving other myelosuppressive medications. Monitor LFTs, PT, alkaline phosphatase, albumin, and bilirubin levels periodically and at approximately 2-week intervals during ALT flare. Monitor TGs, LFTs, electrolytes, chest x-ray, complete and differential WBC count, and platelet count periodically. Perform ECG in patients with preexisting cardiac abnormalities and/or in advanced stages of cancer. Repeat TSH testing at 3 and 6 months during therapy. (Chronic hepatitis B) Monitor CBCs, platelet counts, LFTs (including serum ALT, albumin, bilirubin) at treatment Weeks 1, 2, 4, 8, 12, and 16. Evaluate HBeAg, HBsAg, and ALT at the end of therapy, then at 3 and 6 months post-therapy. Monitor CBC and platelet counts at Weeks 1 and 2 following initiation of therapy and monthly thereafter. (Hepatitis C) Evaluate serum ALT at approximately 3-month intervals to assess response to treatment. Perform periodic ophthalmologic exams in patients who have a preexisting ophthalmologic disorder. Perform complete eye exam if any ocular symptoms develop. If psychiatric problems develop, including clinical depression, monitor during treatment and in the 6 month follow-up period. (Malignant Melanoma) Monitor differential WBC counts and LFTs weekly during induction phase and monthly during maintenance phase of therapy.

Patient Counseling: Inform of risks/benefits associated with treatment. Instruct on proper use of product. Advise to seek medical attention if symptoms indicative of a serious adverse reaction associated with therapy develops (eg, suicidal ideation, chest pain, decrease in/or loss of vision, severe abdominal pain, high persistent fever, bruising, dyspnea). Inform that some side effects, such as fatigue and decreased concentration, may interfere with the ability to perform certain tasks. Advise to remain well hydrated during the initial stages of treatment; inform that use of an antipyretic may ameliorate some of the flu-like symptoms. Instruct self-administering patients on the importance of site selection and rotating inj site, proper disposal of needles/syringes, and caution against reuse of needles/syringes. Inform of the risks to the fetus when therapy is used in combination with ribavirin during pregnancy; encourage to report to Ribavirin Pregnancy Registry to monitor maternal-fetal outcomes. Instruct female patients and female partners of male patients to use 2 forms of birth control during treatment and for 6 months after therapy is discontinued. Instruct to brush teeth thoroughly bid and have regular dental exam. Inform that some patients may experience vomiting. Advise to rinse out the mouth thoroughly afterwards if vomiting occurs.

Storage: 2-8°C (36-46°F). (Powder) Use immediately after reconstitution; may store up to 24 hrs at 2-8°C (36-46°F). (Vial) Do not freeze. Keep away from heat.

INTUNIV – guanfacine **RX**

Class: Alpha$_{2A}$-agonist

PEDIATRIC DOSAGE

Attention-Deficit Hyperactivity Disorder

Monotherapy/Adjunctive Therapy to Stimulant Medications:

6-17 Years:
Initial: 1mg/day
Titrate: Adjust in increments of no more than 1mg/week
Target Dose Range: 0.05-0.12mg/kg/day (total daily dose 1-7mg), depending on clinical response and tolerability
Max: 4mg/day in children 6-12 yrs of age or 7mg/day in adolescents 13-17 yrs of age

Weight-Based Target Dose Range:
25-33.9kg: 2-3mg/kg
34-41.4kg: 2-4mg/kg
41.5-49.4kg: 3-5mg/kg
49.5-58.4kg: 3-6mg/kg
58.5-91kg: 4-7mg/kg
>91kg: 5-7mg/kg

Maint Treatment:
Periodically reevaluate the long-term use of the drug and adjust weight-based dose prn

Missed Dose

When reinitiating to the previous maint dose after ≥2 missed consecutive doses, consider titration based on tolerability

Conversions

Switching from Immediate-Release (IR):
D/C IR, and titrate w/ extended-release following the recommended schedule
Do not substitute for IR tabs on a mg-per-mg basis

DOSE MODIFICATION

Concomitant Medications

Strong CYP3A4 Inhibitors:
(Based on Weight-Based Target Dose Range)
Continue CYP3A4 Inhibitor/Initiate Guanfacine: Decrease guanfacine dose by 1/2
Continue Guanfacine/Initiate CYP3A4 Inhibitor: Decrease guanfacine dose by 1/2
Stop CYP3A4 Inhibitor/Continue Guanfacine: Increase guanfacine to recommended level

Strong CYP3A4 Inducers:
(Based on Weight-Based Target Dose Range)
Continue CYP3A4 Inducer/Initiate Guanfacine: Consider increasing guanfacine up to twice the recommended dose
Continue Guanfacine/Initiate CYP3A4 Inducer: Consider increasing guanfacine up to twice the recommended dose over 1-2 weeks

Stop CYP3A4 Inducer/Continue Guanfacine: Decrease guanfacine dose to recommended level over 1-2 weeks

Renal Impairment

Significant Impairment: May need to reduce dose

Hepatic Impairment

Significant Impairment: May need to reduce dose

Discontinuation

Taper dose in decrements of no more than 1mg every 3-7 days

ADMINISTRATION

Oral route

Take either in am or pm, at approx same time each day
Swallow tabs whole w/ water, milk, or other liquid; do not crush, chew, or break
Do not administer w/ high-fat meals

HOW SUPPLIED

Tab, Extended-Release: 1mg, 2mg, 3mg, 4mg

WARNINGS/PRECAUTIONS

May experience increase in BP and HR following discontinuation of therapy. May cause dose-dependent decreases in BP and HR. Orthostatic hypotension and syncope reported. Titrate slowly in patients w/ a history of hypotension, and those w/ underlying conditions that may be worsened by hypotension and bradycardia (eg, heart block, cardiovascular disease, vascular disease). In patients who have a history of syncope or may have a condition that predisposes to syncope (eg, hypotension, orthostatic hypotension, bradycardia), avoid dehydration or overheating. Somnolence and sedation commonly reported. May impair mental/physical abilities. May worsen sinus node dysfunction and atrioventricular (AV) block; titrate slowly and monitor vital signs frequently in patients w/ cardiac conduction abnormalities.

ADVERSE REACTIONS

Somnolence, fatigue, abdominal pain, hypotension, N/V, lethargy, dizziness, irritability, decreased appetite, dry mouth, insomnia, enuresis, bradycardia.

DRUG INTERACTIONS

See Dose Modification. CYP3A4 inhibitors (eg, ketoconazole) may increase exposure. CYP3A4 inducers (eg, rifampin) may decrease exposure. Monitor BP and HR, and adjust dosages accordingly w/ antihypertensives or other drugs that can reduce BP/HR or increase the risk of syncope. Consider the potential for additive sedative effects before using w/ other centrally active depressants. Avoid w/ alcohol. May worsen sinus node dysfunction and AV block, especially w/ other sympatholytic drugs; titrate slowly and monitor vital signs frequently w/ other sympatholytic drugs.

NURSING CONSIDERATIONS

Assessment: Assess for history of hypotension, underlying conditions that may be worsened by hypotension and bradycardia, history of syncope, condition that predisposes to syncope, cardiac conduction abnormalities, hypersensitivity to drug, renal/hepatic impairment, pregnancy/nursing status, and possible drug interactions. Assess HR and BP.

Monitoring: Monitor for hypotension, bradycardia, syncope, somnolence, sedation, cardiac conduction abnormalities, and other adverse reactions. Monitor HR and BP following dose increases, and periodically while on therapy. Monitor BP and pulse when reducing the dose or discontinuing the drug. Observe human milk-fed infants for sedation and somnolence. Monitor vital signs frequently in patients w/ cardiac conduction abnormalities. Periodically reevaluate the long term use of the drug.

Patient Counseling: Instruct caregiver to supervise the child or adolescent taking the drug. Counsel on how to properly taper the medication, if the physician decides to d/c treatment. Instruct patients not to d/c therapy w/o consulting their physician. Inform of the adverse reactions (eg, sedation, headache, abdominal pain) that may occur; advise to consult physician if any of these symptoms persist or other symptoms occur. Caution patients against operating heavy equipment or driving until accustomed to effects of medication. Advise to avoid becoming dehydrated or overheated, and to avoid use w/ alcohol.

Storage: 20-25°C (68-77°F); excursions permitted to 15-30°C (59-86°F).

INVANZ – ertapenem

RX

Class: Carbapenem

ADULT DOSAGE

Intra-Abdominal Infections

Complicated:
1g qd IV/IM for 5-14 days

Skin and Skin Structure Infections

Complicated Infections, Including Diabetic Foot Infections:
1g qd IV/IM for 7-14 days; patients w/ diabetic foot infections received up to 28 days of treatment (parenteral or parenteral + oral switch therapy)

Community-Acquired Pneumonia

1g qd IV/IM for 10-14 days (duration includes a possible switch to oral therapy, after at least 3 days of parenteral therapy, once clinical improvement has been demonstrated)

Urinary Tract Infections

Complicated UTIs, Including Pyelonephritis:
1g qd IV/IM for 10-14 days (duration includes a possible switch to oral therapy, after at least 3 days of parenteral therapy, once clinical improvement has been demonstrated)

Acute Pelvic Infections

Including Postpartum Endomyometritis, Septic Abortion, and Postsurgical Gynecological Infections:
1g qd IV/IM for 3-10 days

Prophylaxis of Postoperative Infections

Prophylaxis of Surgical-Site Infection, Following Colorectal Surgery:
1g as a single IV dose given 1 hr prior to surgical incision

PEDIATRIC DOSAGE

Intra-Abdominal Infections

Complicated:
3 Months-12 Years:
15mg/kg IV/IM bid for 5-14 days; not to exceed 1g/day
≥13 Years:
1g qd IV/IM for 5-14 days

Skin and Skin Structure Infections

Complicated Infections, Including Diabetic Foot Infections:
3 Months-12 Years:
15mg/kg IV/IM bid for 7-14 days; not to exceed 1g/day
≥13 Years:
1g qd IV/IM for 7-14 days

Community-Acquired Pneumonia

3 Months-12 Years:
15mg/kg IV/IM bid for 10-14 days; not to exceed 1g/day
≥13 Years:
1g qd IV/IM for 10-14 days
Duration includes a possible switch to oral therapy, after at least 3 days of parenteral therapy, once clinical improvement has been demonstrated

Urinary Tract Infections

Complicated UTIs, Including Pyelonephritis:
3 Months-12 Years:
15mg/kg IV/IM bid for 10-14 days; not to exceed 1g/day
≥13 Years:
1g qd IV/IM for 10-14 days
Duration includes a possible switch to oral therapy, after at least 3 days of parenteral therapy, once clinical improvement has been demonstrated

Acute Pelvic Infections

3 Months-12 Years:
15mg/kg IV/IM bid for 3-10 days; not to exceed 1g/day
≥13 Years:
1g qd IV/IM for 3-10 days

DOSE MODIFICATION

Renal Impairment
Adults:
Severe Impairment (CrCl ≤30mL/min)/ESRD (CrCl ≤10mL/min): 500mg/day
Hemodialysis: 500mg/day; if administered w/in 6 hrs prior to hemodialysis, give 150mg supplementary dose following hemodialysis session

ADMINISTRATION

IV/IM route
Do not mix or coinfuse w/ other medications
Do not use diluents containing dextrose

IV
Reconstitute and then dilute prior to administration
Complete infusion w/in 6 hrs of reconstitution; infuse over a period of 30 min
May administer by IV infusion for up to 14 days

Preparation:
Reconstitute 1g vial w/ 10mL of water for inj, 0.9% NaCl for inj, or bacteriostatic water for inj; shake well

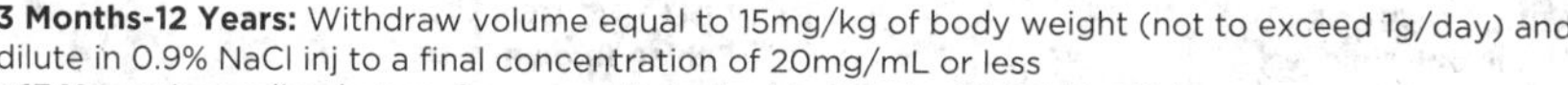

3 Months-12 Years: Withdraw volume equal to 15mg/kg of body weight (not to exceed 1g/day) and dilute in 0.9% NaCl inj to a final concentration of 20mg/mL or less
≥13 Years: Immediately transfer reconstituted sol to 50mL of 0.9% NaCl inj
IM
Reconstitute prior to administration
Use reconstituted sol w/in 1 hr after preparation
May administer by IM inj for up to 7 days
Preparation:
Reconstitute 1g vial w/ 3.2mL of 1% lidocaine HCl inj (w/o epinephrine); shake thoroughly
Immediately withdraw appropriate dose and administer by deep IM inj into a large muscle mass (eg, gluteal muscles or lateral part of thigh)
Refer to PI for ADD-Vantage Vial Instructions

HOW SUPPLIED
Inj: 1g

CONTRAINDICATIONS
(IM) Hypersensitivity to amide-type local anesthetics.

WARNINGS/PRECAUTIONS
Serious and occasionally fatal hypersensitivity (anaphylactic) reactions reported; d/c immediately if an allergic reaction occurs. Seizures and other CNS adverse experiences reported; caution with known factors that predispose to convulsive activity, and continue anticonvulsant therapy with known seizure disorders. If focal tremors, myoclonus, or seizures occur, evaluate neurologically, place on anticonvulsant therapy if not already instituted, and reexamine dosage to determine whether it should be decreased or discontinued. *Clostridium difficile*-associated diarrhea (CDAD) reported; d/c if CDAD is suspected or confirmed. Use caution when administering IM to avoid inadvertent inj into a blood vessel. May result in bacterial resistance with prolonged use in the absence of proven or suspected bacterial infection, or a prophylactic indication; take appropriate measures if superinfection develops. Caution in elderly.

ADVERSE REACTIONS
Diarrhea, infused vein complication, N/V, anemia, headache, edema/swelling, fever, abdominal pain, constipation, altered mental status, insomnia, vaginitis, infusion-site pain, infusion-site erythema.

DRUG INTERACTIONS
Increased plasma concentrations with probenecid; coadministration is not recommended. May reduce concentrations of valproic acid, thereby increasing the risk of breakthrough seizures; concomitant use with valproic acid/divalproex sodium is generally not recommended, but if necessary, consider supplemental anticonvulsant therapy.

NURSING CONSIDERATIONS

Assessment: Assess for factors that predispose to convulsive activity, seizure disorders, renal impairment, pregnancy/nursing status, and possible drug interactions. Carefully assess for previous hypersensitivity reactions to drug, PCN, cephalosporins, other β-lactams, and other allergens. (IM) Assess for hypersensitivity to amide-type local anesthetics.

Monitoring: Monitor for hypersensitivity (anaphylactic) reactions, CNS effects (eg, focal tremors, myoclonus, seizures), CDAD, superinfection, and other adverse reactions. Periodically monitor organ system function (eg, renal, hepatic, hematopoietic) during prolonged therapy.

Patient Counseling: Advise that allergic reactions, including serious allergic reactions, could occur, and that serious reactions may require immediate treatment. Advise to report any previous hypersensitivity reactions to the medication, other β-lactams, or other allergens. Counsel to inform physician if taking valproic acid or divalproex sodium. Counsel that therapy should only be used to treat bacterial, not viral, infections. Instruct to take exactly ud even if the patient feels better early in the course of therapy. Inform that skipping doses or not completing the full course of therapy may decrease effectiveness of treatment and increase bacterial resistance. Inform that diarrhea is a common problem caused by therapy that usually ends when therapy is discontinued. Instruct to immediately contact physician if watery and bloody stools (with or without stomach cramps and fever) occur, even as late as ≥2 months after the last dose.

Storage: ≤25°C (77°F). Reconstituted and Infusion Sol: 25°C (77°F) and use within 6 hrs, or 5°C (41°F) for 24 hrs and use within 4 hrs after removal from refrigeration. Do not freeze sol.

INVEGA – paliperidone — RX

Class: Atypical antipsychotic

Elderly patients with dementia-related psychosis treated with antipsychotic drugs are at an increased risk of death; most deaths appeared to be cardiovascular (CV) (eg, heart failure, sudden death) or infectious (eg, pneumonia) in nature. Not approved for the treatment of patients with dementia-related psychosis.

ADULT DOSAGE

Schizophrenia

6mg qd
Titrate: If indicated, may increase by 3mg/day; dose increases >6mg/day should be made at intervals >5 days
Usual Range: 3-12mg/day
Max: 12mg/day

Schizoaffective Disorder

Monotherapy or Adjunct to Mood Stabilizers and/or Antidepressants:
6mg qd
Titrate: If indicated, may increase by 3mg/day at intervals of >4 days
Usual Range: 3-12mg/day
Max: 12mg/day

PEDIATRIC DOSAGE

Schizophrenia

12-17 Years:
Initial: 3mg qd
Titrate: If indicated, may increase by 3mg/day at intervals of >5 days

DOSE MODIFICATION

Renal Impairment
Mild (CrCl ≥50-<80mL/min):
Initial: 3mg qd
Max: 6mg qd
Moderate to Severe (CrCl ≥10-<50mL/min):
Initial: 1.5mg qd
Max: 3mg qd

Elderly
Adjust dose according to renal function

ADMINISTRATION

Oral route

Take w/ or w/o food
Swallow whole with liquids; do not crush, divide, or chew

HOW SUPPLIED

Tab, ER: 1.5mg, 3mg, 6mg, 9mg

WARNINGS/PRECAUTIONS

Neuroleptic malignant syndrome (NMS) reported; d/c if this occurs. May increase QTc interval; avoid with congenital long QT syndrome and history of cardiac arrhythmias. Tardive dyskinesia (TD) may develop; consider discontinuation if signs/symptoms of TD appear. Hyperglycemia and diabetes mellitus (DM), in some cases extreme and associated with ketoacidosis or hyperosmolar coma or death, reported. Undesirable alterations in lipids and weight gain reported. May elevate prolactin levels. Avoid with preexisting severe GI narrowing. May induce orthostatic hypotension and syncope; caution with known CV disease, cerebrovascular disease, or conditions that predispose to hypotension. Leukopenia, neutropenia, and agranulocytosis reported; d/c in cases of severe neutropenia (absolute neutrophil count <1000/mm^3). Somnolence reported. May impair mental/physical abilities. Seizures reported; caution with history of seizures or conditions that lower the seizure threshold. May cause esophageal dysmotility and aspiration; caution with risk of aspiration pneumonia. May induce priapism; severe cases may require surgical intervention. May disrupt body's ability to reduce core body temperature; caution with conditions that may contribute to an elevated core body temperature. May have an antiemetic effect that may mask signs/symptoms of overdosage with certain drugs or of conditions (eg, intestinal obstruction, Reye's syndrome, brain tumor). Patients with Parkinson's disease or dementia with Lewy bodies may have increased sensitivity to therapy. Caution with suicidal tendencies, renal impairment, and in elderly. Not recommended with CrCl <10mL/min.

ADVERSE REACTIONS

Extrapyramidal symptoms, tachycardia, somnolence, akathisia, dyskinesia, dyspepsia, dizziness, nasopharyngitis, headache, nausea, hyperkinesia, constipation, weight gain, parkinsonism, tremors.

DRUG INTERACTIONS

Consider additive exposure with risperidone. Avoid with other drugs known to prolong QTc interval, including Class 1A (eg, quinidine, procainamide) or Class III (eg, amiodarone, sotalol) antiarrhythmics, antipsychotics (eg, chlorpromazine, thioridazine), and antibiotics (eg, gatifloxacin, moxifloxacin). Caution with other centrally acting drugs, alcohol, and drugs with anticholinergic activity. May antagonize the effect of levodopa and other dopamine agonists. Additive effect may be observed with other agents that cause orthostatic hypotension. Carbamazepine may decrease levels. Paroxetine (a potent CYP2D6 inhibitor) may increase exposure in CYP2D6 extensive metabolizers. Divalproex sodium may increase levels; consider dose reduction with valproate.

NURSING CONSIDERATIONS

Assessment: Assess for dementia-related psychosis, congenital long QT syndrome, history of cardiac arrhythmias, DM, risk factors for DM, severe GI narrowing, history of clinically significant low WBCs or drug-induced leukopenia/neutropenia, Parkinson's disease, dementia with Lewy bodies, renal impairment, any other conditions where treatment is contraindicated or cautioned, pregnancy/nursing status, and possible drug interactions. Obtain baseline FPG in patients at risk for DM.

Monitoring: Monitor for NMS, TD, QT prolongation, hyperprolactinemia, orthostatic hypotension, syncope, cognitive and motor impairment, seizures, esophageal dysmotility, aspiration, priapism, disruption of body temperature, and other adverse reactions. Monitor for signs of hyperglycemia; perform periodic monitoring of FPG levels in patients with DM or at risk for DM. Monitor for signs/symptoms of leukopenia/neutropenia; frequently monitor CBC in patients with a history of clinically significant low WBC or drug-induced leukopenia/neutropenia. Monitor weight and renal function.

Patient Counseling: Inform of the risk of orthostatic hypotension during initiation/reinitiation or dose increases. Inform that therapy has the potential to impair judgment, thinking, or motor skills; advise to use caution when operating hazardous machinery (eg, automobiles). Advise to avoid alcohol during therapy. Instruct to notify physician of all prescription and nonprescription drugs currently taking, and if pregnant, intending to become pregnant, or breastfeeding. Counsel on appropriate care in avoiding overheating and dehydration. Advise that the tab shell, along with insoluble core components, may be found in stool.

Storage: Up to 25°C (77°F); excursions permitted to 15-30°C (59-86°F). Protect from moisture.

INVEGA SUSTENNA – paliperidone palmitate RX

Class: Atypical antipsychotic

Elderly patients with dementia-related psychosis treated with antipsychotic drugs are at an increased risk of death. Not approved for use in patients with dementia-related psychosis.

ADULT DOSAGE

Schizophrenia

Initial: 234mg IM on Day 1, then 156mg on Day 8 (both in deltoid muscle)
Maint: 117mg/month (in deltoid/gluteal muscle), administer 5 weeks after 1st inj; some may benefit from lower or higher dose w/in the available strengths (39-234mg)
Max: 234mg/month
Establish tolerability w/ oral paliperidone/risperidone prior to initiating therapy in oral paliperidone- or oral/injectable risperidone-naive patients

Schizoaffective Disorder

Monotherapy and Adjunctive Therapy to Mood Stabilizers/Antidepressants:
Initial: 234mg IM on Day 1, then 156mg on Day 8 (both in deltoid muscle)
Maint: 78-234mg/month (in deltoid/gluteal muscle), administer 5 weeks after 1st inj
Titrate: May adjust maint dose monthly based on tolerability and/or efficacy using available strengths
Max: 234mg/month

Conversions

Switching from Oral Antipsychotics:
D/C oral antipsychotics at the time of initiation of therapy
Tab, ER to Inj Maint Dose Conversion:
3mg PO qd: 39-78mg IM every 4 weeks
6mg PO qd: 117mg IM every 4 weeks
12mg PO qd: 234mg IV every 4 weeks

Switching from Long-Acting Injectable Antipsychotics:
Initiate therapy in place of the next scheduled inj and continue w/ monthly maint dose

PEDIATRIC DOSAGE

Pediatric use may not have been established

Missed Dose

Avoiding Missed Doses:
May give 2nd initiation dose 4 days before/after 1-week time point
May give 3rd and subsequent monthly inj up to 7 days before/after the monthly time point

Management of a Missed 2nd Initiation Dose:
<4 Weeks Since 1st Inj:
Administer 2nd inj (156mg) as soon as possible. A 3rd inj (117mg) is recommended 5 weeks after 1st inj (regardless of timing of 2nd inj), followed thereafter by normal monthly inj
4-7 Weeks Since 1st Inj:
Resume dosing w/ 2 inj of 156mg IM, administered in the deltoid one week apart, then resume usual monthly inj cycle
>7 Weeks Since 1st Inj:
Restart therapy

Management of a Missed Maint Dose:
4-6 Weeks Since Last Inj:
Resume regular monthly dosing as soon as possible at previously stabilized dose, followed by inj at monthly intervals
>6 Weeks-6 Months Since Last Inj:
Resume the same previously stabilized dose as soon as possible into the deltoid, followed by another deltoid inj at the same dose 1 week later. Resume monthly dosing thereafter. If previous stabilized dose was 234mg, then 1st two inj should be 156mg each
>6 Months Since Last Inj:
Restart therapy

DOSE MODIFICATION
Concomitant Medications
Strong CYP3A4/P-gp Inducers:
May need to increase dose; may need to decrease the dose when the strong inducer is discontinued

Renal Impairment
Mild (CrCl 50-<80mL/min):
Initial: 156mg IM on Day 1, then 117mg 1 week later (both in deltoid muscle)
Maint: 78mg/month IM (in deltoid or gluteal muscle)
Moderate or Severe (CrCl <50mL/min): Not recommended

ADMINISTRATION
IM route

Shake syringe vigorously for 10 sec
Inject slowly, deep into muscle
Administer as a single inj; do not administer dose in divided inj
Avoid inadvertent inj into a blood vessel
Alternate deltoid inj between the 2 deltoid muscles
Administer into the upper outer quadrant of gluteal muscle; alternate gluteal inj between the 2 gluteal muscles

Needle Size Recommendations
Deltoid Muscle:
<90kg: 1-inch, 23-gauge needle
≥90kg: 1.5-inch, 22-gauge needle
Gluteal Muscle:
1.5-inch, 22-gauge needle size regardless of weight

HOW SUPPLIED
Inj, Extended-Release: 39mg, 78mg, 117mg, 156mg, 234mg

WARNINGS/PRECAUTIONS
Recommended to establish tolerability with oral paliperidone or oral risperidone prior to initiating treatment if have never taken oral paliperidone or oral/injectable risperidone. Neuroleptic malignant syndrome (NMS) reported; d/c if this occurs. May increase QTc interval; avoid with congenital long QT syndrome and history of cardiac arrhythmias. May develop tardive dyskinesia (TD); consider discontinuing if this occurs. Hyperglycemia and diabetes mellitus (DM), in some cases extreme

and associated with ketoacidosis or hyperosmolar coma or death, reported. Dyslipidemia, weight gain, and hyperprolactinemia reported. May induce orthostatic hypotension and syncope; caution with known cardiovascular/cerebrovascular disease or conditions that predispose to hypotension. Leukopenia, neutropenia, and agranulocytosis reported; d/c in cases of severe neutropenia (absolute neutrophil count <1000/mm^3). Somnolence, sedation, and dizziness reported. May impair mental/physical abilities. Seizures reported; caution with history of seizures or conditions that lower the seizure threshold. May cause esophageal dysmotility and aspiration; caution with risk of aspiration pneumonia. May induce priapism; severe cases may require surgical intervention. May disrupt body's ability to reduce core body temperature; caution with conditions that may contribute to an elevated core body temperature. Patients with Parkinson's disease or dementia with Lewy Bodies may have increased sensitivity to therapy. Caution with renal impairment and in elderly. Not recommended with moderate or severe renal impairment (CrCl <50mL/min).

ADVERSE REACTIONS
Upper abdominal pain, N/V, inj-site reactions, nasopharyngitis, weight gain, dizziness, akathisia, extrapyramidal disorder, headache, somnolence, agitation, anxiety, toothache, upper respiratory tract infection, back pain.

DRUG INTERACTIONS
See Dosage. May antagonize the effect of levodopa and other dopamine agonists. An additive effect may occur with other agents that also cause orthostatic hypotension. Avoid with other drugs known to prolong QTc interval, including Class 1A (eg, quinidine, procainamide) or Class III (eg, amiodarone, sotalol) antiarrhythmics, antipsychotics (eg, chlorpromazine, thioridazine), or antibiotics (eg, gatifloxacin, moxifloxacin). Carbamazepine may decrease levels. Additive exposure with oral paliperidone or oral/injectable risperidone. Caution with anticholinergics; may contribute to an elevated body temperature. Paroxetine (a potent CYP2D6 inhibitor) may increase exposure in CYP2D6 extensive metabolizers.

NURSING CONSIDERATIONS

Assessment: Assess for known hypersensitivity to drug/risperidone/any of the excipients, dementia-related psychosis, congenital long QT syndrome, history of cardiac arrhythmias, DM, risk factors for DM, history of clinically significant low WBCs or drug-induced leukopenia/neutropenia, Parkinson's disease, dementia with Lewy bodies, renal impairment, any other conditions where treatment is contraindicated or cautioned, pregnancy/nursing status, and possible drug interactions. Obtain baseline FPG in patients at risk for DM.

Monitoring: Monitor for hypersensitivity reactions, NMS, TD, QT prolongation, hyperprolactinemia, orthostatic hypotension, syncope, cognitive and motor impairment, seizures, aspiration, priapism, disruption of body temperature, and other adverse reactions. Monitor for signs of hyperglycemia; perform periodic monitoring of FPG levels in patients with DM or at risk for DM. Monitor for signs/symptoms of leukopenia/neutropenia; frequently monitor CBC in patients with a history of clinically significant low WBC or drug-induced leukopenia/neutropenia. Monitor weight and renal function. Reassess periodically to determine need for continued treatment.

Patient Counseling: Advise patients on risk of orthostatic hypotension. Caution about operating machinery/driving. Advise to avoid overheating and becoming dehydrated. Instruct to inform physician about any concomitant medications. Advise to notify physician if pregnancy occurs or is intended. Instruct not to breastfeed.

Storage: 25°C (77°F); excursions permitted to 15-30°C (59-86°F).

INVIRASE — saquinavir mesylate RX

Class: Protease inhibitor

ADULT DOSAGE

HIV-1 Infection

≥16 Years:

1000mg bid + 100mg ritonavir bid

May administer in combination w/ other antiretroviral agents

When administering in combination w/ 400mg lopinavir + 100mg ritonavir, no additional ritonavir is recommended

PEDIATRIC DOSAGE

Pediatric use may not have been established

ADMINISTRATION
Oral route

Take w/in 2 hrs pc

Refer to ritonavir labeling for dosage and administration

Patients Unable to Swallow Caps

1. Open the caps and place contents into an empty container
2. Add 15mL of either sugar syrup or sorbitol syrup (for patients w/ Type 1 diabetes or glucose intolerance) or 3 tsp of jam to the contents of the caps in the container
3. Stir w/ a spoon for 30-60 sec
4. Administer the full amount prepared for each dose
5. Sus should be at room temperature before administering

HOW SUPPLIED

Cap: 200mg; Tab: 500mg

CONTRAINDICATIONS

Congenital long QT syndrome, refractory hypokalemia or hypomagnesemia, complete atrioventricular (AV) block w/o implanted pacemakers, high risk of complete AV block, severe hepatic impairment, and w/ drugs that both increase saquinavir plasma levels and prolong the QT interval. Coadministration w/ CYP3A substrates (eg, alfuzosin, amiodarone, bepridil, dofetilide, flecainide, lidocaine [systemic], propafenone, quinidine, trazodone, rifampin, dihydroergotamine, ergonovine, ergotamine, methylergonovine, cisapride, lovastatin, simvastatin, pimozide, sildenafil for treatment of pulmonary arterial HTN, triazolam, oral midazolam).

WARNINGS/PRECAUTIONS

Refer to the individual monograph of RTV. Interrupt therapy if serious or severe toxicity occurs until etiology is identified or toxicity resolves. May prolong PR and QT intervals in a dose-dependent fashion. 2nd- or 3rd-degree AV block and torsades de pointes reported. Do not initiate if QT interval >450 msec. If therapy is initiated w/ QT interval <450 msec, monitor ECG after 3-4 days; d/c if QT interval is >480 msec or increased >20 msec over pretreatment. Monitor ECG w/ preexisting conduction system abnormalities, certain heart diseases, electrolyte abnormalities, and hepatic impairment. Correct hypokalemia/hypomagnesemia prior to therapy and monitor periodically. New onset or exacerbation of diabetes mellitus (DM), hyperglycemia, diabetic ketoacidosis, immune reconstitution syndrome, autoimmune disorders (eg, Graves' disease, polymyositis, Guillain-Barre syndrome) in the setting of immune reconstitution, redistribution/accumulation of body fat, and spontaneous bleeding w/ hemophilia A and B reported. Worsening liver disease in patients w/ underlying hepatitis B or C, cirrhosis, chronic alcoholism, and/or other underlying liver abnormalities reported. Elevated cholesterol and/or TG levels observed; marked elevation in TGs is a risk factor for pancreatitis. Various degrees of cross-resistance observed. Caution w/ severe renal impairment, ESRD, and in elderly. Contains lactose; should not induce symptoms of intolerance.

ADVERSE REACTIONS

DM/hyperglycemia, lipodystrophy, N/V, diarrhea, abdominal pain, fatigue, fever, pneumonia, bronchitis, influenza, sinusitis, rash, pruritus.

DRUG INTERACTIONS

See Contraindications. Not recommended w/ garlic cap, fluticasone, salmeterol, ketoconazole or itraconazole >200mg/day, and tipranavir/RTV combination. Avoid w/ colchicine in patients w/ renal/hepatic impairment and tadalafil during initiation. Caution w/ drugs that prolong PR interval (eg, calcium channel blockers [CCBs], β-blockers, digoxin, atazanavir), lopinavir/RTV, ibutilide, sotalol, erythromycin, halofantrine, pentamidine, dexamethasone, methadone, proton pump inhibitors, neuroleptics, and anticonvulsants. Drugs that affect CYP3A and/or P-gp may modify pharmacokinetics. May increase levels of bosentan, maraviroc, warfarin (monitor INR), colchicine, ketoconazole, rifabutin, TCAs, benzodiazepines, IV midazolam, CCBs, digoxin, salmeterol, fluticasone, atorvastatin, immunosuppressants, clarithromycin, and PDE-5 inhibitors. Increases quetiapine levels; consider alternative therapy. May decrease levels of methadone and ethinyl estradiol. Delavirdine, atazanavir, indinavir, clarithromycin, and omeprazole may increase levels. Efavirenz, nevirapine, dexamethasone, St. John's wort, garlic cap, and potent CYP3A inducers (eg, phenobarbital, phenytoin, carbamazepine) may decrease levels. May require initiation or adjustments of insulin or oral hypoglycemics for treatment of DM. Refer to PI for dosing modifications when used w/ certain concomitant therapies.

NURSING CONSIDERATIONS

Assessment: Assess for conditions where treatment is contraindicated or cautioned, renal/hepatic impairment, drug hypersensitivity, pregnancy/nursing status, and possible drug interactions. Obtain serum K^+ and Mg^{2+}, TG and cholesterol levels, and ECG prior to initiation of treatment.

Monitoring: Periodically monitor ECG results, serum K^+ and Mg^{2+} levels, TG and cholesterol levels, and hepatic/renal function. Monitor for signs/symptoms of AV block, PR/QT interval prolongation, cardiac conduction abnormalities, torsades de pointes, bleeding, immune reconstitution syndrome, autoimmune disorders, fat redistribution/accumulation, new onset DM, and other adverse reactions.

Patient Counseling: Inform that therapy is not a cure for HIV-1 infection; opportunistic infections may still occur. Advise to avoid doing things that can spread HIV-1 infection to others. Inform that changes in the ECG (PR interval or QT interval prolongation) may occur; instruct to consult physician if experiencing dizziness, lightheadedness, or palpitations. Advise to report the use of any other prescription/nonprescription medications or herbal products (eg, St. John's wort). Inform that redistribution or accumulation of body fat may occur. Advise that therapy should be used in combination w/ RTV. Counsel about the importance of taking medication every day; instruct not to alter dose or d/c therapy w/o consulting physician.

Storage: 25°C (77°F); excursions permitted to 15-30°C (59-86°F).

INVOKAMET – canagliflozin/metformin hydrochloride RX

Class: Biguanide/sodium-glucose cotransporter 2 (SGLT2) inhibitor

Lactic acidosis may occur due to metformin accumulation; risk increases with conditions such as renal/hepatic impairment, sepsis, dehydration, excess alcohol intake, and acute CHF. If lactic acidosis is suspected, d/c therapy and hospitalize patient immediately.

ADULT DOSAGE

Type 2 Diabetes Mellitus

Not adequately controlled on a regimen containing metformin or canagliflozin, or in patients who are already treated w/ both canagliflozin and metformin

Patients on Metformin:
Switch to Invokamet containing canagliflozin 50mg w/ a similar total daily dose of metformin

Patients on Canagliflozin:
Switch to Invokamet containing metformin 500mg w/ a similar total daily dose of canagliflozin

Patients Already Treated w/ Canagliflozin and Metformin:
Switch to Invokamet containing the same total daily doses of each component

Max: Metformin 2000mg and canagliflozin 300mg

PEDIATRIC DOSAGE

Pediatric use may not have been established

DOSE MODIFICATION

Concomitant Medications

UGT Inducers:

Patients Currently Tolerating 50mg bid w/ eGFR ≥60mL/min/1.73m²:
Consider increasing canagliflozin dose to 150mg bid if additional glycemic control is required

Patients w/ eGFR 45-<60mL/min/1.73m²:
Consider another antihyperglycemic agent

Renal Impairment

Moderate (eGFR 45-<60mL/min/1.73m²):
Limit canagliflozin dose to 50mg bid

SCr Levels ≥1.5mg/dL (Males)/≥1.4mg/dL (Females) or eGFR is Persistently <45mL/min/1.73m²:
Do not initiate or continue treatment

Other Important Modifications

Patients w/ Volume-Depletion Not Previously Treated w/ Canagliflozin:
Correct this condition before initiating treatment

ADMINISTRATION

Oral route

Take bid w/ meals, with gradual dose escalation to reduce GI side effects

HOW SUPPLIED

Tab: (Canagliflozin-Metformin) 50mg-500mg, 50mg-1000mg, 150mg-500mg, 150mg-1000mg

CONTRAINDICATIONS

Renal impairment (eg, SrCr ≥1.5mg/dL [males]/≥1.4mg/dL [females], or eGFR <45mL/min), ESRD, patients on dialysis, acute or chronic metabolic acidosis, including diabetic ketoacidosis.

WARNINGS/PRECAUTIONS

Not recommended in patients with type 1 DM or hepatic impairment, or for treatment of diabetic ketoacidosis. Causes intravascular volume contraction. Symptomatic hypotension may occur, particularly in patients with eGFR <60mL/min, elderly patients, patients on either diuretics or medications that interfere with the renin-angiotensin-aldosterone system (RAAS), or patients with low systolic BP; assess and correct volume status before initiating treatment in patients with ≥1 of these characteristics who were not already on canagliflozin. Increases SrCr and decreases eGFR; caution in patients with hypovolemia. Renal function abnormalities may occur; d/c with evidence of renal impairment. Temporarily d/c at the time of or prior to radiologic studies involving the use of intravascular iodinated contrast materials, withhold for 48 hrs subsequent to the procedure, and reinstitute only if renal function is normal. Temporarily d/c for any surgical procedure (except minor procedures not associated with restricted food and fluid intake); restart when oral intake is resumed and renal function is normal. May lead to hyperkalemia; increased risk in patients with moderate renal impairment who are taking medications that interfere with K^+ excretion or medications that interfere with the RAAS. Caution in patients susceptible to hypoglycemic effects, such as elderly, debilitated/malnourished patients, and those with adrenal/pituitary insufficiency, or alcohol intoxication. Increases risk of genital mycotic infections; caution in uncircumcised males. Hypersensitivity reactions, some serious, reported; d/c and treat if this occurs and monitor until signs/symptoms resolve. May decrease vitamin B12 levels; monitor hematologic parameters annually. D/C in hypoxic states (eg, acute CHF, shock, acute MI). Dose-related increases in LDL levels reported. Monitoring glycemic control with urine glucose tests or 1,5-anhydroglucitol assay is not recommended.

ADVERSE REACTIONS

Lactic acidosis, genital mycotic infections, UTIs, increased urination, N/V, diarrhea, flatulence, vulvovaginal pruritus, asthenia, indigestion, abdominal discomfort, headache.

DRUG INTERACTIONS

See Dosage. Monitor and adjust dose of therapy or concomitant drug in patients taking medication(s) that may affect renal function or result in a significant hemodynamic change or interfere with the disposition of metformin. Hypoglycemia may occur with other glucose-lowering agents (eg, insulin secretagogues [eg, sulfonylureas], insulin) or ethanol; may require a lower dose of insulin or insulin secretagogue. Alcohol potentiates the effect of metformin on lactate metabolism; avoid excessive alcohol intake. Metformin: May be difficult to recognize hypoglycemia with β-adrenergic blocking drugs. Cationic drugs that are eliminated by renal tubular secretion (eg, cimetidine, amiloride, digoxin, morphine, procainamide) may potentially produce an interaction; monitor and adjust dose of Invokamet and/or the interfering drug. Topiramate or other carbonic anhydrase inhibitors (eg, zonisamide, acetazolamide, dichlorphenamide) may induce metabolic acidosis and may increase the risk of lactic acidosis; monitor for signs/symptoms of acidosis. Monitor for loss of blood glucose control with thiazides and other diuretics, corticosteroids, phenothiazines, thyroid products, estrogens, oral contraceptives, phenytoin, nicotinic acid, sympathomimetics, calcium channel blockers, and INH; monitor for hypoglycemia when such drugs are withdrawn during therapy. Canagliflozin: Rifampin lowered exposure, which may reduce efficacy. Increased digoxin exposure; monitor for a need to adjust dose of either drug.

NURSING CONSIDERATIONS

Assessment: Assess for metabolic acidosis, risk factors for lactic acidosis, type of DM, diabetic ketoacidosis, predisposition to hyperkalemia, alcoholism, hypoxemia, presence of malnourishment or debilitation, adrenal/pituitary insufficiency, risk for genital mycotic infections, inadequate vitamin B12 or Ca^{2+} intake/absorption, drug hypersensitivity, any other conditions where treatment is cautioned, pregnancy/nursing status, and possible drug interactions. Assess if patient is planning to undergo any surgical procedure, or radiologic studies involving the use of intravascular iodinated contrast materials. Assess volume status. Obtain baseline FPG and HbA1c levels, renal/hepatic function, and hematologic parameters.

Monitoring: Monitor for signs/symptoms of lactic acidosis, hypotension, genital mycotic infections, hypersensitivity reactions, hypoxic states, and other adverse reactions. Monitor renal function, especially in elderly, at least annually. Monitor hematologic parameters annually. Perform routine serum vitamin B12 measurements at 2- to 3-yr intervals in patients predisposed to developing subnormal vitamin B12 levels. Monitor FPG and HbA1c, and LDL levels. Periodically monitor serum K^+ levels in patients with impaired renal function and in patients predisposed to hyperkalemia due to medications or other medical conditions.

Patient Counseling: Inform of the risk of lactic acidosis; instruct to d/c immediately and notify physician if unexplained hyperventilation, myalgias, malaise, unusual somnolence, or other nonspecific symptoms occur. Counsel against excessive alcohol intake. Inform about the importance of regular testing of renal function and hematological parameters while on therapy. Instruct to seek medical advice promptly during periods of stress (eg, fever, trauma, infection, surgery) as medication requirements may change. Instruct to take only as prescribed. Instruct to report to physician if pregnant, nursing, or experiencing symptoms of hypotension. Instruct to have adequate fluid intake. Counsel on the signs/symptoms of UTI, vaginal yeast infection, balanitis, and balanoposthitis; inform of treatment options and when to seek medical advice. Instruct to d/c therapy and consult physician if any signs/symptoms suggesting an allergic reaction or angioedema develop.

Storage: 20-25°C (68-77°F); excursions permitted between 15-30°C (59-86°F). Protect from moisture. Do not put in pill boxes or pill organizers.

INVOKANA – canagliflozin

RX

Class: Sodium-glucose cotransporter 2 (SGLT2) inhibitor

ADULT DOSAGE

Type 2 Diabetes Mellitus

Initial: 100mg qd before the 1st meal of the day

Titrate: May increase to 300mg qd in patients tolerating therapy who have an eGFR ≥60mL/min/1.73m^2 and require additional glycemic control

PEDIATRIC DOSAGE

Pediatric use may not have been established

DOSE MODIFICATION

Concomitant Medications

UDP-Glucuronosyl Transferase Enzyme Inducers (eg, Rifampin, Phenytoin, Phenobarbital, Ritonavir):

eGFR ≥60mL/min/1.73m^2: Consider increasing canagliflozin dose to 300mg qd in patients tolerating 100mg qd and requiring additional glycemic control

eGFR 45-<60mL/min/1.73m^2: Consider another antihyperglycemic agent

Renal Impairment

Moderate (eGFR 45-<60mL/min/1.73m^2): Limit dose to 100mg qd

eGFR <45mL/min/1.73m^2: Do not initiate treatment

D/C therapy when eGFR is persistently <45mL/min/1.73m^2

ADMINISTRATION

Oral route

HOW SUPPLIED

Tab: 100mg, 300mg

CONTRAINDICATIONS

Severe renal impairment (eGFR <30mL/min/1.73m^2), ESRD, patients on dialysis.

WARNINGS/PRECAUTIONS

Not recommended w/ type 1 DM or severe hepatic impairment, or for treatment of diabetic ketoacidosis. Causes intravascular volume contraction. Symptomatic hypotension may occur, particularly in patients w/ renal impairment (eGFR <60mL/min/1.73m^2), elderly patients, patients on either diuretics or medications that interfere w/ the renin-angiotensin-aldosterone system (RAAS), or patients w/ low systolic BP; assess and correct volume status before initiating treatment in patients w/ ≥1 of these characteristics. Increases SrCr and decreases eGFR; caution in patients w/ hypovolemia. Renal function abnormalities may occur; monitor renal function more frequently in patients w/ an eGFR <60mL/min/1.73m^2. May lead to hyperkalemia; increased risk in patients w/ moderate renal impairment who are taking medications that interfere w/ K^+ excretion or medications that interfere w/ the RAAS. Increases risk of genital mycotic infections; caution in uncircumcised males. Hypersensitivity reactions, some serious, reported; d/c and treat if this occurs and monitor until signs/symptoms resolve. Dose-related increases in LDL levels reported. Monitoring glycemic control w/ urine glucose tests or 1,5-anhydroglucitol assay is not recommended.

ADVERSE REACTIONS

Genital mycotic infections, UTIs, increased urination, vulvovaginal pruritus, hypersensitivity reactions, hypoglycemia, increases in serum K^+ levels.

DRUG INTERACTIONS

See Dose Modification. May increase risk of hypoglycemia when combined w/ insulin or an insulin secretagogue; lower dose of insulin or insulin secretagogue may be required. Rifampin decreases exposure. Increases levels of digoxin; monitor appropriately.

NURSING CONSIDERATIONS

Assessment: Assess for diabetic ketoacidosis, type of DM, volume status, predisposition to hyperkalemia, risk for genital mycotic infections, drug hypersensitivity, pregnancy/nursing status, and possible drug interactions. Assess baseline renal/hepatic function, LDL levels, and BP.

Monitoring: Monitor for signs/symptoms of hypotension, genital mycotic infections, hypersensitivity reactions, and other adverse reactions. Monitor renal function, serum K^+ levels, and LDL levels.

Patient Counseling: Inform of the risks, benefits, and alternative modes of therapy. Advise about the importance of adherence to dietary instructions, regular physical activity, periodic blood glucose monitoring and HbA1C testing, recognition and management of hypoglycemia and hyperglycemia, and assessment for diabetes complications. Instruct to seek medical advice promptly during periods of stress (eg, fever, trauma, infection, surgery) as medication requirements may change. Instruct to report to physician if pregnant, nursing, or experiencing symptoms of hypotension. Instruct to have adequate fluid intake. Counsel on the signs/symptoms of UTI, vaginal yeast infection, balanitis, and balanoposthitis; inform of treatment options and when to seek medical advice. Instruct to d/c therapy and consult physician if any signs/symptoms suggesting an allergic reaction or angioedema develop.

Storage: 25°C (77°F); excursions permitted to 15-30°C (59-86°F).

ISENTRESS – raltegravir

RX

Class: HIV-integrase strand transfer inhibitor

ADULT DOSAGE

HIV-1 Infection

Combination w/ Other Antiretrovirals:

Tab:
400mg bid

In Combination w/ Rifampin:
800mg bid

PEDIATRIC DOSAGE

HIV-1 Infection

Combination w/ Other Antiretrovirals:

≥4 Weeks of Age:

Tab:
≥25kg: 400mg bid

Tab, Chewable:
11-<14kg: 75mg bid
14-<20kg: 100mg bid
20-<28kg: 150mg bid
28-<40kg: 200mg bid
≥40kg: 300mg bid
Max: 300mg bid

Sus:
3-<4kg: 1mL (20mg) bid
4-<6kg: 1.5mL (30mg) bid
6-<8kg: 2mL (40mg) bid
8-<11kg: 3mL (60mg) bid
11-<14kg: 4mL (80mg) bid
14-<20kg: 5mL (100mg) bid
Max: 100mg bid

ADMINISTRATION

Oral route

Take w/ or w/o food

Tab
Swallow whole

Tab, Chewable
Chew or swallow whole

Sus
1. Pour sus pack contents into mixing cup, add 5mL of water, and mix
2. To mix, swirl mixing cup w/ a gentle circular motion for 30-60 sec; do not turn mixing cup upside down
3. Measure the recommended dose w/ provided syringe and administer w/in 30 min of mixing
4. Discard any remaining sus

HOW SUPPLIED

Sus (Powder): 100mg/pkt; Tab: 400mg; Tab, Chewable: 25mg, 100mg* *scored

WARNINGS/PRECAUTIONS

Do not substitute chewable tabs or oral sus for the 400mg film-coated tab; not bioequivalent. Severe, potentially life-threatening, and fatal skin reactions (eg, Stevens-Johnson syndrome, toxic epidermal necrolysis), and hypersensitivity reactions reported; d/c therapy and other suspect agents immediately if signs/symptoms develop. Immune reconstitution syndrome reported. Autoimmune disorders (eg, Graves' disease, polymyositis, Guillain-Barre syndrome) reported in the setting of immune reconstitution and can occur many months after initiation of treatment. Caution in patients at increased risk of myopathy or rhabdomyolysis and in elderly. Avoid dosing before a dialysis session. (Tab, Chewable) Contains phenylalanine.

ADVERSE REACTIONS

Insomnia, headache, nausea, hyperglycemia, ALT/AST elevation, hyperbilirubinemia, low ANC, serum lipase/creatine kinase/pancreatic amylase increase, thrombocytopenia.

DRUG INTERACTIONS

See Dosage. UGT1A1 inhibitors may increase levels. UGT1A1 inducers (eg, rifampin) may decrease levels. Coadministration or staggered administration w/ aluminum- and/or magnesium hydroxide-containing antacids is not recommended.

NURSING CONSIDERATIONS

Assessment: Assess for risk of myopathy or rhabdomyolysis, previous hypersensitivity to the drug, pregnancy/nursing status, and possible drug interactions. Assess if patient is undergoing dialysis session. (Tab, Chewable) Assess for phenylketonuria.

Monitoring: Monitor for signs/symptoms of severe skin/hypersensitivity reactions, immune reconstitution syndrome, autoimmune disorders, and other adverse reactions. If a severe skin reaction or hypersensitivity reaction develops, monitor clinical status, including liver aminotransferases.

Patient Counseling: Instruct to inform physician if any unusual symptom develops, or if any known symptom persists or worsens. Inform that drug is not a cure for HIV-1 infection and that illnesses associated w/ HIV-1 may still be experienced. Advise to avoid doing things that can spread HIV-1 to others. Instruct to always practice safe sex by using a latex or polyurethane condom. Instruct to immediately d/c therapy and seek medical attention if rash develops w/ signs/symptoms of a more serious skin reaction. Instruct to immediately report to physician if any unexplained muscle pain, tenderness, or weakness occurs. Instruct to avoid taking aluminum- and/or magnesium hydroxide-containing antacids. (Tab, Chewable) Inform patients w/ phenylketonuria that product contains phenylalanine. (Sus) Instruct to administer w/in 30 min of mixing.

Storage: 20-25°C (68-77°F); excursions permitted to 15-30°C (59-86°F). (Tab, Chewable) Protect from moisture. (Sus) Do not open foil pkt until ready for use.

ISONIAZID – isoniazid

RX

Class: Isonicotinic acid hydrazide

Severe, fatal hepatitis may develop. Monitor LFTs monthly. D/C drug if signs and symptoms of hepatic damage occur. Patients with tuberculosis (TB) who have isoniazid-induced hepatitis should have appropriate treatment with alternative drugs. Defer preventive treatment in persons with acute hepatic disease.

ADULT DOSAGE

Tuberculosis

Treatment:

Usual:

5mg/kg (up to 300mg/day) in a single dose or 15mg/kg (up to 900mg/day) 2 or 3X/week

Pulmonary Tuberculosis (TB) w/o HIV Infection:

Option 1: Daily isoniazid + rifampin + pyrazinamide for 8 weeks followed by 16 weeks of isoniazid + rifampin, daily or 2 to 3X/week; ethambutol or streptomycin should be added to the initial regimen until sensitivity to isoniazid and rifampin is demonstrated

Option 2: Daily isoniazid + rifampin + pyrazinamide for 2 weeks followed by 2X/week administration of the same drugs for 6 weeks, subsequently 2X/week isoniazid + rifampin for 16 weeks

Option 3: Isoniazid + rifampin + pyrazinamide + ethambutol or streptomycin 3X/week for 6 months

All regimens given 2 or 3X/week should be administered by directly observed therapy

Extrapulmonary TB:

May be effective w/ 6-9 months of short-course regimen; administer therapy for 12 months for miliary TB, or bone/joint TB

Prevention:

>30kg:

300mg/day as a single dose

Concomitant Administration of Pyridoxine (B6):

Recommended in malnourished patients and in those predisposed to neuropathy (eg, alcoholics and diabetics)

PEDIATRIC DOSAGE

Tuberculosis

Treatment:

Usual:

10-15mg/kg (up to 300mg/day) as a single dose or 20-40mg/kg (up to 900mg/day), 2 or 3X/week

Pulmonary Tuberculosis (TB) w/o HIV Infection:

Option 1: Daily isoniazid + rifampin + pyrazinamide for 8 weeks followed by 16 weeks of isoniazid + rifampin, daily or 2 to 3X/week; ethambutol or streptomycin should be added to the initial regimen until sensitivity to isoniazid and rifampin is demonstrated

Option 2: Daily isoniazid + rifampin + pyrazinamide for 2 weeks followed by 2X/week administration of the same drugs for 6 weeks, subsequently 2X/week isoniazid + rifampin for 16 weeks

Option 3: Isoniazid + rifampin + pyrazinamide + ethambutol or streptomycin 3X/week for 6 months

All regimens given 2 or 3X/week should be administered by directly observed therapy

Extrapulmonary TB:

May be effective w/ 6-9 months of short-course regimen; administer therapy for 12 months for miliary TB, bone/joint TB and tuberculous meningitis

Prevention:

10mg/kg (up to 300mg/day) as a single dose or 20-30mg/kg (not to exceed 900mg/day) 2X/week, under the direct observation of a healthcare worker at the time of administration

Concomitant Administration of Pyridoxine (B6):

Recommended in malnourished patients and in those predisposed to neuropathy (eg, alcoholics and diabetics)

ADMINISTRATION
Oral and IM routes

HOW SUPPLIED
Inj: 100mg/mL; Syrup: 50mg/5mL; Tab: 100mg, 300mg

CONTRAINDICATIONS
Severe hypersensitivity reactions, including drug-induced hepatitis, previous INH-associated hepatic injury, severe adverse effects (eg, drug fever, chills, arthritis), acute liver disease of any etiology.

WARNINGS/PRECAUTIONS
D/C if hypersensitivity occurs. Monitor closely with liver or renal disease, daily alcohol users, pregnancy, age >35, and concurrent chronic medications. Precaution with HIV seropositive patients. Take with vitamin B6 in malnourished and those predisposed to neuropathy.

ADVERSE REACTIONS
Peripheral neuropathy, N/V, anorexia, epigastric distress, elevated serum transaminases, bilirubinemia, jaundice, hepatitis, skin eruptions, pyridoxine deficiency.

DRUG INTERACTIONS
Alcohol is associated with hepatitis. May increase phenytoin, theophylline, and valproate serum levels. Do not take with food. Severe acetaminophen toxicity reported. Decreases carbamazepine metabolism and area under the curve of ketoconazole. Avoid tyramine- and histamine-containing foods.

NURSING CONSIDERATIONS

Assessment: Assess for previous isoniazid-associated hepatic injury, acute liver disease, HIV status, pregnancy status, age, and drug interactions. Document reasons for therapy, culture, and susceptibility.

Monitoring: Prior to therapy and periodically thereafter, measure hepatic enzymes (AST, ALT). D/C at 1st sign of hypersensitivity reaction. Monitor for peripheral neuropathy, convulsions, N/V, agranulocytosis, hemolytic anemia, systemic lupus erythematosus-like syndrome, metabolic and endocrine reactions (hyperglycemia, pyridoxine deficiency, pellagra).

Patient Counseling: Instruct to immediately report signs/symptoms consistent with liver damage or other adverse events (unexplained anorexia, N/V, dark urine, icterus, rash, persistent paresthesias of the hands and feet, persistent fatigue, weakness or fever of >3 days duration, and/or abdominal tenderness). Instruct to take drug without food, and to take pyridoxine tabs if peripheral neuropathy develops.

Storage: Tab: 20-25°C (68-77°F). Syrup: 15-30°C (59-86°F). Protect from light and moisture. Dispense in tight, light-resistant container. Inj: 20-25°C (68-77°F). Protect from light. If vial contents crystallize, warm vial to room temperature to redissolve crystals before use.

IXEMPRA – ixabepilone RX

Class: Antimicrotubule agent

In combination with capecitabine, contraindicated in patients with AST/ALT >2.5X ULN or bilirubin >1X ULN due to increased risk of toxicity and neutropenia-related death.

ADULT DOSAGE

Breast Cancer

Combination w/ Capecitabine:
Metastatic or locally advanced breast cancer resistant to treatment w/ an anthracycline and a taxane, or in patients whose cancer is taxane resistant and for whom further anthracycline therapy is contraindicated

40mg/m^2 IV over 3 hrs every 3 weeks
BSA >2.2m^2: Calculate dose based on 2.2m^2

Monotherapy:
Metastatic or locally advanced breast cancer in patients whose tumors are resistant or refractory to anthracyclines, taxanes, and capecitabine

40mg/m^2 IV over 3 hrs every 3 weeks
BSA >2.2m^2: Calculate dose based on 2.2m^2

PEDIATRIC DOSAGE
Pediatric use may not have been established

Retreatment Criteria:
Do not begin a new cycle of treatment unless neutrophil count is ≥1500 cells/mm^3, platelet count is ≥100,000 cells/mm^3, and nonhematologic toxicities have improved to Grade 1 (mild) or resolved

Premedication

All patients must be premedicated approx 1 hr before infusion w/:

An H_1 antagonist (eg, diphenhydramine 50mg PO or equivalent) and an H_2 antagonist (eg, ranitidine 150-300mg PO or equivalent)

Patients who experienced a hypersensitivity reaction require premedication w/ corticosteroids (eg, dexamethasone 20mg IV, 30 min before infusion or PO, 60 min before infusion) in addition to pretreatment w/ H_1 and H_2 antagonists

DOSE MODIFICATION

Concomitant Medications

Strong CYP3A4 Inhibitors (Including Grapefruit Juice): Avoid concomitant use; if coadministration is necessary, reduce dose to 20mg/m^2. If the strong inhibitor is discontinued, allow a washout period of approx 1 week before adjusting the dose upward to the indicated dose

Strong CYP3A4 Inducers: Avoid concomitant use; if coadministration is necessary, gradually increase dose to 60mg/m^2 IV over 4 hrs once patient has been maintained on a strong CYP3A4 inducer. If the strong inducer is discontinued, return to the dose used prior to initiation of the strong inducer

Hepatic Impairment

Monotherapy:

AST and ALT ≤10X ULN and Bilirubin ≤1.5X ULN: 32mg/m^2

AST and ALT ≤10X ULN and Bilirubin >1.5-≤3X ULN: 20-30mg/m^2

Recommendations are for 1st course of therapy; further decreases in subsequent courses should be based on individual tolerance

Adverse Reactions

Monotherapy or Combination Therapy:

Nonhematologic Toxicities:

Grade 2 Neuropathy (Moderate) Lasting ≥7 Days: Decrease dose by 20%

Grade 3 Neuropathy (Severe) Lasting <7 Days: Decrease dose by 20%

Grade 3 Neuropathy (Severe) Lasting ≥7 Days or Disabling Neuropathy: D/C treatment

Any Grade 3 Toxicity (Severe) Other Than Neuropathy: Decrease dose by 20%

Any Grade 4 Toxicity (Disabling): D/C treatment

Hematologic Toxicities:

Neutrophil <500 cells/mm^3 for ≥7 Days: Decrease dose by 20%

Febrile Neutropenia: Decrease dose by 20%

Platelets <25,000/mm^3 or Platelets <50,000/mm^3 w/ Bleeding: Decrease dose by 20%

Refer to PI for capecitabine dose modifications

ADMINISTRATION

IV route

Preparation and Administration

Prior to constituting ixabepilone for inj, remove the kit from the refrigerator and allowed to stand at room temperature for approx 30 min. When the vials are 1st removed from the refrigerator, a white precipitate may be observed in the diluents vial. This precipitate will dissolve to form a clear sol once the diluents warms to room temperature. After constituting w/ the diluent, the concentration of ixabepilone is 2mg/mL

To Constitute:

1. W/ a suitable syringe, withdraw the diluents and slowly inject it into the ixabepilone for inj vial:

15mg Ixempra: Constitute w/ 8mL of diluent

45mg Ixempra: Constitute w/ 23.5mL of diluent

2. Gently swirl and invert the vial until the powder is completely dissolved

To Dilute:

Before administration, the constituted sol must be further diluted w/ 1 of the specified infusion fluids listed below. The infusion must be prepared in a DEHP [di-(2-ethylhexyl) phthalate] free bag

The following infusion fluids have been qualified for use:

1. Lactated Ringer's inj

2. 0.9% NaCl inj (pH adjusted w/ sodium bicarbonate inj)
When using a 250mL or a 500mL bag of 0.9% NaCl inj to prepare the infusion, the pH must be adjusted to a pH between 6.0 and 9.0 by adding 2mEq (eg, 2mL of an 8.4% w/v sol or 4mL of a 4.2% w/v sol) of sodium bicarbonate inj, prior to the addition of the constituted sol
3. PLASMA-LYTE A inj pH 7.4

For most doses, a 250mL bag of infusion fluid is sufficient. However, it is necessary to check the final infusion concentration of each dose based on the volume of infusion fluid to be used. The final concentration for infusion must be between 0.2mg/mL and 0.6mg/mL; refer to PI for how to calculate the final infusion concentration

1. Withdraw the appropriate volume of constituted sol containing 2mg/mL
2. Transfer to an IV bag containing an appropriate volume of infusion fluid to achieve the final desired concentration
3. Thoroughly mix the infusion bag by manual rotation

The infusion sol must be administered through an appropriate in-line filter w/ a microporous membrane of 0.2-1.2 microns. DEHP-free infusion containers and administration sets must be used. Any remaining sol should be discarded according to institutional procedures for antineoplastics

HOW SUPPLIED
Inj: 15mg, 45mg

CONTRAINDICATIONS
History of a severe (CTC Grade 3/4) hypersensitivity reaction to agents containing Cremophor EL or its derivatives (eg, polyoxyethylated castor oil). Neutrophil count <1500 cells/mm^3 or platelet count <100,000 cells/mm^3. In combination with capecitabine, patients with AST/ALT >2.5X ULN or bilirubin >1X ULN.

WARNINGS/PRECAUTIONS
Peripheral neuropathy reported; caution with diabetes mellitus (DM) or preexisting peripheral neuropathy. Myelosuppression, which is dose-dependent and primarily manifested as neutropenia, reported; frequently monitor peripheral blood cell counts. Monotherapy is not recommended in patients with AST/ALT >10X ULN or bilirubin >3X ULN, and should be used with caution in patients with AST/ALT >5X ULN. Observe for hypersensitivity reactions; d/c infusion and start aggressive supportive treatment if severe hypersensitivity reactions occur. May cause fetal harm. Cardiac adverse reactions (eg, myocardial ischemia, ventricular dysfunction) reported during combination therapy; caution with history of cardiac disease, and consider discontinuation of ixabepilone if cardiac ischemia or impaired cardiac function develops. Contains dehydrated alcohol USP; consider possibility of CNS and other effects of alcohol.

ADVERSE REACTIONS
Peripheral sensory neuropathy, fatigue/asthenia, myalgia/arthralgia, alopecia, N/V, stomatitis/mucositis, diarrhea, musculoskeletal pain, palmar-plantar erythrodysesthesia (hand-foot) syndrome, anorexia, abdominal pain, nail disorder, constipation, hematologic abnormalities.

DRUG INTERACTIONS
Strong CYP3A4 inhibitors (eg, ketoconazole, itraconazole, clarithromycin, atazanavir, grapefruit juice) may increase levels; avoid, or if must be coadministered, reduce dose of ixabepilone. Caution with mild/moderate CYP3A4 inhibitors (eg, erythromycin, fluconazole, verapamil). Monitor closely for acute toxicities in patients receiving CYP3A4 inhibitors during treatment. Strong CYP3A4 inducers (eg, rifampin, dexamethasone) may decrease levels; avoid, or if must be coadministered, consider gradual dose adjustment of ixabepilone. St. John's wort may decrease levels unpredictably; avoid concomitant use.

NURSING CONSIDERATIONS

Assessment: Assess for history of a severe hypersensitivity reaction to Cremophor EL or its derivatives (eg, polyoxyethylated castor oil), DM, preexisting peripheral neuropathy, history of cardiac disease, pregnancy/nursing status, and possible drug interactions. Obtain CBC and LFTs.

Monitoring: Monitor for signs/symptoms of neuropathy, myelosuppression, hypersensitivity reactions, cardiac ischemia/impairment, and other adverse reactions. Perform periodic clinical observation and lab tests (eg, CBC, LFTs).

Patient Counseling: Advise to report to physician any numbness and tingling of the hands or feet, chest pain, difficulty breathing, palpitations, or unusual weight gain. Instruct to contact physician if a fever of ≥100.5°F or other evidence of potential infection (eg, chills, cough, burning or pain on urination) develops, or if experiencing urticaria, pruritus, rash, flushing, swelling, dyspnea, chest tightness, or other hypersensitivity-related symptoms following an infusion. Advise to use effective contraceptive measures to prevent pregnancy and to avoid nursing during treatment.

Storage: 2-8°C (36-46°F). Protect from light. Constituted Sol: Dilute as soon as possible or store in the vial (not the syringe) for a max of 1 hr at room temperature and room light. Diluted with Infusion Fluid: Stable at room temperature and room light for a max of 6 hrs.

IZBA — travoprost RX

Class: Prostaglandin analogue

ADULT DOSAGE

Elevated Intraocular Pressure

Open-Angle Glaucoma/Ocular HTN:
1 drop in the affected eye(s) qpm

PEDIATRIC DOSAGE

Elevated Intraocular Pressure

Open-Angle Glaucoma/Ocular HTN:
≥16 Years:
1 drop in the affected eye(s) qpm

DOSE MODIFICATION

Concomitant Medications

Space dosing by at least 5 min if using >1 topical ophthalmic drug

ADMINISTRATION

Ocular route

HOW SUPPLIED

Sol: 0.003% [2.5mL, 5mL]

WARNINGS/PRECAUTIONS

May cause changes to pigmented tissues (eg, increased pigmentation of the iris [may be permanent], periorbital tissue, and eyelashes [may be reversible]); regularly examine patients who develop noticeably increased iris pigmentation. May gradually change eyelashes and vellus hair in the treated eye. Caution with active intraocular inflammation (eg, uveitis); inflammation may be exacerbated. Macular edema, including cystoid macular edema, reported; caution in aphakic patients, pseudophakic patients with a torn posterior lens capsule, or patients with known risk factors for macular edema. Bacterial keratitis associated with the use of multiple-dose containers reported. Contact lenses should be removed prior to instillation and may be reinserted 15 min following administration.

ADVERSE REACTIONS

Ocular hyperemia, decreased visual acuity, eye discomfort, foreign body sensation, pain, pruritus.

NURSING CONSIDERATIONS

Assessment: Assess for active intraocular inflammation, aphakia, pseudophakia with a torn posterior lens capsule, risk factors for macular edema, and pregnancy/nursing status.

Monitoring: Monitor for increased iris/eyelid/eyelash pigmentation, changes in eyelashes/vellus hair in the treated eye, macular edema, bacterial keratitis, and other adverse reactions.

Patient Counseling: Inform of the possibility of increased brown pigmentation of the iris, eyelid skin darkening, and eyelash and vellus hair changes in the treated eye. Instruct to avoid allowing the tip of the dispensing container to contact the eye, surrounding structures, fingers, or any other surface to avoid contamination. Advise to immediately consult physician about the continued use of treatment if an intercurrent ocular condition (eg, trauma, infection) develops, if undergoing ocular surgery, or if any ocular reactions, particularly conjunctivitis and eyelid reactions, develop. Advise that contact lenses should be removed prior to instillation and may be reinserted 15 min following administration. Instruct that if using >1 topical ophthalmic drug, to administer the drugs at least 5 min apart.

Storage: 2-25°C (36-77°F).

JALYN — dutasteride/tamsulosin hydrochloride RX

Class: 5-alpha reductase inhibitor/alpha antagonist

ADULT DOSAGE

Benign Prostatic Hyperplasia

1 cap qd, 30 min after the same meal each day

PEDIATRIC DOSAGE

Pediatric use may not have been established

ADMINISTRATION

Oral route

Swallow cap whole; do not chew, crush, or open

HOW SUPPLIED

Cap: (Dutasteride-Tamsulosin) 0.5mg-0.4mg

CONTRAINDICATIONS

Pregnancy, women of childbearing potential, pediatric patients.

WARNINGS/PRECAUTIONS

Not approved for the prevention of prostate cancer. Orthostatic hypotension/syncope may occur; avoid situations where syncope may result in an injury. May reduce serum prostate specific antigen (PSA) concentration during therapy; establish a new baseline PSA at least 3 months after starting therapy and monitor PSA periodically thereafter. Any confirmed increase from the lowest PSA value during treatment may signal the presence of prostate cancer and should be evaluated. May increase the risk of high-grade prostate cancer. Prior to initiating treatment, consideration should be given to other urological conditions that may cause similar symptoms; BPH and prostate cancer may coexist. Risk to male fetus; cap should not be handled by pregnant women or women who may become pregnant. May cause priapism; may lead to permanent impotence if not properly treated. Avoid blood donation until at least 6 months following the last dose. Intraoperative floppy iris syndrome (IFIS) reported during cataract surgery; initiation of therapy is not recommended in patients for whom cataract surgery is scheduled. Caution w/ sulfa allergy; allergic reaction rarely reported. Reduced total sperm count, semen volume, and sperm motility reported.

ADVERSE REACTIONS

Ejaculation disorders, impotence, decreased libido, breast disorders, dizziness.

DRUG INTERACTIONS

Avoid w/ strong CYP3A4 inhibitors (eg, ketoconazole); may increase tamsulosin exposure. Caution w/ potent, chronic CYP3A4 inhibitors (eg, ritonavir), moderate CYP3A4 inhibitors (eg, erythromycin), strong (eg, paroxetine) or moderate (eg, terbinafine) CYP2D6 inhibitors; potential for significant increase in tamsulosin exposure. Potential for significant increase in tamsulosin exposure when coadministered w/ a combination of both CYP3A4 and CYP2D6 inhibitors. Caution w/ cimetidine and warfarin. Avoid w/ other α-adrenergic antagonists; may increase the risk of symptomatic hypotension. Caution w/ PDE-5 inhibitors; may cause symptomatic hypotension.

NURSING CONSIDERATIONS

Assessment: Assess for urological conditions that may cause similar symptoms, previous hypersensitivity to the drug, sulfa allergy, and possible drug interactions. Assess if patient is planning to undergo cataract surgery.

Monitoring: Monitor for signs/symptoms of prostate cancer, other urological diseases, orthostatic hypotension, syncope, priapism, IFIS, and allergic reactions. Obtain new baseline PSA at least 3 months after starting treatment and monitor PSA periodically thereafter.

Patient Counseling: Inform about the possible occurrence of symptoms related to orthostatic hypotension and the potential risk of syncope; instruct to avoid situations where injury may result if syncope occurs. Inform that an increase in high-grade prostate cancer was reported. Inform females who are pregnant or who may become pregnant not to handle the drug due to potential risk to the fetus. Instruct that if a pregnant woman or woman of childbearing potential comes in contact w/ a leaking cap to wash the area immediately w/ soap and water. Inform that cap may become deformed and/or discolored if kept at high temperatures; instruct to avoid use if this occurs. Advise about the possibility of priapism (rare) that may lead to permanent erectile dysfunction if not brought to immediate medical attention. Advise not to donate blood for at least 6 months following the last dose. Instruct to inform ophthalmologist of drug if considering cataract surgery.

Storage: 25°C (77°F); excursions permitted to 15-30°C (59-86°F).

JANUMET — metformin hydrochloride/sitagliptin RX

Class: Biguanide/dipeptidyl peptidase-4 (DPP-4) inhibitor

Lactic acidosis may occur due to metformin accumulation; risk increases w/ conditions such as sepsis, dehydration, excess alcohol intake, hepatic/renal impairment, and acute CHF. If acidosis is suspected, d/c therapy and hospitalize patient immediately.

ADULT DOSAGE

Type 2 Diabetes Mellitus

Initial:
Not Currently on Metformin: 50mg-500mg bid
Currently on Metformin: 50mg bid of sitagliptin + current metformin dose
Currently on Metformin 850mg bid: 50mg-1000mg bid
Titrate: Gradually escalate dose to reduce GI side effects

Max: 100mg-2000mg/day

PEDIATRIC DOSAGE

Pediatric use may not have been established

DOSE MODIFICATION

Concomitant Medications

Insulin Secretagogue (eg, Sulfonylurea)/Insulin: May require lower doses of insulin secretagogue or insulin

ADMINISTRATION

Oral route

Take bid w/ meals

Do not split or divide tab before swallowing

HOW SUPPLIED

Tab: (Sitagliptin/Metformin) 50mg/500mg, 50mg/1000mg

CONTRAINDICATIONS

Renal impairment (eg, SrCr ≥1.5mg/dL [men], ≥1.4mg/dL [women], or abnormal CrCl), acute or chronic metabolic acidosis, including diabetic ketoacidosis.

WARNINGS/PRECAUTIONS

Not for use in type 1 DM or for treatment of diabetic ketoacidosis. Acute pancreatitis, including fatal and nonfatal hemorrhagic or necrotizing pancreatitis, reported; d/c if pancreatitis is suspected. Avoid in patients w/ clinical or lab evidence of hepatic disease. Worsening renal function, including acute renal failure, reported; d/c w/ evidence of renal impairment. May decrease serum vitamin B12 levels. Temporarily suspend for any surgical procedure (except minor procedures not associated w/ restricted food and fluid intake); restart when oral intake is resumed and renal function is normal. Evaluate patients previously well controlled on therapy who develop lab abnormalities or clinical illness for evidence of ketoacidosis or lactic acidosis; d/c if acidosis occurs. Caution in patients susceptible to hypoglycemic effects, such as elderly/debilitated/malnourished patients, and those w/ adrenal/pituitary insufficiency or alcohol intoxication. Temporarily d/c at the time of or prior to radiologic studies involving the use of intravascular iodinated contrast materials, withhold for 48 hrs subsequent to the procedure, and reinstitute only if renal function is normal. D/C in hypoxic states (eg, acute CHF, shock, acute MI). Temporary loss of glycemic control may occur when exposed to stress (eg, fever, trauma, infection, surgery); may be necessary to withhold therapy and temporarily administer insulin. Caution in elderly. Sitagliptin: Serious hypersensitivity reactions reported; if suspected, d/c therapy, assess for other potential causes, and institute alternative treatment for DM. Caution in patients w/ history of angioedema w/ another DPP-4 inhibitor.

ADVERSE REACTIONS

Lactic acidosis, diarrhea, URTI, headache, nausea, abdominal pain.

DRUG INTERACTIONS

See Dose Modification. Hypoglycemia may occur w/ other glucose-lowering agents (eg, sulfonylureas, insulin) or ethanol. Caution w/ drugs that may affect renal function or result in significant hemodynamic change. Topiramate or other carbonic anhydrase inhibitors (eg, zonisamide, acetazolamide, dichlorphenamide) may induce metabolic acidosis; use w/ caution. Observe for loss of glycemic control w/ thiazides and other diuretics, corticosteroids, phenothiazines, thyroid products, estrogens, oral contraceptives, phenytoin, nicotinic acid, sympathomimetics, calcium channel blockers, and isoniazid. Metformin: May be difficult to recognize hypoglycemia w/ β-adrenergic blocking drugs. Alcohol potentiates the effect of metformin on lactate metabolism; avoid excessive alcohol intake. Cationic drugs (eg, cimetidine, amiloride, digoxin) that are eliminated by renal tubular secretion may potentially produce an interaction; monitor and adjust dose of Janumet and/or the interfering drug.

NURSING CONSIDERATIONS

Assessment: Assess for previous hypersensitivity to the drug, metabolic acidosis including diabetic ketoacidosis, risk factors for lactic acidosis, renal/hepatic impairment, history of pancreatitis, inadequate vitamin B12 or Ca^{2+} absorption, type of DM, alcoholism, hypoxemia, presence of malnourishment or debilitation, adrenal/pituitary insufficiency, history of angioedema w/ another DPP-4 inhibitor, pregnancy/nursing status, and possible drug interactions. Assess if patient is planning to undergo any surgical procedure, radiologic studies involving the use of intravascular iodinated contrast materials, or is under any form of stress. Obtain baseline FPG and HbA1c levels, and hematologic parameters.

Monitoring: Monitor for signs/symptoms of lactic acidosis, pancreatitis, hypoxic states, hypersensitivity reactions, and other adverse reactions. Monitor for changes in clinical status. Monitor renal function, especially in elderly, at least annually. Monitor hematologic parameters annually. Perform routine serum vitamin B12 measurements at 2- to 3-yr intervals in patients predisposed to developing subnormal vitamin B12 levels. Monitor FPG and HbA1c levels, and hepatic function periodically.

Patient Counseling: Inform of the risks, benefits, and alternative modes of therapy. Advise on the importance of adherence to dietary instructions, regular physical activity, periodic blood glucose monitoring and HbA1c testing, recognition/management of hypo/hyperglycemia, and assessment of diabetic complications. Instruct to seek medical advice during periods of stress (eg, fever, trauma, infection, surgery) as medication needs may change. Inform of the risk of lactic acidosis; instruct to d/c therapy immediately and contact physician if unexplained hyperventilation, myalgia, malaise, unusual somnolence, dizziness, slow or irregular heartbeat, sensation of feeling cold (especially in the extremities), or other nonspecific symptoms occur. Counsel against excessive alcohol intake. Inform that GI symptoms and acute pancreatitis may occur; instruct to d/c therapy promptly and contact physician if persistent severe abdominal pain occurs. Inform that allergic reactions may occur; instruct to d/c therapy and seek medical advice promptly if symptoms occur. Counsel to inform physician if any bothersome or unusual symptom develops, or if any symptom persists or worsens.

Storage: 20-25°C (68-77°F); excursions permitted to 15-30°C (59-86°F).

JANUMET XR – metformin hydrochloride/sitagliptin RX

Class: Biguanide/dipeptidyl peptidase-4 (DPP-4) inhibitor

Lactic acidosis may occur due to metformin accumulation; risk increases w/ conditions (eg, sepsis, dehydration, excess alcohol intake, hepatic/renal impairment, acute CHF). If acidosis is suspected, d/c therapy and hospitalize patient immediately.

ADULT DOSAGE

Type 2 Diabetes Mellitus

Initial:

Not Currently on Metformin: (100mg/1000mg)/day

Currently on Metformin: 100mg/day of sitagliptin + current metformin dose

Currently on Metformin IR 850mg bid or 1000mg bid: Two 50mg/1000mg tabs qd

Changing Between Janumet and Janumet XR: Maintain the same total daily dose of sitagliptin and metformin

Max: (100mg/2000mg)/day

PEDIATRIC DOSAGE

Pediatric use may not have been established

DOSE MODIFICATION

Concomitant Medications

Insulin Secretagogue (eg, Sulfonylurea)/Insulin: May require lower doses of insulin secretagogue or insulin

ADMINISTRATION

Oral route

Take qd w/ a meal, preferably in pm
Swallow tab whole; do not split, crush, or chew
Patients taking 2 tabs should take the 2 tabs together qd

HOW SUPPLIED

Tab, ER: (Sitagliptin/Metformin ER) 50mg/500mg, 50mg/1000mg, 100mg/1000mg

CONTRAINDICATIONS

Renal impairment (eg, SrCr ≥1.5mg/dL [men], ≥1.4mg/dL [women], or abnormal CrCl), acute or chronic metabolic acidosis, including diabetic ketoacidosis.

WARNINGS/PRECAUTIONS

Not for use in type 1 DM or for treatment of diabetic ketoacidosis. Acute pancreatitis, including fatal and nonfatal hemorrhagic or necrotizing pancreatitis, reported; d/c if pancreatitis is suspected. Avoid in patients w/ clinical or lab evidence of hepatic disease. Worsening renal function, including acute renal failure, reported; assess renal function before initiation of therapy and at least annually thereafter; d/c w/ evidence of renal impairment. May decrease vitamin B12 levels. Temporarily suspend for any surgical procedure (except minor procedures not associated w/ restricted food and fluid intake); restart when oral intake is resumed and renal function is normal. Evaluate patients previously well controlled on therapy who develop lab abnormalities or clinical illness for evidence of ketoacidosis or lactic acidosis; d/c if acidosis occurs. Caution in patients susceptible to hypoglycemic effects, such as elderly or debilitated/malnourished patients, and those w/ adrenal/pituitary insufficiency or alcohol intoxication. Temporarily d/c at the time of or prior to radiologic studies involving the use of intravascular iodinated contrast materials, withhold for 48 hrs subsequent to the procedure, and reinstitute only if renal function is normal. D/C in hypoxic states (eg, acute CHF, shock, acute MI). Temporary loss of glycemic control may occur when exposed to stress (eg, fever, trauma, infection, surgery); may be necessary to withhold therapy and temporarily administer insulin. Incompletely dissolved tabs being eliminated in the feces reported; assess adequacy of glycemic control if patient reports repeatedly seeing tabs in feces. Caution in elderly. Sitagliptin: Serious hypersensitivity reactions reported; if suspected, d/c therapy, assess for other potential causes, and institute alternative treatment for DM. Caution in patients w/ history of angioedema w/ another dipeptidyl peptidase-4 (DPP-4) inhibitor.

ADVERSE REACTIONS

Lactic acidosis, diarrhea, URTI, headache, nausea, abdominal pain.

DRUG INTERACTIONS

See Dose Modification. Hypoglycemia may occur w/ other glucose-lowering agents (eg, sulfonylureas, insulin) or ethanol. Caution w/ drugs that may affect renal function or result in significant hemodynamic change. Topiramate or other carbonic anhydrase inhibitors (eg, zonisamide, acetazolamide, dichlorphenamide) may induce metabolic acidosis; use w/ caution. Observe for loss of glycemic control w/ thiazides and other diuretics, corticosteroids, phenothiazines, thyroid products, estrogens, oral contraceptives, phenytoin, nicotinic acid, sympathomimetics, calcium channel blockers, and isoniazid. Metformin: May be difficult to recognize hypoglycemia w/ β-adrenergic blocking drugs. Alcohol potentiates the effect of metformin on lactate metabolism; avoid excessive alcohol intake. Cationic drugs (eg, cimetidine, amiloride, digoxin) that are eliminated by renal tubular secretion may potentially produce an interaction; monitor and adjust dose of Janumet XR and/or the interfering drug.

NURSING CONSIDERATIONS

Assessment: Assess for metabolic acidosis, risk factors for lactic acidosis, renal/hepatic impairment, previous hypersensitivity to the drug, history of pancreatitis, inadequate vitamin B12 or Ca^{2+} intake/absorption, type of DM, diabetic ketoacidosis, alcoholism, hypoxemia, presence of malnourishment or debilitation, adrenal/pituitary insufficiency, history of angioedema w/ another DPP-4 inhibitor, pregnancy/nursing status, and possible drug interactions. Assess if patient is planning to undergo any surgical procedure, radiologic studies involving the use of intravascular iodinated contrast materials, or is under any form of stress. Obtain baseline FPG and HbA1c levels, and hematologic parameters.

Monitoring: Monitor for signs/symptoms of lactic acidosis, pancreatitis, hypoxic states, hypersensitivity reactions, and other adverse reactions. Monitor for changes in clinical status. Monitor renal function, especially in elderly, at least annually. Monitor hematologic parameters annually. Perform routine serum vitamin B12 measurements at 2- to 3-yr intervals in patients predisposed to developing subnormal vitamin B12 levels. Monitor FPG and HbA1c levels, and hepatic function periodically.

Patient Counseling: Inform of the risks, benefits, and alternative modes of therapy. Advise on the importance of adherence to dietary instructions, regular physical activity, periodic blood glucose monitoring and HbA1c, renal function, and hematologic parameter testing, recognition/management of hypo/hyperglycemia, and assessment of diabetes complications. Instruct to seek medical advice during periods of stress (eg, fever, trauma, infection, surgery) as medication needs may change. Inform of the risk of lactic acidosis; instruct to d/c therapy immediately and notify physician if unexplained hyperventilation, myalgia, malaise, unusual somnolence, dizziness, slow or irregular heartbeat, sensation of feeling cold (especially in the extremities), or other nonspecific symptoms occur. Counsel against excessive alcohol intake. Inform that GI symptoms and acute pancreatitis may occur; instruct to d/c therapy promptly and contact physician if persistent severe abdominal pain occurs. Inform that allergic reactions may occur; instruct to d/c therapy and seek medical advice promptly if symptoms occur. Counsel to inform physician if any bothersome or unusual symptom develops, or if any known symptom persists or worsens. Inform that incompletely dissolved tabs may be eliminated in the feces; advise to report to physician if patient repeatedly see tabs in feces.

Storage: 20-25°C (68-77°F); excursions permitted to 15-30°C (59-86°F). Store in a dry place.

JANUVIA – sitagliptin RX

Class: Dipeptidyl peptidase-4 (DPP-4) inhibitor

ADULT DOSAGE

Type 2 Diabetes Mellitus

100mg qd

PEDIATRIC DOSAGE

Pediatric use may not have been established

DOSE MODIFICATION

Concomitant Medications

Insulin Secretagogue (eg, Sulfonylurea)/Insulin: May require lower dose of insulin secretagogue or insulin

Renal Impairment

Moderate (CrCl ≥30-<50mL/min): 50mg qd

Severe (CrCl <30mL/min): 25mg qd

ESRD Requiring Hemodialysis/Peritoneal Dialysis: 25mg qd; administer w/o regard to timing of dialysis

ADMINISTRATION

Oral route

May be taken w/ or w/o food

HOW SUPPLIED

Tab: 25mg, 50mg, 100mg

WARNINGS/PRECAUTIONS

Not for use w/ type 1 DM or for treatment of diabetic ketoacidosis. Acute pancreatitis reported; d/c if pancreatitis is suspected. Worsening renal function, including acute renal failure, reported. Serious hypersensitivity reactions reported; if suspected, d/c therapy, assess for other potential causes, and institute alternative treatment. Caution in patients w/ a history of angioedema w/ another DPP-4 inhibitor and in the elderly.

ADVERSE REACTIONS

Nasopharyngitis, URTI, headache.

DRUG INTERACTIONS

See Dose Modification. May slightly increase digoxin levels; monitor appropriately.

NURSING CONSIDERATIONS

Assessment: Assess for previous hypersensitivity to the drug, type of DM, diabetic ketoacidosis, history of pancreatitis, history of angioedema w/ another DPP-4 inhibitor, pregnancy/nursing status, and possible drug interactions. Obtain baseline renal function, FPG, and HbA1c levels.

Monitoring: Monitor for pancreatitis, hypersensitivity reactions, and other adverse reactions. Monitor FPG, HbA1c, and renal function periodically.

Patient Counseling: Inform of risks, benefits, and alternative modes of therapy. Advise on the importance of adherence to dietary instructions, regular physical activity, periodic blood glucose monitoring, HbA1c testing, recognition/management of hypoglycemia/hyperglycemia, and assessment of diabetic complications. Instruct to seek medical advice during periods of stress as medication requirements may change. Instruct to d/c use and notify physician if signs and symptoms of pancreatitis or allergic reactions occur. Instruct to inform physician if any unusual symptom develops, or if any known symptom persists or worsens.

Storage: 20-25°C (68-77°F); excursions permitted to 15-30°C (59-86°F).

JARDIANCE – empagliflozin RX

Class: Sodium-glucose cotransporter 2 (SGLT2) inhibitor

ADULT DOSAGE

Type 2 Diabetes Mellitus

10mg qam

Titrate: May increase to 25mg

PEDIATRIC DOSAGE

Pediatric use may not have been established

DOSE MODIFICATION

Renal Impairment

Baseline eGFR <45mL/min: Do not initiate treatment

eGFR Persistently <45mL/min: D/C treatment

Other Important Modifications

Patients w/ Volume Depletion: Correct this condition prior to initiating therapy

ADMINISTRATION

Oral route

Take w/ or w/o food

HOW SUPPLIED

Tab: 10mg, 25mg

CONTRAINDICATIONS

Severe renal impairment, ESRD, dialysis.

WARNINGS/PRECAUTIONS

Not recommended with type 1 DM or for treatment of diabetic ketoacidosis. Do not initiate in patients with an eGFR <45mL/min and d/c if eGFR is persistently <45mL/min. Causes intravascular volume contraction. Symptomatic hypotension may occur, particularly in patients with renal impairment, the elderly, in patients with low systolic BP, and in patients on diuretics; assess for volume contraction and correct volume status before initiating treatment, if indicated. Increases SrCr and decreases eGFR; caution in elderly patients and patients with moderate renal impairment. Increases risk for genital mycotic infections and UTIs. Increases in LDL levels may occur. Monitoring glycemic control with urine glucose tests or 1,5-anhydroglucitol assay is not recommended.

ADVERSE REACTIONS

UTIs, genital mycotic infections, dyslipidemia, increased urination, URTI.

DRUG INTERACTIONS

Increased risk of hypoglycemia with insulin secretagogues (eg, sulfonylurea) or insulin; a lower dose of the insulin secretagogue or insulin may be required. Coadministration with diuretics resulted in increased urine volume and frequency of voids, which might enhance the potential for volume depletion.

NURSING CONSIDERATIONS

Assessment: Assess for diabetic ketoacidosis, type of DM, volume contraction/status, risk for genital mycotic infections, drug hypersensitivity, pregnancy/nursing status, and possible drug interactions. Assess baseline renal function, LDL levels, and BP.

Monitoring: Monitor for signs/symptoms of hypotension, genital mycotic infections, UTIs, and other adverse reactions. Monitor renal function and LDL levels.

Patient Counseling: Inform of the risks, benefits, and alternative modes of therapy. Advise about the importance of adherence to dietary instructions, regular physical activity, periodic blood glucose monitoring and HbA1c testing, recognition and management of hypoglycemia and hyperglycemia, and assessment for diabetes complications. Instruct to seek medical advice promptly during periods of stress (eg, fever, trauma, infection), as medication requirements may change. Instruct to inform physician if pregnant/nursing, if experiencing symptoms of hypotension, if any unusual symptom develops, or if any known symptom persists or worsens. Instruct to have adequate fluid intake. Counsel on the signs/symptoms of UTIs, vaginal yeast infections, balanitis, and balanoposthitis; inform of treatment options and when to seek medical advice.

Storage: 25°C (77°F); excursions permitted to 15-30°C (59-86°F).

JENTADUETO – linagliptin/metformin hydrochloride — RX

Class: Biguanide/dipeptidyl peptidase-4 (DPP-4) inhibitor

Lactic acidosis may occur due to metformin accumulation; risk increases w/ conditions such as sepsis, dehydration, excess alcohol intake, hepatic/renal impairment, and acute CHF. If acidosis is suspected, d/c therapy and hospitalize patient immediately.

ADULT DOSAGE

Type 2 Diabetes Mellitus

Initial:

Not Currently on Metformin: 2.5mg-500mg bid

Currently on Metformin: 2.5mg linagliptin + current metformin dose taken at each of the 2 daily meals

Max: 2.5mg-1000mg bid

PEDIATRIC DOSAGE

Pediatric use may not have been established

DOSE MODIFICATION

Hepatic Impairment

Avoid in patients w/ clinical/lab evidence of hepatic disease

Concomitant Medications

Insulin Secretagogue (eg, Sulfonylurea)/Insulin: May require lower dose of insulin secretagogue or insulin

ADMINISTRATION
Oral route

Take w/ meals

HOW SUPPLIED
Tab: (Linagliptin-Metformin) 2.5mg-500mg, 2.5mg-850mg, 2.5mg-1000mg

CONTRAINDICATIONS
Renal impairment (eg, SrCr ≥1.5mg/dL [men], ≥1.4mg/dL [women], or abnormal CrCl), acute or chronic metabolic acidosis, including diabetic ketoacidosis.

WARNINGS/PRECAUTIONS
Not for use in type 1 DM or for treatment of diabetic ketoacidosis. Acute pancreatitis, including fatal pancreatitis, reported; d/c if pancreatitis is suspected. Assess renal function before initiation of therapy and at least annually thereafter; d/c w/ evidence of renal impairment. Temporarily d/c at the time of or prior to radiologic studies involving the use of intravascular iodinated contrast materials, withhold for 48 hrs subsequent to the procedure, and reinstitute only if renal function is normal. Temporarily d/c for any surgical procedure (except minor procedures not associated w/ restricted food and fluid intake); restart when oral intake is resumed and renal function is normal. Avoid in patients w/ clinical or lab evidence of hepatic disease. Caution in patients susceptible to hypoglycemic effects, such as elderly, debilitated/malnourished patients, and those w/ adrenal/pituitary insufficiency, or alcohol intoxication. Serious hypersensitivity reactions reported; if suspected, d/c therapy, assess for other potential causes, and institute alternative treatment for DM. Caution in patients w/ history of angioedema to another DPP-4 inhibitor. May decrease serum vitamin B12 levels. Promptly withhold in the presence of any condition associated w/ hypoxic states (eg, acute CHF, shock, acute MI), dehydration, or sepsis. Do not initiate in patients ≥80 yrs of age unless renal function is not reduced. Caution in elderly.

ADVERSE REACTIONS
Lactic acidosis, nasopharyngitis, diarrhea.

DRUG INTERACTIONS
See Dosage. Hypoglycemia may occur w/ other glucose-lowering agents (eg, insulin secretagogues, insulin) or ethanol. Observe for loss of glycemic control w/ thiazides and other diuretics, corticosteroids, phenothiazines, thyroid products, estrogens, oral contraceptives, phenytoin, nicotinic acid, sympathomimetics, calcium channel blockers, and isoniazid; observe for hypoglycemia when such drugs are withdrawn during therapy. Linagliptin: Strong P-gp or CYP3A4 inducers (eg, rifampin) may reduce efficacy; use alternative treatment. Metformin: Cationic drugs that are eliminated by renal tubular secretion (eg, cimetidine, amiloride, digoxin, morphine, procainamide) may potentially produce an interaction; monitor and adjust dose of Jentadueto and/or the interfering drug. Topiramate or other carbonic anhydrase inhibitors (eg, zonisamide, acetazolamide, dichlorphenamide) may induce metabolic acidosis; use w/ caution. Caution w/ drugs that may affect renal function or result in significant hemodynamic change or interfere w/ the disposition of metformin. May be difficult to recognize hypoglycemia w/ β-adrenergic blocking drugs. Alcohol potentiates the effect of metformin on lactate metabolism; avoid excessive alcohol intake.

NURSING CONSIDERATIONS

Assessment: Assess for metabolic acidosis, risk factors for lactic acidosis, renal/hepatic impairment, previous hypersensitivity to the drug, history of pancreatitis, inadequate vitamin B12 or Ca^{2+} intake/absorption, type of DM, diabetic ketoacidosis, alcoholism, hypoxemia, presence of malnourishment or debilitation, adrenal/pituitary insufficiency, history of angioedema w/ another DPP-4 inhibitor, pregnancy/nursing status, and possible drug interactions. Assess if patient is planning to undergo any surgical procedure, radiologic studies involving the use of intravascular iodinated contrast materials, or is under any form of stress. Obtain baseline FPG and HbA1c levels, and hematologic parameters.

Monitoring: Monitor for signs/symptoms of lactic acidosis, pancreatitis, hypoxic states, hypersensitivity reactions, and other adverse reactions. Monitor renal function, especially in elderly, at least annually. Monitor hematologic parameters annually. Perform routine serum vitamin B12 measurement at 2- to 3-yr intervals in patients predisposed to developing subnormal vitamin B12 levels. Monitor FPG and HbA1c levels and hepatic function periodically.

Patient Counseling: Inform of the risks and benefits of therapy. Advise on the importance of adherence to dietary instructions, regular physical activity, periodic blood glucose monitoring and HbA1c, renal function, and hematologic parameter testing, recognition/management of hypo/hyperglycemia, and assessment of diabetes complications. Instruct to seek medical advice promptly during periods of stress as medication needs may change. Inform of the risk of lactic acidosis; instruct to d/c therapy immediately and contact physician if unexplained hyperventilation, malaise, myalgia, unusual somnolence, slow or irregular heartbeat, sensation of feeling cold (especially in the extremities), or other nonspecific symptoms occur. Inform that GI symptoms and acute pancreatitis may occur; instruct to d/c therapy promptly and contact physician if persistent severe abdominal pain occurs. Inform that allergic reactions may occur; instruct to d/c therapy and seek medical advice promptly if symptoms occur. Counsel against excessive alcohol intake. Counsel to inform physician if any bothersome or unusual symptoms develop, or if any symptom persists or worsens.

Storage: 25°C (77°F); excursions permitted to 15-30°C (59-86°F). Protect from exposure to high humidity.

JEVTANA – cabazitaxel RX

Class: Antimicrotubule agent

Neutropenic deaths reported. Perform frequent blood cell counts to monitor for neutropenia. Avoid with neutrophil counts of ≤1500 cells/mm^3. Severe hypersensitivity reactions may occur; d/c immediately if a severe hypersensitivity reaction occurs and administer appropriate therapy. Patients should receive premedication. Must not be given to patients who have a history of severe hypersensitivity reactions to cabazitaxel or other drugs formulated with polysorbate 80.

ADULT DOSAGE

Metastatic Prostate Cancer

Combination w/ prednisone for hormone-refractory metastatic prostate cancer in patients previously treated w/ a docetaxel-containing treatment regimen

25mg/m^2 IV over 1 hr every 3 weeks + prednisone 10mg PO administered daily throughout treatment

Premedication

Premedicate at least 30 min prior to each dose w/ the following IV medications:
Antihistamine: Dexchlorpheniramine 5mg, diphenhydramine 25mg, or equivalent
Corticosteroid: Dexamethasone 8mg or equivalent
H_2 Antagonist: Ranitidine 50mg or equivalent

Antiemetic prophylaxis is recommended and can be given PO or IV prn

PEDIATRIC DOSAGE

Pediatric use may not have been established

DOSE MODIFICATION

Concomitant Medications

Strong CYP3A Inhibitors: Avoid concomitant use; if coadministration is required, consider a 25% cabazitaxel dose reduction

Adverse Reactions

Prolonged Grade ≥3 Neutropenia (>1 Week) Despite Appropriate Medication (Including G-CSF): Delay treatment until neutrophil count is >1500 cells/mm^3, then reduce dose to 20mg/m^2; use G-CSF for secondary prophylaxis
Febrile Neutropenia/Neutropenic Infections: Delay treatment until improvement or resolution, and until neutrophil count is >1500 cells/mm^3, then reduce dose to 20mg/m^2; use G-CSF for secondary prophylaxis
Grade ≥3 Diarrhea or Persisting Diarrhea Despite Appropriate Medication, Fluid and Electrolyte Replacement: Delay treatment until improvement or resolution, then reduce dose to 20mg/m^2
Grade 2 Peripheral Neuropathy: Delay treatment until improvement or resolution, then reduce dose to 20mg/m^2
Grade ≥3 Peripheral Neuropathy: D/C therapy

D/C therapy if patient continues to experience any of the above reactions at 20mg/m^2

ADMINISTRATION

IV route

Do not mix w/ any other drugs
Use an in-line filter of 0.22μm nominal pore size (also referred to as 0.2μm) during administration

Preparation Instructions

Do not use PVC infusion containers or polyurethane infusions sets for preparation and administration of infusion sol
Cabazitaxel requires 2 dilutions prior to administration

1st Dilution:
1. Mix each vial of cabazitaxel 60mg/1.5mL w/ the entire contents of supplied diluents; once reconstituted, the resultant sol contains 10mg/mL
2. When transferring the diluent, direct the needle onto the inside wall of cabazitaxel vial and inject slowly to limit foaming
3. Remove the syringe and needle and gently mix the initial diluted sol by repeated inversions for at least 45 sec to assure full mixing of the drug and diluents; do not shake
4. Let the sol stand for a few min to allow any foam to dissipate, and check that the sol is homogeneous and contains no visible particulate matter; it is not required that all foam dissipate prior to continuing the preparation process
5. The resulting initial diluted sol (cabazitaxel 10mg/mL) requires further dilution before administration; the 2nd dilution should be done immediately (w/in 30 minutes) to obtain the final infusion

2nd (Final) Dilution:
1. Withdraw the recommended dose from the cabazitaxel sol containing 10mg/mL using a calibrated syringe and further dilute into a sterile 250mL PVC-free container of either 0.9% NaCl sol or D5 sol for infusion; if a dose >65mg of cabazitaxel is required, use a larger volume of the infusion vehicle so that a concentration of 0.26mg/mL is not exceeded
2. The concentration of the final infusion sol should be between 0.10mg/mL and 0.26mg/mL
3. Remove the syringe and thoroughly mix the final infusion sol by gently inverting the bag or bottle
4. As the final infusion sol is supersaturated, it may crystallize over time; do not use if this occurs and discard

Handling Precautions

If cabazitaxel inj or dilution for IV infusion comes into contact w/ the skin, immediately and thoroughly wash w/ soap and water

If cabazitaxel inj or dilution for IV infusion comes into contact w/ mucosa, immediately and thoroughly wash w/ water

HOW SUPPLIED

Inj: 60mg/1.5mL

CONTRAINDICATIONS

Neutrophil counts $\leq$1500/mm^3.

WARNINGS/PRECAUTIONS

Should be administered under the supervision of a qualified physician and where adequate diagnostic and treatment facilities are readily available. G-CSF may be administered to reduce risks of neutropenia complications; consider primary prophylaxis with G-CSF in patients with high-risk clinical features (eg, >65 yrs of age, poor performance status, previous episodes of febrile neutropenia, extensive prior radiation ports, poor nutritional status, or other serious comorbidities) that predispose them to increased complications from prolonged neutropenia. N/V and severe diarrhea may occur. Death related to diarrhea and electrolyte imbalance reported; intensive measures may be required for severe diarrhea and electrolyte imbalance. GI hemorrhage and perforation, ileus, enterocolitis, neutropenic enterocolitis, including fatal outcome, reported; risk may be increased with neutropenia, age, steroid use, concomitant use of NSAIDs, antiplatelet therapy, or anticoagulants, and prior history of pelvic radiotherapy, adhesions, ulceration, and GI bleeding. Abdominal pain/tenderness, fever, persistent constipation, diarrhea (with or without neutropenia), may be early manifestations of serious GI toxicity and should be evaluated and treated promptly; treatment delay or discontinuation may be necessary. Renal failure, including cases with fatal outcome, reported; identify causes and treat aggressively. Caution with severe renal impairment (CrCl <30mL/min), end-stage renal disease, and in elderly. Avoid with hepatic impairment (total bilirubin $\geq$ULN, or AST and/or ALT $\geq$1.5X ULN). May cause fetal harm when administered to a pregnant woman.

ADVERSE REACTIONS

Hypersensitivity reactions, neutropenia, anemia, leukopenia, thrombocytopenia, diarrhea, fatigue, N/V, constipation, asthenia, abdominal pain, anorexia, back pain, hematuria, dyspnea.

DRUG INTERACTIONS

See Dosage. Strong CYP3A inhibitors may increase levels.

NURSING CONSIDERATIONS

Assessment: Assess for history of hypersensitivity to drug or to other drugs formulated with polysorbate 80, hepatic/renal impairment, risk of developing GI complications, pregnancy/nursing status, and possible drug interactions. Assess for high-risk clinical features that may predispose to increased complications from prolonged neutropenia. Obtain baseline CBC, including neutrophil count.

Monitoring: Monitor for signs/symptoms of neutropenia, infections, hypersensitivity reactions, severe diarrhea, dehydration, N/V, electrolyte imbalance, renal failure, serious GI toxicity, and other adverse reactions. Monitor CBCs, including neutrophil count, on a weekly basis during cycle 1 and before each treatment cycle thereafter.

Patient Counseling: Counsel about the risk of potential hypersensitivity; instruct to immediately report signs of a hypersensitivity reaction. Advise on the importance of routine blood cell counts. Instruct to immediately report to physician any occurrence of fever, significant vomiting or diarrhea, decreased urinary output, and hematuria. Instruct to report to physician if not compliant with oral corticosteroid regimen. Counsel about side effects associated with exposure, such as severe and fatal infections, dehydration, and renal failure. Advise to inform physician before taking any other medications. Inform elderly patients that certain side effects may be more frequent or severe.

Storage: Undiluted: 25°C (77°F); excursions permitted to 15-30°C (59-86°F). Do not refrigerate. Diluted 1st Sol: Use within 30 min. Diluted 2nd Sol in 0.9% NaCl or D5W: Use within 8 hrs at ambient temperature (including the 1-hr infusion) or for a total of 24 hrs (including the 1-hr infusion) under refrigeration.

JUXTAPID – lomitapide

RX

Class: Lipid-regulating agent

May cause elevations in transaminases; measure ALT, AST, alkaline phosphatase, and total bilirubin prior to therapy, and then ALT/AST regularly as recommended. Adjust dose if ALT/AST is ≥3X ULN. D/C for clinically significant liver toxicity. May increase hepatic fat. Hepatic steatosis associated with lomitapide treatment may be a risk factor for progressive liver disease, including steatohepatitis and cirrhosis. Available only through a restricted program under a Risk Evaluation and Mitigation Strategy (REMS) because of the risk of hepatotoxicity.

ADULT DOSAGE

Homozygous Familial Hypercholesterolemia

Prior to treatment, initiate a low-fat diet supplying <20% of energy from fat

Initial: 5mg qd

Titrate: After ≥2 weeks, may increase dose to 10mg qd; and then at ≥4-week intervals, may increase to 20mg qd, then 40mg qd, and then up to a max of 60mg qd

Max: 60mg qd

PEDIATRIC DOSAGE

Pediatric use may not have been established

DOSE MODIFICATION

Concomitant Medications

Weak CYP3A4 Inhibitors:

Max: 30mg/day

Renal Impairment

ESRD Receiving Dialysis:

Max: 40mg/day

Hepatic Impairment

Mild (Child-Pugh A):

Max: 40mg/day

ALT/AST ≥3X and <5X ULN:

Confirm elevation w/ repeat measurement w/in 1 week

If confirmed, reduce dose and obtain additional liver-related tests if not already measured (eg, alkaline phosphatase, total bilirubin, INR)

Repeat tests weekly and withhold dosing if signs of abnormal liver function (increase in bilirubin/INR) present, if transaminase levels rise above 5X ULN, or if transaminase levels do not fall below 3X ULN w/in 4 weeks; investigate to identify probable cause in these cases of persistent or worsening abnormalities

Consider reducing dose and monitoring liver-related tests more frequently if resuming therapy after transaminases resolve to <3X ULN

ALT/AST ≥5X ULN:

Withhold dosing, obtain additional liver-related tests if not already measured (eg, alkaline phosphatase, total bilirubin, INR), and investigate to identify probable cause

Consider reducing dose and monitoring liver-related tests more frequently if resuming therapy after transaminases resolve to <3X ULN

If transaminase elevations are accompanied by clinical symptoms of liver injury, increases in bilirubin ≥2X ULN, or active liver disease, d/c and investigate to identify probable cause

ADMINISTRATION

Oral route

Take qd w/ a glass of water, w/o food, at least 2 hrs after pm meal

Swallow cap whole; do not open, crush, dissolve, or chew
Take daily supplements containing 400 IU vitamin E and at least 200mg linoleic acid, 210mg alpha-linolenic acid, 110mg eicosapentaenoic acid, and 80mg docosahexaenoic acid

HOW SUPPLIED

Cap: 5mg, 10mg, 20mg

CONTRAINDICATIONS

Pregnancy, moderate or severe hepatic impairment (based on Child-Pugh category B or C), active liver disease including unexplained persistent elevations of serum transaminases, concomitant moderate or strong CYP3A4 inhibitors.

WARNINGS/PRECAUTIONS

If baseline LFTs are abnormal, consider initiating therapy after an appropriate work-up and the baseline abnormalities are explained or resolved. May cause fetal harm; females of reproductive potential should have a negative pregnancy test before initiation of therapy and use effective contraception during therapy. May reduce absorption of fat-soluble nutrients, especially in patients with chronic bowel or pancreatic diseases that predispose to malabsorption; patients should take daily supplements. GI adverse reactions reported; absorption of concomitant oral medications may be affected in patients who develop diarrhea or vomiting. Avoid in patients with rare hereditary problems of galactose intolerance, Lapp lactase deficiency, or glucose-galactose malabsorption; may result in diarrhea and malabsorption. Caution in elderly.

ADVERSE REACTIONS

Hepatic steatosis, increased serum transaminases, diarrhea, N/V, dyspepsia, abdominal pain/discomfort/distention, weight loss, constipation, flatulence, chest pain, influenza, nasopharyngitis, fatigue.

DRUG INTERACTIONS

See Contraindications and Dosage. Not recommended with other LDL-lowering agents that can increase hepatic fat. Avoid grapefruit juice. Alcohol may increase levels of hepatic fat and induce/exacerbate liver injury; avoid consumption of >1 alcoholic drink/day. Caution with other medications known to have potential for hepatotoxicity (eg, isotretinoin, amiodarone, acetaminophen [>4g/day for ≥3 days/week]). Increased exposure with weak CYP3A4 inhibitors (eg, alprazolam, atorvastatin, cimetidine, oral contraceptives). May increase INR and plasma concentrations of both R(+)-warfarin and S(-)-warfarin; regularly monitor INR (particularly after any changes in lomitapide dosage) and adjust dose of warfarin as clinically indicated. May double the exposure of simvastatin; refer to simvastatin PI for dosing recommendations. May increase the exposure of lovastatin; consider reducing dose of lovastatin when initiating therapy. May increase the absorption of P-glycoprotein (P-gp) substrates (eg, aliskiren, colchicine, digoxin, sirolimus); consider dose reduction of the P-gp substrate. Separate dosing by at least 4 hrs with bile acid sequestrants.

NURSING CONSIDERATIONS

Assessment: Assess for active liver disease including unexplained persistent elevations of serum transaminases, bowel/pancreatic disease, galactose intolerance, renal dysfunction, pregnancy/nursing status, and possible drug interactions. Measure ALT/AST, alkaline phosphatase, and serum bilirubin prior to therapy.

Monitoring: Monitor for hepatic steatosis, hepatotoxicity, and GI and other adverse reactions. Monitor renal/hepatic function. During the 1st yr, perform hepatic-related tests (eg, ALT, AST) prior to each increase in dose or monthly, whichever occurs 1st. After the 1st yr, perform these tests at least every 3 months and before any dose increase. Monitor INR with warfarin.

Patient Counseling: Encourage to participate in the registry to monitor/evaluate long-term effects and inform that participation is voluntary. Advise that medication is only available from certified pharmacies enrolled in the REMS program. Discuss the importance of liver-related tests before initiation, prior to each dose escalation, and periodically thereafter. Advise of the potential for increased risk of liver injury if alcohol is consumed and instruct to limit alcohol consumption to not >1 drink/day. Advise to report any symptoms of possible liver injury (eg, fever, jaundice, lethargy, flu-like symptoms). Advise females of reproductive potential to have a negative pregnancy test before starting treatment and to use effective contraception while on therapy. Discuss the importance of taking daily supplements. Inform that GI adverse reactions are common and that strict adherence to a low-fat diet (<20% of total calories from fat) may reduce these reactions. Inform that absorption of oral medications may be affected in patients who develop diarrhea or vomiting; instruct to seek physician's advice if symptoms develop. Instruct to omit grapefruit juice from diet; advise to inform physician about all medications, nutritional supplements, and vitamins taken. If a dose is missed, instruct to take the normal dose at the usual time the next day; if dose is interrupted for more than a week, advise to contact physician before restarting treatment.

Storage: 20-25°C (68-77°F); excursions permitted to 15-30°C (59-86°F). May tolerate brief exposure up to 40°C (104°F), provided the mean kinetic temperature does not exceed 25°C (77°F); however, such exposure should be minimized. Protect from moisture.

KADIAN – morphine sulfate

CII

Class: Opioid analgesic

Exposes users to risks of addiction, abuse, and misuse, leading to overdose and death; assess each patient's risk prior to prescribing, and monitor regularly for development of these behaviors/conditions. Serious, life-threatening, or fatal respiratory depression may occur; monitor during initiation or following a dose increase. Crushing, chewing, or dissolving caps can cause rapid release and absorption of a potentially fatal dose; instruct to swallow whole. Accidental ingestion, especially by children, can result in fatal overdose. Prolonged use during pregnancy can result in neonatal opioid withdrawal syndrome; advise pregnant women of the risk and ensure availability of appropriate treatment. Avoid alcohol consumption or medications containing alcohol; may result in increased plasma levels and potentially fatal overdose of morphine.

ADULT DOSAGE

Severe Pain (Daily, Around-the-Clock Management)

1st Opioid Analgesic:
Initial: Begin treatment using immediate-release (IR) morphine then convert to extended-release formulation

Opioid Intolerant:
Initial: 30mg q24h

Titration/Maint:
Individually titrate to a dose that provides adequate analgesia and minimizes adverse reactions at a frequency of either once or twice daily; dose adjustments may be done every 1-2 days

Breakthrough Pain:
May require a dose increase, or may need rescue medication w/ an IR analgesic

Conversions

From Other Opioids:
Initial: 30mg q24h; d/c all other around-the-clock opioids when therapy is initiated

From Other Oral Morphine:
Initial: Give 1/2 total daily oral morphine dose bid or total daily dose qd

From Parenteral Morphine:
Parenteral to Oral Morphine Ratio: 2-6mg may be required to provide analgesia equivalent to 1mg of parenteral morphine
Usual: Approximately 3X the daily parenteral morphine requirement is typically sufficient

From Other Oral or Parenteral Non-Morphine Opioids:
Initial: 1/2 of the estimated daily requirement
May supplement w/ immediate-release morphine to manage inadequate analgesia

PEDIATRIC DOSAGE

Pediatric use may not have been established

DOSE MODIFICATION

Discontinuation

Use a gradual downward titration every 2-4 days; do not abruptly d/c

ADMINISTRATION

Oral route

Swallow cap whole; do not crush, dissolve, or chew

Alternative Administration

PO:
Sprinkle contents of cap over applesauce then swallow
Rinse mouth to ensure all pellets have been swallowed
Discard any unused portion of caps after contents have been sprinkled on applesauce

Gastrostomy Tube:
Flush gastrostomy tube w/ water
Sprinkle pellets into 10mL of water

Use a swirling motion to pour the pellets and water into the gastrostomy tube through a funnel
Rinse the beaker w/ another 10mL of water and pour into the funnel
Repeat rinsing until no pellets remain in the beaker

HOW SUPPLIED

Cap, Extended-Release: 10mg, 20mg, 30mg, 40mg, 50mg, 60mg, 70mg, 80mg, 100mg, 130mg, 150mg, 200mg

CONTRAINDICATIONS

Significant respiratory depression, acute or severe bronchial asthma in an unmonitored setting or in the absence of resuscitative equipment, known or suspected paralytic ileus.

WARNINGS/PRECAUTIONS

Should be prescribed only by healthcare professionals knowledgeable in the use of potent opioids for management of chronic pain. 100mg, 130mg, 150mg, and 200mg caps are for use in opioid-tolerant patients only. Life-threatening respiratory depression is more likely to occur in elderly, cachectic, or debilitated patients. Consider alternative nonopioid analgesics in patients with significant chronic obstructive pulmonary disease or cor pulmonale, and in patients having a substantially decreased respiratory reserve, hypoxia, hypercapnia, or preexisting respiratory depression. May cause severe hypotension, including orthostatic hypotension and syncope; increased risk in patients whose ability to maintain BP has already been compromised by a reduced blood volume or concurrent administration of certain CNS depressants. Avoid with circulatory shock, impaired consciousness, coma, or GI obstruction. Monitor patients who may be susceptible to intracranial effects of carbon dioxide retention (eg, those with evidence of increased intracranial pressure, brain tumors) for signs of sedation and respiratory depression, particularly when initiating therapy. May obscure clinical course in patients with head injury. May cause spasm of sphincter of Oddi and increases in serum amylase; monitor patients with biliary tract disease, including acute pancreatitis, for worsening symptoms. May lead to acute retention of urine by causing spasm of the bladder sphincter, particularly in men with an enlarged prostate. May aggravate convulsions and induce/aggravate seizures. May impair mental/physical abilities. Not recommended for use during and immediately prior to labor.

ADVERSE REACTIONS

Respiratory depression, drowsiness, constipation, nausea, dizziness, anxiety, confusion, dry mouth, diarrhea, anorexia, pain, dyspnea, peripheral edema, abdominal pain, rash.

DRUG INTERACTIONS

See Boxed Warning. Concomitant use with other CNS depressants (eg, sedatives, anxiolytics, hypnotics, tranquilizers, general anesthetics, antiemetics, phenothiazines, other opioids, neuroleptics) may increase the risk of respiratory depression, profound sedation, hypotension, coma and death; if coadministration is required, consider dose reduction of one or both agents. Monitor use in elderly, cachectic, and debilitated patients when given concomitantly with other drugs that depress respiration. Mixed agonist/antagonists (eg, pentazocine, nalbuphine, butorphanol) and partial agonist (buprenorphine) analgesics may reduce analgesic effect or precipitate withdrawal symptoms; avoid coadministration. May enhance neuromuscular blocking action of skeletal muscle relaxants and produce an increased degree of respiratory depression. MAOIs may potentiate effects of morphine; avoid use with MAOIs or within 14 days of stopping such treatment. Cimetidine may potentiate morphine-induced respiratory depression. Confusion and severe respiratory depression in a patient undergoing hemodialysis reported with concurrent cimetidine. May reduce efficacy of diuretics. Anticholinergics or other medications with anticholinergic activity may increase risk of urinary retention and/or severe constipation and lead to paralytic ileus. Absorption/exposure may be increased with p-glycoprotein inhibitors (eg, quinidine).

NURSING CONSIDERATIONS

Assessment: Assess for abuse/addiction risk, pain intensity, prior analgesic treatment experience, opioid tolerance, respiratory depression, drug hypersensitivity, history of seizure disorders, or any other condition where treatment is contraindicated or cautioned, pregnancy/nursing status, and possible drug interactions.

Monitoring: Monitor for respiratory depression (especially within first 24-72 hrs of initiation), hypotension, seizures/convulsions, and other adverse reactions. Monitor BP and serum amylase levels. Routinely monitor for signs of misuse, abuse, and addiction. Periodically reassess the continued need of therapy.

Patient Counseling: Inform that use of drug can result in addiction, abuse, and misuse; instruct not to share with others and to take steps to protect from theft or misuse. Inform about the risk of respiratory depression and advise how to recognize respiratory depression and to seek medical attention if breathing difficulties develop. Advise to store drug securely and dispose unused caps by flushing down the toilet. Inform women of reproductive potential that prolonged use during pregnancy may result in neonatal opioid withdrawal syndrome and instruct to inform physician if pregnant/planning to become pregnant. Inform that potentially serious additive effects may occur when used with alcohol or other CNS depressants, and not to use such drugs unless supervised by physician. Instruct about proper administration instructions. Inform that drug may cause orthostatic hypotension and syncope; instruct how to recognize symptoms of low BP. Inform that drug may impair the ability to perform potentially hazardous activities; advise not to perform such tasks until patients know how they will react to medication. Advise of the potential for severe constipation, including management instructions. Advise how to recognize anaphylaxis and when to seek medical attention.

Storage: 25°C (77°F); excursions permitted to 15-30°C (59-86°F). Protect from light and moisture.

KALETRA – lopinavir/ritonavir — RX

Class: Protease inhibitor

ADULT DOSAGE

HIV-1 Infection

Combination w/ Other Antiretrovirals:
400mg-100mg bid

<3 Lopinavir Resistance-Associated Substitutions:
800mg-200mg qd

PEDIATRIC DOSAGE

HIV-1 Infection

Combination w/ Other Antiretrovirals:

14 Days-6 Months of Age:

Sol:

Weight-Based: 16mg-4mg/kg bid

BSA-Based: 300mg-75mg/m^2 bid

6 Months of Age-18 Years:

Sol:

Weight-Based:

<15kg: 12mg-3mg/kg bid

≥15-40kg: 10mg-2.5mg/kg bid

Max: 400mg-100mg bid

BSA-Based: 230mg-57.5mg/m^2 bid

Max: 400mg-100mg bid

Tab:

15-25kg/≥0.6-<0.9m^2: 200mg-50mg bid

>25-35kg/≥0.9-<1.4m^2: 300mg-75mg bid

>35kg/≥1.4m^2: 400mg-100mg bid

DOSE MODIFICATION

Concomitant Medications

Combination w/ Efavirenz/Nevirapine/Nelfinavir:

6 Months-18 Years:

Sol:

Weight-Based:

<15kg: 13mg-3.25mg/kg bid

≥15-45kg: 11mg-2.75mg/kg bid

Max: 533mg-133mg bid

BSA-Based: Increase dose to 300mg-75mg/m^2 bid

Max: 533mg-133mg bid

Tab:

15-20kg/≥0.6-<0.8m^2: 200mg-50mg bid

>20-30kg/≥0.8-<1.2m^2: 300mg-75mg bid

>30-45kg/≥1.2-<1.7m^2: 400mg-100mg bid

>45kg/≥1.7m^2: 500mg-125mg bid

Adults:

Tab:
Increase dose to 500mg-125mg bid

Sol:
Increase dose to 533mg-133mg bid

ADMINISTRATION

Oral route

Tab

Take w/ or w/o food
Swallow whole; do not crush, break, or chew

Sol

Take w/ food

HOW SUPPLIED

(Lopinavir-Ritonavir) Sol: 80mg-20mg/mL [160mL]; Tab: 100mg-25mg, 200mg-50mg

CONTRAINDICATIONS

Coadministration with CYP3A substrates for which elevated plasma concentrations are associated with serious and/or life-threatening reactions and with potent CYP3A inducers where significantly reduced lopinavir levels may be associated with the potential for loss of virologic response and possible resistance and cross-resistance (eg, alfuzosin, rifampin, dihydroergotamine, ergotamine, methylergonovine, St. John's wort, cisapride, lovastatin, simvastatin, sildenafil [when used to treat pulmonary arterial HTN], pimozide, triazolam, oral midazolam).

WARNINGS/PRECAUTIONS

Avoid sol in preterm neonates in the immediate postnatal period; preterm neonates may be at increased risk of propylene glycol-associated adverse events and other toxicities. Pancreatitis, including marked TG elevations, reported; evaluate and suspend therapy if clinically appropriate. Patients with underlying hepatitis B or C or marked serum transaminase elevations prior to treatment may be at increased risk for developing or worsening of transaminase elevations or hepatic decompensation; conduct appropriate lab testing prior to therapy and monitor closely during treatment. New onset or exacerbation of diabetes mellitus (DM), hyperglycemia, diabetic ketoacidosis, immune reconstitution syndrome, autoimmune disorders (eg, Graves' disease, polymyositis, Guillain-Barre syndrome) in the setting of immune reconstitution, redistribution/accumulation of body fat, lipid elevations, and increased bleeding with hemophilia A and B reported. PR and QT interval prolongation, torsades de pointes, and cases of 2nd- and 3rd-degree atrioventricular block reported; caution with underlying structural heart disease, preexisting conduction system abnormalities, ischemic heart disease, or cardiomyopathies. Avoid use with congenital long QT syndrome or hypokalemia and with other drugs that prolong QT interval. Once daily regimen not recommended for adults with ≥3 lopinavir resistance-associated substitutions or in pediatric patients <18 yrs. Caution with hepatic impairment and in elderly.

ADVERSE REACTIONS

Diarrhea, N/V, hypertriglyceridemia and hypercholesterolemia, dysgeusia, rash, decreased weight, insomnia.

DRUG INTERACTIONS

See Contraindications. Caution with drugs that prolong the PR interval (eg, calcium channel blockers [CCBs], β-adrenergic blockers, digoxin, atazanavir). Avoid with colchicine in patients with renal/hepatic impairment, tadalafil during initiation, tipranavir/ritonavir combination, and drugs that prolong the QT interval. Not recommended with voriconazole, high doses of itraconazole or ketoconazole, boceprevir, telaprevir, avanafil, and salmeterol. Not recommended with fluticasone or other glucocorticoids that are metabolized by CYP3A unless benefit outweighs the risk of systemic corticosteroid effects. Cushing's syndrome and adrenal suppression reported with budesonide and fluticasone propionate. May increase levels of CYP3A substrates, colchicine, fentanyl, tenofovir, indinavir, nelfinavir, saquinavir, maraviroc, antiarrhythmics, vincristine, vinblastine, dasatinib, nilotinib, trazodone, itraconazole, ketoconazole, rifabutin and rifabutin metabolite, clarithromycin in patients with renal impairment, IV midazolam, dihydropyridine CCB, bosentan, atorvastatin, rosuvastatin, immunosuppressants, salmeterol, rivaroxaban, glucocorticoids, sildenafil, tadalafil, and vardenafil. May decrease levels of methadone, phenytoin, bupropion, atovaquone, ethinyl estradiol, abacavir, zidovudine, lamotrigine, valproate, voriconazole, boceprevir, and amprenavir. Delavirdine and CYP3A inhibitors may increase levels. May alter concentrations of warfarin; monitor INR. Efavirenz, nevirapine, nelfinavir, carbamazepine, phenobarbital, and phenytoin may decrease levels; not for qd dosing regimen. Rifampin, fosamprenavir/ritonavir, systemic corticosteroids, and CYP3A inducers may decrease levels. May require initiation or dose adjustments of insulin or PO hypoglycemics for treatment of DM. (Sol) Contains alcohol; may produce disulfiram-like reactions with disulfiram or metronidazole. Didanosine should be given 1 hr before or 2 hrs after sol. Refer to PI for further information and dosing modifications when used with certain concomitant therapies.

NURSING CONSIDERATIONS

Assessment: Assess for history of hypersensitivity reactions, history of pancreatitis, hepatitis B or C, cirrhosis, DM or hyperglycemia, dyslipidemia, hemophilia type A or B, structural heart disease, preexisting conduction system abnormalities, ischemic heart disease or cardiomyopathies, congenital long QT syndrome, hypokalemia, renal/hepatic impairment, pregnancy/nursing status, and for possible drug interactions. Assess children for the ability to swallow intact tab.

Monitoring: Monitor for signs/symptoms of pancreatitis, hyperglycemia, hepatic dysfunction, immune reconstitution syndrome, autoimmune disorders, fat redistribution/accumulation, hypersensitivity reactions, and other adverse reactions. Monitor lipid profile, glucose levels, total bilirubin levels, ECG changes, serum lipase levels, and serum amylase levels. Monitor infants for increase in serum osmolality, SrCr, and other toxicities.

Patient Counseling: Instruct to take prescribed dose ud. Advise to inform physician if weight changes in children occur. Inform that if a dose is missed, take dose as soon as possible and return to normal schedule; instruct not to double the next dose. Advise that therapy is not a cure for HIV; opportunistic infections may still occur. Instruct to avoid doing things that can spread HIV-1 infection to others. Instruct not to have any kind of sex without protection; advise to always practice safe sex by using a latex or polyurethane condom to lower the chance of sexual contact with semen, vaginal secretions, or blood. Instruct to notify physician if using other prescription/OTC or herbal products, particularly St. John's wort. Inform that skin rashes, liver function changes, ECG changes, redistribution/accumulation of body fat, new onset or worsening of preexisting diabetes, and hyperglycemia may occur. Instruct to seek medical attention if symptoms of worsening liver disease (eg, loss of appetite, abdominal pain, jaundice, itchy skin), dizziness, abnormal heart rhythm, loss of consciousness, or any other adverse reactions develop.

Storage: (Tab) 20-25°C (68-77°F); excursions permitted to 15-30°C (59-86°F). (Sol) 2-8°C (36-46°F). Avoid exposure to excessive heat. If stored at room temperature up to 25°C (77°F), sol should be used within 2 months.

KAPVAY – clonidine hydrochloride RX

Class: Alpha$_2$-agonist

PEDIATRIC DOSAGE

Attention-Deficit Hyperactivity Disorder

Monotherapy or Adjunctive Therapy to Stimulant Medications:
6-17 Years:
Initial: 0.1mg hs
Titrate: Adjust daily dose in increments of 0.1mg/day at weekly intervals until desired response is achieved; doses should be taken bid, w/ either an equal or higher split dosage being given hs
Max: 0.4mg/day
Dosing Guidance:
Total Daily Dose of 0.1mg: 0.1mg qhs
Total Daily Dose of 0.2mg: 0.1mg qam and 0.1mg qhs
Total Daily Dose of 0.3mg: 0.1mg qam and 0.2mg qhs
Total Daily Dose of 0.4mg: 0.2mg qam and 0.2mg qhs

DOSE MODIFICATION

Concomitant Medications
Concomitant Psychostimulant: Adjust psychostimulant dose depending on response to clonidine

Renal Impairment
Give initial dosage based on degree of impairment; titrate to higher doses cautiously

Discontinuation
Taper total daily dose in decrements of no more than 0.1mg every 3-7 days

ADMINISTRATION

Oral route

Take w/ or w/o food
Swallow tabs whole; do not crush, chew, or break

HOW SUPPLIED

Tab, Extended-Release: 0.1mg, 0.2mg

WARNINGS/PRECAUTIONS

Substitution for other clonidine products on mg-per-mg basis is not recommended. May cause dose-related decreases in BP and HR. Titrate slowly in patients with history of hypotension and those with underlying conditions that may be worsened by hypotension and bradycardia (eg, heart block, bradycardia, cardiovascular/vascular/cerebrovascular disease, chronic renal failure). Caution with a history of syncope or with a condition that predisposes to syncope (eg, hypotension, orthostatic hypotension, bradycardia, dehydration); avoid becoming dehydrated or overheated. Somnolence and sedation reported. May impair mental/physical abilities. Abrupt discontinuation may cause rebound HTN; gradually reduce dose when discontinuing therapy. May elicit allergic reactions (eg, generalized rash, urticaria, angioedema) in patients who develop an allergic reaction from clonidine transdermal system. May worsen sinus node dysfunction and atrioventricular (AV) block; titrate slowly and monitor vital signs frequently in patients with cardiac conduction abnormalities.

ADVERSE REACTIONS

Somnolence, fatigue, nausea, dizziness, nasal congestion, nightmare, insomnia, emotional disorder, headache, upper abdominal pain, irritability, constipation, dry mouth, decreased appetite, tremor.

DRUG INTERACTIONS

TCAs increase BP and may counteract hypotensive effects, while antihypertensives potentiate hypotensive effect; monitor BP and adjust dose PRN. Avoid with CNS depressants; may potentiate sedating effects. Avoid with drugs that affect sinus node function or AV node conduction (eg, digitalis, calcium channel blockers, β-blockers); may potentiate bradycardia and risk of AV block. Monitor BP and HR, and adjust dosages accordingly in patients treated concomitantly with antihypertensives or other drugs that can reduce BP/HR or increase risk of syncope. Consider the potential for additive sedative effects with other centrally active depressants (eg, phenothiazines, barbiturates, benzodiazepines). Titrate slowly and monitor vital signs frequently with other sympatholytics. Avoid use with alcohol.

NURSING CONSIDERATIONS

Assessment: Assess for drug hypersensitivity, history of hypotension, underlying conditions that may be worsened by hypotension and bradycardia, history of syncope or conditions that predispose to syncope, cardiac conduction abnormalities, renal impairment, pregnancy/nursing status, and for possible drug interactions. Obtain baseline HR and BP.

Monitoring: Monitor for somnolence, sedation, hypotension, bradycardia, allergic reactions, dehydration, overheating, and for other adverse reactions. Monitor BP and HR following dose increases and periodically while on therapy. Monitor vital signs frequently in patients with cardiac conduction abnormalities.

Patient Counseling: Inform about risks/benefits of therapy and instruct to take ud. If a dose is missed, instruct to skip that dose and take the next dose as scheduled; advise not to take more than the prescribed total daily amount in any 24-hr period. Advise patients with a history of syncope or who may have a condition that predisposes them to syncope (eg, hypotension, orthostatic hypotension, bradycardia, dehydration) to avoid becoming dehydrated or overheated. Instruct to use caution when driving or operating hazardous machinery until they know how they will respond to treatment. Advise to avoid use of therapy with other centrally active depressants and with alcohol. Advise not to d/c therapy abruptly. Instruct to d/c therapy and seek immediate medical attention if any signs/symptoms of a hypersensitivity reaction (eg, generalized rash, urticaria, angioedema) occur.

Storage: 20-25°C (68-77°F).

KAYEXALATE – sodium polystyrene sulfonate RX

Class: Cation-exchange resin

ADULT DOSAGE

Hyperkalemia

PO:

Usual: 15-60g/day administered as 15g qd-qid

Rectal Enema:

30-50g q6h

PEDIATRIC DOSAGE

Hyperkalemia

Smaller Children and Infants:

Use 1mEq of K^+ per 1g of resin as basis of calculation

Avoid oral administration in neonates

ADMINISTRATION

Oral/Rectal routes

Do not heat; may alter exchange properties of the resin
Give sus in a small quantity of water or in syrup, for greater palatability; amount of fluid ranges from 20-100mL or may determine by allowing 3-4mL per gram of resin
Position should be upright while resin is being administered
May introduce resin into the stomach through a plastic tube and, if desired, mixed w/ a diet appropriate for a patient in renal failure

Rectal Enema

Administer each dose as a warm emulsion (at body temperature) in 100mL of aqueous vehicle; gently agitate emulsion during administration
Retain enema as long as possible, followed by a cleansing enema

Preparation:

After initial enema, insert a soft, large size (French 28) rubber tube into the rectum for a distance of about 20cm, w/ the tip well into the sigmoid colon, and taped in place
Suspend resin in the appropriate amount of aqueous vehicle at body temperature and introduce by gravity, while the particles are kept in suspension by stirring
Flush sus w/ 50mL or 100mL of fluid, clamp the tube and leave in place
Keep sus in the sigmoid colon for several hrs, if possible
Then irrigate the colon w/ a nonsodium containing sol at body temperature to remove the resin; 2 quarts of flushing sol may be necessary
Drain the returns constantly through a Y tube connection
Use of sorbitol is not recommended

HOW SUPPLIED
Powder: 453.6g

CONTRAINDICATIONS
Hypokalemia, obstructive bowel disease, neonates with reduced gut motility (post-op or drug-induced), oral administration in neonates.

WARNINGS/PRECAUTIONS
Cases of intestinal necrosis and other serious GI adverse events (eg, bleeding, ischemic colitis, perforation) reported. Avoid use in patients who have not had a bowel movement post-surgery and in patients at risk for developing constipation or impaction. Hypokalemia may occur. May be insufficient for emergency correction of hyperkalemia; consider other definitive measures (eg, dialysis). Monitor for electrolyte disturbances. Caution if intolerant to Na^+ increases (eg, severe CHF or HTN, marked edema). Follow full aspiration precautions during administration. Caution with premature infants or low birth weight infants. If clinically significant constipation occurs d/c until normal bowel movement is resumed.

ADVERSE REACTIONS
Anorexia, N/V, constipation, hypokalemia, hypocalcemia, Na^+ retention, diarrhea, fecal impaction, gastric irritation, intestinal necrosis.

DRUG INTERACTIONS
Avoid nonabsorbable cation-donating antacids and laxatives (eg, magnesium hydroxide, aluminum carbonate); systemic alkalosis may occur. Hypokalemia exaggerates toxic effects of digitalis. Intestinal obstruction reported with aluminum hydroxide. May decrease absorption of lithium and thyroxine. Concomitant use with sorbitol has been implicated in cases of intestinal necrosis; avoid use.

NURSING CONSIDERATIONS

Assessment: Assess for hypokalemia, obstructive bowel disease, CHF, HTN, marked edema, prematurity, history of intestinal disease or surgery, hypovolemia, bowel function, renal insufficiency and failure, pregnancy/nursing status, and for possible drug interactions. Assess neonates for reduced gut motility.

Monitoring: Monitor for signs/symptoms of intestinal necrosis or other GI events (eg, bleeding, ischemic colitis, perforation), hypokalemia, cardiac arrhythmias, electrolyte disturbances, and constipation. Monitor ECG and serum electrolytes.

Patient Counseling: Counsel about potential side effects and advise to seek medical attention if signs/symptoms develop.

Storage: 25°C (77°F); excursions permitted to 15-30°C (59-86°F). Suspension should be freshly prepared and not stored beyond 24 hrs.

KAZANO — alogliptin/metformin hydrochloride RX

Class: Biguanide/dipeptidyl peptidase-4 (DPP-4) inhibitor

Lactic acidosis may occur due to metformin accumulation; risk increases with conditions such as sepsis, dehydration, excess alcohol intake, hepatic impairment, renal impairment, and acute CHF. If acidosis is suspected, d/c therapy and hospitalize patient immediately.

ADULT DOSAGE

Type 2 Diabetes Mellitus

When treatment w/ both alogliptin and metformin is appropriate

Initial: Base on current regimen
May adjust dose based on effectiveness and tolerability; gradually escalate dose to reduce GI side effects of metformin
Max: 25mg-2000mg/day

PEDIATRIC DOSAGE
Pediatric use may not have been established

DOSE MODIFICATION
Hepatic Impairment
Not recommended

ADMINISTRATION
Oral route

Take bid w/ food
Do not split tab before swallowing

HOW SUPPLIED

Tab: (Alogliptin-Metformin) 12.5mg-500mg, 12.5mg-1000mg

CONTRAINDICATIONS

Renal impairment (eg, SrCr ≥1.5mg/dL [men], ≥1.4mg/dL [women], or abnormal CrCl), acute or chronic metabolic acidosis, including diabetic ketoacidosis.

WARNINGS/PRECAUTIONS

Not for use in type 1 DM or for treatment of diabetic ketoacidosis. Acute pancreatitis reported; d/c if suspected and initiate appropriate management. Serious hypersensitivity reactions reported; d/c if suspected, assess for other potential causes, and institute alternative treatment for DM. Caution with history of angioedema to another dipeptidyl peptidase-4 (DPP-4) inhibitor. Fatal and nonfatal hepatic failure reported; interrupt therapy and investigate probable cause if liver enzymes are significantly elevated or if abnormal LFTs persist/worsen, and do not restart without another explanation for the liver test abnormalities. Avoid in patients with clinical or lab evidence of hepatic disease. D/C if evidence of renal impairment is present and do not initiate in patients ≥80 yrs of age unless renal function is normal. Temporarily d/c at time of or prior to radiologic studies involving intravascular iodinated contrast materials, withhold for 48 hrs subsequent to the procedure, and reinstitute only if renal function is normal. Suspend temporarily for any surgical procedure (except minor procedures not associated with restricted food and fluid intake); restart when oral intake is resumed and renal function is normal. D/C in hypoxic states (eg, acute CHF, shock, acute MI). May decrease vitamin B12 levels; monitor hematologic parameters annually. Caution in patients susceptible to hypoglycemic effects, such as elderly, debilitated, or malnourished patients, and those with adrenal/pituitary insufficiency or alcohol intoxication. No conclusive evidence of macrovascular risk reduction.

ADVERSE REACTIONS

Lactic acidosis, URTI, nasopharyngitis, diarrhea, HTN, headache, back pain, UTI, hypoglycemia.

DRUG INTERACTIONS

Topiramate or other carbonic anhydrase inhibitors (eg, zonisamide, acetazolamide, dichlorphenamide) may induce metabolic acidosis; use with caution. Hypoglycemia may occur with other glucose-lowering agents (eg, sulfonylureas, insulin) or ethanol; may require lower doses of sulfonylureas or insulin. Metformin: Cationic drugs that are eliminated by renal tubular secretion (eg, cimetidine, amiloride, digoxin, morphine, procainamide, quinidine, quinine, ranitidine, triamterene, trimethoprim, vancomycin) may potentially produce an interaction; monitor and adjust dose. Observe for loss of glycemic control with thiazides and other diuretics, corticosteroids, phenothiazines, thyroid products, estrogens, oral contraceptives, phenytoin, nicotinic acid, sympathomimetics, calcium channel blockers, and INH. Alcohol may potentiate effect of metformin on lactate metabolism; avoid excessive alcohol intake. Caution with drugs that may affect renal function or result in significant hemodynamic change or may interfere with the disposition of metformin (eg, cationic drugs eliminated by renal tubular secretion). Hypoglycemia may be difficult to recognize with β-adrenergic blocking drugs.

NURSING CONSIDERATIONS

Assessment: Assess for metabolic acidosis, risk factors for lactic acidosis, renal/hepatic impairment, previous hypersensitivity to the drug, history of pancreatitis, inadequate vitamin B12 or calcium absorption, type of DM, diabetic ketoacidosis, history of angioedema with another DPP-4 inhibitor, pregnancy/nursing status, and possible drug interactions. Assess if patient is planning to undergo any surgical procedure. Obtain baseline FPG, HbA1c, and hematologic parameters.

Monitoring: Monitor for lactic acidosis, pancreatitis, hypoxic states, decreases in vitamin B12 levels, and hypersensitivity reactions. Monitor renal function, especially in patients in whom development of renal dysfunction is anticipated, at least annually. Monitor FPG, HbA1c, hepatic function, and hematologic parameters periodically.

Patient Counseling: Inform of risks and benefits of therapy. Advise of the risk of lactic acidosis; instruct to d/c therapy immediately and contact physician if unexplained hyperventilation, myalgia, malaise, unusual somnolence, or other nonspecific symptoms occur. Counsel against excessive alcohol intake. Inform that GI symptoms, acute pancreatitis, and hypoglycemia may occur. Advise to d/c and seek medical advice if signs/symptoms of allergic reactions, liver injury, or persistent severe abdominal pain occur. Inform about the importance of regular testing of renal function and hematological parameters during treatment. Counsel to inform physician if any unusual symptom develops, or if any known symptom persists or worsens. Instruct to take ud.

Storage: 25°C (77°F); excursions permitted to 15-30°C (59-86°F). Keep container tightly closed.

KEPPRA – levetiracetam

RX

Class: Pyrrolidine derivative

ADULT DOSAGE

Partial Onset Seizures

Adjunctive Therapy for Patients w/ Epilepsy:
≥16 Years:
Initial: 500mg bid
Titrate: May increase by 1000mg/day every 2 weeks
Max: 3000mg/day

Myoclonic Seizures

Adjunctive Therapy for Patients w/ Juvenile Myoclonic Epilepsy:
Initial: 500mg bid
Titrate: Increase by 1000mg/day every 2 weeks to recommended dose of 3000mg/day

Tonic-Clonic Seizures

Adjunctive Therapy in the Treatment of Primary Generalized Tonic-Clonic Seizures w/ Idiopathic Generalized Epilepsy:
≥16 Years:
Initial: 500mg bid
Titrate: Increase by 1000mg/day every 2 weeks to recommended dose of 3000mg/day

Conversions

Switching from Oral Dosing:
Initial total daily IV dose should be equivalent to the total daily dose and frequency of oral formulation

Switching to Oral Dosing:
At the end of IV treatment period, switch at equivalent daily dose and frequency of IV administration

PEDIATRIC DOSAGE

Partial Onset Seizures

Adjunctive Therapy for Patients w/ Epilepsy:
1-<6 Months of Age:
Initial: 7mg/kg bid
Titrate: Increase by 14mg/kg/day every 2 weeks to recommended dose of 21mg/kg bid

6 Months-<4 Years:
Initial: 10mg/kg bid
Titrate: Increase by 20mg/kg/day in 2 weeks to recommended dose of 25mg/kg bid; may reduce dose if 50mg/kg/day cannot be tolerated

4-<16 Years:
Initial: 10mg/kg bid
Titrate: Increase by 20mg/kg/day every 2 weeks to recommended dose of 30mg/kg bid; may reduce dose if 60mg/kg/day cannot be tolerated
Max: 3000mg/day

Tab:
20-40kg:
Initial: 250mg bid
Titrate: Increase by 500mg/day every 2 weeks
Max: 750mg bid

>40kg:
Initial: 500mg bid
Titrate: Increase by 1000mg/day every 2 weeks
Max: 1500mg bid

Myoclonic Seizures

Adjunctive Therapy for Patients w/ Juvenile Myoclonic Epilepsy:
≥12 Years:
Initial: 500mg bid
Titrate: Increase by 1000mg/day every 2 weeks to recommended dose of 3000mg/day

Tonic-Clonic Seizures

Adjunctive Therapy in the Treatment of Primary Generalized Tonic-Clonic Seizures w/ Idiopathic Generalized Epilepsy:
6-<16 Years:
Initial: 10mg/kg bid
Titrate: Increase by 20mg/kg/day every 2 weeks to recommended dose of 30mg/kg bid

Conversions

Switching from Oral Dosing:
Initial total daily IV dose should be equivalent to the total daily dose and frequency of oral formulation

Switching to Oral Dosing:
At the end of IV treatment period, switch at equivalent daily dose and frequency of IV administration

DOSE MODIFICATION

Renal Impairment
Adults:
Mild (CrCl 50-80mL/min): 500-1000mg q12h
Moderate (CrCl 30-50mL/min): 250-750mg q12h

Severe (CrCl <30mL/min): 250-500mg q12h
ESRD Using Dialysis: 500-1000mg q24h
Following dialysis, a supplemental dose of 250-500mg is recommended

ADMINISTRATION
Oral/IV route

Oral
Take w/ or w/o food
Prescribe oral sol for pediatric patients ≤20kg
Prescribe oral sol or tabs for pediatric patients >20kg
Tab:
Swallow whole; do not crush or chew
Sol:
Dosing is weight-based using a calibrated measuring device

IV
Use only as an alternative for patients when oral administration is temporarily not feasible
Administer as a 15-min IV infusion following dilution
Dilute in 100mL of a compatible diluent; if smaller volume is required, amount of diluent should be calculated to not exceed a max levetiracetam concentration of 15mg/mL of diluted sol
Consider total daily fluid intake of patient
Stable for ≥24 hrs when mixed w/ compatible diluents and antiepileptic drugs and stored in polyvinyl chloride bags
Compatible Diluents:
0.9% NaCl inj
Lactated Ringer's inj
D5 inj

Compatible Antiepileptic Drugs:
Lorazepam
Diazepam
Valproate sodium

IV/Sol
Refer to PI for weight-based dosing calculation

HOW SUPPLIED
Inj: 100mg/mL [5mL]; Sol: 100mg/mL [16 fl oz]; Tab: 250mg*, 500mg*, 750mg*, 1000mg* *scored

WARNINGS/PRECAUTIONS
May cause behavioral abnormalities, psychotic symptoms, somnolence, fatigue, and coordination difficulties. May impair mental/physical abilities. Serious dermatological reactions (eg, Stevens-Johnson syndrome [SJS], toxic epidermal necrolysis [TEN]), and recurrence of serious skin reactions following rechallenge reported; d/c at the 1st sign of rash, unless the rash is clearly not drug-related. Do not resume, and consider alternative therapy if signs/symptoms suggest SJS/TEN. Increased risk of suicidal thoughts or behavior. Withdraw gradually to minimize the potential of increased seizure frequency. Hematologic abnormalities and agranulocytosis reported. Physiological changes may decrease plasma levels throughout pregnancy; monitor patients during pregnancy and through the postpartum period, especially if the dose was changed during pregnancy. Caution in elderly. (Oral) Increased diastolic BP reported.

ADVERSE REACTIONS
Somnolence, asthenia, infection, dizziness, fatigue, aggression, irritability, neck pain, pharyngitis, vertigo, diarrhea, anorexia, pain, depression, nervousness.

NURSING CONSIDERATIONS

Assessment: Assess for renal impairment, depression, suicidal thoughts/behavior, pregnancy/nursing status, and possible drug interactions.

Monitoring: Monitor for signs/symptoms of psychiatric reactions, behavior abnormalities, somnolence and fatigue, coordination difficulties, suicidal behavior, serious dermatological reactions, hematologic abnormalities, agranulocytosis, and other adverse reactions. Monitor patients during pregnancy and continue close monitoring through the postpartum period, especially if the dose was changed during pregnancy. Monitor for increase in diastolic BP in patients 1 month to <4 yrs of age.

Patient Counseling: Advise patients and their caregivers that the drug may cause behavioral changes and psychotic symptoms. Inform that the drug may increase the risk of suicidal thoughts and behavior; advise to be alert for the emergence or worsening of symptoms of depression, unusual changes in mood/behavior, or the emergence of suicidal thoughts, behavior, or thoughts about self-harm. Instruct to immediately report behaviors of concern to physician. Inform that dizziness and somnolence may occur; advise not to drive, operate heavy machinery, or engage in other hazardous activities until they have gained sufficient experience to gauge whether it adversely affects their performance of these activities. Inform that serious dermatological adverse reactions have been reported; advise to notify physician if a rash develops. Advise to notify physician if patient becomes pregnant or intends to become pregnant; encourage to enroll in the North American Antiepileptic Drug pregnancy registry.

Storage: 25°C (77°F); excursions permitted to 15-30°C (59-86°F).

KEPPRA XR – levetiracetam RX

Class: Pyrrolidine derivative

ADULT DOSAGE

Partial Onset Seizures

Adjunctive Therapy in Patients w/ Epilepsy:
Initial: 1000mg qd
Titrate: Adjust dose in increments of 1000mg every 2 weeks
Max: 3000mg/day

PEDIATRIC DOSAGE

Partial Onset Seizures

Adjunctive Therapy in Patients w/ Epilepsy:
≥12 Years:
Initial: 1000mg qd
Titrate: Adjust dose in increments of 1000mg every 2 weeks
Max: 3000mg/day

DOSE MODIFICATION

Renal Impairment
Adults:
Mild (CrCl 50-80mL/min): 1000-2000mg q24h
Moderate (CrCl 30-50mL/min): 500-1500mg q24h
Severe (CrCl <30mL/min): 500-1000mg q24h
ESRD on Dialysis: Use immediate-release formulation

ADMINISTRATION

Oral route

Swallow tabs whole; do not chew, break, or crush

HOW SUPPLIED

Tab, Extended-Release: 500mg, 750mg

WARNINGS/PRECAUTIONS

Increased risk of suicidal thoughts/behavior. May cause behavioral abnormalities, psychotic symptoms, somnolence, fatigue, and coordination difficulties. May impair mental/physical abilities. Serious dermatological reactions (eg, Stevens-Johnson syndrome [SJS], toxic epidermal necrolysis [TEN]) and recurrence of serious skin reactions following rechallenge reported; d/c at the 1st sign of rash, unless the rash is clearly not drug-related. If signs/symptoms suggest SJS/TEN, do not resume therapy and consider alternative therapy. Withdraw gradually to minimize the potential of increased seizure frequency. Hematologic abnormalities and agranulocytosis reported. Physiological changes may decrease plasma levels throughout pregnancy. Caution in elderly.

ADVERSE REACTIONS

Somnolence, nausea, influenza, nasopharyngitis, dizziness, irritability.

NURSING CONSIDERATIONS

Assessment: Assess for renal impairment, depression, suicidal thoughts/behavior, and pregnancy/nursing status.

Monitoring: Monitor for emergence or worsening of depression, suicidal thoughts/behavior, and/or any unusual changes in mood or behavior, psychotic symptoms, somnolence, fatigue, coordination difficulties, serious dermatological reactions, hematologic abnormalities, agranulocytosis, and other adverse reactions. Monitor patients during pregnancy and continue close monitoring through the postpartum period, especially if the dose was changed during pregnancy.

Patient Counseling: Inform that the drug may increase the risk of suicidal thoughts/behavior; instruct to immediately report the emergence or worsening of symptoms of depression, any unusual changes in mood/behavior, or suicidal thoughts, behavior, or thoughts about self-harm to physician. Counsel that medication may cause changes in behavior (eg, irritability and aggression). Inform that dizziness and somnolence may occur; advise not to drive or operate heavy machinery or engage in other hazardous activities until patients have gained sufficient experience to gauge whether it adversely affects their performance of these activities. Advise that serious dermatological adverse reactions may occur; instruct to notify physician immediately if rash develops. Instruct to take as directed. Advise to notify physician if patient becomes pregnant or intends to become pregnant; encourage to enroll in the North American Antiepileptic Drug pregnancy registry.

Storage: 25°C (77°F); excursions permitted to 15-30°C (59-86°F).

KETEK – telithromycin

RX

Class: Ketolide antibiotic

Contraindicated w/ myasthenia gravis. Fatal and life-threatening respiratory failure reported in patients w/ myasthenia gravis.

ADULT DOSAGE

Community-Acquired Pneumonia

Mild to Moderate:
800mg qd for 7-10 days

PEDIATRIC DOSAGE

Pediatric use may not have been established

DOSE MODIFICATION

Renal Impairment

Severe (CrCl <30mL/min)/Hemodialysis: 600mg qd; give after dialysis session on dialysis days if undergoing hemodialysis

Severe Impairment (CrCl <30mL/min) w/ Hepatic Impairment: 400mg qd

ADMINISTRATION

Oral route
May take w/ or w/o food

HOW SUPPLIED

Tab: 300mg, 400mg

CONTRAINDICATIONS

Myasthenia gravis, history of hepatitis and/or jaundice associated w/ use of telithromycin or any macrolide antibacterial, history of hypersensitivity to macrolide antibacterials, concomitant use w/ cisapride or pimozide, and concomitant use w/ colchicine in patients w/ renal or hepatic impairment.

WARNINGS/PRECAUTIONS

Acute hepatic failure and severe liver injury, including fulminant hepatitis and hepatic necrosis, reported; d/c if any signs/symptoms of hepatitis occur. Permanently d/c if clinical hepatitis or transaminase elevations combined w/ systemic symptoms occur. May prolong QTc interval leading to increased risk for ventricular arrhythmias, including torsades de pointes; avoid in patients w/ congenital prolongation of QTc interval, w/ ongoing proarrhythmic conditions (eg, uncorrected hypokalemia/hypomagnesemia), or w/ clinically significant bradycardia. Visual disturbances and loss of consciousness reported; avoid hazardous activities (eg, driving, operating heavy machinery) if these symptoms occur. *Clostridium difficile*-associated diarrhea (CDAD) reported; may need to d/c if CDAD is suspected or confirmed. May result in bacterial resistance if used in the absence of a proven or suspected bacterial infection.

ADVERSE REACTIONS

Diarrhea, nausea.

DRUG INTERACTIONS

See Contraindications. If coadministration w/ colchicine is necessary in patients w/ normal renal/hepatic function, reduce colchicine dose and monitor for symptoms of colchicine toxicity. CYP3A4 inducers/inhibitors may affect levels, resulting in diminished efficacy or an increase or prolongation of effects; dose adjustments may be necessary for these drugs. Avoid w/ simvastatin, lovastatin, atorvastatin, ergot alkaloid derivatives (eg, ergotamine, dihydroergotamine), Class IA (eg, quinidine, procainamide) or Class III (eg, dofetilide) antiarrhythmics, rifampin and other CYP3A4 inducers (phenytoin, carbamazepine, phenobarbital), itraconazole, and ketoconazole. Hypotension, bradyarrhythmia, and loss of consciousness reported w/ calcium channel blockers (CCBs) that are CYP3A4 substrates (eg, verapamil, amlodipine, diltiazem); monitor for these adverse reactions and toxicity related to CCBs and adjust CCB dosage as necessary. Monitor for benzodiazepine-related adverse reactions and adjust midazolam dosage if necessary; caution w/ other benzodiazepines, which are metabolized by CYP3A4 and undergo a high 1st-pass effect (eg, triazolam). Caution w/ other drugs metabolized by the CYP3A4 (eg, cyclosporine, tacrolimus, sirolimus, hexobarbital); increases or prolongation of effects of these drugs may be observed. Coadministration w/ metoprolol in patients w/ heart failure may lead to metoprolol toxicity; monitor for metoprolol toxicity and adjust metoprolol dosage. Caution w/ digoxin; monitor for digoxin side effects or serum levels. Theophylline may worsen GI side effects, especially in females; administer 1 hr apart to decrease likelihood of GI side effects. May potentiate the effects of oral anticoagulants; consider monitoring PT/INR.

NURSING CONSIDERATIONS

Assessment: Assess for myasthenia gravis, history of hepatitis and/or jaundice associated w/ the use of telithromycin or any macrolides, history of hypersensitivity to telithromycin or any macrolides, renal/hepatic impairment, risk for QTc prolongation, pregnancy/nursing status, and possible drug interactions. Perform culture and susceptibility testing.

Monitoring: Monitor for signs/symptoms of hepatitis, QTc prolongation, visual disturbances, loss of consciousness, CDAD, and other adverse reactions. Monitor LFTs in patients w/ signs and symptoms of hepatitis. Consider monitoring PT/INR w/ oral anticoagulants.

Patient Counseling: Inform that therapy treats only bacterial, not viral, infections. Instruct to take exactly ud even if the patient feels better early in the course of therapy; inform that skipping doses or not completing full course may decrease effectiveness and may increase likelihood of bacterial resistance. Instruct to d/c and seek medical attention immediately if signs/symptoms of liver injury occur. Advise to report any fainting or palpitations occurring during treatment. Counsel on problems w/ vision and loss of consciousness. Advise to minimize engaging in hazardous activities (eg, driving, operating machinery) and to seek physician's advice before taking another dose if visual difficulties, loss of consciousness/fainting, confusion, or hallucination occurs. Advise to inform physician of any other medications concurrently being taken, including OTC products. Inform that diarrhea is a common problem caused by therapy; instruct to contact physician as soon as possible if watery and bloody stools (w/ or w/o stomach cramps and fever) occur, even as late as ≥2 months after taking last dose.

Storage: 25°C (77°F); excursions permitted to 15-30°C (59-86°F).

KETOCONAZOLE TABLETS – ketoconazole RX

Class: Azole antifungal

Serious hepatotoxicity, including cases with a fatal outcome or requiring liver transplantation, reported; monitor closely. Contraindicated with dofetilide, quinidine, pimozide, and cisapride; may cause elevated levels of these drugs and may prolong QT intervals, sometimes resulting in life-threatening ventricular dysrhythmias (eg, torsades de pointes). Should be used only when other effective antifungal therapy is not available or tolerated and potential benefits outweigh potential risks.

ADULT DOSAGE

Fungal Infections

Following systemic infections in patients who have failed or who are intolerant to other therapies: blastomycosis, coccidioidomycosis, histoplasmosis, chromomycosis, and paracoccidioidomycosis

Initial: 200mg qd

Titrate: May be increased to 400mg qd if clinical responsiveness is insufficient w/in the expected time

Usual treatment duration is 6 months; continue until active fungal infection has subsided

PEDIATRIC DOSAGE

Fungal Infections

Following systemic infections in patients who have failed or who are intolerant to other therapies: blastomycosis, coccidioidomycosis, histoplasmosis, chromomycosis, and paracoccidioidomycosis

>2 Years:

3.3-6.6mg/kg single daily dose

Usual treatment duration is 6 months; continue until active fungal infection has subsided

ADMINISTRATION

Oral route

HOW SUPPLIED

Tab: 200mg* *scored

CONTRAINDICATIONS

Coadministration of CYP3A4 substrates (eg, dofetilide, quinidine, cisapride, pimozide), methadone, disopyramide, dronedarone, ergot alkaloids (eg, dihydroergotamine, ergometrine, ergotamine, methylergometrine), irinotecan, lurasidone, oral midazolam, alprazolam, triazolam, felodipine, nisoldipine, ranolazine, tolvaptan, eplerenone, lovastatin, simvastatin, colchicine, and CYP3A4 metabolized HMG-CoA reductase inhibitors (eg, simvastatin, lovastatin). Acute or chronic liver disease.

WARNINGS/PRECAUTIONS

Cases of hepatitis reported in children. Monitor ALT weekly during treatment; interrupt therapy and obtain a full set of liver tests if ALT values increase to a level above the ULN or 30% above baseline, or if symptoms develop. Repeat liver tests to ensure normalization of values. If therapy is restarted, monitor frequently to detect any recurring liver injury. May prolong the QT interval. May decrease adrenal corticosteroid secretion at doses ≥400mg; do not exceed the recommended daily dose of 200-400mg. Monitor adrenal function in patients with adrenal insufficiency or with borderline adrenal function and in patients under prolonged periods of stress (eg, major surgery, intensive care). Not approved for treatment of advanced prostate cancer and Cushing's syndrome. Anaphylaxis and hypersensitivity reactions, including urticaria, reported. May lower serum testosterone levels. Penetrates poorly into the CSF; should not be used for fungal meningitis.

ADVERSE REACTIONS

Hepatotoxicity, diarrhea, gynecomastia, anorexia, insomnia, headache, photophobia, orthostatic hypotension, epistaxis, N/V, abdominal pain, pruritus, myalgia, asthenia, thrombocytopenia.

DRUG INTERACTIONS

See Boxed Warning and Contraindications. Avoid with potentially hepatotoxic drugs. Drugs that reduce the gastric acidity (eg, acid neutralizing medicines [eg, aluminum hydroxide], or acid secretion suppressors [eg, H2-receptor antagonists and proton pump inhibitors]) may impair absorption; use with caution. Administer with an acidic beverage (eg, non-diet cola) upon co-treatment with drugs reducing gastric acidity. Administer acid-neutralizing medicines at least 1 hr before or 2 hrs after taking ketoconazole tabs; upon coadministration, monitor antifungal activity and increase ketoconazole dose as deemed necessary. Potent CYP3A4 inducers (eg, isoniazid, rifabutin, rifampicin, carbamazepine, phenytoin, efavirenz, nevirapine) may decrease bioavailability and reduce efficacy; avoid use of these drugs from 2 weeks before and during treatment, unless the benefits outweigh the risk of potentially reduced ketoconazole efficacy; monitor ketoconazole and increase dose as deemed necessary. Potent CYP3A4 inhibitors (eg, ritonavir, ritonavir-boosted darunavir, ritonavir-boosted fosamprenavir) may increase levels; use with caution and monitor closely for signs or symptoms of increased or prolonged pharmacologic effects of ketoconazole; decrease ketoconazole dose as deemed necessary. May increase levels of tamsulosin, rifabutin, rivaroxaban, carbamazepine, dasatinib, lapatinib, nilotinib, everolimus, rapamycin (also known as sirolimus), temsirolimus, and salmeterol; avoid use of these drugs during and up to 1 week after discontinuation of treatment unless the benefits outweigh the risks of side effects. May also increase levels of alfentanil, buprenorphine IV and SL, fentanyl, oxycodone, sufentanil, digoxin, telithromycin, cilostazol, coumarins, dabigatran, repaglinide, saxagliptin, praziquantel, eletriptan, bortezomib, busulphan, docetaxel, erlotinib, imatinib, ixabepilone, paclitaxel, trimetrexate, vinca alkaloids, aripiprazole, buspirone, haloperidol, quetiapine, ramelteon, risperidone, indinavir, maraviroc, saquinavir, nadolol, verapamil, aliskiren, bosentan, aprepitant, budesonide, ciclesonide, cyclosporine, dexamethasone, fluticasone, methylprednisolone, tacrolimus, atorvastatin, fesoterodine, sildenafil, solifenacin, tadalafil, tolterodine, vardenafil, alcohol, and cinacalcet; use with caution and monitor closely for signs or symptoms of increased or prolonged effects or side effects of the interacting drug, and reduce its dose as deemed necessary. Refer to PI for further information and dosing modifications/ recommendations when used with certain concomitant therapies.

NURSING CONSIDERATIONS

Assessment: Assess for drug hypersensitivity, adrenal insufficiency, conditions where treatment is contraindicated or cautioned, pregnancy/nursing status, and possible drug interactions. Perform lab and clinical documentation of infection prior to therapy. Obtain baseline lab tests (eg, GGT, alkaline phosphatase, ALT/AST, total bilirubin, PT, INR, testing for viral hepatitis) prior to therapy.

Monitoring: Monitor for signs/symptoms of hepatotoxicity, anaphylaxis/hypersensitivity reactions, and other adverse reactions. Monitor serum ALT weekly during treatment. Monitor adrenal function in patients with adrenal insufficiency or with borderline adrenal function and in patients under prolonged periods of stress.

Patient Counseling: Inform patients about risk of hepatotoxicity. Instruct to report any signs/ symptoms of liver dysfunction (eg, unusual fatigue, anorexia, N/V, abdominal pain, jaundice, dark urine, pale stools) to physician. Advise against alcohol consumption while on treatment.

Storage: 20-25°C (68-77°F). Protect from moisture.

KETOROLAC – ketorolac tromethamine — RX

Class: NSAID

For short-term (up to 5 days in adults) use only; total combined duration of oral and inj use should not exceed 5 days. Use tab only as continuation therapy following IV/IM dosing, if necessary. Not indicated for use in pediatric patients and not indicated for minor or chronic painful conditions. Increasing the dose beyond the label recommendations will not provide better efficacy but will increase risk of developing serious adverse events. May cause peptic ulcers, GI bleeding, and/or perforation of the stomach or intestines; contraindicated with active peptic ulcer disease, recent GI bleeding or perforation, and in patients with a history of peptic ulcer disease or GI bleeding. Elderly are at greater risk for serious GI events. May increase risk of serious cardiovascular (CV) thrombotic events, MI, and stroke; risk may increase with duration of use and with CV disease or risk factors for CV disease. Contraindicated for treatment of perioperative pain in the setting of CABG surgery, use as a prophylactic analgesic before any major surgery, with advanced renal impairment, in patients at risk for renal failure due to volume depletion, with suspected or confirmed cerebrovascular bleeding, with hemorrhagic diathesis, incomplete hemostasis, those at high-risk of bleeding, use in labor and delivery, and in patients currently receiving ASA or NSAIDs. Adjust dosage for patients ≥65 yrs of age, <50kg (110 lbs), and with moderately elevated SrCr; doses of inj are not to exceed 60mg/day in these patients. (Inj) Hypersensitivity reactions reported and appropriate counteractive measures must be available when administering the 1st dose. Contraindicated in patients with previously demonstrated allergic manifestations to ASA or other NSAIDs, for intrathecal/epidural administration, and in nursing mothers.

ADULT DOSAGE

Acute Pain

Short-Term (≤5 Days) Management of Moderately Severe Acute Pain:

Inj:

Single-Dose Treatment:

IM Dosing:

<65 Years:

One 60mg dose

≥65 Years:

One 30mg dose

IV Dosing:

<65 Years:

One 30mg dose

≥65 Years:

One 15mg dose

Multiple-Dose Treatment (IV or IM):

<65 Years:

30mg q6h

Max: 120mg/day

≥65 Years:

15mg q6h

Max: 60mg/day

Breakthrough Pain:

Do not increase the dose or frequency of ketorolac; consider supplementing these regimens w/ low doses of opioids prn unless otherwise contraindicated

Oral (Following IV or IM Dosing):

17-64 Years:

20mg once, then 10mg q4-6h prn

Max: 40mg/day

≥65 Years:

10mg once, then 10mg q4-6h prn

Max: 40mg/day

PEDIATRIC DOSAGE

Pediatric use may not have been established

DOSE MODIFICATION

Renal Impairment

Inj:

Single-Dose Treatment:

IM Dosing: One 30mg dose

IV Dosing: One 15mg dose

Multiple-Dose Treatment (IV or IM):

15mg q6h

Max: 60mg/day

Oral (Following IV or IM Dosing):

10mg once, then 10mg q4-6h prn

Max: 40mg/day

Other Important Modifications

Patients <50kg (110 lbs):

Inj:

Single-Dose Treatment:

IM Dosing: One 30mg dose

IV Dosing: One 15mg dose

Multiple-Dose Treatment (IV or IM):

15mg q6h

Max: 60mg/day

Oral (Following IV or IM Dosing):

10mg once, then 10mg q4-6h prn

Max: 40mg/day

ADMINISTRATION

IM/IV/Oral route

Combined duration of use of IV or IM dosing of ketorolac and ketorolac tabs is not to exceed 5 days

Inj

IV bolus must be given over ≥15 sec

IM administration should be given slowly and deeply into muscle

Do not mix in a small volume (eg, in a syringe) w/ morphine sulfate, meperidine HCl, promethazine HCl, or hydroxyzine HCl; this will result in precipitations of ketorolac from sol

Tab

Do not administer as initial dose; use is only indicated as continuation therapy to IV or IM dosing

Do not shorten dosing interval of 4-6 hrs

HOW SUPPLIED

Inj: 15mg/mL [1mL], 30mg/mL [1mL, 2mL, 10mL]; Tab: 10mg

CONTRAINDICATIONS

Active/history of peptic ulcer, recent/history of GI bleeding, recent GI perforation, advanced renal impairment or risk of renal failure due to volume depletion, labor and delivery, cerebrovascular bleeding, hemorrhagic diathesis, incomplete hemostasis, patients at high risk of bleeding. Patients who have experienced asthma, urticaria, or allergic reactions after taking ASA or other NSAIDs. Prophylactic analgesic before major surgery. Treatment of perioperative pain in the setting of CABG surgery. Current ASA or NSAIDs use. Concomitant use of probenecid and pentoxifylline. (Inj) Neuraxial (epidural or intrathecal) administration. Nursing mothers.

WARNINGS/PRECAUTIONS

Do not give oral formulation as an initial dose. Use lowest effective dose for the shortest duration possible. Increased risk for GI bleeding with longer duration of NSAID therapy, older age, and poor general health status. D/C and promptly initiate additional evaluation and treatment if a serious GI adverse event is suspected; consider alternate therapy that does not involve NSAIDs for high risk patients. May exacerbate inflammatory bowel disease (eg, ulcerative colitis, Crohn's disease). Renal papillary necrosis and other renal injury reported with long-term use. Renal toxicity reported; increased risk with renal/hepatic impairment, HF, and in the elderly. Acute renal failure, interstitial nephritis, and nephrotic syndrome reported. Caution with impaired renal function or history of kidney disease. May cause anaphylactoid reactions and serious skin adverse events (eg, exfoliative dermatitis, Stevens-Johnson syndrome, toxic epidermal necrolysis); d/c at 1st appearance of skin rash or any other signs of hypersensitivity. May lead to onset of new HTN or worsening of preexisting HTN; caution in patients with HTN. Monitor BP closely during initiation of therapy and throughout the course of therapy. Fluid retention, edema, retention of NaCl, oliguria, elevations of BUN and SrCr reported; caution with cardiac decompensation, HTN or similar conditions. Avoid in late pregnancy; may cause premature closure of the ductus arteriosus. Not a substitute for corticosteroids or for the treatment of corticosteroid insufficiency. May mask signs of inflammation. Caution with impaired hepatic function or history of liver disease; rare cases of severe hepatic reactions (eg, jaundice, fatal fulminant hepatitis, liver necrosis, hepatic failure) reported. Evaluate patients with signs/symptoms suggesting liver dysfunction, or abnormal LFTs for development of a more severe hepatic reaction; d/c if signs/symptoms of liver disease develop, or systemic manifestations (eg, eosinophilia, rash) occur. Anemia may occur; monitor Hgb or Hct if signs/symptoms of anemia develop with long-term use. May inhibit platelet aggregation and prolong bleeding time; caution with coagulation disorders and in postoperative setting when hemostasis is critical. Caution with preexisting asthma and avoid with ASA-sensitive asthma. Use with extreme caution in the elderly. Caution in debilitated patients. (Inj) Correct hypovolemia prior to administration.

ADVERSE REACTIONS

Hypersensitivity reactions, nausea, headache, dyspepsia, abdominal pain, edema, drowsiness, dizziness, abnormal renal function.

DRUG INTERACTIONS

See Boxed Warning and Contraindications. Binding reduced with concomitant use with salicylate. May increase risk of bleeding with drugs affecting hemostasis (eg, warfarin, dicumarol derivatives, heparin, dextrans). May increase risk of serious GI bleeding with oral corticosteroids, anticoagulants, SSRIs, smoking, and alcohol. May reduce natriuretic effect of furosemide and thiazide diuretics; observe closely for signs of renal failure and diuretic efficacy. May elevate plasma lithium levels and reduce renal lithium clearance; monitor for lithium toxicity. May enhance MTX toxicity; caution with concomitant use. Caution with ACE inhibitors and/or ARBs; may increase risk of renal impairment and diminish antihypertensive effect of ACE inhibitors and/or ARBs. Sporadic cases of seizures reported with concomitant use with antiepileptic drugs (eg, phenytoin, carbamazepine). Hallucinations reported with psychoactive drugs (eg, fluoxetine, thiothixene, alprazolam). (Inj) Apnea reported with nondepolarizing muscle relaxants.

NURSING CONSIDERATIONS

Assessment: Assess that use is not for perioperative pain in the setting of CABG surgery. Assess for previous hypersensitivity to drug, history of asthma, urticaria, or allergic-type reactions with ASA or other NSAIDs, CV disease, risk factors for GI events/CV disease, active/history of peptic ulcer, recent/history of GI bleeding, recent GI perforation, cerebrovascular bleeding, hemorrhagic diathesis, incomplete hemostasis, high risk of bleeding, renal/hepatic impairment, any other conditions where therapy is cautioned or contraindicated, pregnancy/nursing status, and for possible drug interactions. Obtain baseline BP.

Monitoring: Monitor for GI events, anaphylactoid/skin/hypersensitivity reactions, CV events, fluid retention, edema, hematological effects, and other adverse reactions. Monitor BP, LFTs, and renal function. Monitor CBC and chemistry profile periodically during long-term use.

Patient Counseling: Inform about potential risks/benefits of therapy. Advise not to give tab to other family members and to discard any unused drug. Instruct that the duration of use should not exceed 5 days. Inform that therapy is not indicated for use in pediatric patients. Instruct to seek medical attention for signs/symptoms of GI ulceration/bleeding (eg, epigastric pain, dyspepsia, melena, and hematemesis), CV events (eg, chest pain, SOB, weakness, slurring of speech), hepatotoxicity (eg, nausea, fatigue, lethargy, pruritus, jaundice, right upper quadrant tenderness, flu-like symptoms), skin reactions (eg, skin rash/blisters, fever or other signs of hypersensitivity such as itching), anaphylactoid reaction (eg, difficulty breathing, swelling of face/throat), or unexplained weight gain or edema. Instruct to avoid use in late pregnancy.

Storage: 20-25°C (68-77°F). (Inj) Protect from light.

KHEDEZLA – desvenlafaxine

RX

Class: Serotonin and norepinephrine reuptake inhibitor

Antidepressants increased the risk of suicidal thoughts and behavior in children, adolescents, and young adults in short-term studies. Monitor and observe closely for worsening, and emergence of suicidal thoughts and behaviors. Not approved for use in pediatric patients.

ADULT DOSAGE

Major Depressive Disorder

Usual: 50mg qd

Doses up to 400mg/day were effective but w/ no additional benefit; more frequent adverse reactions reported at higher doses

Periodically reassess need for continued treatment

Conversions

Switching from Other Antidepressants:
May need to taper the initial antidepressant to minimize discontinuation symptoms

Dosing Considerations with MAOIs

Switching to/from an MAOI for Psychiatric Disorders:
Allow at least 14 days between discontinuation of an MAOI and initiation of treatment, and conversely allow at least 7 days between discontinuing treatment and initiation of an MAOI

W/ Other MAOIs (eg, Linezolid, IV Methylene Blue):
Do not start desvenlafaxine in patients being treated w/ linezolid or IV methylene blue
In patients already receiving desvenlafaxine, if acceptable alternatives are not available and benefits outweigh risks, d/c desvenlafaxine and administer linezolid or IV methylene blue; monitor for serotonin syndrome for 7 days or until 24 hrs after the last dose of linezolid or IV methylene blue, whichever comes 1st. May resume desvenlafaxine therapy 24 hrs after the last dose of linezolid or IV methylene blue

PEDIATRIC DOSAGE

Pediatric use may not have been established

DOSE MODIFICATION

Renal Impairment

Moderate (CrCl 30-50mL/min):
Max: 50mg/day

Severe (CrCl <30mL/min)/ESRD:
Max: 50mg qod. Do not give supplemental doses after dialysis

Hepatic Impairment

Moderate-Severe:

Usual: 50mg/day

Max: 100mg/day

Discontinuation

Gradually reduce dose whenever possible

If intolerable symptoms occur following a decrease in dose or upon discontinuation of treatment, may consider resuming the previously prescribed dose; subsequently, may continue decreasing dose, but at a more gradual rate

ADMINISTRATION

Oral route

Take at the same time each day, w/ or w/o food

Swallow tab whole w/ fluid; do not divide, crush, chew, or dissolve

HOW SUPPLIED

Tab, Extended-Release: 50mg, 100mg

CONTRAINDICATIONS

Use of an MAOI intended to treat psychiatric disorders either concomitantly or within 7 days of stopping treatment. Treatment within 14 days of stopping an MAOI intended to treat psychiatric disorders. Starting treatment in patients being treated with other MAOIs (eg, linezolid, IV methylene blue).

WARNINGS/PRECAUTIONS

Not approved for the treatment of bipolar depression. Serotonin syndrome reported; d/c immediately if symptoms occur and initiate supportive symptomatic treatment. Caution with preexisting HTN, cardiovascular (CV), or cerebrovascular conditions that might be compromised by increases in BP. Consider dose reduction or discontinuation of therapy if sustained increases in BP occur. May increase risk of bleeding events. Pupillary dilation that occurs following use may trigger an angle-closure attack in a patient with anatomically narrow angles who does not have a patent iridectomy. Activation of mania/hypomania reported; caution with history or family history of mania/hypomania. Discontinuation symptoms reported. Avoid abrupt discontinuation; gradually reduce dose whenever possible. Seizures reported. Hyponatremia may occur; caution in elderly and volume-depleted patients. Consider discontinuation in patients with symptomatic hyponatremia and institute appropriate medical intervention. Interstitial lung disease and eosinophilic pneumonia may occur; consider this diagnosis in patients with progressive dyspnea, cough, or chest discomfort, and consider discontinuing therapy.

ADVERSE REACTIONS

N/V, dry mouth, dizziness, insomnia, somnolence, hyperhidrosis, constipation, anxiety, decreased appetite, tremor, mydriasis, erectile dysfunction, male libido decreased, fatigue, vision blurred.

DRUG INTERACTIONS

See Contraindications. Avoid with other desvenlafaxine-containing products or venlafaxine products; may increase levels and increase dose-related adverse reactions. Avoid alcohol consumption. Increased risk of serotonin syndrome when used concomitantly with other serotonergic drugs (eg, triptans, TCAs, fentanyl) and with drugs that impair metabolism of serotonin; d/c desvenlafaxine and any concomitant serotonergic agent immediately and initiate supportive symptomatic treatment. Caution with NSAIDs, aspirin, warfarin, and other drugs that affect coagulation or bleeding, due to increased risk of bleeding. May increase risk of hyponatremia with diuretics. Potent CYP3A4 inhibitors (eg, ketoconazole) may increase levels. CYP2D6 substrates (eg, desipramine, atomoxetine, dextromethorphan) should be dosed at the original level when coadministered with 100mg desvenlafaxine or lower; reduce dose of these substrates by up to 1/2 if coadministered with 400mg of desvenlafaxine; increase substrate dose to original level when 400mg of desvenlafaxine is discontinued.

NURSING CONSIDERATIONS

Assessment: Assess for seizure disorder, HTN, CV/cerebrovascular conditions, susceptibility to angle-closure glaucoma, volume depletion, hypersensitivity to the drug, hepatic/renal impairment, pregnancy/nursing status, and possible drug interactions. Perform adequate screening to determine if patient is at risk for bipolar disorder; such screening should include a detailed psychiatric history, including a family history of suicide, bipolar disorder, and depression.

Monitoring: Monitor for signs/symptoms of clinical worsening (eg, suicidality, unusual changes in behavior), serotonin syndrome, abnormal bleeding, angle-closure glaucoma, activation of mania/hypomania, seizures, hyponatremia, interstitial lung disease, eosinophilic pneumonia, and other adverse reactions. Monitor BP, LFTs, and renal function. Monitor for discontinuation symptoms (eg, dysphoric mood, irritability, agitation) when discontinuing therapy. Carefully monitor patients receiving concomitant warfarin therapy when treatment with desvenlafaxine is initiated or discontinued. Periodically reassess to determine the need for continued treatment.

Patient Counseling: Advise patients, families, and caregivers about the benefits and risks of treatment and instruct on appropriate use. Counsel patients, families, and caregivers to look for the emergence of suicidality, especially early during treatment and when the dose is adjusted up or down. Caution about the risk of serotonin syndrome. Advise patients that they should have regular BP monitoring, observe for signs/symptoms of activation of mania/hypomania, avoid alcohol, and that they should not d/c therapy without notifying their physician. Advise that therapy may increase the risk of bleeding events. Caution about risk of angle-closure glaucoma. Caution against operating hazardous machinery (including automobiles) until reasonably certain that therapy does not adversely affect ability to engage in such activities. Advise to notify physician if allergic phenomena develop, if pregnant, intending to become pregnant, or if breastfeeding. Inform that an inert matrix tab passing in the stool or via colostomy may be noticed.

Storage: 20-25°C (68-77°F); excursions permitted to 15-30°C (59-86°F).

KITABIS PAK – tobramycin RX

Class: Aminoglycoside

ADULT DOSAGE

Cystic Fibrosis

Patients w/ *Pseudomonas aeruginosa*:
1 single-use ampule (300mg/5mL) bid by oral inh in alternating periods of 28 days on drug followed by 28 days off drug

PEDIATRIC DOSAGE

Cystic Fibrosis

Patients w/ *Pseudomonas aeruginosa*:
≥6 Years:
1 single-use ampule (300mg/5mL) bid by oral inh in alternating periods of 28 days on drug followed by 28 days off drug

ADMINISTRATION

Oral inh route

Take doses as close to 12 hrs apart as possible; not <6 hrs apart
Administer using only the Pari LC Plus Reusable Nebulizer with a DeVilbiss Pulmo-Aide air compressor
Entire treatment should take approximately 15 min to complete; continue treatment until all inh sol has been delivered and there is no longer any mist being produced
Do not dilute/mix inh sol with other drugs in the nebulizer, including dornase alfa

HOW SUPPLIED

Sol, Inh: 300mg/5mL

WARNINGS/PRECAUTIONS

Bronchospasm, ototoxicity (eg, tinnitus), and nephrotoxicity may occur. If ototoxicity is noted, or nephrotoxicity develops, patient should be managed as medically appropriate, including potentially discontinuing tobramycin inh sol. May aggravate muscle weakness because of a potential curare-like effect on neuromuscular function. If neuromuscular blockade occurs, it may be reversed by administration of Ca^{2+} salts but mechanical assistance may be necessary. May cause fetal harm.

ADVERSE REACTIONS

Cough, pharyngitis, increased sputum, dyspnea, hemoptysis, decreased lung function, voice alteration, taste perversion, rash.

DRUG INTERACTIONS

Avoid concurrent and/or sequential use with other drugs with neurotoxic, nephrotoxic, or ototoxic potential. Some diuretics may enhance aminoglycoside toxicity by altering aminoglycoside concentrations in serum and tissue; do not administer with ethacrynic acid, furosemide, urea, or IV mannitol. Monitor for toxicities associated with aminoglycosides if used concomitantly with parenteral aminoglycosides; monitor serum tobramycin levels.

NURSING CONSIDERATIONS

Assessment: Assess for auditory or vestibular dysfunction, renal dysfunction, neuromuscular disorders, drug hypersensitivity, pregnancy/nursing status, and possible drug interactions.

Monitoring: Monitor for bronchospasm, ototoxicity, nephrotoxicity, neuromuscular effects, and other adverse reactions.

Patient Counseling: Advise to inform physician if SOB or wheezing occurs soon after administration, or if ringing in the ears, dizziness, or any changes in hearing develop. Instruct to notify physician if planning to become pregnant or if nursing. Instruct patients on multiple therapies to take their medications prior to inhaling the tobramycin inh sol, or ud by physician.

Storage: 2-8°C (36-46°F). Upon removal from the refrigerator, or if refrigeration is unavailable, may be stored at room temperature (up to 25°C [77°F]) for up to 28 days. Do not expose to intense light.

KLOR-CON M – potassium chloride

RX

Class: K^+ supplement

OTHER BRAND NAMES
Klor-Con

ADULT DOSAGE

Hypokalemia

Prevention:
20mEq/day

Treatment:
≥40-100mEq/day or more; divide dose so that no more than 20mEq is given in a single dose

PEDIATRIC DOSAGE
Pediatric use may not have been established

DOSE MODIFICATION

Elderly
Start at lower end of dosing range

ADMINISTRATION
Oral route

Take w/ meals and w/ a glass of water or other liquid

Klor-Con
Swallow tab whole; do not crush, chew, or suck

Klor-Con M

If Unable to Swallow Whole Tab:
A) Break tab in 1/2 and take each half separately w/ a glass of water, or
B) Prepare an aqueous sus

Aqueous Sus Preparation:
1. Place whole tab in approx 4 fl oz of water
2. Allow 2 min for tab to disintegrate
3. Stir for 30 sec after tab has disintegrated
4. Swirl sus and consume entire contents of the glass immediately by drinking or using a straw
5. Add another 1 fl oz of water, swirl, and consume immediately
6. Then, add an additional 1 fl oz of water, swirl, and consume immediately

HOW SUPPLIED
Tab, Extended-Release (ER): (Klor-Con M) 10mEq, 15mEq, 20mEq; (Klor-Con) 8mEq, 10mEq

CONTRAINDICATIONS
Hyperkalemia, cardiac patients with esophageal compression due to an enlarged left atrium. Structural, pathological (eg, diabetic gastroparesis) or pharmacological (eg, use of anticholinergic agents or other agents with anticholinergic properties) cause for arrest or delay through the GI tract with all solid dosage forms.

WARNINGS/PRECAUTIONS
Potentially fatal hyperkalemia and cardiac arrest may occur; monitor serum K^+ levels and adjust dose appropriately. Extreme caution with acidosis and cardiac and renal disease; monitor ECG and electrolytes. Hypokalemia with metabolic acidosis should be treated with an alkalinizing K^+ salt (eg, potassium bicarbonate, potassium citrate, potassium acetate, potassium gluconate). Solid oral dosage forms may produce ulcerative and/or stenotic lesions of the GI tract; d/c use if severe vomiting, abdominal pain, distention, or GI bleeding occurs. Reserve use for those who cannot tolerate, cannot comply, or refuse to take liquid or effervescent preparations. Caution in elderly.

ADVERSE REACTIONS
Hyperkalemia, GI effects (eg, obstruction, bleeding, ulceration), N/V, abdominal pain/discomfort, flatulence, diarrhea.

DRUG INTERACTIONS
See Contraindications. Risk of hyperkalemia with ACE inhibitors (eg, captopril, enalapril). Risk of hyperkalemia with K^+-sparing diuretics (eg, spironolactone, triamterene, amiloride).

NURSING CONSIDERATIONS

Assessment: Assess for hyperkalemia, chronic renal failure, systemic acidosis, cardiac patients, if patient cannot tolerate, refuses to take, or cannot comply with taking liquid or effervescent K^+ preparations prior to administration of an ER tab formulation. Obtain baseline ECG, serum electrolyte levels, and renal function.

Monitoring: Monitor for signs/symptoms of hyperkalemia and other adverse events that may occur. In patients taking solid oral dosage forms, monitor for signs/symptoms of GI lesions. In patients with cardiac disease, acidosis, or renal disease, monitor acid-base balance and perform appropriate monitoring of serum electrolytes, ECG, renal function, and the clinical status of the patient.

Patient Counseling: Inform about benefits and risks of therapy. Instruct to report to physician if patient develops any type of GI symptoms (eg, tarry stools or other evidence of GI bleeding, vomiting, abdominal pain/distention) or if other adverse events occur. Instruct to contact physician if difficulty in swallowing develops or if the tabs are sticking in the throat. (Klor-Con): Instruct to swallow tabs whole and to take with meals and full glass of water or other liquid. Follow the frequency and amount prescribed by the physician, especially if also taking diuretics and/or digitalis preparations. (Klor-Con M): Instruct to take each dose with meals and with full glass of water or other liquid. Inform that patient may break tabs in half or make an oral aqueous sus with tabs and 4 fl oz of water (see PI for proper preparation). Inform that aqueous sus not taken immediately should be discarded and use of other liquids for suspending is not recommended.

Storage: Klor-Con: 15-30°C (59-86°F). Klor-Con M: 20-25°C (68-77°F); excursions permitted to 15-30°C (59-86°F).

KOMBIGLYZE XR – metformin hydrochloride/saxagliptin RX

Class: Biguanide/dipeptidyl peptidase-4 (DPP-4) inhibitor

Lactic acidosis may occur due to metformin accumulation; risk increases w/ conditions such as sepsis, dehydration, excess alcohol intake, hepatic impairment, renal impairment, and acute CHF. If acidosis is suspected, d/c and hospitalize patient immediately.

ADULT DOSAGE

Type 2 Diabetes Mellitus

Initial:
Patients Requiring 5mg Saxagliptin:
Not Currently on Metformin: 5mg-500mg qd

Patients Requiring 2.5mg Saxagliptin:
Currently on Metformin ER: 2.5mg-1000mg qd
Metformin Naive/Requiring >1000mg Metformin: Use individual components

Max: 5mg-2000mg/day

PEDIATRIC DOSAGE

Pediatric use may not have been established

DOSE MODIFICATION

Concomitant Medications
Strong CYP3A4/5 Inhibitors:
Max: 2.5mg-1000mg qd

Insulin Secretagogue (eg, Sulfonylurea)/Insulin:
May require lower doses of insulin secretagogue or insulin

ADMINISTRATION

Oral route

Swallow tab whole; do not cut, crush, or chew
Give w/ pm meal

HOW SUPPLIED

Tab, ER: (Saxagliptin-Metformin ER) 5mg-500mg, 5mg-1000mg, 2.5mg-1000mg

CONTRAINDICATIONS

Renal impairment (eg, SrCr ≥1.5mg/dL [men], ≥1.4mg/dL [women], or abnormal CrCl), acute or chronic metabolic acidosis, including diabetic ketoacidosis.

WARNINGS/PRECAUTIONS

Not for use for the treatment of type 1 DM or diabetic ketoacidosis. Not studied in patients w/ history of pancreatitis. Acute pancreatitis reported; d/c if pancreatitis is suspected. Assess renal function before initiation of therapy and at least annually thereafter; d/c w/ evidence of renal impairment. Avoid w/ hepatic disease/impairment. May decrease vitamin B12 levels; monitor hematological parameters annually. Suspend temporarily for any surgical procedure (except minor procedures not associated w/ restricted intake of foods and fluids); restart when oral intake is resumed and renal function is normal. Evaluate for evidence of ketoacidosis or lactic acidosis if lab abnormalities or clinical illness develops; d/c if acidosis occurs. Temporarily d/c at time of or prior to intravascular contrast studies w/ iodinated materials, withhold for 48 hrs subsequent to the procedure, and reinstitute only if renal function is normal. D/C in hypoxic states (eg, shock, acute CHF, acute myocardial infarction [MI]). Serious hypersensitivity reactions reported; d/c if suspected, assess for other potential causes, and institute alternative treatment for DM. Avoid in patients ≥80 yrs of age unless renal function is not reduced. Caution in patients susceptible to hypoglycemic effects, such as elderly, debilitated/malnourished patients, and those w/ adrenal/pituitary insufficiency or alcohol intoxication. Caution in patients with history of angioedema to another DPP-4 inhibitor. No conclusive evidence of macrovascular risk reduction.

ADVERSE REACTIONS

Lactic acidosis, diarrhea, N/V, upper respiratory tract infection, urinary tract infection, headache, nasopharyngitis.

DRUG INTERACTIONS

Hypoglycemia may occur w/ other glucose-lowering agents (eg, sulfonylureas, insulin) or ethanol; may require lower dose of sulfonylurea or insulin. Metformin: Cationic drugs that are eliminated by renal tubular secretion (eg, cimetidine, amiloride, digoxin, morphine, procainamide, quinidine, quinine, ranitidine, triamterene, trimethoprim, vancomycin) may potentially produce an interaction; monitor and adjust dose of Kombiglyze XR and/or cationic drug if necessary. Observe for loss of glycemic control w/ thiazides and other diuretics, corticosteroids, phenothiazines, thyroid products, estrogens, oral contraceptives, phenytoin, nicotinic acid, sympathomimetics, calcium channel blockers, and isoniazid. Alcohol may potentiate the effect of metformin on lactate metabolism; avoid excessive alcohol intake. Caution w/ drugs that may affect renal function or result in significant hemodynamic change or may interfere w/ the disposition of metformin (eg, cationic drugs eliminated by renal tubular secretion). May be difficult to recognize hypoglycemia w/ β-adrenergic blocking drugs. Saxagliptin: Increased plasma concentrations w/ ketoconazole and other strong CYP3A4/5 inhibitors (eg, atazanavir, clarithromycin, indinavir, itraconazole, nefazodone, nelfinavir, ritonavir, saquinavir, telithromycin); limit dose of saxagliptin to 2.5mg. Strong CYP3A4/5 inducers and inhibitors may alter pharmacokinetics of saxagliptin and its active metabolite.

NURSING CONSIDERATIONS

Assessment: Assess for metabolic acidosis, risk factors for lactic acidosis, renal/hepatic impairment, previous hypersensitivity to the drug, history of pancreatitis, inadequate vitamin B12 or Ca^{2+} absorption, type of DM, diabetic ketoacidosis, history of angioedema w/ another DPP-4 inhibitor, pregnancy/nursing status, and possible drug interactions. Assess if patient is planning to undergo any surgical procedure or is under any form of stress. Obtain baseline FPG and HbA1c levels, and hematological parameters.

Monitoring: Monitor for signs/symptoms of lactic acidosis, pancreatitis, hypoxic states, hypoglycemia, hypersensitivity reactions, and for other adverse reactions. Monitor for changes in clinical status. Monitor renal function, especially in elderly, at least annually. Perform routine serum vitamin B12 measurements at 2- to 3-yr intervals in patients predisposed to develop subnormal vitamin B12 levels. Monitor FPG and HbA1c levels, hepatic function, and hematologic parameters periodically.

Patient Counseling: Inform of the risks, benefits, and alternative modes of therapy. Advise on the importance of adherence to dietary instructions, regular physical activity, periodic blood glucose monitoring and HbA1c testing, recognition/management of hypo/hyperglycemia, and assessment of diabetes complications. Instruct to seek medical advice promptly during periods of stress as medication needs may change. Inform of the risk of developing lactic acidosis during therapy. Advise to d/c therapy and contact physician if symptoms of allergic reactions, unexplained hyperventilation, myalgia, malaise, unusual somnolence, dizziness, slow or irregular heartbeat, sensation of feeling cold (especially in the extremities) or other nonspecific symptoms occur. Counsel to inform physician if any unusual symptom develops, or if any known symptom persists or worsens. Counsel against excessive alcohol intake. Inform that inactive ingredients may be eliminated in the feces as a soft mass that may resemble the original tab.

Storage: 20-25°C (68-77°F); excursions permitted to 15-30°C (59-86°F).

KYNAMRO – mipomersen sodium **RX**

Class: Lipid-regulating agent

May cause elevations in transaminases; measure ALT, AST, alkaline phosphatase, and total bilirubin prior to therapy, and then ALT/AST regularly as recommended. Withhold dose if ALT/AST is ≥3X ULN. D/C for clinically significant liver toxicity. May increase hepatic fat. Hepatic steatosis is a risk factor for advanced liver disease, including steatohepatitis and cirrhosis. Available only through a restricted program under a Risk Evaluation and Mitigation Strategy because of the risk of hepatotoxicity.

ADULT DOSAGE

Homozygous Familial Hypercholesterolemia

Usual: 200mg SQ once weekly; give on the same day every week, but if dose is missed, give at least 3 days from the next weekly dose

PEDIATRIC DOSAGE

Pediatric use may not have been established

DOSE MODIFICATION

Adverse Reactions

Transaminase Elevations:

ALT/AST ≥3X and <5X ULN:

Confirm elevation w/ repeat measurement w/in 1 week

If confirmed, withhold dosing, and obtain additional liver-related tests if not already measured (eg,

total bilirubin, alkaline phosphatase, INR) and investigate to identify probable cause
If resuming therapy after transaminases resolve to <3X ULN, consider monitoring liver-related tests more frequently

ALT/AST ≥5X ULN:
Withhold dosing, obtain additional liver-related tests if not already measured (eg, total bilirubin, alkaline phosphatase, INR) and investigate to identify probable cause
If resuming therapy after transaminases resolve to <3X ULN, monitor liver-related tests more frequently

If transaminase elevations are accompanied by clinical symptoms of liver injury, increases in bilirubin ≥2X ULN, or active liver disease, d/c therapy and investigate to identify probable cause

ADMINISTRATION
SQ route

Remove from refrigerated storage and allow to reach room temperature for at least 30 min prior to administration
Inject into abdomen, thigh region, or outer area of the upper arm
Do not inject in areas of active skin disease or injury; avoid areas of tattooed skin and scarring

HOW SUPPLIED
Inj: 200mg/mL [1mL]

CONTRAINDICATIONS
Moderate or severe hepatic impairment (Child-Pugh B or C), active liver disease, including unexplained persistent elevations of serum transaminases.

WARNINGS/PRECAUTIONS
Not recommended as an adjunct to LDL apheresis. Not recommended in patients w/ severe renal impairment, clinically significant proteinuria, or on renal dialysis. If baseline LFTs are abnormal, consider initiating therapy after an appropriate work-up and the baseline abnormalities are explained or resolved. D/C therapy and identify the probable cause if transaminase elevations are accompanied by clinical symptoms of liver injury (eg, N/V, abdominal pain, fever), increases in bilirubin ≥2X ULN, or active liver disease. Inj-site reactions (eg, erythema, pain, tenderness) reported; follow proper technique for SQ administration. Flu-like symptoms (eg, influenza-like illness, pyrexia, chills) reported. May cause fetal harm; females of reproductive potential should use effective contraception during therapy.

ADVERSE REACTIONS
Hepatic steatosis, increased serum transaminases, N/V, headache, pain in extremity, inj-site reactions, fatigue, influenza-like illness, HTN, pyrexia, chills, angina pectoris, peripheral edema, musculoskeletal pain, insomnia.

DRUG INTERACTIONS
Not recommended w/ other LDL-lowering agents that can increase hepatic fat. Alcohol may increase levels of hepatic fat and induce/exacerbate liver injury; avoid consumption of >1 alcoholic drink/day. Caution w/ other medications known to have potential for hepatotoxicity (eg, isotretinoin, amiodarone, acetaminophen [>4g/day for ≥3days/week], methotrexate, tetracyclines, tamoxifen); more frequent monitoring of liver-related tests may be warranted.

NURSING CONSIDERATIONS

Assessment: Assess for hepatic/renal impairment, drug hypersensitivity, pregnancy/nursing status, and possible drug interactions. Obtain baseline lipid levels, ALT/AST, alkaline phosphatase, and total bilirubin.

Monitoring: Monitor for inj-site reactions, flu-like symptoms, and other adverse reactions. Monitor LFTs monthly during 1st yr and at least every 3 months after 1st yr of therapy. Monitor lipid levels at least every 3 months for the 1st yr of therapy. Evaluate LDL level after 6 months to determine if LDL reduction achieved is sufficiently robust to warrant the potential risk of liver toxicity.

Patient Counseling: Inform that transaminase elevations and hepatic steatosis may occur; inform of the importance of monitoring LFTs prior to therapy and periodically thereafter. Advise of the potential for increased risk of liver injury if alcohol is consumed; instruct to limit alcohol consumption to ≤1 drink/day. Advise to report any symptoms of possible liver injury (eg, N/V, fever, anorexia). Inform that inj-site reactions and flu-like symptoms have been reported. Instruct patient or caregiver of the proper technique of administration and safe disposal procedures. Instruct females of reproductive potential to use effective contraception during therapy.

Storage: 2-8°C (36-46°F). Protect from light and keep in the original carton until time of use. If refrigeration is unavailable, may store ≤30°C (86°F), away from heat sources, for up to 14 days.

KYPROLIS – carfilzomib RX

Class: Proteasome inhibitor

ADULT DOSAGE

Multiple Myeloma

In patients who received at least 2 prior therapies including bortezomib and an immunomodulatory agent and have demonstrated disease progression on or w/in 60 days of completing last therapy
Cycle 1: 20mg/m^2
Cycle 2: Escalate dose to 27mg/m^2 if dose in Cycle 1 is tolerated
Subsequent Cycles: Continue at 27mg/m^2; continue until disease progression or an unacceptable toxicity occurs
Administer on 2 consecutive days, each week for 3 weeks (Days 1, 2, 8, 9, 15, 16), followed by a 12-day rest period (Days 17-28)
Each 28-day period is 1 treatment cycle
Calculate dose based on actual BSA at baseline; patients w/ BSA >2.2m^2 should receive a dose based on a BSA of 2.2m^2
Weight change of ≤20% do not need to be dose adjusted

Premedication

Hydration and Fluid Monitoring:
Prior to Each Dose in Cycle 1: Give 250mL-500mL of IV normal saline or other appropriate IV fluid; give an additional 250mL-500mL of IV fluids prn following administration
Subsequent Cycles: Continue IV hydration prn
Dexamethasone:
Give dexamethasone 4mg PO/IV prior to all doses during Cycle 1 and during 1st cycle of dose escalation to 27mg/m^2 to reduce infusion reactions
Reinstate dexamethasone premedication if these symptoms develop or reappear during subsequent cycles

PEDIATRIC DOSAGE

Pediatric use may not have been established

DOSE MODIFICATION

Adverse Reactions
Hematologic Toxicity:
Grade 3 or 4 Neutropenia:
Withhold dose; if fully recovered before next scheduled dose, continue at same dose level
If recovered to Grade 2 neutropenia, reduce dose by 1 dose level (from 27mg/m^2 to 20mg/m^2, or from 20mg/m^2 to 15mg/m^2)
If tolerated, the reduced dose may be escalated to the previous dose w/ discretion
Grade 4 Thrombocytopenia:
Withhold dose; if fully recovered before next scheduled dose, continue at same dose level
If recovered to Grade 3 thrombocytopenia, reduce dose by 1 dose level (from 27mg/m^2 to 20mg/m^2, or from 20mg/m^2 to 15mg/m^2)
If tolerated, the reduced dose may be escalated to the previous dose w/ discretion
Non-Hematologic Toxicity:
Cardiac Toxicity:
Grade 3 or 4, New Onset/Worsening of CHF, Decreased Left Ventricular Function, or MI:
Withhold until resolved or returned to baseline
After resolution, consider restarting at a reduced dose if appropriate (from 27mg/m^2 to 20mg/m^2, or from 20mg/m^2 to 15mg/m^2)
If tolerated, the reduced dose may be escalated to the previous dose w/ discretion
Pulmonary HTN:
Withhold until resolved or returned to baseline
Restart at the dose used prior to the event or reduced dose (from 27mg/m^2 to 20mg/m^2, or from 20mg/m^2 to 15mg/m^2) w/ discretion
If tolerated, the reduced dose may be escalated to the previous dose w/ discretion

Pulmonary Complications:
Grade 3 or 4:
Withhold until resolved or returned to baseline
Consider restarting at the next scheduled treatment w/ 1 dose level reduction (from 27mg/m^2 to 20mg/m^2, or from 20mg/m^2 to 15mg/m^2)
If tolerated, the reduced dose may be escalated to the previous dose w/ discretion
Hepatic Toxicity:
Grade 3 or 4 Elevation of Transaminases, Bilirubin, or Other Liver Abnormalities:
Withhold until resolved or returned to baseline
After resolution, consider restarting if appropriate; may be reinitiated at a reduced dose (from 27mg/m^2 to 20mg/m^2, or from 20mg/m^2 to 15mg/m^2) w/ frequent monitoring of liver function
If tolerated, the reduced dose may be escalated to the previous dose w/ discretion
Renal Toxicity:
SrCr ≥2X Baseline:
Withhold until renal function has recovered to Grade 1 or to baseline and monitor renal function
If attributable to therapy, restart at the next scheduled treatment at a reduced dose (from 27mg/m^2 to 20mg/m^2, or from 20mg/m^2 to 15mg/m^2)
If not attributable, restart at the dose used prior to the event
If tolerated, the reduced dose may be escalated to the previous dose w/ discretion
Peripheral Neuropathy:
Grade 3 or 4:
Withhold until resolved or returned to baseline
Restart at the dose used prior to the event or reduced dose (from 27mg/m^2 to 20mg/m^2, or from 20mg/m^2 to 15mg/m^2) w/ discretion
If tolerated, the reduced dose may be escalated to the previous dose w/ discretion
Other Grade 3 or 4 Nonhematological Toxicities:
Withhold until resolved or returned to baseline
Consider restarting at the next scheduled treatment w/ 1 dose level reduction (from 27mg/m^2 to 20 mg/m^2, or from 20mg/m^2 to 15mg/m^2)
If tolerated, the reduced dose may be escalated to the previous dose w/ discretion

ADMINISTRATION
IV route

Only for single use
Administer over 2-10 min
Do not mix w/ or administer as an infusion w/ other medicinal products
Flush IV line w/ normal saline or D5 inj immediately before and after administration; do not administer as a bolus

Reconstitution/Preparation
1. Slowly inject 29mL of sterile water for inj, directing the sol onto the inside wall of the vial to minimize foaming
2. Gently swirl and/or invert vial slowly for about 1 min, or until complete dissolution of any cake or powder occurs; do not shake. If foaming occurs, allow sol to rest for about 2-5 min, until foaming subsides
3. When administering in an IV bag, withdraw calculated dose from vial and dilute into 50mL D5 inj IV bag
4. Immediately discard the vial containing unused portion

HOW SUPPLIED
Inj: 60mg

WARNINGS/PRECAUTIONS
Death due to cardiac arrest has occurred w/in a day of administration. New onset/worsening of preexisting CHF w/ decreased left ventricular function or MI reported. Cardiac failure events (eg, cardiac failure congestive, pulmonary edema, decreased ejection fraction) reported; monitor for cardiac complications and manage promptly. Pulmonary arterial HTN (PAH) and dyspnea reported. Infusion reactions (eg, fever, chills, vomiting) may occur immediately following or up to 24 hrs after treatment; administer dexamethasone prior to treatment to reduce the incidence and severity of reactions. Tumor lysis syndrome (TLS) may occur; interrupt treatment until TLS is resolved. May cause thrombocytopenia; reduce or interrupt dose as clinically indicated. Hepatic failure, including fatal cases, and elevations of serum transaminases and bilirubin reported; monitor liver enzymes frequently. Thrombotic thrombocytopenic purpura/hemolytic uremic syndrome (TTP/HUS) including fatal outcome reported; if diagnosis is suspected, d/c therapy and evaluate. If diagnosis of TTP/HUS is excluded, therapy can be restarted. Posterior reversible encephalopathy syndrome (PRES) reported; d/c if suspected and evaluate. May cause fetal harm; patient should avoid becoming pregnant while on therapy.

ADVERSE REACTIONS
Fatigue, anemia, thrombocytopenia, dyspnea, diarrhea, pyrexia, URTI, headache, cough, N/V, blood creatinine increased, lymphopenia, peripheral edema, constipation.

NURSING CONSIDERATIONS

Assessment: Assess for dehydration, preexisting CHF, hepatic dysfunction, and pregnancy/nursing status. Obtain baseline CBC, LFTs, SrCr, and weight.

Monitoring: Monitor for signs/symptoms of dehydration, cardiac failure events/complications, PAH, dyspnea, TLS, infusion reactions, TTP/HUS, PRES, fluid overload during hydration, and other adverse reactions. Monitor CBC, LFTs, and SrCr.

Patient Counseling: Advise to contact physician if SOB, fever, chills, rigors, chest pain, cough, or swelling of the feet or legs develops. Instruct not to drive or operate machinery if fatigue, dizziness, fainting, and/or drop in BP are experienced. Advise regarding appropriate measures to avoid dehydration. Instruct female patients to use effective contraceptive measures to prevent pregnancy and instruct to inform physician immediately if pregnant. Instruct not to breastfeed while on therapy. Advise to notify physician if using or planning to take other prescription or OTC drugs.

Storage: Unopened Vials: 2-8°C (36-46°F). Store in carton to protect from light. Reconstituted Sol: 2-8°C (36-46°F) for 24 hrs and 15-30°C (59-86°F) for 4 hrs.

LABETALOL INJECTION – labetalol hydrochloride **RX**

Class: Alpha$_1$ blocker/nonselective beta-blocker

ADULT DOSAGE

Severe Hypertension

Repeated IV Inj:
Initial: 20mg slow IV inj over 2 min; measure supine BP immediately before and at 5 and 10 min after inj to evaluate response
Titrate: May give additional 40mg or 80mg inj at 10-min intervals until desired supine BP is achieved or a total of 300mg has been injected

Slow Continuous Infusion:
2mg/min
Titrate: May adjust infusion rate according to BP response
Effective Dose: 50-200mg
Max: 300mg
When a satisfactory response is obtained, d/c and start oral labetalol

Initiation of Dosing w/ Labetalol Tab:
Begin when supine diastolic BP has begun to rise
Initial: 200mg, followed by an additional 200mg or 400mg 6-12 hrs later, depending on BP response
Inpatient Titration: 200mg bid (400mg/day), 400mg bid (800mg/day), 800mg bid (1600mg/day), then 1200mg bid (2400mg/day)
If needed, total daily dose may be given in 3 divided doses
While in hospital, may increase dose of tabs at 1-day intervals

PEDIATRIC DOSAGE

Pediatric use may not have been established

ADMINISTRATION

IV Route

Administer in supine position

Compatibility
Ringers Inj; Lactated Ringers Inj;D5 and Ringers Inj; 5% Lactated Ringers and D5 Inj; D5 Inj; 0.9% NaCl Inj; D5 and 0.2% NaCl; 2.5% Dextrose and 0.45% NaCl inj; D5 and 0.9% NaCl Inj; D5 and 0.33% NaCl Inj

Incompatibility
5% Sodium Bicarbonate Inj
Care should be taken when administering alkaline drugs, including furosemide, in combination w/ labetalol

HOW SUPPLIED

Inj: 5mg/mL [20mL, 40mL]

CONTRAINDICATIONS

Bronchial asthma, overt cardiac failure, >1st-degree heart block, cardiogenic shock, severe bradycardia, other conditions associated with severe and prolonged hypotension, and history of obstructive airway disease.

WARNINGS/PRECAUTIONS

For IV use in hospitalized patients. Severe hepatocellular injury (rare) reported. Caution with hepatic impairment. Perform appropriate lab testing at the 1st symptom/sign of liver dysfunction. D/C and do not restart if with lab evidence of liver injury or jaundice. May precipitate more severe failure in patients with congestive heart failure (CHF); avoid with overt CHF and caution with history of well-compensated heart failure (HF). May lead to cardiac failure in patients without a history of HF; digitalize and/or treat with a diuretic at the 1st sign/symptom of HF and observe carefully; d/c (gradually, if possible) if cardiac failure continues. Exacerbation of angina and, in some cases, myocardial infarction reported after abrupt discontinuation. If angina markedly worsens or acute coronary insufficiency develops, reinstitute therapy promptly, at least temporarily, and take other appropriate measures for the management of unstable angina. Avoid in patients with nonallergic bronchospastic disease. Caution with pheochromocytoma; paradoxical hypertensive responses reported. May prevent appearance of premonitory signs/symptoms of acute hypoglycemia (eg, tachycardia). Chronically administered therapy should not be routinely withdrawn prior to major surgery. Several deaths have occurred during surgery (including when used in cases to control bleeding). Caution when reducing severely elevated BP; cerebral infarction, optic nerve infarction, angina, and ECG ischemic changes reported with other agents. Avoid rapid/excessive falls in BP; achieve desired BP lowering over as long a period of time as is compatible with patient status. Symptomatic postural hypotension may occur if patients are tilted or allowed to assume upright position within 3 hrs of administration; establish patient's ability to tolerate an upright position before permitting any ambulation. Intraoperative floppy iris syndrome (IFIS) observed during cataract surgery. Avoid in patients with low cardiac indices and elevated systemic vascular resistance. Hypotension or bradycardia reported with administration of up to 3g/day as an infusion for up to 2-3 days. Patients with a history of severe anaphylactic reactions to a variety of allergens may be more reactive to repeated challenge and may be unresponsive to usual doses of epinephrine. Lab test interactions may occur.

ADVERSE REACTIONS

Symptomatic postural hypotension, dizziness, N/V, somnolence/yawning, increased sweating, tingling of scalp/skin, transient BUN/SrCr increase.

DRUG INTERACTIONS

Tremors reported with oral labetalol in combination with TCAs. May blunt the bronchodilator effect of β-agonists in patients with bronchospasm; doses greater than the normal antiasthmatic dose may be required. Cimetidine may increase bioavailability of oral labetalol; caution in establishing required dose for BP control in patients with conditions that enhance absorption or alter hepatic metabolism. Synergistic effect with halothane; do not use ≥3% halothane during controlled hypotensive anesthesia. Additional antihypertensive effects with nitroglycerin. Caution with calcium antagonists of the verapamil type. May need to adjust dose of antidiabetic drugs.

NURSING CONSIDERATIONS

Assessment: Assess for hypersensitivity to the drug, bronchospastic disease, heart block, severe bradycardia, cardiogenic shock, overt cardiac failure, diabetes mellitus, pheochromocytoma, ischemic heart disease, hepatic/renal impairment, any other conditions where treatment is contraindicated or cautioned, pregnancy/nursing status, and possible drug interactions. Obtain baseline BP.

Monitoring: Monitor BP. Monitor LFTs periodically. In patients with concomitant illnesses (eg, renal impairment), monitor these conditions. Monitor for signs/symptoms of HF, postural hypotension, exacerbation of ischemic heart disease following abrupt withdrawal, hypersensitivity reactions, IFIS during cataract surgery, and other adverse reactions. Monitor patient when discontinuing therapy.

Patient Counseling: Instruct to remain supine during and immediately following (for up to 3 hrs) inj; advise on how to proceed gradually to become ambulatory. Instruct to consult physician at any sign/symptom of impending HF or hepatic dysfunction. Instruct on appropriate directions for titration of dosage when started on labetalol tabs following adequate BP control with labetalol inj. Inform that transient scalp tingling may occur when treatment with tabs is initiated. Instruct patients being treated with labetalol tabs not to interrupt or d/c therapy without physician's advice. Advise to limit physical activity when discontinuing therapy.

Storage: 2-30°C (36-86°F). Protect from light and freezing.

LAMICTAL – lamotrigine RX

Class: Phenyltriazine

Serious life-threatening rashes, including Stevens-Johnson syndrome, toxic epidermal necrolysis, and/or rash-related death reported. Serious rash occurs more often in pediatric patients than in adults. D/C at 1st sign of rash, unless rash is clearly not drug related. Potential increased risk w/ concomitant valproate (including valproic acid and divalproex sodium) or exceeding the recommended initial dose/dose escalation.

OTHER BRAND NAMES

Lamictal ODT

ADULT DOSAGE

Epilepsy

Adjunctive Therapy for Partial-Onset, Primary Generalized Tonic-Clonic Seizures, or Generalized Seizures of Lennox-Gastaut Syndrome:

Taking Valproate:

Weeks 1 and 2: 25mg qod

Weeks 3 and 4: 25mg qd

Week 5 Onward: Increase every 1-2 weeks by 25-50mg/day

Maint: 100-200mg/day w/ valproate alone or 100-400mg/day w/ valproate and other drugs inducing glucuronidation in 1 or 2 divided doses

Not Taking Carbamazepine, Phenytoin, Phenobarbital, Primidone, or Valproate:

Weeks 1 and 2: 25mg qd

Weeks 3 and 4: 50mg/day

Week 5 Onward: Increase every 1-2 weeks by 50mg/day

Maint: 225-375mg/day in 2 divided doses

Taking Carbamazepine, Phenytoin, Phenobarbital, or Primidone, w/o Valproate:

Weeks 1 and 2: 50mg/day

Weeks 3 and 4: 100mg/day in 2 divided doses

Week 5 Onward: Increase every 1-2 weeks by 100mg/day

Maint: 300-500mg/day in 2 divided doses

Bipolar I Disorder

Maint Treatment to Delay the Time to Occurrence of Mood Episodes in Patients Treated for Acute Mood Episodes w/ Standard Therapy:

Taking Valproate:

Weeks 1 and 2: 25mg qod

Weeks 3 and 4: 25mg/day

Week 5: 50mg/day

Weeks 6 and 7: 100mg/day

Not Taking Carbamazepine, Phenytoin, Phenobarbital, Primidone, or Valproate:

Weeks 1 and 2: 25mg/day

Weeks 3 and 4: 50mg/day

Week 5: 100mg/day

Weeks 6 and 7: 200mg/day

Taking Carbamazepine, Phenytoin, Phenobarbital, or Primidone, w/o Valproate:

Weeks 1 and 2: 50mg/day

Weeks 3 and 4: 100mg/day

Week 5: 200mg/day

Week 6: 300mg/day

Week 7: Up to 400mg/day

Weeks 3-7: Take in divided doses

PEDIATRIC DOSAGE

Epilepsy

Adjunctive Therapy for Partial-Onset, Primary Generalized Tonic-Clonic Seizures, or Generalized Seizures of Lennox-Gastaut Syndrome:

2-12 Years:

Round dose down to the nearest whole tab; give in 1-2 divided doses

Taking Valproate:

Initial Weight-Based Dosing Guide (Weeks 1-4): Refer to PI

Weeks 1 and 2: 0.15mg/kg/day

Weeks 3 and 4: 0.3mg/kg/day

Week 5 Onward: Increase every 1-2 weeks by 0.3mg/kg/day

Maint: 1-5mg/kg/day (max 200mg/day) or 1-3mg/kg/day w/ valproate alone

Not Taking Carbamazepine, Phenytoin, Phenobarbital, Primidone, or Valproate:

Weeks 1 and 2: 0.3mg/kg/day

Weeks 3 and 4: 0.6mg/kg/day

Week 5 Onward: Increase every 1-2 weeks by 0.6mg/kg/day

Maint: 4.5-7.5mg/kg/day

Max: 300mg/day in 2 divided doses

Taking Carbamazepine, Phenytoin, Phenobarbital, or Primidone, w/o Valproate:

Weeks 1 and 2: 0.6mg/kg/day

Weeks 3 and 4: 1.2mg/kg/day

Week 5 Onward: Increase every 1-2 weeks by 1.2mg/kg/day

Maint: 5-15mg/kg/day

Max: 400mg/day in 2 divided doses

>12 Years:

Taking Valproate:

Weeks 1 and 2: 25mg qod

Weeks 3 and 4: 25mg qd

Week 5 Onward: Increase every 1-2 weeks by 25-50mg/day

Maint: 100-200mg/day w/ valproate alone or 100-400mg/day w/ valproate and other drugs inducing glucuronidation in 1 or 2 divided doses

Not Taking Carbamazepine, Phenytoin, Phenobarbital, Primidone, or Valproate:

Weeks 1 and 2: 25mg qd

Weeks 3 and 4: 50mg/day

Week 5 Onward: Increase every 1-2 weeks by 50mg/day

Maint: 225-375mg/day in 2 divided doses

Taking Carbamazepine, Phenytoin, Phenobarbital, or Primidone, w/o Valproate:

Weeks 1 and 2: 50mg/day

Weeks 3 and 4: 100mg/day in 2 divided doses

Conversions

Conversion from Adjunctive Therapy to Monotherapy:
≥16 Years:
Monotherapy Maint: 500mg/day in 2 divided doses

From Adjunctive Therapy w/ Carbamazepine, Phenytoin, Phenobarbital, or Primidone:
After achieving a dose of 500mg/day of lamotrigine, withdraw concomitant antiepileptic drug by 20% decrements each week over a 4-week period

From Adjunctive Therapy w/ Valproate:
1. Maintain lamotrigine at 200mg/day and decrease valproate by decrements no >500mg/day/week to 500mg/day and then maintain for 1 week
2. Increase lamotrigine to 300mg/day and maintain for 1 week; simultaneously decrease valproate to 250mg/day and maintain for 1 week
3. Increase lamotrigine by 100mg/day every week to achieve maint dose of 500mg/day; d/c valproate

Week 5 Onward: Increase every 1-2 weeks by 100mg/day
Maint: 300-500mg/day in 2 divided doses

DOSE MODIFICATION
Concomitant Medications
Taking Estrogen-Containing Oral Contraceptives w/o Other Drugs Known to Induce Glucuronidation:
May need to increase by as much as 2-fold for maint dose of lamotrigine
Starting Estrogen-Containing Oral Contraceptives w/o Other Drugs Known to Induce Glucuronidation:
May need to increase by as much as 2-fold for maint dose of lamotrigine
Increase lamotrigine dose at the same time the oral contraceptive is introduced; no more than 50-100mg/day every week
If adverse reactions occur during the pill-free week due to lamotrigine, may need to adjust overall maint dose; dose adjustments limited to pill-free week not recommended
Stopping Estrogen-Containing Oral Contraceptives w/o Other Drugs Known to Induce Glucuronidation:
May need to decrease maint dose of lamotrigine by as much as 50%; decreases should not exceed 25% of total daily dose/week over a 2-week period, unless clinical response or lamotrigine plasma levels indicate otherwise
Taking Atazanavir/Ritonavir But Not Taking Other Glucuronidation Inducers:
Lamotrigine may need to be increased if atazanavir/ritonavir is added or decreased if atazanavir/ritonavir is discontinued
Bipolar Disorder:
Discontinuation of Psychotropic Drugs Excluding Valproate, Carbamazepine, Phenytoin, Phenobarbital, or Primidone:
Maintain current dose of lamotrigine
After Discontinuation of Valproate w/ Current dose of 100mg/day Lamotrigine:
Week 1: 150mg/day
Week 2 Onward: 200mg/day
After Discontinuation of Carbamazepine, Phenytoin, Phenobarbital, or Primidone w/ Current Dose of 400mg/day Lamotrigine:
Week 1: 400mg/day
Week 2: 300mg/day
Week 3 Onward: 200mg/day
Renal Impairment
Significant: Reduce maint doses
Hepatic Impairment
Moderate/Severe w/o Ascites: Reduce initial, escalation, and maint doses by approx 25%
Severe w/ Ascites: Reduce initial, escalation, and maint doses by 50%
Adjust maint and escalation doses based on clinical response
Elderly
Start at lower end of dosing range
Discontinuation
A step-wise reduction over at least 2 weeks (approx 50% per week) is recommended unless safety concerns require a more rapid withdrawal

Other Important Modifications

<30kg: Maint dose may need to be increased by as much as 50%, based on clinical response

ADMINISTRATION

Oral route

Tab, Chewable

May swallow whole, chewed, or dispersed in water or diluted fruit juice

If tabs are chewed, consume a small amount of water or diluted fruit juice to aid in swallowing

To disperse chewable tabs, add tabs to a small amount of liquid (1 tsp, or enough to cover the medication); approx 1 min later when tabs are completely dispersed, swirl sol and consume entire quantity immediately

Tab, Orally Disintegrating

Place onto the tongue and move around in the mouth

Can be swallowed w/ or w/o water and taken w/ or w/ food

HOW SUPPLIED

Tab: 25mg*, 100mg*, 150mg*, 200mg*; Tab, Chewable: 2mg, 5mg, 25mg; Tab, Disintegrating: (ODT) 25mg, 50mg, 100mg, 200mg *scored

WARNINGS/PRECAUTIONS

Drug reaction w/ eosinophilia and systemic symptoms (DRESS), also known as multiorgan hypersensitivity reactions, reported. Fatalities from acute multiorgan failure and various degrees of hepatic failure reported. Isolated liver failure w/o rash or involvement of other organs reported. D/C if alternative etiology for signs/symptoms of early manifestations of hypersensitivity cannot be established. Blood dyscrasias (eg, neutropenia, leukopenia) reported. Increased risk of suicidal thoughts or behavior. Worsening of depressive symptoms and/or emergence of suicidal ideation and behaviors (suicidality) may be experienced in patients w/ bipolar disorder; consider discontinuation. Increases risk of developing aseptic meningitis; evaluate for other causes of aseptic meningitis and treat appropriately. Avoid abrupt withdrawal due to risk of withdrawal seizures. Treatment-emergent status epilepticus and sudden unexplained death in epilepsy reported. May cause toxicity in the eyes and other melanin-rich tissues due to melanin binding. Medication errors reported. Caution w/ renal impairment. Do not restart therapy in patients who discontinued due to rash associated w/ prior treatment, unless potential benefits outweigh the risks. If restarting after discontinuation, assess the need to restart w/ initial dosing recommendations. May interfere w/ assay used in some rapid urine screens, which can result in false-positive readings, particularly for phencyclidine; use a more specific analytical method to confirm a positive result.

ADVERSE REACTIONS

Rash, dizziness, diplopia, infection, headache, ataxia, blurred vision, N/V, somnolence, fever, pharyngitis, rhinitis, diarrhea, abdominal pain, tremor.

DRUG INTERACTIONS

See Boxed Warning and Dose Modification. Estrogen-containing oral contraceptives, carbamazepine, lopinavir/ritonavir, phenobarbital/primidone, and phenytoin decreased levels. Atazanavir/ritonavir and rifampin decreased exposure. May decrease levels of levonorgestrel. Valproate may increase levels. May increase carbamazepine epoxide levels. Drugs known to induce or inhibit glucuronidation may affect clearance. May increase plasma levels of drugs substantially excreted via organic cationic transporter 2 (OCT2) proteins; avoid w/ OCT2 substrates w/ a narrow therapeutic index (eg, dofetilide).

NURSING CONSIDERATIONS

Assessment: Assess for history of allergy/rash to other AEDs, renal/hepatic impairment, depression, systemic lupus erythematosus or other autoimmune diseases, hypersensitivity to drug, pregnancy/nursing status, and possible drug interactions.

Monitoring: Monitor for signs/symptoms of rash, DRESS, multiorgan failure, status epilepticus, blood dyscrasias, emergence/worsening of depression, suicidal thoughts or behavior, unusual mood/behavior changes, aseptic meningitis, ophthalmologic effects, and other adverse reactions. Monitor effectiveness of long-term use (>16 weeks) w/ bipolar disorder.

Patient Counseling: Inform that a rash or other signs/symptoms of hypersensitivity may herald a serious medical event; instruct to report such symptoms to healthcare providers immediately. Instruct to notify healthcare providers immediately if blood dyscrasias, DRESS, acute multiorgan failure, or aseptic meningitis occur. Inform about increased risk of suicidal thoughts and behavior; instruct to be alert for emergence/worsening of symptoms of depression, any unusual changes in mood/behavior, suicidal thoughts/behavior, or thoughts about self-harm. Instruct to immediately report behaviors of concern to healthcare providers. Instruct to notify healthcare providers if worsening of seizure control occurs. Inform that CNS depression may occur; instruct to avoid operating machinery/driving until effects of the drug are known. Instruct to notify healthcare providers if pregnant, intending to become pregnant, or if breastfeeding. Encourage patients to enroll in the North American Antiepileptic Drug Pregnancy Registry. Instruct women to notify healthcare providers if they plan to start/stop use of oral contraceptives or other hormonal preparations. Instruct to promptly notify healthcare providers of changes in menstrual pattern and adverse reactions. Instruct to notify healthcare providers if medication is discontinued and not to resume therapy w/o consulting healthcare providers. Strongly advise to visually inspect tab to verify if correct drug/formulation was dispensed each time prescription is filled.

Storage: (Tab/Tab, Chewable) 25°C (77°F); excursions permitted to 15-30°C (59-86°F) in a dry place. (Tab) Protect from light. (Tab, Disintegrating) 20-25°C (68-77°F); excursions permitted between 15-30°C (59-86°F).

LAMISIL – terbinafine hydrochloride RX

Class: Allylamine antifungal

ADULT DOSAGE

Tinea Capitis

Granules:

<25kg: 125mg/day qd
25-35kg: 187.5mg/day qd
>35kg: 250mg/day qd

Treatment Duration: 6 weeks

Onychomycosis

Due to Dermatophytes (Tinea Unguium):

Tab:

Fingernail: 250mg qd for 6 weeks
Toenail: 250mg qd for 12 weeks

PEDIATRIC DOSAGE

Tinea Capitis

≥4 Years:

Granules:

<25kg: 125mg/day
25-35kg: 187.5mg/day
>35kg: 250mg/day

Treatment Duration: 6 weeks

DOSE MODIFICATION

Elderly

Tab:

Start at lower end of dosing range

ADMINISTRATION

Oral route

Granules

Take w/ food

Sprinkle contents of 1 pkt on a spoonful of pudding or other soft, nonacidic food (eg, mashed potatoes), and swallow entire spoonful (w/o chewing); do not use applesauce or fruit-based foods

Either the contents of both pkts may be sprinkled on 1 spoonful, or the contents of both pkts may be sprinkled on 2 spoonfuls of nonacidic food if 2 pkts are required/dose

Tab

Take w/ or w/o food

HOW SUPPLIED

Granules: 125mg/pkt, 187.5mg/pkt; Tab: 250mg

WARNINGS/PRECAUTIONS

Cases of liver failure, some leading to liver transplant or death, reported in individuals with and without preexisting liver disease; d/c therapy if evidence of liver injury develops. Hepatotoxicity may occur. Not recommended for patients with chronic or active liver disease; perform LFTs prior to initiating therapy and periodically thereafter. D/C immediately in case of LFTs elevation or if any symptoms of persistent N/V, anorexia, fatigue, right upper abdominal pain, jaundice, dark urine, or pale stools occur. Taste/smell disturbance reported; d/c if symptoms occur. Depressive symptoms reported. Transient decreases in absolute lymphocyte counts and severe neutropenia reported; d/c and start supportive management if neutrophil count is ≤1000 cells/mm^3. Consider monitoring CBCs in patients with known or suspected immunodeficiency if treatment continues for >6 weeks. Serious skin/hypersensitivity reactions (eg, Stevens-Johnson syndrome, toxic epidermal necrolysis, erythema multiforme, exfoliative/bullous dermatitis, drug reaction with eosinophilia and systemic symptoms (DRESS) syndrome) reported; d/c if progressive skin rash or signs/symptoms of DRESS occur. Precipitation and exacerbation of cutaneous and systemic lupus erythematosus reported; d/c in patients with clinical signs/symptoms suggestive of lupus erythematosus.

ADVERSE REACTIONS

Headache, diarrhea. (Granules) Nasopharyngitis, pyrexia, cough, vomiting, URTI, upper abdominal pain. (Tab) Dyspepsia, nausea, rash, liver enzyme abnormalities, pruritus, taste disturbances.

DRUG INTERACTIONS

Coadministration with drugs predominantly metabolized by CYP2D6 (eg, TCAs, β-blockers, SSRIs, antiarrhythmics class 1C [eg, flecainide, propafenone], MAOIs type B, dextromethorphan) should be done with careful monitoring; may require dose reduction of the CYP2D6-metabolized drug. Increased dextromethorphan/dextrorphan metabolite ratio in urine in patients who are extensive metabolizers of dextromethorphan; may convert extensive CYP2D6 metabolizers to poor metabolizer status. Increased levels/exposure of desipramine. Increased clearance of cyclosporine. Decreased clearance of caffeine. Fluconazole may increase levels and exposure. May increase systemic exposure with other inhibitors of both CYP2C9 and CYP3A4 (eg, ketoconazole, amiodarone). Clearance increased by rifampin and decreased by cimetidine. Increased or decreased PT with warfarin.

NURSING CONSIDERATIONS

Assessment: Assess for known hypersensitivity to the drug, active/chronic liver disease, immunodeficiency, lupus erythematosus, pregnancy/nursing status, and possible drug interactions. Confirm diagnosis of onychomycosis (potassium hydroxide preparation, fungal culture, or nail biopsy). Obtain baseline LFTs.

Monitoring: Monitor for signs/symptoms of hepatotoxicity, taste/smell disturbances, progressive skin rash, DRESS, depressive symptoms, lupus erythematosus, and other adverse reactions. Monitor CBC in patients with known or suspected immunodeficiency if therapy continues for >6 weeks, or if signs/symptoms of secondary infection occur. Monitor LFTs periodically.

Patient Counseling: Advise to d/c treatment and report immediately to physician if N/V, right upper abdominal pain, jaundice, dark urine, pale stools, taste/smell disturbance, anorexia, fatigue, depressive symptoms, hives, mouth sores, blistering and peeling of skin, swelling of face, lips, tongue, or throat, difficulty breathing/swallowing, fever, skin eruption, erythema, scaling, loss of pigment, unusual photosensitivity that can result in a rash, and lymph node enlargement occur. Instruct to minimize exposure to natural and artificial sunlight (tanning beds or UVA/B treatment) while on therapy. Advise to call physician if too many doses have been taken. If a dose is missed, advise to take tab as soon as remembered, unless it is <4 hrs before the next dose is due.

Storage: (Tab) <25°C (77°F); in a tight container. Protect from light. (Granules) 25°C (77°F); excursions permitted to 15-30°C (59-86°F).

LANOXIN INJECTION – digoxin RX

Class: Cardiac glycoside

ADULT DOSAGE

Heart Failure

Initiate w/ LD followed by maintenance dosing if rapid titration is desired, or initiate w/ maintenance dosing w/o LD
LD: 8-12mcg/kg
Give 1/2 the total LD, then 1/4 the LD every 6-8 hrs, twice
Initial Maint: 2.4-3.6mcg/kg/day qd
Titrate: May be increased every 2 weeks according to clinical response, serum drug levels, and toxicity
Max: 500mcg in a single site

Atrial Fibrillation

Initiate w/ LD followed by maintenance dosing if rapid titration is desired, or initiate w/ maintenance dosing w/o LD

LD: 8-12mcg/kg
Give 1/2 the total LD, then 1/4 the LD every 6-8 hrs, twice
Initial Maint: 2.4-3.6mcg/kg/day qd
Titrate: May be increased every 2 weeks according to clinical response, serum drug levels, and toxicity
Max: 500mcg in a single site

Conversions

IV to PO Conversion:
50mcg inj = 62.5mcg tab
100mcg inj = 125mcg tab
200mcg inj = 250mcg tab
400mcg inj = 500mcg tab

PEDIATRIC DOSAGE

Heart Failure

Initiate with LD followed by maintenance dosing if rapid titration is desired, or initiate with maintenance dosing without LD
LD: Give 1/2 the total LD, then 1/4 the LD every 6-8 hrs, twice
Premature Infants: 15-25mcg/kg
Full-Term Infants: 20-30mcg/kg
1-24 Months: 30-50mcg/kg
2-5 Years: 25-35mcg/kg
5-10 Years: 15-30mcg/kg
>10 Years: 8-12mcg/kg

Starting Maint:
Premature Infants: 1.9-3.1mcg/kg/dose bid
Full-Term: 3.0-4.5mcg/kg/dose bid
1-24 Months: 4.5-7.5mcg/kg/dose bid
2-5 Years: 3.8-5.3mcg/kg/dose bid
5-10 Years: 2.3-4.5mcg/kg/dose bid
>10 Years: 2.4-3.6mcg/kg/day qd; may be increased every 2 weeks according to clinical response, serum drug levels, and toxicity

Max: 200mcg in a single site

Conversions

IV to PO Conversion:
50mcg inj = 62.5mcg tab
100mcg inj = 125mcg tab
200mcg inj = 250mcg tab
400mcg inj = 500mcg tab

DOSE MODIFICATION

Renal Impairment

Refer to PI for recommended maintenance dose according to lean body weight and renal function

ADMINISTRATION

IV/IM route

IV route is preferred because IM inj may lead to severe pain at the inj site
Inject deep into the muscle followed by massage if administered IM
Administer over a period of ≥5 min
May be administered undiluted or diluted w/ a 4-fold or greater volume of Sterile Water for Inj, 0.9% NaCl, or 5% Dextrose Inj
Use of less than 4-fold volume of diluent could lead to precipitation of digoxin

Refer to PI for detailed instructions

HOW SUPPLIED

Inj: (Lanoxin) 0.25mg/mL, (Lanoxin Pediatric) 0.1mg/mL

CONTRAINDICATIONS

Ventricular fibrillation.

WARNINGS/PRECAUTIONS

Increased risk of ventricular fibrillation in patients with Wolff-Parkinson-White syndrome who develop A-fib. May cause severe sinus bradycardia or sinoatrial block, particularly with preexisting sinus node disease, and may cause advanced or complete heart block with preexisting incomplete atrioventricular (AV) block; consider insertion of a pacemaker before treatment. Signs and symptoms of digoxin toxicity include anorexia, N/V, visual changes, and cardiac arrhythmias. Low body weight, advanced age or impaired renal function, hypokalemia, hypercalcemia, or hypomagnesemia may predispose to digoxin toxicity; assess serum electrolytes and renal function periodically. Reduce dose or d/c therapy 1-2 days prior to electrical cardioversion of A-fib; if digitalis toxicity is suspected, delay elective cardioversion, and if it is not prudent to delay cardioversion, select the lowest possible energy level to avoid provoking ventricular arrhythmias. Not recommended with acute myocardial infarction. Avoid in patients with HF associated with preserved left ventricular ejection fraction (eg, restrictive cardiomyopathy, constrictive pericarditis, amyloid heart disease, acute cor pulmonale), idiopathic hypertrophic subaortic stenosis, and myocarditis. Hypocalcemia may nullify the effects of treatment. Hypothyroidism may reduce the requirements for therapy. HF and/or atrial arrhythmias resulting from hypermetabolic or hyperdynamic states (eg, hyperthyroidism, hypoxia, or arteriovenous shunt) are best treated by addressing the underlying condition. Caution with impaired renal function and in elderly. Should be used only when the need for rapid digitalization is urgent or when the drug cannot be taken orally. Avoid bolus inj.

ADVERSE REACTIONS

Cardiac arrhythmias, N/V, abdominal pain, intestinal ischemia, hemorrhagic necrosis of the intestines, headache, weakness, dizziness, apathy, mental disturbances.

DRUG INTERACTIONS

Drugs that induce/inhibit P-glycoprotein in intestine/kidney may alter digoxin pharmacokinetics. Increased levels with quinidine, ritonavir, amiodarone, propafenone, quinine, spironolactone, and verapamil; refer to PI for recommendations to reduce digoxin concentrations. Drugs that affect renal function (eg, ACE inhibitors, ARBs, NSAIDs, COX-2 inhibitors) may impair excretion. Higher rate of torsades de pointes with dofetilide. Proarrhythmic events were more common with concomitant sotalol. Sudden death was more common with concomitant dronedarone. Teriparatide transiently increases serum calcium. Thyroid supplements may increase digoxin dose requirement. Increased risk of arrhythmias with epinephrine, norepinephrine, dopamine, and succinylcholine. Rapid IV calcium administration can produce serious arrhythmias in digitalized patients. Additive effects on AV node conduction with β-adrenergic blockers and calcium channel blockers.

NURSING CONSIDERATIONS

Assessment: Assess for known hypersensitivity to the drug or other digitalis preparations, ventricular fibrillation, myocarditis, hypermetabolic or hyperdynamic states, sinus node disease, AV block, pregnancy/nursing status, possible drug interactions, and any other conditions where treatment is cautioned. Assess serum electrolytes and renal function. Obtain a baseline digoxin level; serum digoxin concentrations may be falsely elevated by endogenous digoxin-like substances.

Monitoring: Monitor for signs/symptoms of severe sinus bradycardia, sinoatrial block, advanced or complete heart block, digoxin toxicity, vasoconstriction, and other adverse reactions. Monitor serum electrolytes and renal function periodically. Obtain serum digoxin concentrations just before the next dose or at least 6 hours after the last dose. Monitor for clinical response.

Patient Counseling: Advise that digoxin is a cardiac glycoside used to treat HF and heart arrhythmias. Advise to inform physician if taking any OTC medications, including herbal medication, or if started on a new prescription. Inform that blood tests will be necessary to ensure the appropriate digoxin dose. Instruct to contact physician if N/V, persistent diarrhea, confusion, weakness, or visual disturbances occur. Advise parents or caregivers that symptoms of having too high doses may be difficult to recognize in infants and pediatric patients; symptoms such as weight loss, failure to thrive in infants, abdominal pain, and behavioral disturbances may be indications of digoxin toxicity. Suggest to monitor and record HR and BP daily. Instruct women of childbearing potential who become or are planning to become pregnant to consult physician prior to initiation or continuing therapy with digoxin.

Storage: 25°C (77°F); excursions permitted to 15-30°C (59-86°F). Protect from light. Diluted Sol: Use immediately.

LANTUS – insulin glargine (rDNA origin) RX

Class: Insulin

ADULT DOSAGE

Type 1 Diabetes Mellitus

Initial: 1/3 of total daily insulin requirements
Titrate: Adjust dose based on blood glucose measurements

Use short-acting, premeal insulin to satisfy remainder of the daily insulin requirements

Type 2 Diabetes Mellitus

Not Currently Treated w/ Insulin:
Initial: 10 U (or 0.2 U/kg) qd
Titrate: Adjust dose based on blood glucose measurements

Conversions

From QD NPH Insulin:
Initial Lantus dose is the same as the dose of NPH being discontinued

From BID NPH Insulin:
Initial Lantus dose is 80% of total NPH dose being discontinued

PEDIATRIC DOSAGE

Type 1 Diabetes Mellitus

≥6 Years:
Initial: 1/3 of total daily insulin requirements
Titrate: Adjust dose based on blood glucose measurements

Use short-acting, premeal insulin to satisfy remainder of the daily insulin requirements

Conversions

From QD NPH Insulin:
Initial Lantus dose is the same as the dose of NPH being discontinued

From BID NPH Insulin:
Initial Lantus dose is 80% of total NPH dose being discontinued

DOSE MODIFICATION

Renal Impairment
Careful glucose monitoring and dose adjustments may be necessary

Hepatic Impairment
Careful glucose monitoring and dose adjustments may be necessary

Elderly
Dose conservatively

ADMINISTRATION
SQ route

Inject qd at same time every day
Must be used in regimens w/ short-acting insulin in patients w/ type 1 diabetes mellitus
Do not administer IV or via an insulin pump
Rotate inj sites w/in the same region (abdomen, thigh, or deltoid) from 1 inj to the next
Do not dilute or mix w/ any other insulin or sol

HOW SUPPLIED
Inj: 100 U/mL [3mL SoloStar, 10mL vial]

WARNINGS/PRECAUTIONS
Not recommended for the treatment of diabetic ketoacidosis. Insulin pens must never be shared between patients, even if needle is changed; may carry a risk for transmission of blood-borne pathogens. Glucose monitoring is essential for all patients receiving insulin therapy. Changes to an insulin regimen should be made cautiously and only under medical supervision. Changes in insulin strength, manufacturer, type, or method of administration may result in need for a change in insulin dose or adjustment in concomitant oral antidiabetic treatment. Hypoglycemia may occur; caution in patients w/ hypoglycemia unawareness and in patients who may be predisposed to hypoglycemia (eg, pediatric population, patients who fast or have erratic food intake). Hypoglycemia may impair ability to concentrate and react. Severe, life-threatening, generalized allergy, including anaphylaxis, may occur. Careful glucose monitoring and dose adjustments may be necessary w/ renal/hepatic impairment. Not recommended during periods of rapidly declining renal/hepatic function. Caution in elderly.

ADVERSE REACTIONS
Hypoglycemia, allergic reactions, URTI, peripheral edema, HTN, influenza, sinusitis, cataract, bronchitis, arthralgia, infection, pain in extremities, back pain, cough, URI.

DRUG INTERACTIONS
May require dose adjustment and close monitoring w/ drugs that may increase the blood-glucose-lowering effect and susceptibility to hypoglycemia (eg, ACE inhibitors, MAOIs, salicylates, somatostatin analogues, sulfonamide antibiotics), drugs that may decrease the blood-glucose-lowering effect (eg, corticosteroids, niacin, phenothiazine derivatives, thyroid hormones, progestogens [eg, in oral contraceptives]), or drugs that may either potentiate or weaken the blood-glucose-lowering effect (β-blockers, clonidine, lithium salts, alcohol). Pentamidine may cause hypoglycemia, sometimes followed by hyperglycemia. Signs of hypoglycemia may be reduced or absent w/ sympatholytics (eg, β-blockers, clonidine, guanethidine, reserpine). Observe for signs/symptoms of heart failure (HF) if treated concomitantly w/ a peroxisome proliferator-activated receptor (PPAR)-gamma agonist (eg, thiazolidinedione); consider discontinuation or a dose reduction of the PPAR-gamma agonist if HF develops.

NURSING CONSIDERATIONS

Assessment: Assess for diabetic ketoacidosis, predisposition to hypoglycemia, hypersensitivity, renal/hepatic impairment, pregnancy/nursing status, and possible drug interactions. Obtain baseline blood glucose and HbA1c levels.

Monitoring: Monitor for signs/symptoms of hypoglycemia, allergic reactions, and other adverse reactions. Monitor blood glucose and HbA1c levels, and renal/hepatic function.

Patient Counseling: Advise never to share insulin pen w/ another person, even if needle is changed. Inform about potential side effects (eg, lipodystrophy, weight gain, allergic reactions, hypoglycemia). Inform that hypoglycemia may impair ability to concentrate and react; advise to use caution when driving or operating machinery. Instruct to always check the label before each inj to avoid medication errors. Advise to use only if sol is clear and colorless w/ no particles visible. Do not dilute or mix w/ any other insulin or sol. Instruct on self-management procedures, including glucose monitoring, proper inj technique, and management of hypoglycemia and hyperglycemia, and on handling of special situations, such as intercurrent conditions (eg, illness, stress, or emotional disturbances), inadequate or skipped dose, inadvertent administration of increased insulin dose, inadequate food intake, and skipped meals. Advise to inform physician if pregnant or contemplating pregnancy.

Storage: Do not freeze; discard if drug has been frozen. Unopened: 2-8°C (36-46°F) until expiration date. Open (In-Use): 2-8°C (36-46°F) or ≤30°C (86°F) for vials and <30°C (86°F) for SoloStar. Discard after 28 days. Protect from direct heat and light. Do not refrigerate opened (in-use) SoloStar.

LASTACAFT – alcaftadine **RX**

Class: H_1-antagonist

ADULT DOSAGE
Allergic Conjunctivitis
Prevention of Itching:
1 drop in ou qd

PEDIATRIC DOSAGE
Allergic Conjunctivitis
Prevention of Itching:
≥2 Years:
1 drop in ou qd

DOSE MODIFICATION
Concomitant Medications
Space dosing by at least 5 min if using >1 topical ophthalmic drug

ADMINISTRATION
Ocular route

HOW SUPPLIED
Sol: 0.25% [3mL]

WARNINGS/PRECAUTIONS
Caution not to touch the dropper tip to eyelids or surrounding areas to minimize eye injury and contamination. Do not wear contact lens if the eye is red. Not for treatment of contact lens-related irritation. Do not instill while wearing contact lenses; reinsert lenses after 10 min following administration.

ADVERSE REACTIONS
Eye irritation, burning and/or stinging upon instillation, eye redness, eye pruritus.

NURSING CONSIDERATIONS

Assessment: Assess for hypersensitivity to the drug, contact lens-related irritation, and pregnancy/nursing status.

Monitoring: Monitor for possible adverse reactions.

Patient Counseling: Advise to avoid touching the eyelids or surrounding areas with the dropper tip to minimize eye injury and contamination of the dropper tip and sol. Instruct to administer ≥5 min apart if >1 topical ophthalmic drug is being used. Advise not to wear contact lenses if the eye is red. Advise not to use to treat contact lens-related irritation. Advise to remove contact lenses prior to instillation, then reinsert lenses after 10 min following administration. Inform that the drug is for topical ophthalmic administration only.

Storage: 15-25°C (59-77°F). Keep bottle tightly closed when not in use.

LATISSE – bimatoprost **RX**

Class: Prostaglandin analogue

ADULT DOSAGE	PEDIATRIC DOSAGE
Hypotrichosis	**Hypotrichosis**
Eyelashes:	**Eyelashes:**
Apply 1 drop qpm	**≥5 Years:**
	Apply 1 drop qpm

ADMINISTRATION

Topical route

Ensure face is clean, and that makeup and contact lenses are removed

Place one drop on disposable sterile applicator and apply evenly along the skin of the upper eyelid margin at the base of eyelashes; do not apply to lower eyelash line

Upper lid margin in area of lash growth should feel lightly moist w/o runoff; blot any excess sol runoff outside upper eyelid margin w/ a tissue or other absorbent cloth

Dispose of applicator after one use; repeat for the opposite eyelid margin using a new sterile applicator

Do not reuse applicators and do not use any other brush/applicator to apply sol

HOW SUPPLIED

Sol: 0.03% [3mL, 5mL]

WARNINGS/PRECAUTIONS

May lower intraocular pressure (IOP) when instilled directly to the eye. Increased iris pigmentation reported; may continue therapy in patients who develop noticeably increased iris pigmentation. May cause pigment changes (darkening) to periorbital pigmented tissues and eyelashes. May cause hair growth to occur in areas where sol comes in repeated contact with skin surface. Caution with active intraocular inflammation (eg, uveitis); inflammation may be exacerbated. Macular edema (eg, cystoid macular edema) reported during treatment of elevated IOP; caution in aphakic patients, pseudophakic patients with a torn posterior lens capsule, or in patients at risk for macular edema. Do not allow the bottle tip to contact any other surface. Use the accompanying sterile applicators on 1 eye and then discard; reuse of applicators increases the potential for contamination and infections. Bacterial keratitis associated with the use of multiple-dose containers reported. Contains benzalkonium chloride, which may be absorbed by and cause discoloration of soft contact lenses; contact lenses should be removed prior to application and may be reinserted 15 min following administration.

ADVERSE REACTIONS

Eye pruritus, conjunctival hyperemia, skin hyperpigmentation, ocular irritation, dry eye symptoms, periorbital erythema.

DRUG INTERACTIONS

May interfere with the desired reduction in IOP when given with other prostaglandin analogues for the treatment of elevated IOP.

NURSING CONSIDERATIONS

Assessment: Assess for active intraocular inflammation, aphakia, pseudophakia with a torn posterior lens capsule, risk for macular edema, pregnancy/nursing status, and possible drug interactions.

Monitoring: Monitor for IOP changes, increased iris pigmentation, pigment changes (darkening) to periorbital pigmented tissues and eyelashes, macular edema, bacterial keratitis, and other adverse reactions.

Patient Counseling: Instruct to apply medication ud. Counsel that if any sol gets into the eye proper, it will not cause harm, and the eye should not be rinsed. Counsel that the effect is not permanent and can be expected to gradually return to original level upon discontinuation. Instruct that the bottle must be maintained intact and to avoid contaminating the bottle tip or applicator. Advise that serious infections may result from using contaminated sol or applicators. Instruct to consult physician before use if using prostaglandin analogues for IOP reduction.

Inform about the possibility of eyelid skin darkening, increased brown iris pigmentation (may be permanent), hair growth outside of the target treatment area, and disparity between eyes in length, thickness, pigmentation, number of eyelashes or vellus hairs, and/or direction of eyelash growth. Advise to consult physician if patient has ocular surgery, develops a new ocular condition (eg, trauma, infection), experiences a sudden decrease in visual acuity, or if any ocular reactions (eg, conjunctivitis, eyelid reactions) develop. Advise that contact lenses should be removed prior to application, and may be reinserted 15 min following administration.

Storage: 2-25°C (36-77°F).

LATUDA – lurasidone hydrochloride **RX**

Class: Atypical antipsychotic

Elderly patients with dementia-related psychosis treated with antipsychotic drugs are at an increased risk of death. Not approved for use in patients with dementia-related psychosis. Antidepressants increased the risk of suicidal thoughts and behavior in children, adolescents, and young adults in short-term studies. Monitor closely for worsening, and for emergence of suicidal thoughts and behaviors in patients who are started on antidepressant therapy.

ADULT DOSAGE

Schizophrenia

Initial: 40mg qd
Range: 40-160mg/day
Max: 160mg/day
Periodically reevaluate long-term usefulness of therapy for individual patient

Bipolar I Disorder

Treatment of major depressive episodes as monotherapy or as adjunctive therapy w/ either lithium or valproate

Initial: 20mg qd
Range: 20-120mg/day
Max: 120mg/day
Periodically reevaluate long-term usefulness of therapy for individual patient

PEDIATRIC DOSAGE

Pediatric use may not have been established

DOSE MODIFICATION

Concomitant Medications

Moderate CYP3A4 Inhibitors (eg, Diltiazem, Atazanavir, Erythromycin, Fluconazole, Verapamil):
Moderate CYP3A4 Inhibitor Added to Current Therapy w/ Lurasidone: Reduce lurasidone dose to 1/2 of the original dose level
Lurasidone Added to Current Therapy w/ a Moderate CYP3A4 Inhibitor:
Initial: 20mg/day
Max: 80mg/day

Moderate CYP3A4 Inducers:
May need to increase lurasidone dose after chronic treatment (≥7 days) w/ the CYP3A4 inducer

Renal Impairment

Moderate (CrCl 30-<50mL/min) and Severe (CrCl <30mL/min):
Initial: 20mg/day
Max: 80mg/day

Hepatic Impairment

Moderate (Child-Pugh Score 7-9):
Initial: 20mg/day
Max: 80mg/day

Severe (Child-Pugh Score 10-15):
Initial: 20mg/day
Max: 40mg/day

ADMINISTRATION

Oral route

Take w/ food (at least 350 calories)

HOW SUPPLIED

Tab: 20mg, 40mg, 60mg, 80mg, 120mg

CONTRAINDICATIONS

Concomitant use with strong CYP3A4 inhibitors (eg, ketoconazole, clarithromycin, ritonavir, voriconazole, mibefradil) or strong CYP3A4 inducers (eg, rifampin, avasimibe, St. John's wort, phenytoin, carbamazepine).

WARNINGS/PRECAUTIONS

Neuroleptic malignant syndrome (NMS) reported; d/c immediately and institute symptomatic treatment. May cause tardive dyskinesia (TD), especially in the elderly; d/c if this occurs. May cause metabolic changes (eg, hyperglycemia, dyslipidemia, weight gain) that may increase cardiovascular (CV)/cerebrovascular risk. Hyperglycemia, in some cases extreme and associated with ketoacidosis or hyperosmolar coma or death, reported; monitor glucose control regularly in patients with diabetes mellitus (DM) and FPG in patients at risk for DM. May elevate prolactin levels. Leukopenia, neutropenia, and agranulocytosis may occur; monitor CBC frequently during the 1st few months in patients with preexisting low WBCs or history of drug-induced leukopenia/neutropenia, and d/c at 1st sign of decline in WBCs without other causative factors. D/C therapy and follow WBCs until recovery in patients with severe neutropenia (absolute neutrophil count <1000/mm^3). May cause orthostatic hypotension and syncope; consider using a lower starting dose/slower titration and monitor orthostatic vital signs in patients at increased risk of these reactions or at increased risk of developing complications from hypotension (eg, dehydration, hypovolemia, treatment with antihypertensives, history of CV/cerebrovascular disease, antipsychotic-naive patients). Caution with history of seizures or with conditions that lower the seizure threshold. May impair mental/physical abilities. May disrupt body's ability to reduce core body temperature; caution when prescribing for patients who will be experiencing conditions that may contribute to an elevation in core body temperature (eg, concomitant anticholinergics). Closely supervise patients at high risk of suicide. May increase risk of developing a manic or hypomanic episode, particularly in patients with bipolar disorder. May cause esophageal dysmotility and aspiration; caution in patients at risk for aspiration pneumonia. Increased sensitivity reported in patients with Parkinson's disease or dementia with Lewy bodies. Evaluate for history of drug abuse; observe for drug misuse/abuse in these patients.

ADVERSE REACTIONS

Somnolence, akathisia, N/V, extrapyramidal symptoms, agitation, dyspepsia, back pain, dizziness, insomnia, anxiety, restlessness, diarrhea, dry mouth, nasopharyngitis.

DRUG INTERACTIONS

See Contraindications. Grapefruit/grapefruit juice may inhibit CYP3A4 and alter concentrations; avoid concomitant use. Adjust lurasidone dose when used in combination with moderate CYP3A4 inhibitors/inducers.

NURSING CONSIDERATIONS

Assessment: Assess for dementia-related psychosis, DM, renal/hepatic impairment, drug hypersensitivity, any other conditions where treatment is cautioned, pregnancy/nursing status, and possible drug interactions. Obtain baseline FPG in patients with DM or at risk for DM. Obtain baseline CBC if at risk for leukopenia/neutropenia.

Monitoring: Monitor for signs/symptoms of clinical worsening, suicidality, unusual changes in behavior, NMS, TD, hyperglycemia, hyperprolactinemia, orthostatic hypotension/syncope, cognitive/motor impairment, seizures, disruption of body temperature, manic/hypomanic episodes, esophageal dysmotility, aspiration, and other adverse reactions. Monitor FPG in patients with DM or at risk for DM, lipid profile, and weight. Monitor CBC frequently during the 1st few months in patients with preexisting low WBCs or history of drug-induced leukopenia/neutropenia. Monitor for fever or other signs/symptoms of infection in patients with neutropenia. Periodically reevaluate long-term usefulness for individual patient.

Patient Counseling: Advise to monitor for the emergence of suicidal thoughts and behavior, manic/hypomanic symptoms, irritability, agitation, or unusual changes in behavior and to report such symptoms to physician. Counsel about signs/symptoms of NMS (eg, hyperpyrexia, muscle rigidity, altered mental status, autonomic instability), hyperglycemia, and DM. Advise of the risk of dyslipidemia, weight gain, CV reactions, and orthostatic hypotension. Advise patients with preexisting low WBCs or history of drug-induced leukopenia/neutropenia to have their CBC monitored. Instruct to use caution when performing activities requiring mental alertness (eg, operating hazardous machinery, driving) until patients are reasonably certain that therapy does not affect them adversely. Instruct to notify physician if pregnant/intending to become pregnant, or if taking/planning to take any other medications. Advise to avoid alcohol while on treatment. Counsel regarding appropriate care in avoiding overheating and dehydration.

Storage: 25°C (77°F); excursions permitted to 15-30°C (59-86°F).

LAZANDA – fentanyl

CII

Class: Opioid analgesic

Fatal respiratory depression may occur. Contraindicated in the management of acute or postoperative pain (eg, headache/migraine) and in opioid-nontolerant patients. Keep out of reach of children. Concomitant use with CYP3A4 inhibitors may increase plasma levels, and may cause fatal respiratory depression. Do not convert patients on a mcg-per-mcg basis from any other fentanyl products to Lazanda. Do not substitute for any other fentanyl products; may result in fatal overdose. Contains fentanyl with abuse liability similar to other opioid analgesics. Available only through a restricted program called Transmucosal Immediate Release Fentanyl Risk Evaluation Mitigation Strategy (TIRF REMS) Access program, due to risk of misuse, abuse, addiction, and overdose. Outpatients, healthcare professionals who prescribe to outpatients, pharmacies, and distributors must enroll in this program.

ADULT DOSAGE

Pain

Management of Breakthrough Pain in Cancer Patients Already Receiving and Tolerant to Opioid Therapy for Underlying Persistent Cancer Pain:

≥18 Years:

Initial (Including Switching from Another Fentanyl Product):

One 100mcg spray (1 spray in 1 nostril); if adequate analgesia is obtained w/in 30 min, treat subsequent episodes w/ this dose

Titrate:

If adequate analgesia is not achieved w/ the first 100mcg dose, escalate dose in a step-wise manner over consecutive episodes until adequate analgesia w/ tolerable side effects is achieved

100mcg/dose: 1 x 100mcg spray

200mcg/dose: 2 x 100mcg spray (1 in each nostril)

400mcg/dose: 4 x 100mcg spray (2 in each nostril) or 1 x 400mcg spray

800mcg/dose: 2 x 400mcg spray (1 in each nostril)

Confirm dose w/ a 2nd episode of breakthrough pain and review experience if dose is appropriate or further adjustment is warranted

Wait at least 2 hrs before treating another episode of breakthrough cancer pain

Maint:

Use the established dose for each subsequent episode; limit to ≤4 doses/day and wait at least 2 hrs before treating another episode

May use rescue medication if pain relief is inadequate after 30 min following dosing or if a separate episode occurs before the next dose is permitted

Max: 800mcg

PEDIATRIC DOSAGE

Pediatric use may not have been established

DOSE MODIFICATION

Renal Impairment

Severe: Use w/ caution; titrate to clinical effect

Hepatic Impairment

Severe: Use w/ caution; titrate to clinical effect

Discontinuation

No Longer Requires Opioid Therapy: Consider discontinuation along w/ a gradual downward titration of other opioids

Continuing to Take Chronic Opioid Therapy but No Longer Requires Treatment for Breakthrough Pain: Therapy can be discontinued immediately

Other Important Modifications

Dose Readjustment:

Response (Analgesia or Adverse Reactions) to Titrated Dose Markedly Changes: An adjustment may be necessary

>4 Episodes of Breakthrough Pain/Day: Reevaluate the dose of the long-acting opioid used; if the long-acting opioid or dose of long-acting opioid is changed, reevaluate and retitrate the Lazanda dose as necessary

ADMINISTRATION

Intranasal route

Prime device before use by spraying into the pouch (4 sprays total)

If not used for 5 days, reprime by spraying once

Insert nozzle of the bottle a short distance (about 1/2 inch or 1cm) into nose and point towards bridge of nose, tilting bottle slightly

Press down firmly on the finger grips until a click is heard and the number in the counting window advances by 1

Fine mist spray is not always felt; rely on audible click and dose counter to confirm a spray has been administered

Refer to PI for further priming and disposal instructions

HOW SUPPLIED

Spray: 100mcg/spray, 400mcg/spray

CONTRAINDICATIONS

Opioid-nontolerant patients, management of acute or postoperative pain, including headache/migraine or dental pain.

WARNINGS/PRECAUTIONS

Increased risk of respiratory depression in patients with underlying respiratory disorders and in elderly/debilitated. May impair mental and/or physical abilities. Caution with COPD or preexisting medical conditions predisposing to respiratory depression; may further decrease respiratory drive to the point of respiratory failure. Extreme caution in patients who may be susceptible to intracranial effects of CO_2 retention (eg, with evidence of increased intracranial pressure or impaired consciousness). May obscure the clinical course of head injuries. May produce bradycardia; caution with bradyarrhythmias. Avoid use during labor and delivery. Caution in the elderly.

ADVERSE REACTIONS

Respiratory depression, N/V, somnolence, dizziness, headache, constipation, pyrexia.

DRUG INTERACTIONS

See Boxed Warning. Increase dose conservatively when beginning therapy with or increasing dose of CYP3A4 inhibitors. Not recommended with MAOIs or within 14 days of discontinuation of MAOIs. Increased depressant effects with other CNS depressants (eg, other opioids, sedatives/hypnotics, skeletal muscle relaxants); may require adjustment of Lazanda dose. CYP3A4 inducers (eg, barbiturates, carbamazepine, efavirenz) may decrease levels; adjust dose of Lazanda accordingly. Vasoconstrictive nasal decongestants such as oxymetazoline may decrease efficacy; avoid titration while patient is experiencing an acute episode of rhinitis as it could lead to incorrect dose identification. Respiratory depression reported with other drugs that depress respiration.

NURSING CONSIDERATIONS

Assessment: Assess for degree of opioid tolerance, previous opioid dose, level of pain intensity, type of pain, patient's general condition and medical status, and any other conditions where treatment is contraindicated or cautioned. Assess for hypersensitivity to the drug, renal/hepatic impairment, pregnancy/nursing status, and possible drug interactions.

Monitoring: Monitor for signs/symptoms of respiratory depression, impairment of mental/physical abilities, drug abuse/addiction, bradycardia, hypersensitivity reactions, and other adverse reactions.

Patient Counseling: Inform outpatients to enroll in the TIRF REMS Access program. Explain that therapy may be fatal in children, in individuals for whom it was not prescribed, and in those who are not opioid tolerant. Counsel on proper administration and disposal. Advise to take drug as prescribed and to avoid sharing it with anyone else. Instruct not to take medication for acute or postoperative pain, pain from injuries, headache, migraine, or any other short-term pain. Instruct to notify physician if breakthrough pain is not alleviated or worsens after taking the drug. Inform that drug may impair mental/physical abilities; caution against performing activities that require high level of attention (eg, driving/using heavy machinery). Advise not to combine with alcohol, sleep aids, or tranquilizers, except if ordered by the physician. Instruct to notify physician if pregnant or planning to become pregnant.

Storage: Up to 25°C (77°F). Do not freeze. Protect from light.

LESCOL — fluvastatin sodium

Class: HMG-CoA reductase inhibitor

RX

OTHER BRAND NAMES
Lescol XL

ADULT DOSAGE

Primary Hypercholesterolemia/Mixed Dyslipidemia

Initial: 40mg cap qpm or 80mg tab qd or 40mg cap bid
Usual: 20-80mg/day
Titrate: Adjust dose as necessary following periodic lipid determinations w/in 4 weeks of a given dose

LDL Reduction ≥25%:
Initial: 40mg cap qpm or 80mg tab qd or 40mg cap bid
LDL Reduction <25%:
Initial: 20mg cap qpm

Do not take two 40mg caps at 1 time

Secondary Prevention of Cardiovascular Disease

Dose based on current clinical practice

PEDIATRIC DOSAGE

Heterozygous Familial Hypercholesterolemia

Treatment of adolescents w/ the following findings: LDL remains ≥190mg/dL, or LDL remains ≥160mg/dL and there is a positive family history of premature cardiovascular disease or 2 or more other cardiovascular disease risk factors are present

10-16 Years (at Least 1 Year Postmenarche):
Initial: 20mg cap
Titrate: Adjust dose at 6-week intervals
Max: 40mg cap bid or 80mg tab qd

Do not take two 40mg caps at 1 time

DOSE MODIFICATION
Concomitant Medications
W/ Cyclosporine or Fluconazole:
Max: 20mg cap bid

Renal Impairment
Severe: Caution w/ higher doses (>40mg)

ADMINISTRATION
Oral route

Take w/ or w/o food
Do not break, crush, or chew tab, or open cap before administration

HOW SUPPLIED
Cap: (Lescol) 20mg, 40mg; Tab, ER: (Lescol XL) 80mg

CONTRAINDICATIONS
Active liver disease or unexplained, persistent elevations of serum transaminases, women who are pregnant or may become pregnant, nursing mothers.

WARNINGS/PRECAUTIONS
Has not been studied in conditions where the major abnormality is elevation of chylomicrons, VLDL, or IDL (eg, hyperlipoproteinemia Types I, III, IV, or V). Rhabdomyolysis with acute renal failure secondary to myoglobinuria reported; caution in patients with predisposing factors to myopathy (eg, ≥65 yrs, renal impairment, and inadequately treated hypothyroidism). Myopathy (including immune-mediated necrotizing myopathy [IMNM]) reported; d/c if markedly elevated CPK levels occur or myopathy is diagnosed/suspected. Temporarily withhold in any patient experiencing an acute or serious condition predisposing to development of renal failure secondary to rhabdomyolysis. Increases in serum transaminases reported; perform LFTs before initiation and if signs/symptoms of liver injury occur. Fatal and nonfatal hepatic failure reported (rare); promptly interrupt therapy if serious liver injury and/or hyperbilirubinemia or jaundice occurs and do not restart if no alternate etiology found. Caution with heavy alcohol use or history of liver disease and in elderly. Increase in HbA1c and fasting serum glucose levels reported. May blunt adrenal and/or gonadal steroid hormone production. Evaluate if endocrine dysfunction develops. May cause CNS toxicity. Caution with severe renal impairment at doses >40mg.

ADVERSE REACTIONS
Dyspepsia, abdominal pain, headache, sinusitis, nausea, diarrhea, myalgia, flu-like symptoms, abnormal LFTs.

DRUG INTERACTIONS
Increased risk of myopathy and/or rhabdomyolysis with cyclosporine, erythromycin, fibrates, niacin, colchicine, and gemfibrozil; avoid with gemfibrozil, caution with colchicine and fibrates, and consider dose reduction with niacin. Caution with drugs that decrease levels of endogenous steroid hormones (eg, ketoconazole, spironolactone, cimetidine). Cyclosporine and fluconazole

may increase levels. May increase levels of warfarin. Bleeding and/or increased PT reported with coumarin anticoagulants; monitor PT of patients on warfarin-type anticoagulants when therapy is initiated or dosage is changed. Increased glyburide and phenytoin levels.

NURSING CONSIDERATIONS

Assessment: Assess for active liver disease or unexplained, persistent elevations in serum transaminases, pregnancy/nursing status, predisposing factors for myopathy, heavy alcohol intake, history of liver disease, and possible drug interactions. Obtain baseline lipid profile (total-C, LDL, HDL, TG) and LFTs.

Monitoring: Monitor for signs/symptoms of myopathy (including IMNM), rhabdomyolysis, liver/renal/endocrine dysfunction, CNS toxicity, and other adverse reactions. Perform periodic monitoring of lipid profile. Check PT with coumarin anticoagulants.

Patient Counseling: Inform of the substances that should not be taken concomitantly with the drug. Counsel to inform other healthcare professionals that they are taking the drug. Advise to report promptly any unexplained muscle pain, tenderness, or weakness, particularly if accompanied by malaise or fever or if muscle signs/symptoms persist after discontinuation. Advise to report promptly any symptoms that may indicate liver injury (eg, fatigue, anorexia, right upper abdominal discomfort, dark urine, or jaundice). Inform women of childbearing age to use an effective method of birth control, stop taking drug if they become pregnant, and not to breastfeed while on therapy.

Storage: 25°C (77°F); excursions permitted to 15-30°C (15-86°F). Protect from light.

LETAIRIS – ambrisentan RX

Class: Endothelin receptor antagonist

Do not administer to a pregnant female; may cause serious birth defects. Exclude pregnancy before initiation of treatment. Females of reproductive potential must use acceptable methods of contraception during and for 1 month after treatment; obtain monthly pregnancy tests during and 1 month after discontinuation of treatment. Females can only receive the drug through a restricted program called the Letairis Risk Evaluation and Mitigation Strategy (REMS) program.

ADULT DOSAGE

Pulmonary Arterial Hypertension

Treatment of pulmonary arterial HTN (WHO Group 1) to improve exercise ability and delay clinical worsening
Initial: 5mg qd
Titrate: May increase to 10mg qd if 5mg is tolerated
Max: 10mg qd

PEDIATRIC DOSAGE

Pediatric use may not have been established

DOSE MODIFICATION

Hepatic Impairment
Preexisting Impairment:
Moderate/Severe: Not recommended

Elevation of Liver Transaminases:
D/C if elevations of ALT/AST >5X ULN or if elevations are accompanied by bilirubin >2X ULN, or by signs/symptoms of liver dysfunction and other causes are excluded

ADMINISTRATION

Oral route

Take w/ or w/o food
Do not split, crush, or chew tabs

HOW SUPPLIED

Tab: 5mg, 10mg

CONTRAINDICATIONS

Pregnancy, idiopathic pulmonary fibrosis (IPF), including IPF patients w/ pulmonary HTN (WHO Group 3).

WARNINGS/PRECAUTIONS

May cause peripheral edema; reported w/ greater frequency and severity in elderly patients. If clinically significant fluid retention develops, evaluate further to determine the cause and the possible need for specific treatment or discontinuation of therapy. If acute pulmonary edema develops during initiation of therapy, consider the possibility of pulmonary veno-occlusive disease (PVOD); d/c if confirmed. May decrease sperm counts. Decreases in Hgb concentration and Hct reported and may result in anemia requiring transfusion. Initiation of therapy is not recommended w/ clinically significant anemia. Consider discontinuation if a clinically significant Hgb decrease is observed and other causes have been excluded. Fully investigate the cause of liver injury if hepatic impairment develops.

ADVERSE REACTIONS

Peripheral edema, nasal congestion, flushing, sinusitis.

DRUG INTERACTIONS

Cyclosporine may increase exposure; limit dose of ambrisentan to 5mg qd when coadministered w/ cyclosporine.

NURSING CONSIDERATIONS

Assessment: Assess for IPF, anemia, hepatic impairment, pregnancy/nursing status, and possible drug interactions. Obtain baseline Hgb level.

Monitoring: Monitor for fluid retention, pulmonary edema, PVOD, hepatic impairment, and other adverse reactions. Obtain monthly pregnancy tests in females of reproductive potential during therapy and 1 month after discontinuation of treatment. Measure Hgb at 1 month after initiating therapy and periodically thereafter.

Patient Counseling: Instruct on the risk of fetal harm when used in pregnancy and instruct to immediately contact physician if pregnancy is suspected. Inform female patients that drug is only available through a restricted program called the Letairis REMS program. Inform female patients that they must sign an enrollment form and that female patients of reproductive potential must comply w/ pregnancy testing and contraception requirements. Educate and counsel females of reproductive potential on the use of emergency contraception in the event of unprotected sex or known or suspected contraceptive failure. Advise prepubertal females to immediately report to physician any reproductive status changes. Instruct to contact physician if any symptoms of liver injury occur. Advise of the importance of Hgb testing and of other risks associated w/ therapy (eg, decreases in Hgb, Hct, and sperm count; fluid overload).

Storage: 25°C (77°F); excursions permitted to 15-30°C (59-86°F).

LEVAQUIN – levofloxacin RX

Class: Fluoroquinolone

Fluoroquinolones are associated with an increased risk of tendinitis and tendon rupture in all ages. Risk is further increased in patients >60 yrs of age, patients taking corticosteroids, and with kidney, heart, or lung transplants. May exacerbate muscle weakness with myasthenia gravis; avoid in patients with known history of myasthenia gravis.

ADULT DOSAGE

Pneumonia

PO/IV:

Nosocomial Pneumonia: 750mg q24h for 7-14 days

Community-Acquired Pneumonia: 750mg q24h for 5 days or 500mg q24h for 7-14 days

Acute Bacterial Sinusitis

750mg q24h for 5 days or 500mg q24h for 10-14 days

Acute Bacterial Exacerbation of Chronic Bronchitis

500mg q24h for 7 days

Skin and Skin Structure Infections

Complicated: 750mg q24h for 7-14 days

Uncomplicated: 500mg q24h for 7-10 days

Chronic Bacterial Prostatitis

500mg q24h for 28 days

Urinary Tract Infections

Complicated/Acute Pyelonephritis: 750mg q24h for 5 days or 250mg q24h for 10 days

Uncomplicated: 250mg q24h for 3 days

Inhalational Anthrax (Postexposure)

>50kg: 500mg q24h for 60 days

Plague

Pneumonic/Septicemic Plague and Prophylaxis:

500mg q24h for 10-14 days

PEDIATRIC DOSAGE

Inhalational Anthrax (Postexposure)

≥6 Months of Age:

<50kg: 8mg/kg q12h for 60 days

Max: 250mg/dose

>50kg: 500mg q24h for 60 days

Plague

Pneumonic/Septicemic Plague and Prophylaxis:

≥6 Months of Age:

<50kg: 8mg/kg q12h for 10-14 days

Max: 250mg/dose

>50kg: 500mg q24h for 10-14 days

DOSE MODIFICATION

Renal Impairment

750mg q24h:

CrCl 20-49mL/min: 750mg q48h

CrCl 10-19mL/min or Hemodialysis/Chronic Ambulatory Peritoneal Dialysis: 750mg initial dose, then 500mg q48h

500mg q24h:

CrCl 20-49mL/min: 500mg initial dose, then 250mg q24h

CrCl 10-19mL/min or Hemodialysis/Chronic Ambulatory Peritoneal Dialysis: 500mg initial dose, then 250mg q48h

250mg q24h:

CrCl 20-49mL/min: No dose adjustment

CrCl 10-19mL/min: 250mg q48h; if treating uncomplicated UTI, no dose adjustment required

Hemodialysis/Chronic Ambulatory Peritoneal Dialysis: No information on dose adjustment available

ADMINISTRATION

IV/Oral route

Drink fluids liberally

PO

Take antacids, metal cations, and multivitamins at least 2 hrs before or 2 hrs after oral administration

Take at the same time each day

Tab: Take w/ or w/o food

Sol: Take 1 hr before or 2 hrs after eating

IV

Not for rapid or bolus IV infusion

Do not coadminister w/ any sol containing multivalent cations through the same IV line

Infuse over 60 min (250-500mg) or over 90 min (750mg)

Refer to PI for administration, preparation, stability, compatibility, and thawing instructions

HOW SUPPLIED

Inj: 5mg/mL in D5W [50mL, 100mL, 150mL]; Sol: 25mg/mL [480mL]; Tab: 250mg, 500mg, 750mg

WARNINGS/PRECAUTIONS

D/C if patient experiences pain, swelling, inflammation, or rupture of a tendon. Serious and occasionally fatal hypersensitivity and/or anaphylactic reactions reported; d/c immediately at the 1st appearance of a skin rash, jaundice, or any other sign of hypersensitivity, and institute supportive measures. Severe hepatotoxicity, including acute hepatitis and fatal events, reported; d/c immediately if signs and symptoms of hepatitis occur. Convulsions, toxic psychoses, and increased intracranial pressure (including pseudotumor cerebri) reported. CNS stimulation may occur; d/c and institute appropriate measures if CNS events occur. Caution with CNS disorders (eg, severe cerebral arteriosclerosis, epilepsy) or risk factors that may predispose to seizures or lower seizure threshold. *Clostridium difficile*-associated diarrhea (CDAD) reported; may need to d/c if CDAD is suspected or confirmed. Cases of sensory or sensorimotor axonal polyneuropathy resulting in paresthesias, hypoesthesias, dysesthesias, and weakness reported; d/c immediately if symptoms of neuropathy occur. May prolong QT interval; avoid with known QT interval prolongation or uncorrected hypokalemia. Increased incidence of musculoskeletal disorders in pediatric patients. Blood glucose disturbances reported in diabetics; d/c and initiate appropriate therapy if hypoglycemic reaction occurs. May cause photosensitivity/phototoxicity reactions; avoid excessive exposure to sun/UV light and d/c if occurs. May increase risk of bacterial resistance if used in the absence of a proven/suspected bacterial infection or a prophylactic indication. Crystalluria and cylindruria reported; maintain adequate hydration. May produce false-positive urine screening results for opiates. Caution in elderly and with renal impairment.

ADVERSE REACTIONS

Tendinitis, tendon rupture, nausea, diarrhea, constipation, headache, insomnia, dizziness.

DRUG INTERACTIONS

See Boxed Warning. Caution with drugs that may lower the seizure threshold. Avoid with Class IA (eg, quinidine, procainamide) and Class III (eg, amiodarone, sotalol) antiarrhythmics. May enhance effects of warfarin; monitor PT and INR. Disturbances of blood glucose in diabetic patients receiving a concomitant antidiabetic agent reported; monitor glucose levels. NSAIDs may increase risk of CNS stimulation and convulsive seizures. May prolong theophylline $T_{1/2}$ and increase theophylline levels/risk of theophylline-related adverse reactions; monitor theophylline levels closely. Probenecid or cimetidine may increase exposure and reduce renal clearance. (PO) Antacids containing Mg^{2+}, aluminum, as well as sucralfate, metal cations such as iron, and multivitamin preparations with zinc or didanosine chewable/buffered tab or pediatric powder for oral sol may substantially interfere with the GI absorption and lower systemic concentrations; take at least 2 hrs before or 2 hrs after oral levofloxacin.

NURSING CONSIDERATIONS

Assessment: Assess for risk factors for developing tendinitis and tendon rupture, history of myasthenia gravis, drug hypersensitivity, CNS disorders or risk factors that may predispose to seizures or lower seizure threshold, QT interval prolongation, uncorrected hypokalemia, renal/hepatic impairment, pregnancy/nursing status, and possible drug interactions.

Monitoring: Monitor for tendon rupture, tendinitis, exacerbation of myasthenia gravis, hypersensitivity reactions, hepatotoxicity, CNS effects, CDAD, peripheral neuropathy, ECG changes, arrhythmias, musculoskeletal disorders (pediatric patients), photosensitivity/phototoxicity reactions, and other adverse reactions. Monitor hydration status, blood glucose levels, and renal function. Monitor for evidence of bleeding, PT, and INR with warfarin.

Patient Counseling: Inform that drug only treats bacterial, not viral, infections. Advise to take as prescribed; inform that skipping doses or not completing full course of therapy may decrease effectiveness and increase likelihood of drug resistance. Advise to contact physician if pain, swelling, or inflammation of a tendon, or weakness or inability to move joints develops; instruct to d/c therapy and rest/refrain from exercise. Advise to d/c use and notify physician if allergic reaction, skin rash, or signs/symptoms of liver injury occur. Instruct to inform physician if experiencing any symptoms of muscle weakness, including respiratory difficulties. Advise to notify physician of any history of convulsions, QT prolongation, or myasthenia gravis. Inform that peripheral neuropathy has been associated with therapy, and that symptoms may occur soon after initiation of therapy and may be irreversible; instruct to d/c treatment immediately and contact physician if symptoms of peripheral neuropathy develop. Instruct to use caution with activities requiring mental alertness and coordination; advise to notify physician if persistent headache with or without blurred vision occurs. Instruct to contact physician immediately if watery and bloody diarrhea (with or without stomach cramps and fever) develop, even as late as ≥2 months after last dose. Advise to inform physician if child has tendon or joint-related problems prior to, during, or after therapy. Advise to minimize or avoid exposure to natural or artificial sunlight. Instruct diabetic patients being treated with antidiabetic agents to d/c therapy and notify physician if hypoglycemia occurs. Advise to inform physician if taking warfarin.

Storage: (Tab) 15-30°C (59-86°F). (Sol) 25°C (77°F); excursions permitted to 15-30°C (59-86°F). (Inj) Single-use Vials: Controlled room temperature. Protect from light. Premixed Sol: ≤25°C (77°F); brief exposure ≤40°C (104°F) does not adversely affect product. Avoid excessive heat and protect from freezing and light. Diluted Sol (5mg/mL): Stable at ≤25°C (77°F) for 72 hrs; 5°C (41°F) for 14 days; -20°C (-4°F) for 6 months.

LEVEMIR — insulin detemir (rDNA origin) RX

Class: Insulin

ADULT DOSAGE

Type 1 Diabetes Mellitus

Initial: Approx 1/3 of total daily insulin requirements
Titrate: Adjust dose based on blood glucose measurements
Use rapid-acting or short-acting, premeal insulin to satisfy the remainder of the daily insulin requirements

Type 2 Diabetes Mellitus

Inadequately Controlled on Oral Antidiabetics:
Initial: 10 U (or 0.1-0.2 U/kg) qpm or divided bid
Titrate: Adjust dose based on blood glucose measurements

Inadequately Controlled on Glucagon-Like Peptide (GLP)-1 Receptor Agonist:
Initial: 10 U qpm
Titrate: Adjust dose based on blood glucose measurements
Administer as separate inj when using w/ a GLP-1 receptor agonist

Conversions

From Insulin Glargine/NPH Insulin:
Convert on a unit-to-unit basis
In converting from NPH insulin, some type 2 diabetes mellitus patients may require more units of therapy than NPH insulin

PEDIATRIC DOSAGE

Type 1 Diabetes Mellitus

≥2 Years:
Initial: Approx 1/3 of total daily insulin requirements
Titrate: Adjust dose based on blood glucose measurements
Use rapid-acting or short-acting, premeal insulin to satisfy the remainder of the daily insulin requirements

Conversions

From Insulin Glargine/NPH Insulin:
Convert on a unit-to-unit basis
In converting from NPH insulin, some type 2 diabetes mellitus patients may require more units of therapy than NPH insulin

DOSE MODIFICATION

Elderly

Dose conservatively

ADMINISTRATION

SQ route

Rotate inj sites w/in the same region (abdomen, thigh, or deltoid) from 1 inj to the next

Do not dilute or mix w/ any other insulin or sol

QD Dosing

Administer dose w/ pm meal or hs

BID Dosing

Administer pm dose w/ pm meal, hs, or 12 hrs after am dose

HOW SUPPLIED

Inj: 100 U/mL [3mL, FlexTouch; 10mL, vial]

WARNINGS/PRECAUTIONS

Not recommended for treatment of diabetic ketoacidosis. Do not share insulin device between patients, even if the needle is changed; may carry a risk for transmission of blood-borne pathogens. Changes to an insulin regimen should be made cautiously and only under medical supervision. Changes in strength, manufacturer, type, or method of administration may result in the need for a change in dose or an adjustment of concomitant antidiabetic treatment. Not for IV/IM use or use in insulin infusion pumps. Hypoglycemia may occur; caution in patients w/ hypoglycemia unawareness and patients predisposed to hypoglycemia. Hypoglycemia may impair ability to concentrate and react. Severe, life-threatening, generalized allergy, including anaphylaxis, may occur. Caution in renal/hepatic impairment.

ADVERSE REACTIONS

Hypoglycemia, URTI, headache, pharyngitis, influenza-like illness, abdominal pain, back pain, gastroenteritis, bronchitis, pyrexia, cough, viral infection, N/V, rhinitis.

DRUG INTERACTIONS

May require insulin dose adjustment and close monitoring w/ drugs that may increase blood-glucose-lowering effect and susceptibility to hypoglycemia (eg, oral antidiabetic drugs, pramlintide acetate, ACE inhibitors), drugs that may reduce blood-glucose-lowering effect (eg, corticosteroids, niacin, danazol), or drugs that may either increase or decrease blood-glucose-lowering effect (eg, β-blockers, clonidine, lithium salts, alcohol). Pentamidine may cause hypoglycemia, sometimes followed by hyperglycemia. Signs of hypoglycemia may be reduced or absent w/ antiadrenergic drugs (eg, β-blockers, clonidine, guanethidine, reserpine). May need to lower or more conservatively titrate dose when used w/ a GLP-1 receptor agonist to minimize risk of hypoglycemia. Observe for signs/symptoms of heart failure (HF) if treated concomitantly w/ a peroxisome proliferator-activated receptor (PPAR)-gamma agonist (eg, thiazolidinedione); consider discontinuation or dose reduction of the PPAR-gamma agonist if HF develops.

NURSING CONSIDERATIONS

Assessment: Assess for diabetic ketoacidosis, predisposition to hypoglycemia, hypersensitivity, renal/hepatic impairment, pregnancy/nursing status, and possible drug interactions. Obtain baseline blood glucose and HbA1c levels.

Monitoring: Monitor for signs/symptoms of hypoglycemia, allergic reactions, and other adverse reactions. Monitor blood glucose and HbA1c levels, and renal/hepatic function.

Patient Counseling: Inform about the potential side effects, including hypoglycemia, weight gain, lipodystrophy, and allergic reactions. Inform that hypoglycemia may impair ability to concentrate and react; advise to use caution when driving or operating machinery. Instruct to always check the label before each inj to avoid medication errors/accidental mix-ups. Advise to use only if sol is clear and colorless w/ no particles visible. Instruct on self-management procedures, including glucose monitoring, proper inj technique, and management of hypoglycemia and hyperglycemia, and on handling of special situations (eg, intercurrent conditions, inadequate or skipped insulin dose, inadequate food intake). Advise to inform physician if pregnant/contemplating pregnancy. Counsel to never share insulin device w/ another person, even if the needle is changed.

Storage: Unopened: 2-8°C (36-46°F) until expiration date. If refrigeration is not possible, may be kept at room temperature <30°C (86°F) for 42 days. Do not freeze. Protect from direct heat and light. Opened: Vial: 2-8°C (36-46°F) or room temperature <30°C (86°F). Discard refrigerated vials 42 days after initial use and discard unrefrigerated vials 42 days after they are 1st kept out of the refrigerator. Do not freeze. Protect from direct heat and light. FlexTouch: Room temperature <30°C (86°F) for 42 days; do not refrigerate after initial use or store w/ the needle in place. Protect from direct heat and light. Always remove the needle after each inj and use a new needle for each inj.

LEVITRA – vardenafil hydrochloride

RX

Class: Phosphodiesterase type 5 inhibitor

ADULT DOSAGE

Erectile Dysfunction

Initial: 10mg prn, 60 min prior to sexual activity

Titrate: May decrease to 5mg or increase to max of 20mg based on efficacy and side effects

Max: 1 tab/day

PEDIATRIC DOSAGE

Pediatric use may not have been established

DOSE MODIFICATION

Concomitant Medications

Ritonavir:

Max: 2.5mg/72 hrs

Indinavir/Saquinavir/Atazanavir/Clarithromycin/Ketoconazole (400mg/day)/Itraconazole (400mg/day):

Max: 2.5mg/24 hrs

Ketoconazole (200mg/day)/Itraconazole (200mg/day)/Erythromycin:

Max: 5mg/24 hrs

Stable on α-Blocker:

Initial: 5mg; 2.5mg when used w/ certain CYP3A4 inhibitors

Consider a time interval between dosing

Renal Impairment

Dialysis: Avoid use

Hepatic Impairment

Moderate (Child-Pugh B):

Initial: 5mg

Max: 10mg

Severe (Child-Pugh C): Avoid use

Elderly

≥65 Years:

Initial: 5mg

ADMINISTRATION

Oral route

Take w/ or w/o food

HOW SUPPLIED

Tab: 2.5mg, 5mg, 10mg, 20mg

CONTRAINDICATIONS

Concomitant use (regularly or intermittently) with nitrates and nitric oxide donors.

WARNINGS/PRECAUTIONS

Avoid if sexual activity is not recommended due to underlying cardiovascular (CV) status, or if with severe hepatic impairment (Child-Pugh C)/congenital QT prolongation, or if on renal dialysis. Patients with left ventricular outflow obstruction (eg, aortic stenosis, idiopathic hypertrophic subaortic stenosis) may be sensitive to vasodilation. Has vasodilatory properties resulting in transient decreases in supine BP. Not recommended with unstable angina, hypotension (resting systolic BP <90mmHg), uncontrolled HTN (>170/110mmHg), recent history of stroke, life-threatening arrhythmia, or MI (within last 6 months), severe cardiac failure, or hereditary degenerative retinal disorders, including retinitis pigmentosa. Rare reports of prolonged erections >4 hrs and priapism. Caution with bleeding disorders, significant active peptic ulceration, anatomical deformation of the penis (eg, angulation, cavernosal fibrosis, Peyronie's disease) or conditions that predispose to priapism (eg, sickle cell anemia, multiple myeloma, leukemia). Non-arteritic anterior ischemic optic neuropathy (NAION) reported (rare); d/c if sudden loss of vision occurs. Caution in patients with underlying NAION risk factors; increased risk with previous history of NAION and individuals with "crowded" optic disc. Sudden decrease or loss of hearing accompanied by tinnitus and dizziness reported; d/c if this occurs. QT prolongation may occur.

ADVERSE REACTIONS

Headache, flushing, rhinitis, dyspepsia, sinusitis, flu syndrome.

DRUG INTERACTIONS

See Contraindications. Avoid with Class IA (eg, quinidine, procainamide) or Class III (eg, amiodarone, sotalol) antiarrhythmics and other agents for ED. Caution with medications known to prolong QT interval. Increased levels with CYP3A4 inhibitors (eg, ritonavir, ketoconazole, clarithromycin). Caution when coadministering α-blockers; additive effect on BP may be anticipated. CYP3A4/5 or CYP2C9 inhibitors may reduce clearance.

NURSING CONSIDERATIONS

Assessment: Assess for CV disease, left ventricular outflow obstruction, congenital or history of QT prolongation, hereditary degenerative retinal disorders, bleeding disorders, active peptic ulceration, anatomical deformation of the penis, conditions that predispose to priapism, renal/hepatic impairment, potential underlying causes of ED, risk for NAION, and for possible drug interactions. Obtain baseline BP.

Monitoring: Monitor for priapism, changes in vision/hearing, QT prolongation, and other adverse reactions.

Patient Counseling: Instruct to take ud. Inform that regular and/or intermittent use of nitrates may cause BP to suddenly drop to an unsafe level. Inform patients with preexisting CV risk factors of the potential cardiac risk of sexual activity. Inform that concomitant use of α-blockers may lower BP significantly. Instruct to contact physician for dose modification if not satisfied with quality of sexual performance or in case of an unwanted effect. Instruct to seek immediate medical assistance if erection persists >4 hrs; inform that penile tissue damage and permanent loss of potency may result. Instruct to d/c and seek medical attention in the event of sudden loss of vision in 1 or both eyes; inform of the increased risk of NAION with history of NAION in 1 eye and in patients with a "crowded" optic disc. Instruct to d/c treatment and seek prompt medical attention in the event of sudden decrease or loss of hearing that may be accompanied by tinnitus and dizziness. Counsel about protective measures necessary to guard against STDs, including HIV; inform that drug does not protect against STDs.

Storage: 25°C (77°F); excursions permitted to 15-30°C (59-86°F).

LEVOPHED — norepinephrine bitartrate RX

Class: Alpha-adrenergic agonist

To prevent sloughing and necrosis in area of extravasation, area should be infiltrated with 10-15mL saline sol containing 5-10mg of Regitine (brand of phentolamine), an adrenergic blocking agent. Sympathetic blockade with phentolamine causes immediate and conspicuous local hyperemic changes if infiltrated within 12 hrs. Give phentolamine as soon as possible after the extravasation is noted.

ADULT DOSAGE

Acute Hypotension

For BP control in certain acute hypotensive states (eg, pheochromocytomectomy, sympathectomy, poliomyelitis, spinal anesthesia, MI, septicemia, blood transfusion, and drug reactions)

Average Dosage:
Initial: 8-12mcg/min (2-3mL) as IV infusion until low normal BP (80-100mmHg systolic) is established and maintained by adjusting rate of flow
Maint: 2-4mcg/min (0.5-1mL)

High Dosage:
Individualize dose (as high as 68mg/day)

Continue infusion until adequate BP and tissue perfusion are maintained w/o therapy
Reduce dose gradually, avoiding abrupt withdrawal

Adjunct Treatment of Cardiac Arrest and Profound Hypotension:
Average Dosage:
Initial: 8-12mcg/min (2-3mL) as IV infusion until low normal BP (80-100mmHg systolic) is established and maintained by adjusting rate of flow
Maint: 2-4mcg/min (0.5-1mL)

PEDIATRIC DOSAGE

Pediatric use may not have been established

DOSE MODIFICATION

Elderly

Start at lower end of dosing range

ADMINISTRATION

IV route

Inj is a concentrated, potent drug that must be diluted in dextrose containing sol prior to infusion

An infusion should be given into a large vein

Avoid contact w/ iron salts, alkalis, or oxidizing agents

Diluent

Dilute in D5 inj or D5 and NaCl inj

Whole blood or plasma, if indicated to increase blood volume, should be administered separately (eg, Y-tube and individual containers if given simultaneously)

HOW SUPPLIED

Inj: 4mg/4mL

CONTRAINDICATIONS

Hypotension from blood volume deficits, except as an emergency measure to maintain coronary and cerebral artery perfusion until blood volume replacement therapy can be completed, mesenteric or peripheral vascular thrombosis (unless administration is necessary as a life-saving procedure in the opinion of the attending physician), profound hypoxia or hypercarbia, concomitant use of cyclopropane and halothane anesthetics.

WARNINGS/PRECAUTIONS

Contains sodium metabisulfite; may cause allergic-type reactions (eg, anaphylactic symptoms, life-threatening or less severe asthmatic episodes). May produce dangerously high BP with overdoses due to potency and varying response; monitor BP every 2 min from initial administration until desired BP is obtained, then every 5 min if administration is to be continued. Headache may be a symptom of HTN due to overdosage; monitor rate of flow constantly. Infusions should be given into a large vein, particularly an antecubital vein whenever possible. Avoid a catheter tie-in technique if possible. Occlusive vascular diseases (eg, atherosclerosis, arteriosclerosis, diabetic endarteritis, Buerger's disease) more likely to occur in the lower than in the upper extremity; avoid leg veins in elderly or in those suffering from such disorders. Gangrene in lower extremity reported when given in an ankle vein. Check infusion site frequently for free flow. Avoid extravasation into the tissues; local necrosis might ensue. Blanching may occur; consider changing the infusion site at intervals to allow effects of local vasoconstriction to subside. Caution in elderly.

ADVERSE REACTIONS

Ischemic injury, bradycardia, arrhythmias, anxiety, headache, respiratory difficulty, extravasation necrosis at inj site.

DRUG INTERACTIONS

See Contraindications. Caution with MAOI or triptyline/imipramine antidepressants; severe, prolonged HTN may result.

NURSING CONSIDERATIONS

Assessment: Assess hypotension and need for blood volume replacement. Assess use as emergency measure or life-saving procedure (eg, hypotension from blood volume deficits to maintain coronary and cerebral artery perfusion until blood volume replacement therapy can be completed, mesenteric or peripheral vascular thrombosis). Assess for profound hypoxia or hypercarbia, sulfite sensitivity, pregnancy/nursing status, and possible drug interactions. Assess use in elderly and occlusive vascular diseases. Obtain baseline BP.

Monitoring: Monitor for HTN, headache, gangrene, extravasation, blanching, and hypersensitivity/allergic reactions. Monitor infusion site, rate of flow, BP, and central venous pressure.

Patient Counseling: Inform of risks/benefits of therapy. Advise to inform physician if headache occurs.

Storage: 20-25°C (68-77°F); (vial) excursions permitted to 15-30° (59-86°F). Protect from light.

LEVOXYL – levothyroxine sodium — RX

Class: Thyroid replacement hormone

Do not use for the treatment of obesity or weight loss; doses within range of daily hormonal requirements are ineffective for weight reduction in euthyroid patients. Serious or life-threatening manifestations of toxicity may occur when given in larger doses, particularly when given in association with sympathomimetic amines.

ADULT DOSAGE

Hypothyroidism

Replacement/supplemental therapy in hypothyroidism of any etiology, except transient hypothyroidism during the recovery phase of subacute thyroiditis

Adjust dose based on periodic assessment of patient's clinical response and lab parameters

Usual: 1.7mcg/kg/day; >200mcg/day seldom required

Severe Hypothyroidism:
Initial: 12.5-25mcg/day
Titrate: Increase by 25mcg/day every 2-4 weeks until TSH level normalized

Secondary (Pituitary)/Tertiary (Hypothalamic) Hypothyroidism: Titrate until euthyroid and serum free-T4 level is restored to the upper 1/2 of the normal range

Subclinical Hypothyroidism: Lower doses may be adequate to normalize TSH level (eg, 1mcg/kg/day)

Pituitary TSH Suppressant

Used to treat/prevent various types of euthyroid goiters (eg, thyroid nodules, subacute or chronic lymphocytic thyroiditis, multinodular goiter) and to manage thyroid cancer

Well-Differentiated (Papillary and Follicular) Thyroid Cancer:

Usual: >2mcg/kg/day, w/ target TSH level <0.1 mU/L
High-Risk Tumors: Target TSH level <0.01 mU/L

Benign Nodules and Nontoxic Multinodular Goiter:
Suppressed to a higher TSH target than that used for treatment of thyroid cancer (eg, 0.1-0.5 mU/L for nodules, 0.5-1.0 mU/L for multinodular goiter)

PEDIATRIC DOSAGE

Hypothyroidism

Replacement/supplemental therapy in hypothyroidism of any etiology, except transient hypothyroidism during the recovery phase of subacute thyroiditis

Adjust dose based on periodic assessment of patient's clinical response and lab parameters

Usual:
0-3 Months of Age: 10-15mcg/kg/day
3-6 Months of Age: 8-10mcg/kg/day
6-12 Months of Age: 6-8mcg/kg/day
1-5 Years: 5-6mcg/kg/day
6-12 Years: 4-5mcg/kg/day
>12 Years: 2-3mcg/kg/day
Growth/Puberty Complete: 1.7mcg/kg/day

Infants w/ Serum T4 <5mcg/dL or Undetectable T4:
Initial: 50mcg/day

Chronic/Severe Hypothyroidism:
Children:
Initial: 25mcg/day
Titrate: Increase by 25mcg increments every 2-4 weeks until desired effect is achieved

DOSE MODIFICATION

Pregnancy

May increase levothyroxine requirements

Elderly

Hypothyroidism:
>50 Years:
Initial: 25-50mcg/day
Titrate: Increase by 12.5-25mcg increments every 6-8 weeks prn

W/ Underlying Cardiac Disease:
Initial: 12.5-25mcg/day
Titrate: Increase by 12.5-25mg increments every 4-6 weeks

Adverse Reactions

Minimize Hyperactivity in Older Children:
Initial: Give 1/4 of full replacement dose
Titrate: Increase on a weekly basis by 1/4 the full recommended replacement dose until the full recommended replacement dose is reached

Other Important Modifications

Hypothyroidism W/ Underlying Cardiac Disease:
Infants (Risk for Cardiac Failure):
Initial: Consider lower dose (eg, 25mcg/day)
Titrate: Increase dose in 4-6 weeks prn
<50 Years:
Initial: 25-50mcg/day
Titrate: Increase by 12.5-25mcg increments every 6-8 weeks prn

ADMINISTRATION

Oral route

Take in the am on an empty stomach at least 30 min before food
Take w/ water
Take at least 4 hrs apart from drugs that are known to interfere w/ its absorption

Pediatrics

May crush tab and mix w/ 5-10mL of water

HOW SUPPLIED

Tab: 25mcg, 50mcg, 75mcg, 88mcg, 100mcg, 112mcg, 125mcg, 137mcg, 150mcg, 175mcg, 200mcg

CONTRAINDICATIONS

Untreated subclinical (suppressed serum TSH level with normal T3 level and T4 levels) or overt thyrotoxicosis of any etiology, acute myocardial infarction (MI), uncorrected adrenal insufficiency.

WARNINGS/PRECAUTIONS

Should not be used in the treatment of male or female infertility unless associated with hypothyroidism. Contraindicated in patients with nontoxic diffuse goiter or nodular thyroid disease, particularly in elderly or with underlying cardiovascular (CV) disease if serum TSH level is already suppressed; use with caution if TSH level is not suppressed and carefully monitor thyroid function. Has narrow therapeutic index; carefully titrate dose to avoid over- or under-treatment. May decrease bone mineral density (BMD) with long term use; give minimum dose necessary to achieve desired clinical and biochemical response. Caution with CV disorders and the elderly. If cardiac symptoms develop or worsen, reduce or withhold dose for 1 week and then restart at lower dose. Overtreatment may produce CV effects (eg, increase in HR, increase in cardiac wall thickness, increase in cardiac contractility, precipitation of angina or arrhythmias). Monitor patients with coronary artery disease (CAD) closely during surgical procedures; may precipitate cardiac arrhythmias. Caution in patients with diabetes mellitus (DM). Patients with concomitant adrenal insufficiency should be treated with replacement glucocorticoids prior to therapy.

ADVERSE REACTIONS

Fatigue, increased appetite, weight loss, heat intolerance, headache, hyperactivity, irritability, insomnia, palpitations, arrhythmias, dyspnea, hair loss, menstrual irregularities, pseudotumor cerebri (children), slipped capital femoral epiphysis (children).

DRUG INTERACTIONS

Concurrent sympathomimetics may increase effects of sympathomimetics or thyroid hormone; may increase risk of coronary insufficiency with CAD. Upward dose adjustments may be needed for insulin and oral hypoglycemic agents. May decrease absorption with soybean flour, cottonseed meal, walnuts, and dietary fiber. May increase oral anticoagulant activity; adjust dose of anticoagulant and monitor PT. May decrease levels and effects of digitalis glycosides. Transient reduction in TSH secretion with dopamine/dopamine agonists, glucocorticoids, octreotide. Decreased thyroid hormone secretion with aminoglutethimide, amiodarone, iodide (including iodine-containing radiographic contrast agents), lithium, methimazole, propylthiouracil (PTU), sulfonamides, and tolbutamide. May increase thyroid hormone secretion with amiodarone and iodide. May decrease T4 absorption with antacids (aluminum and magnesium hydroxides), simethicone, bile acid sequestrants (cholestyramine, colestipol), calcium carbonate, cation exchange resins (kayexalate), ferrous sulfate, orlistat, and sucralfate; administer at least 4 hrs apart. May increase serum thyroxine-binding globulin (TBG) concentrations with clofibrate, estrogen-containing oral contraceptives, oral estrogens, heroin/methadone, 5-fluorouracil, mitotane, and tamoxifen. May decrease serum TBG concentrations with androgens/anabolic steroids, asparaginase, glucocorticoids, and slow-release nicotinic acid. May cause protein-binding site displacement with furosemide (>80mg IV), heparin, hydantoins, NSAIDs (fenamates, phenylbutazone), and salicylates (>2g/day). May alter T4 and T3 metabolism with carbamazepine, hydantoins, phenobarbital, and rifampin. May decrease T4 5'-deiodinase activity with amiodarone, β-adrenergic antagonists (eg, propranolol >160mg/day), glucocorticoids (eg, dexamethasone >4mg/day), and PTU. Concurrent use with tricyclic (eg, amitriptyline) and tetracyclic (eg, maprotiline) antidepressants may increase the therapeutic and toxic effects of both drugs. Coadministration with sertraline in patients stabilized on levothyroxine may result in increased levothyroxine requirements. Interferon-α may cause development of antithyroid microsomal antibodies and transient hypothyroidism, hyperthyroidism, or both. Interleukin-2 has been associated with transient painless thyroiditis. Excessive use with growth hormones (eg, somatropin, somatrem) may accelerate epiphyseal closure. Ketamine may produce marked HTN and tachycardia. May reduce uptake of radiographic agents. Decreased theophylline clearance may occur in hypothyroid patients. Altered levels of thyroid hormone and/or TSH levels with choral hydrate, diazepam, ethionamide, lovastatin, metoclopramide, 6-mercaptopurine, nitroprusside, para-aminosalicylate sodium, perphenazine, resorcinol (excessive topical use), and thiazide diuretics.

NURSING CONSIDERATIONS

Assessment: Assess for untreated subclinical or overt thyrotoxicosis, acute MI, uncorrected adrenal insufficiency, CAD, CV disorders, nontoxic diffuse goiter, nodular thyroid disease, DM, hypersensitivity, pregnancy/nursing status, and possible drug interactions. In patients with secondary or tertiary hypothyroidism, assess for additional hypothalamic/pituitary hormone deficiencies. Assess TSH levels. In infants with congenital hypothyroidism, assess for other congenital anomalies.

Monitoring: Monitor for CV effects. In patients on long-term therapy, monitor for signs/symptoms of decreased BMD. In patients with nontoxic diffuse goiter or nodular thyroid disease, monitor for precipitation of thyrotoxicosis. In adults with primary hypothyroidism, perform periodic monitoring of serum TSH levels. In pediatric patients with congenital hypothyroidism, perform periodic monitoring of serum TSH levels and total or free T4 levels. In patients with secondary and tertiary hypothyroidism, perform periodic monitoring of serum free T4 levels. Refer to PI for TSH and T4 monitoring parameters. Closely monitor PT if coadministered with an oral anticoagulant.

Patient Counseling: Instruct to notify physician if allergic to any foods or medicines, pregnant or plan to become pregnant, breastfeeding or taking any other drugs, including prescriptions and OTC preparations. Instruct to notify physician of any other medical conditions, particularly heart disease, diabetes, clotting disorders, and adrenal or pituitary gland problems. Instruct not to stop or change dose unless directed by physician. Instruct to take on empty stomach, at least 1/2 hr before eating any food. Advise that partial hair loss may occur during the 1st few months of therapy, but is usually temporary. Instruct to notify physician or dentist prior to surgery about levothyroxine therapy. Inform that drug should not be used for weight control. Inform patients that tabs may rapidly swell and disintegrate resulting in choking, gagging, tab getting stuck in throat or difficulty swallowing; take with a full glass of water. Instruct to notify physician if rapid or irregular heartbeat, chest pain, SOB, leg cramps, headache, or any other unusual medical event occurs. Inform that dose may be increased during pregnancy. Inform that drug should not be administered within 4 hrs of agents such as iron/calcium supplements and antacids.

Storage: 20-25°C (68-77°F); excursions permitted to 15-30°C (59-86°F). Store away from heat, moisture, and light.

LEXAPRO — escitalopram oxalate RX

Class: Selective serotonin reuptake inhibitor

Antidepressants increased the risk of suicidal thinking and behavior (suicidality) in children, adolescents, and young adults in short-term studies of major depressive disorder (MDD) and other psychiatric disorders. Monitor and observe closely for clinical worsening, suicidality, or unusual changes in behavior in patients who are started on antidepressant therapy. Advise families and caregivers of the need for close observation and communication with the prescriber. Not approved for use in pediatric patients <12 yrs of age.

ADULT DOSAGE

Major Depressive Disorder

Initial: 10mg qd
Titrate: May increase to 20mg after a minimum of 1 week

Generalized Anxiety Disorder

Initial: 10mg qd
Titrate: May increase to 20mg after a minimum of 1 week

Dosing Considerations with MAOIs

Switching to/from an MAOI for Psychiatric Disorders:
Allow at least 14 days between discontinuation of an MAOI and initiation of treatment, and allow at least 14 days between discontinuation of treatment and initiation of an MAOI

W/ Other MAOIs (eg, Linezolid, IV Methylene Blue):
Do not start escitalopram in a patient being treated w/ linezolid or IV methylene blue
In patients already receiving escitalopram, if acceptable alternatives are not available and benefits outweigh risks, d/c escitalopram and administer linezolid or IV methylene blue; monitor for serotonin syndrome for 2 weeks or until 24 hrs after the last dose of linezolid or IV methylene blue, whichever comes 1st. May resume escitalopram therapy 24 hrs after the last dose of linezolid or IV methylene blue

PEDIATRIC DOSAGE

Major Depressive Disorder

≥12 Years:
Initial: 10mg qd
Titrate: May increase to 20mg after a minimum of 3 weeks

Dosing Considerations with MAOIs

Switching to/from an MAOI for Psychiatric Disorders:
Allow at least 14 days between discontinuation of an MAOI and initiation of treatment, and allow at least 14 days between discontinuation of treatment and initiation of an MAOI

W/ Other MAOIs (eg, Linezolid, IV Methylene Blue):
Do not start escitalopram in a patient being treated w/ linezolid or IV methylene blue
In patients already receiving escitalopram, if acceptable alternatives are not available and benefits outweigh risks, d/c escitalopram and administer linezolid or IV methylene blue; monitor for serotonin syndrome for 2 weeks or until 24 hrs after the last dose of linezolid or IV methylene blue, whichever comes 1st. May resume escitalopram therapy 24 hrs after the last dose of linezolid or IV methylene blue

DOSE MODIFICATION

Hepatic Impairment

10mg/day

Elderly

10mg/day

Discontinuation

Gradually reduce dose; if intolerable symptoms occur following a decrease in dose or upon discontinuation, consider resuming previously prescribed dose or continue decreasing dose at a more gradual rate

ADMINISTRATION

Oral route

Administer in the am or pm, w/ or w/o food

HOW SUPPLIED

Sol: 5mg/5mL [240mL]; Tab: 5mg, 10mg*, 20mg* *scored

CONTRAINDICATIONS

Use of an MAOI for psychiatric disorders either concomitantly or within 14 days of stopping treatment. Treatment within 14 days of stopping an MAOI for psychiatric disorders. Starting treatment in a patient being treated with other MAOIs (eg, linezolid, IV methylene blue). Concomitant use with pimozide.

WARNINGS/PRECAUTIONS

Not approved for the treatment of bipolar depression. Serotonin syndrome reported; d/c immediately and initiate supportive symptomatic treatment. Avoid abrupt discontinuation; gradual dose reduction is recommended whenever possible. Convulsions reported; caution with history of seizure disorder. Activation of mania/hypomania reported; caution with history of mania. Hyponatremia may occur; caution in elderly and volume-depleted patients. Consider discontinuation in patients with symptomatic hyponatremia and institute appropriate medical intervention. May increase the risk of bleeding events. May impair mental/physical abilities. Pupillary dilation that occurs following use may trigger an angle-closure attack in a patient with anatomically narrow angles who does not have a patent iridectomy. May precipitate mixed/manic episode in patients at risk for bipolar disorder; screen for risk for bipolar disorder prior to initiating treatment. Caution with diseases/conditions that produce altered metabolism or hemodynamic responses, and with severe renal impairment.

ADVERSE REACTIONS

N/V, insomnia, ejaculation disorder, increased sweating, somnolence, fatigue, diarrhea, dry mouth, headache, constipation, decreased appetite, neck/shoulder pain, decreased libido, anorgasmia.

DRUG INTERACTIONS

See Contraindications. Not recommended for use with alcohol. May cause serotonin syndrome with other serotonergic drugs (eg, triptans, TCAs, fentanyl) and with drugs that impair metabolism of serotonin; d/c immediately if this occurs. Caution with other centrally acting drugs, and drugs metabolized by CYP2D6 (eg, desipramine). Increased risk of bleeding with ASA, NSAIDs, warfarin, and other drugs that affect coagulation. May increase levels with cimetidine. Rare reports of weakness, hyperreflexia, and incoordination with sumatriptan. Possible increased clearance with carbamazepine. May decrease levels of ketoconazole. May increase levels of metoprolol. Increased risk of hyponatremia with diuretics. Monitor lithium levels and adjust its dose appropriately.

NURSING CONSIDERATIONS

Assessment: Assess for drug hypersensitivity, risk for bipolar disorder, history of seizure disorder, history of mania, volume depletion, diseases/conditions that produce altered metabolism or hemodynamic response, susceptibility to angle-closure glaucoma, hepatic/renal impairment, pregnancy/nursing status, and possible drug interactions. Obtain detailed psychiatric history.

Monitoring: Monitor for signs/symptoms of clinical worsening, serotonin syndrome, bleeding events, hyponatremia, seizures, cognitive and motor impairment, activation of mania/hypomania, angle-closure glaucoma, and other adverse reactions. If therapy is abruptly discontinued, monitor for discontinuation symptoms. Regularly monitor weight and growth in pediatrics. Periodically reassess the need for maintenance treatment.

Patient Counseling: Inform about the benefits and risks of therapy. Counsel on the appropriate use of the drug. Advise to look for emergence of symptoms associated with an increased risk for suicidal thinking and behavior; instruct to report such symptoms, especially if severe, abrupt in onset, or not part of presenting symptoms. Caution about risk of serotonin syndrome with other serotonergic agents (eg, triptans, buspirone, St. John's wort) and about risk of bleeding with ASA, warfarin, or other drugs that affect coagulation. Caution about risk of angle-closure glaucoma. Instruct to notify physician if taking or planning to take any prescription or OTC drugs. Inform that improvement may be noticed in 1-4 weeks; instruct to continue therapy ud. Caution about operating hazardous machinery, including automobiles. Instruct to avoid alcohol. Instruct to notify physician if pregnant, intending to become pregnant, or if breastfeeding. Inform of the need for comprehensive treatment program.

Storage: 25°C (77°F); excursions permitted to 15-30°C (59-86°F).

LEXIVA – fosamprenavir calcium

Class: Protease inhibitor

RX

ADULT DOSAGE

HIV-1 Infection

Combination w/ Other Antiretrovirals:
Therapy-Naive:
1400mg bid w/o ritonavir (RTV)
1400mg qd + RTV 200mg qd
1400mg qd + RTV 100mg qd
700mg bid + RTV 100mg bid
Protease Inhibitor-Experienced:
700mg bid + RTV 100mg bid

PEDIATRIC DOSAGE

HIV-1 Infection

Combination w/ Other Antiretrovirals:
Sus:
Protease Inhibitor-Naive (≥4 Weeks of Age) and Protease Inhibitor-Experienced (≥6 Months of Age):
<11kg: 45mg/kg bid + ritonavir (RTV) 7mg/kg bid
11-<15kg: 30mg/kg bid + RTV 3mg/kg bid
15-<20kg: 23mg/kg bid + RTV 3mg/kg bid
≥20kg: 18mg/kg bid + RTV 3mg/kg bid
Max: 700mg bid + RTV 100mg bid

Protease Inhibitor-Naive (≥2 Years):
30mg/kg bid w/o RTV
Tab:
Administering w/o RTV:
≥47kg: 1400mg bid

DOSE MODIFICATION

Hepatic Impairment

Mild (Child-Pugh Score 5-6):
Therapy-Naive:
Reduce dose to 700mg bid w/o ritonavir (RTV)
Therapy-Naive/Protease Inhibitor-Experienced:
Reduce dose to 700mg bid + RTV 100mg qd

Moderate (Child-Pugh Score 7-9):
Therapy-Naive:
Reduce dose to 700mg bid w/o RTV
Therapy-Naive/Protease Inhibitor-Experienced:
Reduce dose to 450mg bid + RTV 100mg qd

Severe (Child-Pugh Score 10-15):
Therapy-Naive:
Reduce dose to 350mg bid w/o RTV
Therapy-Naive/Protease Inhibitor-Experienced:
Reduce dose to 300mg bid + RTV 100mg qd

Other Important Modifications

Pediatrics:
Only administer to infants ≥38 weeks gestation and who have attained a postnatal age of 28 days
RTV Combination Treatment:
Tabs: May be used for patients ≥39kg
RTV Caps: May be used for patients ≥33kg

ADMINISTRATION

Oral route

Tab
Take w/ or w/o food

Sus
Shake vigorously before using
Adults: Take w/o food
Pediatrics: Take w/ food
Redose if emesis occurs w/in 30 min after dosing

HOW SUPPLIED

Sus: 50mg/mL [225mL]; Tab: 700mg

CONTRAINDICATIONS

Concomitant use w/ drugs that are highly dependent on CYP3A4 for clearance and for which elevated concentrations are associated w/ serious and/or life-threatening events (eg, alfuzosin, flecainide, propafenone, rifampin, dihydroergotamine, ergonovine, ergotamine, methylergonovine, cisapride, St. John's wort, lovastatin, simvastatin, pimozide, delavirdine, sildenafil when used for pulmonary arterial HTN, midazolam, triazolam). When used w/ ritonavir (RTV), refer to the individual monograph.

WARNINGS/PRECAUTIONS
Severe/life-threatening skin reactions, including Stevens-Johnson syndrome, reported; d/c if severe/life-threatening rashes or moderate rashes w/ systemic symptoms occur. Caution w/ known sulfonamide allergy. Use w/ RTV at higher-than-recommended doses should not be used due to possible transaminase elevations. Increased risk for transaminase elevations in patients w/ hepatitis B or C or marked transaminase elevation prior to treatment. New onset or exacerbation of diabetes mellitus (DM), hyperglycemia, diabetic ketoacidosis reported. Immune reconstitution syndrome, autoimmune disorders (eg, Graves' disease, polymyositis, and Guillain-Barre syndrome) in the setting of immune reconstitution, redistribution/accumulation of body fat, and lipid elevations reported. Acute hemolytic anemia reported w/ amprenavir. Spontaneous bleeding w/ hemophilia A and B reported. Nephrolithiasis reported; consider temporarily interrupting or discontinuing therapy if signs/symptoms occur. Caution in the elderly. Not recommended for qd administration w/ RTV for adult protease inhibitor-experienced patients or any pediatric patients. Not recommended w/ or w/o RTV for protease inhibitor-experienced pediatric patients <6 months of age.

ADVERSE REACTIONS
Diarrhea, N/V, headache, rash, increased AST/ALT, increased serum lipase, decreased ANC.

DRUG INTERACTIONS
See Contraindications. Not recommended w/ CYP3A4 substrates w/ narrow therapeutic windows, nevirapine (w/o RTV), and salmeterol. Fosamprenavir/RTV is not recommended w/ telaprevir, boceprevir, fluticasone and high doses of ketoconazole or itraconazole. Avoid (w/ RTV) concomitant colchicine in patients w/ renal/hepatic impairment. May increase levels of nevirapine, maraviroc, antiarrhythmics, trazodone, ketoconazole, itraconazole, colchicine, rifabutin, (w/ RTV) quetiapine, benzodiazepines, calcium channel blockers, bosentan, atorvastatin, immunosuppressants, salmeterol, fluticasone, PDE-5 inhibitors, TCAs, and esomeprazole. May decrease levels of telaprevir, boceprevir, lopinavir, raltegravir, methadone, ethinyl estradiol, or (w/ RTV) atazanavir, phenytoin, and paroxetine. May alter levels of warfarin; monitor INR. CYP3A4 inhibitors, indinavir, nelfinavir, and phenytoin (w/ RTV) may increase levels. CYP3A4 inducers (eg, rifampin), telaprevir, boceprevir, efavirenz, nevirapine, lopinavir/RTV, saquinavir, raltegravir, maraviroc, carbamazepine, phenobarbital, phenytoin, dexamethasone, H_2-receptor antagonists, and ethinyl estradiol/norethindrone may decrease levels. May require initiation or dose adjustments of insulin or oral hypoglycemics for treatment of DM. Refer to PI for dosing modifications when used w/ certain concomitant therapies.

NURSING CONSIDERATIONS

Assessment: Assess for hypersensitivity to the drug, sulfonamide allergy, hepatitis B or C, hepatic dysfunction, preexisting DM, hemophilia, lipid disorder, pregnancy/nursing status, and possible drug interactions. Obtain serum transaminase, TG, and cholesterol levels.

Monitoring: Monitor for signs/symptoms of skin reactions, hepatic toxicity, new onset or exacerbation of DM, hyperglycemia, diabetic ketoacidosis, immune reconstitution syndrome, autoimmune disorders, redistribution/accumulation of body fat, lipid elevations, nephrolithiasis, hemolytic anemia, and other adverse effects. In patients w/ hemophilia, monitor for spontaneous bleeding events. Monitor TG, cholesterol, and serum transaminase levels periodically.

Patient Counseling: Advise to report to physician the use of other prescription, OTC, or herbal products, particularly St. John's wort. Inform that use w/ PDE-5 inhibitors may increase risk of hypotension, visual changes, and priapism; instruct to contact physician if any of these symptoms occur. Advise that if taking oral contraceptives, an additional contraceptive measure should be used. Instruct to notify physician of any sulfonamide allergy. Inform that redistribution or accumulation of body fat may occur during therapy. Inform that therapy is not a cure for HIV-1 infection and that illnesses associated w/ HIV-1 infection may continue, including opportunistic infections. Advise to avoid doing things that can spread HIV-1 infection to others. Instruct not to breastfeed to prevent postnatal transmission. Advise not to alter the dose or d/c therapy w/o consulting physician. (Sus) Instruct to shake vigorously before each use and inform that refrigeration may improve the taste.

Storage: (Tab) 25°C (77°F); excursions permitted to 15-30°C (59-86°F). (Sus) 5-30°C (41-86°F). Do not freeze.

LIALDA – mesalamine RX

Class: 5-aminosalicylic acid derivative

ADULT DOSAGE

Ulcerative Colitis

Induction of Remission:
Active, Mild to Moderate: 2-4 tabs qd

Maint of Remission:
2 tabs qd

PEDIATRIC DOSAGE

Pediatric use may not have been established

DOSE MODIFICATION

Elderly

Start at lower end of dosing range

ADMINISTRATION

Oral route

Take w/ a meal
Swallow tab whole

HOW SUPPLIED

Tab, Delayed-Release: 1.2g

WARNINGS/PRECAUTIONS

Renal impairment, including minimal change nephropathy, acute/chronic interstitial nephritis, and, rarely, renal failure reported; evaluate renal function prior to therapy and periodically thereafter. Caution with known renal impairment or history of renal disease. Has been associated with an acute intolerance syndrome that may be difficult to distinguish from an exacerbation of ulcerative colitis (UC); observe closely for worsening of symptoms and d/c therapy if acute intolerance syndrome is suspected. Patients with sulfasalazine hypersensitivity may have similar reaction to therapy. Mesalamine-induced cardiac hypersensitivity reactions (eg, myocarditis, pericarditis) reported; caution with conditions that predispose to the development of myocarditis or pericarditis. Hepatic failure reported in patients with preexisting liver disease; caution with liver disease. Pyloric stenosis or other organic/functional obstruction in the upper GI tract may cause prolonged gastric retention of therapy, which could delay drug release in the colon. Caution with sulfasalazine hypersensitivity and in elderly. May interfere with lab tests.

ADVERSE REACTIONS

Headache, flatulence, UC, abnormal LFTs, abdominal pain.

DRUG INTERACTIONS

Nephrotoxic agents, including NSAIDs, may increase risk of renal reactions. Azathioprine or 6-mercaptopurine may increase risk for blood disorders.

NURSING CONSIDERATIONS

Assessment: Assess for hypersensitivity to the drug, salicylates/aminosalicylates, or sulfasalazine, conditions that predispose to the development of myocarditis or pericarditis, pyloric stenosis or other organic/functional upper GI tract obstruction, hepatic impairment, pregnancy/nursing status, and possible drug interactions. Evaluate renal function prior to initiation of therapy.

Monitoring: Monitor for acute intolerance syndrome, hypersensitivity reactions, hepatic failure, and other adverse reactions. Perform periodic monitoring of renal function. Monitor blood cell counts in elderly.

Patient Counseling: Instruct not to take drug if hypersensitive to salicylates (eg, aspirin) or other mesalamines. Inform to notify physician of all medications being taken and if pregnant, planning to become pregnant, or breastfeeding. Instruct to inform physician if allergic to sulfasalazine, if taking NSAIDs or other nephrotoxic agents, azathioprine, or 6-mercaptopurine, and if experiencing cramping, abdominal pain, bloody diarrhea, fever, headache, or rash. Inform to notify physician of history of myocarditis/pericarditis or stomach blockage, and if patient has kidney/liver disease.

Storage: 15-25°C (59-77°F); excursions permitted to 30°C (86°F).

LIBRAX – chlordiazepoxide hydrochloride/clidinium bromide RX

Class: Anticholinergic/benzodiazepine

ADULT DOSAGE

Acute Enterocolitis

Adjunctive Therapy:
Usual: 1-2 caps tid-qid ac and hs
Maint: 1-2 caps tid-qid ac and hs

Peptic Ulcer

Adjunctive Therapy:
Usual: 1-2 caps tid-qid ac and hs
Maint: 1-2 caps tid-qid ac and hs

Irritable Bowel Syndrome

Adjunctive Therapy:
Usual: 1-2 caps tid-qid ac and hs
Maint: 1-2 caps tid-qid ac and hs

PEDIATRIC DOSAGE

Pediatric use may not have been established

DOSE MODIFICATION

Elderly/Debilitated

Initial: Not more than 2 caps/day

Titrate: Increase gradually prn and as tolerated

ADMINISTRATION

Oral route

HOW SUPPLIED

Cap: (Chlordiazepoxide-Clidinium) 5mg-2.5mg

CONTRAINDICATIONS

Glaucoma, prostatic hypertrophy, benign bladder neck obstruction.

WARNINGS/PRECAUTIONS

Use lowest effective dose in debilitated patients. May impair mental/physical abilities. Caution with renal/hepatic impairment and in elderly. Chlordiazepoxide: Increased risk of congenital malformations during 1st trimester of pregnancy; avoid use. Paradoxical reactions (eg, excitement, stimulation, acute rage) reported in psychiatric patients. Caution in the treatment of anxiety states with evidence of impending depression; suicidal tendencies may be present. Avoid abrupt withdrawal after extended therapy; withdrawal symptoms reported following discontinuation. Clidinium: Inhibition of lactation may occur.

ADVERSE REACTIONS

Drowsiness, ataxia, confusion, skin eruptions, edema, extrapyramidal symptoms, dry mouth, nausea, constipation, altered libido, blood dyscrasias, jaundice, hepatic dysfunction, blurred vision, urinary hesitancy.

DRUG INTERACTIONS

Additive effects with alcohol and other CNS depressants. Coadministration with other psychotropic agents is not recommended; caution with MAOIs and phenothiazines. Constipation has occurred more often when coadministered with other spasmolytic agents. Chlordiazepoxide: Altered coagulation effects reported with oral anticoagulants.

NURSING CONSIDERATIONS

Assessment: Assess for glaucoma, prostatic hypertrophy, benign bladder neck obstruction, anxiety, renal/hepatic dysfunction, alcohol intake, history of drug abuse, drug hypersensitivity, pregnancy/nursing status, and possible drug interactions.

Monitoring: Monitor for ataxia, oversedation, drowsiness, confusion, and other adverse reactions. Monitor for paradoxical reactions (eg, excitement, stimulation, acute rage) in psychiatric patients. Periodic blood counts and LFTs are advisable when treatment is protracted. Monitor for signs of impending depression, or any suicidal tendencies.

Patient Counseling: Inform that psychological and physical dependence may develop, and advise to consult physician before increasing dose or discontinuing abruptly. Advise to observe caution when performing hazardous tasks (eg, operating machinery/driving). Advise to notify physician if pregnant/breastfeeding or planning to become pregnant. Inform of potential additive effects with alcohol and other CNS depressants.

Storage: 25°C (77°F); excursions permitted to 15-30°C (59-86°F).

LIDOCAINE VISCOUS – lidocaine hydrochloride RX

Class: Acetamide local anesthetic

ADULT DOSAGE

Topical Anesthetic

Symptomatic Treatment of Irritated/Inflamed Mucous Membranes of Mouth and Pharynx:

Usual: 15mL undiluted at intervals of ≥3 hrs

Max Single Dose: 4.5mg/kg or 300mg

Max Daily Dose: 8 doses/24 hrs

Also useful for reducing gagging during the taking of x-ray and dental impressions

PEDIATRIC DOSAGE

Topical Anesthetic

Symptomatic Treatment of Irritated/Inflamed Mucous Membranes of Mouth and Pharynx:

<3 Years:

Apply no more than 1.2mL to the immediate area

Wait at least 3 hrs before giving the next dose

Max: 4 doses/12 hrs

>3 Years:

Max: Determine by age and weight

Also useful for reducing gagging during the taking of x-ray and dental impressions

ADMINISTRATION
Oral/Topical route

Shake well before use
For use in the mouth, swish sol around in the mouth and spit out
For use in the pharynx, gargle sol and may spit/swallow

HOW SUPPLIED
Sol: 2% [20mL, 100mL]

WARNINGS/PRECAUTIONS
Excessive dosage or short intervals between doses may result in high plasma levels and serious adverse effects. Management of serious adverse reactions may require the use of resuscitative equipment, oxygen, and other resuscitative drugs. Use with extreme caution if mucosa in the area of application has been traumatized; risk of rapid systemic absorption. Safety and effectiveness depend on proper dosage, correct technique, adequate precautions, and readiness for emergencies. Cases of seizures, cardiopulmonary arrest, and death in patients <3 yrs of age reported when administered without strict adherence to the dosing and administration recommendations. Avoid in the setting of teething pain. For other conditions, use in patients <3 yrs of age should be limited to those situations where safer alternatives are not available or have been tried but failed. Repeated doses may cause significant increases in blood levels. Tolerance varies with the status of the patient. Caution in patients with severe shock or heart block and in patients with known drug sensitivities. Acidosis affects the CNS levels of lidocaine required to produce overt systemic effects.

ADVERSE REACTIONS
Lightheadedness, nervousness, confusion, euphoria, dizziness, drowsiness, blurred vision, tremors, convulsions, respiratory depression, bradycardia, hypotension, urticaria, edema, anaphylactoid reactions.

DRUG INTERACTIONS
CNS stimulants and depressants affect the CNS levels of lidocaine required to produce overt systemic effects.

NURSING CONSIDERATIONS

Assessment: Assess for hypersensitivity to local anesthetics of the amide type or to other components of the sol, traumatized mucosa in the area of application, acidosis, debilitation or acute illness, severe shock or heart block, known drug sensitivities, pregnancy/nursing status, and possible drug interactions.

Monitoring: Monitor for signs/symptoms of hypersensitivity reactions, seizures, cardiopulmonary arrest and other adverse reactions.

Patient Counseling: Instruct that for patients <3 yrs of age, special care must be given to accurately measure the prescribed dose and to not administer the product more often than prescribed. Instruct to use a measuring device to carefully measure the correct volume. Inform that the product should only be used for the prescribed indication. Instruct that the product container should be tightly closed and stored well out of reach of all children immediately after each use. Instruct that emergency medical attention should be sought immediately and no additional product should be administered if patient shows signs of systemic toxicity. Instruct that unused product should be discarded in a manner that prevents possible exposure to children and pets. Inform that therapy may impair swallowing and enhance danger of aspiration if used in the mouth or throat; instruct not to ingest food for 60 min following use in the mouth/throat area. Inform that numbness of tongue or buccal mucosa may increase the danger of biting trauma; do not to ingest food and/or chew gum while the mouth or throat area is anesthetized.

Storage: 20-25°C (68-77°F).

LIDODERM PATCH – lidocaine

RX

Class: Acetamide local anesthetic

ADULT DOSAGE

Postherpetic Neuralgia

Relief of Pain:
Apply to intact skin to cover the most painful area
Apply up to 3 patches, only once for up to 12 hrs w/in 24-hr period

PEDIATRIC DOSAGE
Pediatric use may not have been established

DOSE MODIFICATION

Concomitant Medications

Consider total amount absorbed from all formulations when used concomitantly w/ other local anesthetics

Adverse Reactions

Remove patch if irritation or burning occurs; may reapply when irritation subsides

Other Important Modifications

Debilitated/Impaired Elimination:

Treat smaller areas

ADMINISTRATION

Transdermal route

May cut patches into smaller sizes before removal of the release liner
Avoid contact with water (eg, bathing, swimming, or showering)
Wash hands after handling and avoid eye contact
Apply immediately after removal from protective envelope
May wear clothing over the area of application
Fold used patches and discard patches or pieces of patches

HOW SUPPLIED

Patch: 5% [30s]

WARNINGS/PRECAUTIONS

Serious adverse events may occur in children or pets if ingested; keep out of reach. Excessive dosing by applying to larger areas or for longer than the recommended wearing time may result in serious adverse effects. Increased risk of toxicity in patients with severe hepatic disease. Caution with history of drug sensitivities, smaller patients, and patients with impaired elimination. Avoid broken or inflamed skin, placement of external heat (eg, heating pads, electric blankets) and eye contact.

ADVERSE REACTIONS

Application-site reactions (eg, erythema, edema, bruising, papules, vesicles, discoloration, depigmentation, burning sensation, pruritus, dermatitis, petechia, blisters, exfoliation, abnormal sensation).

DRUG INTERACTIONS

Additive toxic effects with concomitant Class I antiarrhythmics (eg, tocainide, mexiletine); use caution. Consider total amount absorbed from all formulations containing other local anesthetics.

NURSING CONSIDERATIONS

Assessment: Assess for history of drug sensitivities to local anesthetics of the amide type and para-aminobenzoic acid derivatives, hepatic disease, pregnancy/nursing status, and for possible drug interactions.

Monitoring: Monitor for local skin reactions, allergic/anaphylactoid reactions, liver function, pain intensity, pain relief (periodically), and other adverse reactions.

Patient Counseling: Instruct to remove patch if irritation or burning sensation occurs during application and not to reapply until irritation subsides. If eye contact occurs, instruct to immediately wash with water or saline and protect eye until sensation returns. Counsel to avoid application to larger areas and for longer than recommended wearing time. Advise to avoid applying to broken or inflamed skin. Instruct to wash hands after handling patch and to fold used patches so adhesive side sticks to itself. Instruct to keep out of reach of children and pets.

Storage: Store at 25°C (77°F); excursions permitted to 15-30°C (59-86°F).

LINZESS – linaclotide RX

Class: Guanylate cyclase-C agonist

Contraindicated in pediatric patients up to 6 yrs of age. Avoid use in pediatric patients 6-17 yrs of age; safety and efficacy has not been established in pediatric patients <18 yrs of age.

ADULT DOSAGE

Irritable Bowel Syndrome with Constipation

290mcg qd

Chronic Idiopathic Constipation

145mcg qd

PEDIATRIC DOSAGE

Pediatric use may not have been established

ADMINISTRATION
Oral route

Take PO on an empty stomach, at least 30 min prior to 1st meal of the day
Swallow cap whole; do not break apart or chew

HOW SUPPLIED
Cap: 145mcg, 290mcg

CONTRAINDICATIONS
Pediatric patients <6 yrs of age, known or suspected mechanical GI obstruction.

WARNINGS/PRECAUTIONS
Diarrhea commonly reported; consider dose suspension and rehydration if severe diarrhea occurs.

ADVERSE REACTIONS
Diarrhea, abdominal pain, flatulence, abdominal distension, viral gastroenteritis, headache, URTI, sinusitis.

NURSING CONSIDERATIONS

Assessment: Assess for known or suspected mechanical GI obstruction and pregnancy/nursing status.

Monitoring: Monitor for diarrhea and other adverse reactions.

Patient Counseling: Advise to seek medical attention if experiencing unusual or severe abdominal pain and/or severe diarrhea, especially if in combination with hematochezia or melena; instruct to d/c treatment and contact physician if severe diarrhea occurs. Instruct to skip dose if the dose is missed, and take next dose at the regular time; advise not to take 2 doses at the same time.

Storage: 25°C (77°F); excursions permitted between 15-30°C (59-86°F). Keep caps in the original container. Do not subdivide or repackage. Protect from moisture. Do not remove desiccant from the container.

LIPITOR – atorvastatin calcium RX

Class: HMG-CoA reductase inhibitor

ADULT DOSAGE

Hyperlipidemia/Mixed Dyslipidemia

Initial: 10mg or 20mg qd (or 40mg qd for LDL reduction >45%)
Titrate: Adjust dose accordingly at 2- to 4-week intervals
Usual: 10-80mg qd

Homozygous Familial Hypercholesterolemia

10-80mg qd

Prevention of Cardiovascular Disease

Dose based on current clinical practice

PEDIATRIC DOSAGE

Heterozygous Familial Hypercholesterolemia

10-17 Years (Boys and Postmenarchal Girls):
Initial: 10mg/day
Titrate: Adjust dose at intervals of ≥4 weeks
Max: 20mg/day

DOSE MODIFICATION

Concomitant Medications

Lopinavir plus Ritonavir:
Use lowest dose necessary

Clarithromycin/Itraconazole/Fosamprenavir/Ritonavir plus Saquinavir, Darunavir, or Fosamprenavir:
Limit to 20mg/day; use lowest dose necessary

Nelfinavir or Boceprevir:
Limit to 40mg/day; use lowest dose necessary

ADMINISTRATION
Oral route

Take PO as a single dose at any time of the day, w/ or w/o food

HOW SUPPLIED
Tab: 10mg, 20mg, 40mg, 80mg

CONTRAINDICATIONS
Active liver disease, which may include unexplained persistent elevations in hepatic transaminases, women who are pregnant or may become pregnant, nursing mothers.

WARNINGS/PRECAUTIONS

Has not been studied in conditions where the major lipoprotein abnormality is elevation of chylomicrons (Fredrickson Types I and V). Rare cases of rhabdomyolysis with acute renal failure secondary to myoglobinuria reported. Increased risk of rhabdomyolysis with history of renal impairment; closely monitor for skeletal muscle effects. May cause myopathy (including immune-mediated necrotizing myopathy [IMNM]); d/c if markedly elevated CPK levels occur or if myopathy is diagnosed or suspected. Temporarily withhold or d/c if acute, serious condition suggestive of myopathy occurs or if with risk factor predisposing to development of renal failure secondary to rhabdomyolysis. Persistent increases in serum transaminases reported; obtain liver enzyme tests prior to initiation and repeat as clinically indicated. Fatal and nonfatal hepatic failure reported (rare); promptly interrupt therapy if serious liver injury with clinical symptoms and/or hyperbilirubinemia or jaundice occurs and do not restart if no alternate etiology found. Caution in patients who consume substantial quantities of alcohol and/or have history of liver disease. Increases in HbA1c and FPG levels reported. May blunt adrenal and/or gonadal steroid production. Increased risk of hemorrhagic stroke in patients with recent stroke or transient ischemic attack (TIA). Caution in elderly.

ADVERSE REACTIONS

Nasopharyngitis, arthralgia, diarrhea, diabetes, pain in extremity, UTI, dyspepsia, nausea, musculoskeletal pain, muscle spasms, myalgia, insomnia.

DRUG INTERACTIONS

Avoid with cyclosporine, telaprevir, gemfibrozil, or combination of tipranavir plus ritonavir. Caution with fibrates and drugs that decrease levels or activity of endogenous steroid hormones (eg, ketoconazole, spironolactone, cimetidine). Increased risk of myopathy with fibric acid derivatives, erythromycin, lipid-modifying doses of niacin, strong CYP3A4 inhibitors (eg, clarithromycin, HIV protease inhibitors), and azole antifungals; consider lower initial and maintenance doses. Strong CYP3A4 inhibitors (eg, clarithromycin, several combinations of HIV protease inhibitors, telaprevir, itraconazole) and grapefruit juice may increase levels. CYP3A4 inducers (eg, efavirenz, rifampin) may decrease levels; simultaneous coadministration with rifampin recommended. May increase digoxin levels; monitor appropriately. May increase area under the curve of norethindrone and ethinyl estradiol. Myopathy, including rhabdomyolysis, reported with colchicine; use with caution. OATP1B1 inhibitors (eg, cyclosporine) may increase bioavailability.

NURSING CONSIDERATIONS

Assessment: Assess for active or history of liver disease, unexplained and persistent elevations in serum transaminase levels, pregnancy/nursing status, history of renal impairment, risk factors predisposing to the development of renal failure secondary to rhabdomyolysis, alcohol intake, recent stroke or TIA, hypersensitivity to the drug, and possible drug interactions. Obtain baseline LFTs.

Monitoring: Monitor for signs/symptoms of rhabdomyolysis and myopathy (including IMNM). Monitor lipid profile and CPK levels. Perform LFTs as clinically indicated.

Patient Counseling: Advise to adhere to the National Cholesterol Education Program-recommended diet, a regular exercise program, and periodic testing of a fasting lipid panel. Inform of the substances that should not be taken concomitantly with the drug. Advise to inform other healthcare professionals that they are taking the drug. Inform of the risk of myopathy; instruct to report promptly any unexplained muscle pain, tenderness, or weakness, particularly if accompanied by malaise or fever or if these muscle signs or symptoms persist after discontinuation. Inform that liver function will be checked prior to initiation and if signs or symptoms of liver injury occur; instruct to report promptly any symptoms that may indicate liver injury. Instruct women of childbearing age to use effective method of birth control to prevent pregnancy. Advise to d/c therapy and contact physician if pregnancy occurs. Instruct not to use the drug if breastfeeding.

Storage: 20-25°C (68-77°F).

LIPOFEN – fenofibrate RX

Class: Fibric acid derivative

ADULT DOSAGE

Primary Hypercholesterolemia/Mixed Dyslipidemia

Usual/Max: 150mg qd

Titrate: May consider reducing dose if lipid levels fall significantly below the targeted range

D/C if no adequate response after 2 months of treatment with max dose

Severe Hypertriglyceridemia

Initial: 50-150mg/day

PEDIATRIC DOSAGE

Pediatric use may not have been established

Titrate: Adjust dose if necessary following repeat lipid determination at 4- to 8-week intervals; may consider reducing dose if lipid levels fall significantly below the targeted range
Max: 150mg qd

D/C if no adequate response after 2 months of treatment with max dose

DOSE MODIFICATION
Renal Impairment
Mild to Moderate:
Initial: 50mg/day
Titrate: Increase only after evaluation of the effects on renal function and lipid levels

ADMINISTRATION
Oral route

Take with meals
Swallow cap whole; do not open, crush, dissolve, or chew

HOW SUPPLIED
Cap: 50mg, 150mg

CONTRAINDICATIONS
Severe renal impairment (including dialysis), active liver disease (including primary biliary cirrhosis and unexplained persistent liver function abnormalities), preexisting gallbladder disease, nursing mothers.

WARNINGS/PRECAUTIONS
Not shown to reduce coronary heart disease morbidity and mortality in patients with type 2 diabetes mellitus. Increased risk of myopathy and rhabdomyolysis; increased risk with diabetes, renal insufficiency, hypothyroidism, and in elderly. D/C therapy if markedly elevated CPK levels occur or myopathy is diagnosed. Increases in serum transaminases, chronic active hepatocellular and cholestatic hepatitis, and cirrhosis (rare) reported; perform baseline and regular monitoring of LFTs, and d/c therapy if enzyme levels persist >3X the normal limit. Elevations in SrCr reported; monitor renal function in patients with renal impairment or at risk for renal insufficiency. May cause cholelithiasis; d/c if gallstones are found. Mild to moderate decreases in Hgb, Hct and WBCs, thrombocytopenia, and agranulocytosis reported; periodically monitor RBC and WBC counts during the first 12 months of therapy. Acute hypersensitivity reactions and pancreatitis reported. May cause venothromboembolic disease (eg, pulmonary embolus [PE], deep vein thrombosis [DVT]). Severe decreases in HDL levels reported; check HDL levels within the 1st few months after initiation of therapy. If a severely depressed HDL level is detected, withdraw therapy, monitor HDL level until it has returned to baseline, and do not reinitiate therapy. Estrogen therapy, thiazide diuretics and β-blockers may be associated with massive rises in plasma TGs; discontinuation of these drugs may obviate the need for specific drug therapy of hypertriglyceridemia.

ADVERSE REACTIONS
Abdominal pain, back pain, headache, abnormal LFTs, respiratory disorder, increased CPK/AST/ALT.

DRUG INTERACTIONS
Increased risk of rhabdomyolysis with HMG-CoA reductase inhibitors (statins); avoid combination unless benefits outweigh risks. May potentiate anticoagulant effects of coumarin anticoagulants; use with caution, adjust anticoagulant dose, and monitor PT/INR frequently. Immunosuppressants (eg, cyclosporine, tacrolimus) may impair renal function; use lowest effective dose and monitor renal function with immunosuppressants and other potentially nephrotoxic agents. Bile acid-binding resins may bind other drugs given concurrently; take at least 1 hr before or 4-6 hrs after the bile acid-binding resin. Cases of myopathy, including rhabdomyolysis, reported when coadministered with colchicine; caution when prescribing with colchicine. Changes in exposure/levels with atorvastatin, pravastatin, fluvastatin, glimepiride, metformin, and rosiglitazone.

NURSING CONSIDERATIONS

Assessment: Assess for renal impairment, active liver disease, preexisting gallbladder disease, other medical conditions (diabetes, hypothyroidism), hypersensitivity to the drug, pregnancy/nursing status, and possible drug interactions. Obtain baseline LFTs.

Monitoring: Monitor for signs/symptoms of myopathy or rhabdomyolysis; measure CPK levels in patients reporting such symptoms. Monitor for cholelithiasis, pancreatitis, hypersensitivity reactions, PE, and DVT. Monitor renal function, LFTs, CBC, and lipid levels. Monitor PT/INR frequently with coumarin anticoagulants.

Patient Counseling: Advise of the potential benefits and risks of therapy, and medications to be avoided during treatment. Instruct to continue to follow an appropriate lipid-modifying diet during therapy, and to take drug ud. Instruct to inform physician of all medications, supplements, and herbal preparations being taken, any changes in medical condition, development of muscle pain, tenderness, or weakness, onset of abdominal pain, or any other new symptoms. Advise to return to the physician's office for routine monitoring.

Storage: 15-30°C (59-86°F). Protect from moisture and light.

LIPTRUZET – atorvastatin/ezetimibe RX

Class: Cholesterol absorption inhibitor/HMG-CoA reductase inhibitor

ADULT DOSAGE

Primary Hyperlipidemia/Mixed Hyperlipidemia

Initial: 10mg-10mg/day or 10mg-20mg/day as a single dose at any time of the day
Usual: 10mg-10mg to 10mg-80mg qd
Titrate: After initiation or titration, analyze lipid levels after ≥2 weeks and adjust dose, if needed

Patients Requiring Larger LDL Reduction (>55%):
Initial: 10mg-40mg/day

Homozygous Familial Hypercholesterolemia

10mg-40mg/day or 10mg-80mg/day

PEDIATRIC DOSAGE

Pediatric use may not have been established

DOSE MODIFICATION
Concomitant Medications
Bile Acid Sequestrants: Take either ≥2 hrs before or ≥4 hrs after bile acid sequestrant

Cyclosporine, Tipranavir Plus Ritonavir, Telaprevir, Gemfibrozil: Avoid therapy w/ Liptruzet

Lopinavir Plus Ritonavir: Use caution; use lowest dose of Liptruzet necessary

Clarithromycin, Itraconazole, Saquinavir Plus Ritonavir, Darunavir Plus Ritonavir, Fosamprenavir, Fosamprenavir Plus Ritonavir:
Max: 10mg-20mg/day

Nelfinavir, Boceprevir:
Max: 10mg-40mg/day

ADMINISTRATION
Oral route

Take w/ or w/o food
Swallow tab whole; do not crush, dissolve, or chew

HOW SUPPLIED
Tab: (Ezetimibe-Atorvastatin) 10mg-10mg, 10mg-20mg, 10mg-40mg, 10mg-80mg

CONTRAINDICATIONS
Active liver disease or unexplained persistent elevations in hepatic transaminase levels, women who are or may become pregnant, nursing mothers.

WARNINGS/PRECAUTIONS
Has not been studied in Fredrickson type I, III, IV, and V dyslipidemias. Myopathy (including immune-mediated necrotizing myopathy [IMNM]) and rhabdomyolysis reported; d/c if markedly elevated CPK levels occur or myopathy is diagnosed or suspected. Temporarily withhold or d/c therapy in any patient with an acute, serious condition suggestive of a myopathy or having a risk factor predisposing to development of renal failure secondary to rhabdomyolysis (eg, severe acute infection, hypotension, major surgery, trauma, severe metabolic/endocrine/electrolyte disorders, uncontrolled seizures). Liver enzyme elevations and fatal and nonfatal hepatic failure reported; obtain LFTs prior to initiating therapy and repeat as clinically indicated; promptly interrupt therapy if serious liver injury and/or hyperbilirubinemia or jaundice occurs and do not restart if no alternative etiology found. Caution in patients who consume substantial quantities of alcohol and/or have a history of liver disease. Increases in HbA1c and FPG levels reported. May blunt adrenal and/or gonadal steroid production. Increased risk of hemorrhagic stroke in patients with recent stroke or transient ischemic attack (TIA). Caution in elderly.

ADVERSE REACTIONS
Increased ALT/AST, musculoskeletal pain, abdominal pain, nausea, arthralgia.

DRUG INTERACTIONS
Avoid with gemfibrozil, cyclosporine, tipranavir plus ritonavir, and telaprevir. Caution with lopinavir plus ritonavir; use lowest dose necessary. Caution with drugs that decrease levels or activity of

endogenous steroid hormones (eg, ketoconazole, spironolactone, cimetidine). Increased risk of myopathy with fibric acid derivatives, erythromycin, lipid-modifying doses of niacin, strong CYP3A4 inhibitors (eg, clarithromycin, HIV protease inhibitors), and azole antifungals; consider lower initial and maint doses. Monitor INR levels when used with warfarin. Atorvastatin: Strong CYP3A4 inhibitors, grapefruit juice, saquinavir plus ritonavir, diltiazem, and amlodipine may increase levels. Itraconazole may increase area under the curve (AUC). Myopathy, including rhabdomyolysis, reported with colchicine; use with caution. OATP1B1 inhibitors may increase bioavailability. May increase levels of digoxin; monitor appropriately. May increase AUC of norethindrone and ethinyl estradiol. CYP3A4 inducers (eg, efavirenz, rifampin) may decrease levels; simultaneous coadministration with rifampin is recommended. Ezetimibe: Cholestyramine may decrease levels.

NURSING CONSIDERATIONS

Assessment: Assess for history of or active liver disease, unexplained persistent elevations in hepatic transaminases, risk factors for developing myopathy (eg, advanced age, hypothyroidism, renal impairment), recent stroke or TIA, hypersensitivity to the drug, pregnancy/nursing status, and possible drug interactions. Assess use in patients who consume substantial quantities of alcohol. Obtain baseline lipid profile (total-C, LDL, HDL, TGs) and LFTs (eg, AST, ALT).

Monitoring: Monitor for signs/symptoms of myopathy, rhabdomyolysis, liver dysfunction, and other adverse reactions. Analyze lipid levels within 2 or more weeks after initiation and/or upon titration. Monitor LFTs as clinically indicated, and for increases in HbA1c and FPG levels.

Patient Counseling: Advise to adhere to the National Cholesterol Education Program recommended diet, a regular exercise program, and periodic testing of a fasting lipid panel. Counsel about risk of myopathy and inform that consuming large quantities (>1L) of grapefruit juice may increase this risk. Advise to discuss with physician all medications, both prescription and OTC, currently taking. Instruct to report to physician any unexplained muscle pain, tenderness, or weakness, particularly if accompanied by malaise or fever, or if signs/symptoms persist after discontinuing therapy. Advise to report promptly any signs of liver injury, including fatigue, anorexia, right upper abdominal discomfort, dark urine, or jaundice. Counsel women of childbearing age to use an effective method of birth control while using the drug and to discuss future pregnancy plans; instruct to d/c therapy and contact physician if pregnancy occurs. Advise not to breastfeed during treatment.

Storage: 20-25°C (68-77°F); excursions permitted to 15-30°C (59-86°F). Store in foil pouch until use. Protect from moisture and light and store in a dry place after the foil pouch is opened. Once a tab is removed, slide blister card back into case. Discard any unused tab 30 days after pouch is opened.

LITHIUM 450MG ER TABLETS – lithium carbonate RX

Class: Antimanic agent

Lithium toxicity is closely related to serum levels, and can occur at doses close to therapeutic levels. Facilities for prompt and accurate serum lithium determinations should be available before initiating therapy.

ADULT DOSAGE

Manic-Depressive Illness

Individualize dose according to serum levels and clinical response

Acute Mania:
Usual/Maint: 1800mg/day in divided doses to achieve desired serum levels of 1-1.5mEq/L
Monitor serum levels 2X/week, and until serum level and clinical condition have been stabilized

Long-Term Control:
Usual: 900-1200mg/day in divided doses to maintain desirable serum levels of 0.6-1.2mEq/L
Monitor serum lithium levels in uncomplicated cases at least every 2 months

Patients unusually sensitive to lithium may exhibit toxic signs at serum levels <1mEq/L

Conversions

Switching from Immediate-Release (IR) Caps to Extended-Release (ER) Tabs:
Give the same total daily dose when possible
When previous dosage of IR lithium is not a

PEDIATRIC DOSAGE

Manic-Depressive Illness

≥12 Years:
Individualize dose according to serum levels and clinical response

Acute Mania:
Usual/Maint: 1800mg/day in divided doses to achieve desired serum levels of 1-1.5mEq/L

Monitor serum levels 2X/week, and until serum level and clinical condition have been stabilized

Long-Term Control:
Usual: 900-1200mg/day in divided doses to maintain desirable serum levels of 0.6-1.2mEq/L

Monitor serum lithium levels in uncomplicated cases at least every 2 months

Patients unusually sensitive to lithium may exhibit toxic signs at serum levels <1mEq/L

Conversions

Switching from Immediate-Release (IR) Caps to Extended-Release (ER) Tabs:

multiple of 450mg (eg, 1500mg), initiate ER tab at the multiple of 450mg nearest to, but below, the original daily dose (eg, 1350mg)
When the 2 doses are unequal, give larger dose in pm (eg, 1350mg/day [450mg am and 900mg pm]); if desired, give total daily dose tid (eg, 1350mg/day [450mg tid])

Monitor at 1- to 2-week intervals and adjust dose if necessary, until stable and satisfactory serum levels and clinical state achieved

When closer titration is required than that available w/ doses of ER tabs in increments of 450mg, use IR caps
Most patients on maint therapy are stabilized on 900mg daily (eg, 450mg bid ER tab)

Give the same total daily dose when possible

When previous dosage of IR lithium is not a multiple of 450mg (eg, 1500mg), initiate ER tab at the multiple of 450mg nearest to, but below, the original daily dose (eg, 1350mg)

When the 2 doses are unequal, give larger dose in pm (eg, 1350mg/day [450mg am and 900mg pm]); if desired, give total daily dose tid (eg, 1350mg/day [450mg tid])

Monitor at 1- to 2-week intervals and adjust dose if necessary, until stable and satisfactory serum levels and clinical state achieved

When closer titration is required than that available w/ doses of ER tabs in increments of 450mg, use IR caps

Most patients on maint therapy are stabilized on 900mg daily (eg, 450mg bid ER tab)

DOSE MODIFICATION

Elderly

May require lower dosages to achieve therapeutic serum levels

ADMINISTRATION

Oral route

Doses are usually given bid (approx 12-hr intervals)

HOW SUPPLIED

Tab, Extended-Release: 450mg* *scored

WARNINGS/PRECAUTIONS

Avoid w/ significant renal or cardiovascular disease (CVD), severe debilitation/dehydration, or Na^+ depletion. Use extreme caution if psychiatric indication is life-threatening, and if such patient fails to respond to other measures. May be associated w/ the unmasking of Brugada syndrome; avoid w/ known or suspected Brugada syndrome. Chronic therapy may be associated w/ diminution of renal concentrating ability; carefully manage to avoid dehydration w/ resulting lithium retention and toxicity. Morphologic changes w/ glomerular and interstitial fibrosis and nephron atrophy reported. Assess kidney function prior to and during therapy. May decrease Na+ reabsorption, which could lead to Na+ depletion; maintain normal diet, including salt, and an adequate fluid intake at least during the initial stabilization period. Decreased tolerance reported to ensue from protracted sweating or diarrhea; if this occurs, administer supplemental fluid and salt. Temporarily reduce dose or d/c therapy w/ sweating, diarrhea, or concomitant infection w/ elevated temperature. Caution w/ thyroid disorders; monitor thyroid function. May impair mental/physical abilities.

ADVERSE REACTIONS

Fine hand tremor, polyuria, mild thirst, general discomfort, diarrhea, N/V, drowsiness, lithium toxicity, blackout spells, ataxia, dry mouth, alopecia, oliguria, albuminuria.

DRUG INTERACTIONS

Encephalopathic syndrome (eg, weakness, lethargy, fever) followed by irreversible brain damage w/ neuroleptics reported; monitor for evidence of neurological toxicity and d/c therapy if such signs appear. May prolong effects of neuromuscular blockers; use w/ caution. Caution w/ diuretics; monitor lithium levels and adjust lithium dose if necessary. Caution w/ calcium channel blockers; may increase risk of neurotoxicity. Increased levels w/ indomethacin, piroxicam, and other NSAIDs (eg, selective COX-2 inhibitors); monitor levels closely when initiating or discontinuing NSAID use. Acetazolamide, urea, xanthine preparations, and alkalinizing agents (eg, sodium bicarbonate) may decrease levels. May provoke lithium toxicity w/ metronidazole; monitor closely. Risk of lithium toxicity w/ ACE inhibitors (eg, enalapril, captopril) and angiotensin II receptor antagonists (eg, losartan); may need to reduce lithium dose and monitor lithium levels more often. Caution w/ SSRIs. May interact w/ methyldopa, phenytoin, and carbamazepine.

NURSING CONSIDERATIONS

Assessment: Assess for CVD, severe debilitation, dehydration, Na^+ depletion, life-threatening psychiatric indication, thyroid disorders, Brugada syndrome or risk factors, pregnancy/nursing status, and for possible drug interactions. Assess baseline renal function (eg, tubular function, glomerular function).

Monitoring: Monitor for diminution of renal concentrating ability (eg, nephrogenic diabetes insipidus), glomerular and interstitial fibrosis, nephron atrophy, decreased tolerance to therapy, decreased Na^+ reabsorption, signs of lithium toxicity, and other adverse reactions. Monitor for renal or thyroid function. Monitor patient's clinical state and serum lithium levels regularly.

Patient Counseling: Inform of the risks and benefits of therapy. Counsel about clinical signs of lithium toxicity (eg, diarrhea, vomiting, tremor); advise to d/c therapy and notify physician if any of these signs occur. Advise to seek immediate emergency assistance if fainting, lightheadedness, abnormal heartbeats, SOB, or other adverse reactions develop. Advise to use caution w/ activities requiring alertness.

Storage: 25°C (77°F); excursions permitted to 15-30°C (59-86°F).

LIVALO – pitavastatin RX

Class: HMG-CoA reductase inhibitor

ADULT DOSAGE

Primary Hypercholesterolemia/Mixed Dyslipidemia

Initial: 2mg qd
Usual: 1-4mg qd
Max: 4mg qd

After initiation or upon titration, analyze lipid levels after 4 weeks and adjust dose accordingly

PEDIATRIC DOSAGE

Pediatric use may not have been established

DOSE MODIFICATION

Concomitant Medications

Erythromycin:
Max: 1mg qd

Rifampin:
Max: 2mg qd

Renal Impairment

Moderate/Severe (GFR 30-59mL/min/1.73m^2 and GFR 15-29mL/min/1.73m^2 Not Receiving Hemodialysis, Respectively)/ESRD Receiving Hemodialysis:
Initial: 1mg qd
Max: 2mg qd

ADMINISTRATION

Oral route

Take PO at any time of the day w/ or w/o food

HOW SUPPLIED

Tab: 1mg, 2mg, 4mg

CONTRAINDICATIONS

Active liver disease, including unexplained persistent elevations of hepatic transaminase levels, women who are pregnant or may become pregnant, nursing mothers, and coadministration with cyclosporine.

WARNINGS/PRECAUTIONS

Increased risk for severe myopathy with doses >4mg qd. Myopathy (including immune-mediated necrotizing myopathy [IMNM]) and rhabdomyolysis with acute renal failure secondary to myoglobinuria reported. Caution with predisposing factors for myopathy (eg, advanced age [≥65 yrs], renal impairment, and inadequately treated hypothyroidism). D/C if markedly elevated creatine kinase (CK) levels occur or myopathy is diagnosed/suspected and temporarily withhold in any patient experiencing an acute or serious condition suggestive of myopathy or predisposing to the development of renal failure secondary to rhabdomyolysis (eg, sepsis, hypotension, dehydration). Increases in serum transaminases (eg, AST, ALT) reported; perform LFTs before the initiation of treatment and if signs or symptoms of liver injury occur. Fatal and nonfatal hepatic failure reported (rare); promptly interrupt therapy if serious liver injury with clinical symptoms and/or hyperbilirubinemia or jaundice occurs; do not restart if no alternative etiology found. Increases in HbA1c and fasting serum glucose levels reported. Caution with substantial alcohol consumption.

ADVERSE REACTIONS

Back pain, constipation, myalgia.

DRUG INTERACTIONS

See Contraindications. Erythromycin and rifampin may increase exposure. Due to an increased risk of myopathy/rhabdomyolysis, avoid coadministration with gemfibrozil and use caution when coadministered with fibrates and colchicine. May enhance risk of skeletal muscle effects with niacin; consider dose reduction with lipid-modifying doses of niacin. Monitor PT and INR with warfarin.

NURSING CONSIDERATIONS

Assessment: Assess for hepatic/renal impairment, inadequately treated hypothyroidism, substantial alcohol consumption, pregnancy/nursing status, possible drug interactions, and other conditions where treatment is cautioned/contraindicated. Obtain baseline lipid profile.

Monitoring: Monitor signs/symptoms of myopathy, rhabdomyolysis, IMNM, acute renal failure, hypersensitivity reactions, and other adverse reactions. Monitor for increases in HbA1c and fasting serum glucose levels. Perform periodic monitoring of lipid profile and CK levels. Analyze lipid levels 4 weeks after initiation/titration. Perform LFTs with signs or symptoms of liver injury. Monitor PT and INR when using warfarin.

Patient Counseling: Advise to promptly notify physician of any unexplained muscle pain, tenderness, or weakness, particularly if accompanied by malaise or fever, or if these muscle signs/symptoms persist after discontinuing treatment. Advise to discuss all medications, both prescription and OTC, with physician. Counsel women of childbearing age to use effective method of birth control to prevent pregnancy during therapy. Instruct pregnant or breastfeeding women to d/c therapy and consult physician. Inform that liver enzymes will be checked before therapy and if signs/symptoms of liver injury occur (eg, fatigue, anorexia, right upper abdominal discomfort, dark urine, or jaundice). Advise to report promptly any symptoms that may indicate liver injury.

Storage: 15-30°C (59-86°F). Protect from light.

LOESTRIN FE – ethinyl estradiol/ferrous fumarate/norethindrone acetate RX

Class: Estrogen/progestogen combination

Cigarette smoking increases the risk of serious cardiovascular (CV) side effects. Risk increases with age and with heavy smoking (≥15 cigarettes/day) and is quite marked in women >35 yrs of age. Women who use oral contraceptives should be strongly advised not to smoke.

OTHER BRAND NAMES

Loestrin Fe 1/20, Loestrin Fe 1.5/30, Gildess Fe 1/20, Gildess Fe 1.5/30, Junel Fe 1/20, Junel Fe 1.5/30, Microgestin Fe 1/20, Microgestin Fe 1.5/30

ADULT DOSAGE

Contraception

1 tab qd for 28 days, then repeat

Start 1st Sunday after menses begins or 1st day of menses

Missed Dose

Miss 1 Active Tab: Take as soon as remembered; take next tab at regular time

Miss 2 Consecutive Active Tabs in Week 1 or 2: Take 2 tabs as soon as remembered and 2 tabs the next day; use another birth control method for 7 days following missed tabs

Miss 2 Consecutive Active Tabs in Week 3 or Miss ≥3 Consecutive Active Tabs: (Sunday Start) Take 1 tab qd until Sunday, then discard remaining tabs and start a new pack immediately on Sunday. (Day 1 Start) Discard remaining tabs and start new pack that same day. (Sunday/Day 1 Start) Use another birth control method for 7 days following missed tabs

Miss Any Inactive Tabs in Week 4: Discard missed tabs and take 1 tab qd until pack is empty; no backup birth control method is needed. A new pack of tabs should be started no later than the 8th day after the last active tab was taken

PEDIATRIC DOSAGE

Contraception

Not indicated for use premenarche; refer to adult dosing

ADMINISTRATION

Oral route

Take regularly with a meal or hs

Take exactly ud and at intervals not exceeding 24 hrs

Use an additional method of protection until after the 1st week of administration in the initial cycle when utilizing the Sunday Start regimen

HOW SUPPLIED

Tab: (Norethindrone-Ethinyl Estradiol [EE]) (1/20) 1mg-20mcg, (1.5/30) 1.5mg-30mcg; Tab: (Ferrous Fumarate) 75mg

CONTRAINDICATIONS

Thrombophlebitis, thromboembolic disorders, past history of deep vein thrombophlebitis or thromboembolic disorders, cerebral vascular or coronary artery disease, known or suspected carcinoma of the breast, carcinoma of the endometrium or other known or suspected estrogen-dependent neoplasia, undiagnosed abnormal genital bleeding, cholestatic jaundice of pregnancy or jaundice with prior pill use, hepatic adenomas or carcinomas, known or suspected pregnancy.

WARNINGS/PRECAUTIONS

When initiating a Sunday Start regimen, use another method of contraception until after the first 7 consecutive days of administration. Increased risk of myocardial infarction (MI), thromboembolism, stroke, hepatic neoplasia, gallbladder disease, and vascular disease. Increased risk of morbidity and mortality if other risk factors (eg, HTN, hyperlipidemias, obesity, diabetes) are present. If feasible, d/c at least 4 weeks prior to and for 2 weeks after elective surgery with an increased risk of thromboembolism and during and following prolonged immobilization. Start use no earlier than 4-6 weeks after delivery in women who elect not to breastfeed. Retinal thrombosis reported; d/c if unexplained partial or complete loss of vision occurs, or if onset of proptosis or diplopia, papilledema, or retinal vascular lesions develop. Should not be used to induce withdrawal bleeding as a test for pregnancy, or to treat threatened or habitual abortion during pregnancy. Rule out pregnancy if 2 consecutive periods are missed. May cause glucose intolerance; monitor prediabetic and diabetic patients. May elevate serum TG and LDL levels and may render the control of hyperlipidemias more difficult. May elevate BP; monitor closely and d/c use if significant BP elevation occurs. D/C and evaluate the cause if new onset/exacerbation of migraine, or recurrent, persistent, severe headache develops. Breakthrough bleeding and spotting reported; rule out malignancy or pregnancy. Post-pill amenorrhea or oligomenorrhea may occur. D/C if jaundice develops. May cause fluid retention. Monitor closely in patients with history of depression; d/c if depression recurs to serious degree. Contact lens wearers who develop visual changes or changes in lens tolerance should be assessed by an ophthalmologist. May affect certain endocrine function tests, LFTs, and blood components in lab tests.

ADVERSE REACTIONS

N/V, GI symptoms, breakthrough bleeding, spotting, amenorrhea, migraine, mental depression, vaginal candidiasis, edema, weight changes, menstrual flow changes, melasma, breast changes, changes in cervical erosion and secretion, rash (allergic).

DRUG INTERACTIONS

Reduced effects, increased breakthrough bleeding, and menstrual irregularities reported with rifampin and phenylbutazone. Increased metabolism and possibly reduced contraceptive effectiveness with anticonvulsants (eg, phenobarbital, phenytoin, carbamazepine). Reduced plasma levels with troglitazone, resulting in possible reduced contraceptive effectiveness. Pregnancy reported with antimicrobials (eg, ampicillin, griseofulvin, tetracycline). Atorvastatin may increase norethindrone and EE exposure. Ascorbic acid and acetaminophen (APAP) may increase EE levels. Increased plasma levels of cyclosporine, prednisolone, and theophylline reported. Decreased levels of APAP and increased clearance of temazepam, salicylic acid, morphine, and clofibric acid reported with concomitant use.

NURSING CONSIDERATIONS

Assessment: Assess for hypersensitivity to drug, thrombophlebitis or thromboembolic disorders, HTN, hyperlipidemia, diabetes, breast cancer, endometrial cancer or other estrogen-dependent neoplasia, undiagnosed abnormal genital bleeding, cholestatic jaundice of pregnancy or jaundice with prior pill use, pregnancy/nursing status, and for any other conditions where treatment is contraindicated/cautioned. Assess for possible drug interactions.

Monitoring: Monitor for MI, thromboembolism, stroke, hepatic neoplasia, and other adverse reactions. Monitor BP with history of HTN, serum glucose levels in diabetic or prediabetic patients, lipid levels with hyperlipidemia, and for signs of worsening depression with previous history. Monitor liver function. Refer patients with contact lenses to an ophthalmologist if visual changes or changes in lens tolerance occur. Monitor women who have breast nodules or a strong family history of breast cancer. Perform annual history and physical exam.

Patient Counseling: Counsel about potential adverse effects. Inform that drug does not protect against HIV infection (AIDS) and other sexually transmitted diseases. Counsel that cigarette smoking increases the risk of serious CV effects and that women who use oral contraceptives should not smoke. Instruct to take exactly ud and at intervals not exceeding 24 hrs. Instruct on what to do if pills are missed. Instruct to use additional method of protection until after the 1st week of administration in the initial cycle when utilizing the Sunday Start Regimen. Inform that spotting or breakthrough bleeding may occur; advise not to d/c medication and instruct to notify physician if symptoms persist. Instruct to d/c if pregnancy is confirmed/suspected during treatment. If scheduled for any lab test, advise to inform physician of use of birth control pills. Instruct to notify physician if breastfeeding. Inform that certain drugs may make therapy less effective and that additional contraception may be needed.

Storage: 20-25°C (68-77°F).

LOFIBRA — fenofibrate **RX**

Class: Fibric acid derivative

ADULT DOSAGE

Primary Hypercholesterolemia/Mixed Dyslipidemia

Cap:
Initial/Max: 200mg/day

Tab:
Initial/Max: 160mg qd

Severe Hypertriglyceridemia

Cap:
Initial: 67-200mg/day
Titrate: Adjust dose if necessary following repeat lipid determinations at 4- to 8-week intervals; consider reducing dose if lipid levels fall significantly below targeted range
Max: 200mg/day

Tab:
Initial: 54-160mg/day
Titrate: Adjust dose if necessary following repeat lipid determinations at 4- to 8-week intervals; consider reducing dose if lipid levels fall significantly below targeted range
Max: 160mg qd

PEDIATRIC DOSAGE

Pediatric use may not have been established

DOSE MODIFICATION

Renal Impairment

Mild to Moderate:
Cap:
Initial: 67mg/day
Titrate: Increase only after evaluation of effects on renal function and lipid levels
Tab:
Initial: 54mg/day
Titrate: Increase only after evaluation of effects on renal function and lipid levels

Elderly

Cap:
Initial: 67mg/day

Cap, Tab:
Dose based on renal function

Discontinuation

D/C if no adequate response after 2 months of treatment w/ max dose

ADMINISTRATION

Oral route

Cap:
Give w/ meals

Tab:
May be given w/o regard to meals

HOW SUPPLIED

Cap: 67mg, 134mg, 200mg; Tab: 54mg, 160mg

CONTRAINDICATIONS

Hepatic or severe renal dysfunction (including primary biliary cirrhosis and unexplained persistent liver function abnormalities), preexisting gallbladder disease. (Tab) Severe renal impairment (including dialysis), active liver disease, nursing mothers.

WARNINGS/PRECAUTIONS

Increased risk of myopathy and rhabdomyolysis; risk increased with diabetes, renal insufficiency, hypothyroidism, and in elderly. D/C if marked CPK elevations occur or myopathy/myositis is suspected or diagnosed. Increases in serum transaminases; hepatocellular, chronic active, and cholestatic hepatitis, and cirrhosis (rare) reported; d/c therapy if enzyme levels persist >3X the normal limit. Elevations in SrCr reported; monitor renal function in patients with renal impairment or at risk for renal insufficiency. May cause cholelithiasis; d/c if gallstones are found. Acute hypersensitivity reactions and pancreatitis reported. Mild to moderate decreases in Hgb, Hct, and WBCs, thrombocytopenia, and agranulocytosis reported. May cause venothromboembolic disease (eg, pulmonary embolus [PE], DVT). Estrogen therapy, thiazide diuretics, and β-blockers may be associated with massive rises in plasma TGs; discontinuation of these drugs may obviate the need for specific drug therapy of hypertriglyceridemia. (Tab) Not shown to reduce coronary heart disease morbidity and mortality in patients with type 2 diabetes mellitus. Severe decreases in HDL levels reported; check HDL levels within the 1st few months after initiation of therapy. If a severely depressed HDL level is detected, withdraw therapy, monitor HDL level until it has returned to baseline, and do not reinitiate therapy.

ADVERSE REACTIONS

Abnormal LFTs, abdominal pain, respiratory disorder, back pain, increased ALT/AST/CPK, headache.

DRUG INTERACTIONS

May potentiate anticoagulant effects of coumarin anticoagulants; use with caution, reduce anticoagulant dosage, and monitor PT/INR frequently. Immunosuppressants (eg, cyclosporine, tacrolimus) may produce nephrotoxicity; consider benefits and risks, use lowest effective dose, and monitor renal function with immunosuppressants and other potentially nephrotoxic agents. Bile-acid-binding resins may bind other drugs given concurrently; take at least 1 hr before or 4-6 hrs after the bile-acid-binding resin. Cases of myopathy, including rhabdomyolysis, reported when coadministered with colchicine; caution when prescribing with colchicine. (Cap) Increased risk of rhabdomyolysis with HMG-CoA reductase inhibitors (statins); avoid combination unless benefit outweighs risk.

NURSING CONSIDERATIONS

Assessment: Assess for renal impairment, active liver disease, gallbladder disease, other medical conditions (eg, diabetes, hypothyroidism), hypersensitivity to the drug, pregnancy/nursing status, and possible drug interactions. Obtain baseline LFTs.

Monitoring: Monitor for myopathy, myositis, or rhabdomyolysis; measure CPK levels in patients reporting such symptoms. Monitor for cholelithiasis, pancreatitis, hypersensitivity reactions, PE, DVT, and other adverse reactions. Monitor renal function, LFTs, and lipid levels periodically. Perform periodic monitoring of RBC and WBC counts during the first 12 months of administration.

Patient Counseling: Advise of potential benefits and risks of therapy, and of medications to avoid during treatment. Instruct to follow appropriate lipid-modifying diet during therapy, and to take drug ud. Instruct to inform physician of all medications, supplements, and herbal preparations being taken, any changes in medical condition, development of muscle pain, tenderness, or weakness, and onset of abdominal pain or any other new symptoms. Advise to return for routine monitoring.

Storage: 20-25°C (68-77°F). Protect from moisture.

LOMOTIL — atropine sulfate/diphenoxylate hydrochloride CV

Class: Anticholinergic/opioid

ADULT DOSAGE

Diarrhea

Adjunctive Therapy:

Initial: 2 tabs or 10mL qid

Titrate: Reduce dose after symptoms are controlled

Maint: 2 tabs or 10mL qd

Max: 20mg/day diphenoxylate

D/C if symptoms not controlled after 10 days at max dose of 20mg/day (diphenoxylate)

PEDIATRIC DOSAGE

Diarrhea

Adjunctive Therapy:

2-12 Years:

Initial: 0.3-0.4mg/kg/day of sol in four divided doses

Titrate: Reduce dose after symptoms are controlled

Maint: May be as low as 25% of initial dose

D/C if no improvement w/in 48 hrs

ADMINISTRATION
Oral route

Plastic dropper should be used when measuring liquid for administration to children

HOW SUPPLIED
(Diphenoxylate-Atropine) Sol: 2.5mg-0.025mg/5mL [60mL]; Tab: 2.5mg-0.025mg

CONTRAINDICATIONS
Obstructive jaundice, diarrhea associated with pseudomembranous enterocolitis or enterotoxin-producing bacteria.

WARNINGS/PRECAUTIONS
Avoid in children <2 yrs. Overdosage may result in severe respiratory depression and coma, leading to brain damage or death. Avoid use with severe dehydration or electrolyte imbalance until corrective therapy is initiated. May induce toxic megacolon with acute ulcerative colitis; d/c if abdominal distention occurs or untoward symptoms develop. May cause intestinal fluid retention. Avoid with diarrhea associated with organisms that penetrate the intestinal mucosa, and with pseudomembranous enterocolitis. Extreme caution with advanced hepatorenal disease and liver dysfunction. Caution in pediatrics, especially with Down's syndrome.

ADVERSE REACTIONS
Numbness of extremities, dizziness, anaphylaxis, drowsiness, toxic megacolon, N/V, urticaria, pruritus, anorexia, pancreatitis, paralytic ileus, euphoria, malaise/lethargy.

DRUG INTERACTIONS
MAOIs may precipitate hypertensive crisis. (Diphenoxylate) May potentiate barbiturates, tranquilizers, and alcohol. Potential to prolong $T_{1/2}$ of drugs for which the rate of elimination is dependent on the microsomal drug metabolizing enzyme system.

NURSING CONSIDERATIONS

Assessment: Assess for hypersensitivity, obstructive jaundice, diarrhea associated with pseudomembranous enterocolitis or enterotoxin-producing bacteria, severe dehydration, electrolyte imbalance, hepatic dysfunction, hepatorenal disease, ulcerative colitis, Down's syndrome, diarrhea (caused by *Escherichia coli*, *Salmonella*, *Shigella*), pregnancy/nursing status, and possible drug interactions.

Monitoring: Monitor for severe dehydration, electrolyte imbalance, renal function, toxic megacolon in ulcerative colitis, abdominal distention, signs of atropinism, and other adverse reactions.

Patient Counseling: Instruct to take ud and not to exceed the recommended dosage. Inform of consequences of overdosage, including severe respiratory depression and coma, possibly leading to permanent brain damage or death. Instruct to exercise caution while operating machinery/driving. Advise to avoid alcohol and other CNS depressants. Advise to keep medicines out of reach of children. Inform patient that drowsiness or dizziness may occur.

Storage: Dispense liquids in original container.

Lopid – gemfibrozil **RX**

Class: Fibric acid derivative

ADULT DOSAGE

Coronary Heart Disease

Adjunctive therapy to diet to reduce risk of developing coronary heart disease only in Type IIb patients w/o history of or symptoms of existing coronary heart disease who have had an inadequate response to weight loss, dietary therapy, exercise, and other pharmacologic agents and who have the triad of low HDL, elevated LDL, and elevated TG levels
1200mg in 2 divided doses 30 min before am and pm meals

Hypertriglyceridemia

Adjunctive therapy to diet for treatment of adults w/ very high elevations of serum TG levels (Types IV and V hyperlipidemia) who present a risk of pancreatitis and who do not respond adequately to diet
1200mg in 2 divided doses 30 min before am and pm meals

PEDIATRIC DOSAGE

Pediatric use may not have been established

ADMINISTRATION
Oral route

Take 30 min before am and pm meals

HOW SUPPLIED
Tab: 600mg* *scored

CONTRAINDICATIONS
Severe renal dysfunction, hepatic dysfunction (including primary biliary cirrhosis), preexisting gallbladder disease, combination therapy with repaglinide or simvastatin.

WARNINGS/PRECAUTIONS
Cholelithiasis reported; perform gallbladder studies if cholelithiasis is suspected and d/c therapy if gallstones are found. May be associated with myositis; d/c if myositis is suspected/diagnosed. Control any medical problems (eg, diabetes mellitus [DM], hypothyroidism) that contribute to lipid abnormalities before initiating therapy. D/C if lipid response is inadequate after 3 months of therapy. Mild Hgb, Hct, and WBC decreases, and severe anemia; leukopenia, thrombocytopenia, and bone marrow hypoplasia reported; periodically monitor blood counts during the first 12 months of therapy. Abnormal LFTs reported; periodically monitor LFTs and d/c if abnormalities persist. Worsening renal insufficiency reported upon the addition of therapy in patients with baseline plasma creatinine >2mg/dL. Estrogen therapy is associated with massive rises in plasma TGs; discontinuation of estrogen therapy may obviate the need for specific drug therapy of hypertriglyceridemia.

ADVERSE REACTIONS
Dyspepsia, abdominal pain, diarrhea, fatigue.

DRUG INTERACTIONS
See Contraindications. Caution with anticoagulants; reduce anticoagulant dose and frequently monitor prothrombin until it has been definitely determined that prothrombin level has stabilized. Increased risk of myopathy and rhabdomyolysis with HMG-CoA reductase inhibitors. Reduced exposure with resin-granule drugs (eg, colestipol); administer ≥2 hrs apart. May potentiate myopathy with colchicine; caution when prescribing with colchicine, especially in elderly patients or patients with renal dysfunction.

NURSING CONSIDERATIONS

Assessment: Assess for hepatic/renal dysfunction, gallbladder disease, other medical conditions (eg, DM, hypothyroidism), hypersensitivity to drug, pregnancy/nursing status, and possible drug interactions. Obtain lipid levels.

Monitoring: Monitor for signs/symptoms of cholelithiasis, myositis, worsening renal insufficiency, and other adverse reactions. Periodically monitor serum lipids levels, CBC, and LFTs. Frequently monitor prothrombin with anticoagulants. Closely observe patients with significantly elevated TGs during therapy.

Patient Counseling: Inform about potential risks/benefits of therapy. Advise to report to physician any muscle pain/tenderness/weakness, or other adverse reactions. Instruct to notify physician if pregnant/nursing or planning to become pregnant.

Storage: 20-25°C (68-77°F). Protect from light and humidity.

LORAZEPAM ORAL – lorazepam CIV

Class: Benzodiazepine

OTHER BRAND NAMES
Ativan

ADULT DOSAGE
Anxiety Disorders

Anxiety Disorders or Short-Term Relief of Symptoms of Anxiety or Anxiety Associated w/ Depressive Symptoms:
Initial: 2-3mg/day given bid or tid
Usual: 2-6mg/day in divided doses; take largest dose before hs
Dosage Range: 1-10mg/day

Increase dose gradually prn; when higher dosage is indicated, increase pm dose before daytime doses

Insomnia Due to Anxiety or Transient Situational Stress:
2-4mg as a single daily dose qhs

PEDIATRIC DOSAGE
Anxiety Disorders

Anxiety Disorders or Short-Term Relief of Symptoms of Anxiety or Anxiety Associated w/ Depressive Symptoms:

≥12 Years:
Initial: 2-3mg/day given bid or tid
Usual: 2-6mg/day in divided doses; take largest dose before hs
Increase dose gradually prn; when higher dosage is indicated, increase pm dose before daytime doses
Dosage Range: 1-10mg/day

Insomnia Due to Anxiety or Transient Situational Stress:
2-4mg as a single daily dose qhs

DOSE MODIFICATION

Elderly/Debilitated

Initial: 1-2mg/day in divided doses; adjust prn and as tolerated

ADMINISTRATION

Oral route

Sol

Dispense only in the bottle and only w/ the calibrated dropper provided

Mix w/ liquid or semi-solid food for a few sec; Intensol formulation blends quickly and completely

Entire amount of mixture, of drug and liquid or drug and food, should be consumed immediately

HOW SUPPLIED

Sol: 2mg/mL; Tab: (Ativan) 0.5mg, 1mg*, 2mg* *scored

CONTRAINDICATIONS

Acute narrow-angle glaucoma.

WARNINGS/PRECAUTIONS

Effectiveness in long-term use (>4 months) has not been assessed; prescribe for short periods only (eg, 2-4 weeks) and periodically reassess usefulness of drug. Continuous long-term use is not recommended. Preexisting depression may emerge or worsen; not for use with primary depressive disorder or psychosis. May lead to potentially fatal respiratory depression. May impair mental/physical abilities. Use may lead to physical and psychological dependence; increased risk with higher doses, longer term use, and in patients with history of alcoholism/drug abuse, or with significant personality disorders. Withdrawal symptoms reported; avoid abrupt d/c and follow a gradual dosage-tapering schedule after extended therapy. May develop tolerance to sedative effects. Paradoxical reactions reported; d/c if these occur. May have abuse potential, especially with a history of drug and/or alcohol abuse. Possible suicide in patients with depression; do not use in such patients without adequate antidepressant therapy. Caution with compromised respiratory function (eg, COPD, sleep apnea syndrome), impaired renal/hepatic function, hepatic encephalopathy, in elderly, and in debilitated patients. May worsen hepatic encephalopathy. Adjust dose with severe hepatic insufficiency; lower doses may be sufficient. Monitor frequently for symptoms of upper GI disease. Leukopenia and elevations of lactate dehydrogenase reported; perform periodic blood counts and LFTs with long-term therapy.

ADVERSE REACTIONS

Sedation, dizziness, weakness, unsteadiness.

DRUG INTERACTIONS

Increased CNS-depressant effects with other CNS depressants (eg, alcohol, barbiturates, antipsychotics, sedative/hypnotics, anxiolytics, antidepressants, narcotic analgesics, sedative antihistamines, anticonvulsants, anesthetics); may lead to potentially fatal respiratory depression. Concomitant use with clozapine may produce marked sedation, excessive salivation, hypotension, ataxia, delirium, and respiratory arrest. Increased plasma concentrations with valproate and more rapid onset or prolonged effect with probenecid; reduce dose by 50%. Decreased sedative effects with theophylline or aminophylline.

NURSING CONSIDERATIONS

Assessment: Assess for acute narrow-angle glaucoma, primary depressive disorder, psychosis, personality disorders, compromised respiratory function, impaired renal/hepatic function, hepatic encephalopathy, history of alcohol/drug abuse, previous hypersensitivity to the drug, pregnancy/nursing status, and possible drug interactions.

Monitoring: Monitor for respiratory depression, physical/psychological dependence, withdrawal symptoms, tolerance, abuse, suicidal thinking, paradoxical reactions, symptoms of upper GI disease, and emergence/worsening of depression. Reassess usefulness of drug periodically. Monitor elderly/debilitated frequently and addiction-prone individuals carefully. Perform periodic blood counts and LFTs with long-term therapy.

Patient Counseling: Inform that psychological/physical dependence may occur; instruct to consult physician before increasing dose or abruptly d/c drug. Warn not to operate dangerous machinery or motor vehicles and that tolerance for alcohol and other CNS depressants will be diminished. Advise to consult physician if pregnancy occurs.

Storage: (Sol) 2-8°C (36-46°F). Protect from light. Discard opened bottle after 90 days. (Tab) 25°C (77°F); excursions permitted to 15-30°C (59-86°F).

LOTEMAX SUSPENSION – loteprednol etabonate RX

Class: Corticosteroid

ADULT DOSAGE

Steroid-Responsive Inflammatory Ocular Conditions

Treatment of palpebral and bulbar conjunctiva, cornea, and anterior segment of the globe, such as allergic conjunctivitis, acne rosacea, superficial punctate keratitis, herpes zoster keratitis, iritis, cyclitis, and selected infective conjunctivitides

Usual: Apply 1-2 drops into the conjunctival sac of the affected eye(s) qid; may increase up to 1 drop qh, if necessary, during initial treatment w/in the 1st week

Reevaluate if signs/symptoms fail to improve after 2 days

Postoperative Inflammation

Usual: Apply 1-2 drops into the conjunctival sac of the operated eye(s) qid beginning 24 hrs after surgery, and continuing throughout the first 2 weeks of the postoperative period

PEDIATRIC DOSAGE

Pediatric use may not have been established

ADMINISTRATION

Ocular route

Shake vigorously before use

HOW SUPPLIED

Sus: 0.5% [5mL, 10mL, 15mL]

CONTRAINDICATIONS

Most viral diseases of the cornea and conjunctiva (eg, epithelial herpes simplex keratitis [dendritic keratitis], vaccinia, varicella), mycobacterial infection of the eye, and fungal diseases of ocular structures.

WARNINGS/PRECAUTIONS

For ophthalmic use only. Prolonged use may result in glaucoma with damage to the optic nerve, defects in visual acuity and fields of vision, and in posterior subcapsular cataract formation; caution with glaucoma. Prolonged use may suppress host response and increase hazard of secondary ocular infections. Perforations reported with diseases causing thinning of cornea/sclera. May mask or enhance existing infection in acute purulent conditions of the eye. Caution with history of herpes simplex; may prolong course and exacerbate severity of many viral infections of the eye. May delay healing and increase incidence of bleb formation after cataract surgery. Initial prescription and renewal of medication order beyond 14 days should only be made after examination of the patient with aid of magnification (eg, slit-lamp biomicroscopy) and, where appropriate, fluorescein staining. Monitor IOP if used for ≥10 days. Fungal infections of the cornea may develop coincidentally with long-term use; consider fungal invasion in any persistent corneal ulceration and take fungal cultures when appropriate. For steroid-responsive diseases, caution not to d/c therapy prematurely. Should not be used for acute anterior uveitis in patients who require a more potent corticosteroid.

ADVERSE REACTIONS

Abnormal vision/blurring, burning on instillation, chemosis, discharge, dry eyes, epiphora, foreign body sensation, itching, photophobia, headache, rhinitis, pharyngitis.

NURSING CONSIDERATIONS

Assessment: Assess for previous drug hypersensitivity, viral diseases of the cornea and conjunctiva, mycobacterial infection of the eye, fungal diseases of ocular structures, glaucoma, thinning of the cornea/sclera, history of herpes simplex, and pregnancy/nursing status. Perform examination of patient with the aid of magnification (eg, slit-lamp biomicroscopy, fluorescein staining). Assess use in patients who have undergone recent cataract surgery.

Monitoring: Monitor for glaucoma and its complications, defects in visual acuity and fields of vision, posterior subcapsular cataract formation, perforation of the cornea/sclera, secondary ocular infections, fungal infections, masking of existing infections, and other adverse reactions. Reevaluate if signs/symptoms fail to improve after 2 days. Monitor IOP during prolonged use (≥10 days). Perform examination of patient with the aid of magnification (eg, slit-lamp biomicroscopy, fluorescein staining) before renewal of medication order beyond 14 days.

Patient Counseling: Advise not to allow dropper tip to touch any surface to avoid contamination of sus. Instruct to consult physician if pain develops or if redness, itching, or inflammation becomes aggravated. Inform not to wear soft contact lenses during treatment.

Storage: 15-25°C (59-77°F); store upright. Do not freeze.

LOTENSIN HCT – benazepril hydrochloride/hydrochlorothiazide RX

Class: ACE inhibitor/thiazide diuretic

D/C when pregnancy is detected. Drugs that act directly on the renin-angiotensin system (RAS) can cause injury/death to the developing fetus.

ADULT DOSAGE

Hypertension

Uncontrolled BP on Benazepril or HCTZ Alone:

Initial: 10mg/12.5mg qd

Titrate: May increase after 2-3 weeks prn to help achieve BP goals

Max: 20mg/25mg

Replacement Therapy: May be substituted for the titrated individual components

PEDIATRIC DOSAGE

Pediatric use may not have been established

ADMINISTRATION

Oral route

HOW SUPPLIED

Tab: (Benazepril/HCTZ) 5mg/6.25mg*, 10mg/12.5mg*, 20mg/12.5mg*, 20mg/25mg* *scored

CONTRAINDICATIONS

Anuria, sulfonamide-derived drug hypersensitivity, history of angioedema. Coadministration with aliskiren in patients with diabetes.

WARNINGS/PRECAUTIONS

Not for initial therapy of HTN. Head/neck angioedema reported; d/c and institute appropriate therapy immediately. Higher incidence of angioedema in blacks than nonblacks. Intestinal angioedema reported; monitor for abdominal pain. Anaphylactoid reactions reported during desensitization with hymenoptera venom, dialysis with high-flux membranes, and LDL apheresis with dextran sulfate absorption. Symptomatic hypotension may occur, most likely in patients with volume and/or salt depletion; correct depletion before initiating therapy. Enhanced effects in postsympathectomy patients. Excessive hypotension, which may be associated with oliguria, azotemia, and (rarely) with acute renal failure and death, may occur in patients with CHF; monitor closely during first 2 weeks of therapy and whenever dose is increased. May cause changes in renal function, including renal failure; consider withholding or discontinuing therapy if clinically significant decrease in renal function develops. May increase BUN or SrCr in patients with renal artery stenosis. May cause agranulocytosis and bone marrow depression. Associated with syndrome that starts with cholestatic jaundice and progresses to fulminant hepatic necrosis and sometimes death (rare); d/c if jaundice or marked hepatic enzyme elevations develop. May cause exacerbation or activation of systemic lupus erythematosus (SLE). May cause idiosyncratic reaction, resulting in acute transient myopia and acute angle-closure glaucoma; d/c as rapidly as possible. May cause serum electrolyte abnormalities. Persistent nonproductive cough reported. Hypotension may occur with surgery or during anesthesia. May decrease serum protein-bound iodine levels without signs of thyroid disturbance. D/C before testing for parathyroid function. HCTZ: May alter glucose tolerance and raise serum cholesterol and TG levels. May cause or exacerbate hyperuricemia and precipitate gout. May elevate serum Ca^{2+}; avoid with hypercalcemia. May precipitate hepatic coma in patients with hepatic impairment or progressive liver disease.

ADVERSE REACTIONS

Dizziness, fatigue, postural dizziness, headache.

DRUG INTERACTIONS

See Contraindications. Caution with other antihypertensives. May affect K^+ levels with K^+ supplements and K^+-sparing diuretics; monitor K^+ periodically. Increased lithium levels and lithium toxicity reported; monitor lithium levels. Dual blockade of the RAS is associated with increased risks of hypotension, hyperkalemia, and changes in renal function (including acute renal failure); closely monitor BP, renal function, and electrolytes with concomitant agents that also affect the RAS. Avoid aliskiren in patients with renal impairment (GFR <60mL/min). NSAIDs, including selective COX-2 inhibitors, may attenuate antihypertensive effect and may cause deterioration of renal function. Benazepril: Nitritoid reactions reported with injectable gold. HCTZ: May potentiate action of other antihypertensives, especially ganglionic/peripheral adrenergic-blocking drugs. Cholestyramine and colestipol resins reduce absorption from GI tract; administer at least 4 hrs before or 4-6 hrs after administration of resins. Drug-induced hypokalemia or hypomagnesemia may predispose patient to digoxin toxicity. May increase responsiveness to skeletal muscle relaxants (eg, curare derivatives). Dosage adjustment of antidiabetic drugs may be required. May reduce renal excretion of cytotoxic agents (eg, cyclophosphamide, methotrexate) and enhance their myelosuppressive effects. Anticholinergics (eg, atropine, biperiden) may increase bioavailability due to decrease in GI motility and stomach emptying rate. Prokinetic drugs may decrease bioavailability. Increased risk of hyperuricemia and gout-type complications with cyclosporine. May potentiate orthostatic hypotension with alcohol, barbiturates, or narcotics. May reduce response to pressor amines (eg, noradrenaline).

NURSING CONSIDERATIONS

Assessment: Assess for anuria, sulfonamide-derived drug hypersensitivity, history of angioedema/allergy/asthma, risk factors for angle-closure glaucoma, volume/salt depletion, CHF, collagen vascular diseases, SLE, hypercalcemia, diabetes, renal/hepatic impairment, postsympathectomy status, pregnancy/nursing status, and possible drug interactions.

Monitoring: Monitor for angioedema, anaphylactoid reactions, exacerbation/activation of SLE, myopia, angle-closure glaucoma, hyperuricemia or precipitation of gout, and other adverse reactions. Monitor BP, LFTs, renal function, serum electrolytes, cholesterol, and TG levels. Monitor WBCs in patients with collagen vascular disease and renal impairment.

Patient Counseling: Inform about fetal risks if taken during pregnancy and discuss treatment options in women planning to become pregnant; instruct to report pregnancy as soon as possible. Instruct to d/c therapy and to immediately report signs/symptoms of angioedema. Instruct to report lightheadedness, especially during the 1st days of therapy; advise to d/c and consult with a physician if syncope occurs. Inform that inadequate fluid intake, excessive perspiration, diarrhea, or vomiting may lead to excessive fall in BP, with the same consequences of lightheadedness and possible syncope. Advise not to use K^+ supplements or salt substitutes containing K^+ without consulting physician. Advise to promptly report any indication of infection.

Storage: ≤30°C (86°F). Protect from moisture and light.

LOTREL – amlodipine besylate/benazepril hydrochloride RX

Class: ACE inhibitor/calcium channel blocker (dihydropyridine)

D/C when pregnancy is detected. Drugs that act directly on the renin-angiotensin system (RAS) can cause injury/death to the developing fetus.

ADULT DOSAGE

Hypertension

Not Adequately Controlled on Monotherapy w/ Either Agent:
Initial: 2.5mg-10mg qd
Titrate: May increase up to 10mg-40mg qd if BP remains uncontrolled

Replacement Therapy: May substitute for titrated components

PEDIATRIC DOSAGE

Pediatric use may not have been established

DOSE MODIFICATION

Hepatic Impairment

Consider using lower doses

Elderly

Consider lower initial doses

ADMINISTRATION

Oral route

HOW SUPPLIED

Cap: (Amlodipine-Benazepril) 2.5mg-10mg, 5mg-10mg, 5mg-20mg, 5mg-40mg, 10mg-20mg, 10mg-40mg

CONTRAINDICATIONS

History of angioedema. Coadministration with aliskiren in patients with diabetes.

WARNINGS/PRECAUTIONS

Symptomatic hypotension may occur, most likely in patients who have been volume- or salt-depleted (eg, diuretic therapy, dietary salt restriction, dialysis, diarrhea, vomiting); correct volume and/or salt depletion before starting therapy. Benazepril: Head and neck angioedema reported; d/c and institute appropriate treatment if angioedema occurs. More reports of angioedema in blacks than in nonblacks. Intestinal angioedema reported; monitor for abdominal pain. Anaphylactoid reactions reported during desensitization with hymenoptera venom, dialysis with high-flux membranes, and LDL apheresis with dextran sulfate absorption. Excessive hypotension, which may be associated with oliguria, azotemia, and (rare) acute renal failure or death, may occur in CHF patients; monitor patients during first 2 weeks of therapy and whenever dose is increased or a diuretic is added/increased. Cholestatic hepatitis and acute liver failure rarely reported; d/c if jaundice or marked elevation of hepatic enzymes develops. Not recommended with severe renal impairment (CrCl ≤30mL/min). May cause changes in renal function, including acute renal failure, and may occur in patients whose renal function depends on the RAS (eg, renal artery stenosis, severe HF, post MI); consider withholding or discontinuing therapy if clinically significant decrease in renal function develops. Hyperkalemia and persistent nonproductive cough reported. Hypotension may occur with surgery or during anesthesia. Amlodipine: Worsening angina and acute MI may develop after starting or increasing the dose, particularly in patients with severe obstructive CAD. Caution with aortic/mitral stenosis, or obstructive hypertrophic cardiomyopathy.

ADVERSE REACTIONS

Cough, headache, dizziness, edema, angioedema.

DRUG INTERACTIONS

See Contraindications. Benazepril: Coadministration with NSAIDs, including selective COX-2 inhibitors, may result in deterioration of renal function and attenuation of antihypertensive effect. Diabetic patients receiving concomitant insulin or oral antidiabetics may develop hypoglycemia. Dual blockade of the RAS is associated with increased risks of hypotension, hyperkalemia, and changes in renal function (including acute renal failure); avoid combined use of RAS inhibitors, or closely monitor BP, renal function, and electrolytes with concomitant agents that also block the RAS. Avoid with aliskiren in patients with renal impairment (GFR <60mL/min). K^+ supplements, K^+-sparing diuretics (eg, spironolactone, amiloride, triamterene), or K^+-containing salt substitutes may increase risk of hyperkalemia; frequently monitor serum K^+. Increased lithium levels and symptoms of lithium toxicity reported; frequently monitor lithium levels. Nitritoid reactions (eg, facial flushing, N/V, hypotension) reported with injectable gold. Amlodipine: May increase exposure of simvastatin; limit dose of simvastatin to 20mg daily. Increased systemic exposure with moderate and strong CYP3A inhibitors (eg, diltiazem); monitor for symptoms of hypotension and edema. Monitor BP when coadministered with CYP3A4 inducers. Strong CYP3A4 inhibitors (eg, ketoconazole, itraconazole, ritonavir) may increase concentrations to a greater extent.

NURSING CONSIDERATIONS

Assessment: Assess for history of angioedema, diabetes, hypersensitivity to drug, aortic/mitral stenosis, obstructive hypertrophic cardiomyopathy, CHF, severe obstructive CAD, volume/salt depletion, hepatic/renal impairment, pregnancy/nursing status, and possible drug interactions.

Monitoring: Monitor for signs/symptoms of hypotension, anaphylactoid or hypersensitivity reactions, head/neck and intestinal angioedema, worsening angina or AMI, and other adverse reactions. Monitor BP, hepatic/renal function, and serum K^+ levels.

Patient Counseling: Inform of the consequences of exposure to the medication during pregnancy and of treatment options in women planning to become pregnant. Advise to report pregnancies as soon as possible. Advise diabetic patients about the possibility of hypoglycemic reactions when drug is used concomitantly with insulin or oral antidiabetics. Advise to seek medical attention if symptoms of hypotension, anaphylactoid or hypersensitivity reactions, angioedema, infection, trouble swallowing, breathing problems, or hepatic dysfunction occurs.

Storage: 25°C (77°F); excursions permitted to 15-30°C (59-86°F). Protect from moisture.

LOTRISONE – betamethasone dipropionate/clotrimazole RX

Class: Azole antifungal/corticosteroid

ADULT DOSAGE

Tinea Corporis

≥17 Years:
Apply a thin film into affected skin areas bid for 1 week
Max: 45g/week

Reevaluate if no improvement seen after 1 week; do not use for >2 weeks

Tinea Cruris

≥17 Years:
Apply a thin film into affected skin areas bid for 1 week
Max: 45g/week

Reevaluate if no improvement seen after 1 week; do not use for >2 weeks

PEDIATRIC DOSAGE

Pediatric use may not have been established

Tinea Pedis

≥17 Years:
Gently massage sufficient amount into affected skin areas bid for 2 weeks
Max: 45g/week

Reevaluate if no improvement seen after 2 weeks; do not use for >4 weeks

ADMINISTRATION
Topical route
Do not use w/ occlusive dressings unless directed by a physician

HOW SUPPLIED
Cre: (Betamethasone/Clotrimazole) 0.05%/1% [15g, 45g]

WARNINGS/PRECAUTIONS
Not for oral, ophthalmic, or intravaginal use. Avoid use with occlusive dressings. May cause reversible hypothalamic-pituitary-adrenal (HPA) axis suppression with the potential for glucocorticosteroid insufficiency during and after withdrawal of treatment. Cushing's syndrome and hyperglycemia may occur. Factors predisposing to HPA axis suppression include use of high-potency steroids, large treatment surface areas, prolonged use, use of occlusive dressings, altered skin barrier, liver failure, and young age. Evaluate periodically for evidence of HPA axis suppression. Gradually withdraw drug, reduce frequency of application, or substitute a less potent corticosteroid if HPA axis suppression is documented. Pediatric patients may be more susceptible to systemic toxicity. Not recommended for treatment of diaper dermatitis. Caution in elderly.

ADVERSE REACTIONS
Paresthesia, rash, edema, secondary infection.

NURSING CONSIDERATIONS

Assessment: Assess for hypersensitivity to drug, predisposing factors to HPA axis suppression, and pregnancy/nursing status.

Monitoring: Monitor for signs/symptoms of HPA axis suppression, Cushing's syndrome, hyperglycemia, and other adverse reactions. Perform periodic monitoring for HPA axis suppression using adrenocorticotropic hormone stimulation test. Review diagnosis if no clinical improvement seen after 1 week of treatment for tinea corporis or tinea cruris, and 2 weeks for tinea pedis.

Patient Counseling: Inform to use externally ud. Advise to avoid intravaginal contact or contact with the eyes or mouth. Advise not to use on the face or underarms. When using in the groin area, counsel to use only for 2 weeks and apply the cream sparingly; advise to wear loose-fitting clothing and to notify physician if condition persists after 2 weeks. Instruct not to bandage, cover, or wrap the treatment area unless directed by physician. Advise to avoid use in the diaper area. Instruct to report any signs of local adverse reactions to physician. Instruct to notify physician if no improvement seen after 1 week of treatment for tinea cruris or tinea corporis, or 2 weeks for tinea pedis.

Storage: 20-25°C (68-77°F); excursions permitted to 15-30°C (59-86°F).

LOVASTATIN — lovastatin RX

Class: HMG-CoA reductase inhibitor

ADULT DOSAGE

Primary Hypercholesterolemia

Initial: 20mg qd w/ pm meal (LDL reductions of ≥20%); may consider 10mg if smaller reductions required
Usual: 10-80mg/day in single or 2 divided doses
Titrate: Adjust at ≥4-week intervals
Max: 80mg/day

Consider dose reduction if cholesterol levels fall significantly below the targeted range

Coronary Artery Disease

Primary prevention of coronary heart disease. Slow progression of coronary atherosclerosis in patients w/ coronary heart disease

Dose based on current clinical practice

PEDIATRIC DOSAGE

Heterozygous Familial Hypercholesterolemia

Treatment of adolescents w/ the following findings: LDL remains >189mg/dL, or LDL remains >160mg/dL and there is a positive family history of premature cardiovascular disease or 2 or more other cardiovascular disease risk factors are present

10-17 Years (at Least 1 Year Postmenarche):
Initial: 20mg/day (LDL reductions of ≥20%); may consider 10mg if smaller reductions required
Usual: 10-40mg/day
Titrate: Adjust at ≥4-week intervals
Max: 40mg/day

DOSE MODIFICATION

Concomitant Medications

W/ Amiodarone:
Max: 40mg/day

W/ Danazol, Diltiazem, Dronedarone, or Verapamil:
Initial: 10mg/day
Max: 20mg/day

Renal Impairment

Severe (CrCl <30mL/min): Carefully consider dosage increases above 20mg/day; give cautiously if deemed necessary

ADMINISTRATION

Oral route

Take w/ meals

HOW SUPPLIED

Tab: 10mg, 20mg, 40mg

CONTRAINDICATIONS

Active liver disease or unexplained persistent elevations of serum transaminases, pregnancy, women of childbearing age who may become pregnant, and nursing mothers. Concomitant administration with strong CYP3A4 inhibitors (eg, itraconazole, ketoconazole, posaconazole, voriconazole, HIV protease inhibitors, boceprevir, telaprevir, erythromycin, clarithromycin, telithromycin, nefazodone, cobicistat-containing products).

WARNINGS/PRECAUTIONS

Myopathy (including immune-mediated necrotizing myopathy [IMNM]) and rhabdomyolysis reported; d/c if markedly elevated CPK levels occur or myopathy is diagnosed/suspected, and temporarily withhold in any patient experiencing acute or serious condition predisposing to development of renal failure secondary to rhabdomyolysis. Risk of myopathy/rhabdomyolysis is dose related. Persistent increases in serum transaminases reported; obtain LFTs prior to initiation and repeat as clinically indicated. Fatal and nonfatal hepatic failure (rare) reported; promptly interrupt therapy if serious liver injury with clinical symptoms and/or hyperbilirubinemia or jaundice occurs and do not restart if no alternate etiology found. Caution in patients who consume substantial quantities of alcohol and/or have history of liver disease. Increases in HbA1c and FPG levels reported. Evaluate patients who develop endocrine dysfunction. Caution in the elderly.

ADVERSE REACTIONS

Headache, constipation, flatulence, myalgia.

DRUG INTERACTIONS

See Contraindications and Dosage. Ranolazine may increase risk of myopathy/rhabdomyolysis; consider dose adjustment of lovastatin. Due to the risk of myopathy, avoid with gemfibrozil, cyclosporine, and grapefruit juice, and caution with fibrates, lipid-lowering doses (≥1g/day) of niacin, colchicine, danazol, diltiazem, dronedarone, verapamil, and amiodarone. Determine PT before initiation and frequently during therapy with coumarin anticoagulants. Caution with drugs that may decrease the levels or activity of endogenous steroid hormones (eg, spironolactone, cimetidine).

NURSING CONSIDERATIONS

Assessment: Assess for history of or active liver disease, unexplained persistent serum transaminase elevations, secondary causes for hypercholesterolemia, alcohol consumption, diabetes, drug hypersensitivity, pregnancy/nursing status, and possible drug interactions. Assess lipid profile, LFTs, and renal function.

Monitoring: Monitor for signs/symptoms of myopathy (including IMNM), rhabdomyolysis, liver/renal/endocrine dysfunction, increases in HbA1c and FPG levels, and other adverse reactions. Monitor lipid profile, creatine kinase, and LFTs. Check PT frequently with coumarin anticoagulants.

Patient Counseling: Advise about substances to be avoided and to report promptly any unexplained muscle pain, tenderness, or weakness, particularly if accompanied by malaise or fever or if muscle signs and symptoms persist after discontinuation. Inform that liver function will be checked prior to therapy and if signs/symptoms of liver injury occur; instruct to report promptly any symptoms that may indicate liver injury (eg, right upper abdominal discomfort, dark urine, jaundice). Instruct women of childbearing age to use an effective method of birth control, to stop taking drug if they become pregnant, and not to breastfeed while on therapy. Advise patients to inform other physicians prescribing a new medication, that they are taking lovastatin.

Storage: 20-25°C (68-77°F). Protect from light.

LOVAZA – omega-3-acid ethyl esters RX

Class: Lipid-regulating agent

ADULT DOSAGE

Severe Hypertriglyceridemia (≥500mg/dL)

Usual: 4g/day (4 caps qd or 2 caps bid)

PEDIATRIC DOSAGE

Pediatric use may not have been established

ADMINISTRATION

Oral route

Swallow caps whole; do not break open, crush, dissolve, or chew

HOW SUPPLIED

Cap: 1g

WARNINGS/PRECAUTIONS

Increases in ALT levels without a concurrent increase in AST levels reported. May increase LDL levels; monitor LDL levels periodically during therapy. Contains ethyl esters of omega-3 fatty acids (eicosapentaenoic acid [EPA] and docosahexaenoic acid [DHA]), obtained from oil of several fish sources; caution with known hypersensitivity to fish and/or shellfish. Recurrent symptomatic atrial fibrillation/flutter (A-fib/flutter) reported in patients with paroxysmal or persistent A-fib, particularly within the first 2-3 months of initiating therapy. Assess TG levels carefully before initiating therapy and monitor TG levels periodically during therapy.

ADVERSE REACTIONS

Eructation, taste perversion, dyspepsia.

DRUG INTERACTIONS

Periodically monitor patients receiving concomitant treatment with an anticoagulant or other drugs affecting coagulation (eg, antiplatelet agents). D/C or change medications known to exacerbate hypertriglyceridemia (eg, β-blockers, thiazides, estrogens), if possible, prior to consideration of therapy.

NURSING CONSIDERATIONS

Assessment: Assess for hypersensitivity to drug, fish and/or shellfish; hepatic impairment; A-fib/flutter; pregnancy/nursing status; and possible drug interactions. Attempt to control serum lipids with appropriate diet, exercise, weight loss in obese patients, and control of any medical problems that are contributing to lipid abnormalities (eg, diabetes mellitus, hypothyroidism). Assess TG and LDL levels.

Monitoring: Monitor for recurrent symptomatic A-fib/flutter in patients with paroxysmal or persistent A-fib. Monitor for allergic reactions and other adverse reactions. Periodically monitor ALT and AST levels in patients with hepatic impairment. Periodically monitor LDL and TG levels.

Patient Counseling: Instruct to notify physician if allergic to fish and/or shellfish. Advise that the use of lipid-regulating agents does not reduce the importance of adhering to diet. Advise not to alter caps in any way and to ingest intact caps only. Instruct to take as prescribed.

Storage: 25°C (77°F); excursions permitted to 15-30°C (59-86°F). Do not freeze.

LOVENOX – enoxaparin sodium RX

Class: Low molecular weight heparin

Epidural or spinal hematomas resulting in long-term or permanent paralysis may occur in patients anticoagulated with low molecular weight heparins (LMWHs) or heparinoids and are receiving neuraxial anesthesia or undergoing spinal puncture. Increased risk with indwelling epidural catheters, concomitant use of other drugs that affect hemostasis (eg, NSAIDs, platelet inhibitors, other anticoagulants), history of traumatic or repeated epidural or spinal punctures, a history of spinal deformity or spinal surgery, or when optimal timing between the administration of enoxaparin and neuraxial procedures is not known. Monitor frequently for signs/symptoms of neurological impairment; if neurological compromise noted, urgent treatment is necessary. Consider benefit and risks before neuraxial intervention in patients anticoagulated or to be anticoagulated for thromboprophylaxis.

ADULT DOSAGE

Deep Vein Thrombosis

Prophylaxis:

Abdominal Surgery:

40mg SQ qd w/ initial dose given 2 hrs prior to surgery for 7-10 days (up to 12 days in clinical trials)

PEDIATRIC DOSAGE

Pediatric use may not have been established

Hip Replacement Surgery:
Twice-Daily Dosing: 30mg SQ q12h w/ initial dose given 12-24 hrs after surgery for 7-10 days (up to 14 days in clinical trials)
Once-Daily Dosing: 40mg SQ qd w/ initial dose given 12 hrs prior to surgery for 7-10 days (up to 14 days in clinical trials)

Continue prophylaxis w/ 40mg SQ qd for 3 weeks following initial phase

Knee Replacement Surgery:
30mg SQ q12h w/ initial dose given 12-24 hrs after surgery for 7-10 days (up to 14 days in clinical trials)

Acute Illness w/ Severely Restricted Mobility:
40mg SQ qd for 6-11 days (up to 14 days in clinical trials)

Acute Treatment:
Outpatient (w/o Pulmonary Embolism):
1mg/kg SQ q12h for 7 days (up to 17 days in clinical trials)

Inpatient (w/ or w/o Pulmonary Embolism):
1mg/kg SQ q12h, or 1.5mg/kg SQ qd at the same time every day for 7 days (up to 17 days in clinical trials)

Outpatient and Inpatient Treatments:
Initiate warfarin therapy when appropriate (usually w/in 72 hrs of enoxaparin); continue enoxaparin for at least 5 days and until therapeutic oral anticoagulant effect has been achieved

Unstable Angina

Prophylaxis:
1mg/kg SQ q12h in conjunction w/ oral aspirin therapy (100-325mg qd) for 2-8 days (up to 12.5 days in clinical trials)

Myocardial Infarction

Non-Q-Wave:
Prophylaxis:
1mg/kg SQ q12h in conjunction w/ oral aspirin therapy (100-325mg qd) for 2-8 days (up to 12.5 days in clinical trials)

Acute ST- Segment Elevation:
Treatment:
<75 Years:
Initial: 30mg single IV bolus plus a 1mg/kg SQ dose, followed by 1mg/kg SQ q12h
Max: 100mg for the first 2 SQ doses only

All patients should receive aspirin (75-325mg qd) as soon as they are identified as having ST-segment elevation MI unless contraindicated

Concomitant Thrombolytic (Fibrin-Specific or Non-Fibrin Specific):
Administer enoxaparin between 15 min before and 30 min after the start of fibrinolytic therapy

Percutaneous Coronary Intervention:
Last SQ Enoxaparin Dose Given <8 hrs Before Balloon Inflation: No additional dosing needed
Last SQ Enoxaparin Dose Given >8 hrs Before Balloon Inflation: Administer 0.3mg/kg IV bolus

DOSE MODIFICATION

Renal Impairment

Severe (CrCl <30mL/min):

Prophylaxis in Abdominal Surgery: 30mg SQ qd

Prophylaxis in Hip/Knee Replacement Surgery: 30mg SQ qd

Prophylaxis in Acute Illness: 30mg SQ qd

Outpatient Treatment of Acute DVT w/o Pulmonary Embolism (w/ Warfarin): 1mg/kg SQ qd

Inpatient Treatment of Acute DVT w/ or w/o Pulmonary Embolism (w/ Warfarin): 1mg/kg SQ qd

Ischemic Prophylaxis in Unstable Angina/Non-Q-Wave MI (w/ Aspirin): 1mg/kg SQ qd

Treatment of Acute ST-Segment Elevation MI in Patients <75 Years (w/ Aspirin): 30mg single IV bolus plus a 1mg/kg SQ dose, followed by 1mg/kg SQ qd

Treatment of Acute ST-Segment Elevation MI in Patients ≥75 Years (w/ Aspirin): 1mg/kg SQ qd (no initial bolus)

Elderly

≥75 Years:

Acute ST-Segment Elevation MI:

Do not use initial IV bolus

Initial: 0.75mg/kg SQ q12h

Max: 75mg for the first 2 doses only

ADMINISTRATION

SQ or IV (for multidose vial) route

Use tuberculin syringe or equivalent when using multidose vials

Prefilled syringes and graduated prefilled syringes are for single, one-time use only and are available w/ a system that shields the needle after inj

SQ Inj Technique

Remove the prefilled syringe from the blister packaging by peeling at the arrow as directed on the blister; do not remove by pulling on the plunger as this may damage the syringe

Patients should be lying down and enoxaparin administered by deep SQ inj

Do not expel the air bubble from the prefilled syringe before the inj

Administration should be alternated between the left and right anterolateral and left and right posterolateral abdominal wall

The whole length of the needle should be introduced into a skin fold held between the thumb and forefinger; the skin fold should be held throughout the inj

Do not rub the inj site after completion of the inj

IV (Bolus) Inj

Use multiple-dose vial and administer through an IV line

Do not mix or coadminister w/ other medications

Flush the chosen IV access w/ a sufficient amount of saline or dextrose sol prior to and following the IV bolus administration of enoxaparin to clear the port of drug; enoxaparin may be safely administered w/ normal saline sol (0.9%) or D5W

HOW SUPPLIED

Inj: (Multidose vial) 300mg/3mL; (Prefilled Syringe) 30mg/0.3mL, 40mg/0.4mL, 60mg/0.6mL, 80mg/0.8mL, 100mg/mL, 120mg/0.8mL, 150mg/mL

CONTRAINDICATIONS

Active major bleeding, thrombocytopenia associated with a positive in vitro test for antiplatelet antibody in the presence of enoxaparin sodium, hypersensitivity to heparin or pork products, hypersensitivity to benzyl alcohol (only with the multidose formulation).

WARNINGS/PRECAUTIONS

Consider pharmacokinetic profile of enoxaparin to reduce the potential risk of bleeding associated with concurrent use with epidural or spinal anesthesia/analgesia or spinal puncture. Placement or removal of catheter should be delayed for at least 12 hrs after administration of lower doses and at least 24 hrs after higher doses. Extreme caution with increased risk of hemorrhage (eg, bacterial endocarditis, congenital or acquired bleeding disorders) and with history of heparin-induced thrombocytopenia. Major hemorrhages, including retroperitoneal and intracranial bleeding, reported. To minimize the risk of bleeding following vascular instrumentation during treatment of unstable angina, non-Q-wave MI, and acute STEMI, adhere precisely to the intervals recommended between doses. Observe for signs of bleeding or hematoma formation at the site of the procedure. Caution in patients with bleeding diathesis, uncontrolled arterial HTN or history of recent GI ulceration, diabetic retinopathy, renal dysfunction, and hemorrhage. Thrombocytopenia reported; d/c if platelet count <100,000/mm^3. Cannot be used interchangeably (unit for unit) with heparin or other LMWH. Pregnant women with mechanical prosthetic heart valves may be at higher risk for thromboembolism and have a higher rate of fetal loss; monitor anti-factor Xa levels, and adjust dosage prn. Multidose vial contains benzyl alcohol that crosses the placenta and has been associated with fatal "gasping syndrome" in premature neonates; use with caution or only when clearly needed in pregnant women. Periodic CBC, including platelet count and stool occult blood tests are recommended during course of treatment. Anti-factor Xa may be used to monitor anticoagulant activity in patients with significant renal impairment or if abnormal coagulation parameters or bleeding occurs. Hyperkalemia reported in patients with renal failure. Increase in exposure with prophylactic dosages (non-weight adjusted) observed in low-weight women (<45kg) and low-weight men (<57kg). Higher risk for thromboembolism in obese patients; observe for signs/symptoms of thromboembolism. Caution with hepatic impairment.

ADVERSE REACTIONS

Epidural or spinal hematoma, hemorrhage, ecchymosis, anemia, peripheral edema, fever, dyspnea, nausea, ALT/AST elevations.

DRUG INTERACTIONS

See Boxed Warning. D/C agents that may enhance the risk of hemorrhage prior to therapy (eg, anticoagulants, platelet inhibitors, such as acetylsalicylic acid, salicylates, NSAIDs [including ketorolac tromethamine], dipyridamole, or sulfinpyrazone). If coadministration is essential, conduct close monitoring. May increase risk of hyperkalemia with K^+-sparing drugs, and administration of K^+.

NURSING CONSIDERATIONS

Assessment: Assess for presence of active major bleeding, thrombocytopenia, hypersensitivity to heparin or pork products, hypersensitivity to benzyl alcohol, renal dysfunction, obesity, any other conditions where treatment is cautioned, nursing/pregnancy status, and for possible drug interactions.

Monitoring: Monitor for signs/symptoms of hemorrhage, thrombocytopenia, hyperkalemia, thromboembolism, and other adverse reactions. Monitor for epidural or spinal hematomas, and for neurological impairment if used concomitantly with spinal/epidural anesthesia or spinal puncture. Periodically monitor CBC, including platelet count, and stool occult blood tests. If bleeding occurs, monitor anti-factor Xa levels.

Patient Counseling: Inform of the benefits and risks of therapy. Instruct to watch for signs/symptoms of spinal or epidural hematoma (tingling, numbness, muscular weakness) if patients have had neuraxial anesthesia or spinal puncture, particularly, if they are taking concomitant NSAIDs, platelet inhibitors, or other anticoagulants; instruct to contact physician if these occur. Advise to seek medical attention if unusual bleeding, bruising, signs of thrombocytopenia, or allergic reactions develop. Counsel that it will take longer than usual to stop bleeding; explain that patient may bruise and/or bleed more easily when treated with enoxaparin. Inform of administration instructions if therapy is to continue after discharge. Instruct to notify physicians and dentists of enoxaparin therapy prior to surgery or taking a new drug.

Storage: 25°C (77°F); excursions permitted to 15-30°C (59-86°F). Do not store multidose vials for >28 days after first use.

LUMIGAN – bimatoprost

RX

Class: Prostaglandin analogue

ADULT DOSAGE

Elevated Intraocular Pressure

Open-Angle Glaucoma/Ocular HTN:
Usual: 1 drop in the affected eye(s) qpm

PEDIATRIC DOSAGE

Elevated Intraocular Pressure

Open-Angle Glaucoma/Ocular HTN:
≥16 Years:
Usual: 1 drop in the affected eye(s) qpm

DOSE MODIFICATION

Concomitant Medications

Space dosing by at least 5 min if using >1 topical ophthalmic drug

ADMINISTRATION

Ocular route

HOW SUPPLIED

Sol: 0.01% [2.5mL, 5mL, 7.5mL]

WARNINGS/PRECAUTIONS

Changes to pigmented tissues, including increased pigmentation of iris (may be permanent), eyelid, and eyelashes (may be reversible) reported. Regularly examine patients with noticeably increased iris pigmentation. May cause changes to eyelashes and vellus hair in the treated eye. Intraocular inflammation reported; caution with active intraocular inflammation (eg, uveitis). Macular edema, including cystoid macular edema, reported; caution with aphakic patients, pseudophakic patients with a torn posterior lens capsule, or patients at risk of macular edema. Bacterial keratitis reported with multidose containers. Remove contact lenses prior to instillation; may reinsert 15 min after administration.

ADVERSE REACTIONS

Conjunctival hyperemia/edema/hemorrhage, eye irritation/pain/pruritus, reduced visual acuity, blurred vision, skin hyperpigmentation, eyelid erythema/pruritus, growth of eyelashes, hypertrichosis, instillation site irritation, punctate keratitis.

NURSING CONSIDERATIONS

Assessment: Assess for active intraocular inflammation, risk of macular edema, contact lens use, and pregnancy/nursing status. Assess use in aphakic patients, and in pseudophakic patients with a torn posterior lens capsule.

Monitoring: Monitor for changes to pigmented tissue, changes in eyelashes and vellus hair, intraocular inflammation, exacerbation of intraocular inflammation, macular edema, bacterial keratitis, and other adverse reactions.

Patient Counseling: Advise about the potential for increased brown pigmentation of iris (may be permanent) and the possibility of darkening of eyelid skin (may be reversible after discontinuation). Inform about the possibility of eyelash and vellus hair changes in the treated eye during treatment. Instruct to avoid touching tip of dispensing container to the eye, surrounding structures, fingers, or any other surface in order to avoid contamination of the sol. Advise to consult physician if having ocular surgery, if an intercurrent ocular condition (eg, trauma or infection) develops, or if any ocular reactions develop. Instruct to remove contact lenses prior to instillation and reinsert 15 min after administration. Instruct to administer at least 5 min apart if using more than 1 topical ophthalmic drug.

Storage: 2-25°C (36-77°F).

LUNESTA – eszopiclone CIV

Class: Nonbenzodiazepine hypnotic agent

ADULT DOSAGE

Insomnia

Initial: 1mg immediately hs

Titrate: May increase to 2mg or 3mg if clinically indicated

Max: 3mg qd immediately hs

Use lowest effective dose

PEDIATRIC DOSAGE

Pediatric use may not have been established

DOSE MODIFICATION

Concomitant Medications

Potent CYP3A4 Inhibitors:

Max: 2mg

Concomitant CNS Depressants: Dose adjustments may be necessary

Hepatic Impairment

Severe:

Max: 2mg

Elderly

Elderly/Debilitated:

Max: 2mg

ADMINISTRATION

Oral route

Take immediately hs with at least 7-8 hrs remaining before planned time of awakening
Do not administer with or immediately after a meal

HOW SUPPLIED

Tab: 1mg, 2mg, 3mg

WARNINGS/PRECAUTIONS

May impair daytime function at the higher dose (2mg or 3mg), even when used as prescribed; monitor for excess depressant effects. May impair physical/mental abilities. Increased risk of next-day psychomotor impairment if taken with less than a full night of sleep remaining (7-8 hrs) or if higher than recommended dose is taken. Initiate only after careful evaluation; failure of insomnia to remit after 7-10 days of treatment may indicate presence of a primary psychiatric and/or medical illness. Use the lowest possible effective dose, especially in elderly. Severe anaphylactic/anaphylactoid reactions reported; do not rechallenge if angioedema develops. Abnormal thinking and behavioral changes (eg, bizarre behavior, agitation, hallucinations, depersonalization) reported. Amnesia and other neuropsychiatric symptoms may occur unpredictably. Worsening of depression, including suicidal thoughts and actions (including completed suicides), reported in primarily depressed patients. Complex behaviors (eg, sleep-driving) reported; consider discontinuation if a sleep-driving episode occurs. Withdrawal signs/symptoms reported following rapid dose decrease or abrupt discontinuation. Should be taken immediately hs; taking medication while still up and about may result in short-term memory impairment, hallucinations, impaired coordination, dizziness, and lightheadedness. Caution with severe hepatic impairment, elderly/debilitated patients, patients with diseases/conditions that could affect metabolism/hemodynamic responses, compromised respiratory function, history of alcohol/drug abuse, history of psychiatric disorders, and in patients exhibiting signs and symptoms of depression.

ADVERSE REACTIONS

Headache, unpleasant taste, somnolence, dry mouth, dizziness, infection, rash, pain, N/V, diarrhea, hallucinations, dyspepsia, nervousness, depression, anxiety.

DRUG INTERACTIONS

See Dosage. Not recommended with other sedative-hypnotics hs or in the middle of the night. Additive effects may occur with other CNS depressants (eg, benzodiazepines, opioids, TCAs, alcohol), including daytime use; consider downward dose adjustment of both drugs. Increased risk of next-day psychomotor impairment if coadministered with other CNS depressants and other drugs that increase blood levels of eszopiclone. Increased risk of complex behaviors with alcohol and other CNS depressants. May produce additive effect on psychomotor performance with ethanol. Decreased digit symbol substitution test scores with olanzapine. Decreased exposure and effects with CYP3A4 inducers (eg, rifampicin). Increased exposure with ketoconazole and other strong CYP3A4 inhibitors (eg, clarithromycin, nefazodone, ritonavir); dose reduction needed.

NURSING CONSIDERATIONS

Assessment: Assess for psychiatric or physical disorder, depression, severe hepatic impairment, diseases/conditions that could affect metabolism/hemodynamic responses, compromised respiratory function, history of alcohol/drug abuse, history of psychiatric disorders, drug hypersensitivity, pregnancy/nursing status, and possible drug interactions.

Monitoring: Monitor for excessive depressant effects, anaphylactic/anaphylactoid reactions, emergence of any new behavioral signs/symptoms, withdrawal symptoms, abnormal thinking, and other adverse reactions.

Patient Counseling: Inform of the risks and benefits of therapy. Inform that therapy may cause next-day impairment even when used as prescribed. Caution patients taking the 3mg dose against driving and other activities requiring complete mental alertness the day after use; inform that impairment may be present despite feeling fully awake. Advise to seek medical attention immediately if any adverse reactions (eg, severe anaphylactic/anaphylactoid reactions, sleep-driving, other complex behaviors) develop. Advise to immediately report any suicidal thoughts. Advise not to use therapy if patient drank alcohol that pm or hs.

Storage: 25°C (77°F); excursions permitted to 15-30°C (59-86°F).

LUXIQ – betamethasone valerate RX

Class: Corticosteroid

ADULT DOSAGE

Inflammatory and Pruritic Manifestations of Corticosteroid-Responsive Dermatoses

Apply small amounts to affected scalp area bid (am and pm)

D/C when control is achieved

Reassess diagnosis if no improvement w/in 2 weeks

PEDIATRIC DOSAGE

Pediatric use may not have been established

ADMINISTRATION

Topical Route

Avoid use w/ occlusive dressing unless directed

Application

Invert can and dispense a small amount of foam onto a saucer or other cool surface; do not dispense directly onto hands as foam will begin to melt immediately upon contact w/ warm skin

Pick up small amounts of foam w/ fingers and gently massage into affected area until foam disappears

Repeat until entire affected scalp area is treated

HOW SUPPLIED

Foam: 0.12% [50g, 100g]

WARNINGS/PRECAUTIONS

Systemic absorption may produce reversible hypothalamic-pituitary-adrenal (HPA) axis suppression, manifestations of Cushing's syndrome, hyperglycemia, and glucosuria. Evaluate periodically for evidence of HPA axis suppression when applying to large surface area or to areas under occlusion; d/c treatment, reduce frequency of application, or substitute a less potent steroid if HPA axis suppression is noted. D/C and institute appropriate therapy if irritation develops. Use appropriate antifungal or antibacterial agent in the presence of dermatological infections; if favorable response does not occur promptly, d/c until infection is controlled. Pediatric patients may be more susceptible to systemic toxicity from equivalent doses.

ADVERSE REACTIONS

Application-site burning/itching/stinging.

NURSING CONSIDERATIONS

Assessment: Assess for hypersensitivity to the drug, dermatological infections, and pregnancy/nursing status.

Monitoring: Monitor for signs/symptoms of HPA axis suppression, Cushing's syndrome, hyperglycemia, glucosuria, skin irritation, allergic contact dermatitis, and other adverse reactions. Monitor for signs of glucocorticosteroid insufficiency after withdrawal. Monitor clinical improvement; if no improvement seen within 2 weeks, reassess diagnosis.

Patient Counseling: Advise to use externally and ud, to avoid contact with eyes, and not to use for any disorder other than that for which it was prescribed. Instruct not to bandage, cover, or wrap treated scalp area unless directed by physician. Advise to report any signs of local adverse reactions to physician. Advise to d/c use when control is achieved, and to notify physician if no improvement is seen within 2 weeks. Instruct to avoid fire, flame, or smoking during and immediately following application.

Storage: 20-25°C (68-77°F). Do not expose to heat or store at >49°C (120°F).

Luzu – luliconazole RX

Class: Azole antifungal

ADULT DOSAGE

Fungal Infections

Caused by *Trichophyton rubrum* and *Epidermophyton floccosum*:

≥18 Years:

Interdigital Tinea Pedis:
Apply a thin layer to affected area and approximately 1 inch of the immediate surrounding area(s) qd for 2 weeks

Tinea Cruris/Tinea Corporis:
Apply to the affected area and approximately 1 inch of the immediate surrounding area(s) qd for 1 week

PEDIATRIC DOSAGE

Pediatric use may not have been established

ADMINISTRATION

Topical route

HOW SUPPLIED

Cre: 1% [60g]

ADVERSE REACTIONS

Application-site reactions.

DRUG INTERACTIONS

May inhibit the activity of CYP2C19 and CYP3A4.

NURSING CONSIDERATIONS

Assessment: Assess pregnancy/nursing status and for possible drug interactions.

Monitoring: Monitor for application-site reactions and other adverse reactions.

Patient Counseling: Instruct to use ud. Inform that the product is for topical use only and not intended for intravaginal or ophthalmic use.

Storage: 20-25°C (68-77°F); excursions permitted from 15-30°C (59-86°F).

LYRICA – pregabalin CV

Class: GABA analogue

ADULT DOSAGE

Neuropathic Pain

Associated w/ Diabetic Peripheral Neuropathy:
Initial: 50mg tid (150mg/day)
Titrate: May increase to 300mg/day w/in 1 week prn
Max: 100mg tid (300mg/day)

Associated w/ Spinal Cord Injury:
Initial: 75mg bid
Titrate: May increase to 150mg bid (300mg/day) w/in 1 week prn
Max: 300mg bid (600mg/day) if no sufficient pain relief experienced following 2-3 weeks of treatment w/ 150mg bid

Postherpetic Neuralgia
Initial: 75mg bid or 50mg tid (150mg/day)
Titrate: May increase to 300mg/day w/in 1 week prn
Max: 600mg/day divided bid or tid if no sufficient pain relief experienced following 2-4 weeks of treatment w/ 300mg/day

Partial Onset Seizures

Adjunctive Therapy:
Initial: 150mg/day divided bid-tid
Titrate: May increase up to max dose of 600mg/day

Fibromyalgia
Initial: 75mg bid
Titrate: May increase to 150mg bid (300mg/day) w/in 1 week prn
Max: 225mg bid (450mg/day)

PEDIATRIC DOSAGE

Pediatric use may not have been established

DOSE MODIFICATION

Renal Impairment

Recommended Dose of 150mg/day bid or tid w/ Normal Renal Function:
CrCl 30-60mL/min: 75mg/day bid or tid
CrCl 15-30mL/min: 25-50mg/day qd or bid
CrCl <15mL/min: 25mg/day qd

Recommended Dose of 300mg/day bid or tid w/ Normal Renal Function:
CrCl 30-60mL/min: 150mg/day bid or tid
CrCl 15-30mL/min: 75mg/day qd or bid
CrCl <15mL/min: 25-50mg/day qd

Recommended Dose of 450mg/day bid or tid w/ Normal Renal Function:
CrCl 30-60mL/min: 225mg/day bid or tid
CrCl 15-30mL/min: 100-150mg/day qd or bid
CrCl <15mL/min: 50-75mg/day qd

Recommended Dose of 600mg/day bid or tid w/ Normal Renal Function:
CrCl 30-60mL/min: 300mg/day bid or tid
CrCl 15-30mL/min: 150mg/day qd or bid
CrCl <15mL/min: 75mg/day qd

Hemodialysis:
25mg qd Regimen: Take 1 supplemental dose of 25mg or 50mg
25-50mg qd Regimen: Take 1 supplemental dose of 50mg or 75mg
50-75mg qd Regimen: Take 1 supplemental dose of 75mg or 100mg
75mg qd Regimen: Take 1 supplemental dose of 100mg or 150mg

Discontinuation
Taper over minimum of 1 week

ADMINISTRATION
Oral route

HOW SUPPLIED

Cap: 25mg, 50mg, 75mg, 100mg, 150mg, 200mg, 225mg, 300mg; Sol: 20mg/mL [16 fl oz]

WARNINGS/PRECAUTIONS

Angioedema reported; d/c immediately if symptoms of angioedema with respiratory compromise occur. Caution in patients who had a previous episode of angioedema. Hypersensitivity reactions reported; d/c immediately if symptoms occur. Avoid abrupt withdrawal; gradually taper over a minimum of 1 week. Increased risk of suicidal thoughts/behavior; monitor for emergence or worsening of depression, suicidal thought/behavior, and/or unusual changes in mood/behavior. May cause weight gain and peripheral edema; caution with CHF. May cause dizziness and somnolence; may impair physical/mental abilities. New or worsening of preexisting tumors reported. Blurred vision, decreased visual acuity, visual field changes, and funduscopic changes reported. Creatine kinase (CK) elevations and rhabdomyolysis reported; d/c if myopathy is diagnosed or suspected or if markedly elevated CK levels occur. Associated with a decrease in platelet counts and PR interval prolongation. Caution in patients with renal impairment.

ADVERSE REACTIONS

Somnolence, dizziness, peripheral edema, ataxia, weight gain, dry mouth, fatigue, asthenia, blurred vision, diplopia, edema, nasopharyngitis, constipation, abnormal thinking, tremor.

DRUG INTERACTIONS

May increase risk of angioedema with other drugs associated with angioedema (eg, ACE inhibitors). Additive effects on cognitive and gross motor functioning with oxycodone, lorazepam, and ethanol. Caution with thiazolidinedione class of antidiabetic drugs; higher frequencies of weight gain and peripheral edema reported. Gabapentin reported to cause a small reduction in absorption rate. Reduced lower GI tract function (eg, intestinal obstruction, paralytic ileus, constipation) reported with medications that have the potential to produce constipation, such as opioid analgesics.

NURSING CONSIDERATIONS

Assessment: Assess for hypersensitivity, renal impairment, preexisting tumors, history of drug abuse, history of depression, previous episode of angioedema, CHF, pregnancy/nursing status, and possible drug interactions. Obtain baseline weight.

Monitoring: Monitor for angioedema, hypersensitivity reactions, peripheral edema, weight gain, new tumors or worsening of preexisting tumors, ophthalmological effects, rhabdomyolysis, dizziness, somnolence, emergence or worsening of depression, suicidal thoughts or behavior, and/or changes in behavior. Monitor CK levels and platelet counts. Monitor ECG for PR interval prolongation.

Patient Counseling: Instruct to d/c therapy and seek medical attention if hypersensitivity reactions or symptoms of angioedema occur. Inform patients and caregivers to be alert for the emergence or worsening of depression, unusual changes in mood or behavior, or the emergence of suicidal thoughts or behavior; immediately report behaviors of concern to physician. Counsel that dizziness, somnolence, blurred vision, and other CNS signs and symptoms may occur; advise to use caution when operating machinery/driving. Inform that weight gain and edema may occur. Instruct not to abruptly/rapidly d/c therapy. Instruct to report unexplained muscle pain, tenderness, or weakness, particularly if accompanied by malaise or fever, to physician. Instruct not to consume alcohol while on therapy. Instruct to notify physician if pregnant, intending to become pregnant, breastfeeding or intending to breastfeed. Inform men on therapy who plan to father a child of the potential risk of male-mediated teratogenicity. Instruct diabetic patients to pay attention to skin integrity while on therapy.

Storage: 25°C (77°F); excursions permitted to 15-30°C (59-86°F).

MACROBID – nitrofurantoin macrocrystals/nitrofurantoin monohydrate RX

Class: Imidazolidinedione antibacterial

ADULT DOSAGE

Urinary Tract Infections

Caused by susceptible strains of *Escherichia coli* or *Staphylococcus saprophyticus*

Acute Uncomplicated (Acute Cystitis): 100mg q12h for 7 days

PEDIATRIC DOSAGE

Urinary Tract Infections

Caused by susceptible strains of *Escherichia coli* or *Staphylococcus saprophyticus*

>12 Years:

Acute Uncomplicated (Acute Cystitis): 100mg q12h for 7 days

ADMINISTRATION

Oral route

Take with food

HOW SUPPLIED

Cap: 100mg

CONTRAINDICATIONS

Anuria, oliguria, significant impairment of renal function (CrCl <60mL/min or clinically significant elevated SrCr), pregnancy at term (38-42 weeks' gestation), during labor and delivery or when onset of labor is imminent, and neonates <1 month of age, and previous history of cholestatic jaundice/hepatic dysfunction associated with nitrofurantoin.

WARNINGS/PRECAUTIONS

Not for treatment of pyelonephritis or perinephric abscesses. Many patients who undergo treatment are predisposed to persistence/reappearance of bacteriuria; if this occurs after treatment, select other therapeutic agents with broader tissue distribution. Acute, subacute, or chronic pulmonary reactions (diffuse interstitial pneumonitis, pulmonary fibrosis, or both) reported; d/c and take appropriate measures if these occur. Closely monitor pulmonary condition if on long-term therapy. Hepatic reactions (eg, hepatitis, cholestatic jaundice, chronic active hepatitis, hepatic necrosis) occur rarely. Monitor periodically for changes in biochemical tests that would indicate liver injury; withdraw immediately and take appropriate measures if hepatitis occurs. Peripheral neuropathy, which may become severe or irreversible, reported; risk may be enhanced with renal impairment, anemia, diabetes mellitus (DM), electrolyte imbalance, vitamin B deficiency, and debilitating disease. Monitor periodically for renal function changes with long-term therapy. Optic neuritis reported rarely. May induce hemolytic anemia of the primaquine-sensitivity type; d/c therapy if hemolysis occurs. *Clostridium difficile*-associated diarrhea (CDAD) reported; d/c therapy is CDAD is suspected/confirmed. Use in the absence of a proven or strongly suspected bacterial infection or prophylactic indication is unlikely to provide benefit and increases the risk of the development of drug-resistant bacteria. Lab test interactions may occur. Caution with impaired renal function and in elderly.

ADVERSE REACTIONS

Nausea, headache.

DRUG INTERACTIONS

Antacids containing magnesium trisilicate reduce both the rate and extent of absorption. Uricosuric drugs (eg, probenecid, sulfinpyrazone) may inhibit renal tubular secretion of nitrofurantoin; resulting increased nitrofurantoin serum levels may increase toxicity, and the decreased urinary levels could lessen its efficacy.

NURSING CONSIDERATIONS

Assessment: Assess for anuria, oliguria, significant renal impairment, history of cholestatic jaundice/hepatic dysfunction associated with nitrofurantoin, G6PD deficiency, DM, anemia, electrolyte imbalance, vitamin B deficiency, debilitating disease, drug hypersensitivity, pregnancy/nursing status, and possible drug interactions. Obtain urine specimens for culture and susceptibility testing prior to therapy.

Monitoring: Monitor for persistence or reappearance of bacteriuria, acute/subacute/chronic pulmonary reactions, hepatic reactions, peripheral neuropathy, optic neuritis, hematologic manifestations, and CDAD. Monitor LFTs periodically. Monitor renal and pulmonary function periodically during long-term therapy. Obtain urine specimens for culture and susceptibility testing after completion of therapy.

Patient Counseling: Inform of the potential risks and benefits of therapy. Advise to take with food (ideally breakfast and dinner) to further enhance tolerance and improve drug absorption. Instruct to complete the full course of therapy and advise to contact physician if any unusual symptoms occur during therapy. Advise not to take antacids containing magnesium trisilicate while on therapy. Inform that therapy treats bacterial, not viral, infections. Advise to take exactly ud; skipping doses or not completing full course may decrease effectiveness and increase drug resistance. Inform that diarrhea is a common problem that usually ends when antibiotic is discontinued. Inform that watery and bloody stools (with/without stomach cramps and fever) may develop even as late as 2 or more months after having taken the last dose; instruct to contact physician as soon as possible if this occurs.

Storage: 15-30°C (59-86°F).

MACRODANTIN – nitrofurantoin macrocrystals RX

Class: Imidazolidinedione antibacterial

ADULT DOSAGE

Urinary Tract Infections

Due to susceptible *Escherichia coli*, enterococci, *Staphylococcus aureus*, and certain susceptible Klebsiella and *Enterobacter* species

PEDIATRIC DOSAGE

Urinary Tract Infections

Due to susceptible *E. coli*, enterococci, *S. aureus*, and certain susceptible *Klebsiella* and *Enterobacter* species

Usual: 50-100mg qid for 1 week or for at least 3 days after sterility of the urine obtained

Long-Term Suppressive Therapy:
Reduce dose to 50-100mg qhs

≥1 Month of Age:
Usual: 5-7mg/kg/day given in 4 divided doses for 1 week or for at least 3 days after sterility of the urine obtained

Long-Term Suppressive Therapy:
1mg/kg/day given in a single dose or in 2 divided doses

ADMINISTRATION
Oral route

Take with food

HOW SUPPLIED
Cap: 25mg, 50mg, 100mg

CONTRAINDICATIONS
Anuria, oliguria, significant impairment of renal function (CrCl <60mL/min or clinically significant elevated SrCr), pregnancy at term (38-42 weeks' gestation), during labor and delivery, or when the onset of labor is imminent, neonates <1 month of age, and previous history of cholestatic jaundice/hepatic dysfunction associated with nitrofurantoin.

WARNINGS/PRECAUTIONS
Not for the treatment of pyelonephritis or perinephric abscesses. Many patients who undergo treatment are predisposed to persistence/reappearance of bacteriuria; if this occurs after treatment, select other therapeutic agents with broader tissue distribution. Acute, subacute, or chronic pulmonary reactions (diffuse interstitial pneumonitis, pulmonary fibrosis, or both) reported; d/c and take appropriate measures if these occur. Closely monitor pulmonary condition if on long-term therapy. Hepatic reactions (eg, hepatitis, cholestatic jaundice, chronic active hepatitis, hepatic necrosis) occur rarely. Monitor periodically for changes in biochemical tests that would indicate liver injury; withdraw immediately and take appropriate measures if hepatitis occurs. Peripheral neuropathy, which may become severe or irreversible, reported; risk may be enhanced with renal impairment, anemia, diabetes mellitus (DM), electrolyte imbalance, vitamin B deficiency, and debilitating disease. Monitor periodically for renal function changes with long-term therapy. Optic neuritis reported rarely. May induced hemolytic anemia of the primaquine-sensitivity type; d/c therapy if hemolysis occurs. *Clostridium difficile*-associated diarrhea (CDAD) reported; d/c therapy if CDAD is suspected/confirmed. Use in the absence of a proven or strongly suspected bacterial infection or prophylactic indication is unlikely to provide benefit and increases the risk of the development of drug-resistant bacteria. Lab test interactions may occur. Caution with impaired renal function and in elderly.

ADVERSE REACTIONS
Pulmonary hypersensitivity reactions, hepatic reactions, peripheral neuropathy, exfoliative dermatitis, erythema multiforme, lupus-like syndrome, nausea, emesis, anorexia, asthenia, vertigo, nystagmus, dizziness, headache, drowsiness.

DRUG INTERACTIONS
Antacids containing magnesium trisilicate reduce both the rate and extent of absorption. Uricosuric drugs (eg, probenecid, sulfinpyrazone) may inhibit renal tubular secretion of nitrofurantoin; resulting increased nitrofurantoin serum levels may increase toxicity, and the decreased urinary levels could lessen its efficacy.

NURSING CONSIDERATIONS

Assessment: Assess for anuria, oliguria, significant renal impairment, history of cholestatic jaundice/hepatic dysfunction associated with nitrofurantoin, G6PD deficiency, DM, anemia, electrolyte imbalance, vitamin B deficiency, debilitating disease, drug hypersensitivity, pregnancy/nursing status, and possible drug interactions. Obtain urine specimen for culture and susceptibility testing prior to therapy.

Monitoring: Monitor for persistence or reappearance of bacteriuria, acute/subacute/chronic pulmonary reactions, hepatic reactions, peripheral neuropathy, optic neuritis, hematologic manifestations, and CDAD. Monitor LFTs periodically. Monitor renal and pulmonary function periodically during long-term therapy. Obtain urine specimens for culture and susceptibility testing after completion of therapy.

Patient Counseling: Inform of the potential risks and benefits of therapy. Advise to take with food to further enhance tolerance and improve drug absorption. Instruct to complete full course of therapy and advise to contact physician if any unusual symptoms occur during therapy. Advise not to take antacid preparations containing magnesium trisilicate while on therapy. Inform that therapy treats bacterial, not viral, infections. Advise to take exactly ud; skipping doses or not completing full course may decrease effectiveness and increase drug resistance. Inform that diarrhea is a common problem that usually ends when antibiotic is discontinued. Inform that watery and bloody stools (with/without stomach cramps and fever) may develop even as late as ≥2 months after having taken the last dose; instruct to contact physician as soon as possible if this occurs.

Storage: 20-25°C (68-77°F).

MAXALT – rizatriptan benzoate

RX

Class: 5-$HT_{1B/1D}$ agonist

OTHER BRAND NAMES
Maxalt-MLT

ADULT DOSAGE
Migraine
W/ or w/o Aura:
Usual: 5mg or 10mg single dose; separate repeat doses by at least 2 hrs if migraine returns
Max: 30mg/24 hrs

PEDIATRIC DOSAGE
Migraine
W/ or w/o Aura:
6-17 Years:
<40kg:
Usual: 5mg single dose
≥40kg:
Usual: 10mg single dose

DOSE MODIFICATION
Concomitant Medications
Propranolol:
6-17 Years:
≥40kg:
Usual: 5mg single dose
Max: 5mg/24 hrs
≥18 Years:
Usual: 5mg single dose
Max: 3 doses/24 hrs
Elderly
Start at lower end of dosing range

ADMINISTRATION
Oral route
Tab, Disintegrating
Do not remove blister from outer pouch until just prior to dosing
Peel open w/ dry hands and place tab on tongue, where it will dissolve and be swallowed w/ saliva

HOW SUPPLIED
Tab: 5mg, 10mg; Tab, Disintegrating: (MLT) 5mg, 10mg

CONTRAINDICATIONS
Ischemic coronary artery disease (CAD) (angina pectoris, history of MI, or documented silent ischemia) or other significant underlying cardiovascular (CV) disease, coronary artery vasospasm (eg, Prinzmetal's angina), history of stroke or transient ischemic attack (TIA), peripheral vascular disease (PVD), ischemic bowel disease, uncontrolled HTN, hemiplegic/basilar migraine. Recent use (within 24 hrs) of another 5-HT_1 agonist or ergotamine-containing/ergot-type medication (eg, dihydroergotamine, methysergide). Concurrent use or recent discontinuation (within 2 weeks) of an MAO-A inhibitor.

WARNINGS/PRECAUTIONS
Use only when diagnosis of migraine has been clearly established. If no response after the 1st migraine attack, reconsider diagnosis before treating subsequent attacks. Not indicated for prevention of migraine attacks. Serious cardiac adverse reactions, including acute MI, reported. May cause coronary artery vasospasm (Prinzmetal's angina). Perform CV evaluation prior to therapy with multiple CV risk factors; consider administering 1st dose in a medically supervised setting and perform ECG immediately following administration in patients with a negative CV evaluation. Consider periodic CV evaluation in intermittent long-term users who have CV risk factors. Life-threatening cardiac rhythm disturbances (eg, ventricular tachycardia/fibrillation leading to death) reported; d/c if these occur. Sensations of tightness, pain, pressure, and heaviness in precordium, throat, neck, and jaw, usually of noncardiac origin, commonly occur after treatment; evaluate if cardiac origin is suspected. Cerebral/subarachnoid hemorrhage and stroke reported; d/c if cerebrovascular event occurs. Evaluate for other potentially serious neurological conditions before treatment. May cause noncoronary vasospastic reactions (eg, peripheral vascular ischemia, GI vascular ischemia, splenic infarction, Raynaud's syndrome); rule out before administering additional doses if experiencing signs/symptoms of noncoronary vasospasms. Transient and permanent blindness and significant partial vision loss reported. Overuse of acute migraine drugs may lead to exacerbation of headache (medication overuse headache); detoxification, including withdrawal of the overused drugs, and treatment of withdrawal symptoms may be necessary. Serotonin syndrome may occur; d/c if serotonin syndrome is suspected. Significant elevation in BP, including hypertensive crisis with acute impairment of organ systems, reported. Caution in elderly. (Tab, Disintegrating) Contains phenylalanine.

ADVERSE REACTIONS

Paresthesia, dry mouth, nausea, dizziness, somnolence, asthenia/fatigue, pain/pressure sensation.

DRUG INTERACTIONS

See Contraindications. Increased plasma area under the curve with propranolol; adjust dose. Serotonin syndrome reported with SSRIs, SNRIs, and TCAs.

NURSING CONSIDERATIONS

Assessment: Assess for ischemic CAD or other significant underlying CV disease, history of stroke or TIA, PVD, ischemic bowel disease, uncontrolled HTN, hemiplegic/basilar migraine, neurological conditions, phenylketonuria, drug hypersensitivity, pregnancy/nursing status, and possible drug interactions. Perform CV evaluation with multiple CV risk factors.

Monitoring: Monitor for coronary artery vasospasm, cardiac rhythm disturbances, cerebrovascular event, noncoronary vasospastic reactions, serotonin syndrome, BP elevation, and other adverse reactions. Consider periodic CV evaluation in intermittent long-term users who have CV risk factors.

Patient Counseling: Inform of possible serious CV side effects, including chest pain, SOB, weakness, and slurring of speech, and to seek medical advice in the presence of such symptoms. Caution about the risk of serotonin syndrome. Advise to notify physician if pregnant, breastfeeding, or planning to breastfeed. Instruct to evaluate their ability to perform complex tasks during migraine attacks and after administration. Inform that overuse (≥10 days/month) may lead to exacerbation of headache; encourage to record headache frequency and drug use. (Tab, Disintegrating) Inform phenylketonuric patients that tab contains phenylalanine.

Storage: 15-30°C (59-86°F).

MAXIPIME – cefepime hydrochloride RX

Class: Cephalosporin (4th generation)

ADULT DOSAGE

Pneumonia

Pneumonia due to *Streptococcus pneumoniae* (including cases associated w/ concurrent bacteremia), *Klebsiella pneumoniae*, or *Enterobacter* species
Moderate to Severe: 1-2g IV q8-12h for 10 days
***Pseudomonas aeruginosa* Infections:** 2g IV q8h

Febrile Neutropenia

Empiric Therapy:
Usual: 2g IV q8h for 7 days or until neutropenia resolves
Reevaluate frequently the need for continued antimicrobial therapy in patients whose fever resolves but remain neutropenic for >7 days

Urinary Tract Infections

Uncomplicated or Complicated Infections, Including Pyelonephritis and Cases Associated w/ Concurrent Bacteremia:
Mild to Moderate Infections Due to *Escherichia coli, Klebsiella pneumoniae*, or *Proteus mirabilis*:
Usual: 0.5-1g IM/IV q12h for 7-10 days
IM administration is only for infections due to *E. coli* when IM route is considered more appropriate
Severe Infections Due to *E. coli* or *K. pneumoniae*:
Usual: 2g IV q12h for 10 days

Skin and Skin Structure Infections

Uncomplicated Infections Due to *Staphylococcus aureus* or *Streptococcus pyogenes*:
Moderate to Severe:
Usual: 2g IV q12h for 10 days

PEDIATRIC DOSAGE

Urinary Tract Infections

Uncomplicated or Complicated Infections, Including Pyelonephritis and Cases Associated w/ Concurrent Bacteremia:
2 Months-16 Years:
Up to 40kg:
Mild to Moderate Infections Due to *Escherichia coli, Klebsiella pneumoniae*, or *Proteus mirabilis*: 50mg/kg q12h IV/IM for 7-10 days
IM administration is only for infections due to *E. coli* when IM route is considered more appropriate
Severe Infections Due to *E. coli* or *K. pneumoniae*: 50mg/kg q12h IV for 10 days
Max: Do not exceed the recommended adult dose

Skin and Skin Structure Infections

Uncomplicated Infections Due to *Staphylococcus aureus* or *Streptococcus pyogenes*:
2 Months-16 Years:
Up to 40kg:
Moderate to Severe: 50mg/kg q12h for 10 days
Max: Do not exceed the recommended adult dose

Pneumonia

Pneumonia due to *Streptococcus pneumoniae* (including cases associated w/ concurrent bacteremia), *Pseudomonas aeruginosa*, *Klebsiella pneumoniae*, or *Enterobacter* species
2 Months-16 Years:
Up to 40kg:
Moderate to Severe: 50mg/kg/dose q12h for 10 days

Intra-Abdominal Infections

Complicated infections due to *Escherichia coli*, viridans group streptococci, *Klebsiella pneumoniae*, *Enterobacter* species, or *Bacteroides fragilis*
2g IV q8-12h for 7-10 days in combination w/ metronidazole
***Pseudomonas aeruginosa* Infections:** 2g IV q8h

***Pseudomonas aeruginosa* Infections:** 50mg/kg/dose q8h for 10 days
Max: Do not exceed the recommended adult dose

Febrile Neutropenia

Empiric Therapy:
2 Months-16 Years:
Up to 40kg:
50mg/kg q8h for 7 days
Max: Do not exceed the recommended adult dose
Reevaluate frequently the need for continued antimicrobial therapy in patients whose fever resolves but remain neutropenic for >7 days

DOSE MODIFICATION
Renal Impairment
Adults:
Recommended maint dose of 500mg q12h:
CrCl 11-60mL/min: 500mg q24h
CrCl <11mL/min: 250mg q24h
Recommended maint dose of 1g q12h:
CrCl 30-60mL/min: 1g q24h
CrCl 11-29mL/min: 500mg q24h
CrCl <11mL/min: 250mg q24h
Recommended maint dose of 2g q12h:
CrCl 30-60mL/min: 2g q24h
CrCl 11-29mL/min: 1g q24h
CrCl <11mL/min: 500mg q24h
Recommended maint dose of 2g q8h:
CrCl 30-60mL/min: 2g q12h
CrCl 11-29mL/min: 2g q24h
CrCl <11mL/min: 1g q24h
Continuous Ambulatory Peritoneal Dialysis: Receive normal recommended doses q48h
Hemodialysis:
Administer at the same time each day and following the completion of hemodialysis on hemodialysis days
All Infections Except Febrile Neutropenia: 1g on Day 1, then 500mg q24h thereafter
Febrile Neutropenia: 1g q24h
Pediatrics:
Changes in dosing regimen proportional to those in adults are recommended

ADMINISTRATION
IV/IM route
Preparation
Reconstitute 500mg single-dose vial w/ 5mL (for IV administration) or 1.3mL (for IM administration) of diluent
Reconstitute 1g single dose vial w/ 10mL (for IV administration) or 2.4mL (for IM administration) of diluent
Reconstitute 2g single vial dose w/ 10mL (for IV administration) of diluent
Reconstitute ADD-Vantage vials only w/ 50mL or 100mL of D5 inj or 0.9% NaCl inj in ADD-Vantage flexible diluent containers
IV
Dilute w/ suitable parenteral vehicle and administer resulting sol over 30 min
May administer intermittent IV infusion w/ a Y-type administration set w/ compatible sol; however, desirable to d/c other sol when infusing sol containing cefepime HCl
Compatible at concentrations between 1-40mg/mL w/ 0.9% NaCl, D5 and D10 inj, M/6 Sodium Lactate inj, D5 and 0.9% NaCl inj, Lactated Ringer's and D5 inj, Normosol-R, and Normosol-M in D5 inj
May store up to 24 hrs at room temperature (20-25°C [68-77°F]) or 7 days in a refrigerator (2-8°C [36-46°F])
ADD-Vantage vials are stable at concentrations between 10-40mg/mL in D5 inj or 0.9% NaCl inj for 24 hrs room temperature (20-25°C [68-77°F]) or 7 days in a refrigerator (2-8°C [36-46°F])
IM
Constitute w/ sterile water for inj, 0.9% NaCl, D5 inj, 0.5% or 1% lidocaine HCl, or sterile bacteriostatic water for inj (w/ parabens or benzyl alcohol)
Constituted sol is stable for 24 hrs at room temperature (20-25°C [68-77°F]) or 7 days in a refrigerator (2-8°C [36-46°F])

Refer to PI for Instructions for Use

HOW SUPPLIED

Inj: 500mg, 1g, 2g

WARNINGS/PRECAUTIONS

Cross-hypersensitivity among β-lactam antibiotics reported; caution in penicillin (PCN)-sensitive patients. D/C if an allergic reaction occurs. Serious adverse reactions reported including life-threatening or fatal occurrences of encephalopathy, myoclonus, seizures, and nonconvulsive status epilepticus. If neurotoxicity associated w/ therapy occurs, consider discontinuation of therapy or make appropriate dose adjustments in patients w/ renal impairment. *Clostridium difficile*-associated diarrhea (CDAD) reported; d/c if CDAD is suspected or confirmed. May result in overgrowth of nonsusceptible organisms w/ prolonged use; take appropriate measures if superinfection develops. Use in the absence of a proven or strongly suspected bacterial infection or a prophylactic indication is unlikely to provide benefit and increases the risk of development of drug-resistant bacteria. May be associated w/ a fall in prothrombin activity; monitor PT in patients at risk (eg, patients w/ renal/hepatic impairment, poor nutritional state, receiving a protracted course of antimicrobial therapy) and administer exogenous vitamin K as indicated. Caution w/ history of GI disease, particularly colitis, renal impairment, and in elderly. Lab test interactions may occur.

ADVERSE REACTIONS

Local reactions, rash, diarrhea, (+) Coombs' test w/o hemolysis.

DRUG INTERACTIONS

Increased potential of nephrotoxicity and ototoxicity w/ high doses of aminoglycosides; monitor renal function. Nephrotoxicity reported w/ potent diuretics (eg, furosemide).

NURSING CONSIDERATIONS

Assessment: Assess for hypersensitivity to drug, cephalosporins, PCNs, or other β-lactam antibiotics, poor nutritional status, history of GI disease, renal/hepatic impairment, pregnancy/nursing status, and possible drug interactions. Perform culture and susceptibility testing.

Monitoring: Monitor for signs/symptoms of hypersensitivity reactions, CDAD, superinfection, encephalopathy, myoclonus, seizures, nonconvulsive status epilepticus, and other adverse reactions. Monitor PT in patients w/ renal/hepatic impairment, poor nutritional state, and in patients receiving a protracted course of antimicrobial therapy.

Patient Counseling: Counsel that therapy should only be used to treat bacterial, not viral infections. Instruct to take exactly ud; inform that skipping doses or not completing the full course of therapy may decrease effectiveness of immediate treatment and increase bacterial resistance. Inform that diarrhea may occur and will usually end if therapy is discontinued. Instruct to contact physician as soon as possible if watery/bloody stools (w/ or w/o stomach cramps, fever) develop even as late as 2 or more months after the last dose. Advise that neurological adverse events may occur; instruct to inform physician at once of any neurological signs and symptoms, including encephalopathy, myoclonus, seizures and nonconvulsive status epilepticus, for immediate treatment, dosage adjustment, or discontinuation of therapy.

Storage: Dry State: 20-25°C (68-77°F). Protect from light.

MAXITROL — dexamethasone/neomycin sulfate/polymyxin B sulfate **RX**

Class: Antibacterial/corticosteroid combination

ADULT DOSAGE

Steroid-Responsive Inflammatory Ocular Conditions

For which a corticosteroid is indicated and where bacterial infection or risk of bacterial infection exists

Oint:

Apply small amount (1/2 inch) in conjunctival sac(s) up to 3-4 times daily

Not more than 8g should be prescribed initially

Sus:

Instill 1-2 drops in conjunctival sac(s) up to 4-6 times daily in mild disease and hourly in severe disease; taper to d/c as inflammation subsides

Not more than 20mL should be prescribed initially

PEDIATRIC DOSAGE

Steroid-Responsive Inflammatory Ocular Conditions

For which a corticosteroid is indicated and where bacterial infection or risk of bacterial infection exists

Sus:

≥2 Years:

Instill 1-2 drops in conjunctival sac(s) up to 4-6 times daily in mild disease and hourly in severe disease; taper to d/c as inflammation subsides

Not more than 20mL should be prescribed initially

ADMINISTRATION
Ocular route

Oint
Tilt head back. Place finger on cheek just under the eye and gently pull down until a "V" pocket is formed between eyeball and lower lid. Place small amount of oint in the "V" pocket. Look downward before closing eye

HOW SUPPLIED
Oint: (Dexamethasone-Neomycin Sulfate-Polymyxin Sulfate) 0.1%-3.5mg-10,000 U/g [3.5g]; Sus: (Dexamethasone-Neomycin Sulfate-Polymyxin Sulfate) 0.1%-3.5mg-10,000 U/mL [5mL]

CONTRAINDICATIONS
Epithelial herpes simplex keratitis (dendritic keratitis), vaccinia, varicella, and other viral diseases of the cornea and conjunctiva, mycobacterial infection of the eye, fungal diseases of ocular structures.

WARNINGS/PRECAUTIONS
For topical ophthalmic use only. Prolonged use may cause glaucoma with damage to the optic nerve, defects in visual acuity and fields of vision, posterior subcapsular cataract formation, suppressed host response, increased risk of secondary ocular infections, or persistent corneal fungal infections. May cause perforations when used with diseases causing thinning of cornea or sclera. May mask infection or enhance existing infection in acute purulent conditions of the eye. Monitor intraocular pressure (IOP) if used for ≥10 days. May cause cutaneous sensitization. Caution in the treatment of herpes simplex. Perform eye exam prior to therapy and renewal of medication. (Sus) Usage after cataract surgery may delay healing and increase incidence of bleb formation. May prolong course and exacerbate severity of ocular viral infections (eg, herpes simplex). Do not inject subconjunctivally, nor directly introduce into anterior chamber of the eye. Reevaluate patient if no improvement seen after 2 days. Suspect fungal invasion in any persistent corneal ulceration during or after therapy; take fungal cultures when appropriate.

ADVERSE REACTIONS
Allergic sensitizations, elevated IOP, posterior subcapsular cataract formation, delayed wound healing, secondary infections.

NURSING CONSIDERATIONS

Assessment: Assess for active viral diseases of the cornea and conjunctiva, epithelial herpes simplex keratitis, vaccinia, varicella, mycobacterial infection of the eye, fungal disease of ocular structures, diseases causing thinning of sclera or cornea, acute purulent conditions, history of cataract surgery, hypersensitivity to the drug or its components, and pregnancy/nursing status. Perform eye exam (eg, slit-lamp biomicroscopy, fluorescein staining) prior to therapy.

Monitoring: Monitor for signs/symptoms of glaucoma, optic nerve damage, visual acuity and visual field defects, subcapsular cataract, ocular/corneal perforations, cutaneous sensitizations, and for bacterial, viral, and fungal infections. Monitor IOP and perform eye exams (eg, slit-lamp biomicroscopy, fluorescein staining) prior to renewal of medication. (Sus) Monitor use after cataract surgery. Perform fungal cultures when fungal invasion is suspected.

Patient Counseling: Advise not to touch dropper tip to any surface; may contaminate drug. Instruct to keep out of reach of children. Instruct to use medication as prescribed. Inform that medication is for topical ophthalmic use only. Instruct to inform physician if pregnant or breastfeeding. (Oint) Advise not to wear contact lenses if signs and symptoms of bacterial ocular infection are present. Instruct not to use product if the imprinted carton seals have been damaged or removed. (Sus) Advise to d/c and consult physician if inflammation or pain persists >48 hrs or becomes aggravated. Warn that use of the same bottle by more than one person may spread infection. Instruct to shake well before use and keep bottle tightly closed when not in use.

Storage: (Oint) 2-25°C (36-77°F). (Sus) 8-27°C (46-80°F). Store upright.

MAXZIDE – hydrochlorothiazide/triamterene — RX

Class: K^+-sparing diuretic/thiazide diuretic

Abnormal elevation of serum K^+ levels (≥5.5mEq/L) may occur with all K^+-sparing diuretic combinations. Hyperkalemia is more likely to occur with renal impairment and diabetes (even without evidence of renal impairment), and in elderly or severely ill; monitor serum K^+ levels at frequent intervals.

OTHER BRAND NAMES
Maxzide-25

ADULT DOSAGE

Hypertension

Treatment when hypokalemia occurs on HCTZ alone, or when a thiazide diuretic is required and cannot risk hypokalemia

Maxzide-25:
1-2 tabs qd, given as a single dose

Maxzide:
1 tab qd

Edema

Treatment when hypokalemia occurs on HCTZ alone, or when a thiazide diuretic is required and cannot risk hypokalemia

Maxzide-25:
1-2 tabs qd, given as a single dose

Maxzide:
1 tab qd

PEDIATRIC DOSAGE

Pediatric use may not have been established

ADMINISTRATION
Oral route

HOW SUPPLIED
Tab: (Triamterene-HCTZ) (Maxzide) 75mg-50mg*, (Maxzide-25) 37.5mg-25mg* *scored

CONTRAINDICATIONS
Elevated serum K^+ (≥5.5mEq/L), anuria, acute or chronic renal insufficiency or significant renal impairment, sulfonamide hypersensitivity, K^+-sparing agents (eg, spironolactone, amiloride, or other formulations containing triamterene), K^+ supplements, K^+ salt substitutes, K^+-enriched diets.

WARNINGS/PRECAUTIONS
Obtain ECG if hyperkalemia is suspected. Avoid in severely ill in whom respiratory or metabolic acidosis may occur; if used, frequent evaluations of acid/base balance and serum electrolytes are necessary. May cause idiosyncratic reaction, resulting in acute transient myopia and acute angle-closure glaucoma; d/c as rapidly as possible. Monitor for fluid/electrolyte imbalances. May manifest latent diabetes mellitus (DM). Caution with hepatic impairment or progressive liver disease; minor alterations in fluid and electrolyte balance may precipitate hepatic coma. May cause hypochloremia. Dilutional hyponatremia may occur in edematous patients in hot weather. Caution with history of renal lithiasis. May increase BUN and SrCr; d/c if azotemia increases. May contribute to megaloblastosis in folic acid deficiency. Hyperuricemia may occur or acute gout may be precipitated. May decrease serum PBI levels. Decreased Ca^{2+} excretion reported. Changes in parathyroid glands with hypercalcemia and hypophosphatemia reported during prolonged use. Sensitivity reactions may occur. May exacerbate or activate systemic lupus erythematosus (SLE). May interfere with the fluorescent measurement of quinidine.

ADVERSE REACTIONS
Hyperkalemia, jaundice, pancreatitis, N/V, taste alteration, drowsiness, dry mouth, depression, anxiety, tachycardia, fluid/electrolyte imbalances.

DRUG INTERACTIONS
See Contraindications. Increased risk of hyperkalemia with ACE inhibitors. Hypokalemia may develop with corticosteroids, adrenocorticotropic hormone, or amphotericin B. Insulin requirements may be increased, decreased, or unchanged. May potentiate other antihypertensives (eg, β-blockers); dosage adjustments may be necessary. Avoid with lithium due to risk of lithium toxicity. Acute renal failure reported with indomethacin; caution with NSAIDs. May increase responsiveness to tubocurarine. May decrease arterial responsiveness to norepinephrine. Alcohol, barbiturates, or narcotics may aggravate orthostatic hypotension. May cause hypokalemia, which can sensitize or exaggerate the response of the heart to the toxic effects of digitalis (eg, increased ventricular irritability).

NURSING CONSIDERATIONS

Assessment: Assess for conditions where treatment is contraindicated or cautioned, DM, risk for respiratory or metabolic acidosis, SLE, pregnancy/nursing status, and for possible drug interactions. Obtain baseline BUN, SrCr, and serum electrolytes.

Monitoring: Monitor for signs/symptoms of hyperkalemia, idiosyncratic reaction, hypokalemia, azotemia, renal stones, hepatic coma, and for fluid/electrolyte imbalances. Monitor BUN, SrCr, and serum K^+ and folic acid levels. Monitor serum and urine electrolytes if vomiting or receiving parenteral fluids.

Patient Counseling: Inform about risks/benefits of therapy. Advise to seek medical attention if symptoms of hyperkalemia, hypokalemia, renal stones, electrolyte imbalance, or hypersensitivity reactions occur. Instruct to notify physician if pregnant/nursing.

Storage: 20-25°C (68-77°F). Protect from light.

MEDROL – methylprednisolone

RX

Class: Glucocorticoid

ADULT DOSAGE

Steroid-Responsive Disorders

Initial: 4-48mg/day, depending on disease and response

Maint: Decrease dose by small amounts to lowest effective dose

Withdraw gradually after long-term therapy

Acute Exacerbations of Multiple Sclerosis:

200mg/day for 1 week followed by 80mg qod for 1 month

Alternate Day Therapy (ADT):

Twice the usual daily dose administered every other am

Refer to PI for detailed information on ADT

PEDIATRIC DOSAGE

Steroid-Responsive Disorders

Initial: 4-48mg/day, depending on disease and response

Maint: Decrease dose by small amounts to lowest effective dose

Withdraw gradually after long-term therapy

Acute Exacerbations of Multiple Sclerosis:

200mg/day for 1 week followed by 80mg qod for 1 month

ADT:

Twice the usual daily dose administered every other am

Refer to PI for detailed information on ADT

ADMINISTRATION

Oral route

HOW SUPPLIED

Tab: 2mg*, 4mg*, 8mg*, 16mg*, 32mg*; (Dose-Pak) 4mg* [21[s]] *scored

CONTRAINDICATIONS

Systemic fungal infections.

WARNINGS/PRECAUTIONS

May need to increase dose before, during, and after stressful situations. May mask signs of infection or cause new infections. Possible benefits should be weighed against potential hazards if used during pregnancy/nursing. Prolonged use may produce glaucoma, optic nerve damage, and secondary ocular infections. May cause BP elevation, increased K^+ excretion, and salt/water retention. More severe/fatal course of infections reported with chickenpox and measles. Caution with *Strongyloides*, latent tuberculosis (TB), hypothyroidism, cirrhosis, ocular herpes simplex, HTN, diverticulitis, fresh intestinal anastomoses, ulcerative colitis, osteoporosis, myasthenia gravis, renal insufficiency, and peptic ulcer disease. Kaposi's sarcoma reported. Growth and development of children on prolonged therapy should be monitored. Monitor for psychic disturbances. Avoid abrupt withdrawal.

ADVERSE REACTIONS

Fluid and electrolyte disturbances, HTN, osteoporosis, muscle weakness, cushingoid state, menstrual irregularities, impaired wound healing, convulsions, ulcerative esophagitis, excessive sweating, increased intracranial pressure, glaucoma, abdominal distention, headache, decreased carbohydrate tolerance.

DRUG INTERACTIONS

Reduced efficacy with hepatic enzyme inducers (eg, phenobarbital, phenytoin, rifampin). Increases clearance of chronic high-dose aspirin (ASA). Caution with ASA in hypoprothrombinemia. Effects on oral anticoagulants are variable; monitor PT. Increased insulin and oral hypoglycemic requirements in diabetics. Avoid live vaccines with immunosuppressive doses. Possible decreased vaccine response with killed or inactivated vaccines with immunosuppressive doses. Mutual inhibition of metabolism with cyclosporine; convulsions reported. Potentiated by ketoconazole and troleandomycin. Concomitant administration with immunosuppressive agents may be associated with development of infections.

NURSING CONSIDERATIONS

Assessment: Assess for systemic fungal infections, current infections, active TB, vaccination history, ulcerative colitis, diverticulitis, peptic ulcer with impending perforation, renal/hepatic insufficiency, septic arthritis/unstable joint, HTN, osteoporosis, myasthenia gravis, thyroid status, psychotic tendencies, drug hypersensitivity, and possible drug interactions.

Monitoring: Monitor for adrenocortical insufficiency, occurrence of infection, psychic derangement, cataracts, acute myopathy, Kaposi's sarcoma, and fluid retention. Monitor serum electrolytes, TSH, LFTs, intraocular pressure, and BP. Monitor urinalysis, blood sugar, weight, chest x-ray, and upper GI x-ray (if ulcer history) regularly during prolonged therapy. Monitor growth and development of infants and children on prolonged corticosteroids therapy.

Patient Counseling: Advise not to d/c abruptly or without medical supervision. Inform that susceptibility to infections may increase. Instruct to avoid exposure to chickenpox or measles and to seek medical advice immediately if exposed. Recommend dietary salt restriction and K^+ supplementation.

Storage: 20-25°C (68-77°F).

MEGACE ES – megestrol acetate RX

Class: Progesterone

OTHER BRAND NAMES

Megace

ADULT DOSAGE

Weight Loss

Anorexia, Cachexia or Unexplained Significant Weight Loss in AIDS Patients:
Megace ES:
Initial: 625mg/day (5mL/day)

Megace:
Initial: 800mg/day (20mL/day)
Daily doses of 400mg/day and 800mg/day found to be effective

PEDIATRIC DOSAGE

Pediatric use may not have been established

DOSE MODIFICATION

Elderly
Start at lower end of dosing range

ADMINISTRATION

Oral route

Shake well before use

HOW SUPPLIED

Sus: (ES) 125mg/mL [150mL]; (Megace) 40mg/mL [240mL]

CONTRAINDICATIONS

Known or suspected pregnancy.

WARNINGS/PRECAUTIONS

Institute only after treatable causes of weight loss are sought and addressed. 125mg/mL strength is not substitutable with other strengths (eg, 40mg/mL). Overt Cushing's syndrome and asymptomatic pituitary-adrenal suppression reported with chronic use. Adrenal insufficiency reported in patients receiving or being withdrawn from chronic therapy; consider use of replacement or stress doses of a rapidly acting glucocorticoid. New onset diabetes mellitus (DM) and exacerbation of preexisting DM reported with chronic use. Breakthrough bleeding reported in women. Caution with history of thromboembolic disease and in elderly.

ADVERSE REACTIONS

Diarrhea, rash, flatulence, N/V, HTN, headache, pain, asthenia, insomnia, anemia, fever, decreased libido, impotence, hyperglycemia.

DRUG INTERACTIONS

(ES) May decrease exposure of indinavir; consider higher dose of indinavir.

NURSING CONSIDERATIONS

Assessment: Assess for preexisting DM, history of thromboembolic disease, hypersensitivity to drug, pregnancy/nursing status, and possible drug interactions.

Monitoring: Monitor for adrenal insufficiency, new onset/exacerbation of DM, vaginal bleeding, and other adverse reactions.

Patient Counseling: Inform about product differences to avoid overdosing or underdosing. Instruct to use ud. Advise to report any adverse reactions. Advise women of childbearing potential to use contraception while on therapy, and to notify physician if pregnancy occurs.

Storage: 15-25°C (59-77°F). Protect from heat.

MERREM – meropenem RX

Class: Carbapenem

ADULT DOSAGE

Skin and Skin Structure Infections

Complicated:
Usual: 500mg q8h
Caused by *Pseudomonas aeruginosa*: 1g q8h

PEDIATRIC DOSAGE

Skin and Skin Structure Infections

Complicated:
≥3 Months of Age:
≥50kg: 500mg q8h
≤50kg: 10mg/kg q8h

Useful as presumptive therapy prior to identification of causative organisms

Intra-Abdominal Infections

Complicated Appendicitis and Peritonitis:
Usual: 1g q8h

Useful as presumptive therapy prior to identification of causative organisms

Max: 500mg q8h
Caused by *P. aeruginosa*: 20mg/kg q8h

Useful as presumptive therapy prior to identification of causative organisms

Intra-Abdominal Infections

Complicated Appendicitis and Peritonitis:
≥3 Months of Age:
≥50kg: 1g q8h
≤50kg: 20mg/kg q8h
Max: 1g q8h

Refer to PI for dosing in infants <3 months of age

Useful as presumptive therapy prior to identification of causative organisms

Bacterial Meningitis

≥3 Months of Age:
≥50kg: 2g q8h
≤50kg: 40mg/kg q8h
Max: 2g q8h

Useful as presumptive therapy prior to identification of causative organisms

DOSE MODIFICATION

Renal Impairment
CrCl >25-50mL/min: Give usual dose q12h
CrCl 10-25mL/min: Give 1/2 usual dose q12h
CrCl <10mL/min: Give 1/2 usual dose q24h

ADMINISTRATION

IV route

Administer by IV infusion over approx 15-30 min; doses of 1g may also be given as an IV bolus inj (5-20mL) over approx 3-5 min

IV Bolus
Add 10mL SWFI to 500mg vial size (20mL for 1g vial size)

IV Infusion
May be directly constituted w/ a compatible infusion fluid
Alternatively, may constitute inj vial and add resulting sol to an IV container and further diluted w/ an appropriate infusion fluid

Compatibility and Stability
Do not mix w/ or physically add to sol containing other drugs
Inj vials reconstituted w/ SWFI for bolus administration (up to 50mg/mL) may be stored for up to 3 hrs at up to 25°C (77°F) or for 13 hrs at up to 5°C (41°F)
Sol prepared for infusion (concentrations ranging from 1-20mg/mL) constituted w/ NaCl Inj 0.9% may be stored for 1 hr at up to 25°C (77°F) or 13 hrs at up to 5°C (41°F); use sol constituted w/ D5 Inj immediately

HOW SUPPLIED

Inj: 500mg, 1g

WARNINGS/PRECAUTIONS

Serious and occasionally fatal hypersensitivity (anaphylactic) reactions reported; d/c immediately if an allergic reaction occurs. Seizures and other adverse CNS effects reported; caution in patients w/ CNS disorders (eg, brain lesions, history of seizures) or w/ bacterial meningitis and/or compromised renal function. Continue anticonvulsant therapy in patients w/ known seizure disorders. If focal tremors, myoclonus, or seizures occur, evaluate neurologically, place on anticonvulsant therapy if not already instituted, and reexamine dosage to determine whether it should be decreased or discontinued. *Clostridium difficile*-associated diarrhea (CDAD) reported; d/c if CDAD is suspected or confirmed. May result in bacterial resistance if used in the absence of proven or suspected bacterial infection, or a prophylactic indication; take appropriate measures if superinfection develops. Thrombocytopenia reported in patients w/ renal impairment. Inadequate information on use in patients on hemodialysis or peritoneal dialysis. May impair mental/physical abilities. Caution in elderly.

ADVERSE REACTIONS

Diarrhea, N/V, headache, constipation, diarrhea, anemia, pain.

DRUG INTERACTIONS

Increased plasma concentrations w/ probenecid; coadministration not recommended. May reduce concentrations of valproic acid, thereby increasing the risk of breakthrough seizures; concomitant use w/ valproic acid or divalproex sodium is generally not recommended, but if necessary, consider supplemental anticonvulsant therapy.

NURSING CONSIDERATIONS

Assessment: Assess for CNS/seizure disorders, factors that predispose to convulsive activity, renal impairment, pregnancy/nursing status, and possible drug interactions. Carefully assess for previous hypersensitivity reactions to drug, penicillins, cephalosporins, other β-lactams, and other allergens.

Monitoring: Monitor for hypersensitivity reactions, CNS effects (eg, focal tremors, myoclonus, seizures), CDAD, superinfection, and other adverse reactions. Periodically monitor organ system functions including renal, hepatic, and hematopoietic, during prolonged therapy.

Patient Counseling: Counsel that therapy should only be used to treat bacterial, not viral, infections. Instruct to take exactly ud, even if patient feels better early in the course of therapy. Inform that skipping doses or not completing the full course of therapy may decrease effectiveness of treatment and increase bacterial resistance. Inform that diarrhea is a common problem caused by therapy, which usually ends when therapy is discontinued. Instruct to immediately contact physician if watery and bloody stools (w/ or w/o stomach cramp and fever) occur, even as late as ≥2 months after the last dose. Counsel to inform physician if taking valproic acid or divalproex sodium. Advise that adverse events (eg, seizures, headaches, and/or paresthesias) may develop that could interfere w/ mental alertness and/or cause motor impairment; instruct not to operate machinery or motorized vehicles until it is reasonably well established that therapy is well tolerated.

Storage: 20-25°C (68-77°F). Constituted Sol: Do not freeze.

METADATE CD – methylphenidate hydrochloride CII

Class: Sympathomimetic amine

Caution with history of drug dependence or alcoholism. Chronic abuse may lead to marked tolerance and psychological dependence with varying degrees of abnormal behavior. Frank psychotic episodes may occur, especially with parenteral abuse. Careful supervision is required during withdrawal from abusive use since severe depression may occur. Withdrawal following chronic use may unmask symptoms of underlying disorder that may require follow-up.

PEDIATRIC DOSAGE

Attention-Deficit Hyperactivity Disorder

≥6 Years:

Initial: 20mg qam

Titrate: May adjust in weekly 10-20mg increments, depending upon tolerability and degree of efficacy observed

Max: 60mg/day

Periodically reevaluate the long-term usefulness of the drug

DOSE MODIFICATION

Adverse Reactions

Reduce dose or d/c if paradoxical aggravation of symptoms or other adverse events occur

D/C if no improvement seen after appropriate dosage adjustment over 1 month

ADMINISTRATION

Oral route

Administer qam before breakfast

May be swallowed whole w/ the aid of liquids, or alternatively, may open caps and sprinkle contents onto a small amount (tbsp) of applesauce and consume immediately

Drinking some fluids (eg, water) should follow the intake of sprinkles w/ applesauce

Do not crush or chew cap or cap contents

HOW SUPPLIED

Cap, Extended-Release: 10mg, 20mg, 30mg, 40mg, 50mg, 60mg

CONTRAINDICATIONS

Marked anxiety, tension, agitation, glaucoma, motor tics, family history or diagnosis of Tourette's syndrome, severe HTN, angina pectoris, cardiac arrhythmias, heart failure, recent myocardial infarction (MI), hyperthyroidism, or thyrotoxicosis. Rare hereditary problems of fructose intolerance, glucose-galactose malabsorption, or sucrase-isomaltase insufficiency. On the day of surgery. Treatment with MAOIs or within a minimum of 14 days following discontinuation of an MAOI.

WARNINGS/PRECAUTIONS

Avoid with known serious structural cardiac abnormalities, cardiomyopathy, serious heart rhythm abnormalities, coronary artery disease, or other serious cardiac problems. Sudden death reported in children and adolescents with structural cardiac abnormalities or other serious heart problems. Sudden deaths, stroke, and MI reported in adults. May increase BP and HR; caution with conditions that might be compromised by increases in BP/HR. Prior to treatment, obtain medical history (including assessment for family history of sudden death or ventricular arrhythmia) and perform physical exam to assess for presence of cardiac disease. Promptly perform cardiac evaluation if symptoms of cardiac disease develop. May exacerbate symptoms of behavior disturbance and thought disorder in patients with preexisting psychotic disorder. Caution in patients with comorbid bipolar disorder; may induce mixed/manic episodes. May cause treatment-emergent psychotic or manic symptoms (eg, hallucinations, delusional thinking, mania) in children and adolescents without prior history of psychotic illness or mania; consider discontinuation if such symptoms occur. Aggressive behavior or hostility reported in children and adolescents. May cause long-term suppression of growth in children; monitor growth, and may need to interrupt treatment in patients not growing or gaining height or weight as expected. May lower convulsive threshold; d/c if seizures occur. Priapism, sometimes requiring surgical intervention, reported. Associated with peripheral vasculopathy, including Raynaud's phenomenon; carefully observe for digital changes. Difficulties with accommodation and blurring of vision reported. May produce a positive result during drug testing.

ADVERSE REACTIONS

Headache, abdominal pain, anorexia, insomnia.

DRUG INTERACTIONS

See Contraindications. Caution with pressor agents. May inhibit metabolism of coumarin anticoagulants, anticonvulsants (eg, phenobarbital, phenytoin, primidone), phenylbutazone, and some antidepressants (eg, TCAs, SSRIs); downward dose adjustment and monitoring of plasma drug concentrations (or coagulation times for coumarin) of these drugs may be necessary when initiating or discontinuing methylphenidate. Clearance might be affected by urinary pH, either being increased with acidifying agents or decreased with alkalinizing agents; caution with agents that alter urinary pH. Avoid with alcohol.

NURSING CONSIDERATIONS

Assessment: Assess for hypersensitivity to the drug, hereditary problems of fructose intolerance, glucose-galactose malabsorption, or sucrase-isomaltase insufficiency, marked anxiety, tension, agitation, glaucoma, motor tics, family history or diagnosis of Tourette's syndrome, cardiovascular conditions, history of drug dependence or alcoholism, psychotic disorder, comorbid bipolar disorder, any other conditions where treatment is contraindicated or cautioned, pregnancy/nursing status, and possible drug interactions.

Monitoring: Monitor for changes in HR and BP, signs/symptoms of cardiac disease, exacerbation of behavior disturbance and thought disorder, psychosis, mania, appearance of or worsening of aggressive behavior or hostility, seizures, priapism, peripheral vasculopathy (including Raynaud's phenomenon), visual disturbances, and other adverse reactions. In pediatric patients, monitor growth. Perform periodic monitoring of CBC, differential, and platelet counts during prolonged therapy. Periodically reevaluate long-term usefulness of drug.

Patient Counseling: Advise to avoid alcohol while taking the drug. Inform about the benefits and risks of therapy. Counsel on the appropriate use of the medication. Instruct to seek immediate medical attention in the event of priapism. Instruct to report to physician any new numbness, pain, skin color change, or sensitivity to temperature in fingers or toes; instruct to contact physician immediately with any signs of unexplained wounds appearing on fingers or toes while taking the drug.

Storage: 25°C (77°F); excursions permitted to 15-30°C (59-86°F).

METADATE ER – methylphenidate hydrochloride CII

Class: Sympathomimetic amine

Caution with history of drug dependence or alcoholism. Chronic abuse may lead to marked tolerance and psychological dependence with varying degrees of abnormal behavior. Frank psychotic episodes may occur, especially with parenteral abuse. Careful supervision is required during withdrawal from abusive use since severe depression may occur. Withdrawal following chronic use may unmask symptoms of underlying disorder that may require follow-up.

ADULT DOSAGE

Attention Deficit Disorders

Immediate-Release (IR) Methylphenidate Tabs:

10-60mg/day given in divided doses bid-tid

Tab, Extended-Release (ER):

May be used in place of the IR tabs when the 8-hr dosage of ER tabs corresponds to the titrated 8-hr dosage of the IR tabs

PEDIATRIC DOSAGE

Attention Deficit Disorders

≥6 Years:

Immediate-Release (IR) Methylphenidate Tabs:

Initial: 5mg bid before breakfast and lunch

Titrate: Increase gradually in increments of 5-10mg weekly

Max: 60mg/day

Narcolepsy

Immediate-Release (IR) Methylphenidate Tabs:
10-60mg/day given in divided doses bid-tid

Tab, Extended-Release (ER):
May be used in place of the IR tabs when the 8-hr dosage of ER tabs corresponds to the titrated 8-hr dosage of the IR tabs

Tab, Extended-Release (ER):
May be used in place of the IR tabs when the 8-hr dosage of ER tabs corresponds to the titrated 8-hr dosage of the IR tabs

D/C periodically to assess the child's condition; therapy should not be indefinite

Narcolepsy

≥6 Years:
Immediate-Release (IR) Methylphenidate Tabs:
Initial: 5mg bid before breakfast and lunch
Titrate: Increase gradually in increments of 5-10mg weekly
Max: 60mg/day

Tab, Extended-Release (ER):
May be used in place of the IR tabs when the 8-hr dosage of ER tabs corresponds to the titrated 8-hr dosage of the IR tabs

D/C periodically to assess the child's condition; therapy should not be indefinite

DOSE MODIFICATION

Adverse Reactions

Children ≥6 Years:
Reduce dose or d/c if paradoxical aggravation of symptoms or other adverse effects occur
D/C if no improvement seen after appropriate dosage adjustment over 1-month period

ADMINISTRATION

Oral route

Tab, Extended-Release

Swallow tabs whole; do not crush or chew

Immediate-Release Methylphenidate Tabs

Administer in divided doses bid-tid, preferably 30-45 min ac
Patients who are unable to sleep if medication is taken late in the day should take last dose before 6pm

HOW SUPPLIED

Tab, ER: 20mg

CONTRAINDICATIONS

Marked anxiety, tension, agitation, glaucoma, motor tics, family history or diagnosis of Tourette's syndrome, severe HTN, angina pectoris, cardiac arrhythmias, heart failure, recent myocardial infarction (MI), hyperthyroidism, or thyrotoxicosis. Rare hereditary problems of galactose intolerance, the Lapp lactase deficiency, or glucose-galactose malabsorption. On the day of surgery. Treatment with MAOIs or within a minimum of 14 days following discontinuation of an MAOI.

WARNINGS/PRECAUTIONS

Avoid with known serious structural cardiac abnormalities, cardiomyopathy, serious heart rhythm abnormalities, coronary artery disease, or other serious cardiac problems. Sudden death reported in children and adolescents with structural cardiac abnormalities or other serious heart problems. Sudden deaths, stroke, and MI reported in adults. May increase BP and HR; caution with conditions that might be compromised by increases in BP/HR. Prior to treatment, obtain medical history (including assessment for family history of sudden death or ventricular arrhythmia) and perform physical exam to assess for presence of cardiac disease. Promptly perform cardiac evaluation if symptoms of cardiac disease develop. May exacerbate symptoms of behavior disturbance and thought disorder in patients with preexisting psychotic disorder. Caution in patients with comorbid bipolar disorder; may induce mixed/manic episodes. May cause treatment-emergent psychotic or manic symptoms (eg, hallucinations, delusional thinking, mania) in children and adolescents without prior history of psychotic illness or mania; consider discontinuation if such symptoms occur. Aggressive behavior or hostility reported in children and adolescents. May cause long-term suppression of growth in children; monitor growth, and may need to interrupt treatment in patients not growing or gaining height or weight as expected. May lower convulsive threshold; d/c if seizures occur. Priapism, sometimes requiring surgical intervention, reported. Associated with peripheral vasculopathy, including Raynaud's phenomenon; carefully observe for digital changes. Difficulties with accommodation and blurring of vision reported. Patients with an element of agitation may react adversely; d/c if necessary. May produce a positive result during drug testing.

ADVERSE REACTIONS

Nervousness, insomnia, hypersensitivity reactions, anorexia, nausea, dizziness, palpitations, headache, dyskinesia, drowsiness, BP and pulse changes, tachycardia, angina, cardiac arrhythmia, abdominal pain.

DRUG INTERACTIONS

See Contraindications. Caution with pressor agents. May decrease effectiveness of drugs used to treat HTN. May inhibit metabolism of coumarin anticoagulants, anticonvulsants (eg, phenobarbital, phenytoin, primidone), phenylbutazone, and TCAs (eg, imipramine, clomipramine, desipramine); downward dose adjustment and monitoring of plasma drug concentration (or coagulation times for coumarin) of these drugs may be necessary when initiating or discontinuing methylphenidate. Clearance might be affected by urinary pH, either being increased with acidifying agents or decreased with alkalinizing agents; caution with agents that alter urinary pH.

NURSING CONSIDERATIONS

Assessment: Assess for hypersensitivity to the drug, hereditary problems of galactose intolerance, the Lapp lactase deficiency, or glucose-galactose malabsorption, marked anxiety, tension, agitation, glaucoma, motor tics, family history or diagnosis of Tourette's syndrome, cardiovascular conditions, history of drug dependence or alcoholism, psychotic disorder, comorbid bipolar disorder, any other conditions where treatment is contraindicated or cautioned, pregnancy/nursing status, and possible drug interactions.

Monitoring: Monitor for changes in HR and BP, signs/symptoms of cardiac disease, exacerbation of behavior disturbance and thought disorder, psychosis, mania, appearance of or worsening of aggressive behavior or hostility, seizures, priapism, peripheral vasculopathy (including Raynaud's phenomenon), visual disturbances, and other adverse reactions. In pediatric patients, monitor growth. Perform periodic monitoring of CBC, differential, and platelet counts during prolonged therapy.

Patient Counseling: Inform about the benefits and risks of therapy. Counsel on the appropriate use of the medication. Instruct to seek immediate medical attention in the event of priapism. Instruct to report to physician any new numbness, pain, skin color change, or sensitivity to temperature in fingers or toes; instruct to contact physician immediately with any signs of unexplained wounds appearing on fingers or toes while taking the drug.

Storage: 20-25°C (68-77°F); excursions permitted to 15-30°C (59-86°F). Protect from moisture.

METHOTREXATE INJECTION – methotrexate RX

Class: Dihydrofolic acid reductase inhibitor

Should be used only by physicians with knowledge and experience in the use of antimetabolite therapy. Use only in life-threatening neoplastic diseases, or in patients with psoriasis or RA with severe, recalcitrant, disabling disease not adequately responsive to other forms of therapy. Deaths reported in the treatment of malignancy, psoriasis, and RA. Closely monitor for bone marrow, liver, lung, and kidney toxicities. Patients should be informed of the risks involved and be under physician's care throughout therapy. Use of high-dose regimens recommended for osteosarcoma requires meticulous care. Formulations and diluents containing preservatives must not be used for intrathecal or high-dose therapy. Fetal death and/or congenital anomalies reported; not recommended for women of childbearing potential unless benefits outweigh risks. Contraindicated in pregnant women with psoriasis or RA. Reduced elimination with impaired renal function, ascites, or pleural effusions; monitor for toxicity and reduce dose or d/c in some cases. Unexpectedly severe (sometimes fatal) bone marrow suppression, aplastic anemia, and GI toxicity reported with coadministration of therapy (usually high dosage) with some NSAIDs. Causes hepatotoxicity, fibrosis, and cirrhosis (generally only after prolonged use); perform periodic liver biopsies in psoriatic patients on long-term therapy. Acutely, liver enzyme elevations frequently seen. Drug-induced lung disease (eg, acute/chronic interstitial pneumonitis) may occur acutely at any time during therapy and reported at low doses. Interrupt therapy if pulmonary symptoms (especially a dry, nonproductive cough), diarrhea, or ulcerative stomatitis occurs. Malignant lymphomas, which may regress following withdrawal of treatment, may occur with low-dose therapy and, thus, may not require cytotoxic treatment; d/c therapy 1st and, if lymphoma does not regress, institute appropriate treatment. May induce tumor lysis syndrome in patients with rapidly growing tumors; may be prevented/alleviated with appropriate supportive and pharmacologic measures. Severe, occasionally fatal, skin reactions reported. Potentially fatal opportunistic infections, especially *Pneumocystis carinii* pneumonia, may occur. Concomitant use with radiotherapy may increase risk of soft tissue necrosis and osteonecrosis.

ADULT DOSAGE

Choriocarcinoma

Gestational Choriocarcinoma, Chorioadenoma Destruens, Hydatidiform Mole, and Similar Trophoblastic Diseases:

15-30mg/day IM for a 5-day course; repeat such courses for 3-5X as required, w/ rest periods of ≥1 week interposed between courses, until manifesting toxic symptoms subside

Acute Lymphoblastic Leukemia

Induction: 3.3mg/m^2/day w/ prednisone 60mg/m^2/day

PEDIATRIC DOSAGE

Acute Lymphoblastic Leukemia

Induction: 3.3mg/m^2/day w/ prednisone 60mg/m^2/day

Remission Maint: 30mg/m^2/week IM given 2X weekly or 2.5mg/kg IV every 14 days

If and when relapse occurs, repeat initial induction regimen to obtain reinduction of remission

Meningeal Leukemia

Prophylaxis/Treatment:

<1 Year:

6mg intrathecally

Remission Maint: 30mg/m^2/week IM given 2X weekly or 2.5mg/kg IV every 14 days

If and when relapse occurs, repeat initial induction regimen to obtain reinduction of remission

Meningeal Leukemia

Prophylaxis/Treatment:
12mg intrathecally

Treatment:
May be given at 2- to 5-day intervals; administer until CSF cell count returns to normal, then give 1 additional dose

Non-Hodgkin's Lymphoma

In combination w/ other chemotherapeutic agents in the treatment of advanced stages

Burkitt's Tumor:
Stages I-II: 10-25mg/day PO for 4-8 days
Lymphosarcomas (Stage III): 0.625-2.5mg/kg/day w/ other antitumor agents
Treatment in all stages usually consists of several courses w/ 7- to 10-day rest periods

Psoriasis

Symptomatic control of severe, recalcitrant, disabling psoriasis not adequately responsive to other forms of therapy, but only when the diagnosis has been established, as by a biopsy and/or after dermatologic consultation

Initial: 10-25mg IM/IV as single dose once weekly until adequate response is achieved, or 2.5mg PO at 12-hr intervals for 3 doses
Titrate: May adjust gradually to achieve optimal response
Max: 30mg/week
Reduce each dosage schedule to lowest possible amount and to longest possible rest period once optimal response has been achieved

Cutaneous T-Cell Lymphoma

Advanced Mycosis Fungoides (Alone or in Combination w/ Other Anticancer Agents):
Early Stages:
5-50mg once weekly, or 15-37.5mg 2X weekly if response is poor to weekly therapy
Dose reduction/cessation is guided by response and hematologic monitoring
Advanced Stages:
Combination chemotherapy regimens that include IV MTX administered at higher doses w/ leucovorin rescue have been utilized

Osteosarcoma

Effective in prolonging relapse-free survival in patients w/ non-metastatic osteosarcoma who have undergone surgical resection or amputation for the primary tumor, when used in high doses followed by leucovorin rescue in combination w/ other chemotherapeutic agents

Initial: 12g/m^2 IV as 4-hr infusion
Titrate: May increase to 15g/m^2 in subsequent treatments if initial dose is not sufficient to produce a peak serum concentration of 1000μM at the end of the infusion

Refer to PI for doses/schedule of chemotherapeutic agents, and guidelines for MTX therapy w/ leucovorin rescue

1 Year:
8mg intrathecally
2 Years:
10mg intrathecally
≥3 Years:
12mg intrathecally

Treatment:
May be given at 2- to 5-day intervals; administer until CSF cell count returns to normal, then give one additional dose

Juvenile Rheumatoid Arthritis

Management of children w/ active polyarticular-course juvenile RA, who have had insufficient therapeutic response to, or are intolerant of, an adequate trial of 1st-line therapy including full-dose NSAIDs
2-16 Years:
Initial: 10mg/m^2 once weekly
Titrate: May adjust gradually to achieve optimal response

Limited data to assess how doses >20mg/m^2/week might affect the risk of serious toxicity; refer to PI for further information

Rheumatoid Arthritis

Management of selected adults w/ severe, active RA (American College of Rheumatology criteria) who have had insufficient therapeutic response to, or are intolerant of, an adequate trial of 1st-line therapy including full-dose NSAIDs

Initial: 7.5mg PO as single dose once weekly, or 2.5mg PO at 12-hr intervals for 3 doses given as a course once weekly
Titrate: May adjust gradually to achieve optimal response. Significant increase in incidence and severity of serious toxic reactions, especially bone marrow suppression, reported at doses >20mg/week.

Other Indications

Treatment of breast cancer, epidermoid cancers of the head and neck, and lung cancer, particularly squamous cell and small cell types, alone or in combination w/ other anticancer agents

DOSE MODIFICATION

Elderly

Consider relatively low doses and closely monitor for early signs of toxicity

ADMINISTRATION

IM/IV/Intra-arterial/Intrathecal route

Reconstitution of Lyophilized Powders

Reconstitute immediately prior to use w/ an appropriate sterile, preservative-free medium such as D5 sol or NaCl inj
The 1g vial should be reconstituted w/ 19.4mL to a concentration of 50mg/mL
When high doses are administered by IV infusion, total dose is diluted in D5 sol
For intrathecal inj, reconstitute to a concentration of 1mg/mL w/ an appropriate sterile, preservative-free medium such as NaCl inj

Dilution of Liquid Inj

If desired, sol may be further diluted immediately prior to use w/ an appropriate sterile, preservative-free medium such as D5 sol or NaCl inj

HOW SUPPLIED

Inj: 25mg/mL [2mL, 4mL, 8mL, 10mL], 1g

CONTRAINDICATIONS

Pregnant women with psoriasis or RA (should be used in treatment of pregnant women with neoplastic diseases only when potential benefit outweighs risk to the fetus), nursing mothers. Psoriasis or RA patients with alcoholism, alcoholic liver disease, chronic liver disease, immunodeficiency syndromes, or preexisting blood dyscrasias (eg, bone marrow hypoplasia, leukopenia, thrombocytopenia, significant anemia).

WARNINGS/PRECAUTIONS

Toxic effects may be related to dose/frequency of administration; if toxicity occurs, reduce dose or d/c therapy and take appropriate corrective measures, which may include use of leucovorin calcium and/or acute, intermittent hemodialysis with high-flux dialyzer, if necessary. If therapy is reinstituted, carry it out with caution, with adequate consideration of further need for the drug and increased alertness as to possible recurrence of toxicity. Caution in elderly/debilitated. Avoid pregnancy if either partner is receiving therapy (during and for a minimum of 3 months after therapy for male patients, and during and for at least 1 ovulatory cycle after therapy for female patients). May impair mental/physical abilities. May cause multiple organ system toxicities (eg, GI, hematologic). May cause impairment of fertility, oligospermia, and menstrual dysfunction during and for a short period after cessation of therapy.

ADVERSE REACTIONS

Bone marrow/liver/lung/kidney toxicities, diarrhea, ulcerative stomatitis, malignant lymphomas, tumor lysis syndrome, skin reactions, opportunistic infections, nausea, abdominal distress, malaise, undue fatigue, chills.

DRUG INTERACTIONS

See Boxed Warning. Do not administer NSAIDs prior to or concomitantly with high doses of therapy (eg, treatment of osteosarcoma); elevated and prolonged levels reported with concomitant NSAIDs. Caution when NSAIDs or salicylates are administered concomitantly with lower doses of therapy. Toxicity may be increased due to displacement by salicylates, phenylbutazone, phenytoin, and sulfonamides. Renal tubular transport diminished by probenecid. In the treatment of patients with osteosarcoma, exercise caution if high-dose therapy is administered with a potentially nephrotoxic chemotherapeutic agent (eg, cisplatin). Increases levels of mercaptopurine; may require dose adjustment. Oral antibiotics (eg, tetracycline, chloramphenicol, nonabsorbable broad spectrum) may decrease intestinal absorption or interfere with enterohepatic circulation. Penicillins may reduce renal clearance; hematologic and GI toxicity observed. Closely monitor for increased risk of hepatotoxicity with hepatotoxins (eg, azathioprine, retinoids, sulfasalazine). May decrease theophylline clearance; monitor theophylline levels. Vitamin preparations containing folic acid or its derivatives may decrease responses to drug; high doses of leucovorin may reduce the efficacy of intrathecally administered drug. Trimethoprim/sulfamethoxazole may increase bone marrow suppression by decreasing tubular secretion and/or additive antifolate effect. Proton pump inhibitors (PPIs) (eg, omeprazole, esomeprazole, pantoprazole) may elevate and prolong levels, possibly leading to toxicities; use caution when administering high-dose therapy with PPIs. Immunization may be ineffective when given during therapy; immunization with live virus vaccines is generally not recommended. Disseminated vaccinia infections after smallpox immunizations reported. Combined use with gold, penicillamine, hydroxychloroquine, sulfasalazine, or cytotoxic agents may increase incidence of adverse effects.

NURSING CONSIDERATIONS

Assessment: Assess for alcoholism, alcoholic/chronic liver disease, immunodeficiency, blood dyscrasias, ascites, pleural effusions, tumors, hypersensitivity to drug, pregnancy/nursing status, any other condition where treatment is cautioned or contraindicated, and possible drug interactions. Obtain baseline CBC with differential and platelet counts, hepatic enzymes, renal function tests, liver biopsy, and chest x-ray.

Monitoring: Monitor for toxicities of bone marrow, liver, lung, kidney, and GI system, diarrhea, ulcerative stomatitis, malignant lymphoma, tumor lysis syndrome, skin reactions, opportunistic infections, and other adverse reactions. Monitor hematology at least monthly and renal/hepatic function every 1-2 months during therapy of RA/psoriasis and more frequently during antineoplastic therapy, during initial/changing doses, or during periods of increased risk of elevated drug levels (eg, dehydration). If drug-induced lung disease is suspected, perform pulmonary function tests.

Patient Counseling: Inform of the early signs/symptoms of toxicity, the need to see physician promptly if they occur, and the need for close follow-up, including periodic lab tests to monitor toxicity. Emphasize that the recommended dose is taken weekly in RA and psoriasis, and that mistaken daily use of recommended dose has led to fatal toxicity. Counsel about risks/benefits of therapy, and effects on reproduction.

Storage: 20-25°C (68-77°F). Protect from light.

METHYLIN — methylphenidate hydrochloride CII

Class: Sympathomimetic amine

Caution with history of drug dependence or alcoholism. Chronic abuse may lead to marked tolerance and physiological dependence with varying degrees of abnormal behavior. Frank psychotic episodes may occur, especially with parenteral abuse. Careful supervision required during withdrawal from abusive use since severe depression may occur. Withdrawal following chronic use may unmask symptoms of underlying disorder that may require follow-up.

ADULT DOSAGE

Attention Deficit Disorders

10-60mg/day given in divided doses bid or tid 30-45 min ac
Last dose should be taken before 6 pm if patient is unable to sleep as a result of taking medication late in the day

Narcolepsy

10-60mg/day given in divided doses bid or tid 30-45 min ac
Last dose should be taken before 6 pm if patient is unable to sleep as a result of taking medication late in the day

PEDIATRIC DOSAGE

Attention Deficit Disorders

≥6 Years:
Initial: 5mg bid before breakfast and lunch
Titrate: Increase gradually in increments of 5-10mg weekly
Max: 60mg/day

D/C if no improvement seen after appropriate dosage adjustment over 1 month
D/C periodically to assess the child's condition; therapy should not be indefinite

Narcolepsy

≥6 Years:
Initial: 5mg bid before breakfast and lunch
Titrate: Increase gradually in increments of 5-10mg weekly
Max: 60mg/day

D/C if no improvement seen after appropriate dosage adjustment over 1 month
D/C periodically to assess the child's condition; therapy should not be indefinite

DOSE MODIFICATION

Adverse Reactions

Children ≥6 Years:

Reduce dose or d/c if paradoxical aggravation of symptoms or other adverse effects occur

ADMINISTRATION

Oral route

Tab, Chewable

Take w/ at least 8 oz (full glass) of water or other fluid

HOW SUPPLIED

Sol: 5mg/5mL [500mL], 10mg/5mL [500mL]; Tab, Chewable: 2.5mg, 5mg, 10mg* *scored

CONTRAINDICATIONS

Marked anxiety, tension, agitation, glaucoma, motor tics, or family history or diagnosis of Tourette's syndrome. Treatment with MAOIs or within a minimum of 14 days following discontinuation of an MAOI.

WARNINGS/PRECAUTIONS

Avoid with known serious structural cardiac abnormalities, cardiomyopathy, serious heart rhythm abnormalities, coronary artery disease or other serious cardiac problems. Sudden death reported in children and adolescents with structural cardiac abnormalities or other serious heart problems. Sudden death, stroke, and myocardial infarction (MI) reported in adults. May cause modest increase in average BP and HR; caution with conditions that might be compromised by increases in BP/HR (eg, preexisting HTN, heart failure, recent MI, ventricular arrhythmias). Prior to treatment, obtain medical history (including assessment for family history of sudden death or ventricular arrhythmia) and perform physical exam to assess for presence of cardiac disease. Promptly perform cardiac evaluation if symptoms suggestive of cardiac disease develop. May exacerbate symptoms of behavior disturbance and thought disorder in patients with a preexisting psychotic disorder. Caution in patients with comorbid bipolar disorder; may induce mixed/manic episode. May cause treatment-emergent psychotic or manic symptoms (eg, hallucinations, delusional thinking, mania) in children and adolescents without prior history of psychotic illness or mania; discontinuation may be appropriate if such symptoms occur. Aggressive behavior or hostility reported in children and adolescents. May lower convulsive threshold; d/c if seizures occur. Priapism, sometimes requiring surgical intervention, reported. May cause long-term suppression of growth in children; monitor growth and may need to interrupt treatment in patients not growing or gaining height or weight as expected. Associated with peripheral vasculopathy, including Raynaud's phenomenon; monitor for digital changes. Difficulties with accommodation and blurring of vision reported. Patients with an element of agitation may react adversely; d/c therapy if necessary. Periodically monitor CBC, differential, and platelet counts during prolonged therapy. Not indicated in all cases of this behavioral syndrome, and in symptoms associated with acute stress reactions. Long-term effects in children not well established.

ADVERSE REACTIONS

Nervousness, insomnia, hypersensitivity, anorexia, nausea, dizziness, palpitations, headache, dyskinesia, drowsiness, BP and pulse changes, tachycardia, weight loss, abdominal pain, loss of appetite.

DRUG INTERACTIONS

See Contraindications. May decrease hypotensive effect of guanethidine. Caution with pressor agents. May inhibit metabolism of coumarin anticoagulants, anticonvulsants (eg, phenobarbital, diphenylhydantoin, primidone), phenylbutazone, and TCAs (eg, imipramine, clomipramine, desipramine); may require downward dose adjustments of these drugs.

NURSING CONSIDERATIONS

Assessment: Assess for previous hypersensitivity to the drug, history of drug dependence or alcoholism, marked anxiety, tension, agitation, glaucoma, motor tics, family history or diagnosis of Tourette's syndrome, preexisting psychotic disorder, comorbid bipolar disorder, cardiac disease, any other conditions where treatment is cautioned or contraindicated, pregnancy/nursing status, and possible drug interactions.

Monitoring: Monitor BP/HR, signs/symptoms of cardiac disease, exacerbations of behavior disturbances and thought disorders, psychosis, mania, appearance of or worsening of aggressive behavior or hostility, seizures, priapism, digital changes, visual disturbances and other adverse reactions. Monitor growth in children. Perform periodic monitoring of CBC, differential, and platelet counts during prolonged therapy.

Patient Counseling: Inform patients/families/caregivers about risks, benefits, and appropriate use of treatment. Instruct to seek immediate medical attention in the event of priapism. Instruct to report to physician if any new numbness, pain, skin color change, sensitivity to temperature in fingers or toes, or any signs of unexplained wounds appearing on fingers or toes develop. (Tab, Chewable) Advise not to take the drug if have difficulty swallowing. Seek immediate medical attention if experience chest pain, vomiting, or difficulty in swallowing or breathing after taking the drug. Inform that drug contains phenylalanine.

Storage: 20-25°C (68-77°F). (Tab, Chewable) Protect from moisture.

METOCLOPRAMIDE – metoclopramide RX

Class: Dopamine antagonist/prokinetic

May cause tardive dyskinesia (TD); d/c if signs/symptoms of TD develop. Avoid use for >12 weeks of therapy unless benefit outweighs risk.

OTHER BRAND NAMES

Reglan Tablets, Reglan Injection

ADULT DOSAGE

Gastroesophageal Reflux Disease

PO:
10-15mg up to qid 30 min ac and hs

Intermittent Symptoms:
Single doses up to 20mg prior to the provoking situation

Esophageal Erosions/Ulcerations:
15mg/dose qid

Therapy should not exceed 12 weeks in duration

Diabetic Gastroparesis

PO:
10mg 30 min ac and hs for 2-8 weeks

Inj:
10mg IV over 1-2 min for up to 10 days, then initiate oral administration

Initial route of administration should be determined by the severity of the presenting symptoms

Postoperative Nausea/Vomiting

Inj:
10mg or 20mg IM near end of surgery

Chemotherapy-Associated Nausea/Vomiting

Inj:
IV infused over at least 15 min, 30 min before chemotherapy and repeated q2h for two doses, then q3h for 3 doses

Initial Two Doses:
Highly Emetogenic Drugs (eg, Cisplatin, Dacarbazine): 2mg/kg
Less Emetogenic Regimens: 1mg/kg

Small Bowel Intubation

Inj:
10mg single dose (undiluted) IV over 1-2 min if the tube has not passed the pylorus w/ conventional maneuvers in 10 min

Aid in Radiological Exam

Inj:
When Delayed Gastric Emptying Interferes w/ Examination of the Stomach/Small Intestine:
10mg single dose (undiluted) IV over 1-2 min

PEDIATRIC DOSAGE

Small Bowel Intubation

Inj:
Administer as a single dose (undiluted) IV over 1-2 min if the tube has not passed the pylorus w/ conventional maneuvers in 10 min

<6 Years: 0.1mg/kg
6-14 Years: 2.5-5mg
>14 Years: 10mg

DOSE MODIFICATION

Renal Impairment

PO/Inj:
CrCl <40mL/min:
Initial: 1/2 the recommended dose; adjust dose as appropriate

Elderly

PO: 5mg/dose

Adverse Reactions

Inj:
Acute Dystonic Reactions: Inject 50mg diphenhydramine IM

ADMINISTRATION
Oral, IV/IM route

Inj
Doses >10mg: Dilute in 50mL of a parenteral sol; preferred sol is normal saline
Refer to PI for Admixture Compatibilities
Admixture Incompatibilities:
Cephalothin Sodium
Chloramphenicol Sodium
Sodium Bicarbonate

HOW SUPPLIED
Inj (Reglan): 5mg/mL [2mL, 10mL, 30mL]; Sol: 5mg/5mL [473mL]; Tab (Reglan): 5mg, 10mg* *scored

CONTRAINDICATIONS
When GI motility stimulation is dangerous (eg, GI hemorrhage, mechanical obstruction, perforation), pheochromocytoma, epilepsy, and concomitant drugs that cause extrapyramidal symptoms (EPS).

WARNINGS/PRECAUTIONS
Mental depression may occur; caution with prior history of depression. EPS, primarily as acute dystonic reactions, may occur. May cause parkinsonian-like symptoms; caution with preexisting Parkinson's disease. May suppress signs of TD; do not use for symptomatic control of TD. Neuroleptic malignant syndrome reported; d/c, monitor, and institute intensive symptomatic treatment. Risk of developing fluid retention and volume overload, especially in patients with cirrhosis or CHF; d/c if these occur. Caution with HTN, renal impairment, and/or in elderly. May increase risk of developing methemoglobinemia and/or sulfhemoglobinemia with NADH-cytochrome b_5 reductase deficiency. May experience withdrawal symptoms after discontinuation. (Inj) Undiluted IV inj should be given slowly since rapid administration may cause anxiety, restlessness, and drowsiness. May increase pressure on suture lines after a gut anastomosis or closure; use caution with PONV.

ADVERSE REACTIONS
TD, restlessness, drowsiness, fatigue, lassitude.

DRUG INTERACTIONS
See Contraindications. GI motility effect antagonized by anticholinergics and narcotic analgesics. Additive sedation with alcohol, sedatives, hypnotics, narcotics, or tranquilizers. Caution with MAOIs. May diminish absorption of drugs from stomach (eg, digoxin) and increase rate and/or extent of absorption of drugs from small bowel (eg, acetaminophen, tetracycline, levodopa, ethanol, cyclosporine). Insulin dose or timing of dose may require adjustment. Rare cases of hepatotoxicity reported with drugs with hepatotoxic potential. Inhibits central and peripheral effects of apomorphine.

NURSING CONSIDERATIONS

Assessment: Assess for conditions when GI motility stimulation is dangerous, pheochromocytoma, epilepsy, sensitivity or tolerance to the drug, CHF, cirrhosis, history of depression, Parkinson's disease, HTN, NADH-cytochrome b_5 reductase and G6PD deficiency, diabetes mellitus, renal impairment, pregnancy/nursing status, and possible drug interactions.

Monitoring: Monitor for signs/symptoms of depression, EPS, parkinsonian-like symptoms, TD, NMS, HTN, fluid retention/volume overload, withdrawal symptoms, hypersensitivity reactions, and other adverse reactions.

Patient Counseling: Inform that drug may impair mental and physical abilities; advise to use caution while operating machinery/driving. Discuss the risks and benefits of treatment.

Storage: 20-25°C (68-77°F). (Inj) If diluted with NaCl, may be stored frozen for up to 4 weeks. Diluted sol may be stored up to 48 hrs (without freezing) if protected from light; 24 hrs in normal lighting conditions.

METOPROLOL – metoprolol tartrate RX

Class: Selective $beta_1$-blocker

OTHER BRAND NAMES
Lopressor

ADULT DOSAGE

Hypertension

Tab:
Initial: 100mg/day PO in single or divided doses given alone or w/ a diuretic
Titrate: May increase at weekly (or longer) intervals until optimum BP reduction is achieved

PEDIATRIC DOSAGE
Pediatric use may not have been established

Effective Range: 100-450mg/day
Max: 450mg/day

Angina Pectoris

Initial: 100mg/day PO in 2 divided doses
Titrate: Gradually increase at weekly intervals until optimum clinical response is achieved or pronounced slowing of HR
Effective Range: 100-400mg/day
Max: 400mg/day
Upon discontinuation, taper gradually over 1-2 weeks

Myocardial Infarction

In Hemodynamically Stable Patients:
Early Phase:
5mg IV bolus every 2 min for 3 doses (monitor BP, HR, and ECG)
Patients Who Tolerate Full IV Dose (15mg):
Give 50mg PO q6h, 15 min after last IV dose and continue for 48 hrs
Maint: 100mg PO bid
Patients Who Cannot Tolerate Full IV Dose:
Give either 25 or 50mg PO q6h (depending on the degree of intolerance) 15 min after the last IV dose or as soon as clinical condition allows; d/c w/ severe intolerance

Late Phase:
100mg PO bid for ≥3 months

DOSE MODIFICATION

Hepatic Impairment
Initiate at low doses w/ cautious gradual dose titration according to clinical response

Elderly
>65 Years:
Start at lower end of dosing range

ADMINISTRATION

Oral/IV route

Tab
Swallow unchewed w/ a glass of water
Always take in standardized relation w/ meals; continue taking w/ the same schedule during the course of therapy

Inj
Parenteral administration should be done in a setting w/ intensive monitoring

HOW SUPPLIED

Tab: 25mg*; (Lopressor) Inj: 1mg/mL [5mL]; Tab: 50mg*, 100mg* *scored

CONTRAINDICATIONS

HR <45 beats/min, 2nd- and 3rd-degree heart block, significant 1st-degree heart block, systolic BP <100mmHg, moderate to severe cardiac failure. (Tab) Sinus bradycardia, >1st-degree heart block, cardiogenic shock, overt cardiac failure, sick sinus syndrome, severe peripheral arterial circulatory disorders.

WARNINGS/PRECAUTIONS

May cause depression of myocardial contractility and may precipitate heart failure (HF) and cardiogenic shock. If signs/symptoms of HF develop, treat patient according to recommended guidelines; lower dose or d/c if necessary. Avoid abrupt discontinuation in patients w/ coronary artery disease (CAD). Severe exacerbation of angina, MI, and ventricular arrhythmias reported in patients w/ CAD following abrupt discontinuation. When discontinuing chronic therapy, particularly w/ coronary heart disease, reduce dose over 1-2 weeks w/ careful monitoring. If angina markedly worsens or acute coronary insufficiency develops, reinstate promptly, at least temporarily, and take other measures for the management of unstable angina. Chronically administered therapy should not be routinely withdrawn prior to major surgery; impaired ability of the heart to respond to reflex adrenergic stimuli may augment the risks of general anesthesia and surgical procedures. Bradycardia, including sinus pause, heart block, and cardiac arrest reported; increased risk in patients w/ 1st degree atrioventricular block, sinus node dysfunction, or conduction disorders. Reduce or d/c if severe bradycardia develops. Avoid w/ bronchospastic diseases; may be used in patients w/ bronchospastic disease who do not respond to or cannot tolerate other antihypertensive treatment. May mask tachycardia occurring w/ hypoglycemia; other manifestations (eg, dizziness, sweating) may not be significantly affected. If used in the setting of pheochromocytoma, should be given in combination w/ an α-blocker, and only after the α-blocker has been initiated; may cause a paradoxical increase in BP if administered alone. May mask certain clinical signs (eg, tachycardia) of hyperthyroidism. Avoid abrupt withdrawal; may precipitate thyroid storm. Patients w/ a history of severe anaphylactic reaction to variety of allergens may be more reactive to repeated challenge and may be unresponsive to usual doses of epinephrine.

ADVERSE REACTIONS

Bradycardia, tiredness, dizziness, depression, SOB, diarrhea, pruritus, rash, heart block, HF, hypotension.

DRUG INTERACTIONS

Additive effects w/ catecholamine-depleting drugs (eg, reserpine). May increase risk of bradycardia w/ digitalis glycosides; monitor HR and PR interval. May produce an additive reduction in myocardial contractility w/ calcium channel blockers. May increase levels w/ potent CYP2D6 inhibitors (eg, antidepressants, antipsychotics, antiarrhythmics). Hydralazine may inhibit presystemic metabolism, leading to increased levels. May potentiate antihypertensive effects of α-blockers (eg, guanethidine, betanidine, reserpine). May potentiate the postural hypotensive effect of 1st dose of prazosin. May potentiate hypertensive response to withdrawal of clonidine; when given concomitantly w/ clonidine, d/c several days before clonidine is withdrawn. May enhance vasoconstrictive action of ergot alkaloids. Withhold therapy before dipyridamole testing, w/ careful monitoring of HR following the dipyridamole inj. (Inj) May enhance cardiodepressant effect w/ some inhalational anesthetics.

NURSING CONSIDERATIONS

Assessment: Assess for hypersensitivity to the drug, sinus bradycardia, heart block, cardiogenic shock, HF, CAD, bronchospastic diseases, hypoglycemia, hyperthyroidism, hepatic impairment, any other conditions where treatment is contraindicated or cautioned, pregnancy/nursing status, and possible drug interactions. Obtain baseline ECG.

Monitoring: Monitor for signs/symptoms of HF, cardiogenic shock, thyrotoxicosis, hypersensitivity reactions, and other adverse reactions. Monitor BP, HR, ECG, and hemodynamic status.

Patient Counseling: Advise to take regularly and continuously, ud, w/ or immediately following meals. Instruct to not interrupt or d/c w/o consulting a physician. Advise to avoid operating automobiles and machinery or engaging in other tasks requiring alertness until response to therapy has been determined. Advise to contact physician if difficulty in breathing or other adverse reactions occur, and to inform physician/dentist of therapy before undergoing any type of surgery.

Storage: 20-25°C (68-77°F). Protect from moisture. (Lopressor) 25°C (77°F); excursions permitted to 15-30°C (59-86°F). Tab: Protect from moisture and heat. Inj: Protect from light and heat.

METOPROLOL TARTRATE/HCTZ – hydrochlorothiazide/metoprolol tartrate

RX

Class: Selective β_1-blocker/thiazide diuretic

Exacerbation of angina and, in some cases, myocardial infarction (MI) reported following abrupt discontinuation. When discontinuing therapy, avoid abrupt withdrawal even without overt angina pectoris. Caution patients against interruption of therapy without physician's advice.

OTHER BRAND NAMES

Lopressor HCT

ADULT DOSAGE

Hypertension

If fixed combination represents dose titrated to patient's needs; therapy with combination may be more convenient than with separate components

Combination Therapy:

100-200mg of metoprolol and HCTZ 25-50mg per day given qd or in divided doses

Max HCTZ: 50mg/day

May gradually add another antihypertensive when necessary, beginning with 50% of the usual recommended starting dose

PEDIATRIC DOSAGE

Pediatric use may not have been established

DOSE MODIFICATION

Elderly

Start at lower end of dosing range

ADMINISTRATION

Oral route

HOW SUPPLIED

Tab: (Metoprolol-HCTZ) 50mg-25mg*, 100mg-25mg*, 100mg-50mg*; (Lopressor HCT) 50mg-25mg*, 100mg-25mg* *scored

CONTRAINDICATIONS

Sinus bradycardia, >1st-degree heart block, cardiogenic shock, overt cardiac failure, sick sinus syndrome, severe peripheral arterial circulatory disorders, anuria, hypersensitivity to sulfonamide-derived drugs.

WARNINGS/PRECAUTIONS

Not for initial therapy. Caution with hepatic dysfunction and in elderly. Metoprolol: May cause/precipitate heart failure; d/c if cardiac failure continues despite adequate treatment. Avoid with bronchospastic diseases, but may use with caution if unresponsive to/intolerant of other antihypertensives. Avoid withdrawal of chronically administered therapy prior to major surgery; however, may augment risks of general anesthesia and surgical procedures. Caution with diabetic patients; may mask tachycardia occurring with hypoglycemia. Paradoxical BP increase reported with pheochromocytoma; give in combination with and only after initiating α-blocker therapy. May mask hyperthyroidism. Avoid abrupt withdrawal in suspected thyrotoxicosis; may precipitate thyroid storm. HCTZ: Caution with severe renal disease; may precipitate azotemia. If progressive renal impairment becomes evident, d/c therapy. May precipitate hepatic coma in patients with liver dysfunction/disease. Sensitivity reactions are more likely to occur with history of allergy or bronchial asthma. May exacerbate/activate systemic lupus erythematosus (SLE). May cause idiosyncratic reaction, resulting in acute transient myopia and acute angle-closure glaucoma; d/c HCTZ as rapidly as possible. Fluid/electrolyte imbalance (eg, hyponatremia, hypochloremic alkalosis, hypokalemia) may develop. May cause hyperuricemia and precipitation of frank gout. Latent diabetes mellitus (DM) may manifest during therapy. Enhanced effects seen in postsympathectomy patients. D/C prior to parathyroid function test. Decreased Ca^{2+} excretion observed. Altered parathyroid gland, with hypercalcemia and hypophosphatemia observed with prolonged therapy. May increase urinary excretion of Mg^{2+}, resulting in hypomagnesemia.

ADVERSE REACTIONS

Fatigue, lethargy, dizziness, vertigo, flu syndrome, drowsiness, somnolence, hypokalemia, headache, bradycardia.

DRUG INTERACTIONS

Metoprolol: May exhibit additive effect with catecholamine-depleting drugs (eg, reserpine). Digitalis glycosides may increase risk of bradycardia. Some inhalation anesthetics may enhance cardiodepressant effect. May be unresponsive to usual doses of epinephrine. Potent CYP2D6 inhibitors (eg, certain antidepressants, antipsychotics, antiarrhythmics, antiretrovirals, antihistamines, antimalarials, antifungals, stomach ulcer drugs) may increase levels. Increased risk for rebound HTN following clonidine withdrawal; d/c metoprolol several days before withdrawing clonidine. Effects can be reversed by β-agonists (eg, dobutamine, isoproterenol). HCTZ: Hypokalemia can sensitize/exaggerate cardiac response to toxic effects of digitalis. Risk of hypokalemia with steroids or adrenocorticotropic hormone. Insulin requirements may change in diabetic patients. May decrease arterial responsiveness to norepinephrine. May increase responsiveness to tubocurarine. May increase risk of lithium toxicity. Rare reports of hemolytic anemia with methyldopa. NSAIDs may reduce diuretic, natriuretic, and antihypertensive effects. Impaired absorption reported with cholestyramine and colestipol. Alcohol, barbiturates, and narcotics may potentiate orthostatic hypotension. May potentiate other antihypertensive drugs (eg, ganglionic or peripheral adrenergic-blocking drugs).

NURSING CONSIDERATIONS

Assessment: Assess for history of heart failure, sulfonamide hypersensitivity, SLE, hyperthyroidism, DM, pheochromocytoma, hepatic/renal impairment, any other conditions where treatment is contraindicated/cautioned, pregnancy/nursing status, and possible drug interactions. Obtain baseline serum electrolytes.

Monitoring: Monitor for signs/symptoms of cardiac failure, hypoglycemia, thyrotoxicosis, electrolyte imbalance, exacerbation/activation of SLE, hyperuricemia or precipitation of gout, hypersensitivity reactions, hepatic/renal dysfunction, myopia, angle-closure glaucoma, and other adverse reactions. Monitor serum electrolytes.

Patient Counseling: Instruct to take regularly and continuously, ud, with or immediately following meals. If dose is missed, instruct to take next dose at scheduled time (without doubling the dose) and not to d/c without consulting physician. Instruct to avoid driving, operating machinery, or engaging in tasks requiring alertness until response to therapy is determined. Advise to contact physician if difficulty in breathing or other adverse reactions occur, and to inform physician/dentist of drug therapy before undergoing any type of surgery.

Storage: (Lopressor HCT) 25°C (77°F); excursions permitted to 15-30°C (59-86°F). (Metoprolol-HCTZ) 20-25°C (68-77°F). Protect from moisture.

METOZOLV ODT – metoclopramide hydrochloride RX

Class: Dopamine antagonist/prokinetic

May cause tardive dyskinesia (TD); d/c if signs/symptoms of TD develop. Avoid use for >12 weeks of therapy unless benefit outweighs risk.

ADULT DOSAGE

Gastroesophageal Reflux Disease

Short-Term (4-12 Weeks) Therapy for Patients w/ Symptomatic, Documented GERD Who Fail to Respond to Conventional Therapy:
10-15mg up to qid

Intermittent Symptoms:
Single doses up to 20mg prior to the symptoms

Esophageal Erosions/Ulcerations:
15mg/dose qid

Therapy should not exceed 12 weeks in duration

Diabetic Gastroparesis

Acute/Recurrent:
10mg up to qid for 2-8 weeks

Therapy should not exceed 12 weeks in duration
Initial route of administration should be determined by the severity of the presenting symptoms; if severe symptoms are present, begin w/ inj. Inj administration may require up to 10 days before symptoms subside, at which time PO administration may be instituted

PEDIATRIC DOSAGE

Pediatric use may not have been established

DOSE MODIFICATION

Renal Impairment
CrCl <40mL/min:
Initial: 1/2 the recommended dose; adjust dose as appropriate

Elderly
Start at lower end of dosing range

ADMINISTRATION

Oral route

Take on an empty stomach at least 30 min ac and hs
Do not repeat dose if inadvertently taken w/ food
Only remove each dose from packaging just prior to taking
Handle tab w/ dry hands and place on tongue; if tab breaks or crumbles while handling, discard and remove a new tab
Disintegrates on tongue in approx 1 min
Take w/o liquid

HOW SUPPLIED

Tab, Disintegrating: 5mg, 10mg

CONTRAINDICATIONS

When GI motility stimulation is dangerous (eg, GI hemorrhage, mechanical obstruction, or perforation), pheochromocytoma, epilepsy, and concomitant drugs that cause extrapyramidal reactions.

WARNINGS/PRECAUTIONS

May cause extrapyramidal symptoms (EPS); usually seen during the 1st 24-48 hrs of treatment. May cause drug-induced parkinsonism; symptoms generally subside within 2-3 months following d/c. Caution with history of Parkinson's disease. Neuroleptic malignant syndrome (NMS) reported; d/c and institute intensive symptomatic treatment and medical monitoring if NMS occurs. Depression may occur; caution with history of depression. Caution with HTN, renal impairment, and in the elderly. May increase risk of developing methemoglobinemia and/or sulfhemoglobinemia with NADH-cytochrome b5 reductase deficiency. Risk of developing fluid retention and volume overload in patients with cirrhosis or congestive heart failure (CHF); d/c if these occur. May experience withdrawal symptoms (eg, dizziness, nervousness, headaches) after d/c.

ADVERSE REACTIONS

N/V, fatigue, somnolence, headache.

DRUG INTERACTIONS

See Contraindications. GI motility effect antagonized by anticholinergics and narcotic analgesics. Additive sedation may occur with alcohol, sedatives, hypnotics, narcotics, or tranquilizers. Caution with MAOIs. May decrease gastric absorption of some drugs (eg, digoxin) and increase intestinal absorption of others (eg, acetaminophen, tetracycline, levodopa, ethanol, cyclosporine). Insulin dose or timing of dose may need adjustment to prevent hypoglycemia. Avoid with antidepressants, antipsychotics, and/or neuroleptics associated with TD or NMS. Rare cases of hepatotoxicity with drugs with hepatotoxic potential. Inhibits the central and peripheral effects of apomorphine.

NURSING CONSIDERATIONS

Assessment: Assess for conditions where treatment is contraindicated or cautioned, pregnancy/nursing status, and for possible drug interactions.

Monitoring: Monitor for signs/symptoms of depression, EPS, Parkinsonism, TD, NMS, HTN, fluid retention/volume overload, withdrawal symptoms, and other adverse reactions.

Patient Counseling: Advise to take drug at least 30 min ac and hs. Inform that drug may impair mental and physical abilities. Inform of serious and potential issues associated with treatment (during and after treatment) and advise to inform physician if symptoms occur.

Storage: 20-25°C (68-77°F).

METROGEL-VAGINAL – metronidazole **RX**

Class: Nitroimidazole

ADULT DOSAGE

Bacterial Vaginosis

Usual: 1 applicatorful (5g) intravaginally qd or bid for 5 days

PEDIATRIC DOSAGE

Pediatric use may not have been established

ADMINISTRATION

Intravaginal route

Administer hs for qd dosing
Refer to PI for administration instructions

HOW SUPPLIED

Gel: 0.75% [70g]

WARNINGS/PRECAUTIONS

Not for ophthalmic, dermal, or PO use. Convulsive seizures and peripheral neuropathy reported; d/c promptly if abnormal neurologic signs appear. Caution with CNS diseases and severe hepatic disease. Known or previously unrecognized vaginal candidiasis may present more prominent symptoms during therapy. May develop symptomatic *Candida* vaginitis during or immediately after therapy. Contains ingredients that may cause burning and irritation of the eye; rinse with copious amounts of cool tap water in the event of accidental contact. May interfere with certain types of serum chemistry values (eg, AST, ALT, LDH, TG, glucose hexokinase).

ADVERSE REACTIONS

Symptomatic *Candida* cervicitis/vaginitis, vaginal discharge, pelvic discomfort, N/V, headache, vulva/vaginal irritation, GI discomfort.

DRUG INTERACTIONS

May potentiate anticoagulant effect of warfarin and other coumarin anticoagulants, resulting in prolongation of PT. Elevation of serum lithium levels and signs of lithium toxicity may occur in short-term therapy with high doses of lithium. Cimetidine may prolong $T_{1/2}$ and decrease plasma clearance. May cause disulfiram-like reaction with alcohol. May cause psychotic reactions in alcoholic patients using disulfiram concurrently; do not administer within 2 weeks of discontinuation of disulfiram.

NURSING CONSIDERATIONS

Assessment: Assess for hypersensitivity to drug, CNS/severe hepatic diseases, vaginal candidiasis, alcohol intake, nursing status, and possible drug interactions. Assess for clinical diagnosis of bacterial vaginosis.

Monitoring: Monitor for convulsive seizures, peripheral neuropathy, *Candida* vaginitis, and other adverse reactions.

Patient Counseling: Caution about drinking alcohol while on therapy. Instruct not to engage in vaginal intercourse during treatment. Inform to avoid contact with eyes and instruct to rinse with copious amounts of cool tap water in the event of accidental contact.

Storage: 15-30°C (59-86°F). Protect from freezing.

METRONIDAZOLE INJECTION – metronidazole RX

Class: Nitroimidazole

Shown to be carcinogenic in mice and rats. Avoid unnecessary use. Should be reserved for the conditions for which it is indicated.

ADULT DOSAGE

General Dosing

Intra-abdominal, skin and skin structure, gynecologic, bone/joint (as adjunctive therapy), CNS, and lower respiratory tract infections, bacterial septicemia, and endocarditis caused by susceptible strains of microorganisms (anaerobic bacteria); effective in *Bacteroides fragilis* infections resistant to clindamycin, chloramphenicol, and penicillin

LD: 15mg/kg IV infusion over 1 hr (approx 1g for a 70kg adult)

Maint: 7.5mg/kg IV infusion over 1 hr q6h (approx 500mg for a 70kg adult), starting 6 hrs after LD initiation

Max: 4g/24 hrs

Usual Duration: 7-10 days; infections of the bone and joint, lower respiratory tract, and endocardium may require longer treatment

May change to oral metronidazole when conditions warrant, based on severity of disease and response

Prophylaxis of Postoperative Infections

In Contaminated or Potentially Contaminated Colorectal Surgery:

15mg/kg IV infusion over 30-60 min (complete 1 hr before surgery), then 7.5mg/kg IV infusion over 30-60 min at 6 and 12 hrs after initial dose

D/C w/in 12 hrs after surgery

PEDIATRIC DOSAGE

Pediatric use may not have been established

DOSE MODIFICATION

Renal Impairment

Hemodialysis: If administration cannot be separated from hemodialysis session, consider supplementation of dosage following the session, depending on patient's clinical situation

Hepatic Impairment

Severe (Child-Pugh C): Reduce dose by 50%

ADMINISTRATION

IV route

No dilution/buffering required

Administer by slow IV drip infusion only (either as continuous or intermittent infusion)

Do not introduce additives into drug sol

If used w/ a primary IV fluid system, the primary sol should be discontinued during metronidazole infusion

Do not use equipment containing aluminum (eg, needles, cannulae) that would come in contact w/ the drug sol

Refer to PI for additional preparation and administration instructions

HOW SUPPLIED

Inj: 5mg/mL [100mL]

CONTRAINDICATIONS

Disulfiram use within the last 2 weeks. Consumption of alcohol or products containing propylene glycol during and for at least 3 days after therapy.

WARNINGS/PRECAUTIONS

Encephalopathy and peripheral neuropathy (including optic neuropathy), convulsive seizures, and aseptic meningitis reported; promptly evaluate benefit/risk ratio of the continuation of therapy if abnormal neurologic signs/symptoms appear. Known or previously unrecognized candidiasis may present more prominent symptoms during therapy and requires treatment with a candicidal agent. Caution with hepatic/renal impairment, evidence of or history of blood dyscrasia, and in the elderly. Mild leukopenia reported; monitor total and differential leukocyte counts before, during, and after prolonged or repeated courses of therapy. May cause Na^+ retention due to Na^+ content; caution in patients receiving corticosteroids or predisposed to edema. May result in bacterial resistance if used in the absence of proven or suspected bacterial infection, or a prophylactic indication. Lab test interactions may occur.

ADVERSE REACTIONS

Headache, syncope, dizziness, vertigo, incoordination, nausea, diarrhea, epigastric distress, abdominal cramping, constipation, unpleasant metallic taste, erythematous rash, pruritus, urticaria, dysuria.

DRUG INTERACTIONS

See Contraindications. May potentiate anticoagulant effect of warfarin and other oral coumarin anticoagulants, resulting in PT prolongation; carefully monitor PT and INR. May increase serum lithium, and may cause lithium toxicity; obtain serum lithium and SrCr levels several days after beginning metronidazole. May increase busulfan concentrations, which can result in increased risk for serious busulfan toxicity; avoid concomitant use or, if coadministration is medically needed, frequently monitor busulfan concentration and adjust busulfan dose accordingly. Simultaneous administration of drugs that decrease microsomal liver enzyme activity (eg, cimetidine) may prolong $T_{1/2}$ and decrease clearance. Simultaneous administration of drugs that induce microsomal liver enzyme activity (eg, phenytoin, phenobarbital) may accelerate elimination, resulting in reduced levels. Impaired clearance of phenytoin reported.

NURSING CONSIDERATIONS

Assessment: Assess for candidiasis, alcohol use, hepatic/renal impairment, evidence/history of blood dyscrasia, predisposition to edema, hypersensitivity to drug or other nitroimidazole derivatives, pregnancy/nursing status, and possible drug interactions. Obtain total and differential leukocyte counts before prolonged/repeated courses of therapy.

Monitoring: Monitor for abnormal neurologic signs/symptoms, candidiasis, Na^+ retention, and other adverse reactions. Monitor total and differential leukocyte counts during and after prolonged or repeated courses of therapy. Monitor PT and INR with oral coumarin anticoagulants (eg, warfarin).

Patient Counseling: Instruct to d/c consumption of alcoholic beverages or products containing propylene glycol while taking the drug and for at least 3 days afterward. Counsel that therapy should only be used to treat bacterial, not viral, infections. Instruct to take exactly ud even if the patient feels better early in the course of therapy. Inform that skipping doses or not completing the full course of therapy may decrease effectiveness of treatment and increase bacterial resistance.

Storage: 25°C (77°F). Protect from light. Do not remove unit from overwrap until ready for use.

MIACALCIN – calcitonin-salmon RX

Class: Hormonal bone resorption inhibitor

ADULT DOSAGE

Paget's Disease

Moderate to Severe Symptomatic Disease:

Inj:

Usual: 100 IU (0.5mL) SQ/IM qd

Periodically reevaluate need for continued therapy

Hypercalcemia

Early treatment of hypercalcemic emergencies, along w/ other appropriate agents, when a rapid decrease in serum Ca^{2+} is required, until more specific treatment of the underlying disease can be accomplished

Inj:

Initial: 4 IU/kg SQ/IM q12h

Titrate: If response is not satisfactory after 1 or 2 days, dose may be increased to 8 IU/kg q12h; if response remains unsatisfactory after 2 more

PEDIATRIC DOSAGE

Pediatric use may not have been established

days, dose may be further increased to a max of 8 IU/kg q6h

Periodically reevaluate need for continued therapy

Postmenopausal Osteoporosis

In Women >5 Years Postmenopause:
Inj:
Usual: 100 IU (0.5mL) SQ/IM qd

Spray:
Usual: 1 spray (200 IU) qd intranasally, alternating nostrils daily

Calcium and Vitamin D Supplementation:
Patients should receive adequate Ca^{2+} (≥1000mg elemental Ca^{2+}/day) and vitamin D (≥400 IU/day)

Periodically reevaluate need for continued therapy

ADMINISTRATION
(Inj) IM/SQ route; (Spray) Intranasal route

Inj
If volume to be injected is >2mL, IM inj is preferable and total dose should be distributed across multiple inj sites

Nasal Spray
Wait until the bottle has reached room temperature before using the 1st dose
To prime the pump before it is used for the 1st time, hold the bottle upright and depress the 2 white side arms of the pump toward the bottle until a full spray is released; the pump is primed once the 1st full spray is emitted
To administer, carefully place the nozzle into the nostril w/ the patient's head in the upright position, then firmly depress the pump toward the bottle
Do not prime the pump before each daily use

HOW SUPPLIED
Inj: 200 IU/mL [2mL]; Spray: 200 IU/actuation [3.7mL]

WARNINGS/PRECAUTIONS
Serious hypersensitivity reactions reported; appropriate medical support and monitoring measures should be readily available. Consider skin testing prior to treatment with suspected sensitivity to therapy. Hypocalcemia associated with tetany and seizure activity reported. Correct hypocalcemia and treat other disorders affecting mineral metabolism (eg, vitamin D deficiency) before initiating therapy. Provisions for parenteral Ca^{2+} administration should be available during the 1st several administrations of therapy in patients at risk for hypocalcemia. Adequate intake of Ca^{2+} and vitamin D is recommended in patients treated for Paget's disease or postmenopausal osteoporosis. Increased risk of malignancies; carefully consider benefits against possible risks. Consider possibility of antibody formation in any patient with an initial response to therapy who later stops responding to treatment. Urinary casts reported; consider periodic exam of urine sediment. (Spray) Nasal adverse reactions (eg, rhinitis, epistaxis) reported; development of mucosal alterations may occur. Periodic nasal exams are recommended prior to start of treatment, periodically during therapy, and at any time nasal symptoms occur. D/C if severe ulceration of the nasal mucosa occurs; d/c temporarily until healing occurs in patients with smaller ulcers.

ADVERSE REACTIONS
Nausea, flushing, malignancy. (Inj) Inj-site local inflammatory reactions, vomiting. (Spray) Nasal symptoms, rhinitis, back pain, epistaxis, headache, arthralgia.

DRUG INTERACTIONS
May reduce plasma lithium concentrations; lithium dose may require adjustment.

NURSING CONSIDERATIONS
Assessment: Assess for hypersensitivity to drug or any of the excipients, hypocalcemia or other disorders affecting mineral metabolism, pregnancy/nursing status, and possible drug interactions. Consider skin testing for patients with suspected sensitivity to therapy. (Spray) Perform baseline nasal exam.

Monitoring: Monitor for signs/symptoms of serious hypersensitivity reactions, malignancy, hypocalcemia associated with tetany and seizure activity, antibody formation, and other adverse reactions. Periodically assess need for continued therapy. Perform periodic exams of urine sediment. (Spray) Perform periodic nasal exams during therapy and when nasal symptoms occur.

Patient Counseling: Inform of the potential increase in risk of malignancy. Advise patients with postmenopausal osteoporosis or Paget's disease of bone to maintain an adequate Ca^{2+} and vitamin D intake. Instruct to seek emergency medical help if any sign/symptoms of a serious allergic reaction develop. (Inj) Instruct about sterile inj technique and to dispose of needles properly. (Spray) Instruct on pump assembly, priming of pump, and nasal introduction of medication. Advise to notify physician if significant nasal irritation develops.

Storage: (Spray) Unopened: 2-8°C (36-46°F). Protect from freezing. In Use: 15-30°C (59-86°F) in an upright position for up to 35 days. Discard after 30 doses. (Inj) 2-8°C (36-46°F).

MICARDIS – telmisartan

RX

Class: Angiotensin II receptor antagonist

D/C when pregnancy is detected. Drugs that act directly on the renin-angiotensin system (RAS) can cause injury/death to the developing fetus.

ADULT DOSAGE

Hypertension

Initial: 40mg qd
Usual: 20-80mg/day
May add diuretic if BP not controlled w/ 80mg

Risk Reduction of Myocardial Infarction, Stroke, Cardiovascular Death

For use in patients ≥55 years of age at high risk of developing major CV events who are unable to take ACE inhibitors

Usual: 80mg qd

PEDIATRIC DOSAGE

Pediatric use may not have been established

DOSE MODIFICATION

Hepatic Impairment

Including Biliary Obstructive Disorders:
Start at low doses and titrate slowly

ADMINISTRATION

Oral route

Take w/ or w/o food

HOW SUPPLIED

Tab: 20mg, 40mg, 80mg

CONTRAINDICATIONS

Coadministration with aliskiren in patients with diabetes.

WARNINGS/PRECAUTIONS

May develop orthostatic hypotension in patients on dialysis. Symptomatic hypotension may occur in patients with an activated RAS (eg, volume- and/or salt-depleted patients receiving high doses of diuretics); correct this condition before therapy or monitor closely. Hyperkalemia may occur, particularly in patients with advanced renal impairment, HF, and on renal replacement therapy; monitor serum electrolytes periodically. Caution in patients with hepatic impairment (eg, biliary obstructive disorders); reduced clearance may be expected. Oliguria and/or progressive azotemia and (rarely) acute renal failure and/or death may occur in patients whose renal function is dependent on the RAS (eg, severe CHF). May increase SrCr/BUN in patients with renal artery stenosis.

ADVERSE REACTIONS

URTI, back pain, sinusitis, diarrhea, intermittent claudication, skin ulcer.

DRUG INTERACTIONS

See Contraindications. Dual blockade of the RAS is associated with increased risk of hypotension, hyperkalemia, and changes in renal function (eg, acute renal failure); avoid combined use of RAS inhibitors. Closely monitor BP, renal function, and electrolytes with concomitant agents that also affect the RAS. Avoid with aliskiren in patients with renal impairment (GFR <60mL/min). Avoid with an ACE inhibitor. Coadministration with ramipril may increase ramipril/ramiprilat levels and decrease telmisartan levels; not recommended with ramipril. Hyperkalemia may occur with K^+ supplements, K^+-sparing diuretics, K^+-containing salt substitutes, or other drugs that increase K^+ levels. May increase digoxin levels; monitor digoxin levels upon initiating, adjusting, and discontinuing therapy. May increase serum lithium levels/toxicity; monitor lithium levels during concomitant use. NSAIDs, including selective COX-2 inhibitors, may attenuate antihypertensive effect and may deteriorate renal function; monitor renal function periodically.

NURSING CONSIDERATIONS

Assessment: Assess for known hypersensitivity to drug, biliary obstructive disorders, CHF, renal artery stenosis, hepatic/renal impairment, volume/salt depletion, dialysis patients, pregnancy/nursing status, and possible drug interactions.

Monitoring: Monitor for symptomatic hypotension and other adverse reactions. Monitor BP, ECG, renal function, and serum electrolytes.

Patient Counseling: Inform women of childbearing age about the consequences of exposure to the medication during pregnancy. Discuss treatment options with women planning to become pregnant. Instruct to report pregnancies to the physician as soon as possible.

Storage: 25°C (77°F); excursions permitted to 15-30°C (59-86°F).

MICARDIS HCT – hydrochlorothiazide/telmisartan RX

Class: Angiotensin II receptor antagonist/thiazide diuretic

D/C when pregnancy is detected. Drugs that act directly on the renin-angiotensin system (RAS) can cause injury/death to the developing fetus.

ADULT DOSAGE

Hypertension

Usual: 80mg-160mg telmisartan/12.5mg-25mg HCTZ qd

Replacement Therapy:
May be substituted for the titrated components

PEDIATRIC DOSAGE

Pediatric use may not have been established

DOSE MODIFICATION

Hepatic Impairment

Biliary Obstruction/Hepatic Insufficiency:
Initial: 40mg-12.5mg qd

ADMINISTRATION

Oral route
Take with or without food

HOW SUPPLIED

Tab: (Telmisartan-HCTZ) 40mg-12.5mg, 80mg-12.5mg, 80mg-25mg

CONTRAINDICATIONS

Anuria, hypersensitivity to sulfonamide-derived drugs. Coadministration with aliskiren in patients with diabetes.

WARNINGS/PRECAUTIONS

Not for initial therapy. Hypotension may occur in patients with activated RAS, such as volume- or Na^+-depleted (eg, vigorously treated with diuretics); correct these conditions prior to therapy and monitor closely. Not recommended with severe renal impairment (CrCl ≤30mL/min) and severe hepatic impairment. HCTZ: Caution with hepatic impairment or progressive liver disease; may precipitate hepatic coma. May cause hypersensitivity reactions, exacerbation or activation of systemic lupus erythematosus (SLE), hyperuricemia or precipitation of frank gout, hyperglycemia, hypomagnesemia, hypercalcemia, and latent diabetes mellitus (DM). May cause an idiosyncratic reaction, resulting in acute transient myopia and acute angle-closure glaucoma; d/c as rapidly as possible. Observe for clinical signs of fluid or electrolyte imbalance (hyponatremia, hypochloremic alkalosis, and hypokalemia). Hypokalemia may develop, especially with brisk diuresis, severe cirrhosis, or after prolonged therapy. Hypokalemia may cause cardiac arrhythmia and may sensitize/exaggerate the response of the heart to toxic effects of digitalis. D/C before testing for parathyroid function. Enhanced effects in postsympathectomy patients. Increased cholesterol and TG levels reported. Caution with severe renal disease; may precipitate azotemia with renal disease. Consider withholding or discontinuing therapy if progressive renal impairment occurs. Telmisartan: Oliguria and/or progressive azotemia and (rare) acute renal failure and/or death may occur in patients whose renal function is dependent on the RAS (eg, severe CHF). May increase SrCr/BUN in patients with renal artery stenosis. Caution in patients with biliary obstructive disorders or hepatic impairment.

ADVERSE REACTIONS

Upper respiratory tract infection, dizziness, sinusitis, fatigue, diarrhea.

DRUG INTERACTIONS

See Contraindications. NSAIDs, including selective COX-2 inhibitors, may decrease effects of diuretics and ARBs and may further deteriorate renal function. May increase risk of lithium toxicity; avoid concurrent use. HCTZ: Alcohol, barbiturates, or narcotics may potentiate orthostatic hypotension. Dosage adjustment of antidiabetic drugs (eg, oral agents, insulin) may be required. Additive effect or potentiation with other antihypertensive drugs. Anionic exchange resins (eg, cholestyramine, colestipol resins) may impair absorption. Corticosteroids and adrenocorticotropic hormone may intensify electrolyte depletion, particularly hypokalemia. May decrease response to pressor amines (eg, norepinephrine). May increase responsiveness to nondepolarizing skeletal muscle relaxants (eg, tubocurarine). Telmisartan: Dual blockade of the RAS is associated with increased risks of hypotension, hyperkalemia, and changes in renal function (including acute renal failure); avoid combined use of RAS inhibitors, or closely monitor BP, renal function, and electrolytes with concomitant agents that also affect the RAS. May increase digoxin levels; monitor digoxin levels. Coadministration with ramipril may increase ramipril and ramiprilat levels and decrease telmisartan levels. May slightly decrease warfarin levels. Possible inhibition of drugs metabolized by CYP2C19.

NURSING CONSIDERATIONS

Assessment: Assess for hypersensitivity to drugs and their components, anuria, sulfonamide-derived hypersensitivity, history of penicillin allergy, volume/salt depletion, SLE, DM, CHF, hepatic/renal impairment, biliary obstructive disorder, renal artery stenosis, postsympathectomy patients, pregnancy/nursing status, and possible drug interactions. Obtain baseline BP.

Monitoring: Monitor for exacerbation/activation of SLE, idiosyncratic reaction, latent DM manifestations, hyperglycemia, hypercalcemia, hyperuricemia or precipitation of gout, hypersensitivity reactions, and other adverse reactions. Monitor BP, serum electrolytes, and renal function periodically.

Patient Counseling: Inform women of childbearing age about the consequences of exposure to the medication during pregnancy. Discuss treatment options with women planning to become pregnant. Instruct to report pregnancies to the physician as soon as possible. Caution that lightheadedness may occur, especially during the 1st days of therapy, and instruct to report to physician. Instruct to d/c therapy and consult physician if syncope occurs. Caution patients that inadequate fluid intake, excessive perspiration, diarrhea, or vomiting can lead to an excessive fall in BP, with the same consequences of lightheadedness and possible syncope. Advise patient not to use K^+ supplements or salt substitutes that contain K^+ without consulting physician.

Storage: 25°C (77°F); excursions permitted to 15-30°C (59-86°F).

MICRO-K – potassium chloride **RX**

Class: K^+ supplement

ADULT DOSAGE

Hypokalemia

Prevention: 20mEq/day

Treatment: 40-100mEq/day or more

Divide dose if >20mEq/day is given such that no more than 20mEq is given in a single dose

PEDIATRIC DOSAGE

Pediatric use may not have been established

DOSE MODIFICATION

Elderly

Start at lower end of dosing range

ADMINISTRATION

Oral route

Take with meals and a full glass of water or other liquid

May sprinkle on a spoonful of soft food (eg, applesauce, pudding) in patients who have difficulty swallowing caps; swallow immediately without chewing and follow with a glass of cool water or juice

HOW SUPPLIED

Cap, Extended-Release: 8mEq, 10mEq

CONTRAINDICATIONS

Hyperkalemia, esophageal ulceration, delay in GI passage (from structural, pathological, pharmacologic causes [eg, anticholinergic agents]), cardiac patients with esophageal compression due to enlarged left atrium.

WARNINGS/PRECAUTIONS

Potentially fatal hyperkalemia may occur. Extreme caution with acidosis, cardiac, and renal disease; monitor ECG and electrolytes. Hypokalemia with metabolic acidosis should be treated with an alkalinizing potassium salt (eg, potassium bicarbonate, potassium citrate). May produce ulcerative or stenotic GI lesions.

ADVERSE REACTIONS
Hyperkalemia, GI effects (obstruction, bleeding, ulceration), N/V, abdominal pain, diarrhea.

DRUG INTERACTIONS
See Contraindications. Risk of hyperkalemia with ACE inhibitors (eg, captopril, enalapril), K^+-sparing diuretics, and K^+ supplements.

NURSING CONSIDERATIONS

Assessment: Assess for conditions that impair excretion of K^+, hyperkalemia, esophageal compression due to enlarged left atrium, conditions causing arrest or delay in passage through GI, renal insufficiency, diabetes mellitus, and possible drug interactions.

Monitoring: Monitor serum K^+ levels regularly; renal function, ECG, and acid-base balance. Monitor for GI ulceration/obstruction/perforation, hyperkalemia, renal dysfunction, and hypersensitivity reactions.

Patient Counseling: Instruct to take with meals; swallow with full glass of water or other suitable liquid. Instruct to not crush, chew, or suck. Instruct to seek medical attention if symptoms of GI ulceration, obstruction, perforation (vomiting, abdominal pain, distention, GI bleeding), hyperkalemia, or hypersensitivity reactions occur.

Storage: 20-25°C (68-77°F).

MICROZIDE – hydrochlorothiazide — RX

Class: Thiazide diuretic

ADULT DOSAGE

Hypertension

Initial: 12.5mg qd
Max: 50mg/day

PEDIATRIC DOSAGE

Pediatric use may not have been established

DOSE MODIFICATION

Elderly
Start at lower end of dosing range, utilizing 12.5mg increments for further titration

ADMINISTRATION
Oral route

HOW SUPPLIED
Cap: 12.5mg

CONTRAINDICATIONS
Anuria, sulfonamide hypersensitivity.

WARNINGS/PRECAUTIONS
May cause idiosyncratic reaction, resulting in acute transient myopia and acute angle-closure glaucoma; d/c as rapidly as possible. May manifest latent diabetes mellitus (DM). May precipitate azotemia with renal impairment. Hypokalemia reported; monitor serum electrolytes and for sign/symptoms of fluid/electrolyte disturbances. Dilutional hyponatremia may occur in edematous patients in hot weather. Hyperuricemia or acute gout may be precipitated. Caution with hepatic impairment; hepatic coma may occur with severe liver disease. Decreased Ca^{2+} excretion and changes in parathyroid glands with hypercalcemia and hypophosphatemia reported during prolonged use. D/C prior to parathyroid test.

ADVERSE REACTIONS
Weakness, hypotension, pancreatitis, jaundice, diarrhea, vomiting, hematologic abnormalities, anaphylactic reactions, electrolyte imbalance, muscle spasm, vertigo, renal failure, erythema multiforme, transient blurred vision, impotence.

DRUG INTERACTIONS
Potentiation of orthostatic hypotension with alcohol, barbiturates, narcotics. Additive effect or potentiation with antihypertensive drugs. Dose adjustment of antidiabetic drugs (oral agents or insulin) may be required. Reduced absorption with cholestyramine or colestipol. Increased risk of electrolyte depletion (eg, hypokalemia) with corticosteroids and adrenocorticotropic hormone. May decrease response to pressor amines (eg, norepinephrine). May increase responsiveness to nondepolarizing skeletal muscle relaxants (eg, tubocurarine). Increased risk of lithium toxicity; avoid with lithium. NSAIDs may reduce diuretic, natriuretic, and antihypertensive effects. May cause hypokalemia, which can sensitize or exaggerate the response of the heart to the toxic effects of digitalis.

NURSING CONSIDERATIONS

Assessment: Assess for anuria, known hypersensitivity to sulfonamide-derived drugs, history of penicillin allergy, DM, risk for developing hypokalemia, impaired renal/hepatic function, edema, pregnancy/nursing status, and for possible drug interactions. Obtain baseline serum electrolytes.

Monitoring: Monitor for signs/symptoms of decreased visual acuity, ocular pain, azotemia, hypokalemia, fluid/electrolyte disturbances, dilutional hyponatremia, hyperuricemia or acute gout, and hepatic coma. Periodically monitor serum electrolytes in patients with risk for developing hypokalemia.

Patient Counseling: Counsel about signs/symptoms of fluid and electrolyte imbalance and advise to seek prompt medical attention.

Storage: 20-25°C (68-77°F). Protect from light, moisture, freezing, -20°C (-4°F). Keep container tightly closed.

MINOCIN – minocycline

RX

Class: Tetracyclines

ADULT DOSAGE

General Dosing

Treatment of the following infections caused by susceptible microorganisms: Rocky Mountain spotted fever, typhus fever and the typhus group, Q fever, rickettsialpox, tick fevers, respiratory tract infections, lymphogranuloma venereum, psittacosis (ornithosis), trachoma, inclusion conjunctivitis, relapsing fever, chancroid (cap), plague, tularemia, cholera, *Campylobacter fetus* infections, brucellosis (in conjunction w/ streptomycin), bartonellosis, granuloma inguinale, UTIs, skin and skin structure infections. Treatment of infections caused by susceptible strains of *Escherichia coli, Enterobacter aerogenes, Shigella* species, and *Acinetobacter* species. When penicillin is contraindicated, treatment of the following infections caused by susceptible microorganisms: infections in women caused by *Neisseria gonorrhoeae* (cap), meningitis (inj), yaws, listeriosis, anthrax, Vincent's infection, actinomycosis, infections caused by *Clostridium* species. Adjunctive therapy in acute intestinal amebiasis and severe acne

Cap:
Initial: 200mg
Maint: 100mg q12h
Alternate Dosing:
Initial: If more frequent doses are preferred, give two or four 50mg caps
Maint: One 50mg cap qid

Inj:
Initial: 200mg
Maint: 100mg q12h
Max: 400mg/24 hrs

Parenteral therapy is indicated only when oral therapy is not adequate or tolerated; institute oral therapy as soon as possible

Gonococcal Infections

Uncomplicated Infections Other Than Urethritis and Anorectal Infections in Men:
Cap:
Initial: 200mg
Maint: 100mg q12h for a minimum of 4 days, w/ post-therapy cultures w/in 2-3 days

Urethral Infections

Cap:
Uncomplicated Gonococcal Urethritis in Men When Penicillin is Contraindicated:
100mg q12h for 5 days

PEDIATRIC DOSAGE

General Dosing

>8 Years:
Cap/IV:
Initial: 4mg/kg
Maint: 2mg/kg q12h, not to exceed usual adult dose

Uncomplicated Infections Caused by *Chlamydia trachomatis/Ureaplasma urealyticum*:
100mg q12h for at least 7 days

Syphilis

When Penicillin is Contraindicated:
Cap:
Initial: 200mg
Maint: 100mg q12h over a period of 10-15 days

Meningococcal Carrier State

Cap:
Usual: 100mg q12h for 5 days

Mycobacterial Infections

***Mycobacterium marinum* Infections:**
Cap:
Optimal doses have not been established; 100mg q12h for 6-8 weeks have been successfully used

Endocervical Infections

Uncomplicated Infections Caused by *Chlamydia trachomatis/Ureaplasma urealyticum*:
Cap:
100mg q12h for at least 7 days

Rectal Infections

Uncomplicated Infections Caused by *Chlamydia trachomatis/Ureaplasma urealyticum*:
Cap:
100mg q12h for at least 7 days

DOSE MODIFICATION

Renal Impairment
CrCl <80mL/min:
Max Dose: 200mg/24 hrs
Elderly
Start at lower end of dosing range

ADMINISTRATION

Oral/IV routes
Cap
Take w/ or w/o food
Swallow whole w/ adequate amounts of fluids
Inj
Avoid rapid administration
Product and diluents are compatible at room temperature for 24 hrs w/o a significant loss of potency; discard any unused portions after that period
IV Reconstitution
Reconstitute w/ 5mL of sterile water for inj and immediately further dilute to 500mL-1000mL w/ NaCl inj, dextrose inj, dextrose and NaCl inj, Ringer's inj, or lactated Ringer's inj, but not w/ other sol containing Ca^{2+}
Final dilutions (500mL-1000mL) should be administered immediately
IV Incompatibilities
Do not mix before or during administration w/ any sol containing: ACTH, aminophylline, amobarbital sodium, amphotericin B, bicarbonate infusion mixtures, calcium gluconate or chloride, carbenicillin, cephalothin sodium, cefazolin sodium, chloramphenicol succinate, colistin sulfate, heparin sodium, hydrocortisone sodium succinate, iodine sodium, methicillin sodium, novobiocin, penicillin, pentobarbital, phenytoin sodium, polymyxin, prochlorperazine, sodium ascorbate, sulfadiazine, sulfisoxazole, thiopental sodium, vitamin K (sodium bisulfate or sodium salt), whole blood

HOW SUPPLIED

Cap: 50mg, 75mg, 100mg; Inj: 100mg

WARNINGS/PRECAUTIONS

May cause fetal harm. May cause permanent discoloration of the teeth (yellow-gray-brown) if used during tooth development (last 1/2 of pregnancy, infancy, and childhood to 8 yrs of age); do not use during tooth development. Enamel hypoplasia reported. May decrease fibula growth rate in premature infants. Drug rash w/ eosinophilia and systemic symptoms (DRESS), including fatal cases, reported; d/c immediately if this syndrome is recognized. May cause an increase in BUN; w/ significant impaired renal function, high levels of therapy may lead to azotemia, hyperphosphatemia, and acidosis. Photosensitivity manifested by an exaggerated sunburn reaction reported. CNS side effects reported; may impair mental/physical abilities. *Clostridium difficile*-associated diarrhea (CDAD) reported; may need to d/c if CDAD is suspected or confirmed. Associated w/ intracranial HTN (pseudotumor cerebri); increased risk in women of childbearing age who are overweight or have a history of intracranial HTN. If visual disturbance occurs, prompt ophthalmologic evaluation is warranted. Intracranial pressure can remain elevated for weeks after drug cessation; monitor patients until they stabilize. May result in bacterial resistance if used in the absence of proven or suspected bacterial infection, or a prophylactic indication; take appropriate measures if superinfection develops. Hepatotoxicity reported. False elevations of urinary catecholamine levels may occur due to interference w/ the fluorescence test. (Cap) Not indicated for the treatment of meningococcal infection; reserve prophylactic use for situations in which the risk of meningococcal meningitis is high.

ADVERSE REACTIONS

Neutropenia, agranulocytosis, lupus-like syndrome, serum sickness-like syndrome, fever, N/V, diarrhea, increased liver enzymes, thyroid cancer, anaphylaxis, exfoliative dermatitis, Stevens-Johnson syndrome, skin and mucous membrane pigmentation, headache.

DRUG INTERACTIONS

Caution w/ other hepatotoxic drugs. Depresses plasma prothrombin activity; may require downward adjustment of anticoagulant dosage. May interfere w/ bactericidal action of PCN; avoid concurrent use. Fatal renal toxicity reported w/ methoxyflurane. May decrease effectiveness of oral contraceptives. Avoid isotretinoin shortly before, during, and after therapy; each drug alone is associated w/ pseudotumor cerebri. Increased risk of ergotism w/ ergot alkaloids or their derivatives. (Cap) Impaired absorption w/ antacids containing aluminum, Ca^{2+}, or Mg^{2+}, and iron-containing preparations.

NURSING CONSIDERATIONS

Assessment: Assess for hypersensitivity to drug, risk for intracranial HTN, hepatic/renal impairment, pregnancy/nursing status, and possible drug interactions. Perform culture and susceptibility tests. (Cap) In venereal disease when coexistent syphilis is suspected, perform a dark-field examination and blood serology. (Inj) Perform serologic test for syphilis (if treating gonorrhea).

Monitoring: Monitor for DRESS, photosensitivity, CNS effects, CDAD, intracranial HTN, superinfection, and other adverse reactions. Perform periodic lab evaluations of organ systems, including hematopoietic, renal, and hepatic studies. (Cap) In venereal disease when coexistent syphilis is suspected, repeat blood serology monthly for at least 4 months. (Inj) In patients w/ gonorrhea, perform a follow-up serologic test for syphilis after 3 months.

Patient Counseling: Apprise of the potential hazard to fetus if used during pregnancy; instruct to notify physician if pregnant. Counsel that therapy should only be used to treat bacterial, not viral, infections. Instruct to take exactly ud even if the patient feels better early in the course of therapy. Inform that skipping doses or not completing the full course of therapy may decrease effectiveness of treatment and increase bacterial resistance. Inform that diarrhea may be experienced; instruct to immediately contact physician if watery and bloody stools (w/ or w/o stomach cramps and fever) occur, even as late as ≥2 months after the last dose. Advise that photosensitivity manifested by an exaggerated sunburn reaction may occur; instruct to d/c treatment at the 1st evidence of skin erythema. Caution patients who experience CNS symptoms about driving vehicles or using hazardous machinery while on therapy. Inform that drug may render oral contraceptives less effective.

Storage: 20-25°C (68-77°F). (Cap) Protect from light, moisture, and excessive heat.

MIRAPEX – pramipexole dihydrochloride RX

Class: Non-ergot dopamine agonist

ADULT DOSAGE

Parkinson's Disease

Initial: 0.125mg tid

Titrate: May increase gradually not more frequently than every 5-7 days (eg, Week 2: 0.25mg tid; Week 3: 0.5mg tid; Week 4: 0.75mg tid; Week 5: 1mg tid; Week 6: 1.25mg tid; Week 7: 1.5mg tid)

Maint: 0.5-1.5mg tid in equally divided doses w/ or w/o levodopa

If a significant interruption in therapy has occurred, retitration may be warranted

PEDIATRIC DOSAGE

Pediatric use may not have been established

Restless Legs Syndrome

Primary, Moderate to Severe:
Initial: 0.125mg qd
Titrate: May increase dose every 4-7 days up to 0.5mg/day, if needed
Titration Step 1: 0.125mg qd
Titration Step 2: 0.25mg qd
Titration Step 3: 0.5mg qd
If a significant interruption in therapy has occurred, retitration may be warranted
Administer 2-3 hrs before hs

DOSE MODIFICATION

Renal Impairment

Parkinson's Disease:
Mild (CrCl >50mL/min):
Initial: 0.125mg tid
Max: 1.5mg tid

Moderate (CrCl 30-50mL/min):
Initial: 0.125mg bid
Max: 0.75mg tid

Severe (CrCl 15-<30mL/min):
Initial: 0.125mg qd
Max: 1.5mg qd

Restless Legs Syndrome:
Moderate and Severe Renal Impairment (CrCl 20-60mL/min):
Increase duration between titration steps to 14 days

Discontinuation

Parkinson's Disease:
Taper off at a rate of 0.75mg/day until daily dose has been reduced to 0.75mg, then reduce dose by 0.375mg/day

ADMINISTRATION

Oral route

Take w/ or w/o food

HOW SUPPLIED

Tab: 0.125mg, 0.25mg*, 0.5mg*, 0.75mg, 1mg*, 1.5mg* *scored

WARNINGS/PRECAUTIONS

Falling asleep during activities of daily living and somnolence reported; reassess for drowsiness or sleepiness, and d/c if significant daytime sleepiness or episodes of falling asleep during activities that require active participation develops. May impair mental/physical abilities. May cause orthostatic hypotension; monitor for signs/symptoms, especially during dose escalation. May cause intense urges to gamble, increased sexual urges, intense urges to spend money uncontrollably, binge eating, and/or other intense urges, and the inability to control these urges while on therapy; consider dose reduction or discontinuation of therapy. Hallucinations and new/worsening mental status and behavioral changes reported; avoid w/ major psychotic disorder. May cause or exacerbate preexisting dyskinesia. Rhabdomyolysis and retinal deterioration reported. Symptom complex resembling the neuroleptic malignant syndrome reported w/ rapid dose reduction, withdrawal of, or changes in dopaminergic therapy; if possible, avoid sudden discontinuation/rapid dose reduction, or taper dose if discontinuing therapy. May cause fibrotic complications (eg, retroperitoneal fibrosis, pulmonary infiltrates, pleural effusion, pleural thickening, pericarditis, cardiac valvulopathy). Monitor for melanomas frequently and regularly; perform periodic skin examinations. Rebound and augmentation in RLS reported.

ADVERSE REACTIONS

Nausea, dizziness, somnolence, insomnia, constipation, asthenia, hallucinations, anorexia, peripheral edema, amnesia, confusion, headache, diarrhea, dreaming abnormalities, fatigue.

DRUG INTERACTIONS

Sedating medications or alcohol, and medications that increase plasma levels of pramipexole (eg, cimetidine) may increase risk of drowsiness. Dopamine antagonists, (eg, neuroleptics [phenothiazines, butyrophenones, thioxanthenes] or metoclopramide) may diminish effectiveness. May potentiate dopaminergic side effects of levodopa; consider dose reduction of levodopa.

NURSING CONSIDERATIONS

Assessment: Assess for preexisting dyskinesia, major psychotic disorder, sleep disorders, renal impairment, pregnancy/nursing status, and possible drug interactions.

Monitoring: Monitor for drowsiness or sleepiness, orthostatic hypotension, impulse control/compulsive behaviors, hallucinations, new/worsening mental status and behavioral changes, signs/symptoms of rhabdomyolysis, retinal deterioration, fibrotic complications, melanomas (frequently and regularly), withdrawal symptoms, and other adverse reactions.

Patient Counseling: Instruct to take as prescribed. If a dose is missed, advise not to double the next dose. Advise that the occurrence of nausea may be reduced if taken w/ food. Instruct not to take both immediate-release pramipexole and extended-release pramipexole. Advise and alert about the potential sedating effects, including somnolence and the possibility of falling asleep while engaged in activities of daily living; instruct not to drive a car or engage in other potentially dangerous activities until the patient has gained sufficient experience w/ pramipexole tabs to gauge whether or not it affects the patient's mental and/or motor performance adversely. Advise to inform physician if taking alcohol or other sedating medications. Inform of the possibility to experience intense urges to spend money uncontrollably, intense urges to gamble, increased sexual urges, binge eating, and/or other intense urges, and of the inability to control these urges. Inform that hallucinations and other psychotic-like behavior may occur. Advise that postural (orthostatic) hypotension may develop w/ or w/o symptoms. Advise to monitor for melanomas frequently and regularly. Instruct to notify physician if pregnant/intending to become pregnant during therapy or breastfeeding/intending to breastfeed.

Storage: 25°C (77°F); excursions permitted to 15-30°C (59-86°F). Protect from light.

MIRAPEX ER – pramipexole dihydrochloride — RX

Class: Non-ergot dopamine agonist

ADULT DOSAGE

Parkinson's Disease

Treatment of Signs/Symptoms of Idiopathic Parkinson's Disease:

Initial: 0.375mg qd
Titrate: Based on efficacy and tolerability, may increase gradually not more frequently than every 5-7 days, first to 0.75mg/day and then by 0.75mg increments
Max: 4.5mg/day

If a significant interruption in therapy occurs, retitration may be warranted

Conversions

Switching from Immediate-Release Tabs:
May switch overnight at the same daily dose; monitor to determine if dosage adjustment is necessary

PEDIATRIC DOSAGE

Pediatric use may not have been established

DOSE MODIFICATION

Renal Impairment

Moderate (CrCl 30-50mL/min):
Initial: Administer qod; carefully assess therapeutic response and tolerability before increasing to daily dosing after 1 week, and before any additional titration in 0.375mg increments
Titrate: Dose adjustment should occur no more frequently than at weekly intervals
Max: 2.25mg/day

Severe (CrCl <30mL/min)/Hemodialysis:
Not recommended

Discontinuation

May taper off at a rate of 0.75mg/day until daily dose has been reduced to 0.75mg; may reduce dose by 0.375mg/day thereafter

ADMINISTRATION

Oral route

Take w/ or w/o food
Swallow tabs whole; do not chew, crush, or divide tab

HOW SUPPLIED

Tab, ER: 0.375mg, 0.75mg, 1.5mg, 2.25mg, 3mg, 3.75mg, 4.5mg

WARNINGS/PRECAUTIONS

Falling asleep during activities of daily living and somnolence reported; continually reassess for drowsiness or sleepiness, and d/c if significant daytime sleepiness or episodes of falling asleep during activities that require active participation develops. May impair mental/physical abilities. May cause orthostatic hypotension; monitor for signs/symptoms, especially during dose escalation. May cause intense urges to gamble/spend money uncontrollably, increased sexual urges, binge eating, and/or other intense urges, and the inability to control these urges while on therapy; consider dose reduction or discontinuation of therapy. Hallucinations reported; risk increases with age. May cause or exacerbate preexisting dyskinesia. May cause rhabdomyolysis. Retinal deterioration reported. Symptom complex resembling the neuroleptic malignant syndrome may occur with rapid dose reduction, withdrawal of, or changes in antiparkinsonian therapy. May cause fibrotic complications (eg, retroperitoneal fibrosis, pulmonary infiltrates, pleural effusion, pleural thickening, pericarditis, cardiac valvulopathy). Monitor for melanomas frequently and regularly; perform periodic skin examinations. Not recommended with severe renal impairment or patients on dialysis.

ADVERSE REACTIONS

Somnolence, N/V, constipation, dizziness, fatigue, hallucinations, dry mouth, muscle spasms, peripheral edema, insomnia, fall, vertigo, dyskinesia, headache.

DRUG INTERACTIONS

Sedating medications or alcohol, and medications that increase plasma levels of pramipexole (eg, cimetidine) may increase risk of drowsiness. May potentiate dopaminergic side effects of levodopa. Dopamine antagonists, such as neuroleptics or metoclopramide may diminish effectiveness.

NURSING CONSIDERATIONS

Assessment: Assess for preexisting dyskinesia, renal impairment, sleep disorders, pregnancy/nursing status, and possible drug interactions.

Monitoring: Monitor signs/symptoms of rhabdomyolysis, orthostatic hypotension, melanomas, fibrotic complications, hallucinations, impulse control/compulsive behaviors, drowsiness or sleepiness, retinal deterioration, and other adverse reactions.

Patient Counseling: Instruct to take therapy as prescribed. If a dose is missed, take as soon as possible, but no later than 12 hrs after the regularly scheduled time. After 12 hrs, skip the missed dose and take the next dose on the following day at the regularly scheduled time. Advise that nausea may be reduced if taken with food. Instruct not to take both IR and ER pramipexole. Advise and alert about the potential sedating effects; instruct not to drive a car or engage in other dangerous activities until the patient has gained sufficient experience with therapy. Advise to inform physician if taking alcohol or other sedating medications. Inform of the possibility to experience intense urges and the inability to control these urges. Inform that hallucinations may occur. Advise that postural (orthostatic) hypotension may develop with or without symptoms. Instruct to notify physician if pregnant/intending to be pregnant during therapy or breastfeeding/intending to breastfeed.

Storage: 25°C (77°F); excursions permitted to 15-30°C (59-86°F). Protect from exposure to high humidity.

MIRTAZAPINE – mirtazapine RX

Class: Piperazino-azepine

Antidepressants increased the risk of suicidal thinking and behavior (suicidality) in children, adolescents, and young adults in short-term studies of major depressive disorder (MDD) and other psychiatric disorders. Monitor and observe closely for clinical worsening, suicidality, or unusual changes in behavior in patients who are started on antidepressant therapy. Not approved for use in pediatric patients.

OTHER BRAND NAMES

Remeron, RemeronSolTab

ADULT DOSAGE

Major Depressive Disorder

Initial: 15mg qhs
Titrate: Dose changes should not be made at intervals of <1-2 weeks
Max: 45mg/day

Dosing Considerations with MAOIs

Switching to/from an MAOI for Psychiatric Disorders:
Allow at least 14 days between discontinuation of an MAOI and initiation of mirtazapine, and allow at least 14 days between discontinuation of mirtazapine and initiation of an MAOI

PEDIATRIC DOSAGE

Pediatric use may not have been established

W/ Other MAOIs (eg, Linezolid, IV Methylene Blue):
Do not start mirtazapine in patients being treated w/ linezolid or IV methylene blue
In patients already receiving mirtazapine, if acceptable alternatives are not available and benefits outweigh risks, d/c mirtazapine and administer linezolid or IV methylene blue; monitor for serotonin syndrome for 2 weeks or until 24 hrs after the last dose of linezolid or IV methylene blue, whichever comes 1st. May resume mirtazapine therapy 24 hrs after the last dose of linezolid or IV methylene blue

DOSE MODIFICATION

Discontinuation
Gradually reduce dose over several weeks whenever possible

ADMINISTRATION
Oral route

RemeronSolTab
Open blister pack w/ dry hands and place tab on the tongue; use immediately after removal from blister
Once removed, it cannot be stored
Tab will disintegrate rapidly on the tongue and can be swallowed w/ saliva; no water is needed
Do not split the tab

HOW SUPPLIED
Tab: 7.5mg; (Remeron) 15mg*, 30mg*, 45mg; Tab, Disintegrating: (RemeronSolTab) 15mg, 30mg, 45mg *scored

CONTRAINDICATIONS
Use of an MAOI for psychiatric disorders either concomitantly or within 14 days of stopping treatment. Treatment within 14 days of stopping an MAOI for psychiatric disorders. Starting treatment in patients being treated with other MAOIs (eg, linezolid, IV methylene blue).

WARNINGS/PRECAUTIONS
Not approved for treatment of bipolar depression. May precipitate a mixed/manic episode in patients at risk for bipolar disorder; screen for risk of bipolar disorder prior to initiating treatment. Agranulocytosis and severe neutropenia reported; d/c if sore throat, fever, stomatitis, or other signs of infection develop, along with low WBC counts. Serotonin syndrome reported; d/c immediately and initiate supportive symptomatic treatment. Pupillary dilation that occurs following use may trigger an angle-closure attack in a patient with anatomically narrow angles who does not have a patent iridectomy. Avoid abrupt discontinuation; gradual dose reduction is recommended. Akathisia/psychomotor restlessness reported; increasing the dose may be detrimental in patients who develop these symptoms. Hyponatremia reported. May impair mental/physical abilities. Somnolence, dizziness, increased appetite, weight gain, and elevation in cholesterol/TG/ALT levels reported. Mania/hypomania and seizures reported. Caution with hepatic/renal impairment, diseases/conditions affecting metabolism or hemodynamic responses, and in the elderly. May cause orthostatic hypotension; caution with cardiovascular (CV) or cerebrovascular disease that could be exacerbated by hypotension and conditions that predispose to hypotension.

ADVERSE REACTIONS
Somnolence, increased appetite, weight gain, dizziness, dry mouth, constipation, asthenia, flu syndrome, abnormal dreams, abnormal thinking.

DRUG INTERACTIONS
See Contraindications. May cause serotonin syndrome with other serotonergic drugs (eg, triptans, TCAs, fentanyl) and with drugs that impair metabolism of serotonin; d/c immediately if this occurs. Caution with antihypertensives and drugs known to cause hyponatremia. Phenytoin, carbamazepine, and other hepatic metabolism inducers (eg, rifampicin) may decrease levels; may need to increase mirtazapine dose. Cimetidine and ketoconazole may increase levels; may need to decrease mirtazapine dose with cimetidine. Avoid alcohol and diazepam or drugs similar to diazepam while on therapy. Caution with potent CYP3A4 inhibitors, HIV protease inhibitors, azole antifungals, erythromycin, or nefazodone. Increased INR with warfarin; monitor INR.

NURSING CONSIDERATIONS

Assessment: Assess for risk of bipolar disorder or hyponatremia, susceptibility to angle-closure glaucoma, CV or cerebrovascular diseases, history of mania/hypomania/seizure, conditions that predispose to hypotension, renal/hepatic impairment, diseases/conditions affecting metabolism or hemodynamic response, hypersensitivity to drug, pregnancy/nursing status, and possible drug interactions.

Monitoring: Monitor for signs/symptoms of clinical worsening, suicidality, unusual changes in behavior, agranulocytosis, neutropenia, serotonin syndrome, angle-closure glaucoma, akathisia, somnolence, dizziness, increased appetite, weight gain, elevation in cholesterol/TG/ALT levels, hyponatremia, seizures, orthostatic hypotension, and other adverse reactions. Monitor INR with warfarin.

Patient Counseling: Inform about the risks, benefits, and appropriate use of therapy. Advise families and caregivers of the need for close observation for signs of clinical worsening and suicidal risks and to report such signs to physician. Warn about risk of developing agranulocytosis and instruct to contact physician if signs of infection (eg, fever, chills, sore throat, mucous membrane ulceration) develop. Advise to use caution when engaging in hazardous activities. Advise that improvement may be noticed in 1-4 weeks of therapy; instruct to continue therapy ud. Advise to inform physician if taking or intending to take any prescription or OTC drugs. Instruct to avoid alcohol while on therapy. Instruct to notify physician if pregnant, intending to become pregnant, or breastfeeding. Caution about the risk of angle-closure glaucoma. (RemeronSolTab) Inform phenylketonuric patients that the tab contains phenylalanine.

Storage: 25°C (77°F); excursions permitted to 15-30°C (59-86°F). Protect from light and moisture.

MOBIC – meloxicam — RX

Class: NSAID

NSAIDs may cause an increased risk of serious cardiovascular (CV) thrombotic events, MI, stroke, and serious GI adverse events, including bleeding, ulceration, and perforation of the stomach or intestines. Elderly patients at greater risk for serious GI events. Contraindicated for the treatment of perioperative pain in the setting of CABG surgery.

ADULT DOSAGE

Osteoarthritis

Initial/Maint: 7.5mg qd
Max: 15mg/day

Rheumatoid Arthritis

Initial/Maint: 7.5mg qd
Max: 15mg/day

PEDIATRIC DOSAGE

Juvenile Rheumatoid Arthritis

Pauciarticular or Polyarticular Course:
≥2 Years:
0.125mg/kg qd
Max: 7.5mg/day

Use of the oral sus is recommended to improve dosing accuracy in smaller weight children

DOSE MODIFICATION

Renal Impairment
Hemodialysis:
Max: 7.5mg/day

ADMINISTRATION

Oral route

Take w/o regard to time of meals
7.5mg/5mL or 15mg/10mL oral sus may be substituted for 7.5mg or 15mg tab, respectively

Sus
Shake gently before using

HOW SUPPLIED

Sus: 7.5mg/5mL; Tab: 7.5mg, 15mg

CONTRAINDICATIONS

ASA or other NSAID allergy that precipitates asthma, urticaria, or allergic-type reactions. Treatment of perioperative pain in the setting of CABG surgery.

WARNINGS/PRECAUTIONS

Use lowest effective dose for the shortest duration possible. Extreme caution with history of ulcer disease or GI bleeding. May cause elevations of LFTs; d/c if liver disease develops, or if systemic manifestations occur. May lead to onset of new HTN, or worsening of preexisting HTN. Fluid retention and edema reported. Renal papillary necrosis, renal insufficiency, acute renal failure, and other renal injury reported after long-term use. Not recommended for use with severe renal impairment (CrCl <20mL/min). Caution in patients with considerable dehydration; rehydrate 1st, then start therapy. Caution in debilitated patients, with preexisting kidney disease, and asthma. Closely monitor patients with significant renal impairment. Avoid with ASA triad/ASA-sensitive asthma. May cause anaphylactoid reactions and serious skin adverse events (eg, exfoliative dermatitis, Stevens-Johnson syndrome, toxic epidermal necrolysis); d/c at 1st appearance of rash or other signs of hypersensitivity. Avoid use starting at 30 weeks gestation; may cause premature closure of ductus arteriosus. Not a substitute for corticosteroids or for treatment of corticosteroid insufficiency. May mask signs of inflammation and fever. Anemia may occur; with long-term use, monitor Hgb/Hct if symptoms of anemia develop. May inhibit platelet aggregation and prolong bleeding time. May be associated with a reversible delay in ovulation; not recommended in women with difficulties conceiving, or who are undergoing investigation of infertility.

ADVERSE REACTIONS

Abdominal pain, diarrhea, dyspepsia, nausea, headache, anemia, arthralgia, insomnia, URTI, UTI, dizziness, pain, pharyngitis, edema, influenza-like symptoms.

DRUG INTERACTIONS

Patients taking ACE inhibitors, thiazides, and loop diuretics (eg, furosemide) may have impaired response to these therapies. Risk of renal toxicity when coadministered with diuretics, ACE inhibitors, and angiotensin II receptor antagonists. Increased risk of GI bleeding with anticoagulants (eg, warfarin), smoking, alcohol, and oral corticosteroids. May diminish antihypertensive effect of ACE inhibitors. Not recommended with ASA; increased rate of GI ulceration or other complications with low-dose ASA. May elevate lithium plasma levels; observe for signs of lithium toxicity. May increase cyclosporine and MTX toxicities. (Sus) Not recommended with sodium polystyrene sulfonate (Kayexalate).

NURSING CONSIDERATIONS

Assessment: Assess for cardiovascular disease (CVD), risk factors for CVD, ASA triad, coagulation disorders, any other conditions where treatment is contraindicated or cautioned, renal/hepatic dysfunction, pregnancy/nursing status, and possible drug interactions. Assess use in elderly and debilitated patients.

Monitoring: Monitor for signs/symptoms of CV thrombotic events, HTN, GI events, fluid retention, edema, and anaphylactoid/skin reactions. Monitor BP, renal function, and LFTs. Perform periodic monitoring of CBC and chemistry profile with long-term use.

Patient Counseling: Advise to seek medical attention if symptoms of CV events (eg, chest pain, SOB, weakness, slurring of speech), GI ulceration and bleeding (eg, epigastric pain, dyspepsia, melena, hematemesis), hepatotoxicity (eg, nausea, fatigue, lethargy, pruritus, jaundice, right upper quadrant tenderness, flu-like symptoms), anaphylactoid reaction (eg, difficulty breathing, swelling of face/throat), skin rash, blisters, fever, hypersensitivity reaction (eg, itching), weight gain, or edema occur. Instruct to avoid use starting at 30 weeks gestation. Advise females of reproductive potential who desire pregnancy that drug may be associated with a reversible delay in ovulation.

Storage: 25°C (77°F); excursions permitted to 15-30°C (59-86°F). Keep tabs in a dry place.

MODERIBA – ribavirin RX

Class: Nucleoside analogue

Not for monotherapy treatment of chronic hepatitis C (CHC) virus infection. Primary toxicity is hemolytic anemia. Anemia associated with therapy may result in worsening of cardiac disease and lead to fatal and nonfatal myocardial infarctions. Avoid with history of significant/unstable cardiac disease. Contraindicated in women who are pregnant and in male partners of pregnant women. Extreme care must be taken to avoid pregnancy during therapy and for 6 months after completion of therapy in both female patients and in female partners of male patients who are taking therapy. Use at least 2 reliable forms of effective contraception during treatment and for 6 months after discontinuation.

ADULT DOSAGE

Chronic Hepatitis C with Compensated Liver Disease

Combination with Peginterferon Alfa-2a:
Not Previously Treated with Interferon Alfa:
Monoinfection:
Genotypes 1, 4:
<75kg: 1000mg/day in 2 divided doses
≥75kg: 1200mg/day in 2 divided doses
Duration: 48 weeks

Genotypes 2, 3:
800mg/day in 2 divided doses
Duration: 24 weeks

HIV Coinfection:
800mg/day in 2 divided doses
Duration: 48 weeks (regardless of genotype)

PEDIATRIC DOSAGE

Pediatric use may not have been established

DOSE MODIFICATION

Renal Impairment

CrCl <50mL/min: Not recommended for use

Adverse Reactions
Without Cardiac Disease:
Hgb <10g/dL: Reduce dose to 600mg/day
Hgb <8.5 g/dL: D/C Moderiba

With History of Stable Cardiac Disease:
Hgb Decrease of ≥2g/dL During Any 4-Week Treatment Period: Reduce dose to 600mg/day
Hgb <12g/dL After 4 Weeks at Reduced Dose: D/C Moderiba

Discontinuation
Consider if at least a 2 $\log_{10}$ HCV RNA reduction from baseline by Week 12 is not achieved
Consider if HCV RNA levels remain detectable after treatment Week 24
D/C if hepatic decompensation develops during treatment

ADMINISTRATION
Oral route

Take with food
Refer to peginterferon alfa-2a labeling for dosage and administration instructions

HOW SUPPLIED
Tab: 200mg, 400mg, 600mg

CONTRAINDICATIONS
Women who are or may become pregnant, men whose female partners are pregnant, hemoglobinopathies (eg, thalassemia major, sickle cell anemia), and in combination with didanosine. When used with peginterferon alfa-2a, refer to the individual monograph.

WARNINGS/PRECAUTIONS
Combination therapy is associated with significant adverse reactions (eg, severe depression and suicidal ideation, hemolytic anemia, suppression of bone marrow function, autoimmune/infectious/ophthalmologic/cerebrovascular disorders, pulmonary dysfunction, colitis, pancreatitis, diabetes). Do not start therapy unless a negative pregnancy test has been obtained immediately prior to therapy. Caution with baseline risk of severe anemia (eg, spherocytosis, history of GI bleeding). Caution with preexisting cardiac disease; suspend or d/c therapy if cardiovascular status deteriorates. Risk of hepatic decompensation and death in CHC patients with cirrhosis. Severe acute hypersensitivity reactions and serious skin reactions reported. D/C with hepatic decompensation, confirmed pancreatitis, severe hypersensitivity, or if signs/symptoms of severe skin reactions develop. Do not use with CrCl <50mL/min. Pulmonary disorders (eg, dyspnea, pulmonary infiltrates, pneumonitis, pulmonary HTN, pneumonia) reported. Closely monitor if pulmonary infiltrates/function impairment develop and d/c if appropriate.

ADVERSE REACTIONS
Hemolytic anemia, fatigue/asthenia, neutropenia, headache, pyrexia, myalgia, irritability/anxiety/nervousness, insomnia, alopecia, rigors, N/V, anorexia.

DRUG INTERACTIONS
See Contraindications. Closely monitor for treatment associated toxicities (eg, hepatic decompensation) with nucleoside reverse transcriptase inhibitors; consider dose reduction or discontinuation of peginterferon alfa-2a and/or ribavirin. Severe neutropenia and severe anemia reported with zidovudine; consider discontinuation of zidovudine if appropriate. Severe pancytopenia and bone marrow suppression reported with azathioprine; d/c peginterferon alfa-2a, ribavirin, and azathioprine if pancytopenia develops.

NURSING CONSIDERATIONS

Assessment: Assess for hemoglobinopathies, autoimmune hepatitis, hepatic decompensation, baseline risk of severe anemia, history of or preexisting cardiac disease, nursing status, and possible drug interactions. Conduct pregnancy test (including in female partners of male patients), standard hematological and biochemical lab tests, ECG in patients with preexisting cardiac abnormalities, renal/thyroid function test, and CD4 count in HIV patients.

Monitoring: Monitor for hepatic decompensation, pancreatitis, hypersensitivity/skin reactions, pulmonary infiltrates/function impairment, and other adverse reactions. Monitor cardiac status, TSH, and HCV RNA. Perform hematological tests at Weeks 2 and 4 and biochemical tests at Week 4; perform additional testing periodically. Perform pregnancy testing monthly and for 6 months after discontinuation (including female partners of male patients).

Patient Counseling: Counsel on risks/benefits associated with treatment. Inform of pregnancy risks; instruct to use at least 2 forms of effective contraception during therapy and for 6 months after discontinuation of therapy (including female partners of male patients). Advise to notify physician immediately in the event of pregnancy. Advise that lab evaluations are required prior to starting therapy and periodically thereafter. Advise to be well-hydrated, especially during the initial stages of treatment. Caution to avoid driving/operating machinery if dizziness, confusion, somnolence, or fatigue develops. Instruct not to drink alcohol; inform that alcohol may exacerbate CHC infection. Inform to take appropriate precautions to prevent HCV transmission.

Storage: 25°C (77°F); excursions permitted between 15-30°C (59-86°F).

Monodox – doxycycline monohydrate

RX

Class: Tetracyclines

ADULT DOSAGE

General Dosing

Initial: 100mg q12h or 50mg q6h on 1st day
Maint: 100mg qd or 50mg q12h
More Severe Infections (eg, Chronic UTIs):
100mg q12h

Streptococcal Infections:
Continue therapy for 10 days

Gonococcal Infections

Uncomplicated Infections (Except Anorectal Infections in Men):
100mg bid for 7 days
Alternate Dosing:
Single visit dose of 300mg stat followed in 1 hr by a second 300mg dose

Acute Epididymo-Orchitis

Caused by *Neisseria gonorrhoeae/Chlamydia trachomatis*:
100mg bid for at least 10 days

Syphilis

Primary and Secondary:
300mg/day in divided doses for at least 10 days

Urethral Infections

Uncomplicated Infections Caused by *Chlamydia trachomatis*:
100mg bid for at least 7 days

Endocervical Infections

Uncomplicated Infections Caused by *Chlamydia trachomatis*:
100mg bid for at least 7 days

Rectal Infections

Uncomplicated Infections Caused by *Chlamydia trachomatis*:
100mg bid for at least 7 days

Nongonococcal Urethritis

Caused by *Chlamydia trachomatis* and *Ureaplasma urealyticum*:
100mg bid for at least 7 days

Inhalational Anthrax (Postexposure)

100mg bid for 60 days

PEDIATRIC DOSAGE

General Dosing

>8 Years:

≤100 lbs:
2mg/lb divided into 2 doses on 1st day, followed by 1mg/lb qd or as 2 divided doses, on subsequent days
More Severe Infections: Up to 2mg/lb

>100 lbs:
Initial: 100mg q12h or 50mg q6h on 1st day
Maint: 100mg qd or 50mg q12h
More Severe Infections (eg, Chronic UTIs):
100mg q12h
Streptococcal Infections:
Continue therapy for 10 days

Inhalational Anthrax (Postexposure)

<100 lbs:
1mg/lb bid for 60 days
≥100 lbs:
100mg bid for 60 days

ADMINISTRATION

Oral route

Administer w/ adequate amounts of fluid
May be given w/ food if gastric irritation occurs

HOW SUPPLIED

Cap: 50mg, 75mg, 100mg

WARNINGS/PRECAUTIONS

May cause permanent discoloration of the teeth (yellow-gray-brown) if used during tooth development (last 1/2 of pregnancy, infancy, and childhood to 8 yrs of age); do not use in this age group, except for anthrax. Enamel hypoplasia reported. *Clostridium difficile*-associated diarrhea (CDAD) reported; d/c if CDAD is suspected or confirmed. May decrease fibula growth rate in prematures. May cause an increase in BUN. Photosensitivity, manifested by an exaggerated sunburn reaction, reported; d/c at the 1st evidence of skin erythema. May result in bacterial resistance if used in the absence of proven or suspected bacterial infection, or a prophylactic indication; take appropriate measures if superinfection develops. Associated w/ intracranial HTN (pseudotumor cerebri); increased risk in women of childbearing age who are overweight or have a history of intracranial HTN. If visual disturbance occurs, prompt ophthalmologic evaluation is warranted. Intracranial pressure can remain elevated for weeks after drug cessation; monitor patients until they stabilize. Incision and drainage or other surgical procedures should be performed in conjunction w/ antibacterial therapy when indicated. False elevations of urinary catecholamine levels may occur due to interference w/ the fluorescence test.

ADVERSE REACTIONS

Diarrhea, hepatotoxicity, maculopapular/erythematous rash, Stevens-Johnson syndrome, toxic epidermal necrolysis, anorexia, N/V, urticaria, serum sickness, pericarditis, hemolytic anemia, thrombocytopenia, neutropenia, eosinophilia.

DRUG INTERACTIONS

Avoid concomitant use w/ isotretinoin; may increase risk of intracranial HTN. Depresses plasma prothrombin activity; may require downward adjustment of anticoagulant dose. May interfere w/ bactericidal action of PCN; avoid concurrent use. Impaired absorption w/ antacids containing aluminum, Ca^{2+}, or Mg^{2+}, and iron-containing preparations. Decreased $T_{1/2}$ w/ barbiturates, carbamazepine, and phenytoin. Fatal renal toxicity reported w/ methoxyflurane. May render oral contraceptives less effective.

NURSING CONSIDERATIONS

Assessment: Assess for hypersensitivity to drug or any tetracyclines, risk for intracranial HTN, pregnancy/nursing status, and possible drug interactions. Perform culture and susceptibility tests. In venereal disease when coexistent syphilis is suspected, perform a dark-field examination and blood serology.

Monitoring: Monitor for CDAD, photosensitivity, skin erythema, superinfection, intracranial HTN, visual disturbance, and other adverse reactions. In long-term therapy, perform periodic lab evaluations of organ systems, including hematopoietic, renal, and hepatic studies. In venereal disease when coexistent syphilis is suspected, repeat blood serology monthly for at least 4 months.

Patient Counseling: Apprise of the potential hazard to fetus if used during pregnancy. Advise to avoid excessive sunlight or artificial UV light, and to d/c therapy if phototoxicity (eg, skin eruptions) occurs; advise to consider use of sunscreen or sunblock. Inform that absorption of drug is reduced when taken w/ bismuth subsalicylate, or w/ foods, especially those that contain Ca^{2+}. Inform that drug may increase incidence of vaginal candidiasis. Inform that diarrhea is a common problem caused by therapy, which usually ends when therapy is discontinued. Instruct to immediately contact physician if watery and bloody stools (w/ or w/o stomach cramps and fever) occur, even as late as ≥2 months after the last dose. Counsel that therapy should only be used to treat bacterial, not viral, infections. Instruct to take exactly ud, even if patient feels better early in the course of therapy. Inform that skipping doses or not completing the full course of therapy may decrease effectiveness of treatment and increase bacterial resistance.

Storage: 20-25°C (68-77°F); excursions permitted to 15-30°C (59-86°F).

MORPHINE — morphine sulfate CII

Class: Opioid analgesic

Oral sol is available in 10mg/5mL, 20mg/5mL, and 100mg/5mL concentrations. The 100mg/5mL (20mg/mL) concentration is indicated for use in opioid-tolerant patients only. Use caution when prescribing and administering to avoid dosing errors due to confusion between different concentrations and between mg and mL, which could result in accidental overdose and death. Ensure the proper dose is communicated and dispensed. Keep sol out of reach of children. Seek emergency medical help immediately in case of accidental ingestion.

ADULT DOSAGE

Moderate to Severe Pain

Acute and Chronic:

Opioid-Naive Patients:

Initial: 10-20mg (sol) or 15-30mg (tab) q4h prn

Titrate: Adjust dose based on response to the initial dose

Opioid-Tolerant Patients:

Use the 100mg/5mL sol only for patients who have already been titrated to a stable analgesic regimen using lower strengths of morphine sulfate and who can benefit from use of a smaller volume of sol

PEDIATRIC DOSAGE

Pediatric use may not have been established

Conversions

From Parenteral Morphine to Oral Morphine Sulfate:
Anywhere from 3-6mg of oral morphine sulfate may be required to provide pain relief equivalent to 1mg of parenteral morphine

From Parenteral/Oral Non-Morphine Opioids to Oral Morphine Sulfate:
Adjust based on response to oral morphine sulfate; refer to published relative potency information

From Controlled-Release Oral Morphine to Oral Morphine Sulfate:
The same total amount of morphine sulfate is available from oral sol, tabs, and controlled-release and ER capsules; the extended duration of release of morphine sulfate results in reduced maximum and increased minimum plasma concentrations as compared to shorter acting morphine sulfate products. Dosage adjustment w/ close observation is necessary

DOSE MODIFICATION

Renal Impairment
Start w/ lower doses and titrate slowly

Hepatic Impairment
Start w/ lower doses and titrate slowly

Elderly
Start at lower end of dosing range

Discontinuation
Gradually taper dose

ADMINISTRATION
Oral route

100mg/5mL Sol
Always use the enclosed calibrated oral syringe

HOW SUPPLIED
Sol: 10mg/5mL [15mL, 100mL, 500mL], 20mg/5mL [100mL, 500mL], 100mg/5mL [15mL, 30mL, 120mL]; Tab: 15mg*, 30mg* *scored

CONTRAINDICATIONS
Respiratory depression in absence of resuscitative equipment, acute or severe bronchial asthma or hypercarbia, confirmed/suspected paralytic ileus.

WARNINGS/PRECAUTIONS
Respiratory depression occurs more frequently in elderly or debilitated patients and in those w/ conditions accompanied by hypoxia, hypercapnia, or upper airway obstruction. Caution and consider alternative nonopioid analgesics w/ COPD or cor pulmonale, and in patients having substantially decreased respiratory reserve (eg, severe kyphoscoliosis), hypoxia, hypercapnia, or preexisting respiratory depression; use only under careful medical supervision at the lowest effective dose. High potential for abuse; is subject to misuse, abuse, or diversion. Possible respiratory depressant effects and potential to elevate CSF pressure may be markedly exaggerated in the presence of head injury, intracranial lesions, or a preexisting increase in intracranial pressure (ICP); may produce effects on pupillary response and consciousness which may obscure neurologic signs of further increases in ICP in patients w/head injuries. May cause severe hypotension in patients whose ability to maintain BP has already been compromised by a depleted blood volume or concurrent administration of drugs (eg, phenothiazines, general anesthetics). May produce orthostatic hypotension and syncope in ambulatory patients. Caution w/ circulatory shock. Avoid w/GI obstruction, especially paralytic ileus; may prolong the obstruction. May obscure diagnosis or clinical course w/ acute abdominal conditions. Caution w/ biliary tract disease, including acute pancreatitis; may cause spasm of the sphincter of Oddi and diminish biliary and pancreatic secretions. Caution w/and reduce dose in patients w/ severe renal or hepatic impairment, Addison's disease, hypothyroidism, prostatic hypertrophy, or urethral stricture, and in elderly or debilitated patients. Caution w/ CNS depression, toxic psychosis, acute alcoholism, and delirium tremens. May aggravate convulsions in patients w/ convulsive disorders and may induce/aggravate seizures. May impair mental/physical abilities. (100mg/5mL Sol) May cause fatal respiratory depression when administered to patients who are not tolerant to the respiratory depressant effects of opioids. Use only for patients who have already been titrated to a stable analgesic regimen using lower strengths and who can benefit from use of a smaller volume of oral sol.

ADVERSE REACTIONS
Respiratory depression, apnea, circulatory depression, respiratory arrest, shock, cardiac arrest, lightheadedness, dizziness, sedation, N/V, sweating, constipation, somnolence.

DRUG INTERACTIONS
Caution w/ CNS depressants (eg, sedatives, hypnotics, general anesthetics, antiemetics, phenothiazines, alcohol); may increase risk of respiratory depression, hypotension, profound sedation, or coma. May enhance neuromuscular-blocking action of skeletal muscle relaxants and produce an increased degree of respiratory depression. Do not administer mixed agonist/antagonist analgesics (eg, pentazocine, nalbuphine, butorphanol) to patients who have received or are receiving a course of therapy w/ morphine; may reduce analgesic effect and/or may precipitate withdrawal symptoms. Apnea, confusion, and muscle twitching reported w/ cimetidine; monitor for increased respiratory and CNS depression. MAOIs potentiate action of morphine; allow at least 14 days after stopping MAOIs before initiating treatment. Anticholinergics or other medications w/ anticholinergic activity may increase risk of urinary retention and/or severe constipation, which may lead to paralytic ileus. Absorption/exposure may be increased w/ P-gp inhibitors (eg, quinidine); use w/ caution.

NURSING CONSIDERATIONS

Assessment: Assess for hypersensitivity to the drug or to any components of the product, drug abuse/addiction risk, prior opioid therapy, opioid tolerance, respiratory depression, or any other conditions where treatment is contraindicated or cautioned, pregnancy/nursing status, and for possible drug interactions.

Monitoring: Monitor for respiratory depression, CSF pressure elevation, orthostatic hypotension, syncope, aggravation of convulsions/seizures, and other adverse reactions. During chronic therapy, especially for noncancer-related pain, periodically reassess the continued need for the use of therapy.

Patient Counseling: Advise to take only ud and not to adjust dose w/o consulting a physician. Inform that the drug may impair the ability to perform potentially hazardous activities (eg, operating machinery/driving); advise to refrain from any potentially dangerous activity until it is established that patient is not adversely affected. Advise to avoid CNS depressants except by the orders of the prescribing physician, and to avoid alcohol during therapy. Instruct women of childbearing potential who become or are planning to become pregnant to consult physician prior to therapy; advise that prolonged use during pregnancy may cause fetal-neonatal physical dependence and neonatal withdrawal may also occur. Counsel on the importance of safely tapering the dose if patient has been receiving therapy for more than a few weeks and cessation of therapy is indicated. Inform that drug has a potential for abuse and should be protected from theft and never be given to anyone other than for whom it was prescribed. Instruct to keep in a secure place out of reach of children, and that when no longer needed, destroy the unused sol/tabs by flushing down the toilet. Inform of the most common adverse events that may occur during therapy and the potential for severe constipation.

Storage: 20-25°C (68-77°F). Protect from moisture.

MoviPrep — ascorbic acid/polyethylene glycol 3350/potassium chloride/sodium ascorbate/sodium chloride/sodium sulfate **RX**

Class: Bowel cleanser

ADULT DOSAGE

Bowel Cleansing

Prior to Colonoscopy:

Split-Dose (2-Day) Regimen (Preferred Method):

Take Dose 1 the pm before the colonoscopy (10-12 hrs before Dose 2), then take Dose 2 the next morning on the day of the colonoscopy, starting at least 3.5 hrs prior to colonoscopy

Evening-Only (1-Day) Regimen (Alternative Method):

Take Dose 1 at least 3.5 hrs before hs the pm before the colonoscopy, then take Dose 2 about 1.5 hrs after starting Dose 1 on the pm before the colonoscopy

PEDIATRIC DOSAGE

Pediatric use may not have been established

ADMINISTRATION
Oral route

Take 2 separate doses in conjunction w/ fluids
Drink only clear liquids up to 2 hrs before the colonoscopy or as prescribed by healthcare provider, then stop drinking liquids until after the colonoscopy
Take w/in 24 hrs after it is mixed in water; do not add other ingredients to the sol

Split-Dose (2-Day) Regimen (Preferred Method)
Dose 1:
1. Empty the contents of 1 pouch A and 1 pouch B into the container
2. Add lukewarm water to the fill line on the container and mix
3. Drink one 8-oz glass (240mL) every 15 min; be sure to drink all of the sol. This should take about 1 hr
4. Fill the container w/ 16-oz (two 8-oz glasses) of clear liquid and drink all of this liquid before going to bed

Dose 2:
1. Repeat steps 1 through 3 from Dose 1 instructions
2. Fill the container w/ 16-oz (two 8-oz glasses) of clear liquid and drink all of this liquid at least 2 hrs before the colonoscopy

Evening only (1-Day) Regimen (Alternative Method)
Dose 1:
1. Empty the contents of 1 pouch A and 1 pouch B into the container
2. Add lukewarm water to the fill line on the container and mix
3. Drink one 8-oz glass (240mL) every 15 min; be sure to drink all of the sol. This should take about 1 hr

Dose 2:
1. Repeat Steps 1 through 3 from Dose 1 instructions
2. Fill the container again to the fill line w/ clear liquid and drink all of this liquid before going to bed

HOW SUPPLIED
Sol (Powder): Pouch A (Polyethylene Glycol 3350/Sodium Sulfate/Sodium Chloride/Potassium Chloride) 100g/7.5g/2.691g/1.015g; Pouch B (Ascorbic Acid/Sodium Ascorbate) 4.7g/5.9g

CONTRAINDICATIONS
GI obstruction, bowel perforation, gastric retention, ileus, toxic colitis or toxic megacolon.

WARNINGS/PRECAUTIONS
Consume only clear liquids (no solid food) from the start of treatment until after the colonoscopy. Do not consume any clear liquids at least 2 hrs before the colonoscopy. Adequately hydrate before, during, and after use. If significant vomiting or signs of dehydration develop, consider performing postcolonoscopy lab tests (electrolytes, SrCr, and BUN). Correct electrolyte abnormalities before treatment. Consider performing predose and postcolonoscopy lab tests in patients with known or suspected hyponatremia. Serious arrhythmias reported (rare); use with caution and consider predose and postcolonoscopy ECGs in patients at increased risk of serious cardiac arrhythmias. Generalized tonic-clonic seizures and/or loss of consciousness reported (rare); caution in patients with a history of or at increased risk of seizures (eg, with known/suspected hyponatremia). Caution with impaired renal function. May produce colonic mucosal aphthous ulcerations; consider this when interpreting colonoscopy findings in patients with known/suspected inflammatory bowel disease. Serious cases of ischemic colitis reported. If severe bloating, abdominal distention/pain occurs, slow administration or temporarily d/c until symptoms abate. Caution with severe ulcerative colitis; impaired gag reflex; in patients prone to regurgitation/aspiration; or with G6PD deficiency, especially in G6PD-deficient patients with an active infection, history of hemolysis, or taking concomitant medications known to precipitate hemolytic reactions. Contains phenylalanine.

ADVERSE REACTIONS
Abdominal distension, anal discomfort, thirst, N/V, abdominal pain, sleep disorder, rigors, hunger, malaise, dizziness.

DRUG INTERACTIONS
Increased risk of colonic mucosal aphthous ulcerations with stimulant laxatives; concurrent use not recommended. Caution with drugs that increase risk of electrolyte abnormalities (eg, diuretics, ACE inhibitors, ARBs) or affect renal function (eg, NSAIDs). Caution with drugs that lower seizure threshold (eg, TCAs) and in patients withdrawing from alcohol or benzodiazepines. Caution with drugs that increase the risk of arrhythmias and prolonged QT in the setting of fluid and electrolyte abnormalities. Consider additional patient evaluations as appropriate. Oral medication administered within 1 hr of the start of administration may be flushed from GI tract and may not be absorbed.

NURSING CONSIDERATIONS

Assessment: Assess for GI obstruction, bowel perforation, gastric retention, ileus, toxic colitis, toxic megacolon, electrolyte abnormalities, G6PD deficiency, renal impairment, drug hypersensitivity, any other conditions where treatment is cautioned, pregnancy/nursing status, and possible drug interactions. Consider performing predose lab tests (electrolytes, SrCr, and BUN) in patients with electrolyte abnormalities or renal impairment. Consider predose ECGs in patients at increased risk of serious cardiac arrhythmias.

Monitoring: Monitor for arrhythmias, generalized tonic-clonic seizures, loss of consciousness, colonic mucosal aphthous ulceration, ischemic colitis, bloating, abdominal distention/pain, and other adverse reactions. Monitor patients with impaired gag reflex and patients prone to regurgitation/aspiration. Consider performing postcolonoscopy lab tests (electrolytes, SrCr, BUN) in patients who develop significant vomiting or signs of dehydration after taking therapy, in patients with electrolyte abnormalities, and in patients with renal impairment. Consider postcolonoscopy ECGs in patients at increased risk of serious cardiac arrhythmias.

Patient Counseling: Inform patients who require a low phenylalanine diet that the product contains a max of 233mg aspartame/treatment (provides 131mg phenylalanine). Instruct to inform physician if patient has trouble swallowing or is prone to regurgitation/aspiration. Inform that each pouch needs to be diluted in water before ingestion and instruct to drink additional clear liquid. Inform that oral medications may not be absorbed properly if taken within 1 hr of starting each dose of the drug. Instruct not to take other laxatives during therapy. Advise to adequately hydrate before, during, and after use. Counsel that clear soup and/or plain yogurt may be taken for dinner, finishing at least 1 hr prior to treatment. Inform that the 1st bowel movement may occur 1 hr after the start of administration, and abdominal bloating and distention may occur before the 1st bowel movement. If severe abdominal discomfort or distention occurs, advise to stop treatment temporarily or drink each portion at longer intervals until symptoms diminish; if severe symptoms persist, instruct to notify physician. Instruct to consume only clear liquids (no solid food) from the start of treatment until after the colonoscopy. Instruct to not consume any clear liquids at least 2 hrs before the colonoscopy.

Storage: 20-25°C (68-77°F); excursions permitted to 15-30°C (59-86°F). Reconstituted Sol: Store upright and keep refrigerated. Use within 24 hrs.

MOXATAG – amoxicillin RX

Class: Semisynthetic ampicillin derivative

ADULT DOSAGE

Tonsillitis and/or Pharyngitis

Secondary to *Streptococcus pyogenes*:
Take 775mg qd for 10 days

PEDIATRIC DOSAGE

Tonsillitis and/or Pharyngitis

Secondary to *Streptococcus pyogenes*:
≥12 Years:
Take 775mg qd for 10 days

ADMINISTRATION

Oral route

Take w/in 1 hr of finishing a meal
Do not chew or crush

HOW SUPPLIED

Tab, ER: 775mg

WARNINGS/PRECAUTIONS

Serious, fatal anaphylactic reactions may occur. *Clostridium difficile*-associated diarrhea (CDAD) reported. May result in bacterial resistance with prolonged use or use in the absence of a proven/suspected bacterial infection or a prophylactic indication; take appropriate measures if superinfection develops. Avoid use in patients with mononucleosis; may cause erythematous skin rash. Not recommended for use in severe renal impairment (CrCl <30mL/min) or hemodialysis. Lab test interactions may occur.

ADVERSE REACTIONS

Vulvovaginal mycotic infection, diarrhea, N/V, abdominal pain, headache.

DRUG INTERACTIONS

Concurrent use with probenecid may increase and prolong blood levels; decreases renal tubular secretion of amoxicillin. Chloramphenicol, macrolides, sulfonamides, and tetracyclines may interfere with bactericidal effects. Lowers estrogen reabsorption and reduces efficacy of combined oral estrogen/progesterone contraceptives.

NURSING CONSIDERATIONS

Assessment: Assess for history of allergic reaction to penicillins, cephalosporins, or other allergens, infectious mononucleosis, phenylketonuria, pregnancy/nursing status, and for possible drug interactions.

Monitoring: Monitor for serious anaphylactic reactions, erythematous skin rash, development of drug resistance or superinfection with mycotic or bacterial pathogen, and for signs/symptoms of CDAD (may range from mild diarrhea to fatal colitis). Monitor for false (+) reactions for urinary glucose test. Caution in dose selection in elderly; monitor renal function.

Patient Counseling: Instruct to not chew or crush. Inform drug treats bacterial, not viral, infections. Instruct to take exactly ud; skipping doses or not completing full course may decrease effectiveness and increase resistance. Inform about potential benefits/risks; notify physician if watery/bloody diarrhea (with/without stomach cramps and fever) is experienced, which may occur as late as 2 months after treatment. Notify physician of serious hypersensitivity reactions, pregnancy, or nursing.

Storage: 25°C (77°F). Excursion permitted to 15-30°C (59-86°).

MOXEZA – moxifloxacin hydrochloride — RX

Class: Fluoroquinolone

ADULT DOSAGE

Bacterial Conjunctivitis

1 drop in the affected eye(s) bid for 7 days

PEDIATRIC DOSAGE

Bacterial Conjunctivitis

≥4 Months of Age:
1 drop in the affected eye(s) bid for 7 days

ADMINISTRATION

Ocular route

HOW SUPPLIED

Sol: 0.5% [3mL]

WARNINGS/PRECAUTIONS

For topical ophthalmic use only; should not be introduced directly into the anterior chamber of the eye. Serious and sometimes fatal hypersensitivity reactions reported with systemic use; d/c and institute appropriate therapy if allergic reaction occurs. Prolonged use may cause overgrowth of nonsusceptible organisms, including fungi. D/C use and consider alternative therapy if superinfection occurs. Avoid wearing contact lenses when signs/symptoms of bacterial conjunctivitis are present.

ADVERSE REACTIONS

Eye irritation, pyrexia, conjunctivitis.

NURSING CONSIDERATIONS

Assessment: Assess severity of infection, symptoms, and pregnancy/nursing status.

Monitoring: Monitor for signs/symptoms of hypersensitivity/anaphylactic reactions and other adverse reactions. Monitor for superinfection; examine with magnification (eg, slit-lamp biomicroscopy) and fluorescein staining, where appropriate.

Patient Counseling: Advise on proper use to prevent bacterial contamination. Instruct to d/c medication and contact physician if rash or allergic reaction occurs. Advise not to wear contact lenses if signs/symptoms of bacterial conjunctivitis are present.

Storage: 2-25°C (36-77°F).

MS CONTIN – morphine sulfate — CII

Class: Opioid analgesic

Exposes users to the risks of opioid addiction, abuse, and misuse, leading to overdose and death; assess each patient's risk prior to prescribing therapy and monitor regularly for the development of these behaviors/conditions. Serious, life-threatening, or fatal respiratory depression may occur; monitor during initiation or following a dose increase. Crushing, chewing, or dissolving tab can cause rapid release and absorption of a potentially fatal dose; instruct to swallow tab whole. Accidental ingestion, especially in children, can result in fatal overdose. Prolonged use during pregnancy can result in neonatal opioid withdrawal syndrome; advise pregnant women of the risk and ensure availability of appropriate treatment.

ADULT DOSAGE

Severe Pain (Daily, Around-the-Clock Management)

Use as 1st Opioid Analgesic:
Initial: 15mg q8h or q12h

PEDIATRIC DOSAGE

Pediatric use may not have been established

Titrate: Dose adjustments may be done every 1-2 days

Opioid Intolerant Patients:
Initial: 15mg q12h
Titrate: Dose adjustments may be done every 1-2 days

Breakthrough Pain:
May require a dose increase, or may need rescue medication w/ an IR analgesic

Conversions

From Other Oral Morphine:
Administer 1/2 of 24 hr requirement on an q12h schedule or administer 1/3 of the daily requirement on an q8h schedule

From Other Opioids:
D/C all other around-the-clock opioids when therapy is initiated and initiate dosing at 15mg q8-12h

From Parenteral Morphine:
Ratio: 2-6mg of oral morphine may be required to provide analgesia equivalent to 1mg of parenteral morphine; typically, a dose of morphine that is approximately 3X the previous daily parenteral morphine requirement is sufficient

From Other Non-Morphine Opioids (Parenteral or Oral):
Begin w/ 1/2 the estimated daily morphine requirement as initial dose, managing inadequate analgesia by supplementation w/ IR morphine

DOSE MODIFICATION

Discontinuation

Use a gradual downward titration of the dose; do not abruptly d/c

ADMINISTRATION

Oral route

Swallow tab whole; do not crush, dissolve, or chew

HOW SUPPLIED

Tab, ER: 15mg, 30mg, 60mg, 100mg, 200mg

CONTRAINDICATIONS

Significant respiratory depression, acute or severe bronchial asthma in an unmonitored setting or in the absence of resuscitative equipment, known or suspected paralytic ileus.

WARNINGS/PRECAUTIONS

Reserve for use in patients for whom alternative treatment options are ineffective, not tolerated, or would be otherwise inadequate to provide sufficient management of pain. Should be prescribed only by healthcare professionals who are knowledgeable in the use of potent opioids for the management of chronic pain. Life-threatening respiratory depression is more likely to occur in elderly, cachectic, or debilitated patients. Consider alternative nonopioid analgesics in patients with significant COPD or cor pulmonale, and in patients having a substantially decreased respiratory reserve, hypoxia, hypercapnia, or preexisting respiratory depression. May cause severe hypotension, orthostatic hypotension, and syncope; increased risk in patients whose ability to maintain BP has already been compromised by a reduced blood volume or concurrent administration of certain CNS depressants. Avoid with circulatory shock, impaired consciousness, or coma. Monitor patients who may be susceptible to intracranial effects of carbon dioxide retention for signs of sedation and respiratory depression, particularly when initiating therapy. Therapy may obscure clinical course in patients with head injury. Avoid with GI obstruction. May cause spasm of sphincter of Oddi and increase in serum amylase; monitor for worsening symptoms with biliary tract disease (eg, acute pancreatitis). May aggravate convulsions in patients with convulsive disorders and may induce or aggravate seizures. May impair mental/physical abilities. Caution in elderly. Not recommended for use during or immediately prior to labor.

ADVERSE REACTIONS
Respiratory depression, constipation, dizziness, sedation, N/V, sweating, dysphoria, euphoric mood.

DRUG INTERACTIONS
Respiratory depression, hypotension, profound sedation, or coma may occur with CNS depressants (eg, sedatives, hypnotics, neuroleptics, alcohol); if coadministration is considered, reduce dose of one or both agents. Mixed agonist/antagonist (eg, pentazocine, nalbuphine, butorphanol) and partial agonist (buprenorphine) may reduce analgesic effect or precipitate withdrawal symptoms; avoid coadministration. May enhance neuromuscular-blocking action of skeletal muscle relaxants and produce increased respiratory depression. MAOIs have been reported to potentiate the effects of morphine anxiety, confusion, and significant depression of respiration or coma; avoid use or within 14 days of MAOI use. Cimetidine may potentiate morphine-induced respiratory depression. May reduce efficacy of diuretics. May lead to acute urine retention, particularly in men with enlarged prostates. Anticholinergics or other drugs with anticholinergic activity may increase risk of urinary retention and/or severe constipation, which may lead to paralytic ileus. Absorption/exposure may be increased with P-gp inhibitors (eg, quinidine) by about 2-fold; monitor for signs of respiratory and CNS depression.

NURSING CONSIDERATIONS

Assessment: Assess for drug abuse/addiction risk, prior opioid therapy, opioid tolerance, respiratory depression, drug hypersensitivity, COPD or other respiratory complications, GI obstruction, paralytic ileus, head injury, history of seizure, pregnancy/nursing status, possible drug interactions, and any other conditions where treatment is contraindicated or cautioned.

Monitoring: Monitor for signs/symptoms of respiratory depression (especially within first 24-72 hrs of initiation), hypotension, symptoms of worsening biliary tract disease, aggravation/induction of seizures, tolerance, physical dependence, mental/physical impairment, and other adverse reactions. Routinely monitor for signs of misuse, abuse, and addiction. Periodically reassess the continued need for therapy.

Patient Counseling: Inform that use of drug can result in addiction, abuse, and misuse; instruct not to share drug with others and to take steps to protect from theft or misuse. Inform about risk of life-threatening respiratory depression; advise how to recognize respiratory depression and to seek medical attention if breathing difficulties develop. Advise to store drug securely; accidental exposure, especially in children, can result in serious harm/death. Instruct to dispose unused drug by flushing down the toilet. Inform females of reproductive potential that prolonged use during pregnancy may result in neonatal opioid withdrawal syndrome. Inform that potentially serious additive effects may occur when used with alcohol or other CNS depressants, and advise not to use such drugs unless supervised by physician. Instruct on how to take the medication properly. Inform that drug may cause orthostatic hypotension and syncope, and may impair the ability to perform potentially hazardous activities; advise to not perform such tasks until they know how they will react to medication. Advise of the potential for severe constipation (including management instructions), on how to recognize anaphylaxis, and when to seek medical attention. Inform females that drug can cause fetal harm; instruct to notify physician if pregnant/planning to become pregnant.

Storage: 25°C (77°F); excursions permitted between 15-30°C (59-86°F).

MULTAQ – dronedarone RX

Class: Class III antiarrhythmic

Doubles the risk of death in patients with symptomatic heart failure (HF), with recent decompensation, requiring hospitalization or NYHA Class IV HF; contraindicated in these patients. Doubles the risk of death, stroke, and hospitalization for HF in patients with permanent A-fib; contraindicated in patients in A-fib who will not or cannot be cardioverted into normal sinus rhythm.

ADULT DOSAGE

Atrial Fibrillation

Reduce Risk of Hospitalization for Patients in Sinus Rhythm w/ History of Paroxysmal/ Persistent A-Fib:
400mg bid (w/ am and pm meal)

PEDIATRIC DOSAGE
Pediatric use may not have been established

ADMINISTRATION
Oral route

Take once w/ am meal and again w/ pm meal

HOW SUPPLIED
Tab: 400mg

CONTRAINDICATIONS
Permanent A-fib, symptomatic HF with recent decompensation requiring hospitalization or NYHA Class IV symptoms, 2nd- or 3rd-degree atrioventricular block or sick sinus syndrome (except when used with a functioning pacemaker), bradycardia <50 bpm, liver or lung toxicity related to previous use of amiodarone, QTc Bazett interval ≥500 msec or PR interval >280 msec, severe hepatic impairment, women who are or may become pregnant, nursing mothers. Concomitant use of strong CYP3A inhibitors (eg, ketoconazole, clarithromycin, nefazodone), drugs or herbal products that prolong QT interval and might increase risk of torsades de pointes (eg, phenothiazine antipsychotics, TCAs, certain oral macrolide antibiotics, Class I and III antiarrhythmics).

WARNINGS/PRECAUTIONS
Monitor cardiac rhythm no less than every 3 months. Cardiovert patients or d/c drug if patients are in A-fib. Only initiate in patients who are receiving appropriate antithrombotic therapy. New onset or worsening of HF reported; d/c if HF develops or worsens and requires hospitalization. Hepatocellular liver injury (including acute liver failure requiring transplant) reported; d/c if hepatic injury is suspected and test serum enzymes, AST, ALT, alkaline phosphatase, and serum bilirubin. Do not restart therapy without another explanation for observed liver injury. Interstitial lung disease (including pneumonitis and pulmonary fibrosis) reported. Onset of dyspnea or nonproductive cough may be related to pulmonary toxicity; evaluate patients carefully. D/C if pulmonary toxicity is confirmed. K^+ levels should be within normal range prior to and during therapy. May induce moderate QTc (Bazett) prolongation. Increase in SrCr, prerenal azotemia, and acute renal failure often in the setting of HF or hypovolemia reported. Premenopausal women who have not undergone hysterectomy/oophorectomy must use effective contraception while on therapy.

ADVERSE REACTIONS
QT prolongation, SrCr increase, diarrhea, N/V, abdominal pain, asthenic conditions, bradycardia, rashes, pruritus, eczema, dermatitis, allergic dermatitis.

DRUG INTERACTIONS
See Contraindications. Hypokalemia/hypomagnesemia may occur with K^+-depleting diuretics. May increase exposure to digoxin. Digoxin may also potentiate electrophysiologic effects; consider discontinuing or 1/2 the dose of digoxin and closely monitor serum levels and for toxicity if digoxin treatment is continued. Calcium channel blockers (CCBs) may potentiate effects on conduction and may increase exposure. Bradycardia more frequently observed with β-blockers. Give a low dose of CCBs or β-blockers initially and increase only after ECG verification of good tolerability. Avoid grapefruit juice, rifampin, or other CYP3A inducers (eg, phenobarbital, carbamazepine, St. John's wort). May increase exposure of simvastatin/simvastatin acid, CCBs, dabigatran, P-glycoprotein substrates, and CYP2D6 substrates (eg, β-blockers, TCAs, SSRIs). Avoid doses >10mg qd of simvastatin. May increase plasma levels of tacrolimus, sirolimus, and other CYP3A substrates with a narrow therapeutic range; monitor concentrations and adjust dosage appropriately. Clinically significant INR elevations with oral anticoagulants and increased S-warfarin exposure reported; monitor INR after initiating therapy in patients taking warfarin.

NURSING CONSIDERATIONS

Assessment: Assess for recent HF decompensation, permanent A-fib, hepatic impairment, any other conditions where treatment is contraindicated/cautioned, pregnancy/nursing status, and possible drug interactions. Assess serum K^+ levels.

Monitoring: Monitor for signs/symptoms of new/worsening HF, hepatic injury, pulmonary toxicity, and QT interval prolongation. Monitor cardiac rhythm no less than every 3 months, hepatic serum enzymes periodically, especially during first 6 months, and renal function periodically.

Patient Counseling: Instruct to take with meals and not to take with grapefruit juice. If a dose is missed, advise to take next dose at the regularly scheduled time and not to double the dose. Counsel to consult physician if signs/symptoms of HF or potential liver injury occur and before stopping the treatment. Advise to inform physician of any history of HF, rhythm disturbance other than A-fib or atrial flutter, or predisposing conditions, such as uncorrected hypokalemia. Advise to report any use of other prescription, nonprescription medication, or herbal products, particularly St. John's wort. Counsel patients of childbearing potential about appropriate contraceptive choices while on therapy.

Storage: 25°C (77°F); excursions permitted to 15-30°C (59-86°F).

MYRBETRIQ — mirabegron RX

Class: Adrenergic/anticholinergic agent

ADULT DOSAGE

Overactive Bladder

Initial: 25mg qd

Titrate: May increase to 50mg qd based on individual efficacy and tolerability

PEDIATRIC DOSAGE

Pediatric use may not have been established

DOSE MODIFICATION

Renal Impairment

Severe (CrCl 15-29mL/min or eGFR 15-29mL/min/1.73m²):
Max: 25mg qd
ESRD: Not recommended

Hepatic Impairment

Moderate (Child-Pugh Class B):
Max: 25mg qd
Severe (Child-Pugh Class C): Not recommended

ADMINISTRATION

Oral route

Take w/ or w/o food and w/ water
Swallow whole; do not chew, divide, or crush

HOW SUPPLIED

Tab, Extended-Release: 25mg, 50mg

WARNINGS/PRECAUTIONS

May increase BP. Not recommended in patients with severe uncontrolled HTN, ESRD, or severe hepatic impairment (Child-Pugh Class C). Worsening of preexisting HTN reported infrequently. Urinary retention in patients with bladder outlet obstruction (BOO) reported.

ADVERSE REACTIONS

HTN, nasopharyngitis, UTI, headache.

DRUG INTERACTIONS

May increase systemic exposure of drugs metabolized by CYP2D6 enzyme (eg, metoprolol, desipramine); monitoring and dose adjustment may be necessary, especially with narrow therapeutic index CYP2D6 substrates (eg, thioridazine, flecainide, propafenone). May increase levels of digoxin; monitor levels and consider using lowest digoxin dose initially. May increase levels of warfarin. Caution with antimuscarinic medications for OAB; urinary retention may occur with concomitant use.

NURSING CONSIDERATIONS

Assessment: Assess for HTN, BOO, renal/hepatic impairment, pregnancy/nursing status, and possible drug interactions.

Monitoring: Monitor for urinary retention in patients with BOO, and other adverse reactions. Monitor BP periodically, especially in hypertensive patients.

Patient Counseling: Inform that therapy may increase BP and may cause infrequent UTI, rapid heartbeat, rash, and pruritus; instruct to contact physician if these effects occur.

Storage: 25°C (77°F); excursions permitted from 15-30°C (59-86°F).

MYSOLINE – primidone RX

Class: Pyrimidinedione derivative

ADULT DOSAGE

Seizures

Grand Mal, Psychomotor, and Focal Epileptic Seizures (Alone or w/ Other Anticonvulsants):

No Prior Antiepileptic Therapy:
Initial:
Days 1-3: 100-125mg qhs
Days 4-6: 100-125mg bid
Days 7-9: 100-125mg tid
Days 10/Maint: 250mg tid
Usual Maint: 250mg tid or qid
Max: 500mg qid

Already Receiving Other Anticonvulsants:
Initial: 100-125mg qhs
Titrate: Increase gradually to maint dose as other drug is gradually decreased. Continue until satisfactory dosage level achieved or other medication is completely withdrawn. When therapy w/ primidone alone is the objective, transition from concomitant therapy should not be completed in <2 weeks

PEDIATRIC DOSAGE

Seizures

Grand Mal, Psychomotor, and Focal Epileptic Seizures (Alone or w/ Other Anticonvulsants):

<8 Years:
Days 1-3: 50mg qhs
Days 4-6: 50mg bid
Days 7-9: 100mg bid
Days 10/Maint: 125-250mg tid
Usual Maint: 125-250mg tid or 10-25mg/kg/day in divided doses

≥8 Years:
No Prior Antiepileptic Therapy:
Initial:
Days 1-3: 100-125mg qhs
Days 4-6: 100-125mg bid
Days 7-9: 100-125mg tid
Days 10/Maint: 250mg tid
Usual Maint: 250mg tid or qid
Max: 500mg qid

Max: 2g/day

May also control grand mal seizures refractory to other anticonvulsant therapy

Already Receiving Other Anticonvulsants:
Initial: 100-125mg qhs
Titrate: Increase gradually to maint dose as other drug is gradually decreased. Continue until satisfactory dosage level achieved or other medication is completely withdrawn. When therapy w/ primidone alone is the objective, transition from concomitant therapy should not be completed in <2 weeks
Max: 2g/day

May also control grand mal seizures refractory to other anticonvulsant therapy

ADMINISTRATION
Oral route

HOW SUPPLIED
Tab: 50mg*, 250mg* *scored

CONTRAINDICATIONS
Porphyria, phenobarbital hypersensitivity.

WARNINGS/PRECAUTIONS
Avoid abrupt withdrawal; may precipitate status epilepticus. Increased risk of suicidal thoughts or behavior; monitor for emergence or worsening of depression, suicidal thoughts/behavior, or any unusual changes in mood or behavior. Increased incidence of birth defects reported; encourage pregnant patients to enroll in the North American Antiepileptic Drug (NAAED) Pregnancy Registry. Neonatal hemorrhage reported in newborns; give pregnant women prophylactic vitamin K1 therapy for 1 month prior to, and during, delivery.

ADVERSE REACTIONS
Ataxia, vertigo, granulocytopenia, agranulocytosis, red-cell hypoplasia, aplasia.

NURSING CONSIDERATIONS

Assessment: Assess for porphyria, hypersensitivity to phenobarbital, prior anticonvulsant therapy, depression, and pregnancy/nursing status.

Monitoring: Monitor for status epilepticus, emergence or worsening of depression, suicidal thoughts/behavior, and any unusual changes in mood or behavior. Monitor CBC, drug serum blood level, and sequential multiple analysis-12 test every 6 months.

Patient Counseling: Counsel patients, their caregivers, and families that the therapy may increase risk of suicidal thoughts and behavior and advise to be alert for the emergence or worsening of symptoms of depression, any unusual changes in mood or behavior, or the emergence of suicidal thoughts, behavior, or thoughts about self-harm. Instruct to immediately report behaviors of concern to healthcare providers. Encourage pregnant patients to enroll in the NAAED Pregnancy Registry (1-888-233-2334).

Storage: 20-25°C (68-77°F).

NABUMETONE – nabumetone RX

Class: NSAID

NSAIDs may increase risk of serious cardiovascular (CV) thrombotic events, MI, stroke and serious GI adverse events including bleeding, ulceration, and perforation of the stomach or intestines. Contraindicated for the treatment of perioperative pain in the setting of CABG surgery.

ADULT DOSAGE

Osteoarthritis

Initial: 1000mg qd
Titrate: Adjust dose/frequency based on individual needs after observing response to initial therapy; some may obtain relief from 1500-2000mg/day
Max: 2000mg/day

May be given qd-bid; use lowest effective dose for chronic treatment

PEDIATRIC DOSAGE

Pediatric use may not have been established

Rheumatoid Arthritis

Initial: 1000mg qd
Titrate: Adjust dose/frequency based on individual needs after observing response to initial therapy; some may obtain relief from 1500-2000mg/day
Max: 2000mg/day

May be given qd-bid; use lowest effective dose for chronic treatment

DOSE MODIFICATION

Renal impairment

Moderate (CrCl 30-49mL/min):
Initial: ≤750mg qd
Max: 1500mg/day

Severe (CrCl <30mL/min):
Initial: ≤500mg qd
Max: 1000mg/day

ADMINISTRATION

Oral route

Take w/ or w/o food

HOW SUPPLIED

Tab: 500mg, 750mg

CONTRAINDICATIONS

History of asthma, urticaria, or allergic-type reactions after taking ASA or other NSAIDs. Treatment of perioperative pain in the setting of CABG surgery.

WARNINGS/PRECAUTIONS

Use lowest effective dose for shortest duration possible to minimize risk for CV events and adverse GI events. May lead to onset of new HTN or worsening of preexisting HTN; caution with HTN and monitor BP closely. Fluid retention and edema reported; caution with fluid retention or HF. Renal papillary necrosis and other renal injury reported after long-term use. Not recommended for use with advanced renal disease; if therapy must be initiated, monitor renal function closely. Anaphylactoid reactions may occur. Should not be given with ASA triad. May cause serious skin adverse events (eg, exfoliative dermatitis, Stevens-Johnson syndrome, and toxic epidermal necrolysis). Avoid in late pregnancy; may cause premature closure of ductus arteriosus. May cause elevations of LFTs; d/c if liver disease develops or systemic manifestations occur. Caution in elderly. Anemia may occur; monitor Hgb/Hct if signs or symptoms of anemia develop. May inhibit platelet aggregation and prolong bleeding time; monitor with coagulation disorders. Caution with asthma and avoid with ASA-sensitive asthma. May induce photosensitivity.

ADVERSE REACTIONS

Diarrhea, dyspepsia, abdominal pain, constipation, flatulence, N/V, positive stool guaiac, dizziness, headache, pruritus, rash, tinnitus, edema.

DRUG INTERACTIONS

Caution with warfarin and other protein-bound drugs. May decrease natriuretic effect of furosemide and thiazides; possible renal failure risk. May elevate lithium and MTX levels. May diminish antihypertensive effect of ACE inhibitors. Avoid concomitant ASA. May increase risk of GI bleeding with concomitant use of oral corticosteroids, anticoagulants, or alcohol.

NURSING CONSIDERATIONS

Assessment: Assess LFTs, renal function, CBC, and coagulation profile. Assess for history of CABG surgery, asthma and allergic reactions to ASA or other NSAIDs, active ulceration or chronic inflammation of GI tract, CV disease, asthma, alcohol intake, pregnancy/nursing status. Note other diseases/conditions and drug therapies.

Monitoring: Monitor for hypersensitivity reactions, CV thrombotic events, MI, stroke, GI bleeding, asthma, and skin adverse effects. Monitor BP, LFTs, renal function, CBC with differential and platelet count, coagulation profile, ocular effects, and photosensitivity.

Patient Counseling: Counsel about potential side effects; instruct seek medical attention if any develop, especially serious CV events or adverse GI events. Counsel about possible drug interactions and to take as prescribed. Advise women not to use in late pregnancy.

Storage: 20-25°C (68-77°F). Dispense in tight, light-resistant container.

NAMENDA – memantine hydrochloride

RX

Class: NMDA receptor antagonist

OTHER BRAND NAMES
Namenda XR

ADULT DOSAGE

Alzheimer's Disease

Moderate to Severe Dementia:
Sol, Tab:
Initial: 5mg qd
Titrate: Increase in 5mg increments to 10mg/day (5mg bid), 15mg/day (5mg and 10mg as separate doses), and 20mg/day (10mg bid) at ≥1-week intervals
Cap, ER:
Initial: 7mg qd
Titrate: Increase in 7mg increments to 28mg qd at ≥1-week intervals
Max/Target Dose: 28mg qd

Conversions

Switching from Tabs to Cap, ER: Switch from 10mg bid tabs to 28mg qd caps the day following last dose of 10mg tab
Severe Renal Impairment: Switch from 5mg bid tabs to 14mg qd caps the day following last dose of 5mg tab

Missed Dose

Sol, Tab
If a single dose is missed, take next dose as scheduled and do not double dose; if missed for several days, resume dose at lower dose and retitrate

PEDIATRIC DOSAGE
Pediatric use may not have been established

DOSE MODIFICATION
Renal Impairment
Severe (CrCl 5-29mL/min): Target Dose:
Sol, Tab: 5mg bid
Cap, ER: 14mg/day

ADMINISTRATION
Oral route

May take w/ or w/o food

Sol
Do not mix w/ any other liquid
Administer w/ a dosing device (syringe, syringe adaptor cap, tubing, other supplies needed) that comes w/ the drug
Use syringe to withdraw correct volume of oral sol and squirt slowly into the corner of the mouth

Cap, ER
Swallow cap whole; do not divide, chew, or crush
May be opened, sprinkled on applesauce, and swallowed

HOW SUPPLIED
Sol: 2mg/mL [360mL]; Tab: 5mg, 10mg; Titration-Pack: 5mg [28^s], 10mg [21^s]. Cap, ER: 7mg, 14mg, 21mg, 28mg; Titration Pack: 7mg [7^s], 14mg [7^s], 21mg [7^s], 28mg [7^s].

WARNINGS/PRECAUTIONS
Conditions that raise urine pH may decrease urinary elimination, resulting in increased plasma levels. Caution in patients with severe renal/hepatic impairment.

ADVERSE REACTIONS
Dizziness, headache, constipation, confusion, HTN, coughing, somnolence, hallucination, vomiting, back pain, (Sol, Tab) pain, (Cap, ER) diarrhea, influenza, weight gain, anxiety.

DRUG INTERACTIONS
Caution with other N-methyl-D-aspartate (NMDA) antagonists (eg, amantadine, ketamine, dextromethorphan) and drugs that alter urine pH towards the alkaline condition (eg, carbonic anhydrase inhibitors, sodium bicarbonate). (Cap, ER) Coadministration with drugs eliminated via

renal (cationic system) mechanism (eg, HCTZ, triamterene, metformin, cimetidine, ranitidine) may result in altered plasma levels of both agents.

NURSING CONSIDERATIONS

Assessment: Assess for hypersensitivity to drug, conditions that raise urine pH, renal/hepatic impairment, pregnancy/nursing status, and possible drug interactions.

Monitoring: Monitor for hypersensitivity reactions and other adverse reactions. Monitor renal/hepatic function.

Patient Counseling: Instruct to take as prescribed. Inform about possible side effects and instruct to notify physician if any develop. (Sol, Tab) Instruct to follow dose titration schedule and not to resume dosing without consulting physician if there has been a failure to take the medication for several days. (Tab) Instruct not to use any damaged or tampered tabs. (Sol) Instruct on how to use the oral sol dosing device.

Storage: 25°C (77°F); excursions permitted to 15-30°C (59-86°F).

NAPRELAN – naproxen sodium RX

Class: NSAID

NSAIDs may increase risk of serious cardiovascular (CV) thrombotic events, MI, and stroke; increased risk w/ duration of use and w/ CV disease (CVD) or risk factors for CVD. Contraindicated for the treatment of perioperative pain in the setting of CABG surgery. May increase risk of serious GI adverse events (eg, bleeding, ulceration, and stomach/intestinal perforation), which can be fatal and can occur at any time during use and w/o warning symptoms; elderly patients are at greater risk.

ADULT DOSAGE

Rheumatoid Arthritis

Initial: 750mg or 1000mg qd
Titrate:
Adjust dose/frequency depending on clinical response
In patients who tolerate lower doses well, may increase to two 750mg tabs or three 500mg tabs once daily for limited periods, as needed

Osteoarthritis

Initial: 750mg or 1000mg qd
Titrate:
Adjust dose/frequency depending on clinical response
In patients who tolerate lower doses well, may increase to two 750mg tabs or three 500mg tabs once daily for limited periods, as needed

Ankylosing Spondylitis

Initial: 750mg or 1000mg qd
Titrate:
Adjust dose/frequency depending on clinical response
In patients who tolerate lower doses well, may increase to two 750mg tabs or three 500mg tabs once daily for limited periods, as needed

Mild to Moderate Pain

Initial: 1000mg qd; may give 1500mg qd for a limited period in patients requiring greater analgesia
Max: 1000mg/day after limited period of 1500mg qd

Primary Dysmenorrhea

Initial: 1000mg qd; may give 1500mg qd for a limited period in patients requiring greater analgesia
Max: 1000mg/day after limited period of 1500mg qd

PEDIATRIC DOSAGE

Pediatric use may not have been established

Bursitis/Tendinitis

Acute:
Initial: 1000mg qd; may give 1500mg qd for a limited period in patients requiring greater analgesia
Max: 1000mg/day after limited period of 1500mg qd

Gout

Acute:
Day 1: 1000-1500mg qd
Succeeding Days: 1000mg qd until attack subsides

DOSE MODIFICATION

Renal Impairment
Start at lower end of dosing range

Hepatic Impairment
Start at lower end of dosing range

Elderly
Start at lower end of dosing range

ADMINISTRATION
Oral route

HOW SUPPLIED
Tab, Controlled-Release: 375mg, 500mg, 750mg

CONTRAINDICATIONS
History of asthma, urticaria, or allergic-type reactions w/ aspirin (ASA) or other NSAIDs. Treatment of perioperative pain in the setting of CABG surgery.

WARNINGS/PRECAUTIONS
Use lowest effective dose for the shortest duration possible. May cause HTN or worsen preexisting HTN; monitor BP closely. Fluid retention and edema reported; caution w/ fluid retention or heart failure (HF). Caution w/ history of ulcer disease, GI bleeding, or risk factors for GI bleeding; monitor for GI ulceration/bleeding and d/c if serious GI event occurs. Renal injury reported w/ long-term use; increased risk w/ renal/hepatic impairment, HF, and elderly. Not recommended w/ advanced renal disease or moderate to severe or severe renal impairment (CrCl <30mL/min); monitor renal function closely if therapy is initiated. Anaphylactoid reactions may occur. Caution w/ asthma and avoid w/ ASA-sensitive asthma and the ASA triad. May cause serious skin reactions (eg, exfoliative dermatitis, Stevens-Johnson syndrome, toxic epidermal necrolysis); d/c at 1st appearance of skin rash/hypersensitivity. Avoid in late pregnancy; may cause premature closure of ductus arteriosus. Not a substitute for corticosteroids nor treatment for corticosteroid insufficiency. May mask signs of inflammation and fever. May cause elevated LFTs or severe hepatic reactions; d/c if liver disease or systemic manifestations occur, and if abnormal LFTs persist/worsen. Anemia reported; monitor Hgb/Hct if anemia develops. May inhibit platelet aggregation and prolong bleeding time; monitor patients w/ coagulation disorders.

ADVERSE REACTIONS
CV thrombotic events, MI, stroke, GI events, headache, dyspepsia, flu syndrome, pain, infection, nausea, diarrhea, constipation, rhinitis, sinusitis, UTI.

DRUG INTERACTIONS
Increased risk of GI bleeding w/ oral corticosteroids, anticoagulants, alcohol use, and smoking. Risk of renal toxicity w/ diuretics and ACE inhibitors. Monitor patients receiving anticoagulants. May diminish antihypertensive effect of ACE inhibitors. Not recommended w/ ASA. May reduce natriuretic effect of loop (eg, furosemide) or thiazide diuretics; monitor for signs of renal failure and diuretic efficacy. May increase lithium levels; monitor for lithium toxicity. May enhance methotrexate toxicity; caution w/ concomitant use. Synergistic effect on GI bleeding w/ warfarin.

NURSING CONSIDERATIONS

Assessment: Assess for history of asthma, urticaria, or allergic-type reactions w/ ASA or other NSAIDs, ASA triad, CVD, risk factors for CVD, HTN, fluid retention, HF, history of ulcer disease, history of/risk factors for GI bleeding, general health status, renal/hepatic function, coagulation disorders, pregnancy/nursing status, and possible drug interactions. Obtain baseline CBC and BP.

Monitoring: Monitor BP, CBC, bleeding time, LFTs, renal function, and chemistry profile periodically. Monitor for GI bleeding/ulceration/perforation, CV thrombotic events, MI, stroke, HTN, fluid retention, edema, and skin/allergic reactions.

Patient Counseling: Inform to seek medical advice if symptoms of CV events, GI ulceration/bleeding, skin/hypersensitivity reactions, unexplained weight gain or edema, hepatotoxicity, or anaphylactoid reactions occur. Instruct to avoid in late pregnancy.

Storage: 20-25°C (68-77°F).

NAPROSYN – naproxen

Class: NSAID

RX

NSAIDs may increase risk of serious cardiovascular thrombotic events, MI, and stroke; increased risk with duration of use and with cardiovascular disease (CVD) or risk factors for CVD. Increased risk of serious GI adverse events (eg, bleeding, ulceration, and stomach/intestinal perforation) that can be fatal and occur anytime during use without warning symptoms; elderly patients are at a greater risk. Contraindicated for treatment of perioperative pain in the setting of CABG surgery.

OTHER BRAND NAMES

EC-Naprosyn, Anaprox, Anaprox DS

ADULT DOSAGE

Gout

Acute Attack:
Naprosyn:
Initial: 750mg, then 250mg q8h until attack subsides

Anaprox:
Initial: 825mg, then 275mg q8h until attack subsides

Bursitis

Anaprox/Anaprox DS:
Initial: 550mg, then 550mg q12h or 275mg q6-8h as required
Max: 1375mg/day initially, 1100mg/day thereafter

Rheumatoid Arthritis

Naprosyn:
250mg, 375mg, or 500mg bid

EC-Naprosyn:
375mg or 500mg bid

Anaprox:
275mg bid

Anaprox DS:
550mg bid
Titrate: Adjust dose/frequency up or down depending on clinical response; may increase to 1500mg/day for ≤6 months if patient can tolerate lower doses well

Ankylosing Spondylitis

Naprosyn:
250mg, 375mg, or 500mg bid

EC-Naprosyn:
375mg or 500mg bid

Anaprox:
275mg bid

Anaprox DS:
550mg bid
Titrate: Adjust dose/frequency up or down depending on clinical response; may increase to 1500mg/day for ≤6 months if patient can tolerate lower doses well

Pain

Anaprox/Anaprox DS:
Initial: 550mg, then 550mg q12h or 275mg q6-8h as required
Max: 1375mg/day initially, 1100mg/day thereafter

Primary Dysmenorrhea

Anaprox/Anaprox DS:
Initial: 550mg, then 550mg q12h or 275mg q6-8h as required

PEDIATRIC DOSAGE

Juvenile Arthritis

≥2 Years:
Sus:
Usual: 5mg/kg bid

Max: 1375mg/day initially, 1100mg/day thereafter

Osteoarthritis

Naprosyn:
250mg, 375mg, or 500mg bid

EC-Naprosyn:
375mg or 500mg bid

Anaprox:
275mg bid

Anaprox DS:
550mg bid

Titrate: Adjust dose/frequency up or down depending on clinical response; may increase to 1500mg/day for ≤6 months if patient can tolerate lower doses well

DOSE MODIFICATION

Renal Impairment
Start w/ lower end of dosing range
Moderate to Severe (CrCl <30mL/min): Not recommended

Hepatic Impairment
Start w/ lower end of dosing range

Elderly
Start w/ lower end of dosing range

ADMINISTRATION
Oral route

EC-Naprosyn
Do not chew, crush, or break

HOW SUPPLIED
Sus: (Naprosyn) 125mg/5mL [473mL]; Tab: (Naprosyn) 250mg*, 375mg, 500mg*, (Anaprox [naproxen sodium]) 275mg, (Anaprox DS [naproxen sodium]) 550mg*; Tab, Delayed-Release: (EC-Naprosyn) 375mg, 500mg *scored

CONTRAINDICATIONS
History of asthma, urticaria, or other allergic-type reactions with ASA or other NSAIDs. Treatment of perioperative pain in the setting of CABG surgery.

WARNINGS/PRECAUTIONS
Use lowest effective dose for the shortest duration possible. May cause HTN or worsen preexisting HTN; monitor BP closely. Fluid retention and edema reported; caution with fluid retention, HTN, or HF. Caution with prior history of ulcer disease, GI bleeding, and risk factors for GI bleeding; monitor for GI ulceration/bleeding and d/c if serious GI event occurs. May exacerbate inflammatory bowel disease. Renal injury reported with long-term use; increased risk with renal/hepatic impairment, hypovolemia, HF, salt depletion, and in elderly. Not recommended with advanced renal disease or moderate to severe renal impairment (CrCl <30mL/min); monitor renal function closely and hydrate adequately. D/C if signs and symptoms consistent with renal disease develop. Anaphylactoid reactions may occur. Caution with asthma and avoid with ASA-sensitive asthma and the ASA triad. May cause serious skin adverse events (eg, exfoliative dermatitis, Stevens-Johnson syndrome, toxic epidermal necrolysis); d/c at 1st appearance of skin rash/hypersensitivity. Avoid in late pregnancy; may cause premature closure of ductus arteriosus. Not a substitute for corticosteroids or for the treatment of corticosteroid insufficiency. May mask signs of inflammation and fever. Periodically monitor Hgb if initial Hgb ≤10g and receiving long-term therapy. Perform ophthalmic studies if visual changes/disturbances occur. May cause elevations of LFTs or severe hepatic reactions; d/c if liver disease or systemic manifestations occur, or if abnormal LFTs persist/worsen. Caution with chronic alcoholic liver disease and other diseases with decreased/abnormal plasma proteins if high doses are administered; dosage adjustment may be required. Anemia reported; monitor Hgb/Hct if anemia develops. May inhibit platelet aggregation and prolong bleeding time; monitor patients with coagulation disorders. Monitor CBC and chemistry profile periodically with long-term treatment. (Sus, Anaprox/Anaprox DS) Contains Na^+; caution with severely restricted Na^+ intake. (EC-Naprosyn) Not recommended for initial treatment of acute pain.

ADVERSE REACTIONS
Cardiovascular (CV) thrombotic events, MI, stroke, GI adverse events, edema, drowsiness, dizziness, constipation, heartburn, abdominal pain, nausea, headache, tinnitus, dyspnea, pruritus.

DRUG INTERACTIONS
Avoid with other naproxen products. Not recommended with ASA. Risk of renal toxicity with diuretics, ACE inhibitors, and ARBs. May reduce natriuretic effect of loop (eg, furosemide)

or thiazide diuretics; monitor for signs of renal failure and diuretic efficacy. May diminish antihypertensive effect of ACE inhibitors, ARBs, or β-blockers (eg, propranolol); monitor changes in BP. May result in deterioration of renal function, including possible acute renal failure with ACE inhibitors or ARBs; monitor closely for signs of worsening renal function. May enhance methotrexate toxicity; caution with concomitant use. May increase lithium levels and reduce renal lithium clearance; monitor for lithium toxicity. Increased risk of GI bleeding with SSRIs, oral corticosteroids, anticoagulants, alcohol, and smoking; monitor carefully. Synergistic effect on GI bleeding with warfarin. Potential for interaction with other albumin-bound drugs (eg, coumarin-type anticoagulants, sulfonylureas, hydantoins, other NSAIDs, ASA); dose adjustment with hydantoin, sulfonamide, or sulfonylurea may be required. Probenecid significantly increases plasma levels and extends $T_{1/2}$. Antacids, sucralfate, and cholestyramine can delay absorption. (EC-Naprosyn) Not recommended with H_2-blockers, sucralfate, or intensive antacid therapy.

NURSING CONSIDERATIONS

Assessment: Assess for history of asthma, urticaria, or allergic-type reactions with ASA or other NSAIDs, ASA triad, CVD, risk factors for CVD, HTN, fluid retention, HF, salt restriction, history of ulcer disease, history of/risk factors for GI bleeding, general health status, history of IBD, renal/hepatic impairment, hypovolemia, decreased/abnormal plasma proteins, coagulation disorders, pregnancy/nursing status, and for possible drug interactions. Obtain baseline CBC and BP.

Monitoring: Monitor for GI bleeding/ulceration/perforation, CV thrombotic events, MI, stroke, HTN, fluid retention, edema, and skin/allergic reactions. Monitor BP, CBC, LFTs, renal function, and chemistry profile periodically.

Patient Counseling: Inform to seek medical advice if symptoms of CV events, GI ulceration/bleeding, skin/hypersensitivity reactions, unexplained weight gain or edema, hepatotoxicity, or anaphylactoid reactions occur. Instruct to avoid use in late pregnancy. Instruct to use caution when performing activities that require alertness if drowsiness, dizziness, vertigo, or depression occurs.

Storage: 15-30°C (59-86°F). (Sus) Avoid excessive heat, >40°C (104°F). Shake gently before use.

NASONEX – mometasone furoate monohydrate RX

Class: Corticosteroid

ADULT DOSAGE

Seasonal/Perennial Allergic Rhinitis

2 sprays/nostril qd

Prophylaxis:
May start 2-4 weeks before pollen season

Nasal Congestion:
2 sprays/nostril qd

Nasal Polyps

2 sprays/nostril qd-bid

PEDIATRIC DOSAGE

Seasonal/Perennial Allergic Rhinitis

2-11 Years:
1 spray/nostril qd

≥12 Years:
2 sprays/nostril qd

Prophylaxis:
May start 2-4 weeks before pollen season (≥12 years)

Nasal Congestion:

2-11 Years:
1 spray/nostril qd

≥12 Years:
2 sprays/nostril qd

ADMINISTRATION
Intranasal route

HOW SUPPLIED
Spray: 50mcg/spray [17g]

WARNINGS/PRECAUTIONS
Local nasal effects (eg, epistaxis, *Candida* infections of nose and pharynx, nasal septum perforation, impaired wound healing) may occur; d/c when infection occurs. Glaucoma and/or cataracts may develop; monitor closely in patients with change in vision, history of increased intraocular pressure (IOP), glaucoma, and/or cataracts. D/C if hypersensitivity reactions, including instances of wheezing, occur. May increase susceptibility to infections; caution with active/quiescent tuberculosis (TB), ocular herpes simplex, or untreated bacterial, fungal, and systemic viral infections. Hypercorticism and adrenal suppression may appear when used at higher than recommended doses or in susceptible individuals at recommended doses; d/c slowly if such changes occur. May reduce growth velocity of pediatrics; monitor growth routinely.

ADVERSE REACTIONS
Headache, viral infection, pharyngitis, epistaxis/blood-tinged mucus, cough, upper respiratory tract infection, dysmenorrhea, musculoskeletal pain, sinusitis, N/V.

DRUG INTERACTIONS

May increase plasma concentrations with ketoconazole.

NURSING CONSIDERATIONS

Assessment: Assess for previous hypersensitivity, active/quiescent TB, infections, ocular herpes simplex, change in vision, history of IOP, glaucoma or cataracts, recent nasal septum ulcers, nasal surgery/trauma, pregnancy/nursing status, and possible drug interactions.

Monitoring: Monitor for acute adrenal insufficiency, hypercorticism, nasal or pharyngeal *Candida* infections, suppression of growth velocity in children, hypersensitivity reactions, wheezing, nasal septum perforation, changes in vision, glaucoma, cataracts, increased IOP, epistaxis, wound healing, worsening of infections, and other adverse reactions.

Patient Counseling: Advise to take ud at regular intervals and not to increase prescribed dosage. Inform patients that treatment may be associated with adverse reactions (eg, epistaxis, nasal septum perforation, *Candida* infection). Inform that glaucoma and/or cataracts may develop. Counsel to avoid exposure to chickenpox or measles and to immediately consult a physician if exposed. Contact physician if symptoms worsen or do not improve. Supervise young children during administration. Advise patient to take missed dose as soon as remembered. Counsel on proper priming and administration techniques.

Storage: 25°C (77°F); excursions permitted to 15-30°C (59-86°F). Protect from light.

NATACYN – natamycin

RX

Class: Tetraene polyene antifungal

ADULT DOSAGE

Ocular Infections

Caused by susceptible organisms, including *Fusarium solani* keratitis

Fungal Keratitis:
Initial: 1 drop in the conjunctival sac q1-2h
Titrate: May reduce to 1 drop 6-8X/day after 3-4 days; continue therapy for 14-21 days or until resolution. May reduce dose gradually at 4- to 7-day intervals

Fungal Blepharitis/Conjunctivitis:
Initial: 1 drop 4-6X/day

PEDIATRIC DOSAGE

Pediatric use may not have been established

ADMINISTRATION

Ocular route

Shake well before using

HOW SUPPLIED

Sus: 5% [15mL]

WARNINGS/PRECAUTIONS

Not for inj. Failure of improvement of keratitis following 7-10 days of administration suggests that the infection may be caused by a microorganism not susceptible to natamycin. Continuation of therapy should be based on clinical reevaluation and additional lab studies. Adherence of sus to areas of epithelial ulceration or retention of the sus in the fornices occurs regularly.

ADVERSE REACTIONS

Allergic reaction, change in vision, chest pain, corneal opacity, dyspnea, eye discomfort/edema/hyperemia/irritation/pain, foreign body sensation, paresthesia, tearing.

NURSING CONSIDERATIONS

Assessment: Assess for history of hypersensitivity to drug, and pregnancy/nursing status.

Monitoring: Monitor for clinical response and development of adverse reactions.

Patient Counseling: Advise not to touch dropper tip to any surface to avoid contamination of sus. Instruct not to wear contact lenses if patient has signs/symptoms of fungal blepharitis, conjunctivitis, and keratitis.

Storage: 2-24°C (36-75°F). Do not freeze. Avoid exposure to light and excessive heat.

NATAZIA – dienogest/estradiol valerate

RX

Class: Estrogen/progestogen combination

Cigarette smoking increases risk of serious cardiovascular (CV) events from combination oral contraceptive (COC) use. Risk increases with age (>35 yrs) and with the number of cigarettes smoked. Should not be used by women who are >35 yrs and smoke.

ADULT DOSAGE

Contraception

1 tab qd at the same time for 28 days, then repeat

Start on Day 1 of menses

Heavy Menstrual Bleeding

In women w/o organic pathology who choose to use oral contraceptives as method of contraception

1 tab qd at the same time for 28 days, then repeat

Start on Day 1 of menses

Conversions

Switching from Combination Hormonal Method:
Another Pill: Start on 1st day of withdrawal bleed. Do not continue pills from previous birth control pack
Vaginal Ring/Transdermal Patch: Start on the day ring/patch is removed

Switching from Progestin-Only Method (eg, Progestin-Only Pill, Implant, Intrauterine System, Injection):
Start on the day the next progestin-only pill/injection would have been taken/administered, or on the day of removal of implant/intrauterine system

Use a nonhormonal backup method (eg, condom, spermicide) for the first 9 days

PEDIATRIC DOSAGE

Contraception

Not indicated for use premenarche; refer to adult dosing

Heavy Menstrual Bleeding

Not indicated for use premenarche; refer to adult dosing

ADMINISTRATION

Oral route

Take in the order directed on the blister pack
Tabs should not be skipped or intake delayed by >12 hrs
Use a nonhormonal contraceptive as back-up during the first 9 days
For postpartum women who do not breastfeed or after a second trimester abortion, start therapy no earlier than 4 weeks postpartum; if patient has not yet had a period, she should use an additional contraceptive method until she has taken 9 consecutive days of therapy
If vomiting/diarrhea occurs w/in 3-4 hrs after taking a colored tab, consider as missed tab

HOW SUPPLIED

Tab: (Estradiol Valerate) 1mg, 3mg; Tab: (Estradiol Valerate-Dienogest) 2mg-2mg, 2mg-3mg

CONTRAINDICATIONS

High risk of arterial/venous thrombotic diseases (eg, smoking if >35 yrs, history/presence of deep vein thrombosis/pulmonary embolism, cerebrovascular disease, coronary artery disease, thrombogenic valvular or thrombogenic rhythm diseases of the heart [eg, subacute bacterial endocarditis with valvular disease, or atrial fibrillation], inherited/acquired hypercoagulopathies, uncontrolled HTN, diabetes mellitus [DM] with vascular disease, headaches with focal neurological symptoms or migraine with/without aura if >35 yrs), undiagnosed abnormal uterine bleeding, history/presence of breast or other estrogen-/progestin-sensitive cancer, benign/malignant liver tumors, liver disease, pregnancy.

WARNINGS/PRECAUTIONS

Increased risk of venous thromboembolism (VTE) and arterial thrombosis (eg, stroke, myocardial infarction [MI]); greatest risk of VTE during the first 6 months of COC use and is present after initially starting COC or restarting (after ≥4 weeks pill-free interval) the same or different COC. D/C if arterial/venous thrombotic event occurs. D/C at least 4 weeks before and through 2 weeks after major surgery or other surgeries known to have an elevated risk of thromboembolism. Start therapy no earlier than 4 weeks postpartum in women who do not breastfeed. Caution with CV disease risk factors. D/C if there is unexplained loss of vision, proptosis, diplopia, papilledema, or retinal vascular lesions; evaluate for retinal vein thrombosis immediately. May increase risk of breast or cervical cancer, intraepithelial neoplasia, gallbladder disease, hepatic adenomas, and hepatocellular carcinoma; d/c if jaundice develops. Cholestasis may occur with history of pregnancy-related cholestasis. Increased BP reported; d/c if BP rises significantly. May decrease glucose tolerance; monitor prediabetic and diabetic women. Consider alternative contraception with uncontrolled dyslipidemia. Increased risk of pancreatitis with hypertriglyceridemia or family history thereof. May increase frequency/severity of migraine; d/c if new headaches that are recurrent, persistent, or severe develop. May cause bleeding irregularities (eg, breakthrough bleeding, spotting, amenorrhea); rule out pregnancy or malignancies. Not for use as a test for pregnancy, or to treat threatened or habitual abortion during pregnancy. Caution with history of depression; d/c if depression recurs to serious degree. May change results of lab tests (eg, coagulation factors, lipids, glucose tolerance, binding proteins). May induce/exacerbate angioedema in patients with hereditary angioedema. Chloasma may occur; women with chloasma should avoid sun exposure or UV radiation. Not for use before menarche or evaluated in women with BMI >30kg/m^2.

ADVERSE REACTIONS

N/V, headache, migraine, menstrual disorders, breast pain/discomfort/tenderness, acne, increased weight, mood changes.

DRUG INTERACTIONS

Agents that induce certain enzymes, including CYP3A4 (eg, barbiturates, bosentan, felbamate, griseofulvin, oxcarbazepine, topiramate) may decrease COC efficacy and/or increase breakthrough bleeding; consider alternative contraceptive or a back-up method when using moderate or weak inducers and continue back-up contraception for 28 days after discontinuation of the inducer. Avoid with strong CYP3A4 inducers (eg, carbamazepine, phenytoin, rifampicin, St. John's wort) and for at least 28 days after discontinuation of these inducers. Strong CYP3A4 inhibitors (eg, ketoconazole) and moderate CYP3A4 inhibitors (eg, erythromycin) may increase dienogest and estradiol levels. Other CYP3A4 inhibitors (eg, azole antifungals, cimetidine, verapamil, macrolides, diltiazem, antidepressants, grapefruit juice) may increase dienogest levels. Significant changes (increase/decrease) in plasma estrogen and progestin levels may occur with some HIV/hepatitis C virus protease inhibitors or with non-nucleoside reverse transcriptase inhibitors. Pregnancy reported with antibiotics. May decrease plasma concentrations of lamotrigine and reduce seizure control; may need dosage adjustment. Increases thyroid-binding globulin; may need to increase dose of thyroid hormone in patients on thyroid hormone replacement therapy.

NURSING CONSIDERATIONS

Assessment: Assess for renal impairment, abnormal uterine bleeding, adrenal insufficiency, and known or suspected pregnancy and other conditions where treatment is cautioned or contraindicated. Assess use in women who are >35 yrs and smoke, have CV disease and arterial/venous thrombosis risk factors, predisposition to hyperkalemia, pregnancy-related cholestasis, HTN, DM, uncontrolled dyslipidemia, history of hypertriglyceridemia, history of depression, hereditary angioedema, and history of chloasma. Assess for possible drug interactions.

Monitoring: Monitor for bleeding irregularities, venous/arterial thrombotic and thromboembolic events, cervical cancer or intraepithelial neoplasia, retinal vein thrombosis or any other ophthalmic changes, jaundice, acute/chronic disturbances in liver function, new/worsening headaches or migraines, serious depression, cholestasis with history of pregnancy-related cholestasis, and pancreatitis. Monitor K^+ levels, thyroid function if receiving thyroid replacement therapy, glucose levels in DM or prediabetes, lipids with dyslipidemia, liver function, and check BP annually.

Patient Counseling: Counsel that cigarette smoking increases the risk of serious CV events from COC use and to avoid use in women who are >35 yrs of age and smoke. Inform that drug does not protect against HIV infection and other sexually transmitted diseases. Instruct to take at the same time every day, preferably pm pc or hs. Counsel on what to do if pills are missed or if vomiting occurs within 4 hrs after tablet-taking. Inform that amenorrhea may occur and pregnancy should be ruled out if amenorrhea occurs in ≥2 consecutive cycles. Advise to inform physician of preexisting medical conditions and/or drugs currently being taken. Counsel to use an additional method of contraception when enzyme inducers are used with COCs. Counsel any patient who starts medication postpartum, and who has not yet had a period, to use an additional method of contraception until have taken medication for 9 consecutive days. Instruct to d/c if pregnancy occurs during treatment.

Storage: 25°C (77°F); excursions permitted to 15-30°C (59-86°F).

NATROBA – spinosad

RX

Class: Pediculocide

ADULT DOSAGE

Head Lice Infestations

Depending on hair length, apply up to 120mL to adequately cover dry scalp and hair; leave on for 10 min, then thoroughly rinse off w/ warm water

Apply 2nd treatment if live lice seen 7 days after the 1st treatment

PEDIATRIC DOSAGE

Head Lice Infestations

≥4 Years:
Depending on hair length, apply up to 120mL to adequately cover dry scalp and hair; leave on for 10 min, then thoroughly rinse off w/ warm water

Apply 2nd treatment if live lice seen 7 days after the 1st treatment

ADMINISTRATION

Topical route

Shake well before use
Avoid contact w/ eyes

HOW SUPPLIED

Sus: 0.9% [120mL]

WARNINGS/PRECAUTIONS

Not for PO, ophthalmic, or intravaginal use. Contains benzyl alcohol; avoid in neonates and infants <6 months of age. Should be used in the context of an overall lice management program (eg, washing of recently worn clothing and personal care items).

ADVERSE REACTIONS

Application-site erythema/irritation, ocular erythema.

NURSING CONSIDERATIONS

Assessment: Assess pregnancy/nursing status.

Monitoring: Monitor for presence of live lice after 7 days of 1st treatment.

Patient Counseling: Advise to use only on dry scalp and hair. Instruct not to swallow. Instruct to rinse thoroughly with water if medication gets in or near the eyes. Advise to wash hands after application. Inform to use on children only under direct supervision of an adult. Advise to consult physician if pregnant/breastfeeding.

Storage: 25°C (77°F); excursions permitted between 15-30°C (59-86°F).

NATURE-THROID – thyroid

RX

Class: Thyroid replacement hormone

ADULT DOSAGE

Hypothyroidism

Replacement/supplemental therapy in hypothyroidism of any etiology, except transient hypothyroidism during the recovery phase of subacute thyroiditis

Initial: 32.5mg/day; 16.25mg/day is recommended in patients w/ myxedema, particularly if cardiovascular impairment is suspected
Titrate: Increase by 16.25mg every 2-3 weeks
Maint: 65-130mg/day

Myxedema Coma:
Initial: 400mcg (100mcg/mL) of levothyroxine sodium (T4) given rapidly; follow by daily supplements of 100-200mcg given IV

Pituitary TSH Suppressant

Used to treat/prevent various types of euthyroid goiters (eg, thyroid nodules, subacute or chronic lymphocytic thyroiditis [Hashimoto's], multinodular goiter) and to manage thyroid cancer

PEDIATRIC DOSAGE

Hypothyroidism

Congenital:
0-6 Months of Age: 4.8-6mg/kg/day (16.25-32.5mg/day)
6-12 Months of Age: 3.6-4.8mg/kg/day (32.5-48.75mg/day)
1-5 Years: 3-3.6mg/kg/day (48.75-65mg/day)
6-12 Years: 2.4-3mg/kg/day (65-97.5mg/day)
>12 Years: 1.2-1.8mg/kg/day (>97.5mg/day)

1.56mg/kg/day of levothyroxine (T4) for 7-10 days

Diagnostic Aid

In Suppression Tests to Differentiate Suspected Mild Hyperthyroidism or Thyroid Gland Anatomy:
1.56mg/kg/day of levothyroxine (T4) for 7-10 days

DOSE MODIFICATION

Adverse Reactions

Hypothyroidism:
Angina: Reduce dose if angina occurs

Elderly
Start at lower end of dosing range

ADMINISTRATION
Oral route

HOW SUPPLIED
Tab: 16.25mg, 32.5mg, 48.75mg, 65mg, 81.25mg, 97.5mg, 113.75mg, 130mg, 146.25mg, 162.5mg, 195mg, 260mg, 325mg

CONTRAINDICATIONS
Uncorrected adrenal cortical insufficiency, untreated thyrotoxicosis.

WARNINGS/PRECAUTIONS
Not for treatment of obesity; larger doses in euthyroid patients can cause serious or even life-threatening toxicity. Not for the treatment of male or female infertility unless accompanied by hypothyroidism. Caution with cardiovascular (CV) disorders (eg, angina pectoris) and elderly with risk of occult cardiac disease; initiate at low doses and reduce dose if aggravation of CV disease suspected. May aggravate diabetes mellitus (DM), diabetes insipidus (DI), or adrenal cortical insufficiency. Treatment of myxedema coma requires simultaneous administration of glucocorticoids. Excessive doses in infants may cause craniosynostosis. Caution with strong suspicion of thyroid gland autonomy. Androgens, corticosteroids, estrogens, iodine-containing preparations, and salicylates may interfere with lab tests.

DRUG INTERACTIONS
Large doses in euthyroid patients may cause serious or even life-threatening toxicity particularly with sympathomimetic amines. Closely monitor PT in patients on oral anticoagulants; dose reduction of anticoagulant may be required. May increase insulin or oral hypoglycemic requirements. Potentially impaired absorption with cholestyramine and colestipol; space dosing by 4-5 hrs. Estrogens may decrease free T4; increase in thyroid dose may be needed.

NURSING CONSIDERATIONS

Assessment: Assess for adrenal cortical insufficiency, thyrotoxicosis, apparent hypersensitivity to the drug, CV disorders (CAD, angina pectoris), DM/DI, myxedema coma, nursing status, and possible drug interactions.

Monitoring: Monitor response to treatment, urinary glucose levels in patients with DM, PT in patients receiving anticoagulants, and for aggravation of CV disease. Monitor thyroid function periodically.

Patient Counseling: Inform that replacement therapy is taken essentially for life except in transient hypothyroidism. Instruct to immediately report to physician any signs/symptoms of thyroid hormone toxicity (eg, chest pain, increased pulse rate, palpitations, excessive sweating, heat intolerance, nervousness). Inform the importance of frequent/close monitoring of PT and urinary glucose and the need for dose adjustment of antidiabetic and/or oral anticoagulant medication. Inform that partial loss of hair may be seen in children in 1st few months of therapy.

Storage: 15-30°C (59-86°F).

NEORAL – cyclosporine

RX

Class: Cyclic polypeptide immunosuppressant

Should only be prescribed by physicians experienced in management of systemic immunosuppressive therapy for indicated diseases. Manage patients in facilities equipped and staffed w/ adequate lab and supportive medical resources. Increased susceptibility to infection and development of neoplasia (eg, lymphoma) may result from immunosuppression. May be coadministered w/ other immunosuppressive agents in kidney, liver, and heart transplant patients. Not bioequivalent to Sandimmune and cannot be used interchangeably w/o physician supervision. Caution in switching from Sandimmune. Monitor cyclosporine blood concentrations in transplant and rheumatoid arthritis (RA) patients to avoid toxicity due to high concentrations. Dose adjustments should be made to minimize possible organ rejection due to low concentrations in transplant patients. Increased risk of developing skin malignancies in psoriasis patients previously treated w/ PUVA, methotrexate (MTX) or other immunosuppressive agents, UVB, coal tar, or radiation therapy. May cause systemic HTN and nephrotoxicity. Monitor for renal dysfunction, including structural kidney damage, during therapy.

ADULT DOSAGE

Organ Transplant

Organ Rejection Prophylaxis in Kidney, Liver, and Heart Allogeneic Transplants:

Newly Transplanted Patients:
Initial dose may be given 4-12 hrs prior to transplant or given postoperatively; dose varies depending on transplanted organ and other immunosuppressive agents included in protocol

Suggested Initial Doses:
Renal Transplant: 933mg/kg/day
Liver Transplant: 834mg/kg/day
Heart Transplant: 733mg/kg/day
Give bid

Subsequently adjust dose to achieve a predefined blood concentration

Adjunct therapy w/ adrenal corticosteroids is recommended initially

Conversion from Sandimmune:
Start w/ same daily dose as was previously used w/ Sandimmune (1:1 dose conversion); subsequently adjust dose to attain the pre-conversion blood trough concentration
After conversion, monitor blood trough concentration every 4-7 days while adjusting to trough levels until concentration attains pre-conversion value

Transplant Patients w/ Poor Sandimmune Absorption:
Patients tend to have higher cyclosporine concentrations after conversion to therapy; caution when converting patients at doses >10mg/kg/day
Titrate dose individually based on trough concentrations, tolerability, and clinical response and measure blood trough concentration at least 2X a week (daily if initial dose >10mg/kg/day) until stabilized w/in desired range

Rheumatoid Arthritis

Severe, active RA where the disease has not adequately responded to Methotrexate (MTX)

W/ or w/o MTX:
Initial: 2.5mg/kg/day, taken bid
Titrate: May increase by 0.5-0.75mg/kg/day after 8 weeks and again after 12 weeks
Max: 4mg/kg/day

Salicylates, NSAIDs, and oral corticosteroids may be continued

D/C if no benefit is seen by 16 weeks

PEDIATRIC DOSAGE

Pediatric use may not have been established

Combination w/ MTX:
Most patients can be treated w/ doses of ≤3mg/kg/day when combined w/ MTX doses of up to 15mg/week

Plaque Psoriasis

In immunocompetent patients w/ severe, recalcitrant, plaque psoriasis who failed to respond to at least 1 systemic therapy (eg, PUVA, retinoids, methotrexate) or for whom other systemic therapies are contraindicated, or cannot be tolerated

Initial: 2.5mg/kg/day, taken bid, for at least 4 weeks
Titrate: If clinical improvement does not occur, increase dose at 2-week intervals by approx 0.5mg/kg/day
Max: 4mg/kg/day

D/C if satisfactory response cannot be achieved after 6 weeks at 4mg/kg/day or the patient's max tolerated dose

DOSE MODIFICATION

Renal Impairment

In Kidney, Liver, and Heart Transplant:
Reduce dose if indicated

In Rheumatoid Arthritis/Plaque Psoriasis:
Not recommended for use

Hepatic Impairment

Severe: Dose reduction may be necessary

Elderly

Start at lower end of dosing range

Adverse Events

Rheumatoid Arthritis/Plaque Psoriasis:
Reduce dose by 25-50% to control adverse events; d/c therapy if dose reduction is not effective or if adverse event or abnormality is severe

Other Important Modifications

Avoid consumption of grapefruit or grapefruit juice during therapy

ADMINISTRATION

Oral route

Always administer daily dose in 2 divided doses (bid); administer on a consistent schedule w/ regard to time of day and relation to meals

Sol

1. Dilute w/ room temperature orange or apple juice to make sol more palatable; avoid switching diluents frequently or diluting w/ grapefruit juice
2. Take the prescribed amount of sol from the container using supplied dosing syringe, after removal of protective cover, and transfer sol to a glass of orange or apple juice (do not use a plastic container)
3. Stir well and drink at once; do not allow diluted oral sol to stand before drinking
4. Rinse the glass w/ more diluent to ensure that the total dose is consumed
5. After use, dry the outside of dosing syringe w/ a clean towel and replace protective cover
6. Do not rinse dosing syringe w/ water or other cleaning agents; if syringe requires cleaning, it must be completely dry before resuming use

HOW SUPPLIED

Cap: 25mg, 100mg; Sol: 100mg/mL [50mL]

CONTRAINDICATIONS

RA/Psoriasis: Abnormal renal function, uncontrolled HTN, malignancies. Psoriasis: Concomitant PUVA or UVB therapy, MTX, other immunosuppressants, coal tar, or radiation therapy.

WARNINGS/PRECAUTIONS

May cause hepatotoxicity and liver injury (eg, cholestasis, jaundice, hepatitis, liver failure). Elevations of SrCr and BUN may occur and reflect a reduction in GFR; closely monitor renal function and frequent dose adjustments may be indicated. Elevations in SrCr and BUN levels do not necessarily indicate rejection; evaluate patient before initiating dose adjustment. Thrombocytopenia and microangiopathic hemolytic anemia, resulting in graft failure, significant hyperkalemia (sometimes associated w/ hyperchloremic metabolic acidosis) and hyperuricemia reported.

Avoid excessive ultraviolet light exposure. Oversuppression of the immune system resulting in increased risk of infection/malignancy may occur; caution w/ a multiple immunosuppressant regimen. Increased risk of developing bacterial, viral, fungal, protozoal, and opportunistic infections (eg, polyomavirus infections). JC virus-associated progressive multifocal leukoencephalopathy and polyomavirus-/BK virus-associated nephropathy reported; consider reduction in immunosuppression if either develops. Convulsions, encephalopathy including posterior reversible encephalopathy syndrome, and rarely, optic disc edema reported. Evaluate before and during treatment for development of malignancies. In RA patients, monitor BP on at least 2 occasions and obtain 2 baseline SrCr levels before treatment, then monitor BP and SrCr every 2 weeks for the first 3 months of therapy, and then monthly if the patient is stable or more frequently during dose adjustments. In psoriasis patients, assess BP on at least 2 occasions and obtain baseline SrCr, BUN, CBC, Mg^{2+}, K^+, uric acid, and lipids before treatment, then monitor every 2 weeks for the first 3 months of therapy, and then monthly if the patient is stable or more frequently during dose adjustments. Monitor CBC and LFTs monthly w/ MTX. Monitor SrCr and BP after initiation or increases in NSAID dose for RA. Consider the alcohol content of the drug when given to patients in whom alcohol intake should be avoided or minimized (eg, pregnant or breastfeeding women, patients presenting w/ liver disease or epilepsy, alcoholic patients, or pediatric patients). HTN may occur and persist, and may require antihypertensive therapy.

ADVERSE REACTIONS

Increased susceptibility to infection, neoplasia, renal dysfunction, HTN, hirsutism/hypertrichosis, tremor, headache, gum hyperplasia, diarrhea, N/V, paresthesia, hypertriglyceridemia, hyperesthesia.

DRUG INTERACTIONS

See Boxed Warning, Dose Modification, and Contraindications. Avoid w/ K^+-sparing diuretics, aliskiren, orlistat, bosentan, or dabigatran. Vaccinations may be less effective; avoid live vaccines during therapy. Frequent gingival hyperplasia reported w/ nifedipine; avoid concomitant use w/ nifedipine in patients in whom gingival hyperplasia develops as a side effect of cyclosporine. Caution w/ rifabutin, nephrotoxic drugs, HIV protease inhibitors (eg, indinavir, nelfinavir, ritonavir, saquinavir), K^+-sparing drugs (eg, ACE inhibitors, ARBs), K^+-containing drugs, and K^+-rich diet. Ciprofloxacin, gentamicin, tobramycin, vancomycin, trimethoprim w/ sulfamethoxazole, melphalan, amphotericin B, ketoconazole, azapropazon, colchicine, diclofenac, naproxen, sulindac, cimetidine, ranitidine, tacrolimus, fibric acid derivatives (eg, bezafibrate, fenofibrate), MTX, and NSAIDs may potentiate renal dysfunction; closely monitor renal function and reduce dose of coadministered drug or consider alternative treatment if significant renal impairment occurs. Diltiazem, nicardipine, verapamil, fluconazole, itraconazole, ketoconazole, voriconazole, azithromycin, clarithromycin, erythromycin, quinupristin/dalfopristin, methylprednisolone, allopurinol, amiodarone, bromocriptine, colchicine, danazol, imatinib, metoclopramide, nefazodone, oral contraceptives, grapefruit, grapefruit juice, HIV protease inhibitors, boceprevir, and telaprevir may increase levels. Nafcillin, rifampin, carbamazepine, oxcarbazepine, phenobarbital, phenytoin, bosentan, octreotide, orlistat, sulfinpyrazone, terbinafine, ticlopidine, and St. John's wort may decrease levels. May increase levels of bosentan, dabigatran, and CYP3A4, P-gp, or organic anion transporter protein substrates. May increase levels of ambrisentan; do not titrate ambrisentan dose to the recommended max daily dose. CYP3A4 and/or P-gp inducers and inhibitors may alter levels; may require dose adjustments of cyclosporine if cyclosporine concentrations are significantly altered. May reduce clearance of digoxin, colchicine, prednisolone, HMG-CoA reductase inhibitors (statins), aliskiren, bosentan, dabigatran, repaglinide, NSAIDs, sirolimus, and etoposide. Digitalis toxicity reported when used w/ digoxin; monitor digoxin levels. May increase levels and enhance toxic effects (eg, myopathy, neuropathy) of colchicine; may reduce colchicine dose. Myotoxicity cases seen w/ lovastatin, simvastatin, atorvastatin, pravastatin, and, rarely fluvastatin; temporarily withhold or d/c statin therapy if signs of myopathy develop or w/ risk factors predisposing to severe renal injury, including renal failure, secondary to rhabdomyolysis. May increase levels of repaglinide, thereby increasing the risk of hypoglycemia; closely monitor blood glucose levels. High doses of cyclosporine may increase the exposure to anthracycline antibiotics (eg, doxorubicin, mitoxantrone, daunorubicin) in cancer patients. May double diclofenac blood levels; dose of diclofenac should be in the lower end of the therapeutic range. May increase MTX levels and decrease levels of active metabolite of MTX. May elevate SrCr and increase levels of sirolimus; give 4 hrs after cyclosporine administration. Convulsions reported w/ high-dose methylprednisolone. Calcium antagonists may interfere w/ cyclosporine metabolism.

NURSING CONSIDERATIONS

Assessment: Assess for hypersensitivity to the drug, renal dysfunction, uncontrolled HTN, presence of malignancies, pregnancy/nursing status, and possible drug interactions. RA: Assess BP (on at least 2 occasions) and obtain 2 SrCr levels. Psoriasis: Perform dermatological and physical examination, including measuring BP. Assess for presence of occult infections and for the presence of tumors. Assess for atypical skin lesions and biopsy them. Obtain baseline SrCr (at least twice), BUN, LFTs, bilirubin, CBC, Mg^{2+}, K^+, uric acid, and lipid levels.

Monitoring: Monitor for signs/symptoms of hepatotoxicity, liver injury, nephrotoxicity, thrombocytopenia, microangiopathic hemolytic anemia, HTN, hyperkalemia, lymphomas and other malignancies, serious/polyoma virus infections, convulsions and other neurotoxicities, and other adverse reactions. Monitor cyclosporine blood concentrations routinely in transplant patients and periodically in RA patients. RA: Monitor BP and SrCr every 2 weeks during the initial 3 months of treatment, then monthly if patient is stable. Monitor SrCr and BP after an increase of the dose of NSAIDs and after initiation of new NSAID therapy. If coadministered w/ MTX, monitor CBC and LFTs monthly. Psoriasis: Monitor for occult infections and tumors. Monitor SrCr, BUN, BP, CBC, uric acid, K^+, lipids, and Mg^{2+} levels every 2 weeks during first 3 months of treatment, then monthly if stable.

Patient Counseling: Instruct to contact physician before changing formulations of cyclosporine, which may require dose changes. Inform that repeated lab tests are required while on therapy. Advise of the potential risks if used during pregnancy and inform of the increased risk of neoplasia, HTN, and renal dysfunction. Inform that vaccinations may be less effective and to avoid live vaccines during therapy. Advise to take the medication on a consistent schedule w/ regard to time and meals, and to avoid grapefruit and grapefruit juice. Inform to avoid excessive sun exposure.

Storage: 20-25°C (68-77°F). (Sol) Use w/in 2 months upon opening. Do not refrigerate. At <20°C (68°F) may form gel; light flocculation, or formation of light sediment may occur; allow to warm to 25°C (77°F) to reverse changes.

NESINA – alogliptin RX

Class: Dipeptidyl peptidase-4 (DPP-4) inhibitor

ADULT DOSAGE

Type 2 Diabetes Mellitus

Usual: 25mg qd

PEDIATRIC DOSAGE

Pediatric use may not have been established

DOSE MODIFICATION

Renal Impairment

Moderate (CrCl 30-<60mL/min): 12.5mg qd

Severe (CrCl 15-<30mL/min): 6.25mg qd

ESRD (CrCl <15mL/min or requiring hemodialysis): 6.25mg qd

ADMINISTRATION

Oral route

May be taken w/ or w/o food

May be administered w/o regard to timing of hemodialysis

HOW SUPPLIED

Tab: 6.25mg, 12.5mg, 25mg

WARNINGS/PRECAUTIONS

Not for use in type 1 DM or for treatment of diabetic ketoacidosis. Acute pancreatitis reported; d/c if pancreatitis is suspected and initiate appropriate management. Serious hypersensitivity reactions reported; d/c if suspected, assess for other potential causes, and institute alternative treatment. Caution with history of angioedema with another DPP-4 inhibitor. Fatal/nonfatal hepatic failure and serum ALT >3X ULN reported; initiate with caution in patients with abnormal LFTs. Interrupt treatment and investigate probable cause if clinically significant liver enzyme elevations and abnormal LFTs persist/worsen; do not restart without another explanation for abnormal LFTs. No conclusive evidence of macrovascular risk reduction.

ADVERSE REACTIONS

Hypoglycemia, nasopharyngitis, headache, URI.

DRUG INTERACTIONS

May require lower dose of insulin therapy or insulin secretagogue (eg, sulfonylurea) to reduce risk of hypoglycemia.

NURSING CONSIDERATIONS

Assessment: Assess renal/hepatic function, previous hypersensitivity to the drug, history of pancreatitis, type of DM, diabetic ketoacidosis, history of angioedema with another DPP-4 inhibitor, pregnancy/nursing status, and possible drug interactions. Obtain baseline FPG and HbA1c.

Monitoring: Monitor for pancreatitis and hypersensitivity reactions. Monitor FPG, HbA1c, renal/hepatic function periodically.

Patient Counseling: Inform of risks/benefits of therapy. Inform of signs/symptoms of pancreatitis; instruct to d/c promptly and contact physician if persistent severe abdominal pain occurs. Inform that allergic reactions and liver injury have been reported; instruct to d/c and seek medical advice promptly if these occur. Inform that hypoglycemia can occur, particularly when therapy is used in combination with insulin or sulfonylurea; explain risks/symptoms/appropriate management of hypoglycemia. Instruct to take only ud; if a dose is missed, advise not to double next dose. Instruct to inform physician if unusual symptom develops or if a symptom persists/worsens.

Storage: 25°C (77°C); excursions permitted to 15-30°C (59-86°F).

NEULASTA – pegfilgrastim RX

Class: Granulocyte colony-stimulating factor

ADULT DOSAGE

Chemotherapy-Associated Neutropenia

To decrease the incidence of infection in patients w/ nonmyeloid malignancies receiving myelosuppressive anticancer drugs associated w/ febrile neutropenia

Usual: 6mg SQ once per chemotherapy cycle; do not administer between 14 days before and 24 hrs after administration of cytotoxic chemotherapy

PEDIATRIC DOSAGE

Pediatric use may not have been established

ADMINISTRATION

SQ route

Administer via a single prefilled syringe for manual use or w/ the On-body Injector

Instructions for On-body Injector

For Physicians:

Fill the On-body Injector w/ pegfilgrastim using prefilled syringe and apply to patient's skin (abdomen or back of arm)

Use back of the arm only if a caregiver is available to monitor the status of the On-body Injector

Approx 27 hrs after the application, pegfilgrastim will be delivered over approx 45 min

May initiate administration on the same day as the administration of cytotoxic chemotherapy, as long as On-body Injector delivers pegfilgrastim no <24 hrs after administration of cytotoxic chemotherapy

Do not use On-body Injector to deliver any other drug product except pegfilgrastim prefilled syringe co-packaged w/ On-body Injector

Apply to intact, nonirritated skin on the arm or abdomen

Missed dose may occur due to an On-body Injector failure/leakage; if a dose is missed, administer new dose by single prefilled syringe for manual use, as soon as possible after detection

Refer to Healthcare Provider Instructions for Use for the On-body Injector for Neulasta for full administration information

For Patients:

Avoid activities (eg, traveling, driving, operating heavy machinery) during 26-29 hrs following application of On-body Injector (this includes the 45-min delivery period plus 1 hr post-delivery)

Patients should have a caregiver nearby for the 1st use

Refer to the dose delivery information written on the Patient Instructions for Use

Provide training to ensure patients understand when the dose delivery of pegfilgrastim will begin and how to monitor the On-body Injector for completed delivery

Ensure patients understand how to identify signs of malfunction of On-body Injector

HOW SUPPLIED

Inj: 6mg/0.6mL [prefilled syringe for manual use, Delivery Kit]

WARNINGS/PRECAUTIONS

Splenic rupture, including fatal cases, may occur; evaluate for an enlarged spleen or splenic rupture if left upper abdominal or shoulder pain occurs. Acute respiratory distress syndrome (ARDS) may occur; evaluate for ARDS if fever and lung infiltrates or respiratory distress develops, and d/c if ARDS develops. Serious allergic reactions (eg, anaphylaxis) may occur; permanently d/c if a serious allergic reaction occurs. Use of On-body Injector may result in a significant reaction in patients who have reactions to acrylic adhesives. Severe and sometimes fatal sickle cell crises may occur in patients w/ sickle cell disorders. May act as a growth factor for any tumor type. Needle cap on prefilled syringe contains latex; do not administer to persons w/ latex allergies. Increased hematopoietic activity of the bone marrow in response to therapy may result in transiently positive bone imaging changes; consider this when interpreting bone-imaging results.

ADVERSE REACTIONS

Bone pain, pain in extremity.

NURSING CONSIDERATIONS

Assessment: Assess for history of hypersensitivity to pegfilgrastim or filgrastim, acrylic/latex allergy, sickle cell disorders, pregnancy/nursing status, and possible drug interactions.

Monitoring: Monitor for enlarged spleen/splenic rupture, ARDS, serious allergic reactions, sickle cell crises (in patients w/ sickle cell disorders), and other adverse reactions.

Patient Counseling: Advise of the risks of therapy (eg, splenic rupture, ARDS, serious allergic reactions, sickle cell crisis). Instruct to immediately contact physician if left upper quadrant or shoulder pain, SOB, signs/symptoms of sickle cell crisis or infection, flushing, dizziness, or rash develops. Advise on the use of the On-body Injector. Encourage women who become pregnant during treatment to enroll in Amgen's Pregnancy Surveillance Program.

Storage: 2-8°C (36-46°F). Prefilled Syringe for Manual Use: Protect from light. Do not shake. Discard syringes stored at room temperature for >48 hrs. Avoid freezing; if frozen, thaw in the refrigerator before administration. Discard syringe if frozen more than once. Delivery Kit: Do not hold Kit at room temperature >12 hrs prior to use; discard if stored at room temperature for >12 hrs.

NEUPOGEN – filgrastim RX

Class: Granulocyte colony-stimulating factor

ADULT DOSAGE

Chemotherapy-Associated Neutropenia

To decrease incidence of infection, as manifested by febrile neutropenia, in patients w/ nonmyeloid malignancies receiving myelosuppressive anticancer drugs associated w/ a significant incidence of severe neutropenia w/ fever; to reduce the time to neutrophil recovery and duration of fever, following induction or consolidation chemotherapy treatment of adults w/ acute myeloid leukemia

Receiving Myelosuppressive Chemotherapy or Induction and/or Consolidation Chemotherapy for Acute Myeloid Leukemia:
Initial: 5mcg/kg/day qd
Titrate: May increase in increments of 5mcg/kg for each chemotherapy cycle, according to duration and severity of ANC nadir
D/C if ANC surpasses 10,000/mm^3 after the expected chemotherapy-induced neutrophil nadir

To reduce the duration of neutropenia and neutropenia-related clinical sequelae in patients w/ nonmyeloid malignancies undergoing myeloablative chemotherapy followed by marrow transplantation

Receiving Bone Marrow Transplant:
10mcg/kg/day by IV infusion no longer than 24 hrs
Titrate:
When ANC >1000/mm^3 for 3 Consecutive Days: Reduce to 5mcg/kg/day then,
If ANC Remains >1000/mm^3 for 3 More Consecutive Days: D/C therapy then,
If ANC Decreases to <1000/mm^3: Resume at 5mcg/kg/day
If ANC decreases to <1000/mm^3 at any time during the 5mcg/kg/day administration, increase to 10mcg/kg/day, and retitrate following the above schedule

Hematopoietic Progenitor Cell Mobilization

For mobilization of hematopoietic progenitor cells into the peripheral blood for collection by leukapheresis
Usual: 10mcg/kg/day SQ for ≥4 days before the 1st leukapheresis procedure and continued until the last leukapheresis

Monitor neutrophil counts after 4 days of therapy, and d/c if WBC count >100,000/mm^3 develops

Administration of therapy for 6-7 days w/ leukapheresis on Days 5, 6, and 7 was found to be safe and effective

PEDIATRIC DOSAGE

Pediatric use may not have been established

Severe Chronic Neutropenia
Initial:
Congenital: 6mcg/kg SQ bid
Idiopathic/Cyclic: 5mcg/kg SQ qd
Titrate: Adjust dose based on clinical course and ANC

ADMINISTRATION
SQ/IV route
Avoid administration of prefilled syringe in people w/ latex allergies; needle cap contains dry natural rubber
Prior to use, remove the vial or prefilled syringe from the refrigerator and allow therapy to reach room temperature for a minimum of 30 min and a max of 24 hrs

SQ Administration
Inject in the outer area of upper arms, abdomen, thighs, or upper outer areas of buttocks

Chemotherapy-Associated Neutropenia
Cancer Patients Receiving Myelosuppressive Chemotherapy:
May administer by SQ bolus inj, by short IV infusion (15-30 min), or by continuous SQ/IV infusion
Do not administer w/in 24 hrs before or after cytotoxic chemotherapy
Administer daily for up to 2 weeks, until ANC has reached 10,000/mm^3 following the expected chemotherapy-induced neutrophil nadir
Cancer Patients Receiving Bone Marrow Transplant:
Administer 1st dose at least 24 hrs after cytotoxic chemotherapy and at least 24 hrs after bone marrow infusion

Dilution
May dilute in D5
Protect diluted concentrations between 5-15mcg/mL from adsorption to plastic materials by the addition of albumin (human) to a final concentration of 2mg/mL
When diluted in D5 or D5 plus albumin (human), compatible w/ glass bottles, PVC and polyolefin IV bags, and polypropylene syringes
Do not dilute to a final concentration <5mcg/mL
Do not dilute w/ saline; product may precipitate

HOW SUPPLIED
Inj: 300mcg/mL, 480mcg/1.6mL [vial]; 300mcg/0.5mL, 480mcg/0.8mL [prefilled syringe]

WARNINGS/PRECAUTIONS
Splenic rupture, including fatal cases, reported. Acute respiratory distress syndrome (ARDS) reported; d/c in patients w/ ARDS. Serious allergic-type reactions, including anaphylaxis, reported; permanently d/c in patients w/ serious allergic reactions. Sickle cell crisis, in some cases fatal, reported in patients w/ sickle cell trait/disease. Not approved for peripheral blood progenitor cell collection mobilization in healthy donors. Capillary leak syndrome (CLS) reported. Myelodysplastic syndrome (MDS) and AML reported to occur in the natural history of congenital neutropenia w/o cytokine therapy. Cytogenetic abnormalities, transformation to MDS, and AML observed in patients treated for severe chronic neutropenia (SCN); carefully consider the risks and benefits of continuing therapy if a patient w/ SCN develops abnormal cytogenetics or myelodysplasia. Thrombocytopenia and leukocytosis reported. Cutaneous vasculitis reported; hold therapy w/ cutaneous vasculitis and may start therapy at a reduced dose when the symptoms resolve and the ANC has decreased. May act as a growth factor for any tumor type. Consider transient positive bone-imaging changes when interpreting bone-imaging results.

ADVERSE REACTIONS
Nausea, pyrexia, thrombocytopenia, bone/back/chest pain, dizziness, pain, fatigue, dyspnea, headache, cough, rash, pain in extremity, arthralgia, increased blood lactate dehydrogenase, increased blood alkaline phosphatase.

DRUG INTERACTIONS
Avoid simultaneous use w/ chemotherapy and radiation therapy.

NURSING CONSIDERATIONS

Assessment: Assess for hypersensitivity to the drug, latex allergy, ARDS, sickle cell disorder, pregnancy/nursing status, and possible drug interactions. Obtain baseline CBC and platelet count in patients receiving myelosuppressive chemotherapy/induction, and/or consolidation chemotherapy for AML.

Monitoring: Monitor for serious allergic-type reactions, splenic rupture, ARDS, sickle cell crisis, CLS, MDS, AML, cytogenetic abnormalities, transformation to MDS, cutaneous vasculitis, thrombocytopenia, leukocytosis, and other adverse reactions. In patients receiving myelosuppressive chemotherapy/induction, and/or consolidation chemotherapy for AML, monitor CBC and platelet count twice weekly. In patients w/ SCN, monitor CBC w/ differential and platelet counts during the initial 4 weeks of therapy and during the 2 weeks following any dose adjustment, and, once patient is clinically stable, monthly during the 1st yr of treatment; thereafter, if clinically stable, less frequent routine monitoring is recommended. Frequently monitor CBCs and platelet counts following marrow transplantation.

Patient Counseling: Inform that rupture or enlargement of the spleen may occur; advise to immediately report to physician if symptoms develop. Advise to seek immediate medical attention if signs/symptoms of hypersensitivity reaction occur. Advise to immediately report to physician if dyspnea develops. Discuss potential risks and benefits for patients w/ sickle cell disease prior to administration. Advise to immediately report to physician signs/symptoms of vasculitis. Advise female of reproductive potential that therapy should be used during pregnancy only if the potential benefit justifies the potential risk to the fetus.

Storage: 2-8°C (36-46°F). Protect from light. Avoid freezing; if frozen, thaw in the refrigerator before administration. Discard if frozen more than once. Avoid shaking. Diluted Sol: May store at room temperature for up to 24 hrs; the 24 hr time period includes the time during room temperature storage of the infusion sol and the duration of the infusion.

NEUPRO — rotigotine

RX

Class: Non-ergoline dopamine agonist

ADULT DOSAGE

Parkinson's Disease

Early-Stage Parkinson's Disease (PD):
Initial: 2mg/24 hrs
Titrate: May increase weekly by 2mg/24 hrs based on response and tolerability, and if additional therapeutic effect is needed
Lowest Effective Dose: 4mg/24 hrs
Max: 6mg/24 hrs

Advanced-Stage PD:
Initial: 4mg/24 hrs
Titrate: May increase weekly by 2mg/24 hrs based on response and tolerability, and if additional therapeutic effect is needed
Max: 8mg/24 hrs

Discontinuation of Therapy:
Reduce daily dose by a max of 2mg/24 hrs preferably qod, until complete withdrawal is achieved

Restless Legs Syndrome

Moderate to Severe Primary Restless Leg Syndrome:
Initial: 1mg/24 hrs
Titrate: May increase weekly by 1mg/24 hrs based on response and tolerability, and if additional therapeutic effect is needed
Lowest Effective Dose: 1mg/24 hrs
Max: 3mg/24 hrs

Discontinuation of Therapy:
Reduce daily dose by 1mg/24 hrs preferably qod, until complete withdrawal is achieved

PEDIATRIC DOSAGE

Pediatric use may not have been established

ADMINISTRATION

Transdermal route

Apply 1 patch qd at approx the same time every day
Apply to clean, dry, intact healthy skin on the front of the abdomen, thigh, hip, flank, shoulder, or upper arm
Do not apply on oily, irritated, or damaged skin or where it will be rubbed by tight clothing
Rotate application site qd
Do not apply to same application site more than once every 14 days
Apply immediately upon removal from the pouch; press firmly in place for 30 sec
If applying to hairy area is necessary, shave area ≥3 days prior to application
Apply another patch if patient forgets to replace patch or if patch becomes dislodged

HOW SUPPLIED

Patch, Extended-Release: 1mg/24 hrs, 2mg/24 hrs, 3mg/24 hrs, 4mg/24 hrs, 6mg/24 hrs, 8mg/24 hrs [30[s]]

WARNINGS/PRECAUTIONS
Contains sodium metabisulfite that may cause allergic-type reactions, including anaphylactic symptoms and life-threatening or less severe asthmatic episodes in certain susceptible people. Falling asleep during activities of daily living and somnolence reported. Should ordinarily d/c if daytime sleepiness or episodes of falling asleep during activities that require active participation occur. May impair mental/physical abilities. Hallucinations and new/worsening mental status and behavioral changes reported; avoid w/ major psychotic disorder. May cause postural/orthostatic hypotension; monitor for signs/symptoms, especially during dose escalation. Syncope reported; patients w/ severe cardiovascular disease (CVD) should be monitored for symptoms of syncope and presyncope. May cause intense urges (eg, to gamble, have sex, to spend money, binge eating); consider dose reduction or discontinuation. BP and HR elevations reported. Weight gain and fluid retention reported; monitor patients w/ concomitant illnesses (eg, CHF, renal insufficiency). May cause or exacerbate preexisting dyskinesia. Application-site reactions reported; d/c if a generalized skin reaction is observed. Monitor for melanomas frequently and on a regular basis. Augmentation and rebound in RLS reported. Backing layer of patch contains aluminum; remove patch prior to MRI or cardioversion. Avoid exposing application site to external sources of direct heat. Symptom complex resembling neuroleptic malignant syndrome reported w/ rapid dose reduction, withdrawal of, or changes in antiparkinsonian therapy. Cases of retroperitoneal fibrosis, pulmonary infiltrates, pleural effusion, pleural thickening, pericarditis, and cardiac valvulopathy reported in some patients treated w/ ergot-derived dopaminergic agents.

ADVERSE REACTIONS
N/V, dizziness, somnolence, application-site reactions, hyperhidrosis, anorexia, headache, disturbances in initiating and maintaining sleep, visual disturbance, peripheral edema, dyskinesia, low Hgb/Hct, elevated serum BUN/CPK, low serum glucose.

DRUG INTERACTIONS
Sedating medications may increase risk of drowsiness. Dopamine antagonists (eg, antipsychotics, metoclopramide) may diminish effectiveness. May potentiate dopaminergic side effects of levodopa.

NURSING CONSIDERATIONS

Assessment: Assess for major psychotic disorder, sleep disorders, dyskinesia, CVD, CHF, renal insufficiency, hypersensitivity to drug or sulfites, pregnancy/nursing status, and possible drug interactions.

Monitoring: Monitor for drowsiness or sleepiness, hallucinations, new/worsening mental status and behavioral changes, symptomatic hypotension, syncope, impulse control/compulsive behaviors, BP and HR elevations, dyskinesia, application-site/generalized skin reactions, melanomas (frequently and regularly), and other adverse reactions.

Patient Counseling: Advise about potential for sulfite sensitivity. Advise and alert about potential for sedating effects, including somnolence and possibility of falling asleep while engaged in activities of daily living; instruct not to drive a car or engage in potentially dangerous activities until effects have been determined. Advise to inform physician if taking alcohol, sedating medications, or other CNS depressants. Inform that hallucinations and other psychosis symptoms, symptomatic hypotension, syncope, BP and HR elevations, weight gain, fluid retention, dyskinesia, N/V, and general GI distress may occur. Instruct to notify physician if experiencing new/increased gambling urges, increased sexual urges, or other intense urges. Instruct not to apply patch to the same site more than once every 14 days and to report persistent application-site reaction (of more than a few days), increases in severity, or skin reactions that spread outside the application site. Advise to monitor for melanomas frequently and regularly. Inform that drug may cause RLS symptoms to have an earlier onset during the day or become worse. Instruct to avoid applying heating pads or other sources of heat to the area of the patch and to avoid direct sun exposure of the patch. Advise to d/c use only under the supervision of a physician to reduce risk for hyperpyrexia and confusion associated w/ sudden discontinuation or dose reduction.

Storage: 20-25°C (68-77°F); excursions permitted between 15-30°C (59-86°F).

NEURONTIN – gabapentin RX

Class: GABA analogue

ADULT DOSAGE

Postherpetic Neuralgia

Initial: 300mg single dose on Day 1, then 300mg bid (600mg/day) on Day 2, and 300mg tid (900mg/day) on Day 3
Titrate: May subsequently increase prn up to 600mg tid (1800mg/day)

PEDIATRIC DOSAGE

Partial Seizures

Adjuvant Therapy for Partial Onset Seizures w/ Epilepsy, w/ and w/o Secondary Generalization:

3-11 Years:
Initial: 10-15mg/kg/day in 3 divided doses
Titrate: Increase to effective dose over a period of 3 days

Partial Seizures

Adjuvant Therapy for Partial Onset Seizures w/ Epilepsy, w/ and w/o Secondary Generalization:

Initial: 300mg tid
Usual: 300-600mg tid
Doses up to 2400mg/day (long-term) and 3600mg/day (short-term) have been well tolerated
Administer tid using 300mg or 400mg caps, or 600mg or 800mg tabs
Dosing intervals should not exceed 12 hrs

3-4 Years:
Usual: 40mg/kg/day in 3 divided doses
5-11 Years:
Usual: 25-35mg/kg/day in 3 divided doses
Doses up to 50mg/kg/day have been well tolerated
Dosing intervals should not exceed 12 hrs
≥12 Years:
Initial: 300mg tid
Usual: 300-600mg tid
Doses up to 2400mg/day (long-term) and 3600mg/day (short-term) have been well tolerated
Administer tid using 300mg or 400mg caps, or 600mg or 800mg tabs
Dosing intervals should not exceed 12 hrs

DOSE MODIFICATION
Renal Impairment
≥12 Years:
CrCl ≥60mL/min: 900-3600mg/day in 3 divided doses
CrCl >30-59mL/min: 400-1400mg/day in 2 divided doses
CrCl >15-29mL/min: 200-700mg single daily dose
CrCl 15mL/min: 100-300mg single daily dose
CrCl <15mL/min: Reduce daily dose in proportion to CrCl
Hemodialysis: Dose adjustment is necessary; see PI
Discontinuation
Dose Reduction/Substitution/Discontinuation: Should be done gradually over a minimum of 1 week

ADMINISTRATION
Oral route

Take w/ or w/o food
Swallow caps whole with plenty of water

HOW SUPPLIED
Cap: 100mg, 300mg, 400mg; Sol: 250mg/5mL [470mL]; Tab: 600mg*, 800mg* *scored

WARNINGS/PRECAUTIONS
Drug reaction with eosinophilia and systemic symptoms (DRESS)/multiorgan hypersensitivity reported; evaluate immediately if signs/symptoms (eg, fever, lymphadenopathy) are present and d/c if an alternative etiology cannot be established. May cause significant driving impairment. Somnolence/sedation and dizziness reported, which could increase the occurrence of accidental injury (fall). Do not abruptly d/c; may increase seizure frequency. Confusion, loss of consciousness, and mental impairment reported. Increases the risk of suicidal thoughts/behavior. Use in pediatric patients with epilepsy 3-12 yrs of age is associated with the occurrence of CNS-related adverse events. May have tumorigenic potential. Sudden and unexplained deaths reported in patients with epilepsy. Lab test interactions may occur. Caution in elderly.

ADVERSE REACTIONS
Dizziness, somnolence, fatigue, peripheral edema, hostility, diarrhea, asthenia, infection, dry mouth, nystagmus, constipation, N/V, ataxia, fever, amblyopia.

DRUG INTERACTIONS
Decreases levels of hydrocodone in a dose-dependent manner. Increased exposure with hydrocodone or controlled-release morphine cap. Decreased bioavailability with Maalox; take gabapentin at least 2 hrs following Maalox administration. Opioids may increase levels; carefully observe for signs of CNS depression (eg, somnolence, sedation, respiratory depression) and reduce gabapentin or opioid dose appropriately.

NURSING CONSIDERATIONS

Assessment: Assess for hypersensitivity to the drug, renal impairment, depression, history of drug abuse, pregnancy/nursing status, and possible drug interactions.

Monitoring: Monitor for DRESS, somnolence/sedation, dizziness, emergence/worsening of depression, suicidal thoughts/behavior, accidental injury (fall), confusion, loss of consciousness, mental impairment, unusual changes in mood/behavior, development/worsening of tumors, increased seizure frequency (upon abrupt discontinuation), signs/symptoms of misuse/abuse, and other adverse reactions.

Patient Counseling: Instruct to take drug only as prescribed. Instruct to immediately report to physician any rash or other signs/symptoms of hypersensitivity, emergence/worsening of depression symptoms, any unusual changes in mood/behavior, emergence of suicidal thoughts/behavior, or thoughts of self-harm. Inform that therapy may cause a significant driving impairment, dizziness, somnolence, and other signs/symptoms of CNS depression; advise not to drive a car or operate other complex machinery until patient has gained sufficient experience on therapy. Instruct to notify physician if pregnant/breastfeeding or intending to become pregnant or to breastfeed during therapy; encourage enrollment in the North American Antiepileptic Drug Pregnancy Registry if patient becomes pregnant.

Storage: (Cap/Tab) 25°C (77°F); excursions permitted to 15-30°C (59-86°F). (Sol) 2-8°C (36-46°F).

NEVANAC – nepafenac RX

Class: NSAID

ADULT DOSAGE

Cataract Surgery

Pain and Inflammation:
Instill 1 drop to affected eye tid beginning 1 day prior to cataract surgery
Continue on day of surgery and throughout first 2 weeks of postoperative period

PEDIATRIC DOSAGE

Cataract Surgery

Pain and Inflammation:
≥10 Years:
Instill 1 drop to affected eye tid beginning 1 day prior to cataract surgery
Continue on day of surgery and throughout first 2 weeks of postoperative period

ADMINISTRATION

Intraocular route

Administer 5 min apart if using >1 topical medication

HOW SUPPLIED

Sus: 0.1% [3mL]

WARNINGS/PRECAUTIONS

Potential for increased bleeding time due to interference with thrombocyte aggregation. Increased bleeding of ocular tissue (eg, hyphemas); caution with known bleeding tendencies that may prolong bleeding time. May slow or delay healing, or result in keratitis. Continued use may be sight threatening due to epithelial breakdown, corneal thinning, erosion, ulceration, or perforation; d/c if corneal epithelial breakdown occurs. Caution with complicated ocular surgeries, corneal denervation, corneal epithelial defects, diabetes mellitus (DM), ocular surface diseases (eg, dry eye syndrome), rheumatoid arthritis (RA), or repeat ocular surgeries within a short period. Increased risk for occurrence and severity of corneal adverse events if used >1 day prior to surgery or use beyond 14 days postsurgery. Avoid use with contact lenses and during late pregnancy.

ADVERSE REACTIONS

Capsular opacity, decreased visual acuity, foreign body sensation, IOP, sticky sensation, conjunctival edema, corneal edema, dry eye, lid margin crusting, ocular discomfort, ocular hyperemia/pain/pruritus, photophobia, tearing.

DRUG INTERACTIONS

Increased potential for healing problems with topical steroids. Caution with agents that may prolong bleeding time.

NURSING CONSIDERATIONS

Assessment: Assess for drug hypersensitivity, bleeding tendencies, complicated or repeated ocular surgeries, corneal denervation, corneal epithelial defects, DM, ocular surface diseases, RA, if using contact lenses, pregnancy/nursing status, and possible drug interactions.

Monitoring: Monitor for hypersensitivity reactions, wound healing problems, keratitis, bleeding time, bleeding of ocular tissues in conjunction with ocular surgery, and evidence of epithelial corneal breakdown.

Patient Counseling: Inform of possibility that slow or delayed healing may occur. Advise on proper use to prevent bacterial contamination, and shake bottle well before use. Instruct if using >1 ophthalmic medication, separate by 5 min, and not use while wearing contact lenses. Instruct to immediately notify physician if intercurrent ocular condition (eg, trauma or infection) occurs or undergoing ocular surgery to assess continuation of therapy.

Storage: 2-25°C (36-77°F).

NEXAVAR – sorafenib

RX

Class: Kinase inhibitors

ADULT DOSAGE

Hepatocellular Carcinoma

Unresectable:

Usual: 400mg (two 200mg tabs) bid

Continue until patient is no longer clinically benefiting from therapy or until unacceptable toxicity occurs

Advanced Renal Cell Carcinoma

Usual: 400mg (two 200mg tabs) bid

Continue until patient is no longer clinically benefiting from therapy or until unacceptable toxicity occurs

Differentiated Thyroid Carcinoma

Locally recurrent or metastatic, progressive, differentiated thyroid carcinoma that is refractory to radioactive iodine treatment

Usual: 400mg (two 200mg tabs) bid

Continue until patient is no longer clinically benefiting from therapy or until unacceptable toxicity occurs

PEDIATRIC DOSAGE

Pediatric use may not have been established

DOSE MODIFICATION

Adverse Reactions

Dermatologic Toxicities:

Hepatocellular/Renal Cell Carcinoma:

Grade 1 (Numbness/Dysesthesia/Paresthesia/Tingling/Painless Swelling/Erythema/Discomfort of Hands or Feet Which Does Not Disrupt Normal Activities):

Any Occurrence: Continue treatment and consider topical therapy for symptomatic relief

Grade 2 (Painful Erythema and Swelling of Hands or Feet and/or Discomfort Affecting Normal Activities):

1st Occurrence: Continue treatment and consider topical therapy for symptomatic relief

No Improvement w/in 7 Days or 2nd/3rd Occurrence: Interrupt treatment until toxicity resolves to Grade 0-1; when resuming treatment, decrease dose by 1 dose level (400mg/day or 400mg qod)

4th Occurrence: D/C treatment

Grade 3 (Moist Desquamation/Ulceration/Blistering/Severe Pain of Hands or Feet, or Severe Discomfort That Causes Inability to Work or Perform Activities of Daily Living):

1st/2nd Occurrence: Interrupt treatment until toxicity resolves to Grade 0-1; when resuming treatment, decrease dose by 1 dose level (400mg/day or 400mg qod)

3rd Occurrence: D/C treatment

Differentiated Thyroid Carcinoma:

Grade 1:

Any Occurrence: Continue treatment

Grade 2:

1st Occurrence: Decrease dose to 600mg/day

No Improvement w/in 7 Days or 2nd/3rd Occurrence: Interrupt treatment until toxicity resolves or improves to Grade 1; if treatment is resumed, decrease dose as follows:

1st Dose Reduction: 600mg/day (400mg and 200mg 12 hrs apart)

2nd Dose Reduction: 400mg/day (200mg bid)

3rd Dose Reduction: 200mg qd

4th Occurrence: D/C treatment permanently

Grade 3:

1st Occurrence: Interrupt treatment until toxicity resolves or improves to Grade 1; if treatment is resumed, decrease dose to 600mg/day (400mg and 200mg 12 hrs apart)

2nd Occurrence: Interrupt treatment until toxicity resolves or improves to Grade 1; if treatment is resumed, decrease dose to 400mg/day (200mg bid)

3rd Occurrence: D/C treatment

Discontinuation

Temporary interruption or permanent discontinuation may be required for the following:

1. Cardiac ischemia or infarction
2. Hemorrhage requiring medical intervention
3. Severe or persistent hypertension despite adequate anti-hypertensive therapy
4. Gastrointestinal perforation
5. QTc prolongation
6. Severe drug-induced liver injury

Other Important Modifications

Patients Undergoing Major Surgical Procedures: Temporarily interrupt therapy

Dose Reductions:

Hepatocellular Carcinoma/Renal Cell Carcinoma:

Reduce to 400mg qd; if additional dose reduction is required, reduce to a single 400mg dose qod

Differentiated Thyroid Carcinoma:

1st Dose Reduction: 600mg/day (400mg and 200mg 12 hrs apart)

2nd Dose Reduction: 400mg/day(200mg bid)

3rd Dose Reduction: 200mg qd

ADMINISTRATION

Oral route

Take w/o food (at least 1 hr ac or 2 hrs pc)

HOW SUPPLIED

Tab: 200mg

CONTRAINDICATIONS

Concomitant use with carboplatin and paclitaxel in patients with squamous cell lung cancer.

WARNINGS/PRECAUTIONS

HTN, cardiac ischemia, and/or infarction reported; temporary or permanent discontinuation should be considered. Increased risk of bleeding may occur; consider permanent discontinuation if bleeding necessitates medical intervention. Hand-foot skin reaction and rash reported; may require topical treatment, temporary interruption, and/or dose modification, or permanent discontinuation in severe or persistent cases. Severe dermatologic toxicities, including Stevens-Johnson syndrome (SJS) and toxic epidermal necrolysis (TEN) reported; d/c if SJS or TEN are suspected. D/C if GI perforation occurs. Temporarily interrupt therapy when undergoing major surgical procedures. May prolong QT/QTc interval; avoid in patients with congenital long QT syndrome. Monitor electrolytes and ECG in patients with congestive heart failure (CHF), bradyarrhythmias, and in patients taking drugs known to prolong QT interval (eg, Class Ia and III antiarrhythmics). Correct electrolyte abnormalities (Mg^{2+}, K^+, Ca^{2+}). Interrupt treatment if QTc interval is >500 msec or for an increase from baseline ≥60 msec. Drug-induced hepatitis, and increased bilirubin and INR may occur; d/c in case of significantly increased transaminases without alternative explanation (eg, viral hepatitis or progressing underlying malignancy). May impair exogenous thyroid suppression; monitor TSH levels monthly and adjust thyroid replacement medication as needed in patients with DTC. May cause fetal harm.

ADVERSE REACTIONS

HTN, fatigue, weight loss, rash, hand-foot skin reaction, alopecia, pruritus, diarrhea, N/V, abdominal pain, anorexia, constipation, hemorrhage, infection, decreased appetite.

DRUG INTERACTIONS

See Contraindications. Avoid with gemcitabine/cisplatin in squamous cell lung cancer patients. Avoid with strong CYP3A4 inducers (eg, carbamazepine, dexamethasone, phenobarbital, phenytoin, rifampin, rifabutin, St. John's wort). Infrequent bleeding or increased INR with warfarin; monitor for changes in PT, INR, or bleeding episodes. Decreased exposure with oral neomycin.

NURSING CONSIDERATIONS

Assessment: Assess for bleeding disorders, upcoming major surgical procedures, CHF, bradyarrhythmias, electrolyte abnormalities, drug hypersensitivity, pregnancy/nursing status, and possible drug interactions.

Monitoring: Monitor BP weekly during the first 6 weeks and periodically thereafter. Monitor for cardiac ischemia/infarction, hemorrhage, HTN, dermatologic toxicities, GI perforation, QT/QTc prolongation, and other adverse reactions. Monitor electrolytes (eg, Mg^{2+}, Ca^{2+}, K^+) and ECG in patients with CHF, bradyarrhythmias, and in patients taking drugs known to prolong QT interval. Monitor LFTs regularly, and TSH levels monthly. Monitor patients taking concomitant warfarin for changes in PT, INR, or clinical bleeding episodes.

Patient Counseling: Counsel about possible side effects and to report any episodes of bleeding, chest pain, or other symptoms of cardiac ischemia. Inform that HTN may develop, especially during the first 6 weeks; and that BP should be monitored regularly during therapy. Inform of possible occurrence of hand-foot skin reaction and rash during therapy and appropriate countermeasures. Advise that GI perforation and drug-induced hepatitis may occur and to report signs/symptoms of hepatitis. Inform that temporary interruption is recommended in patients undergoing major surgical procedures. Counsel patients with history of prolonged QT interval that treatment can worsen the condition. Inform that the drug may cause birth defects or fetal loss during pregnancy; both males and females should use effective birth control during treatment and for at least 2 weeks after stopping therapy. Instruct to notify physician if patient becomes pregnant while on therapy. Advise against breastfeeding.

Storage: 25°C (77°F); excursions permitted to 15-30°C (59-86°F). Store in a dry place.

NEXIUM ORAL – esomeprazole magnesium — RX

Class: Proton pump inhibitor

ADULT DOSAGE

Gastroesophageal Reflux Disease

Healing of Erosive Esophagitis:
20mg or 40mg qd for 4-8 weeks; may consider an additional 4-8 weeks of treatment if not healed

Maint of Healing of Erosive Esophagitis:
20mg qd for up to 6 months

Symptomatic GERD:
20mg qd for 4 weeks; may consider an additional 4 weeks of treatment if symptoms do not resolve completely

NSAID-Associated Gastric Ulcer

Risk Reduction of NSAID-Associated Gastric Ulcer:
20mg or 40mg qd for up to 6 months

***Helicobacter pylori* Eradication**

Triple Therapy:
40mg qd + amoxicillin 1000mg bid + clarithromycin 500mg bid, all for 10 days

Pathological Hypersecretory Conditions

Eg, Zollinger-Ellison Syndrome
40mg bid; adjust dose to individual patient needs

Doses up to 240mg/day have been administered

PEDIATRIC DOSAGE

Gastroesophageal Reflux Disease

Symptomatic GERD
1-11 Years:
10mg qd for up to 8 weeks
Max: 1mg/kg/day
12-17 Years:
20mg qd for 4 weeks

Healing of Erosive Esophagitis:
1-11 Years:
<20kg: 10mg qd for 8 weeks
≥20kg: 10mg or 20mg qd for 8 weeks
Max: 1mg/kg/day
12-17 Years:
20mg or 40mg qd for 4-8 weeks

Erosive Esophagitis due to Acid-Mediated GERD:
1 Month-<1 Year:
3-5kg: 2.5mg qd for up to 6 weeks
>5-7.5kg: 5mg qd for up to 6 weeks
>7.5-12kg: 10mg qd for up to 6 weeks

DOSE MODIFICATION

Hepatic Impairment
Severe (Child-Pugh Class C):
Max Dose: 20mg/day

ADMINISTRATION

Oral route
Take at least 1 hr ac

Cap
Swallow whole, or alternatively, open cap and add granules on 1 tbsp of applesauce, then swallow immediately; do not chew or crush the granules

NG Tube:
1. Open and empty the intact granules into a 60mL catheter tipped syringe and mix w/ 50mL of water
2. Replace the plunger and shake the syringe vigorously for 15 sec
3. Attach the syringe to a NG tube and deliver the contents of the syringe into the stomach
4. Flush the NG tube w/ additional water after use

Sus
1. Empty the contents of a 2.5mg pkt into 5mL of water. For the 10mg, 20mg, and 40mg pkts, empty into 15mL of water
2. Stir and leave 2-3 min to thicken

3. Drink w/in 30 min. If any medicine remains after drinking, add more water, stir and drink immediately
4. In cases where 2 pkts need to be used, may mix in a similar way by adding twice the required amount of water or follow mixing instructions provided

NG/Gastric Tube:
1. Add 5mL of water to a catheter tipped syringe, then add contents of a 2.5mg or 5mg pkt. For 10mg, 20mg, and 40mg pkts, volume of water in the syringe should be 15mL
2. Immediately shake syringe and leave 2-3 min to thicken
3. Shake syringe and inject through NG or gastric tube, French size ≥6, into the stomach w/in 30 min
4. Refill the syringe w/ an equal amount of water (5mL or 15mL)
5. Shake and flush any remaining contents from NG or gastric tube into stomach

HOW SUPPLIED

Cap, Delayed-Release: 20mg, 40mg; Sus, Delayed-Release: 2.5mg, 5mg, 10mg, 20mg, 40mg (granules/pkt)

WARNINGS/PRECAUTIONS

Symptomatic response does not preclude the presence of gastric malignancy. Atrophic gastritis reported with long-term omeprazole use. Acute interstitial nephritis reported; d/c if this develops. Cyanocobalamin (vitamin B12) deficiency may occur due to malabsorption, with daily long-term treatment (eg, >3 yrs) with any acid-suppressing medications. May increase risk of *Clostridium difficile* (CDAD) associated diarrhea, especially in hospitalized patients. May increase risk for osteoporosis-related fractures of the hip, wrist, or spine, especially with high-dose and long-term therapy. Use lowest dose and shortest duration possible. Hypomagnesemia reported and may require Mg^{2+} replacement and discontinuation of therapy. Drug-induced decrease in gastric acidity results in enterochromaffin-like cell hyperplasia and increased chromogranin A (CgA) levels, which may interfere with investigations for neuroendocrine tumors; d/c treatment for at least 14 days before assessing CgA levels and consider repeating test if initial CgA levels are high.

ADVERSE REACTIONS

Headache, diarrhea, abdominal pain.

DRUG INTERACTIONS

CYP2C19 or CYP3A4 inducers may decrease levels; avoid with St. John's wort or rifampin. Reduces pharmacological activity of clopidogrel; avoid concomitant use. May reduce atazanavir and nelfinavir levels; concomitant use not recommended. May change absorption or levels of antiretrovirals. May increase levels of saquinavir, cilostazol, and tacrolimus; consider saquinavir and cilostazol dose reduction. May reduce the absorption of drugs where gastric pH is an important determinant of bioavailability; ketoconazole, atazanavir, iron salts, erlotinib and mycophenolate mofetil (MMF) absorption may decrease, while digoxin absorption may increase. Caution in transplant patients receiving MMF. Monitor for increases in INR and PT with warfarin. Decreases clearance of diazepam. Increased exposure with combined inhibitors of CYP2C19 and CYP3A4 (eg, voriconazole); consider dose adjustment w/ Zollinger-Ellison syndrome. Increased levels of esomeprazole and 14-hydroxyclarithromycin with amoxicillin and clarithromycin. Caution with digoxin or other drugs that may cause hypomagnesemia (eg, diuretics). May elevate and prolong levels of MTX and/or its metabolite, possibly leading to toxicities; consider temporary withdrawal of therapy with high-dose MTX.

NURSING CONSIDERATIONS

Assessment: Assess for hypersensitivity to substituted benzimidazoles or to any component of the formulation, hepatic dysfunction, risk for osteoporosis-related fractures, pregnancy/nursing status, and possible drug interactions. Obtain Mg^{2+} levels in patients expected to be on prolonged therapy.

Monitoring: Monitor for signs/symptoms of atrophic gastritis, acute interstitial nephritis, cyanocobalamin deficiency, bone fractures, hypomagnesemia, CDAD, and other adverse reactions.

Patient Counseling: Advise to notify physician if taking or beginning to take other medications. Inform that antacids may be used while on therapy. Instruct not to chew or crush cap; if opening cap to mix granules with food, mix with applesauce only. Inform about proper technique for administration of opened cap or oral sus. Counsel regarding the correct amount of water to use when mixing dose of oral sus. Advise to immediately report and seek care for diarrhea that does not improve and for any cardiovascular/neurological symptoms.

Storage: 25°C (77°F); excursions permitted to 15-30°C (59-86°F).

NIASPAN – niacin

Class: Nicotinic acid

RX

ADULT DOSAGE

Hyperlipidemia

For use in patients w/ primary hyperlipidemia and mixed dyslipidemia. In combination w/ simvastatin or lovastatin for treatment of primary hyperlipidemia and mixed dyslipidemia when treatment w/ niacin extended-release (ER), simvastatin, or lovastatin monotherapy is inadequate. To reduce the risk of recurrent nonfatal MI in patients w/ a history of MI and hyperlipidemia. To slow progression or promote regression of atherosclerotic disease in patients w/ a history of coronary artery disease and hyperlipidemia in combination w/ a bile acid binding resin. To reduce elevated total cholesterol and LDL levels in patients w/ primary hyperlipidemia in combination w/ a bile acid binding resin. Adjunctive therapy in patients w/ severe hypertriglyceridemia who present a risk of pancreatitis and who do not respond adequately to a determined dietary effort to control them

>16 Years:
Initial: 500mg qhs after a low-fat snack
Titrate: Increase by 500mg every 4 weeks; after Week 8, titrate to patient response and tolerance; increase to 1500mg qd if response to 1000mg qd is inadequate and may subsequently increase to 2000mg qd
Do not increase daily dose by >500mg in any 4-week period
Maint: 1000-2000mg qhs
Max: 2000mg/day

Women may respond at lower doses than men

If therapy is discontinued for an extended period, reinstitution should include a titration phase

In Combination w/ Simvastatin or Lovastatin for Primary Hyperlipidemia and Mixed Dyslipidemia:
Patients Receiving Stable Dose of Lovastatin or Simvastatin Who Require Further TG-Lowering or HDL-Raising:
May receive concomitant dosage titration w/ niacin ER per recommended initial titration schedule
Max: 2000mg/day niacin ER and 40mg/day of lovastatin or simvastatin
Patients Receiving Stable Dose of Niacin ER Who Require Further LDL-Lowering:
Initial: 20mg qd of lovastatin or simvastatin
Titrate: Dose adjustments should be made at intervals of ≥4 weeks
Max: 2000mg/day niacin ER and 40mg/day of lovastatin or simvastatin

PEDIATRIC DOSAGE

Pediatric use may not have been established

DOSE MODIFICATION

Renal Impairment

Use caution

ADMINISTRATION

Oral route

Take at hs after a low-fat snack
Swallow tab whole; do not break, crush, or chew

Avoid administration on an empty stomach and slowly increase niacin dose to reduce flushing, pruritus, and GI distress
May take aspirin (ASA) (up to 325mg) 30 min prior to treatment to reduce flushing
Do not interchange three 500mg tabs w/ two 750mg tabs
Equivalent doses of niacin ER should not be substituted for sustained-release (modified-release, timed-release) niacin preparations or immediate-release (IR) (crystalline) niacin

HOW SUPPLIED
Tab, Extended-Release: 500mg, 750mg, 1000mg

CONTRAINDICATIONS
Active liver disease or unexplained persistent elevations in hepatic transaminases, active peptic ulcer disease (PUD), arterial bleeding.

WARNINGS/PRECAUTIONS
At doses of 1500-2000mg/day, in combination with simvastatin, did not reduce the incidence of cardiovascular (CV) events more than simvastatin in patients with CV disease and mean baseline LDL-C levels of 74mg/dL. Do not substitute for equivalent doses of sustained-release (modified-release, timed-release) niacin or IR (crystalline) niacin; severe hepatic toxicity, including fulminant hepatic necrosis, may occur. If switching from IR niacin, initiate with low doses (500mg at hs) and titrate to desired therapeutic response. Caution in patients with unstable angina or in the acute phase of MI, particularly if also receiving vasoactive drugs (eg, nitrates, calcium channel blockers, adrenergic blocking agents). Caution in patients with renal impairment, or who consume substantial quantities of alcohol, and/or have history of liver disease. Closely observe patients with history of jaundice, hepatobiliary disease, or peptic ulcer. Associated with abnormal LFTs; monitor LFTs (eg, AST, ALT) before treatment, every 6-12 weeks for the 1st yr, and periodically thereafter (eg, 6-month intervals). If elevated serum transaminase levels develop, measurements should be repeated promptly and then performed more frequently. D/C if transaminase levels progress, particularly if they rise to 3X ULN and are persistent, or if associated with nausea, fever, and/or malaise. May increase FPG; closely monitor diabetic/potentially diabetic patients (particularly during 1st few months of therapy or dose adjustment), and adjust diet and/or hypoglycemic therapy if necessary. Associated with dose-related reductions in platelet count and phosphorus (P) levels; periodically monitor P levels in patients at risk for hypophosphatemia. Associated with increases in PT; carefully evaluate patients undergoing surgery. Elevated uric acid levels reported; caution in patients predisposed to gout. Lab test interactions may occur.

ADVERSE REACTIONS
Flushing (warmth, redness, itching, and/or tingling), diarrhea, N/V, increased cough, pruritus, rash.

DRUG INTERACTIONS
Avoid ingestion of alcohol, hot drinks, or spicy foods around the time of administration; may increase flushing and pruritus. Use caution when prescribing niacin (≥1g/day) with statins; may increase risk of myopathy and rhabdomyolysis. Separate dosing from bile acid-binding resins by at least 4-6 hrs. ASA may decrease the metabolic clearance of nicotinic acid. May potentiate the effects of ganglionic blocking agents and vasoactive drugs, resulting in postural hypotension. Vitamins or other nutritional supplements containing large doses of niacin or related compounds (eg, nicotinamide) may potentiate adverse effects. Use caution with anticoagulants; monitor platelet counts and PT.

NURSING CONSIDERATIONS

Assessment: Assess for history of/active liver disease or PUD, unexplained persistent hepatic transaminase elevations, arterial bleeding, history of jaundice or hepatobiliary disease, renal impairment, predisposing factors for myopathy/rhabdomyolysis, risk for hypophosphatemia, drug hypersensitivity, any other conditions where treatment is contraindicated or cautioned, pregnancy/nursing status, and possible drug interactions. Obtain baseline LFTs and lipid levels.

Monitoring: Monitor for signs/symptoms of rhabdomyolysis, liver dysfunction, decreases in platelet counts and P levels, increases in PT and uric acid levels, and other adverse reactions. Monitor LFTs every 6-12 weeks for the 1st yr and periodically thereafter, and lipid levels. Frequently monitor blood glucose. Periodically monitor P levels in patients at risk for hypophosphatemia. Monitor PT and platelet counts with anticoagulants.

Patient Counseling: Advise to adhere to the National Cholesterol Education Program-recommended diet, a regular exercise program, and periodic testing of a fasting lipid panel. Instruct to contact physician before restarting therapy if dosing is interrupted for any length of time. Instruct to notify physician of any unexplained muscle pain, tenderness or weakness, dizziness, changes in blood glucose if diabetic, and all medications being taken (eg, vitamins or other nutritional supplements containing niacin or nicotinamide). Inform that flushing may occur and may subside after several weeks of consistent use of therapy. Instruct that if awakened by flushing at night, to get up slowly, especially if feeling dizzy or faint, or taking BP medications. Advise of the symptoms of flushing and how they differ from the symptoms of MI. Instruct to avoid ingestion of alcohol, hot beverages, and spicy foods around the time of administration to minimize flushing. Advise to d/c use and contact physician if pregnant.

Storage: 20-25°C (68-77°F).

NITRO-DUR – nitroglycerin

RX

Class: Nitrate vasodilator

OTHER BRAND NAMES
Minitran

ADULT DOSAGE

Angina Pectoris

Prevention:

Initial: 0.2-0.4mg/hr patch for 12-14 hrs/day, remove patch for 10-12 hrs/day

PEDIATRIC DOSAGE

Pediatric use may not have been established

DOSE MODIFICATION

Elderly

Start at low end of dosing range

ADMINISTRATION

Transdermal route

HOW SUPPLIED

Patch: 0.1mg/hr, 0.2mg/hr, 0.3mg/hr, 0.4mg/hr, 0.6mg/hr, 0.8mg/hr [30[s]]; (Minitran) 0.1mg/hr, 0.2mg/hr, 0.4mg/hr, 0.6mg/hr [30[s]]

CONTRAINDICATIONS

Concomitant use with phosphodiesterase inhibitors (eg, sildenafil, tadalafil, vardenafil) for erectile dysfunction or pulmonary arterial HTN, or the soluble guanylate cyclase stimulator riociguat.

WARNINGS/PRECAUTIONS

Use careful clinical or hemodynamic monitoring to avoid the hazards of hypotension and tachycardia if treating patients with acute MI (AMI) or CHF. Do not discharge a cardioverter/defibrillator through a paddle electrode that overlies the patch; the arcing that may be seen in this situation is harmless in itself, but it may be associated with local current concentration that can cause damage to the paddles and burns to the patient. Severe hypotension, particularly with upright posture, may occur with even small doses; caution in patients with volume depletion, hypotension, or on multiple medications. Nitroglycerin-induced hypotension may be accompanied by paradoxical bradycardia and increased angina pectoris. May aggravate the angina caused by hypertrophic cardiomyopathy. Tolerance and physical dependence may occur. Caution in elderly.

ADVERSE REACTIONS

Headache, lightheadedness, hypotension, syncope.

DRUG INTERACTIONS

See Contraindications. Vasodilating effects may be additive with those of other vasodilators (eg, alcohol). Marked symptomatic orthostatic hypotension reported when used with calcium channel blockers; dose adjustments of either drug may be necessary.

NURSING CONSIDERATIONS

Assessment: Assess for hypersensitivity to drug, AMI, CHF, volume depletion, hypotension, angina caused by hypertrophic cardiomyopathy, pregnancy/nursing status, and possible drug interactions.

Monitoring: Monitor for hypotension, paradoxical bradycardia, increased/aggravated angina pectoris, tolerance, physical dependence, and other adverse reactions. Perform careful clinical or hemodynamic monitoring in patients with AMI or CHF.

Patient Counseling: Inform that daily headaches sometimes accompany treatment and that the headaches may be a marker of the activity of the drug; advise to resist the temptation to avoid headaches by altering the schedule of treatment, since loss of headache may be associated with simultaneous loss of antianginal efficacy. Inform that therapy may be associated with lightheadedness on standing, especially just after rising from a recumbent or seated position; counsel that lightheadedness may be more frequent in patients who have consumed alcohol. Instruct to properly discard patches.

Storage: 25°C (77°F); excursions permitted to 15-30°C (59-86°F). Do not refrigerate. (Minitran) 15-30°C (59-86°F). Avoid extreme temperatures and/or humidity.

NORCO – acetaminophen/hydrocodone bitartrate CII

Class: Opioid analgesic

Associated w/ cases of acute liver failure, at times resulting in liver transplant and death. Most cases of liver injury are associated w/ APAP use at doses >4000mg/day, and often involve >1 APAP-containing product.

ADULT DOSAGE

Moderate to Moderately Severe Pain

5mg/325mg:
Usual: 1 or 2 tabs q4-6h prn
Max: 8 tabs/day
7.5mg/325mg, 10mg/325mg:
Usual: 1 tab q4-6h prn
Max: 6 tabs/day

PEDIATRIC DOSAGE

Pediatric use may not have been established

DOSE MODIFICATION

Elderly

Start at lower end of dosing range

ADMINISTRATION

Oral route

HOW SUPPLIED

Tab: (Hydrocodone/APAP) 5mg/325mg*, 7.5mg/325mg*, 10mg/325mg* *scored

WARNINGS/PRECAUTIONS

Increased risk of acute liver failure in patients w/ underlying liver disease. May cause serious skin reactions (eg, acute generalized exanthematous pustulosis, Stevens-Johnson syndrome, toxic epidermal necrolysis); d/c at the 1st appearance of skin rash or any other sign of hypersensitivity. Hypersensitivity and anaphylaxis reported; d/c immediately if signs/symptoms occur. May produce dose-related respiratory depression and irregular/periodic breathing. Respiratory depressant effects and CSF pressure elevation capacity may be markedly exaggerated in the presence of head injury, other intracranial lesions, or a preexisting increase in intracranial pressure. May obscure clinical course of head injuries and acute abdominal conditions. Caution w/ hypothyroidism, Addison's disease, prostatic hypertrophy, urethral stricture, severe hepatic/renal impairment, or in elderly/debilitated. Suppresses cough reflex; caution w/ pulmonary disease and in postoperative use. Lab test interactions may occur. May be habit-forming.

ADVERSE REACTIONS

Acute liver failure, lightheadedness, dizziness, sedation, N/V.

DRUG INTERACTIONS

Increased risk of acute liver failure w/ alcohol. Additive CNS depression w/ other narcotics, antihistamines, antipsychotics, antianxiety agents, or other CNS depressants (eg, alcohol); reduce dose of one or both agents. Concomitant use w/ MAOIs or TCAs may increase the effect of either the antidepressant or hydrocodone.

NURSING CONSIDERATIONS

Assessment: Assess for history of hypersensitivity to drug, level of pain intensity, type of pain, patient's general condition and medical status, renal/hepatic impairment, pregnancy/nursing status, any other conditions where treatment is cautioned, and possible drug interactions.

Monitoring: Monitor for signs/symptoms of hypersensitivity or anaphylaxis, serious skin reactions, acute liver failure, respiratory depression, elevations in CSF pressure, drug abuse/dependence/tolerance, and other adverse reactions. In patients w/ severe hepatic/renal disease, monitor effects w/ serial hepatic and/or renal function tests.

Patient Counseling: Instruct to look for APAP on package labels and not to use >1 APAP-containing product. Instruct to seek medical attention immediately upon ingestion of >4000mg/day of APAP, even if feeling well. Advise to d/c use and contact physician immediately if signs of allergy develop. Inform about signs of serious skin reactions. Inform that drug may impair mental/physical abilities, and to use caution if performing potentially hazardous tasks (eg, driving, operating machinery). Instruct to avoid alcohol and other CNS depressants. Inform that drug may be habit-forming; instruct to take only ud.

Storage: (5mg-325mg) 15-30°C (59-86°F). (7.5mg-325mg, 10mg-325mg) 20-25°C (68-77°F).

NORVASC – amlodipine besylate RX

Class: Calcium channel blocker (dihydropyridine)

ADULT DOSAGE

Hypertension

Initial: 5mg qd

Titrate: Adjust according to BP goals; wait 7-14 days between titration steps; if clinically warranted, titrate more rapidly and assess patient frequently

Max: 10mg qd

Coronary Artery Disease

Chronic Stable/Vasospastic Angina; Angiographically Documented CAD w/o HF or Ejection Fraction <40%

Usual: 5-10mg qd

PEDIATRIC DOSAGE

Hypertension

6-17 Years:

Usual: 2.5-5mg qd

Max: 5mg qd

DOSE MODIFICATION

Concomitant Medications

Other Antihypertensives:

Initial: 2.5mg qd

Hepatic Impairment

Initial: 2.5mg qd

Elderly

Initial: 2.5mg qd

Other Important Modifications

Small/Fragile Patients

Initial: 2.5mg qd

ADMINISTRATION

Oral route

HOW SUPPLIED

Tab: 2.5mg, 5mg, 10mg

WARNINGS/PRECAUTIONS

May cause symptomatic hypotension, particularly in patients with severe aortic stenosis. Worsening angina and AMI may develop after starting or increasing the dose, particularly with severe obstructive CAD. Titrate slowly in patients with severe hepatic impairment. Caution in elderly.

ADVERSE REACTIONS

Edema, palpitations, dizziness, fatigue, flushing.

DRUG INTERACTIONS

Diltiazem increased systemic exposure in elderly hypertensive patients. Strong inhibitors of CYP3A4 (eg, ketoconazole, itraconazole, ritonavir, clarithromycin) may increase plasma concentrations to greater extent; monitor for symptoms of hypotension and edema with CYP3A4 inhibitors. Monitor BP if coadministered with CYP3A4 inducers. May increase simvastatin exposure; limit dose of simvastatin to 20mg daily. Increased cyclosporine trough levels reported in renal transplant patients. Risk of increased tacrolimus blood levels with coadministration; monitor tacrolimus blood levels and adjust dose when appropriate.

NURSING CONSIDERATIONS

Assessment: Assess for hypersensitivity to the drug, severe aortic stenosis, severe obstructive CAD, hepatic impairment, pregnancy/nursing status, and possible drug interactions. Obtain baseline BP.

Monitoring: Monitor for worsening of angina, MI, and other adverse reactions. Monitor BP.

Patient Counseling: Inform of the risks/benefits of therapy. Advise to seek medical attention if any adverse effects develop. Instruct to take as prescribed.

Storage: 15-30°C (59-86°F).

NORVIR – ritonavir

RX

Class: Protease inhibitor

Coadministration with several classes of drugs, including sedative hypnotics, antiarrhythmics, or ergot alkaloid preparations, may result in potentially serious and/or life-threatening adverse events due to possible effects of ritonavir (RTV) on the hepatic metabolism of certain drugs. Review medications taken by patients prior to prescribing RTV or when prescribing other medications to patients already taking RTV.

ADULT DOSAGE

HIV-1 Infection

Combination w/ Other Antiretrovirals:
Initial: 300mg bid
Titrate: Increase at 2- to 3-day intervals by 100mg bid
Maint/Max: 600mg bid

PEDIATRIC DOSAGE

HIV-1 Infection

Combination w/ Other Antiretrovirals:
>1 Month of Age:
Initial: 250mg/m^2 bid
Titrate: Increase at 2- to 3-day intervals by 50mg/m^2 bid
Maint: 350-400mg/m^2 bid or highest tolerated dose
Max: 600mg bid

DOSE MODIFICATION

Concomitant Medications
Reduce dose when used w/ other protease inhibitors

Elderly
Start at lower end of dosing range

Other Important Modifications
Do not administer oral sol to neonates before a postmenstrual age (1st day of the mother's last menstrual period to birth plus the time elapsed after birth) of 44 weeks has been attained

ADMINISTRATION

Oral route

Take w/ meals

HOW SUPPLIED

Cap: 100mg; Sol: 80mg/mL [240mL]; Tab: 100mg

CONTRAINDICATIONS

Coadministration with voriconazole or St. John's wort. Coadministration of RTV with several classes of drugs (including sedative hypnotics, antiarrhythmics, or ergot alkaloid preparations) is contraindicated and may result in potentially serious and/or life-threatening adverse events due to possible effects of RTV on the hepatic metabolism of these drugs (eg, alfuzosin HCl, amiodarone, flecainide, propafenone, quinidine, dihydroergotamine, ergonovine, ergotamine, methylergonovine, cisapride, lovastatin, simvastatin, pimozide, sildenafil when used for treatment of pulmonary arterial HTN, triazolam, oral midazolam).

WARNINGS/PRECAUTIONS

Hepatic transaminase elevations >5X ULN, clinical hepatitis, and jaundice reported; increased risk with underlying hepatitis B or C. Caution with preexisting liver diseases, liver enzyme abnormalities, or hepatitis; consider increased AST/ALT monitoring, especially during first 3 months of therapy. Not recommended in severe hepatic impairment. Pancreatitis observed; d/c if diagnosed. Allergic reactions, anaphylaxis, Stevens-Johnson syndrome, and toxic epidermal necrolysis reported; d/c if severe reactions develop. Prolonged PR interval and 2nd- or 3rd-degree atrioventricular (AV) block may occur; caution with underlying structural heart disease, preexisting conduction system abnormalities, ischemic heart disease, and cardiomyopathies. May elevate TG and total cholesterol levels. New onset or exacerbation of diabetes mellitus (DM), hyperglycemia, diabetic ketoacidosis, immune reconstitution syndrome, autoimmune disorders (eg, Graves' disease, polymyositis, Guillain-Barre syndrome) in the setting of immune reconstitution, and redistribution/accumulation of body fat reported. Increased bleeding in patients with hemophilia type A and B reported. Various degrees of cross-resistance observed. Caution in elderly. (Sol) Contains alcohol and propylene glycol; do not administer to preterm neonates in the immediate postnatal period because of possible toxicities; if benefit outweighs potential risk, monitor infants closely for increases in serum osmolality and SrCr, and for drug-related toxicity.

ADVERSE REACTIONS

Diarrhea, N/V, abdominal pain, dizziness, dysgeusia, paresthesia, peripheral neuropathy, rash, fatigue/asthenia, arthralgia, back pain, coughing, oropharyngeal pain, pruritus, flushing.

DRUG INTERACTIONS

See Boxed Warning and Contraindications. Coadministration with CYP3A substrates for which elevated plasma concentrations are associated with serious and/or life-threatening reactions is contraindicated. Not recommended with fluticasone, other glucocorticoids that are metabolized by CYP3A, salmeterol, and high doses of itraconazole or ketoconazole. Avoid with colchicine in patients with renal/hepatic impairment, saquinavir/rifampin/RTV combination, avanafil, and rivaroxaban. Delavirdine may increase levels and rifampin may decrease levels. May increase levels of CYP3A or 2D6 substrates, atazanavir, darunavir, amprenavir, saquinavir, tipranavir, maraviroc, normeperidine, vincristine, vinblastine, dasatinib, nilotinib, antiarrhythmics, rivaroxaban, carbamazepine, clonazepam, ethosuximide, nefazodone, SSRIs, TCAs, desipramine, trazodone, dronabinol, ketoconazole, itraconazole, salmeterol, fluticasone, colchicine, clarithromycin, rifabutin, quinine, β-blockers, avanafil, vardenafil, sildenafil, tadalafil, calcium channel blockers, digoxin, bosentan, atorvastatin, rosuvastatin, immunosuppressants, neuroleptics, sedative/hypnotics, parenteral midazolam, glucocorticoids, methamphetamine, and fentanyl. May decrease levels of voriconazole, raltegravir, meperidine, theophylline, divalproex, lamotrigine, phenytoin, bupropion, atovaquone, methadone, and ethinyl estradiol. Caution with other drugs that prolong the PR interval, particularly with those drugs metabolized by CYP3A. May alter concentrations of warfarin (monitor INR) and indinavir. May need dose decrease of tramadol, and propoxyphene. Refer to PI for dosing modifications when used with certain concomitant therapies. (Cap/Sol) Contains alcohol; may produce disulfiram-like reactions with disulfiram or metronidazole.

NURSING CONSIDERATIONS

Assessment: Assess for previous hypersensitivity to the drug, preexisting liver diseases, hepatitis, DM, hemophilia type A or B, underlying cardiac problems, lipid disorders, pregnancy/nursing status, and possible drug interactions. Obtain baseline ECG, AST, ALT, gamma-glutamyl transferase (GGT), CPK, uric acid, TG, and cholesterol levels.

Monitoring: Monitor for signs/symptoms of anaphylaxis or allergic reactions, hepatitis, jaundice, hepatic dysfunction, new onset or exacerbation of DM, hyperglycemia, diabetic ketoacidosis, pancreatitis, AV block, cardiac conduction abnormalities, immune reconstitution syndrome, autoimmune disorders, fat redistribution or accumulation, and for other adverse reactions. Monitor for bleeding in patients with hemophilia type A or B. Monitor ECG, LFTs, GGT, CPK, uric acid, TG, and cholesterol levels. Frequently monitor INR during coadministration with warfarin.

Patient Counseling: Counsel to take prescribed dose ud. Instruct to inform physician if weight changes in children occur. Inform that therapy is not a cure for HIV-1 infection and illnesses associated with HIV-1 infection may still be experienced. Advise to practice safe sex, use latex or polyurethane condoms, not to share personal items (eg, toothbrush, razor blades), needles, or other inj equipment, and not to breastfeed. Advise to notify physician of any use of Rx, OTC, or herbal products, particularly St. John's wort. Advise to use additional or alternative contraceptive measures if receiving estrogen-based hormonal contraceptives. Inform that use with certain drugs may increase risk of hypotension, visual changes, and priapism; instruct to contact physician if any of these symptoms occur. Counsel about potential adverse effects; instruct to report symptoms such as dizziness, lightheadedness, abnormal heart rhythm, or loss of consciousness.

Storage: Cap: 2-8°C (36-46°F). May not require refrigeration if used within 30 days and stored below 25°C (77°F). Protect from light. Avoid exposure to excessive heat. Sol: 20-25°C (68-77°F). Do not refrigerate. Avoid exposure to excessive heat. Tab: ≤30°C (86°F). Exposure up to 50°C (122°F) for 7 days permitted. Dispense in original container or USP equivalent tight container (≤60mL). Exposure to high humidity outside the original or USP equivalent tight container (≤60mL) for >2 weeks is not recommended.

NOVOLOG – insulin aspart (rDNA origin) RX

Class: Insulin

ADULT DOSAGE

Diabetes Mellitus

SQ/IV:

Total Daily Insulin Requirement:

Usual: 0.5-1 U/kg/day; generally used w/ an intermediate or long-acting insulin

Meal-Related SQ Regimen:

50-70% of total requirement may be provided by insulin aspart; remainder provided by an intermediate- or long-acting insulin

PEDIATRIC DOSAGE

Type 1 Diabetes Mellitus

≥2 Years:

SQ:

Total Daily Insulin Requirement:

Usual: 0.5-1 U/kg/day; generally used w/ an intermediate or long-acting insulin

Meal-Related SQ Regimen:

50-70% of total requirement may be provided by insulin aspart; remainder provided by an intermediate- or long-acting insulin

ADMINISTRATION

SQ/IV route

SQ

Administer in the abdominal region, buttocks, thigh, or upper arm; rotate inj sites w/in the same region
Administer immediately (w/in 5-10 min) ac
May be diluted w/ insulin diluting medium
If mixed w/ NPH insulin, draw insulin aspart into syringe first and inject immediately after mixing

Continuous SQ Insulin Infusion by External Pump

Infuse premeal boluses immediately (w/in 5-10 min) ac
Rotate infusion sites w/in the same region
Do not use diluted or mixed insulins w/ external pump

Initial Programming of External Insulin Infusion Pump:

Base on total daily insulin dose of previous regimen
Approx 50% of total dose given as meal-related boluses; remainder given as basal infusion
Change insulin in the reservoir at least every 6 days; change infusion sets and infusion set insertion site at least every 3 days

IV

Use at concentrations 0.05-1.0 U/mL in infusion systems using polypropylene infusion bags; stable in infusion fluids such as 0.9% NaCl
Do not administer insulin mixtures IV

HOW SUPPLIED

Inj: 100 U/mL [3mL, PenFill cartridge, FlexPen, FlexTouch; 10mL, vial]

CONTRAINDICATIONS

During episodes of hypoglycemia.

WARNINGS/PRECAUTIONS

Insulin delivery devices should never be shared between patients, even if needle is changed; may carry a risk for transmission of blood-borne pathogens. Any change of insulin dose should be made cautiously and under medical supervision. Changing from one insulin product to another or changing the insulin strength may result in the need for a change in dosage. May require dosage adjustment w/ change in physical activity or meal plan. Illness, emotional disturbances, or other stresses may alter insulin requirements. Hypoglycemia may occur and may impair ability to concentrate and react; caution in patients w/ hypoglycemia unawareness and who may be predisposed to hypoglycemia. Hypokalemia, inj-site redness/swelling/itching, and severe, life-threatening, generalized allergy may occur. Contains metacresol as excipient; localized reactions and generalized myalgias reported. Increases in anti-insulin antibodies observed; presence of such insulin antibodies may need to adjust insulin dose to correct a tendency towards hyper/hypoglycemia in rare cases. Malfunction of the insulin pump or infusion set or insulin degradation can lead to a rapid onset of hyperglycemia and ketosis; prompt identification and correction of the cause is necessary. Train patients using continuous SQ infusion pump therapy to administer by inj and have alternate insulin therapy available in case of pump failure. IV administration should be under medical supervision w/ close monitoring of blood glucose and K^+ levels. Caution w/ renal/hepatic impairment.

ADVERSE REACTIONS

Hypoglycemia, headache, hyporeflexia, onychomycosis, sensory disturbance, UTI, nausea, diarrhea, chest pain, abdominal pain, skin disorder, sinusitis.

DRUG INTERACTIONS

May require dose adjustment and increased frequency of glucose monitoring w/ drugs that may increase the risk of hypoglycemia (eg, ACE inhibitors, MAOIs, salicylates, somatostatin analogues [eg, octreotide], sulfonamide antibiotics), drugs that may decrease the glucose-lowering effect (eg, atypical antipsychotics [eg, olanzapine, clozapine], corticosteroids, oral contraceptives, protease inhibitors, sympathomimetic agents [eg, albuterol, epinephrine, terbutaline]), or drugs that may increase or decrease the glucose-lowering effect (eg, alcohol, β-blockers, clonidine, lithium salts). Pentamidine may cause hypoglycemia, sometimes followed by hyperglycemia. Signs and symptoms of hypoglycemia may be blunted w/ β-blockers, clonidine, guanethidine, and reserpine. Caution w/ K^+-lowering drugs or drugs sensitive to serum K^+ concentrations. Observe for signs/symptoms of heart failure (HF) if treated concomitantly w/ a peroxisome proliferator-activated receptor (PPAR)-gamma agonist (eg, thiazolidinedione); consider discontinuation or dose reduction of the PPAR-gamma agonist if HF develops.

NURSING CONSIDERATIONS

Assessment: Assess for predisposition to hypoglycemia, risk of hypokalemia, hypersensitivity, renal/hepatic impairment, pregnancy/nursing status, and possible drug interactions. Obtain baseline blood glucose and HbA1c levels.

Monitoring: Monitor for signs/symptoms of hypoglycemia, hypokalemia, allergic reactions, and other adverse effects. Monitor blood glucose, HbA1c, K^+ levels, and renal/hepatic function.

Patient Counseling: Advise to never share insulin delivery device w/ another person, even if needle is changed. Inform about potential risks and benefits of therapy. Counsel on proper inj technique, lifestyle management, regular glucose monitoring, periodic HbA1c testing, recognition and management of hypo/hyperglycemia, adherence to meal planning, complications of insulin therapy, timing of dose, instruction in the use of inj or SQ insulin infusion pump, and proper storage of insulin. Inform that the ability to concentrate and react may be impaired as a result of hypoglycemia; advise to use caution when driving or operating machinery. Instruct to always carefully check that appropriate insulin is administered to avoid medication errors. Advise to inform physician if pregnant or intending to become pregnant.

Storage: Unused: 2-8°C (36-46°F) until expiration date. Do not freeze or store directly adjacent to the refrigerator cooling element; do not use if it has been frozen. Should not be drawn into a syringe and stored for later use. Opened: <30°C (86°F) for up to 28 days. (Vials) May refrigerate. (PenFill/FlexPen/FlexTouch) Do not refrigerate. Pump: Discard insulin in reservoir after exposure to >37°C (98.6°F). Diluted Sol: <30°C (86°F) for 28 days. Sol in Infusion Fluids: Stable at room temperature for 24 hrs. Protect from direct heat and light.

NovoLog Mix 70/30 – insulin aspart protamine (rDNA origin)/insulin aspart (rDNA origin) RX

Class: Insulin

ADULT DOSAGE

Type 1 Diabetes Mellitus

Individualize dose; inject w/in 15 min ac
Typically dosed bid (w/ each dose intended to cover 2 meals or a meal and snack)

Type 2 Diabetes Mellitus

Individualize dose; inject w/in 15 min ac or pc
Typically dosed bid (w/ each dose intended to cover 2 meals or a meal and snack)

PEDIATRIC DOSAGE

Pediatric use may not have been established

DOSE MODIFICATION

Elderly

Start at lower end of dosing range

ADMINISTRATION

SQ route
Administer in the abdominal region, buttocks, thigh, or upper arm; rotate inj sites w/in the same region
Do not use in insulin infusion pump; do not mix w/ any other insulin product
Always use a new needle for each inj and always remove needle after each inj to prevent contamination

Resuspension

Resuspension is easier when the insulin has reached room temperature

Vial:

1. Roll vial gently between hands in a horizontal position 10X to mix it
2. Repeat rolling procedure until the sus appears uniformly white and cloudy
3. Inject immediately

FlexPen:

1. Roll 10X gently between hands in a horizontal position
2. Turn FlexPen upside down so that the glass ball moves from 1 end of the reservoir to the other at least 10X
3. Repeat rolling and turning procedure until the sus appears uniformly white and cloudy
4. Inject immediately
5. Repeat turning procedure at least 10X before each subsequent inj

HOW SUPPLIED

Inj: (Insulin Aspart Protamine/Insulin Aspart) (70 U/30 U)/mL [3mL, FlexPen; 10mL, vial]

CONTRAINDICATIONS

During episodes of hypoglycemia.

WARNINGS/PRECAUTIONS

Not for IV use. FlexPens must never be shared between patients, even if needle is changed; may carry a risk for transmission of blood-borne pathogens. Any change of insulin dose should be made cautiously and under medical supervision. Changing from 1 insulin product to another or changing the insulin strength may result in the need for a change in dosage; changes may also be necessary during illness, emotional stress, and other physiologic stress in addition to changes in meals and exercise. Hypoglycemia may occur and may impair ability to concentrate and react. Hypokalemia, inj-site reactions (eg, erythema, edema, pruritus), and severe, life-threatening, generalized allergy may occur. Contains metacresol as excipient; localized reactions and generalized myalgias reported. Changes in cross-reactive anti-insulin antibodies reported; may need to adjust dose in order to correct a tendency towards hyper/hypoglycemia. Caution in renal/hepatic impairment.

ADVERSE REACTIONS

Hypoglycemia, headache, influenza-like symptoms, dyspepsia, back pain, diarrhea, pharyngitis, rhinitis, skeletal pain, URTI, neuropathy, abdominal pain.

DRUG INTERACTIONS

May require insulin dose adjustment and close monitoring w/ drugs that may increase blood glucose-lowering effect and susceptibility to hypoglycemia (eg, oral antidiabetic products, pramlintide, ACE inhibitors), drugs that may reduce blood glucose-lowering effect (eg, corticosteroids, niacin, danazol), or drugs that may potentiate or weaken blood glucose-lowering effect (β-blockers, clonidine, lithium salts, alcohol). Pentamidine may cause hypoglycemia, sometimes followed by hyperglycemia. Signs of hypoglycemia may be reduced or absent w/ sympatholytics (eg, β-blockers, clonidine, guanethidine). Caution w/ K^+-lowering drugs or drugs sensitive to K^+ concentrations. Observe for signs/symptoms of heart failure (HF) if treated concomitantly w/ a peroxisome proliferator-activated receptor (PPAR)-gamma agonist (eg, thiazolidinediones); consider discontinuation or dose reduction of the PPAR-gamma agonist if HF develops.

NURSING CONSIDERATIONS

Assessment: Assess for predisposition to hypoglycemia, risk of hypokalemia, renal/hepatic impairment, drug hypersensitivity, pregnancy/nursing status, and possible drug interactions. Obtain baseline blood glucose and HbA1c levels.

Monitoring: Monitor for signs/symptoms of hypoglycemia, hypokalemia, allergic reactions, and other adverse effects. Monitor blood glucose, HbA1c, K^+ levels, and renal/hepatic function.

Patient Counseling: Advise to never share FlexPen w/ another person, even if the needle is changed. Inform about potential risks and benefits of therapy. Counsel on proper inj technique, lifestyle management, regular glucose monitoring, periodic HbA1c testing, recognition and management of hypo/hyperglycemia, adherence to meal planning, complications of insulin therapy, timing of dose, instruction in the use of inj devices, and proper storage of insulin. Inform that the ability to concentrate and react may be impaired as a result of hypoglycemia; advise to use caution when driving or operating machinery. Instruct to always carefully check that appropriate insulin is administered to avoid medication errors. Advise to inform physician if pregnant/intending to become pregnant.

Storage: Unopened: 2-8°C (36-46°F) until expiration date, or room temperature (<30°C [86°F]) for 28 days (vial) or 14 days (FlexPen). Do not freeze; do not use if it has been frozen. Do not store directly adjacent to the refrigerator cooling element. Opened: <30°C (86°F) for 28 days (vial) or 14 days (FlexPen). Do not refrigerate FlexPen; store w/o a needle attached. Protect from excessive heat or sunlight.

NOXAFIL – posaconazole RX

Class: Azole antifungal

ADULT DOSAGE

Invasive *Aspergillus* and *Candida* Infections

Prophylaxis:

Inj/Tab:

LD: 300mg bid on the 1st day

Maint: 300mg qd, starting on the 2nd day

Sus:

Usual: 200mg (5mL) tid

Duration of therapy is based on recovery from neutropenia or immunosuppression

Oropharyngeal Candidiasis

Sus:

LD: 100mg (2.5mL) bid on 1st day

Maint: 100mg qd for 13 days

Refractory to Itraconazole and/or Fluconazole:

400mg (10mL) bid; duration of therapy is based on severity of underlying disease and clinical response

PEDIATRIC DOSAGE

Invasive *Aspergillus* and *Candida* Infections

Prophylaxis:

≥13 Years:

Tab:

LD: 300mg bid on the 1st day

Maint: 300mg qd, starting on the 2nd day

Sus:

Usual: 200mg (5mL) tid

Duration of therapy is based on recovery from neutropenia or immunosuppression

Oropharyngeal Candidiasis

≥13 Years:

Sus:

LD: 100mg (2.5mL) bid on 1st day

Maint: 100mg qd for 13 days

Refractory to Itraconazole and/or Fluconazole:

400mg (10mL) bid; duration of therapy is based on severity of underlying disease and clinical response

DOSE MODIFICATION

Renal Impairment

IV:

Moderate or Severe (eGFR <50mL/min): Avoid use; monitor SrCr levels closely and consider changing to oral therapy if increases occur

ADMINISTRATION

Oral/IV routes

Delayed-release tab and oral sus are not to be used interchangeably

Inj

Administer via a central venous line, including a central venous catheter or peripherally inserted central catheter by slow IV infusion over approx 90 min

If central venous catheter is not available, may administer through a peripheral venous catheter by slow IV infusion over 30 min as a single dose in advance of central venous line placement or to bridge the period during which a central venous line is replaced or is in use for other IV treatment

Infuse through a central venous line when multiple dosing is required

Administer through a 0.22 micron polyethersulfone or polyvinylidene difluoride filter

Do not administer as IV bolus

Preparation:

Once refrigerated vial is equilibrated to room temperature, transfer 16.7mL of sol to IV bag/bottle containing 150mL of D5W or 0.9% NaCl; administer only w/ these diluents

Product is for single use only

Compatibility:

The following products prepared in D5W or 0.9% NaCl can be infused at the same time through the same IV line/cannula: D5W, amikacin sulfate, caspofungin, ciprofloxacin, daptomycin, dobutamine hydrochloride, famotidine, filgrastim, gentamicin sulfate, hydromorphone hydrochloride, levofloxacin, lorazepam, meropenem, micafungin, morphine sulfate, norepinephrine bitartrate, potassium chloride, 0.9% NaCl, vancomycin hydrochloride

Sus

Take during or immediately (eg, w/in 20 min) following a full meal

If unable to eat a full meal, take w/ a liquid nutritional supplement or an acidic carbonated beverage (eg, ginger ale)

Shake well before use

Tab

Take w/ food

Swallow tab whole; do not break, crush, dissolve, or chew before swallowing

HOW SUPPLIED

Inj: 18mg/mL [16.7mL]; Sus: 40mg/mL [105mL]; Tab, Delayed-Release: 100mg

CONTRAINDICATIONS

Coadministration with sirolimus, CYP3A4 substrates that prolong the QT interval (eg, pimozide, quinidine), HMG-CoA reductase inhibitors that are primarily metabolized through CYP3A4 (eg, atorvastatin, lovastatin, simvastatin), and ergot alkaloids.

WARNINGS/PRECAUTIONS

Do not use tab and sus interchangeably. Prolongation of the QT interval and cases of torsades de pointes reported. Rigorous attempts to correct K^+, Mg^{2+}, and Ca^{2+} should be made before initiating treatment. Hepatic reactions reported. More severe hepatic reactions, including cholestasis or hepatic failure, reported in patients with serious underlying medical conditions (eg, hematologic malignancy). Monitor for the development of more severe hepatic injury in patients who develop abnormal LFTs during therapy. Consider discontinuation if signs/symptoms of liver disease develop. Monitor closely for breakthrough fungal infections in patients weighing >120kg. (Inj) Avoid with moderate or severe renal impairment (estimated GFR <50 mL/min), unless an assessment of the benefit/risk justifies the use of inj. Monitor SrCr levels closely in patients with moderate or severe renal impairment; consider changing to oral therapy if increases occur. (Tab/Sus) Monitor closely for breakthrough fungal infections in patients with severe renal impairment and severe diarrhea or vomiting.

ADVERSE REACTIONS

Fever, headache, anemia, thrombocytopenia, diarrhea, N/V, abdominal pain, cough, rash, hypokalemia, constipation, HTN, edema peripheral, hypomagnesemia, epistaxis.

DRUG INTERACTIONS

See Contraindications. May increase whole blood trough concentrations of cyclosporine and tacrolimus; monitor tacrolimus or cyclosporine whole blood trough concentrations frequently during and at discontinuation of posaconazole treatment, and adjust the dose of cyclosporine or tacrolimus accordingly. Avoid with phenytoin, rifabutin, and efavirenz, unless benefit outweighs risk. If phenytoin is required, closely monitor for breakthrough fungal infections and frequently monitor phenytoin concentrations; consider phenytoin dose reduction. If rifabutin is required, frequently monitor CBCs and adverse events due to increased rifabutin plasma concentrations (eg, uveitis, leukopenia); monitor for breakthrough fungal infections. Fosamprenavir may decrease levels; monitor for breakthrough fungal infections. May increase levels of vinca alkaloids; consider dose adjustment of vinca alkaloids. May increase levels of midazolam and other benzodiazepines metabolized by CYP3A4 (eg, alprazolam, triazolam). May increase levels of calcium channel blockers (CCBs) metabolized by CYP3A4 (eg, verapamil, diltiazem, nifedipine), and other drugs that are metabolized through CYP3A4 (eg, atazanavir, ritonavir); monitor for adverse effects and toxicity; dose reduction of CCBs may be needed. Increased digoxin levels reported; monitor digoxin plasma levels. Inhibitors or inducers of UDP glucuronosyltransferase or P-glycoprotein may affect posaconazole levels. Monitor glucose levels with glipizide. (Sus) Avoid with cimetidine and esomeprazole, unless benefit outweighs risks. Cimetidine, esomeprazole, and metoclopramide may decrease levels; monitor for breakthrough fungal infections.

NURSING CONSIDERATIONS

Assessment: Assess for hypersensitivity to any component of the drug or to other azole antifungals, proarrhythmic conditions, renal impairment, serious underlying medical conditions (eg, hematologic malignancy), pregnancy/nursing status, and for possible drug interactions. Obtain baseline LFTs.

Monitoring: Monitor for signs/symptoms of hypersensitivity reactions, hepatic reactions, QT prolongation, torsades de pointes, and other adverse reactions. Monitor LFTs during the course of therapy. Monitor closely for breakthrough fungal infections in patients weighing >120kg. (Tab/Sus) Monitor closely for breakthrough fungal infections in patients with severe renal impairment and severe diarrhea or vomiting.

Patient Counseling: Advise patients to inform physician of all medications being taken and if they have a heart condition or circulatory disease; liver disease; are pregnant, plan to become pregnant, or are breastfeeding; or if have ever had an allergic reaction to other antifungal medications. Advise patients to inform physician if they develop severe diarrhea or vomiting, flu-like symptoms, itching, eyes/skin that turn yellow, swelling of a leg or SOB, notice a change in HR/heart rhythm, or if they feel more tired than usual.

Storage: (Inj) 2-8°C (36-46°F). (Sus) 25°C (77°F); excursions permitted to 15-30°C (59-86°F). Do not freeze. (Tab) 20-25°C (68-77°F); excursions permitted to 15-30°C (59-86°F).

NPLATE – romiplostim **RX**

Class: Thrombopoietin receptor agonist

ADULT DOSAGE

Chronic Immune Thrombocytopenia

Use in patients who have had an insufficient response to corticosteroids, immunoglobulins, or splenectomy

Initial: 1mcg/kg based on actual body weight
Titrate: Adjust weekly dose by increments of 1mcg/kg until platelet count is ≥50 x 10^9/L
Platelet Count >200 x 10^9/L for 2 Consecutive Weeks: Reduce dose by 1mcg/kg
Platelet Count >400 x 10^9/L: Do not dose; continue assessing platelet count weekly. After platelet count falls to <200 x 10^9/L, resume therapy at a dose reduced by 1mcg/kg
Max: 10mcg/kg/week

PEDIATRIC DOSAGE

Pediatric use may not have been established

DOSE MODIFICATION

Concomitant Medications

Concomitant Medical Immune Thrombocytopenia Therapies: May reduce or d/c medical immune thrombocytopenia therapies (eg, corticosteroids, danazol, azathioprine, IV immunoglobulin, and anti-D immunoglobulin) if platelet count is ≥50 x 10^9/L

Discontinuation

D/C if platelet count does not increase to a level sufficient to avoid clinically important bleeding after 4 weeks of therapy at the max weekly dose

ADMINISTRATION

SQ route

Administer as a weekly SQ inj
Use syringe with 0.01mL graduations
Discard any unused portion; do not pool unused portions from vials and do not administer more than 1 dose from a single vial

Preparation

Reconstitute 250mcg single use vial with 0.72mL or 500mcg single use vial with 1.2mL of preservative free sterile water for inj

Gently swirl and invert vial to reconstitute; do not shake

Withdraw appropriate volume of calculated dose from vial and administer SQ

HOW SUPPLIED

Inj: 250mcg, 500mcg [vial]

WARNINGS/PRECAUTIONS

Not for the treatment of thrombocytopenia due to myelodysplastic syndrome (MDS) or any cause of thrombocytopenia other than chronic ITP; progression from MDS to acute myelogenous leukemia has been observed. Use only in patients with ITP whose degree of thrombocytopenia and clinical condition increases the risk for bleeding. Do not use in an attempt to normalize platelet counts. Use lowest dose to achieve and maintain a platelet count $\geq$50 x 10^9/L. Thrombotic/thromboembolic complications may occur. Portal vein thrombosis reported in patients with chronic liver disease. May increase risk for development or progression of reticulin fiber formation within the bone marrow; consider a bone marrow biopsy to include staining for fibrosis if new or worsening morphological abnormalities or cytopenias occur. Worsened thrombocytopenia reported after discontinuation; following discontinuation, obtain weekly CBCs, including platelet counts, for at least 2 weeks, and consider alternative treatments for worsening thrombocytopenia. If hyporesponsiveness or failure to maintain a platelet response occurs, search for causative factors (eg, neutralizing antibodies). Caution with renal/hepatic impairment and in elderly.

ADVERSE REACTIONS

Headache, arthralgia, dizziness, insomnia, myalgia, pain in extremity, abdominal pain, shoulder pain, dyspepsia, development of antibodies, paresthesia.

NURSING CONSIDERATIONS

Assessment: Assess for cause and degree of thrombocytopenia, hepatic/renal impairment, and pregnancy/nursing status.

Monitoring: Obtain CBCs, including platelet counts, weekly during dose adjustment phase, then monthly after establishment of a stable dose, and then weekly for at least 2 weeks after discontinuation. Monitor for thrombotic/thromboembolic complications, bone marrow reticulin fiber formation, new/worsening morphological abnormalities, cytopenias, hyporesponsiveness, and failure to maintain platelet response with therapy.

Patient Counseling: Inform of risks and benefits of therapy. Advise that the risks associated with long-term administration are unknown. Counsel to avoid situations or medications that may increase risk for bleeding. Inform pregnant women that they may enroll in the pregnancy registry.

Storage: 2-8°C (36-46°F). Do not freeze. Protect from light. Reconstituted: 25°C (77°F) or 2-8°C (36-46°F) for up to 24 hrs prior to administration. Protect from light. Discard unused portion.

NUCYNTA — tapentadol CII

Class: Central acting analgesic

ADULT DOSAGE

Acute Pain

Moderate to Severe:

Usual: 50mg, 75mg, or 100mg q4-6h depending upon pain intensity

Day 1: May give 2nd dose 1 hr after 1st dose if pain relief is inadequate, then 50mg, 75mg, or 100mg q4-6h

Adjust dose to maintain adequate analgesia with acceptable tolerability

Max: 700mg on Day 1, then 600mg/day thereafter

Periodically reassess continued need for use during chronic therapy, especially for noncancer-related pain

PEDIATRIC DOSAGE

Pediatric use may not have been established

DOSE MODIFICATION

Hepatic Impairment

Moderate (Child-Pugh Score 7-9):

Initial: 50mg no more frequently than once q8h

Max: 3 doses/24 hrs

Elderly
Start at lower end of dosing range

Discontinuation
Taper dose gradually

ADMINISTRATION

Oral route

Take with or without food

HOW SUPPLIED

Tab: 50mg, 75mg, 100mg

CONTRAINDICATIONS

Significant respiratory depression, acute or severe bronchial asthma or hypercarbia in an unmonitored setting or in the absence of resuscitative equipment, known or suspected paralytic ileus, and patients receiving MAOIs or who have taken them within the last 14 days.

WARNINGS/PRECAUTIONS

Abuse liability similar to other opioid agonists legal or illicit; assess each patient's risk for opioid abuse or addiction prior to prescribing. Routinely monitor all patients for signs of misuse, abuse, and addiction; misuse or abuse by crushing, chewing, snorting, or injecting will pose a significant risk that could result in overdose and death. Respiratory depression, if not immediately recognized and treated, may lead to respiratory arrest and death. Accidental ingestion, especially in children, can result in fatal overdose. Respiratory depression is more likely to occur in elderly, cachectic, or debilitated patients; monitor closely, particularly when given with drugs that depress respiration. Monitor for respiratory depression and consider use of alternative nonopioid analgesics in patients with significant chronic obstructive pulmonary disease (COPD) or cor pulmonale, and in patients with a substantially decreased respiratory reserve, hypoxia, hypercarbia, or preexisting respiratory depression. May cause severe hypotension. Monitor for signs of sedation and respiratory depression in patients susceptible to the intracranial effects of carbon dioxide retention (eg, those with evidence of increased intracranial pressure or brain tumors). May obscure clinical course in patients with a head injury. Avoid with circulatory shock, impaired consciousness, or coma. May aggravate convulsions in patients with convulsive disorders and may induce or aggravate seizures; monitor for worsened seizure control in patients with history of seizure disorders. May cause spasm of sphincter of Oddi; monitor for worsening symptoms in patients with biliary tract disease (eg, acute pancreatitis). Withdrawal symptoms may occur if discontinued abruptly. May impair mental/physical abilities. Monitor for respiratory/CNS depression with moderate hepatic impairment. Avoid use with severe renal/hepatic impairment. Not for use during and immediately prior to labor.

ADVERSE REACTIONS

N/V, dizziness, somnolence, constipation, pruritus, dry mouth, hyperhidrosis, fatigue.

DRUG INTERACTIONS

See Contraindications. Avoid use with alcoholic beverages or medications containing alcohol, other opioids, or drugs of abuse; may have additive effects. CNS depressants (eg, sedatives or hypnotics, general anesthetics, phenothiazines, tranquilizers, alcohol, anxiolytics, neuroleptics, muscle relaxants, other opioids, illicit drugs) may increase risk of respiratory depression, hypotension, profound sedation, or coma; start tapentadol at 1/3 to 1/2 of the usual dose and consider using a lower dose of concomitant CNS depressant. Serotonin syndrome may occur with serotonergic drugs (eg, SSRIs, SNRIs, TCAs, triptans, drugs that affect the serotonergic neurotransmitter system [eg, mirtazapine, trazodone, tramadol]), and drugs that may impair metabolism of serotonin (eg, MAOIs); use with caution. Avoid use with mixed agonist/antagonist analgesics (eg, butorphanol, nalbuphine, pentazocine), and partial agonists (eg, buprenorphine); may precipitate withdrawal symptoms. Anticholinergics may increase risk of urinary retention and/or severe constipation, which may lead to paralytic ileus.

NURSING CONSIDERATIONS

Assessment: Assess for personal/family history or risk factors for drug abuse or addiction, general condition and medical status, opioid experience/tolerance, pain type/severity, previous opioid daily dose, potency and type of prior analgesics used, respiratory depression, COPD or other respiratory complications, GI obstruction, paralytic ileus, renal/hepatic impairment, pregnancy/nursing status, possible drug interactions, and any other condition where treatment is contraindicated or cautioned.

Monitoring: Monitor for improvement of pain, signs/symptoms of respiratory depression, hypotension, symptoms of worsening biliary tract disease, aggravation/induction of seizure, tolerance, physical dependence, mental/physical impairment, serotonin syndrome, and other adverse reactions. Routinely monitor for signs of misuse, abuse, and addiction. Periodically reassess continued need for use during chronic therapy, especially for noncancer-related pain.

Patient Counseling: Instruct to take only as prescribed and not to d/c without first discussing the need for a tapering regimen with prescriber. Inform that drug has potential for abuse; instruct not to share drug with others and to take steps to protect from theft or misuse. Discuss the risks of respiratory depression, orthostatic hypotension, syncope, severe constipation, and anaphylaxis; counsel on how to recognize symptoms and when to seek medical attention. Inform that accidental exposure may result in serious harm or death; advise to dispose unused tabs by flushing them down the toilet. Inform about risks of concomitant use of alcohol, other CNS depressants, MAOIs, and serotonergic drugs; instruct to notify physician if taking/planning to take additional medications. Instruct to not consume alcoholic beverages, or take prescription and OTC products that contain alcohol, during treatment. Counsel that drug may cause seizures if at risk for seizures or if patient has epilepsy; advise to d/c therapy and seek medical attention if seizures occur during therapy. Inform that drug may impair the ability to perform potentially hazardous activities (eg, driving a car or operating heavy machinery); advise not to perform such tasks until patients know how they will react to the medication. Advise females that drug can cause fetal harm; instruct to notify physician if pregnant/planning to become pregnant.

Storage: ≤25°C (77°F); excursions permitted to 15-30°C (59-86°F). Protect from moisture.

NUCYNTA ER – tapentadol CII

Class: Central acting analgesic

Exposes users to risks of addiction, abuse, and misuse, which can lead to overdose and death; assess each patient's risk prior to prescribing and monitor regularly for development of these behaviors/conditions. Serious, life-threatening, or fatal respiratory depression may occur; monitor during initiation or following a dose increase. Crushing, dissolving, or chewing tab can cause rapid release and absorption of potentially fatal dose; instruct patients to swallow tab whole. Accidental ingestion, especially by children, can result in a fatal overdose. Prolonged use during pregnancy can result in neonatal opioid withdrawal syndrome; advise pregnant women of the risk and ensure availability of appropriate treatment. Avoid use with alcoholic beverages or medications containing alcohol; may result in increased levels and potentially fatal overdose of tapentadol.

ADULT DOSAGE

Severe Pain (Daily, Around-the-Clock Management)

Pain severe enough to require daily, around-the-clock, long-term opioid treatment and for which alternative treatment options are inadequate

1st Opioid Analgesic/Opioid Intolerant Patients:
Initial: 50mg bid (q12h)
Titrate: Increase by 50mg no more than twice daily every 3 days

Diabetic Peripheral Neuropathy

Neuropathic pain severe enough to require daily, around-the-clock, long-term opioid treatment and for which alternative treatment options are inadequate

1st Opioid Analgesic/Opioid Intolerant Patients:
Initial: 50mg bid (q12h)
Titrate: Increase by 50mg no more than twice daily every 3 days

Conversions

From Immediate-Release (IR) to (Extended-Release) ER Tapentadol:
Use the equivalent total daily dose of IR tapentadol and divide it into 2 equal doses of ER tapentadol separated by approx 12-hr intervals

From Other Opioids:
D/C all other around-the-clock opioids when therapy is initiated; begin w/ 1/2 of the estimated daily tapentadol requirement as the initial dose, managing inadequate analgesia by supplementation w/ IR rescue medication

PEDIATRIC DOSAGE

Pediatric use may not have been established

DOSE MODIFICATION

Renal Impairment

Severe: Not recommended

Hepatic Impairment

Moderate (Child-Pugh Score 7-9):
Initial: 50mg qd
Max: 100mg/day
Severe (Child-Pugh Score 10-15):
Not recommended

Elderly

Start at lower end of dosing range

Discontinuation

Use gradual downward titration

ADMINISTRATION

Oral route
Swallow tab whole; do not cut, crush, dissolve, or chew
Take 1 tab at a time w/ enough water to ensure complete swallowing

HOW SUPPLIED

Tab, ER: 50mg, 100mg, 150mg, 200mg, 250mg

CONTRAINDICATIONS

Significant respiratory depression, acute or severe bronchial asthma or hypercarbia in an unmonitored setting or in the absence of resuscitative equipment, known or suspected paralytic ileus, patients receiving MAOIs or who have taken them within the last 14 days.

WARNINGS/PRECAUTIONS

Reserve for use in patients for whom alternative treatment options are ineffective, not tolerated, or would be otherwise inadequate to provide sufficient management of pain. Should only be prescribed by healthcare professionals who are knowledgeable in the use of potent opioids for management of chronic pain. D/C all other tapentadol and tramadol products when initiating and during therapy. Life-threatening respiratory depression is more likely to occur in elderly, cachectic, or debilitated patients. Consider alternative nonopioid analgesics in patients with significant COPD or cor pulmonale, and in patients having a substantially decreased respiratory reserve, hypoxia, hypercarbia, or preexisting respiratory depression. May cause severe hypotension; increased risk in patients whose ability to maintain BP is compromised by a reduced blood volume or concurrent administration of certain CNS depressants. Avoid with circulatory shock, impaired consciousness, or coma. Monitor patients who may be susceptible to intracranial effects of carbon dioxide retention for signs of sedation and respiratory depression when initiating therapy. May obscure clinical course in patients with head injury. May aggravate convulsions and induce/aggravate seizures. May cause spasm of sphincter of Oddi; monitor patients with biliary tract disease (eg, acute pancreatitis). May impair mental/physical abilities. Monitor for respiratory/CNS depression with moderate hepatic impairment. Not recommended with severe renal/hepatic impairment.

ADVERSE REACTIONS

Respiratory depression, N/V, dizziness, constipation, headache, somnolence, fatigue, dry mouth, hyperhidrosis, pruritus, insomnia, dyspepsia, diarrhea, decreased appetite, anxiety.

DRUG INTERACTIONS

See Boxed Warning and Contraindications. Hypotension, profound sedation, coma, and respiratory depression may occur with CNS depressants (eg, sedatives, anxiolytics, hypnotics); if coadministration is required, consider dose reduction of one or both agents. Serotonin syndrome may occur with serotonergic drugs (eg, SSRIs, SNRIs, TCAs, triptans, drugs that affect serotonergic neurotransmitter system) and drugs that may impair metabolism of serotonin (eg, MAOIs). Avoid use of mixed agonist/antagonist (eg, nalbuphine, pentazocine, butorphanol) and partial agonists (eg, buprenorphine) analgesics; may reduce analgesic effects and/or precipitate withdrawal symptoms. Enhanced neuromuscular blocking action and increased degree of respiratory depression with skeletal muscle relaxants. Anticholinergics may increase risk of urinary retention and/or severe constipation, which may lead to paralytic ileus.

NURSING CONSIDERATIONS

Assessment: Assess for abuse/addiction risk, opioid experience/tolerance, pain type/severity, pregnancy/nursing status, possible drug interactions, and any other condition where treatment is contraindicated or cautioned.

Monitoring: Monitor for signs/symptoms of respiratory depression, hypotension, symptoms of worsening biliary tract disease, aggravation/induction of seizure, mental/physical impairment, serotonin syndrome, and other adverse reactions. Routinely monitor for signs of misuse, abuse, and addiction.

Patient Counseling: Inform that drug has potential for abuse and addiction; instruct not to share drug with others and to take steps to protect from theft or misuse. Inform about risk of accidental exposure and advise to store securely and to dispose unused tabs by flushing them down the toilet. Inform about the risks of life-threatening respiratory depression, orthostatic hypotension, and syncope. Inform about risks of concomitant use of alcohol, other CNS depressants, MAOIs, and serotonergic drugs; instruct to notify physician if taking/planning to take additional medications. Instruct to not consume alcoholic beverages or take prescription/OTC products that contain alcohol during treatment. Counsel on the risk for seizures and advise to d/c therapy and seek medical attention if seizures occur. Advise to use ud. Inform that drug may impair the ability to perform potentially hazardous activities; advise not to perform such tasks until patients know how they will react to medication. Advise of potential for severe constipation, including management instructions. Advise how to recognize anaphylaxis and when to seek medical attention. Advise females that drug can cause fetal harm; instruct to notify physician if pregnant/planning to become pregnant.

Storage: ≤25°C (77°F); excursions permitted to 15-30°C (59-86°F). Protect from moisture.

NuvaRing — ethinyl estradiol/etonogestrel — RX

Class: Estrogen/progestogen combination

Cigarette smoking increases the risk of serious cardiovascular (CV) events. Risk increases with age and with number of cigarettes smoked. Not for use by women who are >35 yrs of age and smoke.

ADULT DOSAGE

Contraception

1 ring, inserted in the vagina and left in place continuously for 3 weeks, then removed for 1 week. Insert new ring 1 week after the last ring was removed

No Hormonal Contraceptive Use in the Preceding Cycle:
May insert ring on Days 1-5 of menstrual bleeding; if inserted on Days 2-5 of cycle, use an additional barrier method of contraception (eg, male condom w/ spermicide) for the first 7 days

Changing from a Combination Hormonal Contraceptive:
May switch on any day, but at the latest on the day following the usual hormone-free interval

Changing from Progestin-Only Method (Progestin-Only Pill, Implant, Inj, or Progestin-Releasing Intrauterine System):
May switch on any day from the progestin-only pill; start using ring on the day after taking last progestin-only pill
May switch from an implant or intrauterine system on the day of its removal and from an injectable on the day when the next inj is due
In all cases, additional barrier method (eg, male condom w/ spermicide) should be used for the first 7 days

Use After Abortion/Miscarriage:
May start w/in the first 5 days following a complete 1st trimester abortion/miscarriage; no additional method of contraception needed
If not started w/in 5 days, follow instructions for "No Hormonal Contraceptive Use in the Preceding Cycle" and use a non-hormonal contraceptive method in the meantime

Following Childbirth or 2nd Trimester Abortion/Miscarriage:
Use may be initiated no earlier than 4 weeks postpartum in women who elect not to breastfeed, or 4 weeks after a 2nd trimester abortion/miscarriage
If use is begun postpartum, use an additional method of contraception (eg, male condom w/ spermicide) for the first 7 days

PEDIATRIC DOSAGE

Contraception

Not indicated for use premenarche; refer to adult dosing

DOSE MODIFICATION

Other Important Modifications

Inadvertent Removal/Expulsion:

Ring is Left Outside of Vagina for <3 Hrs: Rinse and reinsert as soon as possible, but at the latest w/in 3 hrs. If ring is lost, insert new vaginal ring and continue regimen w/o alteration

Ring is Left Outside of Vagina for >3 Hrs During Weeks 1 and 2: Reinsert ring as soon as remembered and use barrier method (eg, condoms w/ spermicides) until ring has been used continuously for 7 days

Ring is Left Outside of Vagina for >3 Hrs During Week 3: Discard that ring and insert new ring immediately which will start the next 3-week use period. Alternatively, insert new ring no later than 7 days from the time the previous ring was removed/expelled if previous ring was used continuously for at least 7 days. In either case, use a barrier method (eg, condoms w/ spermicides) until new ring has been used continuously for 7 days

Prolonged Ring-Free Interval:

If ring-free interval has been extended beyond 1 week, must use additional method of contraception until ring has been used continuously for 7 days

Prolonged Use of Ring:

Left in Place for Up to 1 Extra Week (up to 4 Weeks Total): Remove ring and insert new ring after 1-week ring-free interval

Left in Place for >4 Weeks: Remove ring, and if pregnancy is ruled out, may restart ring w/ additional method of contraception until ring has been used continuously for 7 days

Ring Breakage:

Discard ring and replace w/ new ring

Use w/ Other Vaginal Products:

Use of diaphragm is not recommended as backup method w/ ring use; ring may interfere w/ correct placement/position of a diaphragm

ADMINISTRATION

Intravaginal route

Compress ring and insert into the vagina; exact position of ring inside the vagina is not critical for its function

Ring must be inserted on the appropriate day and left in place for 3 consecutive weeks

Remove ring 3 weeks later, on the same day of the week and at about the same time as it was inserted

Removal/Reinsertion

Remove by hooking index finger under the forward rim or by grasping the rim between index and middle finger and pulling out

Used ring should be placed in the sachet (foil pouch) and discarded in a waste receptacle; do not flush in toilet

Reinsert new ring exactly 1 week after previous ring was removed, even if menstrual bleeding has not finished

HOW SUPPLIED

Vaginal ring: (Ethinyl Estradiol-Etonogestrel) 0.015mg-0.120mg/day

CONTRAINDICATIONS

A high risk of arterial or venous thrombotic diseases (eg, women who are known to smoke [if >35 yrs of age]), current or history of deep vein thrombosis or pulmonary embolism, cerebrovascular disease, coronary artery disease, thrombogenic valvular or thrombogenic rhythm diseases of the heart (eg, subacute bacterial endocarditis with valvular disease, or atrial fibrillation), inherited or acquired hypercoagulopathies, uncontrolled HTN, diabetes mellitus with vascular disease, headaches with focal neurological symptoms or migraine headaches with aura, >35 yrs of age with any migraine headaches. Benign or malignant liver tumors or liver disease, undiagnosed abnormal uterine bleeding, pregnancy, current or history of breast cancer or other estrogen- or progestin-sensitive cancer.

WARNINGS/PRECAUTIONS

Consider possibility of ovulation and conception prior to 1st use. Increased risk of a venous thromboembolic event (VTE) and arterial thromboses; d/c if these occur. D/C if unexplained loss of vision, proptosis, diplopia, papilledema, or retinal vascular lesions develop; evaluate for retinal vein thrombosis immediately. D/C at least 4 weeks prior to and 2 weeks after major surgery associated with an elevated risk of thromboembolism and during and following prolonged immobilization, if feasible. Caution in women with CV disease risk factors. If patient exhibits signs/symptoms of toxic shock syndrome (TSS), consider possibility of this diagnosis and initiate appropriate medical evaluation and treatment. Acute or chronic disturbances of liver function may necessitate discontinuation until LFTs return to normal and CHC causation has been excluded. D/C if jaundice develops. May increase risk of cervical cancer or intraepithelial neoplasia, hepatic adenoma, hepatocellular carcinoma, and gallbladder disease. Increase in BP reported; monitor BP and d/c if BP rises significantly. May not be suitable for women with conditions that make the vagina more susceptible to vaginal irritation or ulceration; vaginal/cervical erosion or ulceration reported. May increase risk of cholestasis with subsequent CHC use in patients with a history of CHC-related or pregnancy-related cholestasis. May decrease glucose tolerance; monitor prediabetic and diabetic women. Consider alternative contraception with uncontrolled dyslipidemia. May increase risk of pancreatitis with hypertriglyceridemia or a family history thereof. D/C if indicated and evaluate cause if new headaches that are recurrent, persistent, or severe develop. Consider discontinuation in case of increased frequency or severity of migraine during use. Unscheduled (breakthrough or intracyclic) bleeding and spotting reported; check for causes (eg, pregnancy, malignancy) if bleeding persists or occurs after previously regular cycles. Consider possibility of pregnancy if scheduled (withdrawal) bleeding does not occur and patient has not adhered to prescribed dosing schedule or has adhered to prescribed regimen and misses 2 consecutive periods; d/c if pregnancy confirmed. Caution with history of depression; d/c if it recurs to a serious degree. May induce or exacerbate angioedema in patients with hereditary angioedema. Chloasma may occur; avoid exposure to sun or UV radiation in women with a tendency to chloasma. Inadvertent insertion into urinary bladder reported; assess for ring insertion into urinary bladder with persistent urinary symptoms and if unable to locate ring. Cases of disconnection of the ring at the weld joint reported; discard the ring and replace it with a new ring if this occurs. May interfere with correct placement and position of a diaphragm. May influence results of certain lab tests.

ADVERSE REACTIONS

Vaginitis, headache, mood changes, device-related events, vaginal discharge, increased weight, N/V, vaginal discomfort, breast pain, dysmenorrhea, abdominal pain.

DRUG INTERACTIONS

May decrease plasma concentrations and potentially diminish effectiveness or increase breakthrough bleeding when used concomitantly with drugs or herbal products that induce CYP3A4 (eg, phenytoin, barbiturates, products containing St. John's wort); use an alternative method of contraception or a backup method when used concomitantly with enzyme inducers, and continue backup contraception for 28 days after discontinuing enzyme inducers. Atorvastatin, ascorbic acid, acetaminophen, CYP3A4 inhibitors (eg, itraconazole, grapefruit juice, ketoconazole), and vaginal miconazole nitrate may increase plasma hormone levels. HIV protease inhibitors (eg, nelfinavir, ritonavir, indinavir), hepatitis C virus protease inhibitors (eg, boceprevir, telaprevir), and non-nucleoside reverse transcriptase inhibitors (eg, nevirapine, etravirine) may cause significant changes in plasma levels. May inhibit the metabolism of other compounds (eg, cyclosporine, prednisolone, theophylline, tizanidine, voriconazole) and increase their plasma concentrations. May decrease levels of acetaminophen, clofibric acid, morphine, salicylic acid, and temazepam. May decrease levels of lamotrigine and reduce seizure control; dosage adjustments of lamotrigine may be necessary. May raise serum concentrations of thyroxine-binding globulin and cortisol-binding globulin; may need to increase dose of replacement thyroid hormone or cortisol therapy.

NURSING CONSIDERATIONS

Assessment: Assess for high risk of arterial or venous thrombotic diseases; benign or malignant liver tumors; liver disease; undiagnosed, abnormal uterine bleeding; presence or history of breast cancer or other estrogen- or progestin-sensitive cancer; pregnancy; and any other conditions where treatment is contraindicated/cautioned. Assess nursing status and for possible drug interactions.

Monitoring: Monitor for arterial thromboses or VTEs, TSS, hepatic adenomas, hepatocellular carcinoma, gallbladder disease, and other adverse effects. Monitor lipid levels with hyperlipidemia, BP, serum glucose levels in diabetic or prediabetic patients, and for signs of worsening depression with previous history. Have a yearly visit with patient for a BP check and for other indicated healthcare.

Patient Counseling: Inform of risks and benefits of therapy. Inform that cigarette smoking increases risk of serious CV events. Inform of increased risk of VTE. Counsel that therapy does not protect against HIV infection (AIDS) or other STDs. Instruct not to use during pregnancy and to d/c if pregnancy is planned or occurs during use. Instruct to use a barrier method of contraception when ring is out for >3 continuous hrs until ring has been used continuously for at least 7 days. Counsel to use a backup or alternative method of contraception when enzyme inducers are concomitantly used. Inform that breast milk production may be reduced with use. Instruct postpartum women who have not yet had a normal period, to use an additional nonhormonal method of contraception for the first 7 days. Instruct on proper usage and what to do if not compliant with timing of insertion and removal. Inform that ring may be expelled while removing a tampon, during intercourse, or with straining during a bowel movement. Inform that amenorrhea may occur. Advise that pregnancy should be ruled out in the event of amenorrhea, if ring has been out of the vagina for >3 consecutive hrs, if ring-free interval was extended >1 week, if a period was missed for ≥2 consecutive cycles, or if ring has been retained for >4 weeks.

Storage: 2-8°C (36-46°F). After dispensing, store up to 4 months at 25°C (77°F); excursions permitted to 15-30°C (59-86°F). Avoid direct sunlight or >30°C (86°F).

NUVIGIL – armodafinil **CIV**

Class: Wakefulness-promoting agent

ADULT DOSAGE

Excessive Sleepiness

Associated with Narcolepsy/Obstructive Sleep Apnea/Shift Work Disorder:
150-250mg qam

PEDIATRIC DOSAGE

Pediatric use may not have been established

DOSE MODIFICATION

Hepatic Impairment

Severe Impairment with/without Cirrhosis: Reduce dose

Elderly

Consider lower doses

ADMINISTRATION

Oral route

Narcolepsy/Obstructive Sleep Apnea

Take as single dose in am

Shift Work Disorder

Take 1 hr prior to start of work shift

HOW SUPPLIED

Tab: 50mg, 150mg, 200mg, 250mg

WARNINGS/PRECAUTIONS

Use only in patients who have had a complete evaluation of excessive sleepiness, and in whom a diagnosis of narcolepsy, OSA, or SWD has been made in accordance with International Classification of Sleep Disorders (ICSD) or Diagnostic and Statistical Manual of Mental Disorders (DSM) diagnostic criteria. Not indicated as treatment for underlying obstruction in OSA; if continuous positive airway pressure (CPAP) is the treatment of choice, treat with CPAP for an adequate period of time prior to initiation of therapy. Rare cases of serious or life-threatening rash, including Stevens-Johnson syndrome (SJS), toxic epidermal necrolysis (TEN), and drug rash with eosinophilia and systemic symptoms (DRESS) reported; d/c treatment at 1st sign of rash, unless rash is clearly not drug-related. Angioedema, anaphylactoid reactions, multiorgan hypersensitivity reactions, and psychiatric adverse experiences reported; d/c treatment if symptoms develop. Caution with cardiovascular disease (CVD) (eg, recent history of myocardial infarction, unstable angina). Avoid in patients with history of left ventricular hypertrophy or with mitral valve prolapse who have experienced mitral valve prolapse syndrome (eg, ischemic ECG changes, chest pain, arrhythmia) with CNS stimulants. May impair mental/physical abilities. Level of wakefulness may not return to normal in patients with abnormal levels of sleepiness. Potential for abuse. Caution in elderly.

ADVERSE REACTIONS

Headache, nausea, dizziness, insomnia, diarrhea, dry mouth, anxiety, depression, rash.

DRUG INTERACTIONS

Reduced exposure of CYP3A4/5 substrates (eg, cyclosporine, midazolam, triazolam); consider dose adjustment of these drugs. Effectiveness of steroidal contraceptives may be reduced during and for 1 month after discontinuation of therapy; alternative or concomitant methods of contraception are recommended. Cyclosporine levels may be reduced; monitor levels and consider dosage adjustment. Increased exposure of CYP2C19 substrates (eg, omeprazole, diazepam, phenytoin); dosage reduction of these drugs may be required. Frequently monitor PT/INR with warfarin.

NURSING CONSIDERATIONS

Assessment: Assess for hypersensitivity to modafinil or to drug, hepatic impairment, psychosis, depression, mania, left ventricular hypertrophy, mitral valve prolapse, other CVD, pregnancy/nursing status, and possible drug interactions. Perform a complete evaluation of excessive sleepiness and confirm diagnosis of narcolepsy, OSA, and/or SWD in accordance with ICSD or DSM diagnostic criteria.

Monitoring: Monitor for serious rash, SJS, TEN, DRESS, angioedema, anaphylaxis, hypersensitivity reactions, multiorgan hypersensitivity reactions, psychiatric adverse symptoms, and other adverse reactions. Monitor for signs of misuse or abuse. Monitor HR and BP. If used adjunctively with CPAP, monitor for CPAP compliance periodically. Frequently reassess degree of sleepiness; reevaluate long-term usefulness periodically if prescribed for an extended time. Consider close monitoring in elderly. Monitor PT/INR frequently with warfarin.

Patient Counseling: Inform that drug is not a replacement for sleep. Inform that therapy may improve but not eliminate the abnormal tendency to fall asleep; instruct not to alter previous behavior with regard to potentially dangerous activities or other activities requiring appropriate levels of wakefulness, until and unless treatment has shown to produce levels of wakefulness that permit such activities. Inform of importance of continuing previously prescribed treatments. Advise to avoid alcohol during therapy. Advise to notify physician if pregnant, intending to become pregnant, or nursing. Caution about increased risk of pregnancy when using steroidal contraceptives and for 1 month after discontinuation of therapy. Instruct to inform physician if taking/planning to take any prescribed or OTC drugs. Instruct to d/c and notify physician if rash, hives, mouth sores, blisters, peeling skin, trouble swallowing or breathing or related allergic phenomenon, depression, anxiety, or signs of psychosis or mania develop.

Storage: 20-25°C (68-77°F).

NYSTATIN ORAL – nystatin

Class: Polyene antifungal

RX

ADULT DOSAGE

Oral Candidiasis

Oral Cavity Infections Caused by *Candida albicans* (Monilia):

Sus:

4-6mL qid (1/2 of dose in each side of mouth)

Continue treatment for at least 48 hrs after perioral symptoms disappear and cultures demonstrate eradication of *Candida albicans*

Non-Esophageal GI Candidiasis

1-2 tab tid

Continue treatment for at least 48 hrs after clinical cure

Intestinal Candidiasis

Moniliasis:

Sus:

5-10mL tid

Continue treatment for at least 48 hrs after clinical cure

PEDIATRIC DOSAGE

Oral Candidiasis

Oral Cavity Infections Caused by *Candida albicans* (Monilia):

Sus:

Premature/Low Birth Weight Infants: 1mL qid

Infants: 2mL qid

Children: 4-6mL qid (1/2 of dose in each side of mouth)

Continue treatment for at least 48 hrs after perioral symptoms disappear and cultures demonstrate eradication of *C. albicans*

ADMINISTRATION

Oral route

Sus

Shake well before using

Retain in mouth as long as possible before swallowing

In infants and young children, use dropper to place 1/2 of dose in each side of mouth; avoid feeding for 5-10 min

Extemporaneous Preparation of Oral Sus: For adults and older children, add approximately 500,000 U of powder to about 1/2 cup of water and stir well. Use immediately after mixing and do not store

HOW SUPPLIED

Sus: 100,000 U/mL [60mL, 473mL]; Tab: 500,000 U

WARNINGS/PRECAUTIONS

Not for use in treatment of systemic mycoses. D/C if sensitization/irritation occurs.

ADVERSE REACTIONS

Oral irritation/sensitization, diarrhea, N/V, GI upset/disturbances.

NURSING CONSIDERATIONS

Assessment: Assess for history of hypersensitivity to the drug or any of its components, and pregnancy/nursing status. Confirm diagnosis of candidiasis.

Monitoring: Monitor for oral irritation/sensitization, and other adverse reactions.

Patient Counseling: Advise to notify physician if any adverse reactions (eg, sensitization, irritation) occur. Instruct to inform physician if pregnant, planning to become pregnant, or breastfeeding.

Storage: 20-25°C (68-77°F). (Sus) Avoid freezing.

OCUFLOX – ofloxacin

RX

Class: Fluoroquinolone

ADULT DOSAGE

Bacterial Conjunctivitis

Days 1-2:
1-2 drops in the affected eye(s) q2-4h

Days 3-7:
1-2 drops qid

Corneal Ulcers

Days 1-2:
1-2 drops into the affected eye every 30 min while awake; awaken at approx 4 and 6 hrs after retiring and instill 1-2 drops

Days 3 Through 7-9:
1-2 drops every hr while awake

Days 7-9 Through Treatment Completion:
1-2 drops qid

PEDIATRIC DOSAGE

Bacterial Conjunctivitis

≥1 Year:

Days 1-2:
1-2 drops in the affected eye(s) q2-4h

Days 3-7:
1-2 drops qid

Corneal Ulcers

≥1 Year:

Days 1-2:
1-2 drops into the affected eye every 30 min while awake; awaken at approx 4 and 6 hrs after retiring and instill 1-2 drops

Days 3 Through 7-9:
1-2 drops every hr while awake

Days 7-9 Through Treatment Completion:
1-2 drops qid

ADMINISTRATION
Ocular route

HOW SUPPLIED
Sol: 0.3% [5mL]

WARNINGS/PRECAUTIONS
Do not inject subconjunctivally or introduce directly into the eye's anterior chamber. Serious and occasionally fatal hypersensitivity (anaphylactic) reactions reported. Rare Stevens-Johnson syndrome (SJS), which progressed to toxic epidermal necrolysis (TEN) reported. May result in bacterial resistance with prolonged use or use in the absence of a proven/suspected bacterial infection or a prophylactic indication; take appropriate measures if superinfection develops. D/C at 1st appearance of skin rash or other signs of hypersensitivity reaction.

ADVERSE REACTIONS
Transient ocular burning/discomfort, stinging, redness, itching, chemical conjunctivitis/keratitis, ocular/periocular/facial edema, photophobia, blurred vision, tearing, dryness, eye pain, foreign body sensation.

DRUG INTERACTIONS
Systemic quinolone therapy may increase theophylline levels, interfere with caffeine metabolism, enhance effects of warfarin and its derivatives, and elevate SrCr with cyclosporine.

NURSING CONSIDERATIONS

Assessment: Assess for history of hypersensitivity to the drug, other quinolones, or any of its components, pregnancy/nursing status, and possible drug interactions.

Monitoring: Monitor for signs/symptoms of serious hypersensitivity/anaphylactic reactions, SJS, TEN, and other adverse reactions. Monitor for development of superinfection; examine with the aid of magnification (eg, slit lamp biomicroscopy) and fluorescein staining.

Patient Counseling: Instruct to avoid contaminating applicator tip with material from eye, fingers, or other sources. Inform that systemic therapy has been associated with hypersensitivity reactions, even following a single dose; instruct to d/c immediately and contact physician at the 1st sign of a rash/allergic reaction.

Storage: 15-25°C (59-77°F).

OFIRMEV – acetaminophen

RX

Class: Analgesic

Caution when prescribing, preparing, and administering therapy to avoid dosing errors that could result in accidental overdose and death. Ensure that the dose in mg and mL is not confused, the dosing is based on weight for patients <50kg, infusion pumps are properly programmed, and the total daily dose of acetaminophen (APAP) from all sources does not exceed max daily limits. Associated w/ cases of acute liver failure, at times resulting in liver transplant and death. Most cases of liver injury are associated w/ APAP use at doses that exceed the max daily limits, and often involve >1 APAP-containing product.

ADULT DOSAGE

Moderate to Severe Pain

Adjunct to Opioid Analgesics:

<50kg:
Usual: 12.5mg/kg q4h or 15mg/kg q6h
Max: 15mg/kg (up to 750mg)/dose or 75mg/kg (up to 3750mg)/day

≥50kg:
Usual: 650mg q4h or 1000mg q6h
Max: 1000mg/dose or 4000mg/day

Mild to Moderate Pain

<50kg:
Usual: 12.5mg/kg q4h or 15mg/kg q6h
Max: 15mg/kg (up to 750mg)/dose or 75mg/kg (up to 3750mg)/day

≥50kg:
Usual: 650mg q4h or 1000mg q6h
Max: 1000mg/dose or 4000mg/day

Fever

<50kg:
Usual: 12.5mg/kg q4h or 15mg/kg q6h
Max: 15mg/kg (up to 750mg)/dose or 75mg/kg (up to 3750mg)/day

≥50kg:
Usual: 650mg q4h or 1000mg q6h
Max: 1000mg/dose or 4000mg/day

PEDIATRIC DOSAGE

Moderate to Severe Pain

Adjunct to Opioid Analgesics:

2-12 Years:
Usual: 12.5mg/kg q4h or 15mg/kg q6h
Max: 15mg/kg (up to 750mg)/dose or 75mg/kg (up to 3750mg)/day

≥13 Years:

<50kg:
Usual: 12.5mg/kg q4h or 15mg/kg q6h
Max: 15mg/kg (up to 750mg)/dose or 75mg/kg (up to 3750mg)/day

≥50kg:
Usual: 650mg q4h or 1000mg q6h
Max: 1000mg/dose or 4000mg/day

Mild to Moderate Pain

2-12 Years:
Usual: 12.5mg/kg q4h or 15mg/kg q6h
Max: 15mg/kg (up to 750mg)/dose or 75mg/kg (up to 3750mg)/day

≥13 Years:

<50kg:
Usual: 12.5mg/kg q4h or 15mg/kg q6h
Max: 15mg/kg (up to 750mg)/dose or 75mg/kg (up to 3750mg)/day

≥50kg:
Usual: 650mg q4h or 1000mg q6h
Max: 1000mg/dose or 4000mg/day

Fever

2-12 Years:
Usual: 12.5mg/kg q4h or 15mg/kg q6h
Max: 15mg/kg (up to 750mg)/dose or 75mg/kg (up to 3750mg)/day

≥13 Years:

<50kg:
Usual: 12.5mg/kg q4h or 15mg/kg q6h
Max: 15mg/kg (up to 750mg)/dose or 75mg/kg (up to 3750mg)/day

≥50kg:
Usual: 650mg q4h or 1000mg q6h
Max: 1000mg/dose or 4000mg/day

DOSE MODIFICATION

Renal Impairment

Severe (CrCl ≤30mL/min): May need to give at longer dosing intervals and a reduced total daily dose

Hepatic Impairment

May need to reduce total daily dose

ADMINISTRATION

IV route

Minimum dosing interval should be 4 hrs

Adults and Adolescents >50kg Requiring 1000mg Doses

Administer the dose by inserting a vented IV set through the septum of the 100mL vial
May be administered w/o further dilution
Administer contents of the vial IV over 15 min

Doses <1000mg

Withdraw appropriate dose from vial and place into a separate empty, sterile container (eg, glass bottle, plastic IV container, syringe) for IV infusion
The entire 100mL vial is not intended for use in patients weighing <50kg; discard the unused portion
Place small volume pediatric doses up to 60mL in volume in a syringe and administer over 15 min using syringe pump
Once vacuum seal of vial is penetrated, or contents transferred to another container, administer dose w/in 6 hrs
Do not add other medications to sol; diazepam and chlorpromazine are physically incompatible

HOW SUPPLIED

Inj: 10mg/mL [100mL]

CONTRAINDICATIONS

Severe hepatic impairment or severe active liver disease.

WARNINGS/PRECAUTIONS

Caution w/ alcoholism, chronic malnutrition, or severe hypovolemia (eg, due to dehydration or blood loss). May cause serious skin reactions (eg, acute generalized exanthematous pustulosis, Stevens-Johnson syndrome, toxic epidermal necrolysis); d/c at the 1st appearance of skin rash or any other sign of hypersensitivity. Hypersensitivity and anaphylaxis reported; d/c immediately if symptoms occur.

ADVERSE REACTIONS

Liver failure, N/V, headache, insomnia, constipation, pruritus, agitation, atelectasis.

DRUG INTERACTIONS

Substances that induce or regulate CYP2E1 may alter the metabolism and increase hepatotoxic potential. Excessive alcohol use may induce hepatic cytochromes, but ethanol may also inhibit metabolism. Increased INR in some patients stabilized on sodium warfarin; more frequent assessment of INR may be appropriate.

NURSING CONSIDERATIONS

Assessment: Assess for previous hypersensitivity, alcoholism, chronic malnutrition, severe hypovolemia, hepatic/renal impairment, pregnancy/nursing status, and possible drug interactions.

Monitoring: Monitor for signs/symptoms of hypersensitivity and anaphylaxis, acute liver failure, serious skin reactions, and other adverse reactions. Monitor the end of infusion to prevent the possibility of air embolism, especially in cases where therapy is the primary infusion. Monitor INR frequently in patients stabilized on sodium warfarin.

Patient Counseling: Inform about the risks and benefits of therapy. Instruct not to exceed the recommended dose. Instruct to notify physician if any adverse reactions occur or if pregnant/nursing or planning to become pregnant. Counsel about possible drug interactions.

Storage: 20-25°C (68-77°F). Do not refrigerate or freeze.

OFLOXACIN – ofloxacin

RX

Class: Fluoroquinolone

Fluoroquinolones are associated with an increased risk of tendinitis and tendon rupture in all ages. Risk is further increased in patients >60 yrs of age, taking corticosteroids, and with kidney, heart, or lung transplants. May exacerbate muscle weakness with myasthenia gravis; avoid with known history of myasthenia gravis.

ADULT DOSAGE

Acute Bacterial Exacerbation of Chronic Bronchitis

400mg q12h for 10 days

Community-Acquired Pneumonia

400mg q12h for 10 days

Skin and Skin Structure Infections

Uncomplicated:
400mg q12h for 10 days

Gonorrhea

Acute, Uncomplicated Urethral and Cervical:
400mg single dose

Nongonococcal Urethritis

300mg q12h for 7 days

Nongonococcal Cervicitis

300mg q12h for 7 days

Mixed Infection of the Urethra/Cervix

300mg q12h for 7 days

Acute Pelvic Inflammatory Disease

400mg q12h for 10-14 days

Uncomplicated Cystitis

Due to *Escherichia coli/Klebsiella pneumoniae*: 200mg q12h for 3 days

PEDIATRIC DOSAGE

Pediatric use may not have been established

Due to Other Approved Pathogens: 200mg q12h for 7 days

Urinary Tract Infections

Complicated:
200mg q12h for 10 days

Prostatitis

300mg q12h for 6 weeks

DOSE MODIFICATION

Renal Impairment

CrCl 20-50mL/min: Administer usual recommended unit dose q24h
CrCl <20mL/min: Administer 50% of the usual recommended unit dose q24h

Hepatic Impairment

Severe Liver Function Disorders (eg, Cirrhosis w/ or w/o Ascites):
Max: 400mg/day

ADMINISTRATION

Oral route

Administer w/o regard to meals

HOW SUPPLIED

Tab: 200mg, 300mg, 400mg

WARNINGS/PRECAUTIONS

D/C if pain, swelling, inflammation, or rupture of a tendon occurs. Convulsions, increased intracranial pressure (including pseudotumor cerebri), and toxic psychosis reported. CNS stimulation may occur; d/c and institute appropriate measures if reactions occur. Caution with CNS disorder or risk factors that may predispose to seizures or lower seizure threshold. Serious and occasionally fatal hypersensitivity and/or anaphylactic reactions reported; d/c immediately at the 1st appearance of skin rash, jaundice, or any other sign of hypersensitivity and institute supportive measures. Cases of sensory or sensorimotor axonal polyneuropathy resulting in paresthesias, hypoesthesias, dysesthesias, and weakness reported; d/c immediately if symptoms occur. *Clostridium difficile*-associated diarrhea (CDAD) reported; d/c if CDAD suspected or confirmed. May result in bacterial resistance when used in the absence of a proven/strongly suspected bacterial infection or a prophylactic indication. Not shown to be effective in the treatment of syphilis. Maintain adequate hydration to prevent formation of highly concentrated urine. D/C therapy if photosensitivity/phototoxicity occurs. Prolongation of the QT interval on ECG, arrhythmia, and torsades de pointes reported; avoid with known QT interval prolongation or uncorrected hypokalemia. Caution in the presence of renal or hepatic insufficiency/impairment and in elderly, especially those on corticosteroids. Lab test interactions may occur.

ADVERSE REACTIONS

Tendinitis, tendon rupture, N/V, insomnia, headache, dizziness, diarrhea, external genital pruritus in women, vaginitis, abdominal pain, chest pain, decreased appetite, dry mouth, dysgeusia, fatigue.

DRUG INTERACTIONS

See Boxed Warning. Caution with drugs that may lower the seizure threshold. May prolong QT interval; avoid with Class IA (eg, quinidine, procainamide) or Class III (eg, amiodarone, sotalol) antiarrhythmics. Administration with antacids containing Ca^{2+}, Mg^{2+}, or aluminum, with sucralfate, with divalent or trivalent cations (eg, iron), with multivitamins containing zinc or with didanosine, chewable/buffered tabs or pediatric powder for oral sol may result in lower systemic levels; do not take within the 2-hr period before or after ofloxacin administration. Cimetidine may interfere with elimination. May elevate cyclosporine levels. May prolong $T_{1/2}$ of drugs metabolized by CYP450 (eg, cyclosporine, methylxanthines). NSAIDs may increase risk of CNS stimulation and convulsive seizures. Probenecid may affect renal tubular secretion. May increase theophylline levels and increase risk of theophylline-related adverse reactions; monitor theophylline levels closely and adjust theophylline dose, if appropriate. May enhance effects of warfarin or its derivatives; monitor PT or other suitable coagulation test. Disturbances of blood glucose with antidiabetic agents reported; monitor blood glucose levels closely.

NURSING CONSIDERATIONS

Assessment: Assess for risk factors for developing tendinitis and tendon rupture, history of myasthenia gravis, drug hypersensitivity, epilepsy, CNS disorders, risk factors that may predispose to seizures or lower seizure threshold, QT interval prolongation, uncorrected hypokalemia, renal/hepatic dysfunction, pregnancy/nursing status, and possible drug interactions. Obtain baseline culture and susceptibility tests. Perform serologic test for syphilis in patients with gonorrhea.

Monitoring: Monitor for tendinitis or tendon rupture, CNS effects, signs/symptoms of hypersensitivity reactions, CDAD, peripheral neuropathy, photosensitivity/phototoxicity reactions, ECG changes, and other adverse reactions. Monitor renal/hepatic/hematopoietic function with prolonged use. Perform periodic culture and susceptibility testing. Perform follow-up serologic test for syphilis after 3 months in patients with gonorrhea. Monitor PT or other coagulation tests with warfarin or its derivatives.

Patient Counseling: Advise to notify physician if pain, swelling, or inflammation of a tendon, or weakness or inability to move joints develops; instruct to d/c therapy and rest/refrain from exercise. Instruct to notify physician if experiencing worsening muscle weakness or breathing problems, sunburn-like reaction or skin eruption, and of all medications and supplements currently being taken. Inform that drug treats only bacterial, not viral, infections. Counsel to take exactly ud; inform that skipping doses or not completing full course of therapy may decrease effectiveness and increase bacterial resistance. Advise to drink fluids liberally. Instruct to d/c and notify physician if signs/symptoms of hypersensitivity reactions/allergic reactions or peripheral neuropathy develop. Inform that drug may cause dizziness and lightheadedness; advise to assess reaction to therapy before engaging in activities that require mental alertness or coordination. Counsel to minimize or avoid exposure to natural/artificial sunlight. Advise diabetic patients being treated with insulin or oral hypoglycemic drug to d/c therapy immediately if hypoglycemic reaction occurs and consult a physician. Instruct to notify physician of any history of convulsions. Advise to contact physician as soon as possible if watery and bloody stools (with or without stomach cramps and fever) develop. Instruct to notify physician if any symptoms of QT prolongation, including prolonged heart palpitations, or loss of consciousness occur. Advise not to take mineral supplements, vitamins with iron or minerals, antacids containing Ca^{2+}, Mg^{2+}, or aluminum, sucralfate, didanosine, chewable/buffered tabs, or pediatric powder for oral sol within the 2-hr period before or after taking ofloxacin.

Storage: 20-25°C (68-77°F).

OLEPTRO — trazodone hydrochloride

RX

Class: Triazolopyridine derivative

Antidepressants increased the risk of suicidal thinking and behavior (suicidality) in children, adolescents, and young adults in short-term studies of major depressive disorder (MDD) and other psychiatric disorders. Monitor and observe closely for clinical worsening, suicidality, or unusual changes in behavior. Not approved for use in pediatric patients.

ADULT DOSAGE

Major Depressive Disorder

Initial: 150mg qhs
Titrate: May increase by 75mg/day every 3 days (eg, start 225mg on Day 4 of therapy)
Max: 375mg/day
Maint: Generally recommended to continue treatment for several months after an initial response; maintain on the lowest effective dose
Once adequate response is achieved, may reduce dose gradually, w/ subsequent adjustment depending on therapeutic response

Dosing Considerations with MAOIs

Switching to/from an MAOI for Psychiatric Disorders:
Allow at least 14 days between discontinuation of an MAOI and initiation of treatment, and conversely allow at least 14 days between discontinuing treatment before starting an MAOI

Use w/ Other MAOIs (eg, Linezolid, IV Methylene Blue):
Do not start trazodone in patients being treated w/ linezolid or IV methylene blue
If acceptable alternatives are not available and benefits outweigh risks of serotonin syndrome, d/c trazodone promptly and administer linezolid or IV methylene blue; monitor for serotonin syndrome for 2 weeks or until 24 hrs after last dose of linezolid or IV methylene blue, whichever comes 1st. May resume trazodone therapy 24 hrs after last dose of linezolid or IV methylene blue

PEDIATRIC DOSAGE

Pediatric use may not have been established

DOSE MODIFICATION

Discontinuation

Gradually reduce dose whenever possible

ADMINISTRATION

Oral route

Take at the same time every day, in the late pm preferably hs, on an empty stomach
May swallow whole or as a 1/2 tab by breaking the tab along the score line; do not chew or crush

HOW SUPPLIED

Tab, Extended Release: 150mg*, 300mg* *scored

CONTRAINDICATIONS

Use of an MAOI for psychiatric disorders either concomitantly or within 14 days of stopping treatment. Treatment within 14 days of stopping an MAOI for psychiatric disorders. Starting treatment in patients being treated with other MAOIs (eg, linezolid, IV methylene blue).

WARNINGS/PRECAUTIONS

Monitor for withdrawal symptoms when discontinuing treatment; reduce dose gradually. Serotonin syndrome reported; d/c immediately and initiate supportive symptomatic treatment. Pupillary dilation that occurs following use may trigger an angle-closure attack in a patient with anatomically narrow angles who does not have a patent iridectomy. May precipitate mixed/manic episode in patients at risk for bipolar disorder; screen for risk of bipolar disorder prior to initiating treatment. Not approved for treatment of bipolar depression. May cause QT/QTc interval prolongation, torsades de pointes, cardiac arrhythmias, and hypotension, including orthostatic hypotension and syncope. Not recommended for use during the initial recovery phase of myocardial infarction (MI). May increase risk of bleeding events. Priapism reported; caution in men with conditions that may predispose to priapism (eg, sickle cell anemia, multiple myeloma, leukemia) or with penile anatomical deformation; d/c with erection lasting >6 hrs (painful or not). Hyponatremia may occur; caution in elderly and volume-depleted patients. Consider discontinuation in patients with symptomatic hyponatremia and institute appropriate medical intervention. May cause somnolence or sedation and may impair mental/physical abilities. Caution with cardiac disease, hepatic/renal impairment, and in elderly.

ADVERSE REACTIONS

Somnolence, sedation, headache, dry mouth, dizziness, nausea, fatigue, diarrhea, constipation, back pain, blurred vision, sexual dysfunction.

DRUG INTERACTIONS

See Contraindications. May cause serotonin syndrome with other serotonergic drugs (eg, triptans, TCAs, fentanyl) and with drugs that impair serotonin metabolism; d/c immediately if this occurs. May enhance response to alcohol, barbiturates, and other CNS depressants. Increased risk of cardiac arrhythmia with drugs that prolong QT interval or CYP3A4 inhibitors. CYP3A4 inhibitors (eg, ritonavir, ketoconazole, indinavir) may increase levels with the potential for adverse effects. Potent CYP3A4 inhibitors may increase risk of cardiac arrhythmia; consider lower dose of trazodone. Carbamazepine (CYP3A4 inducer) may decrease levels; monitor to determine if a trazodone dose increase is required. Increased serum digoxin or phenytoin levels reported; monitor serum levels and adjust dosages PRN. Concomitant use with an antihypertensive may require a dose reduction of the antihypertensive drug. Monitor for potential risk of bleeding and use caution with NSAIDs, aspirin, and other drugs that affect coagulation or bleeding. Increased risk of hyponatremia with diuretics. Altered PT reported in patients on warfarin.

NURSING CONSIDERATIONS

Assessment: Assess for drug hypersensitivity, risk for bipolar disorder, cardiac disease (eg, recent MI), conditions that may predispose to priapism, penile anatomical deformation, susceptibility to angle-closure glaucoma, volume depletion, hepatic/renal impairment, pregnancy/nursing status, and possible drug interactions.

Monitoring: Monitor for clinical worsening, suicidality, unusual changes in behavior, mania/hypomania, serotonin syndrome, angle-closure glaucoma, QT/QTc interval prolongation, cardiac arrhythmias, hypotension, syncope, bleeding events, priapism, hyponatremia, withdrawal symptoms, and other adverse reactions. Periodically reassess to determine the continued need for maintenance treatment.

Patient Counseling: Inform of the risks, benefits, and appropriate use of therapy. Instruct patients and caregivers to notify physician if signs of clinical worsening, changes in behavior, or suicidality occur. Instruct to report to physician the occurrence of anxiety, agitation, panic attacks, insomnia, irritability, hostility, aggressiveness, impulsivity, akathisia, hypomania, or mania. Instruct to inform physician if patient has history of bipolar disorder, cardiac disease, or MI. Caution about the risks of serotonin syndrome, angle-closure glaucoma, priapism, hypotension, syncope, bleeding, and withdrawal symptoms. Instruct men to immediately d/c use and contact physician if erection lasts >6 hrs, whether painful or not. Caution against performing potentially hazardous tasks (eg, operating machinery) until reasonably certain that treatment does not affect them. Inform that therapy may enhance response to alcohol. Instruct to notify physician if intending to become pregnant, or nursing.

Storage: 15-30°C (59-86°F).

OLUX-E – clobetasol propionate

RX

Class: Corticosteroid

ADULT DOSAGE

Inflammatory and Pruritic Manifestations of Corticosteroid-Responsive Dermatoses

Apply a capful as a thin layer to affected area(s) bid (am and pm), for up to 2 consecutive weeks

Max: 50g/week or 21 capfuls/week

PEDIATRIC DOSAGE

Inflammatory and Pruritic Manifestations of Corticosteroid-Responsive Dermatoses

≥12 Years:

Apply a thin layer to affected area(s) bid (am and pm), for up to 2 consecutive weeks

Max: 50g/week or 21 capfuls/week

ADMINISTRATION

Topical route

Shake can, hold upside down, and depress the actuator
Gently massage into the affected area(s) until foam is absorbed

HOW SUPPLIED

Foam: 0.05% [50g, 100g]

WARNINGS/PRECAUTIONS

May cause reversible hypothalamic-pituitary-adrenal (HPA) axis suppression with the potential for glucocorticosteroid insufficiency, Cushing's syndrome, hyperglycemia, and unmasking of latent diabetes mellitus; withdraw, reduce frequency, or substitute a less potent steroid if HPA axis suppression occurs. Manifestations of adrenal insufficiency may require systemic corticosteroids. Pediatric patients may be more susceptible to systemic toxicity. Local adverse reactions are more likely to occur with occlusive use, prolonged use, or use of higher potency corticosteroids. D/C if irritation occurs. Use appropriate antimicrobial agent with skin infections; d/c until infection is treated. Avoid application to eyes, face, groin, axillae, and area of skin atrophy. Flammable; avoid fire, flame, or smoking during and immediately following application. Do not apply on the chest if used during lactation. D/C if control is achieved.

ADVERSE REACTIONS

Application-site reaction, application-site atrophy, folliculitis, acneiform eruptions, hypopigmentation, perioral dermatitis, allergic contact dermatitis, secondary infection, irritation, striae, miliaria.

DRUG INTERACTIONS

Use of >1 corticosteroid-containing product may increase the total systemic corticosteroid exposure.

NURSING CONSIDERATIONS

Assessment: Assess for presence of concomitant skin infections, severity of dermatoses, factors that predispose to HPA axis suppression, pregnancy/nursing status, and possible drug interactions.

Monitoring: Monitor for signs/symptoms of HPA axis suppression, Cushing's syndrome, hyperglycemia, irritation, allergic contact dermatitis (eg, failure to heal), and skin infections. Monitor for systemic toxicity, linear growth retardation, delayed weight gain, and intracranial HTN in pediatric patients. Monitor response to therapy.

Patient Counseling: Counsel to use externally and exactly ud; avoid use on face, skin folds (eg, underarms, groin), eyes, or other mucous membranes. Advise to wash hands after use. Advise not to bandage or wrap treatment area, unless directed by physician. Counsel to contact physician if any local or systemic adverse reactions occur, if no improvement is seen after 2 weeks, or if surgery is contemplated. Advise that foam is flammable; avoid fire, flame, or smoking during application. Advise to d/c when control is achieved.

Storage: 20-25°C (68-77°F); excursions permitted between 15-30°C (59-86°F). Do not puncture or incinerate container. Do not expose to heat or store above 49°C (120°F).

OLYSIO – simeprevir

Class: HCV NS3/4A protease inhibitor

RX

ADULT DOSAGE

Chronic Hepatitis C (Genotype 1)

Combination w/ Peginterferon Alfa (Peg-IFN-alfa) and Ribavirin (RBV):
150mg qd
Treatment Duration:
Treatment-Naive and Prior Relapsers (Including Those w/ Cirrhosis):
Triple therapy (simeprevir/Peg-IFN-alfa/RBV) x 12 weeks; then dual therapy (Peg-IFN-alfa/RBV) x 12 weeks
Prior Non-Responders, Including Partial and Null Responders (Including Those w/ Cirrhosis):
Triple therapy x 12 weeks; then dual therapy x 36 weeks
Combination w/ Sofosbuvir:
150mg qd
Treatment Duration:
Treatment-Naive and Treatment-Experienced w/o Cirrhosis:
12 weeks
Treatment-Naive and Treatment-Experienced w/ Cirrhosis:
24 weeks

PEDIATRIC DOSAGE

Pediatric use may not have been established

DOSE MODIFICATION

Hepatic Impairment

Severe: Use not recommended
Decompensated Cirrhosis (Moderate or Severe Hepatic Impairment): Do not administer in combination w/ peginterferon alfa and ribavirin

Discontinuation

Hepatitis C Virus (HCV) Ribonucleic Acid (RNA) ≥25 IU/mL at Week 4:
D/C triple therapy
HCV RNA ≥25 IU/mL at Week 12:
D/C dual therapy (treatment w/ simeprevir is complete at Week 12)
HCV RNA ≥25 IU/mL at Week 24:
D/C dual therapy (treatment w/ simeprevir is complete at Week 12)

Other Important Modifications

Do not reinitiate if treatment is discontinued because of adverse reactions or inadequate on-treatment virologic response

ADMINISTRATION

Oral route

Take w/ food
Swallow whole
D/C therapy if any of the antiviral drugs used in combination w/ simeprevir for the treatment of chronic hepatitis C infection are permanently discontinued for any reason

HOW SUPPLIED

Cap: 150mg

CONTRAINDICATIONS

Refer to the individual monographs for peginterferon alfa (Peg-IFN-alfa), ribavirin (RBV), or other antiviral drugs.

WARNINGS/PRECAUTIONS

Efficacy in combination w/ Peg-IFN-alfa and RBV is substantially reduced in patients infected w/ hepatitis C virus (HCV) genotype 1a w/ an NS3 Q80K polymorphism at baseline; consider alternative therapy for these patients. Not recommended as monotherapy. Caution w/ moderate hepatic impairment (Child-Pugh Class B) and in patients of East Asian ancestry. Not recommended in patients who previously failed therapy w/ a treatment regimen that included simeprevir or other HCV protease inhibitors. Fatal cardiac arrest reported w/ sofosbuvir-containing regimen (ledipasvir/sofosbuvir). Photosensitivity reactions and rash observed; consider discontinuation of treatment if a photosensitivity reaction or severe rash occurs and monitor patients until resolved. Contains a sulfonamide moiety; insufficient data to exclude association between sulfa allergy and frequency/severity of adverse reactions. Refer to individual monograph of drugs used in combination w/ simeprevir.

ADVERSE REACTIONS

Rash (including photosensitivity), pruritus, nausea, myalgia, dyspnea, hyperbilirubinemia, fatigue, headache, insomnia, dizziness, diarrhea.

DRUG INTERACTIONS

Coadministration of amiodarone w/ simeprevir in combination w/ sofosbuvir may result in serious symptomatic bradycardia; coadministration is not recommended. If coadministration is required, cardiac monitoring is recommended in an in-patient setting for the first 48 hrs, after which outpatient or self-monitoring of HR should occur on a daily basis for at least the first 2 weeks of treatment. Caution is warranted and therapeutic drug monitoring of amiodarone, if available, is recommended for concomitant use of amiodarone w/ a simeprevir-containing regimen that does not contain sofosbuvir. Concomitant use w/ oral amiodarone may result in mild increases in amiodarone concentrations. Use w/ moderate or strong inducers or inhibitors of CYP3A may lead to significantly lower or higher exposure, respectively, which may result in reduced therapeutic effect or adverse reactions; coadministration is not recommended. May increase concentrations of organic anion-transporting polypeptide 1B1/3 and P-gp substrates, and drugs that are primarily metabolized by CYP3A4. Increased levels of digoxin, oral antiarrhythmics (eg, disopyramide, flecainide, mexiletine, propafenone), oral calcium channel blockers (eg, amlodipine, diltiazem, felodipine), oral midazolam, oral triazolam, and PDE-5 inhibitors (eg, sildenafil, tadalafil, vardenafil). Use w/ caution w/ oral midazolam/triazolam. Concomitant use w/ systemic erythromycin may increase levels of both agents; coadministration is not recommended. May increase cisapride or cyclosporine levels; coadministration is not recommended. May increase levels of darunavir, rosuvastatin, atorvastatin, simvastatin, pitavastatin, pravastatin, and lovastatin. May increase or decrease sirolimus levels. Levels may be decreased w/ anticonvulsants (eg, carbamazepine, oxcarbazepine, phenobarbital), rifampin, rifabutin, rifapentine, systemic dexamethasone, St. John's wort, or efavirenz; coadministration is not recommended. Levels may be increased w/ systemic clarithromycin or telithromycin, systemic antifungals (eg, itraconazole, ketoconazole, posaconazole), milk thistle (Silybum marianum), cobicistat-containing product (elvitegravir/cobicistat/emtricitabine/tenofovir disoproxil fumarate), darunavir/ritonavir, ritonavir, or cyclosporine; coadministration is not recommended. Levels may be increased or decreased w/ delavirdine, etravirine, nevirapine, or other ritonavir-boosted or unboosted HIV protease inhibitors (eg, atazanavir, fosamprenavir, lopinavir); coadministration is not recommended. Refer to PI for dosing modifications and monitoring parameters when used w/ certain concomitant therapies.

NURSING CONSIDERATIONS

Assessment: Assess for presence of HCV genotype 1a w/ NS3 Q80K polymorphism, hepatic impairment, sulfa allergy, pregnancy/nursing status, and possible drug interactions. Obtain baseline HCV-RNA levels.

Monitoring: Monitor for photosensitivity reactions, rash, and other adverse reactions. Monitor HCV RNA levels as clinically indicated.

Patient Counseling: Inform that drug must be used in combination w/ other antiviral drugs. Counsel about the risk of serious symptomatic bradycardia when coadministered w/ amiodarone in combination w/ sofosbuvir; advise to seek medical evaluation immediately if signs/symptoms of bradycardia (eg, near-fainting or fainting, dizziness or lightheadedness, malaise) develop. Advise female patients to use effective contraception during treatment. Inform of the risk of photosensitivity reactions/rash and that these reactions may become severe; instruct to contact physician if a photosensitivity reaction or rash develops and not to stop treatment unless instructed by physician. Advise to use sun protection measures (eg, sunglasses, protective clothing, sunscreen), limit exposure to natural sunlight, and avoid artificial sunlight (tanning beds, phototherapy) during treatment. Advise that reducing or interrupting treatment may increase possibility of treatment failure. Instruct to take missed dose w/ food as soon as possible if a dose is missed and it is w/in 12 hrs of the usual dosing time, and then to take the next dose at the regularly scheduled time. Inform that the effect of treatment of hepatitis C on transmission is unknown; instruct to take appropriate precautions to prevent transmission.

Storage: Room temperature <30°C (86°F). Protect from light.

OMNARIS – ciclesonide

Class: Non-halogenated glucocorticoid

RX

ADULT DOSAGE

Seasonal/Perennial Allergic Rhinitis

2 sprays/nostril qd
Max: 2 sprays/nostril/day (200mcg/day)

PEDIATRIC DOSAGE

Perennial Allergic Rhinitis

≥12 Years:
2 sprays/nostril qd
Max: 2 sprays/nostril/day (200mcg/day)

Seasonal Allergic Rhinitis

≥6 Years:
2 sprays/nostril qd
Max: 2 sprays/nostril/day (200mcg/day)

DOSE MODIFICATION

Elderly
Start at low end of dosing range

ADMINISTRATION

Intranasal route

Priming
Shake bottle gently and prime pump by actuating 8X before initial use
Reprime w/ 1 spray or until fine mist appears if not used for 4 consecutive days

HOW SUPPLIED

Spray: 50mcg/spray [12.5g]

WARNINGS/PRECAUTIONS

Epistaxis reported. *Candida albicans* infections of the nose or pharynx may occur; examine periodically and treat accordingly. Nasal septal perforation may occur; avoid spraying directly onto nasal septum. May impair wound healing; avoid w/ recent nasal septal ulcers, nasal surgery, or nasal trauma until healing has occurred. Glaucoma and/or cataracts may develop. Risk for more severe/fatal course of infections (eg, chickenpox, measles); avoid exposure in patients who have not had these diseases or have not been properly immunized. May increase susceptibility to infections; caution w/ active or quiescent tuberculosis (TB), untreated local or systemic fungal/bacterial infections, systemic viral or parasitic infections, or ocular herpes simplex. D/C slowly if hypercorticism and adrenal suppression occur. Risk of adrenal insufficiency and withdrawal symptoms when replacing systemic corticosteroids w/ topical corticosteroids. May exacerbate symptoms of asthma and other conditions requiring long-term systemic corticosteroid use w/ rapid dose decrease. May reduce growth velocity in pediatric patients. Caution in elderly.

ADVERSE REACTIONS

Headache, epistaxis, nasopharyngitis, back pain, pharyngolaryngeal pain, sinusitis, influenza, nasal discomfort, bronchitis, UTI, cough.

DRUG INTERACTIONS

Ketoconazole may increase exposure of the active metabolite des-ciclesonide.

NURSING CONSIDERATIONS

Assessment: Assess for drug hypersensitivity, TB, any infections, ocular herpes simplex, history of increased IOP, glaucoma, cataracts, recent nasal septal ulcers, nasal surgery/trauma, use of other inhaled or systemic corticosteroids, pregnancy/nursing status, and possible drug interactions. Assess if patients have not been immunized or exposed to infections, such as measles or chickenpox.

Monitoring: Monitor for hypercorticism, adrenal suppression, TB, infections, ocular herpes simplex, chickenpox, and measles. Monitor for epistaxis, nasal septal perforation, growth velocity in children, wound healing, visual changes, hypoadrenalism in infants born to mothers receiving corticosteroids during pregnancy, and hypersensitivity reactions. Monitor for adrenal insufficiency and withdrawal symptoms when replacing systemic w/ topical corticosteroids.

Patient Counseling: Counsel on appropriate priming and administration of spray; avoid spraying in eyes or directly onto nasal septum. Instruct to take ud at regular intervals; not to exceed prescribed dosage. Instruct to contact physician if symptoms do not improve by a reasonable time (over 1-2 weeks in seasonal allergic rhinitis and 5 weeks in perennial allergic rhinitis) or if condition worsens. Counsel about risks of epistaxis, nasal ulceration, *Candida* infections, and other adverse reactions. Instruct to avoid exposure to chickenpox or measles and to consult physician if exposed to chickenpox or measles. Inform that worsening of existing TB infections, fungal/bacterial/viral/parasitic infections, or ocular herpes simplex may occur. Instruct to inform physician if change in vision occurs.

Storage: 25°C (77°F); excursions permitted to 15-30°C (59-86°F). Do not freeze. Discard after 4 months after removal from pouch or after 120 actuations following initial priming, whichever comes 1st.

OMTRYG – omega-3-acid ethyl esters A

RX

Class: Lipid-regulating agent

ADULT DOSAGE

Severe Hypertriglyceridemia (≥500mg/dL)

Usual: 4 caps qd or 2 caps bid

PEDIATRIC DOSAGE

Pediatric use may not have been established

ADMINISTRATION

Oral route

Take with meals

Swallow caps whole; do not break open, crush, dissolve, or chew

HOW SUPPLIED

Cap: 1.2g

WARNINGS/PRECAUTIONS

Increases in ALT levels without a concurrent increase in AST levels reported. May increase LDL levels; monitor LDL levels periodically during therapy. Contains ethyl esters of omega-3 fatty acids (eicosapentaenoic acid [EPA] and docosahexaenoic acid [DHA]) obtained from oil of several fish sources; caution with known hypersensitivity to fish and/or shellfish. Recurrent symptomatic atrial fibrillation/flutter (A-fib/flutter) reported in patients with paroxysmal or persistent A-fib, particularly within the first 2-3 months of initiating therapy. Assess TG levels carefully before initiating therapy and monitor TG levels periodically during therapy.

ADVERSE REACTIONS

Eructation, taste perversion, dyspepsia.

DRUG INTERACTIONS

Periodically monitor patients receiving concomitant treatment with an anticoagulant or other drugs affecting coagulation (eg, antiplatelet agents). D/C or change medications known to exacerbate hypertriglyceridemia (eg, β-blockers, thiazides, estrogens), if possible, prior to consideration of therapy.

NURSING CONSIDERATIONS

Assessment: Assess for hypersensitivity to drug, fish, and/or shellfish; hepatic impairment; A-fib/flutter; pregnancy/nursing status; and possible drug interactions. Attempt to control serum lipids with appropriate diet, exercise, weight loss in obese patients, and control of any medical problems that are contributing to lipid abnormalities. Assess TG and LDL levels.

Monitoring: Monitor for recurrent symptomatic A-fib/flutter in patients with paroxysmal or persistent A-fib. Monitor for allergic reactions and other adverse reactions. Periodically monitor ALT and AST levels in patients with hepatic impairment. Periodically monitor LDL and TG levels.

Patient Counseling: Instruct to notify physician if allergic to fish and/or shellfish. Advise that the use of lipid-regulating agents does not reduce the importance of adhering to diet. Instruct to take ud.

Storage: 25°C (77°F); excursions permitted to 15-30°C (59-86°F). Do not freeze.

ONDANSETRON – ondansetron

RX

Class: 5-HT_3 receptor antagonist

OTHER BRAND NAMES

Zofran, Zofran ODT

ADULT DOSAGE

Chemotherapy-Associated Nausea/Vomiting

Inj:

Prevention of N/V Associated w/ Initial and Repeat Courses of Emetogenic Chemotherapy (Including High-Dose Cisplatin):

Three 0.15mg/kg IV doses (diluted) up to a max of 16mg/dose; infuse over 15 min. Give 1st dose 30 min before the start of chemotherapy, then give subsequent doses 4 and 8 hrs after the 1st dose

PEDIATRIC DOSAGE

Chemotherapy-Associated Nausea/Vomiting

Inj:

Prevention of N/V Associated w/ Initial and Repeat Courses of Emetogenic Chemotherapy (Including High-Dose Cisplatin):

6 Months-18 Years of Age:

Three 0.15mg/kg IV doses (diluted) up to a max of 16mg/dose; infuse over 15 min. Give 1st dose 30 min before the start of chemotherapy, then give subsequent doses 4 and 8 hrs after the 1st dose

Oral:

Prevention of N/V Associated w/ Highly Emetogenic Chemotherapy (Including Cisplatin ≥50mg/m²):
24mg (given as three 8mg tabs) 30 min before start of single-day chemotherapy

Prevention of N/V Associated w/ Moderately Emetogenic Chemotherapy:
8mg bid; give 1st dose 30 min before chemotherapy, then give subsequent dose 8 hrs after 1st dose, then administer 8mg q12h for 1-2 days after completion of chemotherapy

Postoperative Nausea/Vomiting

Prevention:

Inj:
4mg IM/IV undiluted immediately before induction of anesthesia or postoperatively if prophylactic antiemetic was not received and N/V occurs w/in 2 hrs after surgery; infuse IV in not <30 sec, preferably over 2-5 min

Oral:
16mg given 1 hr before induction of anesthesia

Radiotherapy Associated Nausea/Vomiting

Oral:

Prevention in Patients Receiving Either Total Body Irradiation, Single High-Dose Fraction to the Abdomen, or Daily Fractions to the Abdomen:
Usual: 8mg tid

Total Body Irradiation:
8mg should be administered 1-2 hrs before each fraction of radiotherapy administered each day

Single High-Dose Fraction Radiotherapy to the Abdomen:
8mg should be administered 1-2 hrs before radiotherapy, w/ subsequent doses q8h after 1st dose for 1-2 days after completion of radiotherapy

Daily Fractionated Radiotherapy to the Abdomen:
8mg should be administered 1-2 hrs before radiotherapy, w/ subsequent doses q8h after 1st dose for each day radiotherapy is given

Oral:

Prevention of N/V Associated w/ Moderately Emetogenic Cancer Chemotherapy:

4-11 Years:
4mg tid; give 1st dose 30 min before chemotherapy, then give subsequent doses 4 and 8 hrs after 1st dose, then administer 4mg q8h for 1-2 days after completion of chemotherapy

≥12 Years:
8mg bid; give 1st dose 30 min before chemotherapy, then give subsequent dose 8 hrs after 1st dose, then administer 8mg q12h for 1-2 days after completion of chemotherapy

Postoperative Nausea/Vomiting

Prevention:

1 Month-12 Years of Age:

Inj:
≤40kg: 0.1mg/kg IV single dose. Infuse in not <30 sec, preferably over 2-5 min immediately before or after induction of anesthesia or postoperatively if prophylactic antiemetic was not received and N/V occurs shortly after surgery
>40kg: 4mg IV single dose

DOSE MODIFICATION

Hepatic Impairment

Severe (Child-Pugh Score ≥10):

Oral:
Max: 8mg/day

Inj:
Max: 8mg/day infused over 15 min beginning 30 min prior to emetogenic chemotherapy

ADMINISTRATION

IV/M/Oral routes

ODT

Do not attempt to push tabs through the foil backing
Peel back the foil backing of 1 blister and gently remove tab
Immediately place tab on top of the tongue where it will dissolve in seconds, then swallow w/ saliva

Inj

Should be diluted in 50mL of D5 or NaCl before administration
Do not mix w/ alkaline solutions as a precipitate may form

HOW SUPPLIED

Tab: 24mg; (Zofran) Inj: 2mg/mL [20mL], Sol: 4mg base/5mL [50mL], Tab/Tab, Disintegrating (ODT): 4mg, 8mg

CONTRAINDICATIONS

Concomitant use w/ apomorphine.

WARNINGS/PRECAUTIONS

Hypersensitivity reactions reported in patients hypersensitive to other selective 5-HT_3 receptor antagonists. ECG changes, including QT interval prolongation and torsades de pointes, reported; avoid in patients w/ congenital long QT syndrome. Monitor ECG in patients with electrolyte abnormalities (eg, hypokalemia, hypomagnesemia), CHF, bradyarrhythmias, and in patients taking other medications that lead to QT prolongation. Serotonin syndrome reported; d/c and initiate supportive treatment if symptoms occur. Use in patients following abdominal surgery or w/ chemotherapy-induced N/V may mask a progressive ileus and/or gastric distension. Does not stimulate gastric/intestinal peristalsis; do not use instead of NG suction. (ODT) Contains phenylalanine; caution in phenylketonuric patients.

ADVERSE REACTIONS

Headache, diarrhea, constipation, fever, pruritus, dizziness, bradycardia, drowsiness/sedation. (Inj) Inj-site reaction. (PO) Malaise/fatigue, anxiety/agitation, urinary retention.

DRUG INTERACTIONS

See Contraindications. Inducers or inhibitors of CYP3A4, CYP2D6, and CYP1A2 may change the clearance and $T_{1/2}$. Potent CYP3A4 inducers (eg, phenytoin, carbamazepine, rifampin) may significantly increase clearance and decrease blood levels. May reduce analgesic activity of tramadol. May cause serotonin syndrome w/ other serotonergic drugs (eg, SSRIs, SNRIs, MAOIs, mirtazapine, fentanyl, lithium, tramadol, IV methylene blue); d/c and initiate supportive treatment if symptoms occur.

NURSING CONSIDERATIONS

Assessment: Assess for previous hypersensitivity to the drug, congenital long QT syndrome, electrolyte abnormalities, CHF, bradyarrhythmias, hepatic impairment, pregnancy/nursing status, and possible drug interactions. (ODT) Assess for phenylketonuria.

Monitoring: Monitor for QT interval prolongation, torsades de pointes, hypersensitivity reactions, serotonin syndrome, and other adverse reactions. Monitor ECG in patients w/ electrolyte abnormalities, CHF, bradyarrhythmias, and in patients taking other medications that lead to QT prolongation. In patients who recently underwent abdominal surgery or in patients w/ chemotherapy-induced N/V, monitor for masking of a progressive ileus and/or gastric distension.

Patient Counseling: Inform about potential benefits/risks of therapy. Inform that drug may cause serious cardiac arrhythmias (eg, QT prolongation); instruct patients to contact physician if they perceive a change in their HR, if they feel lightheaded, or have a syncopal episode. Inform that chances of developing severe cardiac arrhythmias are higher in patients w/ a personal/family history of abnormal heart rhythms (eg, congenital long QT syndrome), patients taking medications (eg, diuretics) that may cause electrolyte abnormalities, and in patients w/ hypokalemia or hypomagnesemia. Advise of the possibility of serotonin syndrome; instruct to seek immediate medical attention if changes in mental status, autonomic instability, neuromuscular symptoms w/ or w/o GI symptoms occur. Inform that drug may cause hypersensitivity reactions, some as severe as anaphylaxis and bronchospasm; instruct to report any signs/symptoms of hypersensitivity reactions to physician. Advise to report the use of all medications to physician. Inform that drug may cause headache, drowsiness/sedation, constipation, fever, and diarrhea. Inform phenylketonuric patients that ODT contains phenylalanine.

Storage: 20-25°C (68-77°F); excursions permitted to 15-30°C (59-86°F). Protect from light. Zofran: (Inj/ODT/Tab) 2-30°C (36-86°F). (Sol) 15-30°C (59-86°F); store bottles upright in cartons. (Inj/Sol/Tab) Protect from light. (Inj) Diluted Sol: Do not use beyond 24 hrs. Refer to PI for further information on stability and handling.

ONFI – clobazam

CIV

Class: Benzodiazepine

ADULT DOSAGE

Seizures

Associated with Lennox-Gastaut Syndrome:

≤30kg:
Initial: 5mg/day
Starting Day 7: 10mg/day
Starting Day 14: 20mg/day

>30kg:
Initial: 10mg/day
Starting Day 7: 20mg/day
Starting Day 14: 40mg/day

Do not proceed with dose escalation more rapidly than weekly

For doses >5mg/day, administer in divided doses bid

PEDIATRIC DOSAGE

Seizures

Associated with Lennox-Gastaut Syndrome:

≥2 Years:

≤30kg:
Initial: 5mg/day
Starting Day 7: 10mg/day
Starting Day 14: 20mg/day

>30kg:
Initial: 10mg/day
Starting Day 7: 20mg/day
Starting Day 14: 40mg/day

Do not proceed with dose escalation more rapidly than weekly

For doses >5mg/day, administer in divided doses bid

DOSE MODIFICATION

Hepatic Impairment

Mild to Moderate (Child-Pugh Score 5-9):

Initial: 5mg/day

Titrate: Titrate according to weight, but to 1/2 the recommended dose, as tolerated; additional titration to the max dose (20mg/day or 40mg/day, depending on weight) may be started on day 21

Elderly

Initial: 5mg/day

Titrate: Titrate according to weight, but to 1/2 the recommended dose, as tolerated; additional titration to the max dose (20mg/day or 40mg/day, depending on weight) may be started on day 21

Discontinuation

Withdraw gradually; taper by decreasing total daily dose by 5-10mg/day on a weekly basis

Other Important Modifications

CYP2C19 Poor Metabolizers:

Initial: 5mg/day

Titrate: Titrate according to weight, but to 1/2 the recommended dose, as tolerated; additional titration to the max dose (20mg/day or 40mg/day, depending on weight) may be started on day 21

ADMINISTRATION

Oral route

Take with or without food

Tab

May administer whole, break in 1/2 along the score, or crush and mix in applesauce

Sus

Shake well before every administration

Administer using only the dosing syringe provided with the product

To Withdraw a Dose:

1. Insert the provided adapter firmly into the neck of the bottle before first use
2. Insert the dosing syringe into the adapter and invert bottle then slowly pull back plunger to prescribed dose
3. Remove the syringe from the bottle adapter and slowly squirt dose into the corner of the patient's mouth
4. Replace cap after each use (the cap fits over the adapter)

HOW SUPPLIED

Sus: 2.5mg/mL [120mL]; Tab: 10mg*, 20mg* *scored

WARNINGS/PRECAUTIONS

Dose-related somnolence and sedation reported. May impair mental/physical abilities. Withdrawal symptoms reported to occur following abrupt discontinuation; withdraw gradually to minimize risk of precipitating seizures, seizure exacerbation, or status epilepticus. Serious skin reactions (eg, Stevens-Johnson syndrome [SJS], toxic epidermal necrolysis [TEN]) reported; d/c at the 1st sign of rash, unless the rash is clearly not drug-related. If signs/symptoms suggest SJS/TEN, do not resume therapy and consider alternative therapy. Monitor patients with history of substance abuse because of predisposition to habituation and dependence. May increase risk of suicidal thoughts or behavior; monitor for the emergence or worsening of depression, suicidal thoughts/behavior, and/or any unusual changes in mood/behavior.

ADVERSE REACTIONS

Somnolence, pyrexia, upper respiratory tract infection, lethargy, drooling, aggression, vomiting, irritability, constipation, fatigue, sedation, ataxia, insomnia, cough, pneumonia.

DRUG INTERACTIONS

May potentiate effects of other CNS depressants or alcohol; monitor for somnolence and sedation. May decrease effectiveness of hormonal contraceptives; additional nonhormonal forms of contraception are recommended. CYP2D6 substrates may require dose adjustment. Strong (eg, fluconazole, fluvoxamine, ticlopidine) and moderate (eg, omeprazole) inhibitors of CYP2C19 may increase exposure to N-desmethylclobazam; may require dose adjustment of clobazam. Alcohol may increase maximum plasma exposure.

NURSING CONSIDERATIONS

Assessment: Assess for hypersensitivity to drug, hepatic impairment, history of substance abuse, pregnancy/nursing status, and possible drug interactions. Assess if patient is a CYP2C19 poor metabolizer.

Monitoring: Monitor for somnolence, sedation, withdrawal symptoms, habituation, physical/psychological dependence, emergence or worsening of depression, suicidal thoughts/behavior, unusual changes in mood/behavior, and other adverse reactions. Closely monitor for signs/symptoms of SJS/TEN, especially during the first 8 weeks of treatment initiation or when reintroducing therapy.

Patient Counseling: Caution about operating hazardous machinery, including automobiles, until the effect of the treatment is known. Inform to consult physician before increasing the dose or abruptly discontinuing the drug. Instruct to notify physician if a skin reaction occurs. Advise that abrupt withdrawal may increase risk of seizure. Counsel women to also use nonhormonal methods of contraception when clobazam is used with hormonal contraceptives and to continue these alternative methods for 28 days after discontinuation. Inform that clobazam may increase the risk of suicidal thoughts and behavior and counsel to be alert for the emergence or worsening of symptoms of depression, any unusual changes in mood/behavior, or the emergence of suicidal thoughts, behavior, or thoughts of self-harm; instruct to immediately report behaviors of concern to physician. Instruct to notify physician if pregnant/breastfeeding, or if intending to breastfeed or become pregnant during therapy. Encourage to enroll in the North American Antiepileptic Drug Pregnancy Registry if patient becomes pregnant.

Storage: 20-25°C (68-77°F). (Sus) Store in original bottle in an upright position. Use within 90 days of 1st opening the bottle; discard any remainder.

ONGLYZA – saxagliptin RX

Class: Dipeptidyl peptidase-4 (DPP-4) inhibitor

ADULT DOSAGE

Type 2 Diabetes Mellitus

2.5mg or 5mg qd

PEDIATRIC DOSAGE

Pediatric use may not have been established

DOSE MODIFICATION

Concomitant Medications

Strong CYP3A4/5 Inhibitors: 2.5mg qd

Insulin Secretagogue (eg, Sulfonylurea)/Insulin: May require a lower dose of insulin secretagogue or insulin

Renal Impairment

Moderate or Severe/ESRD Requiring Hemodialysis (CrCl ≤50mL/min): 2.5mg qd

Administer following hemodialysis

ADMINISTRATION

Oral route

Take w/ or w/o meals

Do not split or cut tab

HOW SUPPLIED

Tab: 2.5mg, 5mg

WARNINGS/PRECAUTIONS

Not for treatment of type 1 DM or diabetic ketoacidosis. Not studied in patients w/ a history of pancreatitis. Acute pancreatitis reported; d/c if pancreatitis is suspected. Serious hypersensitivity reactions reported; if suspected, d/c therapy, assess for other potential causes, and institute alternative treatment. Caution in patients w/ history of angioedema to another dipeptidyl peptidase-4 (DPP-4) inhibitor and in elderly. No conclusive evidence of macrovascular risk reduction.

ADVERSE REACTIONS

Upper respiratory tract infection, urinary tract infection, headache, peripheral edema.

DRUG INTERACTIONS

May require lower dose of insulin secretagogue (eg, sulfonylurea) or insulin to minimize risk of hypoglycemia. Ketoconazole or other strong CYP3A4/5 inhibitors (eg, atazanavir, clarithromycin, itraconazole, nefazodone) may increase plasma concentrations. Strong CYP3A4/5 inducers and inhibitors may alter pharmacokinetics of saxagliptin and its active metabolite.

NURSING CONSIDERATIONS

Assessment: Assess for previous hypersensitivity to the drug, history of pancreatitis, type of DM, diabetic ketoacidosis, history of angioedema to another DPP-4 inhibitor, pregnancy/nursing status, and possible drug interactions. Obtain baseline renal function, and FPG and HbA1c levels.

Monitoring: Monitor for pancreatitis, hypersensitivity reactions, and other adverse reactions. Monitor FPG, HbA1c, and renal function periodically. Measure lymphocyte count when clinically indicated (eg, settings of unusual or prolonged infection).

Patient Counseling: Inform of the potential risks, benefits, and alternative modes of therapy. Advise on the importance of adherence to dietary instructions, regular physical activity, periodic blood glucose monitoring and HbA1c testing, recognition and management of hypoglycemia and hyperglycemia, and assessment of diabetic complications. Instruct to seek medical advice promptly during periods of stress as medication requirements may change. Instruct to d/c use and notify physician if signs and symptoms of pancreatitis or allergic reactions occur. Counsel to inform physician if any unusual symptom develops, or if any existing symptom persists or worsens. Inform that if a dose was missed, to take the next dose as prescribed, unless otherwise instructed by physician; instruct not to take an extra dose the next day.

Storage: 20-25°C (68-77°F); excursions permitted to 15-30°C (59-86°F).

Opana ER – oxymorphone hydrochloride **CII**

Class: Opioid analgesic

Exposes users to risks of addiction, abuse, and misuse, leading to overdose and death; assess each patient's risk prior to prescribing and monitor regularly for development of these behaviors/conditions. Serious, life-threatening, or fatal respiratory depression may occur; monitor upon initiation or following a dose increase. Crushing, chewing, or dissolving tab can cause rapid release and absorption of potentially fatal dose; instruct patients to swallow tab whole. Accidental ingestion of even 1 dose, especially by children, can result in a fatal overdose. Prolonged use during pregnancy can result in neonatal opioid withdrawal syndrome; advise pregnant women of the risk and ensure availability of appropriate treatment. Avoid use with alcoholic beverages or medications containing alcohol; co-ingestion may result in increased plasma levels and potentially fatal overdose.

ADULT DOSAGE

Severe Pain (Daily, Around-the-Clock Management)

1st Opioid Analgesic/Opioid Intolerant Patients:

Initial: 5mg q12h

Titrate: May adjust dose every 3-7 days in increments of 5-10mg q12h

Conversions

From IR to ER Oxymorphone:
Administer 1/2 the total daily IR dose as ER, q12h

From Parenteral Oxymorphone:
Administer 10X the total daily parenteral oxymorphone dose as ER in 2 equally divided doses

From Other Oral Opioids:
D/C all other around-the-clock opioids when therapy is initiated; refer to PI for conversion factors and dose calculations

PEDIATRIC DOSAGE

Pediatric use may not have been established

DOSE MODIFICATION

Renal Impairment

CrCl <50mL/min:

Opioid-Naive: Initiate treatment w/ 5mg dose

On Prior Opioid Therapy: Initiate at 50% lower than the starting dose for a patient w/ normal renal function on prior opioids and titrate slowly

Hepatic Impairment

Mild:

Opioid-Naive: Initiate treatment w/ 5mg dose

On Prior Opioid Therapy: Initiate at 50% lower than the starting dose for a patient w/ normal hepatic function on prior opioids and titrate slowly

Moderate or Severe:
Contraindicated

Elderly

Opioid-Naive: Initiate treatment w/ 5mg dose

On Prior Opioid Therapy: Initiate at 50% lower than the starting dose for a younger patient on prior opioids and titrate slowly

Discontinuation

Use gradual downward dose titration every 2-4 days

ADMINISTRATION

Oral route

Do not pre-soak, lick, or otherwise wet tab prior to placing in mouth
Swallow tab whole; do not crush, dissolve, or chew

Take 1 tab at a time w/ enough water to ensure complete swallowing
Take on an empty stomach, at least 1 hr ac or 2 hrs pc

HOW SUPPLIED
Tab, ER: 5mg, 7.5mg, 10mg, 15mg, 20mg, 30mg, 40mg

CONTRAINDICATIONS
Significant respiratory depression, acute or severe bronchial asthma or hypercarbia, known or suspected paralytic ileus and GI obstruction, and moderate or severe hepatic impairment.

WARNINGS/PRECAUTIONS
Reserve use in patients for whom alternative treatment options are ineffective, not tolerated, or would be otherwise inadequate to provide sufficient management of pain. Should only be prescribed by healthcare professionals who are knowledgeable in the use of potent opioids for management of chronic pain. Life-threatening respiratory depression is more likely to occur in elderly, cachectic, or debilitated patients. Consider alternative nonopioid analgesics in patients with significant COPD or cor pulmonale, and in patients having a substantially decreased respiratory reserve, hypoxia, hypercapnia, or preexisting respiratory depression. May cause severe hypotension, orthostatic hypotension, and syncope; increased risk in patients whose ability to maintain BP has already been compromised by a reduced blood volume or concurrent administration of certain CNS depressants. Avoid with circulatory shock. Monitor patients who may be susceptible to intracranial effects of carbon dioxide retention for signs of sedation and respiratory depression when initiating therapy. May obscure clinical course in a patient with head injury. Avoid with impaired consciousness or coma. Difficulty in swallowing tab, and intestinal obstruction reported; consider alternative analgesic in patients who have difficulty swallowing or have underlying GI disorders that may predispose them to obstruction. May cause spasm of sphincter of Oddi and increase in serum amylase; monitor patients for worsening symptoms with biliary tract disease. May aggravate convulsions and induce/aggravate seizures. May impair mental/physical abilities. Not for use during and immediately prior to labor.

ADVERSE REACTIONS
Respiratory depression, constipation, N/V, diarrhea, somnolence, headache, dizziness, pruritus, increased sweating, dry mouth, sedation, insomnia, fatigue, decreased appetite, abdominal pain.

DRUG INTERACTIONS
See Boxed Warning. Hypotension, profound sedation, coma, respiratory depression, and death may occur with CNS depressants (eg, sedatives, anxiolytics, neuroleptics); if coadministration is considered, reduce dose of 1 or both agents. Monitor use in elderly, cachectic, and debilitated patients when coadministered with other drugs that depress respiration. Mixed agonist/antagonist analgesics (pentazocine, nalbuphine, butorphanol) and partial agonists (buprenorphine) may reduce analgesic effect or precipitate withdrawal symptoms; avoid concomitant use. May enhance neuromuscular blocking action of skeletal muscle relaxants and increase degree of respiratory depression. Cimetidine may potentiate opioid-induced respiratory depression. Anticholinergics or other drugs with anticholinergic activity may increase risk of urinary retention and/or severe constipation, which may lead to paralytic ileus.

NURSING CONSIDERATIONS

Assessment: Assess for abuse/addiction risk, pain intensity, prior opioid therapy, opioid tolerance, respiratory depression, renal/hepatic impairment, GI obstruction, drug hypersensitivity, pregnancy/nursing status, possible drug interactions, or any other conditions where treatment is contraindicated or cautioned.

Monitoring: Monitor for sedation, respiratory depression (especially within first 24-72 hrs of initiation or following a dose increase), hypotension, seizures/convulsions, and other adverse reactions. Monitor BP and serum amylase levels. Routinely monitor for signs of misuse, abuse, and addiction. Periodically reassess the continued need for therapy.

Patient Counseling: Inform that use of drug can result in addiction, abuse, and misuse; instruct not to share with others and to take steps to protect from theft or misuse. Inform about risk and signs/symptoms of respiratory depression. Advise to store securely and dispose of unused tabs by flushing down the toilet. Inform female patients of reproductive potential that prolonged use during pregnancy may result in neonatal opioid withdrawal syndrome. Advise that drug may cause fetal harm and instruct to inform physician if pregnant/planning to become pregnant. Instruct not to consume alcoholic beverages or prescription and OTC products that contain alcohol during treatment. Inform that potentially serious additive effects may occur when used with alcohol or other CNS depressants, and not to use such drugs unless supervised by physician. Instruct to take drug exactly as prescribed, and not to d/c without 1st discussing the need for a tapering regimen with the physician. Inform that occasionally, inactive ingredients may be eliminated as a soft mass in stool that may resemble the original tab; inform that the active medication has already been absorbed by the time they see the soft mass. Inform that drug may cause orthostatic hypotension and syncope. Inform that drug may impair the ability to perform potentially hazardous activities; advise not to perform such tasks until they know how they will react to medication. Advise of potential for severe constipation, including management instructions. Advise how to recognize anaphylaxis and when to seek medical attention.

Storage: 25°C (77°F); excursions permitted to 15-30°C (59-86°F).

OPSUMIT – macitentan

Class: Endothelin receptor antagonist

RX

Do not administer to a pregnant female; may cause fetal harm. Exclude pregnancy before the start of treatment, monthly during treatment, and 1 month after stopping treatment. Prevent pregnancy during and for 1 month after stopping treatment; use acceptable methods of contraception. For all female patients, available only through a restricted program called the OPSUMIT Risk Evaluation and Mitigation Strategy (REMS) Program.

ADULT DOSAGE

Pulmonary Arterial Hypertension

Treatment of pulmonary arterial HTN (WHO Group I) to delay disease progression

Usual: 10mg qd

Max: 10mg qd

PEDIATRIC DOSAGE

Pediatric use may not have been established

DOSE MODIFICATION

Hepatic Impairment

Elevation of Aminotransferase Levels:

D/C therapy if clinically relevant ALT/AST elevations occur, or if elevations accompanied by increase in bilirubin >2X ULN, or by clinical symptoms of hepatotoxicity

Consider reinitiation of therapy when hepatic enzyme levels normalize in patients who have not experienced clinical symptoms of hepatotoxicity

ADMINISTRATION

Oral route

Take PO w/ or w/o food

Do not split, crush, or chew tabs

HOW SUPPLIED

Tab: 10mg

CONTRAINDICATIONS

Pregnancy.

WARNINGS/PRECAUTIONS

May cause elevations of aminotransferases, hepatotoxicity, and liver failure; obtain liver enzyme tests prior to initiation of treatment and repeat during treatment as clinically indicated. D/C therapy if clinically relevant aminotransferase elevations occur, or if elevations are accompanied by an increase in bilirubin >2X ULN, or by clinical symptoms of hepatotoxicity. Decreases in Hgb concentration and Hct reported; measure Hgb prior to initiation of treatment and repeat during treatment as clinically indicated. Not recommended in patients with severe anemia. If signs of pulmonary edema occur, consider the possibility of associated pulmonary veno-occlusive disease (PVOD); d/c if confirmed. May decrease sperm count.

ADVERSE REACTIONS

Anemia, nasopharyngitis/pharyngitis, bronchitis, headache, influenza, urinary tract infection.

DRUG INTERACTIONS

Strong CYP3A inducers (eg, rifampin) may significantly reduce exposure; avoid use. Strong CYP3A4 inhibitors (eg, ketoconazole, ritonavir) may approximately double exposure; avoid use.

NURSING CONSIDERATIONS

Assessment: Assess for pregnancy/nursing status, and possible drug interactions. Obtain baseline liver enzyme tests and Hgb levels.

Monitoring: Monitor for signs/symptoms of pulmonary edema, PVOD, hepatic impairment, and other adverse reactions. Obtain pregnancy tests monthly during treatment and 1 month after discontinuation of treatment. Monitor liver enzyme tests and Hgb levels as clinically indicated.

Patient Counseling: Counsel on the risk of fetal harm when used during pregnancy; instruct females of reproductive potential to use effective contraception during therapy and for 1 month after stopping treatment. Instruct to contact physician immediately if pregnancy is suspected. Inform female patients that they must enroll in the OPSUMIT REMS Program. Educate and counsel females of reproductive potential on the use of emergency contraception in the event of unprotected sex or contraceptive failure. Advise prepubertal females to immediately report to physician any reproductive status changes. Advise of the importance of Hgb testing. Educate patients on signs of hepatotoxicity.

Storage: 20-25°C (68-77°F); excursions permitted from 15-30°C (59-86°F).

ORACEA – doxycycline

RX

Class: Tetracyclines

ADULT DOSAGE

Rosacea

Inflammatory Lesions (Papules/Pustules):

40mg qam

PEDIATRIC DOSAGE

Pediatric use may not have been established

DOSE MODIFICATION

Elderly

Start at lower end of dosing range

ADMINISTRATION

Oral route

Take on an empty stomach, preferably at least 1 hr ac or 2 hrs pc

Administer w/ adequate amounts of fluid to reduce the risk of esophageal irritation and ulceration

HOW SUPPLIED

Cap: 40mg

WARNINGS/PRECAUTIONS

Do not use for treating bacterial infections, providing antibacterial prophylaxis, or reducing the numbers of (or eliminating) microorganisms associated with any bacterial disease. May cause fetal harm. May cause permanent discoloration of the teeth (yellow-gray-brown) if used during tooth development (last half of pregnancy, infancy, childhood up to 8 yrs of age). Enamel hypoplasia reported. Do not use during tooth development unless other drugs are not likely to be effective or are contraindicated. May decrease fibula growth rate in premature infants. *Clostridium difficile*-associated diarrhea (CDAD) reported; d/c if CDAD is suspected or confirmed. May result in overgrowth of non-susceptible microorganisms, including fungi; d/c and institute appropriate therapy if superinfection occurs. Caution in patients with a history of or predisposition to *Candida* overgrowth. Bacterial resistance may develop; use only as indicated and do not exceed recommended dosage. Photosensitivity manifested by an exaggerated sunburn reaction reported. Development of autoimmune syndromes reported; d/c immediately and perform LFTs, antinuclear antibodies (ANAs), CBC, and other appropriate tests in symptomatic patients. Tissue hyperpigmentation reported. May increase BUN. Caution in patients with renal impairment; may lead to excessive systemic accumulations and possible liver toxicity; lower than usual total dosages are indicated and if therapy is prolonged, serum drug level determinations may be advisable. Associated with pseudotumor cerebri (benign intracranial HTN) in adults and bulging fontanels in infants. Lab test interactions may occur. Caution in elderly.

ADVERSE REACTIONS

Nasopharyngitis, sinusitis, diarrhea, HTN.

DRUG INTERACTIONS

Depresses plasma prothrombin activity; may require downward adjustment of anticoagulant dosage. May interfere with bactericidal action of penicillin; avoid concurrent use. Fatal renal toxicity reported with methoxyflurane. Bismuth subsalicylate, proton pump inhibitors, antacids containing aluminum, Ca^{2+}, or Mg^{2+}, and iron-containing preparations may impair absorption. May interfere with the effectiveness of low dose oral contraceptives. Avoid concurrent use with oral retinoids (eg, isotretinoin, acitretin); pseudotumor cerebri reported. Barbiturates, carbamazepine, and phenytoin decrease the $T_{1/2}$ of doxycycline.

NURSING CONSIDERATIONS

Assessment: Assess for hypersensitivity to drug and other tetracyclines, renal impairment, history of or predisposition to *Candida* overgrowth, visual disturbances, pregnancy/nursing status, and possible drug interactions.

Monitoring: Monitor for signs/symptoms of CDAD, superinfection, photosensitivity, autoimmune syndromes, tissue hyperpigmentation, and other adverse reactions. Monitor serum drug levels in patients with renal impairment if therapy is prolonged. Routinely check for papilledema while on treatment. Perform periodic lab evaluations of organ systems, including hematopoietic, renal, and hepatic studies. If symptoms of autoimmune syndrome occur, perform LFTs, ANAs, CBC, and other appropriate tests.

Patient Counseling: Inform that drug should not be used by pregnant or breastfeeding women nor by individuals of either gender who are attempting to conceive a child. Inform that drug may render oral contraceptives less effective; advise females to use a second form of contraception. Inform that pseudomembranous colitis and pseudotumor cerebri may occur; instruct to seek immediate medical attention if watery/bloody stools, or headache or blurred vision occur. Inform that photosensitivity, manifested by an exaggerated sunburn reaction, was observed; instruct to minimize/avoid exposure to natural or artificial sunlight and d/c at 1st evidence of sunburn, advise to wear loose-fitting clothes, and discuss other sun protection measures. Inform that medication may cause autoimmune syndromes; instruct to d/c and contact physician if arthralgia, fever, rash, or malaise develops. Inform that drug may cause discoloration of skin, scars, teeth, or gums. Instruct to take exactly ud. Inform that increasing doses beyond 40mg qam may increase likelihood that bacteria will develop resistance and will not be treatable by other antibacterial drugs in the future.

Storage: 15-30°C (59-86°F).

ORAPRED – prednisolone sodium phosphate

Class: Glucocorticoid

RX

ADULT DOSAGE

Steroid-Responsive Disorders

Initial: 5-60mg/day (1.67-20mL), depending on disease and response

Maint: Decrease initial dose in small decrements to lowest effective dose

Multiple Sclerosis

Acute Exacerbations:
200mg/day for a week, followed by 80mg qod for 1 month

PEDIATRIC DOSAGE

Steroid-Responsive Disorders

Initial: 0.14-2mg/kg/day in 3 or 4 divided doses (4-60mg/m^2/day)

Nephrotic Syndrome

>2 Years:
60mg/m^2/day given in 3 divided doses for 4 weeks, followed by 4 weeks of single dose alternate-day therapy at 40mg/m^2/day

Asthma

Uncontrolled by Inhaled Corticosteroids and Long-Acting Bronchodilators:
1-2mg/kg/day in single or divided doses; continue short course ("burst") therapy until peak expiratory flow rate of 80% of personal best is achieved or symptoms resolve (usually 3-10 days)

DOSE MODIFICATION

Elderly

Start at lower end of dosing range

Discontinuation

Withdraw gradually after long-term therapy

ADMINISTRATION

Oral route

HOW SUPPLIED

Sol: 15mg/5mL [237mL]

CONTRAINDICATIONS

Systemic fungal infections.

WARNINGS/PRECAUTIONS

May need to increase dose before, during, and after stressful situations. May produce reversible hypothalamic-pituitary-adrenal (HPA) axis suppression with the potential for glucocorticosteroid insufficiency after withdrawal; gradually reduce dose. May impair mineralocorticoid secretion; administer salt and/or mineralocorticoid concurrently. Metabolic clearance is decreased in hypothyroidism and increased in hyperthyroidism; changes in thyroid status may necessitate dose adjustment. May increase susceptibility to infections, mask signs of current infection, activate latent disease, or exacerbate intercurrent infections. Rule out latent or active amebiasis before initiating therapy. May cause more serious/fatal course of chickenpox and measles; avoid exposure, and if exposed, consider prophylaxis/treatment. Caution with *Strongyloides* infestation, active/latent tuberculosis (TB) or tuberculin reactivity, HTN, CHF, and renal insufficiency. May cause BP elevation, salt/water retention, and increased K^+ and Ca^{2+} excretion; dietary salt restriction and K^+ supplementation may be necessary. Not for use in cerebral malaria and active ocular herpes simplex. Signs of GI perforation (eg, peritoneal irritation) may be masked, minimal, or absent. Caution with nonspecific ulcerative colitis; probable impending perforation, abscess, or other pyogenic infections; diverticulitis; fresh intestinal anastomoses; and active/latent peptic ulcers. Psychic derangements may appear and existing emotional instability or psychotic tendencies may be aggravated. May decrease bone formation and increase bone resorption, and may lead to inhibition of bone growth in children/adolescents and the development of osteoporosis at any age; caution with increased risk of osteoporosis. May produce posterior subcapsular cataracts, glaucoma with possible optic nerve damage, and may enhance the establishment of secondary ocular infections; not recommended in optic neuritis treatment. Acute myopathy with high doses reported, most often in patients with disorders of neuromuscular transmission (eg, myasthenia gravis). Elevation of CK or IOP may occur. May suppress reactions to skin tests. Kaposi's sarcoma reported. Enhanced effect in patients with cirrhosis and hypothyroidism. Caution in elderly.

ADVERSE REACTIONS

Fluid retention, HTN, decreased carbohydrate tolerance, abdominal distention, increased appetite, weight gain, glaucoma, osteoporosis, muscle weakness, development of cushingoid state, menstrual irregularities, convulsions, headache, impaired wound healing, increased sweating.

DRUG INTERACTIONS

Live or live, attenuated vaccines are contraindicated with immunosuppressive doses. Killed or inactivated vaccines may be administered, although response is unpredictable. May exhibit a diminished response to toxoids and live or inactivated vaccines. May potentiate replication of some organisms contained in live, attenuated vaccines. Hepatic enzyme inducers (eg, barbiturates, phenytoin, ephedrine) may enhance metabolism and require corticosteroid dosage increase. Increased activity of both drugs may occur with cyclosporine; convulsions reported with concurrent use. Estrogens may decrease hepatic metabolism and increase effect. Ketoconazole may decrease metabolism leading to an increased risk of corticosteroid side effects. May inhibit response to warfarin. ASA or other NSAIDs may increase risk of GI side effects; caution with ASA in hypoprothrombinemia patients. May increase clearance of salicylates. Closely monitor for hypokalemia with K^+-depleting agents (eg, amphotericin B, diuretics). May increase risk of arrhythmias with digitalis glycosides. Concomitant use with anticholinesterase agents may produce severe weakness in patients with myasthenia gravis; d/c anticholinesterase agents at least 24 hrs before initiating therapy. May increase blood glucose levels; dosage adjustments of antidiabetic agents may be required. Acute myopathy reported with neuromuscular blocking drugs (eg, pancuronium).

NURSING CONSIDERATIONS

Assessment: Assess for hypersensitivity to drug or any of its components, unusual stress, current infections, systemic fungal infections, latent/active amebiasis, peptic ulcer and TB, cerebral malaria, ocular herpes simplex, CHF, HTN, renal insufficiency, diverticulitis, intestinal anastomoses, ulcerative colitis, cirrhosis, psychotic tendencies, myasthenia gravis, thyroid disorders, any other conditions where treatment is contraindicated or cautioned, pregnancy/nursing status, and possible drug interactions.

Monitoring: Monitor for HPA axis suppression, infections, changes in thyroid status, cataracts, glaucoma, Kaposi's sarcoma, growth/development (in pediatric patients), osteoporosis, acute myopathy, psychic derangements, emotional instability or psychotic tendencies aggravation, and other adverse reactions. Monitor BP, serum electrolytes, and CK. Monitor IOP if used for >6 weeks. Frequently monitor coagulation indices with warfarin.

Patient Counseling: Instruct not to d/c therapy abruptly or without medical supervision. Instruct to inform any physician of intake of corticosteroids and to seek medical advice at once if fever or other signs of infection develop. Instruct to avoid exposure to chickenpox or measles; instruct to seek medical advice without delay if exposed.

Storage: 2-8°C (36-46°F). Keep tightly closed.

ORAPRED ODT – prednisolone sodium phosphate RX

Class: Glucocorticoid

ADULT DOSAGE

Steroid-Responsive Disorders

Initial: 10-60mg/day, depending on disease and response

Maint: Decrease initial dose in small decrements to lowest effective dose

Multiple Sclerosis

Acute Exacerbations:

200mg/day for a week, followed by 80mg qod for 1 month

PEDIATRIC DOSAGE

Steroid-Responsive Disorders

Initial: 0.14-2mg/kg/day in 3 or 4 divided doses (4-60mg/m²/day)

Nephrotic Syndrome

>2 Years:

60mg/m²/day given in 3 divided doses for 4 weeks, followed by 4 weeks of single dose alternate-day therapy at 40mg/m²/day

Asthma

Uncontrolled by Inhaled Corticosteroids and Long-Acting Bronchodilators:

1-2mg/kg/day in single or divided doses; continue short course ("burst") therapy until peak expiratory flow rate of 80% of personal best is achieved or symptoms resolve (usually 3-10 days)

DOSE MODIFICATION

Elderly

Start at lower end of dosing range

Discontinuation

Withdraw gradually after long-term therapy

ADMINISTRATION

Oral route

Take w/ food

Place tab on tongue; may be swallowed whole or allowed to dissolve in mouth w/ or w/o water

Do not break or use partial tabs

Do not remove tab from blister until just prior to dosing

HOW SUPPLIED

Tab, Disintegrating: 10mg, 15mg, 30mg

WARNINGS/PRECAUTIONS

May produce reversible hypothalamic-pituitary-adrenal (HPA) axis suppression with the potential for glucocorticosteroid insufficiency after withdrawal; gradually reduce dose. May impair mineralocorticoid secretion; administer salt and/or mineralocorticoid concurrently. Metabolic clearance is decreased in hypothyroidism and increased in hyperthyroidism; changes in thyroid status may necessitate dose adjustment. May increase susceptibility to infections, mask signs of current infection, and increase risk of exacerbation, dissemination, or reactivation of latent infection. May exacerbate systemic fungal infections; avoid use in the presence of systemic fungal infections unless needed to control drug reactions. Rule out latent or active amebiasis before initiating therapy. May cause more serious/fatal course of chickenpox or measles; avoid exposure, and if exposed, consider prophylaxis/treatment. Caution with *Strongyloides* infestation, active/latent TB or tuberculin reactivity, HTN, CHF, and renal insufficiency. May cause BP elevation, salt/water retention, and increased K^+ and Ca^{2+} excretion; dietary salt restriction and K^+ supplementation may be necessary. Caution with recent MI. Increased risk of GI perforation with certain GI disorders; signs of GI perforation (eg, peritoneal irritation) may be masked. Caution with probable impending perforation, abscess or other pyogenic infections; diverticulitis; fresh intestinal anastomoses; and active or latent peptic ulcers. Not for use in cerebral malaria and active ocular herpes simplex. May be associated with CNS effects (eg, euphoria, insomnia, psychotic manifestations); existing emotional instability or psychotic tendencies may be aggravated. May decrease bone formation and increase bone resorption, and may lead to inhibition of bone growth in pediatric patients and the development of osteoporosis at any age; caution with increased risk of osteoporosis. May produce posterior subcapsular cataracts, glaucoma with possible optic nerve damage, and may enhance the establishment of secondary ocular infections; not recommended in optic neuritis treatment. Acute myopathy with high doses reported, most often in patients with disorders of neuromuscular transmission (eg, myasthenia gravis). Elevation of CK or IOP may occur. Kaposi's sarcoma reported. Caution with ocular herpes simplex. May have negative effects on growth and development in children. May cause fetal harm. May suppress reactions to skin tests. Caution in elderly.

ADVERSE REACTIONS

Fluid retention, HTN, alteration of glucose tolerance, behavioral changes, increased appetite, weight gain, glaucoma, osteoporosis, muscle weakness, development of cushingoid state, menstrual irregularities, convulsions, headache, impaired wound healing, increased sweating.

DRUG INTERACTIONS

Live or live, attenuated vaccines are contraindicated with immunosuppressive doses. Killed or inactivated vaccines may be administered, although response is unpredictable. May exhibit a diminished response to toxoids and live or inactivated vaccines. May potentiate replication of some organisms contained in live, attenuated vaccines. Aminoglutethimide may lead to a loss of corticosteroid-induced adrenal suppression. Cardiac enlargement and CHF reported following concomitant use of amphotericin B and hydrocortisone. Concomitant use with anticholinesterase agents may produce severe weakness in patients with myasthenia gravis; d/c anticholinesterase agents at least 24 hrs before initiating therapy. May inhibit response to warfarin. May increase blood glucose levels; dosage adjustments of antidiabetic agents may be required. May decrease serum levels of INH. CYP3A4 inducers (eg, barbiturates, phenytoin, carbamazepine, rifampin) may enhance metabolism and require corticosteroid dosage increase. Ketoconazole may decrease metabolism, leading to an increased risk of corticosteroid side effects. Cholestyramine may increase clearance. Increased activity of both drugs may occur with cyclosporine; convulsions reported with concurrent use. May increase risk of arrhythmias with digitalis glycosides. Estrogens, including oral contraceptives, may decrease hepatic metabolism and enhance effect. ASA or other NSAIDs may increase risk of GI side effects; caution with ASA in hypoprothrombinemia patients. May increase clearance of salicylates. Closely monitor for hypokalemia with K^+-depleting agents (eg, amphotericin B, diuretics). Acute myopathy reported with neuromuscular blocking drugs (eg, pancuronium).

NURSING CONSIDERATIONS

Assessment: Assess for hypersensitivity to drug or any of its components, unusual stress, current infections, systemic fungal infections, latent/active amebiasis, peptic ulcer and TB, cerebral malaria, ocular herpes simplex, CHF, HTN, recent MI, renal insufficiency, diverticulitis, intestinal anastomoses, psychotic tendencies, myasthenia gravis, thyroid disorders, any other conditions where treatment is contraindicated or cautioned, pregnancy/nursing status, and possible drug interactions.

Monitoring: Monitor for infections, changes in thyroid status, cataracts, glaucoma, Kaposi's sarcoma, growth/development (in pediatric patients), osteoporosis, acute myopathy, psychic derangements, emotional instability or psychotic tendencies aggravation, and other adverse reactions. Monitor BP, serum electrolytes, and CK. Monitor IOP if used for >6 weeks. Frequently monitor coagulation indices with warfarin. Monitor for HPA axis suppression, Cushing's syndrome, and hyperglycemia with chronic use.

Patient Counseling: Instruct not to d/c therapy abruptly or without medical supervision. Instruct to inform any physician of intake of corticosteroids and to seek medical advice at once if fever or other signs of infection develop. Instruct to avoid exposure to chickenpox or measles; instruct to seek medical advice without delay if exposed. Advise to take exactly as prescribed. Advise to report recent or ongoing infections, vaccination, and concurrent medicines. Counsel about common adverse reactions (eg, fluid retention, altered glucose tolerance, elevated BP, behavioral and mood changes, increased appetite, weight gain). Instruct to take missed dose as soon as remembered, but if it is almost time for next dose, skip missed dose and take at the next regularly scheduled time; advise not to take an extra dose to make up for missed dose.

Storage: 20-25°C (68-77°F); excursions permitted to 15-30°C (59-86°F). Protect from moisture.

ORAVIG – miconazole

RX

Class: Azole antifungal

ADULT DOSAGE

Oropharyngeal Candidiasis

≥16 Years:
Apply 1 tab qd for 14 consecutive days

PEDIATRIC DOSAGE

Pediatric use may not have been established

ADMINISTRATION

Buccal route

Apply in the upper gum region qam w/ dry hands, after brushing the teeth

Either side of tab may be placed against the upper gum just above the incisor tooth (canine fossa), and held in place w/ slight pressure over the upper lip for 30 sec to ensure adhesion

For improved comfort, may apply rounded side surface of tab to gum

Subsequent applications should be made to alternate sides of the mouth; clear away any remaining tab material prior to next application

Do not crush, chew, or swallow

Food and drink can be taken normally when tab is in place

HOW SUPPLIED

Tab, Buccal: 50mg

CONTRAINDICATIONS

Hypersensitivity (eg, anaphylaxis) to milk protein concentrate.

WARNINGS/PRECAUTIONS

Allergic reactions, including anaphylactic reactions and hypersensitivity, reported; d/c immediately at the 1st sign of hypersensitivity. Caution with hepatic impairment.

ADVERSE REACTIONS

Diarrhea, N/V, headache, dysgeusia.

DRUG INTERACTIONS

May enhance anticoagulant effects of warfarin; closely monitor PT, INR, or other suitable anticoagulation tests, and for evidence of bleeding. May interact with drugs metabolized through CYP2C9 and CYP3A4 (eg, oral hypoglycemics, phenytoin, ergot alkaloids).

NURSING CONSIDERATIONS

Assessment: Assess for hypersensitivity to drug, milk protein concentrate, or any other component of the product, hepatic impairment, pregnancy/nursing status, and possible drug interactions.

Monitoring: Monitor for signs/symptoms of hypersensitivity and other adverse reactions. Closely monitor PT, INR, or other suitable anticoagulation tests, and for evidence of bleeding with warfarin.

Patient Counseling: Instruct on proper application of the tab. Inform that subsequent applications should be made to alternate sides of the gum. Advise that if tab does not stick or falls off within first 6 hrs, the same tab should be repositioned immediately; instruct to place a new tab if tab still does not adhere. Instruct to drink a glass of water and apply a new tab only once if tab is swallowed within first 6 hrs. Instruct to not apply a new tab until the next, regularly scheduled dose, if tab falls off or swallowed after it was in place for ≥6 hrs. Counsel to avoid situations that could interfere with the sticking of the tab (eg, touching/pressing tab after placement, wearing upper denture, chewing gum, hitting tab when brushing teeth, rinsing mouth too vigorously). Advise to d/c and contact physician if hives, skin rash, other symptoms of an allergic reaction, or application-site swelling/pain develops. Inform that patients may experience other adverse reactions, including diarrhea, headache, nausea, and change in taste.

Storage: 20-25°C (68-77°F); excursions between 15-30°C (59-86°F) permitted at room temperature. Protect from moisture.

ORBACTIV – oritavancin

Class: Lipoglycopeptide

RX

ADULT DOSAGE

Skin and Skin Structure Infections

Acute bacterial infections caused by *Staphylococcus aureus* (including methicillin-susceptible and methicillin-resistant isolates), *Streptococcus pyogenes, Streptococcus agalactiae, Streptococcus dysgalactiae, Streptococcus anginosus* group (includes *S. anginosus, S. intermedius*, and *S. constellatus*), and *Enterococcus faecalis* (vancomycin-susceptible isolates only)

Usual: Single 1200mg dose by IV infusion over 3 hrs

PEDIATRIC DOSAGE

Pediatric use may not have been established

ADMINISTRATION

IV route

Preparation

Three 400mg vials need to be reconstituted and diluted to prepare a single 1200mg dose

Reconstitution:

1. Add 40mL of SWFI to reconstitute each vial to provide a 10mg/mL sol per vial
2. Gently swirl each vial to avoid foaming and ensure that all powder is completely reconstituted in sol

Dilution:

1. Use only D5W for dilution; do not use normal saline as it is incompatible and may cause precipitation of the drug
2. Withdraw and discard 120mL from a 1000mL IV bag of D5W
3. Withdraw 40mL from each of the 3 reconstituted vials and add to D5W IV bag to bring the bag volume to 1000mL; this yields a concentration of 1.2mg/mL

Incompatibilities

1. IV substances, additives, or other medications mixed in normal saline should not be added to oritavancin single-use vials or infused simultaneously through the same IV line or through a common IV port
2. Drugs formulated at a basic or neutral pH may be incompatible
3. Do not administer simultaneously w/ commonly used IV drugs through a common IV port; if the same IV line is used for sequential infusion of additional medications, the line should be flushed w/ D5W before and after infusion of oritavancin

HOW SUPPLIED

Inj: 400mg

CONTRAINDICATIONS

Use of IV unfractionated heparin sodium for 48 hrs after administration of therapy.

WARNINGS/PRECAUTIONS

Artificially prolongs activated PTT (aPTT) for 48 hrs and the PT and INR for up to 24 hrs by binding to and preventing action of the phospholipid reagents that activate coagulation in commonly used lab coagulation tests. For patients who require aPTT monitoring within 48 hrs of dosing, a non-phospholipid dependent coagulation test (eg, Factor Xa [chromogenic] assay) or an alternative anticoagulant not requiring aPTT monitoring may be considered. Effects on activated clotting time are expected since the phospholipid reagents are also used in this coagulation test. Serious hypersensitivity reactions reported; d/c immediately and institute appropriate supportive care if an acute hypersensitivity reaction occurs. Infusion-related reactions (eg, pruritus, urticaria, flushing) reported; consider slowing or interrupting drug infusion. *Clostridium difficile*-associated diarrhea (CDAD) reported; d/c if CDAD is suspected or confirmed. Osteomyelitis reported; institute appropriate alternate antibacterial therapy if suspected or diagnosed. May result in bacterial resistance if used in the absence of proven or suspected bacterial infection.

ADVERSE REACTIONS

Headache, N/V, limb and SQ abscesses, diarrhea.

DRUG INTERACTIONS

See Contraindications. Nonspecific, weak inhibitor (CYP2C9 and CYP2C19) or inducer (CYP3A4 and CYP2D6) of several CYP isoforms; caution when concomitantly administering with drugs with a narrow therapeutic window that are predominantly metabolized by 1 of the affected CYP450 enzymes (eg, warfarin); coadministration may increase (eg, CYP2C9 substrates) or decrease (eg, CYP2D6 substrates) concentrations of the narrow therapeutic range drug. Coadministration with warfarin may increase the risk of bleeding; frequently monitor for signs of bleeding.

NURSING CONSIDERATIONS

Assessment: Assess for hypersensitivity to drug or other glycopeptides, pregnancy/nursing status, and for possible drug interactions. Perform culture and susceptibility testing.

Monitoring: Monitor for hypersensitivity reactions, infusion-related reactions, CDAD, osteomyelitis, development of drug-resistant bacteria, and other adverse reactions. Frequently monitor for signs of bleeding with warfarin.

Patient Counseling: Advise that allergic reactions may occur and that serious allergic reactions require immediate treatment. Advise to inform the physician about any previous hypersensitivity reactions to the drug, other glycopeptides, or other allergens. Inform that diarrhea is a common problem caused by therapy and usually resolves when therapy is discontinued; instruct to contact physician if severe watery or bloody diarrhea develops.

Storage: 20-25°C (68-77°F); excursions permitted to 15-30°C (59-86°F). Diluted Sol in Infusion Bag: Use within 6 hrs when stored at room temperature or use within 12 hrs when refrigerated at 2-8°C (36-46°F). Combined storage time (reconstituted sol in the vial and the diluted sol in the bag) and 3-hr infusion time should not exceed 6 hrs at room temperature or 12 hrs if refrigerated.

ORENCIA – abatacept

RX

Class: Selective costimulation modulator

ADULT DOSAGE

Rheumatoid Arthritis

To reduce signs and symptoms, induce major clinical response, inhibit progression of structural damage, and improve physical function in adults w/ moderate to severe active rheumatoid arthritis (RA); may be used as monotherapy or concomitantly w/ disease-modifying antirheumatic drugs other than TNF antagonists.

IV Regimen:

Initial:

<60kg: 500mg

60-100kg: 750mg

>100kg: 1000mg

Maint: Give succeeding infusions at 2 and 4 weeks after the 1st infusion and every 4 weeks thereafter

SQ Regimen:

125mg SQ inj once weekly w/ or w/o an IV LD

If initiating w/ an IV LD, initiate w/ a single IV infusion (as per body weight categories listed in the IV regimen), followed by the first 125mg SQ inj w/in a day of the IV infusion

Switching from IV to SQ Regimen:

Give the 1st SQ dose instead of the next scheduled IV dose

PEDIATRIC DOSAGE

Juvenile Idiopathic Arthritis

To reduce signs and symptoms of moderately to severely active polyarticular juvenile idiopathic arthritis (JIA); may be used as monotherapy or concomitantly w/ methotrexate.

6-17 Years:

Initial:

<75kg: 10mg/kg

≥75kg: Follow adult IV dosing regimen; not to exceed 1000mg

Maint: Give succeeding infusions at 2 and 4 weeks after the 1st infusion and every 4 weeks thereafter

ADMINISTRATION
IV/SQ routes

IV
Give as an IV infusion over 30 min
Do not infuse in the same IV line w/ other agents

IV Preparation
Reconstitute w/ 10mL of sterile water for inj; only use silicone-free disposable syringe provided w/ each vial and 18- to 21-gauge needle
Rotate vial w/ gentle swirling until contents are completely dissolved
Vent vial w/ needle to dissipate any foam after complete dissolution of powder
Dilute reconstituted sol w/ 0.9% NaCl Inj using the same silicone-free disposable syringe to a total volume of 100mL
Final concentration of abatacept in the bag or bottle must be ≤10mg/mL
Do not shake bag or bottle

SQ
Administer inj to front thigh or abdomen (except for the 2-inch area around navel) for self-injection, or outer area of the upper arm if a caregiver is administering dose
Rotate inj site (at least 1 inch away from last inj site)
Do not inject into areas where the skin is tender, bruised, red, or hard

HOW SUPPLIED
Inj: 125mg/mL [prefilled syringe], 250mg [vial]

WARNINGS/PRECAUTIONS
Anaphylaxis or anaphylactoid reactions reported w/ IV use; permanently d/c and institute appropriate therapy if an anaphylactic or other serious allergic reaction occurs. Serious infections, including sepsis and pneumonia, reported; caution in patients w/ history of recurrent infections, underlying conditions that may predispose to infections, or chronic, latent, or localized infections. Immunosuppressive therapy may further predispose to infections; d/c if serious infection develops. Screen for latent tuberculosis (TB) infection and viral hepatitis prior to initiation of therapy; treat patients testing (+) for TB prior to therapy. Hepatitis B reactivation may occur. JIA patients should be brought up to date w/ all immunizations prior to initiation of therapy. Caution in patients w/ COPD. May affect host defenses against infections and malignancies. Caution in elderly. (IV) Contains maltose that may react w/ glucose dehydrogenase pyrroloquinolinequinone-based glucose monitoring and may result in falsely elevated blood glucose readings on the day of infusion; consider methods that do not react w/ maltose in patients requiring blood glucose monitoring.

ADVERSE REACTIONS
Headache, URTI, nasopharyngitis, nausea, sinusitis, UTI, influenza, bronchitis, dizziness, cough, back pain, HTN, dyspepsia, rash, pain in extremities.

DRUG INTERACTIONS
May increase risk of serious infections w/ TNF antagonists; concomitant use is not recommended. Concomitant use w/ other biologic RA therapy (eg, anakinra) is not recommended. Do not use live vaccines concurrently w/ therapy or w/in 3 months of its discontinuation.

NURSING CONSIDERATIONS

Assessment: Assess for previous hypersensitivity to drug, history of recurrent infections, chronic/latent/localized infections, underlying conditions that may predispose to infection, COPD, pregnancy/nursing status, and possible drug interactions. Assess immunization history in pediatric patients. Screen for latent TB infection w/ a tuberculin skin test and for viral hepatitis.

Monitoring: Monitor for signs/symptoms of hypersensitivity, infection, hepatitis B reactivation, worsening of respiratory status, immunosuppression, malignancies, and other adverse reactions.

Patient Counseling: Instruct to immediately contact physician if an allergic reaction or infection occurs. Inform that patient may be tested for TB prior to therapy. Counsel not to receive live vaccines during therapy or w/in 3 months of its discontinuation. Inform caregivers that patients w/ JIA should be brought up to date w/ all immunizations prior to therapy and instruct to discuss w/ physician how to best handle future immunizations once therapy has been initiated. Instruct to inform physician if pregnant/nursing or planning to become pregnant. Inform that the formulation for IV administration contains maltose, which can give falsely elevated blood glucose readings on the day of administration w/ certain blood glucose monitors; advise to discuss w/ physician methods that do not react w/ maltose.

Storage: 2-8°C (36-46°F). Protect from light; store in original package until time of use. Do not allow prefilled syringe to freeze. Diluted Sol: Room temperature or 2-8°C (36-46°F); discard if not used w/in 24 hrs.

ORTHO-CEPT – desogestrel/ethinyl estradiol

RX

Class: Estrogen/progestogen combination

Cigarette smoking increases the risk of serious cardiovascular events. Risk increases w/ age (>35 yrs of age) and w/ the number of cigarettes smoked. Should not be used by women who are >35 yrs of age and smoke.

OTHER BRAND NAMES
Desogen, Emoquette, Reclipsen, Apri

ADULT DOSAGE

Contraception

1 tab qd at the same time each day for 28 days, then repeat

Start 1st Sunday after menses begin or 1st day of menses

Conversions

Switching from Another Oral Contraceptive:
Sunday Start (Except Desogen):
Take 1st active tab on the 1st Sunday after the last active tab of the previous product

Desogen:
Start on the same day that a new pack of the previous oral contraceptive would have been started

PEDIATRIC DOSAGE

Contraception

Not indicated for use premenarche; refer to adult dosing

DOSE MODIFICATION
Other Important Modifications
Missed Doses:
Miss 1 Active Tab: Take as soon as dose is remembered
Miss 2 Active Tabs in Week 1 or 2: Take 2 active tabs on the day dose is remembered and 2 active tabs the next day, then continue taking 1 tab qd until pack is finished. Use a backup method of birth control (eg, condom, spermicide) if patient has intercourse in the 7 days after missing pills
Miss 2 Active Tabs in Week 3 or Miss ≥3 Consecutive Active Tabs: (Day 1 Start) Throw out rest of the pack and start a new pack that same day. (Sunday Start) Continue to take 1 tab qd until Sunday, then throw out rest of the pack and start a new pack that same day. (Day 1/Sunday Start) Use a backup method of birth control (eg, condom, spermicide) if patient has intercourse in the 7 days after missing pills

ADMINISTRATION
Oral route

Take at intervals not to exceed 24 hrs
Use another method of contraception until after the first 7 consecutive days of administration when initiating Sunday Start regimen

HOW SUPPLIED
Tab: (Ethinyl Estradiol [EE]-Desogestrel) 0.03mg-0.15mg

CONTRAINDICATIONS
Thrombophlebitis or thromboembolic disorders, past history of deep vein thrombophlebitis or thromboembolic disorders, known thrombophilic conditions, cerebrovascular or coronary artery disease (current or history), valvular heart disease w/ complications, persistent BP values of ≥160mmHg systolic or ≥100mmHg diastolic, diabetes w/ vascular involvement, headaches w/ focal neurological symptoms, major surgery w/ prolonged immobilization, known or suspected breast carcinoma (or personal history), carcinoma of the endometrium or other known or suspected estrogen-dependent neoplasia, undiagnosed abnormal genital bleeding, cholestatic jaundice of pregnancy or jaundice w/ prior pill use, acute or chronic hepatocellular disease w/ abnormal liver function, hepatic adenomas or carcinomas, known/suspected pregnancy.

WARNINGS/PRECAUTIONS
When initiating a Sunday Start regimen, use another method of contraception until after the first 7 consecutive days of administration. Not indicated for use in emergency contraception. Increased risk of thromboembolism, MI, stroke, vascular disease, hepatic neoplasia, and gallbladder disease. Increased risk of morbidity and mortality in the presence of other underlying risk factors (eg, HTN, hyperlipidemias, obesity, diabetes). If feasible, d/c at least 4 weeks prior to and for 2 weeks after elective surgery of a type associated w/ an increased risk of thromboembolism, and during and following prolonged immobilization. May increase risk of breast cancer and cancer of the reproductive organs. Start use no earlier than 4 weeks after delivery in women who elect not to breastfeed. Contact lens wearers who develop visual changes or changes in lens tolerance

should be assessed by an ophthalmologist. Retinal thrombosis reported; d/c if unexplained partial or complete loss of vision, onset of proptosis or diplopia, papilledema, or retinal vascular lesions develop. Should not be used to induce withdrawal bleeding as a test for pregnancy, or to treat threatened or habitual abortion during pregnancy. Rule out pregnancy if 2 consecutive periods are missed. May decrease glucose tolerance; monitor prediabetic and diabetic patients. May elevate BP; monitor closely and d/c use if significant BP elevation occurs and cannot be adequately controlled. D/C and evaluate the cause if new onset/exacerbation of migraine or recurrent, persistent, severe headache w/ a new pattern develops. Breakthrough bleeding and spotting reported; rule out malignancy or pregnancy. Post-pill amenorrhea or oligomenorrhea may occur. Ectopic and intrauterine pregnancy may occur in contraceptive failures. D/C if jaundice develops. May cause fluid retention. Monitor closely in patients w/ history of depression; d/c if depression recurs to a serious degree. May elevate serum TG and LDL levels and may render the control of hyperlipidemias more difficult. May affect certain endocrine, LFTs, and blood components in lab tests.

ADVERSE REACTIONS

N/V, breakthrough bleeding, spotting, amenorrhea, migraine, vaginal candidiasis, edema, weight changes, melasma, breast changes, changes in cervical erosion and secretion, allergic reaction, mental depression, cholestatic jaundice, GI symptoms (eg, abdominal cramps, bloating).

DRUG INTERACTIONS

May decrease levels and potentially diminish effectiveness or increase breakthrough bleeding when used concomitantly w/ drugs or herbal products that induce certain enzymes, including CYP3A4 (eg, bosentan, rifabutin, St. John's wort); use an alternative or backup method of contraception and continue backup contraception for 28 days after discontinuing the enzyme inducer. Atorvastatin or rosuvastatin may increase EE exposure; ascorbic acid and acetaminophen (APAP) may increase EE levels. CYP3A4 inhibitors (eg, itraconazole, voriconazole, ketoconazole) may increase levels. Significant changes (decreased/increased) sometimes noted in estrogen and/or progestin levels when coadministered w/ HIV protease inhibitors (decreased [eg, nelfinavir, darunavir/ritonavir, (fos)amprenavir/ritonavir] or increased [eg, indinavir, atazanavir/ritonavir])/HCV protease inhibitors (decreased [eg, boceprevir, telaprevir]), or w/ non-nucleoside reverse transcriptase inhibitors (decreased [eg, nevirapine] or increased [eg, etravirine]). Colesevelam reported to significantly decrease EE exposure; decreased drug interaction reported when the 2 drug products are given 4 hrs apart. May inhibit metabolism and increase levels of other compounds (eg, cyclosporine, prednisolone, voriconazole). May decrease levels of APAP, clofibric acid, morphine, salicylic acid, and temazepam. May significantly decrease levels of lamotrigine and may reduce seizure control; dosage adjustment of lamotrigine may be needed. May need to increase dose of thyroid hormone in patients on thyroid hormone replacement therapy due to increased thyroid-binding globulin.

NURSING CONSIDERATIONS

Assessment: Assess for hypersensitivity to drug, thrombophlebitis or thromboembolic disorders, HTN, hyperlipidemia, diabetes, breast cancer, endometrial cancer or other estrogen-dependent neoplasia, undiagnosed abnormal genital bleeding, cholestatic jaundice of pregnancy or jaundice w/ prior pill use, pregnancy/nursing status, and for any other conditions where treatment is contraindicated/cautioned. Assess for possible drug interactions.

Monitoring: Monitor for MI, thromboembolism, stroke, hepatic neoplasia, and other adverse effects. Monitor BP w/ history of HTN, serum glucose levels in diabetic or prediabetic patients, lipid levels w/ hyperlipidemia, and for signs of worsening depression w/ previous history. Monitor liver function. Refer contact lens wearers to an ophthalmologist if visual changes or changes in lens tolerance develop. Monitor women who have strong family history of breast cancer or have breast nodules. Perform annual history and physical exam.

Patient Counseling: Inform of the benefits and risks of therapy. Inform that drug does not protect against HIV infection (AIDS) and other sexually transmitted diseases. Counsel that cigarette smoking increases the risk of serious adverse effects on the heart and blood vessels and that women who are >35 yrs of age and smoke, should not use oral contraceptives. Instruct to take exactly ud and at intervals not exceeding 24 hrs. Instruct on what to do if pills are missed. Instruct to use additional method of protection until after the 1st week of administration in the initial cycle when utilizing the Sunday Start regimen. Counsel that efficacy may decrease if vomiting/diarrhea develops; instruct to use a backup method of contraception and notify physician. Inform that spotting, light bleeding, or stomach sickness may occur during first 1-3 packs of pills; advise not to d/c medication and to notify physician if symptoms persist. Instruct to d/c if pregnancy is confirmed/suspected during treatment. Instruct to notify physician if breastfeeding. If scheduled for any lab test, advise patient to inform physician of birth control pills usage. Inform that certain drugs may make therapy less effective and additional contraception may be needed.

Storage: 25°C (77°F); excursions permitted to 15-30°C (59-86°F).

ORTHO EVRA – ethinyl estradiol/norelgestromin

RX

Class: Estrogen/progestogen combination

Cigarette smoking increases risk of serious cardiovascular (CV) events, particularly in women >35 years of age, and with the number of cigarettes smoked. Should not be used by women who are >35 yrs of age and smoke. May increase risk of venous thromboembolism (VTE) among users of Ortho Evra compared to women who use certain oral contraceptives. Has higher steady state concentrations and a lower peak concentration than oral contraceptives.

ADULT DOSAGE

Contraception

Start during the first 24 hrs of menstrual period or on the 1st Sunday after menstrual period begins. Apply patch each week on the same day for 3 weeks. Week 4 is patch-free. On the day after Week 4 ends, a new 4-week cycle is started by applying a new patch. There should not be more than a 7-day patch-free interval between dosing cycles

Use After Childbirth:

Start no sooner than 4 weeks after childbirth in women who elect not to breastfeed. If use is begun postpartum, use an additional method of contraception (eg, condom and spermicide, diaphragm and spermicide) for the first 7 days

Use After Abortion/Miscarriage:

1st Trimester: May start patch use immediately; additional method of contraception is not needed. If patch use is not started w/in 5 days following a 1st trimester abortion, follow instructions for starting patch for the 1st time and use non-hormonal contraceptive method in the meantime

2nd Trimester: Start no earlier than 4 weeks after a 2nd trimester abortion/miscarriage

Conversions

Switching From the Pill or Vaginal Contraceptive Ring:

Complete current pill/ring cycle and apply 1st patch on the day patient would have normally started next pill or inserted next vaginal ring

If patch is applied >1 week after taking last active pill or removal of last vaginal ring, use nonhormonal contraceptive concurrently for the 1st 7 days of patch use

PEDIATRIC DOSAGE

Contraception

Not indicated for use premenarche; refer to adult dosing

ADMINISTRATION

Transdermal route

Apply immediately upon removal from protective pouch

Only 1 patch should be worn at a time

Do not cut, damage, or alter patch in any way

Apply to clean and dry skin on upper outer arm, abdomen, buttock, or back in a place where it will not be rubbed by tight clothing; do not place on breasts, on cut/irritated skin, or on the same location as previous patch

Do not reapply patch if it is no longer sticky, if it has become stuck to itself or another surface, or if it has other material stuck to it

If utilizing Sunday Start regimen, use a non-hormonal backup method of birth control (eg, condom and spermicide, diaphragm and spermicide) for the first 7 days of the 1st cycle only

Refer to PI for further administration instructions

HOW SUPPLIED

Patch: (Ethinyl Estradiol [EE]-Norelgestromin [NGMN]): 0.75mg-6mg [1[s], 3[s]]

CONTRAINDICATIONS

High risk of arterial/venous thrombotic diseases (eg, smoking if >35 yrs of age, history/presence of deep vein thrombosis/pulmonary embolism, inherited or acquired hypercoagulopathies, cerebrovascular disease, coronary artery disease, thrombogenic valvular or thrombogenic rhythm diseases of the heart [eg, subacute bacterial endocarditis with valvular disease, A-fib], uncontrolled HTN; diabetes mellitus with vascular disease, headaches with focal neurological symptoms or migraine headaches with aura, >35 yrs of age with any migraine headaches), benign or malignant liver tumors, liver disease, undiagnosed abnormal uterine bleeding, pregnancy, current or history of breast cancer or other estrogen- or progestin-sensitive cancer.

WARNINGS/PRECAUTIONS

May be less effective in preventing pregnancy in women who weigh ≥198 lbs (90kg). Increased risk of arterial thromboses. D/C if an arterial or deep venous thrombotic event occurs. D/C if unexplained loss of vision, proptosis, diplopia, papilledema, or retinal vascular lesions develop; evaluate for retinal vein thrombosis immediately. If feasible, d/c at least 4 weeks before and through 2 weeks after major surgery or other surgeries associated with an elevated risk of VTE. D/C during prolonged immobilization. Start use no earlier than 4 weeks after delivery in women who are not breastfeeding. D/C if jaundice develops. Hepatic adenomas and increased risk of hepatocellular carcinoma reported. Increase in BP reported. Monitor BP in women with well-controlled HTN; d/c if BP rises significantly. Increased risk of cervical cancer or intraepithelial neoplasia, and gallbladder disease. May decrease glucose tolerance; monitor prediabetic and diabetic women. Consider alternative contraception with uncontrolled dyslipidemia. May increase risk of pancreatitis with hypertriglyceridemia or a family history thereof. D/C if indicated and evaluate cause if new headaches that are recurrent, persistent, or severe develop. Consider discontinuation in case of increased frequency or severity of migraine during use. Unscheduled bleeding and spotting reported. Consider non-hormonal causes and take adequate diagnostic measures to rule out malignancy, other pathology, or pregnancy in the event of unscheduled bleeding. Consider possibility of pregnancy in the event of amenorrhea. Amenorrhea or oligomenorrhea may occur after discontinuation of therapy. Administration of therapy should not be used as a test for pregnancy. Caution with history of depression; d/c if depression recurs to a serious degree. May raise the serum concentrations of sex hormone-binding globulin. May induce or exacerbate symptoms of angioedema in patients with hereditary angioedema. Chloasma may occur; avoid exposure to sun or UV radiation in women with a tendency to chloasma. May influence the results of certain laboratory tests.

ADVERSE REACTIONS

Breast symptoms (eg, breast discomfort, engorgement, pain); dysmenorrhea, vaginal bleeding, and menstrual disorders; mood, affect, and anxiety disorders; diarrhea; headache; application-site disorder; N/V; abdominal pain; dizziness; vaginal yeast infection.

DRUG INTERACTIONS

May decrease plasma concentrations and potentially diminish effectiveness or increase breakthrough bleeding when used concomitantly with drugs or herbal products that induce certain enzymes, including CYP3A4 (eg, phenytoin, barbiturates, products containing St. John's wort); use an alternative method of contraception or a backup method when used concomitantly with enzyme inducers, and continue backup contraception for 28 days after discontinuing the enzyme inducer. Atorvastatin or rosuvastatin may increase EE exposure; ascorbic acid and acetaminophen (APAP) may increase EE levels. CYP3A4 inhibitors (eg, itraconazole, voriconazole, grapefruit juice) may increase plasma hormone levels. Significant changes (decreased/increased) sometimes noted in estrogen and/or progestin levels when coadministered with HIV protease inhibitors (decreased [eg, nelfinavir, darunavir/ritonavir, (fos)amprenavir/ritonavir] or increased [eg, indinavir, atazanavir/ritonavir])/HCV protease inhibitors or with non-nucleoside reverse transcriptase inhibitors (decreased [eg, nevirapine] or increased [eg, etravirine]). May inhibit the metabolism of other compounds (eg, cyclosporine, prednisolone, theophylline) and increase their plasma concentrations. May decrease concentrations of APAP, clofibric acid, morphine, salicylic acid, and temazepam. May decrease levels of lamotrigine and reduce seizure control; dosage adjustments of lamotrigine may be necessary. May raise the serum concentrations of thyroxine-binding globulin and cortisol-binding globulin; dose of replacement thyroid hormone or cortisol therapy may need to be increased.

NURSING CONSIDERATIONS

Assessment: Assess for risk of arterial or venous thrombotic diseases, benign or malignant liver tumors, liver disease, undiagnosed abnormal uterine bleeding, presence or history of breast cancer or other estrogen- or progestin-sensitive cancer, pregnancy/nursing status, and any other conditions where treatment is contraindicated/cautioned. Assess for possible drug interactions.

Monitoring: Monitor for arterial thrombotic or VTE events, hepatic adenomas, hepatocellular carcinoma, gallbladder disease, and other adverse effects. Monitor lipid levels with hyperlipidemia, BP with history of HTN, serum glucose levels in diabetic and prediabetic patients, and for signs of worsening depression with previous history. Conduct a yearly visit with patient for a BP check and for other indicated healthcare.

Patient Counseling: Inform of risks and benefits of therapy. Inform that cigarette smoking increases risk of serious CV events, and that women who are >35 yrs of age and smoke should not use combined hormonal contraceptives. Counsel that therapy does not protect against HIV infection (AIDS) and other sexually transmitted infections. Instruct to d/c if pregnancy occurs during use. Instruct to apply a single patch on the same day every week (Weeks 1-3). Instruct patient on what to do in the event a patch is missed. Instruct women who start combined hormonal contraceptives postpartum, and who have not yet had a period, to use an additional method of contraception until they have used patch for 7 consecutive days. Counsel to use a backup or alternative method of contraception when enzyme inducers are concomitantly used. Inform that breast milk production may be reduced with use. Inform that amenorrhea may occur. Advise that pregnancy should be ruled out in the event of amenorrhea in 2 or more consecutive cycles. Advise that insufficient drug delivery occurs when patch becomes partially or completely detached and remains detached.

Storage: 25°C (77°F); excursions permitted to 15-30°C (59-86°F). Store patches in their protective pouches. Do not store in the refrigerator or freezer.

ORTHO TRI-CYCLEN LO – ethinyl estradiol/norgestimate — RX

Class: Estrogen/progestogen combination

Cigarette smoking increases risk of serious cardiovascular (CV) side effects. Risk increases with age and with heavy smoking (≥15 cigarettes/day) and is quite marked in women over >35 yrs of age. Women who use oral contraceptives are strongly advised not to smoke.

ADULT DOSAGE

Contraception

1 tab qd at the same time each day, for 28 days, then repeat

Start 1st Sunday after menses begin or 1st day of menses

Conversions

Switching from Another Oral Contraceptive: Start on the same day that a new pack of the previous oral contraceptive would have been started

Missed Dose

Miss 1 Active Tab in Weeks 1, 2, or 3: Take as soon as dose is remembered

Miss 2 Active Tabs in Weeks 1 or 2: Take 2 active tabs on the day it is remembered and 2 active tabs the next day, and then continue taking 1 tab qd until pack is finished. Use a backup method of birth control if patient has intercourse in the 7 days after missing pills

Miss 2 Active Tabs in Week 3 or Miss ≥3 Active Tabs in a Row: (Sunday Start) Continue to take 1 tab qd until Sunday, then throw out the rest of the pack and start a new pack that same day. (Day 1 Start) Throw out the rest of the pack and start a new pack that same day. (Sunday Start/Day 1 Start) Use a backup method of birth control if patient has intercourse in the 7 days after missing pills

PEDIATRIC DOSAGE

Contraception

Not indicated for use premenarche; refer to adult dosing

DOSE MODIFICATION

Other Important Modifications

Postpartum Women Who Elect Not to Breastfeed:
May start 4 weeks postpartum

ADMINISTRATION

Oral route

Take exactly ud and at intervals not exceeding 24 hrs
For the 1st cycle of a Sunday Start regimen, use another method of contraception until after the first 7 consecutive days of administration

HOW SUPPLIED

Tab: (Ethinyl Estradiol [EE]-Norgestimate) 0.025mg-0.18mg, 0.025mg-0.215mg, 0.025mg-0.25mg

CONTRAINDICATIONS

Thrombophlebitis or past history of deep vein thrombophlebitis, thromboembolic disorders (current or past history), cerebral vascular or CAD (current or history), valvular heart disease with complications, severe HTN, diabetes with vascular involvement, headaches with focal neurological symptoms, major surgery with prolonged immobilization, known or suspected carcinoma of the breast or personal history of breast cancer, carcinoma of the endometrium or other known or suspected estrogen-dependent neoplasia, undiagnosed abnormal genital bleeding, cholestatic jaundice of pregnancy or jaundice with prior pill use, hepatic adenomas or carcinomas, known or suspected pregnancy.

WARNINGS/PRECAUTIONS

For the first cycle of a Sunday Start regimen, use another method of contraception until after the first 7 consecutive days of administration. Not indicated for use in emergency contraception. Increased risk of MI, vascular disease, thromboembolism, stroke, hepatic neoplasia, and gallbladder disease. Increased risk of morbidity and mortality in the presence of other underlying risk factors (eg, HTN, hyperlipidemias, obesity, diabetes mellitus). If feasible, d/c at least 4 weeks prior to and for 2 weeks after elective surgery of a type associated with an increased risk of thromboembolism, and during and following prolonged immobilization. Start use no earlier than 4 weeks after delivery in women who elect not to breastfeed. May increase risk of breast cancer and cancer of the reproductive organs. Contact lens wearers who develop visual changes or changes in lens tolerance should be assessed by an ophthalmologist. Retinal thrombosis reported; d/c if unexplained partial or complete loss of vision occurs, or if onset of proptosis or diplopia, papilledema, or retinal vascular lesions develop. Should not be used to induce withdrawal bleeding as a test for pregnancy, nor to treat threatened or habitual abortion during pregnancy. May cause glucose intolerance; monitor prediabetic and diabetic patients. May elevate serum TG and LDL levels and may render the control of hyperlipidemias more difficult. May increase BP; monitor closely and d/c if significant elevation of BP occurs. D/C and evaluate the cause if new onset/exacerbation of migraine or recurrent, persistent, severe headache with a new pattern develops. Breakthrough bleeding and spotting reported; rule out malignancy or pregnancy. Post-pill amenorrhea or oligomenorrhea may occur. D/C if jaundice develops. May cause fluid retention. Monitor closely in patients with history of depression; d/c if depression recurs to a serious degree. Ectopic and intrauterine pregnancies may occur in contraceptive failures. May affect certain endocrine, hepatic, and blood components in lab tests. Rule out pregnancy if 2 consecutive periods are missed.

ADVERSE REACTIONS

N/V, breakthrough bleeding, GI symptoms (eg, abdominal cramps, bloating), spotting, amenorrhea, migraine, depression, vaginal candidiasis, edema, weight changes, melasma, breast changes, changes in cervical erosion and secretion.

DRUG INTERACTIONS

Reduced effects resulting in pregnancy or breakthrough bleeding with antibiotics, anticonvulsants, other drugs that increase the metabolism of contraceptive steroids (eg, rifampin, phenytoin, carbamazepine, bosentan). Significant changes (increase/decrease) sometimes noted in estrogen and/or progestin levels when coadministered with anti-HIV protease inhibitors. Herbal products containing St. John's wort may induce hepatic enzymes (cytochrome P450) and P-gp transporter, may reduce the effectiveness of contraceptive steroids, and may also result in breakthrough bleeding. Bosentan may decrease concentrations and may thereby increase the risk of pregnancy and unscheduled bleeding. Atorvastatin may increase EE exposure; ascorbic acid and APAP may increase plasma EE levels. CYP3A4 inhibitors (eg, itraconazole, ketoconazole) may increase plasma hormone levels. May inhibit metabolism of other compounds. Increased levels of cyclosporine, prednisolone, and theophylline reported. Decreased plasma concentration of APAP and increased the clearance of temazepam, salicylic acid, morphine, and clofibric acid. May significantly decrease plasma levels of lamotrigine and may reduce seizure control; dosage adjustment of lamotrigine may be necessary.

NURSING CONSIDERATIONS

Assessment: Assess for hypersensitivity to therapy, thrombophlebitis or thromboembolic disorders, past history of deep vein thrombophlebitis or thromboembolic disorders, cerebral vascular or CAD (current or past history), valvular heart disease with complications, diabetes with vascular involvement, headaches with focal neurological symptoms, pregnancy/nursing status, and for any other conditions where treatment is contraindicated or cautioned. Assess for possible drug interactions.

Monitoring: Monitor for signs/symptoms of MI, thromboembolism, stroke, and other adverse effects. Monitor BP with history of HTN, serum glucose levels in diabetic or prediabetic patients, lipid levels with history of hyperlipidemia, and for signs of worsening depression with previous history. Monitor liver function. Refer contact lens wearers who develop visual changes or changes in lens tolerance to an ophthalmologist. Monitor women who have breast nodules or a strong family history of breast cancer. Perform annual history and physical exam.

Patient Counseling: Inform that the drug does not protect against HIV infection (AIDS) and other sexually transmitted diseases. Counsel about potential adverse effects. Explain that cigarette smoking increases the risk of serious CV effects and that women who use oral contraceptives should not smoke. Instruct to take exactly ud and at intervals not exceeding 24 hrs. Instruct on what to do if pills are missed. Instruct to use additional method of protection until after the 1st week of administration in the initial cycle when utilizing the Sunday Start regimen. Instruct to d/c if pregnancy is confirmed/suspected. Counsel that efficacy may decrease if vomiting/diarrhea develops; instruct to use a backup method of contraception and to notify physician. Inform that spotting, light bleeding, or stomach sickness may occur during the first 1-3 packs of pills; advise not to d/c medication and to notify physician if symptoms persist. Instruct to d/c if pregnancy is confirmed/suspected. Instruct to notify physician if breastfeeding. Inform that certain drugs may make therapy less effective and that additional contraception may be needed. If scheduled for any lab test, advise to inform physician that patient is taking birth control pills.

Storage: 25°C (77°F); excursions permitted to 15-30°C (59-86°F). Protect from light.

OSENI – alogliptin/pioglitazone RX

Class: Dipeptidyl peptidase-4 (DPP-4) inhibitor/thiazolidinedione

Thiazolidinediones, including pioglitazone, cause or exacerbate CHF in some patients. After initiation and dose increases, monitor carefully for signs and symptoms of heart failure (HF); manage accordingly and consider discontinuation or dose reduction if HF develops. Not recommended with symptomatic HF. Contraindicated with established NYHA Class III or IV HF.

ADULT DOSAGE

Type 2 Diabetes Mellitus

Initial:

Inadequately Controlled on Diet and Exercise:
25mg/15mg qd or 25mg/30mg qd

Inadequately Controlled on Metformin Monotherapy:
25mg/15mg qd or 25mg/30mg qd

On Alogliptin and Requiring Additional Glycemic Control:
25mg/15mg qd or 25mg/30mg qd

On Pioglitazone and Requiring Additional Glycemic Control:
25mg/15mg qd, 25mg/30mg qd, or 25mg/45mg qd as appropriate based upon current therapy

Switching from Alogliptin Coadministered w/ Pioglitazone:
Initiate at the dose of alogliptin and pioglitazone based upon current therapy

Patients w/ CHF (NYHA Class I or II):
25mg/15mg qd

Max: 25mg/45mg qd

PEDIATRIC DOSAGE

Pediatric use may not have been established

DOSE MODIFICATION

Concomitant Medications

Strong CYP2C8 Inhibitors (eg, Gemfibrozil):
Max: 25mg/15mg qd

Renal Impairment

Moderate (CrCl ≥30-<60mL/min): 12.5mg/15mg qd, 12.5mg/30mg qd, or 12.5mg/45mg qd
Severe or ESRD: Not recommended for use; coadministration of pioglitazone and alogliptin 6.25mg qd based on individual requirements may be considered

ADMINISTRATION

Oral route

May be taken w/ or w/o food
Do not split tabs before swallowing

HOW SUPPLIED

Tab: (Alogliptin/Pioglitazone) 12.5mg/15mg, 12.5mg/30mg, 12.5mg/45mg, 25mg/15mg, 25mg/30mg, 25mg/45mg

CONTRAINDICATIONS

NYHA Class III or IV HF.

WARNINGS/PRECAUTIONS

Not for use with type 1 DM or for treatment of diabetic ketoacidosis. Not recommended with severe renal impairment or ESRD. No conclusive evidence of macrovascular risk reduction. Fatal and nonfatal hepatic events reported; obtain baseline LFTs, and initiate with caution in patients with abnormal LFTs. Measure LFTs promptly in patients who report symptoms that may indicate liver injury. If abnormal LFTs (ALT >3X ULN) are reported, interrupt treatment and investigate for the probable cause, and do not restart therapy without another explanation for the LFT abnormalities. Alogliptin: Acute pancreatitis reported; d/c if suspected and initiate appropriate management. Serious hypersensitivity reactions reported; d/c if suspected, assess for other potential causes, and institute alternative treatment for diabetes. Caution with history of angioedema to another dipeptidyl peptidase-4 (DPP-4) inhibitor. Pioglitazone: Dose-related edema reported. Increased incidence of bone fractures reported in females. Not for use in patients with active bladder cancer; consider benefits versus risks in patients with a prior history of bladder cancer. Macular edema reported; promptly refer to an ophthalmologist if visual symptoms occur. May result in ovulation in some premenopausal anovulatory women, which may increase risk for pregnancy; adequate contraception is recommended.

ADVERSE REACTIONS

Nasopharyngitis, back pain, URTI, influenza, hypoglycemia, CHF.

DRUG INTERACTIONS

May require lower dose of insulin or insulin secretagogue to minimize risk of hypoglycemia. Pioglitazone: Increased exposure and $T_{1/2}$ with strong CYP2C8 inhibitors (eg, gemfibrozil). CYP2C8 inducers (eg, rifampin) may decrease exposure; if a CYP2C8 inducer is started or stopped during treatment, dose may need to be adjusted based on clinical response. May cause dose-related fluid retention when used with other antidiabetic medications, most commonly with insulin.

NURSING CONSIDERATIONS

Assessment: Assess for HF or risk of HF, edema, renal/hepatic function, bone health, history of pancreatitis, diabetic ketoacidosis, active/history of bladder cancer, history of angioedema to another DPP-4 inhibitor, pregnancy/nursing status, and possible drug interactions. Obtain FPG and HbA1c.

Monitoring: Monitor for signs/symptoms of CHF, pancreatitis, hypersensitivity reactions, fractures, visual symptoms, and other adverse reactions. Monitor LFTs, FPG, and HbA1c. Monitor renal function periodically.

Patient Counseling: Inform of the potential risks and benefits of therapy. Instruct to immediately report to physician any symptoms that may indicate HF. Inform that pancreatitis may occur; instruct to promptly d/c use and contact physician if persistent severe abdominal pain occurs. Instruct to d/c use and seek medical advice promptly if signs/symptoms of allergic reactions, liver injury, or bladder cancer occur. Inform that hypoglycemia can occur; explain the risks, symptoms, and appropriate management. Counsel premenopausal women to use adequate contraception during treatment. Advise not to double the next dose if a dose is missed. Instruct to inform physician if an unusual symptom develops or if a symptom persists or worsens.

Storage: 25°C (77°F); excursions permitted to 15-30°C (59-86°F). Protect from moisture and humidity.

OSMOPREP – sodium phosphate dibasic anhydrous/sodium phosphate monobasic monohydrate

RX

Class: Bowel cleanser

Rare, but serious, acute phosphate nephropathy reported; some cases resulted in permanent renal impairment and some patients required long-term dialysis. Patients at increased risk may include those with increased age, hypovolemia, increased bowel transit time (eg, bowel obstruction), active colitis, or baseline kidney disease, and those using medicines that affect renal perfusion or function (eg, diuretics, ACE inhibitors, ARBs, and possibly NSAIDs). Use the dose and dosing regimen as recommended (pm/am split dose).

ADULT DOSAGE

Bowel Cleansing

Prior to Colonoscopy:

PM Before Colonoscopy:

Take 4 tabs w/ 8 oz of clear liquids every 15 min for a total of 20 tabs

Day of Colonoscopy:

Starting 3-5 hrs before procedure, take 4 tabs w/ 8 oz of clear liquids every 15 min for a total of 12 tabs

PEDIATRIC DOSAGE

Pediatric use may not have been established

ADMINISTRATION
Oral route

Do not drink any liquids colored purple or red
Adequately hydrate before, during, and after administration

HOW SUPPLIED
Tab: (Sodium Phosphate Monobasic Monohydrate/Sodium Phosphate Dibasic Anhydrous) 1.102g/0.398g

CONTRAINDICATIONS
Biopsy-proven acute phosphate nephropathy, GI obstruction, gastric bypass or stapling surgery, bowel perforation, toxic colitis, toxic megacolon.

WARNINGS/PRECAUTIONS
Do not use within 7 days of previous administration. Rare, but serious, renal failure and nephrocalcinosis reported. Caution with renal impairment (CrCl <30mL/min), history of acute phosphate nephropathy, known or suspected electrolyte disturbances (eg, dehydration), or with conditions that increase the risk for fluid and electrolyte disturbances or increase the risk of seizure (eg, hyponatremia). Adequately hydrate before, during, and after use. If significant vomiting or signs of dehydration develop, consider performing postcolonoscopy lab tests (electrolytes, SrCr, and BUN). Correct electrolyte abnormalities before treatment. Do not administer additional laxative or purgative agents, particularly additional sodium phosphate-based purgative or enema products. Serious arrhythmias rarely reported; consider predose and postcolonoscopy ECGs in patients at increased risk of serious cardiac arrhythmias. Generalized tonic-clonic seizures and/or loss of consciousness rarely reported; caution with history of seizures. May induce colonic mucosal aphthous ulcerations; consider this in patients with known or suspected inflammatory bowel disease (IBD). Caution with acute exacerbation of chronic IBD, impaired gag reflex, in patients prone to regurgitation or aspiration, and in elderly.

ADVERSE REACTIONS
Acute phosphate nephropathy, abdominal bloating, abdominal pain, N/V, dizziness, headache, hyperphosphatemia, hypokalemia.

DRUG INTERACTIONS
See Boxed Warning. PO medication administered within 1 hr of the start of each dose may be flushed from GI tract and may not be absorbed properly. Caution with drugs that may affect electrolyte levels (eg, diuretics), increase the risk of arrhythmias, prolong QT interval, and lower the seizure threshold (eg, TCAs). Caution in patients withdrawing from alcohol or benzodiazepines.

NURSING CONSIDERATIONS

Assessment: Assess for biopsy-proven acute phosphate nephropathy, GI obstruction, gastric bypass or stapling surgery, bowel perforation, toxic colitis, toxic megacolon, risk of acute phosphate nephropathy, electrolyte abnormalities, or any other conditions where treatment is cautioned. Assess for hypersensitivity, pregnancy/nursing status, and possible drug interactions. Consider performing baseline lab tests (electrolytes, SrCr, and BUN). Consider predose ECGs in patients at increased risk of serious cardiac arrhythmias.

Monitoring: Monitor for acute phosphate nephropathy, arrhythmias, generalized tonic-clonic seizures, loss of consciousness, colonic mucosal aphthous ulcerations, and other adverse reactions. Consider performing postcolonoscopy lab tests. Consider postcolonoscopy ECGs in patients at increased risk of serious cardiac arrhythmias.

Patient Counseling: Instruct to notify physician if patient has a history of renal disease or takes medication for BP, or cardiac/renal disease. Explain the importance of taking the recommended fluid regimen and advise to hydrate adequately before, during, and after use. Instruct to contact physician if experiencing symptoms of dehydration, or worsening of bloating, abdominal pain, N/V, or headache. Counsel not to take with other laxatives or enemas made with sodium phosphate.

Storage: 25°C (77°F); excursions permitted to 15-30°C (59-86°F).

OSPHENA — ospemifene

RX

Class: Estrogen agonist/antagonist

Has estrogen agonistic effects in the endometrium. Increased risk of endometrial cancer in a woman w/ a uterus who uses unopposed estrogens. Adding a progestin to estrogen therapy reduces the risk of endometrial hyperplasia. Perform adequate diagnostic measures to rule out malignancy in postmenopausal women w/ undiagnosed persistent/recurring abnormal genital bleeding. Increased risk of stroke and deep vein thrombosis (DVT) reported in postmenopausal women (50-79 yrs of age) who received daily oral conjugated estrogens-alone. Should be prescribed for the shortest duration consistent w/ treatment goals and risks.

ADULT DOSAGE

Dyspareunia

Moderate to Severe Dyspareunia, a Symptom of Vulvar and Vaginal Atrophy, Due to Menopause:

Usual: 60mg qd

Reevaluate periodically as clinically appropriate to determine if treatment is still necessary

PEDIATRIC DOSAGE

Pediatric use may not have been established

DOSE MODIFICATION

Hepatic Impairment

Severe (Child-Pugh Class C): Should not be used

ADMINISTRATION

Oral route

Take w/ food

HOW SUPPLIED

Tab: 60mg

CONTRAINDICATIONS

Undiagnosed abnormal genital bleeding; known or suspected estrogen-dependent neoplasia; active DVT, pulmonary embolism (PE) or a history of these conditions; active arterial thromboembolic disease (eg, stroke, MI) or history of these conditions; women who are or may become pregnant.

WARNINGS/PRECAUTIONS

Manage risk factors for cardiovascular disorders, arterial vascular disease (eg, HTN, diabetes mellitus, tobacco use, hypercholesterolemia, obesity), and/or venous thromboembolism (VTE) (eg, personal/family history of VTE, obesity, systemic lupus erythematosus) appropriately. MI reported. D/C immediately if thromboembolic/hemorrhagic stroke or VTE occurs or is suspected. If feasible, d/c therapy at least 4-6 weeks before surgery of the type associated w/ an increased risk of thromboembolism, or during periods of prolonged immobilization. Avoid w/ known/suspected breast cancer or w/ a history of breast cancer. Avoid w/ severe hepatic impairment.

ADVERSE REACTIONS

Hot flush, vaginal discharge, muscle spasms.

DRUG INTERACTIONS

Avoid w/ estrogens and estrogen agonists/antagonists. Fluconazole increases systemic exposure and may increase ospemifene-related adverse reactions; avoid concomitant use. Rifampin, a strong CYP3A4/moderate CYP2C9/moderate CYP2C19 inducer, decreases systemic exposure; coadministration w/ CYP3A4, CYP2C9, and/or CYP2C19 inducers would be expected to decrease systemic exposure, which may decrease clinical effect. Ketoconazole increases systemic exposure; chronic ketoconazole administration may increase risk of ospemifene-related adverse reactions. Use w/ other drug products that are highly protein bound may increase exposure of either that drug or ospemifene. May increase risk of ospemifene-related adverse reactions w/ CYP3A4 and CYP2C9 inhibitors.

NURSING CONSIDERATIONS

Assessment: Assess for drug hypersensitivity, undiagnosed abnormal genital bleeding, known/suspected estrogen-dependent neoplasia, active/history of DVT, active/history of PE, active/history of arterial thromboembolic disease, known/suspected or history of breast cancer, hepatic impairment, pregnancy/nursing status, possible drug interactions, or any other condition where treatment is cautioned or contraindicated.

Monitoring: Monitor for endometrial cancer, thromboembolic/hemorrhagic stroke, DVT, and other adverse reactions. Reevaluate periodically as clinically appropriate to determine if treatment is still necessary. Perform adequate diagnostic measures, including directed and random endometrial sampling when indicated, to rule out malignancy in postmenopausal women w/ undiagnosed persistent/recurring abnormal genital bleeding.

Patient Counseling: Advise of risks and benefits of therapy. Inform that therapy may initiate/increase occurrence of hot flashes in some women. Inform postmenopausal women who have had hypersensitivity reactions to therapy not to take the drug. Inform postmenopausal women of the importance of reporting unusual vaginal bleeding to healthcare provider as soon as possible.

Storage: 20-25°C (68-77°F); excursions permitted to 15-30°C (59-86°F).

OTEZLA – apremilast

RX

Class: Phosphodiesterase 4 (PDE4) inhibitor

ADULT DOSAGE

Psoriatic Arthritis

Initial Dosage Titration:

Day 1: 10mg (am)
Day 2: 10mg bid (am and pm)
Day 3: 10mg (am) and 20mg (pm)
Day 4: 20mg bid (am and pm)
Day 5: 20mg (am) and 30mg (pm)

Maint:
Day 6 and Thereafter: 30mg bid (am and pm)

Plaque Psoriasis

Patients w/ Moderate to Severe Plaque Psoriasis Who are Candidates for Phototherapy or Systemic Therapy:

Initial Dosage Titration:

Day 1: 10mg (am)
Day 2: 10mg bid (am and pm)
Day 3: 10mg (am) and 20mg (pm)
Day 4: 20mg bid (am and pm)
Day 5: 20mg (am) and 30mg (pm)

Maint:
Day 6 and Thereafter: 30mg bid (am and pm)

PEDIATRIC DOSAGE

Pediatric use may not have been established

DOSE MODIFICATION

Renal Impairment

Severe (CrCl <30mL/min):

Initial Dosage Titration:

Days 1 through 3: 10mg qam
Days 4 and 5: 20mg qam

Maint:
Day 6 and Thereafter: 30mg qam

ADMINISTRATION

Oral route

May be administered w/o regard to meals
Do not crush, split, or chew

HOW SUPPLIED

Tab: 10mg, 20mg, 30mg

WARNINGS/PRECAUTIONS

Depression or depressed mood, and suicidal ideation and behavior reported; carefully evaluate the risks and benefits of continuing treatment if such events occur. Weight decrease reported; consider discontinuation if unexplained or clinically significant weight loss occurs.

ADVERSE REACTIONS

Diarrhea, headache/tension headache, N/V, URTI, abdominal pain, fatigue, dyspepsia, decreased appetite.

DRUG INTERACTIONS

Decreased exposure w/ strong CYP450 inducers (eg, rifampin), which may result in loss of efficacy; not recommended w/ CYP450 inducers (eg, rifampin, phenobarbital, carbamazepine).

NURSING CONSIDERATIONS

Assessment: Assess for history of depression and/or suicidal thoughts or behavior, drug hypersensitivity, renal impairment, pregnancy/nursing status, and possible drug interactions.

Monitoring: Monitor for emergence or worsening of depression, suicidal thoughts, or other mood changes, and for other adverse reactions. Monitor weight regularly and monitor renal function.

Patient Counseling: Inform of the risks and benefits of therapy. Advise patients, their caregivers, and families to be alert for emergence or worsening of depression, suicidal thoughts, or other mood changes, and to contact physician if such changes occur. Counsel to monitor weight regularly and to notify physician if unexplained or clinically significant weight loss occurs. Instruct to take only as prescribed.

Storage: <30°C (86°F).

OXTELLAR XR – oxcarbazepine

RX

Class: Dibenzazepine

ADULT DOSAGE

Partial Seizures

Adjunctive Therapy:

Initial: 600mg qd for 1 week

Titrate: May increase at weekly intervals in 600mg/day increments

Usual: 1200-2400mg qd

Conversions

Conversion from Immediate-Release Oxcarbazepine:

Higher doses may be necessary

PEDIATRIC DOSAGE

Partial Seizures

Adjunctive Therapy:

6-17 Years:

Initial: 8-10mg/kg (up to 600mg) qd for 1 week

Titrate: May increase at weekly intervals in 8-10mg/kg increments (up to 600mg) qd

Target Maint Dose (Achieved Over 2-3 Weeks):

20-29kg: 900mg qd

29.1-39kg: 1200mg qd

>39kg: 1800mg qd

Conversions

Conversion from Immediate-Release Oxcarbazepine:

Higher doses may be necessary

DOSE MODIFICATION

Concomitant Medications

Enzyme-Inducing Antiepileptic Drugs:

Dose increases may be necessary; consider initiating therapy at 900mg qd

Renal Impairment

Severe (CrCl <30mL/min):

Initial: 1/2 the usual initial dose (300mg qd)

Titrate: May increase at weekly intervals in 300-450mg/day increments to achieve desired clinical response

ESRD on Dialysis:

Use immediate-release oxcarbazepine

Hepatic Impairment

Severe: Not recommended

Elderly

Initial: Consider starting at 300-450mg qd

Titrate: May increase at weekly intervals in 300-450mg/day increments to achieve desired clinical effect

Discontinuation

Withdraw gradually to minimize potential of increased seizure frequency

ADMINISTRATION

Oral route

Take on an empty stomach (at least 1 hr ac or at least 2 hrs pc)

Take tabs whole w/ water or other liquid; do not cut, crush, or chew

For ease of swallowing in pediatric patients or patients w/ difficulty swallowing, achieve daily dosages w/ multiples of appropriate lower strength tablets (eg, 150mg tabs)

HOW SUPPLIED

Tab, Extended-Release: 150mg, 300mg, 600mg

WARNINGS/PRECAUTIONS

Clinically significant hyponatremia may develop; measure serum Na^+ levels during treatment if symptoms occur, and particularly if receiving concomitant medications known to decrease serum Na^+ levels (eg, drugs associated with inappropriate antidiuretic hormone secretion). Anaphylaxis and angioedema involving the larynx, glottis, lips, and eyelids reported with IR oxcarbazepine; d/c if any of these reactions develop, do not rechallenge and initiate alternative treatment. Treat patients with history of hypersensitivity reactions to carbamazepine only if potential benefit justifies potential risk; d/c immediately if signs/symptoms of hypersensitivity develop. Serious dermatological reactions (eg, Stevens-Johnson syndrome, toxic epidermal necrolysis) reported with IR oxcarbazepine; consider discontinuing and prescribing another AED if a skin reaction develops. Increased risk of suicidal thoughts/behavior; monitor for emergence or worsening of depression, suicidal thoughts/behavior, and/or any unusual changes in mood/behavior. Withdraw gradually to minimize potential of increased seizure frequency. Multiorgan hypersensitivity reactions reported with IR oxcarbazepine; d/c and initiate an alternative treatment if suspected. Pancytopenia, agranulocytosis, and leukopenia reported; consider discontinuing if any evidence of these hematologic events develop. Levels may decrease during pregnancy; monitor during pregnancy and through the postpartum period. IR oxcarbazepine associated with decreases in T4, without changes in T3 or TSH. Caution with severe renal impairment and in the elderly. Not recommended with severe hepatic impairment.

ADVERSE REACTIONS
Dizziness, somnolence, headache, balance disorder, tremor, vomiting, diplopia, asthenia, fatigue, ataxia, nystagmus, blurred vision, visual impairment, dyspepsia, sinusitis.

DRUG INTERACTIONS
AEDs that are CYP450 inducers (eg, carbamazepine, phenobarbital, phenytoin), valproic acid, and verapamil may decrease 10-monohydroxy derivative (MHD) levels. May inhibit CYP2C19 and induce CYP3A4/5 with potentially important effects on levels of other drugs. May decrease levels of dihydropyridine calcium antagonists (eg, felodipine), oral contraceptives (eg, ethinyl estradiol, levonorgestrel), and cyclosporine.

NURSING CONSIDERATIONS

Assessment: Assess for hypersensitivity to drug or history of hypersensitivity to carbamazepine, depression, renal/hepatic impairment, pregnancy/nursing status, and for possible drug interactions.

Monitoring: Monitor for signs/symptoms of hyponatremia, anaphylaxis, angioedema, dermatological/hematologic reactions, emergence/worsening of depression, suicidal thoughts/behavior and/or any unusual changes in mood/behavior, multiorgan hypersensitivity reactions, and other adverse reactions. Monitor patients during pregnancy and through the postpartum period.

Patient Counseling: Advise to report symptoms of low Na^+, and fever associated with other organ system involvement (eg, rash, lymphadenopathy). Instruct to immediately report signs/symptoms suggesting angioedema and to d/c therapy until consulting with physician. Instruct to contact physician immediately if a hypersensitivity reaction, symptoms suggestive of blood disorders, or if a skin reaction occurs. Inform female patients of childbearing age that concurrent use with hormonal contraceptives may render this method of contraception less effective; advise to use additional nonhormonal forms of contraception. Counsel that therapy may increase risk of suicidal thoughts or behavior and to be alert for emergence/worsening of symptoms of depression, any unusual changes in mood/behavior, or emergence of suicidal thoughts/behavior or thoughts about self-harm; instruct to immediately report behaviors of conern to healthcare providers. Advise to use caution if taking alcohol while on therapy, due to possible additive sedative effect. Inform that therapy may cause dizziness and somnolence; advise not to drive/operate machinery until effects have been determined. Encourage to enroll in the North American Antiepileptic Drug Pregnancy Registry if pregnancy occurs.

Storage: 25°C (77°F); excursions permitted to 15-30°C (59-86°F). Protect from light and moisture.

OXYCODONE TABLETS – oxycodone hydrochloride CII

Class: Opioid analgesic

OTHER BRAND NAMES
Roxicodone

ADULT DOSAGE

Moderate to Severe Pain

Opioid-Naive:
Initial: 5-15mg q4-6h PRN
Titrate: Adjust dose based upon response

For chronic pain, give on an around-the-clock basis
For severe chronic pain, give q4-6h at the lowest effective dose

Conversions

From Fixed-Ratio Opioid/Acetaminophen, Opioid/Aspirin, or Opioid/Nonsteroidal Combination Drugs:
Decision should be made whether or not to continue the nonopioid analgesic

Discontinuing Nonopioid Analgesic:
May be necessary to titrate to the minimum effective dose

Continuing Nonopioid Regimen as a Separate Single Entity Agent:
Starting dose should be based upon the most recent dose of opioid as a baseline for further titration of oxycodone
Incremental increases should be gauged according to side effects to an acceptable level of analgesia

PEDIATRIC DOSAGE
Pediatric use may not have been established

From Other Opioids:
Factor the potency of the prior opioid relative to oxycodone to select the total daily dose
Closely observe and adjust dose based on response

DOSE MODIFICATION

Renal Impairment
Initial: Dose conservatively
Titrate: Adjust according to clinical situation

Hepatic Impairment
Initial: Dose conservatively
Titrate: Adjust according to clinical situation

Discontinuation
D/C gradually; decrease by 25-50% per day
Raise dose to previous level and titrate down more slowly if withdrawal symptoms occur

ADMINISTRATION
Oral route

HOW SUPPLIED
Tab: 10mg*, 20mg*; (Roxicodone) 5mg*, 15mg*, 30mg* *scored

CONTRAINDICATIONS
Significant respiratory depression (in unmonitored settings or the absence of resuscitative equipment), paralytic ileus, acute or severe bronchial asthma or hypercarbia.

WARNINGS/PRECAUTIONS
Respiratory depression may occur; extreme caution with significant chronic obstructive pulmonary disease or cor pulmonale, substantially decreased respiratory reserve, hypoxia, hypercapnia, preexisting respiratory depression, and in the elderly/debilitated. May cause severe hypotension; caution with circulatory shock. May produce orthostatic hypotension in ambulatory patients. Respiratory depressant effects and capacity to elevate CSF pressure may be markedly exaggerated in the presence of head injury, other intracranial lesions, or preexisting increased intracranial pressure. May obscure the clinical course of patients with head injuries. Caution with acute alcoholism, adrenocortical insufficiency (eg, Addison's disease), convulsive disorders, CNS depression or coma, delirium tremens, kyphoscoliosis associated with respiratory depression, myxedema or hypothyroidism, prostatic hypertrophy or urethral stricture, severe hepatic/renal/pulmonary impairment, and toxic psychosis. May obscure diagnosis or clinical course in patients with acute abdominal conditions. May aggravate convulsions with convulsive disorders and may induce or aggravate seizures in some clinical settings. Potential for tolerance and physical dependence. May cause spasm of the sphincter of Oddi; caution with biliary tract disease, including acute pancreatitis. May cause increases in serum amylase level. Not recommended for use during or immediately prior to labor. May impair mental/physical abilities.

ADVERSE REACTIONS
Respiratory depression/arrest, circulatory depression, cardiac arrest, hypotension, shock, N/V, constipation, headache, pruritus, insomnia, dizziness, asthenia, somnolence.

DRUG INTERACTIONS
CYP2D6 inhibitors may block the partial metabolism to oxymorphone. May enhance neuromuscular blocking action of skeletal muscle relaxants and increase respiratory depression. Additive CNS depression with other CNS depressants (eg, narcotics, general anesthetics, tranquilizers, alcohol); when combination is contemplated, reduce dose of one or both agents. Mixed agonist/antagonist analgesics (eg, pentazocine, nalbuphine, buprenorphine) may reduce analgesic effect and/or precipitate withdrawal symptoms. Not recommended with MAOIs or within 14 days of stopping such treatment. May cause severe hypotension with phenothiazines or other agents that compromise vasomotor tone. Muscle relaxants (eg, cyclobenzaprine), MAOIs (eg, phenelzine), and antidepressants (eg, TCAs, SSRIs, SNRIs) may enhance serotonergic activity, resulting in the development of serotonin syndrome.

NURSING CONSIDERATIONS

Assessment: Assess for level of pain intensity, type of pain, patient's general condition and medical status, or any other conditions where treatment is contraindicated or cautioned. Assess for drug hypersensitivity, renal/hepatic/pulmonary impairment, pregnancy/nursing status, and possible drug interactions.

Monitoring: Monitor for signs/symptoms of respiratory depression, hypotension, convulsions/seizures, spasm of the sphincter of Oddi, increases in serum amylase levels, tolerance, physical dependence, and other adverse reactions. Reassess the continued need for therapy.

Patient Counseling: Advise to report episodes of breakthrough pain and adverse experiences occurring during therapy. Instruct to not adjust the dose without consulting physician. Inform that drug may impair mental/physical abilities required for the performance of potentially hazardous tasks. Counsel to avoid alcohol or other CNS depressants, except by the order of physician. Advise to consult physician regarding effects when used during pregnancy. Inform that drug has potential for abuse and should be protected from theft and never be given to anyone other than for whom it was prescribed. Counsel that if taking medication for more than a few weeks and need to d/c therapy, to avoid abrupt withdrawal, as dosing will need to be tapered.

Storage: 25°C (77°F); excursions permitted to 15-30°C (59-86°F). Protect from moisture.

OxyContin – oxycodone hydrochloride CII

Class: Opioid analgesic

Exposes users to risks of addiction, abuse, and misuse, leading to overdose and death; assess each patient's risk prior to prescribing and monitor regularly for development of these behaviors/conditions. Serious, life-threatening, or fatal respiratory depression may occur; monitor during initiation or following a dose increase. Crushing, dissolving, or chewing tab can cause rapid release and absorption of potentially fatal dose; instruct patients to swallow tab whole. Accidental ingestion, especially by children, can result in a fatal overdose. Prolonged use during pregnancy can result in neonatal opioid withdrawal syndrome; advise pregnant women of the risk and ensure availability of appropriate treatment. Concomitant use of CYP3A4 inhibitors or discontinuation of CYP3A4 inducers can result in oxycodone overdose; monitor patients receiving concomitant CYP3A4 inhibitors/inducers.

ADULT DOSAGE

Severe Pain (Daily, Around-the-Clock Management)

1st Opioid Analgesic/Opioid Intolerant Patients:
Initial: 10mg q12h
Titrate: Increase total daily dose by 25-50% every 1-2 days

Conversions

From Other Oral Oxycodone Formulations:
Administer 1/2 of total daily dose q12h

From Other Opioids:
D/C all other around-the-clock opioids when therapy is initiated and initiate dosing using 10mg q12h

From Transdermal Fentanyl:
Initiate treatment 18 hrs following removal of patch; 10mg q12h should be initially substituted for each 25mcg/hr fentanyl transdermal patch

PEDIATRIC DOSAGE

Pediatric use may not have been established

DOSE MODIFICATION

Hepatic Impairment
Initiate at 1/3 to 1/2 the usual starting dose, followed by careful dose titration

Elderly
Reduce starting dose to 1/3 to 1/2 the usual dose in debilitated, opioid intolerant patients

Discontinuation
Use gradual downward titration

ADMINISTRATION

Oral route

Do not pre-soak, lick, or otherwise wet tab prior to placing in mouth
Swallow tab whole; do not crush, dissolve, or chew
Take 1 tab at a time w/ enough water to ensure complete swallowing

HOW SUPPLIED

Tab, ER: 10mg, 15mg, 20mg, 30mg, 40mg, 60mg, 80mg

CONTRAINDICATIONS

Significant respiratory depression, acute or severe bronchial asthma in unmonitored settings or in the absence of resuscitative equipment, known or suspected paralytic ileus and GI obstruction.

WARNINGS/PRECAUTIONS

Reserve use in patients for whom alternative treatment options are ineffective, not tolerated, or would be otherwise inadequate to provide sufficient management of pain. Should only be prescribed by healthcare professionals who are knowledgeable in the use of potent opioids for management of chronic pain. 60mg and 80mg tabs, a single dose >40mg, or a total daily dose >80mg are only for use in opioid-tolerant patients. Life-threatening respiratory depression is more likely to occur in elderly, cachectic, or debilitated patients. Consider alternative nonopioid analgesics in patients with significant COPD or cor pulmonale, and in patients having a substantially decreased respiratory reserve, hypoxia, hypercapnia, or preexisting respiratory depression. May cause severe hypotension, orthostatic hypotension, and syncope; increased risk in patients whose ability to maintain BP has already been compromised by a reduced blood volume or concurrent administration of certain CNS depressants. Avoid with circulatory shock. Monitor patients who may be susceptible to intracranial effects of carbon dioxide retention for signs of sedation and respiratory depression when initiating therapy. Therapy may obscure clinical course in patient with head injury. Avoid with impaired consciousness or coma. Difficulty in swallowing tab, intestinal obstruction, and exacerbation of diverticulitis reported; consider alternative analgesic in patients who have difficulty swallowing or have underlying GI disorders that may predispose them to obstruction. May cause spasm of sphincter of Oddi and increase in serum amylase; monitor patients with biliary tract disease. May aggravate convulsions and induce/aggravate seizures. May impair mental or physical abilities. Urine drug test may not detect oxycodone reliably. Not recommended for use immediately prior to labor.

ADVERSE REACTIONS

Respiratory depression, constipation, N/V, somnolence, dizziness, pruritus, headache, dry mouth, asthenia, sweating, apnea, respiratory arrest, circulatory depression, hypotension.

DRUG INTERACTIONS

See Boxed Warning. Respiratory depression, hypotension, and profound sedation or coma may occur with CNS depressants (eg, sedatives, anxiolytics, neuroleptics); if coadministration is required, consider dose reduction of one or both agents. Monitor use in elderly, cachectic, and debilitated patients when coadministered with other drugs that depress respiration. May enhance neuromuscular blocking action of true skeletal muscle relaxants and increase respiratory depression. CYP3A4 inhibitors (eg, erythromycin, ketoconazole, ritonavir) may increase levels of oxycodone and prolong opioid effects; these effects could be more pronounced with concomitant use of CYP2D6 and 3A4 inhibitors. CYP3A4 inducers (eg, rifampin, carbamazepine, phenytoin) may decrease levels and cause lack of efficacy, or development of abstinence syndrome. If coadministration is necessary, use with caution when initiating oxycodone treatment in patients currently taking, or discontinuing CYP3A4 inhibitors/inducers. Mixed agonist/antagonists (eg, pentazocine, nalbuphine, butorphanol) or partial agonist (buprenorphine) may reduce analgesic effect or precipitate withdrawal symptoms; avoid coadministration. May reduce efficacy of diuretics and lead to acute urinary retention. Anticholinergics or other medications with anticholinergic activity may increase risk of urinary retention and/or severe constipation and lead to paralytic ileus.

NURSING CONSIDERATIONS

Assessment: Assess for abuse/addiction risk, pain intensity, prior opioid therapy, opioid tolerance, respiratory depression, drug hypersensitivity, pregnancy/nursing status, possible drug interactions, or any other conditions where treatment is contraindicated or cautioned.

Monitoring: Monitor for respiratory depression (especially within first 24-72 hrs of initiation), hypotension, seizures/convulsions, and other adverse reactions. Monitor BP and serum amylase levels. Routinely monitor for signs of misuse, abuse, and addiction. Periodically reassess the continued need for therapy.

Patient Counseling: Inform that use of drug can result in addiction, abuse, and misuse; instruct not to share with others and to take steps to protect from theft or misuse. Inform patients about risk of respiratory depression. Advise to store securely and dispose unused tabs by flushing down the toilet. Inform female patients of reproductive potential that prolonged use during pregnancy may result in neonatal opioid withdrawal syndrome and instruct to inform physician if pregnant or planning to become pregnant. Inform that potentially serious additive effects may occur when used with CNS depressants, and not to use such drugs unless supervised by healthcare provider. Instruct about proper administration instructions. Inform that drug may cause orthostatic hypotension, syncope, or may impair the ability to perform potentially hazardous activities; advise to not perform such tasks until they know how they will react to medication. Advise of potential for severe constipation, including management instructions. Advise how to recognize anaphylaxis and when to seek medical attention.

Storage: 25°C (77°F); excursions permitted to 15-30°C (59-86°F).

OXYTROL – oxybutynin

RX

Class: Muscarinic antagonist

ADULT DOSAGE

Overactive Bladder

Apply one 3.9mg/day system to dry, intact skin on the abdomen, hip, or buttock twice weekly (every 3 or 4 days)

PEDIATRIC DOSAGE

Pediatric use may not have been established

ADMINISTRATION

Transdermal route

Apply immediately after removal from the protective pouch

Select a new application site w/ each new system to avoid reapplication to the same site w/in 7 days

HOW SUPPLIED

Patch: 3.9mg/day [8[s]]

CONTRAINDICATIONS

Urinary retention, gastric retention, uncontrolled narrow-angle glaucoma.

WARNINGS/PRECAUTIONS

Caution with bladder outflow obstruction, GI obstructive disorders, gastroesophageal reflux disease (GERD), and myasthenia gravis. May decrease GI motility; caution with ulcerative colitis (UC) or intestinal atony. CNS anticholinergic effects reported; consider discontinuation if these occur. May impair mental/physical abilities. Angioedema may occur; d/c and provide appropriate therapy if this occurs. D/C if skin hypersensitivity develops.

ADVERSE REACTIONS

Application-site reactions (pruritus, erythema, vesicles, rash), dry mouth, diarrhea, constipation.

DRUG INTERACTIONS

Concomitant use with other anticholinergic drugs may increase the frequency and/or severity of dry mouth, constipation, somnolence, and/or other anticholinergic-like effects. May alter the absorption of other drugs due to anticholinergic effects on GI motility. Caution with drugs that can cause or exacerbate esophagitis (eg, bisphosphonates).

NURSING CONSIDERATIONS

Assessment: Assess for urinary/gastric retention, uncontrolled narrow-angle glaucoma, bladder outflow obstruction, GI obstructive disorders, UC, intestinal atony, GERD, myasthenia gravis, pregnancy/nursing status, and possible drug interactions.

Monitoring: Monitor for urinary retention, gastric retention, anticholinergic CNS effects (particularly after beginning treatment), angioedema, skin hypersensitivity, exacerbation of symptoms of myasthenia gravis, and other adverse reactions.

Patient Counseling: Instruct to discard used patch in household trash in a manner that prevents accidental application or ingestion by children, pets, or others. Inform that drug may produce adverse reactions related to anticholinergic activity (eg, urinary retention, constipation, dizziness, blurred vision). Advise that heat prostration may occur when the drug is used in a hot environment. Instruct to avoid driving or operating heavy machinery until effects have been determined. Inform that drowsiness may be worsened by alcohol. Advise to promptly d/c therapy and seek immediate medical attention if symptoms consistent with angioedema occur.

Storage: 20-25°C (68-77°F). Protect from moisture and humidity. Do not store outside the sealed pouch.

PACLITAXEL – paclitaxel

Class: Antimicrotubule agent

RX

Should be administered under supervision of a physician experienced in the use of cancer chemotherapeutic agents. Anaphylaxis and severe hypersensitivity reactions reported; pretreat with corticosteroids, diphenhydramine, and H_2 antagonists. Fatal reactions have occurred despite premedication. Do not rechallenge if severe hypersensitivity reaction occurs. Avoid in patients with solid tumors who have baseline neutrophil counts of <1500 cells/mm³ and in patients with AIDS-related Kaposi's sarcoma if the baseline neutrophil count is <1000 cells/mm³. Perform peripheral blood cell counts frequently to monitor occurrence of bone marrow suppression, primarily neutropenia.

ADULT DOSAGE

Ovarian Carcinoma

1st-line (in combination w/ cisplatin) and subsequent therapy for advanced carcinoma of the ovary

Previously Untreated Patients:
175mg/m² IV over 3 hrs, followed by cisplatin 75mg/m²
or
135mg/m² IV over 24 hrs, followed by cisplatin 75mg/m²

Regimen may be administered every 3 weeks

Previously Treated Patients:
135mg/m² or 175mg/m² IV over 3 hrs every 3 weeks

Breast Cancer

Adjuvant Therapy:
Node-positive breast cancer administered sequentially to standard doxorubicin-containing combination chemotherapy

175mg/m² IV over 3 hrs every 3 weeks for 4 courses

After Failure of Combination Chemotherapy for Metastatic Disease or Relapse w/in 6 Months of Adjuvant Chemotherapy:
Prior therapy should have included an anthracycline unless clinically contraindicated

175mg/m² IV over 3 hrs every 3 weeks

Non-Small Cell Lung Cancer

Combination w/ cisplatin for 1st-line treatment in patients who are not candidates for potentially curative surgery and/or radiation therapy

135mg/m² IV over 24 hrs, followed by cisplatin 75mg/m²

Administer regimen every 3 weeks

AIDS-Related Kaposi's Sarcoma

2nd-Line Treatment:
135mg/m² IV over 3 hrs every 3 weeks or 100mg/m² IV over 3 hrs every 2 weeks

Premedication

All patients should be premedicated prior to paclitaxel inj administration w/ dexamethasone 20mg PO approx 12 and 6 hrs before inj, diphenhydramine (or its equivalent) 50mg IV 30-60 min prior to inj, and cimetidine (300mg) or ranitidine (50mg) IV 30-60 min before inj

PEDIATRIC DOSAGE

Pediatric use may not have been established

DOSE MODIFICATION

Hepatic Impairment

24-Hr Infusion:
AST/ALT 2-<10X ULN and Bilirubin ≤1.5mg/dL: 100mg/m²

AST/ALT <10X ULN and Bilirubin 1.6-7.5mg/dL: 50mg/m^2
AST/ALT ≥10X ULN and Bilirubin >7.5mg/dL: Not recommended for use

3-Hr Infusion:
AST/ALT <10X ULN and Bilirubin 1.26-2X ULN: 135mg/m^2
AST/ALT <10X ULN and Bilirubin 2.01-5X ULN: 90mg/m^2
AST/ALT ≥10X ULN and Bilirubin >5X ULN: Not recommended for use

Dose recommendations are for the 1st course of therapy; further dose reduction in subsequent courses should be based on individual tolerance

These recommendations are based on dosages of 135mg/m^2 over 24 hrs or 175mg/m^2 over 3 hrs; data are not available to make adjustment recommendations for other regimens (eg, AIDS-related Kaposi's sarcoma)

Adverse Reactions
Severe Neutropenia (Neutrophils <500 cells/mm^3 for ≥1 Week) or Severe Peripheral Neuropathy:
Reduce dose of subsequent courses by 20%

Other Important Modifications
Patients w/ Advanced HIV Disease:
1. Reduce dexamethasone dose as 1 of the 3 premedication drugs to 10mg PO
2. Initiate or repeat treatment w/ paclitaxel inj only if the neutrophil count is ≥1000 cells/mm^3
3. Reduce the dose of subsequent courses of paclitaxel inj by 20% for patients who experience severe neutropenia (neutrophil < 500 cells/mm^3 for ≥1 week)
4. Initiate concomitant hematopoietic growth factor (G-CSF) as clinically indicated

ADMINISTRATION
IV route

Administration Precautions
The use of plasticized PVC containers and administration sets is not recommended; store diluted paclitaxel inj sol in bottles (glass, polypropylene) or plastic bags (polypropylene, polyolefin) and administer through polyethylene-lined administration sets

Preparation
Paclitaxel inj must be diluted prior to infusion
1. Dilute paclitaxel inj in 0.9% NaCl inj; D5 inj; D5 and 0.9% NaCl inj; or D5 in Ringer's inj to a final concentration of 0.3-1.2mg/mL
2. Upon preparation, sol may show haziness, which is attributed to the formulation vehicle
3. Administer paclitaxel inj through an in-line filter w/ a microporous membrane not >0.22 microns; use of filter devices such as IVEX-2 filters, which incorporate short inlet and outlet PVC-coated tubing has not resulted in significant leaching of di-(2-ethylhexyl)phthalate (DEHP)
4. Do not use the Chemo Dispensing Pin device or similar devices w/ spikes w/ vials of paclitaxel inj since they can cause the stopper to collapse, resulting in loss of sterile integrity of the paclitaxel inj sol

Handling Precautions
If paclitaxel inj sol contacts the skin, wash the skin immediately and thoroughly w/ soap and water
Following topical exposure, events have included tingling, burning, and redness
If paclitaxel inj contacts mucous membranes, the membranes should be flushed thoroughly w/ water
Upon inh, dyspnea, chest pain, burning eyes, sore throat, and nausea have been reported

HOW SUPPLIED
Inj: 6mg/mL [5mL, 16.7mL, 25mL, 50mL]

CONTRAINDICATIONS
Hypersensitivity to drugs formulated in polyoxyl 35 castor oil, NF; solid tumor patients with baseline neutrophils <1500 cells/mm^3, or AIDS-related Kaposi's sarcoma patients with baseline neutrophils <1000 cells/mm^3.

WARNINGS/PRECAUTIONS
Avoid subsequent cycles until neutrophils recover to >1500 cells/mm^3 (>1000 cells/mm^3 with Kaposi's sarcoma) and platelets recover to >100,000 cells/mm^3. Severe conduction abnormalities reported; administer appropriate therapy and perform continuous cardiac monitoring during subsequent therapy. May cause fetal harm. Hypotension, bradycardia, and HTN reported. Contains dehydrated alcohol; consider possible CNS and other alcohol effects. Extreme caution in patients with bilirubin >2X ULN and in elderly. Inj-site reactions and peripheral neuropathy reported.

ADVERSE REACTIONS
Anaphylaxis, bone marrow suppression, neutropenia, infections, bleeding, abnormal ECG, hypotension, peripheral neuropathy, myalgia/arthralgia, N/V, diarrhea, alopecia, inj-site reactions, mucositis.

DRUG INTERACTIONS
Myelosuppression more profound when given after cisplatin than with the alternate sequence. Caution with CYP3A4 substrates (eg, midazolam, buspirone, felodipine), inducers (eg, rifampin, carbamazepine), and inhibitors (eg, atazanavir, clarithromycin, ketoconazole). Caution with CYP2C8

substrates (eg, repaglinide, rosiglitazone), inhibitors (eg, gemfibrozil), and inducers (eg, rifampin). May increase doxorubicin levels.

NURSING CONSIDERATIONS

Assessment: Assess for hypersensitivity to drug or other drugs with polyoxyl 35 castor oil, NF, hepatic impairment, bilirubin levels, pregnancy/nursing status, and possible drug interactions. Obtain baseline neutrophil counts.

Monitoring: Monitor for signs/symptoms of anaphylaxis/hypersensitivity reactions, inj-site reactions, myelosuppression, and other adverse reactions. Monitor peripheral blood cell counts frequently. Monitor vital signs frequently, particularly during 1st hr of infusion. Closely monitor infusion site for possible infiltration during administration. Monitor cardiac function in patients with serious conduction abnormalities and when used in combination with doxorubicin for the treatment of metastatic breast cancer.

Patient Counseling: Inform about risks and benefits of therapy. Inform that drug may cause fetal harm; advise women of childbearing potential to avoid becoming pregnant. Advise to report to physician if signs of an allergic reaction or infection develop. Advise to inform physician of liver/heart problems and breastfeeding status or plans to breastfeed.

Storage: Undiluted: 20-25°C (68-77°F). Retain in original package to protect from light. Diluted Sol: Stable at ambient temperature (25°C [77°F]) and room lighting conditions for up to 27 hrs.

PATANOL — olopatadine hydrochloride

Class: H_1-antagonist and mast cell stabilizer

RX

ADULT DOSAGE

Allergic Conjunctivitis

1 drop bid q6-8h

PEDIATRIC DOSAGE

Allergic Conjunctivitis

≥3 Years:

1 drop bid q6-8h

ADMINISTRATION

Ocular route

HOW SUPPLIED

Sol: 0.1% [5mL]

WARNINGS/PRECAUTIONS

May reinsert contact lens 10 min after dosing if eye is not red. Not for injection or oral use.

ADVERSE REACTIONS

Headache, asthenia, blurred vision, burning, stinging, cold syndrome, dry eye, foreign body sensation, hyperemia, hypersensitivity, keratitis, lid edema, nausea, pharyngitis, pruritus, rhinitis.

NURSING CONSIDERATIONS

Assessment: Assess for drug hypersensitivity.

Monitoring: Monitor for headache and other adverse reactions.

Patient Counseling: Counsel not to wear contact lenses if eye is red; wait at least 10 min after instillation to wear contact lenses. Instruct to avoid touching tip of container to eye or any other surface to avoid contamination.

Storage: 4-25°C (39-77°F). Keep bottle tightly closed.

PAXIL — paroxetine hydrochloride

Class: Selective serotonin reuptake inhibitor

RX

Antidepressants increased the risk of suicidal thinking and behavior (suicidality) in children, adolescents, and young adults in short-term studies of major depressive disorder and other psychiatric disorders. Monitor and observe closely for clinical worsening, suicidality, or unusual changes in behavior in patients who are started on antidepressants. Not approved for use in pediatric patients.

ADULT DOSAGE

Major Depressive Disorder

Initial: 20mg/day

Titrate: May increase in 10mg/day increments at intervals of at least 1 week

PEDIATRIC DOSAGE

Pediatric use may not have been established

Maint: Efficacy is maintained for periods of up to 1 yr w/ doses that averaged about 30mg
Max: 50mg/day

Obsessive Compulsive Disorder

Initial: 20mg/day
Titrate: May increase in 10mg/day increments at intervals of at least 1 week
Usual: 40mg/day
Max: 60mg/day

Panic Disorder

W/ or w/o Agoraphobia:
Initial: 10mg/day
Titrate: May increase in 10mg/day increments at intervals of at least 1 week
Target Dose: 40mg/day
Max: 60mg/day

Anxiety Disorders

Social Anxiety Disorder:
Initial/Usual: 20mg/day
Titrate: May increase in 10mg/day increments at intervals of at least 1 week
Range: 20-60mg/day; no additional benefit for doses >20mg/day
Generalized Anxiety Disorder:
Initial/Usual: 20mg/day
Titrate: May increase in 10mg/day increments at intervals of at least 1 week
Range: 20-50mg/day

Post-traumatic Stress Disorder

Initial: 20mg/day
Titrate: May increase in 10mg/day increments at intervals of at least 1 week
Range: 20-50mg/day

Dosing Considerations with MAOIs

Switching to/from an MAOI for Psychiatric Disorders:
Allow at least 14 days between discontinuation of an MAOI and initiation of treatment, and conversely allow at least 14 days between discontinuing treatment before starting an MAOI

Use w/ Other MAOIs (eg, Linezolid, IV Methylene Blue):
If acceptable alternatives are not available and benefits outweigh risks of serotonin syndrome, d/c paroxetine promptly and administer linezolid or IV methylene blue; monitor for serotonin syndrome for 2 weeks or until 24 hrs after last dose of linezolid or IV methylene blue, whichever comes 1st.
May resume paroxetine therapy 24 hrs after last dose of linezolid or IV methylene blue

DOSE MODIFICATION

Renal Impairment
Initial: 10mg/day
Max: 40mg/day

Severe Hepatic Impairment
Initial: 10mg/day
Max: 40mg/day

Elderly
Elderly/Debilitated:
Initial: 10mg/day
Max: 40mg/day

Discontinuation
Reduce gradually; consider resuming previously prescribed dose if intolerable symptoms occur following a decrease in dose or upon discontinuation. Subsequently, may continue to decrease the dose, but at a more gradual rate

ADMINISTRATION
Oral route

Take w/ or w/o food
Give qd, usually in the am

Tab
Swallow whole; do not chew or crush

Sus
Shake well before use

HOW SUPPLIED
Sus: 10mg/5mL [250mL]; Tab: 10mg*, 20mg*, 30mg, 40mg *scored

CONTRAINDICATIONS
Use of an MAOI for psychiatric disorders either concomitantly or within 14 days of stopping treatment. Treatment within 14 days of stopping an MAOI for psychiatric disorders. Starting treatment in a patient being treated with other MAOIs (eg, linezolid, IV methylene blue). Concomitant use with thioridazine or pimozide.

WARNINGS/PRECAUTIONS
May precipitate mixed/manic episode in patients at risk for bipolar disorder. Not approved for treatment of bipolar depression. Serotonin syndrome reported; d/c immediately and initiate supportive symptomatic treatment. Pupillary dilation that occurs following use may trigger an angle-closure attack in a patient with anatomically narrow angles who does not have a patent iridectomy. Increased risk of congenital malformations reported in 1st trimester of pregnancy; neonates exposed to therapy late in the 3rd trimester have developed complications. Activation of mania/hypomania reported; caution with history of mania. Seizures reported; d/c if seizures develop. Adverse reactions reported upon discontinuation; avoid abrupt withdrawal. Akathisia may develop. Hyponatremia may occur; caution in elderly and volume-depleted patients. Consider discontinuation in patients with symptomatic hyponatremia and institute appropriate medical intervention. May increase risk of bleeding events. Bone fracture risk following exposure to some antidepressants reported. Caution with diseases/conditions affecting hemodynamic responses or metabolism, severe hepatic/renal impairment, and in elderly/debilitated patients. Mydriasis reported; caution with narrow-angle glaucoma.

ADVERSE REACTIONS
Asthenia, nausea, somnolence, headache, insomnia, abnormal ejaculation, dry mouth, constipation, dizziness, diarrhea, decreased libido, sweating, decreased appetite, tremor, impotence.

DRUG INTERACTIONS
See Contraindications. Not recommended with SSRIs, SNRIs, tryptophan, and alcohol. May cause serotonin syndrome with other serotonergic drugs (eg, triptans, TCAs, fentanyl) and with drugs that impair metabolism of serotonin; d/c immediately if this occurs. Metabolism and pharmacokinetics may be affected by the induction or inhibition of drug-metabolizing enzymes. Increased risk of bleeding with aspirin, NSAIDs, warfarin, and other anticoagulants. Increased risk of hyponatremia with diuretics. Increased levels with cimetidine. Decreased levels with phenobarbital, phenytoin, and fosamprenavir/ritonavir. Caution with drugs that are metabolized by CYP2D6 (eg, phenothiazines, risperidone, type 1C antiarrhythmics) and with drugs that inhibit CYP2D6 (eg, quinidine). May increase levels of desipramine, risperidone, procyclidine and theophylline. May increase levels of atomoxetine; may require dose adjustments of atomoxetine. May inhibit metabolism of TCAs. May displace or be displaced by other highly protein-bound drugs. May reduce efficacy of tamoxifen. Caution with warfarin, TCAs, lithium, and digoxin. Severe hypotension reported when added to chronic metoprolol treatment.

NURSING CONSIDERATIONS

Assessment: Assess for drug hypersensitivity, risk of bipolar disorder, history of seizures or mania, volume depletion, diseases/conditions that affect metabolism or hemodynamic responses, hepatic/renal impairment, susceptibility to angle-closure glaucoma or narrow-angle glaucoma, pregnancy/nursing status, and for possible drug interactions.

Monitoring: Monitor for signs/symptoms of clinical worsening, suicidality, unusual changes in behavior, serotonin syndrome, angle-closure glaucoma, seizures, activation of mania/hypomania, akathisia, bone fracture, hyponatremia especially in the elderly, abnormal bleeding, and other adverse reactions. Periodically reevaluate long-term usefulness of therapy.

Patient Counseling: Inform about benefits, risks, and appropriate use of therapy. Caution about risk of serotonin syndrome, angle-closure glaucoma, and bleeding. Counsel to be alert for emergence of unusual changes in behavior, worsening of depression, and suicidal ideation, especially during drug initiation or dose adjustment. Caution against operating hazardous machinery (including automobiles) until reasonably certain that therapy does not adversely affect ability to engage in such activities. Inform that improvement may be noticed in 1-4 weeks; instruct to continue therapy ud. Inform physician if taking, or planning to take, any prescription or OTC drugs. Instruct to notify physician if pregnant/intending to become pregnant, or if breastfeeding. Advise to avoid alcohol.

Storage: Tab: 15-30°C (59-86°F). Sus: ≤25°C (77°F).

PAXIL CR – paroxetine hydrochloride

RX

Class: Selective serotonin reuptake inhibitor

Antidepressants increased the risk of suicidal thinking and behavior (suicidality) in short-term studies in children, adolescents, and young adults with major depressive disorder and other psychiatric disorders. Monitor and observe closely for clinical worsening, suicidality, or unusual changes in behavior in patients who are started on antidepressants. Not approved for use in pediatric patients.

ADULT DOSAGE

Major Depressive Disorder

Initial: 25mg/day
Titrate: May increase by 12.5mg/day increments at intervals of at least 1 week
Max: 62.5mg/day

Panic Disorder

W/ or w/o Agoraphobia:
Initial: 12.5mg/day
Titrate: May increase by 12.5mg/day increments at intervals of at least 1 week
Max: 75mg/day

Social Anxiety Disorder

Initial: 12.5mg/day
Titrate: May increase by 12.5mg/day increments at intervals of at least 1 week
Max: 37.5mg/day

Premenstrual Dysphoric Disorder

Initial: 12.5mg/day; give either qd throughout menstrual cycle or limit to luteal phase of menstrual cycle
Titrate: May increase to 25mg/day at intervals of at least 1 week

Dosing Considerations with MAOIs

Switching to/from an MAOI for Psychiatric Disorders:
Allow at least 14 days between discontinuation of an MAOI and initiation of treatment, and allow at least 14 days between discontinuation of treatment and initiation of an MAOI

Use w/ Other MAOIs (eg, Linezolid, IV Methylene Blue):
Do not start paroxetine in a patient being treated w/ linezolid or IV methylene blue
In patients already receiving paroxetine, if acceptable alternatives are not available and benefits outweigh risks, d/c paroxetine and administer linezolid or IV methylene blue; monitor for serotonin syndrome for 2 weeks or until 24 hrs after the last dose of linezolid or IV methylene blue, whichever comes 1st. May resume paroxetine therapy 24 hrs after the last dose of linezolid or IV methylene blue

PEDIATRIC DOSAGE

Pediatric use may not have been established

DOSE MODIFICATION

Renal Impairment

Severe (CrCl <30mL/min):
Initial: 12.5mg/day
Max: 50mg/day

Hepatic Impairment
Severe:
Initial: 12.5mg/day
Max: 50mg/day

Elderly
And/Or Debilitated:
Initial: 12.5mg/day
Max: 50mg/day

Discontinuation
Gradually reduce dose whenever possible; consider resuming previously prescribed dose if intolerable symptoms occur following a decrease in dose or upon discontinuation. Subsequently, may continue to decrease the dose, but at a more gradual rate

ADMINISTRATION
Oral route

Administer as a single daily dose, usually in the am
Take w/ or w/o food
Swallow whole; do not chew or crush

HOW SUPPLIED
Tab, Controlled-Release: 12.5mg, 25mg, 37.5mg

CONTRAINDICATIONS
Use of MAOIs intended to treat psychiatric disorders either concomitantly or within 14 days of stopping treatment. Treatment within 14 days of stopping an MAOI intended to treat psychiatric disorders. Starting treatment in patients being treated with MAOIs (eg, linezolid, IV methylene blue). Concomitant use with thioridazine or pimozide.

WARNINGS/PRECAUTIONS
May precipitate mixed/manic episode in patients at risk for bipolar disorder. Not approved for treatment of bipolar depression. Serotonin syndrome reported; d/c immediately and initiate supportive symptomatic treatment. Pupillary dilation that occurs following use may trigger an angle-closure attack in a patient with anatomically narrow angles who does not have a patent iridectomy. Increased risk of congenital malformations reported in 1st trimester of pregnancy; neonates exposed to therapy late in the 3rd trimester have developed complications. Activation of mania/hypomania reported; caution with history of mania. Seizures reported; d/c if seizures occur. Adverse reactions upon discontinuation (eg, dysphoric mood, irritability) reported; avoid abrupt withdrawal. Akathisia may develop. Hyponatremia reported; caution in elderly and volume-depleted patients. Consider discontinuation in patients with symptomatic hyponatremia and institute appropriate medical intervention. May increase risk of bleeding events. Bone fracture risk following exposure to some antidepressants reported. Caution with disease/conditions that could affect metabolism or hemodynamic responses, severe renal/hepatic impairment, pregnancy (3rd trimester), and in elderly/debilitated patients. May impair mental/physical abilities. Mydriasis reported; caution with narrow-angle glaucoma.

ADVERSE REACTIONS
Suicidality, somnolence, insomnia, nausea, asthenia, abnormal ejaculation, dry mouth, constipation, dizziness, diarrhea, decreased libido, sweating, abnormal vision, headache, tremor.

DRUG INTERACTIONS
See Contraindications. Serotonin syndrome reported with other serotonergic drugs (eg, triptans, TCAs, fentanyl, lithium, tramadol, tryptophan, buspirone, St. John's wort) and with drugs that impair serotonin metabolism. Use with other SSRIs, SNRIs, or tryptophan is not recommended. Avoid alcohol. Concomitant use with aspirin (ASA), NSAIDs, warfarin, and other anticoagulants may increase risk of bleeding events. Use with diuretics may increase risk of developing hyponatremia. Increased levels with cimetidine. Reduced levels with phenobarbital, phenytoin, and fosamprenavir/ritonavir. Caution with drugs that are metabolized by CYP2D6 (eg, nortriptyline, phenothiazines, risperidone, type 1C antiarrhythmics) and with drugs that inhibit CYP2D6 (eg, quinidine). May increase levels of desipramine, risperidone, atomoxetine, and theophylline. May reduce efficacy of tamoxifen. May displace or be displaced by other highly protein-bound drugs. May increase procyclidine levels; reduce dose if anticholinergic effects are seen. May inhibit metabolism of TCAs. Caution with digoxin, TCAs, and lithium.

NURSING CONSIDERATIONS

Assessment: Assess for drug hypersensitivity, risk of bipolar disorder, history of seizures or mania, volume depletion, diseases/conditions that affect metabolism or hemodynamic response, hepatic/renal impairment, narrow-angle glaucoma, susceptibility to angle-closure glaucoma, pregnancy/nursing status, and for possible drug interactions.

Monitoring: Monitor for signs/symptoms of clinical worsening, suicidality, unusual changes in behavior, serotonin syndrome, seizures, activation of mania/hypomania, akathisia, bone fracture, hyponatremia especially in the elderly, abnormal bleeding, angle-closure glaucoma, and other adverse reactions. Upon discontinuation, monitor for symptoms. Periodically reassess need for continued therapy.

Patient Counseling: Inform about the risks, benefits, and appropriate use of therapy. Advise to avoid alcohol use. Instruct to notify physician of all prescription or OTC drugs currently taking or planning to take. Caution about risk of serotonin syndrome, angle-closure glaucoma, and bleeding. Instruct patient, families, and caregivers to report emergence of anxiety, agitation, panic attacks, insomnia, irritability, hostility, aggressiveness, impulsivity, akathisia, hypomania, mania, unusual changes in behavior, worsening of depression, and suicidal ideation, especially during drug initiation or dose adjustment. Caution operating hazardous machinery (including automobiles) until reasonably certain that therapy does not adversely affect ability to engage in such activities. Inform that improvement may be noticed in 1-4 weeks; instruct to continue therapy ud. Instruct to notify physician if pregnant/intending to become pregnant, or if breastfeeding.

Storage: ≤25°C (77°F).

PEGASYS – peginterferon alfa-2a

RX

Class: Pegylated virus proliferation inhibitor

May cause or aggravate fatal or life-threatening neuropsychiatric, autoimmune, ischemic, and infectious disorders. Monitor closely w/ periodic clinical and lab evaluations. D/C w/ persistently severe or worsening signs/symptoms of these conditions.

ADULT DOSAGE

Chronic Hepatitis C with Compensated Liver Disease

W/O HIV Coinfection:

Monotherapy:
180mcg once weekly for 48 weeks

Combination Treatment:

Genotypes 1, 4:
180mcg once weekly for 48 weeks (if used w/ ribavirin only)

Genotypes 2, 3:
180mcg once weekly for 24 weeks (if used w/ ribavirin only)

W/ HIV Coinfection:
180mcg once weekly for 48 weeks (if used w/ ribavirin only)

Chronic Hepatitis B with Compensated Liver Disease

HBeAg-Positive and HBeAg-Negative:
180mcg once weekly for 48 weeks

PEDIATRIC DOSAGE

Chronic Hepatitis C with Compensated Liver Disease

≥5 Years:

Combination w/ Ribavirin:
180mcg/1.73m^2 x BSA once weekly

Max Dose: 180mcg

Treatment Duration:

Genotypes 2, 3: 24 weeks

Other Genotypes: 48 weeks

Treatment Initiation Prior to 18 Years:
Maintain pediatric dosing through the completion of therapy

DOSE MODIFICATION

Renal Impairment

Adults:

CrCl <30mL/min and/or Hemodialysis: 135mcg once weekly
If severe adverse reactions or lab abnormalities develop, dose can be reduced to 90mcg once weekly until reactions abate; d/c if intolerance persists after dosage adjustment

Hepatic Impairment

Child Pugh-Score >6 (Class B and C): D/C Pegasys

Adverse Reactions

Neutropenia:

Adults:

ANC <750 cells/mm^3: Reduce dose to 135mcg once weekly

ANC <500 cells/mm^3: D/C until ANC values return to >1000 cells/mm^3; restart at 90mcg once weekly

Pediatrics:

ANC 750-999 cells/mm^3:

Weeks 1-2: Reduce dose to 135mcg/1.73m^2 x BSA

Weeks 3-48: No dose modification

ANC 500-749 cells/mm^3:

Weeks 1-2: Hold dose until >750 cells/mm^3 then resume at 135mcg/1.73m^2 x BSA

Weeks 3-48: Reduce dose to 135mcg/1.73m^2 x BSA

ANC 250-499 cells/mm^3:
Weeks 1-2: Hold dose until >750 cells/mm^3 then resume at 90mcg/1.73m^2 x BSA
Weeks 3-48: Hold dose until >750 cells/mm^3 then resume at 135mcg/1.73m^2 x BSA
ANC <250 cells/mm^3 (or Febrile Neutropenia): D/C treatment
Thrombocytopenia:
Adults:
Platelets <50,000 cells/mm^3: Reduce dose to 90mcg once weekly
Platelets <25,000 cells/mm^3: D/C treatment
Pediatrics:
Platelets <50,000 cells/mm^3: 90mcg/1.73m^2 x BSA
Transaminase Elevations:
Adults:
Progressive ALT Increases after Dose Reduction: D/C therapy
ALT Increases w/ Increased Bilirubin/Evidence of Hepatic Decompensation: D/C therapy
Chronic Hepatitis C Patients:
Progressive ALT Increases Above Baseline: Reduce dose to 135mcg; resume therapy after flares subside
Chronic Hepatitis B Patients:
ALT Elevations >5X ULN: Reduce dose to 135mcg or temporarily d/c; resume therapy after flares subside
Persistent, Severe Flares (ALT >10X above ULN): Consider discontinuation
Pediatrics:
Persistent/Increasing ALT Elevations ≥5 but <10X ULN: Modify dose to 135mcg/1.73m^2 x BSA; reduce dose further if necessary
Persistent ALT Elevations ≥10X ULN: D/C treatment
Depression:
Initial Management (4-8 Weeks):
Adults:
Moderate: Decrease dose to 135mcg or 90mcg once weekly
Severe: Permanently d/c treatment
Pediatrics:
Moderate: Decrease dose to 135mcg/1.73m^2 x BSA or 90mcg/1.73m^2 x BSA once weekly
Severe: Permanently d/c treatment
Worsening of Depression Severity After 8 Weeks:
Adults:
Mild: Decrease dose to 135mcg or 90mcg once weekly or d/c
Moderate: Permanently d/c treatment
Pediatrics:
Mild: Decrease dose to 135mcg/1.73m^2 x BSA or 90mcg/1.73m^2 x BSA once weekly
Moderate: Permanently d/c treatment
Refer to PI for psychiatric visit schedule

Discontinuation
Chronic Hepatic C Genotype 1 in Combination w/ Ribavirin or Alone:
D/C if at least a 2 $\log_{10}$ HCV RNA reduction from baseline is not achieved by Week 12
D/C if undetectable HCV RNA is not achieved after 24 weeks

ADMINISTRATION

SQ route

Administer in abdomen or thigh
Discard unused portion in single-use vials or prefilled syringes in excess of the labeled volume

Recommended Volume to be Administered for Different Dosages
180mcg/mL in a Vial:
90mcg Dose: Use 0.5mL
135mcg Dose: Use 0.75mL
180mcg Dose: Use entire 1mL
180mcg/0.5mL in a Prefilled Syringe:
90mcg: Use 0.25mL
135mcg: Use 0.375mL
180mcg: Use entire 0.5mL
180mcg/0.5mL in an Autoinjector:
90mcg: Do not use
135mcg: Do not use
180mcg: May use
135mcg/0.5mL in an Autoinjector:
90mcg: Do not use

135mcg: May use
180mcg: Do not use

HOW SUPPLIED

Inj: 180mcg/0.5mL [prefilled syringe]; 180mcg/0.5mL, 135mcg/0.5mL [ProClick autoinjector]; 180mcg/mL [vial]

CONTRAINDICATIONS

Autoimmune hepatitis, hepatic decompensation (Child-Pugh score >6 [Class B and C]) in cirrhotic patients before treatment, hepatic decompensation w/ Child-Pugh score ≥6 in cirrhotic CHC patients coinfected w/ HIV before treatment, neonates, and infants (contains benzyl alcohol). When used w/ other HCV antiviral drugs, the contraindications applicable to those agents are applicable to combination therapies; refer to PI of the other HCV antiviral drugs, including ribavirin, for a list of their contraindications.

WARNINGS/PRECAUTIONS

Not recommended, alone or in combination w/ ribavirin w/o additional HCV antiviral drugs, in CHC patients who previously failed therapy w/ an interferon-alfa, and in CHC patients who have had a solid organ transplantation. Avoid in combination w/ ribavirin in pregnant women or men whose female partners are pregnant. Extreme caution w/ history of depression; d/c immediately in severe cases and institute psychiatric intervention. HTN, supraventricular arrhythmias, chest pain, and MI reported; caution w/ preexisting cardiac disease. May cause bone marrow suppression and severe cytopenias; d/c, at least temporarily, if severe decrease in neutrophil or platelet count develops. May cause or aggravate hypo/hyperthyroidism, ophthalmologic disorders, and pulmonary disorders. Hypo/hyperglycemia, diabetes mellitus, and ischemic and hemorrhagic cerebrovascular events reported. CHC patients w/ cirrhosis may be at risk for hepatic decompensation and death; d/c immediately w/ hepatic decompensation. Exacerbation of hepatitis B reported; d/c immediately if hepatic decompensation, progressive ALT increases, or increased bilirubin occurs. Ulcerative or hemorrhagic/ischemic colitis, pancreatitis, and severe acute hypersensitivity reactions reported; d/c if any of these develop. Consider discontinuation of treatment and immediately start appropriate anti-infective therapy if serious and severe infections occur. D/C w/ new or worsening ophthalmologic disorders, pulmonary infiltrates or pulmonary function impairment. Peripheral neuropathy reported in combination w/ telbivudine. May inhibit growth in pediatric patients. May impair fertility in women. Caution in renal impairment and in the elderly.

ADVERSE REACTIONS

Neuropsychiatric/autoimmune/ischemic/infectious disorders, inj-site reactions, fatigue/asthenia, diarrhea, pyrexia, rigors, N/V, anorexia, myalgia, headache, irritability/anxiety/nervousness.

DRUG INTERACTIONS

May inhibit CYP1A2 and increase exposure of theophylline; monitor theophylline serum levels and consider dose adjustments. May increase levels of methadone; monitor for toxicity. Hepatic decompensation can occur w/ peginterferon alfa-2a/ribavirin in combination w/ other HCV antiviral drugs and nucleoside reverse transcriptase inhibitors (NRTIs); refer to PI for other HCV antiviral drugs and the respective NRTIs for guidance regarding toxicity management. Concomitant use of peginterferon alfa-2a/ribavirin w/ zidovudine may cause severe neutropenia and severe anemia; consider discontinuation of zidovudine as medically appropriate and also consider dose reduction or discontinuation of peginterferon alfa-2a, ribavirin or both if worsening clinical toxicities are observed, including hepatic decompensation (eg, Child-Pugh >6). Pancytopenia and bone marrow suppression reported to occur w/in 3-7 weeks after the concomitant administration of pegylated interferon/ribavirin and azathioprine; d/c peginterferon alfa-2a, ribavirin, and azathioprine for pancytopenia, and do not re-introduce pegylated interferon/ribavirin w/ concomitant azathioprine.

NURSING CONSIDERATIONS

Assessment: Assess for neuropsychiatric, autoimmune, ischemic or infectious disorders, hepatic/renal impairment, known hypersensitivity reactions, history of treatment failure w/ interferon alfa in CHC patients, history of solid organ transplantation in CHC patients, nursing status, possible drug interactions, or any other conditions where treatment is contraindicated or cautioned. Obtain baseline CBC, TSH, $CD4^+$ (HIV), and eye exam. Perform ECG for preexisting cardiac diseases. Obtain pregnancy test in women of childbearing potential.

Monitoring: Monitor for signs/symptoms of neuropsychiatric, autoimmune, ischemic, infectious, cardiovascular, cerebrovascular, endocrine, and pulmonary disorders; bone marrow toxicities; colitis; pancreatitis; delayed growth in pediatric patients; and other adverse reactions. Monitor hematological (Weeks 2, 4, and periodically thereafter) and biochemical tests (Week 4 and periodically thereafter), and TSH (every 12 weeks). Perform periodic eye exams in patients w/ preexisting ophthalmologic disorders. Perform monthly pregnancy tests if on combination therapy w/ ribavirin and for 6 months after discontinuation. Monitor clinical status and hepatic/renal function.

Patient Counseling: Counsel on benefits and risks of therapy. Advise not to use drug in combination w/ ribavirin for pregnant women or men whose female partners are pregnant. Inform of the teratogenic/embryocidal risks w/ ribavirin; instruct to use 2 forms of effective contraception during ribavirin therapy and for 6 months post-therapy. Inform that drug is not known if drug will prevent transmission of HCV/HBV infection to others. Advise that it is not known if therapy will prevent cirrhosis, liver failure or liver cancer in HBV patients. Advise that laboratory evaluations are required prior to therapy, and periodically thereafter. Counsel to avoid alcohol, and avoid driving or operating machinery if dizziness, confusion, somnolence, or fatigue occurs. Instruct to remain well hydrated, and not to switch to another brand of interferon w/o consulting physician. Instruct on the proper preparation and administration, and disposal techniques for therapy.

Storage: 2-8°C (36-46°F). Do not leave out of the refrigerator for >24 hrs. Do not freeze or shake. Protect from light.

PegIntron — peginterferon alfa-2b **RX**

Class: Pegylated virus proliferation inhibitor

May cause or aggravate fatal or life-threatening neuropsychiatric, autoimmune, ischemic, and infectious disorders. Closely monitor patients with periodic clinical and lab evaluations. D/C with persistently severe or worsening signs/symptoms of these conditions. When used with ribavirin, refer to the individual monograph.

ADULT DOSAGE

Chronic Hepatitis C with Compensated Liver Disease

Combination with Ribavirin:
1.5mcg/kg/week

Treatment Duration:
Interferon Alfa-Naive Patients:
Genotype 1: 48 weeks
Genotypes 2, 3: 24 weeks

Retreatment:
Prior Treatment Failure:
48 weeks (regardless of genotype)

Monotherapy:
1mcg/kg/week (same day of the week) for 1 yr

PEDIATRIC DOSAGE

Chronic Hepatitis C with Compensated Liver Disease

3-17 Years:
Combination with Ribavirin:
60mcg/m^2/week

Remain on pediatric dosing regimen if 18th birthday was reached during therapy

Treatment Duration:
Genotype 1: 48 weeks
Genotype 2, 3: 24 weeks

DOSE MODIFICATION

Renal Impairment

Moderate (CrCl 30-50mL/min): Reduce dose by 25%
Severe (CrCl 10-29mL/min) and/or Hemodialysis: Reduce dose by 50%
Decline in Renal Function During Treatment: D/C therapy

Adverse Reactions

Refer to PI for dose modification/discontinuation and for scheduling visits for patients with depression
Refer to PI for dose modification/ discontinuation based on lab parameters in adults and pediatrics

Discontinuation

Adults:
Genotype 1:
Interferon-Alfa Naive:
D/C if at least a 2 $\log_{10}$ drop or loss of HCV-RNA at 12 weeks of therapy is not achieved
D/C if HCV-RNA remains detectable after 24 weeks of therapy

All Genotypes:
Previously Treated Patients:
D/C if HCV-RNA is detectable at Week 12 or 24

Pediatrics (3-17 Years):
All Genotypes (Excluding Genotype 2 and 3):
D/C therapy at 12 weeks if treatment Week 12 HCV-RNA drops <2 $\log_{10}$ compared to pretreatment
D/C therapy at 24 weeks if HCV-RNA is detectable at treatment Week 24

ADMINISTRATION

SQ route

Do not reuse vial or prefilled pen; discard unused portion
Refer to Rebetol labeling for dosing and administration

HOW SUPPLIED
Inj: 50mcg/0.5mL, 80mcg/0.5mL, 120mcg/0.5mL, 150mcg/0.5mL [vial, Redipen]

CONTRAINDICATIONS
Autoimmune hepatitis, hepatic decompensation (Child-Pugh score >6 [class B and C]) in cirrhotic CHC patients before or during treatment. When used with ribavirin, refer to the individual monograph.

WARNINGS/PRECAUTIONS
Caution with history of psychiatric disorders. Monitor during treatment and in the 6-month follow-up period if psychiatric problems develop; d/c if symptoms persist or worsen, or if suicidal ideation or aggressive behavior is identified. Cases of encephalopathy reported with higher doses. Cardiovascular (CV) events reported; caution with CV disease (CVD) (eg, myocardial infarction [MI], arrhythmia). Hyperglycemia, diabetes mellitus, and new/worsening hypothyroidism and hyperthyroidism reported; do not begin/continue therapy in patients with these conditions who cannot be controlled with medication. Ophthalmologic disorders may be induced or aggravated; conduct baseline eye exam and periodically monitor patients with preexisting ophthalmologic disorders. D/C if new or worsening ophthalmologic disorders occur. Ischemic and hemorrhagic cerebrovascular events reported. Suppresses bone marrow function; d/c if severe decreases in neutrophil or platelet counts develop. May rarely be associated with aplastic anemia. Autoimmune/pulmonary/dental/periodontal disorders, pancreatitis, ulcerative or hemorrhagic/ischemic colitis, increases in ALT/TG levels, and hypersensitivity reactions have been observed. Caution with autoimmune disorders, debilitating medical conditions (eg, history of pulmonary disease), and in elderly. Suspend combination treatment if pulmonary infiltrates or pulmonary function impairment develops. D/C if signs/symptoms of colitis or hypersensitivity reactions occur, or with diagnosis of pancreatitis. CHC patients with cirrhosis may be at risk for hepatic decompensation and death. Monitor patients with renal insufficiency for toxicity (including increases in SrCr); adjust dose or d/c therapy. Use monotherapy with caution and avoid combination therapy with ribavirin in patients with CrCl <50mL/min. Weight loss and growth inhibition (including long-term growth inhibition) reported in pediatric patients during combination therapy with Rebetol.

ADVERSE REACTIONS
Neuropsychiatric/autoimmune/ischemic/infectious disorders, headache, fatigue/asthenia, rigors, N/V, abdominal pain, anorexia, emotional lability/irritability, myalgia, fever, inj-site inflammation/erythema.

DRUG INTERACTIONS
May decrease therapeutic effects of CYP2C8/9 (eg, warfarin, phenytoin) or CYP2D6 (eg, flecainide) substrates. May increase methadone concentrations; monitor for signs/symptoms of increased narcotic effect. Closely monitor for toxicities, especially hepatic decompensation and anemia, with nucleoside reverse transcriptase inhibitors (NRTIs); consider dose reduction or discontinuation of interferon, ribavirin, or both, or discontinuation of NRTIs if worsening clinical toxicities occur. Concomitant use of peginterferon alpha and ribavirin with zidovudine may cause severe neutropenia and severe anemia. Peripheral neuropathy reported when used in combination with telbivudine.

NURSING CONSIDERATIONS

Assessment: Assess for history of MI, arrhythmia, and psychiatric disorders; presence of CVD, endocrine, autoimmune, and ophthalmologic disorders; hepatic/renal impairment; drug hypersensitivity; any other conditions where treatment is contraindicated or cautioned; pregnancy/nursing status; and possible drug interactions. Obtain baseline CBC, blood chemistry, and eye exam. Perform ECG in patients with preexisting cardiac abnormalities.

Monitoring: Monitor CBC, blood chemistry, LFTs, renal function, TG levels, HCV-RNA, and complete eye and dental exams periodically. Monitor for signs/symptoms of autoimmune, cerebrovascular, infectious, endocrine, and pulmonary disorders; CV and neuropsychiatric events; bone marrow toxicity; hepatic decompensation; colitis; pancreatitis; hypersensitivity reactions; and other adverse reactions.

Patient Counseling: Inform of benefits and risks of therapy. Advise to report immediately any symptoms of depression or suicidal ideation to physician. Instruct to use at least 2 forms of contraception and to avoid pregnancy during treatment with combination therapy and for 6 months post-therapy. Instruct to brush teeth thoroughly bid and to have regular dental examinations when used in combination with Rebetol; if vomiting occurs, advise to rinse out mouth afterwards. Counsel that flu-like symptoms associated with treatment may be minimized by hs administration of the drug or by using antipyretics. Inform that chest x-ray or other tests may be needed if fever, cough, SOB, or other symptoms of a lung problem develop. Advise to remain well hydrated. Instruct self-administering patients on the importance of site selection, rotating inj sites, and proper disposal of needles, syringes, and Redipen; caution against reuse.

Storage: (Redipen) 2-8°C (36-46°F). (Vial) 25°C (77°F); excursions permitted to 15-30°C (59-86°F). (Redipen/Vial) Reconstituted Sol: Use immediately, but may store for up to 24 hrs at 2-8°C (36-46°F). Do not freeze. Keep away from heat.

PENICILLIN VK – penicillin V potassium

RX

Class: Penicillin

ADULT DOSAGE

Fusospirochetosis

Mild to Moderately Severe Infections of the Oropharynx:
250-500mg q6-8h

Streptococcal Infections

Mild to Moderately Severe URTIs, Scarlet Fever, and Mild Erysipelas:
125-250mg q6-8h for 10 days

Respiratory Tract Infections

Mild to Moderately Severe Pneumococcal Infections:
250-500mg q6h until patient has been afebrile for at least 2 days

Otitis Media

Mild to Moderately Severe Pneumococcal Infections:
250-500mg q6h until patient has been afebrile for at least 2 days

Skin and Skin Structure Infections

Mild Staphylococcal Infections of the Skin and Soft Tissues:
250-500mg q6-8h
Culture and sensitivity tests should be performed

Endocarditis

Prophylaxis against bacterial endocarditis in patients w/ congenital heart disease/rheumatic/other acquired valvular heart disease when undergoing dental procedures or surgical procedures of the upper respiratory tract
2g 1hr before the procedure, then 1g 6hrs later

Other Indications

Prevention of Recurrence Following Rheumatic Fever and/or Chorea:
125-500mg bid on a continuing basis

PEDIATRIC DOSAGE

Otitis Media

Mild to Moderately Severe Pneumococcal Infections:
≥12 Years:
250-500mg q6h until patient has been afebrile for at least 2 days

Skin and Skin Structure Infections

Mild Staphylococcal Infections of the Skin and Soft Tissues:
≥12 Years:
250-500mg q6-8h
Culture and sensitivity tests should be performed

Fusospirochetosis

Mild to Moderately Severe Infections of the Oropharynx:
≥12 Years:
250-500mg q6-8h

Streptococcal Infections

Mild to Moderately Severe URTIs, Scarlet Fever, and Mild Erysipelas:
≥12 Years:
125-250mg q6-8h for 10 days

Respiratory Tract Infections

Mild to Moderately Severe Pneumococcal Infections:
≥12 Years:
250-500mg q6h until patient has been afebrile for at least 2 days

Other Indications

≥12 Years:
Prevention of Recurrence Following Rheumatic Fever and/or Chorea:
125-500mg bid on a continuing basis
Prophylaxis against bacterial endocarditis in patients w/ congenital heart disease/rheumatic/other acquired valvular heart disease when undergoing dental procedures or surgical procedures of the upper respiratory tract
<60 lbs: 1g 1hr before the procedure, then 500mg 6hrs later

ADMINISTRATION

Oral route

Directions for Mixing Sol

125mg/mL Sol: Reconstitute 100mL or 200mL bottle size w/ 75mL or 150mL of water, respectively
250mg/5mL Sol: Reconstitute 100mL or 200mL bottle size w/ 75mL or 150mL of water, respectively
Add water in 2 portions, shaking vigorously between each aliquot

HOW SUPPLIED

Sol: 125mg/5mL [100mL, 200mL], 250mg/5mL [100mL, 200mL]; Tab: 250mg, 500mg

WARNINGS/PRECAUTIONS

Not for treatment of severe pneumonia, empyema, bacteremia, pericarditis, meningitis, and arthritis during the acute stage. Necessary dental care should be accomplished in infections involving the gum tissue. Oral PCN should not be used in patients at particularly high risk for endocarditis (eg, those w/ prosthetic heart valves or surgically constructed systemic pulmonary shunts). Should not be used as adjunctive prophylaxis for genitourinary instrumentation/surgery, lower intestinal tract surgery, sigmoidoscopy, and childbirth. Serious and fatal anaphylactic reactions reported; caution w/ a history of hypersensitivity to PCN, cephalosporins, and/or multiple allergens. Caution w/ history of significant allergies and/or asthma. D/C if an allergic reaction occurs and institute appropriate therapy. *Clostridium difficile*-associated diarrhea (CDAD) reported; d/c therapy if CDAD is suspected/confirmed. Use in the absence of a proven/strongly suspected bacterial infection or a prophylactic indication is unlikely to provide benefit and increases the risk of drug-resistant bacteria. Prolonged use may promote overgrowth of nonsusceptible organisms; take appropriate measures if superinfection develops. Oral route of administration should not be relied upon w/ severe illness, N/V, gastric dilatation, cardiospasm, or intestinal hypermotility. Obtain cultures following completion of treatment for streptococcal infections.

ADVERSE REACTIONS

Epigastric distress, N/V, diarrhea, black hairy tongue, hypersensitivity reactions (skin eruptions, urticaria, other serum-sickness like reactions, laryngeal edema, anaphylaxis), fever, eosinophilia.

NURSING CONSIDERATIONS

Assessment: Assess for previous hypersensitivity reactions to PCNs/cephalosporins or other allergens, history of asthma, N/V, gastric dilatation, severe illness, cardiospasm, intestinal hypermotility, and pregnancy/nursing status. Obtain cultures and sensitivity tests, especially in suspected staphylococcal infections.

Monitoring: Monitor for signs/symptoms of hypersensitivity reactions, CDAD, superinfections, and other adverse reactions. Obtain cultures following completion of treatment of streptococcal infections.

Patient Counseling: Counsel that therapy only treats bacterial, not viral, infections. Instruct to take ud; inform that skipping doses or not completing the full course of therapy may decrease effectiveness and increase resistance. Inform that diarrhea may occur. Instruct to seek medical attention if watery and bloody stools (w/ or w/o stomach cramps and fever) occur even after ≥2 months of discontinuing therapy.

Storage: 20-25°C (68-77°F). (Reconstituted Sol) Store in a refrigerator. Discard any unused portion after 14 days.

PENLAC – ciclopirox RX

Class: Broad-spectrum antifungal

ADULT DOSAGE

Onychomycosis

Mild to Moderate Onychomycosis w/o Lunula Involvement Due to *Trichophyton rubrum*:
Apply evenly over the entire plate qd (preferably at hs or 8 hrs before washing); when nail plate is free of nail bed (eg, onychomycosis), apply to the nail bed, hyponychium, and under the surface of the nail plate

Repeat regimen for up to 48 weeks

PEDIATRIC DOSAGE

Onychomycosis

Mild to Moderate Onychomycosis w/o Lunula Involvement Due to *Trichophyton rubrum*:
≥12 Years:
Apply evenly over the entire plate qd (preferably at hs or 8 hrs before washing); when nail plate is free of nail bed (eg, onychomycosis), apply to the nail bed, hyponychium, and under the surface of the nail plate

Repeat regimen for up to 48 weeks

ADMINISTRATION

Topical route

Sol should not be removed on a daily basis; apply daily over previous coat and remove w/ alcohol every 7 days

Removal of the unattached, infected nail, as frequently as monthly, by a healthcare professional, weekly trimming by the patient, and daily application of the medication are all integral parts of this therapy

HOW SUPPLIED

Sol: 8% [6.6mL]

WARNINGS/PRECAUTIONS

Not for ophthalmic, oral, or intravaginal use; for use on nails and immediately adjacent skin only. Should be used as a component of a comprehensive management program for onychomycosis and should be used only under medical supervision by a healthcare professional who has special competence in the diagnosis and treatment of nail disorders, including minor nail procedures. D/C and treat appropriately if sensitivity reaction or chemical irritation occurs. Caution with removal of infected nail in patients with a history of insulin-dependent diabetes mellitus (DM) or diabetic neuropathy.

ADVERSE REACTIONS
Periungual erythema, erythema of the proximal nail fold, nail shape change, nail irritation, ingrown toenail, nail discoloration.

DRUG INTERACTIONS
Avoid with systemic antifungal agents for onychomycosis.

NURSING CONSIDERATIONS

Assessment: Assess for insulin-dependent DM, diabetic neuropathy, drug hypersensitivity, pregnancy/nursing status, and possible drug interactions.

Monitoring: Monitor for sensitivity reactions, chemical irritation, and other adverse reactions. Perform frequent (eg, monthly) removal of unattached infected nails, trimming of onycholytic nail, and filing of any excess horny material.

Patient Counseling: Advise to avoid contact with the eyes and mucous membranes. Instruct to apply medication evenly over entire nail plate and 5mm of surrounding skin. Advise that if possible, the medication should be applied to the nail bed, hyponychium, and the under surface of the nail plate when it is free of the nail bed (eg, onycholysis). Instruct to notify physician if signs of increased irritation at the application site develop. Instruct to inform physician if patient has diabetes or problems with numbness in toes or fingers for consideration of appropriate nail management program. Instruct to file away (with emery board) loose nail material and trim nails as required or ud. Advise to not use nail polish or other nail cosmetic products on the treated nails. Instruct not to use medication near open flame. Inform that it may take up to 48 weeks of daily application of the medication (including monthly professional removal of unattached infected nails) to achieve a clear or almost clear nail.

Storage: 15-30°C (59-86°F). Flammable; keep away from heat and flame. Protect from light.

PENNSAID – diclofenac sodium RX

Class: NSAID

NSAIDs may increase risk of serious cardiovascular (CV) thrombotic events, MI, and stroke; increased risk w/ duration of use and w/ CV disease (CVD) or risk factors for CVD. Contraindicated in the perioperative setting of CABG surgery. May increase risk of serious GI adverse events (eg, bleeding, ulceration, stomach/intestinal perforation), which can be fatal and may occur at any time during use w/o warning symptoms; elderly patients are at greater risk.

ADULT DOSAGE
Osteoarthritis
Knee:
1.5%: 40 drops/knee qid
2%: 40mg (2 pump actuations) on each painful knee bid

PEDIATRIC DOSAGE
Pediatric use may not have been established

ADMINISTRATION
Topical route

Apply to clean, dry skin
Avoid showering/bathing ≥30 min after application
Do not apply to open wounds
Avoid contact w/ eyes and mucous membranes
Do not apply external heat and/or occlusive dressings to treated knees; protect treated knees from sunlight
Wait until the treated area is dry before applying any topical product or medication to treated knee

1.5%
Dispense 10 drops at a time directly onto to knee or 1st into hand and then spread onto knee
Spread evenly around front, back, and sides of knee; repeat until 40 drops have been applied, completely covering knee w/ sol
Avoid skin-to-skin contact between others and the treated knee until knee is completely dry

2%
Prime pump before 1st use
Fully depress the pump mechanism (actuation) 4X while holding the bottle in an upright position and discard the dispensed portion
No further priming of the bottle should be required
Pump directly into palms and spread evenly around front, back, and sides of knees

HOW SUPPLIED
Sol: 1.5% [150mL], 2% [112g]

CONTRAINDICATIONS

Patients who have experienced asthma, urticaria, or allergic-type reactions after taking aspirin (ASA) or other NSAIDs. Perioperative setting of CABG surgery.

WARNINGS/PRECAUTIONS

Use the lowest effective dose for the shortest duration possible. Extreme caution w/ history of ulcer disease or GI bleeding, or risk factors for GI bleeding (eg, longer duration of NSAID therapy, older age, poor general health status). May cause elevation of LFTs, hepatotoxicity, severe hepatic reactions, or liver injury. D/C therapy immediately if abnormal LFTs persist/worsen, liver disease develops, or systemic manifestations occur. May lead to new onset or worsening of preexisting HTN. Fluid retention and edema reported; caution w/ heart failure (HF). Use caution when initiating treatment in patients w/ considerable dehydration. Consider correcting fluid status prior to initiation of treatment. Renal papillary necrosis and other renal injury reported w/ long-term use. Renal toxicity reported in patients in whom renal prostaglandins have a compensatory role in the maintenance of renal perfusion; increased risk w/ renal/hepatic impairment, HF, and in elderly. Not recommended w/ advanced renal disease; if therapy must be initiated, closely monitor renal function. D/C if abnormal renal tests persist/worsen. Anaphylactoid reactions may occur; do not prescribe to patients w/ ASA triad. Do not apply to open skin wounds, infections, inflammations, or exfoliative dermatitis; may affect absorption and tolerability of the drug. May cause serious skin adverse events (eg, Stevens Johnson syndrome, toxic epidermal necrolysis); d/c at 1st appearance of skin rash or any other signs of hypersensitivity. Avoid in pregnant/nursing women or those intending to become pregnant. Caution w/ preexisting asthma and avoid w/ ASA-sensitive asthma. Not a substitute for corticosteroids or for the treatment of corticosteroid insufficiency. May mask signs of inflammation and fever. Anemia may occur; check Hgb/Hct if signs/symptoms of anemia or blood loss develop. May inhibit platelet aggregation and prolong bleeding time; monitor patients w/ coagulation disorders. Caution in elderly/debilitated.

ADVERSE REACTIONS

Application-site skin reactions (dry skin, pruritus, contact dermatitis, exfoliation, erythema), dyspepsia, pharyngitis, abdominal pain, infection, flatulence, diarrhea, nausea, constipation, edema, rash.

DRUG INTERACTIONS

Not recommended w/ ASA; potential for increased adverse effects. Increased risk of GI bleeding w/ oral corticosteroids or anticoagulants (eg, warfarin), smoking, and alcohol; monitor patients receiving anticoagulants. Caution w/ drugs that are potentially hepatotoxic (eg, acetaminophen [APAP], certain antibiotics, antiepileptics). May diminish the antihypertensive effect of ACE inhibitors. May reduce the natriuretic effect of thiazide and loop (eg, furosemide) diuretics. Increased risk of renal toxicity w/ diuretics and ACE inhibitors; monitor renal function. May elevate lithium levels; observe for signs of lithium toxicity. May enhance methotrexate toxicity; use caution when coadministered. May increase cyclosporine's nephrotoxicity; monitor renal function. Concomitant use w/ oral NSAIDs resulted in a higher rate of rectal hemorrhage and more frequent abnormal SrCr, urea, and Hgb; avoid combination unless benefit outweighs risk and conduct periodic lab tests.

NURSING CONSIDERATIONS

Assessment: Assess for history of asthma, urticaria, or allergic-type reactions w/ ASA or other NSAIDs, ASA triad, CVD, risk factors for CVD, history of ulcer disease or GI bleeding, risk factors for GI bleeding, coagulation disorders, HTN, fluid retention, renal/hepatic impairment, any other conditions where treatment is contraindicated or cautioned, fluid status, pregnancy/nursing status, and possible drug interactions. Assess application site for open wounds, infections, inflammations, and exfoliative dermatitis.

Monitoring: Monitor for CV/GI events, anaphylactoid/skin/hypersensitivity reactions, hematological effects, and other adverse reactions. Measure LFTs periodically w/ long-term therapy (monitor w/in 4-8 weeks after initiation). Monitor BP, renal function, CBC, and chemistry profile.

Patient Counseling: Instruct to seek medical advice if signs and symptoms of CV events, GI ulceration/bleeding, hepatotoxicity, skin/hypersensitivity reactions, unexplained weight gain or edema, or anaphylactoid reactions occur. Advise to d/c therapy immediately and contact physician if any type of generalized rash develops. Advise to contact physician as soon as possible if any type of localized application-site rash develops. Instruct not to apply to open skin wounds, infections, inflammations, or exfoliative dermatitis. Instruct to wait until the area treated w/ drug is completely dry before applying sunscreen, insect repellant, lotion, moisturizer, cosmetics, or other topical medication. Instruct to minimize or avoid exposure of treated knee(s) to natural or artificial sunlight. Instruct women who are pregnant or intending to become pregnant not to use the product. Instruct to avoid contact w/ the eyes and mucosa; advise that if eye contact occurs, to immediately wash out the eye w/ water or saline and consult physician if irritation persists for >1 hr. Caution to avoid taking unprescribed APAP while using the drug. Advise to avoid showering/bathing for at least 30 min after application, to wash and dry hands after use, to avoid wearing clothing over the treated knee(s) until the treated knee(s) is dry, and not to apply external heat and/or occlusive dressings to treated knee(s). (1.5%) Advise to avoid skin-to-skin contact between other people and the knee(s) to which drug was applied until the knee(s) is completely dry.

Storage: 25°C (77°F); excursions permitted to 15-30°C (59-86°F).

PENTASA – mesalamine RX

Class: 5-aminosalicylic acid derivative

ADULT DOSAGE

Ulcerative Colitis

Mildly to Moderately Active:
Induction of Remission/Treatment: 1g (4 caps of 250mg or 2 caps of 500mg) qid. May be given up to 8 weeks

PEDIATRIC DOSAGE

Pediatric use may not have been established

ADMINISTRATION
Oral route

HOW SUPPLIED
Cap, Controlled-Release: 250mg, 500mg

WARNINGS/PRECAUTIONS
Caution w/ impaired hepatic and renal function. Has been associated w/ an acute intolerance syndrome (eg, acute abdominal pain, cramping, bloody diarrhea) that may be difficult to distinguish from a flare of inflammatory bowel disease; d/c if suspected. If a rechallenge is performed later in order to validate the hypersensitivity, it should be carried out under close medical supervision at reduced dose and only if clearly needed. Nephrotic syndrome and interstitial nephritis reported; monitor patients w/ preexisting renal disease, increased BUN or SrCr, or proteinuria especially during the initial phase of therapy. Nephrotoxicity should be suspected in patients developing renal dysfunction during treatment. May interfere w/ lab tests.

ADVERSE REACTIONS
Diarrhea, nausea.

NURSING CONSIDERATIONS

Assessment: Assess for hypersensitivity to the drug or salicylates, hepatic/renal impairment, and pregnancy/nursing status.

Monitoring: Monitor for acute intolerance syndrome, hypersensitivity reaction, and other adverse reactions. Monitor renal function. Monitor patients w/ preexisting renal disease, increased BUN or SrCr, or proteinuria especially during the initial phase of therapy.

Patient Counseling: Inform of the risks/benefits of therapy. Advise to take ud. Advise to seek medical attention if symptoms of acute intolerance syndrome and hypersensitivity reactions occur.

Storage: 25°C (77°F); excursions permitted to 15-30°C (59-86°F).

PERCOCET – acetaminophen/oxycodone CII

Class: Opioid analgesic

Associated with cases of acute liver failure, at times resulting in liver transplant and death. Most cases of liver injury are associated with APAP use at doses >4000mg/day, and often involve >1 APAP-containing product.

OTHER BRAND NAMES
Endocet

ADULT DOSAGE

Moderate to Moderately Severe Pain

2.5mg-325mg Strength:
Usual: 1 or 2 tabs q6h prn
Max: 12 tabs/day

5mg-325mg Strength:
Usual: 1 tab q6h prn
Max: 12 tabs/day

7.5mg-325mg Strength:
Usual: 1 tab q6h prn
Max: 8 tabs/day

PEDIATRIC DOSAGE

Pediatric use may not have been established

10mg-325mg Strength:
Usual: 1 tab q6h prn
Max: 6 tabs/day

If pain is constant, administer at regular intervals on an around-the-clock schedule
Max APAP Dose: 4g/day

DOSE MODIFICATION
Discontinuation
Taper dose gradually in patients treated for more than a few weeks

ADMINISTRATION
Oral route

HOW SUPPLIED
Tab: (Oxycodone-APAP) 2.5mg-325mg, 5mg-325mg*, 7.5mg-325mg, 10mg-325mg *scored

CONTRAINDICATIONS
Oxycodone: Significant respiratory depression (in unmonitored settings or absence of resuscitative equipment), acute or severe bronchial asthma or hypercarbia, suspected/known paralytic ileus.

WARNINGS/PRECAUTIONS
May be abused in a manner similar to other opioid agonists. Respiratory depression may occur; use extreme caution and consider alternative nonopioid analgesics in patients with acute asthma, chronic obstructive pulmonary disorder, cor pulmonale, preexisting respiratory impairment, or in the elderly or debilitated. Respiratory depressant effects may be markedly exaggerated in the presence of head injury, other intracranial lesions or preexisting increase in intracranial pressure. Produces effects on pupillary response and consciousness that may obscure neurologic signs of worsening in patients with head injuries. May cause severe hypotension; caution with circulatory shock. May produce orthostatic hypotension in ambulatory patients. Increased risk of acute liver failure in patients with underlying liver disease. May cause serious skin reactions (eg, acute generalized exanthematous pustulosis, Stevens-Johnson syndrome, toxic epidermal necrolysis), which can be fatal; d/c at the 1st appearance of skin rash or any other sign of hypersensitivity. Hypersensitivity and anaphylaxis reported; d/c immediately if signs/symptoms occur. May obscure diagnosis or clinical course in patients with acute abdominal conditions. Caution with CNS depression, hypothyroidism, Addison's disease, prostatic hypertrophy, urethral stricture, acute alcoholism, delirium tremens, kyphoscoliosis with respiratory depression, myxedema, toxic psychosis, hepatic/renal/pulmonary impairment, and in elderly/debilitated. May aggravate convulsions with convulsive disorders and may induce or aggravate seizures in some clinical settings. Monitor for decreased bowel motility in postoperative patients. May cause spasm of the sphincter of Oddi; caution with biliary tract disease, including acute pancreatitis. May cause increases in serum amylase level. Physical dependence and tolerance may occur. Do not abruptly d/c. Lab test interactions may occur. Not recommended for use during and immediately prior to labor and delivery.

ADVERSE REACTIONS
Lightheadedness, dizziness, drowsiness/sedation, N/V, respiratory depression, apnea, respiratory arrest, circulatory depression, hypotension, shock.

DRUG INTERACTIONS
Oxycodone: May cause severe hypotension after coadministration with drugs that compromise vasomotor tone (eg, phenothiazines). May enhance neuromuscular-blocking action of skeletal muscle relaxants and increase respiratory depression. Additive CNS depression with CNS depressants (eg, general anesthetics, phenothiazines, tranquilizers, alcohol); use in reduced dosages. Coadministration with anticholinergics may produce paralytic ileus. Agonist/antagonist analgesics (eg, pentazocine, nalbuphine, naltrexone, butorphanol) may reduce the analgesic effect or precipitate withdrawal symptoms; use with caution. APAP: Increased risk of acute liver failure with alcohol; hepatotoxicity reported in chronic alcoholics. Increase in glucuronidation, resulting in increased plasma clearance and decreased $T_{1/2}$ with oral contraceptives. Propranolol and probenecid may increase pharmacologic/therapeutic effects. May decrease effects of loop diuretics, lamotrigine, and zidovudine.

NURSING CONSIDERATIONS

Assessment: Assess for level of pain intensity, type of pain, patient's general condition and medical status, or any other conditions where treatment is contraindicated or cautioned. Assess for drug hypersensitivity, renal/hepatic/pulmonary impairment, pregnancy/nursing status, and possible drug interactions.

Monitoring: Monitor for acute liver failure, respiratory depression, hypotension, skin/hypersensitivity/anaphylactic reactions, convulsions/seizures, decreased bowel motility in postoperative patients, spasm of sphincter of Oddi, increases in serum amylase levels, physical dependence, tolerance, and other adverse reactions.

Patient Counseling: Advise to d/c use and contact physician immediately if signs of allergy develop. Instruct to look for APAP on package labels and not to use >1 APAP-containing product. Instruct to seek medical attention immediately upon ingestion of >4000mg/day of APAP, even if patient is feeling well. Inform about the signs of serious skin reactions. Advise to destroy unused tabs by flushing down the toilet. Inform that drug may impair mental/physical abilities required to perform hazardous tasks. Instruct to avoid alcohol or other CNS depressants. Advise not to adjust dose without consulting physician and not to abruptly d/c if on treatment for more than a few weeks. Inform that drug has potential for abuse and should be protected from theft. Instruct to consult physician if pregnant, planning to become pregnant, or breastfeeding.

Storage: 20-25°C (68-77°F).

PERCODAN – aspirin/oxycodone CII

Class: Opioid analgesic

OTHER BRAND NAMES

Endodan

ADULT DOSAGE

Moderate to Moderately Severe Pain

Usual: 1 tab q6h prn
Max: 4g/day of aspirin or 12 tabs/day

PEDIATRIC DOSAGE

Pediatric use may not have been established

DOSE MODIFICATION

Discontinuation

In patients who have been treated for more than a few weeks, taper gradually; do not d/c abruptly

ADMINISTRATION

Oral route

HOW SUPPLIED

Tab: (ASA/Oxycodone HCl) 325mg/4.8355mg* *scored

CONTRAINDICATIONS

ASA: Hemophilia, children/teenagers with viral infections, NSAID allergy, and syndrome of asthma, rhinitis, and nasal polyps. Oxycodone: Significant respiratory depression (in unmonitored settings or absence of resuscitative equipment), acute/severe bronchial asthma or hypercarbia, and known/suspected paralytic ileus.

WARNINGS/PRECAUTIONS

Oxycodone: May be abused in a manner similar to other opioid agonists. May cause respiratory depression; extreme caution with acute asthma, chronic obstructive pulmonary disorder, cor pulmonale, or preexisting respiratory impairment. Respiratory depressant effects may be markedly exaggerated in the presence of head injury, other intracranial lesions, or preexisting increased intracranial pressure. Produces effects on pupillary response and consciousness, which may obscure neurologic signs of worsening in patients with head injuries. May cause severe hypotension; caution in circulatory shock. May produce orthostatic hypotension in ambulatory patients. Caution with CNS depression, hypothyroidism, Addison's disease, prostatic hypertrophy, urethral stricture, acute alcoholism, delirium tremens, kyphoscoliosis with respiratory depression, myxedema, toxic psychosis, severe hepatic/pulmonary/renal impairment, and in elderly/debilitated. May obscure diagnosis or clinical course of acute abdominal conditions. May induce or aggravate convulsions/seizures. Monitor for decreased bowel motility in postoperative patients. May cause spasm of the sphincter of Oddi; caution with biliary tract disease, including acute pancreatitis. Physical dependence and tolerance may occur. ASA: May inhibit platelet function. GI side effects reported; monitor for signs of ulceration and bleeding. May cause gastric mucosal irritation and bleeding; avoid with history of active peptic ulcer disease. May cause elevated hepatic enzymes, BUN, SrCr, and amylase, hyperkalemia, proteinuria, and prolonged bleeding time. May cause fetal harm; avoid use during pregnancy, especially in the 3rd trimester. Avoid with severe renal failure (GFR <10mL/min), or with severe hepatic insufficiency. May increase protein-bound iodine result. Avoid use 1 week prior to and during labor and delivery.

ADVERSE REACTIONS

Respiratory depression, apnea, respiratory arrest, circulatory depression, hypotension, shock, lightheadedness, dizziness, drowsiness, sedation, N/V.

DRUG INTERACTIONS

ASA: May increase concentrations of acetazolamide, leading to toxicity. May diminish effects of ACE inhibitors, β-blockers, and diuretics. Bleeding risk increased with anticoagulants (eg, warfarin, heparin) and chronic, heavy alcohol use. May decrease total concentration of phenytoin and increase serum valproic acid levels. May enhance serious side effects and toxicity of methotrexate and ketorolac. Avoid with NSAIDs; may increase bleeding or lead to decreased renal function. May increase serum glucose-lowering action of insulin and sulfonylureas, leading to hypoglycemia. Antagonizes uricosuric action of probenecid or sulfinpyrazone. Oxycodone: May enhance neuromuscular-blocking action of skeletal muscle relaxants and increase respiratory depression. Additive CNS depression with opioid analgesics, general anesthetics, centrally acting antiemetics, phenothiazines, tranquilizers, sedative-hypnotics, or other CNS depressants (eg, alcohol); reduce dose of one or both agents. May cause severe hypotension with drugs that compromise vasomotor tone (eg, phenothiazines). Mixed agonist/antagonist analgesics (eg, pentazocine, nalbuphine, naltrexone, butorphanol) may reduce analgesic effect and/or may precipitate withdrawal symptoms. Increased concentrations with CYP3A4 inhibitors (eg, macrolides, azole antifungals, protease inhibitors). Decreased concentrations with CYP450 inducers (eg, rifampin, carbamazepine, phenytoin).

NURSING CONSIDERATIONS

Assessment: Assess for degree of opioid tolerance, level of pain intensity, type of pain, patient's general condition and medical status, any other conditions where treatment is contraindicated or cautioned, renal/hepatic function, pregnancy/nursing status, and possible drug interactions.

Monitoring: Monitor for signs/symptoms of respiratory depression, elevations in CSF pressure, hypotension, seizures/convulsions, decreased bowel motility in postoperative patients, spasm of sphincter of Oddi, GI ulceration and/or bleeding, physical dependence, tolerance, abuse/addiction, and other adverse reactions. Monitor platelet/renal/hepatic function.

Patient Counseling: Instruct to dispose of unused tabs by flushing down the toilet. Instruct not to adjust dose without consulting physician. Advise that drug may impair mental and/or physical abilities. Instruct to avoid alcohol or other CNS depressants. Advise to consult physician if pregnant, planning to become pregnant, or nursing. Inform that if taking medication for more than a few weeks, to avoid abrupt withdrawal; advise that dosing will need to be tapered. Inform that drug has potential for abuse, to protect it from theft, and not to give to anyone. Advise that drug may cause or worsen constipation; instruct to notify physician for any past history of constipation.

Storage: 25°C (77°F); excursions permitted to 15-30°C (59-86°F).

PERFOROMIST – formoterol fumarate **RX**

Class: Beta$_2$-agonist

Long-acting β_2-adrenergic agonists (LABAs) increase the risk of asthma-related death. Contraindicated in asthma without use of a long-term asthma control medication.

ADULT DOSAGE

Chronic Obstructive Pulmonary Disease

Long-Term Maint Treatment of Bronchoconstriction in Patients w/ COPD (eg, Chronic Bronchitis, Emphysema):
Usual: 20mcg bid (am and pm) by nebulization
Max: 40mcg/day

PEDIATRIC DOSAGE

Pediatric use may not have been established

ADMINISTRATION

Oral inh route

Administer via a standard jet nebulizer connected to an air compressor
Store in the foil pouch and only remove immediately before use

HOW SUPPLIED

Sol, Inhalation: 20mcg/2mL [30^s 60^s]

CONTRAINDICATIONS

Asthma without use of a long-term asthma control medication.

WARNINGS/PRECAUTIONS

Not indicated to treat asthma, acute deteriorations of COPD, or for the relief of acute symptoms (eg, as rescue therapy for acute bronchospasm episodes). D/C regular use of inhaled short-acting β_2-agonists (SABAs) when beginning treatment; use only for symptomatic relief of acute respiratory symptoms. Do not use more often or at higher doses than recommended; clinically significant cardiovascular (CV) effects and fatalities reported with excessive use. May produce paradoxical bronchospasm; d/c therapy immediately and institute alternative therapy. CV effects may occur; d/c if such effects occur. Caution with CV disorders, convulsive disorders, thyrotoxicosis, diabetes mellitus (DM), ketoacidosis, and in patients unusually responsive to sympathomimetic amines. May produce significant hypokalemia and transient hyperglycemia. Immediate hypersensitivity reactions may occur.

ADVERSE REACTIONS
Diarrhea, nausea, nasopharyngitis, dry mouth.

DRUG INTERACTIONS
Do not use with other medications containing LABAs. Adrenergic drugs may potentiate sympathetic effects; use with caution. Xanthine derivatives, steroids, or diuretics may potentiate any hypokalemic effect. Caution is advised when coadministered with non-K^+-sparing diuretics (eg, loop, thiazide). Extreme caution with MAOIs, TCAs, or drugs known to prolong the QTc interval; effect on CV system may be potentiated. Drugs known to prolong the QTc interval have an increased risk of ventricular arrhythmias. β-blockers and formoterol may inhibit the effect of each other when administered concurrently. β-blockers may block therapeutic effects and produce severe bronchospasm in COPD patients; if such therapy is needed, consider cardioselective β-blockers and use with caution.

NURSING CONSIDERATIONS

Assessment: Assess for asthma, acute COPD deteriorations, CV disorders, convulsive disorders, thyrotoxicosis, DM, ketoacidosis, pregnancy/nursing status, and possible drug interactions. Assess use in patients unusually responsive to sympathomimetic amines.

Monitoring: Monitor for deteriorating disease, paradoxical bronchospasm, CV effects, hypokalemia, hyperglycemia, immediate hypersensitivity reactions, and other adverse reactions.

Patient Counseling: Counsel about the risks and benefits of therapy. Inform that drug is not for treatment of asthma. Advise not to use to relieve acute symptoms; inform that acute symptoms should be treated with an inhaled SABA. Instruct to seek medical attention if symptoms worsen despite recommended doses, if treatment becomes less effective, or if experiencing a need for more inhalations of a SABA than usual. Advise not to stop therapy unless directed by physician, not to inhale more than the prescribed number of vials at any 1 time, and not to exceed recommended daily dosage. Instruct to d/c the regular use of inhaled SABAs (eg, albuterol) when beginning treatment. Counsel not to use with other inhaled medications containing LABAs, and not to stop or change the dose of other concomitant COPD therapy without medical advice, even if symptoms improve after initiating treatment. Inform of the common adverse reactions associated with therapy. Instruct on how to properly use the medication.

Storage: Prior to Dispensing: 2-8°C (36-46°F). After Dispensing: 2-25°C (36-77°F) for up to 3 months. Protect pouch from heat. Vial should always be stored in the foil pouch, and only removed immediately before use.

PERIDEX – chlorhexidine gluconate — RX

Class: Antimicrobial

ADULT DOSAGE

Gingivitis

For Use Between Dental Visits:

Usual: Rinse w/ 15mL (undiluted) for 30 sec bid (am and pm) after toothbrushing; initiate directly following a dental prophylaxis

Reevaluate and give a thorough prophylaxis at intervals no longer than 6 months

PEDIATRIC DOSAGE

Pediatric use may not have been established

DOSE MODIFICATION
Oral route

Not intended for ingestion; should be expectorated after rinsing

Instruct to not rinse w/ water or other mouthwashes, brush teeth, or eat immediately after using

ADMINISTRATION
Oral route.

HOW SUPPLIED
Sol: 0.12% [15mL, 118mL, 473mL, 1893mL]

WARNINGS/PRECAUTIONS
Has not been tested among patients with acute necrotizing ulcerative gingivitis (ANUG). Effect on periodontitis has not been determined. Presence or absence of gingival inflammation following treatment should not be used as a major indicator of underlying periodontitis in patients having coexisting gingivitis and periodontitis. Increase in supragingival calculus reported. Calculus deposits should be removed by a dental prophylaxis at intervals not greater than six months. Anaphylaxis, as well as serious allergic reactions, reported. May stain oral surfaces (eg, tooth surfaces, restorations, dorsum of tongue), and alter taste perception. Caution in patients with anterior facial restorations with rough surfaces or margins.

ADVERSE REACTIONS

Increase in staining of teeth and other oral surfaces, increase in calculus formation, alteration in taste perception, oral irritation, local allergy-type symptoms.

NURSING CONSIDERATIONS

Assessment: Assess for drug hypersensitivity, ANUG, coexisting periodontitis and gingivitis, anterior facial restorations with rough surfaces or margins, and pregnancy/nursing status.

Monitoring: Monitor for staining of oral surfaces, alteration of taste, anaphylaxis and serious allergic reactions, and other adverse reactions.

Patient Counseling: Advise to use the oral rinse bid (am and pm) for 30 sec after brushing. Instruct to not rinse with water or other mouthwashes, brush teeth, or eat immediately afterward. Instruct to expectorate after rinsing and not to ingest.

Storage: 20-25°C (68-77°F); excursions permitted to 15-30°C (59-86°F).

PerioGard – chlorhexidine gluconate RX

Class: Antimicrobial

ADULT DOSAGE

Gingivitis

≥18 Years:

Initiate directly following a dental prophylaxis

Rinse w/ 15mL (undiluted) for 30 secs bid, am and pm, after toothbrushing

PEDIATRIC DOSAGE

Pediatric use may not have been established

ADMINISTRATION

Oral route

HOW SUPPLIED

Liq: 0.12% (16oz)

WARNINGS/PRECAUTIONS

Effect in periodontitis not known. May increase supragingival calculus. Hypersensitivity, generalized allergic reactions and altered taste reported. May stain oral surfaces (eg, tooth surfaces, restorations, and dorsum of the tongue). Caution with anterior facial restoration. Re-evaluate and give thorough dental prophylaxis at intervals no longer than 6 months.

ADVERSE REACTIONS

Increase in staining of teeth and other oral surfaces, increase in calculus formation, alteration in taste perception, oral irritation, local allergic type symptoms.

NURSING CONSIDERATIONS

Assessment: Assess for coexisting periodontitis and gingivitis, anterior facial restorations with rough surfaces or margins, pregnancy/nursing status.

Monitoring: Monitor for staining of oral surfaces, alteration of taste, minor irritation and superficial desquamation of oral mucosa, and hypersensitivity reactions.

Patient Counseling: Advise to rinse twice daily (am and pm) for 30 sec after brushing. Instruct not to rinse with water or other mouthwashes, brush teeth, or eat immediately after use. Instruct not to ingest; expectorate product after rinsing.

Storage: Store above freezing (32°F).

Perjeta – pertuzumab RX

Class: Monoclonal antibody/HER2-blocker

May result in subclinical and clinical cardiac failure; evaluate left ventricular function prior to and during treatment. D/C treatment for a confirmed clinically significant decrease in left ventricular function. Exposure during pregnancy may result in embryo-fetal death and birth defects; advise patients of these risks and the need for effective contraception.

ADULT DOSAGE

Breast Cancer

Metastatic:

Combination w/ trastuzumab and docetaxel for HER2-positive metastatic breast cancer

PEDIATRIC DOSAGE

Pediatric use may not have been established

in patients who have not received prior anti-HER2 therapy or chemotherapy for metastatic disease

Initial: 840mg IV infusion over 60 min, followed every 3 weeks by 420mg IV infusion over 30-60 min

Trastuzumab:
Initial: 8mg/kg IV infusion over 90 min, followed every 3 weeks by a dose of 6mg/kg IV infusion over 30-90 min

Docetaxel:
Initial: 75mg/m^2 IV infusion
Titrate: May increase to 100mg/m^2 administered every 3 weeks if initial dose is well tolerated

Neoadjuvant Treatment:
Combination w/ trastuzumab and docetaxel for the neoadjuvant treatment of patients w/ HER2-positive, locally advanced, inflammatory, or early stage breast cancer (either >2cm in diameter or node positive) as part of a complete treatment regimen for early breast cancer

Initial: 840mg IV infusion over 60 min, followed every 3 weeks by a dose of 420mg IV infusion over 30-60 min

Trastuzumab:
Initial: 8mg/kg IV infusion over 90 min, followed every 3 weeks by a dose of 6mg/kg IV infusion over 30-90 min

Administer every 3 weeks for 3-6 cycles as part of 1 of the following treatment regimens for early breast cancer:
4 preoperative cycles of pertuzumab in combination w/ trastuzumab and docetaxel, followed by 3 postoperative cycles of fluorouracil, epirubicin, and cyclophosphamide (FEC)
OR
3 preoperative cycles of FEC alone, followed by 3 preoperative cycles of pertuzumab in combination w/ docetaxel and trastuzumab
OR
6 preoperative cycles of pertuzumab in combination w/ docetaxel, carboplatin, and trastuzumab (TCH) (escalation of docetaxel >75mg/m^2 is not recommended)

Following surgery, patients should continue to receive trastuzumab to complete 1 yr of treatment

Missed Dose

Time Between 2 Sequential Infusions is <6 Weeks:
Administer the 420mg pertuzumab dose; do not wait until the next planned dose

Time Between 2 Sequential Infusions is ≥6 weeks:
Readminister initial dose of 840mg pertuzumab as a 60-min IV infusion, followed every 3 weeks thereafter by a dose of 420mg administered as an IV infusion over 30-60 min

DOSE MODIFICATION

Adverse Reactions

Left Ventricular Ejection Fraction (LVEF):

Withhold Pertuzumab and Trastuzumab Dosing for ≥3 Weeks for Either:

A drop in LVEF to <45%

OR

LVEF of 45-49% w/ a ≥10% absolute decrease below pretreatment values

Pertuzumab may be resumed if LVEF recovers to >49% or to 45-49% associated w/ <10% absolute decrease below pretreatment values; if after a repeat assessment w/in approx 3 weeks, LVEF has not improved or has declined further, d/c pertuzumab and trastuzumab, unless the benefits outweigh the risks

Infusion-Related Reactions:

Infusion rate of pertuzumab may be slowed or interrupted

Hypersensitivity Reactions/Anaphylaxis:

D/C infusion immediately if serious hypersensitivity reaction occurs

ADMINISTRATION

IV route

Do not administer as IV push or bolus

Do not mix w/ other drugs

Administer pertuzumab, trastuzumab, and docetaxel sequentially

Pertuzumab and trastuzumab can be given in any order; administer docetaxel after pertuzumab and trastuzumab

An observation period of 30-60 min is recommended after each pertuzumab infusion and before commencement of any subsequent infusion of trastuzumab or docetaxel

D/C pertuzumab if trastuzumab treatment is discontinued

Preparation

1. Withdraw the appropriate volume of pertuzumab sol from the vial(s)
2. Dilute into a 250mL 0.9% NaCl polyvinyl chloride (PVC) or non-PVC polyolefin infusion bag
3. Mix diluted sol by gentle inversion; do not shake
4. Administer immediately once prepared; if not used immediately, store at 2-8°C for up to 24 hrs
5. Dilute w/ 0.9% NaCl inj only; do not use D5 sol

HOW SUPPLIED

Inj: 30mg/mL [14mL]

WARNINGS/PRECAUTIONS

Monitor for oligohydramnios if pregnancy occurs during therapy; if this occurs, perform fetal testing appropriate for gestational age. Infusion-related reactions reported; observe closely for 60 min after the 1st infusion and for 30 min after subsequent infusions. Consider permanent discontinuation in patients w/ severe infusion reactions. Hypersensitivity/anaphylaxis reactions reported; medications/emergency equipment should be available for immediate use. Detection of HER2 protein overexpression is necessary for appropriate patient selection. Patients who have received prior anthracyclines or prior radiotherapy to the chest area may be at higher risk of decreased left ventricular ejection fraction (LVEF).

ADVERSE REACTIONS

Cardiac failure, diarrhea, alopecia, neutropenia, N/V, fatigue, rash, peripheral neuropathy, neutropenia, mucosal inflammation, anemia, myalgia, decreased appetite, headache, dyspepsia.

NURSING CONSIDERATIONS

Assessment: Assess for hypersensitivity to drug and pregnancy/nursing status. Assess LVEF prior to initiation of therapy. Assess HER2 status; should be performed by laboratories w/ demonstrated proficiency in the specific technology being utilized.

Monitoring: Monitor for infusion-related reactions, hypersensitivity/anaphylaxis reactions, and other adverse reactions. Monitor LVEF at regular intervals (eg, every 3 months in the metastatic setting and every 6 weeks in the neoadjuvant setting).

Patient Counseling: Inform that exposure to drug may result in fetal harm, including embryo-fetal death or birth defects; advise females of reproductive potential to use effective contraception while on therapy and for 6 months following the last dose. Instruct to contact physician immediately if pregnancy is suspected. Encourage women exposed to pertuzumab during pregnancy to enroll in the MotHER Pregnancy Registry. Advise not to breastfeed during therapy.

Storage: 2-8°C (36-46°F) until time of use. Protect from light. Do not freeze or shake. Diluted Sol: 2-8°C (36-46°F) for up to 24 hrs.

PHENOBARBITAL – phenobarbital CIV

Class: Barbiturate

ADULT DOSAGE

Sedation

Tab (15mg, 30mg, 60mg, 100mg):
30-120mg in 2-3 divided doses

Tab (16.2mg, 32.4mg, 64.8mg, 97.2mg):
Daytime Sedation: 30-120mg in 2-3 divided doses
Max: 400mg/24 hrs

Elixir:
Daytime Sedation: 30-120mg in 2-3 divided doses
Max: 400mg/24 hrs

Hypnotic:
Tab (15mg, 30mg, 60mg, 100mg):
100-320mg
Tab (16.2mg, 32.4mg, 64.8mg, 97.2mg):
100-200mg
Elixir:
100-200mg

Seizures

Generalized/Partial Seizures:
Tab (16.2mg, 32.4mg, 64.8mg, 97.2mg):
60-200mg/day
Elixir:
60-200mg/day

Also used in the treatment/prophylaxis of febrile seizures

Anticonvulsant:
Tab (15mg, 30mg, 60mg, 100mg):
50-100mg bid or tid

PEDIATRIC DOSAGE

Sedation

Tab (15mg, 30mg, 60mg, 100mg):
6mg/kg/day in 3 divided doses

Seizures

Generalized/Partial Seizures:
Tab (16.2mg, 32.4mg, 64.8mg, 97.2mg):
3-6mg/kg/day
Elixir:
3-6mg/kg/day

Also used in the treatment/prophylaxis of febrile seizures

Anticonvulsant:
Tab (15mg, 30mg, 60mg, 100mg):
15-50mg bid or tid

DOSE MODIFICATION

Renal Impairment
Reduce dose

Hepatic Impairment
Reduce dose

Elderly/Debilitated
Reduce dose

ADMINISTRATION

Oral route

HOW SUPPLIED

Elixir: 20mg/5mL [473mL]; Tab: 15mg, 16.2mg*, 30mg*, 32.4mg*, 60mg, 64.8mg*, 97.2mg*, 100mg*
*scored

CONTRAINDICATIONS

Marked impairment of liver function or respiratory disease in which dyspnea or obstruction is evident. (Elixir/16.2mg, 32.4mg, 64.8mg, 97.2mg Tab) History of manifest/latent porphyria. (15mg, 30mg, 60mg, 100mg Tab) Personal or familial history of acute intermittent porphyria, known previous addiction to sedative/hypnotic group.

WARNINGS/PRECAUTIONS

Caution with borderline hypoadrenal function and history of drug abuse or dependence. Caution in patients who are mentally depressed or with suicidal tendencies. Caution when prescribing large amounts to patients with a history of emotional disturbances. Elderly or debilitated patients may react with marked excitement, depression, or confusion. (15mg, 30mg, 60mg, 100mg Tab) May increase reaction to painful stimuli in small doses; cannot be relied upon to relieve pain or even produce sedation or sleep in the presence of severe pain if taken alone. Caution with decreased liver function. (Elixir/16.2mg, 32.4mg, 64.8mg, 97.2mg Tab) Caution with acute or chronic pain; may induce paradoxical excitement or mask important symptoms. Some persons, especially children, may repeatedly produce excitement rather than depression. Caution in patients with hepatic damage; initiate therapy in reduced doses. Avoid in patients showing premonitory signs of hepatic coma. May cause fetal damage. Use during labor may result in respiratory depression in the newborn. Cognitive deficits reported in children taking drug for complicated febrile seizures. May be habit-forming; limit prescription and dispensing to amount required for the interval until the next appointment. Withdraw gradually in patients taking excessive doses over long periods of time.

ADVERSE REACTIONS

Respiratory/CNS depression, apnea, circulatory collapse, hypersensitivity reactions, N/V, headache, somnolence.

DRUG INTERACTIONS

May produce additive depressant effects with other CNS depressants (eg, other sedatives/hypnotics, antihistamines, tranquilizers, alcohol). May diminish systemic effects of exogenous corticosteroids (eg, hydrocortisone). Decreased anticoagulant response of oral anticoagulants (eg, warfarin, acenocoumarol, dicumarol, phenprocoumon); determine PT frequently. Dose adjustments of anticoagulants may be required if barbiturates are added to or withdrawn from the dosage regimen. (Elixir/16.2mg, 32.4mg, 64.8mg, 97.2mg Tab) Dose adjustments of corticosteroids may be required if barbiturates are added to or withdrawn from the dosage regimen. May decrease griseofulvin levels; avoid concomitant use. May shorten $T_{1/2}$ of doxycycline for as long as 2 weeks after barbiturate therapy is discontinued; monitor response to doxycycline closely if given concurrently. Monitor phenytoin and barbiturate blood levels frequently when given concurrently. Increased levels with sodium valproate and valproic acid; closely monitor barbiturate blood levels and adjust dose as indicated. MAOIs may prolong effects. May decrease effect of estradiol with pretreatment or with concurrent use. Pregnancy reported with oral contraceptives; may suggest use of alternative contraceptive method.

NURSING CONSIDERATIONS

Assessment: Assess for known barbiturate hypersensitivity, history of porphyria, respiratory disease with evident dyspnea or obstruction, hypoadrenal function, suicidal tendencies, history of drug abuse or dependence, mental depression, hepatic impairment, debilitation, pain, pregnancy/nursing status, and possible drug interactions. (Elixir/16.2mg, 32.4mg, 64.8mg, 97.2mg Tab) Assess for renal impairment.

Monitoring: Monitor for marked excitement, depression, and confusion in elderly and debilitated patients. Monitor for tolerance, psychological and physical dependence, and withdrawal symptoms. Monitor PT frequently if used with coumarin anticoagulants. (Elixir/16.2mg, 32.4mg, 64.8mg, 97.2mg Tab) Monitor for paradoxical excitement and for masking of symptoms in patients with acute/chronic pain. Monitor for cognitive deficits in children with complicated febrile seizures. Perform periodic lab evaluation of hematopoietic, renal, and hepatic systems during prolonged therapy.

Patient Counseling: Inform that medication may impair mental/physical abilities required for the performance of potentially hazardous tasks (eg, driving/operating machinery); advise to use caution. (Elixir/16.2mg, 32.4mg, 64.8mg, 97.2mg Tab) Inform of the risk of psychological and/or physical dependence; instruct not to increase dose without consulting physician. Instruct to avoid alcohol while on therapy; inform that use of other CNS depressants (eg, alcohol, narcotics, tranquilizers, antihistamines) may result in additional CNS depressant effects.

Storage: 20-25°C (68-77°F). (15mg, 30mg, 60mg, 100mg Tab) Protect from light and moisture.

PHENYTOIN – phenytoin sodium RX

Class: Hydantoin

The rate of IV inj administration should not exceed 50mg/min in adults and 1-3mg/kg/min (or 50mg/min, whichever is slower) in pediatric patients because of the risk of severe hypotension and cardiac arrhythmias. Careful cardiac monitoring is needed during and after administration. Risk of cardiovascular (CV) toxicity reported at or below the recommended infusion rate; may need to reduce rate of administration or d/c dosing.

ADULT DOSAGE

Seizures

Status Epilepticus:
LD: 10-15mg/kg IV
Max Rate: 50mg/min
Maint: 100mg PO or IV q6-8h

PEDIATRIC DOSAGE

Seizures

Status Epilepticus:
LD: 15-20mg/kg IV
Max Rate: 1-3mg/kg/min or 50mg/min (whichever is slower)

DOSE MODIFICATION

Renal Impairment

Caution when interpreting total phenytoin plasma concentrations; unbound phenytoin concentrations may be more useful

Hepatic Impairment

Caution when interpreting total phenytoin plasma concentrations; unbound phenytoin concentrations may be more useful

Elderly

May require lower or less frequent dosing

Other Important Modifications

IM Administration:

An IM dose 50% greater than the oral dose is necessary to maintain therapeutic plasma levels. When returned to oral administration, reduce dose by 50% of the original oral dose for one week

IV Substitution for Oral Therapy:

When oral treatment is not possible, IV therapy may be substituted at the same total daily dose

Dosage adjustments may be necessary when switching from a free acid formulation to a product formulated with the sodium salt and vice versa, because there is approximately an 8% increase in drug content with the free acid form over that of the sodium salt

ADMINISTRATION

IM/IV route

As non-emergency therapy, administer more slowly as either a LD or by intermittent infusion; use oral phenytoin whenever possible

Administer IV inj directly into a large peripheral or central vein through a large-gauge catheter; follow each parenteral inj by a flush of sterile saline through the same catheter

Inj may be given diluted with normal saline; avoid addition of parenteral inj to dextrose and dextrose-containing solutions

For Infusion Administration

1. Dilute parenteral inj in normal saline with the final concentration in the sol no less than 5mg/mL
2. Commence administration immediately after the mixture has been prepared and complete within 1 to 4 hours (do not refrigerate the infusion mixture)
3. Use an in-line filter (0.22-0.55 microns)

Status Epilepticus

Do not use IM administration

Consider the use of other anticonvulsants, IV barbiturates, general anesthesia, and other appropriate measures if parenteral inj does not terminate seizures

HOW SUPPLIED

Inj: 50mg/mL [2mL, 5mL]

CONTRAINDICATIONS

Sinus bradycardia, sinoatrial block, 2nd- and 3rd-degree atrioventricular (AV) block, Adams-Stokes syndrome. Coadministration with delavirdine.

WARNINGS/PRECAUTIONS

Use only when oral phenytoin administration is not possible. Do not abruptly d/c; may increase seizure frequency, including status epilepticus. In the event of an allergic or hypersensitivity reaction, rapid substitution of alternative (eg, non-hydantoin antiepileptic) therapy may be necessary. Serious and sometimes fatal dermatologic reactions (eg, toxic epidermal necrolysis [TEN], Stevens-Johnson syndrome [SJS]) reported; d/c at the 1st sign of a rash, unless rash is clearly not drug-related. If signs/symptoms suggest SJS/TEN, do not resume therapy and consider alternative treatment. Consider avoiding therapy as an alternative for carbamazepine in patients positive for HLA-B*1502. Drug reaction with eosinophilia and systemic symptoms (DRESS)/multiorgan hypersensitivity reported; evaluate immediately if signs/symptoms (eg, rash, fever, and/or lymphadenopathy, in association with other organ system involvement) are present, and d/c if an alternative etiology cannot be established. Consider alternative therapy if there is a history of hypersensitivity reactions to structurally similar drugs (eg, carboxamides, barbiturates, succinimides, oxazolidinediones) in the patient or immediate family members. Cases of acute hepatotoxicity, including infrequent cases of acute hepatic failure, reported; immediately d/c and do not readminister. Hematopoietic complications and lymphadenopathy reported; in all cases of lymphadenopathy, follow-up observation for an extended period is indicated and every effort should be made to achieve seizure control using alternative antiepileptic drugs. Soft tissue irritation and inflammation occurred at inj-site with and without extravasation of IV therapy. Local toxicity (purple glove syndrome) reported; administer IV inj directly into a large peripheral/central vein through a large-gauge catheter. IM administration may cause pain, necrosis, and abscess formation at inj site. Potentially life-threatening bleeding disorder may occur in newborns exposed to phenytoin in utero; administer vitamin K to the mother before delivery and to the neonate after birth. Caution with renal/hepatic disease, hypoalbuminemia, porphyria, and in elderly or gravely ill patients. Hyperglycemia reported. May increase serum glucose concentrations in diabetic patients. Not indicated for seizures due to hypoglycemic or other metabolic causes; perform appropriate diagnostic procedures as indicated. Not effective for absence seizures; if tonic-clonic and absence seizures are present, combined drug therapy is needed. Serum levels sustained above the optimal range may produce confusional states (delirium, psychosis, encephalopathy, cerebellar dysfunction); determine plasma concentrations at the 1st sign of acute toxicity. Reduce dose if concentrations are excessive; if symptoms persist, termination is recommended. Lab test interactions may occur.

ADVERSE REACTIONS

CV collapse, CNS depression, nystagmus, ataxia, slurred speech, decreased coordination, somnolence, mental confusion, dizziness, vertigo, transient nervousness, motor twitchings, paresthesia, headache, sensory peripheral polyneuropathy.

DRUG INTERACTIONS

See Contraindications. Acute alcohol intake, amiodarone, antiepileptic agents (eg, felbamate, oxcarbazepine, topiramate), azoles (eg, fluconazole, ketoconazole, itraconazole), capecitabine, chloramphenicol, chlordiazepoxide, disulfiram, estrogens, fluorouracil, fluoxetine, fluvastatin, fluvoxamine, H_2-antagonists (eg, cimetidine), halothane, isoniazid, methylphenidate, omeprazole, phenothiazines, salicylates, sertraline, succinimides, sulfonamides (eg, sulfamethizole, sulfaphenazole, sulfadiazine), ticlopidine, tolbutamide, trazodone, and warfarin may increase concentrations. Anticancer drugs usually in combination (eg, bleomycin, carboplatin, cisplatin), carbamazepine, chronic alcohol abuse, diazepam, diazoxide, folic acid, fosamprenavir, nelfinavir, reserpine, rifampin, ritonavir, St. John's wort, theophylline, and vigabatrin may decrease concentrations. Phenobarbital, valproic acid, and sodium valproate may either increase or decrease concentrations; similarly, the effect on concentrations of such drugs is unpredictable. May impair efficacy of azoles, corticosteroids, doxycycline, estrogens, furosemide, irinotecan, oral contraceptives, paclitaxel, paroxetine, quinidine, rifampin, sertraline, teniposide, theophylline, and vitamin D. Increased and decreased PT/INR responses reported with warfarin. May decrease concentrations of certain HIV antivirals (eg, efavirenz, indinavir, ritonavir), antiepileptics, atorvastatin, chlorpropamide, clozapine, cyclosporine, digoxin, fluvastatin, folic acid, methadone, mexiletine, nifedipine, nimodipine, nisoldipine, praziquantel, simvastatin, verapamil, and active metabolites of albendazole. May decrease concentration of amprenavir (active metabolite) when given with fosamprenavir alone. May increase concentration of amprenavir when given with the combination of fosamprenavir and ritonavir. Resistance to the neuromuscular blocking action of the nondepolarizing neuromuscular blocking agents pancuronium, vecuronium, rocuronium, and cisatracurium reported in patients chronically administered phenytoin; monitor closely for more rapid recovery from neuromuscular blockade than expected, and infusion rate requirements may be higher. Avoid with enteral feeding preparations and/or related nutritional supplements.

NURSING CONSIDERATIONS

Assessment: Assess for hypersensitivity to drug or other hydantoins, sinus bradycardia, sinoatrial block, 2nd- and 3rd-degree AV block, Adams-Stokes syndrome, renal/hepatic disease, hypoalbuminemia, porphyria, grave illness, any other conditions where treatment is contraindicated or cautioned, pregnancy/nursing status, and possible drug interactions.

Monitoring: Monitor for allergic/hypersensitivity reactions, dermatologic reactions, DRESS, hepatotoxicity, hematopoietic complications, lymphadenopathy, local toxicity, hyperglycemia, confusional states, and other adverse reactions. Careful cardiac monitoring is needed during and after IV administration. Continuously monitor ECG, BP, and respiratory function.

Patient Counseling: Inform of the risks and benefits of therapy. Advise to consult with physician if pregnant/planning to become pregnant. Instruct not to breastfeed while on therapy. Instruct to notify physician if adverse reactions develop.

Storage: 20-25°C (68-77°F); excursions permitted to 15-30°C (59-86°F).

PLAQUENIL — hydroxychloroquine sulfate RX

Class: Quinine derivative

Before prescribing, physicians should be completely familiar with the complete prescribing information.

ADULT DOSAGE

Rheumatoid Arthritis

Initial: 400-600mg/day

Some patients may require temporary reduction of initial dose due to troublesome side effects; later (usually from 5-10 days), dose may be gradually increased to optimum response level

Maint: When a good response is obtained (usually in 4-12 weeks), reduce dose by 50% and continue at 200-400mg/day

May resume therapy or continue on an intermittent schedule if relapse occurs after drug withdrawal

PEDIATRIC DOSAGE

Malaria

Suppression:

5mg base/kg weekly; begin 2 weeks prior to exposure

Max: 400mg/dose

If Unable to Begin 2 Weeks Prior to Exposure:

10mg base/kg in 2 divided doses, 6 hrs apart

Continue suppressive therapy for 8 weeks after leaving endemic area

Treatment of Acute Attack:

1st Dose: 10mg base/kg

Malaria

Suppression:
400mg on exactly the same day of each week; begin 2 weeks prior to exposure

If Unable to Begin 2 Weeks Prior to Exposure:
800mg in 2 divided doses, 6 hrs apart

Continue suppressive therapy for 8 weeks after leaving endemic area

Treatment of Acute Attack:
800mg, followed by 400mg 6-8 hrs later, then 400mg on each of 2 consecutive days

Alternative Dosing:
800mg single dose, or calculate on the basis of body weight

Lupus Erythematosus

Chronic Discoid and Systemic:
Initial: 400mg qd-bid for several weeks or months
Prolonged Maint: 200-400mg/day

Max: Single dose of 620mg
2nd Dose: 5mg base/kg 6 hrs after 1st dose
Max: Single dose of 310mg base
3rd Dose: 5mg base/kg 18 hrs after 2nd dose
Max: Single dose of 310mg base
4th Dose: 5mg base/kg 24 hrs after 3rd dose
Max: Single dose of 310mg base

ADMINISTRATION
Oral route

Rheumatoid Arthritis
Take w/ a meal or glass of milk

HOW SUPPLIED
Tab: 200mg (200mg tab=155mg base)

CONTRAINDICATIONS
Long-term therapy in children or in the presence of retinal/visual field changes attributable to any 4-aminoquinoline compound.

WARNINGS/PRECAUTIONS
Not effective against chloroquine-resistant strains of *Plasmodium falciparum*. Carefully examine for visual acuity, central visual field and color vision including fundoscopy prior to long-term therapy; repeat exam at least annually. Irreversible retinal damage reported with long-term or high dosage of 4-aminoquinoline therapy. Perform baseline and periodic (every 3 months) ophthalmologic exams with prolonged therapy. Increased risk of retinal toxicity if recommended daily dose is exceeded sharply. D/C therapy immediately if any visual disturbance occurs and closely observe for possible progression of the abnormality. Retinal and visual disturbances may progress even after discontinuation of therapy. Suicidal behavior reported. May precipitate a severe attack of psoriasis and may exacerbate porphyria; avoid use in these conditions unless benefits outweigh possible hazard. Avoid in pregnancy except in the suppression/treatment of malaria if benefit outweighs the risk. Caution with hepatic disease, alcoholism, and G6PD deficiency. Perform periodic blood cell counts with prolonged therapy; d/c therapy if any severe blood disorder appears that is not attributable to the disease under treatment. (Lupus erythematosus/RA) Examine all patients periodically including testing of knee and ankle reflexes; d/c treatment if muscular weakness occurs. Dermatologic reactions may occur with a significant tendency to produce dermatitis. Caution with impaired renal function and/or metabolic acidosis. In treatment of RA, d/c if no improvement occurs after 6 months.

ADVERSE REACTIONS
Dizziness, headache, convulsions, diarrhea, nervousness, emotional lability, psychosis, suicidal behavior, retinopathy with changes in pigmentation, visual field defects, erythema multiforme, Stevens-Jonhson syndrome, toxic epidermal necrolysis, photosensitivity, exfoliative dermatitis.

DRUG INTERACTIONS
Caution with hepatotoxic drugs.

NURSING CONSIDERATIONS

Assessment: Assess for retinal or visual field defects, psoriasis, porphyria, hepatic/renal disease, alcoholism, G6PD deficiency, chloroquine-resistant strains of *P. falciparum*, or any other conditions where treatment is contraindicated or cautioned, pregnancy/nursing status, and possible drug interactions. Perform baseline ophthalmologic exams with prolonged therapy.

Monitoring: Monitor for retinal/visual disturbances, severe psoriasis attack, exacerbation of porphyria, dermatologic reactions, and other adverse reactions. Perform periodic (every 3 months) ophthalmologic exams with prolonged therapy and monitor CBC with differential and platelet count. Periodically test for knee and ankle reflexes in RA patients.

Patient Counseling: Counsel about adverse effects and to d/c drug and seek medical attention if any signs/symptoms develop. Advise about need for periodic follow-up.

Storage: Room temperature up to 30°C (86°F).

PLAVIX — clopidogrel bisulfate RX

Class: Platelet aggregation inhibitor

Effectiveness is dependent on activation to an active metabolite via CYP2C19. Poor metabolizers of CYP2C19 with acute coronary syndrome (ACS) or undergoing percutaneous coronary intervention treated with clopidogrel at recommended doses exhibit higher cardiovascular (CV) event rates than patients with normal CYP2C19 function. Tests are available to identify a patient's CYP2C19 genotype; these tests can be used as an aid in determining therapeutic strategy. Consider alternative treatment or treatment strategies in patients identified as CYP2C19 poor metabolizers.

ADULT DOSAGE

Acute Coronary Syndrome

Unstable Angina/Non-ST-Elevation MI:
LD: 300mg
Maint: 75mg qd. Initiate ASA (75-325mg qd) and continue in combination w/ clopidogrel

ST-Elevation MI:
75mg qd w/ ASA (75-325mg qd), w/ or w/o thrombolytics
May initiate w/ or w/o a LD

Recent Myocardial Infarction/Recent Stroke/ Peripheral Arterial Disease
75mg qd

PEDIATRIC DOSAGE

Pediatric use may not have been established

ADMINISTRATION

Oral route

May be administered w/ or w/o food

HOW SUPPLIED

Tab: 75mg, 300mg

CONTRAINDICATIONS

Active pathological bleeding (eg, peptic ulcer, intracranial hemorrhage).

WARNINGS/PRECAUTIONS

Increases the risk of bleeding; d/c 5 days prior to surgery if an antiplatelet effect is not desired. Avoid lapses in therapy; if therapy must be temporarily discontinued, restart as soon as possible. Premature discontinuation may increase risk of CV events. TTP reported. Hypersensitivity (eg, rash, angioedema, hematologic reaction) reported, including in patients with a history of hypersensitivity or hematologic reaction to other thienopyridines.

ADVERSE REACTIONS

Bleeding.

DRUG INTERACTIONS

Reduced antiplatelet activity with omeprazole or esomeprazole; avoid concomitant use, or consider using another acid-reducing agent with minimal or no CYP2C19 inhibitory effect on the formation of clopidogrel active metabolite when coadministration of a proton pump inhibitor is required. Certain CYP2C19 inhibitors may reduce platelet inhibition. NSAIDs, warfarin, SSRIs, SNRIs, and ASA may increase risk of bleeding.

NURSING CONSIDERATIONS

Assessment: Assess for active pathological bleeding, hypersensitivity to drug or another thienopyridine, CYP2C19 genotype, pregnancy/nursing status, and possible drug interactions. Assess use in patients at risk for increased bleeding (eg, undergoing surgery).

Monitoring: Monitor for bleeding, TTP, hypersensitivity, and other adverse reactions.

Patient Counseling: Inform about the benefits and risks of treatment. Instruct to take exactly as prescribed and not to d/c without consulting the prescribing physician. Inform that they will bruise and bleed more easily and that bleeding will take longer than usual to stop. Advise to report any unanticipated, prolonged, or excessive bleeding, or blood in stool or urine. Instruct to seek prompt medical attention if unexplained fever, weakness, extreme skin paleness, purple skin patches, yellowing of the skin or eyes, or neurological changes occur. Instruct to notify physician or dentist about therapy before scheduling any invasive procedure. Advise to inform physician of all medications they are taking or planning to take.

Storage: 25°C (77°F); excursions permitted to 15-30°C (59-86°F).

PLETAL – cilostazol RX

Class: Phosphodiesterase III inhibitor

Contraindicated w/ CHF of any severity due to possible decrease in survival.

ADULT DOSAGE

Intermittent Claudication

Reduction of Symptoms:

Usual: 100mg bid

D/C if symptoms have not improved after 3 months

PEDIATRIC DOSAGE

Pediatric use may not have been established

DOSE MODIFICATION

Concomitant Medications

Moderate/Strong CYP3A4 or Strong CYP2C19 Inhibitors: Consider reduction to 50mg bid

ADMINISTRATION

Oral route

Take at least 1/2 hr before or 2 hrs after breakfast and dinner

HOW SUPPLIED

Tab: 50mg, 100mg

CONTRAINDICATIONS

CHF of any severity. Hemostatic disorders or active pathologic bleeding (eg, peptic ulcer, intracranial bleeding).

WARNINGS/PRECAUTIONS

Thrombocytopenia/leukopenia progressing to agranulocytosis reported (rare). May induce tachycardia, palpitation, tachyarrhythmia, and/or hypotension. Patients w/ history of ischemic heart disease may be at risk for angina pectoris or MI exacerbation. Special caution w/ moderate/severe hepatic and severe renal impairment (CrCl <25mL/min).

ADVERSE REACTIONS

Headache, palpitation, tachycardia, abnormal stools, diarrhea, peripheral edema, dizziness, infection, rhinitis, pharyngitis, nausea, back pain, dyspepsia, abdominal pain, increased cough.

DRUG INTERACTIONS

See Dose Modification. May increase levels and overall pharmacological activity w/ strong or moderate CYP3A4 inhibitors (eg, ketoconazole, itraconazole, erythromycin, diltiazem) and strong CYP2C19 inhibitors (eg, ticlopidine, fluconazole, omeprazole).

NURSING CONSIDERATIONS

Assessment: Assess for hypersensitivity to drug, CHF, hemostatic disorders, active pathologic bleeding, history of ischemic heart disease, renal/hepatic impairment, pregnancy/nursing status, and possible drug interactions.

Monitoring: Monitor for tachycardia, palpitation, tachyarrhythmia, hypotension, and other adverse reactions. Monitor platelets and WBC counts periodically.

Patient Counseling: Advise to take at least 1/2 hr ac or 2 hrs pc. Inform that benefits of medication may not be immediate and treatment may be required for up to 12 weeks before beneficial effect is experienced.

Storage: 25°C (77°F); excursions permitted to 15-30°C (59-86°F).

PRADAXA – dabigatran etexilate mesylate RX

Class: Direct thrombin inhibitor

Premature discontinuation of therapy increases the risk of thrombotic events. If therapy is discontinued for a reason other than pathological bleeding, consider coverage with another anticoagulant. Epidural or spinal hematomas may occur in patients treated with dabigatran who are receiving neuraxial anesthesia or undergoing spinal puncture; may result in long-term or permanent paralysis. Consider these risks when scheduling for spinal procedures. Increased risk of developing epidural or spinal hematomas with the use of indwelling epidural catheters, concomitant use of other drugs that affect hemostasis (eg, NSAIDs, platelet inhibitors, other anticoagulants), history of traumatic or repeated epidural or spinal punctures, history of spinal deformity or spinal surgery, or unknown optimal timing between the administration of therapy and neuraxial procedures. Monitor frequently for signs/symptoms of neurological impairment; if neurologic compromise is noted, urgent treatment is necessary. Consider benefits and risks before neuraxial intervention in patients anticoagulated or to be anticoagulated.

ADULT DOSAGE

Reduce Risk of Stroke and Systemic Embolism in Nonvalvular Atrial Fibrillation

150mg bid

Reduce Risk of Recurrent Deep Vein Thrombosis/Pulmonary Embolism

Previously Treated Patients:
150mg bid

Deep Vein Thrombosis/Pulmonary Embolism

Patients Treated w/ a Parenteral Anticoagulant for 5-10 Days:
150mg bid

Conversions

Conversion from Warfarin:
D/C warfarin and start therapy when INR <2.0

Conversion to Warfarin:
CrCl ≥50mL/min: Start warfarin 3 days before discontinuing therapy
CrCl 30-50mL/min: Start warfarin 2 days before discontinuing therapy
CrCl 15-30mL/min: Start warfarin 1 day before discontinuing therapy
CrCl <15mL/min: No recommendations

Conversion from Parenteral Anticoagulants:
Start 0-2 hrs before the time that the next dose of the parenteral drug was to have been administered, or at time of discontinuation of a continuously administered parenteral drug (eg, IV unfractionated heparin)

Conversion to Parenteral Anticoagulant:
CrCl ≥30mL/min: Wait 12 hrs after last dose before initiating treatment w/ a parenteral anticoagulant
CrCl <30mL/min: Wait 24 hrs after last dose before initiating treatment w/ a parenteral anticoagulant

PEDIATRIC DOSAGE

Pediatric use may not have been established

DOSE MODIFICATION

Concomitant Medications

Reduction in Risk of Stroke and Systemic Embolism in Nonvalvular A-Fib:
CrCl 30-50mL/min w/ Concomitant Dronedarone/Ketoconazole: Consider reducing dose to 75mg bid
CrCl <30mL/min w/ Concomitant P-gp Inhibitors: Avoid coadministration

Reduction in Risk of Recurrent DVT/PE:
CrCl <50mL/min w/ Concomitant P-gp Inhibitors: Avoid coadministration

Renal Impairment

Reduction in Risk of Stroke and Systemic Embolism in Nonvalvular A-Fib:
CrCl 15-30mL/min: 75mg bid
CrCl <15mL/min or On Dialysis: Dosing recommendations cannot be provided

Treatment and Reduction in the Risk of Recurrent DVT/PE:
CrCl ≤30mL/min or on Dialysis: Dosing recommendations cannot be provided

Other Important Modifications

Surgery/Other Interventions:
CrCl ≥50mL/min: D/C 1-2 days before invasive or surgical procedures, if possible
CrCl <50mL/min: D/C 3-5 days before invasive or surgical procedures, if possible

Consider longer times for patients undergoing major surgery, spinal puncture, or placement of spinal/epidural catheter or port

ADMINISTRATION

Oral route

Take w/ or w/o food w/ a full glass of water
Swallow cap whole; do not break, chew, or empty cap contents

HOW SUPPLIED

Cap: 75mg, 150mg

CONTRAINDICATIONS
Active pathological bleeding, mechanical prosthetic heart valve.

WARNINGS/PRECAUTIONS
Renal impairment may increase anticoagulant activity and $T_{1/2}$. D/C therapy in patients who develop acute renal failure and consider alternative anticoagulant therapy. Increases risk of bleeding and may cause significant and, sometimes, fatal bleeding; promptly evaluate for any signs/symptoms of blood loss. D/C therapy in patients with active pathological bleeding. Consider administration of platelet concentrates in cases where thrombocytopenia is present or long-acting antiplatelet drugs have been used. Use for the prophylaxis of thromboembolic events in patients with A-fib in the setting of other forms of valvular heart disease (including the presence of a bioprosthetic heart valve) is not recommended.

ADVERSE REACTIONS
GI reactions (eg, dyspepsia, gastritis-like symptoms), bleeding.

DRUG INTERACTIONS
See Boxed Warning and Dose Modification. Reduction of Risk of Stroke and Systemic Embolism in Nonvalvular A-fib: P-gp inducers (eg, rifampin) may reduce exposure. Use with P-gp inhibitors (eg, dronedarone, systemic ketoconazole) in patients with renal impairment may increase exposure.

NURSING CONSIDERATIONS

Assessment: Assess for history of serious hypersensitivity reaction to drug, active pathological bleeding, mechanical prosthetic heart valve, A-fib in the setting of other forms of valvular heart disease, risk factors for bleeding and epidural or spinal hematomas, renal impairment, pregnancy/nursing status, and possible drug interactions.

Monitoring: Monitor for bleeding, GI adverse reactions, hypersensitivity reactions, and other adverse events. Periodically monitor renal function as clinically indicated. When necessary, monitor anticoagulant activity by using activated PTT or ecarin clotting time, and not INR. Monitor for signs/symptoms of neurological impairment (eg, midline back pain, sensory/motor deficits [numbness, tingling, weakness in lower limbs], bowel/bladder dysfunction) frequently in patients receiving neuraxial anesthesia or undergoing spinal puncture.

Patient Counseling: Instruct to take exactly as prescribed and not to d/c without talking to physician. Instruct to keep drug in original bottle to protect from moisture and not to put it in pill boxes/organizers. When >1 bottle is dispensed, instruct to open only 1 bottle at a time. Instruct to remove only 1 cap from the opened bottle at the time of use and to immediately and tightly close bottle. Inform that bleeding may be longer and occur more easily. Instruct to call physician if any signs/symptoms of bleeding, dyspepsia, or gastritis occur. Advise patients who have had neuraxial anesthesia or spinal puncture to watch for signs and symptoms of spinal/epidural hematoma, particularly if concomitantly taking NSAIDs or platelet inhibitors; instruct to contact physician immediately if symptoms occur. Instruct to inform physician of intake of dabigatran before any invasive procedure (including dental procedures) is scheduled. Advise patients to list all prescription/OTC medications or dietary supplements they may be taking or planning to take. Instruct that if a dose is missed, to take that dose as soon as possible on the same day or skip it if cannot be taken at least 6 hrs before the next scheduled dose. Instruct not to double dose.

Storage: 25°C (77°F); excursions permitted to 15-30°C (59-86°F). Store in original package to protect from moisture. Once bottle is opened, use within 4 months; keep tightly closed.

PRAVASTATIN – pravastatin sodium RX

Class: HMG-CoA reductase inhibitor

OTHER BRAND NAMES
Pravachol

ADULT DOSAGE

Hyperlipidemia

Primary Hypercholesterolemia/Mixed Dyslipidemia/Primary Dysbetalipoproteinemia:
Initial: 40mg qd
Titrate: Increase to 80mg qd if 40mg qd does not achieve desired cholesterol levels

Prevention of Cardiovascular Disease
Dose based on current clinical practice

PEDIATRIC DOSAGE

Heterozygous Familial Hypercholesterolemia

8-13 Years:
20mg qd
Max: 20mg/day

14-18 Years:
Initial: 40mg qd
Max: 40mg/day

DOSE MODIFICATION

Concomitant Medications

Bile Acid Resins:
Administer pravastatin either 1 hr or more before or at least 4 hrs following the resin

Clarithromycin:
Limit pravastatin dose to 40mg qd

Cyclosporine:
Initial: 10mg qhs
Titrate: Increase dose cautiously
Max: 20mg/day

Renal Impairment

Significant:
Initial: 10mg qd

ADMINISTRATION

Oral route
Administer as a single dose at any time of the day, w/ or w/o food

HOW SUPPLIED

Tab: 10mg; (Pravachol) 20mg, 40mg, 80mg

CONTRAINDICATIONS

Active liver disease or unexplained, persistent elevations of serum transaminases, women who are pregnant or may become pregnant, and nursing mothers.

WARNINGS/PRECAUTIONS

Rare cases of rhabdomyolysis with acute renal failure secondary to myoglobinuria reported; risk factors may include history of renal impairment. Uncomplicated myalgia and myopathy (including immune-mediated necrotizing myopathy [IMNM]) reported; d/c if markedly elevated CPK levels occur or myopathy is diagnosed/suspected. Temporarily withhold in any patient experiencing an acute or serious condition predisposing to development of renal failure secondary to rhabdomyolysis. May cause biochemical liver function abnormalities; perform LFTs prior to initiation of therapy and when clinically indicated. Caution with recent (<6 months) history of liver disease, signs that may suggest liver disease, in heavy alcohol users, and elderly. Fatal and nonfatal hepatic failure reported (rare); promptly interrupt therapy if serious liver injury with clinical symptoms and/or hyperbilirubinemia or jaundice occurs and do not restart if no alternate etiology found. May blunt adrenal or gonadal steroid hormone production. Evaluate patients who display clinical evidence of endocrine dysfunction.

ADVERSE REACTIONS

Musculoskeletal pain/traumatism, URTI, chest pain, influenza, fatigue, cough, N/V, dizziness, sinus abnormality, rash, diarrhea, headache, muscle cramp, anxiety/nervousness.

DRUG INTERACTIONS

See Dosage. Increased risk of myopathy with cyclosporine, fibrates, niacin (nicotinic acid), erythromycin, clarithromycin, colchicine, and gemfibrozil; caution with colchicine and fibrates, and avoid with gemfibrozil. Niacin may enhance risk of skeletal muscle effects; consider dose reduction of pravastatin. Caution with drugs that may diminish levels or activity of steroid hormones (eg, ketoconazole, spironolactone, cimetidine).

NURSING CONSIDERATIONS

Assessment: Assess for history of or active liver disease, unexplained persistent serum transaminase elevations, predisposing factors for myopathy, alcohol consumption, renal impairment, hypersensitivity to the drug, pregnancy/nursing status, and possible drug interactions. Obtain baseline lipid profile and LFTs.

Monitoring: Monitor for signs/symptoms of rhabdomyolysis, myopathy (including IMNM), liver/endocrine dysfunction, and other adverse reactions. Monitor lipid profile, LFTs when clinically indicated, and CPK levels.

Patient Counseling: Advise to report promptly any unexplained muscle pain, tenderness, or weakness, particularly if accompanied by malaise or fever or if these muscle signs or symptoms persist after discontinuation, or any symptoms that may indicate liver injury. Counsel females of childbearing potential on appropriate contraceptive methods while on therapy.

Storage: 20-25°C (68-77°F); excursions permitted to 15-30°C (59-86°F). Protect from light and moisture. (Pravachol) 25°C (77°F); excursions permitted to 15-30°C (59-86°F). Protect from light and moisture.

PRECEDEX – dexmedetomidine hydrochloride

RX

Class: $Alpha_2$-agonist

ADULT DOSAGE

Sedation

Intensive Care Unit Sedation:
Initiation:
LD: 1mcg/kg over 10 min
Conversion from Alternate Sedative Therapy:
LD may not be required

Maint:
0.2-0.7mcg/kg/hr; adjust rate of infusion to achieve desired level of sedation

Procedural Sedation:
Initiation:
LD: 1mcg/kg over 10 min
Less Invasive Procedures (eg, Ophthalmic Surgery):
LD: 0.5mcg/kg over 10 min

Maint:
Initiate at 0.6mcg/kg/hr; titrate to achieve desired clinical effect
Range: 0.2-1mcg/kg/hr; adjust rate of infusion to achieve desired level of sedation

PEDIATRIC DOSAGE

Pediatric use may not have been established

DOSE MODIFICATION

Concomitant Medications

A dose reduction in Precedex or other concomitant anesthetics, sedatives, hypnotics, or opioids may be required when coadministered

Hepatic Impairment

Consider dose reduction

Elderly

>65 Years:
Intensive Care Unit Sedation:
Initiation/Maint: Consider a dose reduction

Procedural Sedation:
Initiation: LD: 0.5mcg/kg over 10 min
Maint: Consider a dose reduction

ADMINISTRATION

IV route

Administer using a controlled infusion device; not indicated for infusions lasting >24 hrs

Preparation of Sol

Precedex Inj, 200mcg/2mL (100mcg/mL):
Dilute with 0.9% NaCl inj to achieve required concentration (4mcg/mL) prior to administration
Preparation is the same, whether for the LD or maintenance infusion
1. Withdraw 2mL of Precedex Inj and add to 48mL of 0.9% NaCl inj to a total of 50mL
2. Shake gently to mix well

Precedex in 0.9% NaCl Inj, 80mcg/20mL (4mcg/mL), 200mcg/50mL (4mcg/mL), and 400mcg/100mL (4mcg/mL):
Precedex in 0.9% NaCl Inj is supplied in glass containers containing a premixed, ready to use dexmedetomidine hydrochloride solution in 0.9% NaCl in water; no further dilution necessary

Administration with Other Fluids

Do not coadminister through the same IV catheter with blood or plasma
Incompatible when administered with the following drugs:
-amphotericin B
-diazepam
Compatible when administered with the following IV fluids:
- 0.9% NaCl in water
- 5% dextrose in water
- 20% mannitol
- Lactated Ringer's solution
- 100mg/mL magnesium sulfate solution
- 0.3% potassium chloride solution

Compatibility with Natural Rubber
Advisable to use administration components made with synthetic or coated natural rubber gaskets

HOW SUPPLIED
Inj: 100mcg/mL [2mL, vial], 4mcg/mL [50mL, 100mL, bottle; 20mL, vial]

WARNINGS/PRECAUTIONS
Should be administered only by persons skilled in the management of patients in the intensive care or operating room setting. Monitor patients continuously during administration. Hypotension, bradycardia, and sinus arrest reported; treat appropriately. Hypotension and/or bradycardia may be more pronounced in patients with hypovolemia, diabetes mellitus (DM), chronic HTN, and in elderly. Caution with advanced heart block and/or severe ventricular dysfunction. Transient HTN observed primarily during the LD; reduction of loading infusion rate may be desirable. Arousability and alertness reported in some patients upon stimulation. Withdrawal events reported with intensive care unit sedation; if tachycardia and/or HTN occurs after discontinuation, supportive therapy is indicated. Use beyond 24 hrs has been associated with tolerance, tachyphylaxis, and a dose-related increase in adverse reactions.

ADVERSE REACTIONS
Hypotension, HTN, bradycardia, dry mouth, tachycardia, N/V, atrial fibrillation, fever, anemia, hypovolemia, hypoxia, atelectasis, agitation, respiratory depression/failure.

DRUG INTERACTIONS
Coadministration with anesthetics, sedatives, hypnotics, and opioids (eg, sevoflurane, isoflurane, propofol, alfentanil, midazolam) may lead to enhancement of effects; may require dose reduction of Precedex or the concomitant drug. Caution with vasodilators or negative chronotropic agents.

NURSING CONSIDERATIONS

Assessment: Assess for advanced heart block, severe ventricular dysfunction, hepatic impairment, hypovolemia, DM, chronic HTN, pregnancy/nursing status, and possible drug interactions.

Monitoring: Monitor for hypotension, bradycardia, sinus arrest, transient HTN, withdrawal events, and other adverse reactions.

Patient Counseling: When infused for >6 hrs, instruct to report nervousness, agitation, and headaches that may occur for up to 48 hrs. Instruct to report symptoms that occur within 48 hrs after administration (eg, weakness, confusion, excessive sweating, weight loss, abdominal pain, salt cravings, diarrhea, constipation, dizziness, lightheadedness).

Storage: 25°C (77°F); excursions allowed from 15-30°C (59-86°F).

PREDNISONE – prednisone   RX

Class: Glucocorticoid

OTHER BRAND NAMES
Prednisone Intensol

ADULT DOSAGE

Steroid-Responsive Disorders

Initial: 5-60mg/day, depending on disease and response
Maint: Decrease initial dose in small decrements to lowest effective dose

Alternate-Day Therapy: Administer twice the usual daily dose every other am; refer to PI for more detailed information

Multiple Sclerosis

Acute Exacerbations:
200mg/day for 1 week, followed by 80mg qod for 1 month

PEDIATRIC DOSAGE

Steroid-Responsive Disorders

Initial: 5-60mg/day, depending on disease and response
Maint: Decrease initial dose in small decrements to lowest effective dose

Alternate-Day Therapy: Administer twice the usual daily dose every other am; refer to PI for more detailed information

Multiple Sclerosis

Acute Exacerbations:
200mg/day for 1 week, followed by 80mg qod for 1 month

DOSE MODIFICATION

Elderly
Start at lower end of dosing range

Discontinuation
Withdraw gradually after long-term therapy

ADMINISTRATION
Oral route
Take before, during, or immediately pc or w/ food or milk to reduce gastric irritation

Administer in the am prior to 9 am; when large doses are given, administer antacids between meals
Multiple dose therapy should be evenly distributed in evenly spaced intervals throughout the day

HOW SUPPLIED

Sol: (Intensol) 5mg/mL [30mL]; 5mg/5mL [120mL, 500mL]; Tab: 1mg*, 2.5mg*, 5mg*, 10mg*, 20mg*, 50mg* *scored

CONTRAINDICATIONS

Systemic fungal infections.

WARNINGS/PRECAUTIONS

Monitor for situations that may make dosage adjustments necessary (eg, change in clinical status secondary to remissions/exacerbations in the disease process, individual drug responsiveness, effect of patient exposure to stress). Anaphylactoid reactions may occur. May need to increase dose before, during, and after stressful situation. May cause BP elevation, salt/water retention, and increased K^+ and Ca^{2+} excretion; dietary salt restriction and K^+ supplementation may be necessary. Caution in patients with left ventricular free wall rupture after a recent MI. May produce reversible hypothalamic-pituitary-adrenal (HPA) axis suppression with the potential for corticosteroid insufficiency after withdrawal of treatment. Changes in thyroid status may necessitate dose adjustment. May increase susceptibility to infections, mask signs of current infection, activate latent disease, or exacerbate intercurrent infections. Avoid use in the presence of systemic fungal infections unless needed to control life-threatening drug reactions. Rule out latent or active amebiasis before initiating therapy. Caution with *Strongyloides* infestation, active/latent TB or tuberculin reactivity, HTN, CHF, and renal insufficiency. Caution with active or latent peptic ulcers, diverticulitis, fresh intestinal anastomoses, and nonspecific ulcerative colitis; may increase risk of perforation. Signs of peritoneal irritation following GI perforation may be minimal/absent. Not for use in cerebral malaria and active ocular herpes simplex. More serious or fatal course of chickenpox and measles reported. May produce posterior subcapsular cataracts, glaucoma with possible optic nerve damage, and enhance establishment of secondary ocular infections due to bacteria, fungi, or viruses. Kaposi's sarcoma reported. Not recommended in optic neuritis treatment. Avoid abrupt withdrawal. Drug-induced secondary adrenocortical insufficiency may be minimized by gradual dose reduction. Enhanced effect in patients with cirrhosis. May decrease bone formation and increase bone resorption, and may lead to inhibition of bone growth in pediatric patients and development of osteoporosis at any age; caution with increased risk of osteoporosis (eg, postmenopausal women). Acute myopathy with high doses reported, most often in patients with neuromuscular transmission disorders (eg, myasthenia gravis). Psychiatric derangements may appear and existing emotional instability or psychotic tendencies may be aggravated. Elevation of CK may occur. May elevate IOP; monitor IOP if used for >6 weeks. May suppress reactions to skin tests. Caution in elderly.

ADVERSE REACTIONS

Anaphylactoid reactions, HTN, osteoporosis, muscle weakness, menstrual irregularities, insomnia, impaired wound healing, ulcerative esophagitis, increased sweating, decreased carbohydrate tolerance, glaucoma, weight gain, nausea, malaise, anemia.

DRUG INTERACTIONS

Live or live, attenuated vaccines are contraindicated with immunosuppressive doses. May diminish response to toxoids and live or inactivated vaccines. Closely monitor for hypokalemia when administered with K^+-depleting agents (eg, amphotericin B, diuretics). Cardiac enlargement and CHF may occur with concomitant use of amphotericin B. Macrolide antibiotics may decrease clearance. May produce severe weakness in myasthenia gravis patients with anticholinesterase agents (eg, neostigmine, pyridostigmine); d/c anticholinesterase agents at least 24 hrs before start of therapy and monitor for possible respiratory support if concomitant therapy must occur. Monitor coagulation indices frequently with warfarin. Dose adjustment of antidiabetic agents may be required. May decrease serum concentration of INH. Extreme caution with bupropion; employ low initial dosing and small gradual increases. Cholestyramine may increase clearance. Increased activity of both drugs may occur with cyclosporine; convulsions reported with concurrent use. May increase risk of arrhythmias due to hypokalemia with digitalis glycosides. Estrogens may decrease hepatic metabolism, thereby increasing their effect. Increased risk of tendon rupture, especially in elderly, with concomitant fluoroquinolones. CYP3A4 inducers (eg, barbiturates, phenytoin, carbamazepine, rifampin) may enhance metabolism and may require increase in corticosteroid dose. CYP3A4 inhibitors (eg, ketoconazole, itraconazole, ritonavir, indinavir, macrolides [erythromycin]) may increase plasma concentrations. Other drugs that are metabolized by CYP3A4 (eg, indinavir, erythromycin) may increase their clearance, resulting in decreased plasma concentration. Increased risk of corticosteroid side effects with ketoconazole. Aspirin (ASA) or other NSAIDs may increase risk of GI side effects. Caution with ASA in hypoprothrombinemia patients. May increase clearance of salicylates. Decreased therapeutic effect with phenytoin. Increased doses of quetiapine may be required to maintain control of schizophrenia symptoms. Caution with thalidomide; toxic epidermal necrolysis reported. Acute myopathy reported with neuromuscular blocking drugs (eg, pancuronium).

NURSING CONSIDERATIONS

Assessment: Assess for hypersensitivity to drug, CHF, HTN, renal impairment, systemic fungal/other current infections, active TB, latent/active amebiasis, cerebral malaria, active ocular herpes simplex, emotional instability or psychotic tendencies, recent MI, vaccination history, thyroid status, any other conditions where treatment is cautioned, pregnancy/nursing status, and for possible drug interactions.

Monitoring: Monitor for anaphylactoid reactions, HPA axis suppression, adrenocortical insufficiency, salt/water retention, infections, change in thyroid status, cataracts, glaucoma, Kaposi's sarcoma, emotional instability or psychotic tendencies aggravation, and other adverse reactions. Monitor IOP, BP, CK, and serum electrolytes. Monitor growth and development of infants/children on prolonged therapy. Frequently monitor coagulation indices with warfarin.

Patient Counseling: Instruct not to d/c therapy abruptly or without medical supervision. Instruct to advise any medical attendants of intake of corticosteroids and to seek medical advice at once if fever or other signs of infection develop. Advise to avoid exposure to chickenpox or measles; instruct to report immediately without delay if exposed.

Storage: 25°C (77°F); excursions permitted to 15-30°C (59-86°F). (Tab) Protect from moisture. (Intensol) Discard opened bottle after 90 days.

PREMARIN TABLETS – conjugated estrogens — RX

Class: Estrogen

Estrogens increase the risk of endometrial cancer. Perform adequate diagnostic measures, including endometrial sampling, to rule out malignancy in postmenopausal women w/ undiagnosed persistent or recurring abnormal genital bleeding. Should not be used for the prevention of cardiovascular (CV) disease or dementia. Increased risks of MI, stroke, invasive breast cancer, pulmonary embolism (PE), and DVT in postmenopausal women (50-79 yrs of age) reported. Increased risk of developing probable dementia in postmenopausal women ≥65 yrs of age reported. Should be prescribed at the lowest effective dose and for the shortest duration consistent w/ treatment goals and risks.

ADULT DOSAGE

Postmenopausal Osteoporosis

Prevention:
Initial: 0.3mg qd continuously or cyclically (eg, 25 days on, 5 days off)
Titrate: Adjust subsequent dose based on clinical and bone mineral density responses
Use lowest effective dose and for the shortest duration consistent w/ treatment goals and risk

Menopause

Symptoms of Moderate to Severe Vasomotor/ Vulvar and Vaginal Atrophy:
Initial: 0.3mg qd continuously or cyclically (eg, 25 days on, 5 days off)
Titrate: Adjust subsequent dose based on response

Use lowest effective dose and for the shortest duration consistent w/ treatment goals and risk

Hypoestrogenism

Female Hypogonadism:
0.3 or 0.625mg qd cyclically (eg, 3 weeks on and 1 week off)
Titrate: Adjust dose based on severity of symptoms and response of the endometrium

Female Castration/Primary Ovarian Failure:
Usual: 1.25mg qd cyclically
Titrate: Adjust dose based on severity of symptoms and response

Use lowest effective dose and for the shortest duration consistent w/ treatment goals and risk

Metastatic Breast Cancer

Palliative Treatment in Appropriately Selected Women and Men:
10mg tid for a minimum of 3 months

PEDIATRIC DOSAGE

Pediatric use may not have been established

Use lowest effective dose and for the shortest duration consistent w/ treatment goals and risk

Prostate Carcinoma

Palliative Treatment of Advanced Androgen-Dependent Carcinoma:
1.25-2.5mg (two 1.25mg tabs) tid
Use lowest effective dose and for the shortest duration consistent w/ treatment goals and risk

ADMINISTRATION
Oral route
May take w/o regard to meals

HOW SUPPLIED
Tab: 0.3mg, 0.45mg, 0.625mg, 0.9mg, 1.25mg

CONTRAINDICATIONS
Undiagnosed abnormal genital bleeding; known/suspected/history of breast cancer except in appropriately selected patients being treated for metastatic disease; known/suspected estrogen-dependent neoplasia; active/history of DVT/PE/arterial thromboembolic disease (eg, stroke, MI); liver impairment/disease; known protein C, protein S, antithrombin deficiency, or other known thrombophilic disorders; known/suspected pregnancy.

WARNINGS/PRECAUTIONS
D/C immediately if stroke, DVT, PE, and MI occurs or is suspected. Caution in patients w/ risk factors for arterial vascular disease and/or venous thromboembolism. If feasible, d/c at least 4-6 weeks before surgery of the type associated w/ an increased risk of thromboembolism, or during periods of prolonged immobilization. May increase risk of ovarian cancer and gallbladder disease requiring surgery. May lead to severe hypercalcemia in patients w/ breast cancer and bone metastases; d/c and take appropriate measures if hypercalcemia occurs. Retinal vascular thrombosis reported; if visual abnormalities or migraine occurs, d/c pending examination. If examination reveals papilledema or retinal vascular lesions, d/c permanently. Anaphylaxis and angioedema involving tongue, larynx, face, hands, and feet requiring medical intervention reported; d/c if anaphylactic reaction w/ or w/o angioedema occurs. Cases of malignant transformation of residual endometrial implants reported in women treated post-hysterectomy w/ estrogen-alone therapy; consider addition of progestin for women known to have residual endometriosis post-hysterectomy. May elevate BP and thyroid-binding globulin levels. May elevate plasma TGs leading to pancreatitis in patients w/ preexisting hypertriglyceridemia; consider discontinuation if pancreatitis occurs. Caution w/ history of cholestatic jaundice associated w/ past estrogen use or w/ pregnancy; d/c in case of recurrence. May cause fluid retention; caution w/ cardiac/renal dysfunction. Caution w/ hypoparathyroidism; estrogen-induced hypocalcemia may occur. May exacerbate symptoms of angioedema in women w/ hereditary angioedema. May exacerbate asthma, diabetes mellitus, epilepsy, migraine, porphyria, systemic lupus erythematosus, and hepatic hemangiomas; use w/ caution. May affect certain endocrine and blood components in lab tests.

ADVERSE REACTIONS
Abdominal pain, asthenia, back pain, headache, pain, depression, insomnia, dizziness, leukorrhea, breast pain, vaginal hemorrhage, vaginitis, flatulence, nausea, weight gain.

DRUG INTERACTIONS
CYP3A4 inducers (eg, St. John's wort, phenobarbital, carbamazepine, rifampin) may decrease levels, which may decrease therapeutic effects and/or change uterine bleeding profile. CYP3A4 inhibitors (eg, erythromycin, clarithromycin, ketoconazole) may increase levels, which may result in side effects. Women concomitantly receiving thyroid hormone replacement therapy may require increased doses of their thyroid replacement therapy; monitor thyroid function.

NURSING CONSIDERATIONS

Assessment: Assess for undiagnosed abnormal genital bleeding, estrogen-dependent neoplasia, presence or history of breast cancer, active/history of DVT/PE/arterial thromboembolic disease, thrombophilic disorders, pregnancy/nursing status, any other conditions where treatment is contraindicated or cautioned, need for progestin therapy, and possible drug interactions.

Monitoring: Monitor for signs/symptoms of CV events, malignant neoplasms, dementia, gallbladder disease, hypercalcemia, visual abnormalities, anaphylaxis, angioedema, BP and serum TG elevations, fluid retention, exacerbation of endometriosis and other conditions, and other adverse reactions. Perform annual breast exam; schedule mammography based on age, risk factors, and prior mammogram results. Monitor thyroid function in women on thyroid replacement therapy. In cases of undiagnosed persistent or recurring genital bleeding, perform adequate diagnostic measures (eg, endometrial sampling) to rule out malignancies. Periodically reevaluate to determine the need of therapy.

Patient Counseling: Inform of the risks/benefits of therapy. Inform of the importance of reporting vaginal bleeding to physician as soon as possible. Inform of possible serious adverse reactions and of possible less serious but common adverse reactions of estrogen therapy.

Storage: 20-25°C (68-77°F); excursions permitted to 15-30°C (59-86°F).

Premarin Vaginal – conjugated estrogens RX

Class: Estrogen

Estrogens increase the risk of endometrial cancer. Perform adequate diagnostic measures, including endometrial sampling, to rule out malignancy with undiagnosed persistent or recurring abnormal genital bleeding. Should not be used for the prevention of cardiovascular disease (CVD) or dementia. Increased risks of MI, stroke, invasive breast cancer, pulmonary embolism (PE), and deep vein thrombosis (DVT) in postmenopausal women (50-79 yrs of age) reported. Increased risk of developing probable dementia in postmenopausal women ≥65 yrs of age reported. Should be prescribed at the lowest effective dose for the shortest duration consistent with treatment goals and risks.

ADULT DOSAGE

Menopause

Atrophic Vaginitis/Kraurosis Vulvae:
Initial: 0.5g intravaginally cyclically (21 days on, then 7 days off)
Titrate: May increase to 0.5-2g based on individual response

Dyspareunia:
Moderate to Severe:
0.5g intravaginally 2X/week (eg, Monday and Thursday) continuously or cyclically (21 days on, then 7 days off)

PEDIATRIC DOSAGE

Pediatric use may not have been established

ADMINISTRATION

Intravaginal route

Instructions for Use of Applicator

Remove cap from tube and screw nozzle end of applicator onto tube
Gently squeeze tube from the bottom to force sufficient cre into barrel of applicator to provide the prescribed dose; use the marked stopping points on applicator to measure correct dose
Unscrew applicator from tube and gently insert applicatory deeply into vagina while lying on back w/ knees drawn up; press plunger downward to original position
To cleanse, pull plunger to remove from barrel and wash w/ mild soap and warm water; do not boil or use hot water

HOW SUPPLIED

Cre: 0.625mg/g [30g, 42.5g]

CONTRAINDICATIONS

Undiagnosed abnormal genital bleeding, known/suspected/history of breast cancer, known/suspected estrogen-dependent neoplasia, active/history of DVT/PE, active/history of arterial thromboembolic disease (eg, stroke, MI), liver dysfunction/disease, thrombophilic disorders (eg, protein C, protein S, or antithrombin deficiency), or known/suspected pregnancy.

WARNINGS/PRECAUTIONS

D/C therapy immediately if stroke, DVT, PE, or MI occurs or are suspected. Caution in patients with risk factors for arterial vascular disease and/or venous thromboembolism (VTE). If feasible, d/c at least 4-6 weeks before surgery of the type associated with an increased risk of thromboembolism, or during periods of prolonged immobilization. May increase risk of gallbladder disease requiring surgery and ovarian cancer. Consider addition of progestin for women with a uterus or with residual endometriosis post-hysterectomy. May lead to severe hypercalcemia in patients with breast cancer and bone metastases; d/c and take appropriate measures if hypercalcemia occurs. Retinal vascular thrombosis reported; if visual abnormalities or migraine occurs, d/c pending examination. If examination reveals papilledema or retinal vascular lesions, d/c permanently. May elevate BP, thyroid-binding globulin levels, and plasma TG. Consider discontinuation if pancreatitis occurs. Caution with history of cholestatic jaundice associated with past estrogen use or pregnancy; d/c in case of recurrence. May cause fluid retention. Caution with hypoparathyroidism; hypocalcemia may occur. Anaphylaxis and angioedema reported with PO treatment. May induce or exacerbate symptoms of angioedema in women with hereditary angioedema. May exacerbate endometriosis, asthma, diabetes mellitus (DM), epilepsy, migraine, porphyria, systemic lupus erythematosus (SLE), and hepatic hemangiomas. May weaken and contribute to the failure of condoms, diaphragms, or cervical caps made of latex or rubber. May affect certain endocrine and blood components in laboratory tests.

ADVERSE REACTIONS

Breast pain, headache.

DRUG INTERACTIONS

CYP3A4 inducers (eg, St. John's wort, phenobarbital, carbamazepine, rifampin) may decrease levels, which may decrease therapeutic effects and/or change uterine bleeding profile. CYP3A4 inhibitors (eg, erythromycin, ketoconazole, ritonavir, grapefruit juice) may increase levels. Women concomitantly receiving thyroid hormone replacement therapy and estrogens may require increased doses of thyroid replacement therapy.

NURSING CONSIDERATIONS

Assessment: Assess for abnormal genital bleeding, estrogen-dependent neoplasia, presence/history of breast cancer, arterial thromboembolic disease, DVT/PE, hereditary angioedema, previous hypersensitivity, thrombophilic disorders, or any other conditions where treatment is contraindicated or cautioned. Assess use in women ≥65 yrs of age, those with DM, asthma, epilepsy, migraines or porphyria, SLE, and hepatic hemangiomas. Assess for cardiac or renal dysfunction, pregnancy/nursing status, need for progestin therapy, and possible drug interactions.

Monitoring: Monitor for signs/symptoms of cardiovascular events, malignant neoplasms, dementia, gallbladder disease, hypercalcemia, visual abnormalities, pancreatitis, hypertriglyceridemia, cholestatic jaundice, hypothyroidism, fluid retention, exacerbation of endometriosis and other conditions. Perform annual breast exam; schedule mammography based on age, risk factors, and prior mammogram results. Regularly monitor BP, thyroid function in women on thyroid replacement therapy, and periodically evaluate to determine need for treatment. Perform adequate diagnostic measures (eg, endometrial sampling) to rule out malignancies if undiagnosed persistent or recurring genital bleeding occurs.

Patient Counseling: Advise to notify physician if signs/symptoms of unusual vaginal bleeding occur. Inform about possible serious adverse reactions (eg, CVD, malignant neoplasms, and probable dementia) and possible less serious but common adverse reactions (eg, headache, breast pain/tenderness, N/V). Instruct on how to use the applicator. Instruct to perform monthly breast self-examination. Inform that medication may weaken barrier contraceptives (eg, latex or rubber condoms, diaphragms, cervical caps).

Storage: 20-25°C (68-77°F); excursions permitted to 15-30°C (59-86°F).

PREMPHASE – conjugated estrogens/medroxyprogesterone acetate — RX

Class: Estrogen/progestogen combination

Estrogens increase the risk of endometrial cancer. Perform adequate diagnostic measures, including endometrial sampling, to rule out malignancy in postmenopausal women with undiagnosed persistent or recurring abnormal genital bleeding. Should not be used for the prevention of cardiovascular disease (CVD) or dementia. Increased risk of MI, stroke, invasive breast cancer, PE, and DVT in postmenopausal women (50-79 yrs of age) reported. Increased risk of developing probable dementia in postmenopausal women ≥65 yrs of age reported. Should be prescribed at the lowest effective dose and for the shortest duration consistent with treatment goals and risks.

OTHER BRAND NAMES

Prempro

ADULT DOSAGE

Menopause

Moderate to Severe Vasomotor Symptoms/ Vulvar and Vaginal Atrophy:
Premphase: One 0.625mg tab qd on Days 1-14, then one 0.625mg-5mg tab qd on Days 15-28
Prempro: 1 tab qd

Periodically reassess need to continue treatment

Postmenopausal Osteoporosis

Prevention:
Premphase: One 0.625mg tab qd on Days 1-14, then one 0.625mg-5mg tab qd on Days 15-28
Prempro: 1 tab qd

Periodically reassess need to continue treatment

PEDIATRIC DOSAGE

Pediatric use may not have been established

ADMINISTRATION
Oral route

HOW SUPPLIED
Tab: (Premphase) (Conjugated Estrogens [CE]) 0.625mg, (CE-Medroxyprogesterone) 0.625mg-5mg; (Prempro) (CE-Medroxyprogesterone) 0.3mg-1.5mg, 0.45mg-1.5mg, 0.625mg-2.5mg, 0.625mg-5mg

CONTRAINDICATIONS
Undiagnosed abnormal genital bleeding, known/suspected/history of breast cancer, known/suspected estrogen-dependent neoplasia, active or history of DVT/PE/arterial thromboembolic disease (eg, stroke, MI), known liver dysfunction/disease, known protein C/protein S/antithrombin deficiency, or other known thrombophilic disorders, known/suspected pregnancy.

WARNINGS/PRECAUTIONS
D/C immediately if PE, DVT, stroke, or MI occurs or is suspected. Caution in patients with risk factors for arterial vascular disease and/or VTE. If feasible, d/c at least 4-6 weeks before surgery of the type associated with an increased risk of thromboembolism, or during periods of prolonged immobilization. May increase risk of gallbladder disease requiring surgery. May lead to severe hypercalcemia in patients with breast cancer and bone metastases; d/c and take appropriate measures if hypercalcemia occurs. Retinal vascular thrombosis reported; d/c pending examination if sudden partial/complete loss of vision or sudden onset of proptosis, diplopia, or migraine occurs. D/C permanently if examination reveals papilledema or retinal vascular lesions. May increase BP and thyroid-binding globulin levels. May be associated with elevations of plasma TGs; consider discontinuation if pancreatitis occurs. Caution with history of cholestatic jaundice associated with past estrogen use or with pregnancy; d/c in case of recurrence. May cause fluid retention. Caution with hypoparathyroidism; hypocalcemia may occur. Anaphylaxis and angioedema reported. May exacerbate symptoms of angioedema in women with hereditary angioedema. May exacerbate endometriosis, asthma, diabetes mellitus, epilepsy, migraine, porphyria, SLE, and hepatic hemangiomas. May affect certain endocrine and blood components in lab tests.

ADVERSE REACTIONS
MI, stroke, invasive breast cancer, PE, DVT, probable dementia, breast pain, headache, abdominal pain, dysmenorrhea, nausea, depression, leukorrhea, flatulence, asthenia.

DRUG INTERACTIONS
CYP3A4 inducers (eg, St. John's wort, phenobarbital, carbamazepine, rifampin) may decrease levels, which may decrease therapeutic effects and/or change uterine bleeding profile. CYP3A4 inhibitors (eg, erythromycin, ketoconazole, ritonavir, grapefruit juice) may increase levels. Aminoglutethimide may significantly depress bioavailability of medroxyprogesterone acetate (MPA). Patients concomitantly receiving thyroid hormone replacement therapy and estrogens may require increased doses of their thyroid replacement therapy; monitor thyroid function.

NURSING CONSIDERATIONS

Assessment: Assess for abnormal genital bleeding, presence/history of breast cancer, estrogen-dependent neoplasia, active or history of DVT/PE/arterial thromboembolic disease, liver dysfunction/disease, thrombophilic disorders, known anaphylactic reaction or angioedema to the drug, cardiac or renal dysfunction, other conditions where treatment is contraindicated or cautioned, pregnancy/nursing status, and possible drug interactions.

Monitoring: Monitor for signs/symptoms of CVD, malignant neoplasms, dementia, gallbladder disease, hypercalcemia, visual abnormalities, BP and plasma TG elevations, pancreatitis, cholestatic jaundice, hypothyroidism, fluid retention, anaphylaxis, angioedema, and exacerbation of endometriosis and other conditions. Perform annual breast examinations; schedule mammography based on patient age, risk factors, and prior mammogram results. Perform adequate diagnostic measures (eg, endometrial sampling) in patients with undiagnosed persistent or recurring genital bleeding. Perform periodic evaluation to determine treatment need.

Patient Counseling: Inform of the importance of reporting abnormal vaginal bleeding to physician as soon as possible. Advise of possible serious adverse reactions of therapy (eg, CVD, malignant neoplasms, probable dementia) and of possible less serious but common adverse reactions (eg, headache, breast pain and tenderness, N/V). Instruct to have yearly breast examinations by a healthcare provider and to perform monthly breast self-examinations.

Storage: 20-25°C (68-77°F); excursions permitted to 15-30°C (59-86°F).

PREPOPIK – anhydrous citric acid/magnesium oxide/sodium picosulfate RX

Class: Bowel cleanser

ADULT DOSAGE

Bowel Cleansing

Prior to Colonoscopy:

Split-Dose Regimen (Preferred Method):

1st Dose: Take during the pm before colonoscopy (eg, 5-9 pm), followed by five 8-oz drinks (upper line on dosing cup) of clear liquids hs. Consume clear liquids w/in 5 hrs

2nd Dose: Take the next day, approx 5 hrs before colonoscopy, followed by at least three 8-oz drinks of clear liquids before the colonoscopy. Consume clear liquids w/in 5 hrs up until 2 hrs before time of the colonoscopy

Day-Before Regimen (Alternative Method):

1st Dose: Take in afternoon or early pm (eg, 4-6 pm) before colonoscopy, followed by five 8-oz drinks of clear liquids before next dose. Consume clear liquids w/in 5 hrs

2nd Dose: Take approx 6 hrs later in the late pm (eg, 10 pm-12 am) the night before colonoscopy, followed by three 8-oz drinks of clear liquids hs. Consume clear liquids w/in 5 hrs

PEDIATRIC DOSAGE

Pediatric use may not have been established

DOSE MODIFICATION

Adverse Reactions

Severe Bloating/Distention/Abdominal Pain Following 1st Dose: Delay 2nd dose until symptoms resolve

ADMINISTRATION

Oral route

Only clear liquids (no solid food or milk) should be consumed on the day before the colonoscopy up until 2 hrs before the time of the colonoscopy

Reconstitution

1. Reconstitute the powder right before each administration; do not prepare sol in advance
2. Fill the supplied dosing cup w/ cold water up to the lower (5 oz) line on the cup and pour in the contents of 1 pkt of powder
3. Stir for 2-3 min; reconstituted sol may become slightly warm as the powder dissolves

HOW SUPPLIED

Sol (Powder): (Sodium Picosulfate/Magnesium Oxide/Anhydrous Citric Acid) 10mg/3.5g/12g [16.1g, 16.2g]

CONTRAINDICATIONS

Severely reduced renal function (CrCl <30mL/min), GI obstruction or ileus, bowel perforation, toxic colitis or toxic megacolon, gastric retention.

WARNINGS/PRECAUTIONS

May cause fluid/electrolyte disturbances, arrhythmias, and generalized tonic-clonic seizures; correct fluid and electrolyte abnormalities prior to treatment. Caution with CHF when replacing fluids. If vomiting or signs of dehydration (including signs of orthostatic hypotension) develop after treatment, perform postcolonoscopy lab tests (eg, electrolytes, SrCr, BUN) and treat accordingly. Caution with patients at risk of seizure (eg, known/suspected hyponatremia). Caution with impaired renal function and severe active ulcerative colitis. May produce colonic mucosal aphthous ulceration. Serious cases of ischemic colitis reported. Caution in patients prone to regurgitation/aspiration or with impaired gag reflex. Direct ingestion of undissolved powder may increase risk of N/V, dehydration, and electrolyte disturbance. Rule out GI obstruction/perforation before administration.

ADVERSE REACTIONS

Headache, N/V.

DRUG INTERACTIONS

Increased risk of colonic mucosal aphthous ulceration with stimulant laxatives. Caution with drugs that increase the risk of fluid and electrolyte abnormalities, drugs that affect renal function (eg, diuretics, ACE inhibitors, ARBs, NSAIDs), drugs associated with hypokalemia (eg, corticosteroid, cardiac glycosides) or hyponatremia, drugs that lower seizure threshold (eg, TCAs), drugs known to induce antidiuretic hormone secretion (eg, SSRIs, antipsychotics, carbamazepine), and in patients withdrawing from alcohol or benzodiazepines. Caution with drugs that increase the risk for arrhythmias and prolonged QT in the setting of fluid and electrolyte abnormalities. Oral medications given within 1 hr of administration may be flushed from GI tract and may not be absorbed. Take tetracycline and fluoroquinolone antibiotics, iron, digoxin, chlorpromazine, and penicillamine at least 2 hrs before and not <6 hrs after administration. Reduced efficacy with antibiotics.

NURSING CONSIDERATIONS

Assessment: Assess for previous hypersensitivity to any of the components, electrolyte abnormalities, risk for arrhythmias, CHF, risk/history of seizures, renal impairment, ileus, GI obstruction/perforation, gastric retention, toxic colitis/megacolon, ulcerative colitis, impaired gag reflex, regurgitation or aspiration tendencies, pregnancy/nursing status, and possible drug interactions. Perform predose lab tests (eg, electrolytes, SrCr, BUN) and ECG.

Monitoring: Monitor for fluid/electrolyte disturbances, arrhythmias, seizures, GI ulceration, colitis, bloating, abdominal distention/pain, and other adverse reactions. Perform postcolonoscopy lab tests and ECG.

Patient Counseling: Advise to adequately hydrate before, during, and after use. Instruct not to take other laxatives during therapy. Inform patients that if they experience severe bloating, distention or abdominal pain following the 1st pkt, delay the 2nd administration until the symptoms resolve. Instruct patients to contact their healthcare provider if they develop signs/symptoms of dehydration, have trouble swallowing, or are prone to regurgitation or aspiration. Inform that product is not for direct ingestion.

Storage: 25°C (77°F); excursions permitted to 15-30°C (59-86°F).

PRESTALIA — amlodipine/perindopril arginine RX

Class: ACE inhibitor/calcium channel blocker (dihydropyridine)

D/C as soon as possible, when pregnancy is detected. Drugs that act directly on the renin-angiotensin system (RAS) can cause injury/death to the developing fetus.

ADULT DOSAGE

Hypertension

In Patients Inadequately Controlled w/ Monotherapy or as Initial Therapy in Patients who Require Multiple Drugs to Achieve BP Goals:

Initial: 3.5mg perindopril/2.5mg amlodipine qd
Titrate: Adjust based on BP goals; wait 7-14 days between titration steps
Max: 14mg/10mg qd

PEDIATRIC DOSAGE

Pediatric use may not have been established

DOSE MODIFICATION

Renal Impairment

CrCl <60mL/min: Not recommended

Hepatic Impairment

Not recommended

Elderly

Not recommended in patients >65 years

ADMINISTRATION

Oral route

Take w/ or w/o food

HOW SUPPLIED

Tab: (Perindopril/Amlodipine) 3.5mg/2.5mg, 7mg/5mg, 14mg/10mg

CONTRAINDICATIONS

Hereditary or idiopathic angioedema, w/ or w/o previous ACE inhibitor treatment. Coadministration w/ aliskiren in patients w/ diabetes.

WARNINGS/PRECAUTIONS

Not recommended w/ CrCl <60mL/min, hepatic impairment, or w/ heart failure (HF). Worsening angina and acute MI may develop after starting or increasing the dose, particularly w/ severe obstructive coronary artery disease (CAD). Symptomatic hypotension may occur and is most likely to occur in patients w/ volume/salt depletion. Closely monitor patients at risk for excessive hypotension; follow patients closely during the first 2 weeks of treatment and whenever dose is increased or a diuretic is added or its dose increased. Patients w/ severe aortic stenosis may be more likely to experience symptomatic hypotension. Hypotension may occur w/ major surgery or during anesthesia; correct by volume expansion. May cause changes in renal function; consider withholding or discontinuing therapy in patients who develop a clinically significant decrease in renal function. Perindopril: Angioedema of the face, extremities, lips, tongue, glottis, or larynx reported; d/c and administer appropriate therapy. Intestinal angioedema reported. Higher incidence of angioedema in blacks than nonblacks. May cause hyperkalemia; risk factors include renal insufficiency and diabetes mellitus (DM). Persistent nonproductive cough reported; consider ACE inhibitor-induced cough in the differential diagnosis of cough.

ADVERSE REACTIONS

Peripheral edema, cough.

DRUG INTERACTIONS

See Contraindications. Perindopril: May occasionally experience an excessive reduction of BP w/ diuretics after initiation of perindopril; closely monitor w/ the 1st dose of perindopril, for at least 2 hrs and until BP has stabilized for another hr. May attenuate K^+ loss caused by thiazide diuretics. Increased risk of hyperkalemia w/ K^+-sparing diuretics (eg, spironolactone, amiloride, triamterene), K^+ supplements, K^+-containing salt substitutes, or other drugs capable of increasing serum K^+ (eg, indomethacin, heparin, cyclosporine); frequently monitor serum K^+. Increased serum lithium levels and symptoms of lithium toxicity reported; frequently monitor serum lithium levels. Nitritoid reactions reported w/ injectable gold (sodium aurothiomalate). Coadministration w/ NSAIDs, including selective COX-2 inhibitors, may attenuate antihypertensive effect of perindopril, and in patients who are elderly, volume-depleted (including those on diuretic therapy), or w/ compromised renal function, coadministration may result in deterioration of renal function, including possible acute renal failure. Dual blockade of the RAS is associated w/ increased risks of hypotension, hyperkalemia, and changes in renal function (including acute renal failure); avoid combined use of RAS inhibitors, or closely monitor BP, renal function, and electrolytes w/ concomitant agents that affect the RAS. Avoid w/ aliskiren in patients w/ renal impairment (GFR <60mL/min). Amlodipine: May increase simvastatin exposure; limit simvastatin dose to 20mg/day. May increase trough cyclosporine levels in renal transplant patients; frequently monitor trough blood levels of cyclosporine. Moderate CYP3A inhibitor diltiazem increases exposure. Strong CYP3A inhibitors (eg, itraconazole) may increase plasma concentrations; monitor for symptoms of hypotension and edema w/ moderate or strong CYP3A inhibitors to determine the need for dose adjustment.

NURSING CONSIDERATIONS

Assessment: Assess for hypersensitivity to the drug, hereditary or idiopathic angioedema, volume/ salt depletion, HF, severe obstructive CAD, severe aortic stenosis, hepatic/renal impairment, DM, pregnancy/nursing status, and possible drug interactions.

Monitoring: Monitor for signs/symptoms of worsening angina, acute MI, anaphylactoid reactions, head/neck/intestinal angioedema, persistent nonproductive cough, and other adverse reactions. Monitor renal function, BP, and K^+ levels periodically.

Patient Counseling: Advise of risks and benefits of therapy. Inform of pregnancy risks and discuss treatment options w/ women planning to become pregnant; advise to report pregnancy to physician as soon as possible. Instruct to resume the usual dose at the next scheduled time in case of a missed dose. Counsel to notify physician if any adverse reactions develop.

Storage: 25°C (77°F); excursions permitted to 15-30°C (59-86°F). Protect from moisture.

PREVACID — lansoprazole

RX

Class: Proton pump inhibitor

OTHER BRAND NAMES

Prevacid SoluTab

ADULT DOSAGE

Pathological Hypersecretory Conditions

Treatment Including Zollinger-Ellison Syndrome:

Initial: 60mg qd
Titrate: Individualize dose
Doses up to 90mg bid have been administered
Divide dose if >120mg/day

PEDIATRIC DOSAGE

Gastroesophageal Reflux Disease

Symptomatic GERD:
1-11 Years:
≤30kg: 15mg qd for up to 12 weeks; may increase up to 30mg bid after ≥2 weeks if still symptomatic
>30kg: 30mg qd for up to 12 weeks; may increase up to 30mg bid after ≥2 weeks if still symptomatic

Active Duodenal Ulcer

Treatment:
15mg qd for 4 weeks

Maint of Healing of Duodenal Ulcer:
15mg qd

NSAID-Associated Gastric Ulcer

Healing:
30mg qd for 8 weeks

Risk Reduction:
15mg qd for up to 12 weeks

***Helicobacter pylori* Eradication**

W/ Duodenal Ulcer Disease to Reduce the Risk of Duodenal Ulcer Recurrence:

Triple Therapy:
30mg cap + clarithromycin 500mg + amoxicillin 1000mg, all bid for 10 or 14 days

Dual Therapy:
Allergic/Intolerant/Resistant to Clarithromycin:
30mg cap + amoxicillin 1000mg, all tid w/ for 14 days

Gastroesophageal Reflux Disease

Symptomatic GERD:
15mg qd for up to 8 weeks

Treatment of Erosive Esophagitis:
30mg qd for up to 8 weeks; may give for 8 more weeks if healing does not occur
May consider an additional 8-week course if there is a recurrence of erosive esophagitis

Maint of Healing of Erosive Esophagitis:
15mg qd

Gastric Ulcers

Benign:
30mg qd for up to 8 weeks

Symptomatic Nonerosive GERD:
12-17 Years:
15mg qd for up to 8 weeks
Treatment of Erosive Esophagitis:
1-11 Years:
≤30kg: 15mg qd for up to 12 weeks; may increase up to 30mg bid after ≥2 weeks if still symptomatic
>30kg: 30mg qd for up to 12 weeks; may increase up to 30mg bid after ≥2 weeks if still symptomatic
12-17 Years:
30mg qd for up to 8 weeks

DOSE MODIFICATION
Hepatic Impairment
Severe: Consider dose adjustment

ADMINISTRATION
Oral route

Take ac
Cap
Swallow whole; do not crush or chew
If trouble swallowing, may sprinkle intact granules on 1 tbsp of either applesauce, Ensure pudding, cottage cheese, yogurt or strained pears, or into 60mL of either apple juice, orange juice, or tomato juice and swallow immediately
NG Tube (≥16 French):
Mix intact granules into 40mL of apple juice; do not use other liquids
Inject through the NG tube into the stomach
Flush w/ additional apple juice to clear the tube
Disintegrating SoluTab
Do not break, crush, chew, or cut
Allow tab to disintegrate on tongue, w/ or w/o water, until particles can be swallowed
Oral Syringe:
Place a 15mg tab in oral syringe and draw up 4mL of water, or place a 30mg tab w/ 10mL of water
Shake gently to allow for a quick dispersal
After the tab has dispersed, administer w/in 15 min
Refill the syringe w/ approx 2mL (5mL for the 30mg tab) of water, shake gently, and administer any remaining contents
NG Tube (≥8 French):
Place a 15mg tab in a syringe and draw up 4mL of water, or place a 30mg tab w/ 10mL of water
Shake gently to allow for a quick dispersal
After the tab has dispersed, inject through the NG tube into the stomach w/in 15 min
Refill the syringe w/ approx 5mL of water, shake gently, and flush the NG tube

HOW SUPPLIED
Cap, Delayed-Release: 15mg, 30mg; Tab, Disintegrating (SoluTab): 15mg, 30mg

WARNINGS/PRECAUTIONS
Symptomatic response does not preclude the presence of gastric malignancy. Acute interstitial nephritis reported; d/c if this develops. Cyanocobalamin (vitamin B12) deficiency may occur due to malabsorption with daily long-term treatment (eg, >3 yrs) with any acid-suppressing medications. May increase risk for *Clostridium difficile*-associated diarrhea (CDAD), especially in hospitalized patients. May increase risk for osteoporosis-related fractures of the hip, wrist, or spine, especially with high-dose and long-term therapy. Use lowest dose and shortest duration appropriate to the condition being treated. Hypomagnesemia reported; Mg^{2+} replacement and discontinuation of therapy may be required. (Tab, Disintegrating) Contains phenylalanine.

ADVERSE REACTIONS
Abdominal pain, constipation, diarrhea, nausea, dizziness, headache.

DRUG INTERACTIONS
May reduce the absorption of drugs where gastric pH is an important determinant of bioavailability; ampicillin esters, ketoconazole, atazanavir, iron salts, erlotinib and mycophenolate mofetil (MMF) absorption may decrease, while digoxin absorption may increase. May substantially decrease atazanavir concentrations; avoid coadministration. Caution in transplant patients receiving MMF. May increase theophylline clearance; may require theophylline dose titration when lansoprazole is started or stopped. Monitor for increases in INR and PT with warfarin. May increase tacrolimus levels. May elevate and prolong levels of MTX leading to toxicities; consider temporary withdrawal of therapy with high-dose MTX. Caution with digoxin or other drugs that may cause hypomagnesemia (eg, diuretics).

NURSING CONSIDERATIONS

Assessment: Assess for hepatic insufficiency, risk for osteoporosis, phenylketonuria, previous hypersensitivity to the drug, pregnancy/nursing status, and possible drug interactions. Obtain baseline Mg^{2+} levels in patients expected to be on prolonged treatment.

Monitoring: Monitor for signs/symptoms of acute interstitial nephritis, cyanocobalamin deficiency, bone fractures, CDAD, hypersensitivity reactions, and other adverse reactions. Monitor Mg^{2+} levels periodically in patients expected to be on prolonged treatment.

Patient Counseling: Advise to seek immediate medical attention if diarrhea does not improve or cardiovascular/neurological symptoms (eg, palpitations, dizziness, seizures, tetany) develop. Instruct to take exactly ud. Inform of alternative methods of administration if patient has swallowing difficulties.

Storage: 25°C (77°F); excursions permitted to 15-30°C (59-86°F).

PreviDent – sodium fluoride RX

Class: Fluoride preparation

OTHER BRAND NAMES
PreviDent 5000 Plus, Denta 5000 Plus

ADULT DOSAGE

Dental Caries Prevention

Apply a thin ribbon to toothbrush and brush thoroughly qd for 2 min, preferably at hs; expectorate after use

PEDIATRIC DOSAGE

Prevention and Control of Dental Caries

6-16 Years:
Apply a thin ribbon to toothbrush and brush thoroughly qd for 2 min, preferably at hs; expectorate and rinse mouth thoroughly after use

ADMINISTRATION
Topical route (teeth)

For best results, do not eat, drink, or rinse for 30 min

HOW SUPPLIED
Gel: (PreviDent) 1.1% [2 oz.(56g)]; Cre: (PreviDent 5000 Plus/Denta 5000 Plus) 1.1% [1.8 oz.(51g)]

CONTRAINDICATIONS
Not for pediatrics <6 yrs unless recommended by dentist or physician.

WARNINGS/PRECAUTIONS
Prolonged ingestion may lead to dental fluorosis in pediatrics <6 yrs. Not for systemic treatment. Do not swallow.

ADVERSE REACTIONS
Allergic reactions.

NURSING CONSIDERATIONS

Assessment: Assess for dental caries, dental fluorosis, patient age, and pregnancy/nursing status.

Monitoring: Monitor for allergic reactions and other idiosyncrasies.

Patient Counseling: Instruct patient not to swallow after use. Adults should not eat, drink, or rinse for 30 min after use; however, pediatrics 6-16 yrs should rinse mouth thoroughly after use. Keep out of reach of children.

Storage: 20-25°C (68-77°F).

PREVPAC – amoxicillin/clarithromycin/lansoprazole — RX

Class: H. pylori treatment combination

ADULT DOSAGE

Helicobacter pylori **Eradication**

H. pylori **Infection and Duodenal Ulcer Disease (Active or 1-Year History):**
Usual: 30mg lansoprazole, 1g amoxicillin, and 500mg clarithromycin administered together bid (am and pm) for 10 or 14 days

PEDIATRIC DOSAGE

Pediatric use may not have been established

DOSE MODIFICATION

Renal Impairment
Severe (w/ or w/o Coexisting Hepatic Impairment): May need to decrease dosage or prolong dosing intervals of clarithromycin
CrCl <30mL/min: Not recommended

Hepatic Impairment
Severe: Consider reduction of lansoprazole dosage

ADMINISTRATION

Oral route

Take each dose ac
Swallow each pill whole

HOW SUPPLIED

Cap: (Amoxicillin) 500mg; Cap, Delayed-Release: (Lansoprazole) 30mg; Tab: (Clarithromycin) 500mg

CONTRAINDICATIONS

History of cholestatic jaundice/hepatic dysfunction associated with prior use of clarithromycin. History of QT prolongation or ventricular cardiac arrhythmia, including torsades de pointes. Concomitant use with cisapride, pimozide, astemizole, terfenadine, ergotamine, or dihydroergotamine, and with HMG-CoA reductase inhibitors (statins) that are extensively metabolized by CYP3A4 (lovastatin or simvastatin). Concomitant use with colchicine in patients with renal/hepatic impairment.

WARNINGS/PRECAUTIONS

Not recommended with CrCl <30mL/min. Lab test interactions may occur. Caution in elderly. Amoxicillin: Serious and occasionally fatal hypersensitivity (anaphylactic) reactions reported in patients on penicillin (PCN) therapy; caution with history of PCN hypersensitivity and/or a history of sensitivity to multiple allergens. Immediately d/c therapy and initiate appropriate treatment if severe acute hypersensitivity reactions occur. Clarithromycin: Use in pregnancy only when there is no appropriate alternative therapy. Exacerbation of symptoms of myasthenia gravis and new onset of myasthenic syndrome reported. Hepatic dysfunction reported; d/c immediately if signs/symptoms of hepatitis occur. May cause QT interval prolongation, arrhythmia, and torsades de pointes; avoid with ongoing proarrhythmic conditions (eg, uncorrected hypokalemia or hypomagnesemia), and clinically significant bradycardia. Lansoprazole: Symptomatic response does not preclude the presence of gastric malignancy. Acute interstitial nephritis (AIN) reported; d/c if AIN develops. Amoxicillin/Clarithromycin: *Clostridium difficile*-associated diarrhea (CDAD) reported; d/c if CDAD is suspected or confirmed. May result in bacterial resistance with prolonged use in the absence of proven or suspected bacterial infection, or a prophylactic indication; d/c if superinfections occur and institute appropriate therapy.

ADVERSE REACTIONS

Diarrhea, taste perversion, headache.

DRUG INTERACTIONS

See Contraindications. Amoxicillin: Probenecid decreases renal tubular secretion. Chloramphenicol, macrolides, sulfonamides, and tetracyclines may interfere with bactericidal effects of PCN. May affect the gut flora, leading to lower estrogen reabsorption and reduced efficacy of combined oral estrogen/progesterone contraceptives. Clarithromycin: Avoid with class IA (quinidine, procainamide) or class III (dofetilide, amiodarone, sotalol) antiarrhythmic agents. Hypotension may occur with calcium channel blockers metabolized by CYP3A4 (eg, verapamil, amlodipine, diltiazem). Concomitant use with oral hypoglycemic agents and/or insulin may result in significant hypoglycemia; monitor glucose levels. May increase theophylline, carbamazepine, digoxin, colchicine, tolterodine, itraconazole, and saquinavir levels. Tolterodine 1mg bid is recommended in patients deficient in CYP2D6 activity (poor metabolizers). Bradyarrhythmias and lactic acidosis observed with verapamil. May decrease zidovudine levels; separate administration by at least 2 hrs. Fluconazole, itraconazole, and saquinavir may increase levels. Ritonavir and atazanavir may increase clarithromycin exposure and significantly decrease 14-OH clarithromycin exposure; consider alternative antibacterial therapy for indications other than infections due to Mycobacterium avium complex. Do not coadminister doses >1000mg/day with protease inhibitors. Decrease dose by 50% when coadministered with atazanavir. May increase concentrations of CYP3A substrates, which may lead to increased/prolonged therapeutic and adverse effects; caution with CYP3A substrates, especially those with narrow safety margin (eg, carbamazepine) and/or extensively metabolized by CYP3A enzyme. CYP3A inducers (eg, efavirenz, nevirapine, rifampicin, rifabutin, rifapentine) may decrease clarithromycin levels and increase 14-OH clarithromycin levels; consider alternative antibacterial treatment. May increase exposure of sildenafil, tadalafil, and vardenafil; coadministration is not recommended. May increase midazolam exposure; dose adjustments may be necessary when oral midazolam is coadministered. Caution and consider appropriate dose adjustments with triazolam or alprazolam. CNS effects reported with triazolam. Torsades de pointes reported with quinidine or disopyramide; monitor ECG. Interactions with drugs not thought to be metabolized by CYP3A (eg, hexobarbital, phenytoin, valproate) reported. Lansoprazole: May elevate and prolong levels of methotrexate (MTX) and/or its metabolite, possibly leading to toxicities; consider temporary withdrawal of therapy with high-dose MTX. May reduce absorption of drugs where gastric pH is an important determinant of bioavailability (eg, absorption of ampicillin esters, ketoconazole, atazanavir, iron salts, erlotinib, and mycophenolate mofetil may decrease, while absorption of digoxin may increase). Caution with mycophenolate mofetil in transplant patients. May interact with drugs metabolized by CYP450 enzymes (CYP1A2, CYP2C9, CYP2C19, CYP2D6, CYP3A). May increase theophylline clearance; may require additional titration of theophylline dosage when lansoprazole is started or stopped. May increase tacrolimus levels, especially in transplant patients who are intermediate or poor metabolizers of CYP2C19. Delayed absorption and reduced bioavailability with sucralfate; give at least 30 min prior to sucralfate. Clarithromycin/Lansoprazole: May alter the anticoagulant effects of warfarin and other anticoagulants; monitor PT and INR. Refer to PI for additional drug interaction information.

NURSING CONSIDERATIONS

Assessment: Assess for history of hypersensitivity to drug, macrolides, β-lactam antibiotics (PCNs, cephalosporins), or other allergens. Assess for ongoing proarrhythmic conditions, bradycardia, myasthenia gravis, renal/hepatic impairment, any other conditions where treatment is contraindicated or cautioned, pregnancy/nursing status, and possible drug interactions.

Monitoring: Monitor for hypersensitivity reactions, hepatic dysfunction, QT prolongation, CDAD, superinfections, exacerbation of myasthenia gravis symptoms, new onset of symptoms of myasthenic syndrome, AIN, and other adverse reactions. Periodically monitor renal/hepatic/hematopoietic function during prolonged therapy. Monitor PT/INR with warfarin and other anticoagulants.

Patient Counseling: Inform about risks/benefits of therapy. Advise to report the use of any other medications. Advise that diarrhea may occur and will usually end if therapy is discontinued. Instruct to contact physician as soon as possible if watery/bloody stools (with/without stomach cramps and fever) develop even as late as 2 or more months after having taken the last dose of therapy. Counsel that therapy should only be used to treat bacterial, not viral, infections. Instruct to take exactly ud; inform that skipping doses or not completing full course may decrease effectiveness and increase antibiotic resistance. Instruct to immediately report and seek care for any cardiovascular/neurological symptoms.

Storage: 20-25°C (68-77°F). Protect from light and moisture.

PREZCOBIX — cobicistat/darunavir RX

Class: CYP3A inhibitor/protease inhibitor

ADULT DOSAGE

HIV-1 Infection

In treatment-naive and treatment-experienced patients w/ no darunavir resistance-associated substitutions

Combination w/ Other Antiretrovirals:
1 tab qd

PEDIATRIC DOSAGE

Pediatric use may not have been established

HIV Genotypic Testing Prior to Initiation of Therapy:
Recommended for antiretroviral treatment-experienced patients; when genotypic testing is not feasible, therapy may be used in protease inhibitor-naive patients, but not in protease inhibitor-experienced patients

DOSE MODIFICATION

Renal Impairment

CrCl <70mL/min: Do not coadminister w/ tenofovir disoproxil fumarate (TDF)

Hepatic Impairment

Severe: Not recommended for use

ADMINISTRATION

Oral route

Take w/ food

HOW SUPPLIED

Tab: (Darunavir-Cobicistat) 800mg-150mg

CONTRAINDICATIONS

Concomitant use w/ alfuzosin, ranolazine, dronedarone, colchicine, rifampin, lurasidone, pimozide, dihydroergotamine, ergotamine, methylergonovine, cisapride, St. John's wort, lovastatin, simvastatin, sildenafil (when used to treat pulmonary arterial HTN), oral midazolam, or triazolam due to the potential for serious and/or life-threatening events or loss of therapeutic effect.

WARNINGS/PRECAUTIONS

Redistribution/accumulation of body fat, immune reconstitution syndrome, and autoimmune disorders (eg, Graves' disease, polymyositis, Guillain-Barre syndrome) in the setting of immune reconstitution reported. Not recommended for use in patients w/ severe hepatic impairment. Caution in elderly. Darunavir: Drug-induced hepatitis and liver injury, including some fatalities, reported. Consider performing increased AST/ALT monitoring in patients w/ underlying chronic hepatitis, cirrhosis, or those w/ pretreatment transaminase elevations, especially during the 1st several months of treatment. Consider interruption or discontinuation of therapy if evidence of new/worsening liver dysfunction occurs. Severe skin reactions (eg, Stevens-Johnson syndrome, toxic epidermal necrolysis, drug rash w/ eosinophilia and systemic symptoms), accompanied by fever and/or transaminase elevations in some cases, reported; d/c immediately if signs/symptoms of severe skin reactions develop. Contains a sulfonamide moiety; monitor patients w/ a known sulfonamide allergy. May develop new onset diabetes mellitus (DM), exacerbation of preexisting DM, hyperglycemia, and diabetic ketoacidosis; may require either initiation or dose adjustments of insulin or oral hypoglycemic agents. Increased bleeding including spontaneous skin hematomas and hemarthrosis reported in patients w/ hemophilia type A and B. Cobicistat: Decreases estimated CrCl; consider effect when interpreting changes in CrCl in patients initiating therapy particularly w/ medical conditions or receiving drugs needing monitoring w/ estimated CrCl. Closely monitor patients w/ confirmed increase in SrCr >0.4mg/dL from baseline for renal safety.

ADVERSE REACTIONS

Darunavir: Diarrhea, N/V, rash, headache, abdominal pain. Cobicistat: Refer to cobicistat PI for adverse reactions reported w/ cobicistat.

DRUG INTERACTIONS

See Dose Modification and Contraindications. Coadministration w/ TDF in combination w/ concomitant or recent use of a nephrotoxic agent is not recommended. Coadministration w/ drugs that are primarily metabolized by CYP3A and/or CYP2D6 or are substrates of P-gp, BCRP, OATP1B1, or OATP1B3 may increase plasma concentrations of such drugs, which could increase or prolong their therapeutic effect and can be associated w/ adverse events. CYP3A inducers may decrease levels, which may lead to loss of therapeutic effect and development of resistance. CYP3A inhibitors may increase levels. Give didanosine 1 hr before or 2 hrs after administration w/ therapy. Not recommended w/ products containing the individual components of Prezcobix, ritonavir (RTV), other antiretroviral drugs that require pharmacokinetic boosting (eg, another protease inhibitor, elvitegravir), efavirenz, etravirine, nevirapine, apixaban, dabigatran etexilate (in specific renal impairment groups), rivaroxaban, rifapentine, boceprevir, simeprevir, telaprevir, everolimus, avanafil, salmeterol, or voriconazole. Caution w/ SSRIs and w/ narcotics used for treatment of opioid dependence (buprenorphine, buprenorphine/naloxone, methadone). May increase levels of maraviroc, antiarrhythmics, digoxin, dasatinib, nilotinib, vinblastine, vincristine, anticonvulsants metabolized by CYP3A (eg, carbamazepine, clonazepam), TCAs, itraconazole, ketoconazole, trazodone, colchicine, rifabutin, β-blockers, calcium channel blockers, corticosteroids, bosentan, atorvastatin, fluvastatin, pravastatin, rosuvastatin, immunosuppressants (cyclosporine, sirolimus, tacrolimus), narcotic analgesics metabolized by CYP3A (eg, fentanyl, oxycodone), tramadol, neuroleptics, PDE-5 inhibitors, sedatives/hypnotics metabolized by CYP3A (eg, buspirone, diazepam, estazolam), clarithromycin, erythromycin, and telithromycin. Itraconazole, ketoconazole, posaconazole, clarithromycin, erythromycin, and telithromycin may increase levels. Monitor INR w/ warfarin. Monitor phenobarbital or phenytoin levels. Monitor for a potential decrease of antimalarial efficacy or potential QT prolongation if coadministered w/ artemether/lumefantrine. Coadministration w/ inhaled/nasal fluticasone or other corticosteroids that are metabolized by CYP3A may result in reduced serum cortisol concentrations. Coadministration w/ corticosteroids that are metabolized by CYP3A, particularly long-term use, may increase the risk of development of systemic corticosteroid effects. Coadministration w/ dexamethasone or other corticosteroids that induce CYP3A may result in loss therapeutic effect and development of resistance to darunavir. Consider additional or alternative (nonhormonal) forms of contraception if taking hormonal contraceptives. Coadministration w/ parenteral midazolam should be done in a setting that ensures close clinical monitoring and appropriate medical management in case of respiratory depression and/or prolonged sedation. Bosentan may decrease levels. Cobicistat: Renal impairment, including cases of acute renal failure and Fanconi syndrome, reported when used in an antiretroviral regimen w/ TDF. Anticonvulsants that induce CYP3A (eg, carbamazepine, oxcarbazepine, phenobarbital) may decrease levels; consider alternative anticonvulsant or antiretroviral therapy, and if coadministration is necessary, monitor for lack or loss of virologic response. Refer to PI for further detailed information on drug interactions, including dosing modifications required when used w/ certain concomitant therapies.

NURSING CONSIDERATIONS

Assessment: Assess for hypersensitivity to drug, sulfonamide allergy, liver dysfunction, autoimmune disorders, hemophilia, preexisting DM, pregnancy/nursing status, and possible drug interactions. Assess estimated CrCl. When coadministering w/ TDF, assess estimated CrCl, urine glucose, and urine protein at baseline. If feasible, perform HIV genotypic testing in antiretroviral treatment-experienced patients.

Monitoring: Monitor for signs/symptoms of hepatotoxicity, severe skin reactions, new onset/worsening renal impairment when coadministered w/ TDF, new onset/exacerbation of DM, hyperglycemia, diabetic ketoacidosis, fat redistribution/accumulation, immune reconstitution syndrome, autoimmune disorders, and other adverse reactions. In patients w/ hemophilia, monitor for bleeding events. Consider performing increased AST/ALT monitoring in patients w/ underlying chronic hepatitis, cirrhosis, or those w/ pretreatment transaminase elevations, especially during the 1st several months of treatment. Monitor INR during coadministration w/ warfarin. Perform routine monitoring of estimated CrCl, urine glucose, and urine protein when used w/ TDF. Measure serum phosphorus in patients w/ or at risk for renal impairment when used w/ TDF.

Patient Counseling: Inform that therapy is not a cure for HIV and that patient may continue to experience illnesses associated w/ HIV-1 infection. Advise to avoid doing things that can spread HIV infection to others. Instruct to take w/ food qd as prescribed. Instruct not to alter dose or d/c w/o consulting physician. Counsel to take drug immediately for missed dose <12 hrs and to take the next dose at regular scheduled time. Instruct that if a dose is missed by >12 hrs, to take the next dose as scheduled; instruct not to double the dose. Advise about the signs/symptoms of liver problems. Inform that mild to severe skin reactions may develop; advise to immediately contact physician if signs/symptoms of severe skin reactions develop. Inform that renal impairment, including cases of acute renal failure and Fanconi syndrome, has been reported when used in combination w/ TDF-containing regimen. Instruct to notify physician of the use of any other prescription, OTC, or herbal medication. Instruct patients receiving hormonal contraceptives to use additional or alternative contraceptive (nonhormonal) measures during therapy. Inform that redistribution and accumulation of body fat may occur.

Storage: 20-25°C (68-77°F); excursions permitted to 15-30°C (59-86°F).

PREZISTA — darunavir

RX

Class: Protease inhibitor

ADULT DOSAGE

HIV-1 Infection

Combination w/ Ritonavir (RTV) and Other Antiretrovirals:

Treatment-Naive:
800mg (8mL) + RTV 100mg (1.25mL) qd

Treatment-Experienced:
No Darunavir Resistance Associated Substitutions:
800mg (8mL) + RTV 100mg (1.25mL) qd

≥1 Darunavir Resistance Associated Substitution:
600mg (6mL) + RTV 100mg (1.25mL) bid

When Genotypic Testing is Not Feasible:
600mg (6mL) + RTV 100mg (1.25mL) bid

PEDIATRIC DOSAGE

HIV-1 Infection

Combination w/ Ritonavir (RTV) and Other Antiretrovirals:

3-<18 Years:
Treatment-Naive/Treatment-Experienced w/ No Darunavir Resistance Associated Substitutions:
≥10-<11kg: 350mg (3.6mL) + RTV 64mg (0.8mL) qd
≥11-<12kg: 385mg (4mL) + RTV 64mg (0.8mL) qd
≥12-<13kg: 420mg (4.2mL) + RTV 80mg (1mL) qd
≥13-<14kg: 455mg (4.6mL) + RTV 80mg (1mL) qd

≥14-<15kg: 490mg (5mL) + RTV 96mg (1.2mL) qd
≥15-<30kg: 600mg (6mL) + RTV 100mg (1.25mL) qd
≥30-<40kg: 675mg (6.8mL) + RTV 100mg (1.25mL) qd
≥40kg: 800mg (8mL) + RTV 100mg (1.25mL) qd

Treatment-Experienced w/ ≥1 Darunavir Resistance Associated Substitution:
≥10-<11kg: 200mg (2mL) + RTV 32mg (0.4mL) bid
≥11-<12kg: 220mg (2.2mL) + RTV 32mg (0.4mL) bid
≥12-<13kg: 240mg (2.4mL) + RTV 40mg (0.5mL) bid
≥13-<14kg: 260mg (2.6mL) + RTV 40mg (0.5mL) bid
≥14-<15kg: 280mg (2.8mL) + RTV 48mg (0.6mL) bid
≥15-<30kg: 375mg (3.8mL) + RTV 48mg (0.6mL) bid
≥30-<40kg: 450mg (4.6mL) + RTV 60mg (0.75mL) bid
≥40kg: 600mg (6mL) + RTV 100mg (1.25mL) bid

DOSE MODIFICATION

Hepatic Impairment

Severe: Not recommended for use

ADMINISTRATION

Oral route

Take w/ food

Tab

Swallow whole w/ drink

Sus

Shake well before each use

HOW SUPPLIED

Sus: 100mg/mL [200mL]; Tab: 75mg, 150mg, 600mg, 800mg

CONTRAINDICATIONS

Concomitant use w/ drugs that are highly dependent on CYP3A for clearance and for which elevated plasma concentrations are associated w/ serious and/or life-threatening events, and w/ certain other drugs that may lead to reduced efficacy of darunavir (eg, alfuzosin, dihydroergotamine, ergotamine, methylergonovine, cisapride, pimozide, oral midazolam, triazolam, St. John's wort, lovastatin, simvastatin, rifampin, sildenafil [when used to treat pulmonary arterial HTN]).

WARNINGS/PRECAUTIONS

Must be coadministered w/ RTV and food to achieve desired effect. Drug-induced hepatitis and liver injury reported; consider performing increased AST/ALT monitoring in patients w/ underlying chronic hepatitis, cirrhosis, or those w/ pretreatment transaminase elevations. Consider interruption or discontinuation of therapy if evidence of new/worsening liver dysfunction occurs. Increased risk for liver function abnormalities in patients w/ preexisting liver dysfunction, including chronic active hepatitis B or C. Severe skin reactions sometimes accompanied by fever and/or transaminase elevations, Stevens-Johnson syndrome (rare), toxic epidermal necrolysis, drug rash w/ eosinophilia and systemic symptoms, and acute generalized exanthematous pustulosis reported; d/c if severe skin reactions develop. Caution in patients w/ a known sulfonamide allergy. New onset diabetes mellitus (DM), exacerbation of preexisting DM, hyperglycemia, and diabetic ketoacidosis reported. Immune reconstitution syndrome, autoimmune disorders (eg, Graves' disease, polymyositis, Guillain-Barre syndrome) in the setting of immune reconstitution, redistribution/accumulation of body fat, and increased bleeding in hemophilia type A and B reported. Caution in elderly.

ADVERSE REACTIONS

Diarrhea, N/V, headache, abdominal pain, rash, asthenia, anorexia, pruritus, fatigue, decreased appetite.

DRUG INTERACTIONS

See Contraindications. Avoid w/ colchicine in patients w/ renal/hepatic impairment and tadalafil during initiation. Not recommended w/ lopinavir/RTV, saquinavir, boceprevir, telaprevir, salmeterol, and other protease inhibitors. Avoid w/ voriconazole unless an assessment of the benefit/risk ratio justifies use of voriconazole. May increase levels of CYP3A and CYP2D6 substrates, indinavir, maraviroc, antiarrhythmics, digoxin, carbamazepine, trazodone, desipramine, clarithromycin, ketoconazole, itraconazole, colchicine, rifabutin, quetiapine, β-blockers, parenteral midazolam, calcium channel blockers, inhaled fluticasone, bosentan, pravastatin, atorvastatin, rosuvastatin, immunosuppressants, salmeterol, norbuprenorphine, neuroleptics, sildenafil for erectile dysfunction, vardenafil, and tadalafil. May decrease levels of phenytoin, phenobarbital, voriconazole, warfarin (monitor INR), methadone, boceprevir, telaprevir, ethinyl estradiol, norethindrone, sertraline, and paroxetine. CYP3A inhibitors, ketoconazole, itraconazole, indinavir, and rifabutin may increase levels. CYP3A inducers, systemic dexamethasone, lopinavir/RTV, saquinavir, boceprevir, and telaprevir may decrease levels. Give didanosine 1 hr before or 2 hrs after administration. Increased lumefantrine exposure may increase the risk of QT prolongation; caution w/ artemether/lumefantrine. May require initiation or dose adjustments of insulin or oral hypoglycemics for treatment of DM. Refer to PI for dosing modifications when used w/ certain concomitant therapies.

NURSING CONSIDERATIONS

Assessment: Assess for sulfonamide allergy, liver dysfunction, hemophilia, preexisting DM, pregnancy/nursing status, and possible drug interactions. Assess ability to swallow tab in children ≥15kg. In treatment-experienced patients, assess treatment history and perform phenotypic or genotypic testing.

Monitoring: Monitor for signs/symptoms of hepatotoxicity, severe skin reactions, new onset/exacerbation of DM, diabetic ketoacidosis, fat redistribution/accumulation, immune reconstitution syndrome, autoimmune disorders, and other adverse reactions. In patients w/ hemophilia, monitor for bleeding events. Consider performing increased AST/ALT monitoring in patients w/ underlying chronic hepatitis, cirrhosis, or those w/ pretreatment transaminase elevations. Monitor INR during coadministration w/ warfarin.

Patient Counseling: Inform that therapy is not a cure for HIV and that illnesses associated w/ HIV may continue. Advise to avoid doing things that can spread HIV infection to others. Instruct not to alter dose or d/c w/o consulting physician. Counsel to take drug immediately for missed dose <6 hrs and <12 hrs, for bid and qd dosing respectively, and to take the next dose at regular scheduled time. Instruct that if a dose is missed by >6 hrs or >12 hrs, for bid and qd dosing respectively, take the next dose as scheduled; instruct not to double the dose. Advise about the signs/symptoms of liver problems. Inform that mild to severe skin reactions may develop; advise to d/c immediately if signs/symptoms of severe skin reactions develop. Instruct to notify physician if taking any other prescription, OTC, or herbal medication. Instruct to use alternative contraceptive measures if on estrogen-based contraceptive during therapy. Inform that redistribution and accumulation of body fat may occur.

Storage: 25°C (77°F); excursions permitted to 15-30°C (59-86°F). (Sus) Do not refrigerate or freeze. Avoid exposure to excessive heat.

PRILOSEC — omeprazole

RX

Class: Proton pump inhibitor

ADULT DOSAGE

***Helicobacter pylori* Eradication**

Triple Therapy:
20mg + clarithromycin 500mg + amoxicillin 1000mg, each given bid x 10 days. Give additional 18 days of omeprazole 20mg qd if ulcer is present at the time of initiation of therapy

Dual Therapy:
40mg qd + clarithromycin 500mg tid x 14 days. Give additional 14 days of omeprazole 20mg qd if ulcer is present at the time of initiation of therapy

Active Duodenal Ulcer

20mg qd for 4-8 weeks

Gastroesophageal Reflux Disease

W/O Esophageal Lesions:
20mg qd for up to 4 weeks

PEDIATRIC DOSAGE

Erosive Esophagitis

Maint:
1-16 Years:
5-<10kg: 5mg/day
10-<20kg: 10mg/day
≥20kg: 20mg/day

Gastroesophageal Reflux Disease

1-16 Years:
5-<10kg: 5mg/day
10-<20kg: 10mg/day
≥20kg: 20mg/day

W/ Erosive Esophagitis and Accompanying Symptoms:
20mg qd x 4-8 weeks

Erosive Esophagitis

Maint:
20mg qd

Gastric Ulcers

40mg qd x 4-8 weeks

Pathological Hypersecretory Conditions

Long-term Treatment:
Initial: 60mg qd
Titrate: Individualize and continue for as long as clinically indicated. Doses up to 120mg tid have been administered
Give >80mg/day in divided doses

DOSE MODIFICATION

Hepatic Impairment

Consider dose reduction, particularly for maint of healing of erosive esophagitis

Other Important Modifications

Asian Population:
Consider dose reduction, particularly for maint of healing of erosive esophagitis

ADMINISTRATION

Oral route

Take ac

Cap

Swallow whole or, alternatively, open cap and sprinkle all pellets on 1 tbsp of applesauce, then swallow immediately w/ a glass of cool water; do not chew or crush the pellets

Sus

Empty the contents of a 2.5mg pkt into 5mL of water or 10mg pkt into 15mL of water
Stir and leave 2-3 min to thicken
Drink w/in 30 min
If any material remains after drinking, add more water, stir and drink immediately

NG/Gastric Tube:
Add 5mL of water to a catheter-tipped syringe and then add the contents of a 2.5mg pkt (or 15mL of water for the 10mg pkt)
Immediately shake the syringe and leave 2-3 min to thicken
Shake the syringe and inject through the NG or gastric tube, French size 6 or larger, into the stomach w/in 30 min
Refill the syringe w/ an equal amount of water; shake and flush any remaining contents into the stomach

HOW SUPPLIED

Cap, Delayed-Release: 10mg, 20mg, 40mg; Sus, Delayed-Release: 2.5mg, 10mg (granules/pkt)

WARNINGS/PRECAUTIONS

Symptomatic response does not preclude the presence of gastric malignancy. Atrophic gastritis reported with long-term use. Acute interstitial nephritis reported; d/c if this develops. Cyanocobalamin (vitamin B12) deficiency may occur due to malabsorption with daily long-term treatment (eg, >3 yrs) with any acid-suppressing medications. May increase risk of *Clostridium difficile*-associated diarrhea (CDAD), especially in hospitalized patients. May increase risk for osteoporosis-related fractures of the hip, wrist, or spine, especially with high-dose and long-term therapy. Use lowest dose and shortest duration appropriate to the condition being treated. Hypomagnesemia reported and may require Mg^{2+} replacement and discontinuation of therapy. Drug-induced decrease in gastric acidity results in enterochromaffin-like cell hyperplasia and increased chromogranin A (CgA) levels, which may interfere with investigations for neuroendocrine tumors; temporarily d/c treatment at least 14 days before assessing CgA levels and consider repeating test if initial CgA levels are high.

ADVERSE REACTIONS

Headache, diarrhea, abdominal pain, N/V, flatulence.

DRUG INTERACTIONS

May reduce atazanavir and nelfinavir levels; concomitant use not recommended. May change absorption or levels of antiretrovirals. May reduce absorption of drugs where gastric pH is an important determinant of their bioavailability; ketoconazole, atazanavir, iron salts, erlotinib, and mycophenolate mofetil (MMF) absorption can decrease, while digoxin absorption can increase. Caution in transplant patients receiving MMF. May prolong elimination of drugs metabolized by oxidation in the liver (eg, diazepam, warfarin, phenytoin). Monitor patients taking drugs metabolized by CYP450 (eg, cyclosporine, disulfiram, benzodiazepines). Monitor for increases in INR and PT with warfarin. Voriconazole (a combined inhibitor of CYP2C19 and CYP3A4) may increase levels; consider dose adjustment with Zollinger-Ellison syndrome. Decreased levels with CYP2C19 or CYP3A4 inducers; avoid with St. John's wort or rifampin. Reduces pharmacological activity of clopidogrel; avoid concomitant use. May increase levels of saquinavir, cilostazol, and tacrolimus; consider saquinavir and cilostazol dose reduction. Caution with digoxin or other drugs that may cause hypomagnesemia (eg, diuretics). May elevate and prolong levels of MTX and/or its metabolite, possibly leading to toxicities; consider temporary withdrawal of therapy with high-dose MTX.

NURSING CONSIDERATIONS

Assessment: Assess for hypersensitivity to the drug or to substituted benzimidazoles, risk for osteoporosis-related fractures, hepatic impairment, pregnancy/nursing status, and possible drug interactions. Obtain baseline Mg^{2+} levels in patients expected to be on prolonged therapy.

Monitoring: Monitor for signs/symptoms of atrophic gastritis, acute interstitial nephritis, cyanocobalamin deficiency, bone fractures, hypersensitivity reactions, CDAD, and other adverse reactions. Monitor Mg^{2+} levels periodically in patients expected to be on prolonged therapy. Monitor INR and PT when given with warfarin.

Patient Counseling: Advise to immediately report and seek care for diarrhea that does not improve and for any cardiovascular/neurological symptoms. Inform of alternative administration options if patient has difficulty swallowing.

Storage: (Cap) 15-30°C (59-86°F). Protect from light and moisture. (Sus) 25°C (77°F); excursions permitted to 15-30°C (59-86°F).

PRINIVIL — lisinopril **RX**

Class: ACE inhibitor

D/C when pregnancy is detected. Drugs that act directly on the renin-angiotensin system can cause injury and death to the developing fetus.

ADULT DOSAGE

Hypertension

Not on Diuretic Therapy:
Initial: 10mg qd
Titrate: Adjust dose according to BP response
Usual: 20-40mg qd
Max: 80mg

May add a low-dose diuretic if BP is not controlled

Heart Failure

Adjunct w/ Diuretics and Digitalis:
Initial: 5mg qd
Usual: 5-20mg qd

Acute Myocardial Infarction

5mg w/in 24 hrs, followed by 5mg after 24 hrs, 10mg after 48 hrs, and then 10mg qd for 6 weeks

PEDIATRIC DOSAGE

Hypertension

≥6 Years:
Initial: 0.07mg/kg qd (up to 5mg total)
Titrate: Adjust dose according to BP response
Max: 0.61mg/kg (or 40mg)

DOSE MODIFICATION

Concomitant Medications

HTN:
Diuretic-Treated Patients:
If possible d/c diuretic 2-3 days prior to therapy to avoid hypotension. If BP is not controlled w/ lisinopril alone, then diuretic therapy should be resumed
Initial: 5mg

Renal Impairment

HTN:
Initial:
CrCl 10-30mL/min: 5mg qd
CrCl <10mL/min: 2.5mg qd
Titrate: May increase until BP is controlled
Max: 40mg/day

Heart Failure:
CrCl ≤30mL/min or SrCr >3mg/dL:
Initial: 2.5mg qd

Pediatrics:
GFR <30mL/min: Not recommended

Other Important Modifications
Heart Failure:
W/ Hyponatremia:
Initial: 2.5mg qd

Acute MI:
Systolic BP ≤120mmHg When Treatment is Started or During First 3 Days After the Infarct: 2.5mg
Maint: 5mg/day w/ temporary reductions to 2.5mg if needed if systolic BP ≤100mmHg occurs
D/C if systolic BP <90mmHg for >1 hr occurs

Elderly
Start at lower end of dosing range

ADMINISTRATION
Oral route

Preparation of Sus (200mL of 1.0mg/mL Sus):
1. Add 10mL of purified water to polyethylene terephthalate bottle containing ten 20mg tabs
2. Shake for at least 1 min
3. Add 30mL Bicitra diluent and 160mL Ora-Sweet SF and shake gently for several sec
4. Store sus at or below 25°C (77°F) for up to 4 weeks
5. Shake sus before each use

HOW SUPPLIED
Tab: 5mg*, 10mg*, 20mg* *scored

CONTRAINDICATIONS
Hereditary or idiopathic angioedema, history of ACE inhibitor-associated angioedema. Coadministration with aliskiren in patients with diabetes.

WARNINGS/PRECAUTIONS
Not recommended in pediatric patients with GFR <30mL/min/1.73m^2. Head/neck angioedema reported; d/c and administer appropriate therapy. Intestinal angioedema reported; monitor for abdominal pain. More reports of angioedema in blacks than nonblacks. Anaphylactoid reactions reported during desensitization with hymenoptera venom, dialysis with high-flux membranes, and LDL apheresis with dextran sulfate absorption. Caution when initiating therapy in AMI patients with renal impairment (SrCr >2mg/dL) and in HF patients. Excessive hypotension, sometimes associated with oliguria and/or progressive azotemia, and rarely with acute renal failure and/or death may occur; monitor closely. If symptomatic hypotension develops, dose reduction or discontinuation of therapy or concomitant diuretic may be necessary. Rare cases of leukopenia/neutropenia and bone marrow depression reported; consider monitoring of WBCs in patients with collagen vascular disease and renal disease. Rarely, syndrome that starts with cholestatic jaundice or hepatitis progressing to fulminant hepatic necrosis and (sometimes) death reported; d/c if jaundice or marked hepatic enzyme elevations occur. Caution with left ventricular outflow obstruction. May cause changes in renal function. May increase BUN and SrCr in patients with renal artery stenosis or with no preexisting renal vascular disease. Hyperkalemia and persistent nonproductive cough reported. Hypotension may occur with major surgery or during anesthesia. Caution in elderly.

ADVERSE REACTIONS
Hypotension, dizziness, headache, diarrhea, cough, chest pain, hyperkalemia.

DRUG INTERACTIONS
See Contraindications. Hypotension risk and increased BUN and SrCr with diuretics. Increased hypoglycemic risk with insulin or oral hypoglycemics. NSAIDs, including selective COX-2 inhibitors, may diminish effect and may cause further deterioration of renal function. Dual blockade of the renin-angiotensin-aldosterone system (RAAS) is associated with increased risks of hypotension, syncope, hyperkalemia, and changes in renal function (including acute renal failure); closely monitor BP, renal function, and electrolytes with concomitant agents that affect the RAAS. Avoid with aliskiren in patients with renal impairment (GFR <60mL/min). Increased risk of hyperkalemia with K^+-sparing diuretics, K^+ supplements, or K^+-containing salt substitutes; use with caution and frequently monitor serum K^+. Concomitant K^+-sparing agents should generally not be used with HF. Lithium toxicity reported; frequently monitor serum lithium levels. Nitritoid reactions reported with injectable gold.

NURSING CONSIDERATIONS

Assessment: Assess for hereditary or idiopathic angioedema, collagen vascular disease, left ventricular outflow obstruction, renal artery stenosis, risk factors for hyperkalemia, risk of excessive hypotension, history of ACE inhibitor-associated angioedema, renal function, hypersensitivity to the drug, pregnancy/nursing status, and possible drug interactions.

Monitoring: Monitor for angioedema, anaphylactoid reactions, hyperkalemia, and other adverse reactions. Monitor WBCs in patients with collagen vascular disease and renal disease. Monitor BP, LFTs, and renal function.

Patient Counseling: Instruct to d/c therapy and to immediately report signs/symptoms of angioedema. Instruct to report lightheadedness, especially during 1st few days of therapy; advise to d/c and to consult with a physician if actual syncope occurs. Advise that excessive perspiration, dehydration, diarrhea, or vomiting may lead to fall in BP; instruct to consult with a physician. Advise not to use salt substitutes containing K^+ without consulting physician. Advise diabetic patients to monitor for hypoglycemia. Instruct to report any indication of infection (eg, sore throat, fever) that may be a sign of leukopenia/neutropenia. Inform about fetal risks if taken during pregnancy and discuss treatment options with women planning to become pregnant; instruct to report pregnancy to physician as soon as possible.

Storage: (Tab) 15-30°C (59-86°F). Protect from moisture. (Sus) $\leq$25°C (77°F) for up to 4 weeks.

PRISTIQ – desvenlafaxine

Class: Serotonin and norepinephrine reuptake inhibitor

Antidepressants increased the risk of suicidal thoughts and behavior in children, adolescents, and young adults in short-term studies. Monitor and observe closely for worsening, and emergence of suicidal thoughts and behaviors. Not approved for use in pediatric patients.

ADULT DOSAGE

Major Depressive Disorder

50mg qd

50-400mg/day were effective; no additional benefit at doses >50mg/day and more frequent adverse reactions reported at higher doses

Switching from Other Antidepressants:
May need to taper initial antidepressant

Dosing Considerations with MAOIs

Switching to/from an MAOI for Psychiatric Disorders:
Allow at least 14 days between discontinuation of an MAOI and initiation of desvenlafaxine, and allow at least 7 days between discontinuation of desvenlafaxine and initiation of an MAOI

W/ Other MAOIs (eg, Linezolid, IV Methylene Blue):
Do not start desvenlafaxine in a patient being treated w/ linezolid or IV methylene blue
In patients already receiving desvenlafaxine, if acceptable alternatives are not available and benefits outweigh risks, d/c desvenlafaxine promptly and administer linezolid or IV methylene blue; monitor for serotonin syndrome for 7 days or until 24 hrs after the last dose of linezolid or IV methylene blue, whichever comes 1st. May resume desvenlafaxine therapy 24 hrs after the last dose of linezolid or IV methylene blue

PEDIATRIC DOSAGE

Pediatric use may not have been established

DOSE MODIFICATION

Renal Impairment

Moderate (CrCl 30-50mL/min):
Max: 50mg/day

Severe (CrCl <30mL/min)/ESRD:
Max: 25mg qd or 50mg qod; do not give supplemental doses after dialysis

Hepatic Impairment

Moderate to Severe:
Usual: 50mg/day
Max: Dose escalation >100mg/day not recommended

Discontinuation
Gradually reduce dose; if intolerable symptoms occur following a decrease in dose or upon discontinuation, consider resuming the previously prescribed dose and continue decreasing the dose at a more gradual rate. The 25mg dose is available for discontinuing therapy

ADMINISTRATION
Oral route

Take at approx the same time each day, w/ or w/o food
Swallow tab whole w/ fluid; do not divide, crush, chew, or dissolve

HOW SUPPLIED
Tab, Extended Release: 25mg, 50mg, 100mg

CONTRAINDICATIONS
Use of an MAOI intended to treat psychiatric disorders either concomitantly or w/in 7 days of stopping treatment. Treatment w/in 14 days of stopping an MAOI to treat psychiatric disorders. Starting treatment in patients being treated w/ other MAOIs (eg, linezolid, IV methylene blue).

WARNINGS/PRECAUTIONS
Not approved for the treatment of bipolar depression. Serotonin syndrome reported; d/c immediately if symptoms occur and initiate supportive symptomatic treatment. Caution w/ preexisting HTN or cardiovascular (CV)/cerebrovascular conditions that might be compromised by increases in BP. Consider dose reduction or discontinuation of therapy if sustained increases in BP occur. May increase risk of bleeding events. Pupillary dilation that occurs following use may trigger an angle-closure attack in a patient w/ anatomically narrow angles who does not have a patent iridectomy. Activation of mania/hypomania reported. Discontinuation symptoms reported. Avoid abrupt discontinuation. Seizures reported. Hyponatremia may occur; caution in elderly and volume-depleted patients. Consider discontinuation in patients w/ symptomatic hyponatremia. Interstitial lung disease and eosinophilic pneumonia may occur; consider diagnosis for either in patients w/ progressive dyspnea, cough, or chest discomfort, and consider discontinuing therapy. False (+) urine immunoassay screening tests for phencyclidine and amphetamines reported.

ADVERSE REACTIONS
N/V, dry mouth, dizziness, insomnia, somnolence, hyperhidrosis, constipation, anxiety, decreased appetite, tremor, mydriasis, erectile dysfunction, anorgasmia, fatigue, vision blurred.

DRUG INTERACTIONS
See Contraindications. Avoid w/ other desvenlafaxine-containing products or venlafaxine products; may increase levels and increase dose-related adverse reactions. Avoid alcohol consumption. May cause serotonin syndrome w/ other serotonergic drugs (eg, triptans, TCAs, fentanyl) and w/ drugs that impair metabolism of serotonin; d/c desvenlafaxine and any concomitant serotonergic agent immediately if serotonin syndrome occurs. Caution w/ NSAIDs, aspirin (ASA), warfarin, and other drugs that affect coagulation or bleeding, due to increased risk of bleeding. May increase risk of hyponatremia w/ diuretics. Potent CYP3A4 inhibitors (eg, ketoconazole) may increase levels. CYP2D6 substrates (eg, desipramine, atomoxetine, dextromethorphan) should be dosed at the original level when coadministered w/ 100mg desvenlafaxine or lower, or when desvenlafaxine is discontinued; reduce the dose of these substrates by up to 1/2 if coadministered w/ 400mg of desvenlafaxine.

NURSING CONSIDERATIONS

Assessment: Assess for risk for bipolar disorder, history of mania/hypomania, seizure disorders, HTN, CV/cerebrovascular conditions, susceptibility to angle-closure glaucoma, volume depletion, hypersensitivity to the drug, hepatic/renal impairment, pregnancy/nursing status, and possible drug interactions.

Monitoring: Monitor for signs/symptoms of clinical worsening (eg, suicidality, unusual changes in behavior), serotonin syndrome, abnormal bleeding, angle-closure glaucoma, activation of mania/hypomania, seizures, hyponatremia, interstitial lung disease, eosinophilic pneumonia, and other adverse reactions. Monitor BP, LFTs, and renal function. Monitor for discontinuation symptoms (eg, dysphoric mood, irritability, agitation) when discontinuing therapy. Carefully monitor patients receiving concomitant warfarin therapy when treatment w/ desvenlafaxine is initiated or discontinued. Periodically reassess to determine the need for continued treatment.

Patient Counseling: Advise patients, families, and caregivers about the benefits and risks of treatment and counsel on its appropriate use. Counsel patients, families, and caregivers to look for the emergence of suicidality, especially early during treatment and when the dose is adjusted up or down. Caution about the risk of serotonin syndrome, particularly w/ the concomitant use w/ other serotonergic agents. Inform that concomitant use w/ ASA, NSAIDs, warfarin, or other drugs that affect coagulation may increase the risk of bleeding. Advise to monitor BP regularly, to observe for signs/symptoms of activation of mania/hypomania, to avoid alcohol, and not to d/c therapy w/o notifying physician. Inform that discontinuation effects may occur when stopping treatment and a dose of 25mg/day is available for discontinuing therapy. Caution about risk of angle-closure glaucoma. Caution against operating hazardous machinery (including automobiles) until reasonably certain that therapy does not adversely affect ability to engage in such activities. Advise to notify physician if allergic phenomena develop, if pregnant, intending to become pregnant, or if breastfeeding. Inform that an inert matrix tab may pass in the stool or via colostomy.

Storage: 20-25°C (68-77°F); excursions permitted to 15-30°C (59-86°F).

ProAir HFA – albuterol sulfate RX

Class: Beta$_2$-agonist

ADULT DOSAGE

Bronchospasm

Treatment/Prevention of Bronchospasm w/ Reversible Obstructive Airway Disease:
2 inh q4-6h; 1 inh q4h may be sufficient in some patients

Exercise-Induced Bronchospasm

Prevention:
2 inh 15-30 min prior to exercise

PEDIATRIC DOSAGE

Bronchospasm

≥4 Years:
Treatment/Prevention w/ Reversible Obstructive Airway Disease:
2 inh q4-6h; 1 inh q4h may be sufficient in some patients

Exercise-Induced Bronchospasm

≥4 Years:
Prevention:
2 inh 15-30 min prior to exercise

DOSE MODIFICATION

Elderly
Start at lower end of dosing range

ADMINISTRATION
Oral inh route

Shake well before each spray

Priming
Prime inhaler before using for the 1st time and when inhaler has not been used for >2 weeks by releasing 3 sprays into the air, away from the face

HOW SUPPLIED
MDI: 90mcg/inh [200 actuations]

WARNINGS/PRECAUTIONS
If more doses than usual are needed, this may be a marker of destabilization of asthma and may require reevaluation of the patient and treatment regimen; anti-inflammatory treatment (eg, corticosteroids) may be needed. May produce paradoxical bronchospasm; d/c immediately and institute alternative therapy if this occurs. D/C if cardiovascular (CV) effects occur. ECG changes and immediate hypersensitivity reactions may occur. Fatalities reported w/ excessive use; do not exceed recommended dose. Caution w/ CV disorders, convulsive disorders, hyperthyroidism, diabetes mellitus (DM), and in patients unusually responsive to sympathomimetic amines. May produce significant hypokalemia and BP changes. Aggravation of preexisting DM and ketoacidosis reported w/ large doses of IV albuterol. Caution in elderly and when administering high doses in patients w/ renal impairment.

ADVERSE REACTIONS
Pharyngitis, headache, rhinitis, dizziness, musculoskeletal pain, tachycardia.

DRUG INTERACTIONS
Avoid w/ other short-acting sympathomimetic aerosol bronchodilators; caution w/ additional adrenergic drugs administered by any route. Use w/ β-blockers may block pulmonary effect and produce severe bronchospasm in asthmatic patients; avoid concomitant use. If needed, consider cardioselective β-blockers. ECG changes and/or hypokalemia caused by non-K^+-sparing diuretics (eg, loop, thiazide) may be worsened; consider monitoring K^+ levels. May decrease digoxin levels; monitor serum digoxin levels. Use extreme caution w/ MAOIs and TCAs, or w/in 2 weeks of discontinuation of such agents; consider alternative therapy in patients taking MAOIs or TCAs.

NURSING CONSIDERATIONS

Assessment: Assess for history of hypersensitivity to drug, CV disorders, convulsive disorders, hyperthyroidism, DM, renal impairment, pregnancy/nursing status, and possible drug interactions. Assess use in patients unusually responsive to sympathomimetic amines.

Monitoring: Monitor for paradoxical bronchospasm, deterioration of asthma, CV effects, ECG changes, hypokalemia, immediate hypersensitivity reactions, and other adverse reactions. Monitor BP, HR, and ECG changes. Monitor renal function in elderly.

Patient Counseling: Counsel not to increase dose/frequency of doses w/o consulting physician. Advise to seek immediate medical attention if treatment becomes less effective for symptomatic relief, symptoms become worse, and/or there is a need to use product more frequently than usual. Inform that drug may cause paradoxical bronchospasm; instruct to d/c if this occurs. Instruct to take concurrent inhaled drugs and other asthma medications only ud. Inform of the common adverse effects of treatment (eg, palpitations, chest pain, rapid HR, tremor, nervousness). Instruct to notify physician if pregnant/nursing.

Storage: 15-25°C (59-77°F). Protect from freezing and direct sunlight. Contents under pressure; do not puncture or incinerate. Exposure to temperatures >49°C (120°F) may cause bursting.

PROCARDIA XL – nifedipine **RX**

Class: Calcium channel blocker (dihydropyridine)

OTHER BRAND NAMES
Nifedical XL

ADULT DOSAGE

Angina

Vasospastic Angina/Chronic Stable Angina (Effort-Associated Angina)
Initial: 30 or 60mg qd
Titrate: Adjust dose over a 7- to 14-day period, but may proceed more rapidly if symptoms warrant
Max: 120mg/day; caution with doses >90mg
Use nearest equivalent total daily dose when switching to extended-release tab from nifedipine caps alone or in combination w/ other antianginal medications; titrate as clinically warranted

Hypertension
Initial: 30 or 60mg qd
Titrate: Adjust dose over a 7- to 14-day period, but may proceed more rapidly if symptoms warrant
Max: 120mg/day

PEDIATRIC DOSAGE
Pediatric use may not have been established

DOSE MODIFICATION
Discontinuation
Gradually decrease w/ close supervision

ADMINISTRATION
Oral route
Swallow tab whole; do not crush, divide, or chew

HOW SUPPLIED
Tab, Extended-Release: 30mg, 60mg, 90mg; (Nifedical XL) 30mg, 60mg

WARNINGS/PRECAUTIONS
May cause excessive hypotension; monitor BP initially and w/ titration. May increase frequency, duration, and/or severity of angina or acute MI (AMI), particularly w/ severe obstructive coronary artery disease (CAD). May develop heart failure (HF) after beginning therapy, w/ a higher risk in patients w/ tight aortic stenosis. GI obstruction and bezoars reported rarely; caution w/ altered GI anatomy (eg, severe GI narrowing, colon cancer, small bowel obstruction), hypomotility disorders, and concomitant medications (eg, H_2-histamine blockers, NSAIDs, laxatives). Mild to moderate peripheral edema, typically associated w/ arterial vasodilation, may occur; differentiate peripheral edema from the effects of increasing left ventricular dysfunction in patients w/ angina or HTN complicated by CHF. Transient elevations of enzymes (eg, alkaline phosphatase, CPK, lactate dehydrogenase, AST, ALT), cholestasis w/ or w/o jaundice, and allergic hepatitis reported (rare). May decrease platelet aggregation and increase bleeding time. Positive direct Coombs test w/ or w/o hemolytic anemia reported. Reversible elevation in BUN and SrCr reported rarely in patients w/ chronic renal insufficiency. (Procardia XL) Tab adherence to GI wall w/ ulceration reported.

ADVERSE REACTIONS
Dizziness, lightheadedness, giddiness, flushing, heat sensation, headache, weakness, nausea, heartburn, muscle cramps, tremor, peripheral edema, nervousness, mood changes, palpitation.

DRUG INTERACTIONS
β-blockers may increase the likelihood of CHF, severe hypotension, or angina exacerbation; avoid abrupt β-blocker withdrawal. Severe hypotension and/or increased fluid volume reported together w/ β-blockers and fentanyl or other narcotic analgesics; if condition permits, allow sufficient time

(at least 36 hrs) for nifedipine to be washed out prior to surgery w/ fentanyl. May increase digoxin levels; monitor digoxin when initiating, adjusting, and discontinuing therapy to avoid possible over- or under-digitalization. May increase PT w/ coumarin anticoagulants. Cimetidine may increase levels; caution during titration. Monitor w/ other medications known to lower BP. (Procardia XL) Phenytoin may lower systemic exposure to nifedipine; avoid w/ phenytoin or any known CYP3A4 inducer. CYP3A inhibitors (eg, fluconazole, itraconazole, clarithromycin) may result in increased exposure to nifedipine when coadministered; monitor carefully and consider initiating nifedipine at the lowest dose available. Grapefruit juice increases levels; avoid ingestion of grapefruit/grapefruit juice while on therapy.

NURSING CONSIDERATIONS

Assessment: Assess for acute coronary syndrome, severe obstructive CAD, aortic stenosis, recent β-blocker withdrawal, renal impairment, altered GI anatomy, hypomotility disorders, hypersensitivity to the drug, pregnancy/nursing status, and possible drug interactions.

Monitoring: Monitor for excessive hypotension, increased frequency, duration, and/or severity of angina and/or AMI, HF, signs/symptoms of GI obstruction, bezoars, peripheral edema, cholestasis w/ or w/o jaundice, allergic hepatitis, and other adverse reactions. Monitor BP, BUN, SrCr, for decreased platelet aggregation, and increased bleeding time.

Patient Counseling: Inform about potential risks/benefits of drug. Instruct to notify physician if pregnant/nursing or if any adverse reactions occur. (Procardia XL) Inform that it is normal to occasionally observe a tab-like material in the stool.

Storage: Protect from moisture and humidity. (Procardia XL) <30°C (86°F). (Nifedical XL) 25°C (77°F); excursions permitted to 15-30°C (59-86°F).

ProCentra – dextroamphetamine sulfate CII

Class: Sympathomimetic amine

High potential for abuse. Prolonged use may lead to drug dependence and must be avoided. Misuse may cause sudden death and serious cardiovascular adverse events.

ADULT DOSAGE

Narcolepsy

Initial: 10mg/day

Titrate: May increase in increments of 10mg at weekly intervals until optimal response is obtained

Usual: 5-60mg/day in divided doses

Give 1st dose on awakening; additional doses (1 or 2) at intervals of 4-6 hrs

PEDIATRIC DOSAGE

Narcolepsy

Usual: 5-60mg/day in divided doses

Give 1st dose on awakening; additional doses (1 or 2) at intervals of 4-6 hrs

6-12 Years:

Initial: 5mg/day

Titrate: May increase in increments of 5mg at weekly intervals until optimal response is obtained

≥12 Years:

Initial: 10mg/day

Titrate: May increase in increments of 10mg at weekly intervals until optimal response is obtained

Attention-Deficit Hyperactivity Disorder

3-5 Years:

Initial: 2.5mg/day

Titrate: May increase in increments of 2.5mg at weekly intervals until optimal response is obtained

≥6 Years:

Initial: 5mg qd or bid

Titrate: May increase in increments of 5mg at weekly intervals until optimal response is obtained. Only in rare cases will it be necessary to exceed a total of 40mg/day

Give 1st dose on awakening; additional doses (1 or 2) at intervals of 4-6 hrs

DOSE MODIFICATION

Adverse Reactions

Narcolepsy:

Reduce dose if bothersome adverse reactions appear (eg, insomnia, anorexia)

ADMINISTRATION

Oral route

Avoid late pm doses

HOW SUPPLIED

Sol: 5mg/5mL (473mL)

CONTRAINDICATIONS

Advanced arteriosclerosis, symptomatic cardiovascular disease (CVD), moderate to severe HTN, hyperthyroidism, glaucoma, agitated states, and history of drug abuse. During or within 14 days following MAOI use.

WARNINGS/PRECAUTIONS

Sudden death reported in children and adolescents with structural cardiac abnormalities or other serious heart problems. Sudden death, stroke, and myocardial infarction (MI) reported in adults. Avoid with known serious structural cardiac abnormalities, cardiomyopathy, serious heart rhythm abnormalities, coronary artery disease, or other serious cardiac problems. May cause a modest increase in average BP and HR. Prior to treatment, obtain medical history and perform physical exam to assess for presence of cardiac disease. Promptly perform cardiac evaluation if symptoms of cardiac disease develop during treatment. May exacerbate symptoms of behavior disturbance and thought disorder in patients with preexisting psychotic disorder. May induce mixed/manic episodes in patients with comorbid bipolar disorder. May cause treatment-emergent psychotic or manic symptoms in children and adolescents without a prior history of psychotic illness or mania; consider discontinuation if such symptoms occur. Aggressive behavior or hostility reported in children and adolescents with ADHD. May cause long-term suppression of growth in children; monitor growth, and may need to interrupt treatment in patients not growing or gaining height or weight as expected. May lower convulsive threshold; d/c if seizures occur. Difficulties with accommodation and blurring of vision reported. May exacerbate motor and phonic tics, and Tourette's syndrome. May elevate plasma corticosteroid levels and interfere with urinary steroid determinations.

ADVERSE REACTIONS

Palpitations, tachycardia, BP elevation, dizziness, insomnia, euphoria, dyskinesia, tremor, headache, dryness of mouth, diarrhea, constipation, urticaria, impotence, changes in libido.

DRUG INTERACTIONS

See Contraindications. GI acidifying agents (eg, guanethidine, reserpine, glutamic acid, ascorbic acid, fruit juices) and urinary acidifying agents (eg, ammonium chloride, sodium acid phosphate) lower blood levels and efficacy. Inhibits adrenergic blockers. GI alkalinizing agents (eg, sodium bicarbonate) and urinary alkalinizing agents (eg, acetazolamide, some thiazides) increase blood levels and therefore potentiate actions. May enhance activity of TCAs or sympathomimetic agents. Desipramine or protriptyline and possibly other TCAs cause striking and sustained increases in the concentration of d-amphetamine in the brain; cardiovascular effects can be potentiated. May counteract sedative effects of antihistamines. May antagonize effect of antihypertensives. Chlorpromazine and haloperidol block dopamine and norepinephrine reuptake, thus inhibiting central stimulant effects. May delay intestinal absorption of ethosuximide, phenobarbital, and phenytoin; coadministration with phenobarbital or phenytoin may produce a synergistic anticonvulsant action. Lithium carbonate may inhibit stimulatory effects. Potentiates analgesic effect of meperidine. Acidifying agents used in methenamine therapy increase urinary excretion and reduce efficacy. Enhances adrenergic effect of norepinephrine. In cases of propoxyphene overdosage, CNS stimulation is potentiated and fatal convulsions can occur. Inhibits hypotensive effect of veratrum alkaloids.

NURSING CONSIDERATIONS

Assessment: Assess for hypersensitivity/idiosyncrasy to sympathomimetic amines, advanced arteriosclerosis, symptomatic CVD, moderate to severe HTN, hyperthyroidism, glaucoma, agitated states, history of drug abuse, tics, Tourette's syndrome, preexisting psychotic disorder, risk for/comorbid bipolar disorder, cardiac disease, medical conditions that might be compromised by increases in BP or HR, any other conditions where treatment is cautioned, pregnancy/nursing status, and possible drug interactions.

Monitoring: Monitor for changes in HR and BP, signs/symptoms of cardiac disease, exacerbation of behavioral disturbance and thought disorder, psychosis, mania, appearance of or worsening of aggressive behavior or hostility, seizures, visual disturbances, exacerbation of motor and phonic tics or Tourette's syndrome, and other adverse reactions. In pediatric patients, monitor growth.

Patient Counseling: Inform about benefits and risks of treatment. Counsel that drug has high potential for abuse. Caution against engaging in potentially hazardous activities.

Storage: 20-25°C (68-77°F).

PROCHLORPERAZINE – prochlorperazine

RX

Class: Phenothiazine derivative

Elderly patients with dementia-related psychosis treated with antipsychotic drugs are at an increased risk of death; most deaths appeared to be cardiovascular (CV) (eg, heart failure, sudden death) or infectious (eg, pneumonia) in nature. Treatment with conventional antipsychotic drugs may similarly increase mortality. Not approved for the treatment of patients with dementia-related psychosis.

ADULT DOSAGE

Nausea/Vomiting

Tab:
Usual: 5mg or 10mg tid-qid
Daily dose >40mg should only be used in resistant cases

IM:
Initial: 5-10mg q3-4h prn
Max: 40mg/day

IV:
2.5-10mg slow inj or infusion at rate ≤5mg/min
Max: 10mg single dose and 40mg/day

N/V w/ Surgery:
IM:
5-10mg 1-2 hrs before induction of anesthesia (repeat once in 30 min if necessary)

IV:
5-10mg as slow inj or infusion 15-30 min before induction of anesthesia. To control acute symptoms during or after surgery, repeat once if necessary
Max: 40mg/day

Psychotic Disorders

Tab:
Nonpsychotic Anxiety
Usual: 5mg tid-qid
Max: 20mg/day, not longer than 12 weeks
Mild Conditions Including Schizophrenia:
Usual: 5 or 10mg tid-qid
Moderate-Severe Conditions (Hospitalized/Supervised):
Initial: 10mg tid-qid.
Titrate: Increase gradually until controlled or bothersome side effects
More Severe Disturbances:
Usual: 100-150mg/day
IM:
Start w/ lowest recommended dose and adjust based on severity
Schizophrenia w/ Severe Symptomatology:
Initial: 10-20mg, may repeat q2-4h if necessary (or, in resistant cases, every hr)
Switch to PO after obtaining control at the same dosage level or higher

Prolonged Parenteral Therapy:
10-20mg IM q4-6h

PEDIATRIC DOSAGE

Nausea/Vomiting

≥2 Years:
Tab:
20-29 lbs:
Usual: 2.5mg qd-bid
Max: 7.5mg/day
30-39 lbs:
Usual: 2.5mg bid-tid
Max: 10mg/day
40-85 lbs:
Usual: 2.5mg tid or 5mg bid
Max: 15mg/day

Severe N/V:
IM:
Usual: 0.06mg/lb; control is usually obtained w/ 1 dose

Schizophrenia

Tab:
2-12 Years:
Initial: 2.5mg bid-tid; do not give >10mg on the 1st day
Titrate: Increase according to response
Max:
2-5 Years: 20mg/day
6-12 Years: 25mg/day

IM:
<12 Years:
Usual: 0.06mg/lb. Control is usually obtained with 1 dose. Switch to PO after obtaining control at the same dosage level or higher

DOSE MODIFICATION

Elderly
Start at lower end of dosing range and increase more gradually

Other Important Modifications
Debilitated or Emaciated Adults:
Increase more gradually

ADMINISTRATION

IV, IM, Oral route

Inj

Inject deeply into upper, outer quadrant of the buttock
SQ is not advisable because of local irritation
May be administered either undiluted or diluted in isotonic sol
When given IV, do not use bolus inj
Do not mix w/ other agents in the syringe
Avoid getting injection sol on hands or clothing because of potential contact dermatitis

HOW SUPPLIED

Inj: (Edisylate) 5mg/mL [2mL, 10mL]; Tab: (Maleate) 5mg, 10mg

CONTRAINDICATIONS

Comatose states, concomitant large doses of CNS depressants (eg, alcohol, barbiturates, narcotics), pediatric surgery, pediatrics <2 yrs of age or <20 lbs.

WARNINGS/PRECAUTIONS

Secondary extrapyramidal symptoms can occur. Tardive dyskinesia (TD) may develop, especially in elderly and during long-term use. Neuroleptic malignant syndrome (NMS) reported; d/c if it occurs and institute appropriate treatment. Caution during reintroduction of therapy as NMS recurrence reported. Avoid in patients with bone marrow depression, previous hypersensitivity reaction, and in pregnant women. May impair mental and/or physical abilities, especially during the 1st few days of therapy. May mask symptoms of overdose of other drugs, and obscure diagnosis of intestinal obstruction, brain tumor, and Reye's syndrome; avoid in children/adolescents whose signs and symptoms suggest Reye's syndrome. May cause hypotension; caution with large doses and parenteral administration in patients with impaired CV system. May interfere with thermoregulation; caution in patients exposed to extreme heat. Evaluate therapy periodically with prolonged use. Leukopenia/neutropenia/agranulocytosis reported; monitor during 1st few months of therapy, and d/c at 1st sign of leukopenia or if severe neutropenia (absolute neutrophil count <1000/mm^3) occurs. Caution with glaucoma, in children with dehydration or acute illness, and in elderly. May produce α-adrenergic blockade, lower seizure threshold, or elevate prolactin levels. D/C 48 hrs before myelography; may resume after 24 hrs postprocedure.

ADVERSE REACTIONS

NMS, cholestatic jaundice, leukopenia, agranulocytosis, drowsiness, dizziness, amenorrhea, blurred vision, skin reactions, hypotension, motor restlessness, extrapyramidal symptoms, TD, dystonia, pseudoparkinsonism.

DRUG INTERACTIONS

See Contraindications. May intensify and prolong action of CNS depressants (eg, alcohol, anesthetics, narcotics), atropine, and organophosphorus insecticides. May decrease oral anticoagulant effects. Thiazide diuretics accentuate orthostatic hypotension. Increased levels of both drugs with propranolol. Anticonvulsants may need dosage adjustment; may lower convulsive threshold. May interfere with metabolism of phenytoin and precipitate toxicity. Risk of encephalopathic syndrome occurs with lithium. May antagonize antihypertensive effects of guanethidine and related compounds. Avoid use prior to myelography with metrizamide; vomiting as a sign of toxicity of cancer chemotherapeutic drugs may be obscured by the antiemetic effect. May reverse effect of epinephrine. May cause paradoxical further lowering of BP with epinephrine and other pressor agents (excluding norepinephrine bitartrate and phenylephrine HCl).

NURSING CONSIDERATIONS

Assessment: Assess for Reye's syndrome, TD, pregnancy/nursing status, possible drug interactions, impaired CV system, breast cancer, glaucoma, bone marrow depression, preexisting low WBC count, history of drug-induced leukopenia/neutropenia, history of psychosis, and seizure disorder. Assess use in children with acute illness or dehydration, elderly, debilitated, or emaciated patients.

Monitoring: Monitor for extrapyramidal symptoms, signs/symptoms of TD, NMS, hypotension, fever, sore throat, infection, jaundice, motor restlessness, dystonia, pseudoparkinsonism, and hypersensitivity reactions. Monitor CBC, WBC, and prolactin levels. Conduct liver studies if fever with grippe-like symptoms occur.

Patient Counseling: Inform about the risks and benefits of therapy. Instruct to avoid engaging in hazardous activities and exposure to extreme heat. Counsel to seek medical attention if symptoms of TD, NMS, hypotension, mydriasis, encephalopathic syndrome, sore throat, infection, deep sleep, or hypersensitivity reactions occur.

Storage: Tab, Inj: 20-25°C (68-77°F). Protect from light. (Inj) Do not freeze.

PROCRIT – epoetin alfa

Class: Erythropoiesis stimulator

RX

Increased risk of death, MI, stroke, venous thromboembolism (VTE), thrombosis of vascular access, and tumor progression or recurrence. Use the lowest dose sufficient to reduce/avoid the need for RBC transfusions. Chronic Kidney Disease (CKD): Greater risks for death, serious adverse cardiovascular (CV) reactions, and stroke when administered to target Hgb level >11g/dL. Cancer: Shortened overall survival and/or increased risk of tumor progression or recurrence in patients with breast, non-small cell lung, head and neck, lymphoid, and cervical cancers. Must enroll in and comply with the ESA APPRISE Oncology Program to prescribe and/or dispense drug to patients. Use only for anemia from myelosuppressive chemotherapy. Not indicated for patients receiving myelosuppressive chemotherapy when anticipated outcome is cure. D/C following completion of chemotherapy course. Perisurgery: Due to increased risk of deep venous thrombosis (DVT), DVT prophylaxis is recommended.

ADULT DOSAGE

Anemia

Chronic Kidney Disease Associated Anemia:
Patients on Dialysis:
Initiate treatment when Hgb is <10g/dL
If Hgb approaches/exceeds 11g/dL, reduce or interrupt dose
Initial: 50-100 U/kg IV/SQ 3X weekly; IV recommended for hemodialysis patients
Patients Not on Dialysis:
Consider initiating treatment when Hgb is <10g/dL AND the following considerations apply:
1. Rate of Hgb decline indicates likelihood of requiring a RBC transfusion AND,
2. Reducing the risk of alloimmunization and/or other RBC transfusion-related risks is a goal
If Hgb exceeds 10g/dL, reduce or interrupt dose and use lowest dose sufficient to reduce the need for RBC transfusion
Initial: 50-100 U/kg IV/SQ 3X weekly
All Patients:
Do not increase dose more frequently than once every 4 weeks; decreases in dose may occur more frequently
If Hgb Rises Rapidly (eg, >1g/dL in any 2-Week Period): Reduce dose by ≥25% prn to reduce rapid responses
If Hgb Has Not Increased by >1g/dL After 4 Weeks: Increase dose by 25%
If adequate response is not achieved over a 12-week escalation period, use lowest dose that will maintain a Hgb level sufficient to reduce need for RBC transfusions and evaluate other causes of anemia; d/c if responsiveness does not improve
Zidovudine Associated Anemia in HIV-Infected Patients:
Initial: 100 U/kg IV/SQ 3X weekly
Titrate:
No Hgb Increase After 8 Weeks: Increase dose by approx 50-100 U/kg at 4- to 8-week intervals until Hgb reaches level needed to avoid RBC transfusions or 300 U/kg
Hgb >12g/dL: Withhold therapy until Hgb <11g/dL; then resume at a dose 25% below previous dose
D/C therapy if an increase in Hgb is not achieved at 300 U/kg for 8 weeks
Chemotherapy Associated Anemia:
Initiate if Hgb <10g/dL and if there is a minimum of 2 additional months of planned chemotherapy
Initial: 150 U/kg SQ 3X weekly or 40,000 U SQ weekly until completion of a chemotherapy course

PEDIATRIC DOSAGE

Anemia

Chronic Kidney Disease Associated Anemia:
1 Month-16 Years on Dialysis:
Initiate treatment when Hgb is <10g/dL
If Hgb approaches/exceeds 11g/dL, reduce or interrupt dose
Initial: 50 U/kg IV/SQ 3X weekly; IV recommended for hemodialysis patients
Do not increase dose more frequently than once every 4 weeks; decreases in dose may occur more frequently
If Hgb Rises Rapidly (eg, >1g/dL in any 2-Week Period): Reduce dose by ≥25% prn to reduce rapid responses
If Hgb Has Not Increased by >1g/dL After 4 Weeks: Increase dose by 25%
If adequate response is not achieved over a 12-week escalation period, use lowest dose that will maintain a Hgb level sufficient to reduce need for RBC transfusions and evaluate other causes of anemia; d/c if responsiveness does not improve
Chemotherapy Associated Anemia:
5-18 Years:
Initiate if Hgb <10g/dL and if there is a minimum of 2 additional months of planned chemotherapy
Initial: 600 U/kg IV weekly until completion of a chemotherapy course
Dose Reduction: Reduce by 25% if
1. Hgb increases >1g/dL in any 2-week period
2. Hgb reaches a level needed to avoid a RBC transfusion
Withhold dose if Hgb exceeds level needed to avoid RBC transfusion; reinitiate at a dose 25% below previous dose when Hgb approaches a level where RBC transfusions may be required
Dose Increase: After initial 4 weeks of therapy, if Hgb increases by <1g/dL and remains below 10g/dL increase dose to 900 U/kg (max 60,000 U) weekly
D/C therapy if there is no response in Hgb levels or if RBC transfusions are still required after 8 weeks

Dose Reduction: Reduce by 25% if:
1. Hgb increases >1g/dL in any 2-week period
2. Hgb reaches a level needed to avoid a RBC transfusion

Withhold dose if Hgb exceeds level needed to avoid RBC transfusion; reinitiate at a dose 25% below previous dose when Hgb approaches a level where RBC transfusions may be required

Dose Increase: After initial 4 weeks of therapy, if Hgb increases by <1g/dL and remains below 10g/dL increase dose to 300 U/kg 3X weekly or 60,000 U weekly

D/C therapy if there is no response in Hgb levels or if RBC transfusions are still required after 8 weeks

Surgery Patients:
300 U/kg/day SQ for 10 days before, on the day of, and for 4 days after surgery; or 600 U/kg SQ in 4 doses administered 21, 14, and 7 days before surgery and on the day of surgery

DVT prophylaxis is recommended

ADMINISTRATION

IV/SQ route

Do not shake; do not use if shaken or frozen

Discard unused portions in preservative-free vials; do not re-enter preservative-free vials

Do not dilute

Preservative-free vials may be admixed in a syringe w/ bacteriostatic 0.9% NaCl Inj, w/ benzyl alcohol 0.9% in a 1:1 ratio

HOW SUPPLIED

Inj: 2000 U/mL, 3000 U/mL, 4000 U/mL, 10,000 U/mL, 40,000 U/mL [single-dose vial]; 10,000 U/mL [2mL], 20,000 U/mL [1mL] [multidose vial]

CONTRAINDICATIONS

Uncontrolled HTN, pure red cell aplasia (PRCA) that begins after treatment with epoetin alfa or other erythropoietin protein drugs. (Multidose Vials) Neonates, infants, pregnant women, and nursing mothers.

WARNINGS/PRECAUTIONS

Not indicated for use in patients with cancer receiving hormonal agents, biologic products, or radiotherapy, unless also receiving concomitant myelosuppressive chemotherapy; in patients scheduled for surgery who are willing to donate autologous blood; in patients undergoing cardiac/vascular surgery, or as a substitute for RBC transfusions in patients requiring immediate correction of anemia. Evaluate transferrin saturation and serum ferritin prior to and during treatment; administer supplemental iron when serum ferritin is <100mcg/L or serum transferrin saturation is <20%. Correct/exclude other causes of anemia (eg, vitamin deficiency, metabolic/chronic inflammatory conditions, bleeding) before initiating therapy. Hypertensive encephalopathy and seizures reported in patients with CKD. Appropriately control HTN prior to initiation of and during treatment; reduce/withhold therapy if BP becomes difficult to control. PRCA and severe anemia, with or without other cytopenias that arise following development of neutralizing antibodies to erythropoietin reported. Withhold and evaluate for neutralizing antibodies to erythropoietin if severe anemia and low reticulocyte count develop; d/c permanently if PRCA develops, and do not switch to other erythropoiesis-stimulating agents. Serious allergic reactions may occur; immediately and permanently d/c therapy. Contains albumin; may carry an extremely remote risk for transmission of viral diseases or Creutzfeldt-Jakob disease. Patients may require adjustments in their dialysis prescriptions after initiation of therapy, or require increased anticoagulation with heparin to prevent clotting of extracorporeal circuit during hemodialysis. Multidose vial contains benzyl alcohol; benzyl alcohol is associated with serious adverse events and death, particularly in pediatric patients.

ADVERSE REACTIONS

MI, stroke, VTE, thrombosis of vascular access, tumor progression/recurrence, pyrexia, N/V, HTN, cough, arthralgia, pruritus, rash, headache, dizziness.

NURSING CONSIDERATIONS

Assessment: Assess for uncontrolled HTN, previous hypersensitivity to the drug, causes of anemia, pregnancy/nursing status, and other conditions where treatment is contraindicated or cautioned. Obtain baseline Hgb levels, transferrin saturation, and serum ferritin.

Monitoring: Monitor for signs/symptoms of an allergic reaction, CV/thromboembolic events, stroke, premonitory neurologic symptoms, PRCA, severe anemia, progression/recurrence of tumor, and other adverse reactions. Monitor BP, transferrin saturation, and serum ferritin. Following initiation of therapy and after each dose adjustment, monitor Hgb weekly until Hgb is stable and sufficient to minimize need for RBC transfusion.

Patient Counseling: Inform of the risks/benefits of therapy and of the increased risks of mortality, serious CV reactions, thromboembolic reactions, stroke, and tumor progression. Advise of the need to have regular lab tests for Hgb. Inform cancer patients that they must sign the patient-physician acknowledgment form prior to therapy. Instruct to undergo regular BP monitoring, adhere to prescribed antihypertensive regimen, and follow recommended dietary restrictions. Advise to contact physician for new-onset neurologic symptoms or change in seizure frequency. Instruct regarding proper disposal of used syringes and caution against the reuse of needles, syringes, or unused portions of single-dose vials.

Storage: 2-8°C (36-46°F). Do not freeze; do not use if it has been frozen. Protect from light. Discard unused portions of multidose vials 21 days after initial entry.

PROCTOFOAM-HC – hydrocortisone acetate/pramoxine hydrochloride **RX**

Class: Anesthetic/corticosteroid

ADULT DOSAGE

Inflammatory and Pruritic Manifestations of Corticosteroid-Responsive Dermatoses

Anal Region:

Apply to affected area tid-qid

D/C if no evidence of improvement w/in 2 or 3 weeks after starting therapy, or if condition worsens

PEDIATRIC DOSAGE

Inflammatory and Pruritic Manifestations of Corticosteroid-Responsive Dermatoses

Anal Region:

Apply to affected area tid-qid; use least amount effective for condition

D/C if no evidence of improvement w/in 2 or 3 weeks after starting therapy, or if condition worsens

ADMINISTRATION

Topical route

For anal administration, use the applicator supplied
For perianal use, transfer a small quantity to a tissue and rub in gently

Directions for Use

1. Shake foam container vigorously for 5-10 sec before each use; do not remove container cap during use of the product
2. Hold container upright on a level surface and gently place the tip of the applicator onto the nose of the container cap; pull plunger past the fill line on the applicator barrel
3. To fill applicator barrel, press down firmly on cap flanges, hold for 1-2 sec, and release
4. Wait 5-10 sec to allow foam to expand in applicator barrel; repeat until foam reaches fill line. It usually requires 3-4 pumps for foam to reach fill line
5. Remove applicator from container cap; if foam goes beyond fill line, it will continue to expand and flow backwards, resulting in foam build-up under cap
6. Gently insert tip into anus; once in place, push plunger to expel foam, then withdraw applicator
7. After each use, applicator parts should be pulled apart for thorough cleaning w/ warm water. Since some foam will appear under the cap, the cap and underlying tip should be pulled apart and rinsed to help prevent build-up of foam and possible blockage

Priming

Prime the container by pressing down firmly on flanges and then release. W/ initial priming, a burst of air may come out of the container; it usually requires 1-2 pumps for foam to appear

HOW SUPPLIED

Foam: (Hydrocortisone-Pramoxine) 1%-1% [10g]

WARNINGS/PRECAUTIONS

Do not insert any part of the aerosol container directly into the anus. Avoid contact with eyes. Contents of the container are under pressure; do not burn or puncture. Systemic absorption may produce reversible hypothalamic-pituitary-adrenal (HPA) axis suppression, manifestations of Cushing's syndrome, hyperglycemia, and glucosuria. Application of more potent steroids, use over large surface areas, prolonged use, and the addition of occlusive dressings may augment systemic absorption. Periodically evaluate for evidence of HPA axis suppression when a large dose is applied to a large surface area or under an occlusive dressing; if noted, withdraw the drug, reduce frequency of application, or substitute with a less potent steroid. Infrequently, signs and symptoms of steroid withdrawal may occur, requiring supplemental systemic corticosteroids. D/C and institute appropriate therapy if irritation develops. Use appropriate antifungal or antibacterial agent in the presence of dermatological infections; if a favorable response does not occur promptly, d/c until infection has been adequately controlled. Pediatric patients may be more susceptible to systemic toxicity. Chronic therapy may interfere with growth and development of pediatric patients. Caution in elderly.

ADVERSE REACTIONS

Burning, itching, irritation, dryness, folliculitis, hypertrichosis, acneiform eruptions, hypopigmentation, perioral dermatitis, allergic contact dermatitis, skin maceration, secondary infection, skin atrophy, striae, miliaria.

NURSING CONSIDERATIONS

Assessment: Assess for drug hypersensitivity, conditions that augment systemic absorption, dermatological infections, and pregnancy/nursing status.

Monitoring: Monitor for signs/symptoms of HPA axis suppression, Cushing's syndrome, hyperglycemia, glucosuria, steroid withdrawal, irritation, dermatological infections, systemic toxicity in pediatric patients, and other adverse reactions. When a large dose is applied to a large surface area or under an occlusive dressing, monitor for HPA axis suppression by using urinary free cortisol and adrenocorticotropic hormone stimulation tests. Monitor for improvement or worsening of condition.

Patient Counseling: Instruct to use ud (anal or perianal use only) and to avoid contact with eyes. Advise not to use for any disorder other than for which it was prescribed. Instruct to report any signs of adverse reactions.

Storage: 20-25°C (68-77°F). Do not store at temperatures >49°C (120°F). Do not refrigerate.

PROGRAF – tacrolimus

RX

Class: Macrolide immunosuppressant

Should only be prescribed by physicians experienced in immunosuppressive therapy and management of organ transplant patients. Manage patients in facilities equipped and staffed with adequate lab and supportive medical resources. Physician responsible for maintenance therapy should have complete information requisite for patient follow-up. Immunosuppression may lead to increased risk of lymphoma and other malignancies, particularly of the skin. Increased susceptibility to infections (bacterial, viral, fungal, protozoal, opportunistic).

ADULT DOSAGE

Hepatic Transplant

Prophylaxis of Organ Rejection in Patients Receiving Allogeneic Liver Transplant:

Cap:
Initial: 0.1-0.15mg/kg/day
Titrate: Based on clinical assessments of rejection and tolerability
Maint: Lower dosages than the initial dosage may be sufficient
Administer no sooner than 6 hrs after liver transplant

Give daily doses as 2 divided doses, q12h

Adjunct therapy w/ adrenal corticosteroids is recommended early post-transplant

If receiving tacrolimus IV infusion, give 1st oral dose 8-12 hrs after discontinuing the IV infusion

Observed Tacrolimus Whole Blood Trough Concentrations w/ Liver Transplant:
Month 1-12: 5-20ng/mL
IV:
Initial: 0.03-0.05mg/kg/day

Renal Transplant

Prophylaxis of Organ Rejection in Patients Receiving Allogeneic Kidney Transplant:

Cap:
Initial: 0.2mg/kg/day in combination w/ azathioprine or 0.1mg/kg/day in combination w/ mycophenolate mofetil/IL-2 receptor antagonist

PEDIATRIC DOSAGE

Hepatic Transplant

Cap:
Initial: 0.15-0.2mg/kg/day as 2 divided doses, q12h

Observed Tacrolimus Whole Blood Trough Concentrations w/ Liver Transplant:
Month 1-12: 5-20ng/mL

Recommended to be used concomitantly w/ adrenal corticosteroids
IV:
Initial: 0.03-0.05mg/kg/day

Titrate: Based on clinical assessments of rejection and tolerability
Maint: Lower dosages than the initial dosage may be sufficient
May administer w/in 24 hrs of kidney transplant, but should be delayed until renal function has recovered

Give daily doses as 2 divided doses, q12h

Adjunct therapy w/ adrenal corticosteroids is recommended early post-transplant
If receiving tacrolimus IV infusion, give 1st oral dose 8-12 hrs after discontinuing the IV infusion

Observed Tacrolimus Whole Blood Trough Concentrations w/ Kidney Transplant:
W/ Azathioprine:
Month 1-3: 7-20ng/mL
Month 4-12: 5-15ng/mL
W/ Mycophenolate Mofetil/IL-2 Receptor Antagonist:
Month 1-12: 4-11ng/mL
IV:
Initial: 0.03-0.05mg/kg/day

Cardiac Transplant

Prophylaxis of Organ Rejection in Patients Receiving Allogeneic Heart Transplant:
Cap:
Initial: 0.075mg/kg/day
Titrate: Based on clinical assessments of rejection and tolerability
Maint: Lower dosages than the initial dosage may be sufficient
Administer no sooner than 6 hrs after heart transplant

Give daily doses as 2 divided doses, q12h

Adjunct therapy w/ adrenal corticosteroids is recommended early post-transplant
Recommended to be used concomitantly w/ azathioprine or mycophenolate mofetil

If receiving tacrolimus IV infusion, give 1st oral dose 8-12 hrs after discontinuing the IV infusion

Observed Tacrolimus Whole Blood Trough Concentrations w/ Heart Transplant:
Month 1-3: 10-20ng/mL
Month ≥4: 5-15ng/mL
IV:
Initial: 0.01mg/kg/day

DOSE MODIFICATION

Renal Impairment

Liver/Heart Transplant:
Preexisting Renal Impairment: Start at lower end of dosing range
Kidney Transplant:
Postoperative Oliguria: Initial dose should be administered no sooner than 6 hrs and w/in 24 hrs of transplantation, but may be delayed until renal function shows evidence of recovery

Hepatic Impairment

Severe (Child-Pugh ≥10): May require lower doses

Elderly

Start at lower end of dosing range

Other Important Modifications

Black patients may require higher doses

ADMINISTRATION

Oral/IV route

Inj should be used only as a continuous IV infusion and when the patient cannot tolerate oral administration of cap

Cap

Take consistently w/ or w/o food

Inj

Dilute product w/ 0.9% NaCl inj or D5 inj to concentration between 0.004mg/mL and 0.02mg/mL prior to use

Diluted infusion sol should be stored in glass or polyethylene containers and should be discarded after 24 hrs; do not store in PVC container due to decreased stability and potential for extraction of phthalates; in situations where more dilute sol are used (eg, pediatric dosing), PVC-free tubing should likewise be used to minimize the potential for significant drug adsorption onto tubing

Should not be mixed or coinfused w/ sol of pH ≥9 (eg, ganciclovir, acyclovir)

HOW SUPPLIED

Cap: 0.5mg, 1mg, 5mg; Inj: 5mg/mL [1mL]

CONTRAINDICATIONS

(Inj) Hypersensitivity to polyoxyl 60 hydrogenated castor oil (HCO-60).

WARNINGS/PRECAUTIONS

Limit exposure to sunlight and UV light in patients at increased risk for skin cancer. Increased risk for polyoma virus infections, cytomegalovirus (CMV) viremia, and CMV disease. Polyoma virus-associated nephropathy (PVAN) reported; may lead to renal function deterioration and kidney graft loss. Progressive multifocal leukoencephalopathy (PML) reported; consider PML in differential diagnosis in patients reporting neurological symptoms and consider consultation with a neurologist. Consider reductions in immunosuppression if CMV viremia and/or CMV disease, or if evidence of PVAN or PML develops. May cause new onset diabetes mellitus; closely monitor blood glucose concentrations. May cause acute/chronic nephrotoxicity; closely monitor patients with renal dysfunction. Consider changing to another immunosuppressive therapy in patients with persistent SrCr elevations unresponsive to dose adjustments. May cause neurotoxicity (eg, posterior reversible encephalopathy syndrome [PRES], delirium, coma); if PRES is suspected or diagnosed, maintain BP control and immediately reduce immunosuppression. Hyperkalemia and HTN reported. May prolong the QT/QTc interval and may cause torsades de pointes; avoid in patients with congenital long QT syndrome and consider obtaining ECGs and monitoring electrolytes (Mg^{2+}, K^+, Ca^{2+}) periodically in patients with congestive heart failure (CHF), bradyarrhythmias, those taking certain antiarrhythmic medications or other medicinal products that lead to QT prolongation, and those with electrolyte disturbances. Myocardial hypertrophy reported; consider dose reduction or discontinuation if diagnosed and consider echocardiographic evaluation in patients who develop renal failure or clinical manifestations of ventricular dysfunction. Pure red cell aplasia (PRCA) reported; consider discontinuation if diagnosed. GI perforation reported; institute appropriate medical/surgical management promptly. Caution in elderly. (Inj) Anaphylactic reactions may occur; should be reserved for patients unable to take cap orally. Patients should be under continuous observation for at least the first 30 min following the start of infusion and at frequent intervals thereafter; d/c infusion if signs/symptoms of anaphylaxis occur.

ADVERSE REACTIONS

Lymphoma, malignancies, infections, tremor, HTN, abnormal renal function, headache, insomnia, hyperglycemia, hyperkalemia, hypomagnesemia, diarrhea, N/V, paresthesia.

DRUG INTERACTIONS

Do not use simultaneously with cyclosporine; d/c tacrolimus or cyclosporine at least 24 hrs before initiating the other. Not recommended with sirolimus in liver and heart transplant; safety and efficacy not established in kidney transplant. Due to potential for additive/synergistic renal impairment, caution with drugs that may be associated with renal dysfunction (eg, aminoglycosides, ganciclovir, amphotericin B). Increased whole blood concentrations with CYP3A inhibitors (eg, antifungals, calcium channel blockers [CCBs], macrolide antibiotics), and magnesium and aluminum hydroxide antacids. Decreased whole blood concentrations with CYP3A inducers. May increase mycophenolic acid (MPA) exposure after crossover from cyclosporine to tacrolimus in patients concomitantly receiving MPA-containing products. Avoid grapefruit or grapefruit juice. Avoid with nelfinavir unless the benefits outweigh the risks. Monitor whole blood concentrations and adjust tacrolimus dose if used concomitantly with protease inhibitors (eg, ritonavir, telaprevir, boceprevir), CCBs (eg, verapamil, diltiazem, nifedipine), erythromycin, clarithromycin, troleandomycin, chloramphenicol, rifampin, rifabutin, phenytoin, carbamazepine, phenobarbital, St. John's wort, magnesium and aluminum hydroxide antacids, bromocriptine, nefazodone, metoclopramide, danazol, ethinyl estradiol, amiodarone, methylprednisolone, or CYP3A inhibitors/inducers. Monitor whole blood concentrations and adjust tacrolimus dose when concomitant use of antifungal drugs (eg, azoles, caspofungin) with tacrolimus is initiated or discontinued; initially reduce tacrolimus dose to 1/3 of the original dose when initiating therapy with voriconazole or posaconazole. May increase levels of phenytoin; monitor phenytoin levels and adjust phenytoin dose as needed. Caution with antihypertensive agents (eg, K^+-sparing diuretics, ACE inhibitors, ARBs) or other agents associated with hyperkalemia. Reduce tacrolimus dose, closely monitor tacrolimus whole blood concentrations, and monitor for QT prolongation when coadministered with CYP3A4 substrates and/or inhibitors that also have the potential to prolong the QT interval. Amiodarone may increase whole blood concentrations with or without concurrent QT prolongation. Avoid live vaccines during therapy. Caution with concomitant immunosuppressants.

NURSING CONSIDERATIONS

Assessment: Assess for drug hypersensitivity, congenital long QT syndrome, CHF, bradyarrhythmias, electrolyte disturbances, renal/hepatic impairment, pregnancy/nursing status, and possible drug interactions. (Inj) Assess for hypersensitivity to HCO-60.

Monitoring: Monitor tacrolimus blood concentrations in conjunction with other laboratory and clinical parameters. Monitor for lymphomas and other malignancies, infections, neurotoxicity, HTN, QT prolongation, PRCA, GI perforation, and other adverse reactions. Monitor serum K^+ and glucose concentrations. (Inj) Monitor for anaphylactic reactions.

Patient Counseling: Inform of the risks and benefits of therapy. Advise to take medicine at the same 12-hr interval every day and not to eat grapefruit or drink grapefruit juice in combination with the drug. Advise to limit exposure to sunlight and UV light by wearing protective clothing and use a sunscreen with a high protection factor. Instruct to contact physician if frequent urination, increased thirst or hunger, vision changes, deliriums, tremors, or any symptoms of infection develop. Advise to attend all visits and complete all blood tests ordered by medical team. Inform that therapy may cause high BP, which may require treatment with antihypertensive therapy. Instruct to inform physician if patient plans to become pregnant or breastfeed or when they start or stop taking all medications (prescription and nonprescription medicines, natural/herbal remedies, nutritional supplements, vitamins). Inform that therapy may interfere with the usual response to immunizations and that live vaccines should be avoided.

Storage: (Cap) 25°C (77°F); excursions permitted to 15-30°C (59-86°F). (Inj) 5-25°C (41-77°F).

PROMACTA – eltrombopag

Class: Thrombopoietin receptor agonist

RX

May increase risk of hepatic decompensation in patients w/ chronic hepatitis C when given in combination w/ interferon and ribavirin.

ADULT DOSAGE

Chronic Immune Thrombocytopenia

W/ Insufficient Response to Corticosteroids, Immunoglobulins, or Splenectomy:

Initial: 50mg qd

Titrate: Adjust to the lowest dose to achieve and maintain a platelet count $\geq 50 \times 10^9$/L

Max: 75mg/day

Dose Adjustment Based on Platelet Counts:

<50 x 10^9/L Following at Least 2 Weeks of Therapy:

Increase daily dose by 25mg to a max of 75mg/day; patients taking 12.5mg qd, increase to 25mg qd before increasing dose amount by 25mg

≥200-≤400 x 10^9/L:

Decrease daily dose by 25mg; wait 2 weeks to assess the effects and any subsequent dose adjustments

>400 x 10^9/L:

Stop therapy and increase frequency of platelet monitoring to twice weekly; once platelet count is <150 x 10^9/L, reinitiate at a daily dose reduced by 25mg or reinitiate at a daily dose of 12.5mg for patients taking 25mg qd

>400 x 10^9/L After 2 Weeks of Therapy at Lowest Dose:

D/C therapy

Chronic Hepatitis C-Associated Thrombocytopenia

To allow the initiation and maint of interferon-based therapy

PEDIATRIC DOSAGE

Pediatric use may not have been established

Initial: 25mg qd
Titrate: Adjust dose in 25mg increments every 2 weeks as necessary to achieve target platelet count required to initiate antiviral therapy. During antiviral therapy, adjust dose to avoid dose reductions of peginterferon
Max: 100mg/day

Dose Adjustment Based on Platelet Counts:
<50 x 10^9/L Following at Least 2 Weeks of Therapy:
Increase daily dose by 25mg to a max of 100mg/day
≥200-≤400 x 10^9/L:
Decrease daily dose by 25mg; wait 2 weeks to assess the effects and any subsequent dose adjustments
>400 x 10^9/L:
Stop therapy and increase frequency of platelet monitoring to twice weekly; once platelet count is <150 x 10^9/L, reinitiate at a daily dose reduced by 25mg or reinitiate at a daily dose of 12.5mg for patients taking 25mg qd
>400 x 10^9/L After 2 Weeks of Therapy at Lowest Dose:
D/C therapy

Severe Aplastic Anemia

W/ Insufficient Response to Immunosuppressive Therapy:
Initial: 50mg qd
Titrate: Adjust dose in 50mg increments every 2 weeks as necessary to achieve the target platelet count ≥50 x 10^9/L
Max: 150mg/day

Dose Adjustment Based on Platelet Counts:
<50 x 10^9/L Following at Least 2 Weeks of Therapy:
Increase daily dose by 50mg to a max of 150mg/day; patients taking 25mg qd, increase to 50mg qd before increasing dose amount by 50mg
≥200-≤400 x 10^9/L:
Decrease daily dose by 50mg; wait 2 weeks to assess the effects and any subsequent dose adjustments
>400 x 10^9/L:
Stop therapy for 1 week; once platelet count is <150 x 10^9/L, reinitiate therapy at a dose reduced by 50mg
>400 x 10^9/L After 2 Weeks of Therapy at Lowest Dose:
D/C therapy

DOSE MODIFICATION

Concomitant Medications

Chronic Immune Thrombocytopenia:
Modify dosage regimen of concomitant medications for therapy to avoid excessive increases in platelet counts; do not administer >1 dose of eltrombopag w/in any 24-hr period

Hepatic Impairment

Mild to Severe (Child-Pugh Class A, B, C):
Chronic Immune Thrombocytopenia:
Initial: 25mg qd; after initiating therapy or after any subsequent dosing increase, wait 3 weeks before increasing the dose
Severe Aplastic Anemia:
Initial: 25mg qd

East Asian Ancestry w/ Hepatic Impairment (Child-Pugh Class A, B, C):
Chronic Immune Thrombocytopenia:
Initial: 12.5mg qd

Discontinuation

Chronic Immune Thrombocytopenia: D/C if platelet count does not increase to a sufficient level after 4 weeks of therapy at max daily dose

Chronic Hepatitis C-Associated Thrombocytopenia: D/C therapy when antiviral therapy is discontinued; important liver test abnormalities may necessitate discontinuation

Severe Aplastic Anemia: D/C therapy if no hematologic response occurs after 16 weeks of therapy. Consider discontinuation if new cytogenetic abnormalities or important liver test abnormalities are observed

Other Important Modifications

Chronic Immune Thrombocytopenia/Severe Aplastic Anemia:
East Asian Ancestry:
Initial: 25mg qd

ADMINISTRATION

Oral route

Take on empty stomach (1 hr ac or 2 hrs pc)
Allow at least a 4-hr interval between therapy and other medications (eg, antacids), Ca^{2+}-rich foods (eg, dairy products, Ca^{2+} fortified juices), or supplements containing polyvalent cations (eg, iron, Ca^{2+}, aluminum, Mg^{2+}, selenium, zinc)

HOW SUPPLIED

Tab: 12.5mg, 25mg, 50mg, 75mg, 100mg

WARNINGS/PRECAUTIONS

Should not be used to normalize platelet counts. Should only be used in patients w/ ITP whose degree of thrombocytopenia and clinical condition increase the risk for bleeding. Liver enzyme elevations and indirect hyperbilirubinemia may occur; if bilirubin is elevated, perform fractionation. D/C if ALT levels increase to ≥3X ULN in patients w/ normal liver function or ≥3X baseline in patients w/ pretreatment elevations in transaminases, and are progressively increasing or persistent for ≥4 weeks, or accompanied by increased direct bilirubin, or by clinical symptoms of liver injury or evidence for hepatic decompensation. Hepatotoxicity may reoccur w/ reinitiation; caution w/ reintroduction of therapy and measure LFTs weekly during the dose adjustment phase. If liver test abnormalities persist, worsen or reoccur, then permanently d/c therapy. Thrombotic/thromboembolic complications may result from increases in platelet counts; caution in patients w/ known risk factors for thromboembolism (eg, factor V Leiden, antithrombin III deficiency, antiphospholipid syndrome, chronic liver disease). Development or worsening of cataracts reported.

ADVERSE REACTIONS

Hepatic decompensation, headache, N/V, diarrhea, URTI, increased ALT/AST, oropharyngeal pain, pharyngitis, back pain, influenza, pyrexia, fatigue, dyspnea, pain in extremity, dizziness.

DRUG INTERACTIONS

See Boxed Warning. Do not take w/in 4 hrs of any medications or products containing polyvalent cations (eg, antacids, dairy products, mineral supplements). Increases rosuvastatin levels; recommended to reduce rosuvastatin by 50%. Caution w/ substrates of organic anion transporting polypeptide 1B1 (eg, atorvastatin, bosentan, glyburide) or breast cancer resistance protein (eg, imatinib, irinotecan, methotrexate); monitor for signs/symptoms of excessive exposure and consider dose reduction of these drugs. Lopinavir/ritonavir may decrease plasma exposure.

NURSING CONSIDERATIONS

Assessment: Assess for degree of thrombocytopenia, risk factors for thromboembolism, renal/hepatic impairment, pregnancy/nursing status, and for possible drug interactions. Obtain baseline CBCs w/ differential, including platelet count, and LFTs. Perform a baseline ocular exam.

Monitoring: Monitor for thrombotic/thromboembolic complications, hepatotoxicity, hepatic decompensation in patients w/ chronic hepatitis C, cataracts, and other adverse reactions. Closely monitor patients w/ renal impairment. Monitor LFTs every 2 weeks during dose adjustment phase, then monthly following establishment of a stable dose. If abnormal LFT levels are detected, repeat tests w/in 3-5 days. If the abnormalities are confirmed, monitor serum LFT tests weekly until resolved or stabilized. Perform a regular ocular exam. Monitor platelet counts every week prior to starting antiviral therapy in patients w/ chronic hepatitis C. Monitor CBCs w/ differentials, including platelets counts, weekly during therapy until a stable platelet count is achieved. Obtain CBCs w/ differentials, including platelet counts, monthly thereafter and then weekly for at least 4 weeks after discontinuation.

Patient Counseling: Inform about the risks and benefits of therapy. Inform that therapy may be associated w/ hepatobiliary lab abnormalities. Advise patients w/ chronic hepatitis C and cirrhosis that hepatic decompensation may occur when receiving alfa interferon therapy. Advise to avoid situations or medications that may increase risk for bleeding and to report to physician any signs/symptoms of liver problems immediately. Inform that thrombocytopenia and risk of bleeding may reoccur upon discontinuation, particularly if therapy is discontinued while on anticoagulants/antiplatelet agents. Inform that excessive dose may result in excessive platelet counts and risk for thrombotic/thromboembolic complications. Advise to have a baseline ocular exam prior to administration of therapy and be monitored for signs/symptoms of cataracts during therapy. Advise to keep at least a 4-hr interval between therapy and foods, mineral supplements, and antacids that contain polyvalent cations.

Storage: 20-25°C (68-77°F); excursions permitted to 15-30°C (59-86°F).

PROMETHAZINE – promethazine hydrochloride RX

Class: Phenothiazine derivative

Do not be use in pediatric patients <2 yrs of age; potential for fatal respiratory depression. Caution when administering to patients ≥2 yrs of age; use lowest effective dose and avoid concomitant administration of other drugs with respiratory depressant effects.

OTHER BRAND NAMES

Phenadoz, Promethegan

ADULT DOSAGE

Nausea/Vomiting

Active Therapy:
12.5-25mg q4-6h, prn

Prophylaxis During Surgery and Postoperative Period:
25mg q4-6h, prn

Sedation

Nighttime, Presurgical, or Obstetrical Sedation:
25-50mg

Pre- and Postoperative Use

Preoperative Medication:
50mg in combination w/ reduced dose of narcotic or barbiturate and the required amount of a belladonna alkaloid

Postoperative Sedation/Adjunctive Use w/ Analgesics:
25-50mg

Allergies

Usual: 25mg qhs or 12.5mg ac and hs; may give 6.25-12.5mg tid

Adjust to lowest effective dose

Motion Sickness

Initial: 25mg 30-60 min before travel and repeat after 8-12 hrs, if necessary
Maint: 25mg bid (on arising and before pm meal)

Other Indications

Perennial and seasonal allergic rhinitis, vasomotor rhinitis, allergic conjunctivitis due to inhalant allergens and foods, mild uncomplicated allergic skin manifestations of urticaria and angioedema, amelioration of allergic reactions to blood or plasma, and dermographism. Adjunct therapy in anaphylactic reactions. Pre/postoperative, or obstetric sedation. Prevention and control of N/V associated w/ certain types of anesthesia and surgery. Adjunct therapy w/ meperidine or other analgesics for control of postoperative pain. Sedation, relief of apprehension, and production of light sleep. Active and prophylactic treatment of motion sickness. Antiemetic in postoperative patients

PEDIATRIC DOSAGE

Allergies

≥2 Years:
Usual: 25mg qhs or 12.5mg ac and hs; may give 6.25-12.5mg tid

Adjust to lowest effective dose

Nausea/Vomiting

≥2 Years:
Active Therapy:
Usual: 0.5mg/lb; adjust dose based on patient age/weight and severity of condition

Prophylaxis During Surgery and the Postoperative Period:
25mg q4-6h, prn

Sedation

≥2 Years:
12.5-25mg qhs

Pre- and Postoperative Use

Preoperative Medication:
0.5mg/lb in combination w/ reduced dose of narcotic or barbiturate and the appropriate dose of an atropine-like drug

Postoperative Sedation/Adjunctive Use w/ Analgesics:
12.5-25mg

Motion Sickness

≥2 Years:
12.5-25mg bid

Other Indications

Perennial and seasonal allergic rhinitis, vasomotor rhinitis, allergic conjunctivitis due to inhalant allergens and foods, mild uncomplicated allergic skin manifestations of urticaria and angioedema, amelioration of allergic reactions to blood or plasma, and dermographism. Adjunct therapy in anaphylactic reactions. Pre/postoperative, or obstetric sedation. Prevention and control of N/V associated w/ certain types of anesthesia and surgery. Adjunct therapy w/ meperidine or other analgesics for control of postoperative pain. Sedation, relief of apprehension, and production of light sleep. Active and prophylactic treatment of motion sickness. Antiemetic in postoperative patients

DOSE MODIFICATION

Elderly

Start at lower end of dosing range

ADMINISTRATION

Oral/rectal route

HOW SUPPLIED

Sup: (Phenadoz) 12.5mg, 25mg, (Promethegan) 50mg; Syrup: 6.25mg/5mL [118mL, 237mL, 473mL] Tab: 12.5mg*, 25mg*, 50mg *scored

CONTRAINDICATIONS

Treatment of lower respiratory tract symptoms (eg, asthma), comatose states. (Promethegan/Syrup/Tab) Pediatric patients <2 yrs of age.

WARNINGS/PRECAUTIONS

Not recommended for uncomplicated vomiting in pediatric patients; should be limited to prolonged vomiting of known etiology. Avoid in pediatric patients whose signs and symptoms may suggest Reye's syndrome or other hepatic diseases. May impair mental/physical abilities. May lead to potentially fatal respiratory depression; avoid with compromised respiratory function. May lower seizure threshold. Caution with bone marrow depression; leukopenia and agranulocytosis reported. Neuroleptic malignant syndrome (NMS) reported alone or with antipsychotics; d/c immediately and monitor. Hallucinations and convulsions may occur in pediatric patients. Acutely ill pediatric patients associated with dehydration may have an increased susceptibility to dystonias. Cholestatic jaundice reported. Caution with narrow-angle glaucoma, prostatic hypertrophy, stenosing peptic ulcer, bladder-neck or pyloroduodenal obstruction, cardiovascular disease, and hepatic impairment. Lab test interactions may occur. Caution in elderly patients.

ADVERSE REACTIONS

Respiratory depression, drowsiness, sedation, blurred vision, dizziness, increased or decreased BP, urticaria, dry mouth, N/V, hallucination, leukopenia, apnea, photosensitivity.

DRUG INTERACTIONS

See Boxed Warning. May increase incidence of extrapyramidal effects with MAOIs. May increase, prolong, or intensify the sedative action of other CNS depressants, (eg, alcohol, sedatives/hypnotics, narcotics, TCAs); avoid such agents or reduce dosage. Reduce dose of barbiturates by at least 50% if given concomitantly. Reduce dose of narcotics by 25-50% if given concomitantly. May reverse vasopressor effect of epinephrine; do not use to treat promethazine overdose. Caution with anticholinergics. Caution with medications that may affect seizure threshold (eg, narcotics, local anesthetics). Leukopenia and agranulocytosis reported when used with other known marrow-toxic agents.

NURSING CONSIDERATIONS

Assessment: Assess for drug hypersensitivity or have had idiosyncratic reaction to phenothiazines, bone marrow depression, narrow-angle glaucoma, pregnancy/nursing status, possible drug interactions, or any other conditions where treatment is contraindicated or cautioned. Assess for signs/symptoms of hepatic diseases, or Reye's syndrome in pediatric patients.

Monitoring: Monitor for signs/symptoms of CNS/respiratory depression, NMS, seizures, cholestatic jaundice, leukopenia, agranulocytosis, and other adverse reactions. Monitor for hallucinations, convulsions, extrapyramidal symptoms, respiratory depression, and dystonias in pediatric patients.

Patient Counseling: Inform that therapy may cause drowsiness and impairment of mental and/or physical abilities. Counsel to report any involuntary muscle movements. Instruct to avoid alcohol use, prolonged sun exposure, and concomitant use of other CNS depressants.

Storage: (Syrup/Tab) 20-25°C (68-77°F). (Sup) 2-8°C (36-46°F). (Syrup) Protect from light.

PROMETHAZINE VC WITH CODEINE – codeine phosphate/phenylephrine hydrochloride/promethazine hydrochloride CV

Class: Antitussive/phenothiazine derivative/sympathomimetic

Contraindicated in pediatric patients <6 yrs of age. Concomitant administration of promethazine products with other respiratory depressants is associated with respiratory depression, and sometimes death, in pediatric patients. Respiratory depression, including fatalities, have been reported with use of promethazine in patients <2 yrs of age. Respiratory depression and death reported in children who received codeine following tonsillectomy and/or adenoidectomy and had evidence of being ultra-rapid metabolizers of codeine due to a CYP2D6 polymorphism.

ADULT DOSAGE

Cough/Cold/Allergy

Temporary Relief of Coughs and Upper Respiratory Symptoms (eg, Nasal Congestion) Associated w/ Allergy or the Common Cold:
5mL q4-6h
Max: 30mL/24 hrs

PEDIATRIC DOSAGE

Cough/Cold/Allergy

Temporary Relief of Coughs and Upper Respiratory Symptoms (eg, Nasal Congestion) Associated w/ Allergy or the Common Cold:

6-<12 Years:
2.5-5mL q4-6h
Max: 30mL/24 hrs

≥12 Years:
5mL q4-6h
Max: 30mL/24 hrs

DOSE MODIFICATION

Elderly

Start at lower end of dosing range

ADMINISTRATION

Oral route

Measure w/ an accurate measuring device

HOW SUPPLIED

Syrup: (Codeine-Promethazine-Phenylephrine) 10mg-6.25mg-5mg/5mL [118mL, 237mL, 473mL]

CONTRAINDICATIONS

Pediatric patients <6 yrs of age, postoperative pain management in children who have undergone tonsillectomy and/or adenoidectomy, comatose states, treatment of lower respiratory tract symptoms (eg, asthma), HTN, peripheral vascular insufficiency, concomitant use with MAOIs.

WARNINGS/PRECAUTIONS

Should only be given to a pregnant woman if clearly needed. Caution in elderly. Lab test interactions may occur. Codeine: Do not increase dose if cough fails to respond to treatment. May cause/aggravate constipation. May release histamine; caution in atopic children. Capacity to elevate CSF pressure and respiratory depressant effects may be markedly exaggerated in head injury, intracranial lesions, or with preexisting increase in intracranial pressure. May obscure clinical course in patients with head injuries. Avoid with acute febrile illness with productive cough or in chronic respiratory disease. May produce orthostatic hypotension in ambulatory patients. Give with caution and reduce initial dose with acute abdominal conditions, convulsive disorders, significant hepatic/renal impairment, fever, hypothyroidism, Addison's disease, ulcerative colitis, prostatic hypertrophy, recent GI or urinary tract surgery, and in very young, elderly, or debilitated patients. Use lowest effective dose for the shortest period of time. Potential for abuse and dependence. Promethazine: May impair mental/physical abilities. May lead to potentially fatal respiratory depression; avoid with compromised respiratory function (eg, COPD, sleep apnea). May lower seizure threshold; caution with seizure disorders. Leukopenia and agranulocytosis reported, especially when given with other marrow-toxic agents; caution with bone-marrow depression. Neuroleptic malignant syndrome (NMS) reported; d/c immediately if NMS occurs. Hallucinations and convulsions reported in pediatric patients. Acutely ill pediatric patients who are dehydrated may have increased susceptibility to dystonias. Cholestatic jaundice reported. Caution with narrow-angle glaucoma, prostatic hypertrophy, stenosing peptic ulcer, pyloroduodenal/bladder-neck obstruction, cardiovascular disease, or impaired liver function. Increased blood glucose reported. Phenylephrine: Caution with diabetes mellitus and thyroid/heart diseases. May cause urinary retention in men with symptomatic BPH. May decrease cardiac output; use extreme caution with arteriosclerosis, in elderly, and/or patients with initially poor cerebral or coronary circulation.

ADVERSE REACTIONS

Respiratory depression, drowsiness, dizziness, somnolence, anxiety, sedation, tremor, blurred vision, dry mouth, increased or decreased BP, N/V, urinary retention, NMS, constipation.

DRUG INTERACTIONS

See Boxed Warning and Contraindications. Promethazine: May increase, prolong, or intensify the sedative action of other CNS depressants (eg, alcohol, narcotics, general anesthetics, tranquilizers); avoid such agents or administer in reduced doses. Reduce dose of barbiturate by at least 1/2 and narcotic analgesics by 1/4 to 1/2; individualize dose. Do not use epinephrine to treat hypotension associated with promethazine overdose; may reverse vasopressor effect of epinephrine. Caution with other agents with anticholinergic properties and drugs that also affect seizure threshold (eg, narcotics, local anesthetics). Phenylephrine: Pressor response increased with TCAs and decreased with prior administration of phentolamine or other α-adrenergic blockers. Ergot alkaloids may cause excessive rise in BP. Tachycardia or other arrhythmias may occur with bronchodilator sympathomimetics, epinephrine, or other sympathomimetics. Reflex bradycardia blocked and pressor response enhanced with atropine sulfate. Cardiostimulating effects blocked with prior administration of propranolol or other β-adrenergic blockers. Synergistic adrenergic response with diet preparations (eg, amphetamines, phenylpropanolamine).

NURSING CONSIDERATIONS

Assessment: Assess for drug hypersensitivity or idiosyncrasy, history of drug abuse/dependence, head injury, compromised respiratory function, poor cerebral/coronary circulation, or any other conditions where treatment is contraindicated or cautioned, pregnancy/nursing status, and for possible drug interactions.

Monitoring: Monitor for signs/symptoms of CNS and respiratory depression, constipation, leukopenia, agranulocytosis, cholestatic jaundice, seizures, NMS, orthostatic hypotension, abuse/dependence, increased blood glucose levels, and other adverse reactions. Monitor for urinary retention in men with BPH. Monitor pediatric patients for hallucinations, convulsions, and dystonias. Reevaluate 5 days or sooner if cough is unresponsive to treatment.

Patient Counseling: Inform that therapy may cause marked drowsiness and may impair mental and/or physical abilities required for performing hazardous tasks; advise to avoid such activities until it is known that they do not become drowsy or dizzy with therapy. Instruct to avoid the use or reduce dose of alcohol and other CNS depressants while on therapy. Advise to report any involuntary muscle movements, and to avoid prolonged sun exposure. Inform that therapy may produce orthostatic hypotension. Advise patients that some people have a genetic variation that results in codeine changing into morphine more rapidly and completely than other people; instruct caregivers of children receiving codeine for other reasons to monitor for signs of respiratory depression. Inform about risks and the signs of morphine overdose. Instruct nursing mothers to notify pediatrician immediately, or get emergency medical attention, if signs of morphine toxicity (eg, increased sleepiness, difficulty breastfeeding, breathing difficulties, limpness) are noticed in their infants.

Storage: 20-25°C (68-77°F).

PROMETHAZINE WITH CODEINE – codeine phosphate/promethazine hydrochloride — CV

Class: Antitussive/phenothiazine derivative

Contraindicated in pediatric patients <6 yrs of age. Concomitant administration of promethazine products with other respiratory depressants is associated with respiratory depression, and sometimes death, in pediatric patients. Respiratory depression, including fatalities, have been reported with use of promethazine in pediatric patients <2 yrs of age. Respiratory depression and death reported in children who received codeine following tonsillectomy and/or adenoidectomy and had evidence of being ultra-rapid metabolizers of codeine due to a CYP2D6 polymorphism.

ADULT DOSAGE

Cough/Cold/Allergy

Temporary Relief of Coughs and Upper Respiratory Symptoms Associated w/ Allergy or the Common Cold:
5mL q4-6h
Max: 30mL/24 hrs

PEDIATRIC DOSAGE

Cough/Cold/Allergy

Temporary Relief of Coughs and Upper Respiratory Symptoms Associated w/ Allergy or the Common Cold:

6-<12 Years:
2.5-5mL q4-6h
Max: 30mL/24 hrs

≥12 Years:
5mL q4-6h
Max: 30mL/24 hrs

DOSE MODIFICATION

Elderly

Start at lower end of dosing range

ADMINISTRATION

Oral route

Measure w/ an accurate measuring device

HOW SUPPLIED

Syrup: (Codeine-Promethazine) 10mg-6.25mg/5mL [473mL]

CONTRAINDICATIONS

Comatose states, treatment of lower respiratory tract symptoms (eg, asthma), pediatric patients <6 yrs of age, postoperative pain management in children who have undergone tonsillectomy and/or adenoidectomy.

WARNINGS/PRECAUTIONS

Should only be given to a pregnant woman if clearly needed. Caution in elderly. Lab test interactions may occur. Codeine: Do not increase dose if cough fails to respond to treatment. May cause/aggravate constipation. May release histamine; caution in atopic children. Capacity to elevate

CSF pressure and respiratory depressant effects may be markedly exaggerated in head injury, intracranial lesions, or with preexisting increase in intracranial pressure. May obscure clinical course in patients with head injuries. Avoid with acute febrile illness with productive cough or in chronic respiratory disease. May produce orthostatic hypotension in ambulatory patients. Give with caution and reduce initial dose with acute abdominal conditions, convulsive disorders, significant hepatic/renal impairment, fever, hypothyroidism, Addison's disease, ulcerative colitis, prostatic hypertrophy, recent GI or urinary tract surgery, and in the very young, elderly, or debilitated patients. Use lowest effective dose for the shortest period of time. Potential for abuse and dependence. Promethazine: May impair mental/physical abilities. May lead to potentially fatal respiratory depression; avoid with compromised respiratory function (eg, COPD, sleep apnea). May lower seizure threshold; caution with seizure disorders. Leukopenia and agranulocytosis reported, especially when given with other marrow-toxic agents; caution with bone-marrow depression. Neuroleptic malignant syndrome (NMS) reported; d/c immediately if NMS occurs. Hallucinations and convulsions reported in pediatric patients. Acutely ill pediatric patients who are dehydrated may have increased susceptibility to dystonias. Cholestatic jaundice reported. Caution with narrow-angle glaucoma, prostatic hypertrophy, stenosing peptic ulcer, pyloroduodenal/bladder-neck obstruction, cardiovascular disease, or impaired liver function. Increased blood glucose reported.

ADVERSE REACTIONS

Drowsiness, dizziness, sedation, blurred vision, dry mouth, increased or decreased BP, N/V, constipation, urinary retention, leukopenia, agranulocytosis, respiratory depression, apnea, NMS.

DRUG INTERACTIONS

See Boxed Warning. Possible interaction with MAOIs (eg, increased incidence of extrapyramidal effects); consider initial small test dose. Promethazine: May increase, prolong, or intensify the sedative action of other CNS depressants (eg, alcohol, narcotics, general anesthetics, tranquilizers); avoid such agents or administer in reduced doses. Reduce dose of barbiturate by at least 1/2 and narcotics by 1/4 to 1/2; individualize dose. Do not use epinephrine to treat hypotension associated with promethazine overdose; may reverse vasopressor effect of epinephrine. Caution with other agents with anticholinergic properties and drugs that also affect seizure threshold (eg, narcotics, local anesthetics).

NURSING CONSIDERATIONS

Assessment: Assess for drug hypersensitivity or idiosyncrasy, history of drug abuse/dependence, head injury, or any other conditions where treatment is contraindicated or cautioned, pregnancy/nursing status, and for possible drug interactions.

Monitoring: Monitor for signs/symptoms of CNS and respiratory depression, constipation, leukopenia, agranulocytosis, cholestatic jaundice, seizures, NMS, orthostatic hypotension, abuse/dependence, increased blood glucose levels, and other adverse reactions. Monitor pediatric patients for hallucinations, convulsions, and dystonias. Reevaluate 5 days or sooner if cough is unresponsive to treatment.

Patient Counseling: Inform that therapy may cause drowsiness and may impair mental and/or physical abilities required for performing potentially hazardous tasks (eg, driving or operating machinery); advise to avoid such activities until it is known that they do not become drowsy or dizzy with therapy. Instruct to avoid the use or reduce dose of alcohol and other CNS depressants while on therapy. Instruct to report any involuntary muscle movements. Instruct to avoid prolonged sun exposure. Inform that therapy may produce orthostatic hypotension. Advise patients that some people have a genetic variation that results in codeine changing into morphine more rapidly and completely than other people; instruct caregivers of children receiving codeine for other reasons to monitor for signs of respiratory depression. Inform about risks and the signs of morphine overdose. Instruct nursing mothers to notify pediatrician immediately, or get emergency medical attention, if signs of morphine toxicity (eg, increased sleepiness, difficulty breastfeeding, breathing difficulties, limpness) are noticed in their infants.

Storage: 20-25°C (68-77°F).

PROPECIA – finasteride RX

Class: Type II 5 alpha-reductase inhibitor

ADULT DOSAGE

Male Pattern Hair Loss

Androgenetic Alopecia:

1 tab (1mg) qd for ≥3 months

Continued use is recommended to sustain benefit; reevaluate periodically

PEDIATRIC DOSAGE

Pediatric use may not have been established

ADMINISTRATION
Oral route
Take w/ or w/o meals

HOW SUPPLIED
Tab: 1mg

CONTRAINDICATIONS
Pregnancy, women of child bearing potential.

WARNINGS/PRECAUTIONS
Withdrawal of treatment may lead to reversal of effect within 12 months. Potential risk to male fetus; broken or crushed tabs should not be handled by pregnant women or women who may potentially be pregnant. May decrease serum prostate specific antigen (PSA) levels during therapy or in the presence of prostate cancer; any confirmed increase from lowest PSA value during treatment may signal presence of prostate cancer and should be evaluated. May increase risk of high-grade prostate cancer. Caution with liver dysfunction.

ADVERSE REACTIONS
Decreased libido, erectile dysfunction, ejaculation disorder.

NURSING CONSIDERATIONS

Assessment: Assess for liver dysfunction and previous hypersensitivity to the drug and its components. Obtain baseline PSA levels.

Monitoring: Monitor for hypersensitivity reactions or other adverse reactions. Monitor PSA levels.

Patient Counseling: Instruct pregnant or potentially pregnant women not to handle crushed or broken tabs due to possible absorption and potential risk to male fetus; advise to immediately wash contact area with soap and water if contact occurs. Inform that there was an increase in high-grade prostate cancer in men treated with 5α-reductase inhibitors indicated for BPH treatment. Instruct to promptly report any changes in breasts (eg, lumps, pain, nipple discharge) to physician.

Storage: 15-30°C (59-86°F). Protect from moisture.

PROPRANOLOL – propranolol hydrochloride RX

Class: Nonselective beta-blocker

ADULT DOSAGE

Hypertension

Sol/Tab:
Initial: 40mg bid
Titrate: May increase gradually until adequate BP control is achieved
Usual Maint: 120-240mg/day

In some instances, 640mg/day may be required

If control is not adequate w/ bid dosing, a larger dose, or tid therapy may achieve better control

Angina Pectoris

Due to coronary atherosclerosis to decrease angina frequency and increase exercise tolerance

Sol/Tab:
Usual: 80-320mg/day given bid, tid or qid
Reduce dose gradually over a period of a few weeks if therapy is to be discontinued

Atrial Fibrillation

Sol/Tab:
Usual: 10-30mg tid or qid ac and hs

Myocardial Infarction

To reduce cardiovascular mortality in patients who have survived the acute phase of MI and are clinically stable
Sol/Tab:
Initial: 40mg tid
Titrate: Increase to 60-80mg tid after 1 month as tolerated

PEDIATRIC DOSAGE

Pediatric use may not have been established

Usual: 180-240mg/day in divided doses (either bid or tid)
Max: 240mg/day

Migraine

Prophylaxis:
Sol/Tab:
Initial: 80mg/day in divided doses
Usual: 160-240mg/day
Titrate: May increase gradually for optimum prophylaxis

D/C gradually if a satisfactory response is not obtained w/in 4-6 weeks after reaching max dose

Essential Tremor

Familial or Hereditary:
Sol/Tab:
Initial: 40mg bid
Usual/Maint: 120mg/day
May be necessary to give 240-320mg/day

Hypertrophic Subaortic Stenosis

Sol/Tab:
Usual: 20-40mg tid or qid ac and hs

Pheochromocytoma

Sol/Tab:
Usual: 60mg/day in divided doses for 3 days before surgery w/ α-adrenergic blocker
Inoperable Tumor:
Usual: 30mg/day in divided doses w/ α-adrenergic blocker

Arrhythmias

Life-threatening or those occurring under anesthesia (supraventricular/ventricular tachycardia, tachyarrhythmia of digitalis intoxication, resistant tachyarrhythmia due to excessive catecholamine action during anesthesia)
Inj:
Usual: 1-3mg IV at ≤1mg/min
May give a 2nd dose if necessary after 2 min then do not give additional drug in <4 hrs

Do not give additional dose when desired alteration in rate/rhythm is achieved

Transfer to oral therapy as soon as possible

DOSE MODIFICATION

Hepatic Insufficiency

Inj:
Consider lower dose

Elderly

Start at lower end of dosing range

ADMINISTRATION

Oral/IV route

HOW SUPPLIED

Inj: 1mg/mL; Sol: 20mg/5mL, 40mg/5mL [500mL]; Tab: 10mg*, 20mg*, 40mg*, 60mg*, 80mg* *scored

CONTRAINDICATIONS

Cardiogenic shock, sinus bradycardia and >1st-degree block, bronchial asthma.

WARNINGS/PRECAUTIONS

Exacerbation of angina and MI following abrupt discontinuation reported; when discontinuation is planned, reduce dose gradually over at least a few weeks. Reinstitute therapy if exacerbation of angina occurs upon interruption and take other measures for management of angina pectoris; follow same procedure in patients at risk of occult atherosclerotic heart disease who are given propranolol for other indication since coronary artery disease may be unrecognized. May precipitate more severe failure in patients w/ CHF; avoid w/ overt CHF and caution in patients w/ history of heart failure (HF) who are well-compensated and are receiving additional therapies. Caution w/

bronchospastic lung disease, hepatic/renal impairment, Wolff-Parkinson-White (WPW) syndrome, and tachycardia. Chronically administered therapy should not be routinely withdrawn prior to major surgery; however, may augment risks of general anesthesia and surgical procedures. May mask acute hypoglycemia and hyperthyroidism signs/symptoms. May be more difficult to adjust insulin dose in labile insulin-dependent diabetics. Abrupt withdrawal may be followed by an exacerbation of symptoms of hyperthyroidism, including thyroid storm. May reduce IOP. Hypersensitivity/anaphylactic/cutaneous reactions reported. Patients w/ history of severe anaphylactic reaction to a variety of allergens may be more reactive to repeated accidental/diagnostic/therapeutic challenge; may be unresponsive to usual doses of epinephrine. Elevated serum K+, transaminases, and alkaline phosphatase levels reported. Increases in BUN reported in patients w/ severe HF. Not for treatment of hypertensive emergencies. (Oral) Not indicated for migraine attack that has started and tremor associated w/ parkinsonism. Continued use in patients w/o history of HF may lead to cardiac failure.

ADVERSE REACTIONS

Bradycardia, CHF, hypotension, lightheadedness, mental depression, N/V, agranulocytosis, respiratory distress.

DRUG INTERACTIONS

Administration w/ CYP450 (2D6, 1A2, 2C19) substrates, inducers, and inhibitors may lead to clinically relevant drug interactions. Increased levels and/or toxicity w/ substrates/inhibitors of CYP2D6 (eg, amiodarone, cimetidine, fluoxetine, ritonavir), CYP1A2 (eg, imipramine, ciprofloxacin, isoniazid, theophylline), and CYP2C19 (eg, fluconazole, teniposide, tolbutamide). Decreased blood levels w/ hepatic enzyme inducers (eg, rifampin, ethanol, phenytoin, phenobarbital). May increase levels of propafenone, lidocaine, nifedipine, zolmitriptan, rizatriptan, diazepam and its metabolites. Increased levels w/ nisoldipine, nicardipine, and chlorpromazine. May decrease theophylline clearance. Increased thioridazine plasma and metabolite (mesoridazine) concentrations w/ doses ≥160mg/day. Decreased levels w/ aluminum hydroxide gel, cholestyramine, and colestipol. May decrease levels of lovastatin and pravastatin. Increased warfarin levels and PT; monitor PT. Additive effect w/ propafenone and amiodarone. Caution w/ drugs that slow atrioventricular (AV) nodal conduction (eg, digitalis, lidocaine, calcium channel blockers); increased risk of bradycardia w/ digitalis. Significant bradycardia, HF, and CV collapse reported w/ concomitant verapamil. Bradycardia, hypotension, high-degree heart block, and HF reported w/ concomitant diltiazem. Concomitant ACE inhibitors may cause hypotension. May antagonize effects of clonidine; administer cautiously to patients withdrawing from clonidine. Prolongation of 1st dose hypotension may occur w/ concomitant prazosin. Postural hypotension reported w/ concomitant terazosin or doxazosin. Monitor for excessive reduction of resting sympathetic nervous activity w/ catecholamine-depleting drugs (eg, reserpine). Patients on long-term therapy may experience uncontrolled HTN w/ concomitant epinephrine. β-receptor agonists (eg, dobutamine, isoproterenol) may reverse effects. NSAIDs (eg, indomethacin) may blunt the antihypertensive effect. Coadministration w/ methoxyflurane and trichloroethylene may depress myocardial contractility. Hypotension and cardiac arrest reported w/ concomitant haloperidol. Thyroxine may result in a lower than expected T3 concentration when coadministered w/ propranolol. May exacerbate hypotensive effects of MAOIs or TCAs. (Inj) Severe bradycardia, asystole, and HF reported w/ concomitant disopyramide. Increased bronchial hyperreactivity w/ ACE inhibitors. (Oral) Increased levels w/ alcohol.

NURSING CONSIDERATIONS

Assessment: Assess for cardiogenic shock, sinus bradycardia, AV heart block, bronchial asthma, CHF, bronchospastic lung disease, hyperthyroidism, diabetes, WPW syndrome, tachycardia, hepatic/renal impairment, history/presence of HF, risk for occult atherosclerotic heart disease, hypersensitivity to drug, pregnancy/nursing status, and possible drug interactions.

Monitoring: Monitor for signs/symptoms of cardiac failure, hypoglycemia, decreased IOP, hyperthyroidism, withdrawal symptoms, hypersensitivity reactions, and other adverse reactions. (Inj) Monitor ECG and central venous pressure. (Oral) For HTN (bid dosing), measure BP near the end of dosing interval to determine satisfactory BP control.

Patient Counseling: Inform of the risk/benefits of therapy. Instruct not to interrupt or d/c therapy w/o physician's advise. Inform that therapy may interfere w/ glaucoma screening test.

Storage: 20-25°C (68-77°F); (Sol) excursions permitted to 15-30°C (59-86°F). (Inj) Protect from freezing and excessive heat. (Tab) Protect from light.

PROSCAR – finasteride

RX

Class: Type II 5 alpha-reductase inhibitor

ADULT DOSAGE

Benign Prostatic Hyperplasia

Monotherapy or in Combination w/ Doxazosin:
1 tab (5mg) qd

PEDIATRIC DOSAGE

Pediatric use may not have been established

ADMINISTRATION
Oral route
Take w/ or w/o meals

HOW SUPPLIED
Tab: 5mg

CONTRAINDICATIONS
Women who are or may potentially be pregnant.

WARNINGS/PRECAUTIONS
Not approved for the prevention of prostate cancer. May decrease serum prostate specific antigen (PSA) concentration during therapy or in the presence of prostate cancer; establish a new baseline PSA at least 6 months after starting treatment and monitor PSA periodically thereafter. Any confirmed increase from lowest PSA value during treatment may signal presence of prostate cancer. May increase risk of high-grade prostate cancer. Potential risk to male fetus; broken or crushed tabs should not be handled by pregnant women or women who may potentially be pregnant. May decrease ejaculate volume and total sperm per ejaculate. Prior to treatment initiation, consider other urological conditions that may cause similar symptoms; BPH and prostate cancer may coexist. Monitor for obstructive uropathy in patients with large residual urinary volume and/or severely diminished urinary flow; such patients may not be candidates for therapy. Caution with liver dysfunction.

ADVERSE REACTIONS
Impotence, decreased libido, decreased ejaculate volume, asthenia, postural hypotension, dizziness, abnormal ejaculation.

NURSING CONSIDERATIONS

Assessment: Assess for liver dysfunction, previous hypersensitivity to the drug, other urological conditions that may cause similar symptoms, residual urinary volume, and diminished urinary flow.

Monitoring: Monitor for obstructive uropathy in patients with large residual urinary volume and/or severely diminished urinary flow. Monitor for signs/symptoms of prostate cancer, hypersensitivity reactions, and other adverse reactions. Obtain baseline PSA levels at least 6 months after starting treatment and monitor PSA periodically thereafter.

Patient Counseling: Inform that therapy may increase risk of high-grade prostate cancer. Instruct pregnant or potentially pregnant females not to handle crushed or broken tabs due to possible absorption and potential risk to male fetus; advise to immediately wash contact area with soap and water if contact occurs. Advise that the volume of ejaculate may be decreased and impotence/decreased libido may occur. Instruct to promptly report to physician any changes in breasts (eg, lumps, pain, nipple discharge).

Storage: Room temperature <30°C (86°F). Protect from light.

PROTONIX – pantoprazole sodium RX

Class: Proton pump inhibitor

OTHER BRAND NAMES
Protonix IV

ADULT DOSAGE

Gastroesophageal Reflux Disease

Short-Term Treatment of Erosive Esophagitis Associated w/ GERD:
40mg qd for up to 8 weeks; may consider additional 8-week course if not healed after 8 weeks of treatment

Maint of Healing of Erosive Esophagitis:
40mg qd; no controlled studies beyond 12 months

GERD Associated w/ History of Erosive Esophagitis:
40mg qd by IV infusion for 7-10 days; D/C as soon as patient is able to receive oral formulation

Pathological Hypersecretory Conditions

Long-term treatment of pathological hypersecretory conditions, including Zollinger-Ellison syndrome

Usual: 40mg bid
Titrate: Adjust to individual needs and continue for as long as clinically indicated; doses up to 240mg have been administered

PEDIATRIC DOSAGE

Gastroesophageal Reflux Disease

Short-Term Treatment of Erosive Esophagitis Associated w/ GERD:

≥5 Years:
≥15kg-<40kg: 20mg qd for up to 8 weeks
≥40kg: 40mg qd for up to 8 weeks

ADMINISTRATION
Oral/IV route

Tab/Sus
Do not split, chew, or crush

Tab
Swallow whole, w/ or w/o food
If patients are unable to swallow a 40mg tab, two 20mg tabs may be taken

Sus
Administer approx 30 min ac via oral administration in apple juice or applesauce or NG tube in apple juice only; do not administer in other liquids/foods
Do not divide the 40mg pkt to create a 20mg dosage

Oral in Applesauce:
Sprinkle granules on 1 tsp of applesauce and take w/in 10 min of preparation
Take sips of water to ensure granules are washed down

Oral in Apple Juice:
Empty granules into a small cup or tsp containing 1 tsp of apple juice
Stir for 5 sec and swallow immediately
Rinse container once or twice w/ apple juice and swallow immediately to ensure entire dose is taken

NG Tube/Gastrostomy Tube Administration:
Connect the catheter tip of the syringe to a 16 French (or larger) tube
Empty the contents of the pkt into the barrel of the syringe
Add 10mL (2 tsp) of apple juice and gently tap and/or shake the barrel of the syringe to help rinse the syringe and tube
Repeat at least twice more using the same amount of apple juice each time; no granules should remain in the syringe

IV
Flush IV line before and after administration

Fifteen-Minute Infusion:
Reconstitute w/ 10mL of 0.9% NaCl and further dilute w/ 80mL of D5W, 0.9% NaCl, or Lactated Ringer's Inj to a total volume of 100mL w/ a final concentration of approx 0.8mg/mL
May store for up to 6 hrs at room temperature prior to further dilution
Admixed sol must be used w/in 24 hrs from the time of initial reconstitution
Administer over approx 15 min at a rate of approx 7mL/min

Two-Minute Infusion:
Reconstitute w/ 10mL of 0.9% NaCl to a final concentration of approx 4mg/mL
The reconstituted sol may be stored for up to 24 hrs at room temperature prior to IV infusion
Administer over at least 2 min

HOW SUPPLIED
Inj: 40mg; Sus, Delayed-Release: 40mg (granules/pkt); Tab, Delayed-Release: 20mg, 40mg

WARNINGS/PRECAUTIONS
Symptomatic response does not preclude the presence of gastric malignancy. Acute interstitial nephritis reported; d/c if this develops. May increase risk of *Clostridium difficile*-associated diarrhea (CDAD), especially in hospitalized patients. May increase risk for osteoporosis-related fractures of the hip, wrist, or spine, especially w/ high-dose and long-term therapy. Use lowest dose and shortest duration appropriate to the condition being treated. Hypomagnesemia reported and may require Mg^{2+} replacement and discontinuation of therapy; consider monitoring Mg^{2+} levels prior to and periodically during therapy w/ prolonged treatment. Anaphylaxis and other serious reactions (eg, erythema multiforme, Stevens-Johnson syndrome, toxic epidermal necrolysis) reported; may require emergency medical treatment. Lab test interactions may occur. (Oral) Atrophic gastritis noted w/ long-term therapy, particularly in patients who were *Helicobacter pylori* positive. Vitamin B12 deficiency caused by hypo- or achlorhydria may occur w/ long-term use (eg, >3 yrs). (IV) Thrombophlebitis reported. Contains EDTA, a chelator of metal ions including zinc; consider zinc supplementation in patients prone to zinc deficiency. Mild, transient transaminase elevations observed in clinical studies.

ADVERSE REACTIONS
Headache, diarrhea, N/V, abdominal pain, flatulence, dizziness, rash, fever, URI, arthralgia.

DRUG INTERACTIONS
Concomitant use w/ atazanavir or nelfinavir is not recommended; may substantially decrease atazanavir or nelfinavir concentrations. Monitor for increases in INR and PT w/ warfarin. May reduce the absorption of drugs where gastric pH is an important determinant of bioavailability; ketoconazole, ampicillin esters, atazanavir, iron salts, erlotinib, mycophenolate mofetil (MMF) absorption may decrease. Caution in transplant patients receiving MMF. Caution w/ digoxin or other drugs that may cause hypomagnesemia (eg, diuretics). May elevate and prolong levels of MTX and/or its metabolite, possibly leading to toxicities; consider temporary withdrawal of therapy w/ high-dose MTX. (IV) Use caution when other EDTA-containing products are also coadministered IV.

NURSING CONSIDERATIONS

Assessment: Assess for hypersensitivity to the drug, risk for osteoporosis-related fractures, pregnancy/nursing status, and possible drug interactions. Obtain baseline Mg^{2+} levels. (IV) Assess if prone to zinc deficiency.

Monitoring: Monitor for signs/symptoms of acute interstitial nephritis, CDAD, bone fractures, hypersensitivity reactions, and other adverse reactions. Monitor Mg^{2+} levels periodically. Monitor INR and PT when given w/ warfarin. (Oral) Monitor for signs/symptoms of atrophic gastritis and vitamin B12 deficiency. (IV) Monitor for thrombophlebitis, zinc deficiency, and transaminase elevations.

Patient Counseling: Instruct to take ud. Inform of the most frequently occurring adverse reactions. Instruct to inform physician if any unusual symptom develops, or if any known symptom persists or worsens; advise to immediately report and seek care for any cardiovascular or neurological symptoms (eg, palpitation, dizziness, seizures, tetany) and for diarrhea that does not improve. Instruct to inform physician of all medications currently being taken, including OTC medications, as well as allergies to any medications. Inform that concomitant administration of antacids does not affect the absorption of the tabs. Advise that oral sus pkt is a fixed dose and cannot be divided to make smaller dose.

Storage: 20-25°C (68-77°F); excursions permitted to 15-30°C (59-86°F). (IV) Protect from light.

PROTOPIC – tacrolimus

RX

Class: Macrolide immunosuppressant

Rare cases of malignancy (eg, skin and lymphoma) reported with topical calcineurin inhibitors, including tacrolimus oint, although causal relationship has not been established. Avoid long-term use, and application should be limited to areas of involvement with atopic dermatitis. Not indicated for children <2 yrs of age; only 0.03% oint is indicated for children 2-15 yrs of age.

ADULT DOSAGE

Atopic Dermatitis

2nd-line therapy for short-term and non-continuous chronic treatment of moderate to severe atopic dermatitis

0.03%/0.1%:

Apply a thin layer to the affected skin bid until signs and symptoms resolve

Reexamine patient if signs and symptoms do not improve w/in 6 weeks

PEDIATRIC DOSAGE

Atopic Dermatitis

2nd-line therapy for short-term and non-continuous chronic treatment of moderate to severe atopic dermatitis

2-15 Years:

0.03%:

Apply a thin layer to the affected skin bid until signs and symptoms resolve

Reexamine patient if signs and symptoms do not improve w/in 6 weeks

ADMINISTRATION

Topical route

Rub minimum amount in gently and completely

Moisturizers can be used w/ oint

HOW SUPPLIED

Oint: 0.03%, 0.1% [30g, 60g, 100g]

WARNINGS/PRECAUTIONS

Long-term safety, beyond 1 yr of noncontinuous use, has not been established. Avoid with premalignant and malignant skin conditions. Not recommended for oral application, or in patients having skin conditions with a skin barrier defect where there is potential for increased systemic absorption (eg, Netherton's syndrome, lamellar ichthyosis, generalized erythroderma, cutaneous graft-versus-host disease). May cause local symptoms, such as skin burning or pruritus and may improve as the lesions of atopic dermatitis resolve. Resolve bacterial or viral infections at treatment sites before starting treatment. Increased risk of varicella zoster and herpes simplex virus (HSV) infection, or eczema herpeticum. Lymphadenopathy reported; d/c if etiology of lymphadenopathy is unknown, or in the presence of acute infectious mononucleosis. Minimize or avoid natural or artificial sunlight exposure during treatment. Rare cases of acute renal failure reported. Not for ophthalmic use. Do not use with occlusive dressings.

ADVERSE REACTIONS

Skin burning, pruritus, flu-like symptoms, allergic reaction, skin erythema, headache, skin infection, fever, herpes simplex, rhinitis, increased cough, asthma, pharyngitis, pustular rash, folliculitis.

DRUG INTERACTIONS

Caution with CYP3A4 inhibitors (eg, erythromycin, ketoconazole, calcium channel blockers, cimetidine) in patients with widespread and/or erythrodermic disease.

NURSING CONSIDERATIONS

Assessment: Assess for history of hypersensitivity to drug, premalignant/malignant skin conditions, conditions where there is potential for increased systemic absorption, bacterial or viral infections at treatment sites, renal impairment, pregnancy/nursing status, and possible drug interactions.

Monitoring: Monitor for skin malignancy, lymphoma, infections, local symptoms, lymphadenopathy, and acute renal failure. Monitor improvement of signs/symptoms of atopic dermatitis within 6 weeks.

Patient Counseling: Instruct to use drug exactly as prescribed, only on areas of skin that have eczema, and not to use continuously for a prolonged period. Advise to d/c medication when signs/symptoms of eczema subside. Instruct to consult physician if symptoms get worse, a skin infection develops, or if symptoms do not improve after 6 weeks. Advise caregivers applying the oint, or patients not treating their hands, to wash hands with soap and water after application. Counsel to not bathe, shower, or swim right after application. Advise to avoid getting oint in the eyes or mouth. Instruct to avoid artificial sunlight exposure during treatment, limit sun exposure, wear loose-fitting clothing that protects treated area from the sun, and not cover treated skin with bandages, dressings, or wraps.

Storage: 25°C (77°F); excursions permitted to 15-30°C (59-86°F).

PROVERA – medroxyprogesterone acetate

RX

Class: Progestogen

Estrogens with progestins should not be used for the prevention of cardiovascular disease (CVD) or dementia. Increased risks of MI, stroke, invasive breast cancer, pulmonary embolism (PE), and DVT reported in postmenopausal women (50-79 yrs of age) treated with daily oral conjugated estrogens (CEs) combined with medroxyprogesterone acetate (MPA). Increased risk of developing probable dementia reported in postmenopausal women ≥65 yrs of age treated with daily CEs combined with MPA. Should be prescribed at the lowest effective dose and for the shortest duration consistent with treatment goals and risks.

ADULT DOSAGE

Abnormal Uterine Bleeding

Due to Hormonal Imbalance in the Absence of Organic Pathology (eg, Fibroids, Uterine Cancer):

5 or 10mg/day for 5-10 days beginning on Day 16 or 21 of cycle; 10mg/day for 10 days, beginning on Day 16 of the cycle is recommended to produce an optimum secretory transformation of an endometrium that has been adequately primed w/ either endogenous or exogenous estrogen

Endometrial Hyperplasia

Reduce Incidence in Non-Hysterectomized Postmenopausal Women Receiving Daily Oral CE 0.625mg Tabs:

5 or 10mg/day for 12-14 consecutive days/month beginning on Day 1 or 16 of cycle

Secondary Amenorrhea

Due to Hormonal Imbalance in the Absence of Organic Pathology (eg, Fibroids, Uterine Cancer):

5 or 10mg/day for 5-10 days. 10mg/day for 10 days is a dose for inducing an optimum secretory transformation of an endometrium that has been adequately primed w/ either endogenous or exogenous estrogen. May start therapy at any time

PEDIATRIC DOSAGE

Pediatric use may not have been established

ADMINISTRATION

Oral route

HOW SUPPLIED

Tab: 2.5mg*, 5mg*, 10mg* *scored

CONTRAINDICATIONS
Undiagnosed abnormal genital bleeding, known/suspected/history of breast cancer, known/suspected estrogen- or progesterone-dependent neoplasia, active or history of DVT/PE, active or recent arterial thromboembolic disease (eg, stroke, MI), known liver dysfunction or disease, missed abortion, known/suspected pregnancy, as a diagnostic test for pregnancy.

WARNINGS/PRECAUTIONS
Increased risk of endometrial cancer reported with use of unopposed estrogen therapy in women with a uterus. Increased risk of ovarian cancer reported with daily CE/MPA. D/C pending exam if there is sudden partial or complete loss of vision, or a sudden onset of proptosis, diplopia or migraine. D/C permanently if exam reveals papilledema or retinal vascular lesions. In cases of undiagnosed abnormal vaginal bleeding, perform adequate diagnostic measures. Monitor BP at regular intervals in patients on estrogen plus progestin therapy. Withdrawal bleeding may occur within 3-7 days after discontinuing therapy. May increase plasma TGs, leading to pancreatitis and other complications in patients with preexisting hypertriglyceridemia. Caution with history of cholestatic jaundice associated with past estrogen use or with pregnancy; d/c in case of recurrence. May cause fluid retention. Caution with severe hypocalcemia. May exacerbate asthma, diabetes mellitus, epilepsy, migraine, porphyria, systemic lupus erythematosus, and hepatic hemangiomas. May affect LFTs and certain endocrine and blood components in lab tests.

ADVERSE REACTIONS
Abnormal uterine bleeding, breast tenderness, galactorrhea, urticaria, pruritus, edema, rash, menstrual changes, change in weight, mental depression, insomnia, somnolence, dizziness, headache, nausea.

DRUG INTERACTIONS
Patients on thyroid replacement therapy may require higher doses of thyroid hormone.

NURSING CONSIDERATIONS

Assessment: Assess for abnormal genital bleeding; cardiac or renal dysfunction; presence or history of breast cancer; estrogen- or progesterone-dependent neoplasias; active or history of DVT or PE; active or recent (within past yr) arterial thromboembolic disease, any other conditions where treatment is contraindicated or cautioned, and for possible drug interactions.

Monitoring: Monitor for signs/symptoms of CVD, malignant neoplasms, visual abnormalities, hypertriglyceridemia, fluid retention, exacerbation of asthma, and other adverse reactions. Perform annual breast exam; schedule mammography based on age, risk factors, and prior mammogram results. Regularly monitor BP in patients on estrogen plus progestin therapy. Monitor thyroid function in patients on thyroid replacement therapy. Periodically reevaluate (every 3-6 months) need for therapy. In cases of undiagnosed, persistent, or recurrent vaginal bleeding in women with a uterus, perform adequate diagnostic measures (eg, endometrial sampling) to rule out malignancy.

Patient Counseling: Advise of risks and benefits of therapy. Inform that therapy may increase risk for breast cancer, uterine cancer, stroke, heart attack, blood clots, and dementia. Instruct to notify physician if breast lumps, unusual vaginal bleeding, dizziness/faintness, changes in speech, severe headaches, chest pain, SOB, leg pain, visual changes, or vomiting develops. Instruct to have an annual pelvic exam, breast exam, and mammogram. Advise to perform monthly breast self-exams.

Storage: 20-25°C (68-77°F).

PROVIGIL – modafinil CIV

Class: Wakefulness-promoting agent

ADULT DOSAGE

Excessive Sleepiness

Associated w/ Narcolepsy/Obstructive Sleep Apnea/Shift Work Disorder:
200mg qd
Max: 400mg/day as a single dose

PEDIATRIC DOSAGE

Pediatric use may not have been established

DOSE MODIFICATION

Hepatic Impairment
Severe: 100mg qd

Elderly
Consider using lower doses

ADMINISTRATION
Oral route

Narcolepsy/Obstructive Sleep Apnea
Take as single dose in am

Shift Work Disorder
Take 1 hr prior to start of work shift

HOW SUPPLIED
Tab: 100mg, 200mg* *scored

WARNINGS/PRECAUTIONS
Not indicated as treatment for underlying obstruction in OSA; if continuous positive airway pressure (CPAP) is the treatment of choice, treat w/ CPAP for an adequate period of time prior to initiating and during treatment. Rare cases of serious or life-threatening rash, including Stevens-Johnson syndrome (SJS), toxic epidermal necrolysis (TEN), and drug rash w/ eosinophilia and systemic symptoms (DRESS), reported; d/c at the 1st sign of rash, unless the rash is clearly not drug-related. Angioedema reported; d/c if angioedema or anaphylaxis occurs. Multiorgan hypersensitivity reactions reported; d/c if suspected. Level of wakefulness may not return to normal in patients w/ abnormal levels of sleepiness. Psychiatric adverse reactions reported; caution w/ history of psychosis, depression, or mania. Consider discontinuation if psychiatric symptoms develop in association w/ drug administration. May impair mental and/or physical abilities. Cardiovascular (CV) adverse reactions reported; not recommended in patients w/ a history of left ventricular hypertrophy (LVH) or in patients w/ mitral valve prolapse who have experienced mitral valve prolapse syndrome (eg, ischemic ECG changes, chest pain, arrhythmia) when previously receiving CNS stimulants. Caution w/ known CV disease (CVD). Caution in elderly. Potential for abuse.

ADVERSE REACTIONS
Headache, nausea, nervousness, anxiety, insomnia, rhinitis, diarrhea, back pain, dizziness, dyspepsia, anorexia, dry mouth, pharyngitis, chest pain, HTN.

DRUG INTERACTIONS
May reduce exposure of CYP3A4/5 substrates (eg, midazolam, triazolam); consider dose adjustment of these drugs. Effectiveness of steroidal contraceptives (eg, ethinyl estradiol) may be reduced when used w/ therapy and for 1 month after discontinuation of therapy; alternative or concomitant methods of contraception are recommended. May reduce levels of cyclosporine; consider dose adjustment for cyclosporine. May increase exposure of CYP2C19 substrates (eg, phenytoin, diazepam, propranolol). In individuals deficient in the CYP2D6 enzyme, levels of CYP2D6 substrates, which have ancillary routes of elimination through CYP2C19 (eg, TCAs, SSRIs) may be increased; dose adjustments of these drugs and other drugs that are substrates for CYP2C19 may be necessary. Consider more frequent monitoring of PT/INR w/ warfarin. Caution w/ MAOIs.

NURSING CONSIDERATIONS

Assessment: Assess for hypersensitivity to the drug, history of psychosis, depression, mania, or LVH, mitral valve prolapse, other CVD, hepatic impairment, pregnancy/nursing status, and possible drug interactions.

Monitoring: Monitor for rash, SJS, TEN, DRESS, angioedema, anaphylaxis, multiorgan hypersensitivity reactions, psychiatric symptoms, CV events (especially in patients w/ a history of MI or unstable angina), and other adverse reactions. Monitor for signs of misuse or abuse. Monitor HR and BP. Frequently reassess degree of sleepiness. Monitor PT/INR frequently w/ warfarin.

Patient Counseling: Instruct to d/c use and notify physician immediately if allergic reactions and other adverse reactions (eg, chest pain, rash, depression, anxiety, signs of psychosis/mania) develop. Advise not to alter previous behavior w/ regard to potentially dangerous activities (eg, driving, operating machinery) or other activities requiring appropriate levels of wakefulness, until and unless treatment has been shown to produce levels of wakefulness that permit such activities. Inform that drug is not a replacement for sleep. Counsel patients that it may be critical that they continue to take their previously prescribed treatments (eg, patients w/ OSA receiving CPAP). Advise to notify physician if pregnancy occurs, if intending to become pregnant, or if breastfeeding. Caution regarding the potential increased risk of pregnancy when using steroidal contraceptives w/ therapy and for 1 month after discontinuation of therapy. Instruct to inform physician if taking/planning to take any prescription/OTC drugs, and to avoid alcohol.

Storage: 20-25°C (68-77°F).

PROZAC — fluoxetine hydrochloride RX

Class: Selective serotonin reuptake inhibitor

Antidepressants increased the risk of suicidal thoughts and behavior in children, adolescents, and young adults in short-term studies. Monitor closely for worsening and for emergence of suicidal thoughts and behaviors in patients who are started on antidepressant therapy. Not approved for use in children <7 yrs of age.

OTHER BRAND NAMES
Prozac Weekly

ADULT DOSAGE

Major Depressive Disorder

Initial: 20mg/day qam
Titrate: Consider a dose increase after several weeks if improvement is insufficient; administer doses >20mg/day qam or bid (am and noon)
Max: 80mg/day

Prozac Weekly:
Initiate 7 days after the last daily dose of 20mg cap
Consider reestablishing a daily dosing regimen if satisfactory response is not maintained

Switching to a TCA:
May need to reduce TCA dose and monitor plasma concentrations temporarily w/ coadministration or when fluoxetine has been recently discontinued

Obsessive Compulsive Disorder

Initial: 20mg/day qam
Titrate: Consider a dose increase after several weeks if improvement is insufficient; administer doses >20mg/day qam or bid (am and noon)
Usual: 20-60mg/day
Max: 80mg/day

Bulimia Nervosa

Initial: 60mg/day qam; may titrate up to this target dose over several days
Max: 60mg/day

Panic Disorder

W/ or w/o Agoraphobia:
Initial: 10mg/day
Titrate: Increase to 20mg/day after 1 week; consider a dose increase after several weeks if no improvement
Max: 60mg/day

Bipolar I Disorder

Depressive Episodes:
In Combination w/ Olanzapine:
Initial: 20mg fluoxetine + 5mg olanzapine qpm
Dose Ranges: 20-50mg fluoxetine + 5-12.5mg olanzapine
Max: 75mg fluoxetine + 18mg olanzapine

Major Depressive Disorder

Use in patients who do not respond to 2 separate trials of different antidepressants of adequate dose and duration in the current episode

In Combination w/ Olanzapine:
Initial: 20mg fluoxetine + 5mg olanzapine qpm
Dose Ranges: 20-50mg fluoxetine + 5-20mg olanzapine
Max: 75mg fluoxetine + 18mg olanzapine

Dosing Considerations with MAOIs

Switching to/from an MAOI for Psychiatric Disorders:
Allow at least 14 days between discontinuation of an MAOI and initiation of treatment, and allow at least 5 weeks between discontinuation of treatment and initiation of an MAOI
W/ Other MAOIs (eg, Linezolid, IV Methylene Blue):
Do not start fluoxetine in patients being treated w/ linezolid or IV methylene blue

PEDIATRIC DOSAGE

Major Depressive Disorder

≥8 Years:
Initial: 10 or 20mg/day
Titrate: After 1 week at 10mg/day, increase to 20mg/day

Lower Weight Children:
Initial/Target: 10mg/day
Titrate: Consider a dose increase to 20mg/day after several weeks if improvement is insufficient

Switching to a TCA:
May need to reduce TCA dose and monitor plasma concentrations temporarily w/ coadministration or when fluoxetine has been recently discontinued

Obsessive Compulsive Disorder

≥7 Years:
Initial: 10mg/day
Titrate: Increase to 20mg/day after 2 weeks; consider additional dose increases after several more weeks if improvement is insufficient
Usual: 20-60mg/day

Lower Weight Children:
Initial: 10mg/day
Titrate: Consider additional dose increases after several weeks if improvement is insufficient
Usual: 20-30mg/day
Max: 60mg/day

Bipolar I Disorder

Depressive Episodes:
In Combination w/ Olanzapine:
10-17 Years:
Initial: 20mg fluoxetine + 2.5mg olanzapine qpm
Max: 50mg fluoxetine + 12mg olanzapine

Dosing Considerations with MAOIs

Switching to/from an MAOI for Psychiatric Disorders:
Allow at least 14 days between discontinuation of an MAOI and initiation of treatment, and allow at least 5 weeks between discontinuation of treatment and initiation of an MAOI
W/ Other MAOIs (eg, Linezolid, IV Methylene Blue):
Do not start fluoxetine in patients being treated w/ linezolid or IV methylene blue
In patients already receiving fluoxetine, if acceptable alternatives are not available and benefits outweigh risks, d/c fluoxetine and administer linezolid or IV methylene blue; monitor for serotonin syndrome for 5 weeks or until 24 hrs after the last dose of linezolid or IV methylene blue, whichever comes 1st. May resume fluoxetine therapy 24 hrs after the last dose of linezolid or IV methylene blue

In patients already receiving fluoxetine, if acceptable alternatives are not available and benefits outweigh risks, d/c fluoxetine and administer linezolid or IV methylene blue; monitor for serotonin syndrome for 5 weeks or until 24 hrs after the last dose of linezolid or IV methylene blue, whichever comes 1st. May resume fluoxetine therapy 24 hrs after the last dose of linezolid or IV methylene blue

DOSE MODIFICATION

Concomitant Medications

Combination w/ Olanzapine:

Patients Predisposed to Hypotensive Reactions w/ Hepatic Impairment, Slow Metabolizers, Pharmacodynamic Olanzapine Sensitivity:

Initial: 20mg fluoxetine + 2.5-5mg olanzapine

Titrate slowly and adjust dosage prn

Hepatic Impairment

Use lower or less frequent dosage

Elderly

Consider lower or less frequent dosage

Other Important Modifications

Concomitant Illness: May require dose adjustments

ADMINISTRATION

Oral route

Take w/ or w/o food

HOW SUPPLIED

Cap: 10mg, 20mg, 40mg; Cap, Delayed-Release (Prozac Weekly): 90mg

CONTRAINDICATIONS

Use of an MAOI for psychiatric disorders either concomitantly or within 5 weeks of stopping treatment. Treatment within 14 days of stopping an MAOI for psychiatric disorders. Starting treatment in patients being treated with other MAOIs (eg, linezolid, IV methylene blue). Concomitant use with pimozide or thioridazine.

WARNINGS/PRECAUTIONS

Serotonin syndrome reported; d/c immediately and initiate supportive symptomatic treatment. Anaphylactoid and pulmonary reactions reported; d/c if unexplained allergic reaction or rash occurs. May precipitate mixed/manic episode in patients at risk for bipolar disorder. Weight loss and anorexia reported. May increase risk of bleeding reactions. Pupillary dilation that occurs following use may trigger an angle-closure attack in a patient with anatomically narrow angles who does not have a patent iridectomy. Hyponatremia may occur; caution in elderly and volume-depleted patients. Consider discontinuation in patients with symptomatic hyponatremia and institute appropriate medical intervention. Convulsions, mania/hypomania, anxiety, insomnia, and nervousness reported. QT interval prolongation and ventricular arrhythmia (eg, torsades de pointes) reported. Caution in patients with congenital long QT syndrome, previous history of QT prolongation, family history of long QT syndrome or sudden cardiac death, and other conditions that predispose to QT prolongation and ventricular arrhythmia. Consider discontinuing treatment and obtaining cardiac evaluation if signs or symptoms of ventricular arrhythmia develop. Caution in patients with diseases/conditions that could affect hemodynamic responses or metabolism. May alter glycemic control in patients with diabetes. May impair mental/physical abilities. Long elimination $T_{1/2}$; changes in dose may not be fully reflected in plasma for several weeks. Adverse reactions reported upon discontinuation; avoid abrupt withdrawal.

ADVERSE REACTIONS

Somnolence, anorexia, anxiety, asthenia, diarrhea, dry mouth, dyspepsia, headache, insomnia, tremor, pharyngitis, flu syndrome, dizziness, nausea, nervousness.

DRUG INTERACTIONS

See Contraindications. Do not use thioridazine within 5 weeks of discontinuing therapy. Caution with CNS-active drugs. Avoid with other drugs that cause QT prolongation (eg, ziprasidone, erythromycin, quinidine). May cause serotonin syndrome with other serotonergic drugs (eg, triptans, TCAs, fentanyl) and with drugs that impair metabolism of serotonin; d/c immediately if this occurs. Increased risk of bleeding with aspirin, NSAIDs, warfarin, and other anticoagulants. Rare reports of prolonged seizures with electroconvulsive therapy. Drugs that are tightly bound to plasma proteins (eg, warfarin, digitoxin) may cause a shift in plasma concentrations, resulting in an adverse effect. Caution with CYP2D6 substrates, including antidepressants (eg, TCAs), antipsychotics (eg, phenothiazines and most atypicals), and antiarrhythmics (eg, propafenone, flecainide). Consider decreasing dose of drugs metabolized by CYP2D6, especially drugs with a narrow therapeutic index (eg, flecainide, propafenone, vinblastine). May prolong $T_{1/2}$ of diazepam. May increase levels of phenytoin, carbamazepine, haloperidol, clozapine, imipramine, and desipramine. Coadministration with alprazolam resulted in increased alprazolam levels and further psychomotor performance decrement. Anticonvulsant toxicity reported with phenytoin and carbamazepine. Antidiabetic drugs (eg, insulin, oral hypoglycemics) may require dose adjustment. May cause lithium toxicity; monitor lithium levels. Increased risk of hyponatremia with diuretics. Increased levels with CYP2D6 inhibitors.

NURSING CONSIDERATIONS

Assessment: Assess for volume depletion, history of seizures, risk for/presence of bipolar disorder, diseases/conditions that affect metabolism or hemodynamic responses, diabetes, susceptibility to angle-closure glaucoma, congenital long QT syndrome, previous history of QT prolongation, family history of long QT syndrome or sudden cardiac death, other conditions that predispose to QT prolongation and ventricular arrhythmia, pregnancy/nursing status, and possible drug interactions. Consider ECG assessment if initiating treatment in patients with risk factors for QT prolongation and ventricular arrhythmia.

Monitoring: Monitor for clinical worsening, suicidality, unusual changes in behavior, allergic reactions, serotonin syndrome, bleeding reactions, angle-closure glaucoma, altered appetite and weight, hyponatremia, seizures, activation of mania/hypomania, hypoglycemia/hyperglycemia, QT interval prolongation, ventricular arrhythmia, and other adverse reactions. Monitor height and weight in children periodically. Consider periodic ECG monitoring if initiating treatment in patients with risk factors for QT prolongation and ventricular arrhythmia. Periodically reassess need for continued/maintenance treatment.

Patient Counseling: Inform of risks, benefits, and appropriate use of therapy. Counsel to be alert for the emergence of suicidality, unusual changes in behavior, or worsening of depression, especially early during treatment and when the dose is adjusted up or down. Inform about risk of serotonin syndrome with concomitant use with other serotonergic agents. Counsel to seek medical care immediately if rash/hives or unusual bruising/bleeding develops, or if experiencing signs/symptoms associated with serotonin syndrome or hyponatremia. Inform that drug may cause mild pupillary dilation, which in susceptible individuals, may lead to an episode of angle-closure glaucoma. Inform that QT interval prolongation and ventricular arrhythmia (eg, torsades de pointes) have been reported. Advise to avoid operating hazardous machinery or driving a car until effects of drug are known. Advise to inform physician if taking or planning to take any prescription or OTC drugs, if pregnant/intending to become pregnant, or if breastfeeding. Instruct to take ud, not to stop taking medication without consulting physician, and to consult physician if symptoms do not improve.

Storage: 15-30°C (59-86°F). (Cap) Protect from light.

PULMICORT – budesonide RX

Class: Corticosteroid

OTHER BRAND NAMES

Pulmicort Respules, Pulmicort Flexhaler

ADULT DOSAGE

Asthma

Flexhaler:
Maint:
Initial: 180-360mcg bid
Max: 720mcg bid

PEDIATRIC DOSAGE

Asthma

1-8 Years:
Respules:
Maint/Prophylaxis:
Previously on Bronchodilators Alone:
Initial: 0.5mg qd or 0.25mg bid
Max: 0.5mg/day
Previously on Inhaled Corticosteroids:
Initial: 0.5mg qd or 0.25mg bid
Max: 1mg/day
Previously on Oral Corticosteroids:
Initial: 1mg qd or 0.5mg bid
Max: 1mg/day
Symptomatic Children Not Responding to Nonsteroidal Therapy:
Initial: 0.25mg qd

≥6 Years:
Flexhaler:
Prophylaxis:
Initial: 180-360mcg bid
Max: 360mcg bid

DOSE MODIFICATION

Elderly

Flexhaler:

Start at lower end of dosing range

ADMINISTRATION

Oral inhalation route

Patients should rinse mouth w/ water w/o swallowing after inh

Flexhaler

Priming is required prior to initial use

Respules

Administer via jet nebulizer connected to air compressor w/ adequate air flow (eg, Pari-LC-Jet Plus Nebulizer [w/ face mask or mouthpiece] connected to a Pari Master compressor)
Administer separately from other nebulizable medications in the nebulizer

HOW SUPPLIED

Powder, Inhalation: (Flexhaler) 90mcg/dose, 180mcg/dose. Sus, Inhalation: (Respules) 0.25mg/2mL, 0.5mg/2mL, 1mg/2mL [2mL]

CONTRAINDICATIONS

Primary treatment of status asthmaticus or other acute episodes of asthma where intensive measures are required. (Flexhaler) Severe hypersensitivity to milk proteins.

WARNINGS/PRECAUTIONS

Candida albicans infections of mouth and pharynx reported; treat and/or d/c if needed. Not indicated for the rapid relief of bronchospasm or other acute episodes of asthma; may require oral corticosteroids. Increased susceptibility to infections (eg, chickenpox, measles), may lead to serious/fatal course; if exposed, consider prophylaxis/treatment. Caution w/ TB, untreated systemic fungal, bacterial, viral or parasitic infections, and ocular herpes simplex. Deaths due to adrenal insufficiency reported w/ transfer from systemic to inhaled corticosteroids (ICS); if oral corticosteroids are required, wean slowly from systemic steroid use after transferring to ICS. Transfer from systemic to inhalation therapy may unmask allergic conditions (eg, rhinitis, conjunctivitis). Observe for systemic corticosteroid withdrawal effects. Hypercorticism and adrenal suppression may appear; reduce dose slowly. Decreases in bone mineral density (BMD) reported; caution w/ chronic use of drugs that can reduce bone mass (eg, anticonvulsants, corticosteroids). May cause reduction in growth velocity in pediatrics. Glaucoma, increased IOP, and cataracts reported. Bronchospasm, w/ immediate increase in wheezing, may occur; d/c immediately. Rare cases of systemic eosinophilic conditions and vasculitis consistent w/ Churg-Strauss syndrome reported. Hypersensitivity reactions reported; d/c if signs and symptoms occur. (Flexhaler) Caution in elderly.

ADVERSE REACTIONS

Respiratory infection. (Flexhaler) Nasopharyngitis, headache, fever, sinusitis, pain, N/V, insomnia, dry mouth, weight gain. (Respules) Rhinitis, otitis media, coughing, viral infection, ear infection, gastroenteritis.

DRUG INTERACTIONS

Oral ketoconazole increases plasma levels of oral budesonide. Inhibition of metabolism and increased exposure w/ CYP3A4 inhibitors. Caution w/ ketoconazole and other known strong CYP3A4 inhibitors (eg, ritonavir, clarithromycin, itraconazole, nefazodone).

NURSING CONSIDERATIONS

Assessment: Assess for concomitant diseases (eg, status asthmaticus, acute bronchospasm, other acute episodes of asthma), infections, major risk factors for decreased bone mineral content, history of eye disorders, hypersensitivity, pregnancy/nursing status, and possible drug interactions. Obtain baseline cortisol production levels. Assess lung function in oral corticosteroids withdrawal. (Flexhaler) Assess for severe milk protein hypersensitivity and hepatic disease.

Monitoring: Monitor for localized oral infections w/ *C. albicans*, worsening or acutely deteriorating asthma, systemic corticosteroid effects, decreased BMD, height in children, vision change, bronchospasm, and hypersensitivity reactions. (Flexhaler) Monitor for hepatic disease.

Patient Counseling: Advise to use at regular intervals and rinse mouth after inhalation; effectiveness depends on regular use. Instruct to d/c if oral candidiasis or hypersensitivity reactions occur. Inform that medication is not meant to relieve acute asthma symptoms and extra doses should not be used for that purpose. Instruct not to d/c w/o physician's guidance; symptoms may recur after discontinuation. Warn to avoid exposure to chickenpox or measles; if exposed, consult physician. Counsel that max benefit may not be achieved for ≥1-2 weeks (Flexhaler) or ≥4-6 weeks (Respules); instruct to notify physician if symptoms worsen or do not improve in that time frame. (Flexhaler) Instruct not to repeat inhalation even if the patient did not feel medication when inhaling; discard whole device after labeled number of inhalations have been used. Advise to carry a warning card indicating need for supplemental systemic corticosteroid during periods of stress or severe asthma attack if chronic systemic corticosteroids have been reduced or withdrawn. Instruct to consult physician if pregnant/breastfeeding or intend to become pregnant.

Storage: (Flexhaler): 20-25°C (68-77°F). Cover tightly. Store in a dry place. (Respules): 20-25°C (68-77°F). Protect from light. Do not freeze. After aluminum foil opened, unused ampules stable for 2 weeks. Once opened, use promptly.

PYRAZINAMIDE — pyrazinamide

RX

Class: Nicotinamide analogue

ADULT DOSAGE

Tuberculosis

Initial treatment of active tuberculosis (TB) when combined w/ other anti-TB agents and for the use after treatment failure w/ other primary drugs in any form of active TB

Usual: 15-30mg/kg qd

Max: 3g/day

Alternate Regimen:

50-70mg/kg twice weekly based on lean body weight

Always administer w/ other effective anti-TB drugs; administer for the initial 2 months of a 6-month or longer treatment regimen

Patients w/ HIV infection may require longer courses of therapy

PEDIATRIC DOSAGE

Tuberculosis

Initial treatment of active tuberculosis (TB) when combined w/ other anti-TB agents and for the use after treatment failure w/ other primary drugs in any form of active TB

Usual: 15-30mg/kg qd

Max: 3g/day

Alternate Regimen:

50-70mg/kg twice weekly based on lean body weight

Always administer w/ other effective anti-TB drugs; administer for the initial 2 months of a 6-month or longer treatment regimen

Patients w/ HIV infection may require longer courses of therapy

DOSE MODIFICATION

Renal Impairment

May start at lower end of dosing range

Elderly

Start at lower end of dosing range

ADMINISTRATION

Oral route

HOW SUPPLIED

Tab: 500mg* *scored

CONTRAINDICATIONS

Severe hepatic damage, acute gout.

WARNINGS/PRECAUTIONS

Should only be used in conjunction with other effective anti-TB agents. Closely monitor patients with preexisting liver disease or those at increased risk for drug-related hepatitis (eg, alcohol abusers). D/C and do not resume therapy if signs of hepatocellular damage or hyperuricemia with acute gouty arthritis appear. Perform in vitro susceptibility tests with recent cultures of *Mycobacterium tuberculosis* against pyrazinamide and the usual primary drugs in cases with known or suspected drug resistance. Interference with Acetest and Ketostix urine tests to produce a pink-brown color reported. Caution with history of diabetes mellitus (DM) and in elderly.

ADVERSE REACTIONS

Gout, hepatotoxicity, N/V, anorexia, arthralgia, myalgia, rash, urticaria, pruritus.

NURSING CONSIDERATIONS

Assessment: Assess for risk for drug-related hepatitis, history of DM, drug hypersensitivity, and pregnancy/nursing status. Obtain baseline serum uric acid levels, LFTs, and renal function.

Monitoring: Monitor for drug resistance, signs of hepatocellular damage, hyperuricemia with acute gouty arthritis, and other adverse reactions. Perform appropriate lab testing periodically and if any clinical signs/symptoms occur.

Patient Counseling: Instruct to notify physician if fever, loss of appetite, malaise, N/V, darkened urine, yellowish discoloration of skin and eyes, or joint pain/swelling occurs. Emphasize compliance with full course of therapy and importance of not missing any doses.

Storage: 20-25°C (68-77°F).

QSYMIA – phentermine/topiramate CIV

Class: Anorectic sympathomimetic amine/sulfamate-substituted monosaccharide

ADULT DOSAGE

Weight Loss

Adjunct to a reduced-calorie diet and increased physical activity for chronic weight management in patients w/ initial BMI ≥30kg/m^2, or ≥27kg/m^2 in the presence of ≥1 weight-related comorbidity

Initial: 3.75mg/23mg qd for 14 days

Titrate: After 14 days, increase to 7.5mg/46mg qd; d/c or escalate dose if patient has not lost at least 3% of baseline weight after 12 weeks

Dose Escalation: Increase to 11.25mg/69mg qd for 14 days, followed by 15mg/92mg qd; d/c if patient has not lost at least 5% of baseline weight after 12 weeks on 15mg/92mg

Use 3.75mg/23mg and 11.25mg/69mg strengths for titration purposes only

Discontinuation: D/C 15mg/92mg gradually by taking a dose qod for at least 1 week prior to stopping treatment

PEDIATRIC DOSAGE

Pediatric use may not have been established

DOSE MODIFICATION

Renal Impairment

Moderate (CrCl ≥30-<50mL/min) to Severe (CrCl <30mL/min):
Max: 7.5mg/46mg qd

ESRD on Dialysis:
Avoid use

Hepatic Impairment

Moderate (Child-Pugh Score 7-9):
Max: 7.5mg/46mg qd

Severe (Child-Pugh Score 10-15):
Avoid use

Elderly

Start at lower end of dosing range

ADMINISTRATION

Oral route

Take w/ or w/o food

Take qam; avoid pm dosing due to the possibility of insomnia

HOW SUPPLIED

Cap, Extended-Release: (Phentermine/Topiramate) 3.75mg/23mg, 7.5mg/46mg, 11.25mg/69mg, 15mg/92mg

CONTRAINDICATIONS

Pregnancy, glaucoma, hyperthyroidism, during or within 14 days of administration of MAOIs.

WARNINGS/PRECAUTIONS

May cause fetal harm; use effective contraception to prevent pregnancy. Available through a limited program under the Risk Evaluation and Mitigation Strategy. May increase resting HR; monitor resting HR regularly in all patients, especially those with cardiac or cerebrovascular disease or when initiating or increasing dose. Reduce dose or d/c if sustained increase in resting HR or persistent SrCr elevations occur. Increased risk of suicidal thoughts/behavior; monitor for emergence/worsening of depression, suicidal thoughts/behavior, and/or any unusual changes in mood or behavior, and d/c if these occur. Avoid with history of suicidal attempts or active suicidal ideation. Acute myopia associated with secondary angle-closure glaucoma reported; d/c immediately to reverse symptoms. Mood/sleep disorders, including anxiety and insomnia, may occur; consider dose reduction or withdrawal for clinically significant or persistent symptoms. May impair physical/mental abilities; consider dose reduction or withdrawal if cognitive dysfunction persists. Hyperchloremic, non-anion gap, metabolic acidosis reported.

Conditions that predispose to acidosis (eg, renal disease, severe respiratory disorders, status epilepticus, diarrhea, surgery, ketogenic diet) may be additive to the bicarbonate lowering effects of topiramate. Weight loss may increase risk of hypoglycemia in patients with type 2 DM treated with insulin and/or insulin secretagogues (eg, sulfonylureas), and risk of hypotension in those treated with antihypertensives; appropriate changes should be made to antidiabetic or antihypertensive therapy if hypoglycemia or hypotension develops. Seizures associated with abrupt withdrawal in individuals without history of seizures or epilepsy; taper dose gradually if using 15mg/92mg and monitor for seizures in situations where immediate termination of therapy is required. Avoid with ESRD on dialysis or severe hepatic impairment (Child-Pugh 10-15). Associated with kidney stone formation; increase fluid intake to increase urine output. Oligohidrosis reported; monitor for decreased sweating and increased body temperature during physical activity, especially in hot weather. May increase risk of hypokalemia. Potential for abuse. Lab test interactions may occur. Caution in elderly.

ADVERSE REACTIONS

Paresthesia, dry mouth, constipation, URTI, headache, dysgeusia, insomnia, nasopharyngitis, dizziness, sinusitis, bronchitis, nausea, back pain, diarrhea, blurred vision.

DRUG INTERACTIONS

See Contraindications. May decrease exposure of ethinyl estradiol and increase exposure of norethindrone with single dose of oral contraceptive. Alcohol or CNS depressants (eg, barbiturates, benzodiazepines, sleep medications) may potentiate CNS depression. May potentiate the K^+ wasting action of non-K^+-sparing diuretics; monitor for hypokalemia. Avoid with other drugs that inhibit carbonic anhydrase (eg, zonisamide, acetazolamide, methazolamide, dichlorphenamide); may increase severity of metabolic acidosis and kidney stone formation. Caution with other drugs that predispose patients to heat-related disorders (eg, other carbonic anhydrase inhibitors, drugs with anticholinergic activity). Phenytoin or carbamazepine may decrease plasma levels. Concurrent administration of valproic acid has been associated with hyperammonemia with or without encephalopathy, and hypothermia.

NURSING CONSIDERATIONS

Assessment: Assess for known hypersensitivity or idiosyncrasy to sympathomimetic amines, glaucoma, hyperthyroidism, cardiac and cerebrovascular disease, history of behavioral/mood disorders, history of seizures, renal/hepatic dysfunction, any other conditions where treatment is contraindicated or cautioned, pregnancy/nursing status, and possible drug interactions. Obtain baseline HR and blood chemistry profile (eg, bicarbonate, creatinine, K^+, glucose).

Monitoring: Monitor for acute myopia, secondary angle-closure glaucoma, emergence/worsening of depression, suicidal thoughts or behavior, mood/sleep disorders, cognitive dysfunction, hyperchloremic metabolic acidosis, seizures, kidney stone formation, oligohidrosis, and hyperthermia. Monitor HR regularly and blood chemistry profile (eg, bicarbonate, creatinine, K^+, glucose) periodically. Assess pregnancy status monthly during therapy.

Patient Counseling: Inform that therapy is for chronic weight management in conjunction with a reduced-calorie diet and increased physical activity. Inform that drug is only available through certified pharmacies. Instruct to inform physician about all medications, nutritional supplements, and vitamins (including any weight loss products) taken while on therapy. Instruct on how to properly take the medication. Instruct to avoid pregnancy/breastfeeding while on therapy and to notify physician immediately if patient becomes pregnant during treatment. Advise to report symptoms of sustained periods of heart pounding or racing while at rest, suicidal behavior/ideation, mood changes, depression, severe/persistent eye pain or significant visual changes, any changes in attention/concentration/memory, and/or difficulty finding words. Advise not to drive/operate machinery until reaction to the medication is known. Instruct to notify physician about any factors that can increase the risk of acidosis (eg, prolonged diarrhea, surgery, high protein/low carbohydrate diet, and/or concomitant medications such as other carbonic anhydrase inhibitors) and to avoid alcohol while on therapy. Instruct diabetic patients to monitor blood glucose levels and to report symptoms of hypoglycemia to physician. Advise not to abruptly d/c therapy without notifying physician. Advise to increase fluid intake and report symptoms of severe side or back pain, and/or blood in urine to physician. Advise to monitor for decreased sweating and increased body temperature during physical activity, especially in hot weather.

Storage: 15-25°C (59-77°F). Protect from moisture.

QUILLIVANT XR – methylphenidate hydrochloride CII

Class: Sympathomimetic amine

High potential for abuse and dependence. Assess the risk of abuse prior to prescribing, and monitor for signs of abuse and dependence while on therapy.

ADULT DOSAGE

Attention-Deficit Hyperactivity Disorder

Initial: 20mg qam
Titrate: May be titrated weekly in increments of 10mg to 20mg
Max: 60mg/day

Maint/Extended Treatment:
Periodically reevaluate long-term usefulness w/ trials off medication to assess functioning w/o pharmacotherapy

D/C if no improvement observed after appropriate dosage adjustments over 1 month

PEDIATRIC DOSAGE

Attention-Deficit Hyperactivity Disorder

≥6 Years:
Initial: 20mg qam
Titrate: May be titrated weekly in increments of 10mg to 20mg
Max: 60mg/day

Maint/Extended Treatment:
Periodically reevaluate long-term usefulness w/ trials off medication to assess functioning w/o pharmacotherapy

D/C if no improvement observed after appropriate dosage adjustments over 1 month

DOSE MODIFICATION

Adverse Reactions
Reduce dose or d/c if necessary, if paradoxical aggravation of symptoms or other adverse events occur

ADMINISTRATION
Oral route

Take w/ or w/o food
Vigorously shake bottle for at least 10 sec before each dose to ensure that the proper dose is administered
Use only w/ the oral dosing dispenser provided

Reconstitution Instructions for Pharmacist
Reconstitute 300mg bottle w/ 53mL water; reconstitute 600mg bottle w/ 105mL water; reconstitute 750mg bottle w/ 131mL water; reconstitute 900mg bottle w/1058mL water
Shake vigorously for at least 10 sec to prepare sus

Refer to PI for further administration instructions

HOW SUPPLIED
Sus, Extended-Release: 5mg/mL [60mL, 120mL, 150mL, 180mL]

CONTRAINDICATIONS
Treatment with or within 14 days following discontinuation of treatment with an MAOI.

WARNINGS/PRECAUTIONS
Sudden death reported in children and adolescents with structural cardiac abnormalities and other serious cardiac problems. Sudden death, stroke, and MI reported in adults. Avoid with known structural cardiac abnormalities, cardiomyopathy, serious cardiac arrhythmias, coronary artery disease, or other serious cardiac problems. May increase BP and HR. May exacerbate symptoms of behavior disturbance and thought disorder in patients with a preexisting psychotic disorder. May induce a manic or mixed episode in patients with bipolar disorder. May cause psychotic or manic symptoms in patients without a prior history of psychotic illness or mania at recommended doses; consider discontinuation if such symptoms occur. Priapism reported; seek immediate medical attention if abnormally sustained or frequent and painful erections develop. Associated with peripheral vasculopathy, including Raynaud's phenomenon; monitor for digital changes. May cause long-term suppression of growth in pediatric patients; may need to interrupt treatment in patients not growing or gaining height or weight as expected.

ADVERSE REACTIONS
Affect lability, excoriation, initial insomnia, tic, decreased appetite, vomiting, motion sickness, eye pain, rash.

DRUG INTERACTIONS
See Contraindications.

NURSING CONSIDERATIONS

Assessment: Assess for drug hypersensitivity, cardiac problems, psychotic disorders, bipolar disorder, pregnancy/nursing status, and for possible drug interactions. Obtain baseline height/weight in children. Screen patients for risk factors for developing a manic episode and the risk of abuse before starting therapy.

Monitoring: Monitor for stroke, MI, HTN, tachycardia, exacerbations of behavior disturbances and thought disorders, psychotic or manic symptoms, digital changes, priapism, and other adverse reactions. Monitor growth in children. Monitor for signs of abuse and dependence. Periodically reevaluate long-term usefulness.

Patient Counseling: Inform about risks, benefits, and appropriate use of treatment. Counsel that drug has potential for abuse or dependence; instruct to keep medication in a safe place to prevent abuse. Advise of the potential for serious cardiovascular risks, including sudden death, MI, and stroke; instruct to contact physician immediately if symptoms, such as exertional chest pain, unexplained syncope, or other symptoms suggestive of cardiac disease develop. Advise that the drug can elevate BP and HR, can cause psychotic or manic symptoms even in patients without a prior history of psychotic symptoms or mania, and in pediatric patients can cause slowing of growth and weight loss. Advise of the possibility of priapism; instruct to seek immediate medical attention in the event of priapism. Inform about the risk of peripheral vasculopathy, including Raynaud's phenomenon; instruct to report to the physician any numbness, pain, skin color change, sensitivity to temperature in fingers or toes, and any signs of unexplained wounds appearing on fingers or toes. Instruct to inform physician if pregnant/intending to become pregnant during therapy. Advise of the potential fetal effects from use during pregnancy.

Storage: 25°C (77°F); excursions permitted from 15-30°C (59-86°F). Stable for up to 4 months after reconstitution.

QUIXIN – levofloxacin **RX**

Class: Fluoroquinolone

ADULT DOSAGE

Bacterial Conjunctivitis

Days 1-2:
1-2 drops in the affected eye(s) q2h while awake, up to 8X/day
Days 3-7:
1-2 drops in the affected eye(s) q4h while awake, up to qid

PEDIATRIC DOSAGE

Bacterial Conjunctivitis

≥1 Year:
Days 1-2:
1-2 drops in the affected eye(s) q2h while awake, up to 8X/day
Days 3-7:
1-2 drops in the affected eye(s) q4h while awake, up to qid

ADMINISTRATION
Ocular route

HOW SUPPLIED
Sol: 0.5% [5mL]

WARNINGS/PRECAUTIONS
Should not be injected subconjunctivally nor introduced directly to anterior chamber of the eye. D/C if allergic reaction or superinfection occurs; prolonged use may cause overgrowth of nonsusceptible organisms. Avoid wearing contact lenses if signs/symptoms of conjunctivitis present.

ADVERSE REACTIONS
Transient ocular burning, transient decreased vision, fever, foreign body sensation, headache, ocular pain/discomfort, pharyngitis, photophobia.

DRUG INTERACTIONS
Systemic quinolone therapy may increase theophylline levels, interfere with caffeine metabolism, enhance warfarin effects, and elevate SrCr with cyclosporine.

NURSING CONSIDERATIONS

Assessment: Assess for hypersensitivity to the drug or to other quinolones, use of contact lenses, pregnancy/nursing status, possible drug interactions, or any other conditions where treatment is contraindicated or cautioned.

Monitoring: Monitor for signs/symptoms of hypersensitivity or anaphylactic reaction, and overgrowth of nonsusceptible organisms. Perform eye exam using magnification (eg, slit-lamp biomicroscopy, fluorescein staining) if necessary.

Patient Counseling: Instruct to avoid contaminating applicator tip with material from eye, fingers, or other sources. Advise to not wear contact lenses if there are signs/symptoms of bacterial conjunctivitis. Instruct to d/c medication and contact physician if signs of hypersensitivity reaction (eg, rash) develop.

Storage: 15-25°C (59-77°F).

QVAR – beclomethasone dipropionate

Class: Corticosteroid

RX

ADULT DOSAGE

Asthma

Previously on Bronchodilators Alone:
Initial: 40-80mcg bid
Max: 320mcg bid

Previously on Inhaled Corticosteroids:
Initial: 40-160mcg bid
Max: 320mcg bid

PEDIATRIC DOSAGE

Asthma

5-11 Years:
Previously on Bronchodilators Alone or Inhaled Corticosteroids:
Initial: 40mcg bid
Max: 80mcg bid

≥12 Years:
Previously on Bronchodilators Alone:
Initial: 40-80mcg bid
Max: 320mcg bid

Previously on Inhaled Corticosteroids:
Initial: 40-160mcg bid
Max: 320mcg bid

DOSE MODIFICATION

Concomitant Medications

Systemic Corticosteroids (eg, Prednisone):
Slowly wean patient beginning after at least 1 week of therapy

Elderly

Start at lower end of dosing range

ADMINISTRATION

Oral inh route

Advise patient to rinse mouth after inh

Priming

Actuate into the air twice before using for the 1st time or if not used for >10 days

HOW SUPPLIED

MDI: 40mcg/inh, 80mcg/inh [120 actuations]

CONTRAINDICATIONS

Primary treatment of status asthmaticus or other acute episodes of asthma where intensive measures are required.

WARNINGS/PRECAUTIONS

Candida albicans infections of mouth and pharynx may occur; treat and/or interrupt therapy if needed. Not indicated for relief of acute bronchospasm. Deaths due to adrenal insufficiency have occurred during and after transfer from systemic to inhaled corticosteroids; wean slowly from systemic corticosteroid use after transferring to therapy. Resume oral corticosteroids (in large doses) immediately during periods of stress or a severe asthmatic attack in patients previously withdrawn from systemic corticosteroids. Transfer from systemic to inhaled corticosteroids may unmask allergic conditions previously suppressed by systemic therapy (eg, rhinitis, conjunctivitis, eczema). Increased susceptibility to infections. May lead to more serious/fatal course of chickenpox or measles; avoid exposure, and if exposed, consider prophylaxis/treatment. Caution w/ active or quiescent TB, untreated systemic fungal/bacterial/parasitic/viral infections, or ocular herpes simplex. Paradoxical bronchospasm, w/ immediate increase in wheezing, may occur after dosing; treat immediately w/ a short-acting inhaled bronchodilator; d/c and institute alternative therapy. Hypersensitivity reactions (eg, urticaria, angioedema, rash) may occur; d/c if these occur. Monitor for systemic corticosteroid effects; reduce dose slowly if hypercorticism and adrenal suppression occur. Caution should be taken in observing patients postoperatively or during periods of stress for evidence of inadequate adrenal response. May cause reduction in growth velocity in pediatric patients; monitor growth. Decreases in bone mineral density (BMD) reported w/ long-term use; monitor in patients w/ major risk factors (eg, prolonged immobilization, family history of osteoporosis, chronic use of drugs that can reduce bone mass). Glaucoma, increased intraocular pressure (IOP), and cataracts reported w/ long-term use. Caution in elderly.

ADVERSE REACTIONS

Headache, pharyngitis, URTI, rhinitis, increased asthma symptoms, oral symptoms (inhalation route), sinusitis, dysphonia, dysmenorrhea, coughing.

NURSING CONSIDERATIONS

Assessment: Assess for status asthmaticus, acute asthma episodes, acute bronchospasm, active/quiescent TB, untreated systemic infections, ocular herpes simplex, known hypersensitivity to drug or to any of the ingredients, risk factors for BMD, history of increased IOP/glaucoma/cataracts, and pregnancy/nursing status.

Monitoring: Monitor for paradoxical bronchospasm, hypercorticism, adrenal suppression/insufficiency, BMD, changes in vision, glaucoma, increased IOP, cataracts, infections, hypersensitivity reactions, asthma instability, and other adverse reactions. Monitor growth in pediatric patients.

Patient Counseling: Advise to contact physician if oropharyngeal candidiasis develops. Instruct to avoid exposure to chickenpox or measles, and, if exposed, to consult physician w/o delay. Inform about risks of immunosuppression, hypercorticism, adrenal suppression, reduction in bone mineral density, reduced growth velocity in pediatric patients, glaucoma, and cataracts. Advise that drug is not intended for use in the treatment of acute asthma; instruct to immediately contact physician if asthma deteriorates. Advise to use medication at regular intervals since its effectiveness depends on regular use. Instruct to contact physician if symptoms do not improve after 2 weeks of therapy or if condition worsens. Counsel about the proper priming/use of inhaler. Instruct not to stop abruptly and to immediately contact physician if drug is discontinued.

Storage: 25°C (77°F); excursions permitted to 15-30°C (59-86°F). For optimal results, canister should be at room temperature when used. Do not puncture, use/store near heat or open flame, or throw container into fire/incinerator. Exposure to temperatures >49°C (120°F) may cause bursting.

RANEXA – ranolazine RX

Class: Miscellaneous antianginal

ADULT DOSAGE

Chronic Angina

Initial: 500mg bid
Titrate: Increase to 1000mg bid prn
Max: 1000mg bid

May be used w/ β-blockers, nitrates, calcium channel blockers, antiplatelet therapy, lipid-lowering therapy, ACE inhibitors, and ARBs

PEDIATRIC DOSAGE

Pediatric use may not have been established

DOSE MODIFICATION

Concomitant Medications

Moderate CYP3A Inhibitors (eg, Diltiazem, Verapamil, Erythromycin):
Max Dose: 500mg bid
P-gp Inhibitors (eg, Cyclosporine):
Titrate ranolazine based on clinical response

Elderly

Start at lower end of dosing range

ADMINISTRATION

Oral route

Take w/ or w/o meals
Swallow tab whole; do not crush, break, or chew

HOW SUPPLIED

Tab, Extended-Release: 500mg, 1000mg

CONTRAINDICATIONS

Liver cirrhosis, concomitant use w/ CYP3A inducers (eg, rifampin, rifabutin, rifapentine, phenobarbital, phenytoin, carbamazepine, St. John's wort) or strong CYP3A inhibitors (eg, ketoconazole, itraconazole, clarithromycin, nefazodone, nelfinavir, ritonavir, indinavir, saquinavir).

WARNINGS/PRECAUTIONS

May prolong QTc interval in a dose-related manner. Acute renal failure reported in patients w/ severe renal impairment (CrCl <30mL/min); d/c and treat appropriately if acute renal failure develops. Monitor renal function after initiation and periodically in patients w/ moderate to severe renal impairment (CrCl <60mL/min) for increases in SrCr accompanied by an increase in BUN. Caution in elderly.

ADVERSE REACTIONS

Dizziness, headache, constipation, N/V, abdominal pain, dyspepsia, anorexia, asthenia, peripheral edema, bradycardia, palpitations, confusion, dyspnea, hematuria, hyperhidrosis.

DRUG INTERACTIONS

See Contraindications and Dosage. P-gp inhibitors (eg, cyclosporine) may increase concentrations. May increase levels of simvastatin; limit simvastatin dose to 20mg qd. May increase concentrations of other sensitive CYP3A substrates (eg, lovastatin) and CYP3A substrates w/ a narrow therapeutic range (eg, cyclosporine, tacrolimus, sirolimus); may require dose adjustment of these drugs. May increase exposure to digoxin and CYP2D6 substrates (eg, TCAs, antipsychotics); may require digoxin dose adjustment and lower doses of CYP2D6 substrates. May increase levels of metformin; do not exceed 1700mg/day of metformin if coadministered w/ ranolazine 1000mg bid and monitor blood glucose levels and risks associated w/ high metformin exposure.

NURSING CONSIDERATIONS

Assessment: Assess for liver cirrhosis, QT interval prolongation, renal impairment, pregnancy/nursing status, and possible drug interactions.

Monitoring: Monitor for ECG changes (eg, QT interval prolongation) and other adverse reactions. Monitor renal function (eg, SrCr, BUN) after initiation and periodically in patients w/ moderate to severe renal impairment.

Patient Counseling: Inform that drug will not abate an acute angina episode. Advise to inform physician of any other concurrent medications, including OTC drugs, and of any history of QTc prolongation, congenital long QT syndrome, or renal impairment. Inform about the risk of renal failure in patients w/ severe renal impairment. Instruct to limit grapefruit juice/products. Instruct to contact physician if fainting spells occur. Advise that therapy may cause dizziness and lightheadedness; instruct patients to know how they react to the drug before engaging in activities requiring mental alertness or coordination (eg, operating machinery, driving).

Storage: 25°C (77°F); excursions permitted to 15-30°C (59-86°F).

RANITIDINE – ranitidine hydrochloride

Class: H_2-blocker

RX

OTHER BRAND NAMES

Zantac Oral, Zantac Injection

ADULT DOSAGE

General Dosing

Inj:

For hospitalized patients w/ pathological hypersecretory conditions or intractable duodenal ulcers, or as an alternative to the oral dosage form for short-term use in patients who are unable to take oral medication

IM:

50mg q6-8h

IV:

Usual: 50mg q6-8h as intermittent bolus/infusion or 6.25mg/hr continuous IV infusion
Max: 400mg/day

Gastric Ulcers

Short-Term Treatment of Active, Benign Ulcers:
PO:
Usual: 150mg bid
Maint: 150mg hs

Gastroesophageal Reflux Disease

PO:
150mg bid

Erosive Esophagitis

Endoscopically Diagnosed:
PO:
Usual: 150mg qid
Maint: 150mg bid

Duodenal Ulcers

Short-Term Treatment of Active Ulcers:
PO:
Usual: 150mg bid or 300mg qd after pm meal or hs
Maint: 150mg hs

Pathological Hypersecretory Conditions

Treatment of pathological hypersecretory conditions (eg, Zollinger-Ellison syndrome, systemic mastocytosis)
PO:
150mg bid; adjust dose according to patient needs and continue as long as clinically

PEDIATRIC DOSAGE

Erosive Esophagitis

Endoscopically Diagnosed:
1 Month-16 Years:
PO:
5-10mg/kg/day given as 2 divided doses

Duodenal Ulcers

Short-Term Treatment of Active Ulcers:
1 Month-16 Years:
PO:
Usual: 2-4mg/kg bid
Maint: 2-4mg/kg qd
Max: 300mg/day (treatment), 150mg/day (maint)

Inj:
Usual: 2-4mg/kg/day IV given q6-8h
Max: 50mg IV q6-8h

Gastric Ulcers

Short-Term Treatment of Active, Benign Ulcers:
1 Month-16 Years:
PO:
Usual: 2-4mg/kg bid
Maint: 2-4mg/kg qd
Max: 300mg/day (treatment), 150mg/day (maint)

Gastroesophageal Reflux Disease

1 Month-16 Years:
PO:
5-10mg/kg/day given as 2 divided doses

Other Indications

Inj:
<1 Month of Age:
Limited data in neonatal patients receiving extracorporeal membrane oxygenation suggest that ranitidine may be useful and safe for increasing gastric pH for patients at risk of GI hemorrhage

2mg/kg given q12-24h or as a continuous infusion should be considered indicated. Doses up to 6g/day have been employed w/ severe disease

Continuous IV Infusion:
Zollinger-Ellison Syndrome:
Initial: 1mg/kg/hr
Titrate: May increase after 4 hrs by 0.5mg/kg/hr increments if gastric acid output is >10mEq/hr or patient becomes symptomatic
Doses up to 2.5mg/kg/hr and infusion rates as high as 220mg/hr have been used

DOSE MODIFICATION

Renal Impairment
CrCl <50mL/min: 150mg PO q24h or 50mg IV/IM q18-24h; may increase dosing frequency to q12h or even further, w/ caution
Hemodialysis: Give dose at the end of treatment

ADMINISTRATION

Oral/IM/IV routes

PO
Administer concomitant antacids prn for pain relief to patients w/ active duodenal ulcer; active, benign gastric ulcer; hypersecretory states; GERD; or erosive esophagitis

Inj
IV:
Intermittent Bolus:
Dilute ranitidine 50mg inj in 0.9% NaCl inj or other compatible IV sol to a concentration ≤2.5mg/mL (20mL)
Inject at a rate ≤4mL/min (5 min)
Intermittent Infusion:
Dilute ranitidine 50mg inj in D5 inj or other compatible IV sol to a concentration ≤0.5mg/mL (100mL)
Infuse at a rate ≤5-7mL/min (15-20 min)
Continuous Infusion:
Add ranitidine inj to D5 inj or other compatible IV sol; deliver at a rate of 6.25mg/hr (eg, 150mg of ranitidine inj in 250mL of D5 inj at 10.7mL/hr)
For Zollinger-Ellison patients, dilute ranitidine inj in D5 inj or other compatible IV sol to a concentration ≤2.5mg/mL
IM:
No dilution necessary

Stability:
Stable for 48 hrs at room temperature when added to or diluted w/ most commonly used IV sol (eg, 0.9% NaCl inj, D5 inj, 10% dextrose inj, lactated Ringer's inj, 5% sodium bicarbonate inj)

HOW SUPPLIED

Cap: 150mg, 300mg; Syrup: 15mg/mL [16 fl oz]; (Zantac) Inj: 25mg/mL [2mL, 6mL]; Tab: 150mg, 300mg

WARNINGS/PRECAUTIONS

Symptomatic response does not preclude the presence of gastric malignancy. Caution w/ hepatic/renal dysfunction. May precipitate acute porphyric attacks in patients w/ acute porphyria; avoid w/ history of acute porphyria. False (+) tests for urine protein w/ Multistix may occur. Caution in elderly. D/C immediately if hepatocellular, cholestatic, or mixed hepatitis occurs. (Inj) Do not exceed recommended administration rates; bradycardia reported w/ rapid infusion. ALT elevations may occur; monitor if on IV therapy for ≥5 days at doses ≥100mg qid.

ADVERSE REACTIONS

Headache, constipation, diarrhea, N/V, abdominal discomfort/pain, rash.

DRUG INTERACTIONS

Affects bioavailability of other drugs through several mechanisms (eg, competition for renal tubular secretion, alteration of gastric pH, CYP450 inhibition). Increased plasma levels of procainamide w/ high doses of ranitidine; monitor for procainamide toxicity when administered w/ oral ranitidine at a dose >300mg/day. Altered PT w/ warfarin; closely monitor PT. May alter absorption of drugs in which gastric pH is an important determinant of bioavailability; may increase absorption of triazolam, midazolam, and glipizide and decrease absorption of ketoconazole, atazanavir, delavirdine, and gefitinib. Monitor for excessive/prolonged sedation w/ oral midazolam and triazolam. Chronic use w/ delavirdine is not recommended.

NURSING CONSIDERATIONS

Assessment: Assess for hypersensitivity to the drug, renal/hepatic impairment, history of acute porphyria, pregnancy/nursing status, and possible drug interactions.

Monitoring: Monitor for signs/symptoms of hepatic effects (eg, hepatitis, elevations in ALT values), hypersensitivity reactions, and other adverse reactions. Monitor PT in patients receiving warfarin.

Patient Counseling: Inform that antacids may be taken prn for relief of pain. Instruct to notify physician if any adverse events develop.

Storage: Cap: 20-25°C (68-77°F) in a dry place. Protect from light. Tab: 15-30°C (59-86°F) in a dry place. Protect from light. Syrup: 4-25°C (39-77°F). Do not freeze. Inj: 4-25°C (39-77°F); excursions permitted to 30°C (86°F). Protect from light. Avoid excessive heat; brief exposure up to 40°C (104°F) does not adversely affect the product. Protect from freezing.

RAPAFLO — silodosin

RX

Class: Alpha$_1$-antagonist

ADULT DOSAGE

Benign Prostatic Hypertrophy

8mg qd w/ a meal

PEDIATRIC DOSAGE

Pediatric use may not have been established

DOSE MODIFICATION

Renal Impairment

CrCl 30-50mL/min: 4mg qd w/ a meal

ADMINISTRATION

Oral route

Take w/ a meal

Patients who have difficulty swallowing caps may sprinkle the cap powder on a tbsp of applesauce (should not be hot)

Swallow immediately (w/in 5 min) w/o chewing and follow with 8 oz of cool water

Do not subdivide the contents of cap or store any powder/applesauce mixture for future use

HOW SUPPLIED

Cap: 4mg, 8mg

CONTRAINDICATIONS

Severe renal impairment (CrCl <30mL/min), severe hepatic impairment (Child-Pugh score ≥10), and concomitant administration with strong CYP3A4 inhibitors (eg, ketoconazole, clarithromycin, itraconazole, ritonavir).

WARNINGS/PRECAUTIONS

Not for treatment of HTN. Postural hypotension and syncope may occur; may impair mental/ physical abilities. Caution in patients with moderate renal impairment. Examine patients prior to therapy to rule out prostate cancer. Intraoperative floppy iris syndrome (IFIS) observed during cataract surgery in some patients on α_1-blockers or previously treated with α_1-blockers.

ADVERSE REACTIONS

Retrograde ejaculation, dizziness, diarrhea, orthostatic hypotension, headache, nasopharyngitis, nasal congestion.

DRUG INTERACTIONS

See Contraindications. Avoid with other α-blockers and strong P-glycoprotein (P-gp) inhibitors (eg, cyclosporine). Caution with antihypertensives. Coadministration with PDE-5 inhibitors may cause symptomatic hypotension; caution with use. Increased concentrations with P-gp inhibitors and moderate CYP3A4 inhibitors (eg, diltiazem, erythromycin, verapamil). UGT2B7 inhibitors (eg, probenecid, valproic acid, fluconazole) may potentially increase exposure.

NURSING CONSIDERATIONS

Assessment: Assess for drug hypersensitivity, renal/hepatic impairment, prostate cancer, and possible drug interactions.

Monitoring: Monitor for signs/symptoms of postural hypotension, syncope, IFIS during cataract surgery, and other adverse reactions.

Patient Counseling: Counsel about possible occurrence of symptoms related to postural hypotension (eg, dizziness); advise to use caution when driving, operating machinery, or performing hazardous tasks, particularly in patients with low BP or taking antihypertensives. Inform that most common side effect seen is an orgasm with reduced or no semen; inform that this side effect does not pose a safety concern and is reversible when drug is discontinued. Advise to notify ophthalmologist about the use of the drug before cataract surgery or other eye procedures, even if no longer taking silodosin.

Storage: 25°C (77°F); excursions permitted to 15-30°C (59-86°F). Protect from light and moisture.

RAPIVAB – peramivir

RX

Class: Neuraminidase inhibitor

ADULT DOSAGE

Influenza

Treatment of Acute Uncomplicated Influenza:
≥18 Years:
Usual: Single 600mg dose, via IV infusion for 15-30 min

PEDIATRIC DOSAGE

Pediatric use may not have been established

DOSE MODIFICATION

Renal Impairment

CrCl 30-49mL/min: 200mg
CrCl 10-29mL/min: 100mg

ADMINISTRATION

IV route

Administer w/in 2 days of onset of symptoms of influenza
In patients w/ chronic renal impairment maintained on hemodialysis, administer after dialysis

Dilute an appropriate dose of peramivir 10mg/mL sol in 0.9% or 0.45% NaCl, D5, or Lactated Ringer's to a max volume of 100mL
Administer diluted sol via IV infusion for 15-30 min

Compatible w/ 0.9% or 0.45% NaCl, D5, or lactated Ringer's
Do not mix or coinfuse w/ other IV medications
If diluted sol refrigerated, allow to reach room temperature then administer immediately
Refer to PI for further administration instructions

HOW SUPPLIED

Inj: 10mg/mL [20mL]

WARNINGS/PRECAUTIONS

Emergence of resistance substitutions can decrease drug effectiveness; consider available information on influenza drug susceptibility patterns and treatment effects when deciding whether to use peramivir. Rare cases of serious skin reactions (eg, erythema multiforme, Stevens-Johnson syndrome) reported; institute appropriate treatment if a serious skin reaction occurs or is suspected. Neuropsychiatric events (eg, hallucinations, delirium, abnormal behavior), in some cases resulting in fatal outcomes, reported; monitor for signs of abnormal behavior. Serious bacterial infections may begin with influenza-like symptoms or may coexist with or occur during the course of influenza; peramivir does not prevent these complications.

ADVERSE REACTIONS

Diarrhea, increased alanine aminotransferase/serum glucose/CPK, decreased neutrophils.

DRUG INTERACTIONS

Avoid use of live attenuated influenza vaccine within 2 weeks before or 48 hrs after administration of peramivir, unless medically indicated.

NURSING CONSIDERATIONS

Assessment: Assess for renal impairment, pregnancy/nursing status, and possible drug interactions.

Monitoring: Monitor for signs/symptoms of serious skin/hypersensitivity reactions, neuropsychiatric events, and other adverse reactions.

Patient Counseling: Advise of the risk of serious skin reactions and to seek immediate medical attention if a skin reaction occurs. Advise of the risk of neuropsychiatric events in patients with influenza and to contact physician if experiencing signs of abnormal behavior after receiving treatment.

Storage: 20-25°C (68-77°F); excursions permitted to 15-30°C (59-86°F). Diluted Sol: 2-8°C (36-46°F) for up to 24 hrs.

RAYOS – prednisone

Class: Glucocorticoid

RX

ADULT DOSAGE

Steroid-Responsive Disorders

Initial: 5-60mg/day depending on disease being treated

If currently on immediate-release prednisone, prednisolone, or methylprednisolone, switch to an equivalent dose based on relative potency

Maintain/adjust initial dose until response is satisfactory

If no satisfactory clinical response after a reasonable period, D/C and transfer to other appropriate therapy

Maint: Decrease initial dosage in small decrements at appropriate time intervals to lowest effective dose

D/C if a period of spontaneous remission occurs in a chronic condition

PEDIATRIC DOSAGE

Steroid-Responsive Disorders

Initial: 5-60mg/day depending on disease being treated

If currently on immediate-release prednisone, prednisolone, or methylprednisolone, switch to an equivalent dose based on relative potency

Maintain/adjust initial dose until response is satisfactory

If no satisfactory clinical response after a reasonable period, D/C and transfer to other appropriate therapy

Maint: Decrease initial dosage in small decrements at appropriate time intervals to lowest effective dose

D/C if a period of spontaneous remission occurs in a chronic condition

DOSE MODIFICATION

Elderly

Start at lower end of dosing range

Discontinuation

Withdraw gradually after long-term therapy

ADMINISTRATION

Oral route

Take PO w/ food

Do not break, divide, or chew tab

HOW SUPPLIED

Tab, Delayed-Release: 1mg, 2mg, 5mg

WARNINGS/PRECAUTIONS

Monitor for situations which may make dosage adjustments necessary (eg, change in clinical status secondary to remissions/exacerbations in the disease process, individual drug responsiveness, effect of patient exposure to stress). May need to increase dose for a period of time consistent with patient's condition during stressful situations. May produce reversible hypothalamic-pituitary adrenal (HPA) axis suppression with potential for corticosteroid insufficiency after withdrawal. Drug-induced secondary adrenocortical insufficiency may be minimized by gradual dose reduction. Changes in thyroid status may necessitate dose adjustment. May mask signs of infection, and increase risk of dissemination, reactivation, or exacerbation of latent infection. May reduce resistance to new infections. More serious or fatal course of chickenpox and measles in non-immune patients reported; avoid exposure. May exacerbate systemic fungal infections; avoid use unless needed to control drug reactions. May activate latent amebiasis; rule out latent or active amebiasis before initiating therapy. Not for use in cerebral malaria and active ocular herpes simplex. Increased risk of GI perforation in patients with certain GI disorders; Signs of GI perforation may be masked. Caution with known or suspected *Strongyloides* (threadworm) infestation, active/latent tuberculosis (TB) or tuberculin reactivity, diverticulitis, fresh intestinal anastomoses, active or latent peptic ulcer, left ventricular free wall rupture after a recent myocardial infarction, probable impending perforation, abscess or other pyogenic infections. May cause BP elevation, salt/water retention, increased K^+ and Ca^{2+} excretion; caution with congestive heart failure (CHF), HTN, or renal insufficiency. May be associated with CNS effects and may aggravate existing emotional instability or psychotic tendencies. May decrease bone formation and increase bone resorption, and may lead to inhibition of bone growth in pediatric patients and development of osteoporosis at any age; caution with increased risk of osteoporosis (eg, postmenopausal women). May produce posterior subcapsular cataracts, glaucoma with possible optic nerve damage, and enhance establishment of secondary ocular infections. Not recommended in optic neuritis treatment. May elevate intraocular pressure (IOP); monitor IOP if used for >6 weeks. Caution with ocular herpes simplex. Monitor growth and development of pediatric patients on prolonged therapy. May cause fetal harm. Acute myopathy reported with use of high doses, most often occurring in patients with neuromuscular transmission disorders (eg, myasthenia gravis). Creatine kinase elevation and Kaposi's sarcoma may occur. May suppress reactions to skin tests. Caution in elderly.

ADVERSE REACTIONS

Fluid retention, glucose tolerance alteration, BP elevation, behavioral/mood changes, increased appetite, weight gain.

DRUG INTERACTIONS

Live or live, attenuated vaccines are contraindicated with immunosuppressive doses. May diminish response to toxoids and live or inactivated vaccines. Aminoglutethimide may lead to loss of corticosteroid-induced adrenal suppression. Cardiac enlargement and CHF may occur with concomitant use of amphotericin B. May produce severe weakness in myasthenia gravis patients with anticholinesterase agents; d/c anticholinesterase agents at least 24 hrs before initiating therapy. Monitor coagulation indices frequently with warfarin. Dose adjustment of antidiabetic agents may be required. May decrease serum concentrations of isoniazid. CYP3A4 inducers (eg, barbiturates, phenytoin, carbamazepine, ephedrine, rifampin) may enhance metabolism and may require increase in corticosteroid dose. CYP3A4 inhibitors (eg, ketoconazole, macrolide antibiotics) may decrease metabolism leading to increased risk of corticosteroid side effects. Cholestyramine may increase clearance. Increased activity of both drugs may occur with cyclosporine; convulsions reported with concurrent use. May increase risk of arrhythmias due to hypokalemia with digitalis glycosides. Estrogens may decrease hepatic metabolism, thereby increasing the effect. Aspirin (ASA) or other NSAIDs may increase risk of GI side effects. Caution with ASA in hypoprothrombinemia patients. May increase clearance of salicylates. Closely monitor for hypokalemia when administered with K^+-depleting agents (eg, amphotericin B, diuretics). Acute myopathy reported with neuromuscular blocking drugs (eg, pancuronium).

NURSING CONSIDERATIONS

Assessment: Assess for systemic fungal/other current infections, active TB, latent/active amebiasis, cerebral malaria, active ocular herpes simplex, emotional instability or psychotic tendencies, hypersensitivity to drug, and for any other condition where treatment is contraindicated or cautioned. Assess pregnancy/nursing status, vaccination history, thyroid status, and for possible drug interactions.

Monitoring: Monitor for HPA axis suppression, adrenocortical insufficiency, salt/water retention, infections/secondary ocular infections, change in thyroid status, posterior subcapsular cataracts, glaucoma with optic nerve damage, Kaposi's sarcoma, emotional instability or psychotic tendencies aggravation, and other adverse reactions. Monitor BP, body weight, routine laboratory studies (eg, 2-hr postprandial blood glucose and serum K^+ levels), and chest X-ray at regular intervals during prolonged therapy. Monitor growth and development of pediatric patients on prolonged therapy. Monitor for hypoadrenalism in infants born to mothers who received substantial doses during pregnancy. Monitor bone density in patients on long term therapy.

Patient Counseling: Instruct to take exactly as prescribed, not to d/c therapy abruptly or without medical supervision, to advise any medical attendants that taking the drug, and to seek medical advice if fever or other signs of infection develop. Instruct to discuss with physician if had recent or ongoing infections or if have recently received a vaccine. Advise if on immunosuppressant doses, to avoid exposure to chickenpox or measles; instruct to seek medical advice if exposed. Instruct to inform physician of all the medicines being taken, including OTC and prescription drugs, dietary supplements, and herbal products. Inform that for missed doses, take the missed dose as soon as remember; counsel that if it is almost time for the next dose, instruct to skip the missed dose and take medicine at the next regularly schedule time. Advise about common adverse reactions that could occur with therapy.

Storage: 25°C (77°F); excursions permitted to 15-30°C (59-86°F). Protect from light and moisture.

RAZADYNE ER – galantamine hydrobromide — RX

Class: Acetylcholinesterase inhibitor

OTHER BRAND NAMES

Razadyne

ADULT DOSAGE

Alzheimer's Disease

Mild to Moderate Dementia of the Alzheimer's Type:

Sol/Tab:
Initial: 4mg bid (8mg/day)
Titrate: Increase to initial maint dose of 8mg bid (16mg/day) after ≥4 weeks, then may increase to 12mg bid (24mg/day) after ≥4 weeks
Usual: 16-24mg/day

If therapy is interrupted for >3 days, restart at the lowest dose and escalate to current dose

PEDIATRIC DOSAGE

Pediatric use may not have been established

Cap, Extended-Release (ER):
Initial: 8mg/day
Titrate: Increase to initial maint dose of 16mg/day after ≥4 weeks, then increase to 24mg/day after ≥4 weeks
Usual: 16-24mg/day

Converting from Immediate-Release (IR) Tab/Sol:
Use same total daily dose of IR; take last dose of IR tab/sol in pm and start ER cap the next am

DOSE MODIFICATION

Renal Impairment
CrCl 9-59mL/min: Do not exceed 16mg/day
<9mL/min: Not recommended

Hepatic Impairment
Child-Pugh 7-9: Do not exceed 16mg/day
Child-Pugh 10-15: Not recommended

ADMINISTRATION

Oral route

Take w/ food
Cap, ER: Administer once daily in the am
Tab/Sol: Administer twice a day, w/ am and pm meals
Ensure adequate fluid intake during treatment

HOW SUPPLIED

Cap, ER: 8mg, 16mg, 24mg; Sol: 4mg/mL [100mL]; Tab: 4mg, 8mg, 12mg

WARNINGS/PRECAUTIONS

Serious skin reactions (Stevens-Johnson syndrome and acute generalized exanthematous pustulosis) reported; d/c at the 1st appearance of skin rash, unless the rash is clearly not drug-related. Do not resume, and consider alternative therapy if signs/symptoms suggest a serious skin reaction. Bradycardia and all types of heart block reported in patients w/ and w/o known underlying cardiac conduction abnormalities; all patients should be considered at risk. May increase gastric acid secretion. May produce N/V, diarrhea, anorexia, or weight loss. May cause bladder outflow obstruction. Potential to cause generalized convulsions. Caution in patients w/ history of severe asthma or obstructive pulmonary disease. Deaths reported w/ mild cognitive impairment.

ADVERSE REACTIONS

N/V, dizziness, decreased appetite, anorexia, diarrhea, headache, decreased weight, depression, fatigue.

DRUG INTERACTIONS

Potential to interfere w/ anticholinergics. Expected synergistic effect w/ succinylcholine, other cholinesterase inhibitors, similar neuromuscular blockers, or cholinergic agonists (eg, bethanechol). Monitor closely for symptoms of active/occult GI bleeding w/ concurrent NSAIDs.

NURSING CONSIDERATIONS

Assessment: Assess for known hypersensitivity to drug, cardiovascular conditions, history of ulcer disease, severe asthma or obstructive pulmonary disease, renal/hepatic impairment, pregnancy/nursing status, and possible drug interactions.

Monitoring: Monitor closely for symptoms of active/occult GI bleeding, serious skin reactions, bradycardia, heart block, bladder outflow obstruction, seizures, and other adverse reactions. Closely monitor respiratory function. Monitor weight during therapy.

Patient Counseling: Advise patients and caregivers to d/c therapy and seek immediate medical attention at the 1st appearance of skin rash. Instruct to take ud in order to minimize adverse reactions. Inform that dose escalation should follow a minimum of 4 weeks at prior dose. Inform that if therapy has been interrupted for >3 days, patient should be restarted w/ the lowest dose and then retitrated to an appropriate dosage. Advise to ensure adequate fluid intake during treatment. (Sol) Inform that there is an Instruction Sheet describing how sol should be given; urge to read prior to administration.

Storage: 25°C (77°F); excursions permitted to 15-30°C (59-86°F). (Sol) Do not freeze.

REBETOL – ribavirin RX

Class: Nucleoside analogue

Not for monotherapy treatment of chronic hepatitis C virus infection. Primary toxicity is hemolytic anemia. Anemia associated with therapy may result in worsening of cardiac disease and lead to fatal and nonfatal MIs. Avoid with history of significant/unstable cardiac disease. Contraindicated in women who are pregnant and in male partners of pregnant women. Extreme care must be taken to avoid pregnancy during therapy and for 6 months after completion of therapy. Use at least 2 reliable forms of effective contraception during treatment and for 6 months after discontinuation.

ADULT DOSAGE

Chronic Hepatitis C with Compensated Liver Disease

Combination Therapy w/ PegIntron:
Treat w/ PegIntron 1.5mcg/kg/week SQ

<66kg: 400mg qam and 400mg qpm
66-80kg: 400mg qam and 600mg qpm
81-105kg: 600mg qam and 600mg qpm
>105kg: 600mg qam and 800mg qpm

Interferon Alfa-Naive:
Genotype 1: Treat for 48 weeks
Genotype 2 or 3: Treat for 24 weeks

Retreatment:
Treat for 48 weeks, regardless of hepatitis C virus (HCV) genotype

Combination Therapy w/ Intron A:
Treat w/ Intron A 3 million IU 3X weekly SQ
≤75kg: 400mg qam and 600mg qpm
>75kg: 600mg qam and 600mg qpm

Interferon Alfa-Naive:
Treat for 24-48 weeks

Retreatment:
Treat for 24 weeks

PEDIATRIC DOSAGE

Chronic Hepatitis C with Compensated Liver Disease

Combination Therapy w/ PegIntron/Intron A:
≥3 Years:
Sol:
<47kg: 15mg/kg/day divided into two doses; may use sol regardless of body weight

Cap:
47-59kg: 400mg qam and 400mg qpm
60-73kg: 400mg qam and 600mg qpm
>73kg: 600mg qam and 600mg qpm

Treat w/ PegIntron 60mcg/m²/week SQ or Intron A 3 million IU/m² 3X weekly SQ for 25-61kg (refer to adult dosing for >61kg)

Genotype 1: Treat for 48 weeks
Genotype 2 or 3: Treat for 24 weeks

Remain on pediatric dosing while receiving therapy in combination w/ PegIntron when 18th birthday is reached

DOSE MODIFICATION

Renal Impairment
CrCl <50mL/min: Not recommended

Elderly
Start at lower end of dosing range

Discontinuation
D/C Therapy if:
WBC Count: $<1.0 \times 10^9$/L
Neutrophils: $<0.5 \times 10^9$/L
Platelets: $<25 \times 10^9$/L (adults) or $<50 \times 10^9$/L (peds)
Creatinine: >2mg/dL (peds)
Hgb w/o History of Cardiac Disease: <8.5g/dL
Hgb w/ History of Stable Cardiac Disease: <8.5g/dL or <12g/dL after four weeks of dose reduction

3-17 Years:
D/C PegIntron/Rebetol Combo (HCV Genotype 1):
At 12 Weeks if: Week 12 HCV-RNA dropped less than 2 $\log_{10}$ compared to a pretreatment; or
At 24 Weeks: HCV-RNA levels remain detectable

≥18 Years:
D/C PegIntron/Rebetol combo if Interferon Alfa-Naive (HCV Genotype 1):
At 12 Weeks if: Not at least a 2 $\log_{10}$ drop or loss of HCV-RNA; or
At 24 Weeks: HCV-RNA levels remain detectable

Other Important Modifications
Reduce Rebetol if:
Hgb w/o History of Cardiac Disease: 8.5 to <10g/dL

≤17 Years:
1st Reduction: 12mg/kg/day
2nd Reduction: 8mg/kg/day

≥18 Years:
1st Reduction: By 200mg/day (except in patients receiving 1400mg, reduction should be by 400mg/day)

2nd Reduction: By additional 200mg/day (if needed)
If dose is reduced to 600mg/day, give one 200mg cap am and two 200mg caps pm

Rebetol (by 200mg/day) and PegIntron or Intron A (by half) if:
Hgb w/ History of Stable Cardiac Disease: ≥2g/dL decrease in Hgb during any 4-week period during treatment

Refer to PI for reduction of Intron A or PegIntron

ADMINISTRATION
Oral route

Take w/ food

Cap
Do not open, crush, or break

HOW SUPPLIED
Cap: 200mg; Sol: 40mg/mL [100mL]

CONTRAINDICATIONS
Women who are or may become pregnant, men whose female partners are pregnant, autoimmune hepatitis, hemoglobinopathies (eg, thalassemia major, sickle cell anemia), CrCl <50mL/min, coadministration with didanosine.

WARNINGS/PRECAUTIONS
Do not start therapy unless a negative pregnancy test has been obtained immediately prior to therapy. Suspend therapy in patients with signs and symptoms of pancreatitis; d/c therapy with confirmed pancreatitis. Pulmonary symptoms (eg, dyspnea, pulmonary infiltrates, pneumonitis, pulmonary HTN, pneumonia, sarcoidosis or exacerbation of sarcoidosis) reported; closely monitor and, if appropriate, d/c if pulmonary infiltrates or pulmonary function impairment develops. Alfa interferons may induce or aggravate ophthalmologic disorders (eg, decrease or loss of vision, retinopathy); perform eye exam in all patients prior to therapy, periodically with preexisting ophthalmologic disorders (eg, diabetic or hypertensive retinopathy), and if ocular symptoms develop during therapy. D/C if new or worsening ophthalmologic disorders develop. Severe decreases in neutrophil and platelet counts, and hematologic, endocrine (eg, TSH), and hepatic abnormalities may occur in combination with PegIntron; perform hematology and blood chemistry testing prior to therapy and periodically thereafter. Dental/periodontal disorders reported. Weight changes and growth inhibition (including long-term growth inhibition) reported in pediatric patients. Associated with significant adverse reactions (eg, severe depression and suicidal ideation, suppression of bone marrow function, autoimmune and infectious disorders, diabetes). Caution with preexisting cardiac disease; d/c if cardiovascular (CV) status deteriorates. Caution in the elderly. (Cap) Not for treatment of HIV infection, adenovirus, respiratory syncytial virus, parainfluenza, or influenza infections.

ADVERSE REACTIONS
Hemolytic anemia, inj-site reactions, headache, fatigue, rigors, fever, N/V, anorexia, myalgia, arthralgia, insomnia, irritability, depression, neutropenia, alopecia.

DRUG INTERACTIONS
See Contraindications. Closely monitor for toxicities, especially hepatic decompensation and anemia, with nucleoside reverse transcriptase inhibitors (NRTIs); consider dose reduction or discontinuation of interferon, ribavirin, or both, or discontinuation of NRTI if worsening clinical toxicities occur. May inhibit phosphorylation of lamivudine, stavudine, and zidovudine. Severe pancytopenia, bone marrow suppression, and myelotoxicity reported with azathioprine.

NURSING CONSIDERATIONS

Assessment: Assess for autoimmune hepatitis, hemoglobinopathies, depression, preexisting ophthalmologic disorders, history of or preexisting cardiac disease, hypersensitivity, and possible drug interactions. Assess nursing status and hepatic/renal/pulmonary function. Conduct pregnancy test (including female partners of male patients), standard hematologic tests, blood chemistries, ECG in patients with preexisting cardiac disease, and eye examination.

Monitoring: Monitor for anemia, worsening of cardiac disease, pancreatitis, renal/hepatic dysfunction, CV deterioration, pulmonary function impairment, new/worsening ophthalmologic disorders, and other adverse reactions. Monitor height and weight in pediatric patients. Perform standard hematologic tests, blood chemistries (eg, TSH), ECG, and HCV-RNA periodically. Obtain Hct and Hgb (Week 2 and 4 of therapy, and as clinically appropriate). Perform pregnancy test monthly during therapy and for 6 months after discontinuation of therapy (including female partners of male patients). Schedule regular dental exams.

Patient Counseling: Counsel on risk/benefits associated with treatment. Inform that anemia may develop. Advise that lab evaluations are required prior to starting therapy and periodically thereafter. Advise to be well-hydrated, especially during the initial stages of treatment. Inform of pregnancy risks. Instruct to use at least 2 forms of contraception and perform a monthly pregnancy test during therapy and for 6 months post-therapy (including female partners of male patients); advise to notify physician in the event of a pregnancy. Inform that appropriate precautions to prevent HCV transmission should be taken. Instruct to take missed doses as soon as possible during the same day and not to double next dose. Instruct to brush teeth bid and have regular dental exams; if vomiting occurs, advise to rinse out mouth afterwards.

Storage: (Cap) 25°C (77°F); excursions permitted to 15-30°C (59-86°F). (Sol) 2-8°C (36-46°F) or at 25°C (77°F); excursions permitted to 15-30°C (59-86°F).

REBIF – interferon beta-1a RX

Class: Biological response modifier

ADULT DOSAGE

Multiple Sclerosis

Treatment of Relapsing Forms:
22mcg or 44mcg 3X/week

Titration Schedule for 22mcg Prescribed Dose:
Week 1: 4.4mcg (half of 8.8mcg syringe)
Week 2: 4.4mcg (half of 8.8mcg syringe)
Week 3: 11mcg (half of 22mcg syringe)
Week 4: 11mcg (half of 22mcg syringe)
Week 5 and After: 22mcg
Use only prefilled syringes to titrate to the 22mcg Prescribed Dose

Titration Schedule for 44mcg Prescribed Dose:
Week 1: 8.8mcg
Week 2: 8.8mcg
Week 3: 22mcg
Week 4: 22mcg
Week 5 and After: 44mcg
Prefilled syringes or autoinjectors can be used to titrate to the 44mcg Prescribed Dose

Premedication for Flu-Like Symptoms:
Concurrent use of analgesics and/or antipyretics may help ameliorate flu-like symptoms on treatment days

PEDIATRIC DOSAGE

Pediatric use may not have been established

DOSE MODIFICATION

Elderly
Start at lower end of dosing range

Adverse Reactions
Decreased Peripheral Blood Counts: May necessitate dose reduction or discontinuation until toxicity is resolved
Elevated LFTs: May necessitate dose reduction or discontinuation until toxicity is resolved

ADMINISTRATION

SQ route

Administer at the same time (preferably late afternoon or pm) on the same 3 days at least 48 hrs apart each week
Rotate site of inj w/ each dose
Refer to PI for additional instructions

HOW SUPPLIED

Inj: 22mcg/0.5mL, 44mcg/0.5mL [prefilled syringe, Rebidose autoinjector]; (Titration Pack) 8.8mcg/0.2mL, 22mcg/0.5mL [prefilled syringe, Rebidose autoinjector]

CONTRAINDICATIONS

History of hypersensitivity to human albumin.

WARNINGS/PRECAUTIONS

Depression, suicidal ideation, and suicide attempts reported; consider cessation of treatment if depression develops. Severe liver injury reported rarely; d/c immediately if jaundice or other symptoms of liver dysfunction appear. Asymptomatic elevation of hepatic transaminases (particularly ALT) may occur; caution with active liver disease, alcohol abuse, increased serum ALT (>2.5X ULN), or history of significant liver disease. Consider dose reduction if ALT rises >5X ULN; may gradually re-escalate dose when enzyme levels have normalized. Anaphylaxis (rare) and other allergic reactions (eg, skin rash, urticaria) reported; d/c if anaphylaxis occurs. Inj-site reactions (eg, necrosis), decreased peripheral blood counts in all cell lines (including pancytopenia), seizures, and new or worsening thyroid abnormalities reported. Caution in patients with preexisting seizure disorders, and in elderly.

ADVERSE REACTIONS

Inj-site disorders, headache, fatigue, fever, rigors, chest pain, back pain, myalgia, abdominal pain, depression, elevation of liver enzymes, hematologic abnormalities.

DRUG INTERACTIONS

Consider the potential for hepatic injury when used in combination with known hepatotoxic products, or when new agents are added to the regimen.

NURSING CONSIDERATIONS

Assessment: Assess for depression, history of or active liver disease, alcohol abuse, preexisting seizure disorder, thyroid dysfunction, myelosuppression, history of hypersensitivity to drug or to human albumin, pregnancy/nursing status, and possible drug interactions.

Monitoring: Monitor for depression, suicidal ideation, jaundice, anaphylaxis, allergic reactions, inj-site reactions, seizures, and other adverse reactions. Perform CBC and LFTs at regular intervals (1, 3, and 6 months) following initiation of therapy and then periodically thereafter in the absence of clinical symptoms; patients with myelosuppression may require more intensive monitoring of CBC, with differential and platelet counts. Perform thyroid function tests every 6 months in patients with a history of thyroid dysfunction, or as clinically indicated.

Patient Counseling: Inform of the symptoms of depression, suicidal ideation, hepatic injury, decreased peripheral blood counts, and seizures, and instruct to immediately report any of these symptoms to physician. Instruct to seek immediate medical attention if symptoms of allergic reactions and anaphylaxis occur. Advise patients that inj-site reactions may occur and to promptly report any signs of necrosis at inj site. Instruct on the use of aseptic technique when self-administering the drug and on the importance of rotating inj sites. Explain the importance of proper disposal of prefilled syringes and autoinjectors, and caution against reuse of these items. Inform about the risks/benefits of treatment during pregnancy.

Storage: 2-8°C (36-46°F). Do not freeze. If needed, may store at 2-25°C (36-77°F) for up to 30 days and away from heat and light, but refrigeration is preferred.

RECLAST — zoledronic acid

Class: Bisphosphonate

RX

ADULT DOSAGE

Osteoporosis

Treatment in Men and Postmenopausal Women:
5mg IV once a yr

Prevention in Postmenopausal Women:
5mg IV once every 2 yrs

Glucocorticoid-Induced Osteoporosis:
In men and women who are either initiating or continuing systemic glucocorticoids in a daily dosage ≥7.5mg of prednisone and who are expected to remain on glucocorticoids for ≥12 months

Treatment/Prevention:
5mg IV once a yr

Paget's Disease

Usual: 5mg IV

May consider retreatment in patients who have relapsed (based on increases in serum alkaline phosphatase), failed to achieve normalization of serum alkaline phosphatase, or those w/ symptoms

PEDIATRIC DOSAGE

Pediatric use may not have been established

ADMINISTRATION

IV route

Infuse IV over ≥15 min at a constant rate
Hydrate patients appropriately prior to administration
IV infusion should be followed by a 10mL normal saline flush of the IV line
Do not allow sol to come in contact with any Ca^{2+} or other divalent cation-containing sol
Administer as a single IV sol through a separate vented infusion line
May give acetaminophen following administration to reduce incidence of acute-phase reaction symptoms

Recommended Intake of Ca^{2+} and Vitamin D

In Osteoporosis: At least 1200mg of Ca^{2+} daily and 800-1000 IU of vitamin D daily
In Paget's Disease: 1500mg of Ca^{2+} daily in divided doses (750mg bid or 500mg tid) and 800 IU of vitamin D daily, particularly in the 2 weeks following administration

HOW SUPPLIED

Inj: 5mg/100mL

CONTRAINDICATIONS

Hypocalcemia, CrCl <35mL/min, acute renal impairment.

WARNINGS/PRECAUTIONS

Consider discontinuation after 3-5 yrs of use in patients at low-risk for fracture; periodically reevaluate risk for fracture in patients who d/c therapy. Contains same active ingredient as Zometa; do not treat w/ Reclast if on concomitant therapy w/ Zometa. Treat preexisting hypocalcemia and disturbances of mineral metabolism prior to treatment. Risk of hypocalcemia in Paget's disease. Withhold therapy until normovolemic status has been achieved if history or physical signs suggest dehydration. Caution w/ chronic renal impairment. Acute renal impairment, including renal failure, reported, especially in patients w/ preexisting renal compromise, advanced age, concomitant nephrotoxic medications or diuretic therapy, or severe dehydration. Transient increase in SrCr may be greater w/ impaired renal function; interim monitoring or CrCl should be performed in at-risk patients. Assess fluid status in patients at increased risk of acute renal failure (ARF) (eg, elderly, concomitant diuretic therapy). Osteonecrosis of the jaw (ONJ) reported; risk may increase w/ duration of exposure to drug or w/ concomitant administration of drugs associated w/ ONJ. Consider a dental examination w/ appropriate preventive dentistry prior to treatment in patients w/ a history of concomitant risk factors (eg, cancer, chemotherapy, angiogenesis inhibitors, radiotherapy, corticosteroids, poor oral hygiene, preexisting dental disease or infection, anemia, coagulopathy) and if possible, avoid invasive dental procedures while on treatment. Atypical, low-energy, or low-trauma fractures of the femoral shaft reported; evaluate any patient w/ a history of bisphosphonate exposure who presents w/ thigh/groin pain to rule out an incomplete femur fracture, and consider interruption of therapy. Avoid use in pregnancy; may cause fetal harm. Severe and occasionally incapacitating bone, joint, and/or muscle pain reported; consider withholding future treatment if severe symptoms develop. Caution w/ ASA sensitivity; bronchoconstriction reported.

ADVERSE REACTIONS

Pain, chills, dizziness, osteoarthritis, fatigue, dyspnea, headache, HTN, influenza-like illness, myalgia, arthralgia, pyrexia, N/V.

DRUG INTERACTIONS

Caution w/ aminoglycosides; may have an additive effect to lower serum Ca^{2+} levels for prolonged periods. Caution w/ loop diuretics; may increase risk of hypocalcemia. Caution w/ other potentially nephrotoxic drugs (eg, NSAIDs). In patients w/ renal impairment, exposure to concomitant medications that are primarily renally excreted (eg, digoxin) may increase.

NURSING CONSIDERATIONS

Assessment: Assess for hypocalcemia, disturbances of mineral metabolism, risk factors for developing renal impairment and ONJ, ASA sensitivity, previous hypersensitivity to the drug, pregnancy/nursing status, and possible drug interactions. Obtain SrCr and calculate CrCl based on actual body weight before each dose. Assess fluid status in patients at increased risk of ARF. Perform routine oral exam, and consider appropriate preventive dentistry in patients w/ a history of risk factors for ONJ.

Monitoring: Monitor for ONJ, atypical femur fracture, musculoskeletal pain, bronchoconstriction, and other adverse events. Monitor renal function and serum Ca^{2+}/mineral levels. Reevaluate the need for continued therapy on a periodic basis.

Patient Counseling: Inform about benefits/risks of therapy, the symptoms of hypocalcemia, and the importance of Ca^{2+} and vitamin D supplementation. Instruct to notify physician if patient had surgery to remove some or all of parathyroid glands, had sections of intestine removed, takes any other medications, or is unable to take Ca^{2+} supplements. Advise to avoid becoming pregnant during treatment. Advise to eat and drink normally (at least 2 glasses of fluid, such as water, w/in a few hrs prior to infusion) on the day of treatment, w/in a few hrs prior to infusion. Inform of the most commonly associated side effects of therapy and to consult physician if these symptoms persist. Instruct to inform physician or dentist if experiencing persistent pain and/or nonhealing sore of the mouth or jaw.

Storage: 25°C (77°F); excursions permitted to 15-30°C (59-86°F). Stable for 24 hrs at 2-8°C (36-46°F) after opening. If refrigerated, allow to reach room temperature before administration.

RECTIV – nitroglycerin

RX

Class: Nitrate vasodilator

ADULT DOSAGE

Moderate to Severe Pain

Associated w/ Chronic Anal Fissure:

Usual: Apply 1 inch (375mg) intra-anally q12h for up to 3 weeks

PEDIATRIC DOSAGE

Pediatric use may not have been established

ADMINISTRATION

Intra-anal route

Gently squeeze tube until a line of ointment the length of the measuring line is expressed onto a covered finger

Insert the ointment into the anal canal using a covered finger no further than to the 1st finger joint

Apply ointment around the side of the anal canal

If unable to reach the anal canal due to pain, application should be made directly to the outside of the anus

HOW SUPPLIED

Oint: 0.4% (4mg/g) [30g tube]

CONTRAINDICATIONS

Concomitant use with phosphodiesterase type 5 (PDE5) (eg, sildenafil, vardenafil, and tadalafil), severe anemia and increased intracranial pressure (ICP).

WARNINGS/PRECAUTIONS

Not for oral, ophthalmic, or intravaginal use. Venous and arterial dilatation reported; may decrease venous blood return and reduce arterial vascular resistance and systolic pressure. Caution with blood volume depletion, existing hypotension, cardiomyopathies, congestive heart failure (CHF), acute myocardial infarction (MI), or poor cardiac function for other reasons; monitor cardiovascular (CV) status and clinical condition. May produce dose-related headaches, which may be severe.

ADVERSE REACTIONS

Headache, dizziness, hypotension, flushing, allergic reactions, application-site reactions, methemoglobinemia.

DRUG INTERACTIONS

See Contraindications. Marked orthostatic hypotension reported with calcium channel blockers. Additive hypotensive effects with antihypertensive drugs, β-adrenergic blockers, and other nitrates. May increase levels with aspirin. Monitor anticoagulation status when administered with IV heparin. Decreased 1st-pass metabolism of dihydroergotamine. Consider the possibility of ergotism with ergotamine. Caution with tissue-type plasminogen activator; may decrease thrombolytic effect. May potentiate additive effects with alcohol.

NURSING CONSIDERATIONS

Assessment: Assess for known hypersensitivity, anemia, ICP, blood volume depletion, existing hypotension, cardiomyopathies, CHF, acute MI, cardiac function, pregnancy/nursing status, and possible drug interactions.

Monitoring: Monitor for CV status, clinical conditions, headaches, and other adverse reactions.

Patient Counseling: Advise patients that treatment may be associated with lightheadedness on standing, especially just after rising from lying or seated position. Inform patient that headaches and dizziness has been reported. Tolerance to headaches occurs. Instruct to avoid driving or operating machinery immediately after applying the ointment. Advise not to use medications for erectile dysfunction (eg, sildenafil, vardenafil, tadalafil); may increase hypotensive effects of nitroglycerin.

Storage: 20-25°C (68-77°F); excursions permitted to 15-30°C (59-85°F). Keep tube tightly closed; use within 8 weeks of 1st opening.

RELPAX – eletriptan hydrobromide

RX

Class: $5\text{-}HT_{1B/1D}$ agonist

ADULT DOSAGE

Migraine

W/ or w/o Aura:
Single Dose: 20mg or 40mg
Max Single Dose: 40mg
May give a 2nd dose at least 2 hrs after 1st dose if migraine has not resolved by 2 hrs or returns after transient improvement
Max Daily Dose: 80mg

Safety of treating >3 migraine attacks/30 days not known

PEDIATRIC DOSAGE

Pediatric use may not have been established

ADMINISTRATION

Oral route

Take w/ or w/o food

HOW SUPPLIED

Tab: 20mg, 40mg

CONTRAINDICATIONS

Ischemic coronary artery disease (CAD) (eg, angina pectoris, history of MI, documented silent ischemia), coronary artery vasospasm (eg, Prinzmetal's angina), Wolff-Parkinson-White syndrome or arrhythmias associated with other cardiac accessory conduction pathway disorders, history of stroke, transient ischemic attack, hemiplegic/basilar migraine or history thereof, peripheral vascular disease, ischemic bowel disease, uncontrolled HTN. Recent use (within 24 hrs) of another $5\text{-}HT_1$ agonist, ergotamine-containing or ergot-type medication (eg, dihydroergotamine, methysergide). Recent use (within 72 hrs) of the following potent CYP3A4 inhibitors: ketoconazole, itraconazole, nefazodone, troleandomycin, clarithromycin, ritonavir, or nelfinavir.

WARNINGS/PRECAUTIONS

If no treatment response for the 1st migraine attack, reconsider diagnosis before treating any subsequent attacks. Not intended for prevention of migraine attacks. Serious cardiac adverse reactions (eg, acute MI) reported. May cause coronary artery vasospasm (Prinzmetal's angina). Perform cardiovascular (CV) evaluation in triptan-naive patients who have multiple CV risk factors (eg, increased age, diabetes, HTN, smoking, obesity, strong family history of CAD) prior to therapy; if CV evaluation is negative, consider administering 1st dose in a medically-supervised setting and performing an ECG immediately following administration. Consider periodic CV evaluation in long-term intermittent users with risk factors for CAD. Life-threatening cardiac rhythm disturbances, including ventricular tachycardia and ventricular fibrillation leading to death, reported; d/c if these occur. Sensations of tightness, pain, and pressure in the chest, throat, neck, and jaw commonly occur, usually noncardiac in origin. Cerebral/subarachnoid hemorrhage and stroke reported; exclude other potentially serious neurological conditions prior to therapy in patients not previously diagnosed as migraineurs, and in migraineurs who present with atypical symptoms. May cause noncoronary vasospastic reactions (eg, peripheral vascular ischemia, GI vascular ischemia/infarction, Raynaud's syndrome). Overuse of acute migraine drugs may lead to exacerbation of headache; detoxification, including drug withdrawal and treatment of withdrawal symptoms may be necessary. Serotonin syndrome may occur; d/c if suspected. Significant elevation in BP, including hypertensive crisis with acute impairment of organ systems, reported. Anaphylaxis, anaphylactoid, and hypersensitivity reactions reported. Not recommended with severe hepatic impairment.

ADVERSE REACTIONS

Asthenia, dizziness, somnolence, nausea, headache, paresthesia, dry mouth, chest tightness/pain/pressure.

DRUG INTERACTIONS

See Contraindications. Serotonin syndrome reported with SSRIs, SNRIs, TCAs, or MAOIs.

NURSING CONSIDERATIONS

Assessment: Confirm diagnosis of migraine and exclude other potentially serious neurological conditions prior to therapy. Assess for ischemic CAD, HTN, hemiplegic/basilar migraine, hypersensitivity to drug, or any other conditions where treatment is contraindicated or cautioned. Assess for hepatic dysfunction, pregnancy/nursing status, and possible drug interactions. Perform a CV evaluation for patients who have multiple CV risk factors.

Monitoring: Monitor for signs/symptoms of cardiac events, cerebrovascular events, noncoronary vasospastic reactions, serotonin syndrome, hypersensitivity reactions, HTN, and other adverse reactions. Perform periodic CV evaluation in intermittent long-term users with risk factors for CAD.

Patient Counseling: Inform that therapy may cause serious CV side effects and anaphylactic/anaphylactoid reactions. Instruct to seek medical attention if signs/symptoms of chest pain, SOB, weakness, slurring of speech, or other vasospastic reactions occur. Inform that use of acute migraine drugs for ≥10 days/month may lead to an exacerbation of headache; encourage to record headache frequency and drug use (eg, by keeping a headache diary). Inform about the risk of serotonin syndrome. Inform that medication should not be used during pregnancy and instruct to notify physician if breastfeeding or planning to breastfeed.

Storage: 20-25°C (68-77°F); excursions permitted to 15-30°C (59-86°F).

REMICADE – infliximab **RX**

Class: Monoclonal antibody/TNF-blocker

Increased risk for developing serious infections (eg, active tuberculosis [TB], latent TB reactivation, invasive fungal infections, bacterial/viral infections, opportunistic infections) leading to hospitalization or death, mostly with concomitant use with immunosuppressants (eg, methotrexate [MTX], corticosteroids). D/C if serious infection or sepsis develops. Active/latent reactivation TB may present with disseminated or extrapulmonary disease; test for latent TB before and during therapy and initiate treatment for latent TB prior to infliximab use. Invasive fungal infections reported; consider empiric antifungal therapy in patients at risk who develop severe systemic illness. Consider risks and benefits prior to therapy in patients with chronic or recurrent infection. Monitor patients for development of infection during and after treatment, including development of TB in patients who tested (-) for latent TB infection prior to therapy. Lymphoma and other malignancies, some fatal, reported in children and adolescents. Postmarketing cases of aggressive and fatal hepatosplenic T-cell lymphoma (HSTCL) reported, and the majority of cases were in patients with Crohn's disease (CD) or ulcerative colitis (UC) and mostly in adolescent and young adult males; almost all of these patients were treated concomitantly with azathioprine or 6-mercaptopurine.

ADULT DOSAGE

Rheumatoid Arthritis

Moderately to Severely Active:

For reducing signs/symptoms, inhibiting progression of structural damage, and improving physical function

In Combination w/ Methotrexate:
Induction: 3mg/kg at 0, 2, and 6 weeks
Maint: 3mg/kg every 8 weeks
Incomplete Response: May give up to 10mg/kg or treat every 4 weeks

Ankylosing Spondylitis

Active:
Induction: 5mg/kg at 0, 2, and 6 weeks
Maint: 5mg/kg every 6 weeks

Psoriatic Arthritis

For reducing signs/symptoms of active arthritis, inhibiting progression of structural damage, and improving physical function

W/ or w/o Methotrexate:
Induction: 5mg/kg at 0, 2, and 6 weeks
Maint: 5mg/kg every 8 weeks

Plaque Psoriasis

Chronic Severe (eg, Extensive and/or Disabling):
Induction: 5mg/kg at 0, 2, and 6 weeks
Maint: 5mg/kg every 8 weeks

Crohn's Disease

Moderately to Severely Active w/ Inadequate Response to Conventional Therapy:

For reducing signs/symptoms and inducing/maintaining clinical remission

Induction: 5mg/kg at 0, 2, and 6 weeks
Maint: 5mg/kg every 8 weeks

May give 10mg/kg to patients who respond and then lose their response
Consider discontinuation if no response by Week 14

PEDIATRIC DOSAGE

Crohn's Disease

Moderately to Severely Active w/ Inadequate Response to Conventional Therapy:

For reducing signs/symptoms and inducing/maintaining clinical remission

≥6 Years:
Induction: 5mg/kg at 0, 2, and 6 weeks
Maint: 5mg/kg every 8 weeks

Ulcerative Colitis

Moderately to Severely Active w/ Inadequate Response to Conventional Therapy:

For reducing signs/symptoms and inducing/maintaining clinical remission

≥6 Years:
Induction: 5mg/kg at 0, 2, and 6 weeks
Maint: 5mg/kg every 8 weeks

Also indicated for reducing number of draining enterocutaneous and rectovaginal fistulas and maintaining fistula closure in patients w/ fistulizing Crohn's disease.

Ulcerative Colitis

Moderately to Severely Active w/ Inadequate Response to Conventional Therapy:

For reducing signs/symptoms, inducing/maintaining clinical remission and mucosal healing, and eliminating corticosteroid use

Induction: 5mg/kg at 0, 2, and 6 weeks
Maint: 5mg/kg every 8 weeks

ADMINISTRATION

IV route

Begin infusion w/in 3 hrs of reconstitution and dilution
Administer infusion over a period of not less than 2 hrs
Do not infuse concomitantly in the same IV line w/ other agents
Refer to PI for further instructions

HOW SUPPLIED

Inj: 100mg

CONTRAINDICATIONS

Hypersensitivity to murine proteins. Moderate to severe heart failure (HF) (NYHA Class III/IV) with doses >5mg/kg.

WARNINGS/PRECAUTIONS

Do not initiate with an active infection. Increased risk of infection in patients >65 yrs of age and in patients with comorbid conditions; consider risks and benefits prior to therapy for those who have resided or traveled in areas of endemic TB or mycoses, and with any underlying conditions predisposing to infection. Cases of acute/chronic leukemia, melanoma, and Merkel cell carcinoma reported. Caution in patients with moderate to severe chronic obstructive pulmonary disease (COPD), history of malignancy, or in continuing treatment in patients who develop malignancy during therapy. Hepatitis B virus (HBV) reactivation reported; if reactivation occurs, d/c and initiate antiviral therapy with appropriate supportive treatment. Severe hepatic reactions (eg, acute liver failure, jaundice, hepatitis, cholestasis) reported; d/c if jaundice or marked elevations of liver enzymes (eg, ≥5X ULN) develop. New onset (rare) HF and worsening of HF reported; d/c if new or worsening symptoms of HF occur. Leukopenia, neutropenia, thrombocytopenia, and pancytopenia reported; consider discontinuation of therapy if significant hematologic abnormalities occur. Caution in patients who have ongoing or history of significant hematologic abnormalities. Hypersensitivity reactions reported; d/c for severe hypersensitivity reactions. CNS manifestation of systemic vasculitis, seizures, and new onset/exacerbation of CNS demyelinating disorders reported (rare); caution in patients with these neurologic disorders and consider discontinuation if these disorders develop. Caution when switching from one biologic disease-modifying antirheumatic drug to another; overlapping biological activity may further increase risk of infection. May cause autoantibody formation and, rarely, may develop lupus-like syndrome; d/c if lupus-like syndrome develops. Caution in administration of live vaccines to infants born to female patients treated with infliximab during pregnancy. All pediatric patients should be up to date with all vaccinations prior to therapy. Caution in elderly.

ADVERSE REACTIONS

Serious infections, malignancies, infusion reactions, nausea, URTI, anemia, rash, headache, sinusitis, pharyngitis, coughing, abdominal pain, diarrhea, bronchitis, leukopenia.

DRUG INTERACTIONS

See Boxed Warning. Avoid with live vaccines or therapeutic infectious agents. Avoid use with tocilizumab; possible increased immunosuppression and increased risk of infection. Not recommended with anakinra or abatacept; may increase risk of serious infections. Not recommended with other biological therapeutics used to treat the same conditions. MTX may decrease the incidence of anti-infliximab antibody production and increase infliximab concentrations. Upon initiation or discontinuation of infliximab in patients being treated with CYP450 substrates with a narrow therapeutic index, monitor therapeutic effect (eg, warfarin) or drug concentration (eg, cyclosporine, theophylline) and adjust individual dose of the drug product as needed.

NURSING CONSIDERATIONS

Assessment: Assess for active/chronic/recurrent infection (eg, TB, HBV), history of an opportunistic infection, recent travel to areas of endemic TB or endemic mycoses, underlying conditions that may predispose to infection, HF, history of malignancy, moderate to severe COPD, presence or history of significant hematologic abnormalities, neurologic disorders, previous hypersensitivity to drug or to murine proteins, risk factors for skin cancer, pregnancy/nursing status, and for possible drug interactions. Assess vaccination history in pediatric patients. Perform test for latent TB infection.

Monitoring: Monitor for sepsis, TB (active, reactivation, or latent), invasive fungal infections, or bacterial, viral, and other infections caused by opportunistic pathogens during and after therapy. Monitor for development of lymphoma, HSTCL, or other malignancies. Monitor for nonmelanoma skin cancers in psoriasis patients, melanoma and Merkel cell carcinoma, new or worsening symptoms of HF, HBV infection reactivation, hepatotoxicity, hematological events, hypersensitivity reactions, CNS demyelinating disorders, lupus-like syndrome, and other adverse reactions. Monitor LFTs. Perform periodic skin examination, particularly in patients with risk factors for skin cancer.

Patient Counseling: Advise of potential risks and benefits of therapy. Inform that therapy may lower the ability of immune system to fight infections; instruct to immediately contact physician if any signs/symptoms of an infection develop, including TB and HBV reactivation. Counsel about the risks of lymphoma and other malignancies while on therapy. Advise to report to physician signs of new or worsening medical conditions (eg, heart disease, neurological disease, autoimmune disorders) and symptoms of cytopenia.

Storage: 2-8°C (36-46°F).

RENVELA – sevelamer carbonate RX

Class: Phosphate binder

ADULT DOSAGE

Hyperphosphatemia

Chronic Kidney Disease on Dialysis:
Not Taking a Phosphate Binder:
Initial:
800mg Tab:
Serum Phosphorus:
>5.5 and <7.5mg/dL: 1 tab tid
≥7.5mg/dL: 2 tabs tid
Powder:
Serum Phosphorus:
>5.5 and <7.5mg/dL: 0.8g tid
≥7.5mg/dL: 1.6g tid

Dose Titration (All Patients):
Titrate by 0.8g tid w/ meals at 2-week intervals as necessary

Conversions

Switching from Sevelamer HCl Tabs/ Switching Between Sevelamer Carbonate Tabs and Powder:
Use the same dose in grams; further titration may be necessary to achieve desired phosphorus levels

Switching from Calcium Acetate:
Initial:
1 Calcium Acetate 667mg Tab/Meal: 1 sevelamer carbonate 800mg tab/meal
2 Calcium Acetate 667mg Tabs/Meal: 2 sevelamer carbonate 800mg tabs/meal
3 Calcium Acetate 667mg Tabs/Meal: 3 sevelamer carbonate 800mg tabs/meal

1 Calcium Acetate 667mg Tab/Meal: 0.8g sevelamer carbonate powder
2 Calcium Acetate 667mg Tabs/Meal: 1.6g sevelamer carbonate powder
3 Calcium Acetate 667mg Tabs/Meal: 2.4g sevelamer carbonate powder

PEDIATRIC DOSAGE

Pediatric use may not have been established

DOSE MODIFICATION

Elderly

Start at low end of dosing range

ADMINISTRATION

Oral route

Take w/ meals

Powder Preparation Instructions

The entire contents of each pkt should be placed in a cup and mixed thoroughly w/ the appropriate amount of water

Minimum Amount of Water for Dose Preparation:

0.8g Powder Pkt: Use 30mL water

2.4g Powder Pkt: Use 60mL water

Multiple pkt may be mixed together w/ the appropriate amount of water

Stir the mixture vigorously (it does not dissolve) and drink the entire preparation w/in 30 min and resuspend the preparation right before drinking

HOW SUPPLIED

Tab: 800mg; Powder: 0.8g/pkt, 2.4g/pkt

CONTRAINDICATIONS

Bowel obstruction.

WARNINGS/PRECAUTIONS

Dysphagia and esophageal tab retention reported with use of tab formulation; consider use of sus formulation in patients with a history of swallowing disorders. Bowel obstruction and perforation reported. Caution in elderly.

ADVERSE REACTIONS

N/V, diarrhea, dyspepsia, abdominal pain, flatulence, constipation.

DRUG INTERACTIONS

Consider separating administration of therapy and an oral medication where a reduction in bioavailability of that medication would have a clinically significant effect on its safety or efficacy (eg, cyclosporine, tacrolimus, levothyroxine). Take oral ciprofloxacin at least 2 hrs before or 6 hrs after therapy. Take oral mycophenolate mofetil at least 2 hrs before therapy. Where possible, consider monitoring clinical response and/or blood levels of concomitant drugs that have a narrow therapeutic range.

NURSING CONSIDERATIONS

Assessment: Assess for presence of bowel obstruction and other GI disorders (eg, dysphagia, swallowing disorders), pregnancy/nursing status, and possible drug interactions.

Monitoring: Monitor for bowel obstruction and perforation, dysphagia, esophageal tab retention, and other adverse reactions. Monitor bicarbonate and Cl^- levels, and for reduced vitamin D, E, K (clotting factors), and folic acid levels.

Patient Counseling: Advise to take with meals and adhere to prescribed diet. If taking an oral medication where reduced bioavailability would produce a clinically significant effect on safety or efficacy, advise to take medication ≥1 hr before or 3 hrs after dosing. Inform that drug may cause constipation and if left untreated, may lead to severe complications; caution to report new onset or worsening of existing constipation promptly to physician.

Storage: 25°C (77°C); excursions permitted to 15-30°C (59-86°F). Protect from moisture.

REQUIP – ropinirole

RX

Class: Non-ergoline dopamine agonist

OTHER BRAND NAMES

Requip XL

ADULT DOSAGE

Parkinson's Disease

Tab:

Week 1: 0.25mg tid

Week 2: 0.5mg tid

Week 3: 0.75mg tid

Week 4: 1mg tid

After Week 4: May increase by 1.5mg/day on a weekly basis up to a 9mg/day, and then by up to 3mg/day weekly

Max: 24mg/day (8mg tid)

PEDIATRIC DOSAGE

Pediatric use may not have been established

Discontinuation:
D/C gradually over a 7-day period; reduce frequency of administration from tid to bid for 4 days, then to qd for the remaining 3 days

Tab, ER:
Initial: 2mg qd for 1-2 weeks
Titrate: May increase by 2mg/day at ≥1-week intervals
Max: 24mg/day

Discontinuation:
D/C gradually over a 7-day period

Restless Legs Syndrome

Moderate to Severe Primary Restless Legs Syndrome:
Tab:
Days 1 and 2: 0.25mg qd 1-3 hrs before hs
Days 3-7: 0.5mg qd 1-3 hrs before hs
Week 2: 1mg qd 1-3 hrs before hs
Week 3: 1.5mg qd1-3 hrs before hs
Week 4: 2mg qd 1-3 hrs before hs
Week 5: 2.5mg qd 1-3 hrs before hs
Week 6: 3mg qd 1-3 hrs before hs
Week 7: 4mg qd 1-3 hrs before hs
Max: 4mg/day

Conversions

Switching from IR to ER Tabs:
0.75-2.25mg/day IR: 2mg/day ER
3-4.5mg/day IR: 4mg/day ER
6mg/day IR: 6mg/day ER
7.5-9mg/day IR: 8mg/day ER
12mg/day IR: 12mg/day ER
15mg/day IR: 16mg/day ER
18mg/day IR: 18mg/day ER
21mg/day IR: 20mg/day ER
24mg/day IR: 24mg/day ER

DOSE MODIFICATION

Renal Impairment

Tab:
Parkinson's Disease:
ESRD on Hemodialysis:
Initial: 0.25mg tid
Patients Receiving Regular Dialysis:
Max: 18mg/day; supplemental doses after dialysis are not required

Restless Legs Syndrome:
ESRD on Hemodialysis:
Initial: 0.25mg qd
Patients Receiving Regular Dialysis:
Max: 3mg/day; supplemental doses after dialysis are not required

Tab, ER:
ESRD on Hemodialysis:
Initial: 2mg qd
Patients Receiving Regular Dialysis:
Max: 18mg/day; supplemental doses after dialysis are not required

ADMINISTRATION

Oral route

Take w/ or w/o food
If a significant interruption in therapy has occurred, retitration may be warranted

Tab, ER

Swallow whole; do not chew, crush, or divide

HOW SUPPLIED

Tab: 0.25mg, 0.5mg, 1mg, 2mg, 3mg, 4mg, 5mg; Tab, Extended-Release (XL): 2mg, 4mg, 6mg, 8mg, 12mg

WARNINGS/PRECAUTIONS

Falling asleep during activities of daily living and somnolence reported; d/c if significant daytime sleepiness or episodes of falling asleep develop during activities that require active participation. May impair mental/physical abilities. Syncope, sometimes associated with bradycardia reported; caution in patients with significant cardiovascular disease (CVD). May cause orthostatic hypotension. Hallucinations reported; risk increases in the elderly treated with XL tab. May experience new or worsening mental status and behavioral changes, which may be severe, including psychotic-like behavior during treatment or after starting or increasing the dose. Avoid with major psychotic disorder due to risk of exacerbating psychosis. Intense urges to gamble, increased sexual urges, intense urges to spend money, binge or compulsive eating, and/or other intense urges, and the inability to control these urges while on therapy reported; consider dose reduction or stopping medication if such urges develop. May cause or exacerbate preexisting dyskinesia. Symptom complex resembling neuroleptic malignant syndrome (NMS) reported in association with rapid dose reduction, withdrawal of, or changes in dopaminergic therapy; tapering dose at the end of treatment for Parkinson's disease is recommended as a prophylactic measure. Increased risk of developing melanoma. Fibrotic complications (eg, retroperitoneal fibrosis, pulmonary infiltrates, pleural effusion, pleural thickening, pericarditis, cardiac valvulopathy) reported. (Tab) Augmentation or early-am rebound in RLS patients reported; review use of medication and consider dosage adjustment or discontinuation of treatment if this occurs. (Tab, XL) May cause BP elevation and changes in HR; caution in patients with CVD. Risk of incomplete release of medication and medication residue being passed in stool if rapid GI transit occurs.

ADVERSE REACTIONS

N/V, somnolence, abdominal pain, dizziness, headache, constipation, syncope, hallucination, dyskinesia, diarrhea. (Tab) viral infection, dyspepsia, leg edema, confusion, asthenic condition.

DRUG INTERACTIONS

Adjustment of ropinirole dose may be required if estrogen or a potent CYP1A2 inducer/inhibitor is stopped or started during treatment. Increased plasma levels of IR tab with ciprofloxacin. Increased clearance with cigarette smoking. Dopamine antagonists, such as neuroleptics (eg, phenothiazines, butyrophenones, thioxanthenes) or metoclopramide may diminish effectiveness. May potentiate dopaminergic side effects of L-dopa and may cause and/or exacerbate preexisting dyskinesia in patients treated with L-dopa for Parkinson's disease; decreasing dose of the dopaminergic drug may ameliorate this adverse reaction. May increase risk of drowsiness with concomitant sedating medications or medications that increase ropinirole plasma levels.

NURSING CONSIDERATIONS

Assessment: Assess for presence of sleep disorders (other than RLS), known hypersensitivity/allergic reaction to drug or to any of the excipients, CVD, dyskinesia, major psychotic disorder, renal impairment, pregnancy/nursing status, and possible drug interactions.

Monitoring: Monitor for hypersensitivity reactions, psychotic-like behavior, impulse control/compulsive behaviors, syncope, bradycardia, hallucinations, dyskinesia, fibrotic complications, symptom complex resembling NMS, melanomas, and other adverse reactions. Monitor for signs/symptoms of hypotension, especially during dose escalation. Continually reassess for drowsiness or sleepiness. Perform periodic skin examinations. (Tab) Monitor for augmentation or early-am rebound in RLS patients. (Tab, XL) Monitor for BP elevation and HR changes.

Patient Counseling: Instruct to take only as prescribed. Advise not to double next dose if a dose is missed. Advise about the potential for developing a hypersensitivity/allergic reaction; instruct patients to immediately contact physician if they experience these or similar reactions. Advise and alert about potential sedating effects; instruct patients not to drive a car, operate machinery, or engage in other dangerous activities until they have gained sufficient experience with therapy. Advise of possible additive effects when taking other sedating medications, alcohol, or other CNS depressants concomitantly, or when taking a concomitant medication (eg, ciprofloxacin) that increases ropinirole plasma levels. Advise patients that they may experience syncope and that hypotension/orthostatic hypotension may develop with/without symptoms; caution against standing rapidly after sitting or lying down, especially at treatment initiation. Inform that hallucinations or other psychotic-like behavior may occur; advise patients to promptly report these to physician should they develop. Inform that medication may cause and/or exacerbate preexisting dyskinesia. Advise to inform physician if new or increased gambling urges, sexual urges, uncontrolled spending, binge or compulsive eating, or other urges develop while on therapy. Advise patients to contact physician if they wish to d/c drug or decrease its dose. Advise of the higher risk of developing melanoma; instruct to have skin examined on a regular basis by a qualified healthcare provider when using medication. Instruct to notify physician if pregnant/intending to become pregnant during therapy. Advise that drug may inhibit lactation. (Tab) Inform RLS patients that augmentation and/or rebound may occur after starting treatment. (Tab, XL) Alert to the possibility of increases in BP and that significant increases/decreases in HR may be experienced during treatment.

Storage: (Tab) 20-25°C (68-77°F). Protect from light and moisture. (Tab, XL) 25°C (77°F); excursions permitted to 15-30°C (59-86°F).

RESCRIPTOR – delavirdine mesylate

Class: Non-nucleoside reverse transcriptase inhibitor

RX

ADULT DOSAGE

HIV-1 Infection

Combination with at Least 2 Other Antiretrovirals:
400mg (four 100mg or two 200mg tabs) tid

PEDIATRIC DOSAGE

HIV-1 Infection

Combination with at Least 2 Other Antiretrovirals:

≥16 Years:
400mg (four 100mg or two 200mg tabs) tid

DOSE MODIFICATION

Concomitant Medications

Antacids: Take at least 1 hr apart

ADMINISTRATION

Oral route

Take with or without food
Take with acidic beverage if achlorhydric
Take 200mg tabs intact; not dispersible in water

Dispersion of 100mg Tab

1. Add four 100mg tabs to at least 3 oz. of water
2. Allow to stand for a few minutes
3. Stir until a uniform dispersion occurs
4. Consume dispersion promptly
5. Rinse glass with water and swallow the rinse

HOW SUPPLIED

Tab: 100mg, 200mg

CONTRAINDICATIONS

Coadministration with CYP3A substrates that are associated with serious and/or life-threatening events at elevated plasma concentrations (eg, astemizole, terfenadine, dihydroergotamine, ergonovine, ergotamine, methylergonovine, cisapride, pimozide, alprazolam, midazolam, triazolam).

WARNINGS/PRECAUTIONS

Immune reconstitution syndrome reported. Autoimmune disorders (eg, Graves' disease, polymyositis, Guillain-Barre syndrome) have been reported to occur in the setting of immune reconstitution. Redistribution/accumulation of body fat reported. May confer cross-resistance to the other non-nucleoside reverse transcriptase inhibitors (NNRTIs). Severe rash (eg, erythema multiforme, Stevens-Johnson syndrome) reported; d/c use if this occurs. Caution with hepatic impairment and in elderly.

ADVERSE REACTIONS

Headache, fatigue, N/V, diarrhea, increased ALT/AST, rash, maculopapular rash, pruritus, erythema, insomnia, upper respiratory infection, depressive symptoms, generalized abdominal pain.

DRUG INTERACTIONS

See Contraindications. Avoid with another NNRTI. Not recommended with lovastatin, simvastatin, St. John's wort, phenytoin, phenobarbital, carbamazepine, rifabutin, rifampin, or chronic use of H_2-receptor antagonists or PPIs. Increased risk of myopathy with HMG-CoA reductase inhibitors metabolized by CYP3A4 (eg, atorvastatin, cerivastatin). May increase levels of nelfinavir, lopinavir, ritonavir, amphetamines, trazodone, antiarrhythmics, warfarin (monitor INR), calcium channel blockers, atorvastatin, cerivastatin, fluvastatin, immunosuppressants, CYP3A substrates, fluticasone, methadone, and ethinyl estradiol. May increase levels of maraviroc; maraviroc dose should be reduced. May increase levels of indinavir; consider dose reduction of indinavir. May increase levels of saquinavir; consider dose reduction of saquinavir (soft gelatin cap). May decrease levels of didanosine. Ketoconazole, fluoxetine, and CYP3A inhibitors may increase levels. Nelfinavir, didanosine, antacids, CYP3A inducers, H_2-receptor antagonists, PPIs, and dexamethasone may decrease levels. May increase levels of clarithromycin; adjust clarithromycin dose in patients with impaired renal function. May increase levels of sildenafil; do not exceed a max single sildenafil dose of 25mg in a 48-hr period. Doses of an antacid and didanosine (buffered tabs) should be separated by at least 1 hr.

NURSING CONSIDERATIONS

Assessment: Assess for hypersensitivity, achlorhydria, hepatic impairment, pregnancy/nursing status, and possible drug interactions.

Monitoring: Monitor for severe rash or rash accompanied by symptoms (eg, fever, blistering, oral lesions, conjunctivitis, swelling, muscle joint aches), immune reconstitution syndrome, cross-resistance to other NNRTIs, fat redistribution, and other adverse reactions.

Patient Counseling: Inform patient that drug is not a cure for HIV-1 infection and that they may continue to experience illnesses associated with HIV-1 infection. Advise to avoid doing things that can spread HIV-1 infection to others. Inform to take as prescribed and to not alter the dose without consulting the physician. Advise patients with achlorhydria to take with acidic beverage (eg, orange or cranberry juice). Inform to take at least 1 hr apart if taking antacids. Advise to d/c and seek medical attention if severe rash or rash with symptoms such as fever, blistering, oral lesions, conjunctivitis, swelling, muscle or joint aches occur. Counsel that fat redistribution may occur. Advise to report use of any prescription or nonprescription medication or herbal products, particularly St. John's wort. Inform patients receiving sildenafil about increased risk of sildenafil-associated adverse events (eg, hypotension, visual changes, prolonged penile erection), and instruct to promptly report any symptoms to the physician. Counsel to notify physician if pregnant or breastfeeding.

Storage: 20-25°C (68-77°F). Protect from high humidity.

RESTASIS – cyclosporine — RX

Class: Topical immunomodulator

ADULT DOSAGE

Keratoconjunctivitis Sicca

Instill 1 drop in ou q12h

PEDIATRIC DOSAGE

Keratoconjunctivitis Sicca

≥16 Years:

Instill 1 drop in ou q12h

ADMINISTRATION

Ocular route

Invert unit dose vial a few times to obtain uniform, white, opaque emulsion before using

Can be used concomitantly with artificial tears, allowing 15-min interval between products

HOW SUPPLIED

Emulsion: 0.05% [0.4mL]

WARNINGS/PRECAUTIONS

Increased tear production not seen in patients currently taking topical anti-inflammatory drugs or using punctal plugs. Do not touch vial tip to the eye or other surfaces to avoid the potential for eye injury and contamination. Do not administer in patients wearing contact lenses. Remove contact lenses prior to administration; may reinsert 15 min after administration.

ADVERSE REACTIONS

Ocular burning, conjunctival hyperemia, discharge, epiphora, eye pain, foreign body sensation, pruritus, stinging, visual disturbance (eg, blurring).

NURSING CONSIDERATIONS

Assessment: Assess for hypersensitivity, contact lens use, and pregnancy/nursing status.

Monitoring: Monitor for signs/symptoms of ocular burning and other adverse reactions.

Patient Counseling: Instruct not to allow the vial tip to touch the eye or any surface. Advise to remove contact lenses before administration; inform that lenses may be reinserted 15 min following administration. Advise to use single-use vial immediately after opening and to discard the remaining contents immediately after administration.

Storage: 15-25°C (59-77°F).

RESTORIL – temazepam — CIV

Class: Benzodiazepine

ADULT DOSAGE

Insomnia

Short-Term Treatment (Generally 7 to 10 Days):

Usual: 15mg before retiring

7.5mg may be sufficient for some patients and others may need 30mg

Transient Insomnia:

7.5mg before retiring

PEDIATRIC DOSAGE

Pediatric use may not have been established

DOSE MODIFICATION

Elderly/Debilitated Patients

Initial: 7.5mg before retiring

ADMINISTRATION

Oral route

HOW SUPPLIED

Cap: 7.5mg, 15mg, 22.5mg, 30mg

CONTRAINDICATIONS

Women who are or may become pregnant.

WARNINGS/PRECAUTIONS

Initiate only after careful evaluation; failure of insomnia to remit after 7-10 days of treatment may indicate primary psychiatric and/or medical illness. Worsening of insomnia and emergence of thinking or behavior abnormalities may occur, especially in elderly; use lowest possible effective dose. Behavioral changes (eg, decreased inhibition, bizarre behavior, agitation, hallucinations, depersonalization) and complex behavior (eg, sleep-driving) reported; strongly consider discontinuation if sleep-driving episode occurs. Amnesia and other neuropsychiatric symptoms may occur unpredictably. Worsening of depression, including suicidal thinking, reported. Withdrawal symptoms may occur after abrupt discontinuation. Rare cases of angioedema and anaphylaxis reported; do not rechallenge. Oversedation, confusion, and/or ataxia may develop w/ large doses in elderly and debilitated patients. Caution w/ hepatic/renal impairment, chronic pulmonary insufficiency, debilitated, severe or latent depression, and in elderly. Abnormal LFTs, renal function tests, and blood dyscrasias reported.

ADVERSE REACTIONS

Drowsiness, headache, fatigue, nervousness, lethargy, dizziness, nausea.

DRUG INTERACTIONS

Increased risk of complex behaviors w/ alcohol and CNS depressants. Potential additive effects w/ hypnotics and CNS depressants. Possible synergistic effect w/ diphenhydramine.

NURSING CONSIDERATIONS

Assessment: Assess for physical and/or psychiatric disorder, medical illness, severe or latent depression, renal/hepatic dysfunction, chronic pulmonary insufficiency, pregnancy/nursing status, alcohol use, and possible drug interactions.

Monitoring: Monitor for signs/symptoms of withdrawal, tolerance, abuse, dependence, abnormal thinking, behavioral changes, agitation, depersonalization, hallucinations, complex behaviors, amnesia, anxiety, neuropsychiatric symptoms, worsening of depression, suicidal thoughts and actions, angioedema, driving/psychomotor impairment, worsening of insomnia, thinking or behavioral abnormalities, and possible abuse/dependence.

Patient Counseling: Inform about the benefits and risks of treatment. Instruct patient to take as prescribed. Inform about the risks and possibility of physical/psychological dependence, memory problems, and complex behaviors (eg, sleep-driving). Caution against hazardous tasks (eg, operating machinery/driving). Advise not to drink alcohol. Instruct to notify physician if pregnant/planning to become pregnant.

Storage: 20-25°C (68-77°F).

RETIN-A – tretinoin **RX**

Class: Retinoid

OTHER BRAND NAMES

Retin-A Micro

ADULT DOSAGE

Acne Vulgaris

Apply qpm/qhs, to the skin where acne lesions appear, using enough to cover the entire affected area lightly

PEDIATRIC DOSAGE

Acne Vulgaris

≥12 Years:

Retin-A Micro:

Apply qpm/qhs, to the skin where acne lesions appear, using enough to cover the entire affected area in a thin layer

DOSE MODIFICATION

Adverse Reactions

If the degree of local irritation warrants, d/c use temporarily, or d/c use altogether

ADMINISTRATION

Topical route

Thoroughly cleanse the areas to be treated before applying the medication

Wash hands after each application

HOW SUPPLIED

(Retin-A) Cre: 0.025%, 0.05%, 0.1% [20g, 45g]; Gel: 0.01%, 0.025% [15g, 45g]; (Retin-A Micro) Gel: 0.04%, 0.1% [20g, 45g, 50g], 0.08% [50g]

WARNINGS/PRECAUTIONS

D/C therapy if a reaction suggesting sensitivity or chemical irritation occurs. Avoid or minimize unprotected exposure to sunlight, including sunlamps; avoid use with sunburn until fully recovered. Caution in patients who may be required to have considerable sun exposure and those with inherent sensitivity to sun. Use of sunscreen products and protective clothing over treated areas is recommended when exposure cannot be avoided. Extreme weather (eg, cold, wind) may irritate skin. Avoid eyes, lips, paranasal creases/angles of the nose, and mucous membranes. May cause transitory feeling of warmth or slight stinging. Reported to cause severe irritation on eczematous skin; use caution in patients with this condition. An apparent exacerbation of inflammatory lesions may occur during early weeks of therapy. (Retin-A) May induce severe local erythema and peeling at application site. Gels are flammable.

ADVERSE REACTIONS

Burning/stinging, itching, erythema, peeling, hyper/hypopigmentation.

DRUG INTERACTIONS

Caution with topical medications, medicated/abrasive soaps and cleansers, products with strong drying effect, products with high concentrations of alcohol, astringents, limes, or spices. (Retin-A/Retin-A Micro 0.04%, 0.1%) Caution with preparations containing sulfur, resorcinol, or salicylic acid; allow effects of these agents to subside before initiation of treatment. (Retin-A Micro 0.04%, 0.1%) Caution with OTC acne preparations containing benzoyl peroxide.

NURSING CONSIDERATIONS

Assessment: Assess for drug hypersensitivity, sun exposure, sensitivity to sun, sunburn, eczematous skin, pregnancy/nursing status, and possible drug interactions.

Monitoring: Monitor for sensitivity reactions, irritation, local erythema or peeling at application site, and other adverse reactions. Closely monitor alterations of vehicle, drug concentration, or dose frequency by carefully observing therapeutic response and skin tolerance.

Patient Counseling: Instruct to d/c use and consult physician if irritation occurs. Instruct not to use more than the recommended amount and not to apply more than once daily. Advise to minimize exposure to sunlight, including sunlamps, and to use sunscreen products and protective clothing over treated areas when exposure to sun cannot be avoided. Inform that weather extremes may be irritating to treated skin. Instruct to use ud, and to keep away from eyes, mouth, angles of the nose, and mucous membranes. Advise to inform physician of other acne preparations being used and if pregnant or breastfeeding. Inform that during the early weeks of therapy, an apparent exacerbation of inflammatory lesions may occur, which should not be considered a reason for discontinuation. (Retin A Micro) Advise to apply moisturizer if dryness is bothersome.

Storage: (Retin-A) Cre: <27°C (80°F). Gel: <30°C (86°F). (Retin-A Micro) Gel: 20-25°C (68-77°F); excursions permitted from 15-30°C (59-86°F). Store pump upright.

REVATIO – sildenafil

RX

Class: Phosphodiesterase type 5 inhibitor

ADULT DOSAGE

Pulmonary Arterial Hypertension

Treatment of pulmonary arterial HTN (WHO Group I) in adults to improve exercise ability and delay clinical worsening

PO:

5mg or 20mg tid, 4-6 hrs apart

Max: 20mg tid

IV:

2.5mg or 10mg IV bolus tid

PEDIATRIC DOSAGE

Pediatric use may not have been established

ADMINISTRATION
Oral, IV route
Refer to PI for reconstitution of the powder for oral sus

Incompatibilities
Do not mix w/ any other medication or additional flavoring agent

HOW SUPPLIED
Inj: 10mg [12.5mL]; Sus: 10mg/mL [112mL]; Tab: 20mg

CONTRAINDICATIONS
Organic nitrates in any form, either regularly/intermittently.

WARNINGS/PRECAUTIONS
Adding sildenafil to bosentan therapy does not result in any beneficial effect on exercise capacity. Not recommended in children. Vasodilatory effects may adversely affect patients with resting hypotension (BP <90/50), fluid depletion, severe left ventricular outflow obstruction, or autonomic dysfunction. Not recommended with pulmonary veno-occlusive disease (PVOD); consider possibility of associated PVOD if signs of pulmonary edema occur. Non-arteritic anterior ischemic optic neuropathy (NAION) reported. Caution with previous NAION in 1 eye and with retinitis pigmentosa. Cases of sudden decrease or loss of hearing, possibly accompanied by tinnitus and dizziness, reported. Caution in patients with anatomical penile deformation (eg, angulation, cavernosal fibrosis, Peyronie's disease) or with predisposition to priapism (eg, sickle-cell anemia, multiple myeloma, leukemia). Penile tissue damage and permanent loss of potency may result if priapism is not immediately treated. Vaso-occlusive crises requiring hospitalization reported in patients with pulmonary HTN secondary to sickle-cell disease. Caution in elderly. (Inj) Used as continued treatment in patients currently taking tab/sus and who are temporarily unable to take oral medication.

ADVERSE REACTIONS
Headache, dyspepsia, gastritis, epistaxis, paresthesia, flushing, diarrhea, insomnia, dyspnea exacerbation, myalgia, nausea, sinusitis, erythema, pyrexia, rhinitis.

DRUG INTERACTIONS
See Contraindications. Vasodilatory effects may adversely affect patients on antihypertensive therapy; monitor BP when given with antihypertensives. Reports of epistaxis with oral vitamin K antagonists. Retinal and eye hemorrhage reported with anticoagulants. Avoid with other PDE-5 inhibitors. Not recommended with ritonavir and other potent CYP3A inhibitors. Symptomatic postural hypotension with doxazosin reported. Additional reduction of supine BP with oral amlodipine reported.

NURSING CONSIDERATIONS

Assessment: Assess for hypotension, fluid depletion, left ventricular outflow obstruction, autonomic dysfunction, PVOD, "crowded disc", age >50, diabetes, HTN, coronary artery disease, hyperlipidemia, smoking, previous NAION in 1 eye, retinitis pigmentosa, anatomical deformities of the penis, conditions predisposing to priapism, pulmonary HTN secondary to sickle-cell disease, hypersensitivity to drug, pregnancy/nursing status, and possible drug interactions. Obtain baseline BP.

Monitoring: Monitor for signs of pulmonary edema, decreased/sudden loss of vision or hearing, tinnitus, dizziness, epistaxis, priapism, vaso-occlusive crises, and hypersensitivity reactions. Monitor BP.

Patient Counseling: Counsel about risks and benefits of the drug. Inform that drug is also marketed as Viagra for male erectile dysfunction. Advise not to take Viagra or other PDE-5 inhibitors and organic nitrates during therapy. Advise to notify physician if sudden decrease/loss of vision or hearing occurs. Instruct to seek immediate medical attention if an erection persists >4 hrs.

Storage: (Tab/Inj) 20-25°C (68-77°F); excursions permitted to 15-30°C (59-86°F). (Sus) <30°C (86°F). Protect from moisture. Constituted: <30°C (86°F) or 2-8°C (36-46°F). Do not freeze. Shelf-life: 60 days.

REVLIMID — lenalidomide RX

Class: Thalidomide analogue

Do not use during pregnancy; may cause birth defects or embryo-fetal death. Females of reproductive potential should have 2 negative pregnancy tests prior to treatment and must use 2 forms of contraception or continuously abstain from heterosexual sex during and for 4 weeks after treatment. Available only through a restricted distribution program, the Revlimid REMS program. May cause significant neutropenia and thrombocytopenia. Patients on therapy for del 5q myelodysplastic syndrome (MDS) should have their CBC monitored weekly for the first 8 weeks of therapy and at least monthly thereafter; may require dose interruption and/or reduction and use of blood product support and/or growth factors. Increased risk of deep vein thrombosis (DVT) and pulmonary embolism (PE), as well as risk of MI and stroke, reported in patients w/ multiple myeloma (MM) treated w/ lenalidomide and dexamethasone; monitor for and advise patients about signs/symptoms of thromboembolism. Advise patients to seek immediate medical care if symptoms such as SOB, chest pain, or arm or leg swelling develop. Thromboprophylaxis is recommended and the choice of regimen should be based on assessment of individual's underlying risks.

ADULT DOSAGE

Multiple Myeloma

Initial: 25mg qd on Days 1-21 of repeated 28-day cycles. Give in combination w/ dexamethasone May reduce initial dose if >75 years

Continue until disease progression or unacceptable toxicity

In patients who are not eligible for autologous stem cell transplantation (ASCT), continue treatment until disease progression or unacceptable toxicity

For patients who are ASCT-eligible, hematopoietic stem cell mobilization should occur w/in 4 cycles of a lenalidomide-containing therapy

Myelodysplastic Syndromes

Patients w/ transfusion-dependent anemia due to low- or intermediate-1-risk myelodysplastic syndromes associated w/ a deletion 5q cytogenetic abnormality w/ or w/o additional cytogenetic abnormalities

Initial: 10mg/day

Continue or modify treatment based upon clinical and lab findings

Mantle Cell Lymphoma

Mantle cell lymphoma (MCL) in patients whose disease has relapsed or progressed after 2 prior therapies, 1 of which included bortezomib

Initial: 25mg/day on Days 1-21 of repeated 28-day cycles for relapsed or refractory MCL

Continue until disease progression or unacceptable toxicity

PEDIATRIC DOSAGE

Pediatric use may not have been established

DOSE MODIFICATION

Renal Impairment

MM:
Moderate (CrCl 30-50mL/min): Initial: 10mg q24h
Severe (CrCl <30mL/min Not Requiring Dialysis): Initial: 15mg q48h
ESRD (CrCl <30mL/min Requiring Dialysis): Initial: 5mg qd. On dialysis days, administer dose following dialysis

MDS:
Moderate (CrCl 30-60mL/min): Initial: 5mg q24h
Severe (CrCl <30mL/min Not Requiring Dialysis): Initial: 2.5mg q24h
ESRD (CrCl <30mL/min Requiring Dialysis): Initial: 2.5mg qd. On dialysis days, administer dose following dialysis

Mantle Cell Lymphoma (MCL):
Moderate (CrCl 30-60mL/min): Initial: 10mg q24h
Severe (CrCl <30mL/min Not Requiring Dialysis): Initial: 15mg q48h
ESRD (CrCl <30mL/min Requiring Dialysis): Initial: 5mg qd. On dialysis days, administer dose following dialysis

Other Important Modifications

MM:
Thrombocytopenia:
Platelets:
Fall to <30,000/mcL: Interrupt treatment and follow CBC weekly
Return to ≥30,000/mcL: Resume at next lower dose. Do not dose <2.5mg/day
For Each Subsequent Drop <30,000/mcL: Interrupt treatment
Return to ≥30,000/mcL: Resume at next lower dose; do not dose <2.5mg/day

Neutropenia:
Neutrophils:
Fall to <1000/mcL: Interrupt treatment, follow CBC weekly
Return to ≥1000/mcL and Neutropenia is Only Toxicity: Resume at 25mg/day or initial starting dose
Return to ≥1000/mcL and if Other Toxicity: Resume at next lower dose. Do not dose <2.5mg/day

For Each Subsequent Drop <1000/mcL: Interrupt treatment
Return to ≥1000/mcL: Resume at next lower dose. Do not dose <2.5mg/day

Other Toxicities in MM:
For other Grade 3/4 toxicities judged to be related to treatment, hold treatment and restart at physician's discretion at next lower dose level when toxicity has resolved to ≤ Grade 2

MDS:
Thrombocytopenia w/in 4 Weeks at Starting Dose 10mg/day (Baseline ≥100,000/mcL):
Platelets:
Fall to <50,000/mcL: Interrupt treatment
Return to ≥50,000/mcL: Resume at 5mg/day

Thrombocytopenia w/in 4 Weeks at Starting Dose 10mg/day (Baseline <100,000/mcL):
Platelets:
Falls to 50% of Baseline: Interrupt treatment
If Baseline ≥60,000/mcL and Return to ≥50,000/mcL: Resume at 5mg/day
If Baseline <60,000/mcL and Return to ≥30,000/mcL: Resume at 5mg/day

Thrombocytopenia after 4 Weeks at Starting Dose 10mg/day:
Platelets:
<30,000/mcL or <50,000/mcL w/ Platelet Transfusions: Interrupt treatment
Return to ≥30,000/mcL (w/o Hemostatic Failure): Resume at 5mg/day
Thrombocytopenia During Treatment at 5mg/day:
Platelets:
<30,000/mcL or <50,000/mcL w/ Platelet Transfusions: Interrupt treatment
Return to ≥30,000/mcL (w/o Hemostatic Failure): Resume at 2.5mg/day

Neutropenia w/in 4 Weeks of Starting Treatment at 10mg/day (Baseline ANC ≥1000/mcL):
Neutrophils:
Fall to <750/mcL: Interrupt treatment
Return to ≥1000/mcL: Resume at 5mg/day
Neutropenia w/in 4 Weeks of Starting Treatment at 10mg/day (Baseline ANC <1000/mcL):
Neutrophils:
Fall to <500/mcL: Interrupt treatment
Return to ≥500/mcL: Resume at 5mg/day
Neutropenia After 4 Weeks of Starting Treatment at 10mg/day:
Neutrophils:
<500/mcL for ≥7 days or <500/mcL Associated w/ Fever (≥38.5°C): Interrupt treatment
Return to ≥500/mcL: Resume at 5mg/day
Neutropenia During Treatment at 5mg/day:
Neutrophils:
<500/mcL for ≥7 Days or <500/mcL Associated w/ Fever (≥38.5°C): Interrupt treatment
Return to ≥500/mcL: Resume at 2.5mg/day
Other Toxicities in MDS:
For other Grade 3/4 toxicities judged to be related to treatment, hold treatment and restart at the physician's discretion at next lower dose level when toxicity has resolved to ≤Grade 2

MCL:
Thrombocytopenia During Treatment:
Platelets:
Fall to <50,000/mcL: Interrupt treatment and follow CBC weekly
Return to ≥50,000/mcL: Resume at 5mg less than the previous dose. Do not dose <5mg daily
Neutropenia During Treatment:
Neutrophils:
Fall to <1000/mcL for at Least 7 Days or Falls to <1000/mcL w/ an Associated Temperature ≥38.5°C or Fall to <500/mcL:
Interrupt treatment and follow CBC weekly
Return to ≥1000/mcL: Resume at 5mg less than previous dose. Do not dose <5mg/day
Other Toxicities in MCL:
For other Grade 3/4 toxicities judged to be related to treatment, hold treatment and restart at physician's discretion at next lower dose level when toxicity has resolved to ≤Grade 2

ADMINISTRATION
Oral route

Take at about the same time each day, w/ or w/o food
Swallow cap whole w/ water; do not open, crush, break, or chew
Wash skin immediately and thoroughly w/ soap and water if powder from cap contacts the skin
If drug contacts the mucous membranes, flush thoroughly w/ water

HOW SUPPLIED
Cap: 2.5mg, 5mg, 10mg, 15mg, 20mg, 25mg

CONTRAINDICATIONS
Pregnancy.

WARNINGS/PRECAUTIONS

Not indicated and not recommended for the treatment of patients w/ chronic lymphocytic leukemia outside of controlled clinical trials; increased risk of death and serious adverse cardiovascular (CV) reactions reported. Avoid pregnancy for at least 4 weeks before beginning therapy, during therapy, during dose interruptions, and for at least 4 weeks after completing therapy. Male patients (including those who had a vasectomy) must always use a latex/synthetic condom during any sexual contact w/ females of reproductive potential during therapy and for up to 28 days after discontinuing therapy. Avoid sperm donation during therapy. Avoid blood donation during treatment and for 1 month following discontinuation. Greater risk of MI or stroke in patients w/ known risk factors, including prior thrombosis; minimize all modifiable factors (eg, hyperlipidemia, HTN, smoking). Increase of invasive 2nd primary malignancies notably acute myelogenous leukemia and MDS reported in patients w/ MM, predominantly in those receiving therapy in combination w/ oral melphalan or immediately following high dose IV mephalan and ASCT. Hepatic failure, including fatal cases, reported in combination w/ dexamethasone. D/C treatment upon elevation of liver enzymes and consider treatment at a lower dose after values return to baseline. Angioedema and serious dermatologic reactions reported; d/c if angioedema, Stevens-Johnson syndrome (SJS), toxic epidermal necrolysis (TEN), Grade 4 rash, or exfoliative or bullous rash is suspected and do not resume following discontinuation for these reactions. Consider treatment interruption or discontinuation for Grade 2-3 skin rash. Avoid w/ a prior history of Grade 4 rash associated w/ thalidomide treatment. Contains lactose. Fatal instances of tumor lysis syndrome reported; caution in patients w/ high tumor burden prior to treatment. Tumor flare reaction (TFR) reported in patients w/ MCL; withhold treatment in patients w/ Grade 3 or 4 TFR until TFR resolves to ≤Grade 1. A decrease in the number of CD34+ cells collected after treatment (>4 cycles) reported; in patients who are ASCT candidates, referral to a transplant center should occur early in treatment to optimize the timing of the stem cell collection. Consider granulocyte-colony stimulating factor (G-CSF) w/ cyclophosphamide or the combination of G-CSF w/ a CXCR4 inhibitor in patients who received >4 cycles of a lenalidomide-containing treatment or for whom inadequate numbers of CD34+ cells have been collected w/ G-CSF alone.

ADVERSE REACTIONS

Thrombocytopenia, neutropenia, PE, pruritus, rash, diarrhea, constipation, nausea, anemia, fatigue, cough, back pain, pyrexia, muscle cramp, asthenia.

DRUG INTERACTIONS

May increase levels of digoxin; monitor digoxin levels periodically. Closely monitor PT and INR w/ warfarin in MM patients. Caution w/ erythropoietic agents or other agents that may increase the risk of thrombosis (eg, estrogen-containing therapies).

NURSING CONSIDERATIONS

Assessment: Assess for renal/hepatic impairment, history of Grade 4 rash, risk factors for MI and stroke, prior thrombosis, high tumor burden, lactose intolerance, hypersensitivity to the drug, pregnancy/nursing status, and possible drug interactions. Perform pregnancy test 10-14 days before and 24 hrs prior to therapy. Obtain baseline CBC.

Monitoring: Monitor for signs/symptoms of thromboembolism, neutropenia, thrombocytopenia, angioedema, SJS, TEN, tumor lysis syndrome, TFR, 2nd primary malignancies, serious adverse CV reactions, and other adverse reactions. Perform pregnancy test weekly during 1st month, then repeat monthly (regular menstrual cycle) or every 2 weeks (irregular menstrual cycle) and perform pregnancy test if period is missed or if there is any abnormal menstrual bleeding. Monitor CBC periodically; every 7 days (weekly) for the first 2 cycles, on Days 1 and 15 of cycle 3, and every 28 days (4 weeks) thereafter (MM patients taking concomitant dexamethasone); weekly for the first 8 weeks of therapy and at least monthly thereafter (MDS); and weekly for the 1st cycle (28 days), every 2 weeks during cycles 2-4, and monthly thereafter (MCL). Monitor patients w/ neutropenia for signs of infection. Monitor renal/hepatic function. Closely monitor patients w/ high tumor burden. Closely monitor PT and INR w/ warfarin in MM patients.

Patient Counseling: Instruct females of reproductive potential to avoid pregnancy, have monthly pregnancy tests, and to use 2 different forms of contraception, including at least 1 highly effective form, simultaneously during therapy, during dose interruption, and for 4 weeks after completing therapy. Instruct to immediately d/c and contact physician if patient becomes pregnant, misses her menstrual period, experiences unusual menstrual bleeding, stops taking birth control, or believes for any reason that she is pregnant. Instruct males (including those who had a vasectomy) to always use a latex/synthetic condom during any sexual contact w/ females of reproductive potential during therapy and for up to 28 days after discontinuing therapy. Advise males not to donate sperm. Instruct not to donate blood during therapy, during dose interruptions, and for 1 month following discontinuation. Inform of the other risks associated w/ therapy. Instruct that if a dose is missed, may still take dose up to 12 hrs after the time dose is normally taken. Advise that if >12 hrs have elapsed, the dose for that day should be skipped, and the dose for the next day should be taken at the usual time. Advise to observe for bleeding/bruising, especially w/ use of concomitant medication that may increase risk of bleeding.

Storage: 20-25°C (68-77°F); excursions permitted to 15-30°C (59-86°F).

REYATAZ – atazanavir

RX

Class: Protease inhibitor

ADULT DOSAGE

HIV-1 Infection

Combination w/ Other Antiretrovirals:
Treatment-Naive:
300mg + Ritonavir (RTV) 100mg qd
Intolerant to RTV:
400mg qd (w/o RTV)
Combination w/ Efavirenz:
400mg + RTV 100mg qd
Treatment-Experienced:
300mg + RTV 100mg qd
Combination w/ H_2-Receptor Antagonists and Tenofovir:
400mg + RTV 100mg qd

PEDIATRIC DOSAGE

HIV-1 Infection

Combination w/ Other Antiretrovirals:
Powder:
≥3 Months of Age:
Treatment-Naive/Treatment-Experienced:
10-<15kg: 200mg + Ritonavir (RTV) 80mg qd
15-<25kg: 250mg + RTV 80mg qd
Cap:
6-<18 Years:
Treatment-Naive/Treatment-Experienced:
15-<20kg: 150mg + RTV 100mg qd
20-<40kg: 200mg + RTV 100mg qd
≥40kg: 300mg + RTV 100mg qd
≥13 Years:
Treatment-Naive & Intolerant to RTV:
≥40kg: 400mg qd (w/o RTV)

DOSE MODIFICATION

Concomitant Medications
H_2-Receptor Antagonists/Proton-Pump Inhibitors:
Dose separation may be required

Renal Impairment
ESRD w/ Hemodialysis:
Treatment-Naive: 300mg + Ritonavir (RTV) 100mg qd
Treatment-Experienced: Not recommended for use

Hepatic Impairment
Treatment-Naive:
Mild (Child-Pugh Class A): 400mg qd (w/o RTV)
Moderate (Child-Pugh Class B): 300mg qd (w/o RTV)
Severe (Child-Pugh Class C): Not recommended for use

Pregnancy
Treatment-Naive and Treatment-Experienced:
300mg + RTV 100mg qd
Treatment-Experienced During 2nd/3rd Trimester w/ Either H_2-Receptor Antagonist or Tenofovir:
400mg + RTV 100mg qd

ADMINISTRATION

Oral route

Take w/ food

Cap
Do not open
Do not administer w/o ritonavir (RTV) in treatment-experienced patients w/ prior virologic failure

Instructions for Mixing Oral Powder
Preferred Method:
1. Mix the recommended number of pkts w/ a minimum of 1 tbsp of food (eg, applesauce or yogurt)
2. Feed the mixture to the infant or young child
3. Add an additional 1 tbsp of food to the container, mix, and feed the child the residual mixture

For Infants Who Can Drink From a Cup:
1. Mix the recommended number of pkts w/ a minimum of 30mL of a beverage (eg, milk or water)
2. Have the child drink the mixture
3. Add an additional 15mL of beverage to the cup, mix, and have the child drink the residual mixture. If water is used, food should also be taken at the same time

For Infants <6 Months Who Cannot Eat Solid Food or Drink From a Cup:
1. Mix the recommended number of pkts w/ 10mL of prepared liquid infant formula
2. Draw up the full amount of the mixture into an oral syringe and administer into either right or left inner cheek of infant
3. Pour another 10mL of formula into the medicine cup to rinse off remaining oral powder in cup
4. Draw up residual mixture into the syringe and administer into either inner cheek again

Administer RTV immediately after powder administration

Administer the entire dose of oral powder (mixed in the food or beverage) w/in 1 hr (may leave the mixture at room temperature during this 1-hr period)

Ensure that the patient eats or drinks all the food or beverage that contains the powder Additional food may be given after consumption of the entire mixture

HOW SUPPLIED

Cap: 150mg, 200mg, 300mg; Powder: 50mg/pkt [30^s]

CONTRAINDICATIONS

Coadministration w/ drugs that are highly dependent on CYP3A or UGT1A1 for clearance, and for which elevated plasma concentrations are associated w/ serious and/or life-threatening events, and w/ strong CYP3A inducers (eg, alfuzosin, rifampin, irinotecan, triazolam, oral midazolam, dihydroergotamine, ergotamine, ergonovine, methylergonovine, cisapride, St. John's wort, lovastatin, simvastatin, pimozide, sildenafil when used for pulmonary arterial HTN, indinavir, nevirapine).

WARNINGS/PRECAUTIONS

Not recommended w/o ritonavir (RTV) for treatment-experienced adults/pediatric patients w/ prior virologic failure and during pregnancy or postpartum period. Atazanavir (ATV)/RTV is not recommended w/ any degree of hepatic impairment. May prolong PR interval; consider ECG monitoring w/ preexisting conduction system disease. Rash and cases of Stevens-Johnson syndrome, erythema multiforme, and toxic skin eruptions, including drug rash w/ eosinophilia and systemic symptoms (DRESS) syndrome, reported; d/c if severe rash develops. May cause hyperbilirubinemia; dose reduction is not recommended. Powder contains phenylalanine; caution w/ phenylketonuria. Increased risk for further transaminase elevations or hepatic decompensation in patients w/ underlying hepatitis B or C infections or marked transaminase elevations; obtain LFTs prior to and during treatment. Nephrolithiasis and/or cholelithiasis reported; consider temporary interruption or discontinuation of therapy if signs/symptoms occur. New onset or exacerbation of diabetes mellitus (DM), hyperglycemia, diabetic ketoacidosis, immune reconstitution syndrome, autoimmune disorders (eg, Graves' disease, polymyositis, Guillain-Barre syndrome) in the setting of immune reconstitution, redistribution/accumulation of body fat, and increased bleeding w/ hemophilia A and B reported. Various degrees of cross-resistance observed. Caution in elderly.

ADVERSE REACTIONS

N/V, jaundice/scleral icterus, rash, myalgia, headache, abdominal pain, insomnia, peripheral neurologic symptoms, diarrhea, cough, fever, AST/ALT elevations, neutropenia, hypoglycemia, extremity pain.

DRUG INTERACTIONS

See Contraindications and Dose Modification. Not recommended w/ salmeterol. Use w/o RTV not recommended w/ drugs highly dependent on CYP2C8 w/ narrow therapeutic indices (eg, paclitaxel, repaglinide), carbamazepine, phenytoin, phenobarbital, bosentan, and buprenorphine. ATV/RTV is not recommended w/ other protease inhibitors, voriconazole, fluticasone propionate, and boceprevir. Not recommended w/ efavirenz or proton pump inhibitors (PPIs) in treatment-experienced patients. Avoid w/ colchicine in patients w/ renal/hepatic impairment. Caution w/ oral contraceptives. CYP3A4 inducers, tenofovir, carbamazepine, boceprevir, phenytoin, phenobarbital, bosentan, efavirenz, PPIs, antacids, buffered medications, and H_2-receptor antagonists may decrease levels. Telaprevir, RTV, and clarithromycin may increase levels. Administer ≥2 hrs before or 1 hr after buffered formulations (eg, didanosine buffered or enteric-coated formulations) and antacids, and 12 hrs after PPIs. May increase levels of CYP3A or UGT1A1 substrates, tenofovir, nevirapine, saquinavir, amiodarone, bepridil, lidocaine (systemic), quinidine, TCAs, trazodone, itraconazole, ketoconazole, colchicine, rifabutin, quetiapine, parenteral midazolam, warfarin (monitor INR), diltiazem and other calcium channel blockers, bosentan, atorvastatin, rosuvastatin, norgestimate, norethindrone, fluticasone propionate, clarithromycin, buprenorphine, norbuprenorphine, immunosuppressants, and PDE-5 inhibitors. ATV/RTV may increase levels of carbamazepine. Rosuvastatin dose should not exceed 10mg/day. May decrease levels of didanosine, 14-OH clarithromycin (clarithromycin active metabolite), and telaprevir. ATV/RTV may decrease levels of phenytoin, phenobarbital, and lamotrigine. Voriconazole may alter levels. May alter levels of ethinyl estradiol. Initiation of medications that inhibit or induce CYP3A may increase or decrease concentrations of ATV/RTV, respectively. Refer to PI for dosing modifications when used w/ certain concomitant therapies.

NURSING CONSIDERATIONS

Assessment: Assess for treatment history, known hypersensitivity, DM, hemophilia, conduction system disease, phenylketonuria, renal/hepatic impairment, pregnancy/nursing status, and possible drug interactions. Obtain baseline LFTs in patients w/ underlying hepatitis B or C infections or marked transaminase elevations.

Monitoring: Monitor for cardiac conduction abnormalities, PR interval prolongation, rash, DRESS, hyperbilirubinemia, nephrolithiasis, cholelithiasis, new onset or exacerbation of DM, hyperglycemia, diabetic ketoacidosis, autoimmune disorders, immune reconstitution syndrome, fat redistribution/accumulation, cross-resistance among protease inhibitors, and other adverse reactions. Monitor LFTs in patients w/ underlying hepatitis B or C infections or marked transaminase elevations. Monitor for bleeding in patients w/ hemophilia. Closely monitor for adverse events during the first 2 months postpartum.

Patient Counseling: Inform that therapy is not a cure for HIV infection, and patients may continue to experience illnesses associated w/ HIV infections. Advise to avoid doing things that can spread HIV infection to others. Advise to take ud and to take w/ food. Instruct not to alter the dose or d/c therapy w/o consulting physician. Advise caregiver on how to mix oral powder w/ a food or beverage, and to carefully follow the instructions for use and storage of powder formulation. Inform caregivers of patients w/ phenylketonuria that oral powder contains phenylalanine, and advise to call healthcare providers if they have any questions. Instruct to report use of any other medications or herbal products. Advise to consult physician if dizziness or lightheadedness occurs. Inform that mild rashes w/o other symptoms, redistribution or accumulation of body fat, or yellowing of the skin or whites of the eyes may occur. Inform that kidney stones and/or gallstones have been reported. Advise to d/c and seek medical evaluation immediately if signs or symptoms of severe skin reactions or hypersensitivity reactions develop.

Storage: (Cap) 25°C (77°F); excursions permitted to 15-30°C (59-86°F). (Powder) <30°C (86°F). Mixed w/ Food/Beverages: 20-30°C (68-86°F) for ≤1 hr prior to administration. Store in original pkt and do not open until ready to use.

RHINOCORT AQUA – budesonide

RX

Class: Corticosteroid

ADULT DOSAGE

Seasonal/Perennial Allergic Rhinitis

Initial: 1 spray/nostril qd
Max: 4 sprays/nostril qd

PEDIATRIC DOSAGE

Seasonal/Perennial Allergic Rhinitis

6-<12 Years:
Initial: 1 spray/nostril qd
Max: 2 sprays/nostril qd

≥12 Years:
Initial: 1 spray/nostril qd
Max: 4 sprays/nostril qd

ADMINISTRATION

Intranasal route

Shake gently before each use

Priming

Prior to initial use, container must be shaken gently and pump must be primed by actuating 8 times
If not used for 2 consecutive days, reprime w/ 1 spray or until a fine spray appears
If not used for >14 days, rinse applicator and reprime w/ 2 sprays or until a fine spray appears

HOW SUPPLIED

Spray: 32mcg/spray [8.6g]

WARNINGS/PRECAUTIONS

Local nasal effects (eg, epistaxis, *Candida* infections of the nose and pharynx, nasal septal perforation, impaired wound healing) may occur. May need to d/c treatment when *Candida* infection develops. Avoid in patients with recent nasal surgery, trauma, or septal ulcers until healing has occurred. Hypersensitivity reactions may occur. May cause immunosuppression; caution with active or quiescent tuberculosis (TB), untreated fungal, bacterial, systemic viral, or parasitic infections; or ocular herpes simplex. Hypercorticism and adrenal suppression may appear with higher than recommended dose or in susceptible individuals at recommended dose; d/c slowly. Adrenal insufficiency and withdrawal symptoms may occur when replacing a systemic with a topical corticosteroid. May reduce growth velocity in pediatric patients. Glaucoma, increased intraocular pressure (IOP), and cataracts reported. Caution with hepatic dysfunction.

ADVERSE REACTIONS

Pharyngitis, epistaxis, cough, bronchospasm, nasal irritation.

DRUG INTERACTIONS

Oral ketoconazole and other known strong CYP3A4 inhibitors (eg, ritonavir, clarithromycin, itraconazole, nefazodone) may increase plasma levels.

NURSING CONSIDERATIONS

Assessment: Assess for history of hypersensitivity, increased IOP, glaucoma, and/or cataracts. Assess for recent nasal ulcers, surgery/trauma, active or quiescent TB, untreated local or systemic fungal or bacterial infections, systemic viral or parasitic infections, ocular herpes simplex, suppressed immune system, asthma or other conditions requiring chronic systemic corticosteroid therapy, pregnancy/nursing status, and possible drug interactions.

Monitoring: Monitor for acute adrenal insufficiency and withdrawal symptoms when replacing systemic corticosteroid with topical corticosteroid. Monitor for hypercorticism and/or HPA-axis suppression, disseminated infections (eg, chickenpox, measles), nasal or pharyngeal *Candida* infections, suppression of growth velocity in children, nasal septal perforation, epistaxis, change in vision, glaucoma, increased IOP, and cataracts.

Patient Counseling: Inform about the benefits and risks of the treatment. Take ud at regular intervals. Avoid exposure to chickenpox or measles. Instruct to consult physician immediately if exposed to chickenpox or measles, if existing infection worsens, or if episodes of epistaxis or nasal discomfort occur. Inform physician if a change in vision occurs.

Storage: 20-25°C (68-77°F) with the valve up. Do not freeze. Protect from light.

RILUTEK – riluzole — RX

Class: Benzothiazole

ADULT DOSAGE

Amyotrophic Lateral Sclerosis

Usual: 50mg q12h

PEDIATRIC DOSAGE

Pediatric use may not have been established

ADMINISTRATION

Oral route

Take 1 hr ac or 2 hrs pc

HOW SUPPLIED

Tab: 50mg

WARNINGS/PRECAUTIONS

Caution with hepatic impairment; monitor LFTs. D/C if ALT levels ≥5 x ULN or clinical jaundice develops. Clinical hepatitis reported. Neutropenia may occur; monitor WBC count with febrile illness. Interstitial lung disease reported; perform chest radiography if respiratory symptoms develop. May impair mental/physical abilities. Caution in elderly.

ADVERSE REACTIONS

Asthenia, N/V, dizziness, decreased lung function, diarrhea, abdominal pain, vertigo, circumonal paresthesia, anorexia, somnolence, headache, anorexia, rhinitis, HTN.

DRUG INTERACTIONS

Caution with concomitant use with potentially hepatotoxic drugs (eg, allopurinol, methyldopa, sulfasalazine). CYP1A2 inhibitors may decrease elimination. CYP1A2 inducers may increase elimination.

NURSING CONSIDERATIONS

Assessment: Assess for hepatic impairment, pregnancy/nursing status, alcohol intake, hypersensitivity, and possible drug interactions. Perform baseline LFTs.

Monitoring: Perform baseline LFTs before therapy, every month during first 3 months, every 3 months for the remainder of the 1st year, then periodically thereafter. Take WBC count and chest radiography if necessary. Monitor for signs/symptoms of febrile illness, liver toxicity, and hypersensitivity reactions.

Patient Counseling: Instruct to notify healthcare professional of any signs of febrile illness. Caution about hazardous tasks. Advise to notify healthcare professional if cough or SOB occur. Instruct to avoid use with excessive intake of alcohol. Instruct patient if a dose is missed, to take next tablet as originally planned.

Storage: 20-25°C (68-77°F); protect from bright light.

RIOMET – metformin hydrochloride — RX

Class: Biguanide

Lactic acidosis may occur due to metformin accumulation; risk increases with conditions such as sepsis, dehydration, excess alcohol intake, hepatic/renal impairment, and acute congestive heart failure (CHF). If acidosis is suspected, d/c therapy and hospitalize patient immediately.

ADULT DOSAGE

Type 2 Diabetes Mellitus

Initial: 500mg (5mL) bid or 850mg (8.5mL) qd

Titrate: Increase in increments of 500mg weekly or 850mg every 2 weeks, up to a total of 2000mg/day (20mL/day), in divided doses; may also increase from 500mg bid to 850mg bid after 2 weeks

PEDIATRIC DOSAGE

Type 2 Diabetes Mellitus

10-16 Years:

Initial: 500mg (5mL) bid

Titrate: Increase in increments of 500mg weekly

Max: 2000mg/day (20mL/day) in divided doses

Max: 2550mg/day (25.5mL/day)

Doses >2000mg may be better tolerated given tid w/ meals

Transfer from Other Antidiabetic Therapy:
From Standard Oral Hypoglycemic Agents Other Than Chlorpropamide: No transition period necessary
From Chlorpropamide: Exercise care during the first 2 weeks for overlapping drug effects and possible hypoglycemia

Transfer from Other Antidiabetic Therapy:
From Standard Oral Hypoglycemic Agents Other Than Chlorpropamide: No transition period necessary
From Chlorpropamide: Exercise care during the first 2 weeks for overlapping drug effects and possible hypoglycemia

DOSE MODIFICATION

Concomitant Medications

Oral Sulfonylurea Therapy in Adults:
If unresponsive to 4 weeks of max dose of metformin HCl monotherapy, consider gradual addition of an oral sulfonylurea while continuing metformin HCl at the max dose
If patients have not satisfactorily responded to 1-3 months of concomitant therapy (max dose of metformin HCl and max dose of an oral sulfonylurea), consider therapeutic alternatives (eg, switching to insulin w/ or w/o metformin HCl)

Insulin Therapy in Adults:
Initial: 500mg (5mL) qd while continuing current insulin dose
Titrate: Increase by 500mg after approx 1 week and by 500mg every week thereafter
Max: 2500mg/day (25mL/day)
Decrease insulin dose by 10-25% when FPG <120mg/dL

Hepatic Impairment
Avoid in patients w/ clinical or laboratory evidence of hepatic disease

Elderly
Initial/Maint: Dose conservatively
Do not titrate to max dose

Other Important Modifications
Debilitated/Malnourished Patients:
Do not titrate to max dose

ADMINISTRATION
Oral route

Give in divided doses w/ meals

HOW SUPPLIED
Sol: 500mg/5mL [118mL, 473mL]

CONTRAINDICATIONS
Renal disease/dysfunction (eg, SrCr ≥1.5mg/dL [males], ≥1.4mg/dL [females], or abnormal CrCl). Acute/chronic metabolic acidosis, including diabetic ketoacidosis, with or without coma. Use in patients undergoing radiologic studies involving intravascular administration of iodinated contrast materials.

WARNINGS/PRECAUTIONS
Do not initiate in patients ≥80 yrs of age unless renal function is not reduced. Avoid in patients with clinical or lab evidence of hepatic disease. Assess renal function before initiation of therapy and at least annually thereafter; d/c with evidence of renal impairment. Promptly withhold in the presence of any condition associated with hypoxemia, dehydration, or sepsis. Temporarily d/c at the time of or prior to radiologic studies involving the use of intravascular iodinated contrast materials, withhold for 48 hrs subsequent to the procedure, and reinstitute only if renal function is normal. May decrease serum vitamin B12 levels. Temporarily suspend for any surgical procedure (except minor procedures not associated with restricted intake of food and fluids); restart when oral intake is resumed and renal function is normal. Evaluate patients previously well controlled on therapy who develop lab abnormalities or clinical illness for evidence of ketoacidosis or lactic acidosis; d/c if acidosis occurs. Caution in patients susceptible to hypoglycemic effects, such as elderly, debilitated/malnourished patients, and those with adrenal/pituitary insufficiency, or alcohol intoxication. Temporary loss of glycemic control may occur when exposed to stress (eg, fever, trauma, infection, surgery); may be necessary to withhold therapy and temporarily administer insulin. Secondary failure may occur; combined therapy with sulfonylurea may result in a response. Caution in elderly. Not recommended for use in pregnancy.

ADVERSE REACTIONS
Lactic acidosis, diarrhea, N/V, flatulence, asthenia, indigestion, abdominal discomfort, headache.

DRUG INTERACTIONS
See Dosage. Alcohol potentiates the effect of metformin on lactate metabolism; avoid excessive alcohol intake. Hypoglycemia may occur with other glucose-lowering agents (eg, sulfonylurea, insulin) or ethanol. May be difficult to recognize hypoglycemia with β-adrenergic blocking drugs. May decrease glyburide and furosemide levels and may decrease furosemide $T_{1/2}$. Furosemide, nifedipine, and oral

cimetidine may increase levels. Caution with drugs that may affect renal function or result in significant hemodynamic change or may interfere with the disposition of metformin, such as cationic drugs eliminated by renal tubular secretion (eg, cimetidine, amiloride, digoxin, morphine); monitor and adjust dose of metformin and/or the interfering drug. Observe for loss of blood glucose control with thiazides and other diuretics, corticosteroids, phenothiazines, thyroid products, estrogens, oral contraceptives, phenytoin, nicotinic acid, sympathomimetics, calcium channel blockers, and isoniazid; observe for hypoglycemia when such drugs are withdrawn during therapy.

NURSING CONSIDERATIONS

Assessment: Assess for metabolic acidosis, diabetic ketoacidosis, risk factors for lactic acidosis, renal/hepatic impairment, inadequate vitamin B12 or Ca^{2+} intake/absorption, presence of malnourishment or debilitation, adrenal/pituitary insufficiency, alcoholism, hypoxemia, drug hypersensitivity, any other conditions where treatment is cautioned, pregnancy/nursing status, and possible drug interactions. Assess if patient is planning to undergo any surgical procedure, radiologic studies involving the use of intravascular iodinated contrast materials, or is under any form of stress. Obtain baseline FPG and HbA1c levels, and hematologic parameters.

Monitoring: Monitor for signs/symptoms of lactic acidosis, hypoxic states, and other adverse reactions. Monitor for changes in clinical status. Monitor renal function, especially in elderly, at least annually. Monitor hematologic parameters annually. Perform routine serum vitamin B12 measurements at 2- to 3-yr intervals in patients predisposed to developing subnormal vitamin B12 levels. Monitor FPG and HbA1c levels periodically.

Patient Counseling: Inform of the potential risks, benefits, and alternative modes of therapy. Advise on the importance of adherence to dietary instructions, regular exercise program, and regular testing of blood glucose, HbA1c, renal function, and hematologic parameters. Inform of the risk of lactic acidosis; instruct to d/c therapy immediately and notify physician if unexplained hyperventilation, myalgia, malaise, unusual somnolence, or other nonspecific symptoms occur. Counsel against excessive alcohol intake. Inform of the risk of hypoglycemia when initiating combination therapy with oral sulfonylureas and insulin.

Storage: 15-30°C (59-86°F).

RISPERDAL CONSTA – risperidone

RX

Class: Atypical antipsychotic

Elderly patients with dementia-related psychosis treated with antipsychotic drugs are at an increased risk of death; most deaths appeared to be cardiovascular (CV) (eg, heart failure, sudden death) or infectious (eg, pneumonia) in nature. Not approved for the treatment of patients with dementia-related psychosis.

ADULT DOSAGE

Schizophrenia

Risperidone-Naive Patients:
Establish tolerability w/ oral risperidone prior to initiating treatment w/ inj in patients who have never taken oral risperidone

Usual: 25mg every 2 weeks
Titrate: May increase to 37.5mg or 50mg; upward dose adjustment should not be made more frequently than every 4 weeks
Max: 50mg every 2 weeks

Oral risperidone (or another antipsychotic) should be given w/ the 1st inj, continued for 3 weeks, and then discontinued

May give lower initial dose of 12.5mg if clinically warranted (eg, history of poor tolerability to psychotropic medications)

Bipolar I Disorder

Monotherapy or Adjunctive Therapy to Lithium or Valproate for Maint Treatment:
Risperidone-Naive Patients:
Establish tolerability w/ oral risperidone prior to initiating treatment w/ inj in patients who have never taken oral risperidone

Usual: 25mg every 2 weeks

PEDIATRIC DOSAGE

Pediatric use may not have been established

Titrate: May increase to 37.5mg or 50mg; upward dose adjustment should not be made more frequently than every 4 weeks
Max: 50mg every 2 weeks

Oral risperidone (or another antipsychotic) should be given w/ the 1st inj, continued for 3 weeks, and then discontinued

May give lower initial dose of 12.5mg if clinically warranted (eg, history of poor tolerability to psychotropic medications)

Conversions

Switching from Other Antipsychotics:
Continue previous antipsychotic for 3 weeks after 1st inj of risperidone

DOSE MODIFICATION

Concomitant Medications

Carbamazepine or Other CYP3A4 Inducers (eg, Phenytoin, Rifampin, Phenobarbital):
Initiation of CYP3A4 Inducers:
Consider dose increase or administration of additional oral risperidone
Discontinuation of CYP3A4 Inducers:
Reevaluate risperidone inj dose and decrease, if necessary. May place on lower dose of risperidone inj 2-4 weeks before the planned discontinuation of CYP3A4 inducer. Patients treated w/ 25mg dose and discontinuing from carbamazepine/other CYP3A4 inducers should continue 25mg dose unless a lower dose of 12.5mg or treatment interruption is necessary

CYP2D6 Inhibitors (eg, Fluoxetine, Paroxetine):
Initiation of Therapy in Patients Receiving Fluoxetine/Paroxetine:
Initial: 12.5mg
Initiation of Fluoxetine/Paroxetine:
May place on lower dose of risperidone 2-4 weeks before the planned start of concomitant therapy. When fluoxetine/paroxetine is initiated in patients receiving 25mg risperidone, it is recommended to continue treatment w/ 25mg dose unless a lower dose of 12.5mg or treatment interruption is necessary

Renal Impairment

Titrate w/ oral risperidone prior to initiating treatment w/ inj
Initial: 0.5mg oral risperidone bid during 1st week
Titrate: May increase to 1mg bid or 2mg qd during 2nd week. If total daily oral dose of ≥2mg is tolerated, may administer 25mg IM every 2 weeks (or alternatively, an initial dose 12.5mg may be appropriate)
Continue oral supplementation for 3 weeks after 1st inj

Hepatic Impairment

Titrate w/ oral risperidone prior to initiating treatment w/ inj
Initial: 0.5mg oral risperidone bid during 1st week
Titrate: May increase to 1mg bid or 2mg qd during 2nd week. If total daily oral dose of ≥2mg is tolerated, may administer 25mg IM every 2 weeks (or alternatively, an initial dose 12.5mg may be appropriate)
Continue oral supplementation for 3 weeks after 1st inj

Other Important Modifications

Reinitiation of Treatment in Patients Previously Discontinued:
Administer supplementation w/ oral risperidone (or another antipsychotic)

ADMINISTRATION

IM route

Administer by deep IM deltoid or gluteal inj
Do not combine 2 different dose strengths in a single administration

Preparation

Remove dose pack from refrigerator and allow it to come to room temperature for approximately 30 min prior to reconstitution
Attach the SmartSite Needle-Free Vial Access Device to the vial appropriately; assemble and connect the prefilled syringe to the vial
Inject entire contents of syringe into vial
Shake vigorously for a minimum of 10 sec; do not store vial after reconstitution as sus may settle
Invert vial completely and slowly withdraw the entire sus into the syringe
Select appropriate needle provided w/ the kit based on inj site
Resuspension will be necessary prior to administration; shake vigorously
Refer to PI for complete instructions for use

HOW SUPPLIED

Inj: 12.5mg, 25mg, 37.5mg, 50mg

WARNINGS/PRECAUTIONS

Each inj should be administered by a healthcare professional. Neuroleptic malignant syndrome (NMS) reported; immediately d/c and treat. May cause tardive dyskinesia (TD), especially in the elderly; consider discontinuation if signs/symptoms appear. Associated with metabolic changes (eg, hyperglycemia, dyslipidemia, weight gain) that may increase CV/cerebrovascular risk. Hyperglycemia and diabetes mellitus (DM), in some cases extreme and associated with ketoacidosis or hyperosmolar coma or death, reported; monitor for worsening of glucose control in patients with DM and FPG in patients at risk for DM. Somnolence, seizures, and prolactin level elevations reported. May induce orthostatic hypotension; consider dose reduction if hypotension occurs. Caution with known CV disease (CVD), cerebrovascular disease, and conditions that predispose to hypotension. Elderly patients and those with a predisposition to hypotensive reactions should avoid Na^+ depletion or dehydration, and circumstances that accentuate hypotension (alcohol intake, high ambient temperature). Leukopenia, neutropenia, and agranulocytosis reported; d/c with severe neutropenia (absolute neutrophil count <1000/mm^3). Monitor CBC and consider discontinuation at the 1st sign of a clinically significant decline in WBC count in the absence of other causative factors in patients with a history of a clinically significant low WBC count or a drug-induced leukopenia/neutropenia. May impair mental/physical abilities. Associated with esophageal dysmotility and aspiration; caution in patients at risk for aspiration pneumonia. Priapism and thrombotic thrombocytopenic purpura (TTP) reported. May cause disruption of body temperature regulation; caution when exposed to temperature extremes. May be associated with an antiemetic effect and may mask signs/symptoms of overdosage with certain drugs or of conditions (eg, intestinal obstruction, Reye's syndrome, brain tumor). Closely supervise patients at high-risk of suicide. Increased sensitivity reported in patients with Parkinson's disease or dementia with Lewy bodies. Caution with diseases/conditions affecting metabolism or hemodynamic responses, renal/hepatic impairment, and in elderly. Avoid inadvertent inj into a blood vessel. Women should not breastfeed for at least 12 weeks after last inj.

ADVERSE REACTIONS

Headache, dizziness, constipation, dyspepsia, akathisia, parkinsonism, weight increased, dry mouth, fatigue, pain in extremity, tremor, nausea, sedation, cough, pain.

DRUG INTERACTIONS

Caution with other centrally-acting drugs or alcohol. May enhance hypotensive effects of other therapeutic agents with this potential. May antagonize effects of levodopa and dopamine agonists. Cimetidine or ranitidine may increase bioavailability. Ranitidine may increase exposure. Chronic administration of clozapine may decrease clearance. May increase valproate peak plasma concentration. Fluoxetine, paroxetine, and other CYP2D6 inhibitors may increase levels. Carbamazepine and other CYP3A4 enzyme inducers may decrease levels.

NURSING CONSIDERATIONS

Assessment: Assess for known hypersensitivity to drug, dementia-related psychosis, DM, risk for hypotension, history of seizures, hepatic/renal impairment, any other conditions where treatment is cautioned, pregnancy/nursing status, and for possible drug interactions. Obtain baseline FPG in patients at risk for DM.

Monitoring: Monitor for NMS, TD, hyperprolactinemia, orthostatic hypotension, cognitive and motor impairment, seizures, esophageal dysmotility, aspiration, priapism, TTP, metabolic changes, disruption of body temperature, and other adverse reactions. Monitor for signs of hyperglycemia; perform periodic FPG in patients at risk for DM. Monitor for signs/symptoms of leukopenia, neutropenia, and agranulocytosis; perform frequent monitoring of CBC in patients with history of clinically significant low WBC count or drug-induced leukopenia/neutropenia. Periodically reevaluate long-term risks and benefits of the drug.

Patient Counseling: Advise of risk of orthostatic hypotension and of nonpharmacologic interventions that help to reduce its occurrence. Inform that therapy has the potential to impair judgment, thinking, or motor skills; advise to use caution when operating hazardous machinery. Instruct to notify physician if pregnant/intending to become pregnant during therapy and for at least 12 weeks after last inj. Instruct not to breastfeed while on therapy and for at least 12 weeks after last inj. Advise to inform physician if taking/planning to take, any prescription or OTC drugs, and to avoid alcohol during treatment.

Storage: 2-8°C (36-46°F). Protect from light. If refrigeration is unavailable, may store at ≤25°C (77°F) for no more than 7 days prior to administration.

RISPERIDONE – risperidone

RX

Class: Atypical antipsychotic

Elderly patients with dementia-related psychosis treated with antipsychotic drugs are at an increased risk of death. Not approved for the treatment of patients with dementia-related psychosis.

OTHER BRAND NAMES

Risperdal, Risperdal M-Tab

ADULT DOSAGE

Schizophrenia

May be administered qd or bid
Initial: 2mg/day
Titrate: May increase at intervals of ≥24 hrs, by 1-2mg/day
Target: 4-8mg/day; efficacy demonstrated in a range of 4-16mg/day
Maint: 2-8mg/day
Max: 16mg/day

If experiencing persistent somnolence, may administer 1/2 daily dose bid

Bipolar Mania

Acute Manic or Mixed Episodes Associated w/ Bipolar I Disorder:
Monotherapy:
Initial: 2-3mg/day
Titrate: May increase at intervals of ≥24 hrs, by 1mg/day
Target: 1-6mg/day
Max: 6mg/day

If experiencing persistent somnolence, may administer 1/2 daily dose bid

Also indicated as adjunctive therapy w/ lithium or valproate for the treatment of acute manic or mixed episodes associated w/ bipolar I disorder

PEDIATRIC DOSAGE

Schizophrenia

13-17 Years:
Initial: 0.5mg qd in am or pm
Titrate: May increase at intervals of ≥24 hrs, by 0.5-1mg/day
Target: 3mg/day; efficacy demonstrated in a range of 1-6mg/day
Max: 6mg/day

If experiencing persistent somnolence, may administer 1/2 daily dose bid

Bipolar Mania

Acute Manic or Mixed Episodes Associated w/ Bipolar I Disorder:
Monotherapy:
10-17 Years:
Initial: 0.5mg qd in am or pm
Titrate: May increase at intervals of ≥24 hrs, by 0.5-1mg/day
Target: 1-2.5mg/day; efficacy demonstrated in range of 0.5-6mg
Max: 6mg/day

If experiencing persistent somnolence, may administer 1/2 daily dose bid

Autistic Disorder

Irritability Associated w/ Autistic Disorder (eg, Symptoms of Aggression Towards Others, Deliberate Self-Injuriousness, Temper Tantrums, Quickly Changing Moods):
5-17 Years:
Total daily dose may be administered qd or divided bid
Initial:
<20kg: 0.25mg/day
≥20kg: 0.5mg/day
Titrate: May increase after a minimum of 4 days
Target:
<20kg: 0.5mg/day
≥20kg: 1mg/day
Maintain target dose for a minimum of 14 days. If not achieving sufficient response, may increase at intervals of ≥2 weeks, by 0.25mg/day (<20kg) or 0.5mg/day (≥20kg)
Range: 0.5-3mg/day

Once sufficient response is achieved and maintained, consider gradually lowering the dose
If experiencing persistent somnolence, may give qd dose hs, divide daily dose bid, or reduce dose

DOSE MODIFICATION

Concomitant Medications

Enzyme Inducers (eg, Carbamazepine, Phenytoin, Rifampin): Increase risperidone dose up to double usual dose when coadministered; may need to decrease dose when enzyme inducers are discontinued

Enzyme Inhibitors (eg, Fluoxetine, Paroxetine): Reduce risperidone dose during coadministration; may need to increase dose when enzyme inhibitors are discontinued
Max: 8mg/day of risperidone in adults during coadministration

Renal Impairment

Adults:

Severe (CrCl <30mL/min):

Initial: 0.5mg bid

Titrate: May increase by ≤0.5mg, administered bid. For doses >1.5mg bid, increase in intervals of ≥1 week

Hepatic Impairment

Adults:

10-15 Points on Child-Pugh System:

Initial: 0.5mg bid

Titrate: May increase by ≤0.5mg, administered bid. For doses >1.5mg bid, increase in intervals of ≥1 week

Elderly

Start at lower end of dosing range

Other Important Modifications

Reinitiation of Treatment in Patients Previously Discontinued:
After an interval off risperidone, follow initial titration schedule

ADMINISTRATION

Oral route

May be given w/ or w/o meals

Sol

May be administered directly from calibrated pipette, or may be mixed w/ a beverage prior to administration (not compatible w/ cola or tea)

Tab, Disintegrating

Immediately place the entire tab on the tongue after removing from blister
Swallow w/ or w/o liquid
Do not split or chew

HOW SUPPLIED

Tab, Disintegrating: 0.25mg, (Risperdal M-Tab) 0.5mg, 1mg, 2mg, 3mg, 4mg; (Risperdal) Sol: 1mg/mL [30mL]; Tab: 0.25mg, 0.5mg, 1mg, 2mg, 3mg, 4mg

WARNINGS/PRECAUTIONS

May cause neuroleptic malignant syndrome (NMS); d/c and treat immediately if this occurs. Tardive dyskinesia (TD) may develop; consider discontinuation if signs/symptoms appear. Associated with metabolic changes (eg, hyperglycemia, dyslipidemia, weight gain) that may increase cardiovascular (CV)/cerebrovascular risk. Hyperglycemia and diabetes mellitus (DM), in some cases extreme and associated with ketoacidosis or hyperosmolar coma or death, reported; monitor for worsening of glucose control in patients with DM, and perform FPG testing in patients at risk for DM. Somnolence, seizures, and elevation of prolactin levels reported. May induce orthostatic hypotension; consider dose reduction if hypotension occurs. Caution with known CV disease (CVD), cerebrovascular disease, and conditions that predispose to hypotension. Leukopenia, neutropenia, and agranulocytosis reported; monitor CBC in patients with history of clinically significant low WBC counts or drug-induced leukopenia/neutropenia, and consider discontinuation at 1st sign of clinically significant decline in WBC counts without other causative factors. D/C and follow WBC counts until recovery in patients with severe neutropenia (absolute neutrophil count <1000/mm^3). May impair mental/physical abilities. Esophageal dysmotility and aspiration reported; caution in patients at risk for aspiration pneumonia. Priapism reported. May disrupt body temperature regulation; caution when prescribing for patients who will be exposed to temperature extremes. Patients with Parkinson's disease or dementia with Lewy bodies may experience increased sensitivity. Caution in elderly. (Tab, Disintegrating) Contains phenylalanine.

ADVERSE REACTIONS

Parkinsonism, akathisia, dystonia, tremor, sedation, dizziness, anxiety, blurred vision, N/V, upper abdominal pain, stomach discomfort, salivary hypersecretion, increased appetite, fatigue, constipation.

DRUG INTERACTIONS

Adjust dose when used with CYP2D6 inhibitors (eg, fluoxetine, paroxetine) and enzyme inducers (eg, carbamazepine). May increase valproate peak plasma concentrations. Caution with other centrally-acting drugs and alcohol. May enhance hypotensive effects of other therapeutic agents with this potential. May antagonize effects of levodopa and dopamine agonists. Chronic administration of clozapine may decrease clearance.

NURSING CONSIDERATIONS

Assessment: Assess for dementia-related psychosis, DM, risk for hypotension, history of seizures, drug hypersensitivity or any other conditions where treatment is cautioned, hepatic/renal function, pregnancy/nursing status, and possible drug interactions. Obtain FPG in patients at risk for DM.

Monitoring: Monitor for NMS, TD, hyperglycemia, hyperprolactinemia, orthostatic hypotension, leukopenia, neutropenia, agranulocytosis, cognitive/motor impairment, seizures, esophageal dysmotility, aspiration, priapism, disruption of body temperature, metabolic changes, and other adverse reactions. Monitor for worsening of glucose control in patients with DM and FPG in patients at risk for DM. Monitor CBC frequently during the 1st few months of therapy in patients with history of clinically significant low WBC or drug-induced leukopenia/neutropenia. In patients with clinically significant neutropenia, monitor for fever or other symptoms or signs of infection. Periodically reevaluate long-term risks and benefits of the drug.

Patient Counseling: Advise about the risk of orthostatic hypotension, especially during the period of initial dose titration. Inform that therapy has the potential to impair judgment, thinking, or motor skills; advise to use caution when operating hazardous machinery. Instruct to notify physician if pregnant/planning to become pregnant, nursing, and if taking/planning to take any prescription or OTC drugs. Advise to avoid alcohol during treatment. Inform that orally disintegrating tab contains phenylalanine. Inform that treatment can be associated with hyperglycemia and DM, dyslipidemia, and weight gain. Inform about risk of TD.

Storage: 20-25°C (68-77°F). (Risperdal/Risperdal M-Tab) 15-25°C (59-77°F). Sol: Protect from light and freezing. Tab: Protect from light and moisture.

RITALIN – methylphenidate hydrochloride CII

Class: Sympathomimetic amine

Caution with history of drug dependence or alcoholism. Chronic abuse may lead to marked tolerance and psychological dependence with varying degrees of abnormal behavior. Frank psychotic episodes may occur, especially with parenteral abuse. Careful supervision is required during withdrawal from abusive use since severe depression may occur. Withdrawal following chronic use may unmask symptoms of underlying disorder that may require follow-up.

OTHER BRAND NAMES

Ritalin-SR

ADULT DOSAGE

Attention Deficit Disorders

Tab:

20-30mg/day given in divided doses bid-tid, preferably 30-45 min ac; some patients may require 40-60mg/day and others, 10-15mg/day may be adequate

Last dose should be taken before 6 pm if patient is unable to sleep as a result of taking medication late in the day

Tab, Sustained-Release (SR):

May be used in place of methylphenidate IR tabs when the 8-hr dosage of SR tab corresponds to the titrated 8-hr dosage of methylphenidate IR tabs

Narcolepsy

Tab:

20-30mg/day given in divided doses bid-tid, preferably 30-45 min ac; some patients may require 40-60mg/day and others, 10-15mg/day may be adequate

Last dose should be taken before 6 pm if patient is unable to sleep as a result of taking medication late in the day

Tab, Sustained-Release (SR):

May be used in place of methylphenidate IR tabs when the 8-hr dosage of SR tab corresponds to the titrated 8-hr dosage of methylphenidate IR tabs

PEDIATRIC DOSAGE

Attention Deficit Disorders

≥6 Years:

Tab:

Initial: 5mg bid before breakfast and lunch

Titrate: Increase gradually by 5-10mg weekly

Max: 60mg/day

Tab, Sustained-Release (SR):

May be used in place of methylphenidate IR tabs when the 8-hr dosage of SR tab corresponds to the titrated 8-hr dosage of methylphenidate IR tabs

D/C if no improvement seen after appropriate dosage adjustment over 1 month

D/C periodically to assess the child's condition; therapy should not be indefinite

Narcolepsy

≥6 Years:

Tab:

Initial: 5mg bid before breakfast and lunch

Titrate: Increase gradually by 5-10mg weekly

Max: 60mg/day

Tab, Sustained-Release (SR):

May be used in place of methylphenidate IR tabs when the 8-hr dosage of SR tab corresponds to the titrated 8-hr dosage of methylphenidate IR tabs

D/C if no improvement seen after appropriate dosage adjustment over 1 month

D/C periodically to assess the child's condition; therapy should not be indefinite

DOSE MODIFICATION

Adverse Reactions

Children ≥6 Years:
Reduce dose or d/c if paradoxical aggravation of symptoms or other adverse effects occur

ADMINISTRATION

Oral route

Tab, SR
Swallow tabs whole; do not crush or chew

HOW SUPPLIED

Tab: (Ritalin) 5mg, 10mg*, 20mg*; Tab, Sustained-Release (SR): (Generic) 10mg, (Ritalin-SR) 20mg
*scored

CONTRAINDICATIONS

Marked anxiety, tension, agitation, glaucoma, motor tics, or family history or diagnosis of Tourette's syndrome. Treatment with MAOIs or within a minimum of 14 days following discontinuation of an MAOI.

WARNINGS/PRECAUTIONS

Avoid with known serious structural cardiac abnormalities, cardiomyopathy, serious heart rhythm abnormalities, coronary artery disease, or other serious cardiac problems. Sudden death reported in children and adolescents with structural cardiac abnormalities or other serious heart problems. Sudden death, stroke, and MI reported in adults. May increase BP and HR. Prior to treatment, obtain medical history (including assessment for family history of sudden death or ventricular arrhythmia) and perform physical exam to assess for presence of cardiac disease. Promptly perform cardiac evaluation if symptoms of cardiac disease develop. May exacerbate symptoms of behavior disturbance and thought disorder in patients with preexisting psychotic disorder. Caution in patients with comorbid bipolar disorder; may induce mixed/manic episode. May cause treatment-emergent psychotic or manic symptoms (eg, hallucinations, delusional thinking, mania) in children and adolescents without prior history of psychotic illness or mania; consider discontinuation if such symptoms occur. Aggressive behavior or hostility reported in children and adolescents. May cause long-term suppression of growth in children; monitor growth, and may need to interrupt treatment in patients not growing or gaining height or weight as expected. May lower convulsive threshold; d/c if seizures occur. Priapism, sometimes requiring surgical intervention, reported. Associated with peripheral vasculopathy, including Raynaud's phenomenon. Difficulties with accommodation and blurring of vision reported. Patients with an element of agitation may react adversely; d/c if necessary.

ADVERSE REACTIONS

Nervousness, insomnia, hypersensitivity reactions, anorexia, nausea, dizziness, palpitations, headache, dyskinesia, drowsiness, BP and pulse changes, tachycardia, angina, cardiac arrhythmia, abdominal pain.

DRUG INTERACTIONS

See Contraindications. Caution with pressor agents. May decrease effectiveness of drugs used to treat HTN. May inhibit metabolism of coumarin anticoagulants, anticonvulsants, and TCAs; downward dose adjustment and monitoring of plasma drug concentration (or coagulation times for coumarin) of these drugs may be necessary when initiating or discontinuing methylphenidate.

NURSING CONSIDERATIONS

Assessment: Assess for hypersensitivity to the drug, marked anxiety, tension, agitation, glaucoma, motor tics, family history or diagnosis of Tourette's syndrome, cardiovascular conditions, history of drug dependence or alcoholism, psychotic disorder, comorbid bipolar disorder, any other conditions where treatment is contraindicated or cautioned, pregnancy/nursing status, and possible drug interactions.

Monitoring: Monitor for changes in HR and BP, signs/symptoms of cardiac disease, exacerbation of behavior disturbance and thought disorder, psychosis, mania, appearance of or worsening of aggressive behavior or hostility, seizures, priapism, digital changes, visual disturbances, and other adverse reactions. In pediatric patients, monitor growth. Perform periodic monitoring of CBC, differential, and platelet counts during prolonged therapy.

Patient Counseling: Inform about the benefits and risks of therapy and counsel about appropriate use. Instruct to seek immediate medical attention in the event of priapism. Instruct to report to physician any new numbness, pain, skin color change, or sensitivity to temperature in fingers or toes, and to contact physician immediately if any signs of unexplained wounds appear on fingers or toes while taking the drug.

Storage: (Ritalin/Ritalin-SR) 25°C (77°F); excursions permitted to 15-30°C (59-86°F). (Generic) 20-25°C (68-77°F). (Ritalin) Protect from light. (Tab, SR) Protect from moisture.

RITUXAN – rituximab

RX

Class: Monoclonal antibody/CD20-blocker

Serious infusion reactions and severe mucocutaneous reactions, some fatal (death has occurred within 24 hrs of infusion), may occur. Monitor patients closely. D/C infusion for severe reaction and treat for Grade 3/4 infusion reactions. Hepatitis B virus (HBV) reactivation can occur, in some cases resulting in fulminant hepatitis, hepatic failure, and death. Screen all patients for HBV infection before treatment initiation; monitor patients during and after treatment. D/C therapy and concomitant medications in the event of HBV reactivation. Fatal progressive multifocal leukoencephalopathy (PML) may occur.

ADULT DOSAGE

Non-Hodgkin's Lymphoma

375mg/m^2 as an IV infusion

Relapsed/Refractory, Low-Grade/Follicular, CD20-Positive, B-Cell Non-Hodgkin's Lymphoma (NHL) as a Single Agent:
Administer once weekly for 4 or 8 doses
Retreatment: Administer once weekly for 4 doses

Previously Untreated Follicular, CD20-Positive, B-Cell NHL:
In Combination w/ Chemotherapy: Administer on Day 1 of each chemotherapy cycle for up to 8 doses
Maint in Complete/Partial Responders: Administer as a single agent every 8 weeks for 12 doses; initiate 8 weeks following completion of combination treatment w/ chemotherapy

Non-Progressing, Low-Grade, CD20-Positive, B-Cell NHL as a Single Agent After 1st Line Cyclophosphamide, Vincristine, and Prednisone (CVP) Chemotherapy:
Administer once weekly for 4 doses at 6-month intervals following completion of 6-8 CVP chemotherapy cycles
Max: 16 doses

Previously Untreated Diffuse Large B-Cell, CD20-Positive NHL in Combination w/ Cyclophosphamide, Doxorubicin, Vincristine, and Prednisone (CHOP) or Other Anthracycline-Based Chemotherapy:
Administer on Day 1 of each chemotherapy cycle for up to 8 infusions

As a Component of Zevalin:
Infuse 250mg/m^2 w/in 4 hrs prior to the administration of Indium-111 (In-111) Zevalin and w/in 4 hrs prior to the administration of Yttrium-90 (Y-90) Zevalin; administer rituximab and In-111 Zevalin 7-9 days prior to rituximab and Y-90 Zevalin

Refer to the Zevalin PI for additional information

Chronic Lymphocytic Leukemia

In combination w/ fludarabine and cyclophosphamide, for previously untreated and previously treated CD20-positive chronic lymphocytic leukemia

375mg/m^2 the day prior to initiation of fludarabine and cyclophosphamide chemotherapy, then 500mg/m^2 on Day 1 of cycles 2-6 (every 28 days)

Pneumocystis jiroveci pneumonia and anti-herpetic viral prophylaxis is recommended during treatment and for up to 12 months following treatment as appropriate

PEDIATRIC DOSAGE

Pediatric use may not have been established

Rheumatoid Arthritis

In combination w/ methotrexate for moderately to severely active rheumatoid arthritis in patients who have had an inadequate response to ≥1 TNF antagonist therapies

Two 1000mg IV infusions separated by 2 weeks

Administer subsequent courses every 24 weeks or based on evaluation, but not sooner than every 16 weeks

Granulomatosis with Polyangiitis and Microscopic Polyangiitis

In Combination w/ Glucocorticoids:
375mg/m^2 IV infusion once weekly for 4 weeks
Glucocorticoid Administration:
Methylprednisolone 1000mg/day IV for 1-3 days, followed by oral prednisone 1mg/kg/day (not to exceed 80mg/day and tapered per clinical need); begin regimen w/in 14 days prior to or w/ initiation of rituximab and continue during and after the 4-week course of treatment

Pneumocystis jiroveci pneumonia prophylaxis is recommended during treatment and for at least 6 months following the last infusion

Premedication

Premedicate before each infusion w/ acetaminophen and an antihistamine

For patients administered rituximab according to the 90-min infusion rate, the glucocorticoid component of their chemotherapy regimen should be administered prior to infusion

Rheumatoid Arthritis Patients:
Methylprednisolone 100mg IV (or its equivalent) 30 min prior to each infusion

DOSE MODIFICATION

Adverse Reactions

Infusion Reactions: Interrupt or slow the infusion; continue at 1/2 the previous rate upon improvement of symptoms

ADMINISTRATION

IV route

For IV infusion only; do not administer as IV push or bolus
Do not mix or dilute w/ other drugs
Single-use vial; discard any unused portion left in vial

1st Infusion

Initiate at a rate of 50mg/hr; in the absence of infusion toxicity, increase rate by 50mg/hr increments every 30 min, to a max of 400mg/hr

Subsequent Infusions

Standard Infusion: Initiate at a rate of 100mg/hr; in the absence of infusion toxicity, increase by 100mg/hr increments every 30 min, to a max of 400mg/hr

Previously Untreated Follicular and Diffuse Large B-Cell Non-Hodgkin's Lymphoma Patients:
Grade 3 or 4 Infusion-Related Adverse Event Not Experienced During Cycle 1:
Administer a 90-min infusion in Cycle 2 w/ a glucocorticoid-containing chemotherapy regimen; initiate at a rate of 20% of the total dose given in the first 30 min and the remaining 80% of the total dose given over the next 60 min. If 90-min infusion is tolerated in cycle 2, use the same rate when administering the remainder of the treatment regimen (through Cycle 6 or 8)
Clinically Significant Cardiovascular Disease/Circulating Lymphocyte Count ≥5000/mm^3 Before Cycle 2:
Do not administer the 90-min infusion

Preparation

1. Withdraw the necessary amount of rituximab and dilute to a final concentration of 1-4mg/mL in an infusion bag containing either 0.9% normal saline or D5W
2. Gently invert bag to mix the sol

HOW SUPPLIED

Inj: 100mg/10mL, 500mg/50mL

WARNINGS/PRECAUTIONS

Should only be administered by a healthcare professional with appropriate medical support to manage severe infusion reactions that can be fatal if they occur. Not recommended for use with severe, active infections. *Pneumocystis jiroveci* pneumonia (PCP) and antiherpetic viral prophylaxis is recommended for patients with CLL during treatment and for up to 12 months following treatment as appropriate. PCP prophylaxis is recommended for patients with GPA and MPA during treatment and for at least 6 months following last infusion. Potential for immunogenicity. Acute renal failure, hyperkalemia, hypocalcemia, hyperuricemia, and/or hyperphosphatemia from tumor lysis may occur within 12-24 hrs after the 1st infusion. A high number of circulating malignant cells ($\geq$25,000/mm^3) or high tumor burden confers greater risk of tumor lysis syndrome (TLS); administer aggressive IV hydration and antihyperuricemic therapy in patients at high risk of TLS. Correct electrolyte abnormalities, monitor renal function and fluid balance, and administer supportive care, including dialysis as indicated. Serious, including fatal, bacterial, fungal, and new/reactivated viral infections may occur during and following the completion of therapy; d/c for serious infections and institute anti-infective therapy. Infections reported in some patients with prolonged hypogammaglobulinemia (>11 months after rituximab exposure). D/C if severe mucocutaneous reactions, PML, or serious/life-threatening cardiac arrhythmias occur. Perform cardiac monitoring during and after all infusions if arrhythmias develop or with history of arrhythmia/angina. Severe renal toxicity may occur in NHL patients; d/c if SrCr rises or oliguria occurs. Abdominal pain, bowel obstruction, and perforation may occur in combination with chemotherapy. Follow current immunization guidelines and administer non-live vaccines at least 4 weeks prior to therapy for RA patients. Obtain CBC and platelet count prior to each course in lymphoid malignancy patients, at weekly to monthly intervals (more frequently if cytopenia develops) during treatment with rituximab and chemotherapy, and at 2- to 4-month intervals during therapy in RA, GPA, or MPA patients. Not recommended in patients with RA who have not had prior inadequate response to one or more TNF antagonists.

ADVERSE REACTIONS

Infusion reactions, mucocutaneous reactions, hepatitis B reactivation, PML, infections, fever, lymphopenia, chills, asthenia, neutropenia, headache, leukopenia, diarrhea, muscle spasms.

DRUG INTERACTIONS

Renal toxicity reported with cisplatin. Vaccination with live viral vaccines not recommended. Observe closely for signs of infection if biologic agents and/or disease-modifying antirheumatic drugs are used concomitantly.

NURSING CONSIDERATIONS

Assessment: Assess for severe active infections, preexisting cardiac/pulmonary conditions, prior experience of cardiopulmonary adverse reactions, high number of circulating malignant cells ($\geq$25,000/mm^3), high tumor burden, electrolyte abnormalities, risk/preexisting HBV infection, hypogammaglobulinemia, any other conditions where treatment is cautioned, pregnancy/nursing status, and possible drug interactions. Perform HBsAg and anti-HBc measurement before initiating treatment. Obtain CBC and platelet count.

Monitoring: Monitor fluid and electrolyte balance, cardiac/renal function, CBC, and platelet counts periodically. Monitor for signs/symptoms of infusion reactions, mucocutaneous reactions, hepatitis B reactivation, PML, new-onset neurologic manifestations, TLS, infections, arrhythmias, bowel obstruction/perforation, cytopenias, and other adverse reactions. Closely monitor for infusion reactions in patients with preexisting cardiac/pulmonary conditions, those who experienced prior cardiopulmonary adverse reactions, and those with high numbers of circulating malignant cells. Monitor patients with evidence of current or prior HBV infection for clinical and lab signs of hepatitis or HBV reactivation during and for several months following therapy.

Patient Counseling: Inform of risks of therapy and importance of assessing overall health status at each visit. Inform that drug is detectable in serum for up to 6 months following completion of therapy. Advise to use effective contraception during and for 12 months after therapy.

Storage: 2-8°C (36-46°F). Protect from direct sunlight. Do not freeze or shake. Sol for Infusion: 2-8°C (36-46°F) for 24 hrs. Stable for additional 24 hrs at room temperature; however, store diluted solutions at 2-8°C (36-46°F).

ROBAXIN – methocarbamol

Class: Muscular analgesic (central-acting)

RX

OTHER BRAND NAMES
Robaxin Injection, Robaxin-750

ADULT DOSAGE

Musculoskeletal Conditions

Adjunct for relief of discomfort associated w/ acute, painful musculoskeletal conditions

Oral:
≥16 Years:
Robaxin:
Initial: 3 tabs qid
Maint: 2 tabs qid
Robaxin-750:
Initial: 2 tabs qid
Maint: 1 tab q4h or 2 tabs tid

6g/day are recommended for the first 48-72 hrs; 8g/day may be administered for severe conditions. Thereafter, the dose can usually be reduce to approx 4g/day

Inj:
Moderate Symptoms:
Single 1g (10mL) dose IV/IM; administration of oral form will usually sustain relief initiated by the inj
Max: 3g/day for no more than 3 consecutive days

Severe Cases/Postop Conditions:
Single 1g (10mL) dose IV/IM; may administer additional doses of 1g q8h
Max: 3g/day for no more than 3 consecutive days

Tetanus

Inj:
1 or 2 vials directly into the tubing of the previously inserted indwelling needle; additional 10mL or 20mL may be added to infusion bottle so that a total of up to 30mL (3 vials) is given as initial dose

Repeat q6h until conditions allow for insertion of NG tube; crushed methocarbamol tabs suspended in water or saline may then be given through this tube

Total oral doses up to 24g/day may be required

PEDIATRIC DOSAGE

Tetanus

Inj:
Initial: 15mg/kg or 500mg/m^2; repeat q6h prn
Max: 1.8g/m^2 for 3 consecutive days

Maint dose may be administered by inj into tubing or by IV infusion w/ an appropriate quantity of fluid

ADMINISTRATION
Oral/IV/IM route

Directions for IV Use
Inj may be administered undiluted at a max rate of 3mL/min or added to an IV drip of NaCl inj or D5 inj
One vial given as a single dose should not be diluted to more than 250mL for IV infusion
Do not refrigerate after mixing w/ IV infusion fluids
Avoid vascular extravasation of this hypertonic sol, which may result in thrombophlebitis
Patient should be in a recumbent position during and for at least 10-15 min following inj

Directions for IM Use
Not more than 5mL (1/2 vial) should be injected into each gluteal region
Inj may be repeated at 8-hr intervals, if necessary
When satisfactory relief of symptoms is achieved, it can usually be maintained w/ tabs
Not recommended for SQ administration

HOW SUPPLIED
Inj: 100mg/mL [10mL]; Tab: 500mg, 750mg

CONTRAINDICATIONS
(Inj) Renal pathology with injection due to propylene glycol content.

WARNINGS/PRECAUTIONS
May impair mental/physical abilities. May cause color interference in certain screening tests for 5-hydroxy-indoleacetic acid (5-HIAA) and vanillylmandelic acid (VMA). Caution in epilepsy with the inj. Inj rate should not exceed 3mL/min. Avoid extravasation with inj. Avoid use in women who are or may become pregnant and particularly during early pregnancy.

ADVERSE REACTIONS
Lightheadedness, dizziness, drowsiness, nausea, urticaria, pruritus, rash, conjunctivitis, nasal congestion, blurred vision, headache, fever, seizures, syncope, flushing.

DRUG INTERACTIONS
Additive adverse effects with alcohol and other CNS depressants. May inhibit effect of pyridostigmine; caution in patients with myasthenia gravis receiving anticholinergics.

NURSING CONSIDERATIONS

Assessment: Assess for renal/hepatic impairment, myasthenia gravis, seizures, pregnancy/nursing status, alcohol intake, and drug interactions.

Monitoring: Monitor for congenital and fetal abnormalities if taken during pregnancy, for color interference in certain screening tests for 5-HIAA using nitrosonaphthol reagent, and in screening tests for urinary VMA using Gitlow method.

Patient Counseling: Instruct to use caution while performing hazardous tasks. Warn to avoid alcohol or other CNS depressants. Instruct to notify physician if pregnant/nursing or if planning to become pregnant.

Storage: 20-25°C (68-77°F), in tight container; excursions permitted to 15-30°C (59-86°F).

ROCALTROL – calcitriol

RX

Class: Vitamin D analogue

ADULT DOSAGE

Hypoparathyroidism

Initial: 0.25mcg/day qam
Titrate: May increase at 2- to 4-week intervals
Usual: 0.5-2mcg/day

Secondary Hyperparathyroidism

In Predialysis Patients:
Initial: 0.25mcg/day
Titrate: May increase to 0.5mcg/day

Hypocalcemia

In Chronic Renal Dialysis Patients:
Initial: 0.25mcg/day
Titrate: May increase by 0.25mcg/day at 4- to 8-week intervals
Usual: 0.5-1mcg/day

Slightly Reduced Serum Calcium:
May respond to 0.25mcg qod

PEDIATRIC DOSAGE

Hypoparathyroidism

1-5 Years:
Usual: 0.25-0.75mcg/day qam
≥6 Years:
Usual: 0.5-2mcg/day qam

Secondary Hyperparathyroidism

In Predialysis Patients:
<3 Years:
Initial: 10-15ng/kg/day
≥3 Years:
Initial: 0.25mcg/day
Titrate: May increase to 0.5mcg/day

DOSE MODIFICATION

Elderly
Start at lower end of dosing range

Adverse Reactions
Hypercalcemia: Immediately d/c until normocalcemia ensues; when normal levels return, continue treatment at a daily dose 0.25mcg lower than that previously used

ADMINISTRATION
Oral route

HOW SUPPLIED
Cap: 0.25mcg, 0.5mcg; Sol: 1mcg/mL [15mL]

CONTRAINDICATIONS
Hypercalcemia or evidence of vitamin D toxicity.

WARNINGS/PRECAUTIONS
Administration in excess of daily requirements may cause hypercalcemia, hypercalciuria, and hyperphosphatemia. Chronic hypercalcemia may lead to generalized vascular calcification,

nephrocalcinosis, and other soft tissue calcification. Serum Ca^{2+} times phosphate (Ca x P) product should not exceed $70mg^2/dL^2$. May increase serum inorganic phosphate levels, leading to ectopic calcification in patients with renal failure; use non-aluminum phosphate binders and low phosphate diet to control serum phosphate in dialysis patients. Caution in elderly and immobilized patients. If treatment switched from ergocalciferol, may take several months for ergocalciferol level in blood to return to baseline. In patients with normal renal function, chronic hypercalcemia may be associated with an increase in SrCr. Avoid dehydration in patients with normal renal function. When indicated, estimate daily dietary Ca^{2+} intake and adjust accordingly.

ADVERSE REACTIONS

Hypercalcemia, hypercalciuria, SrCr elevation, weakness, N/V, dry mouth, constipation, muscle and bone pain, metallic taste, polyuria, polydipsia, weight loss, hypersensitivity reactions.

DRUG INTERACTIONS

Avoid pharmacological doses of vitamin D products and derivatives during therapy. Avoid uncontrolled intake of additional Ca^{2+}-containing preparations. Avoid with Mg^{2+}-containing preparations (eg, antacids) in patients on chronic renal dialysis; use may lead to hypermagnesemia. May impair intestinal absorption with cholestyramine. Reduced blood levels with phenytoin or phenobarbital. Caution with thiazides; may cause hypercalcemia. Reduced serum endogenous concentrations with ketoconazole reported. Hypercalcemia may precipitate cardiac arrhythmias in patients on digitalis; use with caution. Functional antagonism with corticosteroids. Adjust dose of concomitant phosphate-binding agent.

NURSING CONSIDERATIONS

Assessment: Assess for hypercalcemia, evidence of vitamin D toxicity, renal function, presence of immobilization, pregnancy/nursing status, and possible drug interactions. Obtain baseline levels of serum Ca^{2+}, phosphorus (P), alkaline phosphatase, creatinine, and intact parathyroid hormone (iPTH).

Monitoring: Monitor for hypercalcemia, hypercalciuria, and hyperphosphatemia. For dialysis patients, perform periodic monitoring of serum Ca^{2+}, P, Mg^{2+}, and alkaline phosphatase. For hypoparathyroid patients, perform periodic monitoring of serum Ca^{2+}, P, and 24-hr urinary Ca^{2+}. For predialysis patients, perform monthly monitoring of serum Ca^{2+}, P, alkaline phosphatase, and creatinine for 6 months; then periodically, and periodic monitoring of iPTH every 3- to 4-months. Monitor serum Ca^{2+} levels $\geq$2X/week after all dosage changes and during titration periods.

Patient Counseling: Inform about compliance with dosage instructions, adherence to instructions about diet and Ca^{2+} supplementation, and avoidance of the use of unapproved nonprescription drugs. Carefully inform about symptoms of hypercalcemia. Advise to maintain adequate Ca^{2+} intake at a minimum of 600mg/day.

Storage: 15-30°C (59-86°F). Protect from light.

ROTATEQ – rotavirus vaccine, live, oral, pentavalent **RX**

Class: Vaccine

PEDIATRIC DOSAGE

Rotavirus Gastroenteritis Prevention

Caused by the Serotypes G1, G2, G3, and G4:
6-32 Weeks of Age:
Administer series of 3 (2mL) doses PO starting at 6-12 weeks of age, w/ subsequent doses administered at 4- to 10-week intervals; 3rd dose should not be given after 32 weeks of age

ADMINISTRATION

Oral route

Administer as soon as possible after being removed from refrigeration
No restrictions on food/liquid consumption (eg, breast milk) either before or after vaccination
Do not mix w/ any other vaccines or sol
Do not reconstitute or dilute
Gently squeeze liquid into infant's mouth toward inner cheek until dosing tube is empty
A replacement dose is not recommended if an incomplete dose is administered (eg, infant spits or regurgitates vaccine); infant should continue to receive any remaining doses in the recommended series

HOW SUPPLIED

Sol: 2mL

CONTRAINDICATIONS

Severe combined immunodeficiency disease (SCID) and history of intussusception.

WARNINGS/PRECAUTIONS
For PO use only. Appropriate treatment and supervision must be available to manage possible anaphylactic reactions following administration. Safety and efficacy data not available for administration to infants who are potentially immunocompromised. Caution in infants with a history of GI disorders (eg, active acute GI illness, chronic diarrhea, failure to thrive, history of congenital abdominal disorders, abdominal surgery). Intussusception reported. Shedding of vaccine virus in stool reported. Transmission of vaccine virus from vaccinees to unvaccinated contacts reported; caution when administering to individuals with immunodeficient close contacts. Consider delaying use with febrile illness. May not protect all vaccine recipients against rotavirus. Clinical data not available for postexposure prophylaxis or for level of protection provided with administration of an incomplete regimen. If an incomplete dose is administered (eg, infant spits or regurgitates vaccine), do not give replacement dose; continue to give any remaining doses in the recommended series.

ADVERSE REACTIONS
Irritability, fever, diarrhea, vomiting, nasopharyngitis, otitis media.

DRUG INTERACTIONS
Immunosuppressive therapies, including irradiation, antimetabolites, alkylating agents, cytotoxic drugs, and corticosteroids (used in greater than physiologic doses) may reduce immune response to vaccine.

NURSING CONSIDERATIONS
Assessment: Assess for previous hypersensitivity to the vaccine, SCID, history of intussusception, immunization history, immunocompromised conditions, history of GI disorders, febrile illness, and possible drug interactions.

Monitoring: Monitor for hypersensitivity/anaphylactic reactions, intussusception, and other adverse events.

Patient Counseling: Inform parent/guardian of potential benefits/risks of vaccine. Instruct parent/guardian to inform physician of the current health status of patient and to report if patient has close contact with a family/household member who has a weak immune system. Advise to contact physician immediately if patient develops vomiting, diarrhea, severe stomach pain, or blood in the stool and advise to contact physician if any other adverse reactions develop.

Storage: 2-8°C (36-46°F). Protect from light.

ROXICET — acetaminophen/oxycodone CII

Class: Opioid analgesic

Associated with cases of acute liver failure, at times resulting in liver transplant and death. Most cases of liver injury are associated with acetaminophen (APAP) use at doses >4000mg/day, and often involve >1 APAP-containing product.

ADULT DOSAGE
Moderate to Moderately Severe Pain

Usual: 1 tab or 5mL (1 tsp) q6h PRN
Max: 12 tabs/day or 60mL/day (12 tsp/day)

If pain is constant, give at regular intervals on an around-the-clock schedule
Max: 4g/day of APAP

PEDIATRIC DOSAGE
Pediatric use may not have been established

DOSE MODIFICATION
Discontinuation

Taper dose gradually in patients treated for more than a few weeks

ADMINISTRATION
Oral route

HOW SUPPLIED
(Oxycodone-APAP) Sol: 5mg-325mg/5mL [500mL]; Tab: 5mg-325mg* *scored

CONTRAINDICATIONS
Oxycodone: Significant respiratory depression (in unmonitored settings or absence of resuscitative equipment), acute or severe bronchial asthma or hypercarbia, suspected/known paralytic ileus.

WARNINGS/PRECAUTIONS
May be abused in a manner similar to other opioid agonists. Respiratory depression may occur; use extreme caution and consider alternative nonopioid analgesics in patients with acute asthma, chronic obstructive pulmonary disorder (COPD), cor pulmonale, preexisting respiratory impairment, or in the elderly or debilitated. Respiratory depressant effects may be markedly exaggerated in the presence of head injury, other intracranial lesions, or preexisting increase in intracranial pressure. Produces effects on pupillary response and consciousness, which may obscure neurologic signs of worsening

in patients with head injuries. May cause severe hypotension; caution with circulatory shock. May produce orthostatic hypotension in ambulatory patients. Increased risk of acute liver failure in patients with underlying liver disease. May cause serious skin reactions (eg, acute generalized exanthematous pustulosis, Stevens-Johnson syndrome, toxic epidermal necrolysis), which can be fatal; d/c at the 1st appearance of skin rash or any other sign of hypersensitivity/anaphylaxis. Hypersensitivity and anaphylaxis reported. May obscure diagnosis or clinical course in patients with acute abdominal conditions. Caution with CNS depression, hypothyroidism, Addison's disease, prostatic hypertrophy, urethral stricture, acute alcoholism, delirium tremens, kyphoscoliosis with respiratory depression, myxedema, toxic psychosis, hepatic/renal/pulmonary impairment, and in elderly/debilitated. May aggravate convulsions with convulsive disorders and may induce or aggravate seizures in some clinical settings. Monitor for decreased bowel motility in postoperative patients. May cause spasm of the sphincter of Oddi; caution with biliary tract disease, including acute pancreatitis. May cause increases in serum amylase level. Physical dependence and tolerance may occur. Do not abruptly d/c. Lab test interactions may occur. Not recommended for use during and immediately prior to labor and delivery.

ADVERSE REACTIONS

Acute liver failure, respiratory depression, apnea, respiratory arrest, circulatory depression, hypotension, shock, lightheadedness, dizziness, drowsiness/sedation, N/V.

DRUG INTERACTIONS

Oxycodone: May cause severe hypotension with drugs that compromise vasomotor tone (eg, phenothiazines). May enhance neuromuscular-blocking action of skeletal muscle relaxants and increase respiratory depression. Additive CNS depression with CNS depressants (eg, general anesthetics, phenothiazines, tranquilizers, alcohol); reduce dose of one or both agents. Coadministration with anticholinergics may produce paralytic ileus. Agonist/antagonist analgesics (eg, pentazocine, nalbuphine, butorphanol) may reduce analgesic effect and/or precipitate withdrawal symptoms; use with caution. APAP: Increased risk of acute liver failure with alcohol; hepatotoxicity occurred in chronic alcoholics. Increase in glucuronidation and plasma clearance and decreased $T_{1/2}$ with oral contraceptives. Probenecid and propranolol may increase pharmacologic/therapeutic effects. May decrease effects of loop diuretics, lamotrigine, and zidovudine.

NURSING CONSIDERATIONS

Assessment: Assess for risks for opioid abuse, addiction, or misuse, patient's general condition and medical status, severity and type of pain, respiratory depression, bronchial asthma, COPD, cor pulmonale, hypercarbia, paralytic ileus, acute alcoholism, drug hypersensitivity, renal/hepatic impairment, pregnancy/nursing status, or any other conditions where treatment is contraindicated or cautioned, and possible drug interactions.

Monitoring: Monitor for development of addiction, abuse, or misuse, physical dependence, tolerance, acute liver failure, respiratory depression, altered consciousness, hypotension, convulsions, hypersensitivity/anaphylactic/serious skin reactions, decreased bowel motility in postoperative patients, spasm of the sphincter of Oddi, and other adverse reactions. Monitor serum amylase levels.

Patient Counseling: Inform that drug contains oxycodone, which is a morphine-like substance. Instruct to keep in a secure place out of reach of children or from theft; advise to seek emergency medical care immediately in case of accidental ingestions. Advise to destroy the unused tabs/oral sol by flushing down the toilet. Advise not to adjust dosing without consulting physician. Inform that drug may impair mental/physical abilities required to perform potentially hazardous tasks (eg, driving, operating heavy machinery). Instruct not to combine with alcohol, opioid analgesics, tranquilizers, sedatives, or other CNS depressants unless under recommendation and guidance of a physician. Inform that drug may cause dangerous additive CNS or respiratory depression if coadministered with another CNS depressant. Instruct to consult physician if pregnant, planning to become pregnant, or if breastfeeding. Advise not to adjust dose without consulting physician and not to abruptly d/c if on treatment for more than a few weeks. Advise to d/c and contact physician immediately if signs of allergy develop. Inform about signs of serious skin reactions. Instruct to look for APAP on package labels and not to use >1 APAP-containing product. Instruct to seek medical attention immediately upon ingestion of >4000mg/day of APAP, even if patient is feeling well.

Storage: 20-25°C (68-77°F). (Tab) Protect from moisture.

ROZEREM — ramelteon

RX

Class: Melatonin receptor agonist

ADULT DOSAGE

Insomnia

Difficulty w/ Sleep Onset:

Usual: 8mg within 30 min of hs

Max: 8mg/day

PEDIATRIC DOSAGE

Pediatric use may not have been established

ADMINISTRATION
Oral route
Do not take w/ or immediately after high-fat meal

HOW SUPPLIED
Tab: 8mg

CONTRAINDICATIONS
Coadministration with fluvoxamine.

WARNINGS/PRECAUTIONS
Angioedema reported; do not rechallenge if angioedema develops. Sleep disturbances may manifest as a physical and/or psychiatric disorder; symptomatic treatment of insomnia should be initiated only after careful evaluation. Failure of insomnia to remit after 7-10 days of therapy may indicate presence of psychiatric and/or medical illness. Cognitive and behavior changes, hallucinations, amnesia, anxiety, other neuropsychiatric symptoms, and complex behaviors reported; d/c if complex sleep behavior occurs. Worsening of depression reported in primarily depressed patients. May impair physical/mental abilities. May affect reproductive hormones (eg, decreased testosterone levels, increased prolactin levels). Not recommended with severe sleep apnea. Do not use with severe hepatic impairment. Caution with moderate hepatic impairment.

ADVERSE REACTIONS
Dizziness, somnolence, fatigue, nausea, exacerbated insomnia.

DRUG INTERACTIONS
See Contraindications. Decreased efficacy with strong CYP inducers (eg, rifampin). Caution with less strong CYP1A2 inhibitors, strong CYP3A4 inhibitors (eg, ketoconazole), and strong CYP2C9 inhibitors (eg, fluconazole). Increased levels with donepezil and doxepin; monitor patients closely. Increased T_{max} of zolpidem; avoid use. Increased risk of complex behaviors with alcohol and other CNS depressants. Additive effect with alcohol; avoid alcohol use.

NURSING CONSIDERATIONS

Assessment: Assess for hepatic impairment, manifestations of physical and/or psychiatric disorder, depression, sleep apnea, other comorbid diagnoses, hypersensitivity, pregnancy/nursing status, and possible drug interactions.

Monitoring: Monitor for signs/symptoms of angioedema, exacerbations of insomnia, emergence of cognitive or behavioral abnormalities, worsening of depression, complex sleep behaviors, and anaphylactic/anaphylactoid reactions.

Patient Counseling: Inform patients, families, and caregivers about benefits and risks associated with treatment. Counsel for appropriate use and instruct to read Medication Guide. Inform that severe anaphylactic and anaphylactoid reactions may occur; advise to seek immediate medical attention. Instruct to report sleep-driving to doctor immediately. Instruct to consult healthcare provider if cessation of menses, galactorrhea in females, decreased libido, or fertility problems occur. Instruct to take within 30 min prior to hs and confine activities to those necessary to prepare for bed. Instruct to swallow tab whole and to not break tab.

Storage: 25°C (77°F); excursions permitted to 15-30°C (59-86°F). Protect from moisture and humidity.

RYTARY — carbidopa/levodopa RX

Class: Dopa-decarboxylase inhibitor/dopamine precursor

ADULT DOSAGE

Parkinson's Disease

Levodopa Naive:
Initial: 23.75mg/95mg tid for the first 3 days. On the 4th day of treatment, may increase to 36.25mg/145mg tid
Titrate: May increase up to 97.5mg/390mg tid to 5X/day based on clinical response and tolerability
Max: (612.5mg/2450mg)/day

Parkinsonism

Postencephalitic Parkinsonism and Parkinsonism Following Carbon Monoxide/ Manganese Intoxication:
Levodopa Naive:
Initial: 23.75mg/95mg tid for the first 3 days. On the 4th day of treatment, may increase to 36.25mg/145mg tid

PEDIATRIC DOSAGE
Pediatric use may not have been established

Titrate: May increase up to 97.5mg/390mg tid to 5X/day based on clinical response and tolerability
Max: (612.5mg/2450mg)/day

Conversions

From Immediate Release Carbidopa-Levodopa:
Total Daily Dose of Levodopa in Immediate Release (IR) Combination:
400-549mg IR: Three 23.75mg/95mg cap tid
550-749mg IR: Four 23.75mg/95mg cap tid
750-949mg IR: Three 36.25mg/145mg cap tid
950-1249mg IR: Three 48.75mg/195mg cap tid
>1250mg IR: Four 48.7mg/195mg cap tid or three 61.25mg/245mg cap tid

DOSE MODIFICATION

Concomitant Medications

Currently Treated w/ Carbidopa and Levodopa Plus Catechol-O-Methyl Transferase Inhibitors:
Initial: May need to increase initial total daily dose of levodopa

Discontinuation

Avoid sudden discontinuation or rapid dose reduction; taper daily dose at time of treatment discontinuation

ADMINISTRATION

Oral route

Swallow whole w/ or w/o food
Do not chew, divide or crush cap
May administer by carefully opening cap and sprinkling entire contents on a small amount of applesauce (1-2 tbsp) and consuming immediately; do not store drug/food mixture for future use

HOW SUPPLIED

Cap, Extended-Release: (Carbidopa/Levodopa) 23.75mg/95mg, 36.25mg/145mg, 48.75mg/195mg, 61.25mg/245mg

CONTRAINDICATIONS

Patients who are currently taking a nonselective MAOI (eg, phenelzine, tranylcypromine) or have recently (within 2 weeks) taken a nonselective MAOI.

WARNINGS/PRECAUTIONS

A symptom complex resembling neuroleptic malignant syndrome (hyperpyrexia and confusion) reported in association with rapid dose reduction, withdrawal of, or changes in dopaminergic therapy; avoid sudden discontinuation/rapid dose reduction, or taper dose if discontinuing therapy. Cardiovascular ischemic events reported; monitor cardiac function in an intensive cardiac care facility during the period of initial dosage adjustment, in patients with a history of MI who have residual atrial, nodal, or ventricular arrhythmias. Increased risk for hallucinations and psychosis; do not use in patients with a major psychotic disorder. Intense urge to gamble, increased sexual urges, intense urges to spend money, binge eating, and/or other intense urges, and the inability to control these urges may occur; consider dose reduction or discontinuation if such urges develop. May cause dyskinesias; may require dose reduction of Rytary or other medications used for the treatment of Parkinson's disease. May increase the possibility of upper GI hemorrhage in patients with history of peptic ulcer. May cause increased intraocular pressure (IOP) in patients with glaucoma. Perform periodic skin examinations to monitor for melanoma. Levodopa: Falling asleep while engaged in activities of daily living and somnolence reported; consider discontinuation if significant daytime sleepiness or episodes of falling asleep during activities that require active participation occur. May impair mental/physical abilities.

ADVERSE REACTIONS

N/V, dizziness, headache, insomnia, abnormal dreams, dry mouth, dyskinesia, anxiety, constipation, orthostatic hypotension.

DRUG INTERACTIONS

See Contraindications. Selective MAO-B inhibitors (eg, rasagiline, selegiline) may be associated with orthostatic hypotension; monitor patients who are taking these drugs concurrently. Iron salts or multivitamins containing iron salts may form chelates and may cause a reduction in bioavailability; monitor patients for worsening Parkinson's symptoms. Levodopa: Caution with concomitant use of sedating medications; may increase the risk for somnolence. Dopamine D2 receptor antagonists (eg, phenothiazines, butyrophenones, risperidone, metoclopramide) and isoniazid may reduce the effectiveness of levodopa; monitor patients for worsening Parkinson's symptoms.

NURSING CONSIDERATIONS

Assessment: Assess for major psychotic disorder, glaucoma, risk factors that may increase risk for somnolence (eg, presence of sleep disorders), history of peptic ulcer, history of MI with residual atrial, nodal, or ventricular arrhythmias, pregnancy/nursing status, and possible drug interactions.

Monitoring: Monitor for hallucinations, psychosis, control/compulsive behaviors, dyskinesias, drowsiness/sleepiness, somnolence, upper GI hemorrhage in patients with a history of peptic ulcer, increased IOP in patients with glaucoma, and other adverse reactions. Monitor cardiac function in an intensive cardiac care facility during the initial dosage adjustment period in patients with a history of MI who have residual atrial, nodal, or ventricular arrhythmias. Monitor for hyperpyrexia and confusion if sudden discontinuation or rapid dose reduction occurs. Perform periodic skin examinations to monitor for melanoma.

Patient Counseling: Instruct to take ud. Instruct to call physician before stopping therapy and to call physician if withdrawal symptoms (eg, fever, confusion, severe muscle stiffness) develop. Advise that certain side effects (eg, sleepiness and dizziness) that have been reported may affect some patients' ability to drive and operate machinery safely. Inform that hallucinations may occur with levodopa products. Inform of the potential for experiencing intense urges to gamble, increased sexual urges, and other intense urges, and the inability to control these urges while on therapy. Instruct to notify physician if abnormal involuntary movements appear or get worse during treatment. Advise that may develop orthostatic hypotension with or without symptoms (eg, dizziness, nausea, syncope, sweating); advise to rise slowly after sitting or lying down, especially if patient has been doing so for a prolonged period. Advise of the possible additive sedative effects when taking other CNS depressants in combination with therapy. Instruct to notify physician if pregnant/breastfeeding an infant, or intend to breastfeed/become pregnant.

Storage: 25°C (77°F); excursions permitted to 15-30°C (59-86°F). Protect from light and moisture.

RYTHMOL SR — propafenone hydrochloride

RX

Class: Class IC antiarrhythmic

Increased rate of death or reversed cardiac arrest rate reported in patients treated with encainide or flecainide (Class 1C antiarrhythmics) in a study of patients with asymptomatic non-life-threatening ventricular arrhythmias who had a MI >6 days but <2 yrs previously. Consider any 1C antiarrhythmics to have significant proarrhythmic risk in patients with structural heart disease. Avoid in patients with non-life-threatening ventricular arrhythmias, even if experiencing unpleasant, but not life-threatening signs/symptoms.

ADULT DOSAGE

Atrial Fibrillation

In Patients w/ No Structural Heart Disease:

Initial: 225mg q12h

Titrate: May increase at a minimum of 5-day intervals to 325mg q12h. May increase to 425mg q12h if additional therapeutic effect is needed

PEDIATRIC DOSAGE

Pediatric use may not have been established

DOSE MODIFICATION

Hepatic Impairment

Reduce dose

Other Important Modifications

Significant QRS Widening/2nd- or 3rd-degree Atrioventricular Block: Reduce dose

ADMINISTRATION

Oral route

Take w/ or w/o food

Do not crush or further divide cap contents

HOW SUPPLIED

Cap, Extended-Release: 225mg, 325mg, 425mg

CONTRAINDICATIONS

Heart failure (HF), cardiogenic shock, known Brugada syndrome, bradycardia, marked hypotension, bronchospastic disorders or severe obstructive pulmonary disease, marked electrolyte imbalance, and sinoatrial, AV and intraventricular disorders of impulse generation or conduction (eg, sick sinus node syndrome, AV block) in the absence of an artificial pacemaker.

WARNINGS/PRECAUTIONS

Do not use to control ventricular rate during A-fib. Concomitant treatment with drugs that increase the functional AV nodal refractory period is recommended. May cause new or worsened arrhythmias;

evaluate ECG prior to and during therapy. Brugada syndrome may be unmasked after exposure to therapy; perform ECG after initiation of treatment and d/c if changes are suggestive of Brugada syndrome. May provoke overt HF. Proarrhythmic effects more likely occur in patients with HF or severe MI. Conduction disturbances (eg, 1st-degree AV block), agranulocytosis, positive antinuclear antibody (ANA) titers, and exacerbation of myasthenia gravis reported. D/C if persistent or worsening elevation of ANA titers detected. May alter pacing and sensing thresholds of implanted pacemakers and defibrillators; monitor and reprogram devices accordingly during and after therapy. Reversible, short-term drop (within normal range) in sperm count may occur. Caution with renal/hepatic dysfunction.

ADVERSE REACTIONS

Dizziness, palpitations, chest pain, dyspnea, taste disturbance, nausea, fatigue, anxiety, constipation, URTI, edema, influenza.

DRUG INTERACTIONS

Avoid with Class Ia and III antiarrhythmics (eg, quinidine, amiodarone) and withhold these agents for at least 5 half-lives prior to therapy. Inhibitors of CYP2D6 (eg, desipramine, paroxetine, ritonavir) and CYP3A4 (eg, ketoconazole, ritonavir, erythromycin, grapefruit juice) may increase levels; avoid simultaneous use with both a CYP2D6 and a CYP3A4 inhibitor. Amiodarone can affect conduction and repolarization; coadministration is not recommended. Fluoxetine may increase levels in extensive metabolizers. Rifampin may decrease levels and may increase norpropafenone (active metabolite) levels. May increase levels of digoxin, propranolol, metoprolol, and warfarin; monitor digoxin levels and INR. May result in severe adverse events (eg, convulsions, AV block, acute circulatory failure) with abrupt cessation of orlistat. May increase risk of CNS side effects of lidocaine. CYP1A2 inhibitors (eg, amiodarone, tobacco smoke) and cimetidine may increase levels.

NURSING CONSIDERATIONS

Assessment: Assess for HF, cardiogenic shock, sinoatrial/AV/intraventricular disorders, implanted pacemaker/defibrillator, bradycardia, marked hypotension, bronchospastic disorders or severe obstructive pulmonary disease, marked electrolyte imbalance, MI, renal/hepatic dysfunction, known Brugada syndrome, pregnancy/nursing status, and possible drug interactions. Evaluate ECG prior to therapy.

Monitoring: Monitor for proarrhythmic effects, signs/symptoms of conduction disturbances, agranulocytosis, HF, unmasking of Brugada syndrome, exacerbation of myasthenia gravis, and other adverse reactions. Monitor implanted pacemakers and defibrillators during and after therapy and reprogram accordingly. Evaluate ECG during therapy. Monitor ANA titers, LFTs, and renal/hepatic function.

Patient Counseling: Inform about risks/benefits of therapy. Advise to report symptoms that may be associated with electrolyte imbalance (eg, excessive/prolonged diarrhea, sweating, vomiting, loss of appetite, thirst). Inform to notify physician of all prescription, herbal/natural preparations, and OTC medications currently being taken or of any changes with these products. Instruct not to double the next dose if a dose is missed and to take next dose at the usual time.

Storage: 25°C (77°F); excursions permitted to 15-30°C (59-86°F).

SABRIL — vigabatrin **RX**

Class: GABA analogue

Causes permanent bilateral concentric visual field constriction; in some cases, treatment may also damage central retina and may decrease visual acuity. Onset of vision loss is unpredictable. Risk of vision loss increases with increasing dose and cumulative exposure, but there is no dose or exposure known to be free of risk of vision loss. Vision loss may not be recognized until it is severe. Unless a patient is formally exempted from periodic ophthalmologic assessment, vision should be assessed at baseline (no later than 4 weeks after starting therapy), at least every 3 months during therapy, and about 3-6 months after therapy is discontinued. Once detected, vision loss due to treatment is not reversible. Consider discontinuation, balancing benefit and risk, if visual loss is documented. Vision loss may worsen despite discontinuation of therapy. D/C in patients who fail to show clinical benefit within 2-4 weeks (infantile spasms) or 3 months (refractory complex partial seizures) of initiation, or sooner if treatment failure is obvious. Unless benefit clearly outweighs the risk, avoid use with other drugs associated with serious adverse ophthalmic effects (eg, retinopathy, glaucoma) and in patients with, or at high risk of, other types of irreversible vision loss. Use lowest dose and shortest exposure to treatment. Available only through a restricted program under a Risk Evaluation and Mitigation Strategy called the Support, Help And Resources for Epilepsy (SHARE) Program.

ADULT DOSAGE

Refractory Complex Partial Seizures

Adjunctive Therapy:
>16 Years:
Initial: 1000mg/day (500mg bid)
Titrate: May increase total daily dose in 500mg increments at weekly intervals depending on response
Usual: 3000mg/day (1500mg bid)

PEDIATRIC DOSAGE

Refractory Complex Partial Seizures

Adjunctive Therapy:
10-16 Years:
25-60kg:
Initial: 500mg/day (250mg bid)
Titrate: May increase weekly to a total maintenance dose of 2000mg/day (1000mg bid)

>60kg: Dose according to adult recommendations

Infantile Spasms

Monotherapy:

1 Month-2 Years:

Initial: 50mg/kg/day in 2 divided doses

Titrate: Subsequent dosing can be titrated by 25-50mg/kg/day increments every 3 days

Max: 150mg/kg/day in 2 divided doses

DOSE MODIFICATION

Renal Impairment

Adults and Pediatric Patients ≥10 Years:

Mild (CrCl >50-80mL/min): Decrease dose by 25%

Moderate (CrCl >30-50mL/min): Decrease dose by 50%

Severe (CrCl >10-30mL/min): Decrease dose by 75%

Discontinuation

Reduce dose gradually to d/c

ADMINISTRATION

Oral route

Take w/ or w/o food

Either tab or powder for oral sol can be used for complex partial seizures

Use powder for oral sol for infantile spasms; do not use tabs

Preparation/Administration of Oral Sol

Mix powder for oral sol w/ water prior to administration

Empty entire contents of each pkt into a clean cup, and dissolve in 10mL of cold or room temperature water per pkt

Administer the resulting sol using the 10mL oral syringe supplied w/ medication

The concentration of the final sol is 50mg/mL

Each individual dose should be prepared and used immediately; discard any unused portion of sol

HOW SUPPLIED

Sol: 500mg/pkt [50^s]; Tab: 500mg* *scored

WARNINGS/PRECAUTIONS

Not indicated as a 1st line agent for complex partial seizures. Abnormal magnetic resonance imaging (MRI) signal changes involving the thalamus, basal ganglia, brain stem, and cerebellum observed in some infants. May increase risk of suicidal thoughts/behavior. May cause anemia, somnolence, fatigue, peripheral neuropathy, weight gain, and edema. Should be withdrawn gradually. May impair physical/mental abilities. May decrease ALT and AST plasma activity and may preclude the use of these markers, especially ALT, to detect early hepatic injury. May increase amount of amino acids in the urine, possibly leading to false (+) test for certain rare genetic metabolic diseases (eg, alpha aminoadipic aciduria). Caution with renal impairment and in elderly.

ADVERSE REACTIONS

Vision loss, vomiting, upper respiratory tract infection, rash, somnolence, irritability, diarrhea, fever, influenza, headache, fatigue, dizziness, convulsion, nasopharyngitis, weight increased.

DRUG INTERACTIONS

See Boxed Warning. May decrease phenytoin plasma levels; consider dose adjustment of phenytoin if clinically indicated. May increase C_{max} of clonazepam resulting in an increase of clonazepam-associated adverse reactions.

NURSING CONSIDERATIONS

Assessment: Assess for renal impairment, underlying suicidal behavior/ideation, pregnancy/nursing status, and possible drug interactions. Perform baseline vision assessment (no later than 4 weeks after starting therapy).

Monitoring: Monitor for abnormal MRI signal changes, suicidal thoughts/behavior, emergence/worsening of depression, unusual changes in thoughts or behavior, anemia, somnolence, fatigue, peripheral neuropathy, weight gain, edema, and other adverse reactions. Perform vision assessment at least every 3 months during therapy and about 3-6 months after discontinuation of therapy. Periodically reassess response to and continued need for treatment.

Patient Counseling: Inform of the risk of permanent vision loss, particularly loss of peripheral vision, and the need for vision monitoring. Instruct to notify physician if changes in vision are suspected. Inform caregiver(s) of the possibility that infants may develop an abnormal MRI signal of unknown clinical significance. Counsel that therapy may increase risk of suicidal thoughts and behavior; advise of the need to be alert for the emergence or worsening of symptoms of depression, any unusual changes in mood or behavior, or the emergence of suicidal thoughts, behavior, or thoughts of self-harm. Instruct to report immediately to physician behaviors of concern. Instruct to notify physician if pregnant, intending to become pregnant during therapy, or if breastfeeding or intending to breastfeed during therapy; encourage to enroll in the North American Antiepileptic Drug (NAAED) Pregnancy Registry if pregnant. Advise not to drive a car or operate other complex machinery until familiar with the effects of therapy on ability to perform such activities. Instruct not to abruptly d/c therapy.

Storage: 20-25°C (68-77°F).

SANCTURA XR – trospium chloride RX

Class: Muscarinic antagonist

OTHER BRAND NAMES
Sanctura

ADULT DOSAGE

Overactive Bladder

Tab:
Usual: 20mg bid w/ water on an empty stomach, at least 1 hr before a meal

Cap, Extended Release:
60mg qam w/ water on an empty stomach, at least 1 hr before a meal

PEDIATRIC DOSAGE
Pediatric use may not have been established

DOSE MODIFICATION
Renal Impairment
CrCl <30mL/min:
Tab: 20mg qd hs
Cap, Extended-Release: Not recommended
Elderly
Tab:
≥75 Years: May be titrated down to 20mg qd

ADMINISTRATION
Oral route

HOW SUPPLIED
Cap, Extended-Release: 60mg; Tab: 20mg

CONTRAINDICATIONS
Urinary retention, gastric retention, uncontrolled narrow-angle glaucoma.

WARNINGS/PRECAUTIONS
Angioedema reported; d/c if the tongue, hypopharynx, or larynx is involved. Caution with clinically significant bladder outflow obstruction, GI obstructive disorders, moderate and severe hepatic impairment, and patients treated for controlled narrow-angle glaucoma. May decrease GI motility; caution with ulcerative colitis, intestinal atony, and myasthenia gravis. Associated with anticholinergic CNS effects; consider dose reduction or d/c if effects occur. (Cap) Not recommended with severe renal impairment (CrCl <30mL/min). Alcohol should not be consumed within 2 hrs of administration.

ADVERSE REACTIONS
Dry mouth, constipation, urinary tract infection. (Tab) Headache.

DRUG INTERACTIONS
May increase frequency and/or severity of dry mouth, constipation, and other anticholinergic pharmacologic effects with other antimuscarinic agents. May potentially alter the absorption of some concomitantly administered drugs due to effects on GI motility. May interact with other drugs that are eliminated by active tubular secretion (eg, procainamide, pancuronium, morphine, vancomycin, tenofovir). May enhance drowsiness with alcohol. Reduced levels with metformin. (Cap) Antacids containing aluminum hydroxide and magnesium carbonate may alter exposure.

NURSING CONSIDERATIONS

Assessment: Assess for drug hypersensitivity, other conditions where treatment is contraindicated or cautioned, hepatic/renal impairment, pregnancy/nursing status, and for possible drug interactions.

Monitoring: Monitor for angioedema, anticholinergic CNS effects, urinary retention, gastric retention, and decreased GI motility. Monitor renal/hepatic function.

Patient Counseling: Inform that angioedema may occur and could result in life-threatening airway obstruction; instruct to d/c and seek medical attention if edema of the tongue/laryngopharynx or difficulty breathing occurs. Inform about the most common side effects (eg, dry mouth, constipation) and less common side effects (eg, trouble emptying the bladder, blurred vision, heat prostration). Advise not to drive or operate heavy machinery until patient knows how the drug affects him or her. Advise that alcohol may enhance drowsiness. (Cap) Advise that use of alcoholic beverages within 2 hrs of dosing is not recommended.

Storage: 20-25°C (68-77°F); (Cap) excursions permitted between 15-30°C (59-86°F).

SANDIMMUNE — cyclosporine

RX

Class: Cyclic polypeptide immunosuppressant

Should only be prescribed by physicians experienced in immunosuppressive therapy and management of organ transplant patients. Manage patients in facilities equipped and staffed w/ adequate laboratory and supportive medical resources. Give w/ adrenal corticosteroids but not w/ other immunosuppressive agents. Increased susceptibility to infection and development of lymphoma may result from immunosuppression. Not bioequivalent to Neoral; not interchangeable w/o physician supervision. Monitor cyclosporine blood concentrations at repeated intervals during chronic administration of sol/cap; adjust subsequent dose to avoid toxicity due to high levels and possible organ rejection due to low absorption.

ADULT DOSAGE

Organ Rejection Prophylaxis

Kidney, Liver, and Heart Allogeneic Transplants:

Oral:

Initial: 15mg/kg single dose given 4-12 hrs prior to transplant

Continue postoperatively for 1-2 weeks, then taper by 5%/week to a maintenance dose of 5-10mg/kg/day

IV:

For patients unable to take caps or oral sol pre- or postoperatively

Administer at 1/3 the oral dose

Initial: 5-6mg/kg/day single dose given 4-12 hrs prior to transplant

Continue postoperatively until the patient can tolerate caps or oral sol; patients should be switched to caps or oral sol as soon as possible after surgery

Adjunct therapy w/ adrenal corticosteroids is recommended

Other Indications

Treatment of chronic rejection in patients previously treated w/ other immunosuppressive agents

PEDIATRIC DOSAGE

Organ Rejection Prophylaxis

Kidney, Liver, and Heart Allogeneic Transplants:

≥6 Months of Age:

Oral:

Initial: 15mg/kg single dose given 4-12 hrs prior to transplant

Continue postoperatively for 1-2 weeks, then taper by 5%/week to a maintenance dose of 5-10mg/kg/day

Higher doses may be required in pediatric patients

IV:

For patients unable to take caps or oral sol pre- or postoperatively

Administer at 1/3 the oral dose

Initial: 5-6mg/kg/day single dose given 4-12 hrs prior to transplant

Continue postoperatively until the patient can tolerate caps or oral sol; patients should be switched to caps or oral sol as soon as possible after surgery

Higher doses may be required in pediatric patients

Adjunct therapy w/ adrenal corticosteroids is recommended

Other Indications

Treatment of chronic rejection in patients previously treated w/ other immunosuppressive agents

DOSE MODIFICATION

Renal Impairment

Reduce dose if indicated

Hepatic Impairment

Severe: Dose reduction may be necessary

Elderly

Start at lower end of dosing range

ADMINISTRATION

Oral/IV route

Cap/Sol

Administer on a consistent schedule w/ regard to time of day and relation to meals

Sol
May dilute w/ milk, chocolate milk, or orange juice preferably at room temperature; avoid switching diluents frequently
Once opened, use contents w/in 2 months

Instructions:
1. Take the prescribed amount of cyclosporine from the container using the dosage syringe supplied, and transfer the sol to a glass of milk, chocolate milk, or orange juice
2. Stir well and drink at once; do not allow to stand before drinking
3. It is best to use a glass container and rinse it w/ more diluent to ensure that the total dose is taken
4. After use, replace dosage syringe in the protective cover
5. Do not rinse the dosage syringe w/ water or other cleaning agents either before or after use; if the dosage syringe requires cleaning, it must be completely dry before resuming use
6. Introduction of water into the product by any means will cause variation in dose

Inj
Immediately before use, dilute 1mL cyclosporine inj in 20-100mL 0.9% NaCl inj or D5 inj
Administer in a slow IV infusion over approx 2-6 hrs
Discard diluted infusion sol after 24 hrs
The polyoxyethylated castor oil contained in the concentrate for IV infusion can cause phthalate stripping from PVC

HOW SUPPLIED
Cap: 25mg, 100mg; Inj: 50mg/mL [5mL]; Sol: 100mg/mL [50mL]

CONTRAINDICATIONS
(Inj) Hypersensitivity to polyoxyethylated castor oil.

WARNINGS/PRECAUTIONS
Due to risk of anaphylaxis, only use inj if unable to take cap/sol. May cause nephrotoxicity, hepatotoxicity, and liver injury (eg, cholestasis, jaundice, hepatitis, liver failure). Elevations in SrCr and BUN levels do not necessarily indicate rejection in renal transplant patients; evaluate patient before initiating dose adjustment. Impaired renal function at any time requires close monitoring, and frequent dose adjustment may be indicated. Consider switching to other immunosuppressive therapy w/ persistent high elevations of BUN/SrCr unresponsive to dosage adjustments. Convulsions, encephalopathy (including posterior reversible encephalopathy syndrome), and rarely, optic disc edema reported. Thrombocytopenia and microangiopathic hemolytic anemia, resulting in graft failure, hyperuricemia, and hyperkalemia (sometimes associated w/ hyperchloremic metabolic acidosis) may develop. Increased risk for development of lymphomas and other malignancies. Consider the alcohol content of the drug when given to patients in whom alcohol intake should be avoided or minimized (eg, pregnant or breastfeeding women, patients presenting w/ liver disease or epilepsy, alcoholic patients, or pediatric patients). Caution w/ malabsorption. HTN may occur requiring antihypertensive therapy. Increased risk of developing bacterial, viral, fungal, protozoal, and opportunistic infections (eg, polyoma virus infections). JC virus-associated progressive multifocal leukoencephalopathy (PML) and polyoma virus-associated nephropathy (PVAN) reported; consider reduction in immunosuppression if evidence of PML or PVAN develops. (Inj) Contains polyoxyethylated castor oil. Anaphylactic reactions reported rarely w/ IV administration; observe for 30 min after start of infusion and frequently thereafter. D/C infusion if anaphylaxis occurs.

ADVERSE REACTIONS
Increased susceptibility to infection, lymphoma, renal dysfunction, tremor, hirsutism, HTN, gum hyperplasia, headache, diarrhea, hepatotoxicity, convulsions, abdominal discomfort, flushing, N/V, sinusitis.

DRUG INTERACTIONS
See Boxed Warning. Avoid w/ K^+-sparing diuretics, compounds that decrease drug absorption (eg, orlistat), aliskiren, grapefruit, grapefruit juice, bosentan, or dabigatran. Avoid in psoriasis patients receiving other immunosuppressive agents or radiation therapy (including PUVA and UVB). Vaccination may be less effective; avoid live vaccines during therapy. Caution w/ rifabutin, nephrotoxic drugs, HIV protease inhibitors (eg, indinavir, nelfinavir, ritonavir, saquinavir), K^+-sparing drugs (eg, ACE inhibitors, ARBs), K^+-containing drugs, and K^+-rich diet. Ciprofloxacin, gentamicin, tobramycin, vancomycin, trimethoprim w/ sulfamethoxazole, amphotericin B, ketoconazole, melphalan, diclofenac, azapropazon, sulindac, naproxen, colchicine, cimetidine, ranitidine, tacrolimus, fibric acid derivatives (eg, bezafibrate, fenofibrate), methotrexate (MTX), and NSAIDs may potentiate renal dysfunction; closely monitor renal function and reduce dose of cyclosporine and/or coadministered drug or consider alternative treatment. CYP3A4 or P-gp inhibitors/inducers may alter levels; adjust cyclosporine dose appropriately. Diltiazem, nicardipine, verapamil, fluconazole, itraconazole, ketoconazole, voriconazole, azithromycin, clarithromycin, erythromycin, quinupristin/dalfopristin, allopurinol, amiodarone, bromocriptine, colchicine, danazol, imatinib, nefazodone, metoclopramide, oral contraceptives, methylprednisolone, grapefruit, grapefruit juice, HIV protease inhibitors, boceprevir, and telaprevir may increase levels. St. John's wort, carbamazepine, oxcarbazepine, phenobarbital, phenytoin, bosentan, sulfinpyrazone, octreotide,

orlistat, terbinafine, ticlopidine, rifampin, and nafcillin may decrease levels. May increase plasma concentration of CYP3A4, P-gp, or organic anion transporter protein substrates. May reduce clearance of digoxin, colchicine, prednisolone, HMG-CoA reductase inhibitors (statins), aliskiren, bosentan, dabigatran, repaglinide, NSAIDs, sirolimus, and etoposide. Digitalis toxicity reported when used w/ digoxin; monitor digoxin levels. May increase levels and enhance toxic effects (eg, myopathy, neuropathy) of colchicine; reduce colchicine dose. Myotoxicity cases seen lovastatin, simvastatin, atorvastatin, pravastatin, and rarely fluvastatin; temporarily withhold or d/c statin if signs of myopathy develop or w/ risk factors predisposing to severe renal injury. May increase levels of repaglinide and thereby, increasing the risk of hypoglycemia; closely monitor blood glucose levels. May increase levels of ambrisentan; do not titrate ambrisentan dose to the recommended max daily dose. May increase levels of bosentan or dabigatran. High doses of cyclosporine may increase the exposure to anthracycline antibiotics (eg, doxorubicin, mitoxantrone, daunorubicin) in cancer patients. Frequent gingival hyperplasia w/ nifedipine; avoid concomitant use w/ nifedipine in patients in whom gingival hyperplasia develops as a side effect of cyclosporine. Convulsions reported w/ high-dose methylprednisolone. Concomitant use of high-dose corticosteroids may predispose to developing encephalopathy. Increases levels of sirolimus w/ elevations of SrCr; give 4 hrs after cyclosporine. May double diclofenac blood levels. May increase levels of MTX and decrease levels of MTX metabolite. Dose adjustment may be required w/ calcium antagonists; use w/ caution.

NURSING CONSIDERATIONS

Assessment: Prior to IV administration, assess ability to take oral formulations. Assess for hypersensitivity to the drug or to polyoxyethylated castor oil, malabsorption, pregnancy/nursing status, and possible drug interactions. Obtain baseline SrCr, BUN, LFTs, and serum bilirubin.

Monitoring: Continuously monitor patients receiving IV formulation for anaphylactic reactions for at least the first 30 min following start of infusion and at frequent intervals thereafter. Monitor for signs/symptoms of hepatotoxicity, nephrotoxicity, thrombocytopenia, microangiopathic hemolytic anemia, HTN, hyperkalemia, hyperuricemia, lymphomas and other malignancies, serious/opportunistic/polyoma virus infections, convulsions and other neurotoxicities, and other adverse reactions. Frequently monitor cyclosporine blood levels, especially when converting from Neoral to Sandimmune. Monitor renal/hepatic function (eg, BUN, SrCr, serum bilirubin, LFTs).

Patient Counseling: Instruct to contact physician before changing formulations of cyclosporine. Inform that repeated laboratory tests are required while on therapy. Advise of the potential risks if used during pregnancy and inform of the increased risk of neoplasia. Instruct patients using the oral syringe not to rinse before or after use as the introduction of water will cause variation in dosage.

Storage: Cap: 25°C (77°F); excursions permitted to 15-30°C (59-86°F). Sol: <30°C (86°F). Do not refrigerate. Protect from freezing. Inj: <30°C (86°F). Protect from light.

SANDOSTATIN LAR – octreotide acetate RX

Class: Somatostatin analogue

ADULT DOSAGE

Acromegaly

Long-Term Maint Therapy in Patients Who Have Had an Inadequate Response to Surgery and/or Radiotherapy, or if Surgery and/or Radiotherapy is Not an Option:

Not Currently Receiving Octreotide:
Begin therapy w/ Sandostatin SQ (initial dose of 50mcg tid; most patients require doses of 100-200mcg tid but some patients require up to 500mcg tid) and maintain for at least 2 weeks to determine tolerance

Patients considered to be responders to the drug and who tolerate it may be switched to Sandostatin LAR

Currently Receiving Sandostatin Inj:
Initial: 20mg at 4-week intervals for 3 months

Titrate:
Growth Hormone (GH) ≤2.5ng/mL, Normal Insulin-Like Growth Factor-1 (IGF-1), and Controlled Clinical Symptoms: Maintain at 20mg every 4 weeks

PEDIATRIC DOSAGE

Pediatric use may not have been established

GH >2.5ng/mL, Elevated IGF-1, and/or Uncontrolled Clinical Symptoms: Increase to 30mg every 4 weeks
GH ≤1ng/mL, Normal IGF-1, and Controlled Clinical Symptoms: Reduce to 10mg every 4 weeks
GH, IGF-1, or Symptoms are not Adequately Controlled at 30mg: May increase to 40mg every 4 weeks

Max: 40mg every 4 weeks

In patients who have received pituitary irradiation, withdraw therapy yearly for 8 weeks to assess disease activity; may resume therapy if GH or IGF-1 levels increase and signs/symptoms recur

Carcinoid Tumors

Long-Term Treatment of Severe Diarrhea and Flushing Episodes Associated w/ Metastatic Carcinoid Tumors:

Not Currently Receiving Octreotide:
Begin therapy w/ Sandostatin SQ (100-600mcg/day in 2-4 divided doses; some patients may require doses up to 1500mcg/day) and maintain for at least 2 weeks to determine tolerance

Patients considered to be responders to the drug and who tolerate it may be switched to Sandostatin LAR

Currently Receiving Sandostatin Inj:
Initial: 20mg at 4-week intervals for 2 months; patients should continue to receive Sandostatin SQ for at least 2 weeks in the same dosage taken before the switch

Titrate:
If Symptoms are Adequately Controlled: Consider reducing to 10mg for a trial period; if symptoms recur, then increase to 20mg every 4 weeks
If Symptoms are Not Adequately Controlled: Increase to 30mg every 4 weeks; lower to 10mg for a trial period if good control is achieved on 20mg dose and if symptoms recur, increase to 20mg every 4 weeks

Max: 30mg every 4 weeks

For exacerbation of symptoms, may give Sandostatin SQ for a few days at the dosage received prior to switching to Sandostatin LAR; d/c when symptoms are again controlled

Vasoactive Intestinal Peptide-Secreting Tumors

Long-Term Treatment of Profuse Watery Diarrhea Associated W/ Vasoactive Intestinal Peptide-Secreting Tumors:

Not Currently Receiving Octreotide:
Begin therapy w/ Sandostatin SQ (200-300mcg in 2-4 divided doses [range 150-750mcg]; doses >450mcg/day are usually not required) and maintain for at least 2 weeks to determine tolerance

Patients considered to be responders to the drug and who tolerate it may be switched to Sandostatin LAR

Currently Receiving Sandostatin Inj:
Initial: 20mg at 4-week intervals for 2 months; patients should continue to receive

Sandostatin SQ for at least 2 weeks in the same dosage taken before the switch
Titrate:
If Symptoms are Adequately Controlled:
Consider reducing to 10mg for a trial period; if symptoms recur, then increase to 20mg every 4 weeks
If Symptoms are Not Adequately Controlled:
Increase to 30mg every 4 weeks; lower to 10mg for a trial period if good control is achieved on 20mg dose and if symptoms recur, increase to 20mg every 4 weeks

Max: 30mg every 4 weeks

For exacerbation of symptoms, may give Sandostatin SQ for a few days at the dosage received prior to switching to Sandostatin LAR; d/c when symptoms are again controlled

DOSE MODIFICATION
Renal Impairment
Renal Failure Requiring Dialysis:
Initial: 10mg every 4 weeks

Hepatic Impairment
Cirrhotic Patients:
Initial: 10mg every 4 weeks

Elderly
Start at lower end of dosing range

ADMINISTRATION
IM route

Administer in the gluteal region; avoid deltoid inj
Rotate inj sites to avoid irritation
Administer immediately after reconstitution; do not directly inject diluent w/o preparing sus
Refer to PI for further administration instructions

HOW SUPPLIED
Inj, Depot: 10mg, 20mg, 30mg

WARNINGS/PRECAUTIONS
Should be administered by a trained healthcare provider. Rotate inj sites in a systematic manner to avoid irritation. May inhibit gallbladder contractility and decrease bile secretion, which may lead to gallbladder abnormalities or sludge. Alters balance between the counter-regulatory hormones, insulin, glucagon, and GH, which may result in hypo/hyperglycemia. Hypothyroidism may occur. Bradycardia, arrhythmias, and cardiac conduction abnormalities reported. May alter dietary fat absorption. Depressed vitamin B12 levels and abnormal Schilling test reported. Serum zinc may rise excessively when fluid loss is reversed in patients on TPN. Caution in elderly.

ADVERSE REACTIONS
Diarrhea, N/V, abdominal pain, flatulence, constipation, inj-site pain, influenza-like symptoms, fatigue, dizziness, headache, cholelithiasis, back pain, anemia, URTI.

DRUG INTERACTIONS
Associated with nutrient absorption alterations; may alter absorption of orally administered drugs. May decrease cyclosporine levels and result in transplant rejection. May need dose adjustments of insulin, oral hypoglycemics, and drugs with bradycardic effects (eg, β-blockers). Increases availability of bromocriptine. May decrease metabolic clearance of drugs metabolized by CYP450; caution with other drugs mainly metabolized by CYP3A4 and which have a low therapeutic index (eg, quinidine, terfenadine).

NURSING CONSIDERATIONS

Assessment: Assess for renal/hepatic impairment, cardiac dysfunction, pregnancy/nursing status, and possible drug interactions. Obtain baseline thyroid function tests (TSH, total and/or free T4). Obtain baseline plasma vasoactive intestinal peptide levels with VIPoma.

Monitoring: Monitor for signs/symptoms of gallbladder abnormalities or sludge, hypo/hyperglycemia, hypothyroidism, bradycardia, arrhythmia, cardiac conduction abnormalities, and other adverse reactions. Monitor zinc levels if receiving TPN. Monitor vitamin B12 levels. Monitor thyroid function periodically during chronic therapy. Monitor GH and IGF-1 levels with acromegaly. Monitor urinary 5-hydroxyindole acetic acid, plasma serotonin, and plasma substance P levels with carcinoids.

Patient Counseling: Inform of the risks and benefits of treatment. Advise patients with carcinoid tumors and VIPomas to adhere closely to scheduled return visits for reinjection to minimize exacerbation of symptoms. Instruct patients with acromegaly to adhere to return visit schedule to help assure steady control of GH and IGF-1 levels.

Storage: 2-8°C (36-46°F). Protect from light until time of use. Drug product kit should remain at room temperature for 30-60 min prior to preparation of drug sus.

SAPHRIS – asenapine

RX

Class: Atypical antipsychotic

Elderly patients with dementia-related psychosis treated with antipsychotic drugs are at an increased risk of death. Not approved for treatment of dementia-related psychosis.

ADULT DOSAGE

Schizophrenia

Acute Treatment:
Initial/Usual: 5mg bid
Max: 10mg bid

Maint Treatment:
Initial: 5mg bid
Titrate: May increase to 10mg bid after 1 week
Max: 10mg bid

Bipolar I Disorder

Acute Treatment of Manic or Mixed Episodes Associated w/ Bipolar I Disorder:

Monotherapy:
Initial/Usual: 10mg bid; may decrease to 5mg bid if warranted by adverse effects or based on individual tolerability
Max: 10mg bid

Adjunctive Therapy (w/ Lithium or Valproate):
Initial: 5mg bid
Titrate: May increase to 10mg bid
Max: 10mg bid

Continue treatment beyond acute response in responding patients

Conversions

Switching from Other Antipsychotics:
Minimize period of overlapping antipsychotics

PEDIATRIC DOSAGE

Pediatric use may not have been established

DOSE MODIFICATION

Hepatic Impairment
Severe (Child-Pugh C): Not recommended

ADMINISTRATION

SL route

Place tab under tongue and allow to dissolve completely
Do not split, crush, chew, or swallow
Do not eat/drink for 10 min after administration

HOW SUPPLIED

Tab, SL: 5mg, 10mg

WARNINGS/PRECAUTIONS

Neuroleptic malignant syndrome (NMS) reported; d/c therapy and institute symptomatic treatment. May cause tardive dyskinesia (TD), especially in the elderly; consider discontinuation of therapy if this occurs. Associated with metabolic changes (eg, hyperglycemia sometimes associated with ketoacidosis or hyperosmolar coma, dyslipidemia, weight gain) that may increase cardiovascular (CV) and cerebrovascular risk. Hypersensitivity reactions reported usually after the 1st dose. May induce orthostatic hypotension and syncope; consider dose reduction if hypotension occurs. Caution with known CV disease, cerebrovascular disease, or conditions that predispose to hypotension. Leukopenia, neutropenia, and agranulocytosis may occur; monitor CBC frequently during 1st few months in patients with preexisting low WBCs or history of drug-induced leukopenia/

neutropenia, and d/c at 1st sign of decline in WBCs without causative factors. D/C therapy and follow WBC count until recovery in patients with severe neutropenia (ANC <1000/mm^3). May prolong QTc interval; avoid use with history of cardiac arrhythmias or in circumstances that may increase risk of torsades de pointes. May elevate prolactin levels. Seizures and somnolence reported. May impair mental/physical abilities. May disrupt body's ability to reduce core body temperature. Caution with those at risk for suicide and in elderly patients. May cause esophageal dysmotility and aspiration; avoid in patients at risk for aspiration pneumonia.

ADVERSE REACTIONS

Somnolence, insomnia, headache, dizziness, extrapyramidal symptoms, akathisia, vomiting, oral hypoesthesia, constipation, weight increase, fatigue, increased appetite, anxiety, arthralgia, dyspepsia.

DRUG INTERACTIONS

Avoid use with other drugs known to prolong QTc, including Class 1A antiarrhythmics (eg, quinidine, procainamide), Class 3 antiarrhythmics (eg, amiodarone, sotalol), antipsychotics (eg, ziprasidone, chlorpromazine, thioridazine), and antibiotics (eg, gatifloxacin, moxifloxacin). Caution with other centrally acting drugs, alcohol, CYP2D6 substrates/inhibitors, drugs that can induce hypotension/bradycardia/respiratory or CNS depression, and drugs with anticholinergic activity. May enhance effects of certain antihypertensive agents. Fluvoxamine may increase levels; use with caution. Imipramine may increase levels. Paroxetine, cimetidine, and carbamazepine may decrease levels. May enhance inhibitory effects of paroxetine on its own metabolism.

NURSING CONSIDERATIONS

Assessment: Assess for dementia-related psychosis, history of cardiac arrhythmias, factors that may increase risk of torsades de pointes, risk for aspiration pneumonia, hepatic impairment, known hypersensitivity to the drug, history of seizures/conditions that lower seizure threshold, any other conditions where treatment is contraindicated or cautioned, pregnancy/nursing status, and possible drug interactions. Obtain baseline FPG in patients with diabetes mellitus (DM) or at risk for DM. Obtain baseline CBC if at risk for leukopenia/neutropenia.

Monitoring: Monitor for QT prolongation, NMS, TD, hyperglycemia, orthostatic hypotension, seizures, esophageal dysmotility, aspiration, suicidal ideation, hypersensitivity reactions, metabolic changes, and other adverse reactions. Monitor CBC frequently in patients with preexisting low WBC or history of drug-induced leukopenia/neutropenia. Monitor for fever or other signs/symptoms of infection in patients with neutropenia. Monitor hepatic function. Monitor worsening of glucose control in patients with DM or FPG in patients at risk for DM. Reassess periodically to determine need for maintenance treatment.

Patient Counseling: Inform of the risks/benefits and appropriate administration instructions of therapy. Inform of the signs/symptoms of serious allergic reaction; instruct to seek immediate medical attention if these develop. Inform that application-site reactions, including oral ulcers, blisters, peeling/sloughing, and inflammation, have been reported; instruct to monitor for these reactions. Inform about risk of developing NMS and counsel about its signs and symptoms. Counsel about the risk of metabolic changes and the need for specific monitoring. Inform of the need to monitor blood glucose in patients with DM or with risk factors for DM. Advise that weight should be monitor regularly. Inform about risk of developing orthostatic hypotension. Advise patients with preexisting low WBC counts or history of drug-induced leukopenia/neutropenia to have their CBC monitored. Caution about performing activities requiring mental alertness. Instruct regarding appropriate care in avoiding overheating or dehydration. Advise to notify physician if taking/planning to take any prescription or OTC medications, or if pregnant/intending to become pregnant during therapy. Instruct to avoid breastfeeding and alcohol use while on therapy.

Storage: 15-30°C (59-86°F).

SAVAYSA – edoxaban

RX

Class: Selective factor Xa inhibitor

Reduced efficacy reported in nonvalvular A-fib patients (NVAF) w/ CrCl >95 mL/min; should not be used in NVAF patients w/ CrCl >95mL/min; use another anticoagulant. Increased risk of ischemic events w/ premature discontinuation of any oral anticoagulant in the absence of adequate alternative anticoagulation; consider coverage w/ another anticoagulant if therapy is discontinued for a reason other than pathological bleeding or completion of a course of therapy. Epidural or spinal hematomas may occur in patients treated w/ edoxaban who are receiving neuraxial anesthesia or undergoing spinal puncture; hematomas may result in long-term or permanent paralysis. Increased risk of developing epidural or spinal hematomas in patients using indwelling epidural catheters, concomitant use of other drugs that affect hemostasis (eg, NSAIDs, platelet inhibitors, other anticoagulants), history of traumatic or repeated epidural or spinal punctures, history of spinal deformity or spinal surgery, or unknown optimal timing between the administration of edoxaban and neuraxial procedures. Monitor frequently for signs/symptoms of neurologic impairment; if neurologic compromise noted, urgent treatment is necessary. Consider benefits and risks before neuraxial intervention in patients anticoagulated or to be anticoagulated.

ADULT DOSAGE

Reduce Risk of Stroke and Systemic Embolism in Nonvalvular Atrial Fibrillation

Usual: 60mg qd

Deep Vein Thrombosis/Pulmonary Embolism

Treatment:
Usual: 60mg qd following 5-10 days of initial therapy w/ a parenteral anticoagulant

Conversions

Transition to Edoxaban:
From Warfarin/Other Vitamin K Antagonists: D/C warfarin and start edoxaban when INR ≤2.5
From Oral Anticoagulants Other Than Warfarin/Other Vitamin K Antagonists: D/C current oral anticoagulant and start edoxaban at the time of next scheduled dose of the other oral anticoagulant
From Low Molecular Weight Heparin (LMWH): D/C LMWH and start edoxaban at the time of next schedule administration of LMWH
From Unfractionated Heparin: D/C infusion and start edoxaban 4 hrs later

Transition from Edoxaban:
To Warfarin:
Oral Option: For patients taking 60mg, reduce dose to 30mg and begin warfarin concomitantly. For patients taking 30mg, reduce dose to 15mg and begin warfarin concomitantly. INR must be measured at least weekly and just prior to the daily dose of edoxaban to minimize the influence of edoxaban on INR measurements.
D/C edoxaban and continue warfarin once a stable INR ≥2 is achieved
Parenteral Option: D/C and administer a parenteral anticoagulant and warfarin at the time of next scheduled edoxaban dose. Once a stable INR ≥2.0 is achieved, d/c parenteral anticoagulant and continue warfarin
To Non-Vitamin-K Dependent Oral Anticoagulants or Parenteral Anticoagulants: D/C edoxaban and start other PO/parenteral anticoagulant at the time the next dose of edoxaban

PEDIATRIC DOSAGE

Pediatric use may not have been established

DOSE MODIFICATION

Concomitant Medications
DVT and PE:
Certain P-gp Inhibitors: 30mg qd

Renal Impairment
Nonvalvular A-Fib:
CrCl >95mL/min: Do not use
CrCl 15-50mL/min: 30mg qd

DVT and PE:
CrCl 15-50mL/min: 30mg qd

Discontinuation
D/C at least 24 hrs before invasive/surgical procedure. May restart edoxaban after the procedure as soon as adequate hemostasis has been established noting that the time to onset of pharmacodynamic effect is 1-2 hrs. Administer a parenteral anticoagulant and then switch to edoxaban if oral medication cannot be taken during/after surgical intervention

Other Important Modifications
DVT and PE:
≤60kg: 30mg qd

ADMINISTRATION
Oral route

May take w/o regard to food

HOW SUPPLIED
Tab: 15mg, 30mg, 60mg

CONTRAINDICATIONS
Active pathological bleeding.

WARNINGS/PRECAUTIONS
Increases risk of bleeding and can cause serious and potentially fatal bleeding; promptly evaluate any signs or symptoms of blood loss. D/C in patients w/ active pathological bleeding. No established way to reverse anticoagulant effects of edoxaban; effects can be expected to persist for approx 24 hrs after last dose. Indwelling epidural or intrathecal catheters should not be removed earlier than 12 hrs after the last administration of edoxaban; next dose of edoxaban should not be administered earlier than 2 hrs after removal of the catheter. Not recommended w/ mechanical heart valves or moderate to severe mitral stenosis, CrCl <15mL/min, moderate/severe hepatic impairment (Child-Pugh B and C). Increased risk for ischemic stroke in patients w/ NVAF, as renal function improves and edoxaban blood levels decrease.

ADVERSE REACTIONS
Bleeding, rash, abnormal LFTs.

DRUG INTERACTIONS
See Boxed Warning and Dosing Modifications. May increase risk of bleeding w/ drugs affecting hemostasis (eg, ASA and other antiplatelet agents, anticoagulants, fibrinolytics, thrombolytics, chronic use of NSAIDs); promptly evaluate any signs or symptoms of blood loss if patients are treated concomitantly w/ anticoagulants, ASA, other platelet aggregation inhibitors, and/or NSAIDs. Long-term concomitant treatment w/ other anticoagulants is not recommended; short-term coadministration may be needed for patients transitioning to or from edoxaban. Avoid use w/ rifampin. Dose reduction in NVAF patients concomitantly receiving P-gp inhibitors resulted in edoxaban blood levels that were lower than in patients who were given the full dose; no dose reduction is recommended for concomitant P-gp inhibitor use.

NURSING CONSIDERATIONS

Assessment: Assess for active pathological bleeding, risk factors of developing epidural/spinal hematomas, mechanical heart valves, moderate to severe mitral stenosis, renal/hepatic impairment, pregnancy/nursing status, and possible drug interactions. Assess if patient is receiving neuraxial anesthesia or scheduled to undergo spinal puncture.

Monitoring: Monitor for signs/symptoms of ischemic events w/ premature discontinuation of therapy, bleeding, and other adverse reactions.

Patient Counseling: Inform of the risks and benefits of therapy. Advise that may bleed/bruise more easily or may bleed longer while on therapy. Instruct to report any unusual bleeding immediately to physician. Advise to take exactly as prescribed. Counsel not to d/c therapy w/o talking to physician. Advise to inform all healthcare providers and dentists that patient is taking edoxaban before any surgery, medical or dental procedure is scheduled. Instruct to inform all healthcare providers and dentists if patient is taking/planning to take any prescription medications, OTC drugs, or herbal products. Counsel to inform physician immediately if pregnant/breastfeeding or intending to become pregnant/breastfeed during treatment. Advise patients who are having neuraxial anesthesia or spinal puncture to watch for signs and symptoms of spinal/epidural hematoma; instruct to contact physician immediately if symptoms occur.

Storage: 20-25°C (68-77°F); excursions permitted to 15-30°C (59-86°F).

SAVELLA – milnacipran hydrochloride

RX

Class: Serotonin and norepinephrine reuptake inhibitor

Savella is a selective SNRI, similar to some drugs used for the treatment of depression and other psychiatric disorders. Antidepressants increased the risk of suicidal thinking and behavior (suicidality) in children, adolescents, and young adults in short-term studies of major depressive disorder (MDD) and other psychiatric disorders. Monitor appropriately and observe closely for clinical worsening, suicidality, or unusual behavioral changes in patients who are started on milnacipran. Not approved for use in the treatment of MDD and in pediatric patients.

ADULT DOSAGE

Fibromyalgia

Usual: 50mg bid

Titrate:

Day 1: 12.5mg

PEDIATRIC DOSAGE

Pediatric use may not have been established

Days 2-3: 12.5mg bid
Days 4-7: 25mg bid
After Day 7: 50mg bid
Max: 100mg bid

Dosing Considerations with MAOIs

Switching to/from an MAOI for Psychiatric Disorders:
Allow at least 14 days between discontinuation of an MAOI and initiation of treatment, and allow at least 5 days between discontinuation of treatment and initiation of an MAOI

W/ Other MAOIs (eg, Linezolid, IV Methylene Blue):
Do not start milnacipran in patients being treated w/ linezolid or IV methylene blue
In patients already receiving milnacipran, if acceptable alternatives are not available and benefits outweigh risks, d/c milnacipran and administer linezolid or IV methylene blue; monitor for serotonin syndrome for 5 days or until 24 hrs after the last dose of linezolid or IV methylene blue, whichever comes 1st. May resume milnacipran therapy 24 hrs after the last dose of linezolid or IV methylene blue

DOSE MODIFICATION
Renal Impairment
Moderate: Use w/ caution
Severe (CrCl 5-29mL/min): Reduce maint dose by 50% to 25mg bid; may increase to 50mg bid based on individual response
ESRD: Not recommended

Discontinuation
Taper gradually and do not abruptly d/c after extended use

ADMINISTRATION
Oral route

Take w/ or w/o food
Taking w/ food may improve tolerability

HOW SUPPLIED
Tab: 12.5mg, 25mg, 50mg, 100mg

CONTRAINDICATIONS
Use of an MAOI for psychiatric disorders either concomitantly or w/in 5 days of stopping treatment. Treatment w/in 14 days of stopping an MAOI for psychiatric disorders. Starting treatment in patients being treated w/ other MAOIs (eg, linezolid, IV methylene blue).

WARNINGS/PRECAUTIONS
Serotonin syndrome reported; d/c immediately and initiate supportive symptomatic treatment. Associated w/ increase in BP and HR; treat preexisting HTN, preexisting tachyarrhythmias, and other cardiac diseases before starting therapy. Caution w/ significant HTN or cardiac disease. Consider dose reduction or discontinuation of therapy if sustained increase in BP or HR occurs. Increased liver enzymes and severe liver injury reported; d/c if jaundice or other evidence of liver dysfunction develops. Withdrawal symptoms and physical dependence reported; taper gradually. Hyponatremia may occur; elderly and volume-depleted patients may be at greater risk. Consider discontinuation in patients w/ symptomatic hyponatremia. May increase risk of bleeding events. Caution w/ history of a seizure disorder or mania. May affect urethral resistance and micturition; caution w/ history of dysuria, notably in male patients w/ prostatic hypertrophy, prostatitis, and other lower urinary tract obstructive disorders. Male patients may experience testicular pain or ejaculation disorders. Pupillary dilation that occurs following use may trigger an angle-closure attack in a patient w/ anatomically narrow angles who does not have a patent iridectomy. May aggravate preexisting liver disease; avoid w/ substantial alcohol use or chronic liver disease. Caution in the elderly.

ADVERSE REACTIONS
N/V, headache, constipation, hot flush, insomnia, hyperhidrosis, palpitations, URTI, increased HR, dry mouth, HTN, anxiety, dizziness, migraine, abdominal pain.

DRUG INTERACTIONS
See Contraindications. May cause serotonin syndrome w/ other serotonergic drugs (eg, triptans, TCAs, fentanyl, lithium, tramadol, tryptophan, buspirone, St. John's wort) and w/ drugs that impair

metabolism of serotonin; d/c immediately if this occurs. If treatment w/ other serotonergic drugs is clinically warranted, patient should be made aware of potential risk for serotonin syndrome, particularly during dose initiation and dose increases. Paroxysmal HTN and possible arrhythmia may occur w/ epinephrine and norepinephrine. Increase in euphoria and postural hypotension observed in patients who switched from clomipramine; caution w/ other centrally acting drugs. Concomitant use w/ digoxin may potentiate adverse hemodynamic effects. Avoid w/ IV digoxin; postural hypotension and tachycardia reported. May inhibit antihypertensive effect of clonidine. Caution w/ NSAIDs, aspirin (ASA), warfarin, and other drugs that affect coagulation due to potential increased risk of bleeding. Caution w/ drugs that increase BP and HR. May increase risk of hyponatremia w/ diuretics.

NURSING CONSIDERATIONS

Assessment: Assess for HTN, tachyarrhythmias, cardiac diseases, depression, history of seizure disorder/mania/dysuria, prostatic hypertrophy, prostatitis, lower urinary tract obstructive disorders, volume depletion, susceptibility to angle-closure glaucoma, renal/hepatic impairment, pregnancy/nursing status, and possible drug interactions. Assess alcohol use. Obtain baseline BP and HR.

Monitoring: Monitor for clinical worsening, suicidality, unusual changes in behavior, serotonin syndrome, hyponatremia, bleeding events, withdrawal symptoms, physical dependence, liver dysfunction, angle-closure glaucoma, and other adverse reactions. Monitor for urethral resistance and micturition, testicular pain, and ejaculation disorders in male patients. Monitor BP and HR.

Patient Counseling: Inform about risks/benefits of therapy and counsel on its appropriate use. Advise to look for the emergence of suicidality, especially early during treatment and when the dose is adjusted up or down. Inform about the risk of serotonin syndrome, particularly w/ concomitant use w/ other serotonergic agents. Instruct to consult physician if symptoms of serotonin syndrome and emergence of suicidality occur. Advise to have BP and HR monitored regularly. Caution about the increased risk of abnormal bleeding w/ concomitant use of NSAIDs, ASA, and other drugs that affect coagulation. Caution w/ risk of angle closure glaucoma. Inform that drug may impair mental/physical abilities; caution against operating machinery/driving motor vehicles until effects of drug are known. Instruct to discuss alcohol intake w/ physician prior to initiating therapy. Advise that withdrawal symptoms may occur w/ abrupt discontinuation. Advise that if a dose is missed, to skip the dose and take the next dose at the regular time. Instruct to notify physician if pregnant, intending to become pregnant, or if breastfeeding; encourage to enroll in the Savella Pregnancy Registry if patient becomes pregnant.

Storage: 25°C (77°F); excursions permitted to 15-30°C (59-86°F).

SELZENTRY – maraviroc

RX

Class: CCR5 co-receptor antagonist

Hepatotoxicity reported; may be preceded by severe rash or evidence of systemic allergic reaction (eg, fever, eosinophilia, elevated IgE). Immediately evaluate patients with signs or symptoms of hepatitis or allergic reaction.

ADULT DOSAGE

CCR5-Tropic HIV-1

Concomitant Potent CYP3A Inhibitors (with/without Potent CYP3A Inducer):
150mg bid

Concomitant Potent CYP3A Inducers (without Potent CYP3A Inhibitor):
600mg bid

Other Concomitant Medications (Eg, Tipranavir/Ritonavir, Nevirapine, Raltegravir, All NRTIs, Enfuvirtide):
300mg bid

PEDIATRIC DOSAGE

Pediatric use may not have been established

DOSE MODIFICATION

Renal Impairment

Concomitant Potent CYP3A Inhibitors (with/without a CYP3A Inducer):
CrCl <30 mL/min or ESRD on Regular Hemodialysis: Not recommended for use

Concomitant Potent CYP3A Inducers (without a Potent CYP3A Inhibitor):
CrCl <30 mL/min or ESRD on Regular Hemodialysis: Not recommended for use

Other Concomitant Medications:
CrCl <30 mL/min or ESRD on Regular Hemodialysis: Reduce dose to 150mg bid if symptoms of postural hypotension develop

ADMINISTRATION

Oral route

Take with or without food

HOW SUPPLIED

Tab: 150mg, 300mg

CONTRAINDICATIONS

In patients with severe renal impairment or end-stage renal disease (ESRD) (CrCl <30mL/min) who are taking potent CYP3A inhibitors or inducers.

WARNINGS/PRECAUTIONS

Caution in patients with preexisting liver dysfunction or who are coinfected with viral hepatitis B or C. Consider discontinuation in patients with signs or symptoms of hepatitis, or with increased liver transaminases combined with rash or other systemic symptoms. Severe, potentially life-threatening skin and hypersensitivity reactions reported (eg, Stevens-Johnson syndrome, toxic epidermal necrolysis, drug rash with eosinophilia and systemic symptoms); d/c therapy and other suspected agents immediately if signs and symptoms develop. Cardiovascular (CV) events (eg, myocardial ischemia/infarction) and postural hypotension reported; caution in patients at increased risk for CV events and with history of or risk factors for postural hypotension or CV comorbidities. Increased risk of postural hypotension in patients with severe renal insufficiency or ESRD. Immune reconstitution syndrome reported. Autoimmune disorders (eg, Graves' disease, polymyositis, Guillain-Barre syndrome) reported in the setting of immune reconstitution and can occur many months after initiation of treatment. May increase risk of developing infections. May affect immune surveillance and lead to increased risk of malignancy. In treatment-naive patients, more subjects treated with maraviroc experienced virologic failure and developed lamivudine resistance compared with efavirenz. Caution in elderly.

ADVERSE REACTIONS

Hepatotoxicity, upper respiratory tract infections, cough, pyrexia, rash, dizziness.

DRUG INTERACTIONS

See Contraindications and dosage. Not recommended with St. John's wort or products containing St. John's wort; may substantially decrease levels and lead to loss of virologic response and possible resistance. Dose adjustment may be required with CYP3A inhibitors/inducers and P-glycoprotein inhibitors/inducers. Caution with medications known to lower BP.

NURSING CONSIDERATIONS

Assessment: Assess for renal and liver dysfunction, coinfection with hepatitis B or C, risk for CV events, history of or risk factors for postural hypotension and CV comorbidities, pregnancy/nursing status, and possible drug interactions. Conduct tropism testing to identify appropriate patients. Obtain baseline LFTs.

Monitoring: Monitor for signs/symptoms of hepatotoxicity, allergic reactions, skin/hypersensitivity reactions, immune reconstitution syndrome, CV events, postural hypotension, infections, malignancy, and other adverse reactions. Monitor LFTs as clinically indicated.

Patient Counseling: Inform that liver problems have been reported and advise to d/c therapy and seek medical attention if signs/symptoms of hepatitis or allergic reaction develop. Inform that therapy is not a cure for HIV-1 infection and patients may continue to experience illnesses associated with HIV-1 infection, including opportunistic infections. Instruct to avoid driving/operating machinery if dizziness occurs. Advise to remain under the care of a physician, to take all anti-HIV medicines as prescribed, and not to change dose or d/c therapy without consulting physician. Instruct to take missed dose as soon as possible; advise not to take missed dose if it is <6 hours before next scheduled dose and to take next dose at the regular time. Counsel to avoid doing things that can spread HIV-1 infection to others (eg, sharing of needles/inj equipment or personal items that can have blood/body fluids on them). Advise to always practice safe sex by using latex or polyurethane condoms. Instruct to avoid breastfeeding.

Storage: 25°C (77°F); excursions permitted between 15-30°C (59-86°F).

SENSIPAR – cinacalcet

RX

Class: Calcimimetic agent

ADULT DOSAGE

Secondary Hyperparathyroidism

In Patients w/ Chronic Kidney Disease on Dialysis:
Initial: 30mg qd
Titrate: Increase no more frequently than every 2-4 weeks through sequential doses of

PEDIATRIC DOSAGE

Pediatric use may not have been established

30mg, 60mg, 90mg, 120mg, and 180mg qd to target intact parathyroid (iPTH) hormone of 150-300pg/mL

Measure serum Ca^{2+} and phosphorus w/in 1 week and measure iPTH hormone 1-4 weeks after initiation/dose adjustment; serum iPTH levels should be assessed no earlier than 12 hrs after dosing

Once maint dose is established, measure serum Ca^{2+} monthly

May be used alone or in combination w/ vitamin D sterols and/or phosphate binders

Hypercalcemia

In Patients w/ Primary Hyperparathyroidism who are Unable to Undergo Parathyroidectomy and Patients w/ Parathyroid Carcinoma:
Initial: 30mg bid
Titrate: Increase every 2-4 weeks through sequential doses of 30mg bid, 60mg bid, 90mg bid, and 90mg tid-qid as necessary to normalize serum Ca^{2+} levels

Measure serum Ca^{2+} w/in 1 week after initiation/dose adjustment; once maint dose is established, measure serum Ca^{2+} every 2 months

DOSE MODIFICATION

Adverse Reactions

Secondary Hyperparathyroidism in Patients w/ Chronic Kidney Disease on Dialysis:
If serum Ca^{2+} falls <7.5mg/dL, or if hypocalcemia symptoms persist and vitamin D dose cannot be increased, withhold administration until Ca^{2+} levels reach 8.0mg/dL and/or symptoms of hypocalcemia resolve. Treatment should be reinitiated using next lowest dose of cinacalcet

ADMINISTRATION

Oral route

Take whole; do not divide
Take w/ food or shortly after a meal

HOW SUPPLIED

Tab: 30mg, 60mg, 90mg

CONTRAINDICATIONS

Hypocalcemia.

WARNINGS/PRECAUTIONS

Avoid use in patients with CKD not on dialysis. Lowers serum Ca^{2+}; monitor for occurrence of hypocalcemia during treatment. Life-threatening events and fatal outcomes associated with hypocalcemia reported in patients treated with the drug, including pediatric patients. QT prolongation and ventricular arrhythmia secondary to hypocalcemia reported. Seizures reported; monitor serum Ca^{2+}, particularly in patients with history of seizure disorder. Hypotension, worsening HF, and/or arrhythmia reported in patients with impaired cardiac function. Adynamic bone disease may develop with iPTH levels <100pg/mL; reduce dose or d/c therapy if iPTH levels <150pg/mL. Monitor patients with moderate and severe hepatic impairment throughout treatment.

ADVERSE REACTIONS

N/V, diarrhea, myalgia, dizziness, HTN, asthenia, anorexia, paresthesia, fatigue, fracture, hypercalcemia, dehydration, anemia, arthralgia, depression.

DRUG INTERACTIONS

May require dose adjustment with CYP2D6 substrates (eg, desipramine, metoprolol, carvedilol) and particularly those with narrow therapeutic index (eg, flecainide, most TCAs). May require dose adjustment if a patient initiates or discontinues therapy with strong CYP3A4 inhibitors (eg, ketoconazole, itraconazole); closely monitor iPTH and serum Ca^{2+} levels.

NURSING CONSIDERATIONS

Assessment: Assess for hypocalcemia, history of seizure disorder, hepatic impairment, cardiac function, pregnancy/nursing status, and possible drug interactions. Assess serum Ca^{2+} levels prior to administration.

Monitoring: Monitor for signs/symptoms of hypocalcemia, adynamic bone disease, and other adverse reactions. In patients with impaired cardiac function, monitor for hypotension, worsening HF, and/or arrhythmias. Monitor iPTH/Ca^{2+}/phosphorus levels with moderate and severe hepatic impairment. Monitor serum Ca^{2+} carefully for the occurrence of hypocalcemia during treatment.

Patient Counseling: Inform of the importance of regular blood tests. Advise to report to physician if N/V and potential symptoms of hypocalcemia occur. Advise to report to their physician if taking medication to prevent seizures, have had seizures in the past, and experience any seizure episodes while on therapy. Encourage patients who are nursing during treatment to enroll in Amgen's Lactation Surveillance Program.

Storage: 25°C (77°F); excursions permitted to 15-30°C (59-86°F).

SEREVENT DISKUS – salmeterol xinafoate — RX

Class: $Beta_2$-agonist

Long-acting β_2-adrenergic agonists (LABAs) increase the risk of asthma-related death. Contraindicated in asthma without use of a concomitant long-term asthma control medication (eg, inhaled corticosteroid). Do not use if asthma is adequately controlled on low- or medium-dose inhaled corticosteroids. LABAs may increase the risk of asthma-related hospitalization in pediatric and adolescent patients.

ADULT DOSAGE

Asthma

Use only as concomitant therapy w/ a long-term asthma control medication (eg, inhaled corticosteroid) in patients with reversible obstructive airway disease, including patients w/ symptoms of nocturnal asthma

Usual: 1 inh bid (12 hrs apart)

Chronic Obstructive Pulmonary Disease

Maint Treatment of Bronchospasm (eg, Emphysema, Chronic Bronchitis):
1 inh bid (12 hrs apart)

Exercise-Induced Bronchospasm

Prevention:
1 inh ≥30 min before exercise (additional doses should not be used for 12 hrs after administration or if already on bid dose)

PEDIATRIC DOSAGE

Asthma

≥4 Years:
1 inh bid (12 hrs apart)

Exercise-Induced Bronchospasm

Prevention:
≥4 Years:
1 inh ≥30 min before exercise (additional doses should not be used for 12 hrs after administration or if already on bid dose)

ADMINISTRATION

Oral inh route

HOW SUPPLIED

Disk: 50mcg/inh [28, 60 blisters]

CONTRAINDICATIONS

Treatment of asthma without concomitant use of long-term asthma control medication (eg, inhaled corticosteroid). Primary treatment of status asthmaticus or other acute episodes of asthma/COPD where intensive measures are required. Milk protein hypersensitivity.

WARNINGS/PRECAUTIONS

Not indicated for acute bronchospasm relief. Do not initiate during rapidly deteriorating or potentially life-threatening episodes of asthma or COPD; serious acute respiratory events reported. D/C regular use of oral/inhaled short-acting β_2-agonist (SABA) when beginning treatment. Not a substitute for corticosteroids. Do not use more often or at higher doses than recommended; clinically significant cardiovascular (CV) effects and fatalities reported with excessive use. May produce paradoxical bronchospasm; treat immediately with an inhaled, short acting bronchodilator; d/c and institute alternative therapy. Upper airway symptoms reported. Immediate hypersensitivity reactions and CV/CNS effects may occur. Caution with CV disorders, convulsive disorders, thyrotoxicosis, hepatic disease, diabetes mellitus (DM), ketoacidosis, and in patients unusually responsive to sympathomimetic amines. Clinically significant and dose-related changes in blood glucose and/or serum K^+ reported.

ADVERSE REACTIONS

Nasal/sinus congestion, pharyngitis, cough, viral respiratory infection, musculoskeletal pain, rhinitis, headache, tracheitis/bronchitis, influenza, throat irritation.

DRUG INTERACTIONS

Do not use with other medicines containing a LABA. Not recommended with strong CYP3A4 inhibitors (eg, ketoconazole, ritonavir, clarithromycin); increased CV adverse effects may occur. Extreme caution with MAOIs or TCAs, or within 2 weeks of discontinuation of such agents; action on the vascular system may be potentiated. β-blockers may block pulmonary effects and produce severe bronchospasm; if such therapy is needed, consider cardioselective β-blockers and use with caution. Caution is advised when coadministered with non-K^+-sparing diuretics (eg, loop, thiazide).

NURSING CONSIDERATIONS

Assessment: Assess for hypersensitivity to milk proteins, status asthmaticus, asthma/COPD status, CV disorders, convulsive disorders, thyrotoxicosis, DM, ketoacidosis, hepatic disease, pregnancy/nursing status, and possible drug interactions.

Monitoring: Monitor for deteriorating disease, paradoxical bronchospasm, upper airway symptoms, immediate hypersensitivity reactions, CV and CNS effects, changes in blood glucose and/or serum K^+, and other adverse reactions.

Patient Counseling: Counsel about the risks and benefits of therapy. Inform that the medication should only be used as additional therapy when long-term asthma control medications do not adequately control asthma symptoms. Inform that drug is not meant to relieve acute asthma or exacerbations of COPD symptoms and extra doses should not be used for that purpose; advise to treat acute symptoms with an inhaled SABA (eg, albuterol). Instruct to seek medical attention immediately if experiencing a decrease in effectiveness of inhaled SABA, a need for more inhalations than usual of inhaled SABA, or a significant decrease in lung function. Advise not to d/c therapy without physician guidance and not to use other LABA. Advise that therapy is not a substitute for oral or inhaled corticosteroids; instruct not to change dosage or stop therapy without consulting physician. Advise that immediate hypersensitivity reactions may occur; instruct to d/c if such reactions occur. Inform of adverse effects (eg, palpitations, chest pain, rapid HR, tremor, nervousness). Inform patients treated for EIB not to use additional doses for 12 hrs and not to use additional doses for prevention of EIB if receiving therapy bid. Inform that the inhaler is not reusable and advise not to take the inhaler apart.

Storage: 20-25°C (68-77°F); excursions permitted from 15-30°C (59-86°F). Store in a dry place away from direct heat or sunlight. Store inside the unopened moisture-protective foil pouch and only remove from the pouch immediately before initial use. Discard 6 weeks after opening the foil pouch or when the counter reads "0," whichever comes 1st.

SEROQUEL — quetiapine fumarate **RX**

Class: Atypical antipsychotic

Elderly patients with dementia-related psychosis treated with antipsychotic drugs are at an increased risk of death. Not approved for the treatment of patients with dementia-related psychosis. Antidepressants increased the risk of suicidal thoughts and behavior in children, adolescents, and young adults in short-term studies. Monitor closely for worsening, and for emergence of suicidal thoughts and behaviors in patients who are started on antidepressant therapy. Not approved for use in pediatric patients <10 yrs of age.

ADULT DOSAGE

Schizophrenia

Day 1: 25mg bid
Days 2-3: Increase by 25-50mg divided bid or tid to a range of 300-400mg by Day 4
Titrate: Further adjustments can be made in increments of 25-50mg bid, in intervals of ≥2 days
Usual: 150-750mg/day
Max: 750mg/day

Maint:
Usual: 400-800mg/day
Max: 800mg/day

Switching from Depot Antipsychotics:
Initiate quetiapine therapy in place of the next scheduled inj if medically appropriate

Bipolar I Disorder

Mania:
Monotherapy/Adjunct to Lithium or Divalproex:
Day 1: 100mg/day given bid

PEDIATRIC DOSAGE

Schizophrenia

13-17 Years:
Day 1: 25mg bid
Day 2: 100mg/day given bid
Day 3: 200mg/day given bid
Day 4: 300mg/day given bid
Day 5: 400mg/day given bid
Titrate: Further adjustments should be in increments ≤100mg/day; may administer tid based on response and tolerability
Usual: 400-800mg/day
Max: 800mg/day

Switching from Depot Antipsychotics:
Initiate quetiapine therapy in place of the next scheduled inj if medically appropriate

Bipolar I Disorder

Mania:
10-17 Years:
Monotherapy:
Day 1: 25mg bid
Day 2: 100mg/day given bid

Day 2: 200mg/day given bid
Day 3: 300mg/day given bid
Day 4: 400mg/day given bid
Titrate: Further adjustments up to 800mg/day by Day 6 should be in increments of ≤200mg/day
Usual: 400-800mg/day
Max: 800mg/day

Maint:
Adjunct to Lithium or Divalproex:
400-800mg/day given bid
Max: 800mg/day

Bipolar Disorder
Depression:
Monotherapy:
Day 1: 50mg qhs
Day 2: 100mg qhs
Day 3: 200mg qhs
Day 4: 300mg qhs
Usual/Max: 300mg/day

Day 3: 200mg/day given bid
Day 4: 300mg/day given bid
Day 5: 400mg/day given bid
Titrate: Further adjustments should be in increments ≤100mg/day; may administer tid based on response and tolerability
Usual: 400-600mg/day
Max: 600mg/day

DOSE MODIFICATION
Concomitant Medications
CYP3A4 Inhibitors:
Reduce dose of quetiapine to 1/6 of original dose; when CYP3A4 inhibitor is discontinued, increase quetiapine dose by 6-fold

CYP3A4 Inducers:
Increase quetiapine dose up to 5-fold of the original dose when used in combination w/ a chronic treatment (eg, >7-14 days) of a potent CYP3A4 inducer; when CYP3A4 inducer is discontinued, reduce quetiapine dose to original level w/in 7-14 days

Hepatic Impairment
Initial: 25mg/day
Titrate: Increase by 25-50mg/day

Elderly
Initial: 50mg/day
Titrate: May increase by 50mg/day

Other Important Modifications
Debilitated Patients/Predisposed to Hypotension:
Consider slower rate of titration and lower target dose

Reinitiation of Treatment:
Discontinued <1 Week: Reinitiate maint dose
Discontinued for >1 Week: Follow initial dosing schedule

ADMINISTRATION
Oral route

Take w/ or w/o food

HOW SUPPLIED
Tab: 25mg, 50mg, 100mg, 200mg, 300mg, 400mg

WARNINGS/PRECAUTIONS
Initiate in pediatric patients only after a thorough diagnostic evaluation is conducted and careful consideration is given to the risks of therapy. Neuroleptic malignant syndrome (NMS) reported; d/c and institute symptomatic treatment. Hyperglycemia, in some cases extreme and associated with ketoacidosis or hyperosmolar coma or death, reported; monitor glucose regularly in patients with diabetes mellitus (DM) and FPG in patients at risk for DM. Alterations in lipids and weight gain observed. May cause tardive dyskinesia (TD), especially in the elderly; consider discontinuation if this occurs. May induce orthostatic hypotension. Leukopenia, neutropenia, and agranulocytosis reported; monitor CBC frequently during 1st few months in patients with preexisting low WBC count or history of drug-induced leukopenia/neutropenia, and d/c at 1st sign of decline in WBC count without causative factors. D/C therapy and follow WBC count until recovery in patients with severe neutropenia (ANC <1000/mm^3). QT prolongation reported. Avoid in circumstances that may increase the risk of torsades de pointes and/or sudden death. Seizures reported; caution with conditions that lower seizure threshold. Decrease in thyroid hormone levels reported; measure TSH and free T4 at baseline and at follow-up in addition to clinical assessment. May elevate prolactin levels. May impair physical/mental abilities. May disrupt body's ability to reduce core body temperature. May cause esophageal dysmotility and aspiration; caution in patients at risk for

aspiration pneumonia. Acute withdrawal symptoms (eg, N/V, insomnia) may occur after abrupt cessation; d/c gradually.

ADVERSE REACTIONS

Headache, somnolence, dizziness, dry mouth, constipation, dyspepsia, tachycardia, asthenia, agitation, pain, weight gain, ALT increased, abdominal pain, back pain, N/V.

DRUG INTERACTIONS

Caution with other centrally acting drugs and alcohol. Increased exposure with CYP3A4 inhibitors (eg, ketoconazole, ritonavir, nefazodone) and decreased exposure with CYP3A4 inducers (eg, phenytoin, carbamazepine, rifampin, St. John's wort); dose adjustment of quetiapine may be necessary. May enhance the effects of certain antihypertensives. May antagonize the effects of levodopa and dopamine agonists. QT prolongation reported with drugs known to cause electrolyte imbalance. Avoid with other drugs that are known to prolong QTc interval (eg, quinidine, amiodarone, ziprasidone, gatifloxacin, methadone). Caution with anticholinergic medications.

NURSING CONSIDERATIONS

Assessment: Assess for history of dementia-related psychosis, risk for hypotension, drug hypersensitivity, psychiatric disorders, hepatic impairment, other conditions where treatment is cautioned, pregnancy/nursing status, and possible drug interactions. Obtain baseline FPG in patients with DM or at risk for DM. Obtain baseline CBC if at risk for leukopenia/neutropenia. Obtain baseline TSH, and free T4. Obtain baseline BP in children and adolescents. Assess for cataracts by performing lens exam (eg, slit-lamp exam).

Monitoring: Monitor for clinical worsening, suicidality, unusual changes in behavior, NMS, TD, hyperglycemia, orthostatic hypotension, hypothyroidism, seizures, aspiration, and other adverse effects. Monitor CBC frequently in patients with preexisting low WBC or history of drug-induced leukopenia/neutropenia. Monitor for fever or other signs/symptoms of infection in patients with neutropenia. Monitor weight regularly; monitor lipids, hepatic function, and FPG periodically. Monitor for cataract formation shortly after start of treatment, and at 6-month intervals during chronic treatment. Monitor BP periodically during treatment in children and adolescents. Periodically reassess for continued need for maintenance treatment.

Patient Counseling: Inform of the risks and benefits of therapy. Instruct caregivers and patients to contact physician if signs of agitation, anxiety, panic attacks, insomnia, hostility, aggressiveness, impulsivity, akathisia, hypomania, mania, irritability, worsening of depression, changes in behavior, or suicidal ideation develop. Advise about signs/symptoms of NMS, symptoms of hyperglycemia and DM, weight gain, and risk of orthostatic hypotension. Instruct to avoid overheating and dehydration. Caution about performing activities requiring mental alertness. Instruct to notify physician if patient becomes pregnant or intends to become pregnant during therapy, and if patient is taking or plans to take any prescription or OTC drugs.

Storage: 25°C (77°F); excursions permitted to 15-30°C (59-86°F).

SEROQUEL XR – quetiapine fumarate RX

Class: Atypical antipsychotic

Elderly patients with dementia-related psychosis treated with antipsychotic drugs are at an increased risk of death. Not approved for the treatment of patients with dementia-related psychosis. Antidepressants increased the risk of suicidal thoughts and behavior in children, adolescents, and young adults in short-term studies. Monitor closely for worsening, and for emergence of suicidal thoughts and behaviors in patients who are started on antidepressant therapy. Not approved for use in pediatric patients <10 yrs of age.

ADULT DOSAGE

Schizophrenia

Day 1: 300mg/day
Titrate: May increase at intervals as short as 1 day and in increments of up to 300mg/day
Usual: 400-800mg/day
Max: 800mg/day

Maint:
Monotherapy:
Usual: 400-800mg/day
Max: 800mg/day

Bipolar I Disorder

Manic/Mixed Episodes:
Acute Monotherapy/Adjunct to Lithium or Divalproex:
Day 1: 300mg/day

PEDIATRIC DOSAGE

Schizophrenia

13-17 Years:
Day 1: 50mg/day
Day 2: 100mg/day
Day 3: 200mg/day
Day 4: 300mg/day
Day 5: 400mg/day
Usual: 400-800mg/day
Max: 800mg/day

Bipolar I Disorder

Mania:
10-17 Years:
Acute Monotherapy:
Day 1: 50mg/day
Day 2: 100mg/day

Day 2: 600mg/day
Day 3: 400-800mg/day
Usual: 400-800mg/day
Max: 800mg/day

Maint:
Adjunct to Lithium or Divalproex:
Usual: 400-800mg/day
Max: 800mg/day

Bipolar Disorder

Depressive Episodes:
Day 1: 50mg/day
Day 2: 100mg/day
Day 3: 200mg/day
Day 4: 300mg/day
Usual/Max: 300mg/day

Major Depressive Disorder

Adjunctive Therapy to Antidepressants:
Days 1 & 2: 50mg/day
Day 3: 150mg/day
Usual: 150-300mg/day
Max: 300mg/day

Conversions

Switching from IR to ER Quetiapine:
Switch at the equivalent total daily dose taken qd

Switching from Depot Antipsychotics:
Initiate quetiapine therapy in place of next scheduled inj if medically appropriate

Day 3: 200mg/day
Day 4: 300mg/day
Day 5: 400mg/day
Usual: 400-600mg/day
Max: 600mg/day

Conversions

Switching from IR to ER Quetiapine:
Switch at the equivalent total daily dose taken qd

Switching from Depot Antipsychotics:
Initiate quetiapine therapy in place of next scheduled inj if medically appropriate

DOSE MODIFICATION

Concomitant Medications

Potent CYP3A4 Inhibitors (eg, Ketoconazole, Itraconazole, Indinavir):
Reduce dose of quetiapine to one sixth of original dose; when CYP3A4 inhibitor is discontinued, increase quetiapine dose by 6-fold

Potent CYP3A4 Inducers (eg, Phenytoin, Carbamazepine, Rifampin):
Increase quetiapine dose up to 5-fold of the original dose when used in combination w/ a chronic treatment (eg, >7-14 days) of a potent CYP3A4 inducer; when CYP3A4 inducer is discontinued, reduce quetiapine dose to original level w/in 7-14 days

Hepatic Impairment
Initial: 50mg/day
Titrate: May increase in increments of 50mg/day

Elderly
Initial: 50mg/day
Titrate: May increase in increments of 50mg/day

Other Important Modifications

Debilitated Patients/Predisposed to Hypotension:
Consider slower rate of titration and lower target dose

Reinitiation of Treatment in Patients Previously Discontinued:
Discontinued <1 Week: Reinitiate maint dose
Discontinued for >1 Week: Follow initial dosing schedule

ADMINISTRATION

Oral route

Swallow tab whole; do not split, crush, or chew
Take w/o food or w/ a light meal (approx 300 calories)
Administer qd, preferably in the pm

HOW SUPPLIED

Tab, ER: 50mg, 150mg, 200mg, 300mg, 400mg

WARNINGS/PRECAUTIONS

Initiate in pediatric patients only after a thorough diagnostic evaluation is conducted and careful consideration is given to the risks of therapy. Neuroleptic malignant syndrome (NMS) reported; d/c and institute symptomatic treatment. Hyperglycemia, in some cases extreme and associated with ketoacidosis or hyperosmolar coma or death, reported; monitor glucose regularly in patients with diabetes mellitus (DM) and FPG in patients at risk for DM. Alterations in lipids and weight gain observed. May cause tardive dyskinesia (TD), especially in the elderly; consider discontinuation if this occurs. May induce orthostatic hypotension. Leukopenia, neutropenia, and agranulocytosis reported; monitor CBC frequently during 1st few months in patients with preexisting low WBC count or history of drug-induced leukopenia/neutropenia, and d/c at 1st sign of decline in WBC count without causative factors. D/C therapy and follow WBC count until recovery in patients with severe neutropenia (ANC <1000/mm^3). QT prolongation reported. Avoid in circumstances that may increase the risk of torsades de pointes and/or sudden death. Seizures reported; caution with conditions that lower seizure threshold. Decrease in thyroid hormone levels reported; measure TSH and free T4 at baseline and at follow-up in addition to clinical assessment. May elevate prolactin levels. May impair physical/mental abilities. May disrupt body's ability to reduce core body temperature. May cause esophageal dysmotility and aspiration; caution in patients at risk for aspiration pneumonia. Acute withdrawal symptoms (eg, N/V, insomnia) may occur after abrupt cessation; d/c gradually.

ADVERSE REACTIONS

Dry mouth, constipation, dyspepsia, somnolence, dizziness, orthostatic hypotension, weight gain, fatigue, dysarthria, nasal congestion, extrapyramidal symptoms, increased appetite, back pain, abnormal dreams, irritability.

DRUG INTERACTIONS

Caution with other centrally acting drugs and alcohol. Increased exposure with CYP3A4 inhibitors (eg, ketoconazole, ritonavir, nefazodone) and decreased exposure with CYP3A4 inducers (eg, phenytoin, carbamazepine, rifampin, St. John's wort); dose adjustment of quetiapine may be necessary. May enhance the effects of certain antihypertensives. May antagonize the effects of levodopa and dopamine agonists. QT prolongation reported with drugs known to cause electrolyte imbalance. Avoid with other drugs that are known to prolong QTc interval (eg, quinidine, amiodarone, ziprasidone, gatifloxacin, methadone). Caution with anticholinergic medications.

NURSING CONSIDERATIONS

Assessment: Assess for history of dementia-related psychosis, risk for hypotension, drug hypersensitivity, psychiatric disorders, hepatic impairment, other conditions where treatment is cautioned, pregnancy/nursing status, and possible drug interactions. Obtain baseline FPG in patients with DM or at risk for DM. Obtain baseline CBC if at risk for leukopenia/neutropenia. Obtain baseline TSH, and free T4. Obtain baseline BP in children and adolescents. Assess for cataracts by performing lens exam (eg, slit-lamp exam).

Monitoring: Monitor for clinical worsening, suicidality, unusual changes in behavior, NMS, TD, hyperglycemia, orthostatic hypotension, hypothyroidism, seizures, aspiration, and other adverse effects. Monitor CBC frequently in patients with preexisting low WBC count or history of drug-induced leukopenia/neutropenia. Monitor for fever or other signs/symptoms of infection in patients with neutropenia. Monitor weight regularly, and lipids, hepatic function, and FPG periodically. Monitor for cataract formation at 6-month intervals during chronic treatment. Monitor BP periodically during treatment in children and adolescents. Periodically reassess for continued need for maintenance treatment.

Patient Counseling: Inform of the risks and benefits of therapy. Instruct caregivers and patients to contact physician if signs of agitation, anxiety, panic attacks, insomnia, hostility, aggressiveness, impulsivity, akathisia, hypomania, mania, irritability, worsening of depression, changes in behavior, or suicidal ideation develop. Advise about signs/symptoms of NMS, symptoms of hyperglycemia and DM, weight gain, or risk of orthostatic hypotension. Counsel to avoid overheating and dehydration. Caution about performing activities requiring mental alertness. Counsel to notify physician if patient becomes pregnant or intends to become pregnant during therapy, and if patient is taking or plans to take any prescription or OTC drugs.

Storage: 25°C (77°F); excursions permitted to 15-30°C (59-86°F).

SILENOR – doxepin

Class: H_1-antagonist

RX

ADULT DOSAGE

Insomnia

Difficulty w/ Sleep Maintenance:

Initial: 6mg qd w/in 30 min of hs; may use 3mg qd if clinically indicated

Max: 6mg/day

PEDIATRIC DOSAGE

Pediatric use may not have been established

DOSE MODIFICATION

Concomitant Medications

Concomitant Use w/ Cimetidine:
Max: 3mg

Hepatic Impairment

Initial: 3mg

Elderly

≥65 Years:
Initial: 3mg qd; may increase to 6mg

ADMINISTRATION

Oral route

Do not take w/in 3 hrs of a meal

HOW SUPPLIED

Tab: 3mg, 6mg

CONTRAINDICATIONS

W/ or w/in 2 weeks of MAOIs. Untreated narrow-angle glaucoma, severe urinary retention.

WARNINGS/PRECAUTIONS

Evaluate comorbid diagnoses prior to initiation of treatment. Failure of remission after 7-10 days may indicate the presence of primary psychiatric and/or medical illness that should be evaluated. Complex behaviors (eg, sleep-driving), amnesia, anxiety, and other neuropsychiatric symptoms reported; consider discontinuation if sleep-driving episode occurs. Worsening of depression reported. May impair physical/mental abilities. Caution in patients w/ compromised respiratory function. Avoid in patients w/ severe sleep apnea.

ADVERSE REACTIONS

Somnolence/sedation, URTI/nasopharyngitis, HTN.

DRUG INTERACTIONS

See Contraindications and Dose Modification. Sedative effects of alcohol, CNS depressants, and sedating antihistamines may be potentiated w/ concomitant use. Increased exposure w/ inhibitors of CYP2C19, CYP2D6, CYP1A2, and CYP2C9. Exposure doubled w/ cimetidine. Hypoglycemia reported when therapy added to tolazamide regimen.

NURSING CONSIDERATIONS

Assessment: Assess for drug hypersensitivity, untreated narrow-angle glaucoma, urinary retention, presence of a primary psychiatric and/or medical illness that may cause insomnia, depression, hepatic impairment, sleep apnea, pregnancy/nursing status, and possible drug interactions.

Monitoring: Monitor for treatment response, complex behaviors/neuropsychiatric symptoms, worsening of depression, and other adverse reactions.

Patient Counseling: Inform of benefits and risks associated w/ therapy. Counsel on appropriate use of medication. Instruct to contact physician if sleep-driving occurs or if patient performs other complex behaviors while not fully awake. Instruct to seek medical attention if symptoms of cognitive or behavioral abnormalities or if worsening of insomnia occurs. Inform that medication may cause sedation; caution against operating machinery (eg, automobiles) during therapy. Advise to avoid alcohol consumption during therapy.

Storage: 20-25°C (68-77°F). Protect from light.

SILVADENE – silver sulfadiazine

RX

Class: Sulfonamide

OTHER BRAND NAMES

SSD

ADULT DOSAGE

Burns

Adjunct for the Prevention and Treatment of Wound Sepsis in Patients With 2nd- and 3rd-Degree Burns:
Apply under sterile conditions qd-bid to a thickness of approximately 1/16 inch
Whenever necessary, reapply to any areas from which it has been removed due to patient activity
Reapply immediately after hydrotherapy
Continue treatment until satisfactory healing

PEDIATRIC DOSAGE

Pediatric use may not have been established

has occurred or until the burn site is ready for grafting; do not withdraw from therapeutic regimen while there remains possibility of infection, except if a significant adverse reaction occurs

ADMINISTRATION
Topical route

Cleanse and debride burn wounds prior to application, under sterile conditions
Burn areas should be covered with cre at all times
Administration may be accomplished in minimal time because dressings are not required; however, if individual patient requirements make dressings necessary, they may be used

HOW SUPPLIED
Cre: 1% [50g, 400g, 1000g (jar); 20g, 85g (tube)]; (SSD) 1% [50g, 400g (jar); 25g, 50g, 85g (tube)]

CONTRAINDICATIONS
Pregnant women approaching or at term, premature infants, newborns during the first 2 months of life.

WARNINGS/PRECAUTIONS
Potential cross-sensitivity with other sulfonamides; if allergic reactions attributable to treatment occur, weigh continuation of therapy against potential hazards of the particular allergic reaction. Fungal proliferation in and below the eschar may occur. Caution with G6PD deficiency; hemolysis may occur. Drug accumulation may occur if hepatic and renal functions become impaired and elimination of drug decreases; weigh discontinuation of therapy against the therapeutic benefit being achieved. In the treatment of burn wounds involving extensive areas of the body, serum sulfa concentrations may approach adult therapeutic levels (8-12mg%); monitor serum sulfa concentrations in these patients. Monitor renal function and check urine for sulfa crystals. Lab test interactions may occur. Adverse reactions associated with sulfonamides (eg, blood dyscrasias, dermatologic and allergic reactions, GI reactions, hepatitis and hepatocellular necrosis, CNS reactions, toxic nephrosis) may occur.

ADVERSE REACTIONS
Transient leukopenia, skin necrosis, erythema multiforme, skin discoloration, burning sensation, rash, interstitial nephritis.

DRUG INTERACTIONS
May inactivate topical proteolytic enzymes.

NURSING CONSIDERATIONS

Assessment: Assess for hypersensitivity to drug, G6PD deficiency, renal/hepatic impairment, pregnancy/nursing status, and possible drug interactions.

Monitoring: Monitor for allergic reactions, fungal proliferation, renal/hepatic dysfunction, and other adverse reactions. Check urine for sulfa crystals. Monitor serum sulfa concentrations in patients with wounds involving extensive areas of the body.

Patient Counseling: Inform of the risks and benefits of therapy. Instruct to use ud. Advise to notify physician if adverse reactions occur.

Storage: 15-30°C (59-86°F).

SIMBRINZA – brimonidine tartrate/brinzolamide RX

Class: $Alpha_2$-agonist/carbonic anhydrase inhibitor

ADULT DOSAGE

Elevated Intraocular Pressure

Open-Angle Glaucoma/Ocular HTN:
1 drop in the affected eye(s) tid

PEDIATRIC DOSAGE

Elevated Intraocular Pressure

Open-Angle Glaucoma/Ocular HTN:
≥2 Years:
1 drop in the affected eye(s) tid

ADMINISTRATION
Ocular route

Shake well before use
Space dosing by at least 5 min if using >1 topical ophthalmic drug

HOW SUPPLIED
Sus: (Brinzolamide-Brimonidine) 1%-0.2% [8mL]

CONTRAINDICATIONS
Neonates and infants (<2 yrs of age).

WARNINGS/PRECAUTIONS
Systemically absorbed. Fatalities occurred due to severe reactions to sulfonamides, including Stevens-Johnson syndrome, toxic epidermal necrolysis, fulminant hepatic necrosis, agranulocytosis, aplastic anemia, and other blood dyscrasias. Sensitization may recur when a sulfonamide is readministered irrespective of route. D/C if signs of serious reactions or hypersensitivity occur. Caution with low endothelial cell counts; increased potential for corneal edema. Not recommended with severe renal impairment (CrCl <30mL/min). Contains benzalkonium chloride, which may be absorbed by soft contact lenses; contact lenses should be removed during instillation, but may be reinserted 15 min after instillation. Caution with severe cardiovascular disease (CVD), severe hepatic impairment, depression, cerebral or coronary insufficiency, Raynaud's phenomenon, orthostatic hypotension, or thromboangiitis obliterans. Bacterial keratitis reported with multidose containers.

ADVERSE REACTIONS
Blurred vision, eye irritation, dysgeusia, dry mouth, eye allergy.

DRUG INTERACTIONS
Potential additive systemic effects with oral carbonic anhydrase inhibitors; coadministration is not recommended. Acid-base alterations reported with high-dose salicylate therapy in patients treated with oral carbonic anhydrase inhibitors. Possible additive or potentiating effect with CNS depressants (eg, alcohol, opiates, barbiturates, sedatives, anesthetics). Caution with antihypertensives and/or cardiac glycosides. Caution with TCAs and MAOIs, which can affect the metabolism and uptake of circulating amines.

NURSING CONSIDERATIONS

Assessment: Assess for hypersensitivity to drug or to sulfonamides, low endothelial cell counts, renal/hepatic impairment, contact lens use, severe CVD, depression, cerebral or coronary insufficiency, Raynaud's phenomenon, orthostatic hypotension, thromboangiitis obliterans, pregnancy/nursing status, and possible drug interactions.

Monitoring: Monitor for sulfonamide hypersensitivity reactions, potentiation of syndromes associated with vascular insufficiency, bacterial keratitis, and other adverse reactions.

Patient Counseling: Advise to d/c use and consult physician if serious or unusual ocular or systemic reactions or signs of hypersensitivity occur. Inform that vision may be temporarily blurred following dosing and fatigue and/or drowsiness may be experienced; instruct to use caution in operating machinery, driving a motor vehicle, and engaging in other hazardous activities. Instruct that ocular sol, if handled improperly or if the tip of dispensing container contacts the eye or surrounding structures, can become contaminated by common bacteria known to cause ocular infections. Advise that using contaminated sol may result in serious eye damage and subsequent loss of vision. Instruct to always replace cap after using. Advise not to use if sol changes color or becomes cloudy. Instruct to consult physician about the continued use of the present multidose container if having ocular surgery or if an intercurrent ocular condition (eg, trauma, infection) develops. If using >1 topical ophthalmic drug, instruct to administer the drugs at least 5 min apart. Advise that contact lenses should be removed during instillation, but may be reinserted 15 min after instillation.

Storage: 2-25°C (36-77°F).

SIMCOR — niacin/simvastatin — RX

Class: HMG-CoA reductase inhibitor/nicotinic acid

ADULT DOSAGE

Hypertriglyceridemia

Not Currently on Niacin ER or Switching from Non-ER Niacin:
Initial: 500mg-20mg qd at hs
Titrate (Niacin ER Component): Increase by no more than 500mg qd every 4 weeks; after Week 8, titrate to patient response and tolerance
Maint: 1000mg-20mg to 2000mg-40mg qd depending on tolerability and lipid levels
Max: 2000mg-40mg qd

If discontinued for >7 days, retitrate as tolerated

Additional Lipid Level Management Needed Despite Simvastatin 20-40mg Only:
Initial: 500mg-40mg qd at hs

PEDIATRIC DOSAGE
Pediatric use may not have been established

Primary Hypercholesterolemia/Mixed Dyslipidemia

Not Currently on Niacin ER or Switching from Non-ER Niacin:
Initial: 500mg-20mg qd at hs
Titrate (Niacin ER Component): Increase by no more than 500mg qd every 4 weeks; after Week 8, titrate to patient response and tolerance
Maint: 1000mg-20mg to 2000mg-40mg qd depending on tolerability and lipid levels
Max: 2000mg-40mg qd

If discontinued for >7 days, retitrate as tolerated

Additional Lipid Level Management Needed Despite Simvastatin 20-40mg Only:
Initial: 500mg-40mg qd at hs

DOSE MODIFICATION

Concomitant Medications

Amiodarone, Amlodipine, or Ranolazine:
Max: 1000mg-20mg/day

Renal Impairment

Severe:
Do not start unless already tolerated ≥10mg simvastatin

Other Important Modifications

Chinese Patients:
Caution w/ doses >1000mg-20mg/day

ADMINISTRATION

Oral route

Take at hs w/ a low-fat snack
Swallow whole; do not break, crush, or chew
Avoid administration on an empty stomach to reduce flushing, pruritus, and GI distress
May take aspirin (up to 325mg) 30 min prior to treatment to reduce flushing

HOW SUPPLIED

Tab: (Niacin ER-Simvastatin) 500mg-20mg, 500mg-40mg, 750mg-20mg, 1000mg-20mg, 1000mg-40mg

CONTRAINDICATIONS

Active liver disease or unexplained persistent elevations in hepatic transaminase levels, active peptic ulcer disease (PUD), arterial bleeding, women who are or may become pregnant, and nursing mothers. Concomitant administration with strong CYP3A4 inhibitors (eg, itraconazole, ketoconazole, posaconazole, HIV protease inhibitors, boceprevir, telaprevir, erythromycin, clarithromycin, telithromycin, nefazodone), gemfibrozil, cyclosporine, danazol, verapamil, or diltiazem.

WARNINGS/PRECAUTIONS

No incremental benefit of Simcor on cardiovascular (CV) morbidity and mortality over and above that demonstrated for simvastatin monotherapy and niacin monotherapy has been established. Niacin ER, at doses of 1500-2000mg/day, in combination with simvastatin, did not reduce the incidence of CV events more than simvastatin in patients with CV disease and mean baseline LDL levels of 74mg/dL. Should be substituted only for equivalent doses of niacin ER (Niaspan); do not substitute for equivalent doses of IR (crystalline) niacin. Dose-related myopathy and/or rhabdomyolysis reported; predisposing factors include advanced age (≥65 yrs of age), female gender, uncontrolled hypothyroidism, and renal impairment. Immune-mediated necrotizing myopathy (IMNM) reported. D/C if markedly elevated CPK levels occur or myopathy is diagnosed/suspected, and temporarily withhold in any patient experiencing an acute or serious condition predisposing to development of renal failure secondary to rhabdomyolysis. Stop treatment for a few days before elective major surgery and when any major acute medical/surgical condition supervenes. Severe hepatic toxicity, including fulminant hepatic necrosis, reported when substituting sustained-release niacin for IR niacin at equivalent doses. Caution with substantial alcohol consumption and/or history of liver disease. May cause abnormal LFTs; obtain LFTs prior to initiation and repeat as clinically indicated. Fatal and nonfatal hepatic failure (rare) reported; promptly interrupt therapy if serious liver injury with clinical symptoms and/or hyperbilirubinemia or jaundice occurs and do not restart if no alternate etiology found. Increases in HbA1c and FPG levels reported; closely monitor diabetic/potentially diabetic patients (particularly during 1st few months of therapy), and adjust diet and/or hypoglycemic therapy or d/c Simcor if necessary.

May reduce platelet count or phosphorus (P) levels, and increase PT or uric acid levels. Caution in patients predisposed to gout, with renal impairment, and in elderly.

ADVERSE REACTIONS

Flushing, headache, back pain, diarrhea, nausea, pruritus.

DRUG INTERACTIONS

See Contraindications. Avoid ingestion of alcohol, hot drinks, or spicy foods around the time of administration; may increase flushing and pruritus. Simvastatin: Due to the risk of myopathy, avoid with large quantities of grapefruit juice (>1 quart/day) and drugs that cause myopathy/rhabdomyolysis when given alone (eg, fibrates); caution with colchicine; do not exceed 1000mg-20mg/day with amiodarone, amlodipine, and ranolazine. Voriconazole may increase concentration; consider dose adjustment of Simcor to reduce risk of myopathy/rhabdomyolysis. Decreased C_{max} with propranolol. May increase digoxin concentrations; monitor patients taking digoxin when therapy is initiated. May potentiate effect of coumarin anticoagulants; determine PT before initiation and frequently during therapy. Niacin: ASA may decrease metabolic clearance. May potentiate effects of ganglionic blocking agents and vasoactive drugs, resulting in postural hypotension. Separate administration from bile acid-binding resins (eg, colestipol, cholestyramine) by at least 4-6 hrs. Nutritional supplements containing large doses of niacin or related compounds may potentiate adverse effects.

NURSING CONSIDERATIONS

Assessment: Assess for history of/active liver disease, unexplained persistent hepatic transaminase elevations, active PUD, arterial bleeding, predisposing factors for myopathy, renal impairment, diabetes, any other conditions where treatment is contraindicated or cautioned, drug hypersensitivity, pregnancy/nursing status, and possible drug interactions. Assess lipid profile and LFTs.

Monitoring: Monitor for signs/symptoms of myopathy (including IMNM), rhabdomyolysis, liver/renal dysfunction, decreases in platelet counts and P levels, increases in PT and uric acid levels, and other adverse reactions. Monitor lipid profile, LFTs, blood glucose, and CPK levels. Check PT with coumarin anticoagulants.

Patient Counseling: Advise to adhere to their National Cholesterol Education Program-recommended diet, a regular exercise program, and periodic testing of a fasting lipid panel. Inform about substances that should be avoided during therapy, and advise to discuss all medications, both prescription and OTC, including vitamins or other nutritional supplements containing niacin or nicotinamide, with their physician. Instruct to report promptly any unexplained muscle pain, tenderness, or weakness, particularly if accompanied by malaise or fever or if these muscle signs or symptoms persist after discontinuation, any symptoms that may indicate liver injury, or if symptoms of dizziness occur. Advise to notify physician prior to restarting therapy if dosing is interrupted for any length of time, and of changes in blood glucose if diabetic. Inform that flushing may occur but may subside after several weeks of consistent use of therapy. If awakened by flushing at night, instruct to get up slowly, especially if feeling dizzy or faint, or taking BP medications. Instruct women to use an effective method of birth control to prevent pregnancy while on therapy, to d/c therapy and call physician if pregnant, and not to breastfeed while on therapy.

Storage: 20-25°C (68-77°F).

SIMPONI – golimumab

RX

Class: Monoclonal antibody/TNF-blocker

Increased risk for developing serious infections (eg, active TB, latent TB reactivation, invasive fungal infections, bacterial/viral infections, opportunistic infections) leading to hospitalization or death, mostly w/ concomitant use of immunosuppressants (eg, methotrexate [MTX] or corticosteroids). D/C if serious infection develops. Active TB/latent TB reactivation may present w/ disseminated or extrapulmonary disease; test for latent TB before and during therapy and initiate treatment for latent TB prior to therapy. Invasive fungal infections reported; consider empiric antifungal therapy in patients at risk who develop severe systemic illness. Monitor patients for development of infection during and after treatment, including development of TB in patients who tested (-) for latent TB infection prior to therapy. Lymphoma and other malignancies, some fatal, reported in children and adolescents.

ADULT DOSAGE

Ulcerative Colitis

Moderately to Severely Active:
Initial (Week 0): 200mg SQ
Week 2: 100mg SQ
Maint: 100mg SQ every 4 weeks

Rheumatoid Arthritis

Moderately to Severely Active in Combination w/ MTX:
50mg SQ once a month

PEDIATRIC DOSAGE

Pediatric use may not have been established

Psoriatic Arthritis

W/ or w/o MTX or Other Nonbiologic Disease Modifying Antirheumatic Drugs:
50mg SQ once a month

Ankylosing Spondylitis

W/ or w/o MTX or Other Nonbiologic Disease Modifying Antirheumatic Drugs:
50mg SQ once a month

ADMINISTRATION

SQ route
Allow the prefilled syringe or autoinjector to sit at room temperature outside the carton for 30 min prior to SQ inj. Do not warm in any other way
If multiple inj are required, administer the inj at different sites on the body
Rotate inj sites; avoid areas where skin is tender, bruised, red, or hard
Refer to PI for further instructions

HOW SUPPLIED

Inj: 50mg/0.5mL, 100mg/mL [prefilled SmartJect autoinjector, prefilled syringe]

WARNINGS/PRECAUTIONS

Do not initiate in patients w/ an active infection. Increased risk of infection in patients >65 yrs of age and in patients w/ comorbid conditions. Hepatitis B virus (HBV) reactivation reported in chronic carriers; closely monitor for signs of active HBV infection during and for several months after therapy. D/C if reactivation occurs and initiate antiviral therapy. Consider risks and benefits prior to initiating therapy in patients w/ a known malignancy other than a successfully treated nonmelanoma skin cancer or when considering continuing therapy in patients who develop a malignancy. Rare postmarketing cases of hepatosplenic T-cell lymphoma reported. All patients w/ ulcerative colitis (UC) who are at increased risk for dysplasia or colon carcinoma, or who had a prior history of dysplasia or colon carcinoma should be screened for dysplasia at regular intervals before therapy and throughout their disease course. Melanoma and Merkel cell carcinoma reported. Worsening/new onset CHF reported; d/c if new or worsening symptoms of CHF appear. New onset or exacerbation of CNS (eg, multiple sclerosis)/peripheral (eg, Guillain-Barre syndrome) demyelinating disorders reported; consider discontinuation if these disorders develop. Caution when switching from one biological product to another biological product; overlapping biological activity may further increase risk of infection. Hematologic cytopenias (eg, neutropenia, aplastic anemia) reported. Serious systemic hypersensitivity reactions reported; d/c immediately if these reactions occur. Caution in elderly.

ADVERSE REACTIONS

Serious infection, malignancies, upper respiratory tract infection, inj-site reactions, HTN, increased ALT/AST.

DRUG INTERACTIONS

See Boxed Warning. Not recommended w/ anakinra, abatacept, or biologics approved to treat RA, psoriatic arthritis, or ankylosing spondylitis; may increase risk of serious infections. Avoid w/ live vaccines and therapeutic infectious agents (eg, live attenuated bacteria [eg, BCG bladder instillation for the treatment of cancer]). Avoid administration of live vaccines to infants for 6 months following the mother's last golimumab inj during pregnancy. Upon initiation or discontinuation of therapy in patients being treated w/ CYP450 substrates w/ a narrow therapeutic index, monitor effect (eg, warfarin) or drug concentration (eg, cyclosporine, theophylline) and may adjust individual dose of the drug product as needed.

NURSING CONSIDERATIONS

Assessment: Assess for active/chronic/recurrent infection, history of an opportunistic infection, recent travel to areas of endemic TB or endemic mycoses, underlying conditions that may predispose to infection, malignancies, dysplasia (in UC patients), CHF, demyelinating disorders, significant cytopenias, latex sensitivity, risk factors for skin cancer, pregnancy/nursing status, and possible drug interactions. Test for latent TB infection and for HBV infection.

Monitoring: Monitor for development of infection during and after treatment. Monitor for HBV reactivation, malignancies, dysplasia, new or worsening CHF, demyelinating disorders, hematological events, hypersensitivity reactions, and other adverse reactions. Periodically evaluate for active TB and test for latent TB infection. Perform periodic skin examination, particularly in patients w/ risk factors for skin cancer.

Patient Counseling: Advise of the potential risks and benefits of therapy. Inform that therapy may lower the ability of immune system to fight infections; instruct to contact physician if any symptoms of infection develop. Counsel about the risk of lymphoma and other malignancies. Instruct patients sensitive to latex to not handle the needle cover on the prefilled syringe as well as the needle cover of the prefilled syringe w/in the autoinjector cap because it contains dry natural rubber (a derivative of latex). Advise to report any signs of new/worsening medical conditions (eg, CHF, demyelinating disorders, autoimmune diseases, liver disease, cytopenias, psoriasis).

Storage: 2-8°C (36-46°F). Protect from light. Do not freeze or shake.

SIMPONI ARIA – golimumab RX

Class: Monoclonal antibody/TNF-blocker

Increased risk for developing serious infections (eg, active tuberculosis [TB], latent TB reactivation, invasive fungal infections, bacterial/viral infections, and opportunistic infections) leading to hospitalization or death, mostly with concomitant use with immunosuppressants (eg, methotrexate [MTX] or corticosteroids). D/C if serious infection develops. Active/latent reactivation TB may present with disseminated or extrapulmonary disease; test for latent TB before and during therapy and initiate treatment for latent TB prior to therapy. Invasive fungal infections reported; consider empiric antifungal therapy in patients at risk who develop severe systemic illness. Consider risks and benefits prior to therapy in patients with chronic or recurrent infection. Monitor patients for development of infection during and after treatment, including development of TB in patients who tested (-) for latent TB infection prior to therapy. Lymphoma and other malignancies, some fatal, reported in children and adolescents.

ADULT DOSAGE

Rheumatoid Arthritis

Moderately to Severely Active in Combination w/ MTX:
2mg/kg IV at Weeks 0 and 4, then every 8 weeks thereafter

PEDIATRIC DOSAGE

Pediatric use may not have been established

ADMINISTRATION

IV route

Use only an infusion set w/ an in-line, sterile, non-pyrogenic, low protein-binding filter (pore size 0.22μM or less)
Dilute w/ 0.9% w/v NaCl to a final volume of 100mL. Gently mix
Infuse diluted sol over 30 min
Do not infuse concomitantly in the same IV line w/ other agents
Refer to PI for further administration instructions

HOW SUPPLIED

Inj: 50mg/4mL

WARNINGS/PRECAUTIONS

Do not initiate in patients with an active infection. Increased risk of infection in patients >65 yrs of age and in patients with comorbid conditions; consider the risks and benefits prior to therapy in patients who have resided or traveled in areas of endemic TB or endemic mycoses, and with any underlying conditions predisposing to infection. Hepatitis B virus (HBV) reactivation reported in chronic carriers; closely monitor for signs of active HBV infection during and for several months after therapy. D/C if reactivation occurs and initiate antiviral therapy. Consider risks and benefits prior to initiating therapy in patients with a known malignancy other than a successfully treated non-melanoma skin cancer or when considering continuing therapy in patients who develop a malignancy. Rare postmarketing cases of hepatosplenic T-cell lymphoma reported. Melanoma and Merkel cell carcinoma reported. Worsening and new onset congestive heart failure (CHF) reported; caution with CHF, d/c if new/worsening symptoms appear. Associated with rare cases of new onset or exacerbation of CNS (eg, multiple sclerosis) and peripheral (eg, Guillain-Barre syndrome) demyelinating disorders; consider discontinuation if these disorders develop. Caution when switching from one biologic product to another biologic product; overlapping biological activity may further increase risk of infection. Pancytopenia, leukopenia, neutropenia, aplastic anemia, and thrombocytopenia reported; caution in patients who have or have had significant cytopenias. Serious systemic hypersensitivity reactions may occur; d/c immediately and institute appropriate therapy if these reactions occur. Caution in elderly.

ADVERSE REACTIONS

Serious infection, malignancies, upper respiratory tract infection, viral infections, bronchitis, HTN, rash.

DRUG INTERACTIONS

See Boxed Warning. MTX decreases clearance. Not recommended with anakinra, abatacept, or biologics approved to treat RA; may increase risk of serious infections. Avoid with live vaccines and therapeutic infectious agents (eg, live attenuated bacteria [eg, BCG bladder instillation for the treatment of cancer]). Avoid administration of live vaccines to infants for 6 months following the mother's last golimumab infusion during pregnancy. Upon initiation or discontinuation of therapy in patients being treated with CYP450 substrates with a narrow therapeutic index, monitor effect (eg, warfarin) or drug concentration (eg, cyclosporine, theophylline) and adjust individual dose of the drug product as needed.

NURSING CONSIDERATIONS

Assessment: Assess for active/chronic/recurrent infection, history of an opportunistic infection, recent travel to areas of endemic TB or endemic mycoses, underlying conditions that may predispose to infection, malignancies, CHF, demyelinating disorders, significant cytopenias, risk factors for skin cancer, pregnancy/nursing status, and possible drug interactions. Test for latent TB infection and for HBV infection.

Monitoring: Monitor for development of infection during and after treatment. Monitor for HBV reactivation, malignancies, new or worsening CHF, demyelinating disorders, hematological events, hypersensitivity reactions, and other adverse reactions. Periodically evaluate for active TB and test for latent TB infection. Perform periodic skin examination, particularly in patients with risk factors for skin cancer.

Patient Counseling: Advise of the potential risks and benefits of therapy. Inform that therapy may lower the ability of immune system to fight infections; instruct to contact physician if any symptoms of infection develop. Counsel about the risk of lymphoma and other malignancies. Advise to report any signs of new/worsening medical conditions (eg, CHF, demyelinating disorders, autoimmune diseases, liver disease, cytopenias, psoriasis).

Storage: 2-8°C (36-46°F). Protect from light. Do not freeze or shake. Diluted Sol: May be stored for 4 hrs at room temperature.

SINEMET CR – carbidopa/levodopa

RX

Class: Dopa-decarboxylase inhibitor/dopamine precursor

OTHER BRAND NAMES

Sinemet

ADULT DOSAGE

Parkinsonism

Treatment of Parkinson's Disease, Postencephalitic Parkinsonism, and Symptomatic Parkinsonism Following Carbon Monoxide/Manganese Intoxication:

Tab:

Usual Dose:

Initial: One 25mg-100mg tab tid or one 10mg-100mg tab tid-qid

Titrate: May increase by 1 tab (25mg-100mg or 10mg-100mg) qd or qod, as necessary, until a dose of 8 tabs/day is reached

Transfer from Levodopa:

D/C levodopa at least 12 hrs before starting therapy; choose a daily dose of therapy that will provide approx 25% of the previous levodopa dose

Previously Taking <1500mg/day of Levodopa:

Initial: One 25mg-100mg tab tid or qid

Previously Taking >1500mg/day of Levodopa:

Initial: One 25mg-250mg tab tid or qid

Maint:

At least 70-100mg/day of carbidopa should be provided; may substitute one 25mg-100mg tab for each 10mg-100mg tab when greater proportion of carbidopa is required

When more levodopa is required, substitute 25mg-250mg tab for 25mg-100mg or 10mg-100mg; may increase dose of 25mg-250mg by 1/2 or 1 tab qd or qod to a max of 8 tabs/day if necessary

Max: 200mg/day of carbidopa

Tab, Sustained-Release (SR):

Initial Dosage:

Currently Treated w/ Conventional Carbidopa Levodopa Preparations:

Dosage w/ SR tabs should be substituted at an amount that provides approx 10% more levodopa per day. May need to increase to a

PEDIATRIC DOSAGE

Pediatric use may not have been established

dose that provides up to 30% more levodopa per day depending on clinical response; interval between doses should be 4-8 hrs during the waking day

Initial Conversion from IR to SR Tabs (Based on Levodopa Component):
300-400mg: 200mg bid
500-600mg: 300mg bid or 200mg tid
700-800mg: Total of 800mg in ≥3 divided doses (eg, 300mg am, 300mg early pm, and 200mg later pm)
900-1000mg: Total of 1000mg in ≥3 divided doses (eg, 400mg am, 400mg early pm, and 200mg later pm)

Currently Treated w/ Levodopa w/o a Decarboxylase Inhibitor:
D/C levodopa at least 12 hrs before starting therapy; substitute at a dose that will provide approx 25% of the previous levodopa dose

Mild to Moderate Disease:
Initial: One 50mg-200mg tab bid

Patients Not Receiving Levodopa:
Mild to Moderate Disease:
Initial: One 50mg-200mg tab bid at ≥6-hr intervals

Titration:
Following therapy initiation, may increase/decrease doses and dosing intervals depending on response
Most patients have been adequately treated w/ doses that provide 400-1600mg/day of levodopa given in divided doses at 4- to 8-hr intervals during the waking day
When given at intervals of <4 hrs, and/or if the divided doses are not equal, give the smaller doses at the end of the day
An interval of at least 3 days between dosage adjustments is recommended

DOSE MODIFICATION

Concomitant Medications

Addition of Other Antiparkinsonian Medications:
Tab/Tab, Sustained-Release (SR):
Standard drugs for Parkinson's disease, other than levodopa w/o a decarboxylase inhibitor, may be used concomitantly w/ therapy, although their dosage may have to be adjusted

Tab, SR:
Anticholinergic agents, dopamine agonists, and amantadine may be given w/ therapy; dosage adjustment of therapy may be necessary when these agents are added
A dose of 25mg-100mg IR or 10mg-100mg IR (1/2 tab or whole tab) may be added to the dosage regimen in selected patients w/ advanced disease who need additional IR levodopa for a brief time during daytime hrs

Interruption of Therapy:
Tab/Tab, SR:
If general anesthesia is required, may continue therapy as long as patient is permitted to take fluids and medication by mouth. If therapy is interrupted temporarily, observe for symptoms resembling neuroleptic malignant syndrome and administer usual daily dose as soon as patient is able to take oral medication

Adverse Reactions
Tab:
Involuntary movements may require dosage reduction

ADMINISTRATION

Oral route

Tab
Tabs w/ different ratios of carbidopa to levodopa may be given separately or combined as needed to provide the optimum dosage

Tab, Sustained-Release
Do not chew or crush

HOW SUPPLIED
(Carbidopa-Levodopa) Tab, Sustained-Release (SR) (CR): 25mg-100mg, 50mg-200mg; (Sinemet) Tab: 10mg-100mg, 25mg-100mg, 25mg-250mg

CONTRAINDICATIONS
During or within 2 weeks of using nonselective MAOIs. Narrow-angle glaucoma.

WARNINGS/PRECAUTIONS
May cause or increase dyskinesias; may require dose reduction. Monitor for depression with concomitant suicidal tendencies. Caution with severe cardiovascular (CV) or pulmonary disease, bronchial asthma, renal/hepatic/endocrine disease, chronic wide-angle glaucoma, or history of MI with residual atrial, nodal, or ventricular arrhythmias. May increase the possibility of upper GI hemorrhage in patients with history of peptic ulcer. Falling asleep during activities of daily living and somnolence reported; consider discontinuation if significant daytime sleepiness or episodes of falling asleep during activities that require active participation occur. May impair mental/physical abilities. Sporadic cases of a symptom complex resembling neuroleptic malignant syndrome (hyperpyrexia and confusion) reported during dose reductions or withdrawal; observed carefully when the dosage of levodopa is reduced abruptly or discontinued, especially if the patient is receiving neuroleptics. Hallucinations and psychotic-like behavior reported; do not use in patients with a major psychotic disorder. Intense urge to gamble, increased sexual urges, intense urges to spend money, binge eating, and/or other intense urges, and the inability to control these urges may occur; consider dose reduction or discontinuation if such urges develop. Monitor for melanomas frequently and on a regular basis. Abnormalities in lab tests, including elevations of LFTs, and abnormalities in BUN and (+) Coombs test reported. Lab test interactions may occur. Cases of falsely diagnosed pheochromocytoma reported very rarely; caution when interpreting the plasma and urine levels of catecholamines and their metabolites. Caution in elderly.

ADVERSE REACTIONS
Dyskinesias (eg, choreiform, dystonic, other involuntary movements), nausea, hallucinations, confusion.

DRUG INTERACTIONS
See Contraindications. Caution with concomitant use of sedating medications; may increase the risk for somnolence. Certain medications used to treat psychosis may exacerbate the symptoms of Parkinson's disease and may decrease effectiveness of carbidopa-levodopa. Symptomatic postural hypotension reported with concomitant use of some antihypertensive drugs; dosage adjustment of the antihypertensive drug may be required. Use with selegiline may cause severe orthostatic hypotension. Adverse reactions, including HTN and dyskinesia, reported rarely with TCAs. Dopamine D_2 receptor antagonists (eg, phenothiazines, butyrophenones, risperidone) and isoniazid may reduce effects of levodopa. Beneficial effects of levodopa in Parkinson's disease reported to be reversed by phenytoin and papaverine; monitor for loss of therapeutic response. Not recommended with dopamine-depleting agents (eg, reserpine, tetrabenazine) or other drugs known to deplete monoamine stores. Iron salts may reduce bioavailability; caution with iron salts or multivitamins containing iron salts. Metoclopramide may increase bioavailability of levodopa and may also adversely affect disease control.

NURSING CONSIDERATIONS

Assessment: Assess for hypersensitivity to drug; narrow-angle/chronic wide-angle glaucoma; major psychotic disorder; history of peptic ulcer; risk factors that may increase risk for somnolence (eg, presence of sleep disorders); severe CV or pulmonary disease; bronchial asthma; renal/hepatic/endocrine disease; history of MI with residual atrial, nodal, or ventricular arrhythmias; pregnancy/nursing status; and possible drug interactions.

Monitoring: Monitor for dyskinesias, depression with suicidal tendencies, drowsiness/sleepiness, somnolence, hyperpyrexia and confusion, hallucinations/psychotic-like behavior, impulse control/compulsive behaviors, upper GI hemorrhage in patients with a history of peptic ulcer, and other adverse reactions. In patients with a history of MI who have residual atrial, nodal, or ventricular arrhythmias, monitor cardiac function with particular care during the period of initial dosage adjustment. Monitor for LFT elevations and BUN abnormalities. For patients on extended therapy, perform periodic evaluation of hepatic, hematopoietic, CV, and renal function. Monitor for melanomas frequently and on a regular basis. Monitor for changes in intraocular pressure in patients with chronic wide-angle glaucoma. Monitor closely during the dose adjustment period.

Patient Counseling: Instruct to take ud and not to change the prescribed dosage regimen or add any additional antiparkinson medications, including other carbidopa-levodopa preparations, without 1st consulting the physician. Inform that, occasionally, dark color (red, brown, or black) may appear in saliva, urine, or sweat after ingestion of therapy. Inform that high protein diet, excessive acidity, and iron salts may reduce clinical effectiveness. Instruct to exercise caution while driving or operating machinery, and that if somnolence and/or sudden sleep onset is experienced, to refrain from these activities. Instruct to inform physician if new/increased gambling urges, increased sexual urges, or other intense urges develop. (Tab, IR) Advise that sometimes a "wearing-off" effect may occur at the end of the dosing interval; instruct to notify physician if such response poses a problem to lifestyle. (Tab, SR) Instruct to notify physician if abnormal involuntary movements appear or get worse during treatment. Advise that sometimes the onset of effect of the 1st am dose may be delayed for up to 1 hr compared with the response usually obtained from the 1st am dose of IR tab; instruct to notify physician if such delayed responses pose a problem in treatment.

Storage: 25°C (77°F); excursions permitted to 15-30°C (59-86°F). Protect from light and moisture.

SINGULAIR – montelukast sodium RX

Class: Leukotriene receptor antagonist

ADULT DOSAGE

Asthma

Prophylaxis/Chronic Treatment:
10mg tab qpm
Patients w/ both asthma and allergic rhinitis should take only 1 dose qpm

Perennial Allergic Rhinitis

10mg tab qd
Patients w/ both asthma and allergic rhinitis should take only 1 dose qpm

Seasonal Allergic Rhinitis

10mg tab qd

Patients w/ both asthma and allergic rhinitis should take only 1 dose qpm

Exercise-Induced Bronchospasm

Prevention:
10mg tab at least 2 hrs before exercise
Do not take an additional dose w/in 24 hrs of a previous dose

PEDIATRIC DOSAGE

Asthma

Prophylaxis/Chronic Treatment:
12-23 Months:
4mg granules qpm
2-5 Years:
4mg chewable tab or 4mg granules qpm
6-14 Years:
5mg chewable tab qpm
≥15 Years:
10mg tab qpm

Patients w/ both asthma and allergic rhinitis should take only 1 dose qpm

Perennial Allergic Rhinitis

6-23 Months:
4mg granules qd
2-5 Years:
4mg chewable tab or 4mg granules qd
6-14 Years:
5mg chewable tab qd
≥15 Years:
10mg tab qd

Patients w/ both asthma and allergic rhinitis should take only 1 dose qpm

Seasonal Allergic Rhinitis

2-5 Years:
4mg chewable tab or 4mg granules qd
6-14 Years:
5mg chewable tab qd
≥15 Years:
10mg tab qd
Patients w/ both asthma and allergic rhinitis should take only 1 dose qpm

Exercise-Induced Bronchospasm

Prevention:
6-14 Years:
5mg chewable tab at least 2 hrs before exercise
≥15 Years:
10mg tab at least 2 hrs before exercise
Do not take an additional dose w/in 24 hrs of a previous dose

ADMINISTRATION

Oral route

Refer to PI for instructions for administration of granules

HOW SUPPLIED

Granules: 4mg/pkt; Tab, Chewable: 4mg, 5mg; Tab: 10mg

WARNINGS/PRECAUTIONS

Not for use in the reversal of bronchospasm in acute asthma attacks, including status asthmaticus; have appropriate rescue medication available. Therapy may be continued during acute exacerbations of asthma. Patients who have exacerbations of asthma after exercise should have short-acting inhaled β-agonist available for rescue. Should not be abruptly substituted for inhaled or oral corticosteroids. Eosinophilic conditions reported. Neuropsychiatric events reported; evaluate risks and benefits of continuing treatment if such events occur. Chewable tabs contain phenylalanine; caution with phenylketonuria. Avoid aspirin (ASA) and NSAIDs with known ASA sensitivity; has not been shown to truncate bronchoconstrictor response to ASA and other NSAIDs in ASA-sensitive asthmatic patients.

ADVERSE REACTIONS

Headache, pharyngitis, influenza, fever, sinusitis, diarrhea, URTI, cough, abdominal pain, otitis media, rhinorrhea, otitis.

NURSING CONSIDERATIONS

Assessment: Assess for hypersensitivity to drug, phenylketonuria, asthma status, pregnancy/nursing status, and possible drug interactions.

Monitoring: Monitor for signs/symptoms of eosinophilia, vasculitic rash, worsening pulmonary symptoms, cardiac complications, neuropathy, neuropsychiatric events, hypersensitivity reactions, and other adverse reactions.

Patient Counseling: Advise to take daily as prescribed, even when asymptomatic, as well as during periods of worsening asthma; instruct to contact physician if asthma is not well controlled. Inform that drug is not for treatment of acute asthma attacks; advise to have appropriate short-acting inhaled β-agonist medication available to treat asthma exacerbations. Advise to seek medical attention if short-acting inhaled bronchodilators are needed more than usual while on therapy or if more than the max number of inhalations of short-acting bronchodilator treatment prescribed for a 24-hr period are needed. Instruct not to decrease dose or d/c other antiasthma medications unless instructed by physician. Instruct to notify physician if symptoms of neuropsychiatric events occur. Advise patients with ASA sensitivity to continue avoiding ASA and NSAIDs while on therapy. Inform phenylketonuric patients that the 4mg and 5mg chewable tabs contain phenylalanine.

Storage: 25°C (77°F); excursions permitted to 15-30°C (59-86°F). Protect from light and moisture.

SIRTURO – bedaquiline — RX

Class: Antibacterial agent

Increased risk of death reported; only use when an effective treatment regimen cannot otherwise be provided. QT prolongation may occur. Use with drugs that prolong the QT interval may cause additive QT prolongation.

ADULT DOSAGE

Tuberculosis

As part of combination therapy in adults w/ pulmonary multidrug resistant tuberculosis, for use when an effective treatment regimen cannot otherwise be provided

Usual:

Weeks 1-2: 400mg qd w/ food

Weeks 3-24: 200mg 3X/week w/ food (w/ at least 48 hrs between doses)

Total Treatment Duration: 24 weeks

Missed Dose

If a dose is missed during the first 2 weeks of treatment, do not make up the missed dose but continue the usual dosing schedule

From Week 3 onwards, if 200mg dose is missed, take the missed dose as soon as possible, and then resume the 3X/week regimen

PEDIATRIC DOSAGE

Pediatric use may not have been established

ADMINISTRATION

Oral route

Take w/ food; swallow tab whole w/ water

HOW SUPPLIED

Tab: 100mg

WARNINGS/PRECAUTIONS

Not recommended for the treatment of latent infection due to *Mycobacterium tuberculosis*, drug-sensitive TB, extra-pulmonary TB, and infections caused by non-TB mycobacteria. Therapy should only be administered by directly observed therapy and in combination with at least 3 other drugs to which the patient's MDR-TB isolate is susceptible. If in vitro testing results are unavailable, may initiate treatment in combination with at least 4 other drugs to which patient's MDR-TB isolate is likely susceptible. Throughout treatment, and following the last intake, continue to take the companion drugs ud. Obtain serum electrolytes (serum K^+, Ca^+, and Mg^+) at baseline, correct levels if abnormal, and monitor if QT prolongation is detected. Caution with history of torsades de pointes, congenital long QT syndrome, hypothyroidism and bradyarrhythmias, uncompensated heart failure (HF), serum Ca^+, Mg^+, or K^+ levels below the lower limits of normal; monitor ECG closely. D/C treatment and all other QT prolonging drugs if clinically significant ventricular arrhythmia or QTcF interval of >500ms (confirmed by repeat ECG) develops. If syncope occurs, obtain an ECG to detect QT prolongation. Hepatic-related adverse drug reactions reported. Test for viral hepatitis and d/c other hepatotoxic drugs if serum aminotransferases >3X ULN (repeat testing within 48 hours). D/C if aminotransferase elevations with total bilirubin >2X ULN, aminotransferase elevations >8X ULN, or aminotransferase elevations persist >2 weeks. Isolates from patients who fail to convert or relapse following treatment should be tested for bedaquiline minimum inhibitory concentrations. Caution with severe hepatic impairment, and/or severe renal impairment requiring hemodialysis or peritoneal dialysis.

ADVERSE REACTIONS

QT prolongation, nausea, arthralgia, headache, increased transaminases, hemoptysis, chest pain, anorexia, rash.

DRUG INTERACTIONS

See Boxed Warning. More hepatic-related adverse drug reactions were reported with the addition of other drugs used to treat TB. Avoid use with alcohol, other hepatotoxic drugs, rifamycins (eg, rifampin, rifapentine, rifabutin) or other strong CYP3A4 inducers, and use for >14 consecutive days of strong CYP3A4 inhibitors (eg, ketoconazole) unless benefit outweighs the risk. Caution when coadministered with lopinavir/ritonavir. Refer to PI for additional drug interaction information.

NURSING CONSIDERATIONS

Assessment: Assess for history of torsades de pointes, congenital long QT syndrome, hypothyroidism, bradyarrhythmias, uncompensated HF, low serum electrolyte (Ca^+, Mg^+, or K^+) levels, severe hepatic impairment, or severe renal impairment requiring hemodialysis or peritoneal dialysis, pregnancy/nursing status, and possible drug reactions. Obtain baseline ECG, serum electrolytes, ALT, AST, alkaline phosphatase, and bilirubin.

Monitoring: Monitor for evidence of new/worsening liver dysfunction, syncope, QT interval prolongation and other adverse reactions. Obtain ECG at least 2, 12, and 24 weeks after starting treatment. Monitor ECGs frequently to confirm that the QTc interval has returned to baseline. Perform follow-up monitoring of electrolytes. Perform laboratory tests (ALT, AST, alkaline phosphatase, and bilirubin) monthly while on treatment, and PRN.

Patient Counseling: Advise of the need to take ud; emphasize compliance with the full course of therapy. Inform about serious adverse reactions (eg, death, heart rhythm abnormalities, and/or hepatitis) and other potential side effects (eg, nausea, joint pain, headache). Advise about instruction for missed dose. Instruct to abstain from alcohol, hepatotoxic drugs, or herbal products. Advise to consult with physician about other drugs taken, other medical conditions, or if patient has a personal/family history of congenital QT prolongation or HF.

Storage: 25°C (77°F); excursions permitted to 15-30°C (59-86°F).

SIVEXTRO – tedizolid phosphate — RX

Class: Oxazolidinone class antibacterial

ADULT DOSAGE

Skin and Skin Structure Infections

Acute bacterial infections caused by *Staphylococcus aureus* (including methicillin-resistant and methicillin-susceptible isolates), *Streptococcus pyogenes, Streptococcus agalactiae, Streptococcus anginosus* Group (including *Streptococcus anginosus, Streptococcus intermedius,* and *Streptococcus constellatus*), and *Enterococcus faecalis*

IV:
200mg qd infused over 1 hr for 6 days

Oral:
200mg qd for 6 days

PEDIATRIC DOSAGE

Pediatric use may not have been established

ADMINISTRATION
Oral/IV route

No dose adjustment is necessary when changing from IV to oral route
If patients miss a dose, they should take it as soon as possible anytime up to 8 hrs prior to their next scheduled dose; if <8 hrs remain before the next dose, wait until their next scheduled dose

Preparation of IV Sol
1. Reconstitute the vial w/ 4mL of SWFI
2. Gently swirl the contents and let the vial stand until the cake has completely dissolved and any foam disperses
3. Inspect the vial to ensure the sol contains no particulate matter and no cake or powder remains attached to the sides of the vial; if necessary, invert the vial to dissolve any remaining powder and swirl gently to prevent foaming
4. Tilt the upright vial and insert a syringe w/ appropriately sized needle into the bottom corner of the vial and remove 4mL of the reconstituted sol; do not invert the vial during extraction
5. The reconstituted sol must be further diluted in 250mL of 0.9% NaCl Inj. Slowly inject the 4mL of reconstituted sol into a 250mL bag of 0.9% NaCl Inj and invert the bag gently to mix; do not shake the bag

Administration of IV Sol
Administer as an IV infusion only
Incompatibilities:
1. Any sol containing divalent cations (eg, Ca^{2+}, Mg^{2+}), including Lactated Ringer's Inj and Hartmann's Sol
2. Do not add other IV substances, additives, or other medications to the single-use vials or infuse simultaneously; if the same IV line is used for sequential infusion of several different drugs, the line should be flushed before and after infusion of tedizolid phosphate w/ 0.9% NaCl Inj

HOW SUPPLIED
Inj/Tab: 200mg

WARNINGS/PRECAUTIONS
Consider alternative therapies when treating patients with neutropenia and acute bacterial skin and skin structure infections. *Clostridium difficile*-associated diarrhea (CDAD) reported; d/c if CDAD is suspected or confirmed. May result in bacterial resistance if used in the absence of proven or suspected bacterial infection or a prophylactic indication.

ADVERSE REACTIONS
N/V, headache, diarrhea.

NURSING CONSIDERATIONS

Assessment: Assess for neutropenia, pregnancy/nursing status, and possible drug interactions.

Monitoring: Monitor for CDAD and other adverse reactions.

Patient Counseling: Counsel that therapy should only be used to treat bacterial, not viral, infections. Instruct to take exactly ud even if the patient feels better early in the course of therapy. Inform that skipping doses or not completing full course of therapy may decrease effectiveness of immediate treatment and increase bacterial resistance. Inform that diarrhea is a common problem caused by therapy and usually resolves when therapy is discontinued. Instruct to contact physician if severe watery or bloody diarrhea develops.

Storage: 20-25°C (68-77°F); excursions permitted to 15-30°C (59-86°F). (Inj) Reconstituted Sol: Do not exceed 24 hrs at room temperature or under 2-8°C (36-46°F).

SKELAXIN – metaxalone RX

Class: Muscular analgesic (central-acting)

ADULT DOSAGE
Musculoskeletal Pain
Relief of Discomforts Associated w/ Acute Conditions:
800mg tid-qid

PEDIATRIC DOSAGE
Musculoskeletal Pain
Relief of Discomforts Associated w/ Acute Conditions:
>12 Years:
800mg tid-qid

ADMINISTRATION
Oral route

Taking w/ food may enhance general CNS depression

HOW SUPPLIED
Tab: 800mg* *scored

CONTRAINDICATIONS
Known tendency to drug-induced, hemolytic, and other anemias. Significantly impaired renal/hepatic function.

WARNINGS/PRECAUTIONS
Caution with preexisting liver damage; perform serial LFTs. False-(+) Benedict's tests reported; glucose-specific test will differentiate findings. Taking with food may enhance general CNS depression, especially in elderly patients.

ADVERSE REACTIONS
Drowsiness, dizziness, headache, nervousness, irritability, N/V, GI upset.

DRUG INTERACTIONS
Additive sedative effects with other CNS depressants (eg, alcohol, benzodiazepines, opioids, TCAs); use with caution if taking >1 CNS depressant simultaneously.

NURSING CONSIDERATIONS

Assessment: Assess for known tendency to drug-induced, hemolytic, or other anemias, significant renal/hepatic impairment, hypersensitivity to the drug, pregnancy/nursing status, and possible drug interactions.

Monitoring: Perform serial LFTs with preexisting liver damage. Monitor for signs/symptoms of CNS depression.

Patient Counseling: Inform that drug may impair mental and/or physical abilities required to perform hazardous tasks, especially when used with alcohol or other CNS depressants.

Storage: 15-30°C (59-86°F).

SKLICE – ivermectin **RX**

Class: Avermectin derivative

ADULT DOSAGE

Head Lice Infestations

Apply sufficient amount (up to 1 tube) to dry hair to thoroughly coat the hair and scalp

PEDIATRIC DOSAGE

Head Lice Infestations

≥6 Months:
Apply sufficient amount (up to 1 tube) to dry hair to thoroughly coat the hair and scalp

ADMINISTRATION
Topical route

Leave on hair and scalp for 10 min, then rinse off with water
The tube is intended for single use; discard any unused portion

HOW SUPPLIED
Lot: 0.5% [117g]

WARNINGS/PRECAUTIONS
Not for PO, ophthalmic, or intravaginal use. Pediatric use should be done under the direct supervision of an adult in order to prevent ingestion.

ADVERSE REACTIONS
Conjunctivitis, ocular hyperemia, eye irritation, dandruff, dry skin, skin burning sensation.

NURSING CONSIDERATIONS

Assessment: Assess for pregnancy and nursing status.

Monitoring: Monitor for conjunctivitis, ocular hyperemia, eye irritation, dandruff, dry skin, skin burning sensation, and other adverse reactions.

Patient Counseling: Instruct to apply lot to dry scalp and dry scalp hair. Instruct to avoid contact with the eyes. Instruct not to swallow lot and keep out of reach of children. Advise that use on children should be under the direct supervision of an adult. Inform that lot is for single use only; instruct not to retreat and to discard tube after use. Instruct to wash hands after application. Instruct to wash all recently worn clothing and personal care items.

Storage: 20-25°C (68-77°F); excursions permitted to 15-30°C (59-86°F). Do not freeze. Discard any unused portion.

SKYLA – levonorgestrel

Class: Progestin contraceptive

RX

ADULT DOSAGE

Contraception

Insert w/ the provided inserter into the uterine cavity during the first 7 days of the menstrual cycle or immediately after a 1st trimester abortion

Conversions

Switching to a Different Birth Control Method:

Regular Cycle:

Remove implant during the first 7 days of menstrual cycle and start the new method, or start the new method at least 7 days prior to removing implant if removal is to occur at other times during the cycle

Irregular Cycle/Amenorrhea:

Start new method at least 7 days before removal

PEDIATRIC DOSAGE

Contraception

Not indicated for use premenarche; refer to adult dosing

DOSE MODIFICATION

Other Important Modifications

Postpartum/2nd Trimester Abortions: Postpone insertion for a minimum of 6 weeks or until uterus is fully involuted

ADMINISTRATION

Intrauterine route

Consider administering analgesics prior to insertion

Remove implant if it is not positioned completely w/in the uterus; do not reinsert device once it is removed

Remove by the end of the 3rd year

If pregnancy is not desired, removal should be carried out during menstruation, provided patient is still experiencing regular menses

If removal occurs at other times during the cycle, consider starting a new contraceptive method a week prior to removal

Refer to PI for additional insertion and removal instructions

HOW SUPPLIED

Intrauterine Insert: 13.5mg

CONTRAINDICATIONS

Pregnancy or suspicion of pregnancy, congenital or acquired uterine anomaly (including fibroids if they distort the uterine cavity), acute or history of pelvic inflammatory disease (PID) (unless there has been a subsequent intrauterine pregnancy), postpartum endometritis or infected abortion in the past 3 months, known/suspected uterine or cervical neoplasia, known/suspected or history of breast cancer or other progestin-sensitive cancer, uterine bleeding of unknown etiology, untreated acute cervicitis or vaginitis (including bacterial vaginosis or other lower genital tract infections until infection is controlled), acute liver disease or liver tumor (benign or malignant), conditions associated w/ increased susceptibility to pelvic infections, and previously inserted IUD that has not been removed.

WARNINGS/PRECAUTIONS

Not for use for post-coital contraception. Should be inserted by a trained healthcare provider. Evaluate for ectopic pregnancy and remove device if pregnancy occurs w/ device in place. Increased risk of septic abortion, miscarriage, sepsis, premature delivery/labor, and possible congenital anomalies if pregnancy occurs and device is left in place. Severe infection or sepsis, including Group A streptococcal sepsis may occur; use aseptic technique during insertion of device. Associated w/ increased risk of PID and actinomycosis. May alter bleeding pattern and result in spotting, irregular bleeding, heavy bleeding, oligomenorrhea, and amenorrhea; perform appropriate diagnostic measures to rule out endometrial pathology if bleeding irregularities develop during prolonged use. Consider possibility of pregnancy if menstruation does not occur w/in 6 weeks of the onset of a previous menstruation. Perforation may occur and may reduce contraceptive effectiveness; risk increased if inserted in lactating women and may be increased if inserted when the uterus is fixed retroverted or not completely involuted during the postpartum period. Postpone insertion for a minimum of 6 weeks or until uterine involution is complete following delivery or 2nd trimester abortion. Partial or complete expulsion may occur; may be replaced w/in 7 days of a menstrual period after ruling out pregnancy. Ovarian cysts reported. Breast cancer reported w/ another levonorgestrel-releasing intrauterine system. Caution in patients w/ coagulopathy or receiving anticoagulants, migraine, focal migraine w/ asymmetrical visual loss or other symptoms indicating transient cerebral ischemia, exceptionally severe headache, marked increase in BP, and in patients w/ severe arterial disease. Consider removing device if uterine/cervical malignancy or jaundice arises during use and consider removing device if the threads are not visible or are significantly shortened; consider possibility that device may have been displaced (eg, expelled or perforated the uterus); exclude pregnancy and verify location of device. May be safely scanned on MRI only under specific conditions. MRI quality may be compromised if area of interest is in exact same area or relatively close to position of the device.

ADVERSE REACTIONS

Increased bleeding, vulvovaginitis, abdominal/pelvic pain, acne/seborrhea, ovarian cyst, headache, dysmenorrhea, breast pain/discomfort, nausea, genital discharge, device expulsion, depression.

DRUG INTERACTIONS

Drugs or herbal products that induce enzymes, including CYP3A4 that metabolize progestins (eg, barbiturates, bosentan, carbamazepine), may decrease levels. HIV protease inhibitors or non-nucleoside reverse transcriptase inhibitors may significantly increase or decrease plasma levels. CYP3A4 inhibitors (eg, itraconazole, ketoconazole) may increase plasma hormone levels.

NURSING CONSIDERATIONS

Assessment: Assess for congenital or acquired uterine anomaly, acute or history of PID, known/suspected or history of breast cancer or other progestin-sensitive cancer, acute liver disease or liver tumor, pregnancy/nursing status, any other conditions where treatment is contraindicated or cautioned, and for possible drug interactions. Perform a complete medical and social history and if indicated, a physical examination, and appropriate tests for any forms of genital or other sexually transmitted infections (STIs).

Monitoring: Monitor for intrauterine/ectopic pregnancy, sepsis, PID, actinomycosis, bleeding pattern alterations, perforation, migraine/exceptionally severe headache, jaundice, marked BP increase, and other adverse reactions. Reexamine and evaluate 4-6 weeks after insertion and once a yr thereafter, or more frequently if clinically indicated. Monitor if thread is still visible and length of thread.

Patient Counseling: Inform that product does not protect against HIV infection (AIDS) and other STDs. Inform of the risks/benefits/side effects of the device. Inform of the risk of ectopic pregnancy, including loss of fertility; instruct to promptly report symptoms of ectopic pregnancy to physician. Inform of the possibility of PID and of the symptoms of PID; instruct to promptly notify physician if any symptoms of PID develop. Inform that irregular/prolonged bleeding and spotting, and/or cramps may occur during the 1st few weeks after insertion; instruct to report to physician if symptoms continue or are severe. Instruct on how to check if the device's threads still protrude from the cervix and caution not to pull on the threads and displace device. Inform that no contraceptive protection exists if device is displaced or expelled. Instruct to contact physician if any adverse reactions develop, if pregnancy is suspected or occurs, if HIV positive seroconversion occurs in the patient or her partner, or if possible exposure to STIs occurs. Inform that device may be safely scanned w/ MRI only under specific conditions; instruct patients who will have an MRI to notify their physician that they have an IUD.

Storage: 25°C (77°F); excursions permitted to 15-30°C (59-86°F).

SOLU-CORTEF — hydrocortisone sodium succinate RX

Class: Glucocorticoid

ADULT DOSAGE

Steroid-Responsive Disorders

When oral therapy is not feasible

Initial: 100-500mg IV/IM, depending on disease being treated; administer IV over 30 sec (eg, 100mg)-10 min (eg, ≥500mg)
May repeat dose at intervals of 2, 4, or 6 hrs
High-dose therapy should be continued only until patient is stabilized, usually not beyond 48-72 hrs
Maint: After a favorable response is noted, decrease initial dose in small decrements at appropriate time intervals until lowest effective dose
Withdraw gradually after long-term therapy

Acute Exacerbations of Multiple Sclerosis:
Usual: 800mg/day for 1 week followed by 320mg qod for 1 month

PEDIATRIC DOSAGE

Steroid-Responsive Disorders

When oral therapy is not feasible

Initial: 0.56-8mg/kg/day IV/IM in 3 or 4 divided doses (20-240mg/m²BSA/day), depending on disease being treated
Maint: After a favorable response is noted, decrease initial dose in small decrements at appropriate time intervals until lowest effective dose
Withdraw gradually after long-term therapy

DOSE MODIFICATION

Elderly

Start at lower end of dosing range

ADMINISTRATION

IM/IV routes

IV inj preferred for initial emergency use; consider longer acting inj preparation or oral preparation after initial emergency period

Avoid inj into deltoid muscle

Should not be diluted or mixed w/ other sol

Preparation

IV or IM Inj:

Add not more than 2mL of bacteriostatic water for inj or bacteriostatic NaCl inj to contents of one 100mg vial

IV Infusion:

1. Add not more than 2mL of bacteriostatic water for inj to vial
2. 100mg sol may then be added to 100-1000mL of D5W (or isotonic saline sol or D5 in isotonic saline sol if patient is not on Na^+ restriction); 250mg sol may be added to 250-1000mL; 500mg sol may be added to 500-1000mL; and 1000mg sol may be added to 1000mL of same diluents
3. If administration of small volume of fluid is desirable, 100mg-3000mg may be added to 50mL of above diluents

Act-O-Vial System:

Refer to PI for directions

HOW SUPPLIED

Inj: 100mg, 250mg, 500mg, 1000mg

CONTRAINDICATIONS

Systemic fungal infections, idiopathic thrombocytopenic purpura (IM preparations), intrathecal administration.

WARNINGS/PRECAUTIONS

Serious neurologic events reported with epidural inj; not approved for epidural administration. May result in dermal and/or subdermal changes forming depressions in the skin at the inj site; avoid inj into the deltoid muscle. Anaphylactoid reactions may occur. May need to increase dose before, during, and after stressful situations. High doses should not be used for the treatment of traumatic brain injury. May cause elevation of BP, salt/water retention, and increased excretion of K^+ and Ca^{2+}; dietary salt restriction and K^+ supplementation may be necessary. Caution in patients with recent MI. Hypothalamic-pituitary-adrenal (HPA) axis suppression, Cushing's syndrome, and hyperglycemia reported; monitor with chronic use. May produce reversible HPA axis suppression with the potential for glucocorticosteroid insufficiency after withdrawal of treatment; reduce dose gradually. May cause decreased resistance and inability to localize infection. May mask some signs of current infection or cause new infections; do not use intra-articularly, intrabursally, or for intratendinous administration for local effect in the presence of acute local infection. May exacerbate systemic fungal infections; avoid use in the presence of such infections unless needed to control drug reactions. Rule out latent or active amebiasis before initiating therapy. Caution with *Strongyloides* infestation, active or latent tuberculosis (TB), CHF, HTN, renal insufficiency, osteoporosis, and ocular herpes simplex. Not for use in cerebral malaria or active ocular herpes simplex. May cause more serious/fatal course of chickenpox and measles. Severe medical events associated with intrathecal route of administration reported. May produce posterior subcapsular cataracts, glaucoma with possible damage to the optic nerves, and may enhance the establishment of secondary ocular infections due to bacteria, fungi, or viruses. Sensitive to heat; should not be autoclaved when it is desirable to sterilize the exterior of the vial. Kaposi's sarcoma reported. Caution with active or latent peptic ulcers, diverticulitis, fresh intestinal anastomoses, and nonspecific ulcerative colitis; may increase risk of perforation. Signs of peritoneal irritation following GI perforation may be minimal or absent. Enhanced effect in patients with cirrhosis. May decrease bone formation and increase bone resorption, which may lead to inhibition of bone growth in pediatric patients and development of osteoporosis at any age. Local inj into a previously infected site is not recommended. Acute myopathy with high doses reported most often in patients with disorders of neuromuscular transmission (eg, myasthenia gravis). Elevation of creatine kinase (CK) may occur. Changes in thyroid status may necessitate dose adjustment. Psychic derangements may appear and existing emotional instability or psychotic tendencies may be aggravated. May elevate intraocular pressure (IOP); monitor IOP if steroid therapy is continued for >6 weeks. May suppress reactions to skin tests. Caution in elderly.

ADVERSE REACTIONS

Bradycardia, cardiac arrest, acne, allergic dermatitis, decreased carbohydrate and glucose tolerance, fluid retention, abdominal distention, bowel/bladder dysfunction, negative nitrogen balance, aseptic necrosis of femoral and humeral heads, convulsions, emotional instability, exophthalmoses, glaucoma, abnormal fat deposits.

DRUG INTERACTIONS

Aminoglutethimide may lead to a loss of corticosteroid-induced adrenal suppression. Closely monitor for the development of hypokalemia with K^+-depleting agents (eg, amphotericin B, diuretics). Reports of cardiac enlargement and CHF with amphotericin B. Macrolide antibiotics may decrease clearance. Concomitant use with anticholinesterase agents may produce severe weakness in patients with myasthenia gravis; d/c anticholinesterase agents at least 24 hrs before initiating therapy. May inhibit response to warfarin; frequently monitor coagulation indices. May increase blood glucose levels; may require dose adjustments of antidiabetic agents. May decrease serum levels of isoniazid. Cholestyramine may increase clearance. Increased activity of both drugs may occur with cyclosporine; convulsions reported with concurrent use. May increase risk of arrhythmias with digitalis glycosides. Estrogens, including oral contraceptives, may decrease hepatic metabolism and increase effect. Drugs that induce CYP3A4 (eg, barbiturates, phenytoin, carbamazepine) may enhance metabolism and require corticosteroid dosage increase. Drugs that inhibit CYP3A4 (eg, ketoconazole, macrolide antibiotics) may increase plasma levels. Ketoconazole may increase risk of corticosteroid side effects. Aspirin (ASA) or other NSAIDs may increase risk of GI side effects; caution with ASA in hypoprothrombinemia. May increase clearance of salicylates. Administration of live or live, attenuated vaccines is contraindicated in patients receiving immunosuppressive doses. Killed or inactivated vaccines may be administered, although response is unpredictable. Acute myopathy reported with neuromuscular blocking drugs (eg, pancuronium).

NURSING CONSIDERATIONS

Assessment: Assess for hypersensitivity to drug, traumatic brain injury, CHF, renal insufficiency, systemic fungal infections, active/latent TB, vaccination status, unusual stress, ulcerative colitis, diverticulitis, HTN, recent MI, intestinal anastomoses, active or latent peptic ulcer, myasthenia gravis, psychotic tendencies, cerebral malaria, active ocular herpes simplex, any other conditions where treatment is contraindicated or cautioned, pregnancy/nursing status, and possible drug interactions.

Monitoring: Monitor for anaphylactoid reactions, dermal and/or subdermal changes, growth/development (in pediatric patients), intestinal perforation, Kaposi's sarcoma, cataracts, glaucoma, osteoporosis, and other adverse reactions. Monitor for HPA axis suppression, Cushing's syndrome, and hyperglycemia with chronic use. Monitor BP, CK, serum electrolytes, and IOP. Frequently monitor coagulation indices with warfarin.

Patient Counseling: Warn not to d/c abruptly or without medical supervision. Advise patients to inform any medical attendants that they are taking corticosteroids. Instruct to seek medical advice at once if fever or other signs of infection develop. Warn to avoid exposure to chickenpox or measles; advise to report immediately if exposed.

Storage: 20-25°C (68-77°F). Protect from light. Discard unused sol after 3 days.

SOMA – carisoprodol RX

Class: Skeletal muscle relaxant (central-acting)

ADULT DOSAGE

Musculoskeletal Conditions

Relief of Discomforts Associated w/ Acute Painful Conditions:

≥16 Years:

250-350mg tid and hs for up to 2-3 weeks

PEDIATRIC DOSAGE

Pediatric use may not have been established

ADMINISTRATION

Oral route

HOW SUPPLIED

Tab: 250mg, 350mg

CONTRAINDICATIONS

History of acute intermittent porphyria.

WARNINGS/PRECAUTIONS

May impair mental/physical abilities. Drug abuse, dependence, and withdrawal reported with prolonged use. Withdrawal symptoms reported following abrupt cessation after prolonged use. Seizures reported in postmarketing surveillance. Caution with hepatic or renal dysfunction and in addiction-prone patients. Not studied in patients >65 yrs of age.

ADVERSE REACTIONS

Drowsiness, dizziness, headache.

DRUG INTERACTIONS

Additive sedative effects with other CNS depressants (eg, alcohol, benzodiazepines, opioids, TCAs); caution when coadministering. Concomitant use with meprobamate is not recommended. Increased exposure of carisoprodol and decreased exposure of meprobamate with CYP2C19 inhibitors (eg, omeprazole, fluvoxamine). Decreased exposure of carisoprodol and increased exposure of meprobamate with CYP2C19 inducers (eg, rifampin, St. John's wort). Induction effect on CYP2C19 seen with low-dose aspirin.

NURSING CONSIDERATIONS

Assessment: Assess for acute intermittent porphyria, renal/hepatic impairment, seizures, history of addiction, use of alcohol/illegal drugs/drugs of abuse, pregnancy/nursing status, and possible drug interactions.

Monitoring: Monitor for signs/symptoms of CNS depression, drug abuse/dependence, and seizures.

Patient Counseling: Advise that drug may cause drowsiness and/or dizziness; instruct to avoid taking carisoprodol before engaging in hazardous tasks. Instruct to avoid alcohol, illegal drugs, drugs of abuse, or other CNS depressants. Inform that drug is limited to acute use. Instruct to notify physician if musculoskeletal symptoms persist. Inform of drug dependence/abuse potential.

Storage: 20-25°C (68-77°F).

SONATA — zaleplon CIV

Class: Pyrazolopyrimidine (non-benzodiazepine)

ADULT DOSAGE

Insomnia

Short-Term Treatment:

Usual: 10mg qhs; for certain low weight individuals, 5mg may be a sufficient dose

Max: 20mg

PEDIATRIC DOSAGE

Pediatric use may not have been established

DOSE MODIFICATION

Concomitant Medications

Concomitant Use w/ Cimetidine:

Initial: 5mg

Hepatic Impairment

Mild to Moderate Impairment: 5mg

Severe Impairment: Not recommended

Elderly

Elderly/Debilitated:

Usual: 5mg

Max: 10mg

ADMINISTRATION

Oral route

Take immediately before hs or after patient has gone to bed and has experienced difficulty falling asleep.

HOW SUPPLIED

Cap: 5mg, 10mg

WARNINGS/PRECAUTIONS

Initiate only after careful evaluation; failure of insomnia to remit after 7-10 days of treatment may indicate presence of a primary psychiatric and/or medical illness. Use lowest effective dose, especially in elderly. Abnormal thinking and behavior changes reported. Complex behaviors (eg, sleep-driving) reported; consider discontinuation if sleep-driving occurs. Amnesia and other neuropsychiatric symptoms may occur unpredictably. Worsening of depression, including suicidal thoughts and actions, reported in primarily depressed patients; caution with signs/symptoms of depression. Withdrawal signs/symptoms reported following rapid dose decrease or abrupt discontinuation. May impair mental/physical abilities. Severe anaphylactic and anaphylactoid reactions reported; do not rechallenge if angioedema develops. May result in short-term memory impairment, hallucinations, impaired coordination, dizziness, and lightheadedness when taken while still up and about. Caution with diseases or conditions affecting metabolism or hemodynamic responses, or with compromised respiratory function. Carefully monitor patients with compromised respiration due to preexisting illness. Not recommended for use in patients with severe hepatic impairment or in women during pregnancy. Contains tartrazine, which may cause allergic-type reactions (including bronchial asthma) in certain susceptible persons. Has an abuse potential.

Monitor patients at risk of habituation and dependence (eg, history of addiction to, or abuse of, drugs or alcohol).

ADVERSE REACTIONS
Headache, dizziness, nausea, asthenia, abdominal pain, somnolence, amnesia, eye pain, dysmenorrhea, paresthesia.

DRUG INTERACTIONS
Additive CNS depression with other psychotropic medications, anticonvulsants, antihistamines, narcotic analgesics, anesthetics, ethanol, and other CNS depressants; dosage adjustment may be necessary. Do not take with alcohol. Increased risk of complex behaviors with alcohol and other CNS depressants. Decreased C_{max} with promethazine. Decreased levels with rifampin (a potent CYP3A4 inducer); coadministration of a potent CYP3A4 inducer can lead to ineffectiveness of zaleplon. May consider alternative non-CYP3A4 substrate hypnotic agent in patients taking CYP3A4 inducers (eg, phenytoin, carbamazepine, phenobarbital). Strong selective CYP3A4 inhibitors (eg, erythromycin, ketoconazole) may increase levels. Increased levels with cimetidine; give an initial dose of 5mg.

NURSING CONSIDERATIONS

Assessment: Assess for physical and/or psychiatric disorders, medical illness, depression, diseases/conditions affecting metabolism or hemodynamic responses, compromised respiratory function, hepatic impairment, risk of habituation and dependence, hypersensitivity, pregnancy/nursing status, and possible drug interactions.

Monitoring: Monitor for complex behaviors, emergence of any new behavioral signs/symptoms, anaphylactic/anaphylactoid reactions, angioedema, abuse, habituation, dependence, withdrawal symptoms, and other adverse reactions. Monitor elderly and/or debilitated patients closely.

Patient Counseling: Inform of the risks and benefits of therapy. Caution against engaging in hazardous occupations requiring complete mental alertness (eg, operating machinery, driving). Instruct to immediately report to physician if any adverse reactions (eg, sleep-driving or other complex behaviors) occur. Instruct to notify physician if pregnant/nursing or planning to become pregnant. Instruct not to take with alcohol. Inform that taking the drug with or immediately after a heavy, high-fat meal results in slower absorption and may reduce the effect of the drug on sleep latency.

Storage: 20-25°C (68-77°F).

SOVALDI – sofosbuvir **RX**

Class: HCV nucleotide analogue NS5B polymerase inhibitor

ADULT DOSAGE

Chronic Hepatitis C

HCV Mono-Infected and HCV/HIV-1 Coinfected:

Genotype 1 or 4:
400mg qd in combination w/ peginterferon alfa and ribavirin for 12 weeks

Genotype 1 Ineligible for Interferon-Based Regimen:
400mg qd in combination w/ ribavirin for 24 weeks

Genotype 2:
400mg qd in combination w/ ribavirin for 12 weeks

Genotype 3:
400mg qd in combination w/ ribavirin for 24 weeks

Hepatocellular Carcinoma Awaiting Liver Transplantation:
400mg qd in combination w/ ribavirin for up to 48 weeks or until time of transplant, whichever occurs 1st

PEDIATRIC DOSAGE
Pediatric use may not have been established

DOSE MODIFICATION

Adverse Reactions

Genotype 1 and 4

Serious Reaction Potentially Related to Peginterferon Alfa and/or Ribavirin:
Reduce dose of or d/c peginterferon alfa and/or ribavirin; refer to each respective PI for instructions

Genotype 2 and 3
Ribavirin Dose Modification:
No Cardiac Disease:
Hgb <10g/dL: Reduce ribavirin dose to 600mg/day
Hgb <8.5g/dL: D/C ribavirin
History of Stable Cardiac Disease:
≥2g/dL Decrease in Hgb During Any 4-Week Treatment Period: Reduce ribavirin dose to 600mg/day
Hgb <12g/dL Despite 4 Weeks at Reduced Dose: D/C ribavirin

ADMINISTRATION
Oral route

Take w/ or w/o food
D/C sofosbuvir if concomitant agents are permanently discontinued

HOW SUPPLIED
Tab: 400mg

CONTRAINDICATIONS
Women who are pregnant or may become pregnant and men whose female partners are pregnant. Refer to the individual monographs for peginterferon alfa and ribavirin.

WARNINGS/PRECAUTIONS
Fatal cardiac arrest reported w/ sofosbuvir-containing regimen (ledipasvir/sofosbuvir). Women of childbearing potential and their male partners must use 2 forms of effective contraception during treatment and for at least 6 months after discontinuation; perform routine monthly pregnancy tests during this time.

ADVERSE REACTIONS
Fatigue, headache, nausea, insomnia, anemia, pruritus, asthenia, rash, decreased appetite, chills, influenza-like illness, pyrexia, diarrhea, myalgia, irritability.

DRUG INTERACTIONS
Coadministration of amiodarone w/ sofosbuvir in combination w/ another direct-acting antiviral (DAA) may result in serious symptomatic bradycardia; coadministration is not recommended. If coadministration is required, cardiac monitoring is recommended in an in-patient setting for the first 48 hrs, after which outpatient or self-monitoring of HR should occur on a daily basis for at least the first 2 weeks. Potent P-gp inducers in the intestine (eg, rifampin, St. John's wort) may significantly decrease concentration and may lead to a reduced therapeutic effect; do not use w/ rifampin and St. John's wort. P-gp and/or breast cancer resistance protein inhibitors may increase concentration. Carbamazepine, phenytoin, phenobarbital, oxcarbazepine, rifabutin, rifapentine, and tipranavir/ritonavir may decrease concentration, leading to reduced therapeutic effects; coadministration is not recommended.

NURSING CONSIDERATIONS

Assessment: Assess for pregnancy/nursing status and possible drug interactions.

Monitoring: Monitor for adverse reactions. Perform routine monthly pregnancy tests.

Patient Counseling: Advise women of childbearing potential and their male partners to use at least 2 forms of effective contraception during therapy and for at least 6 months after treatment discontinuation. Instruct to notify physician immediately in the event of a pregnancy. Encourage patients to enroll in the Ribavirin Pregnancy Registry, or the Antiretroviral Pregnancy Registry for patients who are HCV/HIV-1 coinfected and taking concomitant antiretrovirals. Inform that the effect of treatment of hepatitis C on transmission is unknown and that appropriate precautions should be taken to prevent HCV transmission during treatment or in the event of treatment failure. Advise to take ud and not to reduce dose. Advise to take drug on a regular dosing schedule. Counsel about the risk of serious symptomatic bradycardia when coadministered w/ amiodarone and another DAA; instruct to seek medical evaluation immediately if signs/symptoms of bradycardia (eg, near-fainting or fainting, dizziness or lightheadedness, malaise) develop.

Storage: Room temperature <30°C (86°F).

SPIRIVA — tiotropium bromide RX

Class: Anticholinergic bronchodilator

ADULT DOSAGE

Chronic Obstructive Pulmonary Disease

Maint Treatment of Bronchospasm Associated w/ COPD, Including Chronic Bronchitis and Emphysema/Reduction of COPD Exacerbations:

2 inh of the powder contents of 1 cap qd via HandiHaler device

PEDIATRIC DOSAGE

Pediatric use may not have been established

ADMINISTRATION

Orally inhaled powder

Do not swallow caps

Use w/ HandiHaler device only and inhale through the mouth

Do not use HandiHaler device to take any other medicine

Instructions

1. Place cap into the center chamber of the HandiHaler device
2. Spiriva cap is pierced by pressing and releasing the green piercing button on the side of the device
3. The formulation will be dispersed into the air stream when the patient inhales through the mouthpiece

HOW SUPPLIED

Cap, Inhalation: 18mcg

WARNINGS/PRECAUTIONS

Not for initial treatment of acute episodes of bronchospasm (eg, rescue therapy). D/C and consider alternative treatments if immediate hypersensitivity reactions (eg, angioedema, itching, rash) or paradoxical bronchospasm occurs. Caution with hypersensitivity to milk proteins or to atropine. Caution with narrow-angle glaucoma; observe for signs and symptoms of acute narrow-angle glaucoma. Caution with urinary retention; observe for signs and symptoms of prostatic hyperplasia or bladder-neck obstruction (eg, difficulty passing urine, painful urination). Monitor for anticholinergic effects in patients with moderate to severe renal impairment (CrCl ≤50mL/min).

ADVERSE REACTIONS

Dry mouth, sinusitis, constipation, abdominal pain, UTI, URTI, chest pain, edema, vomiting, myalgia, moniliasis, rash, dyspepsia, pharyngitis, rhinitis.

DRUG INTERACTIONS

Avoid with other anticholinergic-containing drugs; may lead to an increase in anticholinergic adverse effects.

NURSING CONSIDERATIONS

Assessment: Assess for hypersensitivity to atropine or its derivatives, narrow-angle glaucoma, urinary retention, renal impairment, pregnancy/nursing status, and possible drug interactions.

Monitoring: Monitor for signs and symptoms of prostatic hyperplasia or bladder neck obstruction, worsening narrow-angle glaucoma, paradoxical bronchospasm, and hypersensitivity reactions.

Patient Counseling: Inform that contents of cap are for oral inhalation only and must not be swallowed. Advise to administer only via the HandiHaler device and that the device should not be used for other medications. Advise not to use as a rescue medication for immediate relief of breathing problems. Advise to seek medical attention if acute eye pain/discomfort, blurring of vision, visual halos or colored images, difficulty in passing urine or dysuria develop. Advise to use caution when engaging in activities such as driving a vehicle or operating appliances/machinery. Inform that paradoxical bronchospasm may occur; d/c if this develops. Instruct not to allow the powder to enter into the eyes.

Storage: 25°C (77°F); excursions permitted to 15-30°C (59-86°F). Do not expose to extreme temperatures or moisture. Do not store caps in the HandiHaler device.

SPRYCEL – dasatinib RX

Class: Kinase inhibitors

ADULT DOSAGE

Ph+ Chronic Phase CML

Newly Diagnosed Philadelphia Chromosome-Positive Chronic Myeloid Leukemia in Chronic Phase:

Initial: 100mg qd

Titrate: If no response, increase to 140mg qd

Accelerated Phase CML/Myeloid or Lymphoid Blast Phase CML/Ph+ ALL

Chronic, accelerated, or myeloid or lymphoid blast phase Philadelphia Chromosome-Positive chronic myeloid leukemia with resistance or intolerance to prior therapy, including imatinib. Also, treats adults with Ph+ acute lymphoblastic leukemia w/ resistance or intolerance to prior therapy

Initial: 140mg qd

Titrate: If no response, increase to 180mg qd

PEDIATRIC DOSAGE

Pediatric use may not have been established

DOSE MODIFICATION

Concomitant Medications

Strong CYP3A4 Inducers:

Avoid use; if necessary, consider dose increase of dasatinib with careful monitoring for toxicity

Strong CYP3A4 Inhibitors:

Avoid use; if necessary, consider dose decrease of dasatinib to 20mg if taking 100mg qd, and to 40mg if taking 140mg qd, with careful monitoring for toxicity
If therapy is not tolerated after dose reduction, either d/c concomitant inhibitor and allow 1-week washout period before increasing dasatinib dose, or d/c dasatinib until end of treatment with inhibitor

Adverse Reactions

Neutropenia and Thrombocytopenia:

Chronic Phase CML:

ANC <0.5 x 10^9/L or Platelets <50 x 10^9/L:

1. Stop until ANC ≥1.0 x 10^9/L and platelets ≥50 x 10^9/L
2. Resume at the original starting dose if recovery occurs in ≤7 days
3. If platelets <25 x 10^9/L or recurrence of ANC <0.5 x 10^9/L for >7 days, repeat Step 1 and resume at a reduced dose of 80mg qd for second episode. For third episode, further reduce dose to 50mg qd (for newly diagnosed patients) or d/c (for patients resistant or intolerant to prior therapy including imatinib)

Accelerated Phase CML, Blast Phase CML and Ph+ ALL:

ANC <0.5 x 10^9/L or Platelets <10 x 10^9/L:

1. If cytopenia is unrelated to leukemia, stop until ANC ≥1.0 x 10^9/L and platelets ≥20 x 10^9/L and resume at the original starting dose
2. If recurrence of cytopenia, repeat Step 1 and resume at a reduced dose of 100mg qd (second episode) or 80mg qd (third episode)
3. If cytopenia is related to leukemia, consider dose escalation to 180mg qd

Severe Non-Hematological Adverse Reaction:

Withhold until the event has resolved or improved
May resume at a reduced dose depending on the initial severity of the event

ADMINISTRATION

Oral route

Take with or without meal, either in am or pm
Swallow whole; do not crush or cut

HOW SUPPLIED

Tab: 20mg, 50mg, 70mg, 80mg, 100mg, 140mg

WARNINGS/PRECAUTIONS

Severe thrombocytopenia, neutropenia, and anemia reported; monitor CBCs weekly for first 2 months and monthly thereafter, or as clinically indicated. Manage myelosuppression by temporarily withholding therapy or by dose reduction. Severe CNS and GI hemorrhage, including fatalities and other cases of severe hemorrhage, reported. Severe fluid retention, ascites, pulmonary edema, and generalized edema reported; perform chest x-ray if symptoms suggestive of pleural effusion develop (eg, dyspnea, dry cough). QT prolongation reported; correct hypokalemia or hypomagnesemia prior to therapy. Cardiac adverse reactions reported; monitor for signs/symptoms consistent with cardiac dysfunction and treat appropriately. May increase risk of developing pulmonary arterial HTN (PAH); d/c permanently if PAH is confirmed. May cause fetal harm. Caution with hepatic impairment.

ADVERSE REACTIONS

Myelosuppression, fluid retention, diarrhea, N/V, headache, musculoskeletal pain, abdominal pain, hemorrhage, pneumonia, pyrexia, pleural effusion, dyspnea, skin rash, fatigue, myalgia.

DRUG INTERACTIONS

See Dosage. CYP3A4 inhibitors (eg, ketoconazole, clarithromycin, ritonavir) and grapefruit juice may increase levels. CYP3A4 inducers (eg, dexamethasone, phenytoin, carbamazepine) and St. John's wort may decrease levels. Avoid with antacids (eg, aluminum hydroxide/magnesium hydroxide); if use is necessary, administer antacid dose at least 2 hrs prior to or after dasatinib dose. H_2 antagonists (eg, famotidine) or proton pump inhibitors (eg, omeprazole) may reduce exposure; concomitant use is not recommended. May increase levels of simvastatin (a CYP3A4 substrate); caution with CYP3A4 substrates with narrow therapeutic index (eg, alfentanil, astemizole, ergotamine). Caution with anticoagulants or medications that inhibit platelet function. Antiarrhythmics or other QT-prolonging agents, and cumulative high-dose anthracycline therapy may increase risk of QT prolongation.

NURSING CONSIDERATIONS

Assessment: Assess for signs/symptoms of underlying cardiopulmonary disease, hepatic impairment, presence or risk of QT prolongation, hypokalemia, hypomagnesemia, pregnancy/nursing status, and possible drug interactions.

Monitoring: Monitor for hemorrhage, cardiac dysfunction, myelosuppression, pleural effusion, fluid retention, QT prolongation, PAH, and other adverse reactions. Perform chest x-ray if symptoms of pleural effusion develop. Monitor CBCs weekly for first 2 months and monthly thereafter.

Patient Counseling: Inform of pregnancy risks; advise to avoid becoming pregnant during therapy and to contact physician if patient becomes pregnant, or if pregnancy is suspected. Instruct to seek medical attention if symptoms of hemorrhage, myelosuppression, fluid retention, significant N/V, diarrhea, headache, musculoskeletal pain, fatigue, or rash develop. Inform that product contains lactose.

Storage: 20-25°C (68-77°F); excursions permitted between 15-30°C (59-86°F).

Stalevo – carbidopa/entacapone/levodopa — RX

Class: COMT inhibitor/dopa-decarboxylase inhibitor/dopamine precursor

ADULT DOSAGE

Parkinson's Disease

May be used:
1. To substitute (w/ equivalent strengths of each of the 3 components) carbidopa/levodopa and entacapone previously administered as individual products
2. To replace carbidopa/levodopa therapy (w/o entacapone) for patients experiencing signs/symptoms of end-of-dose "wearing-off" and who have been taking a total daily dose of levodopa of ≤600mg and have not been experiencing dyskinesias

Converting from Carbidopa, Levodopa, and Entacapone:
In patients currently treated w/ entacapone 200mg w/ each dose of non-extended release carbidopa/levodopa tab may switch to corresponding strength of Stalevo w/ same amounts of carbidopa and levodopa

Converting from Carbidopa and Levodopa Products:
Titrate patients initially to a dose that is tolerated and that meets individual therapeutic need using a separate carbidopa/levodopa tab (1:4 ratio) plus an entacapone tab; switch to the corresponding single tab of Stalevo once the individual dose of carbidopa/levodopa plus entacapone has been established

When less levodopa is required, reduce the total daily dose of carbidopa/levodopa either by decreasing the strength of Stalevo at each administration or by decreasing the frequency of administration by extending time between doses

Max: 8 tabs/day (Stalevo 50, 75, 100, 125, 150); 6 tabs/day (Stalevo 200)

Determine optimum daily dose by careful titration in each patient

Administer only 1 tab at each dosing interval

PEDIATRIC DOSAGE

Pediatric use may not have been established

DOSE MODIFICATION

Concomitant Medications

Other Anti-Parkinson's Disease Drugs: May need to adjust concomitant medication or Stalevo

Other Important Modifications

Decrease or Interruption of Dosing: Avoid interruption of Stalevo dosing; hyperpyrexia reported when levodopa is discontinued or reduced

ADMINISTRATION
Oral route

Do not split, crush, or chew tabs
Take w/ or w/o food; a high-fat, high-calorie meal may delay absorption of levodopa by about 2 hrs

HOW SUPPLIED
Tab: (Carbidopa-Levodopa-Entacapone): Stalevo 50: 12.5mg-50mg-200mg; Stalevo 75: 18.75mg-75mg-200mg; Stalevo 100: 25mg-100mg-200mg; Stalevo 125: 31.25mg-125mg-200mg; Stalevo 150: 37.5mg-150mg-200mg; Stalevo 200: 50mg-200mg-200mg

CONTRAINDICATIONS
Narrow-angle glaucoma. Nonselective MAOIs (eg, phenelzine, tranylcypromine); d/c nonselective MAOIs at least 2 weeks prior to therapy.

WARNINGS/PRECAUTIONS
Falling asleep suddenly without prior warning of sleepiness while engaged in activities of daily living and somnolence reported; reassess for drowsiness or sleepiness, and should ordinarily be discontinued if significant daytime sleepiness or episodes of falling asleep during activities that require active participation occur. May impair mental/physical abilities. Dyskinesia may occur or be exacerbated at lower dosages and sooner than with carbidopa/levodopa; may require dose reductions. Monitor for depression with concomitant suicidal tendencies. Caution with past or current psychoses. May cause intense urges to gamble/spend money uncontrollably, increased sexual urges, and other intense urges; consider dose reduction or discontinuation if such urges develop. Caution with biliary obstruction or hepatic disease/impairment. Cases of hyperpyrexia and confusion resembling neuroleptic malignant syndrome (NMS) reported in association with dose reduction or withdrawal; decrease dose slowly if a patient needs to d/c or reduce daily dose. Syncope, orthostatic hypotension, hypotension, hallucinations and/or psychotic-like behavior, and rhabdomyolysis reported. Cases of retroperitoneal fibrosis, pulmonary infiltrates, pleural effusion, and pleural thickening reported in patients treated with ergot derived dopaminergic agents. Diarrhea and colitis reported with entacapone use; d/c and consider appropriate medical therapy if prolonged diarrhea is suspected to be related to therapy. Monitor for melanomas frequently and regularly; perform periodic skin examination. May increase the possibility of upper GI hemorrhage in patients with history of peptic ulcer. Lab test abnormalities, including elevations of LFTs, BUN abnormalities, and (+) Coombs test reported. May cause a false-positive reaction for urinary ketone bodies or false-negative glucose oxidase test. Cases of falsely diagnosed pheochromocytoma in patients on carbidopa/levodopa reported very rarely; caution when interpreting the plasma and urine levels of catecholamines and their metabolites. Levodopa is known to depress prolactin secretion and increase growth hormone levels.

ADVERSE REACTIONS
Dyskinesia, N/V, hyperkinesia, diarrhea, urine discoloration, hypokinesia, dizziness, abdominal pain, constipation, fatigue, back pain, dry mouth, dyspnea.

DRUG INTERACTIONS
See Contraindications. Caution with concomitant use of alcohol, sedating medications, and other CNS depressants (eg, benzodiazepines, antipsychotics, antidepressants); may increase the risk of somnolence. Iron salts may reduce bioavailability; caution with iron salts or multivitamins containing iron salts. Adjust dose as clinically needed with other CYP2C9 substrates. Entacapone: Caution with drugs metabolized by catechol-O-methyltransferase (COMT) (eg, epinephrine, dopamine, α-methyldopa, isoetherine); increased HR, possibly arrhythmias, and excessive changes in BP may occur. Caution with drugs known to interfere with biliary excretion, glucuronidation, and intestinal β-glucuronidase (eg, probenecid, cholestyramine, erythromycin, ampicillin). Increased R-warfarin exposure and INR values reported with warfarin. Levodopa: Beneficial effects of levodopa in Parkinson's disease reported to be reversed by phenytoin and papaverine; monitor for loss of therapeutic response and increase dosage of Stalevo as clinically needed. Isoniazid and dopamine D_2 receptor antagonists (eg, phenothiazines, butyrophenones, risperidone) may reduce therapeutic effects. Carbidopa/Levodopa: Symptomatic postural hypotension reported when added with antihypertensives; dosage adjustment of the antihypertensive drug may be required when starting therapy. Adverse reactions, including HTN and dyskinesia, reported with TCAs.

NURSING CONSIDERATIONS

Assessment: Assess for narrow-angle glaucoma, past/current psychoses, history of peptic ulcer, hypotension, biliary obstruction, dyskinesias, alcoholism, hepatic impairment, pregnancy/nursing status, any other conditions where treatment is contraindicated or cautioned, and possible drug interactions.

Monitoring: Monitor for signs and symptoms of falling asleep during activities of daily living, hypotension/orthostatic hypotension, syncope, dyskinesia, depression, suicidal tendencies, hallucinations/psychotic-like behavior, impulse control/compulsive behaviors, withdrawal-emergent hyperpyrexia and confusion, diarrhea, colitis, melanoma, rhabdomyolysis, peptic ulcer, and other adverse reactions. Perform skin examination periodically. Monitor INR with warfarin.

Patient Counseling: Inform of the risks and benefits of therapy. Advise about the potential for sedating effects including somnolence and the possibility of falling asleep while engaged in activities of daily living; instruct not to drive or participate in potentially dangerous activities until aware of how medication affects mental and/or motor performance. Advise to speak with physician before taking alcohol, sedating medications, or other CNS depressants because of the possible additive effects in combination with therapy. Inform that symptomatic (or asymptomatic) postural (orthostatic) hypotension or non-orthostatic hypotension may develop; advise not to rise rapidly after sitting or lying down, especially if doing so for prolonged periods and at the initiation of treatment. Inform about the possibility of syncope. Inform that therapy may cause and/or exacerbate preexisting dyskinesias. Inform that hallucinations and other psychotic-like behavior may occur. Instruct to inform physician of new or increased gambling urges, sexual urges, or other intense urges while on therapy. Advise that fever and confusion may develop as part of a syndrome resembling NMS, possibly with other clinical features; instruct to contact physician if wishing to d/c or decrease dose, or if fever and confusion develop. Inform that diarrhea, colitis, rhabdomyolysis, myalgia, and N/V may occur. Inform of higher risk of developing melanoma; instruct to have skin examined on a regular basis by a qualified healthcare provider (eg, dermatologist) and to monitor for melanomas frequently and on a regular basis when using therapy.

Storage: 25°C (77°F); excursions permitted to 15-30°C (59-86°F).

STAXYN – vardenafil hydrochloride RX

Class: Phosphodiesterase type 5 inhibitor

ADULT DOSAGE

Erectile Dysfunction

10mg prn, 60 min before sexual activity
Max: 1 tab/day

PEDIATRIC DOSAGE

Pediatric use may not have been established

DOSE MODIFICATION

Concomitant Medications

α-blocker:
Initiate vardenafil at the lowest recommended dose
Use lower doses of vardenafil film-coated tab as initial therapy
Consider a time interval between dosing

Potent or Moderate CYP3A4 Inhibitors: Avoid use

Renal Impairment

Dialysis: Avoid use

Hepatic Impairment

Moderate to Severe (Child-Pugh B or C): Avoid use

ADMINISTRATION

Oral route
Place on tongue to disintegrate
Take w/o liquid and immediately upon removal from blister
Take w/ or w/o food

HOW SUPPLIED

Tab, Disintegrating: 10mg

CONTRAINDICATIONS

Concomitant use (regularly or intermittently) with nitrates or nitric oxide donors.

WARNINGS/PRECAUTIONS

Not interchangeable with vardenafil 10mg film-coated tab (Levitra); prescribe film-coated tab if requiring a lower/higher dose. Do not use in men for whom sexual activity is not recommended due to underlying cardiovascular (CV) status. Patients with left ventricular outflow obstruction (eg, aortic stenosis, idiopathic hypertrophic subaortic stenosis) may be sensitive to vasodilation. Has systemic vasodilatory properties that resulted in transient decreases in supine BP. Prolonged erections >4 hrs (rare) and priapism (painful erections >6 hrs in duration) reported; caution with anatomical deformation of the penis (eg, angulation, cavernosal fibrosis, Peyronie's disease) or predispositions to priapism (eg, sickle cell anemia, multiple myeloma, leukemia). Avoid with moderate or severe hepatic impairment (Child-Pugh B or C), congenital QT prolongation, or if on renal dialysis. Not recommended with unstable angina, hypotension (resting SBP <90mmHg), uncontrolled HTN (>170/110mmHg), recent history of stroke, life-threatening arrhythmia, or myocardial infarction (within last 6 months), severe cardiac failure, or hereditary degenerative retinal disorders (including retinitis pigmentosa). Caution with bleeding disorders, or significant active peptic ulceration. Non-arteritic anterior ischemic optic neuropathy (NAION) reported (rare); d/c therapy if sudden loss of vision occurs. Caution with underlying NAION risk factors; increased risk in patients with "crowded" optic disc or with previous history of NAION. D/C if sudden decrease or loss of hearing occurs. QT prolongation may occur; caution with known history of QT prolongation. Contains aspartame; may be harmful in phenylketonurics. Contains sorbitol; avoid with hereditary problems of fructose intolerance. Does not protect against sexually transmitted diseases (STDs).

ADVERSE REACTIONS

Headache, flushing, nasal congestion.

DRUG INTERACTIONS

See Contraindications. Avoid use with Class IA (eg, quinidine, procainamide) or Class III (eg, amiodarone, sotalol) antiarrhythmics and other treatments for ED. Avoid with potent or moderate CYP3A4 inhibitors (eg, ketoconazole, ritonavir, clarithromycin). Step-wise increase in α-blocker dose may be associated with further lowering of BP; caution when coadministering. Additive hypotensive effect with other antihypertensive agents. Caution with medications known to prolong QT interval.

NURSING CONSIDERATIONS

Assessment: Assess for left ventricular outflow obstruction, CV disease, congenital or history of QT prolongation, hereditary degenerative retinal disorders, bleeding disorders, active peptic ulceration, anatomical deformation of the penis, predisposition to priapism, phenylketonuria, renal/hepatic impairment, potential underlying causes of ED, "crowded" optic disc, any other conditions where treatment is contraindicated or cautioned, and for possible drug interactions. Obtain baseline BP.

Monitoring: Monitor for priapism, changes in vision/hearing, QT prolongation, and other adverse reactions.

Patient Counseling: Instruct to take ud. Inform that drug is not interchangeable with vardenafil film-coated tab (Levitra). Inform that regular and/or intermittent use of nitrates may cause BP to suddenly drop to an unsafe level, resulting in dizziness, syncope, or even heart attack or stroke. Inform patients with preexisting CV risk factors of the potential cardiac risk of sexual activity. Inform that concomitant use of α-blockers may lower BP significantly, leading to symptomatic hypotension; instruct to use drug only when previous treatment with vardenafil film-coated tab has been well tolerated. Instruct to contact physician if not satisfied with quality of sexual performance or in case of unwanted effect. Instruct to seek immediate medical assistance if erection persists >4 hrs; inform that penile tissue damage and permanent loss of potency may result. Instruct to d/c and seek medical attention in the event of sudden loss of vision in 1 or both eyes; inform of the increased risk of NAION with history of NAION in 1 eye or with a "crowded" optic disc. Instruct to d/c treatment and seek prompt medical attention in the event of sudden decrease or loss of hearing. Counsel about protective measures necessary to guard against STDs, including HIV; inform that drug does not protect against STDs. Advise to examine blister pack before use and not to use if blisters are torn, broken, or missing.

Storage: 25°C (77°F); excursions permitted to 15-30°C (59-86°F).

STELARA – ustekinumab

RX

Class: Monoclonal antibody

ADULT DOSAGE

Psoriasis

Patients w/ Moderate to Severe Plaque Psoriasis who are Candidates for Phototherapy or Systemic Therapy:

≤100kg (≤220 lbs): 45mg initially and 4 weeks later, followed by 45mg every 12 weeks

>100kg (>220 lbs): 90mg initially and 4 weeks later, followed by 90mg every 12 weeks

Psoriatic Arthritis

Active:

45mg initially and 4 weeks later, followed by 45mg every 12 weeks

Coexistent Moderate to Severe Plaque Psoriasis:

>100kg (>220 lbs): 90mg initially and 4 weeks later, followed by 90mg every 12 weeks

Can be used alone or in combination w/ methotrexate

PEDIATRIC DOSAGE

Pediatric use may not have been established

ADMINISTRATION

SQ route

Administer each inj at a different anatomic location (eg, upper arms, gluteal regions, thighs, any quadrant of abdomen) than the previous inj; do not administer into areas where the skin is tender, bruised, erythematous, or indurated

When using the single-use vial, a 27 gauge, 1/2 inch needle is recommended

Administration Instructions

1. To prevent premature activation of the needle safety guard, do not touch the NEEDLE GUARD ACTIVATION CLIPS at any time during use
2. Hold body and remove needle cover; do not hold plunger or plunger head while removing needle cover and do not use prefilled syringe if it is dropped w/o needle cover in place
3. Inject SQ as recommended; inject all of the medication by pushing in plunger until plunger head is completely between needle guard wings; inj of entire prefilled syringe contents is necessary to activate needle guard
4. After injection, maintain pressure on plunger head and remove needle from skin
5. Slowly take your thumb off plunger head to allow empty syringe to move up until entire needle is covered by needle guard; discard used syringes in puncture-resistant container

HOW SUPPLIED

Inj: 45mg/0.5mL, 90mg/mL [prefilled syringe, vial]

WARNINGS/PRECAUTIONS

Serious bacterial, fungal, and viral infections, and infections requiring hospitalization reported. Do not give to patients with any clinically important active infection or until infection resolves or is adequately treated. Caution with chronic infection or a history of recurrent infection. Individuals genetically deficient in interleukin (IL)-12/IL-23 are particularly vulnerable to disseminated infections from mycobacteria (eg, nontuberculous, environmental mycobacteria), salmonella (eg, nontyphi strains), and Bacillus Calmette-Guerin (BCG) vaccinations; consider appropriate diagnostic testing. Evaluate for tuberculosis (TB) infection prior to, during, and after treatment; do not administer to patients with active TB. Consider anti-TB therapy prior to initiation in patients with history of latent or active TB when an adequate course of treatment cannot be confirmed. Rapid appearance of multiple cutaneous squamous cell carcinomas reported in patients who had preexisting risk factors for developing non-melanoma skin cancer; closely monitor patients with history of prolonged immunosuppressant therapy, history of PUVA treatment, and patients >60 yrs of age. Hypersensitivity reactions (eg, anaphylaxis, angioedema) reported; institute appropriate therapy and d/c. Reversible posterior leukoencephalopathy syndrome (RPLS) reported; administer appropriate treatment and d/c if suspected. Prior to initiating therapy, patients should receive all immunizations appropriate for age as recommended by current immunization guidelines. Needle cover on prefilled syringe contains dry natural rubber and should not be handled by latex-sensitive individuals. Should only be given to patients who will be closely monitored and have regular follow-up visits with a physician.

ADVERSE REACTIONS

Infection, nasopharyngitis, upper respiratory tract infection, headache, fatigue, arthralgia, nausea.

DRUG INTERACTIONS

Do not give with live vaccines; caution when administering live vaccines to household contacts of patients receiving ustekinumab. BCG vaccines should not be given during, for 1 yr prior to initiating, or 1 yr following discontinuation of treatment. Non-live vaccinations received during course of therapy may not elicit an immune response sufficient to prevent disease. Consider monitoring for therapeutic effect (eg, for warfarin) or drug concentration (eg, for cyclosporine) with concomitant CYP450 substrates, particularly those with a narrow therapeutic index; adjust individual dose prn. May decrease protective effect of allergen immunotherapy (decrease tolerance), which may increase the risk of an allergic reaction to a dose of allergen immunotherapy; caution in patients receiving or who have received allergen immunotherapy.

NURSING CONSIDERATIONS

Assessment: Assess for drug hypersensitivity, active/chronic/serious infections, history of recurrent infection, IL-12/IL-23 genetic deficiency, TB, immunization history, pregnancy/nursing status, and possible drug interactions.

Monitoring: Monitor for signs/symptoms of infection, appearance of non-melanoma skin cancer, TB during and after treatment, malignancies, hypersensitivity reactions, RPLS, and other adverse reactions.

Patient Counseling: Advise that therapy may lower the ability of the immune system to fight infections. Inform of the importance of communicating any history of infections to physician and instruct to contact physician if any signs/symptoms of infection develop. Counsel about the risk of malignancies while on therapy. Advise to seek immediate medical attention if experiencing any symptoms of a serious allergic reaction. Inform of inj techniques and procedures. Advise not to reuse needles/syringes and instruct on proper disposal procedures.

Storage: 2-8°C (36-46°F). Store vials upright. Protect from light. Do not freeze or shake.

STENDRA – avanafil

RX

Class: Phosphodiesterase type 5 inhibitor

ADULT DOSAGE

Erectile Dysfunction

Initial: 100mg prn, as early as 15 min before sexual activity

Titrate: May increase to 200mg as early as 15 min before, or decrease to 50mg 30 min before sexual activity, based on individual efficacy and tolerability

Max Dosing Frequency: QD

Use lowest effective dose

Sexual stimulation is required for response to treatment

PEDIATRIC DOSAGE

Pediatric use may not have been established

DOSE MODIFICATION

Concomitant Medications

α-Blocker:

Initial: 50mg

Moderate CYP3A4 Inhibitors (eg, Erythromycin, Amprenavir, Diltiazem):

Max: 50mg/24 hrs

Strong CYP3A4 Inhibitors (Eg, Ketoconazole, Ritonavir, Atazanavir):

Do not use

ADMINISTRATION

Oral route

Take w/ or w/o food

HOW SUPPLIED

Tab: 50mg, 100mg, 200mg

CONTRAINDICATIONS

Concomitant use (regularly and/or intermittently) with organic nitrates.

WARNINGS/PRECAUTIONS

In a patient who has taken avanafil, where nitrate administration is necessary, allow at least 12 hrs to elapse after the last dose of therapy before considering nitrate administration; only administer under close medical supervision with appropriate hemodynamic monitoring. Potential for cardiac risk during sexual activity in patients with preexisting cardiovascular (CV) disease; avoid if sexual activity is inadvisable due to underlying CV status. Patients with left ventricular outflow obstruction (eg, aortic stenosis, idiopathic hypertrophic subaortic stenosis) and those with severely impaired autonomic control of BP may be sensitive to therapy. Not recommended in patients with myocardial infarction, stroke, life-threatening arrhythmia, or coronary revascularization within the last 6 months; resting hypotension (BP <90/50mmHg) or HTN (BP >170/100mmHg), or unstable angina, angina with sexual intercourse, or NYHA Class 2 or greater congestive heart failure. Has vasodilatory properties resulting in transient decreases in sitting BP. Prolonged erection >4 hrs and priapism reported; caution with anatomical deformation of the penis (eg, angulation, cavernosal fibrosis, Peyronie's disease), or conditions that may predispose to priapism (eg, sickle cell anemia, multiple myeloma, leukemia). Non-arteritic anterior ischemic optic neuropathy (NAION) reported (rare); d/c if sudden loss of vision in 1 or both eyes occurs. Caution with underlying NAION risk factors; increased risk with previous history of NAION and in individuals with "crowded" optic disc. Sudden decrease or loss of hearing that may be accompanied by tinnitus or dizziness reported; d/c if this occurs. Avoid in patients with severe renal disease, on renal dialysis, or with severe hepatic disease.

ADVERSE REACTIONS

Headache, flushing, nasopharyngitis, nasal congestion, back pain, upper respiratory infection, ECG abnormal.

DRUG INTERACTIONS

See Contraindications and Dosage. Not recommended with other PDE-5 inhibitors or ED therapy combinations. Not recommended with CYP inducers. Caution with α-blockers; may augment BP-lowering effect of α-blockers and other antihypertensives. May increase BP-lowering effect of each compound with concomitant alcohol use and the risk of orthostatic signs/symptoms with substantial alcohol consumption. Do not use with strong CYP3A4 inhibitors (eg, ketoconazole, ritonavir, clarithromycin, nefazodone). Increased levels with strong, moderate, and other CYP3A4 inhibitors (eg, grapefruit juice). May increase levels of desipramine or omeprazole. May affect rosiglitazone levels. Amlodipine may increase levels and prolong $T_{1/2}$. May decrease amlodipine levels. May potentiate the antiaggregatory effect of sodium nitroprusside.

NURSING CONSIDERATIONS

Assessment: Assess for hypersensitivity to the drug, CV disease, left ventricular outflow obstruction, anatomical deformation of the penis, conditions that predispose to priapism, potential underlying causes of ED, risk for NAION, renal/hepatic impairment, any other conditions where treatment is contraindicated/cautioned, and possible drug interactions. Obtain baseline BP.

Monitoring: Monitor for hypersensitivity reactions, CV risk, priapism, changes in vision/hearing, and other adverse reactions.

Patient Counseling: Instruct to take ud and explain that sexual stimulation is required for an erection to occur. Inform about the contraindication of avanafil with regular and/or intermittent use of organic nitrates; instruct patients who experience anginal chest pain after taking medication to seek immediate medical attention. Inform patients with preexisting CV risk factors of the potential cardiac risk of sexual activity; advise patients who experience symptoms upon initiation of sexual activity to refrain from further sexual activity and seek immediate medical attention. Advise to contact prescribing physician if new medications that may interact with therapy are prescribed by another healthcare provider. Instruct to seek emergency medical attention if erection persists >4 hrs; inform that priapism, if not treated promptly, may result in irreversible erectile tissue damage. Inform of the increased risk of NAION with history of NAION in 1 eye and in patients with a "crowded" optic disc. Instruct to d/c and seek medical attention in the event of sudden loss of vision in 1 or both eyes, or if a sudden decrease or loss of hearing that may be accompanied by tinnitus and dizziness occurs. Inform that substantial alcohol consumption (eg, >3 units) in combination with medication may increase the potential for orthostatic signs/symptoms. Inform that drug does not protect against sexually transmitted diseases (STDs); counsel about protective measures necessary to guard against STDs, including HIV.

Storage: 20-25°C (68-77°F); excursions permitted to 30°C (86°F). Protect from light.

STIVARGA – regorafenib

RX

Class: Kinase inhibitors

Severe and sometimes fatal hepatotoxicity reported. Monitor hepatic function prior to and during treatment. Interrupt and then reduce or d/c treatment for hepatotoxicity as manifested by elevated LFTs or hepatocellular necrosis, depending upon severity and persistence.

ADULT DOSAGE

Metastatic Colorectal Cancer

Previously treated w/ fluoropyrimidine-, oxaliplatin-, and irinotecan-based chemotherapy, an antivascular endothelial growth factor therapy, and, if KRAS wild type, an anti-epidermal growth factor receptor therapy

Usual: 160mg qd for the first 21 days of each 28-day cycle until disease progression or unacceptable toxicity

Locally Advanced, Unresectable or Metastatic Gastrointestinal Stromal Tumor

Previously treated w/ imatinib mesylate and sunitinib malate

Usual: 160mg qd for the first 21 days of each 28-day cycle until disease progression or unacceptable toxicity

PEDIATRIC DOSAGE

Pediatric use may not have been established

DOSE MODIFICATION

Hepatic Impairment

Severe (Child-Pugh Class C): Not recommended

Adverse Reactions

Interruption:

NCI CTCAE Grade 2 hand-foot skin reaction (HFSR) that is recurrent or does not improve w/in 7 days despite dose reduction; interrupt therapy for a minimum of 7 days for Grade 3 HFSR

Symptomatic Grade 2 HTN

Any NCI CTCAE Grade 3 or 4 adverse reaction

Reduce to 120mg if:

For the first occurrence of Grade 2 HFSR of any duration

After recovery of any Grade 3 or 4 adverse reaction

For Grade 3 AST/ALT elevation; only resume if the potential benefit outweighs the risk of hepatotoxicity

Reduce to 80mg if:
For reoccurrence of Grade 2 HFSR at the 120mg dose
After recovery of any Grade 3 or 4 adverse reaction at the 120mg dose (except hepatotoxicity)

Discontinuation
Failure to tolerate 80mg dose
Any occurrence of AST or ALT >20X ULN
Any occurrence of AST or ALT >3X ULN w/ concurrent bilirubin >2X ULN
Reoccurrence of AST or ALT >5X ULN despite dose reduction to 120mg
For any Grade 4 adverse reaction; only resume if the potential benefit outweighs the risks

ADMINISTRATION
Oral route
Swallow tab whole w/ a low-fat breakfast that contains <30% fat

HOW SUPPLIED
Tab: 40mg

WARNINGS/PRECAUTIONS
Increased incidence of hemorrhage reported; permanently d/c with severe or life-threatening hemorrhage. May increase incidence of adverse reactions involving the skin and SQ tissues (eg, HFSR, toxic epidermal necrolysis, Stevens Johnson syndrome, severe rash); withhold, reduce dose, or permanently d/c treatment depending on severity and persistence of dermatologic toxicity. Increased incidence of HTN reported; temporarily or permanently withhold for severe or uncontrolled HTN. Avoid initiation unless BP is adequately controlled. May increase incidence of myocardial ischemia and infarction; withhold if new or acute onset cardiac ischemia or infarction develops. Resume treatment only after resolution of acute cardiac ischemic events, if benefits outweigh risks of further cardiac ischemia. Reversible posterior leukoencephalopathy syndrome (RPLS) reported; perform evaluation for RPLS in any patient presenting with seizures, headache, visual disturbances, confusion, or altered mental function. D/C if RPLS develops. Permanently d/c if GI perforation or fistula develops. May impair wound healing; d/c at least 2 weeks prior to scheduled surgery. D/C in patients with wound dehiscence. May cause fetal harm; women and men of reproductive potential should use effective contraception during treatment and up to 2 months after completion of therapy. Not recommended with severe hepatic impairment (Child-Pugh Class C).

ADVERSE REACTIONS
Hepatotoxicity, asthenia, HFSR, fatigue/diarrhea, decreased appetite/food intake, HTN, mucositis, dysphonia, infection, pain, decreased weight, GI/abdominal pain, rash, fever, nausea.

DRUG INTERACTIONS
Avoid with strong CYP3A4 inducers (eg, rifampin, phenytoin, carbamazepine) and strong CYP3A4 inhibitors (eg, clarithromycin, grapefruit juice, itraconazole). Monitor INR levels more frequently in patients receiving warfarin.

NURSING CONSIDERATIONS

Assessment: Assess for scheduled/recent surgical procedures, hepatic impairment, HTN, pregnancy/nursing status, and possible drug interactions. Obtain baseline LFTs (ALT, AST, and bilirubin).

Monitoring: Monitor for hepatotoxicity, hemorrhage, dermatologic toxicity, HTN, myocardial ischemia or infarction, RPLS, wound dehiscence, GI perforation or fistula, and other adverse reactions. Monitor BP weekly for the first 6 weeks of treatment and then every cycle, or more frequently, as clinically indicated. Monitor LFTs at least every 2 weeks during the first 2 months of treatment, then monthly or more frequently as clinically indicated; monitor weekly in patients experiencing elevated LFTs until improvement to <3X ULN or baseline. Monitor INR levels more frequently in patients receiving warfarin.

Patient Counseling: Inform about the need to undergo monitoring for liver damage and instruct to immediately report to physician any signs or symptoms of severe liver damage. Advise to contact physician for any episode of bleeding, or if experiencing skin changes associated with redness, pain, blisters, bleeding, or swelling. Advise of the need for BP monitoring and to contact physician if BP is elevated, or if HTN symptoms occur. Instruct to seek immediate emergency help if experiencing chest pain, SOB, dizziness, or feeling like passing out. Advise to contact physician immediately if experiencing severe pain in the abdomen, persistent swelling of the abdomen, high fever, chills, N/V, severe diarrhea, or dehydration. Instruct to inform physician if patient plans to undergo a surgical procedure or had recent surgery. Advise women of reproductive potential and men of the need for effective contraception during treatment and for up to 2 months after completion of treatment. Instruct women of reproductive potential to immediately contact physician if pregnancy is suspected or confirmed during or within 2 months of completing treatment. Advise nursing mothers that it is not known whether the drug is present in breast milk and discuss whether to d/c nursing or to d/c treatment. Instruct to take any missed dose on the same day, as soon as they remember, and to not take 2 doses on the same day to make up for a dose missed on the previous day.

Storage: 25°C (77°F); excursions permitted to 15-30°C (59-86°F). Store tabs in original bottle and do not remove the desiccant. Keep the bottle tightly closed after 1st opening. Discard any unused tabs 7 weeks after opening the bottle.

STRATTERA – atomoxetine RX

Class: Selective norepinephrine reuptake inhibitor

Increased risk of suicidal ideation in short-term studies in children or adolescents with attention-deficit hyperactivity disorder (ADHD); balance this risk with the clinical need. Closely monitor for suicidality (suicidal thinking and behavior), clinical worsening, or unusual changes in behavior. Not approved for major depressive disorder.

ADULT DOSAGE

Attention-Deficit Hyperactivity Disorder

Initial: 40mg/day
Titrate: Increase after a minimum of 3 days to target dose of approx 80mg/day; may increase after 2-4 additional weeks if optimal response is not achieved
Max: 100mg/day

Periodically reevaluate long-term usefulness

May d/c w/o tapering

PEDIATRIC DOSAGE

Attention-Deficit Hyperactivity Disorder

≤70kg:
Initial: 0.5mg/kg/day
Titrate: Increase after a minimum of 3 days to target dose of approx 1.2mg/kg/day
Max: 1.4mg/kg/day or 100mg/day, whichever is less

>70kg:
Initial: 40mg/day
Titrate: Increase after a minimum of 3 days to target dose of approx 80mg/day; may increase after 2-4 additional weeks if optimal response is not achieved
Max: 100mg/day

Periodically reevaluate long-term usefulness

May d/c w/o tapering

DOSE MODIFICATION

Concomitant Medications

Strong CYP2D6 Inhibitors:
<70kg:
Initial: 0.5mg/kg/day
Titrate: Only increase to target dose of 1.2mg/kg/day if symptoms fail to improve after 4 weeks and initial dose is well tolerated

>70kg or Adults:
Initial: 40mg/day
Titrate: Only increase to target dose of 80mg/day if symptoms fail to improve after 4 weeks and initial dose is well tolerated

Hepatic Impairment

Moderate Impairment (Child-Pugh Class B):
Initial/Target: Reduce to 50% of normal dose

Severe Impairment (Child-Pugh Class C):
Initial/Target: Reduce to 25% of normal dose

Other Important Modifications

CYP2D6 Poor Metabolizers:
Initial: 0.5mg/kg/day
Titrate: Only increase to target dose of 1.2mg/kg/day if symptoms fail to improve after 4 weeks and initial dose is well tolerated

ADMINISTRATION

Oral route

Take whole, w/ or w/o food; do not open cap
Take as a single dose in the am or as evenly divided doses in the am and late afternoon/early pm

HOW SUPPLIED

Cap: 10mg, 18mg, 25mg, 40mg, 60mg, 80mg, 100mg

CONTRAINDICATIONS

Narrow-angle glaucoma, presence/history of pheochromocytoma, and severe cardiac/vascular disorders that would deteriorate with increases in BP/HR that would be clinically important (eg,

15-20mmHg in BP or 20 beats/min in HR). Use of an MAOI either concomitantly or within 2 weeks of stopping treatment. Treatment within 2 weeks of stopping an MAOI.

WARNINGS/PRECAUTIONS

May cause severe liver injury; d/c in patients with jaundice or lab evidence of liver injury, and do not restart therapy. Perform LFTs upon the 1st sign/symptom of liver dysfunction. Sudden death reported in children and adolescents with structural cardiac abnormalities or other serious heart problems. Sudden death, stroke, and MI reported in adults. Avoid in patients with known serious structural cardiac abnormalities, cardiomyopathy, serious heart rhythm abnormalities, coronary artery disease, or other serious cardiac problems. Promptly perform cardiac evaluation if symptoms suggestive of cardiac disease develop. May increase BP/HR; caution in patients whose underlying medical conditions could be worsened by increases in BP or HR. Orthostatic hypotension and syncope reported; caution with conditions predisposing to hypotension, or conditions associated with abrupt HR/BP changes. Caution in patients with comorbid bipolar disorder; may induce mixed/manic episode. May cause treatment-emergent psychotic or manic symptoms in children/adolescents without prior history of psychotic illness or mania; consider discontinuation if such symptoms occur. Monitor for appearance/worsening of aggressive behavior or hostility. Allergic reactions and priapism reported. May cause urinary retention/hesitation. Monitor growth in children.

ADVERSE REACTIONS

Abdominal pain, N/V, fatigue, decreased appetite, somnolence, headache, dry mouth, dizziness, insomnia, constipation, urinary hesitation, erectile dysfunction, irritability, weight decreased, hyperhidrosis.

DRUG INTERACTIONS

See Contraindications. Caution with systemically administered albuterol or other β_2 agonists; may potentiate cardiovascular (CV) effects of albuterol. Caution with antihypertensive drugs and pressor agents (eg, dopamine, dobutamine) or other drugs that increase BP. CYP2D6 inhibitors (eg, paroxetine, fluoxetine, quinidine) increase levels in extensive metabolizers (EMs).

NURSING CONSIDERATIONS

Assessment: Assess for hypersensitivity to drug, narrow-angle glaucoma, presence/history of pheochromocytoma, comorbid bipolar disorder, CV disorders, hepatic impairment, any other conditions where treatment is contraindicated or cautioned, pregnancy/nursing status, and possible drug interactions. Obtain baseline pulse and BP.

Monitoring: Monitor for signs/symptoms of CV events, liver injury, allergic reactions, emergence of psychosis/mania, suicidality, clinical worsening, aggressive or unusual changes in behavior, hostility, urinary retention/hesitation, priapism, and other adverse reactions. Monitor growth in children. Monitor pulse and BP following dose increases and periodically during therapy. Periodically reevaluate long-term usefulness.

Patient Counseling: Inform about risks, benefits, and appropriate use of therapy. Encourage patients, families, and caregivers to be alert for the emergence of agitation, irritability, and unusual changes in behavior, as well as the emergence of suicidality, especially early during treatment and when dose is adjusted; advise to report such symptoms to physician, especially if severe, abrupt in onset, or not part of presenting symptoms. Advise to contact physician if symptoms of liver injury develop. Inform that priapism requires prompt medical attention. Inform that drug is an ocular irritant; if content of cap comes in contact with eye, instruct to immediately flush affected eye with water and obtain medical advice. Tell to notify physician if taking or planning to take any prescription or OTC medicines, dietary supplements, or herbal remedies. Instruct to notify physician if nursing, pregnant, or thinking of becoming pregnant. Advise to use caution when driving a car/operating hazardous machinery until reasonably certain that performance is not affected by therapy.

Storage: 25°C (77°F); excursions permitted to 15-30°C (59-86°F).

STRIBILD — cobicistat/elvitegravir/emtricitabine/tenofovir disoproxil fumarate RX

Class: CYP3A inhibitor/HIV integrase strand transfer inhibitor/nucleoside analogue combination

Lactic acidosis and severe hepatomegaly w/ steatosis, including fatal cases, reported w/ the use of nucleoside analogues in combination w/ other antiretrovirals. Not approved for the treatment of chronic hepatitis B virus (HBV) infection. Severe acute exacerbations of hepatitis B reported in patients coinfected w/ HBV and HIV-1 upon discontinuation of therapy; closely monitor hepatic function w/ both clinical and lab follow-up for at least several months. If appropriate, initiation of anti-hepatitis B therapy may be warranted.

ADULT DOSAGE

HIV-1 Infection

For use as a complete regimen for the treatment of HIV-1 infection in adults who have no antiretroviral treatment history or to replace the current antiretroviral regimen in those who are virologically-suppressed (HIV-1

PEDIATRIC DOSAGE

Pediatric use may not have been established

RNA <50 copies/mL) on a stable antiretroviral regimen for at least 6 months w/ no history of treatment failure and no known substitutions associated w/ resistance to the individual components of the drug

Usual: 1 tab qd

DOSE MODIFICATION

Renal Impairment

CrCl <70mL/min: Initiation of treatment not recommended

CrCl Declines <50mL/min During Treatment: D/C therapy

Hepatic Impairment

Severe (Child-Pugh Class C): Not recommended

ADMINISTRATION

Oral route

Take w/ food

HOW SUPPLIED

Tab: (Cobicistat/Elvitegravir/Emtricitabine/Tenofovir Disoproxil Fumarate [TDF]) 150mg/150mg/200mg/300mg

CONTRAINDICATIONS

Concomitant use w/ drugs that are highly dependent on CYP3A for clearance and for which elevated plasma concentrations are associated w/ serious and/or life-threatening reactions and w/ other drugs that may lead to reduced efficacy and possible resistance (eg, alfuzosin, rifampin, dihydroergotamine, ergotamine, methylergonovine, cisapride, St. John's wort, lovastatin, simvastatin, pimozide, sildenafil [when used to treat pulmonary arterial HTN], triazolam, oral midazolam).

WARNINGS/PRECAUTIONS

Test for HBV infection and document estimated CrCl, urine glucose, and urine protein prior to initiation of therapy. Not recommended for use in patients w/ severe hepatic impairment. Renal impairment, including cases of acute renal failure and Fanconi syndrome, reported; d/c if estimated CrCl <50mL/min. Do not initiate therapy in patients w/ estimated CrCl <70mL/min. Immune reconstitution syndrome, autoimmune disorders (eg, Graves' disease, polymyositis, Guillain-Barre syndrome) in the setting of immune reconstitution, and redistribution/accumulation of body fat reported. Caution in elderly. Cobicistat: May cause modest increases in SrCr and modest declines in estimated CrCl w/o affecting renal glomerular function; closely monitor patients w/ confirmed increase in SrCr >0.4mg/dL from baseline for renal safety. TDF: Obesity and prolonged nucleoside exposure may be risk factors for lactic acidosis and severe hepatomegaly. Caution w/ known risk factors for liver disease. D/C if lactic acidosis or pronounced hepatotoxicity occurs. Decreased bone mineral density (BMD), increased biochemical markers of bone metabolism, and osteomalacia reported. Consider hypophosphatemia and osteomalacia secondary to proximal renal tubulopathy in patients at risk of renal dysfunction who present w/ persistent/worsening bone or muscle symptoms.

ADVERSE REACTIONS

Lactic acidosis, severe hepatomegaly w/ steatosis, diarrhea, nausea, fatigue, headache, dizziness, insomnia, abnormal dreams, rash, CK/amylase elevation, hematuria.

DRUG INTERACTIONS

See Contraindications. Avoid w/ cobicistat, elvitegravir, adefovir dipivoxil, rifabutin, rifapentine, salmeterol, nephrotoxic agents (eg, high dose or multiple NSAIDs), other antiretrovirals, or with products containing emtricitabine, TDF, lamivudine, or ritonavir. Avoid w/ colchicine in patients w/ renal or hepatic impairment. Antacids (eg, aluminum and magnesium hydroxide) may decrease elvitegravir levels; separate administration by at least 2 hrs. May increase levels of antiarrhythmics (eg, digoxin), carbamazepine, clonazepam, ethosuximide, ketoconazole, itraconazole, voriconazole, colchicine, β-blockers, calcium channel blockers, fluticasone (inhaled or nasal), bosentan, atorvastatin, immunosuppressants, salmeterol, neuroleptics, PDE-5 inhibitors, and sedative/hypnotics (eg, benzodiazepines). May increase norgestimate and decrease ethinyl estradiol levels; caution w/ contraceptives containing norgestimate/ethinyl estradiol. Consider alternative (nonhormonal) methods of contraception. May increase levels of buprenorphine and norbuprenorphine and may decrease levels of naloxone; monitor for sedation and cognitive effects upon coadministration w/ buprenorphine/naloxone. Monitor INR upon coadministration w/ warfarin. May increase levels of antidepressants (eg, SSRIs, TCAs, trazodone); carefully titrate antidepressant dose and monitor response. May increase levels of clarithromycin; reduce clarithromycin dose by 50% in patients w/ CrCl 50-60mL/min. Anticonvulsants (eg, carbamazepine, oxcarbazepine, phenobarbital, phenytoin) may decrease elvitegravir and cobicistat levels; consider alternative anticonvulsants. Rifabutin, rifapentine, and dexamethasone may decrease elvitegravir and cobicistat levels. Ketoconazole, itraconazole, or voriconazole may increase levels of elvitegravir and cobicistat.

May increase levels of drugs that are primarily metabolized by CYP3A/2D6, or are substrates of P-gp, breast cancer resistance protein, or organic anion transporting polypeptides 1B1/1B3. Elvitegravir may decrease levels of CYP2C9 substrates. CYP3A inducers may decrease elvitegravir and cobicistat levels and may result in loss of therapeutic effect and development of resistance. Drugs that reduce renal function or compete for active tubular secretion (eg, acyclovir, cidofovir, gentamicin) may increase levels of emtricitabine, TDF, and other renally eliminated drugs and may increase risk of adverse reactions. CYP3A inhibitors and clarithromycin may increase plasma levels of cobicistat. Cases of acute renal failure after initiation of high dose or multiple NSAIDs reported in patients w/ risk factors for renal dysfunction who appeared stable on TDF; consider alternatives to NSAIDs, if needed. Refer to PI for dosing modifications when used w/ certain concomitant therapies.

NURSING CONSIDERATIONS

Assessment: Assess for obesity, prolonged nucleoside exposure, risk factors for liver disease, renal/hepatic impairment, pregnancy/nursing status, and possible drug interactions. Assess BMD in patients who have a history of pathological bone fracture or w/ other risk factors for osteoporosis or bone loss. Obtain baseline estimated CrCl, urine glucose, urine protein, and SrCr. Perform test for HBV infection prior to therapy.

Monitoring: Monitor for signs/symptoms of lactic acidosis, severe hepatomegaly w/ steatosis, new onset/worsening renal impairment, immune reconstitution syndrome, autoimmune disorders, fat redistribution/accumulation, decreased BMD, increased biochemical markers for bone metabolism, osteomalacia, and other adverse reactions. Monitor for exacerbations of hepatitis B in patients w/ coinfection for at least several months upon discontinuation of therapy. Monitor BMD, estimated CrCl, urine glucose, urine protein, and SrCr. Monitor serum phosphorus levels in patients at risk for renal impairment. Monitor INR upon coadministration w/ warfarin.

Patient Counseling: Advise to remain under care of a physician during therapy. Inform that therapy does not cure HIV-1 infection and continuous therapy is necessary to control HIV-1 infection and decrease HIV-related illnesses. Advise to practice safe sex, to use latex or polyurethane condoms, not to share personal items (eg, toothbrush, razor blades), needles, or other inj equipment, and not to breastfeed. Instruct to take on a regular dosing schedule w/ food and to avoid missing doses. Instruct to contact physician if symptoms of lactic acidosis/pronounced hepatotoxicity, or any symptoms of infection occur. Advise that fat redistribution/accumulation, renal impairment, and decreases in BMD may occur. Inform patients that hepatitis B testing is recommended prior to initiating therapy. Advise to report use of any prescription or nonprescription medication or herbal products, including St. John's wort.

Storage: 25°C (77°F); excursions permitted to 15-30°C (59-86°F).

STRIVERDI RESPIMAT – olodaterol

RX

Class: Beta$_2$-agonist

Long-acting β_2-adrenergic agonists (LABAs) increase the risk of asthma-related death. Not indicated for the treatment of asthma.

ADULT DOSAGE

Chronic Obstructive Pulmonary Disease

Airflow Obstruction (Including Chronic Bronchitis and/or Emphysema):
Maint: 2 inh qd at the same time of day
Max: 2 inh/24 hrs

PEDIATRIC DOSAGE

Pediatric use may not have been established

ADMINISTRATION

Oral inh route

Insert cartridge into inhaler and prime the unit prior to 1st use

Priming Instructions

1. Actuate the inhaler toward the ground until the aerosol cloud is visible
2. Repeat 3 more times

If Not Used >3 Days: Actuate inhaler once to prepare for use
If Not Used >21 Days: Repeat priming instructions

HOW SUPPLIED

Spray, Inh: 2.5mcg/actuation [28, 60 actuations]

CONTRAINDICATIONS

Asthma without use of a long-term asthma control medication.

WARNINGS/PRECAUTIONS

Do not initiate in acutely deteriorating COPD patients or use for the relief of acute symptoms. D/C regular use of inhaled short-acting β_2-agonists (SABAs) when beginning treatment; use only for symptomatic relief of acute respiratory symptoms. Do not use more often or at higher doses than recommended; clinically significant cardiovascular (CV) effects and fatalities reported with excessive use. May produce paradoxical bronchospasm; d/c therapy immediately and institute alternative therapy. CV effects may occur; d/c if such effects occur. Caution with CV disorders, convulsive disorders, thyrotoxicosis, diabetes mellitus (DM), ketoacidosis, and in patients unusually responsive to sympathomimetic amines. May produce significant hypokalemia and increases in plasma glucose. Immediate hypersensitivity reactions may occur; d/c therapy immediately and consider alternative treatment.

ADVERSE REACTIONS

Nasopharyngitis, URTI, bronchitis, cough, back pain.

DRUG INTERACTIONS

Do not use with other medications containing LABAs. Adrenergic drugs may potentiate sympathetic effects; use with caution. Xanthine derivatives, steroids, or diuretics may potentiate any hypokalemic effect. Caution is advised when coadministered with non-K^+-sparing diuretics (eg, loop, thiazide). Extreme caution with MAOIs, TCAs, or drugs known to prolong the QTc interval; action on CV system may be potentiated. Drugs known to prolong the QTc interval may be associated with an increased risk of ventricular arrhythmias. β-blockers and olodaterol may interfere with the effect of each other when administered concurrently. β-blockers may block therapeutic effects and produce severe bronchospasm in COPD patients; if such therapy is needed, consider cardioselective β-blockers and use with caution. Ketoconazole (a strong dual CYP and P-gp inhibitor) may increase levels.

NURSING CONSIDERATIONS

Assessment: Assess for asthma, acute COPD deteriorations, CV disorders, convulsive disorders, thyrotoxicosis, DM, ketoacidosis, pregnancy/nursing status, and possible drug interactions. Assess use in patients unusually responsive to sympathomimetic amines.

Monitoring: Monitor for deteriorating disease, paradoxical bronchospasm, CV effects, hypokalemia, hyperglycemia, immediate hypersensitivity reactions, and other adverse reactions.

Patient Counseling: Counsel about the risks and benefits of therapy. Inform that drug is not for treatment of asthma. Advise not to use to relieve acute symptoms; inform that acute symptoms should be treated with an inhaled SABA. Instruct to notify physician immediately if experiencing worsening of symptoms, decreasing effectiveness of inhaled SABA, a need for more inhalations than usual of inhaled SABA, or a significant decrease in lung function. Advise not to stop therapy without physician guidance, not to use additional LABA, and not to use more than the recommended once-daily dose. Instruct to d/c the regular use of inhaled SABAs when beginning treatment. Inform of adverse effects associated with therapy.

Storage: 25°C (77°F); excursions permitted to 15-30°C (59-86°F). Avoid freezing.

STROMECTOL — ivermectin RX

Class: Avermectin derivative

ADULT DOSAGE

Intestinal Strongyloidiasis (*Strongyloides stercoralis*)

Usual: 200mcg/kg single dose

Weight-Based Dosing Recommendations:
15-24kg: 3mg single dose
25-35kg: 6mg single dose
36-50kg: 9mg single dose
51-65kg: 12mg single dose
66-79kg: 15mg single dose
≥80kg: 200mcg/kg single dose

Onchocerciasis (*Onchocerca volvulus*)

No activity against adult Onchocerca volvulus parasites

Usual: 150mcg/kg single dose

Weight-Based Dosing Recommendations:
15-25kg: 3mg single dose
26-44kg: 6mg single dose
45-64kg: 9mg single dose

PEDIATRIC DOSAGE

Intestinal Strongyloidiasis (*Strongyloides stercoralis*)

Usual: 200mcg/kg single dose

Weight-Based Dosing Recommendations:
15-24kg: 3mg single dose
25-35kg: 6mg single dose
36-50kg: 9mg single dose
51-65kg: 12mg single dose
66-79kg: 15mg single dose
≥80kg: 200mcg/kg single dose

Onchocerciasis (*Onchocerca volvulus*)

No activity against adult Onchocerca volvulus parasites

Usual: 150mcg/kg single dose

Weight-Based Dosing Recommendations:
15-25kg: 3mg single dose
26-44kg: 6mg single dose
45-64kg: 9mg single dose

65-84kg: 12mg single dose
≥85kg: 150mcg/kg single dose
For mass distribution in international treatment programs, the usual dosing interval is 12 months
Usual dosing interval for retreatment for individual patients can be as short as 3 months

65-84kg: 12mg single dose
≥85kg: 150mcg/kg single dose
For mass distribution in international treatment programs, the usual dosing interval is 12 months
Usual dosing interval for retreatment for individual patients can be as short as 3 months

ADMINISTRATION
Oral route
Take on empty stomach w/ water

HOW SUPPLIED
Tab: 3mg

WARNINGS/PRECAUTIONS
Cutaneous and/or systemic reactions of varying severity (the Mazzotti reaction) and ophthalmological reactions may develop in onchocerciasis treatment. Caution in hyperreactive onchodermatitis (sowda); severe adverse reactions (eg, edema, aggravation of onchodermatitis) are more likely to occur. Rarely, serious or even fatal encephalopathy may develop spontaneously or following treatment in patients with onchocerciasis who are also heavily infected with *Loa loa*. Implement pretreatment assessment for loiasis and post-treatment follow-up in patients who were exposed to *Loa loa*-endemic areas. Repeated courses of therapy may be required in immunocompromised (including HIV-infected) patients treated for intestinal strongyloidiasis. Caution in elderly.

ADVERSE REACTIONS
Pruritus, edema, papular/pustular/frank urticarial rash, fever, axillary/cervical/inguinal lymphadenopathy, arthralgia/synovitis, limbitis, tachycardia, peripheral edema, leukopenia, eosinophilia.

DRUG INTERACTIONS
Increased INR with warfarin has been rarely reported.

NURSING CONSIDERATIONS

Assessment: Assess for strongyloidiasis, onchocerciasis and loiasis. Assess for immunocompromised state (eg, HIV-infection), pregnancy/nursing status, and for possible drug interactions.

Monitoring: Monitor for cutaneous and/or systemic reactions, ophthalmological reactions, hyperreactive onchodermatitis, and other adverse reactions (eg, edema, dyspnea, urinary/fecal incontinence, neurologic changes, Stevens-Johnson syndrome, hypotension). Conduct at least three stool exams over 3 months to ensure *Strongyloides* eradication. Monitor LFTs and serum bilirubin levels.

Patient Counseling: Advise to take tab on empty stomach with water. Counsel on need for repeated stool exams to document clearance of infection with strongyloidiasis. Inform that with onchocerciasis, repeated follow up and retreatment is usually needed; drug does not kill adult *Onchocerca* parasite. Instruct to notify physician if pregnant, breastfeeding, or intend to breastfeed.

Storage: <30°C (86°F).

SUBOXONE FILM – buprenorphine/naloxone CIII

Class: Partial opioid agonist/opioid antagonist

ADULT DOSAGE

Opioid Dependence

Part of a complete treatment plan that includes counseling and psychosocial support

Prior to Induction:
Consider type of opioid dependence (eg, long- or short-acting opioid products), the time since last opioid use, and degree or level of opioid dependence. The 1st dose of therapy should be started only when objective signs of moderate withdrawal appear

Induction:
Day 1:
Initial: 2mg-0.5mg or 4mg-1mg

PEDIATRIC DOSAGE

Pediatric use may not have been established

Titrate: May titrate upwards in 2mg or 4mg increments of buprenorphine, at approx 2-hr intervals to 8mg-2mg based on the control of acute withdrawal symptoms. Induction dosage of up to 8mg-2mg is recommended

Day 2:
Up to 16mg-4mg as single daily dose

On Methadone/Long-Acting Opioids:
May be more susceptible to precipitated and prolonged withdrawal during induction therapy; buprenorphine monotherapy is recommended when used according to approved administration instructions. Following induction, may then be transitioned to qd SL film dose

On Heroin/Other Short-Acting Opioids:
May be inducted w/ SL film or w/ SL buprenorphine monotherapy
Administer 1st dose when objective signs of moderate opioid withdrawal appear, and not <6 hrs after last opioid use. Achieve adequate maintenance dose, titrated to clinical effectiveness as soon as possible

Maint:

Day 3 Onwards:
Progressively adjust dose in increments/decrements of 2mg-0.5mg or 4mg-1mg to a level that maintains treatment and suppresses opioid withdrawal signs/symptoms. After treatment induction and stabilization, the maintenance dose is generally in the range of 4mg-1mg to 24mg-6mg/day depending on the patient/response

Target Dose: 16mg-4mg/day as single daily dose

Max: 24mg-6mg/day

Conversions

Switching Between Buprenorphine or Buprenorphine/Naloxone SL Tabs and Buprenorphine/Naloxone SL Film:
Start on the corresponding dosage of the previously administered product; adjust dose prn. Refer to PI for switching between SL film strengths

DOSE MODIFICATION

Hepatic Impairment

Moderate: Use may not be appropriate

Severe: Avoid use

Elderly

Start at lower end of dosing range

Discontinuation

Should be made as part of a comprehensive treatment plan; taper patients to avoid opioid withdrawal signs/symptoms

Other Important Modifications

Unstable Patients:
Patients who continue to misuse, abuse, or divert buprenorphine products or other opioids should be provided w/, or referred to, more intensive and structured treatment

ADMINISTRATION

SL route

Do not cut, chew, or swallow film
If an additional SL film is necessary, place it on the opposite side from the 1st film in a manner to minimize overlapping
Keep under the tongue until completely dissolved; should not be moved after placement

HOW SUPPLIED

Film, SL: (Buprenorphine-Naloxone) 2mg-0.5mg, 4mg-1mg, 8mg-2mg, 12mg-3mg

WARNINGS/PRECAUTIONS
Not appropriate as an analgesic. Hypersensitivity reactions, bronchospasm, angioneurotic edema, and anaphylactic shock reported. May precipitate opioid withdrawal signs and symptoms if administered before the agonist effects of the opioid have subsided. Not recommended in patients with severe hepatic impairment and not recommended for initiation of treatment in patients with moderate hepatic impairment. May be used with caution for maintenance treatment in patients with moderate hepatic impairment who have initiated treatment on a buprenorphine product without naloxone. May impair mental/physical abilities. May produce orthostatic hypotension in ambulatory patients. Caution with myxedema, hypothyroidism, adrenal cortical insufficiency (eg, Addison's disease), CNS depression/coma, toxic psychoses, prostatic hypertrophy, urethral stricture, acute alcoholism, delirium tremens, kyphoscoliosis, and in elderly/debilitated patients. Caution in patients with compromised respiratory function (eg, chronic obstructive pulmonary disease, cor pulmonale, decreased respiratory reserve, hypoxia, hypercapnia, preexisting respiratory depression). Buprenorphine: Potential for abuse. Significant respiratory depression and death reported. Reestablish adequate ventilation in case of overdose; may use higher than normal doses and repeated administration of naloxone PRN to manage buprenorphine overdose. Accidental pediatric exposure can cause severe, possibly fatal respiratory depression. Chronic use produces physical dependence. Cytolytic hepatitis and hepatitis with jaundice reported. If a hepatic event is suspected, biological and etiological evaluation is recommended; careful discontinuation may be needed depending on the case. Caution with preexisting liver enzyme abnormalities, hepatitis B or C infection, use with other potentially hepatotoxic drugs, and ongoing injecting drug use. Neonatal withdrawal reported when used during pregnancy. May elevate CSF pressure; caution with head injury, intracranial lesions, and other circumstances when CSF pressure may be increased. May produce miosis and changes in the level of consciousness that may interfere with patient evaluation. May increase intracholedochal pressure; caution with biliary tract dysfunction. May obscure the diagnosis or clinical course of patients with acute abdominal conditions.

ADVERSE REACTIONS
Oral hypoesthesia, constipation, glossodynia, oral mucosal erythema, vomiting, intoxication, disturbance in attention, palpitations, insomnia, withdrawal syndrome, hyperhidrosis, blurred vision, restlessness.

DRUG INTERACTIONS
May cause respiratory depression, coma, and death with benzodiazepines or other CNS depressants (eg, alcohol); use with caution. Opioid analgesics, general anesthetics, benzodiazepines, phenothiazines, other tranquilizers, sedative/hypnotics, or other CNS depressants (eg, alcohol) may increase CNS depression; consider dose reduction of 1 or both agents. Concomitant use with CYP3A4 inhibitors (eg, azole antifungals such as ketoconazole, macrolides such as erythromycin, HIV protease inhibitors) should be monitored and may require dose reduction of 1 or both agents. Monitor for signs and symptoms of opioid withdrawal with CYP3A4 inducers (eg, efavirenz, phenobarbital, carbamazepine, phenytoin, rifampicin). Monitor dose of patients who are on chronic buprenorphine treatment if non-nucleoside reverse transcriptase inhibitors are added to treatment regimen. Atazanavir and atazanavir/ritonavir may increase levels and sedation; monitor and consider dose reduction of buprenorphine.

NURSING CONSIDERATIONS

Assessment: Assess for history of hypersensitivity to drug, myxedema, hypothyroidism, adrenal cortical insufficiency, CNS depression or coma, toxic psychoses, prostatic hypertrophy, urethral stricture, acute alcoholism, delirium tremens, kyphoscoliosis, debilitation, compromised respiratory function, hepatic impairment, hepatitis B or C infection, head injury, intracranial lesions and other circumstances in which CSF pressure may be increased, biliary tract dysfunction, acute abdominal conditions, pregnancy/nursing status, and possible drug interactions. Obtain baseline LFTs prior to therapy.

Monitoring: Monitor for hypersensitivity reactions, signs/symptoms of precipitated opioid withdrawal, impaired mental/physical ability, orthostatic hypotension, respiratory depression, drug abuse/dependence, cytolytic hepatitis, hepatitis with jaundice, elevation of CSF pressure and intracholedochal pressure, miosis, changes in consciousness levels, and other adverse reactions. Monitor LFTs periodically. Monitor for symptoms related to over-dosing or under-dosing when switching between buprenorphine or other buprenorphine/naloxone products.

Patient Counseling: Warn about danger of self-administration of benzodiazepines and other CNS depressants, including alcohol, while on therapy. Advise that drug contains opioid that can be a target for abuse; instruct to keep film in a safe place protected from theft and children. Instruct to seek medical attention immediately if a child is exposed to the drug. Caution that drug may impair mental/physical abilities and cause orthostatic hypotension. Advise to take film qd and to not change dose without consulting physician. Inform that treatment can cause dependence and withdrawal syndrome may occur upon discontinuation. Advise patients seeking to d/c treatment with buprenorphine for opioid dependence to work closely with physician on a tapering schedule, and apprise of the potential to relapse to illicit drug use associated with discontinuation of treatment. Advise to report to physician all medications prescribed or currently being used. Advise women regarding possible effects during pregnancy. Advise women who are breastfeeding to monitor the infant for drowsiness and difficulty breathing. Advise to instruct family members that, in event of emergency, the treating physician or staff should be informed that patient is physically dependent on an opioid and that the patient is being treated with SL film.

Storage: 25°C (77°F); excursions permitted to 15-30°C (59-86°F).

Subsys – fentanyl CII

Class: Opioid analgesic

Fatal respiratory depression may occur. Contraindicated in the management of acute or postoperative pain (eg, headache/ migraine) and in opioid-nontolerant patients. Death reported upon accidental ingestion in children; keep out of reach of children. Concomitant use w/ CYP3A4 inhibitors may increase plasma levels, and may cause fatal respiratory depression. Do not convert patients on a mcg-per-mcg basis from any other fentanyl product to Subsys. Do not substitute for any other fentanyl products; may result in fatal overdose. Contains fentanyl w/ an abuse liability similar to other opioid analgesics. Available only through a restricted program called the Transmucosal Immediate-Release Fentanyl Risk Evaluation and Mitigation Strategy (TIRF REMS) Access program due to risk for misuse, abuse, addiction, and overdose. Outpatients, healthcare professionals who prescribe to outpatients, pharmacies, and distributors must enroll in the program.

ADULT DOSAGE

Cancer Pain

Breakthrough Pain in Patients Already Receiving and Tolerant to Around-the-Clock Opioid Therapy:

Initial: 100mcg

Titrate: May take only 1 additional dose of the same strength for each breakthrough pain episode if pain is not relieved after 30 min

100mcg: 1 x100mcg unit
200mcg: 1 x 200mcg unit
400mcg: 1 x 400mcg unit
600mcg: 1 x 600mcg unit
800mcg: 1 x 800mcg unit
1200mcg: 2 x 600mcg unit
1600mcg: 2 x 800mcg unit

Maint: Once titrated to an effective dose, use only 1 dose of the appropriate strength per breakthrough pain episode; only increase dose when single administration of current dose fails to adequately treat the breakthrough pain episode for several consecutive episodes

Max: 2 doses for any breakthrough pain episode; limit consumption to ≤4 doses/day

Wait at least 4 hrs before treating another episode of breakthrough pain

If >4 breakthrough pain episodes/day are experienced, reevaluate maint dose (around-the-clock) used for persistent pain

Conversions

Switching from Actiq to Subsys:

Initial:
200 or 400mcg Actiq: 100mcg Subsys
600 or 800mcg Actiq: 200mcg Subsys
1200 or 1600mcg Actiq: 400mcg Subsys

Titrate:
≤400mcg Actiq: Proceed using multiples of 100mcg Subsys
600 and 800mcg Actiq: Proceed using multiples of 200mcg Subsys
1200 and 1600mcg Actiq: Proceed using multiples of 400mcg Subsys

PEDIATRIC DOSAGE

Pediatric use may not have been established

DOSE MODIFICATION

Adverse Reactions

Oral Mucositis:

Grade 1: Monitor closely for respiratory depression and CNS depression particularly during initiation of therapy

Grade ≥2: Avoid use unless benefits outweigh potential risk

Excessive Opioid Effects: Decrease subsequent doses

ADMINISTRATION

SL route

Open blister package w/ scissors immediately prior to use

Carefully spray contents into mouth underneath the tongue

Disposal

Use the charcoal-lined disposal pouch to dispose of the contents of any unneeded unit dose systems

HOW SUPPLIED

Spray: 100mcg/spray, 200mcg/spray, 400mcg/spray, 600mcg/spray, 800mcg/spray

CONTRAINDICATIONS

Opioid-nontolerant patients, management of acute or postoperative pain (eg, headache/migraine).

WARNINGS/PRECAUTIONS

Increased risk of respiratory depression in patients w/ underlying respiratory disorders and in elderly/debilitated. May impair mental and/or physical abilities. Caution w/ COPD or preexisting medical conditions predisposing to respiratory depression; may further decrease respiratory drive to the point of respiratory failure. Extreme caution in patients who may be susceptible to intracranial effects of carbon dioxide retention (eg, those w/ evidence of increased intracranial pressure or impaired consciousness). May obscure clinical course of head injuries; use only if clinically warranted. Caution w/ bradyarrhythmias. Avoid use during labor and delivery. Caution w/ renal/hepatic impairment.

ADVERSE REACTIONS

Respiratory depression, circulatory depression, hypotension, shock, N/V, constipation, somnolence, dizziness, asthenia, dyspnea, anxiety.

DRUG INTERACTIONS

See Boxed Warning. Monitor for an extended period of time w/ concomitant use w/ moderate or strong CYP3A4 inhibitors. Not recommended w/ an MAOI or w/in 14 days of MAOI discontinuation. Increased depressant effects w/ other CNS depressants (eg, other opioids, sedatives/hypnotics, general anesthetics); adjust dose of Subsys if warranted and monitor for a change in opioid effects. CYP3A4 inducers (eg, barbiturates, carbamazepine, efavirenz) may decrease levels; monitor and adjust dose of Subsys accordingly. Respiratory depression may be more likely to occur when given in conjunction w/ other drugs that depress respiration.

NURSING CONSIDERATIONS

Assessment: Assess for degree of opioid tolerance, previous opioid dose, level of pain intensity, type of pain, patient's general condition and medical status, underlying respiratory disorders, or any other conditions where treatment is contraindicated or cautioned. Assess for intolerance or previous hypersensitivity, renal/hepatic function, pregnancy/nursing status, and possible drug interactions.

Monitoring: Monitor for signs/symptoms of respiratory depression, impairment of mental/physical abilities, drug abuse/addiction, and other adverse reactions. Closely monitor patients w/ Grade 1 mucositis or hepatic/renal impairment, and monitor elderly for respiratory depression and CNS effects.

Patient Counseling: Inform outpatients to enroll in the TIRF REMS Access program; instruct to sign a patient-prescriber agreement form to confirm understanding. Instruct to properly dispose of consumed units. Instruct not to take medication for acute or postoperative pain, pain from injuries, headache, migraine, or any other short-term pain. Advise to take drug as prescribed and avoid sharing it w/ anyone else. Inform of the high risk of fatal respiratory depression in children if exposed to therapy. Instruct to notify physician if breakthrough pain is not alleviated or worsens after taking the medication. Inform that medication use may impair mental/physical abilities; caution against performing activities that require a high level of attention. Advise not to combine w/ alcohol, sleep aids, or tranquilizers, except if ordered by physician. Instruct to inform physician if pregnant or planning to become pregnant.

Storage: 20-25°C (68-77°F); excursions permitted between 15-30°C (59-86°F) until ready to use.

SULFAMETHOXAZOLE/TRIMETHOPRIM – sulfamethoxazole/trimethoprim RX

Class: Sulfonamide/tetrahydrofolic acid inhibitor

OTHER BRAND NAMES

Bactrim, Bactrim DS, Sulfatrim

ADULT DOSAGE

Traveler's Diarrhea

Sus/Tab:
Usual: One 800mg-160mg tab or two 400mg-80mg tabs or 4 tsp sus q12h for 5 days

Urinary Tract Infections

Inj:
Severe Infections: 8-10mg/kg/day (based on the trimethoprim component) given in equally divided doses q6h, q8h, or q12h for up to 14 days
Max: 60mL/day

Sus/Tab:
Usual: One 800mg-160mg tab or two 400mg-80mg tabs or 4 tsp (20mL) sus q12h for 10-14 days

Acute Bacterial Exacerbation of Chronic Bronchitis

Usual: One 800mg-160mg tab or two 400mg-80mg tabs or 4 tsp sus q12h for 14 days

Shigellosis

Inj:
8-10mg/kg/day (based on the trimethoprim component) given in equally divided doses q6h, q8h, or q12h for up to 5 days
Max: 60mL/day

Sus/Tab:
Usual: One 800mg-160mg tab or two 400mg-80mg tabs or 4 tsp (20mL) sus q12h for 5 days

Pneumonia

***Pneumocystis jiroveci* pneumonia (PCP)**
Treatment:
Inj:
15-20mg/kg/day (based on the trimethoprim component) given in 3 or 4 equally divided doses q6-8h for up to 14 days
Sus/Tab:
75-100mg/kg sulfamethoxazole and 15-20mg/kg trimethoprim per 24 hrs given in equally divided doses q6h for 14-21 days

PCP Prophylaxis in Immunosuppressed Patients:
Sus/Tab:
One 800mg-160mg tab or 4 tsp sus daily

PEDIATRIC DOSAGE

Pneumonia

***Pneumocystis jiroveci* pneumonia (PCP)**
Treatment:
≥2 Months of Age:
Inj:
15-20mg/kg/day (based on the trimethoprim component) given in 3 or 4 equally divided doses q6-8h for up to 14 days
Sus/Tab:
75-100mg/kg sulfamethoxazole and 15-20mg/kg trimethoprim per 24 hrs given in equally divided doses q6h for 14-21 days

PCP Prophylaxis in Immunosuppressed Patients:
Sus/Tab:
750mg/m^2/day sulfamethoxazole w/ 150mg/m^2/day trimethoprim given in equally divided doses bid, on 3 consecutive days/week. Not to exceed 1600mg/day sulfamethoxazole and 320mg/day trimethoprim

Acute Otitis Media

Use only when sulfamethoxazole/trimethoprim could offer some advantage over the use of a single antimicrobial agent
≥2 Months of Age:
Sus/Tab:
40mg/kg sulfamethoxazole and 8mg/kg trimethoprim per 24 hrs, given in 2 divided doses q12h for 10 days

Shigellosis

≥2 Months of Age:
Inj:
8-10mg/kg/day (based on the trimethoprim component) given in equally divided doses q6h, q8h, or q12h for up to 5 days
Max: 60mL/day

Sus/Tab:
40mg/kg sulfamethoxazole and 8mg/kg trimethoprim per 24 hrs, given in 2 divided doses q12h for 5 days

Urinary Tract Infections

≥2 Months of Age:

Inj:
Severe Infections: 8-10mg/kg/day (based on the trimethoprim component) given in equally divided doses q6h, q8h, or q12h for up to 14 days
Max: 60mL/day
Sus/Tab:
40mg/kg sulfamethoxazole and 8mg/kg trimethoprim per 24 hrs, given in 2 divided doses q12h for 10 days

DOSE MODIFICATION

Renal Impairment

Inj/Sus/Tab:

CrCl 15-30mL/min: 1/2 the usual regimen

CrCl <15mL/min: Use not recommended

ADMINISTRATION

IV/Oral route

Inj

Administer by IV infusion over 60-90 min; avoid rapid infusion or bolus inj

Do not mix w/ other drugs or sol

IV Preparation/Dilution

Dilute prior to administration

Each 5mL of sulfamethoxazole-trimethoprim should be added to 125mL D5W; use w/in 6 hrs after dilution and do not refrigerate

If 5mL/100mL D5W dilution is desired, use w/in 4 hrs

If fluid restriction is desired, each 5mL of sulfamethoxazole-trimethoprim may be added to 75mL D5W; administer w/in 2 hrs

Multidose vials must be used w/in 48 hrs after initial entry into vial

Compatible Infusion Systems

Unit-dose glass containers

Unit-dose polyvinyl chloride and polyolefin containers

Sus

Shake well before using

Refer to PI for specific weight-dose recommendations for sus/tab use in pediatrics

HOW SUPPLIED

Sulfamethoxazole-Trimethoprim (SMX-TMP) Inj: 80mg-16mg/mL [5mL, 10mL]; Sus: (Sulfatrim) 200mg-40mg/5mL [473mL]; Tab: (Bactrim) 400mg-80mg*, (Bactrim DS) 800mg-160mg* *scored

CONTRAINDICATIONS

Documented megaloblastic anemia due to folate deficiency, history of drug-induced immune thrombocytopenia with use of TMP and/or sulfonamides, and pediatrics <2 months of age. (Inj/Sus) Pregnant and nursing women. (Sus/Tab) Marked hepatic damage, and severe renal insufficiency when renal function status cannot be monitored.

WARNINGS/PRECAUTIONS

Fatalities, although rare, have occurred due to severe reactions, including Stevens-Johnson syndrome, toxic epidermal necrolysis, fulminant hepatic necrosis, agranulocytosis, aplastic anemia, thrombocytopenia, and other blood dyscrasias; d/c at the 1st appearance of skin rash or any sign of adverse reaction. Cough, SOB, and pulmonary infiltrates reported. Do not use for treatment of group A β-hemolytic streptococcal infections. *Clostridium difficile*-associated diarrhea (CDAD) reported; d/c if CDAD is suspected or confirmed. May result in bacterial resistance if used in the absence of proven or suspected bacterial infection or a prophylactic indication. Caution with hepatic/renal impairment, possible folate deficiency (eg, in the elderly, chronic alcoholics, those receiving anticonvulsant therapy, with malabsorption syndrome, and in malnutrition states), severe allergies or bronchial asthma, porphyria, and thyroid dysfunction. Hematological changes indicative of folic acid deficiency may occur in the elderly, or with preexisting folic acid deficiency or kidney failure; effects are reversible by folinic acid therapy. Hemolysis may occur in patients with G6PD deficiency. Cases of hypoglycemia in nondiabetic patients reported rarely. TMP may impair phenylalanine metabolism. AIDS patients may not tolerate or respond to therapy in the same manner as non-AIDS patients; increased incidence of side effects, particularly rash, fever, leukopenia, elevated transaminase values, and hyperkalemia, in AIDS patients being treated for *P. jiroveci* pneumonia; reevaluate therapy if skin rash or any sign of adverse reaction develops. May cause hyperkalemia in patients receiving high dosage of TMP, with underlying disorders of K^+ metabolism, with renal insufficiency, or when used concomitantly with drugs known to induce hyperkalemia; closely monitor serum K^+. Ensure adequate fluid intake and urinary output during treatment to prevent crystalluria. Slow acetylators may be more prone to idiosyncratic reactions to sulfonamides. D/C if a significant reduction in the count of any formed blood element is noted. Lab test interactions may occur. (Inj) Contains sodium metabisulfite, which may cause allergic-type reactions, including anaphylactic symptoms and life-threatening or less severe asthmatic episodes in certain susceptible people. Contains benzyl alcohol, which has been associated with an increased incidence of neurological and other complications (sometimes fatal) in newborns. Local irritation and inflammation due to extravascular infiltration of the infusion reported; d/c infusion and restart at another site if these occur. (Tab) Severe and symptomatic hyponatremia may occur, particularly in patients treated for *P. jiroveci* pneumonia; evaluation for hyponatremia and appropriate correction is necessary in symptomatic patients to prevent life-threatening complications. Use during pregnancy may be associated with an increased risk of congenital malformations.

ADVERSE REACTIONS

GI disturbances (N/V, anorexia), allergic skin reactions (eg, rash, urticaria).

DRUG INTERACTIONS

Increased incidence of thrombocytopenia with purpura reported in elderly concurrently receiving certain diuretics, primarily thiazides. May prolong PT with warfarin; caution with anticoagulants. May inhibit the hepatic metabolism of phenytoin; monitor for possible excessive phenytoin effect. May increase MTX concentrations. Marked but reversible nephrotoxicity reported with cyclosporine in renal transplant recipients. May increase digoxin levels, especially in the elderly; monitor digoxin levels. Increased SMX levels with indomethacin. Megaloblastic anemia may develop if used in patients receiving pyrimethamine as malaria prophylaxis in doses >25mg/week. May decrease efficacy of TCAs. Potentiates the effect of oral hypoglycemics. Toxic delirium reported with amantadine. Hyperkalemia in elderly patients reported after concomitant use with an ACE inhibitor. (Inj/Tab) Treatment failure and excess mortality reported when used concomitantly with leucovorin for the treatment of HIV positive patients with P. jiroveci pneumonia; avoid coadministration during treatment of P. jiroveci pneumonia. (Tab) Caution with drugs that are substrates of CYP2C8 (eg, pioglitazone, repaglinide, rosiglitazone), CYP2C9 (eg, glipizide, glyburide), or OCT2 (eg, memantine, metformin).

NURSING CONSIDERATIONS

Assessment: Assess for hypersensitivity to the drug, megaloblastic anemia, history of drug-induced immune thrombocytopenia, hepatic/renal impairment, folate deficiency, severe allergies, bronchial asthma, G6PD deficiency, porphyria, thyroid dysfunction, underlying disorders of K^+ metabolism, pregnancy/nursing status, and possible drug interactions.

Monitoring: Monitor for hypersensitivity and other fatal reactions, CDAD, folate deficiency, hypoglycemia, hyperkalemia, and other adverse reactions. Monitor hydration status. Perform CBC frequently, and urinalyses with careful microscopic exam and renal function tests. (Inj) Monitor for infusion reactions. (Tab) Monitor for hyponatremia.

Patient Counseling: Counsel that therapy should only be used to treat bacterial, not viral (eg, common cold), infections. Instruct to take exactly ud even if patient feels better early in the course of therapy. Inform that skipping doses or not completing the full course of therapy may decrease effectiveness of treatment and increase bacterial resistance. Instruct to maintain an adequate fluid intake. Inform that diarrhea is a common problem caused by therapy, which usually ends when therapy is discontinued. Instruct to immediately contact physician if watery and bloody stools (with or without stomach cramps and fever) occur, even as late as ≥2 months after having taken the last dose.

Storage: 20-25°C (68-77°F). (Inj) Do not refrigerate. (Sus) Protect from light.

SUMAVEL DOSEPRO – sumatriptan RX

Class: 5-$HT_{1B/1D}$ agonist

ADULT DOSAGE

Migraine

W/ or w/o Aura:

Max Single Dose: 6mg; if side effects are dose limiting, 4mg may be used

Max Cumulative Dose: 12mg/24 hrs; separate doses by ≥1 hr

Only consider 2nd dose if there is some response to the 1st dose observed

Cluster Headache

Acute Treatment:

Max Single Dose: 6mg

Max Cumulative Dose: 12mg/24 hrs; separate doses by ≥1 hr

Only consider 2nd dose if there is some response to the 1st dose observed

PEDIATRIC DOSAGE

Pediatric use may not have been established

DOSE MODIFICATION

Elderly

Use caution; start at lower end of dosing range

ADMINISTRATION

SQ route

HOW SUPPLIED

Inj: 4mg/0.5mL, 6mg/0.5mL

CONTRAINDICATIONS

Ischemic coronary artery disease (CAD) (eg, angina pectoris, history of MI, documented silent ischemia), coronary artery vasospasm (eg, Prinzmetal's variant angina), Wolff-Parkinson-White syndrome or arrhythmias associated with other cardiac accessory conduction pathway disorders, history of stroke or transient ischemic attack (TIA), history of hemiplegic/basilar migraine, peripheral vascular disease, ischemic bowel disease, uncontrolled HTN. Recent (eg, within 24 hrs) use of another 5-HT_1 agonist, or of ergotamine-containing or ergot-type medication (eg, dihydroergotamine, methysergide). Concurrent administration or recent use (within 2 weeks) of an MAO-A inhibitor.

WARNINGS/PRECAUTIONS

May cause coronary artery vasospasm. Perform a cardiovascular (CV) evaluation in triptan-naive patients with multiple CV risk factors (eg, diabetes, HTN, smoking) prior to therapy; if negative, consider administering 1st dose under medical supervision and obtain ECG immediately following administration. Perform periodic CV evaluation in these patients if on long-term intermittent use. Life-threatening cardiac rhythm disturbances reported; d/c if these occur. Sensations of tightness, pain, pressure, and heaviness in the precordium, throat, neck, and jaw may occur. Cerebral/subarachnoid hemorrhage, stroke, other cerebrovascular events, noncoronary vasospastic reactions (eg, peripheral vascular ischemia, GI vascular ischemia/infarction, Raynaud's syndrome, splenic infarction) reported. Rule out a vasospastic reaction in patients who experience symptoms/signs suggestive of noncoronary vasospasm reaction following any 5-HT_1 agonist use before receiving additional doses. Exclude other potentially serious neurologic conditions before treating headaches in patients not previously diagnosed as migraineurs, and in migraineurs who present with atypical symptoms. May cause transient and permanent blindness and significant partial vision loss. Overuse of acute migraine drugs may lead to exacerbation of headache; detoxification, including withdrawal of the overused drugs and treatment of withdrawal symptoms may be necessary. Serotonin syndrome may occur; d/c if serotonin syndrome is suspected. Significant elevation in BP, including hypertensive crisis, reported; monitor BP. Anaphylaxis, anaphylactoid, and hypersensitivity reactions may occur; caution with history of sensitivity to multiple allergens. Seizures reported; caution with history of epilepsy or a lowered seizure threshold. Reconsider the diagnosis of migraine before giving a 2nd dose if patient does not respond to the 1st dose of therapy. Not recommended for use in patients with severe hepatic impairment. Not indicated for prevention of migraine attacks. Use only if clear diagnosis of migraine or cluster headache has been established. Caution in elderly.

ADVERSE REACTIONS

Inj-site reaction, tingling, warm sensation, burning sensation, feeling of heaviness, pressure sensation, feeling of tightness, numbness, flushing, chest discomfort, weakness, dizziness, neck pain, paresthesia, N/V.

DRUG INTERACTIONS

See Contraindications. Serotonin syndrome reported with SSRIs, SNRIs, TCAs, or MAOIs.

NURSING CONSIDERATIONS

Assessment: Assess for CV disease, HTN, hemiplegic or basilar migraine, hypersensitivity to drug, hepatic impairment, any other conditions where treatment is contraindicated or cautioned, pregnancy/nursing status, and possible drug interactions. Perform CV evaluation with multiple CV risk factors. Confirm diagnosis of migraine or cluster headache and exclude other potentially serious neurological conditions.

Monitoring: Monitor for signs/symptoms of cardiac events (eg, coronary vasospasm, acute MI, arrhythmia, ECG changes), cerebrovascular events (eg, hemorrhage, stroke, TIA), noncoronary vasospastic reactions, blindness, vision loss, serotonin syndrome, anaphylactic/anaphylactoid/hypersensitivity reactions, HTN, seizures, and other adverse reactions. Perform periodic CV evaluation in patients on long-term intermittent use with risk factors for CAD. Reassess diagnosis if clinical response does not occur following 1st dose of therapy.

Patient Counseling: Inform that therapy may cause CV side effects and anaphylactic/anaphylactoid reactions. Instruct to seek medical attention if signs/symptoms of chest pain, SOB, irregular heartbeat, significant rise in BP, weakness, and slurring of speech occur. Inform that use of acute migraine drugs for ≥10 days/month may lead to an exacerbation of headache; encourage to record headache frequency and drug use (eg, by keeping a headache diary). Inform about the risk of serotonin syndrome, particularly during combined use with SSRIs, SNRIs, TCAs, and MAOIs. Inform that drug may cause somnolence and dizziness; instruct to evaluate ability to perform complex tasks during migraine attacks and after administration of drug. Inform that medication should not be used during pregnancy and instruct to notify physician if breastfeeding or plan to breastfeed. Instruct on proper use of product and to avoid IM or IV use. Instruct to use inj sites on the abdomen (but not within 2 inches of the navel) or thigh with adequate SQ thickness to accommodate penetration of drug into the SQ space, and not on the arms or other areas of the body.

Storage: 20-25°C (68-77°F); excursions permitted between 15-30°C (59-86°F). Do not freeze. Protect from light.

SUPRAX – cefixime

RX

Class: Cephalosporin (3rd generation)

ADULT DOSAGE

General Dosing

Uncomplicated UTIs, Otitis Media, Pharyngitis, Tonsillitis, and Acute Exacerbation of Chronic Bronchitis:

400mg tab/cap qd or 1/2 tab q12h

***Streptococcus pyogenes* Infection:**

Administer for at least 10 days

Gonorrhea

Uncomplicated Cervical/Urethral Infections:

400mg single dose

PEDIATRIC DOSAGE

General Dosing

Uncomplicated UTIs, Otitis Media, Pharyngitis, Tonsillitis, and Acute Exacerbation of Chronic Bronchitis:

≥6 Months of Age:

Sus:

8mg/kg qd or 4mg/kg q12h

>12 Years or >45kg:

Use adult dose

Refer to PI for Pediatric Dosage Chart

***Streptococcus pyogenes* Infection:**

Administer for at least 10 days

Otitis Media:

Treat w/ chewable tab/sus

DOSE MODIFICATION

Renal Impairment

CrCl 21-59mL/min or on Hemodialysis: 13mL/day of 100mg/5mL sus; 6.5mL/day of 200mg/5mL sus; 2.6mL/day of 500mg/5mL sus

CrCl ≤20mL/min or on Continuous Peritoneal Dialysis: 8.6mL of 100mg/5mL sus; 4.4mL/day of 200mg/5mL sus; 1.8mL/day of 500mg/5mL sus; 200mg/day of tab; or 200mg of tab, chewable

ADMINISTRATION

Oral route

Cap/Tab

Take w/ or w/o food

Tab, Chewable

Chew or crush before swallowing

Sus

Refer to PI for reconstitution directions

HOW SUPPLIED

Cap: 400mg; Sus: 100mg/5mL [50mL, 75mL, 100mL], 200mg/5mL [25mL, 37.5mL, 50mL, 75mL, 100mL], 500mg/5mL [10mL, 20mL]; Tab, Chewable: 100mg, 150mg, 200mg; Tab: 400mg* *scored

WARNINGS/PRECAUTIONS

Do not substitute tab/cap for chewable tab or sus in the treatment of otitis media. Anaphylactic/anaphylactoid reactions reported. Cross hypersensitivity among β-lactam antibiotics reported; caution in patients with penicillin (PCN) sensitivity. D/C if an allergic reaction occurs. *Clostridium difficile*-associated diarrhea (CDAD) reported; d/c if CDAD is suspected or confirmed. Carefully monitor patients on dialysis. May be associated with fall in prothrombin activity; caution in patients with renal/hepatic impairment, poor nutritional state, protracted course of antimicrobial therapy, and those previously stabilized on anticoagulant therapy. May result in bacterial resistance if used in the absence of proven/suspected bacterial infection. Lab test interactions may occur.

ADVERSE REACTIONS

Diarrhea, loose or frequent stools, abdominal pain, nausea, dyspepsia, flatulence.

DRUG INTERACTIONS

May increase levels of carbamazepine. Increased PT, with or without bleeding, with anticoagulants (eg, warfarin).

NURSING CONSIDERATIONS

Assessment: Assess for previous hypersensitivity to cephalosporins, PCNs, or other drugs. Assess renal/hepatic function, nutritional status, history of antimicrobial or anticoagulants use, pregnancy/nursing status, and for possible drug interactions.

Monitoring: Monitor for signs/symptoms of anaphylactic/anaphylactoid reactions and CDAD. Monitor PT and renal function.

Patient Counseling: Inform that therapy only treats bacterial, not viral, infections. Instruct to take exactly ud; inform that skipping doses or not completing full course of therapy may decrease effectiveness and increase risk of bacterial resistance. Inform that diarrhea may be experienced as late as 2 or more months after last dose; instruct to contact physician if watery/bloody stools (with/without stomach cramps and fever) occur. Inform that chewable tabs contain phenylalanine.

Storage: 20-25°C (68-77°F). (Sus) After reconstitution, store for 14 days either at room temperature, or under refrigeration; keep tightly closed. Shake well before use. Discard unused portion after 14 days.

SUPREP – magnesium sulfate/potassium sulfate/sodium sulfate RX

Class: Bowel cleanser

ADULT DOSAGE

Bowel Cleansing

Prior to Colonoscopy:

Split-Dose (2-Day) Regimen:

Day Prior to Colonoscopy:

1. A light breakfast may be consumed, or have only clear liquids; avoid red and purple liquids, milk, and alcoholic beverages
2. Early in the pm, pour the contents of 1 bottle into the mixing container provided, fill the container w/ water to the 16 oz fill line, and drink the entire amount
3. Drink 2 additional containers filled to the 16 oz line w/ water over the next hr

Day of Colonoscopy:

1. Have only clear liquids until after the colonoscopy; avoid red and purple liquids, milk, and alcoholic beverages
2. The morning of colonoscopy (10-12 hrs after the evening dose), pour the contents of the 2nd bottle into the mixing container provided, fill the container w/ water to the 16 oz fill line, and drink the entire amount
3. Drink 2 additional containers filled to the 16 oz line w/ water over the next hr
4. Complete all Suprep Bowel Prep Kit and required water at least 1 hr prior to colonoscopy

PEDIATRIC DOSAGE

Pediatric use may not have been established

ADMINISTRATION

Oral route

HOW SUPPLIED

Sol: (Sodium Sulfate/Potassium Sulfate/Magnesium Sulfate) 17.5g/3.13g/1.6g

CONTRAINDICATIONS

GI obstruction, bowel perforation, gastric retention, ileus, toxic colitis, or toxic megacolon.

WARNINGS/PRECAUTIONS

Hydrate adequately before, during, and after use. If significant vomiting or signs of dehydration occur, consider performing postcolonoscopy tests (eg, electrolytes, creatinine, BUN). Correct electrolyte abnormalities prior to use. Caution w/ conditions that may increase the risk of fluid/electrolyte disturbances and renal impairment. May increase uric acid levels. Serious arrhythmias reported rarely; caution in patients at increased risk of arrhythmias. Generalized tonic-clonic seizures and/or loss of consciousness reported; caution in patients at increased risk of seizures (eg, hyponatremia, alcohol or benzodiazepine withdrawal). May produce colonic mucosal aphthous ulcerations and ischemic colitis. If suspected, rule out GI obstruction or perforation prior to administration. Caution in patients w/ impaired gag reflex and patients prone to regurgitation/aspiration; observe during administration. Not for direct ingestion.

ADVERSE REACTIONS

Overall discomfort, abdominal distention, abdominal pain, N/V.

DRUG INTERACTIONS

Caution w/ concomitant use of medications that increase the risk for fluid and electrolyte disturbances or increase the risk of seizures (eg, TCAs), arrhythmias and prolonged QT. Caution w/ medications that may affect renal function (eg, diuretics, ACE inhibitors, ARBs, NSAIDs). Concurrent use w/ stimulant laxatives may increase risk of colonic mucosal ulcerations and ischemic colitis. Absorption of oral medications may not occur if administered w/in an hr of the start of a Suprep dose.

NURSING CONSIDERATIONS

Assessment: Assess for GI obstruction, bowel perforation, or any other conditions where treatment is contraindicated or cautioned. Assess for pregnancy/nursing status, and for possible drug interactions. Obtain baseline electrolytes, creatinine, and BUN in patients w/ renal impairment. Perform baseline ECGs in patients at risk for arrhythmias.

Monitoring: Monitor for electrolyte abnormalities, cardiac arrhythmias, seizures, loss of consciousness, colonic mucosal ulcerations, ischemic colitis, and aspiration. Perform ECG in patients at increased risk of serious cardiac arrhythmias. Monitor electrolytes, creatinine, and BUN in patients w/ renal impairment.

Patient Counseling: Instruct to notify physician if patient has difficulty swallowing or is prone to regurgitation/aspiration. Instruct to dilute each bottle w/ water prior to ingestion and drink additional water ud by instructions. Advise that ingestion of undiluted solution may increase risk of N/V and dehydration. Inform that oral medications may not be absorbed properly if they are taken w/in 1 hr of starting each dose of Suprep Bowel Kit. Instruct not to take additional laxatives.

Storage: 20-25°C (68-77°F); excursions permitted between 15-30°C (59-86°F).

SUSTIVA – efavirenz

RX

Class: Non-nucleoside reverse transcriptase inhibitor

ADULT DOSAGE
HIV-1 Infection

Combination w/ Protease Inhibitor and/or Nucleoside Analogue Reverse Transcriptase Inhibitors:
600mg qd

PEDIATRIC DOSAGE
HIV-1 Infection

Combination w/ Other Antiretrovirals:
≥3 Months of Age:
3.5-<5kg: 100mg qd
5-<7.5kg: 150mg qd
7.5-<15kg: 200mg qd
15-<20kg: 250mg qd
20-<25kg: 300mg qd
25-<32.5kg: 350mg qd
32.5-<40kg: 400mg qd
≥40kg: 600mg qd

DOSE MODIFICATION
Concomitant Medications

Voriconazole: Increase voriconazole maintenance dose to 400mg q12h and decrease Sustiva dose to 300mg qd (use one 200mg and two 50mg caps or six 50mg caps)

Rifampin:
≥50kg: Increase Sustiva dose to 800mg qd

Hepatic Impairment
Moderate to Severe (Child-Pugh Class B or C): Not recommended for use

ADMINISTRATION
Oral route

Take on empty stomach, preferably hs
Swallow caps and tabs whole w/ liquid
Tabs must not be broken

Cap Sprinkle Method
Use if unable to swallow caps/tabs whole
1. Gently mix entire cap contents w/ 1-2 tsp of an age-appropriate soft food (eg, applesauce, grape jelly, yogurt, or infant formula) and administer
2. Add an additional small amount (approx 2 tsp) of food or formula to the empty mixing container, stir, and administer
3. Administer entire mixture w/in 30 min of mixing; do not consume additional food for 2 hrs after administration

Young Infants Receiving Cap Sprinkle-Infant Formula Mixture:
1. Gently mix entire cap contents into 2 tsp of reconstituted room temperature infant formula in a small container by carefully stirring w/ a small spoon
2. Draw up the mixture into a 10mL oral dosing syringe for administration

HOW SUPPLIED
Cap: 50mg, 200mg; Tab: 600mg

WARNINGS/PRECAUTIONS
Do not use as monotherapy or add on as a sole agent to a failing regimen. Not recommended w/ other efavirenz-containing products, unless needed for dose adjustment. Serious

psychiatric events reported; immediate medical evaluation is recommended if symptoms occur. CNS symptoms reported; dosing hs may improve tolerability. May impair mental/physical abilities. May cause fetal harm if administered during 1st trimester of pregnancy; avoid pregnancy during use. Skin rash reported; d/c and administer appropriate treatment if severe rash associated w/ blistering, desquamation, mucosal involvement, or fever develops. Consider alternative therapy in patients who have had a life-threatening cutaneous reaction (eg, Stevens-Johnson syndrome). Consider prophylaxis w/ appropriate antihistamines before initiating therapy in pediatric patients. Caution w/ mild hepatic impairment and in elderly. Hepatotoxicity reported; monitor liver enzymes before and during treatment w/ underlying hepatic disease, marked transaminase elevations, and w/ other medications associated w/ liver toxicity, and consider monitoring in patients w/ preexisting hepatic dysfunction/risk factors. Convulsions reported; caution w/ history of seizures. Lipid elevations, immune reconstitution syndrome, fat redistribution/accumulation, and autoimmune disorders (eg, Graves' disease, polymyositis, Guillain-Barre syndrome) in the setting of immune reconstitution reported. False-(+) urine cannabinoid test results reported; confirm positive results by a more specific method.

ADVERSE REACTIONS

Rash, dizziness, N/V, headache, fatigue, insomnia, anxiety, diarrhea, depression, increased ALT/AST levels, hypercholesterolemia, CNS symptoms.

DRUG INTERACTIONS

See Dose Modification. Avoid w/ other non-nucleoside reverse transcriptase inhibitors (NNRTIs). Potential additive CNS effects w/ alcohol or psychoactive drugs. CYP3A substrates, inhibitors, or inducers may alter levels. May alter levels of warfarin and drugs metabolized by CYP3A or CYP2B6. Ritonavir (RTV) and voriconazole may increase levels. CYP3A inducers (eg, phenobarbital, rifampin, rifabutin), carbamazepine, and anticonvulsants may decrease levels. May increase levels of RTV. May decrease levels of amprenavir, atazanavir (avoid combination in treatment-experienced patients), indinavir, lopinavir, saquinavir, maraviroc, boceprevir, simeprevir, carbamazepine, anticonvulsants (monitor levels), bupropion, sertraline, voriconazole, itraconazole, ketoconazole, clarithromycin, rifabutin, artemether, lumefantrine, diltiazem or other calcium channel blockers, atorvastatin, pravastatin, simvastatin, norgestimate, norelgestromin, levonorgestrel, etonogestrel, immunosuppressants, and methadone. Not recommended w/ simeprevir. May decrease posaconazole levels; avoid concomitant use unless benefit outweighs risks. Refer to PI for further dosing modifications when used w/ certain concomitant therapies.

NURSING CONSIDERATIONS

Assessment: Assess for underlying hepatic disease, history of inj drug use/seizures/cutaneous reaction, psychiatric history, hypersensitivity to the drug, pregnancy/nursing status, and possible drug interactions. Assess baseline LFTs and lipid profile (eg, cholesterol, TGs).

Monitoring: Monitor for psychiatric events, CNS symptoms, skin rash, convulsions, immune reconstitution syndrome (eg, opportunistic infections), fat redistribution/accumulation, and other adverse reactions. Monitor LFTs and lipid profile.

Patient Counseling: Inform that therapy is not a cure for HIV-1 infection and illnesses associated w/ HIV-1 infection may still be experienced. Advise to practice safer sex by using latex or polyurethane condoms, not to share or reuse needles or other inj equipment or personal items (eg, toothbrush, razor blades), and not to breastfeed. Advise to take medication ud and provide appropriate instructions for missed doses. Inform that CNS symptoms may occur during 1st weeks of therapy. Counsel that rash, psychiatric symptoms, and redistribution/accumulation of body fat may occur. Advise to avoid potentially hazardous tasks if experiencing CNS symptoms. Inform of the potential additive effects of the drug when used concomitantly w/ alcohol or psychoactive drugs. Instruct to seek medical attention if symptoms of rash and serious psychiatric events occur. Advise to inform physician of any history of mental illness or substance abuse. Advise females of reproductive potential to use effective contraception as well as a barrier method during treatment and for 12 weeks after discontinuing therapy; instruct to contact physician if planning to become pregnant, become pregnant, or if pregnancy is suspected during treatment. Advise that there is a pregnancy exposure registry that monitors pregnancy outcomes in women exposed to therapy during pregnancy. Advise to report use of any prescription or OTC medication.

Storage: 25°C (77°F); excursions permitted to 15-30°C (59-86°F).

Sutent – sunitinib malate RX

Class: Kinase inhibitors

Hepatotoxicity has been observed; may be severe, and deaths have been reported.

ADULT DOSAGE

Gastrointestinal Stromal Tumor

After Disease Progression or Intolerance to Imatinib Mesylate:
50mg qd, on a schedule of 4 weeks on, followed by 2 weeks off

Advanced Renal Cell Carcinoma

50mg qd, on a schedule of 4 weeks on, followed by 2 weeks off

Advanced Pancreatic Neuroendocrine Tumors

Progressive, Well-Differentiated Tumors w/ Unresectable Locally Advanced or Metastatic Disease:

37.5mg qd continuously w/o a scheduled off-treatment period

PEDIATRIC DOSAGE

Pediatric use may not have been established

DOSE MODIFICATION

Concomitant Medications

Strong CYP3A4 Inhibitors:

GI Stromal Tumors/Advanced Renal Cell Carcinoma: Consider dose reduction to a minimum of 37.5mg qd

Advanced Pancreatic Neuroendocrine Tumors: Consider dose reduction to a minimum of 25mg qd

CYP3A4 Inducers:

GI Stromal Tumors/Advanced Renal Cell Carcinoma: Consider dose increase to a max of 87.5mg qd

Advanced Pancreatic Neuroendocrine Tumors: Consider dose increase to a max of 62.5mg qd

Other Important Modifications

Interruption and/or modification in 12.5mg increments or decrements is recommended based on individual safety and tolerability

ADMINISTRATION

Oral route

Take w/ or w/o food

HOW SUPPLIED

Cap: 12.5mg, 25mg, 37.5mg, 50mg

WARNINGS/PRECAUTIONS

Interrupt therapy for Grade 3/4 hepatic adverse events; d/c if no resolution. Do not restart treatment if subsequent severe changes in LFTs or other signs/symptoms of liver failure occur. May cause fetal harm; avoid pregnancy. Cardiovascular (CV) events, including decline in left ventricular ejection fraction (LVEF) to below lower limit of normal, reported; d/c in the presence of clinical manifestations of CHF, and interrupt and/or reduce dose in patients w/o clinical evidence of CHF but w/ ejection fraction <50% and >20% below baseline. Dose-dependent QT interval prolongation and torsades de pointes observed; caution w/ history of QT interval prolongation or preexisting cardiac disease, bradycardia, or electrolyte disturbances. Monitor for HTN and treat prn; suspend temporarily in cases of severe HTN. Hemorrhagic events, including tumor-related hemorrhage, reported. Serious, sometimes fatal GI complications (eg, GI perforation) may occur in patients w/ intra-abdominal malignancies. Osteonecrosis of the jaw (ONJ) reported; exposure to risk factors (eg, dental disease) may increase the risk of ONJ. Tumor lysis syndrome (TLS) reported; closely monitor patients presenting w/ a high tumor burden prior to treatment and treat as clinically indicated. Observe closely for signs/symptoms of thyroid dysfunction (eg, hypo/hyperthyroidism, thyroiditis). Associated w/ symptomatic hypoglycemia, resulting in loss of consciousness, or requiring hospitalization; reductions in blood glucose may be worse in diabetic patients. Impaired wound healing reported; interrupt temporarily in patients undergoing major surgical procedures. Proteinuria and nephrotic syndrome reported; interrupt and reduce dose for 24-hr urine protein ≥3g. D/C therapy for patients w/ nephrotic syndrome or repeat episodes of urine protein ≥3g despite dose reductions. Severe cutaneous reactions (eg, erythema multiforme, Stevens Johnson syndrome [SJS], toxic epidermal necrolysis [TEN]) reported; d/c therapy if signs/symptoms are present and do not restart treatment if a diagnosis of SJS or TEN is suspected. Necrotizing fasciitis reported; d/c therapy in patients who develop necrotizing fasciitis. Monitor for adrenal insufficiency in patients w/ stress, trauma, or severe infection.

ADVERSE REACTIONS

Hepatotoxicity, fatigue, fever, asthenia, diarrhea, N/V, mucositis/stomatitis, abdominal pain, HTN, rash, hand-foot syndrome, skin discoloration, altered taste, anorexia, bleeding.

DRUG INTERACTIONS

See Dose Modification. Caution w/ antiarrhythmics. Strong CYP3A4 inhibitors (eg, ketoconazole, nefazodone, ritonavir) and grapefruit may increase levels. CYP3A4 inducers (eg, dexamethasone, phenytoin, rifampin) may decrease levels. Avoid w/ St. John's wort. Concomitant use w/ bisphosphonates may increase the risk of ONJ.

NURSING CONSIDERATIONS

Assessment: Assess for cardiac events, electrolyte disturbances, dental disease, high tumor burden, diabetes, pregnancy/nursing status, and possible drug interactions. Obtain baseline LFTs, LVEF, thyroid function, CBC w/ platelet count, serum chemistries (eg, phosphate), and urinalysis.

Monitoring: Monitor for signs/symptoms of CV events, HTN, hemorrhagic events, ONJ, TLS, adrenal insufficiency, hepatotoxicity, nephrotic syndrome, severe cutaneous reactions, necrotizing fasciitis, and other adverse reactions. Monitor LFTs, LVEF (in patients w/ cardiac risk factors), ECG, electrolytes (Mg^{2+}, K^+), thyroid function, CBC w/ platelet count, and serum chemistries (eg, phosphate). Monitor blood glucose levels regularly during and after discontinuation of treatment. Perform periodic urinalysis w/ follow-up measurement of 24-hr urine protein as clinically indicated.

Patient Counseling: Inform about the most commonly reported GI disorders and other adverse reactions that may occur. Advise that depigmentation of the hair or skin, and other possible dermatologic effects may occur during treatment. Inform that severe dermatologic toxicities (eg, SJS, TEN) have been reported; advise to immediately inform physician if severe dermatologic reactions occur. Advise to consider a dental examination and appropriate preventive dentistry prior to treatment. Advise of the signs, symptoms, and risks associated w/ hypoglycemia that may occur while on therapy; instruct to immediately inform physician if severe signs/symptoms of hypoglycemia occur. Instruct to avoid invasive dental procedures if previously or concomitantly taking bisphosphonates. Advise to inform physician of all concomitant medications, including OTC medications and dietary supplements. Inform of pregnancy risks; advise women of childbearing potential to avoid becoming pregnant.

Storage: 25°C (77°F); excursions permitted to 15-30°C (59-86°F).

SYMBICORT — budesonide/formoterol fumarate dihydrate RX

Class: Beta$_2$-agonist/corticosteroid

Long-acting β_2-adrenergic agonists (LABAs), such as formoterol, increase the risk of asthma-related death. LABAs may increase the risk of asthma-related hospitalization in pediatric patients and adolescents. Use only for patients not adequately controlled on a long-term asthma-control medication or whose disease severity clearly warrants initiation of treatment with both inhaled corticosteroids and LABA. Do not use if asthma is adequately controlled on low- or medium-dose inhaled corticosteroids.

ADULT DOSAGE

Asthma

2 inh bid (am and pm, approx q12h)
Initial: Based on severity
Max: 160mcg-4.5mcg/inh bid

Not Responding After 1-2 Weeks of Therapy w/ 80mcg-4.5mcg/inh:
Replace w/ 160mcg-4.5mcg/inh for better asthma control

Chronic Obstructive Pulmonary Disease

Maint Treatment of Airflow Obstruction in Patients w/ COPD, Including Chronic Bronchitis and Emphysema:
2 inh (160mcg-4.5mcg/inh) bid

PEDIATRIC DOSAGE

Asthma

≥12 Years:
2 inh bid (am and pm, approx q12h)
Initial: Based on severity
Max: 160mcg-4.5mcg/inh bid

Not Responding After 1-2 Weeks of Therapy w/ 80mcg-4.5mcg/inh:
Replace w/ 160mcg-4.5mcg/inh for better asthma control

ADMINISTRATION

Oral inh route

After inh, rinse mouth w/ water w/o swallowing
Shake well for 5 sec before use

Priming

1. Shake the inhaler well for 5 sec
2. Hold the inhaler pointing away from the face and then release a test spray
3. Shake it again for 5 sec and release a 2nd test spray
4. Depending on which size was provided, the counter will read either 120 or 60 after it has been primed

If inhaler is not used for more than 7 days or if it is dropped, prime again

HOW SUPPLIED

MDI: (Budesonide-Formoterol) 80mcg-4.5mcg/inh, 160mcg-4.5mcg/inh [60 inhalations, 120 inhalations]

CONTRAINDICATIONS

Primary treatment of status asthmaticus or other acute episodes of asthma or COPD where intensive measures are required.

WARNINGS/PRECAUTIONS

Not indicated for the relief of acute bronchospasm; take inhaled short-acting β_2-agonists (SABAs) for immediate relief. Do not initiate during rapidly deteriorating/potentially life-threatening asthma or COPD. D/C regular use of oral/inhaled SABAs when beginning treatment. Cardiovascular (CV) effects and fatalities reported with excessive use; do not use more often or at higher doses than recommended. *Candida albicans* infections of the mouth and pharynx reported; treat with appropriate local or systemic (eg, antifungal) therapy or, interrupt therapy if needed. Lower respiratory tract infections (eg, pneumonia) reported in patients with COPD. Increased susceptibility to infections. May lead to serious/fatal course of chickenpox or measles; avoid exposure and, if exposed, consider prophylaxis/treatment. Caution with active/quiescent tuberculosis (TB); untreated systemic fungal, bacterial, viral, or parasitic infections; or ocular herpes simplex. Deaths due to adrenal insufficiency reported with transfer from systemic to inhaled corticosteroids; if systemic corticosteroids are required, wean slowly from systemic steroid after transferring to therapy. Resume oral corticosteroids during periods of stress or a severe asthma attack if patient was previously withdrawn from systemic corticosteroid. Carefully monitor during withdrawal of oral corticosteroid. Transferring from systemic to inhalation therapy may unmask previously suppressed allergic conditions (eg, rhinitis, conjunctivitis, eczema, arthritis, eosinophilic conditions); monitor for systemic corticosteroid withdrawal effects. Observe carefully for any evidence of systemic corticosteroid effects; caution should be taken in observing patients postoperatively or during periods of stress for evidence of inadequate adrenal response. Reduce dose slowly if hypercorticism or adrenal suppression (including adrenal crisis) appears. May produce paradoxical bronchospasm; d/c immediately and institute alternative therapy. Immediate hypersensitivity reactions (eg, urticaria, angioedema, rash, bronchospasm) may occur. Caution with CV disorders (eg, coronary insufficiency, cardiac arrhythmias, HTN). Decreases in bone mineral density (BMD) reported; caution with major risk factors for decreased bone mineral content (eg, prolonged immobilization, family history of osteoporosis, postmenopausal status, tobacco use, advanced age, poor nutrition). May reduce growth velocity in pediatrics; use lowest effective dose. Glaucoma, increased IOP, cataracts, rare cases of systemic eosinophilic conditions, and vasculitis consistent with Churg-Strauss syndrome reported. Caution with convulsive disorders, thyrotoxicosis, diabetes mellitus (DM), ketoacidosis, hepatic impairment, and in patients unusually responsive to sympathomimetic amines. Clinically significant changes in blood glucose and/or serum K^+ reported. Caution in elderly.

ADVERSE REACTIONS

Nasopharyngitis, headache, URTI, pharyngolaryngeal pain, sinusitis, influenza, back pain, nasal congestion, stomach discomfort, oral candidiasis, bronchitis, vomiting.

DRUG INTERACTIONS

Do not use with other medications containing LABAs (eg, salmeterol, formoterol fumarate, arformoterol tartrate); increased risk of CV effects. Caution with ketoconazole, other known strong CYP3A4 inhibitors (eg, ritonavir, nefazodone, telithromycin, itraconazole), and non-K^+-sparing diuretics (eg, loop, thiazide). Caution with MAOIs or TCAs, or within 2 weeks of discontinuation of such agents. Concomitant use with β-blockers may produce severe bronchospasm in patients with asthma; consider cardioselective β-blockers and administer with caution. Caution with chronic use of drugs that can reduce bone mass (eg, anticonvulsants, oral corticosteroids).

NURSING CONSIDERATIONS

Assessment: Assess use of long-term asthma control medication (eg, inhaled corticosteroids), status asthmaticus, acute asthma episodes, rapidly deteriorating asthma, bronchospasm, known hypersensitivity to any component of drug, risk factors for decreased bone mineral content, CV or convulsive disorders, other conditions where treatment is contraindicated or cautioned, pregnancy/nursing status, and possible drug interactions. Assess use in patients unusually responsive to sympathomimetic amines. Obtain baseline BMD, eye exam, and lung function.

Monitoring: Monitor for localized oral *C. albicans* infections, worsening or acutely deteriorating asthma, development of glaucoma, increased IOP, cataracts, CV/CNS effects, inhalation induced paradoxical bronchospasm, pneumonia, lower respiratory tract in patients with COPD, hypercorticism, adrenal suppression, hypersensitivity reactions, signs of increased drug exposure with hepatic impairment, and other adverse reactions. Monitor lung function, pulse rate, BP, ECG changes, blood glucose, and serum K^+ levels. Monitor BMD periodically. Monitor growth in children.

Patient Counseling: Inform about increased risk of asthma-related death/hospitalization in pediatrics and adolescents. Instruct not to use to relieve acute asthma symptoms; treat acute symptoms with an inhaled SABA for immediate relief. Instruct to notify physician immediately if experiencing decreased effectiveness of inhaled SABA, need for more inhalations of inhaled SABA than usual, or significant decrease in lung function. Instruct not to d/c without physician's guidance. Instruct not to use with other LABA for asthma and COPD. Advise that localized infections with *C. albicans* may occur in the mouth and pharynx. Instruct to contact physician if symptoms of pneumonia develop. Instruct to avoid exposure to chickenpox or measles and to consult physician without delay, if exposed. Inform of potential worsening of existing TB, fungal, bacterial, viral, or parasitic infections, or ocular herpes simplex. Inform about risks of hypercorticism and adrenal suppression, decreased BMD, cataracts or glaucoma, and reduced growth velocity in pediatric patients. Instruct to taper slowly from systemic corticosteroids if transferring to budesonide-formoterol. Inform of adverse effects associated with β_2-agonists (eg, palpitations, chest pain, rapid HR, tremor, nervousness).

Storage: 20-25°C (68-77°F). Store with mouthpiece down. Contents under pressure; do not puncture, incinerate, or store near heat or open flame. Discard when labeled number of inhalations have been used or within 3 months after removal from pouch.

SYMBYAX – fluoxetine/olanzapine RX

Class: Selective serotonin reuptake inhibitor/thienobenzodiazepine

Antidepressants increased the risk of suicidal thoughts and behavior in children, adolescents, and young adults in short-term studies. Monitor closely for worsening and emergence of suicidal thoughts and behaviors in patients who are started on antidepressant therapy. Elderly patients with dementia-related psychosis treated with antipsychotic drugs are at an increased risk of death. Not approved for use in children <10 yrs of age or for the treatment of dementia-related psychosis.

ADULT DOSAGE

Bipolar I Disorder

Acute Depressive Episodes:
Initial: 6mg-25mg qpm
Titrate: Adjust dosage, if indicated, according to efficacy and tolerability
Effective Range: 6-12mg (olanzapine) and 25-50mg (fluoxetine)
Max: 18mg-75mg

Periodically reexamine need for continued pharmacotherapy

Depression

Treatment Resistant:
Initial: 6mg-25mg qpm
Titrate: Adjust dosage, if indicated, according to efficacy and tolerability
Effective Range: 6-18mg (olanzapine) and 25-50mg (fluoxetine)
Max: 18mg-75mg

Periodically reexamine need for continued pharmacotherapy

Dosing Considerations with MAOIs

Switching to/from an MAOI for Psychiatric Disorders:
Allow at least 14 days between discontinuation of an MAOI and initiation of treatment, and allow at least 5 weeks between discontinuation of treatment and initiation of an MAOI

With Other MAOIs (eg, Linezolid, IV Methylene Blue):
Do not start in a patient being treated with linezolid or IV methylene blue
If acceptable alternatives are not available, d/c and administer linezolid or IV methylene blue; monitor for serotonin syndrome for 5 weeks or until 24 hours after the last dose of linezolid or IV methylene blue, whichever comes first. May resume therapy 24 hours after the last dose of linezolid or IV methylene blue

PEDIATRIC DOSAGE

Bipolar I Disorder

Acute Depressive Episodes:
10-17 Years:
Initial: 3mg-25mg qpm
Usual/Target Dosing Range: 6mg-25mg to 12mg-50mg
Max: 12mg-50mg

DOSE MODIFICATION

Hepatic Impairment

Initial: 3mg-25mg or 6mg-25mg qpm

Elderly

Use with caution and start at lower end of dosing range

Discontinuation

Gradually reduce dose

Other Important Modifications

Predisposition to Hypotension Risk/Slow Metabolizers (Female, Geriatric Age, Nonsmoker)/ Olanzapine-Sensitive:

Initial: 3mg-25mg or 6mg-25mg qpm

Titrate: Increase slowly and adjust dose prn in slow metabolizers

ADMINISTRATION

Oral route

HOW SUPPLIED

Cap: (Olanzapine-Fluoxetine) 3mg-25mg, 6mg-25mg, 6mg-50mg, 12mg-25mg, 12mg-50mg

CONTRAINDICATIONS

Use of an MAOI intended to treat psychiatric disorders either concomitantly or within 5 weeks of stopping treatment. Treatment within 14 days of stopping an MAOI intended to treat psychiatric disorders. Starting treatment in patients being treated with other MAOIs (eg, linezolid or IV methylene blue). Concomitant use with pimozide or thioridazine.

WARNINGS/PRECAUTIONS

Associated with metabolic changes (eg, hyperglycemia, dyslipidemia, weight gain [dose-related]) that may increase cardiovascular/cerebrovascular risk. Hyperglycemia, in some cases extreme and associated with ketoacidosis/hyperosmolar coma/death reported; caution in patients with diabetes mellitus (DM) or borderline increased blood glucose level. Dose-related hyperprolactinemia reported. Pupillary dilation that occurs following use may trigger an angle-closure attack in a patient with anatomically narrow angles who does not have a patent iridectomy. Anaphylactoid and pulmonary reactions reported; d/c if unexplained allergic reaction occurs. May increase precipitation of a manic episode in patients at risk for bipolar disorder. Tardive dyskinesia (TD) may develop; consider discontinuation if signs and symptoms appear. May induce orthostatic hypotension; caution with cardiovascular disease (CVD), cerebrovascular disease, or conditions that would predispose to hypotension. Leukopenia, neutropenia, and agranulocytosis reported; consider discontinuing at 1st sign of clinically significant decline in WBC count without causative factors, or discontinuing if severe neutropenia (ANC <1000/mm^3) develops. May cause esophageal dysmotility and aspiration. Not approved for treatment of patients with Alzheimer's disease. Seizures reported; caution with history of seizures or with conditions that potentially lower the seizure threshold. May impair physical/mental abilities. May disrupt body's ability to reduce core body temperature; caution with conditions that may elevate core temperature (eg, strenuous exercise, extreme heat exposure, dehydration). Caution with conditions affecting hemodynamic responses, hepatic impairment, in cardiac patients, and in the elderly. Fluoxetine: Serotonin syndrome reported; d/c immediately and initiate supportive symptomatic treatment. May increase risk of bleeding reactions. Hyponatremia reported; consider discontinuation in patients with symptomatic hyponatremia. QT interval prolongation and ventricular arrhythmia, including torsades de pointes, reported; caution in patients with congenital long QT syndrome, a previous history of QT prolongation, a family history of long QT syndrome or sudden cardiac death, and other conditions that predispose to QT prolongation and ventricular arrhythmia. Consider discontinuing treatment and obtaining a cardiac evaluation if signs/symptoms of ventricular arrhythmia develop. Because of long elimination $T_{1/2}$, changes in dose will not be fully reflected for several weeks. Adverse reactions reported upon discontinuation; avoid abrupt withdrawal. Olanzapine: Neuroleptic malignant syndrome (NMS) reported; d/c and instill intensive symptomatic treatment and monitoring. Caution with clinically significant prostatic hypertrophy, angle-closure glaucoma, history of paralytic ileus or related conditions.

ADVERSE REACTIONS

Asthenia, somnolence, weight gain, increased appetite, disturbance in attention, peripheral edema, tremor, dry mouth, arthralgia, blurred vision, sedation, fatigue, flatulence, restlessness, hypersomnia.

DRUG INTERACTIONS

See Contraindications. Caution with CNS-active drugs and anticholinergic drugs. May potentiate sedation and orthostatic hypotension with alcohol. Fluoxetine: May cause serotonin syndrome with other serotonergic drugs (eg, triptans, tramadol, St. John's wort) and with drugs that impair metabolism of serotonin; d/c immediately if this occurs. Increased risk of bleeding with ASA, NSAIDs, warfarin, and other anticoagulants. Rare reports of prolonged seizures with combined use of electroconvulsive therapy. Caution with drugs that cause QT prolongation (eg, specific antipsychotics [eg, ziprasidone, iloperidone, chlorpromazine], specific antibiotics [eg, erythromycin, moxifloxacin, sparfloxacin], class 1A antiarrhythmics [eg, quinidine, procainamide], class III antiarrhythmics [eg, amiodarone, sotalol], and others [eg, pentamidine, methadone, tacrolimus]).

May increase levels of TCAs (eg, imipramine, desipramine). May prolong $T_{1/2}$ of diazepam. May increase levels of carbamazepine, alprazolam, clozapine, phenytoin, and haloperidol. Caution with CYP2D6 substrates, including antidepressants (eg, TCAs), antipsychotics (eg, phenothiazines, most atypicals), vinblastine, and antiarrhythmics (eg, propafenone, flecainide). May cause lithium toxicity; monitor lithium levels. May cause a shift in plasma concentration with drugs that are tightly bound to protein (eg, warfarin, digitoxin), resulting in an adverse effect. CYP2D6 inhibitors or other highly protein-bound drugs may increase levels. Olanzapine: May potentiate orthostatic hypotension with diazepam. Inducers of CYP1A2 or glucuronyl transferase (eg, carbamazepine, omeprazole, rifampin) may increase clearance. Fluvoxamine may increase levels; consider lower doses of the olanzapine component when used concomitantly. May enhance effects of certain antihypertensive agents. May antagonize effects of levodopa and dopamine agonists.

NURSING CONSIDERATIONS

Assessment: Assess for DM, susceptibility to angle-closure glaucoma, CVD, cerebrovascular disease, history of seizures, or any other conditions where treatment is contraindicated or cautioned. Assess for bipolar disorder, dementia-related psychosis, Alzheimer's disease, pregnancy/nursing status, and possible drug interactions. Assess for predisposition to hypotension, hepatic impairment, slow metabolism, and pharmacodynamic sensitivity to olanzapine. Obtain baseline FPG, CBC, and lipid levels. Consider ECG assessment if initiating treatment in patients with risk factors for QT prolongation and ventricular arrhythmia. Consider potential consequences of weight gain.

Monitoring: Monitor for signs/symptoms of NMS, serotonin syndrome, TD, clinical worsening, suicidality, unusual changes in behavior, hyperglycemia, hyperlipidemia, rash or other possible allergic phenomena, orthostatic hypotension, mania/hypomania, QT prolongation, angle-closure glaucoma, and other adverse reactions. Frequently monitor CBC in patients with a history of clinically significant low WBC counts or drug-induced leukopenia/neutropenia. Monitor FPG, lipid levels, and weight of patient. In patients with clinically significant neutropenia, monitor for fever or other signs/symptoms of infection. Consider periodic ECG monitoring in patients with risk factors for QT prolongation and ventricular arrhythmia. Periodically reassess need for continued treatment.

Patient Counseling: Inform about risks and benefits of therapy. Advise patient, family, and caregivers to be alert for signs of behavioral changes, worsening of depression, suicidal ideation, and signs/symptoms of NMS. Inform patient of the potential risk of hyperglycemia, dyslipidemia, weight gain, and hyponatremia. Caution about risk of serotonin syndrome with other serotonergic agents (eg, triptans, buspirone, St. John's wort); instruct to seek medical care immediately if experiencing symptoms of serotonin syndrome. Inform about risk of bleeding with ASA, warfarin, or other drugs that affect coagulation; advise to seek medical care immediately if experiencing any increased or unusual bruising or bleeding. Caution about risk of angle-closure glaucoma. Counsel to seek medical care immediately if a rash or hives, or signs/symptoms associated with orthostatic hypotension occur. Explain that drug may impair physical/mental abilities and instruct to use caution when operating hazardous machinery, including automobiles. Advise about appropriate care in avoiding overheating and dehydration and instruct to notify physician if sever illness or symptoms of dehydration develop. Instruct to notify physician if taking other drugs or if pregnant/planning to become pregnant. Instruct to avoid breastfeeding and alcohol. Instruct to take exactly as prescribed and to continue even if symptoms improve.

Storage: 25°C (77°F); excursions permitted to 15-30°C (59-86°F). Protect from moisture.

SYNTHROID — levothyroxine sodium RX

Class: Thyroid replacement hormone

Do not use for the treatment of obesity or weight loss; doses within range of daily hormonal requirements are ineffective for weight reduction in euthyroid patients. Serious or life-threatening manifestations of toxicity may occur when given in larger doses, particularly when given in association with sympathomimetic amines.

ADULT DOSAGE

Hypothyroidism

Replacement/supplemental therapy in hypothyroidism of any etiology, except transient hypothyroidism during the recovery phase of subacute thyroiditis

Usual: 1.7mcg/kg/day; >200mcg/day seldom required

Severe:

Initial: 12.5-25mcg/day

Titrate: Increase by 25mcg/day every 2-4 weeks until TSH level normalized

PEDIATRIC DOSAGE

Hypothyroidism

Usual:

0-3 Months of Age: 10-15mcg/kg/day

3-6 Months of Age: 8-10mcg/kg/day

6-12 Months of Age: 6-8mcg/kg/day

1-5 Years: 5-6mcg/kg/day

6-12 Years: 4-5mcg/kg/day

>12 Years:

Growth/Puberty Incomplete: 2-3mcg/kg/day

Growth/Puberty Complete: 1.7mcg/kg/day

Secondary (Pituitary) or Tertiary (Hypothalamic) Hypothyroidism:
Titrate: Increase until clinically euthyroid and serum free-T4 level is restored to the upper half of the normal range

Subclinical Hypothyroidism:
Lower doses (eg, 1mcg/kg/day) may be adequate to normalize serum TSH level

Pituitary TSH Suppressant

Used to treat/prevent various types of euthyroid goiters (eg, thyroid nodules, subacute or chronic lymphocytic thyroiditis, multinodular goiter) and to manage thyroid cancer

Well-Differentiated (Papillary and Follicular) Thyroid Cancer:
Adjunct to Surgery and Radioiodine Therapy:
Usual: >2mcg/kg/day, w/ target TSH level <0.1 mU/L
High-Risk Tumors: Target TSH level <0.01 mU/L

Benign Nodules and Nontoxic Multinodular Goiter:
TSH is suppressed to a higher target (eg, 0.1 to 0.5 or 1.0 mU/L)

Infants w/ Very Low (<5mcg/dL) or Undetectable Serum T4:
Initial: 50mcg/day

Chronic/Severe Hypothyroidism:
Initial: 25mcg/day
Titrate: Increase by 25mcg every 2-4 weeks

DOSE MODIFICATION

Pregnancy
May increase levothyroxine requirements

Elderly
Hypothyroidism:
>50 Years:
Initial: 25-50mcg/day
Titrate: Increase by 12.5-25mcg increments every 6-8 weeks prn

W/ Underlying Cardiac Disease:
Initial: 12.5-25mcg/day
Titrate: Increase by 12.5-25mg increments every 4-6 weeks

Adverse Reactions
Minimize Hyperactivity in Older Children:
Initial: Give 1/4 of full replacement dose
Titrate: Increase on a weekly basis by 1/4 the full recommended replacement dose until the full recommended replacement dose is reached

Other Important Modifications
Underlying Cardiac Disease:
Hypothyroidism:
Infants (Risk for Cardiac Failure):
Initial: Consider lower dose (eg, 25mcg/day)
Titrate: Increase dose in 4-6 weeks prn

<50 Years:
Initial: 25-50mcg/day
Titrate: Increase by 12.5-25mcg increments every 6-8 weeks prn

ADMINISTRATION

Oral route

Administer as a single daily dose, preferably 30-60 min before breakfast
Take at least 4 hrs apart from drugs that are known to interfere w/ its absorption

Pediatrics
Unable to Swallow Intact Tab:
1. Crush tab and suspend in small amount (5-10mL or 1-2 tsp) of water
2. Administer using a spoon or dropper
3. Do not store susp for later use
4. Do not use foods that decrease absorption of levothyroxine (eg, soybean infant formula) to administer

HOW SUPPLIED

Tab: 25mcg*, 50mcg*, 75mcg*, 88mcg*, 100mcg*, 112mcg*, 125mcg*, 137mcg*, 150mcg*, 175mcg*, 200mcg*, 300mcg* *scored

CONTRAINDICATIONS
Untreated subclinical (suppressed serum TSH level with normal T3 level and T4 levels) or overt thyrotoxicosis of any etiology, acute MI, and uncorrected adrenal insufficiency.

WARNINGS/PRECAUTIONS
Should not be used in the treatment of male or female infertility unless associated with hypothyroidism. Contraindicated in patients with nontoxic diffuse goiter or nodular thyroid disease, particularly in the elderly or with underlying cardiovascular (CV) disease if serum TSH level is already suppressed; use with caution if TSH level is not suppressed and carefully monitor thyroid function. Has narrow therapeutic index; carefully titrate dose to avoid over- or under-treatment. May decrease bone mineral density (BMD) with long-term use; give minimum dose necessary to achieve desired clinical and biochemical response. Caution with CV disorders and the elderly. If cardiac symptoms develop or worsen, reduce or withhold dose for 1 week and then restart at lower dose. Overtreatment may produce CV effects (eg, increase in HR, increase in cardiac wall thickness, increase in cardiac contractility, precipitation of angina or arrhythmias). Monitor patients with CAD closely during surgical procedures; may precipitate cardiac arrhythmias. Caution in patients with diabetes mellitus (DM). Patients with concomitant adrenal insufficiency should be treated with replacement glucocorticoids prior to therapy.

ADVERSE REACTIONS
Fatigue, increased appetite, weight loss, heat intolerance, headache, hyperactivity, irritability, insomnia, palpitations, arrhythmias, dyspnea, hair loss, menstrual irregularities, pseudotumor cerebri (children), slipped capital femoral epiphysis (children).

DRUG INTERACTIONS
Concurrent sympathomimetics may increase effects of sympathomimetics or thyroid hormone; may increase risk of coronary insufficiency with CAD. Upward dose adjustments may be needed for insulin and oral hypoglycemic agents. May decrease absorption with soybean flour, cottonseed meal, walnuts, and dietary fiber. May increase oral anticoagulant activity; adjust dose of anticoagulant and monitor PT. May decrease levels and effects of digitalis glycosides. Transient reduction in TSH secretion with dopamine/dopamine agonists, glucocorticoids, octreotide. Decreased thyroid hormone secretion with aminoglutethimide, amiodarone, iodide (including iodine-containing radiographic contrast agents), lithium, methimazole, propylthiouracil (PTU), sulfonamides, and tolbutamide. May increase thyroid hormone secretion with amiodarone and iodide. May decrease T4 absorption with antacids (aluminum and magnesium hydroxides), simethicone, bile acid sequestrants (cholestyramine, colestipol), calcium carbonate, cation exchange resins (kayexalate), ferrous sulfate, orlistat, and sucralfate; administer at least 4 hrs apart. May increase serum thyroxine-binding globulin (TBG) concentrations with clofibrate, estrogen-containing oral contraceptives, oral estrogens, heroin/methadone, 5-fluorouracil, mitotane, and tamoxifen. May decrease serum TBG concentrations with androgens/anabolic steroids, asparaginase, glucocorticoids, and slow-release nicotinic acid. May cause protein-binding site displacement with furosemide (>80mg IV), heparin, hydantoins, NSAIDs (fenamates, phenylbutazone), and salicylates (>2g/day). May alter T4 and T3 metabolism with carbamazepine, hydantoins, phenobarbital, and rifampin. May decrease T4 5'-deiodinase activity with amiodarone, β-adrenergic antagonists (eg, propranolol >160mg/day), glucocorticoids (eg, dexamethasone >4mg/day), and PTU. Concurrent use with tricyclic (eg, amitriptyline) and tetracyclic (eg, maprotiline) antidepressants may increase the therapeutic and toxic effects of both drugs. Coadministration with sertraline in patients stabilized on levothyroxine may result in increased levothyroxine requirements. Interferon-α may cause development of antithyroid microsomal antibodies and transient hypothyroidism, hyperthyroidism, or both. Interleukin-2 has been associated with transient painless thyroiditis. Excessive use with growth hormones (eg, somatropin, somatrem) may accelerate epiphyseal closure. Ketamine may produce marked HTN and tachycardia. May reduce uptake of radiographic agents. Decreased theophylline clearance may occur in hypothyroid patients. Altered levels of thyroid hormone and/or TSH levels with choral hydrate, diazepam, ethionamide, lovastatin, metoclopramide, 6-mercaptopurine, nitroprusside, para-aminosalicylate sodium, perphenazine, resorcinol (excessive topical use), and thiazide diuretics.

NURSING CONSIDERATIONS

Assessment: Assess for untreated subclinical or overt thyrotoxicosis, acute MI, uncorrected adrenal insufficiency, CAD, CV disorders, nontoxic diffuse goiter, nodular thyroid disease, DM, hypersensitivity, pregnancy/nursing status, and for possible drug interactions. In patients with secondary or tertiary hypothyroidism, assess for additional hypothalamic/pituitary hormone deficiencies. Assess TSH levels. In infants with congenital hypothyroidism, assess for other congenital anomalies.

Monitoring: Monitor for CV effects. In patients on long-term therapy, monitor for signs/symptoms of decreased BMD. In patients with nontoxic diffuse goiter or nodular thyroid disease, monitor for precipitation of thyrotoxicosis. In adults with primary hypothyroidism, perform periodic monitoring of serum TSH levels. In pediatric patients with congenital hypothyroidism, perform periodic monitoring of serum TSH levels and total or free T4 levels. In patients with secondary and tertiary hypothyroidism, perform periodic monitoring of serum free-T4 levels. Refer to PI for TSH and T4 monitoring parameters. Closely monitor PT if coadministered with an oral anticoagulant.

Patient Counseling: Instruct to notify physician if allergic to any foods or medicines, pregnant/planning to become pregnant, breastfeeding, or taking any other drugs, including prescriptions and OTC preparations. Instruct to notify physician of any other medical conditions, particularly heart disease, diabetes, clotting disorders, and adrenal or pituitary gland problems. Instruct not to stop or change dose unless directed by physician. Instruct to take on empty stomach, at least 30-60 min before eating breakfast. Advise that partial hair loss may occur during the 1st few months of therapy, but is usually temporary. Instruct to notify physician or dentist prior to surgery about levothyroxine therapy. Inform that drug should not be used for weight control. Instruct to notify physician if rapid or irregular heartbeat, chest pain, SOB, leg cramps, headache, or any other unusual medical event occurs. Inform that dose may be increased during pregnancy. Inform that drug should not be administered within 4 hrs of agents such as iron/calcium supplements and antacids.

Storage: 25°C (77°F); excursions permitted to 15-30°C (59-86°F). Protect from light and moisture.

TAFINLAR – dabrafenib **RX**

Class: Kinase inhibitors

ADULT DOSAGE

Unresectable or Metastatic Melanoma with BRAF V600E Mutation

Usual: 150mg bid, approximately 12 hrs apart, as a single agent or in combination with trametinib 2mg qd until disease progression or unacceptable toxicity occurs

Combination with Trametinib:
Take the once-daily dose of trametinib at the same time each day with either the am dose or pm dose of dabrafenib

PEDIATRIC DOSAGE

Pediatric use may not have been established

DOSE MODIFICATION

Dose Reductions

Dabrafenib when Administered as a Single Agent or in Combination:
First Dose Reduction: 100mg bid
Second Dose Reduction: 75mg bid
Third Dose Reduction: 50mg bid
Subsequent Modification: Permanently d/c if unable to tolerate 50mg bid

Trametinib when Administered in Combination with Dabrafenib:
Refer to PI

Adverse Reactions

New Primary Noncutaneous Malignancies:
Permanently d/c if RAS mutation-positive noncutaneous malignancies develop

Febrile Drug Reaction:
Fever of 101.3°F to 104°F: Withhold until fever resolves, then resume at same or lower dose level
Fever >104°F or Fever Complicated by Rigors, Hypotension, Dehydration, or Renal Failure: Withhold until fever resolves, then resume at a lower dose level or permanently d/c

Cutaneous:
Grade 3 or 4 Skin Toxicity or Intolerable Grade 2 Skin Toxicity: Withhold for up to 3 weeks; resume at a lower dose level if improved or permanently d/c if not improved

Cardiac:
Symptomatic Congestive Heart Failure: Withhold; if improved, then resume at the same dose
Absolute Decrease in LVEF >20% from Baseline that is Below LLN: Withhold; if improved, then resume at the same dose

Venous Thromboembolism:
Life Threatening PE: Permanently d/c

Ocular Toxicities:
Uveitis and Iritis: Withhold for up to 6 weeks; resume at the same dose if improved to Grade 0-1 or permanently d/c if not improved

Other:
Any Grade 3 Adverse Reaction or Intolerable Grade 2 Adverse Reactions: Withhold; resume at a lower dose level if improved to Grade 0-1, or permanently d/c if not improved

First Occurrence of Any Grade 4 Adverse Reaction: Withhold until adverse reaction improves to Grade 0-1, then resume at a lower dose level; or permanently d/c
Recurrent Grade 4 Adverse Reaction: Permanently d/c

ADMINISTRATION

Oral route

Take at least 1 hr ac or 2 hrs pc
Do not take a missed dose within 6 hrs of the next dose
Do not open, crush, or break

HOW SUPPLIED

Cap: 50mg, 75mg

WARNINGS/PRECAUTIONS

Not indicated for treatment of patients with wild-type BRAF melanoma. Retinal vein occlusion and interstitial lung disease may occur with trametinib. New primary cutaneous and noncutaneous malignancies may occur; perform dermatologic evaluations prior to initiation, every 2 months while on therapy, and for up to 6 months following discontinuation. Hemorrhages (eg, major hemorrhages) and venous thromboembolism (VTE) may occur with trametinib. Cardiomyopathy may occur with trametinib; assess left ventricular ejection fraction (LVEF) by echocardiogram or multigated acquisition (MUGA) scan before initiation with trametinib, 1 month after initiation, and then at 2- to 3-month intervals while on treatment with the combination. Retinal pigment epithelial detachments (RPED) may occur with trametinib; perform ophthalmological evaluation if visual disturbances develop. Uveitis and iritis may occur; monitor for visual signs/symptoms (eg, change in vision, photophobia, eye pain). Serious febrile reactions and fever of any severity complicated by hypotension, rigors/chills, dehydration, or renal failure, may occur. Serious skin toxicity may occur with trametinib. Hyperglycemia may occur; monitor serum glucose levels in patients with preexisting diabetes or hyperglycemia. Potential risk of hemolytic anemia in patients with G6PD deficiency; closely observe such patients for signs of hemolytic anemia. May cause fetal harm. May impair fertility in female patients with trametinib.

ADVERSE REACTIONS

Hyperkeratosis, headache, pyrexia, arthralgia, papilloma, alopecia, palmar-plantar erythrodysesthesia syndrome, hypophosphatemia, chills, fatigue, peripheral edema, rash, N/V, diarrhea, abdominal pain.

DRUG INTERACTIONS

Strong inhibitors of CYP3A4 or CYP2C8 may increase concentrations and strong inducers of CYP3A4 or CYP2C8 may decrease concentrations; substitution of these medications is recommended during treatment. If concomitant use of strong inhibitors (eg, ketoconazole, nefazodone, clarithromycin, gemfibrozil) or strong inducers (eg, rifampin, phenytoin, carbamazepine, phenobarbital, St. John's wort) of CYP3A4 or CYP2C8 is unavoidable, monitor closely for adverse reactions when taking strong inhibitors or loss of efficacy when taking strong inducers. May decrease systemic exposures of midazolam (CYP3A4 substrate), S-warfarin (CYP2C9 substrate), and R-warfarin (CYP3A4/CYP1A2 substrate). Monitor INR levels more frequently in patients receiving warfarin during initiation or discontinuation of dabrafenib. Coadministration with CYP3A4 and CYP2C9 substrates (eg, dexamethasone, hormonal contraceptives) may result in decreased concentrations and loss of efficacy; substitute for these medications or monitor for loss of efficacy if use of these medications is unavoidable.

NURSING CONSIDERATIONS

Assessment: Assess for diabetes, hyperglycemia, G6PD deficiency, pregnancy/nursing status, and possible drug interactions. Assess for presence of BRAF V600E or V600K mutation in tumor specimens. Perform dermatologic evaluations. Assess LVEF by echocardiogram or MUGA scan before initiation with trametinib.

Monitoring: Monitor for retinal vein occlusion, interstitial lung disease, new primary malignancies, hemorrhagic events, VTE, cardiomyopathy, RPED, uveitis, iritis, febrile reactions, fever, skin toxicity, hyperglycemia, and other adverse reactions. Perform dermatologic evaluations every 2 months during therapy and for up to 6 months following discontinuation. Monitor LVEF by echocardiogram and MUGA scan 1 month after initiation and at 2- to 3-month intervals during therapy with trametinib. Perform ophthalmological evaluation if visual disturbances develop and compare with baseline, if available. Monitor serum glucose levels in patients with preexisting diabetes or hyperglycemia. Closely observe patients with G6PD deficiency for signs of hemolytic anemia. Monitor INR levels more frequently in patients receiving warfarin during initiation or discontinuation.

Patient Counseling: Inform that evidence of BRAF V600E or V600K mutation within the tumor specimen is necessary to identify patients for whom treatment is indicated. Inform that combined use with trametinib may cause intracranial and GI hemorrhage, PE/DVT, cardiomyopathy, and serious skin toxicities; advise to contact physician for signs/symptoms of unusual bleeding/hemorrhage, sudden onset of SOB, leg pain, or swelling, signs/symptoms of heart failure, and for progressive or intolerable rash. Instruct to contact physician immediately for any new lesions, changes to existing lesions on the skin, or signs and symptoms of other malignancies, if experiencing any changes in vision or fever, and to report symptoms of severe hyperglycemia (eg, excessive thirst or any increase in the volume or frequency of urination). Advise patients with known G6PD deficiency to contact physician to report signs/symptoms of anemia or hemolysis. Instruct female patients to use nonhormonal, highly effective contraception during treatment and for 2 weeks after discontinuation of treatment as a single agent, or for 4 months after discontinuation of treatment in combination with trametinib; advise to contact physician if pregnancy occurs, or is suspected, while on therapy. Advise breastfeeding mothers to d/c nursing while on therapy. Inform female patients of reproductive potential that treatment in combination with trametinib may impair fertility in female patients. Advise male patients of the potential risk for impaired spermatogenesis, and to seek counseling on fertility and family planning options prior to starting treatment.

Storage: 25°C (77°F); excursions permitted to 15-30°C (59-86°F).

TAMIFLU – oseltamivir phosphate RX

Class: Neuraminidase inhibitor

ADULT DOSAGE

Influenza

Treatment:
Symptomatic for ≤2 days:
75mg bid for 5 days

Prophylaxis:
75mg qd for at least 10 days

Community Outbreak:
Immunocompetent: 75mg qd for up to 6 weeks
Immunocompromised: 75mg qd for up to 12 weeks

PEDIATRIC DOSAGE

Influenza

Treatment:
Symptomatic for ≤2 days:
2 Weeks of Age-<1 Year:
3mg/kg bid for 5 days

1-12 Years:
≤15kg: 30mg bid for 5 days
15.1-23kg: 45mg bid for 5 days
23.1-40kg: 60mg bid for 5 days
≥40.1kg: 75mg bid for 5 days

≥13 Years:
75mg bid for 5 days

Prophylaxis:
1-12 Years:
≤15kg: 30mg qd for 10 days
15.1-23kg: 45mg qd for 10 days
23.1-40kg: 60mg qd for 10 days
≥40.1kg: 75mg qd for 10 days

≥13 Years:
75mg qd for at least 10 days

Community Outbreak:
Continue for up to 6 weeks

DOSE MODIFICATION

Renal Impairment

Moderate (CrCl >30-60mL/min):
Treatment: 30mg bid for 5 days
Prophylaxis: 30mg qd for at least 10 days

Severe (CrCl >10-30mL/min):
Treatment: 30mg qd for 5 days
Prophylaxis: 30mg qod for at least 10 days

ESRD on Hemodialysis (CrCl ≤10mL/min):
Treatment: 30mg after every hemodialysis cycle; treatment duration not to exceed 5 days
Prophylaxis: 30mg after alternate hemodialysis cycles; initial dose can be given prior to start of hemodialysis

ESRD on Continuous Ambulatory Peritoneal Dialysis (CrCl ≤10mL/min):
Treatment: Single 30mg dose immediately after dialysis exchange
Prophylaxis: 30mg once weekly immediately after dialysis exchange

ADMINISTRATION

Oral route

Take w/ or w/o food
Oral sus is the preferred formulation for patients who cannot swallow caps
Shake oral sus well before use

Preparation of Oral Sus

1. Add 55mL of water to the bottle
2. Close the bottle and shake well for 15 sec

Storage:
Refrigerated: Use w/in 17 days
Room Temperature: Use w/in 10 days

Emergency Compounding of Oral Sus from Caps

Refer to PI for number of capsules and amount of water and vehicle needed
1. Place the specified amount of water into a polyethyleneterephthalate (PET) or glass bottle
2. Open the required number of caps and pour the contents of into the PET or glass bottle
3. Gently swirl the sus for at least 2 min
4. Slowly add the specified amount of vehicle to the bottle
5. Close the bottle and shake well for 30 sec

Storage:
Refrigerated: Stable for 5 weeks (35 days)
Room Temperature: Stable for 5 days

HOW SUPPLIED

Cap: 30mg, 45mg, 75mg; Sus: 6mg/mL [60mL]

WARNINGS/PRECAUTIONS

Not a substitute for early influenza vaccination on an annual basis. Emergence of resistance mutations can decrease drug effectiveness; consider available information on influenza drug susceptibility patterns and treatment effects when deciding whether to use treatment. Anaphylaxis and serious skin reactions (eg, toxic epidermal necrolysis, Stevens-Johnson syndrome, erythema multiforme) reported; d/c and institute appropriate treatment if an allergic-like reaction occurs or is suspected. Neuropsychiatric events (eg, hallucinations, delirium, abnormal behavior), in some cases resulting in fatal outcomes, reported; monitor for abnormal behavior and evaluate risks and benefits of continuing treatment if neuropsychiatric symptoms occur. Serious bacterial infections may begin with influenza-like symptoms or may coexist with or occur during the course of influenza; treatment does not prevent these complications.

ADVERSE REACTIONS

N/V, diarrhea, abdominal pain.

DRUG INTERACTIONS

Avoid administration of live attenuated influenza vaccine within 2 weeks before or 48 hrs after oseltamivir, unless medically indicated. Probenecid may increase exposure.

NURSING CONSIDERATIONS

Assessment: Assess for drug hypersensitivity, renal impairment, pregnancy/nursing status, and possible drug interactions.

Monitoring: Monitor for signs/symptoms of neuropsychiatric events, anaphylaxis/serious skin reactions, and other adverse reactions.

Patient Counseling: Advise of the risk of severe allergic reactions or serious skin reactions and to d/c and seek immediate medical attention if an allergic-like reaction occurs or is suspected. Advise of the risk of neuropsychiatric events and to contact physician if experiencing signs of abnormal behavior during treatment. Instruct to begin treatment as soon as possible from the 1st appearance of flu symptoms, and as soon as possible after exposure (for prevention). Instruct to take missed doses as soon as remembered, unless next scheduled dose is within 2 hrs, and then to continue at the usual times. Inform that the medication is not a substitute for flu vaccination. Inform that oral sus delivers 2g sorbitol/75mg dose; inform that this is above the daily max limit of sorbitol for patients with hereditary fructose intolerance and may cause dyspepsia and diarrhea.

Storage: Cap/Dry Powder: 25°C (77°F); excursions permitted to 15-30°C (59-86°F). Constituted Sus: 2-8°C (36-46°F) for up to 17 days, or 25°C (77°F) for up to 10 days with excursions permitted to 15-30°C (59-86°F). Do not freeze.

TAMOXIFEN – tamoxifen citrate

RX

Class: Antiestrogen

Serious and life-threatening uterine malignancies (endometrial adenocarcinoma and uterine sarcoma), stroke, and pulmonary embolism (PE) reported in the risk-reduction setting; some of these events were fatal. Discuss the potential benefits versus the potential risks of these serious events with women at high-risk for breast cancer and women with ductal carcinoma in situ (DCIS) considering therapy for breast cancer risk reduction.

ADULT DOSAGE

Breast Cancer

Treatment of metastatic breast cancer in women and men. Treatment of node-positive or axillary node-negative breast cancer

PEDIATRIC DOSAGE

Pediatric use may not have been established

in women following total or segmental mastectomy, axillary dissection, and breast irradiation. To reduce risk of invasive breast cancer in women with DCIS following breast surgery and radiation. To reduce incidence of breast cancer in high-risk women (those at least 35 yrs of age with a 5-yr predicted risk of breast cancer ≥1.67%, as calculated by the Gail Model)

Treatment:
Usual: 20-40mg/day
Give dosages >20mg/day in divided doses (am and pm)

Incidence Reduction in High-Risk Women/ DCIS:
20mg qd for 5 years

ADMINISTRATION
Oral route

HOW SUPPLIED
Tab: 10mg, 20mg

CONTRAINDICATIONS
(Breast Cancer Incidence Reduction in High-Risk Women/Women with DCIS) Women who require coumarin-type anticoagulant therapy or with history of deep vein thrombosis (DVT) or PE.

WARNINGS/PRECAUTIONS
Hypercalcemia reported in patients with bone metastases; take appropriate measures if hypercalcemia occurs, and, if severe, d/c therapy. Increased incidence of uterine malignancies reported; promptly evaluate any patient receiving or who has previously received therapy who reports abnormal vaginal bleeding. Perform annual gynecological examinations in patients receiving or who have previously received therapy. Increased incidence of endometrial changes, including hyperplasia and polyps, reported. Endometriosis, uterine fibroids, ovarian cysts (in premenopausal patients with advanced breast cancer), and menstrual irregularity or amenorrhea reported. Increased incidence of thromboembolic events (eg, DVT, PE) reported; for treatment of breast cancer, carefully consider risks and benefits of therapy with history of thromboembolic events. Malignant and nonmalignant (eg, changes in liver enzyme levels) effects on the liver, secondary primary tumors (non-uterine), ocular disturbances, increased incidence of cataracts and risk of having cataract surgery, thrombocytopenia, leukopenia, neutropenia, and pancytopenia reported. May cause fetal harm. Hyperlipidemias reported; may consider periodic monitoring of plasma TGs and cholesterol in patients with preexisting hyperlipidemias.

ADVERSE REACTIONS
Uterine malignancies, stroke, PE, hot flashes, vaginal discharge, fatigue/asthenia, weight loss, flush, skin changes, N/V, irregular menses, fluid retention, pain.

DRUG INTERACTIONS
See Contraindications. For treatment of breast cancer, carefully monitor patient's PT with coumarin-type anticoagulants. Increased risk of thromboembolic events with cytotoxic agents or with chemotherapy. May reduce letrozole concentrations. Reduced concentrations with rifampin, aminoglutethimide, and phenobarbital. Medroxyprogesterone reduces concentrations of N-desmethyl tamoxifen (active metabolite). Increased levels with bromocriptine. May reduce anastrozole concentrations; avoid with anastrozole. Erythromycin, cyclosporine, nifedipine, and diltiazem may inhibit metabolism.

NURSING CONSIDERATIONS

Assessment: Assess for history of thromboembolic events, preexisting hyperlipidemias, known hypersensitivity, pregnancy/nursing status, and possible drug interactions.

Monitoring: Monitor for signs/symptoms of uterine malignancies, stroke, thromboembolic events, hypercalcemia, ocular disturbances, and other adverse reactions. Periodically monitor plasma TG and cholesterol levels in patients with preexisting hyperlipidemias, and CBCs, including platelet counts and LFTs. Perform annual gynecological examinations.

Patient Counseling: Inform about potential risks and benefits of treatment. Advise premenopausal women not to become pregnant and to use nonhormonal contraception during therapy and for 2 months after discontinuation if sexually active. Instruct women to seek prompt medical attention if new breast lumps, vaginal bleeding, gynecologic symptoms (eg, menstrual irregularities, changes in vaginal discharge, pelvic pain/pressure), symptoms of leg swelling/tenderness, unexplained SOB, or changes in vision occur.

Storage: 20-25°C (68-77°F).

TAPAZOLE – methimazole

Class: Thyroid hormone synthesis inhibitor

RX

ADULT DOSAGE

Hyperthyroidism

Associated w/ Graves' Disease or in preparation for thyroidectomy or radioactive iodine therapy

Initial:
Mild: 15mg/day in 3 divided doses (q8h)
Moderately Severe: 30-40mg/day in 3 divided doses (q8h)
Severe: 60mg/day in 3 divided doses (q8h)

Maint: 5-15mg/day

PEDIATRIC DOSAGE

Hyperthyroidism

Associated w/ Graves' Disease or in preparation for thyroidectomy or radioactive iodine therapy

Initial: 0.4mg/kg/day in 3 divided doses (q8h)
Maint: 1/2 of initial dose

DOSE MODIFICATION

Adverse Reactions

Hepatotoxicity: D/C treatment promptly w/ evidence of liver abnormality, including hepatic transaminases >3X ULN

ADMINISTRATION

Oral route

HOW SUPPLIED

Tab: 5mg*, 10mg* *scored

WARNINGS/PRECAUTIONS

May cause fetal harm, particularly during the 1st trimester of pregnancy; congenital defects and GI malformations reported (rare). May cause hypothyroidism; routinely monitor TSH and free T4 levels and adjust dose to maintain a euthyroid state. Use lower maintenance dose once clinical evidence of hyperthyroidism has resolved. May cause fetal goiter and cretinism; lowest possible dose should be given during pregnancy. Agranulocytosis, leukopenia, thrombocytopenia, and aplastic anemia (pancytopenia) may occur. D/C therapy in the presence of agranulocytosis, aplastic anemia, ANCA-positive vasculitis, hepatitis, or exfoliative dermatitis, and monitor bone marrow indices. Hepatotoxicity (including acute liver failure) reported; promptly evaluate liver function (bilirubin, alkaline phosphatase) and hepatocellular integrity (ALT, AST) if symptoms suggestive of hepatic dysfunction occur. D/C treatment promptly with evidence of liver abnormality including hepatic transaminases >3X ULN. May cause hypoprothrombinemia and bleeding; monitor PT during therapy, especially before surgical procedures.

ADVERSE REACTIONS

Agranulocytosis, granulocytopenia, thrombocytopenia, aplastic anemia, drug fever, lupus-like syndrome, insulin autoimmune syndrome, hepatitis, periarteritis, hypoprothrombinemia, skin rash, urticaria, N/V, arthralgia, paresthesia.

DRUG INTERACTIONS

May increase oral anticoagulant (eg, warfarin) activity; consider additional PT/INR monitoring, especially before surgical procedures. β-blockers, digitalis, and theophylline may need dose reduction when patient becomes euthyroid. Caution with other drugs that cause agranulocytosis.

NURSING CONSIDERATIONS

Assessment: Assess for hypersensitivity to drug, pregnancy/nursing status, and possible drug interactions. Obtain baseline TSH and free T4 levels, CBC, and LFTs.

Monitoring: Monitor for agranulocytosis, leukopenia, thrombocytopenia, aplastic anemia, hepatic dysfunction, hypersensitivity reactions, and other adverse reactions. Monitor bone marrow indices in patients with agranulocytosis, aplastic anemia, ANCA-positive vasculitis, hepatitis, or exfoliative dermatitis. Monitor WBC and differential counts. Monitor PT, especially before surgical procedures. Monitor TSH and free T4 levels periodically.

Patient Counseling: Inform of the benefits/risks of therapy. Instruct to inform physician if pregnant/nursing or planning to become pregnant. Instruct to immediately report to physician any symptoms suggestive of agranulocytosis (eg, fever, sore throat) or any signs/symptoms of illness (eg, skin eruptions, headache, general malaise).

Storage: 15-30°C (59-86°F).

TARCEVA – erlotinib

RX

Class: Kinase inhibitors

ADULT DOSAGE

Non-Small Cell Lung Cancer

1st-line treatment of patients w/ metastatic non-small cell lung cancer (NSCLC) whose tumors have epidermal growth factor receptor exon 19 deletions or exon 21 (L858R) substitution mutations; treatment of locally advanced or metastatic NSCLC after failure of at least 1 prior chemotherapy regimen; maint treatment of locally advanced or metastatic NSCLC that has not progressed after 4 cycles of platinum-based 1st-line chemotherapy

Usual: 150mg qd

Pancreatic Cancer

1st-Line Treatment of Locally Advanced, Unresectable, or Metastatic Pancreatic Cancer:

Usual: 100mg qd in combination w/ gemcitabine until disease progression or unacceptable toxicity occurs

PEDIATRIC DOSAGE

Pediatric use may not have been established

DOSE MODIFICATION

Concomitant Medications

Reduce by 50mg Decrements if:

If severe reactions occur w/ concomitant use of strong CYP3A4 inhibitors or w/ concomitant use of both a CYP3A4 and CYP1A2 inhibitor (eg, ciprofloxacin); avoid concomitant use if possible

Increase by 50mg Increments As Tolerated for:

Concomitant use w/ CYP3A4 inducers; increase by 50mg increments at 2-week intervals to a max of 450mg; avoid concomitant use if possible

Concurrent cigarette smoking; increase by 50mg increments at 2-week intervals to a max of 300mg; immediately reduce the dose to the recommended dose (150mg or 100mg qd) upon cessation of smoking

Drugs Affecting Gastric pH:

Avoid concomitant use w/ proton pump inhibitors if possible

If treatment w/ an H_2-receptor antagonist is required, dose must be taken 10 hrs after the H_2-receptor antagonist dosing and at least 2 hrs before the next dose of the H_2-receptor antagonist

If an antacid is necessary, dose should be separated by several hrs

Adverse Reactions:

D/C for:

Interstitial Lung Disease (ILD)

Severe hepatic toxicity that does not improve significantly or resolve w/in 3 weeks

GI perforation

Severe bullous, blistering, or exfoliating skin conditions

Corneal perforation or severe ulceration

Withhold for:

During diagnostic evaluation for possible ILD

For severe (CTCAE Grade 3 to 4) renal toxicity, and consider discontinuation

In patients w/o preexisting hepatic impairment for total bilirubin levels >3X ULN or transaminases >5X ULN, and consider discontinuation

In patients w/ preexisting hepatic impairment or biliary obstruction for doubling of bilirubin or tripling of transaminases values over baseline and consider discontinuation

For persistent severe diarrhea not responsive to medical management (eg, loperamide)

For severe rash not responsive to medical management

For keratitis of (NCI-CTC version 4.0) Grade 3-4 or for Grade 2 lasting more than 2 weeks

For acute/worsening ocular disorders such as eye pain, and consider discontinuation

Reduce by 50mg Decrements if:

When restarting therapy following withholding treatment for a dose-limiting toxicity that has resolved to baseline or Grade ≤1

ADMINISTRATION

Oral route

Take on an empty stomach (at least 1 hr ac or 2 hrs pc)

HOW SUPPLIED
Tab: 25mg, 100mg, 150mg

WARNINGS/PRECAUTIONS
Not recommended for use in combination with platinum-based chemotherapy. Serious interstitial lung disease (ILD) may occur; withhold for acute onset of new/progressive unexplained pulmonary symptoms. Renal failure; hepatotoxicity with or without hepatic impairment; hepatorenal syndrome; bullous, blistering, and exfoliative skin conditions; MI/ischemia; cerebrovascular accidents (CVA); microangiopathic hemolytic anemia with thrombocytopenia; and fetal harm may occur. Decreased tear production, abnormal eyelash growth, keratoconjunctivitis sicca, or keratitis may occur and can lead to corneal perforation/ulceration. GI perforation may occur; increased risk in patients with prior history of peptic ulceration or diverticular disease.

ADVERSE REACTIONS
Rash, diarrhea, anorexia, fatigue, dyspnea, cough, N/V, infection, stomatitis, pruritus, dry skin, conjunctivitis, keratoconjunctivitis sicca, back pain, chest pain.

DRUG INTERACTIONS
Concomitant use with antiangiogenic agents, corticosteroids, NSAIDs, and/or taxane-based chemotherapy may increase risk of GI perforation. Increased levels with potent CYP3A4 inhibitors (eg, ketoconazole), and with inhibitors of both CYP3A4 and CYP1A2 (eg, ciprofloxacin). Decreased levels with CYP3A4 inducers (eg, rifampicin). Cigarette smoking and drugs affecting gastric pH (eg, omeprazole, ranitidine) may decrease levels. INR elevations and bleeding events reported with coumarin-derived anticoagulants (eg, warfarin); monitor PT/INR regularly.

NURSING CONSIDERATIONS

Assessment: Assess for hepatic/renal impairment, dehydration, history of peptic ulceration or diverticular disease, pregnancy/nursing status, and possible drug interactions.

Monitoring: Monitor for signs and symptoms of ILD, hepatotoxicity, GI perforation, MI/ischemia, renal failure/insufficiency, CVA, microangiopathic hemolytic anemia with thrombocytopenia, ocular disorders, bullous and exfoliative skin disorders, and other adverse reactions. Monitor LFTs, renal function, and serum electrolytes.

Patient Counseling: Inform of risks/benefits of therapy. Instruct to notify physician if onset or worsening of skin rash or development of bullous lesions or desquamation; severe/persistent diarrhea, N/V, anorexia; unexplained SOB or cough; or eye irritation occurs. Instruct to stop smoking and advise to contact physician for any changes in smoking status. Advise on the presentation of skin, hair, and nail disorders. Instruct on initial management of rash or diarrhea. Counsel on pregnancy planning and prevention; advise females of reproductive potential to use highly effective contraception during treatment and for at least 2 weeks after the last dose. Advise to contact physician if pregnant or if pregnancy is suspected and to d/c nursing during treatment.

Storage: 25°C (77°F); excursions permitted to 15-30°C (59-86°F).

TASIGNA – nilotinib RX

Class: Kinase inhibitors

Prolongs QT interval. Monitor for hypokalemia or hypomagnesemia and correct deficiencies prior to administration and periodically. Obtain ECGs to monitor QTc at baseline, 7 days after initiation, and periodically thereafter, and following any dose adjustments. Sudden deaths reported. Do not administer to patients w/ hypokalemia, hypomagnesemia, or long QT syndrome. Avoid w/ drugs known to prolong the QT interval and strong CYP3A4 inhibitors. Avoid food 2 hrs before and 1 hr after taking the dose.

ADULT DOSAGE

Ph+ Chronic Myeloid Leukemia

Newly Diagnosed and in Chronic Phase:
300mg bid

Chronic and Accelerated Phase, Resistant or Intolerant to Prior Therapy that Included Imatinib:
400mg bid
May be given in combination w/ hematopoietic growth factors (eg, erythropoietin, granulocyte colony-stimulating factor), hydroxyurea, or anagrelide if clinically indicated

PEDIATRIC DOSAGE
Pediatric use may not have been established

DOSE MODIFICATION

Concomitant Medications

Strong CYP3A4 Inhibitors:

Avoid use

If necessary, consider dose reduction to 300mg qd w/ resistant or intolerant Ph+ CML or to 200mg qd w/ newly diagnosed Ph+ CML

If strong inhibitor is discontinued, allow a washout period of approx 1 week before dose is adjusted upward to the indicated dose

Strong CYP3A4 Inducers:

Avoid use

Hepatic Impairment

Newly Diagnosed Ph+ CML:

Mild, Moderate, or Severe (Child-Pugh Class A, B, or C): 200mg bid initially, escalate to 300mg bid based on tolerability

Resistant or Intolerant Ph+ CML:

Mild or Moderate (Child-Pugh Score A or B): 300mg bid initially, escalate to 400mg bid based on tolerability

Severe (Child-Pugh Score C): 200mg bid escalated sequentially to 300mg bid and then to 400mg bid based on tolerability

Adverse Reactions

ECGs w/ a QTc >480msec:

1. Withhold nilotinib, and perform an analysis of serum K^+ and Mg^{2+}, and if below lower limit of normal, correct w/ supplements to w/in normal limits. Concomitant medication usage must be reviewed
2. Resume w/in 2 weeks at prior dose if QTcF returns to <450msec and to w/in 20msec of baseline
3. If QTcF is between 450msec and 480msec after 2 weeks, reduce dose to 400mg qd
4. If, following dose-reduction to 400mg qd, QTcF returns to >480msec, d/c therapy
5. An ECG should be repeated approx 7 days after any dose adjustment

Neutropenia and Thrombocytopenia:

Newly Diagnosed Ph+ CML/Resistant or Intolerant Ph+ CML:

ANC<1.0 x 10^9/L and/or Platelet Counts <50 x 10^9/L:

1. Stop nilotinib, and monitor blood counts
2. Resume w/in 2 weeks at prior dose if ANC >1.0 x 10^9/L and platelets >50 x 10^9/L
3. If blood counts remain low for >2 weeks, reduce dose to 400mg qd

Selected Nonhematologic Lab Abnormalities:

Elevated Serum Lipase or Amylase ≥Grade 3:

1. Withhold nilotinib, and monitor serum lipase or amylase
2. Resume at 400mg qd if serum lipase or amylase returns to ≤Grade 1

Elevated Bilirubin ≥Grade 3:

1. Withhold nilotinib, and monitor bilirubin
2. Resume at 400mg qd if bilirubin returns to ≤Grade 1

Elevated Hepatic Transaminases ≥Grade 3:

1. Withhold nilotinib, and monitor hepatic transaminases
2. Resume at 400mg qd if hepatic transaminases returns to ≤Grade 1

Other Nonhematologic Toxicities:

Grade 3 to 4 Lipase Elevations, Grade 3 to 4 Bilirubin, or Hepatic Transaminase Elevations:

Withhold dose and may resume at 400mg qd

Other Significant Moderate or Severe Toxicities:

Withhold dose and resume at 400mg once qd when the toxicity has resolved

If clinically appropriate, consider escalating dose back to 300mg (newly diagnosed Ph+ CML) or 400mg (resistant or intolerant Ph+ CML) bid

ADMINISTRATION

Oral route

Take on an empty stomach

Avoid food for at least 2 hrs before and 1 hr after taking the dose

Take at approx 12-hr intervals

Swallow whole w/ water

May disperse contents of each cap in 1 tsp of applesauce if unable to swallow; take immediately (w/in 15 min) and do not store for future use

HOW SUPPLIED

Cap: 150mg, 200mg

CONTRAINDICATIONS

Hypokalemia, hypomagnesemia, long QT syndrome.

WARNINGS/PRECAUTIONS

Myelosuppression (eg, neutropenia, thrombocytopenia, anemia) may occur; perform CBCs every 2 weeks for the first 2 months, then monthly thereafter, or as clinically indicated. Cardiovascular (CV) events, including arterial vascular occlusive events, reported; evaluate CV status and monitor and actively manage CV risk factors during therapy. May increase serum lipase; increased risk in patients w/ history of pancreatitis. Interrupt dosing and consider appropriate diagnostics to exclude pancreatitis if lipase elevations are accompanied by abdominal symptoms. May result in hepatotoxicity as measured by elevations in bilirubin, AST/ALT, and alkaline phosphatase. May cause hypophosphatemia, hypo/hyperkalemia, hypocalcemia, and hyponatremia; correct electrolyte abnormalities prior to initiation and during therapy. Exposure is increased in patients w/ impaired hepatic function. Tumor lysis syndrome cases reported; maintain adequate hydration and correct uric acid levels prior to initiation. Hemorrhage reported in patients w/ newly diagnosed CML. Reduced exposure in patients w/ total gastrectomy; perform more frequent monitoring and consider dose increase or alternative therapy. Contains lactose; not recommended w/ galactose intolerance, severe lactase deficiency w/ a severe degree of intolerance to lactose-containing products, or glucose-galactose malabsorption. May cause fetal harm. Severe fluid retention, effusions (eg, pleural effusion, pericardial effusion, ascites) or pulmonary edema reported; evaluate etiology and treat patients accordingly. Caution w/ relevant cardiac disorders.

ADVERSE REACTIONS

QT prolongation, rash, pruritus, headache, muscle spasms, fatigue, N/V, alopecia, myalgia, arthralgia, abdominal pain, constipation, URTI, diarrhea, cough.

DRUG INTERACTIONS

See Boxed Warning and Dose Modification. Avoid w/ strong CYP3A4 inducers (eg, dexamethasone, phenytoin, carbamazepine, rifampin, rifabutin, rifapentine, phenobarbital), grapefruit products and other foods that inhibit CYP3A4, St. John's wort, and antiarrhythmic drugs. May increase concentrations of drugs eliminated by CYP3A4 (eg, midazolam, certain HMG-CoA reductase inhibitors), CYP2C8, CYP2C9, CYP2D6, and UGT1A1 enzymes; dose adjustment may be necessary for CYP3A4 substrates, especially those that have narrow therapeutic indices (eg, alfentanil, cyclosporine, dihydroergotamine, ergotamine, fentanyl, sirolimus, tacrolimus). May decrease concentrations of drugs eliminated by CYP2B6, CYP2C8, and CYP2C9 enzymes; monitor patients closely when coadministered w/ drugs that have a narrow therapeutic index and are substrates for these enzymes. May increase concentrations of P-gp substrates; use w/ caution. P-gp inhibitors may increase concentrations; use w/ caution. Decreased solubility and reduced bioavailability w/ drugs that inhibit gastric acid secretion to elevate the gastric pH; concomitant use w/ proton pump inhibitors is not recommended. Administer an H_2 blocker approx 10 hrs before and 2 hrs after the dose of nilotinib. Administer an antacid approx 2 hrs before or 2 hrs after the dose of nilotinib.

NURSING CONSIDERATIONS

Assessment: Assess for electrolyte abnormalities, history of pancreatitis, long QT syndrome, cardiac disorders, total gastrectomy, hepatic impairment, galactose intolerance, lactase deficiency, glucose-galactose malabsorption, pregnancy/nursing status, and possible drug interactions. Obtain baseline ECG, uric acid levels, and chemistry panels, including lipid profile and glucose.

Monitoring: Monitor for myelosuppression; perform CBCs every 2 weeks for the first 2 months of therapy, then monthly thereafter or as clinically indicated. Perform chemistry panels, including electrolytes and liver enzymes periodically. Monitor lipid profiles and glucose periodically during 1st yr of therapy and at least yearly during chronic therapy. Monitor for signs/symptoms of QT prolongation; obtain ECG 7 days after initiation, periodically thereafter, and after any dose adjustments. Monitor for hydration status, and CV status/risk factors. Monitor serum lipase levels and LFTs monthly or as clinically indicated. Monitor for signs of severe fluid retention, symptoms of respiratory/cardiac compromise, tumor lysis syndrome, hemorrhage, and other adverse reactions.

Patient Counseling: Instruct to take ud. Advise to seek immediate medical attention w/ any symptoms suggestive of a CV event. Instruct not to consume grapefruit products at any time during treatment. Instruct to inform physician of other medicines being taken, including OTC drugs or herbal supplements (eg, St. John's wort). Advise women of childbearing potential to use highly effective contraceptives while on therapy. Instruct not to d/c or change dose w/o consulting physician.

Storage: 25°C (77°F); excursions permitted between 15-30°C (59-86°F).

TAZICEF – ceftazidime

RX

Class: Cephalosporin (3rd generation)

ADULT DOSAGE

General Dosing

Lower respiratory tract and CNS infections, bacterial septicemia, and sepsis caused by susceptible strains of microorganisms
Usual: 1g IM/IV q8-12h

Urinary Tract Infections

Uncomplicated:
250mg IM/IV q12h
Complicated:
500mg IM/IV q8-12h

Bone/Joint Infections

2g IV q12h

Pneumonia

Uncomplicated:
500mg-1g IM/IV q8h

Skin and Skin Structure Infections

500mg-1g IM/IV q8h

Gynecologic Infections

Serious Infections:
2g IV q8h

Intra-Abdominal Infections

Serious Infections:
2g IV q8h

Meningitis

2g IV q8h

Life-Threatening Infections

Very Severe Infections, Especially in Immunocompromised Patients:
2g IV q8h

Lung Infection

Caused by *Pseudomonas* species in patients w/ cystic fibrosis w/ normal renal function
30-50mg/kg IV q8h
Max: 6g/day

Treatment Duration

Continue for 2 days after signs/symptoms of infection disappear; may require longer therapy w/ complicated infections

PEDIATRIC DOSAGE

General Dosing

Neonates (0-4 Weeks of Age):
30mg/kg IV q12h
Infants and Children (1 Month-12 Years):
30-50mg/kg IV q8h
Max: 6g/day

Reserve higher doses for immunocompromised, cystic fibrosis, or meningitis
Continue for 2 days after signs/symptoms of infection disappear; may require longer therapy w/ complicated infections

DOSE MODIFICATION

Renal Impairment
Adults:
LD: May give 1g
Maint:
CrCl 31-50mL/min: 1g q12h
CrCl 16-30mL/min: 1g q24h
CrCl 6-15mL/min: 500mg q24h
CrCl <5mL/min: 500mg q48h
If usual dose is lower than recommended dose for renal impairment, the lower dose should be used
Renal Impairment and Severe Infection: May increase dose by 50% or the dosing frequency may be increased appropriately
Hemodialysis: Give 1g LD, followed by 1g after each hemodialysis period
Intraperitoneal Dialysis/Continuous Ambulatory Peritoneal Dialysis: Give 1g LD, followed by 500mg q24h, or add to dialysis fluid at 250mg/2L
Pediatrics:
Adjust CrCl for BSA or lean body mass; reduce dosing frequency in renal insufficiency

ADMINISTRATION

IV/IM routes

Avoid intra-arterial administration
Do not add to sol of aminoglycoside; administer separately
May administer as intermittent IV infusion w/ a Y-type administration set w/ compatible sol; during infusion of ceftazidime, desirable to d/c other sol

ADD-Vantage

Not intended for direct IV/IM inj
Intended for single dose administration w/ ADD-Vantage flexible diluent container
Constitute ADD-Vantage vials w/ 50mL or 100mL of D5 inj, 0.9% NaCl inj, or 50mL of 0.45% NaCl inj in ADD-Vantage diluent; constitute only when it is certain patient is ready to receive drug

Refer to PI for further administration procedures, direction for use of inj in ADD-Vantage vials, compatibility, and stability

HOW SUPPLIED

Inj: 1g, 2g. Also available as a Pharmacy Bulk Package. Refer to individual package insert for more information.

WARNINGS/PRECAUTIONS

Caution in penicillin (PCN)-sensitive patients; determine whether patient has had previous hypersensitivity reactions to cephalosporins, PCN, or other drugs. D/C if an allergic reaction occurs. *Clostridium difficile*-associated diarrhea (CDAD) reported; d/c if CDAD is suspected or confirmed. May result in overgrowth of nonsusceptible organisms with prolonged use or use in the absence of a proven or strongly suspected bacterial infection or prophylactic indication; take appropriate measures if superinfection develops. High and prolonged serum concentrations may occur in patients with transient or persistent reduction of urinary output. Elevated levels with renal insufficiency can lead to seizures, encephalopathy, coma, asterixis, neuromuscular excitability, and myoclonia. Risk of decreased prothrombin activity in patients with renal/hepatic impairment, poor nutritional state, and patients receiving a protracted course of therapy; monitor PT. Distal necrosis may occur after inadvertent intra-arterial administration. Lab test interactions may occur. Caution with impaired renal function, history of GI disease, particularly colitis, and in elderly.

ADVERSE REACTIONS

Phlebitis and inflammation at inj site, pruritus, rash, fever, diarrhea, N/V, abdominal pain, increased ALT/AST/GGT/LDH, eosinophilia.

DRUG INTERACTIONS

Nephrotoxicity reported with concomitant aminoglycosides or potent diuretics (eg, furosemide). Avoid with chloramphenicol; may antagonize effect of β-lactam antibiotics. May affect the gut flora, leading to lower estrogen reabsorption and reduced efficacy of combined estrogen/progesterone oral contraceptives.

NURSING CONSIDERATIONS

Assessment: Assess for previous hypersensitivity reaction to cephalosporins, PCNs or other drugs, renal/hepatic impairment, poor nutritional status, patients receiving protracted course of antibiotics, history of GI disease (eg, colitis), pregnancy/nursing status, and possible drug interactions.

Monitoring: Monitor for signs/symptoms of allergic reactions, CDAD, superinfection, and other adverse reactions. Monitor for seizures, encephalopathy, coma, asterixis, neuromuscular excitability, and myoclonia with renal impairment. Monitor renal function and PT. Perform periodic susceptibility testing.

Patient Counseling: Inform that drug only treats bacterial, not viral, infections. Instruct to take exactly ud; skipping doses or not completing full course of therapy may decrease effectiveness and increase the likelihood of bacterial resistance. Inform that diarrhea may occur and will usually end when therapy is discontinued. Instruct to contact physician as soon as possible if watery/bloody stools (with/without stomach cramps, fever) develop even as late as 2 months or more after having taken the last dose of therapy.

Storage: (Dry state) 20-25°C (68-77°F). Protect from light.

TECFIDERA — dimethyl fumarate **RX**

Class: Immunomodulatory agent

ADULT DOSAGE

Multiple Sclerosis

Relapsing Forms:
Initial: 120mg bid
Titrate: Increase to 240mg bid after 7 days

PEDIATRIC DOSAGE

Pediatric use may not have been established

Maint: 240mg bid. Consider temporary reduction to 120mg bid if not tolerated; resume maint dose of 240mg bid w/in 4 weeks and consider discontinuation if unable to tolerate return to maint dose

ADMINISTRATION
Oral route
Take w/ or w/o food
Swallow whole and intact; do not crush or chew
Do not sprinkle cap contents on food
To reduce flushing, take w/ food or take up to 325mg of non-enteric coated aspirin 30 min prior to therapy

HOW SUPPLIED
Cap, Delayed-Release: 120mg, 240mg

WARNINGS/PRECAUTIONS
May cause anaphylaxis and angioedema; d/c if signs/symptoms occur. Progressive multifocal leukoencephalopathy (PML) reported; withhold treatment and perform appropriate diagnostic evaluation at the 1st sign/symptom suggestive of PML. May decrease lymphocyte counts; consider interruption of therapy w/ lymphocyte counts <0.5 x 10^9/L persisting for >6 months and monitor lymphocyte count until lymphopenia is resolved. Consider withholding treatment in patients w/ serious infections until resolved; decisions about whether or not to restart therapy should be individualized based on clinical circumstances. May cause flushing; administration w/ food may reduce the incidence. Alternatively, administration of non-enteric coated ASA (up to a dose of 325mg) 30 min prior to dosing may reduce the incidence or severity of flushing.

ADVERSE REACTIONS
Flushing, abdominal pain, diarrhea, N/V, pruritus, rash, albuminuria, erythema, dyspepsia, increased AST.

NURSING CONSIDERATIONS

Assessment: Assess for known hypersensitivity to drug or any of the excipients, infection, and pregnancy/nursing status. Obtain baseline CBC including lymphocyte count.

Monitoring: Monitor for anaphylaxis, angioedema, PML, lymphopenia, flushing, and other adverse reactions. Monitor CBC including lymphocyte count after 6 months of treatment, every 6-12 months thereafter, and as clinically indicated.

Patient Counseling: Advise to d/c therapy and seek medical care if signs/symptoms of anaphylaxis or angioedema develop. Inform that PML is characterized by progression of deficits and usually leads to death or severe disability; instruct to contact physician if any symptoms suggestive of PML develop. Inform that therapy may decrease lymphocyte counts. Advise to contact physician if patient experiences persistent and/or severe flushing or GI reactions. Instruct to inform physician if patient is pregnant or plans to become pregnant while on therapy; encourage enrollment in the pregnancy registry if patient becomes pregnant while on therapy.

Storage: 15-30°C (59-86°F). Protect from light.

TEFLARO – ceftaroline fosamil — RX
Class: Cephalosporin

ADULT DOSAGE
Skin and Skin Structure Infections
Acute:
Usual: 600mg q12h IV for 5-14 days
Community-Acquired Pneumonia
Usual: 600mg q12h IV for 5-7 days

PEDIATRIC DOSAGE
Pediatric use may not have been established

DOSE MODIFICATION
Renal Impairment
CrCl >30-50mL/min: 400mg IV q12h
CrCl ≥15-30mL/min: 300mg IV q12h
CrCl <15mL/min/Hemodialysis: 200mg IV q12h; administered after hemodialysis on hemodialysis days
Elderly
Adjust dosage based on renal function

ADMINISTRATION
IV route

Administer infusion over 1 hr
Do not mix w/ or physically add to sol containing other drugs

Preparation
Reconstitute contents of vial w/ 20mL of sterile water for inj (SWFI), 0.9% NaCl inj, D5 inj, or lactated Ringer's inj
Further dilute constituted sol in range between 50mL to 250mL before infusion
Use the same diluent for the further dilution, unless SWFI was used earlier; if SWFI was used earlier, then appropriate infusion sol include 0.9% NaCl inj, D5 inj, 2.5% dextrose inj, 0.45% NaCl inj, or lactated Ringer's inj
Preparation of 600mg or 400mg Dose in 50mL:
Withdraw 20mL of diluent from 50mL infusion bag and inject entire contents of reconstituted vial into bag

Refer to PI for stability information

HOW SUPPLIED
Inj: 400mg, 600mg

WARNINGS/PRECAUTIONS
Serious and occasionally fatal hypersensitivity and skin reactions reported; d/c if an allergic reaction occurs. Caution with penicillin (PCN) or other β-lactam allergy; cross-sensitivity may occur. *Clostridium difficile*-associated diarrhea (CDAD) reported; d/c if CDAD is suspected or confirmed. May result in bacterial resistance if used in the absence of a proven/suspected bacterial infection. Seroconversion from negative to a positive direct Coombs' test reported. If anemia develops, drug-induced hemolytic anemia should be considered. If drug-induced hemolytic anemia is suspected, consider discontinuation of therapy and administer supportive care if clinically indicated. Caution with renal impairment and in elderly.

ADVERSE REACTIONS
Diarrhea, nausea, rash.

NURSING CONSIDERATIONS

Assessment: Assess for cephalosporin or other β-lactam allergy, drug hypersensitivity, renal impairment, pregnancy/nursing status, and possible drug interactions. Obtain appropriate specimens for microbiological examination to identify pathogen and determine susceptibility.

Monitoring: Monitor for signs/symptoms of hypersensitivity reactions, skin reactions, CDAD, drug-induced hemolytic anemia, and other adverse reactions. Monitor renal function, especially in elderly.

Patient Counseling: Advise that allergic reactions could occur and that serious reactions require immediate treatment. Advise to inform the physician about any previous hypersensitivity reactions to the drug, other β-lactams (including cephalosporins), or other allergens. Advise that antibacterial drugs should be used to treat only bacterial, not viral (eg, common cold), infections. Instruct to take ud; inform that skipping doses or not completing the full course may decrease effectiveness of treatment and increase bacterial resistance. Advise that diarrhea may occur; instruct to notify physician if severe watery or bloody diarrhea develops.

Storage: Unreconstituted: 25°C (77°F); excursions permitted to 15-30°C (59-86°F).

TEKAMLO – aliskiren/amlodipine RX

Class: Calcium channel blocker (dihydropyridine)/renin inhibitor

D/C when pregnancy is detected. Drugs that act directly on the renin-angiotensin system can cause injury/death to the developing fetus.

ADULT DOSAGE

Hypertension

Initial: 150mg/5mg qd
Titrate: Adjust dose prn; increase ≤300mg/10mg qd if BP remains uncontrolled after 2-4 weeks
Max: 300mg/10mg qd
Add-On Therapy:
Use if not adequately controlled w/ aliskiren alone or another dihydropyridine calcium channel blocker alone
W/ dose-limiting adverse reactions to either component alone, switch to aliskiren/

PEDIATRIC DOSAGE
Pediatric use may not have been established

amlodipine containing a lower dose of that component

Replacement Therapy:
Switch from separate tabs to a single tab of aliskiren/amlodipine containing the same doses
May increase dose of one or both components if BP control has not been satisfactory

DOSE MODIFICATION

Hepatic Impairment
Consider lower doses

Elderly
Consider lower initial doses

ADMINISTRATION

Oral route

Establish a routine pattern for taking the drug either w/ or w/o a meal; high-fat meals decrease absorption substantially

HOW SUPPLIED

Tab: (Aliskiren/Amlodipine) 150mg/5mg, 150mg/10mg, 300mg/5mg, 300mg/10mg

CONTRAINDICATIONS

Concomitant use w/ ARBs or ACE inhibitors in patients w/ diabetes.

WARNINGS/PRECAUTIONS

Symptomatic hypotension may occur (eg, patients w/ marked volume/salt depletion, w/ severe aortic stenosis); correct volume/salt depletion prior to administration, or start treatment under close supervision. May cause changes in renal function, including acute renal failure; consider withholding or discontinuing therapy if significant decrease in renal function develops. Patients whose renal function may depend in part on the activity of the renin-angiotensin-aldosterone system (RAAS) (eg, renal artery stenosis, severe heart failure [HF], post-MI, volume depletion) may be at risk for developing acute renal failure. Aliskiren: Hypersensitivity reactions and head/neck angioedema reported; d/c therapy immediately if anaphylactic reactions or edema occur and do not readminister. May cause hyperkalemia. Amlodipine: May develop worsening of angina and acute MI after starting or increasing dose, particularly w/ severe obstructive coronary artery disease (CAD).

ADVERSE REACTIONS

Peripheral edema.

DRUG INTERACTIONS

See Contraindications. Aliskiren: Cyclosporine or itraconazole may increase levels; avoid concomitant use. NSAIDs (eg, selective COX-2 inhibitors) may deteriorate renal function and attenuate antihypertensive effect. Dual blockade of the RAAS is associated w/ increased risks of hypotension, hyperkalemia, and changes in renal function (including acute renal failure); avoid combined use w/ ACE inhibitors or ARBs, particularly in patients w/ CrCl <60ml/min. Oral coadministration w/ furosemide reduced exposure to furosemide; monitor diuretic effects. Risk of developing hyperkalemia w/ NSAIDs (eg, selective COX-2 inhibitors), K^+ supplements, or K_+-sparing diuretics. Amlodipine: May increase simvastatin exposure; limit simvastatin dose to 20mg/day. Increased systemic exposure w/ CYP3A inhibitors (moderate and strong) warranting dose reduction; monitor for symptoms of hypotension and edema to determine need for dose adjustment. Monitor BP when coadministered w/ CYP3A4 inducers.

NURSING CONSIDERATIONS

Assessment: Assess for drug hypersensitivity, diabetes, volume/salt depletion, renal artery stenosis, HF, post-MI status, severe aortic stenosis, CAD, renal/hepatic impairment, pregnancy/nursing status, and possible drug interactions.

Monitoring: Monitor for signs/symptoms of hypotension, worsening of angina, acute MI, hyperkalemia, hypersensitivity reactions, airway obstruction, angioedema, and other adverse reactions. Monitor BP and renal function periodically.

Patient Counseling: Inform female patients of childbearing age of the consequences of exposure during pregnancy and of the treatment options for women planning to become pregnant. Advise to report pregnancies as soon as possible. Caution that lightheadedness may occur, especially during the 1st days of therapy; advise to contact physician if lightheadedness occurs. Advise to d/c until physician has been consulted if syncope occurs. Caution that inadequate fluid intake, excessive perspiration, diarrhea, or vomiting can lead to an excessive fall in BP. Advise to d/c and immediately report any signs/symptoms of a severe allergic reaction or angioedema. Inform that angioedema (eg, laryngeal edema) may occur anytime during treatment. Instruct not to use K^+ supplements or salt substitutes containing K^+ w/o consulting physician.

Storage: 25°C (77°F); excursions permitted to 15-30°C (59-86°F) in original container. Protect from heat and moisture.

TEKTURNA – aliskiren

RX

Class: Renin inhibitor

D/C when pregnancy is detected. Drugs that act directly on the renin-angiotensin system can cause injury/death to the developing fetus.

ADULT DOSAGE

Hypertension

Initial: 150mg qd

Titrate: May increase to 300mg qd if BP is not adequately controlled

Max: 300mg/day

PEDIATRIC DOSAGE

Pediatric use may not have been established

ADMINISTRATION

Oral route

Establish a routine pattern for taking drug w/ regard to meals; high-fat meals decrease absorption substantially

HOW SUPPLIED

Tab: 150mg, 300mg

CONTRAINDICATIONS

Coadministration w/ ARBs or ACE inhibitors in patients w/ diabetes.

WARNINGS/PRECAUTIONS

Hypersensitivity reactions and head/neck angioedema reported; d/c therapy immediately and do not readminister if anaphylactic reactions or angioedema develop. Symptomatic hypotension may occur in patients w/ marked volume depletion or w/ salt depletion; correct volume/salt depletion prior to administration, or start treatment under close medical supervision. May cause changes in renal function, including acute renal failure; caution in patients whose renal function may depend in part on the activity of the renin-angiotensin-aldosterone system (RAAS) (eg, renal artery stenosis, severe heart failure [HF], post-MI, volume depletion). Consider withholding or discontinuing therapy if clinically significant decrease in renal function develops. May cause hyperkalemia.

ADVERSE REACTIONS

Angioedema, diarrhea, cough, seizures, rash, elevated uric acid, gout, renal stones, increased BUN/SrCr.

DRUG INTERACTIONS

See Contraindications. Cyclosporine or itraconazole may increase levels; avoid concomitant use. NSAIDs, including selective COX-2 inhibitors, may deteriorate renal function and may attenuate antihypertensive effect. Dual blockade of the RAAS is associated w/ increased risk of hypotension, hyperkalemia, and changes in renal function (including acute renal failure); avoid combined use w/ ACE inhibitors or ARBS, particularly in patients w/ CrCl <60mL/min. Reduced furosemide exposure w/ concomitant use. May develop hyperkalemia w/ NSAIDs, K^+ supplements, or K^+-sparing diuretics.

NURSING CONSIDERATIONS

Assessment: Assess for hypersensitivity to the drug, diabetes, volume/salt depletion, renal artery stenosis, HF, post-MI status, pregnancy/nursing status, and possible drug interactions.

Monitoring: Monitor for hypersensitivity reactions, angioedema, airway obstruction, and other adverse reactions. Monitor BP, renal function, and serum K^+ periodically.

Patient Counseling: Inform female patients of childbearing age of the consequences of exposure during pregnancy and of the treatment options for women planning to become pregnant. Advise to report pregnancies to physicians as soon as possible. Advise to d/c therapy and to report immediately any signs/symptoms of a severe allergic reaction or angioedema. Advise that lightheadedness may occur, especially during the 1st days of therapy; instruct to contact physician if lightheadedness occurs. Advise to d/c treatment until physician has been consulted if syncope occurs. Caution that inadequate fluid intake, excessive perspiration, diarrhea, or vomiting can lead to an excessive fall in BP. Advise not to use K^+ supplements or salt substitutes containing K^+ w/o consulting physician.

Storage: 25°C (77°F); excursions permitted to 15-30°C (59-86°F). Protect from moisture.

TEKTURNA HCT – aliskiren/hydrochlorothiazide RX

Class: Renin inhibitor/thiazide diuretic

D/C when pregnancy is detected. Drugs that act directly on the renin-angiotensin system can cause injury/death to the developing fetus.

ADULT DOSAGE

Hypertension

Usual: Dose qd

Add-On/Initial Therapy:
Patients whose BP is not adequately controlled w/ aliskiren alone or hydrochlorothiazide (HCTZ) alone may be switched to Tekturna HCT, patients whose BP is controlled w/ HCTZ alone but who experience hypokalemia may be switched to Tekturna HCT, or patients who experience dose-limiting adverse reactions on either component alone may be switched to Tekturna HCT containing a lower dose of that component in combination w/ the other. May be used as initial therapy in patients likely to need multiple drugs to achieve BP goals
Initial: 150mg/12.5mg qd prn to control BP
Titrate: May increase if BP remains uncontrolled after 2-4 weeks
Max: 300mg/25mg qd

Replacement Therapy:
May substitute for individually titrated components

PEDIATRIC DOSAGE

Pediatric use may not have been established

ADMINISTRATION

Oral route

Establish a routine pattern for taking drug w/ regard to meals; high-fat meals decrease absorption substantially

HOW SUPPLIED

Tab: (Aliskiren/HCTZ) 150mg/12.5mg, 150mg/25mg, 300mg/12.5mg, 300mg/25mg

CONTRAINDICATIONS

Coadministration w/ ARBs or ACE inhibitors in patients w/ diabetes. Anuria, sulfonamide-derived drug hypersensitivity.

WARNINGS/PRECAUTIONS

Not for initial therapy w/ intravascular volume depletion. Symptomatic hypotension may occur in patients w/ marked volume depletion or w/ salt depletion; correct volume/salt depletion prior to administration or begin therapy under close medical supervision. Renal function changes may occur, including acute renal failure; caution in patients whose renal function depend in part on the activity of the renin-angiotensin-aldosterone system (RAAS) (eg, renal artery stenosis, severe heart failure [HF], post-MI, or volume depletion). Consider withholding or discontinuing therapy if clinically significant decrease in renal function develops. May cause serum electrolyte abnormalities (eg, hyper/hypokalemia, hyponatremia, hypomagnesemia); correct hypokalemia and any coexisting hypomagnesemia prior to initiation. D/C if hypokalemia is accompanied by clinical signs (eg, muscular weakness, paresis, ECG alterations). Aliskiren: Hypersensitivity reactions (eg, anaphylactic reactions) and head/neck angioedema reported; d/c therapy immediately and do not readminister if anaphylactic reactions or angioedema develop. HCTZ: May cause hypersensitivity reactions, w/ or w/o bronchial asthma, and exacerbation or activation of systemic lupus erythematosus (SLE). May cause idiosyncratic reaction, resulting in acute transient myopia and acute angle-closure glaucoma; d/c as rapidly as possible. May alter glucose tolerance and increase serum cholesterol and TG levels. May cause or exacerbate hyperuricemia and precipitate gout in susceptible patients. May cause hypercalcemia. Minor alterations of fluid and electrolyte balance may precipitate hepatic coma in patients w/ hepatic impairment or progressive liver disease.

ADVERSE REACTIONS

Dizziness, influenza, diarrhea, cough, vertigo, asthenia, arthralgia.

DRUG INTERACTIONS

See Contraindications. Aliskiren: Cyclosporine or itraconazole may increase levels; avoid concomitant use. NSAIDs (eg, selective COX-2 inhibitors) may deteriorate renal function and may attenuate antihypertensive effect. Dual blockade of the RAAS is associated w/ increased risk of hypotension, hyperkalemia, and changes in renal function (including acute renal failure); in general, avoid combined use w/ ACE inhibitors or ARBS, particularly in patients w/ CrCl <60mL/min. Reduced furosemide exposure w/ concomitant use. May develop hyperkalemia w/ NSAIDs (eg, selective COX-2 inhibitors), K^+ supplements, or K^+-sparing diuretics. HCTZ: Dosage adjustment of antidiabetic drugs (oral agents and insulin) may be required. May increase risk of lithium toxicity; monitor serum lithium levels. Observe patients closely to determine if the desired effect of the diuretic is obtained when used concomitantly w/ NSAIDs and COX-2 selective agents. Administer ≥4 hrs before or 4-6 hrs after the administration of ion exchange resins (eg, cholestyramine, colestipol).

NURSING CONSIDERATIONS

Assessment: Assess for diabetes, anuria, sulfonamide-derived drug hypersensitivity, history of penicillin allergy, volume/salt depletion, renal artery stenosis, HF, post-MI status, SLE, hepatic/renal impairment, pregnancy/nursing status, and possible drug interactions. Correct electrolyte abnormalities (eg, hypokalemia, hypomagnesia) prior to initiating therapy.

Monitoring: Monitor for signs/symptoms of idiosyncratic reactions, hypersensitivity reactions, angioedema, airway obstruction, exacerbation/activation of SLE, hyperuricemia, precipitation of gout, and other adverse reactions. Monitor BP, renal function, serum electrolytes, cholesterol, and TG levels.

Patient Counseling: Inform female patients of childbearing age of the consequences of exposure during pregnancy and of the treatment options for women planning to become pregnant. Advise to report pregnancies to physicians as soon as possible. Inform that lightheadedness may occur, especially during the 1st days of therapy; instruct to contact physician if lightheadedness occurs. Advise to d/c treatment until physician has been consulted if syncope occurs. Caution that inadequate fluid intake, excessive perspiration, diarrhea, or vomiting can lead to an excessive fall in BP. Advise to d/c therapy and immediately report any signs/symptoms of a severe allergic reaction or angioedema. Advise not to use K^+ supplements or salt substitutes containing K^+ w/o consulting physician.

Storage: 25°C (77°F); excursions permitted to 15-30°C (59-86°F). Protect from moisture.

TENEX – guanfacine hydrochloride RX

Class: Alpha$_2$-agonist

ADULT DOSAGE

Hypertension

Initial: 1mg at hs

Titrate: If result is not satisfactory after 3-4 weeks, may increase dose to 2mg

Higher daily doses have been used, but adverse reactions increase significantly w/ doses >3mg/day

PEDIATRIC DOSAGE

Hypertension

≥12 Years:

Initial: 1mg at hs

Titrate: If result is not satisfactory after 3-4 weeks, may increase dose to 2mg

Higher daily doses have been used, but adverse reactions increase significantly w/ doses >3mg/day

DOSE MODIFICATION

Elderly

Start at lower end of dosing range

ADMINISTRATION

Oral route

HOW SUPPLIED

Tab: 1mg, 2mg

WARNINGS/PRECAUTIONS

Caution with severe coronary insufficiency, recent MI, cerebrovascular disease, or chronic renal or hepatic failure. May cause sedation or drowsiness, especially when beginning therapy. Abrupt cessation of therapy may be associated with increases in plasma and urinary catecholamines, symptoms of "nervousness/anxiety," and increases in BP to levels significantly greater than those prior to therapy. Caution in elderly.

ADVERSE REACTIONS

Dry mouth, somnolence, asthenia, dizziness, headache, impotence, constipation, fatigue, insomnia.

DRUG INTERACTIONS

Additive sedative effects with other centrally active depressants (eg, phenothiazines, barbiturates, benzodiazepines). Concomitant use with known microsomal enzyme inducers (eg, phenobarbital, phenytoin) in patients with renal impairment may decrease levels; more frequent dosing may be required to achieve/maintain hypotensive response; taper guanfacine dose upon discontinuation to avoid rebound phenomena.

NURSING CONSIDERATIONS

Assessment: Assess for previous hypersensitivity to the drug, recent MI, severe coronary insufficiency, cerebrovascular disease, chronic renal/hepatic failure, pregnancy/nursing status, and possible drug interactions.

Monitoring: Monitor for drowsiness, sedation, and other adverse reactions. Monitor BP, LFTs, and renal function.

Patient Counseling: Advise to exercise caution when operating dangerous machinery or driving motor vehicles. Inform that tolerance for alcohol and other CNS depressants may be diminished. Instruct not to d/c therapy abruptly.

Storage: 20-25°C (68-77°F).

TENORETIC – atenolol/chlorthalidone RX

Class: Monosulfamyl diuretic/selective $beta_1$-blocker

ADULT DOSAGE

Hypertension

Initial: 50mg-25mg tab qd

Titrate: May increase to 100mg-25mg tab qd, if optimal response not achieved

PEDIATRIC DOSAGE

Pediatric use may not have been established

DOSE MODIFICATION

Renal Impairment

CrCl 15-35mL/min:

Max: 50mg atenolol/day

CrCl <15mL/min:

Max: 50mg atenolol qod

Elderly

Start at lower end of dosing range

ADMINISTRATION

Oral route

HOW SUPPLIED

Tab: (Atenolol-Chlorthalidone) 50mg-25mg*, 100mg-25mg *scored

CONTRAINDICATIONS

Sinus bradycardia, >1st-degree heart block, cardiogenic shock, overt cardiac failure, anuria, hypersensitivity to sulfonamide-derived drugs.

WARNINGS/PRECAUTIONS

Not for initial therapy. Avoid with untreated pheochromocytoma. May aggravate peripheral arterial circulatory disorders. Caution in elderly. Atenolol: May cause/precipitate HF; d/c if cardiac failure continues despite adequate treatment. Caution in patients with impaired renal function. Avoid abrupt discontinuation; exacerbation of angina and MI reported. Avoid with bronchospastic disease, but may use with caution if unresponsive/intolerant of other antihypertensive treatment. Chronically administered therapy should not be routinely withdrawn prior to major surgery; however, may augment risks of general anesthesia and surgical procedures. Caution in diabetic patients; may mask tachycardia occurring with hypoglycemia. May mask clinical signs of hyperthyroidism and precipitate thyroid storm with abrupt discontinuation. May cause fetal harm. Chlorthalidone: May precipitate azotemia with renal disease. If progressive renal impairment becomes evident, d/c therapy. Caution with impaired hepatic function or progressive liver disease; may precipitate hepatic coma. D/C prior to parathyroid function test. Decreased Ca^{2+} excretion observed. Altered parathyroid glands, with hypercalcemia and hypophosphatemia, seen with prolonged therapy. Hyperuricemia may occur, or acute gout may be precipitated. Fluid/electrolyte imbalance may develop. Sensitivity reactions may occur. Exacerbation/activation of systemic lupus erythematous (SLE) reported. May enhance effects in postsympathectomy patients.

ADVERSE REACTIONS

Bradycardia, dizziness, fatigue, nausea.

DRUG INTERACTIONS

May potentiate other antihypertensive agents. Observe for hypotension and/or marked bradycardia with catecholamine-depleting drugs (eg, reserpine). Additive effects with calcium channel blockers. Atenolol: Bradycardia, heart block, and rise of left ventricular end diastolic pressure may occur with verapamil or diltiazem. May cause severe bradycardia, asystole, and HF with disopyramide. Additive effects with amiodarone. Prostaglandin synthase inhibitors (eg, indomethacin) may decrease hypotensive effects. Exacerbates rebound HTN with clonidine withdrawal. May be unresponsive to usual doses of epinephrine. Digitalis glycosides may slow AV conduction and increase risk of bradycardia. Chlorthalidone: May alter insulin requirements in diabetic patients; latent diabetes mellitus (DM) may manifest. May develop hypokalemia with concomitant corticosteroids or adrenocorticotropic hormone. May decrease arterial response to norepinephrine. May increase responsiveness to tubocurarine. Avoid with lithium; risk of lithium toxicity.

NURSING CONSIDERATIONS

Assessment: Assess for bradycardia, cardiogenic shock, >1st-degree heart block, overt cardiac failure, impaired renal/hepatic function, bronchospastic disease, peripheral vascular disease, DM, hyperthyroidism, pheochromocytoma, anuria, hypersensitivity to sulfonamide-derived drugs, serum electrolytes, parathyroid disease, pregnancy/nursing status, SLE, CAD, and possible drug interactions.

Monitoring: Monitor for cardiac failure, hepatic/renal function, withdrawal symptoms, hypersensitivity reactions, hyperuricemia or acute gout, and signs/symptoms of electrolyte imbalance. Monitor serum glucose, serum electrolytes, and BP.

Patient Counseling: Instruct not to interrupt or d/c therapy without consulting physician. Instruct to notify physician if signs/symptoms of impending congestive HF or unexplained respiratory symptoms develop. Counsel about signs/symptoms of electrolyte imbalance, and advise to seek prompt medical attention. Inform that drug may cause potential harm to fetus; instruct to inform physician if pregnant/planning to become pregnant.

Storage: 20-25°C (68-77°F).

TENORMIN — atenolol

RX

Class: Selective $beta_1$-blocker

Avoid abrupt discontinuation of therapy in patients with coronary artery disease (CAD). Severe exacerbation of angina and occurrence of MI and ventricular arrhythmias reported in angina patients following abrupt discontinuation of β-blockers. If plan to d/c therapy, carefully observe and advise to limit physical activity. Promptly reinstitute therapy, at least temporarily, if angina worsens or acute coronary insufficiency develops. CAD may be unrecognized; may be prudent to avoid abrupt discontinuation in patients only treated for HTN.

ADULT DOSAGE

Hypertension

Initial: 50mg qd, either alone or w/ diuretic therapy
Titrate: May increase to 100mg qd after 1-2 weeks
Max: 100mg qd

Angina Pectoris

Long-term Management:
Initial: 50mg qd
Titrate: May increase to 100mg qd after 1 week
Max: 200mg qd

Acute Myocardial Infarction

Management of Hemodynamically Stable Patients w/ Definite/Suspected Acute Myocardial Infarction to Reduce Cardiovascular Mortality:
Initial: 5mg IV over 5 min, repeat 10 min later; if tolerated, give 50mg PO 10 min after the last IV dose, followed by another 50mg PO 12 hrs later
Maint: 100mg qd or 50mg bid for 6-9 days or until discharge from the hospital

PEDIATRIC DOSAGE

Pediatric use may not have been established

DOSE MODIFICATION

Renal Impairment

HTN:
Initial: 25mg qd

HTN/Angina/AMI:
Max:
CrCl 15-35mL/min: 50mg/day
CrCl <15mL/min: 25mg/day

Hemodialysis:
25-50mg after each dialysis

Elderly
HTN:
Initial: 25mg qd

ADMINISTRATION

Oral route

HOW SUPPLIED

Tab: 25mg, 50mg*, 100mg *scored

CONTRAINDICATIONS

Sinus bradycardia, >1st-degree heart block, cardiogenic shock, overt cardiac failure.

WARNINGS/PRECAUTIONS

May cause/precipitate heart failure (HF); d/c if cardiac failure continues despite adequate treatment. Avoid with bronchospastic disease; may use with caution if unresponsive to/intolerant of other antihypertensive treatment. Chronically administered therapy should not be routinely withdrawn prior to major surgery; however, may augment risks of general anesthesia and surgical procedures. Caution in diabetic patients; may mask tachycardia occurring with hypoglycemia. May mask clinical signs of hyperthyroidism and may precipitate thyroid storm with abrupt discontinuation. Avoid with untreated pheochromocytoma. May cause fetal harm. May aggravate peripheral arterial circulatory disorders. Caution in elderly and those with renal impairment.

ADVERSE REACTIONS

Tiredness, dizziness, cold extremities, depression, fatigue, dyspnea, postural hypotension, bradycardia, leg pain, lightheadedness, lethargy, diarrhea, nausea, wheeziness.

DRUG INTERACTIONS

Additive effects with thiazide-type diuretics, catecholamine-depleting drugs (eg, reserpine), calcium channel blockers, and amiodarone. May cause severe bradycardia, asystole, and HF with disopyramide. Bradycardia and heart block can occur and left ventricular end diastolic pressure can rise with verapamil or diltiazem. Exacerbates rebound HTN with clonidine withdrawal. Prostaglandin synthase inhibitors (eg, indomethacin) may decrease hypotensive effects. May be unresponsive to usual doses of epinephrine. Concomitant use with digitalis glycosides may increase risk of bradycardia.

NURSING CONSIDERATIONS

Assessment: Assess for history of hypersensitivity, bradycardia, cardiogenic shock, >1st-degree heart block, overt cardiac failure, AMI, renal dysfunction, bronchospastic disease, conduction abnormalities, left ventricular dysfunction, peripheral arterial circulatory disorders, diabetes mellitus, hyperthyroidism, pheochromocytoma, pregnancy/nursing status, and for possible drug interactions.

Monitoring: Monitor for signs/symptoms of cardiac failure, and for masking of hyperthyroidism/hypoglycemia. Monitor renal function, pulse, and BP. Following abrupt discontinuation, monitor for thyroid storm and in patients with angina, monitor for severe exacerbation of angina, MI, and ventricular arrhythmias.

Patient Counseling: Instruct to take as prescribed. Advise not to interrupt or d/c therapy without first consulting physician. Counsel to notify physician if signs/symptoms of congestive HF or unexplained respiratory symptoms develop. Inform that drug may cause fetal harm; instruct to notify physician if pregnant or if considering becoming pregnant.

Storage: 20-25°C (68-77°F).

TERAZOSIN — terazosin hydrochloride

RX

Class: Alpha$_1$-blocker (quinazoline)

ADULT DOSAGE

Hypertension

Initial: 1mg hs
Usual: 1-5mg qd
If response is substantially diminished at 24 hrs, may slowly increase dose or use bid regimen
Max: 40mg/day

PEDIATRIC DOSAGE

Pediatric use may not have been established

If discontinued for several days or longer, restart using the initial dosing regimen

Benign Prostatic Hyperplasia

Initial: 1mg hs
Titrate: Increase stepwise to 2mg, 5mg, or 10mg qd
Max: 20mg/day

If discontinued for several days or longer, restart using the initial dosing regimen

ADMINISTRATION
Oral route

HOW SUPPLIED
Cap: 1mg, 2mg, 5mg, 10mg

WARNINGS/PRECAUTIONS
May cause marked lowering of BP, especially postural hypotension, and syncope with the 1st dose or 1st few days of therapy; similar effect may be anticipated if therapy is interrupted for several days and then restarted. May impair physical/mental abilities. Examine patients with BPH to rule out prostate cancer prior to initiation of therapy. Priapism reported. Intraoperative floppy iris syndrome observed during cataract surgery. Decreases in Hct, Hgb, WBCs, total protein, and albumin reported.

ADVERSE REACTIONS
Asthenia, postural hypotension, headache, dizziness, dyspnea, nasal congestion, somnolence, palpitations, nausea, peripheral edema, pain in extremities.

DRUG INTERACTIONS
Caution with other antihypertensive agents, especially verapamil; may need dose reduction or retitration of either agent. Increased levels with captopril. Hypotension reported with PDE-5 inhibitors.

NURSING CONSIDERATIONS

Assessment: Assess BP, pregnancy/nursing status, and possible drug interactions. Rule out prostate cancer with BPH.

Monitoring: Monitor for signs/symptoms of hypotension, priapism, and other adverse reactions. Monitor Hct, Hgb, WBCs, total protein/albumin, and BP periodically.

Patient Counseling: Inform of possibility of syncope and orthostatic symptoms, especially at initiation of therapy. Caution against driving or hazardous tasks for 12 hrs after 1st dose, dosage increase, or when resuming therapy after interruption. Avoid situations where injury could result, should syncope occur. Advise to sit or lie down when symptoms of low BP occur. Inform of possibility of priapism; advise to seek medical attention if this occurs and inform that priapism can lead to permanent erectile dysfunction if not brought to immediate medical attention.

Storage: 20-25°C (68-77°F).

TESTIM — testosterone CIII

Class: Androgen

Virilization reported in children secondarily exposed to testosterone gel. Children should avoid contact with unwashed or unclothed application sites in men using testosterone gel. Advise patients to strictly adhere to recommended instructions for use.

ADULT DOSAGE

Testosterone Replacement Therapy

Congenital/Acquired Primary Hypogonadism or Hypogonadotropic Hypogonadism in Males:

Initial: Apply 50mg (1 tube) qd
Measure am, predose serum testosterone levels approx 14 days after initiation of therapy
Titrate: May increase to 100mg (2 tubes) qd if serum testosterone levels are below normal range
Max: 100mg (2 tubes) qd

PEDIATRIC DOSAGE

Pediatric use may not have been established

ADMINISTRATION

Topical route

Apply qd at approx the same time (preferably in am) each day to clean, dry skin of the shoulders and/or upper arms; do not apply to scrotum, penis, or abdomen

Avoid swimming, showering, or washing the administration site for a minimum of 2 hrs after application

Refer to PI for further administration instructions

HOW SUPPLIED

Gel: 1% [5g, 30[s]]

CONTRAINDICATIONS

Breast carcinoma or known/suspected prostate carcinoma in men; women who are or may become pregnant, and women who are breastfeeding.

WARNINGS/PRECAUTIONS

Topical testosterone products may have different doses, strengths, or application instructions that may result in different systemic exposure. Application site and dose are not interchangeable with other topical testosterone products. Patients with BPH are at an increased risk for worsening of signs/symptoms of BPH. May increase risk for prostate cancer. Increases in Hct/RBC mass may increase risk for thromboembolic events; may require lowering of dose or discontinuation of therapy. Venous thromboembolic events (VTE) reported; d/c treatment and initiate appropriate workup and management if VTE is suspected. Suppression of spermatogenesis may occur with large doses. Prolonged use of high doses of orally active 17-α-alkyl androgens has been associated with serious hepatic effects; promptly d/c while cause is evaluated if signs/symptoms of hepatic dysfunction develop. Edema, with or without CHF in patients with preexisting cardiac, renal, or hepatic disease; may require diuretic therapy in addition to discontinuation of therapy. Gynecomastia may develop and persist. May potentiate sleep apnea. Changes in serum lipid profile may occur. Caution in cancer patients at risk of hypercalcemia and associated hypercalciuria. May decrease concentrations of thyroxine-binding globulins, resulting in decreased total T4 concentrations and increased resin uptake of T3 and T4. Flammable; avoid fire, flame, or smoking until the gel has dried.

ADVERSE REACTIONS

Application-site reactions.

DRUG INTERACTIONS

Changes in insulin sensitivity or glycemic control may occur; may decrease blood glucose and therefore, may necessitate a decrease in the dose of antidiabetic medications. Changes in anticoagulant activity may occur; frequently monitor INR and PT in patients taking warfarin, especially at initiation and termination of androgen therapy. Corticosteroids may increase fluid retention; carefully monitor, especially in patients with cardiac, renal, or hepatic disease.

NURSING CONSIDERATIONS

Assessment: Assess for breast carcinoma, prostate cancer, BPH, cardiac/renal/hepatic disease, risk factors for sleep apnea, and any other conditions where treatment is contraindicated or cautioned, and possible drug interactions. Obtain baseline Hct level, lipid levels, and serum testosterone level.

Monitoring: Monitor for worsening of BPH, prostate cancer, edema with or without CHF, sleep apnea, VTE, gynecomastia, and other adverse reactions. Monitor prostate specific antigen, serum lipid profile, and LFTs periodically. Monitor serum Ca^{2+} levels regularly in cancer patients at risk of hypercalcemia. Obtain Hct 3-6 months after starting therapy, then annually. Measure am, predose serum testosterone levels 14 days after initiation of therapy and periodically thereafter.

Patient Counseling: Inform that men with known or suspected prostate/breast cancer should not use this therapy. Advise to report signs and symptoms of hepatic dysfunction and secondary exposure in children and women to physician. Inform about possible adverse reactions. Inform that children and women should avoid contact with unwashed or unclothed application sites of men. Instruct to apply ud and to wash hands with soap and water immediately after application, cover application site with clothing after gel dries, and wash application site thoroughly with soap and water prior to direct skin-to-skin contact with others. Advise to read Medication Guide before therapy and reread each time the prescription is renewed. Inform that drug is flammable; instruct to avoid fire, flame, or smoking until the gel has dried. Advise not to share the medication with anyone. Advise about the importance of adhering to all the recommended monitoring, to report changes in state of health, and to wait 2 hrs before swimming or washing.

Storage: 20-25°C (68-77°F); excursions permitted to 15-30°C (59-86°F).

TETRACYCLINE – tetracycline hydrochloride

RX

Class: Tetracyclines

ADULT DOSAGE

General Dosing

Upper/lower respiratory tract, skin and soft tissue, and UTIs caused by susceptible microorganisms; psittacosis or ornithosis; granuloma inguinale; relapsing fever; bartonellosis; chancroid; tularemia; plague; cholera; infections caused by rickettsia, *Campylobacter fetus*, and other susceptible gram-negative organisms; adjunct therapy in intestinal amebiasis; and alternative treatment of the following infections caused by susceptible microorganisms when penicillin is contraindicated: yaws, Vincent's infection, anthrax, actinomycosis, and infections due to *Listeria monocytogenes* and *Clostridium* species

Usual: 500mg bid or 250mg qid; may require higher doses (eg, 500mg qid) for severe infections or for those infections not responsive to smaller doses

Continue for at least 24-48 hrs after symptoms and fever subside

Streptococcal Infections: Treat for at least 10 days

Brucellosis

500mg qid for 3 weeks, accompanied by 1g streptomycin IM bid for 1st week and qd the 2nd week

Syphilis

In Patients Allergic to Penicillin:

<1 Year Duration:
500mg qid for 15 days

>1 Year Duration (Except Neurosyphilis):
500mg qid for 30 days

Gonorrhea

Usual: 500mg qid for 7 days

Acne

Moderate to Severe:

Initial: 1g/day in divided doses

Maint: Reduce dose to 125-500mg/day when improvement is noted

May be possible to maintain adequate remission of lesions w/ alternate day or intermittent therapy

***Chlamydia trachomatis* Infections**

Uncomplicated Urethral, Endocervical, or Rectal Infections:
500mg qid for at least 7 days

PEDIATRIC DOSAGE

General Dosing

>8 Years:

Usual: 25-50mg/kg/day divided in 4 equal doses

Continue for at least 24-48 hrs after symptoms and fever subside

Streptococcal Infections: Treat for at least 10 days

DOSE MODIFICATION

Renal Impairment

Decrease total dosage by reduction of recommended individual doses and/or by extending time intervals between doses

ADMINISTRATION

Oral route

Take caps w/ adequate amount of fluids; avoid taking w/ food and some dairy products as it may interfere w/ absorption

HOW SUPPLIED

Cap: 250mg, 500mg

WARNINGS/PRECAUTIONS

May cause permanent teeth discoloration during tooth development (last half of pregnancy, infancy and childhood to 8 yrs of age); avoid use in this age group unless other drugs are not likely to be effective or are contraindicated. Enamel hypoplasia reported. May cause fetal harm. Decrease in fibula growth rate in premature infants reported. May lead to excessive systemic accumulation and possible liver toxicity if renal impairment exists; lower than usual doses are indicated, and if therapy is prolonged, determine serum levels. Photosensitivity reported; d/c at first evidence of skin erythema. May increase BUN levels. Higher serum drug levels may lead to azotemia, hyperphosphatemia, and acidosis in patients with renal impairment. May result in bacterial resistance with prolonged use in the absence of proven/strongly suspected bacterial infection or a prophylactic indication; d/c and take appropriate measures if superinfection develops. Bulging fontanels in infants and benign intracranial HTN in adults reported.

ADVERSE REACTIONS

Anorexia, N/V, epigastric distress, diarrhea, maculopapular/erythematous rashes, urticaria, angioneurotic edema, hemolytic anemia, thrombocytopenia.

DRUG INTERACTIONS

May interfere with bactericidal action of PCN; do not coadminister. May depress plasma prothrombin activity; may require downward adjustment of anticoagulant dose. Fatal renal toxicity reported with concurrent methoxyflurane. Antacids containing aluminum, Ca^{2+}, or Mg^{2+}, and preparations containing iron, zinc, or sodium bicarbonate may impair absorption. Food and dairy products may interfere with absorption. May render oral contraceptives less effective.

NURSING CONSIDERATIONS

Assessment: Assess for hypersensitivity to any tetracyclines, renal impairment, pregnancy/nursing status, and possible drug interactions. Perform culture and susceptibility tests. In venereal diseases, when coexistent syphilis is suspected, perform dark-field examinations and blood serology.

Monitoring: Monitor for hypersensitivity reactions, photosensitivity, superinfection, liver toxicity, intracranial HTN, and other adverse reactions. Perform periodic lab evaluations of organ systems, including hematopoietic, renal, and hepatic studies in long-term therapy. In venereal disease when coexistent syphilis is suspected, repeat blood serology monthly for at least 4 months.

Patient Counseling: Inform about potential risks/benefits of therapy. Apprise of the potential hazard to fetus if used during pregnancy; instruct to notify if pregnant. Advise to avoid direct sunlight and d/c if skin erythema occurs. Inform that drug only treats bacterial, not viral, infections. Instruct to take exactly ud; inform that skipping doses or not completing full course of therapy may decrease effectiveness and increase the likelihood of bacterial resistance.

Storage: 20-25°C (68-77°F).

TEVETEN – eprosartan mesylate RX

Class: Angiotensin II receptor antagonist

D/C when pregnancy is detected. Drugs that act directly on the renin-angiotensin system (RAS) can cause injury/death to the developing fetus.

ADULT DOSAGE

Hypertension

Initial: 600mg qd
Usual: 400-800mg/day, given qd or bid
Max: 800mg/day
Twice-a-day regimen at the same total daily dose or an increase in dose may give a more satisfactory response

PEDIATRIC DOSAGE

Pediatric use may not have been established

DOSE MODIFICATION

Renal Impairment
Moderate and Severe:
Max: 600mg/day

ADMINISTRATION

Oral route

Take with or without food

HOW SUPPLIED

Tab: 400mg, 600mg

CONTRAINDICATIONS
Coadministration with aliskiren in patients with diabetes.

WARNINGS/PRECAUTIONS
Symptomatic hypotension may occur in patients with an activated RAS (eg, volume- and/or salt-depleted patients [eg, those being treated with diuretics]); correct volume or salt depletion prior to therapy or monitor closely. Changes in renal function reported. Oliguria and/or progressive azotemia and (rarely) acute renal failure and/or death may occur in patients whose renal function may depend on the renin-angiotensin-aldosterone system activity (eg, severe congestive heart failure [CHF]). Increases in SrCr or BUN reported in patients with renal artery stenosis.

ADVERSE REACTIONS
Upper respiratory tract infection, rhinitis, pharyngitis, cough.

DRUG INTERACTIONS
See Contraindications. Dual blockade of the RAS is associated with increased risks of hypotension, hyperkalemia, and changes in renal function (including acute renal failure); avoid combined use of RAS inhibitors, or closely monitor BP, renal function, and electrolytes with concomitant agents that also affect the RAS. Avoid with aliskiren in patients with renal impairment (GFR <60mL/min). NSAIDs, including selective COX-2 inhibitors, may attenuate antihypertensive effect and may deteriorate renal function. Increases in serum lithium concentrations and lithium toxicity may occur; monitor lithium levels.

NURSING CONSIDERATIONS

Assessment: Assess for hypersensitivity to the drug, volume/salt depletion, renal impairment, CHF, renal artery stenosis, diabetes, pregnancy/nursing status, and possible drug interactions.

Monitoring: Monitor for signs/symptoms of hypotension, renal dysfunction, and other adverse reactions.

Patient Counseling: Inform about the consequences of exposure during pregnancy in females of childbearing age. Discuss treatment options with women planning to become pregnant. Instruct to report pregnancies to physician as soon as possible.

Storage: 20-25°C (68-77°F).

TEVETEN HCT – eprosartan mesylate/hydrochlorothiazide RX

Class: Angiotensin II receptor antagonist/thiazide diuretic

D/C when pregnancy is detected. Drugs that act directly on the renin-angiotensin system (RAS) can cause injury/death to the developing fetus.

ADULT DOSAGE

Hypertension

Replacement Therapy:
May be substituted for individual components

Usual (Not Volume-Depleted): 600mg-12.5mg qd
Titrate: May increase to 600mg-25mg qd
Max: 600mg-25mg qd

If additional BP control required, or to maintain a bid dosing schedule of monotherapy, 300mg eprosartan may be added as pm dose

PEDIATRIC DOSAGE
Pediatric use may not have been established

DOSE MODIFICATION
Renal Impairment
Moderate and Severe:
Max Eprosartan: 600mg/day

ADMINISTRATION
Oral route
Take with or without food

HOW SUPPLIED
Tab: (Eprosartan-HCTZ) 600mg-12.5mg, 600mg-25mg

CONTRAINDICATIONS
Anuria, sulfonamide-derived drug hypersensitivity. Coadministration with aliskiren in patients with diabetes.

WARNINGS/PRECAUTIONS

Not indicated for initial therapy. Symptomatic hypotension may occur in patients with an activated RAS (eg, volume- and/or salt-depleted patients [eg, those being treated with diuretics]); correct volume or salt depletion prior to therapy or monitor closely. Changes in renal function reported. Oliguria and/or progressive azotemia and (rare) acute renal failure and/or death may occur in patients whose renal function may depend on the renin-angiotensin-aldosterone system activity (eg, severe congestive heart failure [CHF]). Increases in SrCr or BUN reported in patients with renal artery stenosis. Consider withholding or discontinuing therapy if progressive renal impairment becomes evident. HCTZ: Caution with severe renal disease; may precipitate azotemia. Caution with hepatic impairment or progressive liver disease; may precipitate hepatic coma. May cause hypersensitivity reactions (with or without a history of allergy or bronchial asthma), exacerbation or activation of systemic lupus erythematosus (SLE), hyperuricemia or precipitation of frank gout, hypomagnesemia, hypercalcemia, hyperglycemia, and manifestations of latent diabetes mellitus (DM). May cause idiosyncratic reaction, resulting in acute transient myopia and acute angle-closure glaucoma; d/c as rapidly as possible. D/C before testing for parathyroid function. Enhanced effects in postsympathectomy patients. Observe for signs of fluid/electrolyte imbalance (eg, hyponatremia, hypochloremic alkalosis, hypokalemia). Hypokalemia may sensitize/exaggerate the response of the heart to toxic effects of digitalis.

ADVERSE REACTIONS

Dizziness, headache.

DRUG INTERACTIONS

See Contraindications. Dual blockade of the RAS is associated with increased risks of hypotension, hyperkalemia, and changes in renal function (including acute renal failure); avoid combined use of RAS inhibitors, or closely monitor BP, renal function, and electrolytes with concomitant agents that also affect the RAS. Avoid with aliskiren in patients with renal impairment (GFR <60mL/min). NSAIDs, including selective COX-2 inhibitors, may decrease effects of diuretics and angiotensin II receptor antagonists and may deteriorate renal function. Increases in serum lithium concentrations and lithium toxicity reported; monitor lithium levels. Eprosartan: K^+-sparing diuretics (eg, spironolactone, triamterene, amiloride), K^+ supplements, or K^+-containing salt substitutes may increase serum K^+. HCTZ: Potentiation of orthostatic hypotension may occur with alcohol, barbiturates, or narcotics. Dose adjustment of antidiabetic drugs (oral agents and insulin) may be required. Additive effect or potentiation with other antihypertensives. Anionic exchange resins (eg, cholestyramine, colestipol) may impair absorption. Corticosteroids and adrenocorticotropic hormone may intensify electrolyte depletion, particularly hypokalemia. May decrease response to pressor amines (eg, norepinephrine). May increase responsiveness to nondepolarizing skeletal muscle relaxants (eg, tubocurarine).

NURSING CONSIDERATIONS

Assessment: Assess for hypersensitivity to the drug or sulfonamide-derived drugs, anuria, volume/salt depletion, CHF, renal artery stenosis, SLE, DM, postsympathectomy status, renal/hepatic impairment, pregnancy/nursing status, and possible drug interactions.

Monitoring: Monitor for signs/symptoms of hypotension, renal/hepatic impairment, hypersensitivity reactions, exacerbation/activation of SLE, hyperuricemia, precipitation of gout, fluid/electrolyte imbalance, latent DM, idiosyncratic reaction, and other adverse reactions. Monitor BP and serum electrolytes periodically.

Patient Counseling: Inform about the consequences of exposure during pregnancy in females of childbearing age. Discuss treatment options with women planning to become pregnant. Instruct to report pregnancies to physician as soon as possible. Caution that lightheadedness may occur, especially during the 1st days of therapy; instruct to report to physician. Instruct to d/c therapy and consult physician if syncope occurs. Caution that inadequate fluid intake, excessive perspiration, diarrhea, or vomiting may lead to an excessive fall in BP, with the same consequences of lightheadedness and possible syncope. Instruct not to use K^+ supplements or salt substitutes containing K^+ without consulting physician.

Storage: 20-25°C (68-77°F).

THYROLAR – liotrix (T3;T4) RX

Class: Thyroid replacement hormone

ADULT DOSAGE

Hypothyroidism

Replacement/supplemental therapy in hypothyroidism of any etiology, except transient hypothyroidism during the recovery phase of subacute thyroiditis

PEDIATRIC DOSAGE

Hypothyroidism

0-6 Months of Age: 3.1mcg/12.5mcg to 6.25mcg/25mcg qd

6-12 Months of Age: 6.25mcg/25mcg to 9.35mcg/37.5mcg qd

Initial: 6.25mcg/25mcg qd or 3.1mcg/12.5mcg qd (in long-standing myxedema, particularly if cardiovascular impairment suspected)
Titrate: Readjust dose w/in the first 4 weeks; increase by 3.1mcg/12.5mcg every 2-3 weeks
Maint: 12.5mcg/50mcg/day to 25mcg/100mcg/day
Failure to respond to 37.5mcg/150mcg dose suggests lack of compliance or malabsorption

Pituitary TSH Suppressant

Treatment or prevention of various types of euthyroid goiters including thyroid nodules, subacute or chronic lymphocytic thyroiditis (Hashimoto's), multinodular goiter, and to manage thyroid cancer

Thyroid Cancer: Give higher doses than those used for replacement therapy

Thyroid Suppression Therapy: 1.56mg/kg/day T4 for 7-10 days

1-5 Years: 9.35mcg/37.5mcg to 12.5mcg/50mcg qd
6-12 Years: 12.5mcg/50mcg to 18.75mcg/75mcg qd
>12 Years: >18.75mcg/75mcg qd

DOSE MODIFICATION

Elderly
Initial: 3.1mcg/12.5mcg to 6.25mcg/25mcg
Adverse Reactions
Hypothyroidism:
Angina: Reduce dose to 3.1mcg/12.5mcg to 6.25mcg/25mcg

ADMINISTRATION

Oral route

HOW SUPPLIED

Tab: (Liothyronine/Levothyroxine) 3.1mcg/12.5mcg, 6.25mcg/25mcg, 12.5mcg/50mcg, 25mcg/100mcg, 37.5mcg/150mcg

CONTRAINDICATIONS

Uncorrected adrenal cortical insufficiency, untreated thyrotoxicosis.

WARNINGS/PRECAUTIONS

Not for treatment of obesity; larger doses in euthyroid patients can cause serious or even life-threatening toxicity. Not for the treatment of male or female infertility unless accompanied by hypothyroidism. Caution with CV disorders (eg, angina pectoris) and in elderly with risk of occult cardiac disease; initiate at low doses and reduce dose if aggravation of CV disease suspected. May aggravate diabetes mellitus (DM), diabetes insipidus (DI), or adrenal cortical insufficiency. Treatment of myxedema coma requires simultaneous administration of glucocorticoids. Excessive doses in infants may cause craniosynostosis. Caution with strong suspicion of thyroid gland autonomy. Androgens, corticosteroids, estrogens, iodine-containing preparations, and salicylates may interfere with laboratory tests.

ADVERSE REACTIONS

Fatigue, sluggishness, weight increase, alopecia, palpitations, dry skin, urticaria, headache, hyperhidrosis, pruritus, asthenia, BP increase, arthralgia, myalgia, tremor.

DRUG INTERACTIONS

Large doses in euthyroid patients may cause serious or even life-threatening toxicity, particularly with sympathomimetic amines. Closely monitor PT in patients on oral anticoagulants; dose reduction of anticoagulant may be required. May increase insulin or oral hypoglycemic requirements. Potentially impaired absorption with cholestyramine and colestipol; space dosing by 4-5 hrs. Estrogens may increase thyroxine-binding globulin and may decrease free T4; increase in thyroid dose may be needed.

NURSING CONSIDERATIONS

Assessment: Assess for adrenal cortical insufficiency, untreated thyrotoxicosis, apparent hypersensitivity to the drug, CV disorders (coronary artery disease, angina pectoris), DM/DI, myxedema coma, pregnancy/nursing status, and possible drug interactions.

Monitoring: Monitor response to treatment, urinary glucose levels in patients with DM, aggravation of CV disease, and other adverse reactions. Monitor thyroid function periodically. Closely monitor PT in patients on oral anticoagulants.

Patient Counseling: Inform that replacement therapy is taken essentially for life, except in transient hypothyroidism. Instruct to immediately report to physician any signs/symptoms of thyroid hormone toxicity (eg, chest pain, increased pulse rate, palpitations, excessive sweating, heat intolerance, nervousness). Inform the importance of frequent/close monitoring of PT and urinary glucose and the need for dose adjustment of antidiabetic and/or oral anticoagulant medication. Inform that partial loss of hair may be seen in children in 1st few months of therapy. Inform that drug is not for treatment of obesity or weight loss.

Storage: 2-8°C (36-46°F). Protect from light.

TIAZAC – diltiazem hydrochloride RX

Class: Calcium channel blocker (nondihydropyridine)

OTHER BRAND NAMES
Taztia XT

ADULT DOSAGE

Hypertension

Initial (Monotherapy): 120-240mg qd
Titrate: Max effect usually observed by 14 days of therapy; schedule dose adjustments accordingly
Usual Range: 120-540mg qd
Max: 540mg qd

Angina

Chronic Stable:
Initial: 120-180mg qd
Titration should be carried out over 7-14 days, when necessary
Max: 540mg qd

Conversions

Hypertensive/Anginal Patients Treated w/ Other Diltiazem Formulations:
May be switched to therapy at the nearest equivalent total daily dose

PEDIATRIC DOSAGE
Pediatric use may not have been established

DOSE MODIFICATION
Elderly
Start at lower end of dosing range

ADMINISTRATION
Oral route
May sprinkle cap contents on a spoonful of applesauce
Swallow applesauce immediately w/o chewing and follow w/ a glass of cool water; do not store for future use
Subdividing contents of cap is not recommended

HOW SUPPLIED
Cap, Extended-Release: 120mg, 180mg, 240mg, 300mg, 360mg, 420mg; (Taztia XT) 120mg, 180mg, 240mg, 300mg, 360mg

CONTRAINDICATIONS
Sick sinus syndrome and 2nd- or 3rd-degree atrioventricular (AV) block (except with a functioning ventricular pacemaker), severe hypotension (<90mmHg systolic), acute myocardial infarction (AMI) and pulmonary congestion documented by x-ray on admission.

WARNINGS/PRECAUTIONS
Prolongs AV node refractory periods without significantly prolonging sinus node recovery time, except in patients with sick sinus syndrome. Periods of asystole reported in a patient with Prinzmetal's angina. Worsening of congestive heart failure (CHF) reported in patients with preexisting ventricular dysfunction. Symptomatic hypotension may occur. Mild elevations of transaminases with and without concomitant alkaline phosphatase and bilirubin elevation reported. Significant elevations in enzymes (eg, alkaline phosphatase, LDH, AST, ALT) and other phenomena consistent with acute hepatic injury reported in rare instances. Monitor LFTs and renal function at regular intervals; caution with renal/hepatic dysfunction. Transient dermatological reactions and skin eruptions progressing to erythema multiforme and/or exfoliative dermatitis have been reported; d/c if a dermatologic reaction persists. Caution in elderly.

ADVERSE REACTIONS
Peripheral edema, dizziness, headache, infection, pain, pharyngitis, dyspepsia, dyspnea, bronchitis, AV block, asthenia, vasodilation.

DRUG INTERACTIONS

Potential additive effects with other agents known to affect cardiac contractility and/or conduction; caution and careful titration are warranted. Additive effects in prolonging cardiac conduction with β-blockers or digitalis. CYP3A4 substrates, inhibitors, or inducers may have a significant impact on the efficacy and side effect profile of diltiazem; patients taking CYP3A4 substrates, especially patients with renal and/or hepatic impairment, may require dosage adjustment when starting or stopping concomitantly administered diltiazem. May potentiate depression of cardiac contractility, conductivity and automaticity, and vascular dilation associated with anesthetics; carefully titrate anesthetics and calcium channel blockers (CCBs) when used concomitantly. May increase levels of midazolam, triazolam, carbamazepine, quinidine, and lovastatin. May increase levels of propranolol; adjustment of the propranolol dose may be warranted. May increase levels of buspirone; dose adjustments may be necessary. Increased levels with cimetidine; adjustment of diltiazem dose may be warranted. Sinus bradycardia resulting in hospitalization and pacemaker insertion reported with clonidine; monitor HR. Monitor cyclosporine/digoxin concentrations, especially when diltiazem therapy is initiated, adjusted, or discontinued. Rifampin may decrease concentrations; avoid rifampin or any CYP3A4 inducer when possible, and consider alternative therapy. May increase simvastatin exposure; limit daily doses of simvastatin to 10mg and diltiazem to 240mg if coadministration is required. Risk of myopathy and rhabdomyolysis with statins metabolized by CYP3A4 may be increased. When possible, use a non-CYP3A4-metabolized statin; otherwise, consider dose adjustments for both agents and closely monitor for signs and symptoms of any statin-related adverse events. Additive antihypertensive effect when used with other antihypertensive agents; dosage of diltiazem or the concomitant antihypertensive may need to be adjusted.

NURSING CONSIDERATIONS

Assessment: Assess for sick sinus syndrome, 2nd- or 3rd-degree AV block, hypotension, AMI, pulmonary congestion, ventricular/renal/hepatic dysfunction, drug hypersensitivity, pregnancy/nursing status, and possible drug interactions.

Monitoring: Monitor for bradycardia, AV block, worsening of CHF, symptomatic hypotension, dermatological reactions, and other adverse reactions. Monitor LFTs and renal function at regular intervals. Monitor HR with clonidine.

Patient Counseling: Inform of risks and benefits of therapy. Instruct to take ud. Counsel to report any adverse reactions to physician. Inform that when administering with applesauce, it should not be hot and it should be soft enough to be swallowed without chewing.

Storage: 25°C (77°F); excursions permitted to 15-30°C (59-86°F). Avoid excessive humidity. (Taztia XT) 20-25°C (68-77°F). Avoid excessive humidity.

TIKOSYN – dofetilide

RX

Class: Class III antiarrhythmic

To minimize risk of induced arrhythmia, for a minimum of 3 days, place patients initiated or reinitiated on therapy in a facility that can provide calculations of CrCl, continuous ECG monitoring, and cardiac resuscitation. Available only to hospitals and prescribers who have received appropriate dofetilide dosing and treatment initiation education.

ADULT DOSAGE

Atrial Fibrillation

Conversion of A-Fib/A-Flutter to Normal Sinus Rhythm and Maint of Normal Sinus Rhythm in Patients w/ Highly Symptomatic A-fib/A-flutter of >1 Week Duration Who Were Converted to Normal Sinus Rhythm:

Reserve for patients in whom A-fib/A-flutter is highly symptomatic

Hypokalemia should be corrected before initiation; maintain serum potassium levels >3.6-4.0mEq/L

Initial:

Individualize dose based on CrCl and QTc (use QT interval if HR <60bpm); QTc must be ≤440 msec to proceed

CrCl >60mL/min: 500mcg bid

CrCl 40-60mL/min: 250mcg bid

CrCl 20-<40mL/min: 125mcg bid

CrCl <20mL/min: Contraindicated

PEDIATRIC DOSAGE

Pediatric use may not have been established

Post Dose Adjustment:
After 2-3 hrs if the QTc has increased ≤15%, continue current dose; if QTc has increased>15% compared to the baseline or if the QTc is >500 msec (550 msec w/ ventricular conduction abnormalities), adjust subsequent doses as such:
Initial Dose of 500mcg bid: Reduce dose to 250mcg bid
Initial Dose of 250mcg bid: reduce dose to 125mcg bid
Initial Dose of 125mcg bid: reduce dose to 125mcg qd

Maint:
If at any time after the 2nd dose the QTc increases >500msec (550msec in patients w/ ventricular conduction abnormalities), d/c dofetilide
If renal function deteriorates, adjust dose based on CrCl as seen above

Max:
CrCl >60mL/min: 500mcg bid

Cardioversion:
If patients do not convert to normal sinus rhythm w/in 24 hrs of initiation, electrical conversion should be considered. Patients continuing on dofetilide after successful electrical cardioversion should continue to be monitored by electrocardiography for 12 hrs post cardioversion, or a minimum of 3 days after initiation of dofetilide therapy, whichever is greater

Conversions

Switching from Class I or Other Class III Antiarrhythmics:
Withdraw previous antiarrhythmic therapy under careful monitoring for a minimum of 3 plasma half-lives before initiating therapy; do not initiate dofetilide following amiodarone therapy until amiodarone plasma levels are <0.3mcg/mL or until withdrawn for at least 3 months

DOSE MODIFICATION

Discontinuation

If dofetilide needs to be discontinued to allow dosing of other potentially interacting drugs, a washout period of ≥2 days should be followed before starting the other drug.

ADMINISTRATION

Oral route

Take PO w/ or w/o food
Initiate/titrate in presence of continuous ECG monitoring and personnel trained in management of serious ventricular arrhythmias

HOW SUPPLIED

Cap: 125mcg, 250mcg, 500mcg

CONTRAINDICATIONS

Congenital or acquired long QT syndromes, baseline QT interval or QTc >440 msec (500 msec with ventricular conduction abnormalities), severe renal impairment (CrCl <20mL/min). Concomitant verapamil, HCTZ (alone/in combinations [eg, triamterene]), and inhibitors of renal cation transport system (eg, cimetidine, trimethoprim [alone/combination with sulfamethoxazole], ketoconazole, prochlorperazine, dolutegravir, megestrol).

WARNINGS/PRECAUTIONS

May cause serious ventricular arrhythmias, primarily torsades de pointes (TdP); risk of TdP can be reduced by controlling the plasma concentration through adjustment of the initial dofetilide dose according to CrCl and by monitoring the ECG. Calculate CrCl before 1st dose. Caution in patients with severe hepatic impairment. Do not discharge patients within 12 hrs of conversion to normal sinus rhythm. Maintain normal K^+ levels prior to and during administration. Patients with A-fib should be anticoagulated prior to cardioversion and may continue to use after cardioversion. Rehospitalize patient for 3 days anytime dose is increased. Consider electrical cardioversion if patient does not convert to normal sinus rhythm within 24 hrs of initiation of therapy. If dofetilide needs to be discontinued to allow dosing of other potentially interacting drug(s), a washout period of at least 2 days should be followed before starting the other drug(s). Caution in elderly.

ADVERSE REACTIONS

Headache, chest pain, dizziness, ventricular arrhythmia, ventricular tachycardia, TdP, respiratory tract infection, dyspnea, nausea, flu syndrome, insomnia, back pain, diarrhea, rash, abdominal pain.

DRUG INTERACTIONS

See Contraindications. Hypokalemia or hypomagnesemia may occur with K^+-depleting diuretics, increasing the potential for TdP. CYP3A4 inhibitors (eg, macrolides, protease inhibitors, serotonin reuptake inhibitors) and drugs actively secreted by cationic secretion (eg, triamterene, metformin, amiloride) may increase levels; caution when coadministered. Not recommended with drugs that prolong the QT interval (eg, phenothiazines, TCAs, certain oral macrolides). Withhold Class I and III antiarrhythmics for at least 3 half-lives prior to dosing with dofetilide. Do not initiate therapy until amiodarone levels are <0.3mcg/mL or until amiodarone has been withdrawn for at least 3 months. Higher occurrence of TdP with digoxin.

NURSING CONSIDERATIONS

Assessment: Assess for previous hypersensitivity to drug, congenital or acquired long QT syndrome, renal/hepatic impairment, pregnancy/nursing status, and possible drug interactions. Correct K^+ levels prior to therapy. Obtain baseline ECG and CrCl prior to therapy.

Monitoring: Monitor serum K^+ levels and for development of ventricular arrhythmias (eg, TdP). After initiation or cardioversion, continuously monitor by ECG for a minimum of 3 days, or for a minimum of 12 hrs after electrical/pharmacological conversion to normal sinus rhythm, whichever is greater. Reevaluate renal function and QTc every 3 months, as medically warranted.

Patient Counseling: Inform about risks/benefits, need for compliance with prescribed dosing, potential drug interactions, and the need for periodic monitoring of QTc and renal function. Instruct to notify physician of any changes in medications and supplements or if hospitalized or prescribed a new medication for any condition. Counsel to report immediately any symptoms associated with electrolyte imbalance (eg, excessive/prolonged diarrhea, sweating, vomiting, loss of appetite, thirst). Instruct not to double the next dose if a dose is missed and take the next dose at the usual time.

Storage: 15-30°C (59-86°F). Protect from humidity and moisture.

TIMENTIN — clavulanate potassium/ticarcillin disodium RX

Class: Beta-lactamase inhibitor/broad-spectrum penicillin

ADULT DOSAGE

Systemic Infections

Lower respiratory, bone and joint, skin and skin structure infections; septicemia (including bacteremia); endometritis; and peritonitis

Usual: 3.1g (3g ticarcillin, 100mg clavulanate) IV q4-6h

Urinary Tract Infections

Usual: 3.1g (3g ticarcillin, 100mg clavulanate) IV q4-6h

Gynecologic Infections

Based on ticarcillin content

Moderate Infections: 200mg/kg/day in divided doses q6h

Severe Infections: 300mg/kg/day in divided doses q4h

Treatment Duration

10 to 14 days; more prolonged therapy may be required in difficult and complicated infections

PEDIATRIC DOSAGE

General Dosing

≥3 Months:

<60kg:

Based on ticarcillin content

Mild to Moderate Infections: 200mg/kg/day IV in divided doses q6h

Severe Infections: 300mg/kg/day IV in divided doses q4h

≥60kg:

Mild to Moderate Infections: 3.1g (3g ticarcillin, 100mg clavulanate) IV q6h

Severe Infections: 3.1g IV q4h

DOSE MODIFICATION

Renal Impairment

Initial LD: 3.1g followed by doses based on CrCl and type of dialysis

Maint (Based on Ticarcillin Content):

CrCl >60mL/min: 3g IV q4h

CrCl 30-60mL/min: 2g IV q4h

CrCl 10-30mL/min: 2g IV q8h

CrCl <10mL/min: 2g IV q12h

CrCl <10mL/min w/ Hepatic Dysfunction: 2g IV q24h

Peritoneal Dialysis: 3g IV q12h

Hemodialysis: 2g IV q12h, supplemented w/ 3g after each dialysis

Other Important Modifications

Adults <60kg:

200-300mg/kg/day in divided doses q4-6h

ADMINISTRATION

IV route

Administer by IV infusion over a 30-min period

May administer by direct infusion or through Y-type infusion set; advisable to temporarily d/c administration of any other sol during infusion

When given w/ another antimicrobial (eg, aminoglycoside), administer each drug separately

Do not use plastic containers in series connections

Reconstitution and Dilution

3.1g Glass Vials:

Add approx 13mL of sterile water for inj (SWFI) or NaCl inj for a concentration of 200mg/mL ticarcillin and 6.7mg/mL clavulanic acid

Further dilute to desired volume using recommended sol to a concentration between 10-100mg/mL

Pharmacy Bulk Package:

Add 76mL of SWFI or NaCl inj to 31g bulk package for a concentration of 300mg/mL ticarcillin and 10mg/mL clavulanic acid; may add diluent in 2 portions for ease of reconstitution

Reconstituted contents should be withdrawn immediately; if this is not possible, aliquoting operations must be completed w/in 4 hrs of reconstitution

Withdraw desired dose from stock sol and further dilute to a concentration between 10-100mg/mL

Compatible Diluents

3.1g Glass Vials: D5 inj, NaCl inj, lactated Ringer's inj

Pharmacy Bulk Package: D5 inj, NaCl inj, lactated Ringer's inj, SWFI

Refer to PI for further administration and directions for use

HOW SUPPLIED

Inj: (Ticarcillin/Clavulanate) 3g/100mg [vial], (3g/100mg)/100mL [Galaxy]. Also available as a Pharmacy Bulk Package.

WARNINGS/PRECAUTIONS

Serious and occasionally fatal hypersensitivity (anaphylactic) reactions reported; d/c and institute appropriate therapy if an allergic reaction occurs. *Clostridium difficile*-associated diarrhea (CDAD) reported; d/c if CDAD is suspected or confirmed. May cause convulsions when the recommended dose is exceeded, especially in the presence of renal impairment. Bleeding associated with abnormalities in coagulation tests may occur, especially in patients with renal impairment; d/c and institute appropriate therapy if bleeding manifestations appear. May result in bacterial resistance if used in the absence of proven or suspected bacterial infection; take appropriate measures if superinfection develops. Lab test interactions may occur. Hypokalemia reported. Consider the Na^+ content of the drug (4.51mEq/g) in patients requiring restricted salt intake. Caution in elderly.

ADVERSE REACTIONS

Elevated eosinophils/AST/ALT, rash, nausea, diarrhea, phlebitis at inj site.

DRUG INTERACTIONS

Probenecid may increase serum concentrations and prolong $T_{1/2}$ of ticarcillin. May reduce efficacy of combined oral estrogen/progesterone contraceptives.

NURSING CONSIDERATIONS

Assessment: Assess for previous hypersensitivity reactions to the drug, other β-lactam antibacterials (eg, PCNs, cephalosporins), or other allergens; renal/hepatic impairment; fluid/electrolyte imbalance; restricted salt intake; pregnancy/nursing status; and possible drug interactions.

Monitoring: Monitor for signs/symptoms of anaphylactic/allergic reactions, CDAD, convulsions, bleeding, superinfection, and other adverse reactions. Monitor serum K^+ in patients with fluid and electrolyte imbalance and in patients receiving prolonged therapy.

Patient Counseling: Inform that drug should only be used to treat bacterial, not viral, infections. Instruct to take exactly ud, even if patient feels better early in the course of therapy. Inform that skipping doses or not completing the full course of therapy may decrease effectiveness of immediate treatment and increase bacterial resistance. Inform that diarrhea is a common problem caused by therapy, which usually ends when therapy is discontinued. Instruct to immediately contact physician if watery and bloody stools (with or without stomach cramps and fever) occur, even as late as ≥2 months after the last dose. Inform that drug contains a PCN that can cause allergic reactions in some individuals.

Storage: Vial/Pharmacy Bulk Package: ≤25°C (77°F). Galaxy: ≤-20°C (-4°F). Thawed Sol: 22°C (72°F) for 24 hrs or 4°C (39°F) for 7 days. Do not refreeze. Refer to PI for stability and handling instructions.

TIMOPTIC – timolol maleate

RX

Class: Nonselective beta-blocker

OTHER BRAND NAMES

Timoptic-XE, Timoptic in Ocudose

ADULT DOSAGE

Elevated Intraocular Pressure

Ocular HTN/Open-Angle Glaucoma:
Timoptic/Timoptic in Ocudose:
1 drop of 0.25% sol in the affected eye(s) bid; may change to 1 drop of 0.5% sol bid if inadequate response. May decrease to 1 drop qd if IOP maintained at satisfactory levels

May use Timoptic in Ocudose when patient is sensitive to preservative in Timoptic

Timoptic-XE:
1 drop of either 0.25% or 0.5% sol in the affected eye(s) qd

PEDIATRIC DOSAGE

Pediatric use may not have been established

DOSE MODIFICATION

Concomitant Medications

Administer other topically applied ophthalmic medications at least 10 min before Timoptic-XE

ADMINISTRATION

Ocular route

Timoptic-XE

Instruct to invert closed container and shake once before each use

HOW SUPPLIED

Sol: (Timoptic) 0.25% [5mL], 0.5% [5mL, 10mL]; Sol: (Timoptic in Ocudose) 0.25%, 0.5% [0.2mL, 60s]; Sol, Gel-Forming: (Timoptic-XE) 0.25%, 0.5% [5mL]

CONTRAINDICATIONS

Bronchial asthma, history of bronchial asthma, severe COPD, sinus bradycardia, 2nd- or 3rd-degree AV block, overt cardiac failure, cardiogenic shock.

WARNINGS/PRECAUTIONS

Severe respiratory and cardiac reactions, including death, due to bronchospasm in patients with asthma and, rarely, death associated with cardiac failure, reported. Caution with cardiac failure; d/c at 1st sign/symptom of cardiac failure. May mask the signs and symptoms of acute hypoglycemia; caution in patients subject to spontaneous hypoglycemia or diabetes mellitus (DM). May mask certain clinical signs (eg, tachycardia) of hyperthyroidism; carefully manage patients suspected of developing thyrotoxicosis. Avoid with COPD (eg, chronic bronchitis, emphysema), and history/known bronchospastic disease. Not for use alone in angle-closure glaucoma. May potentiate muscle weakness consistent with myasthenic symptoms (eg, diplopia, ptosis, generalized weakness); caution with myasthenia gravis or patients with myasthenic symptoms. Caution with cerebrovascular insufficiency; consider alternative therapy if signs/symptoms of reduced cerebral blood flow develop. Choroidal detachment after filtration procedures reported. May be more reactive to repeated challenge with history of atopy or severe anaphylactic reactions to variety of allergens; may be unresponsive to usual doses of epinephrine. (Sol/XE) Bacterial keratitis with the use of multiple-dose containers reported.

ADVERSE REACTIONS

Burning/stinging upon instillation. (XE) Ocular: blurred vision, pain, conjunctivitis, discharge, foreign-body sensation, itching, tearing. Systemic: headache, dizziness, URIs.

DRUG INTERACTIONS

May potentially produce additive effects if used concomitantly with systemic β-blockers. Concomitant use of two topical β-adrenergic blocking agents is not recommended. Caution with oral/IV calcium antagonists because of possible AV conduction disturbances, left ventricular failure, or hypotension. Avoid oral/IV calcium antagonists with impaired cardiac function. Possible additive effects, production of hypotension, and/or marked bradycardia may occur when used concomitantly with catecholamine-depleting drugs (eg, reserpine). Concomitant use with calcium antagonists and digitalis may cause additive effects in prolonging AV conduction time. Potentiated systemic β-blockade reported with concomitant use of CYP2D6 inhibitors (eg, quinidine, SSRIs). Mydriasis reported occasionally with epinephrine. May augment risks of general anesthesia in surgical procedures; protracted severe hypotension and difficulty in restarting and maintaining heartbeat reported; gradual withdrawal recommended. Caution with insulin or oral hypoglycemic agents.

NURSING CONSIDERATIONS

Assessment: Assess for presence or history of bronchial asthma, COPD (eg, bronchitis, emphysema), or any other conditions where treatment is contraindicated or cautioned. Assess for pregnancy/nursing status and possible drug interactions. Assess if planning to undergo major surgery. (Sol/XE) Assess for corneal disease or disruption of the ocular epithelial surface.

Monitoring: Monitor for signs/symptoms of cardiac failure, masking of signs/symptoms of hypoglycemia, masking of hyperthyroidism, thyrotoxicosis, reduced cerebral blood flow, choroidal detachment, anaphylaxis, keratitis, and other adverse reactions. Evaluate IOP after 4 weeks of treatment.

Patient Counseling: Advise not to use product if patient has a presence or history of bronchial asthma, severe COPD, sinus bradycardia, 2nd- or 3rd-degree AV block, or cardiac failure. (Sol/XE) Instruct to avoid touching tip of container to eye or surrounding structures. Counsel to seek physician's advice on continued use of product if patient had prior ocular surgery or develops intercurrent ocular condition (eg, trauma or infection). Instruct to handle ocular sol properly to avoid contamination; inform that using contaminated sol may result in serious eye damage. (Sol) Inform that drug contains benzalkonium chloride, which may be absorbed by soft contact lenses. Instruct to remove contact lenses prior to administration and reinsert 15 min following administration. (Ocudose) Instruct about proper administration. Advise to use immediately after opening, and discard the individual unit and any remaining contents immediately after use. (XE) Instruct to invert the closed container and shake once before each use. Instruct to administer at least 10 min apart with other topical ophthalmic medications. Inform that ability to perform hazardous tasks (eg, operating machinery, driving motor vehicle) may be impaired.

Storage: 15-30°C (59-86°F). Avoid freezing. Protect from light. (Ocudose) Keep unit dose container in protective foil overwrap and use within 1 month after opening.

TINDAMAX – tinidazole RX

Class: Antiprotozoal agent

Carcinogenicity has been seen in mice and rats treated chronically with metronidazole. Although not reported for tinidazole, the two drugs are structurally related and have similar biologic effects. Use only for approved indications.

ADULT DOSAGE

Trichomoniasis

Usual: 2g single dose
Sexual partners should be treated w/ the same dose at the same time

Giardiasis

Usual: 2g single dose taken w/ food

Amebiasis

Intestinal:
Usual: 2g/day for 3 days taken w/ food
Amebic Liver Abscess:
Usual: 2g/day for 3-5 days taken w/ food

Bacterial Vaginosis

In Nonpregnant Woman:
Usual: 2g qd for 2 days taken w/ food or 1g qd for 5 days taken w/ food

PEDIATRIC DOSAGE

Giardiasis

>3 Years:
Usual: 50mg/kg single dose taken w/ food
Max: 2g/day

Amebiasis

>3 Years:
Intestinal:
Usual: 50mg/kg/day for 3 days taken w/ food
Max: 2g/day
Amebic Liver Abscess:
Usual: 50mg/kg/day for 3-5 days taken w/ food; closely monitor when treatment duration is >3 days
Max: 2g/day

DOSE MODIFICATION

Renal Impairment

Hemodialysis: If given on same day and prior to hemodialysis, give additional dose equivalent to 1/2 of recommended dose at the end of dialysis

ADMINISTRATION

Oral route

Take w/ food

Avoid alcoholic beverages when taking tinidazole and for 3 days afterwards

May crush tabs in artificial cherry syrup to be taken w/ food if unable to swallow whole tab; shake well before use

Pharmacy Compounding

Pulverize four 500mg tabs w/ a mortar and pestle

Add approx 10mL of cherry syrup to the powder and mix until smooth; transfer sus to a graduated amber container

Use small rinses of cherry syrup to transfer remaining drug to final sus for a final volume of 30mL

HOW SUPPLIED

Tab: 250mg*, 500mg* *scored

CONTRAINDICATIONS

Treatment during 1st trimester of pregnancy, nursing mothers during therapy and 3 days following last dose.

WARNINGS/PRECAUTIONS

Seizures, peripheral neuropathy reported. D/C if abnormal neurologic signs occur. Caution with hepatic impairment or blood dyscrasias. May develop vaginal candidiasis. May develop drug resistance if prescribed in absence of proven or strongly suspected bacterial infection. Caution in elderly.

ADVERSE REACTIONS

Metallic/bitter taste, N/V, vaginal fungal infection, anorexia, headache, dizziness, constipation, dyspepsia, cramps/epigastric discomfort, weakness, fatigue, malaise, convulsions, peripheral neuropathy.

DRUG INTERACTIONS

Avoid alcohol during therapy and for 3 days after use. Do not give if patient has taken disulfiram within the last 2 weeks. May potentiate oral anticoagulants. May prolong $T_{1/2}$ and reduce clearance of phenytoin (IV). May decrease clearance of fluorouracil, causing increased side effects; if concomitant use needed, monitor for toxicities. May increase levels of lithium, cyclosporine, and tacrolimus. Separate dosing with cholestyramine. Phenobarbital, rifampin, phenytoin, fosphenytoin, and other CYP3A4 inducers may decrease levels. Cimetidine, ketoconazole, and other CYP3A4 inhibitors may increase levels. Therapeutic effect antagonized by oxytetracycline.

NURSING CONSIDERATIONS

Assessment: Assess for blood dyscrasias, seizures, pregnancy/nursing status, hypersensitivity and possible drug interactions. Assess for proven or strongly suspected bacterial infection to avoid drug resistance.

Monitoring: Monitor for convulsive seizures, peripheral neuropathy, vaginal candidiasis, drug resistance, hypersensitivity reactions (urticaria, pruritis, angioedema, erythema multiforme, Stevens-Johnson syndrome).

Patient Counseling: Advise to take with food to minimize epigastric discomfort and other GI side effects. Instruct to avoid alcohol and preparations containing ethanol and propylene glycol during therapy and for 3 days afterward to prevent abdominal cramps, N/V, headache, and flushing. Inform that therapy only treats bacterial, not viral (eg, common cold), infections. Instruct to take ud; skipping doses or not completing full course may decrease effectiveness and increase resistance.

Storage: 20-25°C (68-77°F); excursions permitted to 15-30°C (59-86°F). Protect contents from light.

TIZANIDINE – tizanidine **RX**

Class: Alpha$_2$-agonist

OTHER BRAND NAMES

Zanaflex

ADULT DOSAGE

Spasticity

Management:

Initial: 4mg, (Zanaflex) 2mg

May repeat at 6- to 8-hr intervals, prn, up to a max of 3 doses in 24 hrs

Titrate: May gradually increase by 2-4mg/dose, w/ 1-4 days between increases, until a satisfactory reduction in muscle tone is achieved

Max: 36mg/day

PEDIATRIC DOSAGE

Pediatric use may not have been established

DOSE MODIFICATION

Renal Impairment

CrCl <25mL/min:

Reduce individual doses during titration
If higher doses are required, increase individual doses

Hepatic Impairment

Reduce individual doses during titration
If higher doses are required, increase individual doses

Discontinuation

Decrease dose slowly, particularly in patients who have been receiving high doses for long periods or who may be on concomitant treatment w/ narcotics

ADMINISTRATION

Oral route

Take w/ or w/o food
Do not alter regimen once formulation has been selected and the decision to take w/ or w/o food has been made

HOW SUPPLIED

Tab: 2mg* (Zanaflex) Cap: 2mg, 4mg, 6mg; Tab: 4mg* *scored

CONTRAINDICATIONS

Concomitant use with potent CYP1A2 inhibitors (eg, fluvoxamine, ciprofloxacin).

WARNINGS/PRECAUTIONS

May cause hypotension; may be minimized by dose titration and by focusing attention on signs/symptoms of hypotension prior to dose advancement. May cause hepatocellular liver injury; avoid or caution with hepatic impairment. May cause sedation. Associated with hallucinations/psychosis; consider discontinuation if hallucinations develop. Caution with renal insufficiency (CrCl <25mL/min); monitor closely for the onset or increase in severity of the common adverse events (dry mouth, somnolence, asthenia, dizziness). Withdrawal adverse reactions (eg, rebound HTN, tachycardia, hypertonia) may occur; decrease dose slowly. Caution in elderly. (Zanaflex) May cause anaphylaxis; d/c if signs/symptoms of anaphylaxis occur.

ADVERSE REACTIONS

Dry mouth, somnolence, asthenia, dizziness, UTI, infection, constipation, LFT abnormality, vomiting, speech disorder, amblyopia (blurred vision), urinary frequency, dyskinesia, nervousness, pharyngitis.

DRUG INTERACTIONS

See Contraindications and Dosage. Avoid with other CYP1A2 inhibitors (eg, zileuton, amiodarone, mexiletine, cimetidine); if use is clinically necessary, use with caution. Avoid with oral contraceptives; if use is clinically necessary, the starting dose and subsequent titration rate of tizanidine should be reduced. May have additive sedative effects with alcohol and other CNS depressants (eg, benzodiazepines, opioids, TCAs); monitor for symptoms of excess sedation. Monitor for hypotension in patients receiving concurrent antihypertensive therapy. Not recommended with other α_2-adrenergic agonists. Withdrawal symptoms are more likely to occur with concomitant use of narcotics. May delay T_{max} of acetaminophen.

NURSING CONSIDERATIONS

Assessment: Assess for hypersensitivity to drug, hypotension, hepatic/renal impairment, pregnancy/nursing status, and possible drug interactions. Obtain baseline aminotransferase levels.

Monitoring: Monitor for hypotension, hepatocellular liver injury, anaphylaxis, sedation, hallucinations/psychosis, syncope, and other adverse reactions. Monitor aminotransferase levels at 1 month after max dose is achieved, or if hepatic injury is suspected. Monitor renal function with renal impairment and in elderly.

Patient Counseling: Instruct to inform physician of all medications being taken, including if starting/stopping any medication. Instruct to take exactly ud, and not to switch between tab and cap. Advise not to suddenly d/c therapy, because rebound HTN and tachycardia may occur. Inform that hypotension may occur; advise to be careful when changing from lying/sitting to standing position. Inform that medication may cause somnolence or sedation; instruct to be careful when performing activities that require alertness (eg, driving/operating machinery). Inform that sedation may be additive when taken with drugs (baclofen, benzodiazepines) or substances (eg, alcohol) that act as CNS depressants. Inform that medication decreases spasticity; advise to use caution if dependent on spasticity to sustain posture and balance in locomotion, or whenever spasticity is utilized to obtain increased function. Inform of the signs/symptoms of severe allergic reactions; instruct to d/c and seek immediate medical care if these occur.

Storage: 20-25°C (68-77°F). (Zanaflex) 25°C (77°F); excursions permitted to 15-30°C (59-86°F).

TobraDex – dexamethasone/tobramycin RX

Class: Aminoglycoside/corticosteroid

OTHER BRAND NAMES
TobraDex ST

ADULT DOSAGE

Steroid-Responsive Inflammatory Ocular Conditions

Use for conditions for which a corticosteroid is indicated and where superficial bacterial ocular infection or a risk of bacterial ocular infection exists

Sus:
1-2 drops into the conjunctival sac(s) q4-6h
Titrate: May increase to 1-2 drops q2h during the initial 24-48 hrs; decrease frequency gradually as condition improves

ST:
1 drop into the conjunctival sac(s) q4-6h
Titrate: May increase to 1 drop q2h during the initial 24-48 hrs; decrease frequency gradually as condition improves

Sus/ST:
Do not prescribe more than 20mL initially

Care should be taken not to d/c therapy prematurely

Oint:
Apply a small amount (1/2 inch ribbon) into the conjunctival sac(s) up to tid-qid

Do not prescribe more than 8g initially

PEDIATRIC DOSAGE

Steroid-Responsive Inflammatory Ocular Conditions

Use for conditions for which a corticosteroid is indicated and where superficial bacterial ocular infection or a risk of bacterial ocular infection exists

≥2 Years:

Sus:
1-2 drops into the conjunctival sac(s) q4-6h
Titrate: May increase to 1-2 drops q2h during the initial 24-48 hrs; decrease frequency gradually as condition improves

ST:
1 drop into the conjunctival sac(s) q4-6h
Titrate: May increase to 1 drop q2h during the initial 24-48 hrs; decrease frequency gradually as condition improves

Sus/ST:
Do not prescribe more than 20mL initially

Care should be taken not to d/c therapy prematurely

Oint:
Apply a small amount (1/2 inch ribbon) into the conjunctival sac(s) up to tid-qid

Do not prescribe more than 8g initially

ADMINISTRATION
Ocular route

Sus/ST
Shake well before use

Oint
Tilt head back
Place finger on cheek just under the eye and gently pull down until a "V" pocket is formed between eyeball and lower lid
Apply recommended dose, making sure to avoid touching tip of tube to eye
Look downward before closing the eye

HOW SUPPLIED
Oint: (Tobramycin-Dexamethasone) 0.3%-0.1% [3.5g]; Sus: 0.3%-0.1% [2.5mL, 5mL, 10mL]; Sus (ST): 0.3%-0.05% [2.5mL, 5mL, 10mL]

CONTRAINDICATIONS
Viral diseases of the cornea and conjunctiva, epithelial herpes simplex keratitis (dendritic keratitis), vaccinia, varicella, mycobacterial infection, and fungal diseases of the eye.

WARNINGS/PRECAUTIONS
Prolonged use may result in glaucoma with optic nerve damage, visual acuity and field of vision defects, posterior subcapsular cataract formation, and may suppress host response and increase risk of secondary ocular infections. Perforations may occur with diseases causing thinning of the cornea or sclera. May mask/enhance existing infection in acute purulent conditions. Fungal infections of the cornea may occur; consider fungal invasion in any persistent corneal ulceration. (Oint/Sus) Not for injection into the eye. Routinely monitor intraocular pressure (IOP). D/C if sensitivity occurs. Cross-sensitivity to other aminoglycoside antibiotics may occur; d/c and institute appropriate therapy if hypersensitivity develops. May result in overgrowth of nonsusceptible organisms, including fungi; initiate appropriate therapy if superinfection occurs. (ST) Monitor IOP if to be used for ≥10 days. Reevaluate after 2 days if patient fails to improve. Use may prolong the course and may exacerbate the severity of many viral infections of the eye (including herpes simplex). May delay healing and increase the incidence of bleb formation after cataract surgery. (Oint) May retard corneal wound healing.

ADVERSE REACTIONS
Hypersensitivity, localized ocular toxicity, secondary infection, increased IOP, posterior subcapsular cataract formation, impaired wound healing.

DRUG INTERACTIONS
Monitor total serum concentrations if used concomitantly with systemic aminoglycoside antibiotics.

NURSING CONSIDERATIONS

Assessment: Assess for epithelial herpes simplex keratitis (dendritic keratitis), vaccinia, varicella, other viral diseases of cornea or conjunctiva, mycobacterial infection and fungal diseases of eye, diseases that may cause thinning of cornea or sclera, other existing infections, pregnancy/nursing status, and for drug interactions. (ST) Assess for history of herpes simplex.

Monitoring: Monitor for signs/symptoms of hypersensitivity reactions, glaucoma, defects in visual acuity and fields of vision, posterior subcapsular cataracts, perforations, secondary infections, delayed wound healing. (ST) Monitor for IOP if used for ≥10 days, exacerbation of ocular viral infections, and bleb formation. (Oint/Sus) Routinely monitor IOP, and for development of superinfections.

Patient Counseling: Instruct not to touch dropper tip to any surface to avoid contaminating contents and not to wear contact lenses during therapy.

Storage: (Sus) 8-27°C (46-80°F); store upright. (Oint/ST): 2-25°C (36-77°F); protect ST from light.

TOBREX – tobramycin RX

Class: Aminoglycoside

ADULT DOSAGE
Ocular Infections

External infections of the eye and its adnexa

Mild to Moderate Infection:

Oint:
Apply 1/2 inch ribbon into the affected eye(s) bid-tid

Sol:
1-2 drops into the affected eye(s) q4h

Severe Infection:

Oint:
Apply 1/2 inch ribbon into the affected eye(s) q3-4h until improvement, then reduce treatment prior to discontinuation

Sol:
2 drops into the affected eye(s) qh until improvement, then reduce treatment prior to discontinuation

PEDIATRIC DOSAGE
Ocular Infections

External infections of the eye and its adnexa

≥2 Months of Age:

Mild to Moderate Infection:

Oint:
Apply 1/2 inch ribbon into the affected eye(s) bid-tid

Sol:
1-2 drops into the affected eye(s) q4h

Severe Infection:

Oint:
Apply 1/2 inch ribbon into the affected eye(s) q3-4h until improvement, then reduce treatment prior to discontinuation

Sol:
2 drops into the affected eye(s) qh until improvement, then reduce treatment prior to discontinuation

ADMINISTRATION
Ocular route

Oint

Tilt head back

Place finger on cheek just under the eye and gently pull down until a "V" pocket is formed between eyeball and lower lid

Apply recommended dose in the "V" pocket, making sure to avoid touching tip of tube to eye

Look downward before closing the eye

HOW SUPPLIED
Oint: 0.3% [3.5g]; Sol: 0.3% [5mL]

WARNINGS/PRECAUTIONS
Not for inj into the eye. Prolonged use may result in overgrowth of nonsusceptible organisms (eg, fungi); initiate appropriate therapy if superinfection occurs. Sensitivity reactions and cross-sensitivity to other aminoglycoside antibiotics may occur; d/c and institute appropriate therapy if hypersensitivity develops. Avoid wearing contact lenses if signs/symptoms of ocular infection exist. (Oint) May retard corneal wound healing.

ADVERSE REACTIONS
Hypersensitivity, localized ocular toxicity (eg, lid itching/swelling, conjunctival erythema).

DRUG INTERACTIONS
Monitor total serum concentration if used concomitantly with systemic aminoglycoside antibiotics.

NURSING CONSIDERATIONS

Assessment: Assess for known hypersensitivity to the drug, causative organisms, pregnancy/nursing status, and possible drug interactions.

Monitoring: Monitor for superinfection, hypersensitivity, and other adverse reactions. Monitor for response to therapy.

Patient Counseling: Advise not to wear contact lenses if signs/symptoms of ocular infection exist. Instruct not to touch tube/dropper tip to any surface to avoid contamination.

Storage: 2-25°C (36-77°F).

TOPAMAX – topiramate RX

Class: Sulfamate-substituted monosaccharide antiepileptic

OTHER BRAND NAMES
Topamax Sprinkle

ADULT DOSAGE

Epilepsy

Monotherapy:
Partial Onset/Primary Generalized Tonic-Clonic Seizures:
Week 1: 25mg bid (am and pm)
Week 2: 50mg bid (am and pm)
Week 3: 75mg bid (am and pm)
Week 4: 100mg bid (am and pm)
Week 5: 150mg bid (am and pm)
Week 6 & Onward: 200mg bid (am and pm)

Adjunctive Therapy:
Partial Onset Seizure/Primary Generalized Tonic-Clonic Seizures/Lennox-Gastaut Syndrome:
≥17 Years:
Initial: 25-50mg/day
Titrate: Increase in increments of 25-50mg/day every week

Partial Onset Seizures:
Usual: 200-400mg/day in 2 divided doses

Primary Generalized Tonic-Clonic:
Usual: 400mg/day in 2 divided doses

Migraine

Prophylaxis:
Week 1: 25mg qpm
Week 2: 25mg bid
Week 3: 25mg qam and 50mg qpm
Week 4 & Onward: 50mg bid

PEDIATRIC DOSAGE

Epilepsy

Monotherapy:
Partial Onset/Primary Generalized Tonic-Clonic Seizures:
2-<10 Years:
Up to 11kg:
Minimum Maint Dose: 150mg/day
Max Maint Dose: 250mg/day
12-22kg:
Minimum Maint Dose: 200mg/day
Max Maint Dose: 300mg/day
23-31kg:
Minimum Maint Dose: 200mg/day
Max Maint Dose: 350mg/day
32-38kg:
Minimum Maint Dose: 250mg/day
Max Maint Dose: 350mg/day
>38kg:
Minimum Maint Dose: 250mg/day
Max Maint Dose: 400mg/day

Administer in 2 equally divided doses; refer to PI for titration instructions

≥10 Years:
Week 1: 25mg bid (am and pm)
Week 2: 50mg bid (am and pm)
Week 3: 75mg bid (am and pm)
Week 4: 100mg bid (am and pm)
Week 5: 150mg bid (am and pm)
Week 6 & Onward: 200mg bid (am and pm)

Adjunctive Therapy:
Partial Onset Seizure/Primary Generalized Tonic-Clonic Seizures/Lennox-Gastaut Syndrome:
2-16 Years:
Week 1: 1-3mg/kg/day (≤25mg/day) qpm
Titrate: Increase dose at 1- or 2-week intervals by increments of 1-3mg/kg/day (administered in 2 divided doses)
Usual: 5-9mg/kg/day in 2 divided doses

Migraine

Prophylaxis:
≥12 Years:
Week 1: 25mg qpm
Week 2: 25mg bid
Week 3: 25mg qam and 50mg qpm
Week 4 & Onward: 50mg bid

DOSE MODIFICATION

Renal Impairment

CrCl <70mL/min: Administer 50% of usual adult dose

Patients Undergoing Hemodialysis: May require a supplemental dose

ADMINISTRATION

Oral route

Take w/o regard to meals

Sprinkle Caps

May be swallowed whole or administered by carefully opening the capsule and sprinkling entire contents on a small amount (tsp) of soft food; swallow drug/food mixture immediately and do not chew or store mixture for later use

HOW SUPPLIED

Cap: (Sprinkle) 15mg, 25mg; Tab: 25mg, 50mg, 100mg, 200mg

WARNINGS/PRECAUTIONS

Acute myopia associated with secondary angle-closure glaucoma reported; d/c immediately to reverse symptoms. Elevated IOP of any etiology may lead to serious adverse events (eg, permanent loss of vision) if left untreated. Visual field defects (independent of elevated IOP) reported; consider discontinuing therapy if visual problems occur. Oligohidrosis and hyperthermia reported, mostly in pediatric patients. Hyperchloremic, non-anion gap, metabolic acidosis reported; d/c or reduce dose if metabolic acidosis develops/persists. If decision is to continue therapy, consider alkali treatment. Conditions or therapies that predispose to acidosis (eg, renal disease, severe respiratory disorders, status epilepticus, diarrhea, ketogenic diet, specific drugs) may be additive to the bicarbonate lowering effects. Increased risk of suicidal thoughts/behavior. Cognitive-related dysfunction, psychiatric/behavioral disturbances, and somnolence or fatigue reported. May cause cleft lip and/or palate in infants if used during pregnancy. D/C gradually to minimize the potential for seizure or increased seizure frequency; appropriate monitoring is recommended when rapid withdrawal is required. Sudden unexplained deaths in epilepsy reported. Patients with inborn errors of metabolism or reduced hepatic mitochondrial activity may be at an increased risk for hyperammonemia with or without encephalopathy; consider hyperammonemic encephalopathy and measure ammonia levels in patients who develop unexplained lethargy, vomiting, or changes in mental status associated with therapy. Kidney stone formation reported; hydration is recommended to reduce new stone formation. Paresthesia may occur. Lab abnormalities may occur. Caution with renal/hepatic impairment and in elderly.

ADVERSE REACTIONS

Anorexia, anxiety, diarrhea, fatigue, fever, infection, weight decrease, cognitive problems, paresthesia, somnolence, taste perversion, mood problems, nausea, nervousness, confusion.

DRUG INTERACTIONS

Phenytoin or carbamazepine may decrease levels. Increase in systemic exposure of lithium observed following topiramate doses of ≤600mg/day; monitor lithium levels. May cause CNS depression and cognitive/neuropsychiatric adverse events with alcohol and other CNS depressants; use with extreme caution. May decrease contraceptive efficacy and increase breakthrough bleeding with combination oral contraceptives. Concurrent administration of valproic acid has been associated with hyperammonemia with or without encephalopathy, and hypothermia. Other carbonic anhydrase inhibitors (eg, zonisamide, acetazolamide, dichlorphenamide) may increase the severity of metabolic acidosis and may also increase the risk of kidney stone formation. Caution with agents that predispose patients to heat-related disorders (eg, carbonic anhydrase inhibitors, anticholinergics).

NURSING CONSIDERATIONS

Assessment: Assess for renal/hepatic dysfunction, predisposing factors for metabolic acidosis, inborn errors of metabolism, reduced hepatic mitochondrial activity, pregnancy/nursing status, and possible drug interactions. Obtain baseline serum bicarbonate and blood ammonia levels.

Monitoring: Monitor for signs/symptoms of acute myopia, secondary angle-closure glaucoma, visual field defects, oligohidrosis, hyperthermia, cognitive or neuropsychiatric adverse reactions, kidney stones, renal dysfunction, metabolic acidosis, paresthesia, hyperammonemia, and other adverse reactions. Monitor serum bicarbonate and blood ammonia levels.

Patient Counseling: Instruct to seek immediate medical attention if blurred vision, visual disturbances, periorbital pain, changes in mood/behavior, or suicidal thoughts/behavior occur and to closely monitor for decreased sweating or high/persistent fever. Warn about risk for metabolic acidosis. Advise to use caution when engaging in activities where loss of consciousness may result in serious danger. Inform about risk for hyperammonemia with or without encephalopathy; instruct to contact physician if unexplained lethargy, vomiting, or mental status changes develop. Instruct to maintain adequate fluid intake to minimize risk of kidney stones. Inform of pregnancy risks. Encourage to enroll in the North American Antiepileptic Drug Pregnancy Registry if patient becomes pregnant. Instruct that if a single dose is missed, to take that dose as soon as possible, skip it if cannot be taken at least 6 hrs before the next scheduled dose, and not to double the dose. Advise to contact physician if >1 dose is missed.

Storage: Protect from moisture. (Tab) 15-30°C (59-86°F). (Cap) ≤25°C (77°F).

TOPROL-XL – metoprolol succinate

RX

Class: Selective $beta_1$-blocker

Exacerbations of angina and MI reported following abrupt discontinuation. When discontinuing chronic therapy, particularly w/ ischemic heart disease, taper over 1-2 weeks w/ careful monitoring. If worsening of angina or acute coronary insufficiency develops, reinstate therapy promptly, at least temporarily, and take other appropriate measures. Caution patients against interruption or discontinuation of therapy w/o physician's advice.

ADULT DOSAGE

Hypertension

Initial: 25-100mg qd
Titrate: May increase at weekly (or longer) intervals
Max: 400mg/day

Angina Pectoris

Initial: 100mg qd
Titrate: May gradually increase weekly
Max: 400mg/day
Reduce dose gradually over a period of 1-2 weeks if to be discontinued

Heart Failure

Initial:
NYHA Class II HF: 25mg qd for 2 weeks
Severe HF: 12.5mg qd for 2 weeks
Titrate: Double dose every 2 weeks to the highest dose level tolerated
Max: 200mg
Dose should not be increased until symptoms of worsening HF have been stabilized
Reduce dose if experiencing symptomatic bradycardia

PEDIATRIC DOSAGE

Hypertension

≥6 Years:
Initial: 1mg/kg qd up to 50mg qd
Titrate: Adjust dose according to BP response
Max: 2mg/kg (or up to 200mg) qd

DOSE MODIFICATION

Hepatic Impairment
May require lower initial dose; gradually increase dose to optimize therapy

Elderly
Start at low initial dose

ADMINISTRATION

Oral route
Tab may be divided; do not crush or chew whole or half tab

HOW SUPPLIED

Tab, ER: 25mg*, 50mg*, 100mg*, 200mg* *scored

CONTRAINDICATIONS

Severe bradycardia, 2nd- or 3rd-degree heart block, cardiogenic shock, decompensated cardiac failure, sick sinus syndrome (unless w/ a permanent pacemaker).

WARNINGS/PRECAUTIONS

Worsening cardiac failure may occur during up-titration; lower dose or temporarily d/c therapy. Avoid w/ bronchospastic disease; may be used only w/ those who do not respond to or cannot tolerate other antihypertensive treatment. If used in the setting of pheochromocytoma, should be given in combination w/ α-blockers, and only after α-blocker has been initiated; may cause a paradoxical increase in BP if administered alone. Avoid initiation of a high-dose regimen in patients undergoing noncardiac surgery. Chronically administered therapy should not be routinely withdrawn prior to major surgery; however, the impaired ability of the heart to respond to reflex adrenergic stimuli may augment the risks of general anesthesia and surgical procedures. May mask tachycardia occurring w/ hypoglycemia. May mask signs of hyperthyroidism (eg, tachycardia); abrupt withdrawal may precipitate thyroid storm. Patients w/ a history of severe anaphylactic reactions to variety of allergens may be more reactive to repeated challenge and may be unresponsive to usual doses of epinephrine. May precipitate or aggravate symptoms of arterial insufficiency w/ peripheral vascular disease (PVD). Caution w/ hepatic impairment and in elderly.

ADVERSE REACTIONS

Tiredness, dizziness, depression, diarrhea, SOB, bradycardia, rash.

DRUG INTERACTIONS

Additive effects w/ catecholamine-depleting drugs (eg, reserpine, MAOIs). CYP2D6 inhibitors (eg, quinidine, fluoxetine, propafenone) may increase levels. Caution when used w/ verapamil and diltiazem. May increase the risk of bradycardia w/ digitalis glycosides, clonidine, diltiazem, and verapamil. When given concomitantly w/ clonidine, d/c several days before clonidine is gradually withdrawn; may exacerbate rebound HTN.

NURSING CONSIDERATIONS

Assessment: Assess for severe bradycardia, 2nd- or 3rd-degree heart block, cardiogenic shock, decompensated cardiac failure, sick sinus syndrome, presence of pacemaker, ischemic heart disease, bronchospastic disease, diabetes, hyperthyroidism, PVD, hepatic impairment, pheochromocytoma, history of anaphylactic reactions, pregnancy/nursing status, and possible drug interactions.

Monitoring: Monitor for signs/symptoms of worsening cardiac failure during up-titration, hypoglycemia, precipitation of thyroid storm, precipitation/aggravation of arterial insufficiency in patients w/ PVD, anaphylactic reactions, and other adverse reactions. Monitor patients w/ ischemic heart disease.

Patient Counseling: Advise to take drug regularly and continuously, ud, preferably w/ or immediately following meals. Counsel that if dose is missed, take only the next scheduled dose (w/o doubling). Instruct not to interrupt or d/c therapy w/o consulting physician. Advise to avoid operating automobiles and machinery or engaging in other tasks requiring alertness. Instruct to contact physician if any difficulty in breathing occurs. Instruct to inform physician or dentist of medication use before any type of surgery. Advise HF patients to consult physician if experience signs/symptoms of worsening HF.

Storage: 25°C (77°F); excursions permitted to 15-30°C (59-86°F).

TORSEMIDE – torsemide

RX

Class: Loop diuretic

OTHER BRAND NAMES

Demadex

ADULT DOSAGE

Edema

IV/PO:

CHF:

Initial: 10 or 20mg qd

Titrate: Double dose until desired response is obtained

Max Single Dose: 200mg

Chronic Renal Failure:

Initial: 20mg qd

Titrate: Double dose until desired response is obtained

Max Single Dose: 200mg

Hepatic Cirrhosis:

Initial: 5 or 10mg qd w/ an aldosterone antagonist or K^+-sparing diuretic

Titrate: Double dose until desired response is obtained

Max Single Dose: 40mg

Hypertension

IV/PO:

Initial: 5mg qd

Titrate: May increase to 10mg qd after 4-6 weeks if BP reduction is inadequate

An additional antihypertensive agent should be added to the treatment regimen if response to 10mg is insufficient

PEDIATRIC DOSAGE

Pediatric use may not have been established

DOSE MODIFICATION

IV to PO Conversion

May switch to/from IV form w/ no change in dose

ADMINISTRATION

IV/Oral route

Inj

Administer either slowly as a bolus over 2 min or as continuous infusion
Flush IV line w/ normal saline before and after administration
Refer to PI for further administration instructions

Compatibility

D5W; 0.9% NaCl; 0.45% NaCl

Tab

May be given at any time in relation to a meal

HOW SUPPLIED

Inj: 10mg/mL [2mL, 5mL]; Tab: (Demadex) 5mg*, 10mg*, 20mg*, 100mg* *scored

CONTRAINDICATIONS

Anuria.

WARNINGS/PRECAUTIONS

Caution in patients with hepatic disease with cirrhosis and ascites as sudden alterations of fluid/electrolyte balance may precipitate hepatic coma; diuresis is best initiated in a hospital. Tinnitus and hearing loss (usually reversible) reported. Excessive diuresis may cause dehydration, blood-volume reduction, and possible thrombosis and embolism, especially in elderly. Monitor for electrolyte imbalance, hypovolemia, or prerenal azotemia; d/c until situation is corrected and may restart at a lower dose, if signs/symptoms occur. Increased risk of hypokalemia with liver cirrhosis, brisk diuresis, and inadequate oral intake of electrolytes. Diuretic-induced hypokalemia may be a risk factor for the development of arrhythmias in patients with cardiovascular disease (CVD), especially with concomitant digitalis glycosides. Hyperglycemia, hypomagnesemia, hypercalcemia, and symptomatic gout reported. May increase BUN, SrCr, serum uric acid, total cholesterol, and TGs. Associated with small decreases in Hgb, Hct, erythrocyte count, and small increases in WBC count, platelet count, and alkaline phosphatase.

ADVERSE REACTIONS

Headache, excessive urination, dizziness, hypotension, chest pain, atrial fibrillation, diarrhea, GI hemorrhage, rectal bleeding, rash, shunt thrombosis, syncope, ventricular tachycardia, hyperglycemia, hyperuricemia.

DRUG INTERACTIONS

Reduced renal clearance and increased levels of spironolactone. Salicylate toxicity may occur with concomitant high-dose salicylates. Possible renal dysfunction with NSAIDs (including aspirin). Indomethacin partially inhibits natriuretic effect. Digoxin may increase exposure by 50%. Simultaneous administration with cholestyramine is not recommended. Probenecid may decrease diuretic activity. Caution with lithium; high risk of lithium toxicity. Increased ototoxic potential of aminoglycoside antibiotics and ethacrynic acid reported, especially in the presence of renal impairment. Increased risk of hypokalemia with adrenocorticotropic hormone or corticosteroids.

NURSING CONSIDERATIONS

Assessment: Assess for history of hypersensitivity to the drug or to sulfonylureas, anuria, CVD, renal/hepatic impairment, pregnancy/nursing status, and possible drug interactions.

Monitoring: Monitor for hypovolemia, prerenal azotemia, tinnitus, hearing loss, hypersensitivity reactions, renal/hepatic impairment, arrhythmias in patients with CVD, and other adverse reactions. Monitor serum electrolytes periodically.

Patient Counseling: Inform of risks and benefits of therapy. Advise to seek medical attention if symptoms of hypokalemia, fluid/electrolyte imbalance, hypersensitivity reactions, hearing loss, or tinnitus occur.

Storage: (Inj) 20-25°C (68-77°F). Do not freeze. Continuous Infusion Sol: Stable for 24 hrs at room temperature in plastic containers. Refer to PI for IV fluids and concentrations. (Tab) 15-30°C (59-86°F).

TOVIAZ – fesoterodine fumarate **RX**

Class: Muscarinic antagonist

ADULT DOSAGE

Overactive Bladder

Initial: 4mg qd

Titrate: May increase to 8mg qd based on individual response and tolerability

PEDIATRIC DOSAGE

Pediatric use may not have been established

DOSE MODIFICATION
Concomitant Medications
Strong CYP3A4 Inhibitors:
Max: 4mg/day

Renal Impairment
CrCl <30mL/min:
Max: 4mg/day

ADMINISTRATION
Oral route

Take w/ or w/o food
Take tab w/ liquid and swallow whole; do not crush, chew, or divide

HOW SUPPLIED
Tab, Extended-Release (ER): 4mg, 8mg

CONTRAINDICATIONS
Urinary/gastric retention, uncontrolled narrow-angle glaucoma, hypersensitivity to tolterodine tartrate tab/ER cap.

WARNINGS/PRECAUTIONS
Not recommended with severe hepatic impairment (Child-Pugh C). Angioedema of the face, lips, tongue, and/or larynx reported; d/c and promptly provide appropriate therapy if angioedema occurs. Risk of urinary retention; caution with clinically significant bladder outlet obstruction. Caution with decreased GI motility (eg, severe constipation), controlled narrow-angle glaucoma, and myasthenia gravis. CNS anticholinergic effects (eg, headache, dizziness, somnolence) reported; monitor for signs, particularly after beginning treatment or increasing the dose, and consider dose reduction or discontinuation if such effects occur.

ADVERSE REACTIONS
Dry mouth, constipation, urinary tract infection, dry eyes.

DRUG INTERACTIONS
May increase the frequency and/or severity of dry mouth, constipation, urinary retention, and other anticholinergic pharmacologic effects with other antimuscarinic agents that produce such effects. May potentially alter the absorption of some concomitantly administered drugs due to anticholinergic effects on GI motility. CYP3A4 inhibitors may increase levels; doses >4mg are not recommended in patients taking potent CYP3A4 inhibitors (eg, ketoconazole, itraconazole, clarithromycin). CYP2D6 inhibitors may increase levels. Rifampin or rifampicin may decrease levels.

NURSING CONSIDERATIONS

Assessment: Assess for hypersensitivity to the drug or tolterodine tartrate, urinary/gastric retention, narrow-angle glaucoma, bladder outlet obstruction, decreased GI motility, severe constipation, myasthenia gravis, severe hepatic/renal impairment, pregnancy/nursing status, and possible drug interactions.

Monitoring: Monitor for angioedema, upper airway swelling, urinary retention, CNS anticholinergic effects, and other adverse reactions.

Patient Counseling: Inform that therapy may produce angioedema; instruct to promptly d/c therapy and seek immediate medical attention if edema of the tongue/laryngopharynx or difficulty in breathing occurs. Counsel that therapy may produce clinically significant adverse effects (eg, constipation, urinary retention). Inform that blurred vision may occur; advise to exercise caution in decisions to engage in potentially dangerous activities until effects have been determined. Inform that heat prostration (due to decreased sweating) may occur when used in a hot environment. Inform that alcohol may enhance drowsiness caused by therapy.

Storage: 20-25°C (68-77°F); excursions permitted between 15-30°C (59-86°F). Protect from moisture.

TRADJENTA – linagliptin RX

Class: Dipeptidyl peptidase-4 (DPP-4) inhibitor

ADULT DOSAGE
Type 2 Diabetes Mellitus
5mg qd

PEDIATRIC DOSAGE
Pediatric use may not have been established

DOSE MODIFICATION
Concomitant Medications
W/ Insulin Secretagogue (eg, Sulfonylurea)/Insulin:
May require lower dose of insulin secretagogue or insulin

ADMINISTRATION
Oral route

Take w/ or w/o food

HOW SUPPLIED
Tab: 5mg

WARNINGS/PRECAUTIONS
Not for use in patients w/ type 1 DM or for the treatment of diabetic ketoacidosis. Acute pancreatitis reported; d/c if pancreatitis is suspected. Serious hypersensitivity reactions reported; if suspected, d/c therapy, assess for other potential causes for the event, and institute alternative treatment for diabetes. Caution in patients w/ a history of angioedema w/ another dipeptidyl peptidase-4 (DPP-4) inhibitor.

ADVERSE REACTIONS
Hypoglycemia, nasopharyngitis, diarrhea.

DRUG INTERACTIONS
Strong inducers of P-glycoprotein or CYP3A4 (eg, rifampin) may reduce efficacy; use of alternative treatments is strongly recommended. May require lower dose of insulin secretagogue (eg, sulfonylurea) or insulin to reduce risk of hypoglycemia.

NURSING CONSIDERATIONS

Assessment: Assess for history of hypersensitivity, type of DM, diabetic ketoacidosis, history of pancreatitis, history of angioedema w/ another DPP-4 inhibitor, pregnancy/nursing status, and possible drug interactions. Obtain baseline FPG and HbA1c levels.

Monitoring: Monitor for pancreatitis, hypersensitivity reactions, and other adverse reactions. Monitor FPG and HbA1c levels periodically.

Patient Counseling: Inform of the potential risks/benefits and alternative modes of therapy. Advise on the importance of adherence to dietary instructions, regular physical activity, periodic blood glucose monitoring and HbA1c testing, recognition/management of hypo/hyperglycemia, and assessment for diabetes complications. Instruct to seek medical advice promptly during periods of stress as medication requirements may change. Inform that acute pancreatitis and serious allergic reactions reported; instruct to d/c use and notify physician if signs and symptoms of pancreatitis or allergic reactions occur. Instruct to take as prescribed. Instruct to inform physician or pharmacist if any unusual symptom develops, or if any known symptom persists or worsens.

Storage: 25°C (77°F); excursions permitted to 15-30°C (59-86°F).

TRANSDERM SCOP – scopolamine

RX

Class: Anticholinergic

ADULT DOSAGE

Motion Sickness

Prevention of N/V:
1 patch at least 4 hrs before the antiemetic effect is required
Replace patch after 3 days if therapy is required for >3 days

Postoperative Nausea/Vomiting

Prevention of N/V Associated w/ Recovery from Anesthesia and/or Opiate Analgesia and Surgery:
1 patch on the pm before surgery or 1 hr prior to cesarean section
Remove patch 24 hrs following surgery

PEDIATRIC DOSAGE
Pediatric use may not have been established

ADMINISTRATION
Transdermal route

Apply only to skin in the postauricular area
After application, wash hands thoroughly w/ soap and water and dry
Wear only 1 patch at anytime
Do not cut patch
Discard patch if displaced and replace w/ a fresh patch

HOW SUPPLIED
Patch: 1.5mg [4[s]]

CONTRAINDICATIONS
Angle-closure glaucoma.

WARNINGS/PRECAUTIONS
May increase IOP with open-angle glaucoma; monitor therapy and adjust during use. May cause temporary dilation of pupils and blurred vision if contact with eyes occurs. Caution with pyloric obstruction, urinary bladder neck obstruction, and intestinal obstruction. May aggravate seizures or psychosis. Idiosyncratic reactions may occur with ordinary therapeutic doses. Increased CNS effects may occur in elderly and with hepatic/renal impairment. May impair physical/mental abilities. Remove patch before undergoing a MRI scan; skin burns at the patch site reported. May interfere with gastric secretion test.

ADVERSE REACTIONS
Dry mouth, dizziness, somnolence, urinary retention, agitation, visual impairment, confusion, mydriasis, pharyngitis.

DRUG INTERACTIONS
May decrease absorption of oral medications due to decreased gastric motility and delayed gastric emptying. Caution with other drugs with CNS effects (eg, sedatives, tranquilizers, alcohol) and anticholinergic properties (eg, meclizine, TCAs, muscle relaxants).

NURSING CONSIDERATIONS

Assessment: Assess for known hypersensitivity to the drug, glaucoma, pyloric obstruction, urinary bladder neck obstruction, intestinal obstruction, history of seizures or psychosis, hepatic/renal impairment, pregnancy/nursing status, and for possible drug interactions.

Monitoring: Monitor for aggravation of seizures or psychosis, idiosyncratic reactions (eg, agitation, hallucinations, paranoid behaviors, delusions), CNS effects, drowsiness, disorientation, confusion, withdrawal symptoms, and other adverse reactions. Monitor IOP in patients with open-angle glaucoma.

Patient Counseling: Inform elderly that patch may cause a greater likelihood of CNS effects and to seek medical care if patient becomes confused, disoriented, or dizzy while wearing the patch or after removing. Inform that patch may cause drowsiness, disorientation, and confusion; advise to use caution when engaging in activities that require mental alertness. Instruct to avoid alcohol. Instruct to seek medical care if withdrawal symptoms occur following abrupt discontinuation. Inform that patch may cause temporary dilation of pupils and blurred vision. Instruct to wash hands thoroughly with soap and water immediately after handling patch. Instruct to dispose the patch properly to avoid contact with children or pets. Advise to remove patch before undergoing an MRI to avoid skin burns. Instruct to use ud. Advise to remove the patch immediately and promptly contact physician if symptoms of acute angle-closure glaucoma or difficulty in urinating is experienced.

Storage: 20-25°C (68-77°F).

TRAVATAN Z – travoprost

RX

Class: Prostaglandin analogue

ADULT DOSAGE

Elevated Intraocular Pressure

Open-Angle Glaucoma/Ocular HTN:
1 drop in affected eye(s) qd in pm

PEDIATRIC DOSAGE

Elevated Intraocular Pressure

Open-Angle Glaucoma/Ocular HTN:
≥16 Years:
1 drop in affected eye(s) qd in pm

DOSE MODIFICATION

Concomitant Medications
Space by at least 5 min if using >1 topical ophthalmic drug

ADMINISTRATION
Ocular route

HOW SUPPLIED
Sol: 0.004% [2.5mL, 5mL]

WARNINGS/PRECAUTIONS
Changes to pigmented tissues, including increased pigmentation of iris (may be permanent), eyelid, and eyelashes (may be reversible) reported. Regularly examine patients with noticeably increased iris pigmentation. May cause changes to eyelashes and vellus hair in the treated eye. May exacerbate active intraocular inflammation (eg, uveitis). Macular edema, including cystoid macular edema, reported; caution with aphakic patients, pseudophakic patients with torn posterior lens capsule, or patients at risk of macular edema. Treatment of angle-closure, inflammatory, or

neovascular glaucoma has not been evaluated. Bacterial keratitis reported with multidose container. Remove contact lenses prior to instillation; may reinsert 15 min after administration.

ADVERSE REACTIONS

Ocular hyperemia, foreign body sensation, decreased visual acuity, eye discomfort/pruritus/pain.

NURSING CONSIDERATIONS

Assessment: Assess for active intraocular inflammation (uveitis), active macular edema, aphakic/pseudophakic patients with torn posterior lens capsule, angle-closure, inflammatory, or neovascular glaucoma, and pregnancy/nursing status.

Monitoring: Monitor for increased pigmentation of the iris and periorbital tissue (eyelid), changes in eyelashes, macular edema, and bacterial keratitis.

Patient Counseling: Inform about risk of brown pigmentation of iris and darkening of eyelid skin. Inform about the possibility of eyelash and vellus hair changes. Advise to avoid touching tip of dispensing container to eye, surrounding structures, fingers, or any other surface, in order to avoid contamination of the sol. Advise to consult physician if having ocular surgery or if intercurrent ocular conditions (eg, trauma or infection) or ocular reactions develop. Instruct to remove contact lenses prior to instillation; reinsert 15 min after administration. Instruct to administer at least 5 min apart if using >1 topical ophthalmic drugs.

Storage: 2-25°C (36-77°F).

TRAZODONE – trazodone hydrochloride — RX

Class: Triazolopyridine derivative

Antidepressants increased the risk of suicidal thinking and behavior (suicidality) in children, adolescents, and young adults in short-term studies of major depressive disorder and other psychiatric disorders. Monitor and observe closely for clinical worsening, suicidality, or unusual changes in behavior. Not approved for use in pediatric patients.

ADULT DOSAGE

Major Depressive Disorder

Initial: 150mg/day in divided doses

Titrate: Increase by 50mg/day every 3-4 days

Max:

Outpatient: 400mg/day in divided doses

Inpatient: 600mg/day in divided doses

Once adequate response is achieved, gradually reduce dose, w/ subsequent adjustment depending on therapeutic response; continue treatment for several months after initial response

PEDIATRIC DOSAGE

Pediatric use may not have been established

DOSE MODIFICATION

Adverse Reactions

Drowsiness: Administer major portion of daily dose hs or reduce dose

ADMINISTRATION

Oral route

Take shortly after a meal or light snack

Swallow tab whole or administer as a 1/2 tab by breaking along the score line

HOW SUPPLIED

Tab: 50mg*, 100mg*, 150mg*, 300mg* *scored

WARNINGS/PRECAUTIONS

Monitor for withdrawal symptoms when discontinuing treatment; gradually reduce dose. May cause serotonin syndrome or neuroleptic malignant syndrome (NMS)-like reactions; d/c immediately and initiate supportive symptomatic treatment. May precipitate a mixed/manic episode in patients at risk for bipolar disorder; screen for risk of bipolar disorder prior to initiating treatment. Not approved for treatment of bipolar depression. May cause QT/QTc interval prolongation, torsades de pointes, cardiac arrhythmias, and hypotension, including orthostatic hypotension and syncope. Not recommended for use during initial recovery phase of MI. May increase risk of bleeding events. Priapism reported; caution in men with conditions that may predispose to priapism (eg, sickle cell anemia, multiple myeloma, leukemia) or with penile anatomical deformation; d/c with erection lasting >6 hrs (painful or not). Hyponatremia may occur; caution in elderly and volume-depleted patients. Consider discontinuation in patients with symptomatic hyponatremia and institute appropriate medical intervention. May cause somnolence or sedation and may impair mental/

physical abilities. Pupillary dilation that occurs following use may trigger an angle-closure attack in a patient with anatomically narrow angles who does not have a patent iridectomy. Caution with cardiac disease, hepatic/renal impairment, and in elderly.

ADVERSE REACTIONS

Somnolence/sedation, dizziness, constipation, blurred vision, dry mouth, headache, nervousness, N/V, fatigue, abdominal/gastric disorder, nasal/sinus congestion, musculoskeletal aches/pains.

DRUG INTERACTIONS

May cause serotonin syndrome or NMS-like reactions with other serotonergic drugs (eg, SSRIs, SNRIs, triptans), drugs that impair serotonin metabolism (eg, MAOIs), antipsychotics, or other dopamine antagonists; d/c immediately if these occur. Caution with other drugs that may affect the neurotransmitter systems. Not recommended with serotonin precursors (eg, tryptophan). CYP3A4 inhibitors (eg, ritonavir, ketoconazole, indinavir) may increase levels with the potential for adverse effects. Potent CYP3A4 inhibitors may increase risk of cardiac arrhythmia; consider lower dose of trazodone. CYP3A4 inducers (eg, carbamazepine) may decrease levels; monitor to determine if a trazodone dose increase is required. Increased serum digoxin or phenytoin levels reported; monitor serum levels and adjust dosages as needed. Should not be used with an MAOI or within 14 days of discontinuing an MAOI; allow at least 14 days after stopping trazodone before starting an MAOI. May enhance response to alcohol, barbiturates, and other CNS depressants. May alter PT in patients on warfarin. Concomitant use with an antihypertensive may require a dose reduction of the antihypertensive drug. Monitor for potential risk of bleeding and use caution with NSAIDs, aspirin, and other drugs that affect coagulation or bleeding. Increased risk of hyponatremia with diuretics. Increased risk of cardiac arrhythmia with drugs that prolong QT interval or CYP3A4 inhibitors.

NURSING CONSIDERATIONS

Assessment: Assess for risk for bipolar disorder, cardiac disease (eg, recent MI), conditions that may predispose to priapism, penile anatomical deformation, volume depletion, susceptibility to angle-closure glaucoma, hepatic/renal impairment, pregnancy/nursing status, and possible drug interactions.

Monitoring: Monitor for signs/symptoms of clinical worsening, suicidality, unusual changes in behavior, mania/hypomania, serotonin syndrome, NMS-like reactions, QT/QTc interval prolongation, cardiac arrhythmias, hypotension, syncope, bleeding events, priapism, hyponatremia, angle-closure glaucoma, withdrawal symptoms, and other adverse reactions. Periodically reassess to determine the continued need for maintenance treatment.

Patient Counseling: Inform of the risks, benefits, and appropriate use of therapy. Instruct patients and caregivers to notify physician if signs of clinical worsening, changes in behavior, or suicidality occur. Instruct to report to physician the occurrence of anxiety, agitation, panic attacks, insomnia, irritability, hostility, aggressiveness, impulsivity, akathisia, hypomania, or mania. Instruct to inform physician if patient has history of bipolar disorder, cardiac disease, or MI. Caution about the risks of serotonin syndrome, angle-closure glaucoma, priapism, hypotension, syncope, bleeding, and withdrawal symptoms. Instruct men to immediately d/c use and seek emergency medical attention if erection lasts >6 hrs, whether painful or not. Caution against performing potentially hazardous tasks (eg, operating machinery) until reasonably certain that treatment does not affect them. Inform that therapy may enhance response to alcohol. Instruct to notify physician if intending to become pregnant, or breastfeeding.

Storage: 20-25°C (68-77°F); excursions permitted from 15-30°C (59-86°F).

TREANDA — bendamustine hydrochloride RX

Class: Alkylating agent

ADULT DOSAGE

Chronic Lymphocytic Leukemia

100mg/m² IV over 30 min on Days 1 and 2 of a 28-day cycle, up to 6 cycles

B-Cell Non-Hodgkin Lymphoma

Indolent B-Cell Non-Hodgkin Lymphoma That Has Progressed During or w/in 6 Months of Treatment w/ Rituximab or a Rituximab-Containing Regimen:

120mg/m² IV over 60 min on Days 1 and 2 of a 21-day cycle, up to 8 cycles

PEDIATRIC DOSAGE

Pediatric use may not have been established

DOSE MODIFICATION

Renal Impairment

CrCl <40mL/min: Not recommended for use

Hepatic Impairment

Moderate (AST or ALT 2.5-10X ULN and Total Bilirubin 1.5-3X ULN): Not recommended for use
Severe (Total Bilirubin >3X ULN): Not recommended for use

Adverse Reactions

Chronic Lymphocytic Leukemia:
Grade 4 Hematologic Toxicity: Delay
Clinically Significant ≥Grade 2 Nonhematologic Toxicity: Delay
Nonhematologic Toxicity Has Recovered to ≤Grade 1 and/or the Blood Counts Have Improved (ANC ≥1 x 10^9/L, Platelets ≥75 x 10^9/L): Reinitiate; dose reduction may be warranted
≥Grade 3 Hematologic Toxicity: Reduce to 50mg/m^2 on Days 1 and 2 of each cycle
≥Grade 3 Hematologic Toxicity Recurs: Reduce to 25mg/m^2 on Days 1 and 2 of each cycle
≥Grade 3 Nonhematologic Toxicity: Reduce to 50mg/m^2 on Days 1 and 2 of each cycle; may consider dose re-escalation in subsequent cycles

B-Cell Non-Hodgkin Lymphoma:
Grade 4 Hematologic Toxicity: Delay
Clinically Significant ≥Grade 2 Nonhematologic Toxicity: Delay
Nonhematologic Toxicity Has Recovered to ≤Grade 1 and/or the Blood Counts Have Improved (ANC ≥1 x 10^9/L, Platelets ≥75 x 10^9/L): Reinitiate; dose reduction may be warranted
Grade 4 Hematologic Toxicity: Reduce to 90mg/m^2 on Days 1 and 2 of each cycle
Grade 4 Hematologic Toxicity Recurs: Reduce to 60mg/m^2 on Days 1 and 2 of each cycle
≥Grade 3 Nonhematologic Toxicity: Reduce to 90mg/m^2 on Days 1 and 2 of each cycle
≥Grade 3 Nonhematologic Toxicity Recurs: Reduce to 60mg/m^2 on Days 1 and 2 of each cycle

ADMINISTRATION

IV route

Selection/Preparation

Do not mix or combine the 2 formulations
Admixture should be prepared as close as possible to the time of patient administration; administer diluted sol w/in 2 hrs (sol) or 3 hrs (powder)

Sol:
Withdraw and transfer for dilution in a biosafety cabinet or containment isolator using only a polypropylene syringe w/ a metal needle and a polypropylene hub
Do not use w/ devices containing polycarbonate or acrylonitrile-butadiene-styrene (eg, closed system transfer devices [CSTDs], adapters, syringes)
1. Withdraw the volume needed for the required dose (from the 90mg/mL sol)
2. Immediately transfer to a 500mL infusion bag of 0.9% NaCl. As an alternative, a 500mL infusion bag of 2.5% Dextrose/0.45% NaCl may be considered. The resulting final concentration should be w/in 0.2-0.7mg/mL

Powder:
Only use powder for inj if a CSTD or adaptor is used as supplemental protection during preparation
1. Reconstitute 25mg vial w/ 5mL of sterile water for inj and 100mg vial w/ 20mL of sterile water for inj
2. Shake well to yield a clear, colorless to a pale yellow sol w/ a concentration of 5mg/mL; should completely dissolve in 5 min and transfer reconstituted sol to infusion bag w/in 30 min of reconstitution
3. Withdraw the volume needed for the required dose and immediately transfer to 500mL infusion bag of 0.9% NaCl; as an alternative, a 500mL infusion bag of 2.5% Dextrose/0.45% NaCl may be considered
4. The resulting final concentration should be w/in 0.2-0.6mg/mL; thoroughly mix the contents of the infusion bag after transferring

HOW SUPPLIED

Inj: (Powder) 25mg, 100mg; (Sol) 45mg/0.5mL, 180mg/2mL

WARNINGS/PRECAUTIONS

Severe myelosuppression reported; may require dose delays and/or subsequent dose reductions if recovery to the recommended values has not occurred by the 1st day of the next scheduled cycle. Monitor leukocytes, platelets, Hgb, and neutrophils frequently if treatment-related myelosuppression occurs. Infection (eg, pneumonia, sepsis, septic shock) and death reported. Infusion reactions and severe anaphylactic/anaphylactoid reactions reported; monitor clinically and d/c for severe reactions. Consider measures to prevent severe reactions (eg, antihistamines, antipyretics, corticosteroids) in subsequent cycles in patients who have experienced Grade 1 or 2 infusion reactions. Consider discontinuation for Grade 3 infusion reactions as clinically appropriate; d/c for Grade 4 infusion reactions. Do not rechallenge in patients who experience

≥Grade 3 allergic-type reactions. Tumor lysis syndrome reported; preventive measures include vigorous hydration and close monitoring of blood chemistry, particularly K^+ and uric acid levels. Skin reactions (eg, rash, toxic skin reactions, and bullous exanthema) reported; monitor closely and withhold or d/c if skin reactions are severe or progressive. Premalignant and malignant diseases (eg, myelodysplastic syndrome, myeloproliferative disorders, acute myeloid leukemia, bronchial carcinoma) reported. Extravasations reported; assure good venous access prior to starting infusion and monitor for infusion-site redness, swelling, pain, infection, and necrosis during and after administration. May cause fetal harm. Caution w/ mild/moderate renal impairment and w/ mild impairment.

ADVERSE REACTIONS

Anemia, thrombocytopenia, neutropenia, lymphopenia, leukopenia, N/V, fatigue, diarrhea, pyrexia, constipation, anorexia, cough, headache, decreased weight, stomatitis.

DRUG INTERACTIONS

CYP1A2 inhibitors (eg, fluvoxamine, ciprofloxacin) may increase plasma concentrations of bendamustine and may decrease plasma concentrations of active metabolites. CYP1A2 inducers (eg, omeprazole, smoking) may decrease plasma concentrations of bendamustine and may increase plasma concentrations of active metabolites. Use caution or consider alternative treatments if treatment w/ CYP1A2 inhibitors/inducers is needed. Increased risk of severe skin toxicity w/ allopurinol.

NURSING CONSIDERATIONS

Assessment: Assess for renal/hepatic impairment, hypersensitivity to drug, pregnancy/nursing status, and possible drug interactions.

Monitoring: Monitor for signs/symptoms of myelosuppression, infections, anaphylaxis/infusion reactions, tumor lysis syndrome, skin reactions, premalignant/malignant diseases, extravasation, lab abnormalities, and other adverse reactions. Monitor CBCs and blood chemistry, particularly K^+ and uric acid levels.

Patient Counseling: Inform of the possibility of mild/serious allergic reactions and to immediately report rash, facial swelling, or difficulty breathing during or soon after infusion. Inform that therapy may cause a decrease in WBCs, platelets, and RBCs, and of the need for frequent monitoring of blood counts; instruct to report SOB, significant fatigue, bleeding, fever, or other signs of infection. Advise that therapy may cause tiredness; instruct to avoid driving or operating dangerous tools or machinery if tiredness occurs. Inform that therapy may cause N/V, diarrhea, and mild rash or itching; instruct to report any adverse reactions immediately to physician. Advise women to avoid becoming pregnant and men to use reliable contraception throughout treatment and for 3 months after discontinuation of therapy; instruct to immediately report pregnancy and to avoid nursing while on therapy.

Storage: (Sol) 2-8°C (36-47°F). Protect from light. (Powder) Up to 25°C (77°F); excursions permitted up to 30°C (86°F). Protect from light. Final Admixture: Stable for 24 hrs at 2-8°C (36-47°F) or for 2 hrs (sol) or 3 hrs (powder) at 15-30°C (59-86°F).

TREXALL – methotrexate **RX**

Class: Dihydrofolic acid reductase inhibitor

Should be used only by physicians with knowledge and experience in the use of antimetabolite therapy. Use only in life-threatening neoplastic diseases, or in patients with psoriasis or rheumatoid arthritis (RA) with severe, recalcitrant, disabling disease not adequately responsive to other forms of therapy. Deaths reported in the treatment of malignancy, psoriasis, and RA. Closely monitor for bone marrow, liver, lung, and kidney toxicities. Patients should be informed of the risks involved and be under physician's care throughout therapy. Fetal death and/or congenital anomalies reported; not recommended for women of childbearing potential unless benefits outweigh risks. Contraindicated in pregnant women with psoriasis or RA. Reduced elimination with impaired renal function, ascites, or pleural effusions; monitor for toxicity and reduce dose or d/c in some cases. Unexpectedly severe (sometimes fatal) bone marrow suppression, aplastic anemia, and GI toxicity reported with coadministration of therapy (usually high dosage) with some NSAIDs. Causes hepatotoxicity, fibrosis, and cirrhosis (generally only after prolonged use); perform periodic liver biopsies in psoriatic patients on long-term therapy. Acutely, liver enzyme elevations frequently seen. Drug-induced lung disease may occur acutely at any time during therapy and reported at low doses. Interrupt therapy if pulmonary symptoms (especially a dry, nonproductive cough), diarrhea, or ulcerative stomatitis occurs. Malignant lymphomas, which may regress following withdrawal of treatment, may occur with low-dose therapy and, thus, may not require cytotoxic treatment; d/c therapy 1st and, if lymphoma does not regress, institute appropriate treatment. May induce tumor lysis syndrome in patients with rapidly growing tumors; may be prevented/alleviated by appropriate supportive and pharmacologic measures. Severe, occasionally fatal, skin reactions reported. Potentially fatal opportunistic infections, especially *Pneumocystis carinii* pneumonia, may occur. Concomitant use with radiotherapy may increase risk of soft tissue necrosis and osteonecrosis.

ADULT DOSAGE

Choriocarcinoma/Trophoblastic Diseases

Gestational choriocarcinoma, chorio-adenoma destruens, and hydatidiform mole

15-30mg/day for a 5-day course

Courses are usually repeated 3-5X as required, w/ rest periods of one or more weeks interposed between courses, until any manifesting toxic symptoms subside

Acute Lymphoblastic Leukemia

Induction: 3.3mg/m^2/day + prednisone 60mg/m^2/day
Maint of Remission: 30mg/m^2/week, administered 2X weekly

If and when relapse occurs, repeat the initial induction regimen to obtain reinduction of remission

Lymphomas

Burkitt's Tumor:
Stages I-II:
Usual: 10-25mg/day for 4-8 days
Stage III:
Methotrexate is commonly given concomitantly w/ other anti-tumor agents

Treatment in all stages usually consists of several courses of the drug interposed w/ 7- to 10-day rest periods

Lymphosarcoma:
Stage III: May respond to combined drug therapy w/ methotrexate given in doses of 0.625-2.5mg/kg/day

Mycosis Fungoides (Cutaneous T-Cell Lymphoma)

Early Stages:
Usual: 5-50mg once weekly

Methotrexate has also been administered twice weekly in doses ranging from 15-37.5mg in patients who have responded poorly to weekly therapy

Rheumatoid Arthritis

Severe, active rheumatoid arthritis (ACR criteria) in patients who have had an insufficient therapeutic response to, or are intolerant of, an adequate trial of 1st-line therapy including full-dose NSAIDs

Initial:
Single-Dose Schedule: 7.5mg once weekly
Divided-Dose Schedule: 2.5mg at 12-hr intervals for 3 doses given as a course once weekly
Titrate: Adjust dose gradually to achieve optimal response; significant increase in incidence and severity of serious toxic reactions, especially bone marrow suppression, reported at doses >20 mg/week

Psoriasis

Symptomatic control of severe, recalcitrant, disabling psoriasis not adequately responsive to other forms of therapy, but only when the diagnosis has been established, as by a biopsy and/or after dermatologic consultation

Initial:
Single-Dose Schedule: 10-25mg/week until adequate response is achieved

PEDIATRIC DOSAGE

Acute Lymphoblastic Leukemia

Induction: 3.3mg/m^2/day + prednisone 60mg/m^2/day
Maint of Remission: 30mg/m^2/week, administered 2X weekly

If and when relapse occurs, repeat the initial induction regimen to obtain reinduction of remission

Juvenile Rheumatoid Arthritis

Active polyarticular-course juvenile rheumatoid arthritis in patients who have had an insufficient therapeutic response to, or are intolerant of, an adequate trial of 1st-line therapy including full dose NSAIDs

2-16 Years:
Initial: 10mg/m^2 once weekly
Titrate: Adjust dose gradually to achieve optimal response; there is experience w/ doses up to 30mg/m^2/week, however there are too few published data to assess how doses >20mg/m^2/week might affect the risk of serious toxicity

Divided-Dose Schedule: 2.5mg at 12-hr intervals for 3 doses

Titrate: Adjust dose gradually to achieve optimal response; 30mg/week should not ordinarily be exceeded

Once optimal response is achieved, each dosage schedule should be reduced to the lowest possible amount of drug and to the longest possible rest period

Other Indications

Alone or in combination w/ other anticancer agents in the treatment of breast cancer, epidermoid cancers of the head and neck, and lung cancer, particularly squamous cell and small cell types. Methotrexate is also used in combination w/ other chemotherapeutic agents in the treatment of advanced stage non-Hodgkin's lymphomas

DOSE MODIFICATION

Elderly

Consider relatively low doses and closely monitor for early signs of toxicity

ADMINISTRATION

Oral route

HOW SUPPLIED

Tab: 5mg*, 7.5mg*, 10mg*, 15mg* *scored

CONTRAINDICATIONS

Pregnant women with psoriasis or RA (should be used in treatment of pregnant women with neoplastic diseases only when potential benefit outweighs risk to the fetus), nursing mothers. Psoriasis or RA patients with alcoholism, alcoholic liver disease, chronic liver disease, immunodeficiency syndromes, or preexisting blood dyscrasias (eg, bone marrow hypoplasia, leukopenia, thrombocytopenia, significant anemia).

WARNINGS/PRECAUTIONS

Toxic effects may be related to dose/frequency of administration; if toxicity occurs, reduce dose or d/c therapy and take appropriate corrective measures, which may include use of leucovorin calcium and/or acute, intermittent hemodialysis with high-flux dialyzer, if necessary. If therapy is reinstituted, carry it out with caution, with adequate consideration of further need for the drug and increased alertness as to possible recurrence of toxicity. Caution in elderly/debilitated. Avoid pregnancy if either partner is receiving therapy (during and for a minimum of 3 months after therapy for male patients, and during and for at least 1 ovulatory cycle after therapy for female patients). May cause multiple organ system toxicities (eg, GI, hematologic). May cause impairment of fertility, oligospermia, and menstrual dysfunction during and for a short period after cessation of therapy.

ADVERSE REACTIONS

Bone marrow/liver/lung/kidney toxicities, diarrhea, ulcerative stomatitis, malignant lymphomas, tumor lysis syndrome, skin reactions, opportunistic infections, nausea, abdominal distress, malaise, undue fatigue, chills.

DRUG INTERACTIONS

See Boxed Warning. Elevated and prolonged levels with coadministration of high-dose therapy with NSAIDs; caution when NSAIDs or salicylates are administered concomitantly with lower doses of therapy. Toxicity may be increased due to displacement by salicylates, phenylbutazone, phenytoin, and sulfonamides. Renal tubular transport diminished by probenecid. Oral antibiotics (eg, tetracycline, chloramphenicol, nonabsorbable broad spectrum antibiotics) may decrease intestinal absorption or interfere with enterohepatic circulation. Penicillins may reduce renal clearance; hematologic and GI toxicity observed. Closely monitor for increased risk of hepatotoxicity with hepatotoxins (eg, azathioprine, retinoids, sulfasalazine). May decrease theophylline clearance; monitor theophylline levels. Vitamin preparations containing folic acid or its derivatives may decrease responses; high doses of leucovorin may reduce efficacy of intrathecally administered drug. Trimethoprim/sulfamethoxazole may increase bone marrow suppression by an additive antifolate effect. Immunization may be ineffective when given during therapy; immunization with live virus vaccines is generally not recommended. Disseminated vaccinia infections after smallpox immunizations reported. Combined use with gold, penicillamine, hydroxychloroquine, sulfasalazine, or cytotoxic agents may increase incidence of adverse effects.

NURSING CONSIDERATIONS

Assessment: Assess for alcoholism, alcoholic/chronic liver disease, immunodeficiency, blood dyscrasias, ascites, pleural effusions, tumors, hypersensitivity to drug, pregnancy/nursing status, any other condition where treatment is cautioned or contraindicated, and possible drug interactions. Obtain baseline CBC with differential and platelet counts, hepatic enzymes, renal function tests, liver biopsy, and chest x-ray.

Monitoring: Monitor for toxicities of bone marrow, liver, lung, kidney and GI, diarrhea, ulcerative stomatitis, malignant lymphoma, tumor lysis syndrome, skin reactions, opportunistic infections, and other adverse reactions. Monitor hematology at least monthly and renal/hepatic function every 1-2 months during therapy of RA/psoriasis and more frequently during antineoplastic therapy, during initial/changing doses, or during periods of increased risk of elevated drug levels (eg, dehydration). If drug-induced lung disease is suspected, perform pulmonary function tests.

Patient Counseling: Inform of the early signs/symptoms of toxicity, the need to see physician promptly if toxicity occurs, and the need for close follow-up, including periodic lab tests to monitor toxicity. Emphasize that the recommended dose is taken weekly in RA and psoriasis, and that mistaken daily use of recommended dose has led to fatal toxicity. Counsel about risks/benefits of therapy, and effects on reproduction.

Storage: 20-25°C (68-77°F). Protect from light.

TREXIMET – naproxen sodium/sumatriptan RX

Class: 5-HT_1-agonist/NSAID

May increase risk of serious cardiovascular (CV) thrombotic events, myocardial infarction (MI), and stroke; increased risk with duration of use and with cardiovascular disease (CVD) or risk factors for CVD. Increased risk of serious GI adverse events (eg, bleeding, ulceration, stomach/intestinal perforation) that can be fatal and occur anytime during use without warning symptoms; elderly patients are at greater risk.

ADULT DOSAGE

Migraine

Attacks w/ or w/o Aura:
Usual: 1 tab
Max: 2 tabs/24 hrs

Dosing should be at least 2 hrs apart

PEDIATRIC DOSAGE

Pediatric use may not have been established

ADMINISTRATION

Oral route

Give 1st dose in physician's office or similar medically staffed and equipped facility unless patient has previously received sumatriptan
Take w/ or w/o food
Do not split, crush, or chew

HOW SUPPLIED

Tab: (Naproxen-Sumatriptan): 500mg-85mg

CONTRAINDICATIONS

History, symptoms, or signs of ischemic cardiac syndromes (eg, angina pectoris, MI, silent myocardial ischemia), cerebrovascular syndromes (eg, strokes, transient ischemic attacks), or peripheral vascular syndromes (eg, ischemic bowel disease). Other significant CVD, coronary artery bypass graft (CABG) surgery, hepatic impairment, uncontrolled HTN, hemiplegic or basilar migraine, concurrent administration of MAO-A inhibitors or use within 2 weeks of discontinuation of an MAO-A inhibitor, use within 24 hrs of any ergotamine-containing or ergot-type drugs (eg, dihydroergotamine, methysergide) or other 5-HT_1 agonists. Patients who have experienced asthma, rhinitis, nasal polyps, or allergic-type reactions after taking aspirin (ASA) or other NSAIDs.

WARNINGS/PRECAUTIONS

May cause coronary artery vasospasm; do not give with documented ischemic/vasospastic coronary artery disease (CAD). Avoid in patients whom unrecognized CAD is predicted by the presence of risk factors (eg, HTN, hypercholesterolemia, smoker, obesity, diabetes, strong CAD family history, menopause, males >40 yrs) unless with a satisfactory CV evaluation; administer 1st dose under medical supervision and consider obtaining an ECG immediately following administration. Signs and symptoms suggestive of decreased arterial flow should be evaluated for atherosclerosis or predisposition to vasospasm. Chest discomfort, jaw or neck tightness, peripheral vascular ischemia, and colonic ischemia reported. Transient and permanent blindness and significant partial vision loss have been reported with the use of sumatriptan. Caution with controlled HTN, fluid retention, and heart failure (HF). Serotonin syndrome may occur. Anaphylactic/anaphylactoid reactions may occur; avoid in patients with ASA triad. May cause serious skin reactions (eg, exfoliative dermatitis, Stevens-Johnson syndrome, toxic epidermal necrolysis); d/c at 1st appearance of skin rash/hypersensitivity. Avoid in late pregnancy; may cause premature closure of ductus arteriosus. Caution with diseases that may alter absorption/metabolism/excretion, preexisting asthma, history of epilepsy or conditions associated with a lowered seizure threshold. Renal injury reported with long-term use; increased risk with renal/hepatic impairment, HF, and in elderly. Not recommended in patients with CrCl <30mL/min. Exclude potentially serious neurologic conditions before treatment in patients not previously diagnosed with migraine headache or who experience headache that is atypical for them. Anemia may occur; monitor Hgb/Hct if signs/symptoms of anemia develop. May prolong bleeding time; caution with coagulation disorders. D/C if signs and symptoms of liver/renal disease develop, systemic manifestations (eg, eosinophilia) occur, or abnormal LFTs persist or worsen. Use lowest effective dose for the shortest duration possible. Caution with prior history of ulcer disease, GI bleeding, risk factors for GI bleeding, history of inflammatory bowel disease. Overuse may lead to exacerbation of headache.

ADVERSE REACTIONS

CV thrombotic events, MI, stroke, GI events, dizziness, somnolence, nausea, chest discomfort/pain, neck/throat/jaw pain/tightness/pressure.

DRUG INTERACTIONS

See Contraindications. Avoid with other naproxen-containing products. Caution with methotrexate; may prolong serum methotrexate levels. Not recommended with ASA. Increased plasma lithium levels; monitor for lithium toxicity. May reduce natriuretic effect of loop (eg, furosemide) or thiazide diuretics; monitor for signs of renal failure and diuretic efficacy. Probenecid may increase levels. May reduce the antihypertensive effect of ACE inhibitors and β-blockers (eg, propranolol). Increased risk of renal toxicity with diuretics and ACE inhibitors. Increased risk of GI bleeding with PO corticosteroids or anticoagulants, warfarin, alcohol use, and smoking. Serotonin syndrome reported, particularly during combined use with SSRIs or SNRIs.

NURSING CONSIDERATIONS

Assessment: Assess for conditions where treatment is contraindicated or cautioned, pregnancy/nursing status, and possible drug interactions. Obtain ECG after 1st administration for those with CAD risk factors.

Monitoring: Monitor for signs/symptoms of cardiac events, colonic ischemia, bloody diarrhea, serotonin syndrome, hypersensitivity reactions, jaw/neck tightness, seizures, headache, signs and symptoms of GI adverse events, and clinical response. For long-term therapy or with CAD risk factors, perform periodic monitoring of CV function. Monitor vital signs, CBC, LFTs, bleeding time, renal function, and ECG periodically.

Patient Counseling: Inform to seek medical advice if symptoms of CV events, GI ulcerations/bleeding, skin/hypersensitivity reactions, unexplained weight gain or edema, hepatotoxicity, anaphylactic/anaphylactoid reactions occur. Instruct to notify physician if pregnant, planning to become pregnant, or nursing. Inform about the risk of serotonin syndrome, particularly during combined use with SSRIs or SNRIs. Advise to use caution with activities that require alertness if they experience drowsiness, dizziness, vertigo, or depression during therapy.

Storage: 25°C (77°F); excursions permitted to 15-30°C (59-86°F).

TREZIX – acetaminophen/caffeine/dihydrocodeine bitartrate CIII

Class: Opioid analgesic

Respiratory depression and death have occurred in children who received codeine following tonsillectomy and/or adenoidectomy and had evidence of being ultra-rapid metabolizers of codeine due to a CYP2D6 polymorphism. Acetaminophen (APAP) has been associated with cases of acute liver failure, at times resulting in liver transplant and death. Most cases of liver injury are associated with APAP use at doses >4000mg/day, and often involve >1 APAP-containing product.

ADULT DOSAGE

Moderate to Moderately Severe Pain

Usual: 2 caps q4h PRN
Max: 2 caps/4 hr; 5 doses (10 caps)/24 hrs

PEDIATRIC DOSAGE

Pediatric use may not have been established

DOSE MODIFICATION

Renal Impairment

Reduce dose

ADMINISTRATION

Oral route

HOW SUPPLIED
Cap: (APAP-Caffeine-Dihydrocodeine) 320.5mg-30mg-16mg

CONTRAINDICATIONS
Postoperative pain management in children who have undergone tonsillectomy and/or adenoidectomy; significant respiratory depression (in unmonitored settings or in the absence of resuscitative equipment); acute or severe bronchial asthma or hypercapnia; paralytic ileus.

WARNINGS/PRECAUTIONS
May produce orthostatic hypotension in ambulatory patients; caution in patients in circulatory shock. May aggravate convulsions in patients with convulsive disorders. Caution in elderly or debilitated patients or those with acute alcoholism, adrenocortical insufficiency (eg, Addison's disease), asthma, CNS depression or coma, chronic obstructive pulmonary disease, decreased respiratory reserve (eg, emphysema, severe obesity, cor pulmonale, kyphoscoliosis), delirium tremens, head injury, hypotension, increased intracranial pressure (ICP), myxedema or hypothyroidism, prostatic hypertrophy or urethral stricture, toxic psychosis, and hepatic/renal impairment. May obscure diagnosis or clinical course of acute abdominal conditions. Not recommended for use by women during and immediately before labor and delivery; may cause respiratory depression in the newborn. APAP: Increased risk of acute liver failure in patients with underlying liver disease. Rarely, may cause serious skin reactions (eg, acute generalized exanthematous pustulosis, Stevens-Johnson syndrome, toxic epidermal necrolysis), which can be fatal; d/c at the 1st appearance of skin rash or any other sign of hypersensitivity. Hypersensitivity and anaphylaxis reported; avoid in patients with APAP allergy. Caution when using large doses in malnourished patients or those with history of chronic alcohol abuse; may be more susceptible to hepatic damage. Dihydrocodeine: Deaths reported in nursing infants exposed to high levels of morphine because their mothers were ultra-rapid metabolizers of codeine. Ultra-rapid metabolizers, due to specific CYP2D6 genotype (gene duplications denoted as *1/*1xN or *1/*2xN), may have life-threatening or fatal respiratory depression or experience signs of overdose (eg, extreme sleepiness, confusion, shallow breathing). Use lowest effective dose for the shortest period. May impair mental and/or physical abilities. May cause respiratory depression, most frequently in elderly or debilitated patients, usually after large initial doses in nontolerant patients; caution in patients with cor pulmonale, hypoxia hypercapnia, or respiratory depression; consider alternative nonopioid analgesics and administer opioids only under careful medical supervision. May obscure neurologic signs of increases in ICP in patients with head injuries. Respiratory depressant effects and secondary elevation of CSF pressure may be markedly exaggerated in the presence of head injury, intracranial lesions, or other causes of increased ICP. May cause hypotension in patients whose ability to maintain BP has been compromised by a depleted blood volume. May produce drug dependence and has potential for abuse. May cause spasms of the sphincter of Oddi; caution with biliary tract disease, including pancreatitis. Caffeine: May produce CNS and cardiovascular (CV) stimulation and GI irritation.

ADVERSE REACTIONS
Respiratory depression, acute liver failure, light-headedness, dizziness, drowsiness, headache, fatigue, sedation, sweating, N/V, constipation, pruritus, skin reactions, anxiety, excitement.

DRUG INTERACTIONS
Agonist/antagonist analgesics (eg, pentazocine, nalbuphine, butorphanol, buprenorphine) may reduce analgesic effect. Dihydrocodeine: Concomitant administration with other opioid analgesics, sedatives or hypnotics, muscle relaxants, general anesthetics, centrally acting antiemetics, phenothiazines or other tranquilizers, or alcohol may cause additive CNS depressant effects; when combination is contemplated, reduce dose of one or both agents. May cause respiratory depression with other agents that depress respiration. Concurrent use with phenothiazines or other agents that compromise vasomotor tone may cause hypotension. Caution with MAOIs; may cause CNS excitation and HTN. APAP: Chronic/excessive alcohol consumption may increase hepatotoxic risk. Risk may also be increased in patients receiving anticonvulsants that induce hepatic microsomal enzymes (eg, phenytoin, barbiturates, carbamazepine) or isoniazid. Chronic ingestion of large doses may slightly potentiate the effects of warfarin- and indandione-derivative anticoagulants. Severe hypothermia is possible with phenothiazines. Caffeine: May enhance the cardiac inotropic effects of β-adrenergic stimulating agents. Coadministration with disulfiram may decrease clearance. May increase the metabolism of phenobarbital and aspirin. Caffeine accumulation may occur when products or foods containing caffeine are consumed concomitantly with quinolones (eg, ciprofloxacin).

NURSING CONSIDERATIONS

Assessment: Assess for severity of pain, hypersensitivity to drug, significant respiratory depression, bronchial asthma, hypercapnia, paralytic ileus, hepatic/renal impairment, head injury, intracranial lesions, acute abdominal conditions, history of drug abuse or seizures, any other conditions where treatment is cautioned, pregnancy/nursing status, and possible drug interactions.

Monitoring: Monitor for signs/symptoms of hepatotoxicity, respiratory depression, hypotension, skin reactions, hypersensitivity, anaphylaxis, elevation in CSF pressure, drug abuse, tolerance, dependence, GI irritation, and other adverse reactions.

Patient Counseling: Instruct to d/c therapy and contact physician immediately if signs of allergy develop. Instruct to look for APAP on package labels and not to use >1 APAP-containing product. Instruct to seek medical attention immediately upon ingestion of >4000mg/day APAP, even if feeling well. Advise that drug may impair mental/physical abilities. Advise to report adverse experiences occurring during therapy. Advise not to adjust dose without consulting prescribing physician. Instruct not to combine medication with alcohol or other CNS depressants (sleep aids, tranquilizers) except by the orders of the prescribing physician, because additive effects may occur. Advise women of childbearing potential who become or are planning to become pregnant to consult their physician regarding the effects of analgesics and other drug use during pregnancy on themselves and their unborn child. Advise of the potential for abuse; instruct to protect drug from theft and never to give to anyone other than the individual for whom it was prescribed.

Storage: 20-25°C (68-77°F). Dispense in a tight, light-resistant container with a child-resistant closure. Protect from moisture.

TRIBENZOR – amlodipine/hydrochlorothiazide/olmesartan medoxomil RX

Class: ARB/calcium channel blocker (dihydropyridine)/thiazide diuretic

D/C when pregnancy is detected. Drugs that act directly on the renin-angiotensin system (RAS) can cause injury/death to the developing fetus.

ADULT DOSAGE

Hypertension

Usual: Dose qd
Titrate: May increase dose after 2 weeks
Max: 40mg/10mg/25mg qd

Replacement Therapy:
May substitute for individually titrated components

Add-On/Switch Therapy:
May use for patients not adequately controlled on any 2 of the following classes: ARBs, calcium channel blockers (CCBs), and diuretics
Patients w/ dose-limiting adverse reactions to an individual component while on any dual combination of the components of therapy may be switched to therapy containing a lower dose of that component

PEDIATRIC DOSAGE

Pediatric use may not have been established

DOSE MODIFICATION

Hepatic Impairment
Severe:
Initial: 2.5mg amlodipine

Elderly
≥75 Years:
Initial: 2.5mg amlodipine

ADMINISTRATION

Oral route
Take w/ or w/o food

HOW SUPPLIED

Tab: (Olmesartan/Amlodipine/HCTZ) 20mg/5mg/12.5mg, 40mg/5mg/12.5mg, 40mg/5mg/25mg, 40mg/10mg/12.5mg, 40mg/10mg/25mg

CONTRAINDICATIONS

Anuria, sulfonamide-derived drug hypersensitivity. Coadministration with aliskiren in patients with diabetes.

WARNINGS/PRECAUTIONS

Not for initial therapy. Avoid use with severe renal impairment (CrCl ≤30mL/min). Renal impairment reported; consider withholding or discontinuing either diuretic or ARBs if progressive renal impairment becomes evident. Sprue-like enteropathy with symptoms of severe, chronic diarrhea with substantial weight loss reported; exclude other etiologies if these symptoms develop and consider discontinuation in cases where no other etiology is identified. Olmesartan: Symptomatic hypotension may occur in patients with an activated RAS (eg, volume- and/or salt-depleted patients [eg, those being treated with high doses of diuretics]). Oliguria or progressive azotemia and (rarely) with acute renal failure and/or death may occur in patients whose renal function may depend upon the activity of the renin-angiotensin-aldosterone system (eg, with severe CHF). May increase SrCr and BUN levels in patients with renal artery stenosis. Increased blood creatinine levels and hyperkalemia reported. Amlodipine: May develop increased frequency, duration, or severity of angina or acute MI, particularly with severe obstructive coronary artery disease (CAD). Rare reports of acute hypotension; caution with severe aortic stenosis. Hepatic enzyme elevations reported. HCTZ: May precipitate azotemia with renal disease and hepatic coma due to fluid and electrolyte imbalance. Observe for clinical signs of fluid or electrolyte imbalance (eg, hyponatremia, hypochloremic alkalosis, hypokalemia). Hypokalemia may sensitize/exaggerate the response of the heart to toxic effects of digitalis. May cause metabolic acidosis, hyperuricemia or precipitation of frank gout, hyperglycemia, manifestation of latent diabetes mellitus (DM), hypomagnesemia, hypersensitivity reactions (with or without a history of allergy or bronchial asthma), exacerbation/activation of systemic lupus erythematosus (SLE), and increased cholesterol and TG levels. Enhanced effects in postsympathectomy patients. D/C before carrying out tests for parathyroid function. May cause idiosyncratic reaction, resulting in acute transient myopia and acute angle-closure glaucoma; d/c as rapidly as possible.

ADVERSE REACTIONS

Dizziness, peripheral edema, headache, fatigue, nasopharyngitis, muscle spasms, nausea.

DRUG INTERACTIONS

See Contraindications. Olmesartan: NSAIDs, including selective COX-2 inhibitors, may attenuate antihypertensive effect and result in deterioration of renal function, including possible acute renal failure; monitor renal function periodically. Dual blockade of the RAS is associated with increased risk of hypotension, hyperkalemia, and changes in renal function (including acute renal failure); avoid combined use of RAS inhibitors or closely monitor BP, renal function, and electrolytes with concomitant agents that affect the RAS. Avoid with aliskiren in patients with renal impairment (GFR <60mL/min). Reduced systemic exposure and levels with colesevelam; administer at least 4 hrs before colesevelam dose. Amlodipine: May increase simvastatin exposure; limit simvastatin dose to 20mg daily. HCTZ: Alcohol, barbiturates, or narcotics may potentiate orthostatic hypotension. Dose adjustment of antidiabetic drugs (eg, oral agents, insulin) may be required. Additive effect or potentiation with other antihypertensives. Anionic exchange resins (eg, cholestyramine, colestipol) may impair absorption. Corticosteroids and adrenocorticotropic hormone may intensify electrolyte depletion, particularly hypokalemia. May decrease response to pressor amines (eg, norepinephrine). May increase response to nondepolarizing skeletal muscle relaxants (eg, tubocurarine). NSAIDs may reduce diuretic, natriuretic, and antihypertensive effects. Olmesartan/HCTZ: Increases in serum lithium concentrations and lithium toxicity reported; monitor lithium levels.

NURSING CONSIDERATIONS

Assessment: Assess for anuria, sulfonamide-derived drug hypersensitivity, aortic stenosis, renal artery stenosis, SLE, CHF, volume/salt depletion, electrolyte imbalances, postsympathectomy status, DM, CAD, renal/hepatic impairment, pregnancy/nursing status, any other conditions where treatment is cautioned, and possible drug interactions.

Monitoring: Monitor for signs/symptoms of hypotension, angina, MI, fluid/electrolyte imbalance, latent DM, sprue-like enteropathy, exacerbation/activation of SLE, hypersensitivity/idiosyncratic reactions, metabolic disturbances, myopia and angle-closure glaucoma, and other adverse reactions. Monitor BP, serum electrolytes, cholesterol and TG levels, and renal/hepatic function.

Patient Counseling: Inform female of childbearing potential of the consequences of exposure during pregnancy and of the treatment options for women planning to become pregnant; instruct to report pregnancy to physician as soon as possible. Counsel that lightheadedness may occur, especially during the 1st days of therapy; instruct to report to physician. Instruct to d/c therapy and consult physician if syncope occurs. Advise that inadequate fluid intake, excessive perspiration, diarrhea, or vomiting may lead to an excessive fall in BP, which may result in lightheadedness and possible syncope.

Storage: 25°C (77°F); excursions permitted to 15-30°C (59-86°F).

TRICOR – fenofibrate RX

Class: Fibric acid derivative

ADULT DOSAGE

Primary Hypercholesterolemia/Mixed Dyslipidemia

Initial/Max: 145mg qd

Titrate: May consider reducing dose if lipid levels fall significantly below the targeted range

D/C if no adequate response after 2 months of treatment w/ max dose

Severe Hypertriglyceridemia

Initial: 48-145mg/day

Titrate: Adjust dose if necessary following repeat lipid determinations at 4- to 8-week intervals; may consider reducing dose if lipid levels fall significantly below the targeted range

Max: 145mg qd

D/C if no adequate response after 2 months of treatment w/ max dose

PEDIATRIC DOSAGE

Pediatric use may not have been established

DOSE MODIFICATION

Renal Impairment

Mild to Moderate:

Initial: 48mg/day

Titrate: Increase only after evaluation of effects on renal function and lipid levels

ADMINISTRATION

Oral route

May be taken w/o regard to meals

Swallow tab whole

HOW SUPPLIED

Tab: 48mg, 145mg

CONTRAINDICATIONS

Severe renal impairment (including dialysis), active liver disease (including primary biliary cirrhosis and unexplained persistent liver function abnormalities), preexisting gallbladder disease, and nursing mothers.

WARNINGS/PRECAUTIONS

Not shown to reduce coronary heart disease morbidity and mortality in patients with type 2 diabetes mellitus (DM). Increased risk of myopathy and rhabdomyolysis; risk increased with DM, renal insufficiency, hypothyroidism, and in elderly. D/C therapy if marked CPK elevation occurs or myopathy/myositis is suspected or diagnosed. Increases in serum transaminases, hepatocellular, chronic active and cholestatic hepatitis, and cirrhosis (rare) reported; perform baseline and regular periodic monitoring of LFTs, and d/c therapy if enzyme levels persist >3X the normal limit. Elevations in SrCr reported; monitor renal function in patients with renal impairment or at risk for renal insufficiency. May cause cholelithiasis; d/c if gallstones are found. Acute hypersensitivity reactions and pancreatitis reported. Mild to moderate decreases in Hgb, Hct and WBCs, thrombocytopenia, and agranulocytosis reported; periodically monitor RBC and WBC counts during the first 12 months of therapy. May cause venothromboembolic disease. Severe decreases in HDL levels reported; check HDL levels within the 1st few months after initiation of therapy. If a severely depressed HDL level is detected, withdraw therapy, monitor HDL level until it has returned to baseline, and do not reinitiate therapy. Estrogen therapy, thiazide diuretics, and β-blockers may be associated with massive rises in plasma TG; discontinuation of these drugs may obviate the need for specific drug therapy of hypertriglyceridemia.

ADVERSE REACTIONS

Abnormal LFTs, respiratory disorder, abdominal pain, back pain, increased AST/ALT/CPK, headache.

DRUG INTERACTIONS

Increased risk of rhabdomyolysis with HMG-CoA reductase inhibitors (statins); avoid combination unless benefit outweighs risk. May potentiate anticoagulant effects of coumarin anticoagulants; use with caution, reduce anticoagulant dosage, and monitor PT/INR frequently. Immunosuppressants (eg, cyclosporine, tacrolimus) may produce nephrotoxicity; consider benefits and risks, use lowest effective dose, and monitor renal function with immunosuppressants and other potentially nephrotoxic agents. Bile acid-binding resins may bind other drugs given concurrently; take at least 1 hr before or 4-6 hrs after the bile acid-binding resin to avoid impeding its absorption. Cases of myopathy, including rhabdomyolysis, reported when coadministered with colchicine; caution when prescribing with colchicine.

NURSING CONSIDERATIONS

Assessment: Assess for renal impairment, active liver disease, preexisting gallbladder disease, other medical conditions (eg, DM, hypothyroidism), hypersensitivity to drug, pregnancy/nursing status, and possible drug interactions. Obtain baseline LFTs.

Monitoring: Monitor for signs/symptoms of myositis, myopathy, or rhabdomyolysis; measure CPK levels in patients reporting such symptoms. Monitor for cholelithiasis, pancreatitis, hypersensitivity reactions, pulmonary embolism, and deep vein thrombosis. Monitor renal function, LFTs, CBC, and lipid levels. Monitor PT/INR frequently with coumarin anticoagulants.

Patient Counseling: Advise of potential benefits and risks of therapy, and of medications to avoid during treatment. Instruct to follow appropriate lipid-modifying diet during therapy and to take drug qd, at the prescribed dose. Instruct to inform physician of all medications, supplements, and herbal preparations being taken, any changes in medical condition, development of muscle pain, tenderness, or weakness, and onset of abdominal pain or any other new symptoms. Advise to return for routine monitoring.

Storage: 25°C (77°F); excursions permitted to 15-30°C (59-86°F). Protect from moisture.

TRIGLIDE – fenofibrate RX

Class: Fibric acid derivative

ADULT DOSAGE

Primary Hypercholesterolemia/Mixed Dyslipidemia

Usual/Max: 160mg qd

Titrate: May consider reducing dose if lipid levels fall significantly below the targeted range

D/C if no adequate response after 2 months of treatment w/ max dose

Severe Hypertriglyceridemia

Initial: 50-160mg/day

Titrate: Adjust dose if necessary following repeat lipid determinations at 4- to 8-week intervals; may consider reducing dose if lipid levels fall significantly below the targeted range

Max: 160mg qd

D/C if no adequate response after 2 months of treatment w/ max dose

PEDIATRIC DOSAGE

Pediatric use may not have been established

DOSE MODIFICATION

Renal Impairment

Mild to Moderate:

Initial: 50mg/day

Titrate: Increase only after evaluation of effects on renal function and lipid levels

ADMINISTRATION

Oral route

May be taken w/o regard to meals

Swallow tab whole; do not crush, dissolve, or chew

HOW SUPPLIED

Tab: 50mg, 160mg

CONTRAINDICATIONS

Severe renal impairment (including dialysis), active liver disease (including primary biliary cirrhosis and unexplained persistent liver function abnormalities), preexisting gallbladder disease, and nursing mothers.

WARNINGS/PRECAUTIONS

Not shown to reduce coronary heart disease morbidity and mortality in patients with type 2 diabetes mellitus (DM). Increased risk of myopathy and rhabdomyolysis; risk increased with DM, renal insufficiency, hypothyroidism, and in elderly. D/C if marked CPK elevation occurs or myopathy/myositis is suspected. Increases in serum transaminases, hepatocellular, chronic active and cholestatic hepatitis, and cirrhosis (rare) reported; perform baseline and regular periodic monitoring of LFTs, and d/c therapy if enzyme levels persist >3X the normal limit. Elevations in SrCr reported. May cause cholelithiasis; d/c if gallstones are found. Acute hypersensitivity reactions and pancreatitis reported. Mild to moderate decreases in Hgb, Hct and WBCs, thrombocytopenia, and agranulocytosis reported; periodically monitor RBC and WBC counts during the first 12 months of therapy. May cause venothromboembolic disease. Severe decreases in HDL levels reported; check HDL levels within the 1st few months after initiation of therapy. If a severely depressed HDL level is detected, withdraw therapy, monitor HDL level until it has returned to baseline, and do not reinitiate therapy. Estrogen therapy, thiazide diuretics, and β-blockers may be associated with massive rises in plasma TG; d/c of these drugs may obviate the need for specific drug therapy of hypertriglyceridemia.

ADVERSE REACTIONS

Abnormal LFTs, respiratory disorder, abdominal pain, back pain, increased AST/ALT/CPK, headache.

DRUG INTERACTIONS

Increased risk of rhabdomyolysis with HMG-CoA reductase inhibitors (statins); avoid combination unless benefit outweighs risk. May potentiate anticoagulant effects of coumarin anticoagulants; use with caution, reduce anticoagulant dosage, and monitor PT/INR frequently. Immunosuppressants (eg, cyclosporine, tacrolimus) may produce nephrotoxicity; consider benefits and risks, use lowest effective dose, and monitor renal function with immunosuppressants and other potentially nephrotoxic agents. Bile acid-binding resins may bind other drugs given concurrently; take at least 1 hr before or 4-6 hrs after the bile acid-binding resin to avoid impeding its absorption. Cases of myopathy, including rhabdomyolysis, reported when coadministered with colchicine; caution when prescribing with colchicine. Changes in exposure/levels with atorvastatin, pravastatin, fluvastatin, glimepiride, metformin, and rosiglitazone.

NURSING CONSIDERATIONS

Assessment: Assess for renal impairment, active liver disease, preexisting gallbladder disease, other medical conditions (eg, DM, hypothyroidism), hypersensitivity to the drug, pregnancy/nursing status, and possible drug interactions. Obtain baseline LFTs.

Monitoring: Monitor for signs/symptoms of myositis, myopathy, or rhabdomyolysis; measure CPK levels in patients reporting such symptoms. Monitor for cholelithiasis, pancreatitis, hypersensitivity reactions, pulmonary embolism, and deep vein thrombosis. Monitor renal function, LFTs, CBC, and lipid levels.

Patient Counseling: Advise of potential benefits and risks of therapy, and medications to be avoided during treatment. Instruct to follow appropriate lipid-modifying diet during therapy, and to take drug ud. Instruct to notify physician of all medications, supplements, and herbal preparations being taken, any changes in medical condition, development of muscle pain, tenderness, or weakness, and onset of abdominal pain, or any other new symptoms. Advise to return for routine monitoring.

Storage: 20-25°C (68-77°F); excursions permitted to 15-30°C (59-86°F). Protect from light and moisture.

TRILEPTAL – oxcarbazepine RX

Class: Dibenzazepine

ADULT DOSAGE

Partial Seizures

Adjunctive Therapy:
Initial: 300mg bid
Titrate: Increase by a max of 600mg/day at weekly intervals
Usual: 1200mg/day

Conversion to Monotherapy:
Initial: 300mg bid
Titrate: Increase by a max of 600mg/day at weekly intervals
Usual: 2400mg/day

PEDIATRIC DOSAGE

Partial Seizures

Adjunctive Therapy:
2-<4 Years:
Initial: 8-10mg/kg/day, not to exceed 600mg/day; may consider 16-20mg/kg for patients <20kg
Titrate: Increase to max maint dose over 2-4 weeks
Max: 60mg/kg/day

4-16 Years:
Initial: 8-10mg/kg/day, not to exceed 600mg/day

Reduce dose and withdraw concomitant antiepileptic drugs over 3-6 weeks, while reaching max oxcarbazepine dose in about 2-4 weeks
Initiation of Monotherapy:
Initial: 300mg bid
Titrate: Increase by 300mg/day every third day
Usual: 1200mg/day

Maint: Increase to target dose over 2 weeks
20-29kg: 450mg bid
29.1-39kg: 600mg bid
>39kg: 900mg bid
W/ Epilepsy:
Conversion to Monotherapy:
4-16 Years:
Initial: 8-10mg/kg/day
Titrate: Increase by a max of 10mg/kg/day at weekly intervals
Reduce dose and withdraw concomitant antiepileptic drugs over 3-6 weeks
Initiation of Monotherapy:
4-16 Years:
Initial: 8-10mg/kg/day
Titrate: Increase by 5mg/kg/day every third day
Conversion to/Initiation of Monotherapy:
Maint:
20kg: 600-900mg/day
25-30kg: 900-1200mg/day
35-40kg: 900-1500mg/day
45kg: 1200-1500mg/day
50-55kg: 1200-1800mg/day
60-65kg: 1200-2100mg/day
70kg: 1500-2100mg/day

DOSE MODIFICATION
Renal Impairment
CrCl <30mL/min:
Initial: 1/2 the usual starting dose (300mg/day)
Titrate: Increase slowly

ADMINISTRATION
Oral route

All dosing should be given in a bid regimen
Sus and tabs may be interchanged at equal doses
Take w/ or w/o food

Sus
1. Before use, shake well and prepare dose immediately afterwards
2. Use the supplied oral dosing syringe to withdraw the prescribed amount from the bottle
3. Sus may be mixed in a small glass of water just prior to administration or may be swallowed directly from the syringe
4. Close the bottle and rinse the syringe w/ warm water and allow it to dry thoroughly after each use

HOW SUPPLIED
Sus: 300mg/5mL [250mL]; Tab: 150mg*, 300mg*, 600mg* *scored

WARNINGS/PRECAUTIONS
Clinically significant hyponatremia may develop; consider measurement of serum Na^+ levels during maintenance treatment, particularly if patient is receiving other medications known to decrease serum Na^+ levels (eg, drugs associated w/ inappropriate antidiuretic hormone secretion) or if symptoms indicating hyponatremia develop. Anaphylaxis and angioedema involving the larynx, glottis, lips, and eyelids reported; d/c therapy if any of these reactions develop, start alternative treatment, and do not rechallenge. Caution in patients w/ history of hypersensitivity reactions to carbamazepine; d/c immediately if signs/symptoms of hypersensitivity develop. Serious dermatological reactions (eg, Stevens-Johnson syndrome [SJS], toxic epidermal necrolysis [TEN]) reported; consider discontinuing use and prescribing another antiepileptic drug (AED) if a skin reaction develops. Patients carrying the human leukocyte antigen (HLA)-B*1502 allele may be at increased risk for SJS/TEN; consider testing for presence of HLA-B*1502 allele in patients w/ ancestry in genetically at-risk populations, and avoid use in patients positive for HLA-B*1502 unless benefits clearly outweigh risks. Increased risk of suicidal thoughts or behavior. Withdraw gradually to minimize the potential of increased seizure frequency. Associated w/ CNS-related adverse events (cognitive symptoms, somnolence or fatigue, coordination abnormalities). Drug reaction w/ eosinophilia and systemic symptoms (DRESS)/multiorgan hypersensitivity reported; evaluate immediately if signs/symptoms (eg, rash, fever, lymphadenopathy) are present, and d/c

if an alternative etiology cannot be established. Pancytopenia, agranulocytosis, and leukopenia reported; consider discontinuation if any evidence of hematologic events develop. Levels may decrease during pregnancy; monitor patients during pregnancy and through the postpartum period. Associated w/ decreases in T4, without changes in T3 or TSH. Caution w/ severe hepatic impairment.

ADVERSE REACTIONS
Dizziness, somnolence, diplopia, fatigue, N/V, ataxia, abnormal vision, tremor, abnormal gait, dyspepsia, abdominal pain.

DRUG INTERACTIONS
Verapamil, valproic acid, and strong CYP450 inducers (eg, carbamazepine, phenytoin, phenobarbital) may decrease levels. May decrease levels of dihydropyridine calcium antagonists, oral contraceptives (eg, ethinylestradiol, levonorgestrel), cyclosporine, and felodipine. May increase levels of phenytoin, phenobarbital, and CYP2C19 substrates; may require dose reduction of phenytoin when using oxcarbazepine doses >1200mg/day. Decreased levels w/ AEDs that are CYP450 inducers.

NURSING CONSIDERATIONS

Assessment: Assess for history of hypersensitivity to drug or to carbamazepine, presence of HLA-B*1502 allele, depression, renal/hepatic impairment, pregnancy/nursing status, and possible drug interactions.

Monitoring: Monitor for signs/symptoms of hyponatremia, angioedema, anaphylactic/hypersensitivity/dermatological reactions, emergence/worsening of depression, suicidal thoughts/behavior, unusual changes in mood/behavior, cognitive/neuropsychiatric events, DRESS, hematologic events, and other adverse reactions. Monitor patients during pregnancy and through the postpartum period.

Patient Counseling: Advise to report symptoms of low Na^+, and fever to physician. Instruct to d/c and contact physician immediately if signs/symptoms suggesting angioedema develop. Advise to consult physician immediately if experiencing a hypersensitivity reaction, skin reaction, or symptoms suggestive of blood disorders. Warn female patients of childbearing age that concurrent use w/ hormonal contraceptives may render this method of contraception less effective; advise to use additional nonhormonal forms of contraception. Advise of the need to be alert for the emergence/worsening of symptoms of depression, any unusual changes in mood/behavior, or the emergence of suicidal thoughts, behavior, or thoughts about self-harm; instruct to immediately report behaviors of concern to physician. Instruct to use caution if taking alcohol while on therapy. Advise that drug may cause dizziness and somnolence, and not to drive or operate machinery until effects have been determined. Encourage to enroll in the North American Antiepileptic Drug Pregnancy Registry if patient becomes pregnant.

Storage: 25°C (77°F); excursions permitted to 15-30°C (59-86°F). (Sus) Use w/in 7 weeks of 1st opening the bottle.

TRILIPIX – fenofibric acid — RX

Class: Fibric acid derivative

ADULT DOSAGE

Severe Hypertriglyceridemia

Initial: 45-135mg qd
Titrate: Adjust dose if necessary following repeat lipid determinations at 4- to 8-week intervals
Max: 135mg qd

Primary Hypercholesterolemia/Mixed Dyslipidemia

Usual: 135mg qd
Coadministration Therapy w/ Statins for Mixed Dyslipidemia:
In patients w/ mixed dyslipidemia and coronary heart disease (CHD) or a CHD risk equivalent who are on optimal statin therapy
May be taken at the same time as a statin.
Avoid max dose of statin unless benefits outweigh the risks

PEDIATRIC DOSAGE

Pediatric use may not have been established

DOSE MODIFICATION
Renal Impairment
Mild to Moderate:
Initial: 45mg qd
Titrate: Increase only after evaluation of effects on renal function and lipid levels

ADMINISTRATION
Oral route
May be taken w/o regard to meals
Swallow cap whole; do not open, crush, dissolve, or chew

HOW SUPPLIED
Cap, Delayed-Release: 45mg, 135mg

CONTRAINDICATIONS
Severe renal impairment (including dialysis), active liver disease (including primary biliary cirrhosis and unexplained persistent liver function abnormalities), preexisting gallbladder disease, and nursing mothers.

WARNINGS/PRECAUTIONS
No incremental benefit of fenofibric acid on cardiovascular morbidity and mortality over and above that demonstrated for statin monotherapy has been established. Not shown to reduce CHD morbidity and mortality in patients with type 2 diabetes mellitus (DM). Not indicated for patients who have elevations of chylomicrons and plasma TGs, but have normal VLDL levels. Increased risk of myositis/myopathy and rhabdomyolysis; risk increased with DM, renal failure, hypothyroidism, and in elderly. D/C therapy if markedly elevated CPK levels occur or myopathy/myositis is suspected or diagnosed. Increases in serum transaminases, hepatocellular, chronic active and cholestatic hepatitis, and cirrhosis (rare) reported; perform baseline and regular monitoring of LFTs, and d/c therapy if enzyme levels persist >3X ULN. Reversible elevations in SrCr reported. May cause cholelithiasis; d/c if gallstones are found. Acute hypersensitivity reactions and pancreatitis reported. Mild to moderate decreases in Hgb, Hct and WBCs, thrombocytopenia, and agranulocytosis reported; periodically monitor RBC and WBC counts during the first 12 months of therapy. May cause venothromboembolic disease. Severe decreases in HDL levels reported; check HDL levels within the 1st few months after initiation of therapy. If a severely depressed HDL level is detected, withdraw therapy, monitor HDL level until it has returned to baseline, and do not reinitiate therapy. D/C or change medications known to exacerbate hypertriglyceridemia (eg, β-blockers, thiazides, estrogens) if possible before considering therapy.

ADVERSE REACTIONS
Headache, back pain, nasopharyngitis, nausea, myalgia, diarrhea, upper respiratory tract infection, abnormal LFTs, pain in extremity, arthralgia, dizziness, dyspepsia, sinusitis, constipation, pain.

DRUG INTERACTIONS
Increased risk of rhabdomyolysis with HMG-CoA reductase inhibitors (statins). May potentiate anticoagulant effects of coumarin anticoagulants; use with caution, reduce anticoagulant dosage, and monitor PT/INR frequently. Bile acid-binding resins may bind other drugs given concurrently; take at least 1 hr before or 4-6 hrs after the bile acid resin to avoid impeding its absorption. Immunosuppressants (eg, cyclosporine, tacrolimus) may produce nephrotoxicity; consider benefits and risks, and use lowest effective dose with immunosuppressants and other potentially nephrotoxic agents. Cases of myopathy, including rhabdomyolysis, reported when coadministered with colchicine; caution when prescribing with colchicine.

NURSING CONSIDERATIONS

Assessment: Assess for renal impairment, active liver disease, preexisting gallbladder disease, other medical conditions (eg, DM, hypothyroidism), hypersensitivity to drug, pregnancy/nursing status, and possible drug interactions. Obtain baseline LFTs.

Monitoring: Monitor for signs/symptoms of myositis, myopathy, or rhabdomyolysis; measure CPK levels in patients reporting such symptoms. Monitor for cholelithiasis, pancreatitis, hypersensitivity reactions, pulmonary embolism, and deep vein thrombosis. Monitor renal function, LFTs, CBC, and lipid levels. Monitor PT/INR frequently with coumarin anticoagulants.

Patient Counseling: Advise of the potential benefits and risks of therapy, and of medications to avoid during treatment. Instruct to follow appropriate lipid-modifying diet during therapy, and to take drug ud. Inform that if drug is coadministered with a statin, they may be taken together. Advise to return for routine monitoring. Instruct to inform physician of all medications, supplements, and herbal preparations being taken, any changes in medical condition, development of muscle pain, tenderness, or weakness, and onset of abdominal pain or any other new symptoms.

Storage: 25°C (77°F); excursions permitted to 15-30°C (59-86°F). Protect from moisture.

TRIZIVIR – abacavir sulfate/lamivudine/zidovudine

RX

Class: Nucleoside reverse transcriptase inhibitor

Lactic acidosis and severe hepatomegaly with steatosis, including fatal cases, reported with nucleoside analogues. Abacavir: Serious and sometimes fatal hypersensitivity reactions (multiorgan clinical syndrome) reported; d/c as soon as suspected and never restart therapy or any other abacavir-containing product. Patients with HLA-B*5701 allele are at high risk for hypersensitivity; screen for HLA-B*5701 allele prior to therapy. Zidovudine: Associated with hematologic toxicity (eg, neutropenia, severe anemia), particularly with advanced HIV-1 disease. Symptomatic myopathy associated with prolonged use. Lamivudine: Severe acute exacerbations of hepatitis B reported in patients coinfected with hepatitis B virus (HBV) and HIV-1 and have discontinued therapy; closely monitor hepatic function for at least several months. If appropriate, initiation of antihepatitis B therapy may be warranted.

ADULT DOSAGE

HIV-1 Infection

1 tab bid

PEDIATRIC DOSAGE

HIV-1 Infection

>40kg:
1 tab bid

DOSE MODIFICATION

Renal Impairment

CrCl <50mL/min: Not recommended for use

Hepatic Impairment

Not recommended for use

ADMINISTRATION

Oral route

Take with or without food

HOW SUPPLIED

Tab: (Abacavir Sulfate-Lamivudine-Zidovudine) 300mg-150mg-300mg

CONTRAINDICATIONS

Hepatic impairment.

WARNINGS/PRECAUTIONS

Obesity and prolonged nucleoside exposure may be risk factors for lactic acidosis and severe hepatomegaly with steatosis; suspend therapy if clinical or lab findings suggestive of lactic acidosis or pronounced hepatotoxicity develop. Immune reconstitution syndrome reported. Autoimmune disorders (eg, Graves' disease, polymyositis, Guillain-Barre syndrome) reported to occur in the setting of immune reconstitution and can occur many months after initiation of treatment. Redistribution/accumulation of body fat may occur. Cross-resistance potential with nucleoside reverse transcriptase inhibitors reported. Caution with any known risk factors for liver disease and in elderly. Avoid use in adolescents weighing <40kg and in patients requiring dose adjustments (eg, renal impairment [CrCl <50mL/min]). Abacavir: Increased risk of myocardial infarction (MI) reported; consider underlying risk of coronary heart disease (CHD) when prescribing therapy. Lamivudine: Emergence of lamivudine-resistant HBV reported. Zidovudine: Caution with compromised bone marrow evidenced by granulocyte count <1000 cells/mm^3 or Hgb <9.5g/dL; monitor blood counts frequently with advanced HIV-1 disease and periodically in other HIV-1 infected patients. Interrupt therapy if anemia or neutropenia develops.

ADVERSE REACTIONS

Lactic acidosis, severe hepatomegaly with steatosis, hematologic toxicity, myopathy, N/V, headache, malaise, fatigue, hypersensitivity reaction, diarrhea, fever, chills, depressive disorders.

DRUG INTERACTIONS

Avoid with other abacavir-, lamivudine-, zidovudine-, and/or emtricitabine-containing products. Hepatic decompensation may occur in HIV-1/hepatitis C virus (HCV) coinfected patients receiving interferon alfa with or without ribavirin; closely monitor for treatment-associated toxicities. Abacavir: Ethanol may decrease elimination, causing an increase in overall exposure. May increase oral methadone clearance. Zidovudine: Avoid with stavudine, doxorubicin, and nucleoside analogues that affect DNA replication (eg, ribavirin). Atovaquone, fluconazole, methadone, probenecid, and valproic acid may increase levels. Clarithromycin, nelfinavir, rifampin, and ritonavir may decrease levels. May increase hematologic toxicity with ganciclovir, interferon alfa, ribavirin, and other bone marrow suppressive or cytotoxic agents. Lamivudine: Nelfinavir and trimethoprim/sulfamethoxazole may increase levels.

NURSING CONSIDERATIONS

Assessment: Assess for history of hypersensitivity reactions, advanced HIV disease, hepatic/renal impairment, risk factors for lactic acidosis, risk factors for liver and CHD, bone marrow compromise, HBV infection, pregnancy/nursing status, and possible drug interactions. Screen for HLA-B*5701 allele prior to initiation of therapy. Assess medical history for prior exposure to any abacavir-containing product.

Monitoring: Monitor for signs/symptoms of hypersensitivity reactions, hematologic toxicity, lactic acidosis, hepatomegaly with steatosis, myopathy, immune reconstitution syndrome (eg, opportunistic infections), autoimmune disorders, fat redistribution/accumulation, MI, and other adverse reactions. Monitor hepatic/renal function and blood counts. Monitor hepatic function closely for at least several months in patients who d/c therapy and are coinfected with HIV-1 and HBV.

Patient Counseling: Inform about hypersensitivity reactions; instruct to contact physician immediately if symptoms develop and not to restart or replace with any drug containing abacavir without medical consultation. Inform about risk for hematologic toxicities and advise on importance of close blood count monitoring while on therapy. Counsel about the possible occurrence of myopathy and myositis with pathological changes during prolonged use and that therapy may cause a rare but serious condition called lactic acidosis with liver enlargement (hepatomegaly). Inform patients coinfected with HBV that deterioration of liver disease has occurred in some cases when treatment was discontinued; instruct to discuss any changes in regimen with physician. Inform that hepatic decompensation has occurred in HIV-1/HCV-coinfected patients receiving combination antiretroviral therapy and interferon alfa with or without ribavirin. Inform that redistribution/accumulation of body fat may occur. Advise that drug is not a cure for HIV-1 infection and that illness associated with HIV-1 may still be experienced. Advise to avoid doing things that can spread HIV-1 infection to others. Inform patients to take all HIV medications exactly as prescribed.

Storage: 25°C (77°F); excursions permitted to 15-30°C (59-86°F).

TROKENDI XR – topiramate

RX

Class: Sulfamate-substituted monosaccharide antiepileptic

ADULT DOSAGE

Epilepsy

Partial Onset Seizures or Primary Generalized Tonic-Clonic Seizures:

Monotherapy:

Usual: 400mg qd

Titration Schedule:
Week 1: 50mg qd
Week 2: 100mg qd
Week 3: 150mg qd
Week 4: 200mg qd
Week 5: 300mg qd
Week 6: 400mg qd

Partial Onset Seizures, Primary Generalized Tonic-Clonic Seizures, or Lennox-Gastaut Syndrome:

Adjunctive Therapy:

≥17 Years:
Initial: 25-50mg qd
Titrate: Increase in increments of 25-50mg every week to achieve effective dose
Usual:
Partial Onset Seizures or Lennox-Gastaut Syndrome: 200-400mg qd
Primary Generalized Tonic-Clonic Seizures: 400mg qd

PEDIATRIC DOSAGE

Epilepsy

Partial Onset Seizures or Primary Generalized Tonic-Clonic Seizures:

Monotherapy:

≥10 Years:
Usual: 400mg qd
Titration Schedule:
Week 1: 50mg qd
Week 2: 100mg qd
Week 3: 150mg qd
Week 4: 200mg qd
Week 5: 300mg qd
Week 6: 400mg qd

Partial Onset Seizures, Primary Generalized Tonic-Clonic Seizures, or Lennox-Gastaut Syndrome:

Adjunctive Therapy:

6-16 Years:
Usual: 5-9mg/kg qd
Titrate: Begin titration at 25mg qpm (based on a range of 1-3mg/kg/day) for 1st week. Subsequently, increase at 1- or 2-week intervals by increments of 1-3mg/kg to achieve optimal clinical response; longer intervals between dose adjustments may be used if required

DOSE MODIFICATION

Concomitant Medications

Phenytoin and/or Carbamazepine:
May require an adjustment of the dose of phenytoin to achieve optimal clinical outcome
Addition or withdrawal of phenytoin and/or carbamazepine during adjunctive therapy may require dose adjustment of topiramate

Renal Impairment

CrCl <70mL/min: Use 1/2 the usual starting and maint dose
Hemodialysis: Supplemental dose may be required

ADMINISTRATION

Oral route

May be taken w/o regard to meals
Swallow cap whole and intact; do not sprinkle on food, chew, or crush
Completely avoid alcohol use w/in 6 hrs prior to and 6 hrs after administration

HOW SUPPLIED

Cap, Extended-Release: 25mg, 50mg, 100mg, 200mg

CONTRAINDICATIONS

Patients with recent alcohol use (eg, within 6 hrs prior to and 6 hrs after use), patients with metabolic acidosis taking concomitant metformin.

WARNINGS/PRECAUTIONS

Acute myopia associated with secondary angle-closure glaucoma reported; d/c immediately to reverse symptoms. Oligohydrosis and hyperthermia reported, mostly in pediatric patients; monitor closely for decreased sweating and increased body temperature. Hyperchloremic, non-anion gap, metabolic acidosis reported; conditions or therapies that predispose to acidosis may be additive to the bicarbonate lowering effects. D/C or reduce dose if metabolic acidosis develops/persists. If decision is made to continue therapy, consider alkali treatment. Increased risk of suicidal thoughts/behavior; monitor for the emergence/worsening of depression, suicidal thoughts/behavior, and/or any unusual changes in mood or behavior. Cognitive-related dysfunction, psychiatric/behavioral disturbances, somnolence, or fatigue reported. May cause cleft lip and/or cleft palate in infants if used during pregnancy. D/C gradually to minimize the potential for seizures or increased seizure frequency; appropriate monitoring is recommended when rapid withdrawal is required. Patients with inborn errors of metabolism or reduced hepatic mitochondrial activity may be at an increased risk for hyperammonemia with or without encephalopathy; consider hyperammonemic encephalopathy and measure ammonia levels in patients who develop unexplained lethargy, vomiting, or changes in mental status associated with therapy. Kidney stones formation reported; hydration recommended to reduce new stone formation. Paresthesia may occur. Lab abnormalities may occur.

ADVERSE REACTIONS

Paresthesia, weight decrease, somnolence, anorexia, dizziness, difficulty with memory, upper respiratory tract infection, diarrhea, mood problems, fatigue, nervousness, difficulty with concentration, aggressive reaction, confusion, depression.

DRUG INTERACTIONS

See Contraindications. May decrease contraceptive efficacy and increase breakthrough bleeding with combination oral contraceptives. Phenytoin or carbamazepine may decrease levels. Concurrent administration of valproic acid has been associated with hyperammonemia with or without encephalopathy, and hypothermia. Concomitant administration with other CNS depressant drugs or alcohol can result in significant CNS depression. Other carbonic anhydrase inhibitors (eg, zonisamide, acetazolamide, dichlorphenamide) may increase the severity of metabolic acidosis and may also increase the risk of kidney stone formation. Increase in systemic exposure of lithium observed following topiramate doses of ≤600mg/day; monitor lithium levels. Caution with agents that predispose patients to heat-related disorders (eg, carbonic anhydrase inhibitors, anticholinergics).

NURSING CONSIDERATIONS

Assessment: Assess for recent alcohol use, metabolic acidosis in patients taking concomitant metformin, predisposing factors for metabolic acidosis, renal dysfunction, inborn errors of metabolism, reduced hepatic mitochondrial activity, pregnancy/nursing status, and possible drug interactions. Obtain baseline serum bicarbonate and blood ammonia levels. Obtain baseline estimated GFR measurement in patients at high risk for renal insufficiency.

Monitoring: Monitor for signs/symptoms of acute myopia, secondary-angle glaucoma, oligohydrosis, hyperthermia, cognitive or neuropsychiatric adverse reactions, kidney stones, renal dysfunction, metabolic acidosis, paresthesias, hyperammonemia, and other adverse reactions. Monitor serum bicarbonate and blood ammonia levels.

Patient Counseling: Instruct to take ud. Advise to completely avoid consumption of alcohol at least 6 hrs prior to and 6 hrs after taking the drug. Instruct to seek immediate medical attention if blurred vision, visual disturbances, periorbital pain, decreased sweating, or increased body temperature occurs. Inform about the potentially significant risk for metabolic acidosis that may be asymptomatic and may be associated with adverse effects on kidneys, bones, and growth in pediatric patients, and on the fetus. Instruct to immediately report to the physician if emergence or worsening of depression, unusual changes in mood/behavior, emergence of suicidal thoughts, or behavior/thoughts about self-harm occurs. Instruct to use caution when engaging in any activities where loss of consciousness may result in serious danger. Inform of pregnancy risks; encourage pregnant women to enroll in the North American Antiepileptic Drug Pregnancy Registry. Warn about the possible development of hyperammonemia with or without encephalopathy; instruct to contact physician if unexplained lethargy, vomiting, or mental status changes develop. Instruct to maintain an adequate fluid intake to minimize risk of kidney stones. Inform that therapy may cause a reduction in body temperature that can lead to alterations in mental status; if changes are noted, instruct patients to measure their body temperature and to contact physician. Instruct to consult physician if tingling in the arms and legs occurs.

Storage: 25°C (77°F); excursions permitted to 15-30°C (59-86°F). Protect from moisture and light.

TRULICITY — dulaglutide

RX

Class: Glucagon-like peptide-1 receptor agonist

Causes dose-related and treatment-duration-dependent increase in the incidence of thyroid C-cell tumors (adenomas, carcinomas) after lifetime exposure in animal studies. It is unknown whether drug causes thyroid C-cell tumors (eg, medullary thyroid carcinoma [MTC]) in humans; human relevance of dulaglutide-induced thyroid C-cell tumors in rodents has not been determined. Contraindicated in patients w/ a personal or family history of MTC and in patients w/ multiple endocrine neoplasia syndrome type 2 (MEN 2). Routine monitoring of serum calcitonin or using thyroid ultrasound is of uncertain value for early detection of MTC in patients treated w/ therapy.

ADULT DOSAGE

Type 2 Diabetes Mellitus

Initial: 0.75mg once weekly; may increase to 1.5mg once weekly
Max: 1.5mg once weekly
Day of weekly administration may be changed if necessary as long as the last dose was administered ≥3 days before

Missed Dose

If a dose is missed, administer as soon as possible if there are ≥3 days (72 hrs) until the next scheduled dose; if <3 days remain before the next scheduled dose, skip the missed dose and administer the next dose on the regularly scheduled day
Patients may then resume regular once weekly dosing schedule in each case

PEDIATRIC DOSAGE

Pediatric use may not have been established

DOSE MODIFICATION

Concomitant Medications

Insulin Secretagogue (eg, Sulfonylurea)/Insulin: Consider reducing dose of insulin secretagogues or insulin when initiating therapy

ADMINISTRATION

SQ route
Administer once weekly, any time of day, w/ or w/o food
Inject in the abdomen, thigh, or upper arm

Use w/ Insulin

Administer as separate inj; never mix products
May inject in the same body region; inj should not be adjacent to each other
If injecting in the same body region, use a different inj site each week

HOW SUPPLIED

Inj: 0.75mg/0.5mL, 1.5mg/0.5mL [pen, prefilled syringe]

CONTRAINDICATIONS

Personal or family history of MTC, MEN 2.

WARNINGS/PRECAUTIONS

Not recommended as 1st-line therapy for patients who have inadequate glycemic control on diet and exercise; weigh potential benefits/risks. Not recommended w/ preexisting severe GI disease (eg, gastroparesis). Not a substitute for insulin; do not use in type 1 DM or for treatment of diabetic ketoacidosis. Pancreatitis related adverse reactions reported; d/c promptly if suspected, and do not restart therapy if confirmed. Consider other antidiabetic therapies in patients w/ a history of pancreatitis. Systemic hypersensitivity reactions reported; d/c and promptly seek medical advice if reaction occurs. Acute renal failure and worsening of chronic renal failure reported; caution when initiating/escalating doses in patients w/ renal impairment. Caution w/ hepatic impairment.

ADVERSE REACTIONS

N/V, diarrhea, abdominal pain, decreased appetite, dyspepsia, fatigue.

DRUG INTERACTIONS

See Dose Modification. May slow gastric emptying and thus has the potential to reduce the rate of absorption of concomitant oral medications; use w/ caution. Adequately monitor drug levels of oral medications w/ a narrow therapeutic index.

NURSING CONSIDERATIONS

Assessment: Assess for previous hypersensitivity reactions, MEN 2, personal or family history of MTC, history of pancreatitis, renal/hepatic impairment, GI disease, pregnancy/nursing status, and possible drug interactions. Further evaluate patients w/ thyroid nodules and/or elevated calcitonin levels.

Monitoring: Monitor for signs/symptoms of thyroid tumor, pancreatitis, elevated serum calcitonin levels, hypoglycemia, systemic hypersensitivity reactions, renal impairment, and other adverse reactions. Monitor renal function in patients w/ renal impairment reporting severe adverse GI reactions.

Patient Counseling: Counsel regarding the potential risk of MTC and inform patient of symptoms of thyroid tumors (eg, mass in the neck, dysphagia, persistent hoarseness). Inform of the potential risks/benefits of therapy and of alternative modes of therapy. Instruct to report symptoms of thyroid tumors to physician. Instruct to d/c therapy promptly, and contact physician if persistent severe abdominal pain and/or symptoms of hypersensitivity reactions occur. Advise of the potential risk of dehydration due to GI adverse reactions and instruct to take precautions to avoid fluid depletion. Inform patients treated w/ therapy of the potential risk of worsening renal function and explain the associated signs and symptoms of renal impairment, as well as the possibility of dialysis as a medical intervention if renal failure occurs. Instruct to inform physician if pregnant/intending to become pregnant. Inform about the importance of adherence to dietary instructions, regular physical activity, periodic blood glucose monitoring and HbA1c testing, proper inj technique, recognition and management of hypo/hyperglycemia, and assessment for diabetes complications. Inform that medication requirements may change during periods of stress; advise to seek medical advice promptly. Advise that if a dose is missed, administer as soon as noticed, provided that the next regularly scheduled dose is due at least 3 days later. Instruct to then resume the usual dosing schedule thereafter. Instruct that if a dose is missed and the next regularly scheduled dose is due in 1 or 2 days, not to administer the missed dose and instead resume w/ the next regularly scheduled dose. Advise of the potential risk of GI side effects. Advise to inform physician if any unusual symptom develops, or if any known symptom persists or worsens.

Storage: 2-8°C (36-46°F). If needed, keep at room temperature, not to exceed 30°C (86°F) for a total of 14 days. Do not freeze. Do not use if it has been frozen. Protect from light. Discard after use in a puncture-resistant container.

TRUMENBA – meningococcal group B vaccine RX

Class: Vaccine

ADULT DOSAGE

Meningococcal Vaccine

Active Immunization to Prevent Invasive Disease Caused by *Neisseria meningitidis* Serogroup B:

≤25 Years:

0.5mL IM as a 3-dose series according to a 0-, 2-, and 6-month schedule

PEDIATRIC DOSAGE

Meningococcal Vaccine

Active Immunization to Prevent Invasive Disease Caused by *Neisseria meningitidis* Serogroup B:

≥10 Years:

0.5mL IM as a 3-dose series according to a 0-, 2-, and 6-month schedule

ADMINISTRATION

IM route

Shake syringe vigorously; do not use if vaccine cannot be re-suspended

Preferred site for inj is the deltoid muscle of the upper arm

Do not mix with any other vaccine in the same syringe

HOW SUPPLIED

Inj: 0.5mL

WARNINGS/PRECAUTIONS

Epinephrine and other appropriate agents used to manage immediate allergic reactions must be immediately available should an acute anaphylactic reaction occur. Individuals with altered immunocompetence may have reduced immune responses to therapy.

ADVERSE REACTIONS

Pain at inj site, fatigue, headache, muscle pain, chills.

NURSING CONSIDERATIONS

Assessment: Assess for hypersensitivity/vaccination history, altered immunocompetence, and pregnancy/nursing status.

Monitoring: Monitor for allergic/anaphylactic reactions, and other adverse reactions.

Patient Counseling: Inform of the importance of completing the 3-dose immunization series. Instruct to report any suspected adverse reactions to physician.

Storage: 2-8°C (36-46°F). Store syringes in the refrigerator horizontally (laying flat on the shelf) to minimize the re-dispersion time. Do not freeze; discard if the vaccine has been frozen.

TRUSOPT — dorzolamide hydrochloride RX

Class: Carbonic anhydrase inhibitor

ADULT DOSAGE

Elevated Intraocular Pressure

Ocular HTN/Open-Angle Glaucoma:
1 drop in the affected eye(s) tid

PEDIATRIC DOSAGE

Elevated Intraocular Pressure

Ocular HTN/Open-Angle Glaucoma:
1 drop in the affected eye(s) tid

DOSE MODIFICATION

Concomitant Medications

Administer at least 5 min apart if >1 topical ophthalmic drug is being used

ADMINISTRATION

Ocular route

HOW SUPPLIED

Sol: 2% [10mL]

WARNINGS/PRECAUTIONS

Systemically absorbed. Rare fatalities have occurred due to severe sulfonamide reactions (eg, Stevens-Johnson syndrome, toxic epidermal necrolysis, fulminant hepatic necrosis, agranulocytosis, aplastic anemia, other blood dyscrasias); d/c if signs of hypersensitivity or other serious reactions occur. Sensitization may recur when readministered irrespective of the route of administration. Bacterial keratitis reported with use of multiple-dose containers of topical ophthalmic products that had been inadvertently contaminated by patients with a concurrent corneal disease or a disruption of the ocular epithelial surface. Caution in patients with low endothelial cell counts; increased potential for corneal edema. Local ocular adverse effects (eg, conjunctivitis, lid reactions) reported with chronic use; d/c use and evaluate patient before considering restarting therapy. The management of acute angle-closure glaucoma requires therapeutic interventions in addition to ocular hypotensive agents. Not recommended with severe renal impairment (CrCl <30mL/min). Caution with hepatic impairment.

ADVERSE REACTIONS

Ocular burning/stinging/discomfort, bitter taste, superficial punctate keratitis, ocular allergic reactions, conjunctivitis, lid reactions, blurred vision, eye redness, tearing, dryness, photophobia.

DRUG INTERACTIONS

Concomitant administration of oral carbonic anhydrase inhibitor is not recommended due to potential for additive effects. Acid-base and electrolyte disturbances reported with oral carbonic anhydrase inhibitors; drug interactions (eg, toxicity associated with high-dose salicylate therapy) may occur.

NURSING CONSIDERATIONS

Assessment: Assess for hypersensitivity to drug, acute angle-closure glaucoma, low endothelial cell counts, renal/hepatic impairment, pregnancy/nursing status, and possible drug interactions.

Monitoring: Monitor for sulfonamide hypersensitivity reactions, ocular reactions, bacterial keratitis, and other adverse reactions. Monitor for improvement in IOP.

Patient Counseling: Advise to d/c use if serious or unusual reactions (eg, severe skin reactions, signs of hypersensitivity) occur. Instruct to immediately seek physician's advice concerning the continued use of present multidose container if patients have ocular surgery or develop an intercurrent ocular condition (eg, trauma, infection). Advise to d/c use and seek physician's advice if patient develops any ocular reactions (eg, conjunctivitis, lid reactions). Instruct to avoid allowing tip of dispensing container to contact eye or surrounding structures. Inform that ocular sol can become contaminated by common bacteria known to cause ocular infections if handled improperly or if the tip of the dispensing container contacts the eye or surrounding structures, and may result in serious damage to the eye and subsequent loss of vision. Instruct to administer at least 5 min apart if >1 topical ophthalmic drug is being used. Instruct to remove contact lenses prior to administration and inform that they may be reinserted 15 min after administration.

Storage: 15-30°C (59-86°F). Protect from light.

TRUVADA – emtricitabine/tenofovir disoproxil fumarate RX

Class: Nucleoside analogue combination

Lactic acidosis and severe hepatomegaly w/ steatosis, including fatal cases, reported w/ the use of nucleoside analogues in combination w/ other antiretrovirals. Not approved for treatment of chronic hepatitis B virus (HBV) infection. Severe acute exacerbations of hepatitis B reported in patients coinfected w/ HBV and HIV-1 and who have discontinued therapy; closely monitor hepatic function w/ both clinical and lab follow-up for at least several months. If appropriate, initiation of anti-hepatitic B therapy may be warranted. Drug resistant HIV-1 variants have been identified w/ use for preexposure prophylaxis (PrEP) indication following undetected acute HIV-1 infection. PrEP use must only be prescribed to individuals confirmed to be HIV-negative immediately prior to initiating and periodically (at least every 3 months) during use; do not initiate if signs/symptoms of acute HIV-1 infection are present unless negative infection status is confirmed.

ADULT DOSAGE

HIV-1 Infection

Combination w/ Other Antiretrovirals:
1 tab qd

HIV-1 Pre-Exposure Prophylaxis

Combination w/ Safer Sex Practices for High-Risk Patients:
1 tab qd

PEDIATRIC DOSAGE

HIV-1 Infection

Combination w/ Other Antiretrovirals:
≥12 Years:
≥35kg: 1 tab qd

DOSE MODIFICATION

Renal Impairment

HIV-1 Infection:
CrCl 30-49mL/min: 1 tab q48h
CrCl <30mL/min (Including Hemodialysis): Not recommended for use

HIV-1 PrEP:
CrCl <60mL/min: Not recommended for use

ADMINISTRATION

Oral route

Take w/ or w/o food

HOW SUPPLIED

Tab: (Emtricitabine/Tenofovir Disoproxil Fumarate [TDF]) 200mg/300mg

CONTRAINDICATIONS

Individuals w/ unknown or positive HIV-1 status when used for PrEP. Use in HIV-infected patients w/o other concomitant antiretroviral agents.

WARNINGS/PRECAUTIONS

Obesity and prolonged nucleoside exposure may be risk factors for lactic acidosis and severe hepatomegaly w/ steatosis. Caution w/ known risk factors for liver disease. D/C if findings suggestive of lactic acidosis or pronounced hepatotoxicity develop. Test for the presence of chronic HBV before initiating therapy; offer vaccination to HBV-uninfected individuals. Renal impairment (eg, acute renal failure, Fanconi syndrome) reported; caution in patients at risk of renal dysfunction, including patients who have previously experienced renal events while receiving adefovir dipivoxil. Do not administer in patients w/ CrCl <30mL/min or requiring hemodialysis (HIV-1 treatment) or w/ CrCl <60mL/min (PrEP). Redistribution/accumulation of body fat and immune reconstitution syndrome reported. Autoimmune disorders (eg, Graves' disease, polymyositis, Guillain-Barre syndrome) reported in the setting of immune reconstitution and can occur many months after initiation of treatment. Early virological failure and high rates of resistance substitutions reported w/ certain regimens that only contain 3 nucleoside reverse transcriptase inhibitors; consider treatment modification in these patients. Use for PrEP only as part of a comprehensive prevention strategy that includes other prevention measures (eg, safer sex practices). Delay starting PrEP therapy for at least 1 month and reconfirm HIV-1 status or use an FDA-approved test to diagnose acute or primary HIV-1 infection if symptoms of acute viral infection are present and recent (<1 month) exposures are suspected. D/C PrEP therapy if symptoms of acute HIV-1 infection develop following potential exposure event until negative status is confirmed using an FDA-approved test. Caution in elderly. TDF: Decreased bone mineral density (BMD) and increased biochemical markers of bone metabolism reported. Osteomalacia associated w/ proximal renal tubulopathy reported; consider hypophosphatemia and osteomalacia secondary to proximal renal tubulopathy in patients at risk of renal dysfunction who present w/ persistent or worsening bone/muscle symptoms.

ADVERSE REACTIONS

Lactic acidosis, hepatomegaly w/ steatosis, diarrhea, nausea, fatigue, headache, dizziness, depression, insomnia, abnormal dreams, rash, abdominal pain, pharyngitis, syphilis.

DRUG INTERACTIONS

Avoid w/ concurrent or recent use of nephrotoxic agents (eg, high-dose or multiple NSAIDs). Do not coadminister w/ emtricitabine- or TDF-containing products, drugs containing lamivudine, or w/ adefovir dipivoxil. May increase levels of didanosine; d/c didanosine if didanosine-associated adverse effects develop. TDF decreases atazanavir levels; do not coadminister w/ atazanavir w/o RTV. Lopinavir/RTV, atazanavir w/ RTV, and darunavir w/ RTV may increase TDF levels; d/c treatment if TDF-associated adverse reactions develop. P-gp and breast cancer resistance protein transporter inhibitors may increase absorption. Coadministration w/ drugs eliminated by active tubular secretion (eg, acyclovir, cidofovir, ganciclovir, valacyclovir, aminoglycosides [eg, gentamicin], high-dose or multiple NSAIDs) may increase levels of emtricitabine, TDF, and/or the coadministered drug. Drugs that decrease renal function may increase levels of emtricitabine and/or TDF. Refer to PI for dosing modifications when used w/ concomitant therapies.

NURSING CONSIDERATIONS

Assessment: Assess for risk factors for lactic acidosis or liver disease, renal dysfunction, HBV infection, pregnancy/nursing status, and possible drug interactions. Confirm a negative HIV-1 test immediately prior to initiating PrEP therapy. In patients at risk of renal dysfunction, assess CrCl, serum phosphorus (P), urine glucose, and urine protein. Assess BMD in patients w/ history of pathologic bone fracture or other risk factors for osteoporosis or bone loss.

Monitoring: Monitor for signs/symptoms of lactic acidosis, hepatomegaly w/ steatosis, hepatotoxicity, new onset or worsening renal impairment, bone effects, redistribution/accumulation of body fat, immune reconstitution syndrome (eg, opportunistic infections), autoimmune disorders, and other adverse reactions. Closely monitor hepatic function w/ both clinical and laboratory follow-up for at least several months in patients coinfected w/ HBV and HIV-1 and have discontinued therapy. Screen for HIV-1 infection at least once every 3 months when using for PrEP. In patients at risk of renal dysfunction, monitor CrCl, serum P, urine glucose, and urine protein periodically.

Patient Counseling: Inform about the risks/benefits of therapy. Inform that medication is not a cure for HIV-1 and patients may continue to experience illness associated w/ HIV-1 infection (eg, opportunistic infections). Counsel about the importance of adhering to recommended dosing schedule. Counsel about safe sex practices. Instruct not to breastfeed, share needles or personal items that can have blood or body fluids on them, or d/c w/o informing physician. For PrEP, inform patients/partners about the importance of knowing their HIV-1 status, obtaining HIV-1 test at least every 3 months, getting tested for other sexually transmitted infections, and immediate reporting to physician if any symptoms of acute HIV-1 infection develop.

Storage: 25°C (77°F); excursions permitted to 15-30°C (59-86°F).

TUDORZA PRESSAIR – aclidinium bromide RX

Class: Anticholinergic bronchodilator

ADULT DOSAGE

Chronic Obstructive Pulmonary Disease

Maint Treatment of Bronchospasm Associated w/ COPD, Including Chronic Bronchitis and Emphysema:
1 inh (400mcg) bid

PEDIATRIC DOSAGE

Pediatric use may not have been established

ADMINISTRATION

Orally inhaled powder

Refer to PI for instructions on proper use

HOW SUPPLIED

MDI: 400mcg/actuation [30 doses, 60 doses]

WARNINGS/PRECAUTIONS

Not for initial treatment of acute episodes of bronchospasm (eg, rescue therapy). D/C and consider alternative treatments if paradoxical bronchospasm or immediate hypersensitivity reactions (eg, anaphylaxis, angioedema, urticaria, rash, bronchospasm, itching) occur. Caution w/ hypersensitivity to atropine and/or milk proteins. Caution w/ narrow-angle glaucoma; observe for signs and symptoms of acute narrow-angle glaucoma (eg, eye pain or discomfort, blurred vision, visual halos or colored images in association w/ red eyes from conjunctival congestion and corneal edema). Caution w/ urinary retention; observe for signs and symptoms of prostatic hyperplasia or bladder neck obstruction.

ADVERSE REACTIONS

Headache, nasopharyngitis, cough.

DRUG INTERACTIONS

Avoid w/ other anticholinergic-containing drugs; may lead to an increase in anticholinergic effects.

NURSING CONSIDERATIONS

Assessment: Assess for hypersensitivity to the drug, milk proteins, and/or atropine, narrow-angle glaucoma, urinary retention, pregnancy/nursing status, and possible drug interactions.

Monitoring: Monitor for hypersensitivity reactions, paradoxical bronchospasm, acute narrow-angle glaucoma, prostatic hyperplasia, bladder neck obstruction, and other adverse reactions.

Patient Counseling: Inform that the medication is a bid maintenance bronchodilator and should not be used for immediate relief of breathing problems (eg, as a rescue medication). Advise to d/c treatment if paradoxical bronchospasm occurs. Instruct to consult physician immediately if signs/symptoms of acute narrow-angle glaucoma occur; advise that miotic eye drops alone are not considered to be effective treatment. Inform not to allow the powder to enter into the eyes, as this may cause blurring of vision and pupil dilation. Instruct to consult physician immediately if signs/symptoms of new or worsening prostatic hyperplasia or bladder outlet obstruction occur. Advise to immediately d/c treatment and consult physician if signs/symptoms of immediate hypersensitivity reactions develop. Instruct on how to correctly use the inhaler.

Storage: 25°C (77°F); excursions permitted to 15-30°C (59-86°F). Store in a dry place. Store inhaler inside the sealed pouch and only open immediately before use. Discard inhaler 45 days after opening the pouch, after the marking "0" w/ a red background shows, or when the device locks out, whichever comes 1st.

TUSSIONEX PENNKINETIC — chlorpheniramine polistirex/hydrocodone polistirex CII

Class: Antihistamine/opioid antitussive

ADULT DOSAGE

Cough/Cold/Allergy

Relief of Cough and Upper Respiratory Symptoms Associated w/ Allergy or a Cold:
5mL q12h
Max: 10mL/24 hrs

PEDIATRIC DOSAGE

Cough/Cold/Allergy

Relief of Cough and Upper Respiratory Symptoms Associated w/ Allergy or a Cold:
6-11 Years:
2.5mL q12h
Max: 5mL/24 hrs

≥12 Years:
5mL q12h
Max: 10mL/24 hrs

DOSE MODIFICATION

Elderly

Start at lower end of dosing range

ADMINISTRATION

Oral route

Measure w/ an accurate measuring device
Shake well before using

HOW SUPPLIED

Sus, ER: (Hydrocodone-Chlorpheniramine) 10mg-8mg/5mL [115mL]

CONTRAINDICATIONS

Children <6 yrs of age.

WARNINGS/PRECAUTIONS

May produce dose-related respiratory depression and irregular/periodic breathing; if respiratory depression occurs, it may be antagonized by the use of naloxone HCl and other supportive measures when indicated. May markedly exaggerate respiratory depressant effects and CSF pressure elevation capacity in patients with head injury, other intracranial lesions, or a preexisting increased intracranial pressure. May obscure clinical course of head injuries and acute abdominal conditions. Chronic use may result in obstructive bowel disease, especially in patients with underlying intestinal motility disorder. Suppresses cough reflex. Caution in postoperative use; pulmonary disease, depressed ventilatory function, narrow-angle glaucoma, asthma, prostatic hypertrophy, severe hepatic/renal impairment, hypothyroidism, Addison's disease, or urethral stricture; in pediatric patients ≥6 yrs of age or with respiratory embarrassment (eg, croup); or in elderly/debilitated.

ADVERSE REACTIONS

Sedation, drowsiness, mental clouding, lethargy, anxiety, dysphoria, euphoria, dizziness, rash, pruritus, N/V, ureteral spasm, urinary retention, psychic dependence, mood changes.

DRUG INTERACTIONS

Coadministration with other respiratory depressants may increase risk of respiratory depression in pediatric patients. Additive CNS depression with narcotics, antihistaminics, antipsychotics, antianxiety agents, or other CNS depressants (eg, alcohol); reduce dose of one or both agents. Concomitant use with MAOIs or TCAs may increase the effect of either the antidepressant or hydrocodone. Concurrent use with other anticholinergics may produce paralytic ileus.

NURSING CONSIDERATIONS

Assessment: Assess for hepatic/renal impairment, drug hypersensitivity, any other conditions where treatment is cautioned or contraindicated, pregnancy/nursing status, and possible drug interactions. Assess use in postoperative/elderly/debilitated patients.

Monitoring: Monitor for signs/symptoms of respiratory depression, elevations in CSF pressure, obstructive bowel disease, and other adverse reactions.

Patient Counseling: Inform that medication may produce marked drowsiness and impair mental/physical abilities required for the performance of potentially hazardous tasks (eg, operating machinery, driving). Instruct not to dilute with fluids or mix with other drugs.

Storage: 20-25°C (68-77°F); excursions permitted to 15-30°C (59-86°F).

TWYNSTA — amlodipine/telmisartan RX

Class: ARB/calcium channel blocker (dihydropyridine)

D/C when pregnancy is detected. Drugs that act directly on the renin-angiotensin system (RAS) can cause injury/death to the developing fetus.

ADULT DOSAGE

Hypertension

Initial Therapy:

Initial: 40mg-5mg qd or, if requiring larger BP reductions, 80mg-5mg qd

Titrate: May be increased after at least 2 weeks

Max: 80mg-10mg qd

Replacement Therapy:

May substitute for individual components; increase dose if BP control is unsatisfactory

Add-On Therapy:

May be used if BP not adequately controlled with amlodipine (or another dihydropyridine calcium channel blocker [CCB]) alone or with telmisartan (or another ARB) alone

Patients with dose-limiting adverse reactions to amlodipine 10mg may be switched to telmisartan-amlodipine 40mg-5mg qd

PEDIATRIC DOSAGE

Pediatric use may not have been established

DOSE MODIFICATION

Renal Impairment

Severe: Titrate slowly

Hepatic Impairment

Amlodipine:

Initial: 2.5mg; titrate slowly

Elderly

≥75 Years:

Amlodipine:

Initial: 2.5mg; titrate slowly

ADMINISTRATION

Oral route

Take with or without food

HOW SUPPLIED

Tab: (Telmisartan-Amlodipine) 40mg-5mg, 40mg-10mg, 80mg-5mg, 80mg-10mg

CONTRAINDICATIONS

Coadministration with aliskiren in patients with diabetes.

WARNINGS/PRECAUTIONS

Symptomatic hypotension may occur in patients with an activated RAS (eg, volume- or salt-depleted patients) and in patients with severe aortic stenosis. Correct volume/salt depletion prior to therapy or start therapy under close medical supervision with a reduced dose. Not recommended for use as initial therapy in patients ≥75 yrs or with hepatic impairment. Amlodipine: Worsening angina and acute MI may develop after starting or increasing the dose, particularly in patients with severe obstructive coronary artery disease (CAD). Closely monitor patients with HF. Caution in elderly. Telmisartan: Hyperkalemia may occur, particularly in patients with advanced renal impairment, renal replacement therapy, or HF; periodically monitor serum electrolytes. Clearance is reduced in patients with biliary obstructive disorders or hepatic insufficiency. Changes in renal function may occur; oliguria and/or progressive azotemia and (rare) acute renal failure and/or death reported in patients whose renal function may depend on RAS (eg, severe congestive HF or renal dysfunction). May increase SrCr/BUN with renal artery stenosis.

ADVERSE REACTIONS

Peripheral edema, dizziness, back pain.

DRUG INTERACTIONS

See Contraindications. Amlodipine: Increased exposure to simvastatin reported; limit dose of simvastatin to 20mg daily. Diltiazem may increase systemic exposure. Strong CYP3A4 inhibitors (eg, ketoconazole, itraconazole, ritonavir) may increase concentrations to a greater extent; monitor for symptoms of hypotension and edema. Monitor for adequate clinical effect when coadministered with CYP3A4 inducers. Telmisartan: Dual blockade of the RAS is associated with increased risks of hypotension, hyperkalemia, and changes in renal function (eg, acute renal failure); avoid combined use of RAS inhibitors and closely monitor BP, renal function, and electrolytes with concomitant agents that affect the RAS. Avoid with aliskiren in patients with renal impairment (GFR <60mL/min). May increase digoxin concentrations; monitor digoxin levels upon initiation, adjustment, and discontinuation of therapy. Increases in lithium concentrations/toxicity reported; monitor lithium levels during concurrent use. NSAIDs, including selective COX-2 inhibitors, may attenuate antihypertensive effect and may deteriorate renal function. Coadministration with ramipril may increase ramipril/ramiprilat levels and decrease telmisartan levels; not recommended with ramipril. Increased risk of hyperkalemia with K^+-sparing diuretics, K^+ supplements, K^+-containing salt substitutes, or other drugs that increase K^+ levels. May possibly inhibit metabolism of drugs metabolized by CYP2C19.

NURSING CONSIDERATIONS

Assessment: Assess for severe obstructive CAD, severe aortic stenosis, HF, volume/salt depletion, biliary obstructive disorders, renal artery stenosis, diabetes, hepatic/renal dysfunction, hypersensitivity to drug, pregnancy/nursing status, and possible drug interactions.

Monitoring: Monitor for worsening angina and acute MI, particularly in patients with severe obstructive CAD, and for other adverse reactions. Monitor BP, renal function, and serum electrolytes (especially K^+ levels).

Patient Counseling: Inform of consequences if exposure occurs during pregnancy, and of treatment options in women planning to become pregnant. Instruct to report pregnancies to physician as soon as possible.

Storage: 25°C (77°F); excursions permitted to 15-30°C (59-86°F). Do not remove from blisters until immediately before administration. Protect from light and moisture.

TYBOST — cobicistat **RX**

Class: CYP3A inhibitor

ADULT DOSAGE

HIV-1 Infection

To increase systemic exposure of atazanavir or darunavir (once daily dosing regimen) in combination w/ other antiretroviral agents

Treatment-Naive/Experienced:
150mg qd + atazanavir 300mg qd

Treatment-Naive/Treatment-Experienced w/ No Darunavir Resistance Associated Substitutions:
150mg qd + darunavir 800mg qd

PEDIATRIC DOSAGE

Pediatric use may not have been established

DOSE MODIFICATION

Renal Impairment

CrCl <70mL/min: Do not coadminister w/ tenofovir DF

ADMINISTRATION

Oral route

Take w/ food

Must be coadministered at the same time as atazanavir or darunavir

HOW SUPPLIED

Tab: 150mg

CONTRAINDICATIONS

Concomitant use with alfuzosin, dronedarone, rifampin, irinotecan (when coadministered with atazanavir only), dihydroergotamine, ergotamine, methylergonovine, cisapride, St. John's wort, lovastatin, simvastatin, pimozide, nevirapine (when coadministered with atazanavir only), sildenafil (when used to treat pulmonary arterial HTN), indinavir (when coadministered with atazanavir only), triazolam, and oral midazolam.

WARNINGS/PRECAUTIONS

Not interchangeable with ritonavir to increase systemic exposure of darunavir 600mg bid, fosamprenavir, saquinavir, or tipranavir. Decreases estimated CrCl due to inhibition of tubular secretion of creatinine without affecting actual renal glomerular function; consider this effect when interpreting changes in estimated CrCl in patients initiating therapy, particularly in patients with medical conditions or receiving drugs needing monitoring with estimated CrCl. Consider alternative medications that do not require dosage adjustments in patients with renal impairment. Closely monitor patients who experience a confirmed increase in SrCr of >0.4mg/dL from baseline for renal safety.

ADVERSE REACTIONS

Jaundice, ocular icterus, nausea.

DRUG INTERACTIONS

See Contraindications. Renal impairment, including cases of acute renal failure and Fanconi syndrome, reported with tenofovir disoproxil fumarate (TDF); coadministration is not recommended in patients with estimated CrCl <70mL/min. Coadministration with TDF in combination with concomitant or recent use of a nephrotoxic agent is not recommended. Not recommended with >1 antiretroviral that requires pharmacokinetic enhancement (eg, 2 protease inhibitors or a protease inhibitor in combination with elvitegravir); darunavir in combination with efavirenz, nevirapine, or etravirine; atazanavir in combination with etravirine; atazanavir in combination with efavirenz in treatment-experienced patients; darunavir 600mg bid; other HIV-1 protease inhibitors (eg, fosamprenavir, saquinavir, tipranavir); elvitegravir/cobicistat/emtricitabine/TDF fixed-dose combination; and lopinavir/ritonavir or regimens containing ritonavir. Not recommended with HCV protease inhibitors (eg, boceprevir, telaprevir, simeprevir), salmeterol, avanafil, voriconazole, or with colchicine in patients with renal/hepatic impairment. May increase concentration of drugs that are primarily metabolized by CYP3A (eg, maraviroc, clonazepam, carbamazepine, corticosteroids [eg, dexamethasone, inhaled/nasal fluticasone or budesonide], cyclosporine, everolimus, sirolimus, tacrolimus) or CYP2D6, or are substrates of P-gp, BCRP, OATP1B1 or OATP1B3. CYP3A inducers (eg, carbamazepine, oxcarbazepine, phenytoin, phenobarbital, dexamethasone) may decrease concentrations of cobicistat, atazanavir, and darunavir, which may lead to loss of efficacy and development of resistance. CYP3A inhibitors may increase concentrations. Coadministration with atazanavir in combination with antacids (eg, aluminum and magnesium hydroxide) may decrease atazanavir levels; administer a minimum of 2 hrs apart. May increase levels of antiarrhythmics (eg, amiodarone, quinidine, digoxin), dasatinib, nilotinib, vinblastine, vincristine, itraconazole, ketoconazole, colchicine, rifabutin, β-blockers, calcium channel blockers, bosentan, HMG-CoA reductase inhibitors (eg, atorvastatin, rosuvastatin), fentanyl, tramadol, neuroleptics (eg, perphenazine, risperidone), PDE-5 inhibitors (eg, sildenafil, tadalafil), and sedatives/hypnotics (eg, buspirone, diazepam, parenteral midazolam). Coadministration with macrolide/ketolide antibiotics (clarithromycin, erythromycin, telithromycin) may increase levels of both the antibiotic, and cobicistat, atazanavir, and darunavir; consider alternative antibiotics. Monitor for hematologic or GI side effects with vincristine and vinblastine. Monitor INR with warfarin. Avoid with rivaroxaban. Monitor phenobarbital or phenytoin concentrations. Caution with SSRIs (eg, paroxetine), TCAs (eg, amitriptyline, desipramine), and trazodone; may increase levels of TCAs and trazodone. Ketoconazole and itraconazole may increase levels. Bosentan may decrease levels. Coadministration with atazanavir in combination with H_2-receptor antagonists (eg, famotidine) may decrease atazanavir levels; administer atazanavir/cobicistat coadministration either at the same time or a minimum of 10 hrs after administering H_2-receptor antagonists. Consider additional or alternative (nonhormonal) forms of contraception if to be used with oral/hormonal contraceptives. Caution with buprenorphine, buprenorphine/naloxone, and methadone. Coadministration with atazanavir in combination with proton pump inhibitors (eg, omeprazole), may decrease atazanavir levels; administer cobicistat with atazanavir a minimum of 12 hrs after administering proton pump inhibitors in treatment-naive patients. Refer to PI for further information including dosing modifications when used with certain concomitant therapies.

NURSING CONSIDERATIONS

Assessment: Assess pregnancy/nursing status, and for possible drug interactions. Assess estimated CrCl. When used with TDF, assess estimated CrCl, urine glucose, and urine protein.

Monitoring: Monitor for adverse reactions. Monitor CrCl. When used with TDF, perform routine monitoring of estimated CrCl, urine glucose, and urine protein, and measure serum phosphorus in patients with or at risk for renal impairment.

Patient Counseling: Inform of the risks and benefits of therapy. Inform patients that they should remain under the care of a physician when using therapy. Counsel about the risks of developing resistance to HIV-1 medications. Instruct that if a dose of the drug and atazanavir or darunavir is missed by <12 hrs, take the missed dose of the drug with atazanavir or darunavir together right away, and the next dose together as usual; if a dose of the drug with atazanavir or darunavir is missed by >12 hrs, instruct to wait and take the next dose at the usual time. If a dose of the drug with atazanavir or darunavir is skipped, instruct not to double the next dose. Inform that therapy may interact with many drugs with potential serious implications and that some drugs should not be taken with therapy; advise to report to physician the use of any other prescription or nonprescription medication or herbal products, including St. John's wort.

Storage: 25°C (77°F); excursions permitted to 15-30°C (59-86°F). Keep tightly closed.

TYKERB – lapatinib RX

Class: Kinase inhibitors

Hepatotoxicity observed; may be severe and deaths have been reported.

ADULT DOSAGE

HER2-Positive Metastatic Breast Cancer

In combination w/ capecitabine in patients who have received prior therapy, including an anthracycline, a taxane, and trastuzumab

Usual: 1250mg qd on Days 1-21 continuously w/ capecitabine 2000mg/m²/day (administered PO in 2 doses approx 12 hrs apart) on Days 1-14 in a repeating 21-day cycle; take capecitabine w/ food or w/in 30 min after food

Continue until disease progression or unacceptable toxicity occurs

Hormone Receptor-Positive, HER2-Positive Metastatic Breast Cancer

In combination w/ letrozole for the treatment of postmenopausal women for whom hormonal therapy is indicated

Usual: 1500mg qd continuously w/ letrozole 2.5mg qd

PEDIATRIC DOSAGE

Pediatric use may not have been established

DOSE MODIFICATION

Concomitant Medications

Strong CYP3A4 Inhibitors:

Avoid use; if coadministration is required, reduce lapatinib dose to 500mg/day

If strong inhibitor is discontinued, a washout period of approx 1 week should be allowed before the lapatinib dose is adjusted upward to the indicated dose

Avoid w/ grapefruit

Strong CYP3A4 Inducers:

Avoid use; if coadministration is required, titrate dose gradually as follows:

HER2-Positive Metastatic Breast Cancer: Titrate up to 4500mg/day

Hormone Receptor-Positive, HER2-Positive Metastatic Breast Cancer: Titrate up to 5500mg/day

If strong inducer is discontinued, reduce lapatinib dose to the indicated dose

Hepatic Impairment

Severe (Child-Pugh Class C):

HER2-Positive Metastatic Breast Cancer: Reduce dose to 750mg/day

Hormone Receptor-Positive, HER2-Positive Metastatic Breast Cancer: Reduce dose to 1000mg/day

Adverse Reactions

Cardiac Events:

D/C Therapy in Patients w/:
1. Decreased left ventricular ejection fraction (LVEF) ≥Grade 2 by National Cancer Institute Common Terminology Criteria for Adverse Events (NCI CTCAE v3)
2. LVEF that drops below the lower limit of normal
If LVEF Recovers to Normal and Patient is Asymptomatic for ≥2 Weeks:
In Combination w/ Capecitabine: Restart dose at 1000mg/day
In Combination w/ Letrozole: Restart dose at 1250mg/day
Diarrhea:
NCI CTCAE Grade 3 or Grade 1 or 2 w/ Complicating Features: Interrupt therapy
When Diarrhea Resolves to ≤Grade 1:
HER2-Positive Metastatic Breast Cancer: Reduce dose to 1000mg/day
Hormone Receptor-Positive, HER2-Positive Metastatic Breast Cancer: Reduce dose to 1250mg/day
NCI CTCAE Grade 4: Permanently d/c therapy
Other Toxicities:
≥Grade 2 NCI CTCAE Toxicity: Consider discontinuation/dose interruption
When Toxicity Improves to ≤Grade 1: Restart at standard dose
If Toxicity Recurs:
In Combination w/ Capecitabine: Restart at 1000mg/day
In Combination w/ Letrozole: Restart at 1250mg/day

ADMINISTRATION
Oral route

Take at least 1 hr ac or 1 hr pc
Do not divide the daily dose

HOW SUPPLIED
Tab: 250mg

WARNINGS/PRECAUTIONS
Patients should have disease progression on trastuzumab prior to initiation of treatment w/ lapatinib in combination w/ capecitabine. Decreased LVEF reported; confirm normal LVEF prior to therapy. D/C if severe liver function changes occur, and do not retreat. Diarrhea, including severe cases and deaths, reported; early identification and intervention is critical. Prompt treatment of diarrhea w/ antidiarrheals (eg, loperamide) after the 1st unformed stool is recommended. Severe diarrhea may require administration of oral or IV electrolytes/fluids, use of antibiotics such as fluoroquinolones (especially if diarrhea persists >24 hrs, there is fever, or Grade 3 or 4 neutropenia), and interruption or discontinuation of therapy. Associated w/ interstitial lung disease and pneumonitis; d/c if pulmonary symptoms indicative of interstitial lung disease/pneumonitis (≥Grade 3) occur. QT prolongation observed; caution in patients who have or may develop prolongation of QTc (eg, taking antiarrhythmics or other drugs that prolong the QT interval, cumulative high-dose anthracycline therapy). Correct hypokalemia and hypomagnesemia before administration. Severe cutaneous reactions reported; d/c treatment if life-threatening reactions (eg, erythema multiforme, Stevens-Johnson syndrome, toxic epidermal necrolysis) are suspected. May cause fetal harm.

ADVERSE REACTIONS
Hepatotoxicity, diarrhea, N/V, stomatitis, dyspepsia, palmar-plantar erythrodysesthesia, rash, dry skin, mucosal inflammation, pain in extremity, back pain, dyspnea, fatigue, headache, alopecia.

DRUG INTERACTIONS
See Dose Modification. Caution w/ substrates of CYP3A4, CYP2C8, and P-gp; consider dose reduction of the concomitant substrate drug when dosing lapatinib concurrently w/ concomitant substrate drugs w/ narrow therapeutic windows. Increased levels w/ P-gp inhibitors; use w/ caution. Increased levels w/ grapefruit. May increase exposure of paclitaxel and midazolam. May increase exposure of digoxin; monitor serum digoxin concentrations prior to initiation of lapatinib and throughout coadministration. If digoxin level is >1.2ng/mL, reduce digoxin dose by 1/2.

NURSING CONSIDERATIONS

Assessment: Assess for severe hepatic impairment, decreased LVEF or conditions that may impair left ventricular function, QT prolongation, hypokalemia, hypomagnesemia, pregnancy/nursing status, drug hypersensitivity, and possible drug interactions. Obtain baseline ECG, LFTs, serum K^+, and Mg^{2+} levels.

Monitoring: Monitor for hepatotoxicity, diarrhea, bowel changes, pulmonary symptoms indicative of interstitial lung disease or pneumonitis, decreased LVEF, QT prolongation, severe cutaneous reactions, and other adverse reactions. Consider ECG and electrolyte monitoring. Monitor LFTs every 4-6 weeks during therapy and as clinically indicated.

Patient Counseling: Instruct to notify physician if SOB, palpitations, or fatigue occurs. Advise that diarrhea is a common side effect and instruct on how it should be managed/prevented; instruct to contact physician immediately if any change in bowel patterns or severe diarrhea occurs. Counsel to report use of any prescription/nonprescription drugs or herbal products. Instruct not to take w/ grapefruit products. Advise women not to become pregnant while on therapy.

Storage: 25°C (77°F); excursions permitted to 15-30°C (59-86°F).

TYSABRI – natalizumab

RX

Class: Monoclonal antibody/integrin receptor antagonist

Increases risk of progressive multifocal leukoencephalopathy (PML). Risk factors for development of PML include duration of therapy, prior use of immunosuppressants, and presence of anti-JCV antibodies. Monitor for any new signs/symptoms of PML; withhold therapy at the 1st sign/symptom suggestive of PML. Available only through a special restricted distribution program called the TOUCH Prescribing Program.

ADULT DOSAGE

Multiple Sclerosis

Monotherapy for the Treatment of Relapsing Forms:

Usual: 300mg IV infusion over 1 hr every 4 weeks

Crohn's Disease

To induce and maintain clinical response and remission in patients w/ moderately to severely active Crohn's disease (CD) w/ evidence of inflammation who have had an inadequate response to, or are unable to tolerate, conventional CD therapies and TNF-α inhibitors

Usual: 300mg IV infusion over 1 hr every 4 weeks

In patients starting therapy while on chronic oral corticosteroids, commence steroid tapering as soon as therapeutic benefit has occurred

PEDIATRIC DOSAGE

Pediatric use may not have been established

DOSE MODIFICATION

Discontinuation

Crohn's Disease (CD):

D/C therapy if no therapeutic benefit by 12 weeks of induction therapy, if patient cannot be tapered off of corticosteroids w/in 6 months of starting therapy, and consider discontinuation in patients who require additional steroid use that exceeds 3 months in a calendar yr to control their CD

ADMINISTRATION

IV route

Dilution

1. To prepare sol, withdraw 15mL from the vial using a sterile needle and syringe. Inject the concentrate into 100mL 0.9% NaCl inj; no other IV diluents may be used to prepare the sol
2. Gently invert sol to mix completely; do not shake
3. The final dosage sol has a concentration of 2.6mg/mL
4. Following dilution, infuse sol immediately, or refrigerate at 2-8°C (36-46°F), and use w/in 8 hrs; if refrigerated, allow sol to warm to room temperature prior to infusion. Do not freeze

Administration

1. Infuse 300mg in 100mL 0.9% NaCl inj, over approx 1 hr (infusion rate approx 5mg/min)
2. Do not administer as an IV push or bolus inj
3. After the infusion is complete, flush w/ 0.9% NaCl inj
4. Do not inject other medications into infusion set side ports or mix w/ therapy

HOW SUPPLIED

Inj: 300mg/15mL

CONTRAINDICATIONS

PML or history of PML.

WARNINGS/PRECAUTIONS

Anti-JCV antibody testing should not be used to diagnose PML. Avoid anti-JCV antibody testing for at least 2 weeks following plasma exchange due to the removal of antibodies from the serum. Retest patients with negative anti-JCV antibody test result periodically. PML reported following discontinuation in patient who do not have findings suggestive of PML at the time of discontinuation; monitor for any new signs or symptoms that may be suggestive of PML for at least 6 months following discontinuation. Immune reconstitution inflammatory syndrome (IRIS) reported in patients with PML, who have subsequently discontinued natalizumab; monitor for development of IRIS and treat appropriately. Increases the risk of developing encephalitis and meningitis caused by herpes simplex and varicella zoster viruses; d/c and treat appropriately if herpes encephalitis and meningitis occurs. Liver injury, including acute liver failure requiring transplant, reported; d/c with jaundice or other evidence of significant liver injury (eg, lab evidence). Hypersensitivity reactions, including serious systemic reactions (eg, anaphylaxis) reported; d/c, institute appropriate therapy, and do not retreat. May increase risk for infections. Avoid in patients with systemic medical conditions resulting in significantly compromised immune system function. Induces increases in circulating lymphocytes, monocytes, eosinophils, basophils, and nucleated RBCs or transient decreases in Hgb levels.

ADVERSE REACTIONS

Headache, fatigue, arthralgia, urinary tract infection, depression, lower/upper respiratory tract infection, abdominal discomfort, rash, gastroenteritis, vaginitis, urinary urgency/frequency, diarrhea, abnormal LFTs.

DRUG INTERACTIONS

Avoid with immunomodulatory therapy, immunosuppressants (eg, 6-mercaptopurine, azathioprine, cyclosporine, methotrexate) or TNF-α inhibitors. Taper corticosteroids in CD patients when starting natalizumab therapy. Antineoplastic, immunosuppressive, or immunomodulating agents may further increase risk of infections, including PML and other opportunistic infections.

NURSING CONSIDERATIONS

Assessment: Assess for risk of PML, history of chronic immunosuppressant or immunomodulatory therapy, immunosuppression, drug hypersensitivity, pregnancy/nursing status, and possible drug interactions. Perform magnetic resonance imaging and CSF analysis. Test for anti-JCV antibody status; retest periodically in patients with negative result.

Monitoring: Monitor for PML, anaphylactic/hypersensitivity reactions, infections, hepatotoxicity, development of IRIS and other adverse reactions. Antibody testing recommended if presence of persistent antibodies is suspected. Evaluate patients 3 and 6 months after the 1st infusion, every 6 months thereafter, and for at least 6 months after discontinuing treatment

Patient Counseling: Inform about TOUCH Prescribing Program. Educate on risks/benefits of therapy. Counsel about the follow-up schedule (3 and 6 months after 1st infusion, every 6 months thereafter, and for at least 6 months after discontinuation). Instruct to seek medical attention if symptoms suggestive of PML develop, including progressive weakness on one side of the body or clumsiness of the limbs, disturbance of vision, and changes in thinking, memory, and orientation leading to confusion and personality changes. Instruct to report symptoms of infections, hypersensitivity reactions, and hepatotoxicity.

Storage: 2-8°C (36-46°F). Administer within 8 hrs of preparation. Do not shake or freeze. Protect from light.

Uloric – febuxostat RX

Class: Xanthine oxidase inhibitor

ADULT DOSAGE

Hyperuricemia

Chronic Management in Patients w/ Gout:
Initial: 40mg qd
Titrate: If serum uric acid is not <6mg/dL after 2 weeks, increase dose to 80mg qd

PEDIATRIC DOSAGE

Pediatric use may not have been established

ADMINISTRATION

Oral route

May be taken w/o regard to food or antacid use

HOW SUPPLIED

Tab: 40mg, 80mg

CONTRAINDICATIONS

Patients being treated with azathioprine or mercaptopurine.

WARNINGS/PRECAUTIONS

Not recommended for treatment of asymptomatic hyperuricemia. Increase in gout flares observed after initiation; concurrent prophylactic treatment with NSAIDs or colchicine is recommended. Cardiovascular (CV) thromboembolic events (eg, CV deaths, myocardial infarctions [MI], strokes) reported; monitor for signs and symptoms of MI and stroke. Fatal and nonfatal hepatic failure reported; obtain baseline LFTs before initiation. Measure LFTs promptly in patients who report symptoms that may indicate liver injury; d/c if LFTs are abnormal (ALT >3X ULN) and do not restart if no alternative etiology is found. D/C permanently in patients with ALT >3X ULN with serum total bilirubin >2X ULN without alternative etiologies; use with caution in patients with lesser ALT or bilirubin elevations and with an alternate probable cause. Caution with severe hepatic impairment (Child-Pugh Class C) and severe renal impairment (CrCl <30mL/min). Avoid use in patients whom the rate of urate formation is greatly increased (eg, malignant disease and its treatment, Lesch-Nyhan syndrome).

ADVERSE REACTIONS
Liver function abnormalities, nausea, arthralgia, rash.

DRUG INTERACTIONS
See Contraindications. Caution with theophylline.

NURSING CONSIDERATIONS

Assessment: Assess for asymptomatic hyperuricemia, hepatic/renal impairment, malignant disease, Lesch-Nyhan syndrome, pregnancy/nursing status, and possible drug interactions. Obtain baseline serum uric acid (sUA) and LFTs.

Monitoring: Monitor sUA levels as early as 2 weeks after initiation of therapy. Monitor for signs/symptoms of liver injury, MI, and stroke.

Patient Counseling: Advise of the potential benefits and risks of therapy. Inform that gout flares, elevated liver enzymes, and adverse CV events may occur. Instruct to notify physician if rash, chest pain, SOB, or neurologic symptoms suggesting a stroke occur. Instruct to inform physician of any other medications, including OTC drugs, currently being taken.

Storage: 25°C (77°F); excursions permitted to 15-30°C (59-86°F). Protect from light.

ULTRACET – acetaminophen/tramadol hydrochloride CIV

Class: Central acting analgesic

Associated with cases of acute liver failure, at times resulting in liver transplant and death. Most cases of liver injury are associated with acetaminophen (APAP) use at doses >4000mg/day and often involve >1 APAP-containing product.

ADULT DOSAGE
Acute Pain
Short-Term (≤5 Days) Management:
2 tabs q4-6h prn for ≤5 days
Max: 8 tabs/day

PEDIATRIC DOSAGE
Pediatric use may not have been established

DOSE MODIFICATION
Renal Impairment
CrCl <30mL/min:
Max: 2 tabs q12h

ADMINISTRATION
Oral route

HOW SUPPLIED
Tab: (Tramadol-APAP) 37.5mg-325mg

CONTRAINDICATIONS
Any situation where opioids are contraindicated, including acute intoxication with alcohol, hypnotics, narcotics, centrally acting analgesics, opioids, or psychotropic drugs.

WARNINGS/PRECAUTIONS
Do not exceed recommended dose. May complicate clinical assessment of acute abdominal conditions. Not recommended in patients with hepatic impairment; increased risk of acute liver failure in patients with underlying liver disease. Not for use in pregnant women prior to or during labor unless benefits outweigh risks. Not recommended for obstetrical preoperative medication or for postdelivery analgesia in nursing mothers. Caution in elderly. Serious and fatal anaphylactic reactions reported; avoid use in patients with a history of anaphylactoid reactions to codeine or other opioids. D/C use if anaphylaxis develops. APAP: Avoid in patients with APAP allergy. May cause serious skin reactions (eg, acute generalized exanthematous pustulosis, Stevens-Johnson syndrome, toxic epidermal necrolysis), which can be fatal; d/c at the 1st appearance of skin rash or any other sign of hypersensitivity. Tramadol: Seizures reported; risk increases in patients with epilepsy, history/risk of seizures, and with naloxone coadministration. Avoid in patients who are suicidal or addiction-prone; caution with emotional disturbances or depression. Reports of tramadol-related deaths with previous history of emotional disturbances, suicidal ideation/attempts, and misuse of tranquilizers/alcohol/CNS-active drugs. Potentially life-threatening serotonin syndrome, including mental status changes, autonomic instability, neuromuscular aberrations, and GI symptoms, may occur. Caution if at risk for respiratory depression; consider alternative nonopioid analgesic. Caution with CNS depression, head injury, and increased intracranial pressure (ICP). May impair mental/physical abilities. May cause withdrawal symptoms; do not d/c abruptly.

ADVERSE REACTIONS

Acute liver failure, constipation, somnolence, increased sweating, diarrhea, nausea, anorexia, dizziness.

DRUG INTERACTIONS

See Contraindications. Do not use concomitantly with alcohol, other APAP- or tramadol-containing products; increased risk of acute liver failure with alcohol ingestion. May alter effects of warfarin; periodically monitor PT with warfarin-like compounds. Tramadol: Increased seizure risk with SSRIs, TCAs, other tricyclic compounds (eg, cyclobenzaprine, promethazine), MAOIs, other opioids, neuroleptics, and drugs that reduce seizure threshold. Serotonin syndrome may occur when coadministered with SSRIs, SNRIs, TCAs, MAOIs, triptans, α_2-adrenergic blockers, linezolid, lithium, St. John's wort, or drugs that impair tramadol metabolism; observe carefully, especially during initiation and dose increases. Caution and reduce dose with CNS depressants (eg, alcohol, opioids, anesthetics); increased risk of CNS/respiratory depression. Caution with antidepressants and muscle relaxants; additive CNS depressant effects. CYP2D6 inhibitors (eg, quinidine, fluoxetine, paroxetine, amitriptyline) and/or CYP3A4 inhibitors (eg, ketoconazole, erythromycin) may reduce metabolic clearance; increased risk of serious adverse effects. CYP3A4 inhibitors or inducers (eg, rifampin, St. John's wort) may alter drug exposure. Digoxin toxicity may occur with concomitant use. Carbamazepine may reduce analgesic effect; avoid coadministration.

NURSING CONSIDERATIONS

Assessment: Assess for known hypersensitivity to the drug and other opioids, acute intoxication with alcohol, hypnotics, narcotics, centrally acting analgesics, opioids, or psychotropic drugs, epilepsy, seizure and respiratory depression risks, suicidal ideation, emotional disturbance or depression, increased ICP, head injury, drug abuse potential, suicidal or addiction proneness, renal/hepatic impairment, pregnancy/nursing status, and possible drug interactions.

Monitoring: Monitor for acute liver failure, skin hypersensitivity/anaphylactic reactions, respiratory/CNS depression, physical dependence/abuse, misuse, tolerance, seizures, development of serotonin syndrome, withdrawal symptoms with abrupt discontinuation, and other adverse reactions. Periodically monitor PT with warfarin-like compounds.

Patient Counseling: Instruct to d/c therapy and notify physician if signs of allergy occur. Advise patients of dose limits. Instruct to seek medical attention immediately upon ingestion of >4000mg/day APAP, even if feeling well. Counsel not to use with other tramadol or APAP-containing products, including OTC preparations. Inform that seizures and serotonin syndrome may occur when used with serotonergic agents or drugs that reduce the clearance of tramadol. Inform that therapy may impair physical/mental abilities. Instruct to notify physician if pregnant or planning to become pregnant. Instruct to avoid alcohol-containing beverages while on therapy. Inform about the signs of serious skin reactions and of possible drug interactions.

Storage: 25°C (77°F); excursions permitted to 15-30°C (59-86°F).

ULTRAM — tramadol hydrochloride CIV

Class: Central acting analgesic

ADULT DOSAGE

Moderate to Moderately Severe Pain

≥17 Years:

Initial: 25mg/day qam

Titrate: Increase in 25mg increments every 3 days to reach 100mg/day (25mg qid), then may be increased by 50mg as tolerated every 3 days to reach 200mg/day (50mg qid)

After Titration/Rapid Onset Required: 50-100mg q4-6h prn

Max: 400mg/day

PEDIATRIC DOSAGE

Pediatric use may not have been established

DOSE MODIFICATION

Renal Impairment

CrCl <30mL/min:

Increase dosing interval to 12 hrs

Dialysis patients may receive regular dose on the day of dialysis

Max: 200mg/day

Hepatic Impairment

Cirrhosis: 50mg q12h

Elderly

Start at lower end of dosing range

>75 Years:

Max: 300mg/day

ADMINISTRATION

Oral route

Administer w/o regard to food

HOW SUPPLIED

Tab: 50mg* *scored

CONTRAINDICATIONS

Any situation where opioids are contraindicated, including acute intoxication with alcohol, hypnotics, narcotics, centrally acting analgesics, opioids, or psychotropic drugs.

WARNINGS/PRECAUTIONS

Do not exceed recommended dose. Seizures reported; risk increases in patients with epilepsy, history of seizures, recognized risk for seizures, and with naloxone coadministration. Anaphylactoid reactions and potentially life-threatening serotonin syndrome may occur. Avoid in patients who are suicidal or addiction-prone, and with history of anaphylactoid reactions to codeine and other opioids. Caution with emotional disturbances or depression, and in elderly. Tramadol-related deaths reported with previous histories of emotional disturbances, suicidal ideation/attempts, and misuse of tranquilizers, alcohol, and other CNS active drugs. Caution in patients at risk for respiratory depression; consider alternative nonopioid analgesics. Caution with increased intracranial pressure (ICP) or head injury. May impair mental/physical abilities. Withdrawal symptoms may occur if discontinued abruptly. May complicate clinical assessment of acute abdominal conditions. Not for use in pregnant women prior to or during labor unless benefits outweigh risks. Not recommended for obstetrical preoperative medication or for postdelivery analgesia in nursing mothers.

ADVERSE REACTIONS

Dizziness/vertigo, N/V, constipation, headache, somnolence, sweating, asthenia, dyspepsia, dry mouth, diarrhea, pruritus.

DRUG INTERACTIONS

See Contraindications. Caution and reduce dose with CNS depressants (eg, alcohol, opioids, anesthetics); increased risk of CNS/respiratory depression. CYP2D6 inhibitors (eg, quinidine, fluoxetine, paroxetine, amitriptyline) and CYP3A4 inhibitors (eg, ketoconazole, erythromycin) may reduce metabolic clearance and increase risk for serious adverse events including seizures and serotonin syndrome. Altered exposure with CYP3A4 inducers (eg, rifampin, St. John's wort). Increased seizure risk with SSRIs, TCAs, other tricyclic compounds (eg, cyclobenzaprine, promethazine), MAOIs, other opioids, neuroleptics, and drugs that reduce seizure threshold. Caution with SSRIs, SNRIs, TCAs, MAOIs, α2-adrenergic blockers, triptans, linezolid, lithium, St. John's wort, and drugs that impair tramadol metabolism, due to potential serotonin syndrome. Not recommended with carbamazepine; may significantly reduce analgesic effect. Digoxin toxicity and alteration of warfarin effect, including elevation of PT, reported rarely.

NURSING CONSIDERATIONS

Assessment: Assess for previous hypersensitivity to the drug and other opioids, acute intoxication with alcohol/hypnotics/narcotics/centrally acting analgesics/opioids/psychotropic drugs, epilepsy, seizure and respiratory depression risks, suicidal ideation, emotional disturbance or depression, increased ICP, head injury, drug abuse potential, suicidal/addiction proneness, pain severity, renal/hepatic impairment, pregnancy/nursing status, any other conditions where treatment is contraindicated or cautioned, and possible drug interactions.

Monitoring: Monitor for signs/symptoms of anaphylactoid reactions, respiratory/CNS depression, tolerance, physical dependence, seizures, serotonin syndrome, withdrawal symptoms, and other adverse reactions.

Patient Counseling: Inform of the risks and benefits of therapy. Inform that drug may cause seizures and/or serotonin syndrome with concomitant use of serotonergic agents or drugs that significantly reduce the metabolic clearance of therapy. Inform that drug may impair physical/mental abilities required for the performance of hazardous tasks (eg, driving a car, operating machinery). Instruct not to take drug with alcohol containing beverages. Inform to use drug with caution when taking tranquilizers, hypnotics, other opiate containing analgesics). Instruct to inform physician if pregnant, think or trying to become pregnant. Educate about single-dose and 24-hr dose limits and time interval between doses; advise not to exceed the recommended dose.

Storage: 25°C (77°F); excursions permitted to 15-30°C (59-86°F).

ULTRAM ER – tramadol hydrochloride

CIV

Class: Central acting analgesic

ADULT DOSAGE

Chronic Pain

Moderate to Moderately Severe Pain Requiring Around-the-Clock Treatment for an Extended Period:

Not Currently on Tramadol IR:

Initial: 100mg qd

Titrate: Increase as necessary by 100mg increments every 5 days

Max: 300mg/day

Currently on Tramadol IR:

Initial: Calculate 24-hr tramadol IR dose and initiate total daily dose rounded down to next lowest 100mg increment

Titrate: Individualize according to patients need

Max: 300mg/day

PEDIATRIC DOSAGE

Pediatric use may not have been established

DOSE MODIFICATION

Renal Impairment

CrCl <30mg/mL: Do not use

Hepatic Impairment

Severe (Child-Pugh Class C): Do not use

Elderly

Start at low end of dosing range

ADMINISTRATION

Oral route

Swallow whole; do not chew, crush, or split

HOW SUPPLIED

Tab, Extended-Release: 100mg, 200mg, 300mg

CONTRAINDICATIONS

Any situation where opioids are contraindicated, including acute intoxication w/ alcohol, hypnotics, narcotics, centrally acting analgesics, opioids, or psychotropic drugs.

WARNINGS/PRECAUTIONS

Do not exceed recommended dose. Seizures reported; risk increases in patients w/ epilepsy, history of seizures, recognized risk for seizures, and w/ naloxone coadministration. Anaphylactoid reactions and potentially life-threatening serotonin syndrome may occur. Avoid in patients who are suicidal or addiction-prone, and w/ history of anaphylactoid reactions to codeine and other opioids. Tramadol-related deaths reported w/ previous histories of emotional disturbances, suicidal ideation/attempts, and misuse of tranquilizers, alcohol, and other CNS-active drugs. Caution in patients at risk for respiratory depression; consider alternative nonopioid analgesics. Caution w/ increased intracranial pressure (ICP) or head injury. May impair mental/physical abilities. Withdrawal symptoms may occur if discontinued abruptly. May complicate clinical assessment of acute abdominal conditions. Not for use in pregnant women prior to or during labor unless benefits outweigh risks. Not recommended for obstetrical preoperative medication or for postdelivery analgesia in nursing mothers.

ADVERSE REACTIONS

Dizziness, N/V, constipation, headache, somnolence, flushing, insomnia, increased sweating, asthenia, dry mouth, diarrhea, pruritus, postural hypotension.

DRUG INTERACTIONS

See Contraindications. Caution and reduce dose w/ CNS depressants (eg, alcohol, opioids, anesthetics); increased risk of CNS/respiratory depression. CYP2D6 inhibitors (eg, quinidine, fluoxetine, paroxetine, amitriptyline) and CYP3A4 inhibitors (eg, ketoconazole, erythromycin) may reduce metabolic clearance and increase risk for serious adverse events, including seizures and serotonin syndrome. Altered exposure w/ CYP3A4 inducers (eg, rifampin, St. John's wort) and inhibitors (ketoconazole, erythromycin). Increased seizure risk w/ SSRIs, TCAs, other tricyclic compounds (eg, cyclobenzaprine, promethazine), MAOIs, other opioids, neuroleptics, and drugs that reduce seizure threshold. Caution w/ SSRIs, SNRIs, TCAs, MAOIs, α2-adrenergic blockers, triptans, linezolid, lithium, St. John's wort, and drugs that impair tramadol metabolism, due to potential serotonin syndrome. Not recommended w/ carbamazepine; may significantly reduce analgesic effect. Digoxin toxicity and alterations of warfarin effect, including elevation of PT, reported rarely. Use w/ other tramadol products is not recommended.

NURSING CONSIDERATIONS

Assessment: Assess for previous hypersensitivity to the drug and other opioids, acute intoxication w/ alcohol/hypnotics/narcotics/centrally acting analgesics/opioids/psychotropic drugs, epilepsy, seizure and respiratory depression risks, suicidal ideation, emotional disturbance or depression, increased ICP, head injury, drug abuse potential, suicidal/addiction proneness, pain severity, renal/hepatic impairment, pregnancy/nursing status, any other conditions where treatment is contraindicated or cautioned, and possible drug interactions.

Monitoring: Monitor for signs/symptoms of anaphylactoid reactions, respiratory/CNS depression, tolerance, physical dependence, seizures, serotonin syndrome, withdrawal symptoms, and other adverse reactions.

Patient Counseling: Inform of the risks/benefits of therapy. Inform that drug may cause seizures and/or serotonin syndrome w/ concomitant use of serotonergic agents or drugs that significantly reduce the metabolic clearance of therapy. Inform that drug may impair physical/mental abilities required for the performance of hazardous tasks (eg, driving a car, operating machinery). Instruct not to take drug w/ alcohol containing beverages. Inform to use drug w/ caution when taking tranquilizers, hypnotics, and other opiate containing analgesics. Instruct to inform physician if pregnant, thinking/trying to become pregnant. Educate regarding the single-dose and 24-hr dosing regimen; advise not to exceed the recommended dose.

Storage: 25°C (77°F); excursions permitted to 15-30°C (59-86°F).

ULTRAVATE – halobetasol propionate

RX

Class: Corticosteroid

ADULT DOSAGE

Inflammatory and Pruritic Manifestations of Corticosteroid-Responsive Dermatoses

Apply a thin layer to affected skin qd or bid ud and rub in gently and completely

Max Dose: 50g/week

Max Duration: 2 weeks; reassess diagnosis if no improvement w/in 2 weeks

D/C when control is achieved

PEDIATRIC DOSAGE

Inflammatory and Pruritic Manifestations of Corticosteroid-Responsive Dermatoses

≥12 Years:
Apply a thin layer to affected skin qd or bid ud and rub in gently and completely

Max Dose: 50g/week

Max Duration: 2 weeks; reassess diagnosis if no improvement w/in 2 weeks

D/C when control is achieved

ADMINISTRATION

Topical route

Avoid w/ occlusive dressings

HOW SUPPLIED

Cre, Oint: 0.05% [50g]

WARNINGS/PRECAUTIONS

For dermatologic use only; not for ophthalmic use. May produce reversible hypothalamic-pituitary-adrenal (HPA) axis suppression, manifestations of Cushing's syndrome, hyperglycemia or glucosuria; evaluate periodically for evidence of HPA axis suppression when applying to a large surface area or to areas under occlusion. Attempts should be made to withdraw treatment, reduce frequency of application, or substitute to a less potent corticosteroid if HPA axis suppression is noted. Signs and symptoms of glucocorticosteroid insufficiency may occur (infrequent), requiring supplemental systemic corticosteroids. Pediatric patients may be more susceptible to systemic toxicity. D/C and treat appropriately if irritation develops. Allergic contact dermatitis reported. Use appropriate antibacterial or antifungal agent if skin infections are present or develop; if no favorable prompt response, may need to d/c until infection is controlled. Not for use in rosacea or perioral dermatitis. Do not use on the face, groin, or in the axillae.

ADVERSE REACTIONS

Stinging, burning, itching, dry skin, erythema, skin atrophy, leukoderma, rash.

NURSING CONSIDERATIONS

Assessment: Assess for previous hypersensitivity to any components of the drug, dermatological conditions, pregnancy/nursing status, and conditions that increase systemic absorption of the medication.

Monitoring: Monitor for HPA axis suppression, manifestations of Cushing's syndrome, hyperglycemia, glucosuria, skin irritation, allergic contact dermatitis (eg, failure to heal), skin infections (eg, bacterial, fungal), and other adverse reactions. Monitor for glucocorticosteroid insufficiency following withdrawal from therapy.

Patient Counseling: Instruct to use externally and ud. Instruct to avoid contact with eyes. Advise not to use for any disorder other than for which it was prescribed. Instruct not to bandage, cover, or wrap treated skin, unless directed by physician. Instruct to report any signs of local adverse reactions to physician.

Storage: 15-30°C (59-86°F).

ULTRESA — pancrelipase

Class: Pancreatic enzyme supplement

RX

ADULT DOSAGE

Exocrine Pancreatic Insufficiency

Due to Cystic Fibrosis or Other Conditions:
Individualize dose based on clinical symptoms, degree of steatorrhea present, and fat content of diet; start at lowest recommended dose and increase gradually

Initial: 500 lipase U/kg/meal
Max: 2500 lipase U/kg/meal (or ≤10,000 lipase U/kg/day) or <4000 lipase U/g fat ingested/day

Refer to PI for dosing limitations

PEDIATRIC DOSAGE

Exocrine Pancreatic Insufficiency

Due to Cystic Fibrosis or Other Conditions:
Individualize dose based on clinical symptoms, degree of steatorrhea present, and fat content of diet; start at lowest recommended dose and increase gradually

≤12 Months of Age:
May give 4000 lipase U (1 cap)/120mL of formula or per breastfeeding immediately prior to each feeding

>12 Months-<4 Years:
Initial: 1000 lipase U/kg/meal
Max: 2500 lipase U/kg/meal (or ≤10,000 lipase U/kg/day) or <4000 lipase U/g fat ingested/day

≥4 Years:
Initial: 500 lipase U/kg/meal
Max: 2500 lipase U/kg/meal (or ≤10,000 lipase U/kg/day) or <4000 lipase U/g fat ingested/day

Refer to PI for dosing limitations

DOSE MODIFICATION

Elderly

Start at lower end of dosing range

ADMINISTRATION

Oral route

Infants ≤12 Months of Age

Do not mix cap contents directly into formula or breast milk
Contents of cap may be administered w/ small amounts of applesauce, or other acidic food w/ ≤4.5 pH or may also be administered directly to the mouth
Follow administration by breast milk or formula
Drug should not be crushed, chewed, or retained in mouth

Children and Adults

Take during meals or snacks, w/ sufficient fluid
Swallow whole; do not crush or chew caps and cap contents
Patients unable to swallow intact caps may carefully open caps and sprinkle contents on a small amount of soft acidic food w/ a pH of ≤4.5 (eg, applesauce, yogurt) at room temperature; swallow soft food mixture immediately w/o crushing or chewing, and follow w/ water or juice
Do not retain drug in mouth
1/2 of the dose used for an individualized full meal should be given w/ each snack

HOW SUPPLIED

Cap, Delayed-Release: (Lipase/Protease/Amylase) 4000 U/8000 U/8000 U; 13,800 U/27,600 U/27,600 U; 20,700 U/41,400 U/41,400 U; 23,000 U/46,000 U/46,000 U

WARNINGS/PRECAUTIONS

Not interchangeable w/ other pancrelipase products. Fibrosing colonopathy reported; monitor closely for progression to stricture formation. Doses >6000 lipase U/kg/meal have been associated w/ colonic stricture in children <12 yrs of age. May cause irritation to oral mucosa; ensure that no drug is retained in the mouth. Do not crush or chew caps, or mix in foods w/ pH >4.5; may disrupt enteric coating of cap resulting in early release of enzymes, irritation of oral mucosa, and/or loss of enzyme activity. Caution w/ in patients w/ gout, renal impairment, or hyperuricemia; may increase blood uric acid levels. Risk for transmission of viral diseases. Caution w/ known allergy to proteins of porcine origin; severe allergic reactions reported.

ADVERSE REACTIONS

Nasal congestion, neck pain, β-hemolytic streptococcal infection, ear pain, lymphadenopathy, headache, pharyngolaryngeal pain, epistaxis, abdominal pain, diarrhea, flatulence, constipation, nausea, pruritus, urticaria.

NURSING CONSIDERATIONS

Assessment: Assess for allergy to porcine protein, gout, renal impairment, hyperuricemia, and pregnancy/nursing status.

Monitoring: Monitor for fibrosing colonopathy, stricture formation, oral mucosa irritation, hyperuricemia, viral diseases, allergic reactions, and other adverse reactions.

Patient Counseling: Instruct to take ud and w/ food and fluids. Inform that if a dose is missed, take the next dose w/ the next meal/snack ud; instruct not to double doses. Inform that cap contents can also be sprinkled on soft acidic foods (eg, applesauce) if necessary. Advise to contact physician immediately if an allergic reaction develops, if pregnant/breastfeeding, or if planning to become pregnant/breastfeed during therapy.

Storage: 20-25°C (68-77°F). Avoid excessive heat. Store in a dry place in the original container. Protect from moisture.

UNASYN – ampicillin sodium/sulbactam sodium — RX

Class: Beta-lactamase inhibitor/semisynthetic penicillin

ADULT DOSAGE

General Dosing

Skin and skin structure infections, intra-abdominal infections, and gynecological infections caused by susceptible strains of microorganisms

Usual: 1.5g (1g ampicillin + 0.5g sulbactam)-3g (2g ampicillin + 1g sulbactam) IM/IV q6h

Max: 4g sulbactam/day

PEDIATRIC DOSAGE

Skin and Skin Structure Infections

≥1 Year:

Usual: 300mg/kg/day (200mg ampicillin + 100mg sulbactam) IV in equally divided doses q6h

≥40kg: 1.5g (1g ampicillin + 0.5g sulbactam)-3g (2g ampicillin + 1g sulbactam) IV q6h

Max: 4g sulbactam/day

Therapy should not routinely exceed 14 days

DOSE MODIFICATION

Renal Impairment

CrCl ≥30mL/min: 1.5-3g q6-8h

CrCl 15-29mL/min: 1.5-3g q12h

CrCl 5-14mL/min: 1.5-3g q24h

ADMINISTRATION

IV/IM route

Do not reconstitute/administer w/ aminoglycosides

IM

Administer by deep IM inj

IV

Administer slowly over at least 10-15 min or 15-30 min in greater dilutions

Refer to PI for directions for use, preparation, compatibility, and stability

HOW SUPPLIED

Inj: (Ampicillin/Sulbactam) 1g/0.5g, 2g/1g. Also available as a Pharmacy Bulk Package. Refer to individual package insert for more information

CONTRAINDICATIONS

Previous history of cholestatic jaundice/hepatic dysfunction associated with therapy.

WARNINGS/PRECAUTIONS

Serious and occasionally fatal hypersensitivity reactions reported; d/c and institute appropriate therapy if allergic reaction occurs. Hepatic dysfunction (eg, hepatitis, cholestatic jaundice) reported. *Clostridium difficile*-associated diarrhea (CDAD) reported and may range in severity from mild diarrhea to fatal colitis; may need to d/c if CDAD is suspected or confirmed. Ampicillin class antibacterial should not be administered to patients with mononucleosis. May result in bacterial resistance in the absence of proven or suspected bacterial infection or a prophylactic indication; d/c and/or take appropriate measures if superinfection develops. Decrease in total conjugated estriol, estriol-glucuronide, conjugated estrone, and estradiol reported in pregnant women. Lab test interactions may occur. Caution with renal impairment.

ADVERSE REACTIONS

Inj-site pain, thrombophlebitis, diarrhea.

DRUG INTERACTIONS
Probenecid decreases renal tubular secretion and may increase and prolong blood levels. Ampicillin: Increased incidence of rash with allopurinol.

NURSING CONSIDERATIONS

Assessment: Assess for history of hypersensitivity to drug, PCNs, cephalosporins, or other allergens, history of cholestatic jaundice/hepatic dysfunction, mononucleosis, renal impairment, pregnancy/nursing status, and for possible drug interactions. Perform culture and susceptibility testing.

Monitoring: Monitor for signs/symptoms of hypersensitivity reactions, CDAD, superinfection, and other adverse reactions. Monitor for changes in estrogen levels in pregnant women. Monitor hepatic function at regular intervals in patients with hepatic impairment.

Patient Counseling: Inform that therapy should only be used to treat bacterial and not viral infections (eg, common cold). Advise to take exactly ud even if patient feels better early in the course of therapy. Inform that skipping doses or not completing full course may decrease effectiveness and increase resistance. Inform that diarrhea is a common problem caused by therapy and will usually end upon discontinuation of therapy. Inform that diarrhea may occur as late as ≥2 months after last dose of therapy; instruct to notify physician as soon as possible if watery/bloody stools (with or without stomach cramps and fever) occur.

Storage: Prior to Reconstitution: ≤30°C (86°F). Reconstituted: Refer to PI for storage requirements.

UNITHROID — levothyroxine sodium RX

Class: Thyroid replacement hormone

Do not use for the treatment of obesity or weight loss; doses within range of daily hormonal requirements are ineffective for weight reduction in euthyroid patients. Serious or life-threatening manifestations of toxicity may occur when given in larger doses, particularly when given in association with sympathomimetic amines.

ADULT DOSAGE

Hypothyroidism

Replacement/supplemental therapy in hypothyroidism of any etiology, except transient hypothyroidism during the recovery phase of subacute thyroiditis

Usual: 1.7mcg/kg/day; >200mcg/day seldom required

Severe:
Initial: 12.5-25mcg/day
Titrate: Increase by 25mcg/day every 2-4 weeks until TSH level normalized

Secondary (Pituitary)/Tertiary (Hypothalamic) Hypothyroidism:
Titrate: Increase until euthyroid and serum free-T4 level is restored to the upper 1/2 of the normal range

Subclinical Hypothyroidism:
Lower doses (eg, 1mcg/kg/day) may be adequate to normalize the serum TSH level

Pituitary TSH Suppressant

Used to treat/prevent various types of euthyroid goiters (eg, thyroid nodules, subacute or chronic lymphocytic thyroiditis, multinodular goiter) and to manage thyroid cancer

Well-Differentiated (Papillary and Follicular) Thyroid Cancer:
Adjunct to Surgery and Radioiodine Therapy:

Usual: >2 mcg/kg/day, w/ target TSH level <0.1 mU/L
High-Risk Tumors: Target TSH level <0.01 mU/L

Benign Nodules and Nontoxic Multinodular Goiter:
TSH is suppressed to a higher target (eg, 0.1 to 0.5 for nodules and 1.0 mU/L for multinodular goiter)

PEDIATRIC DOSAGE

Hypothyroidism

Usual:
0-3 Months of Age: 10-15mcg/kg/day
3-6 Months of Age: 8-10mcg/kg/day
6-12 Months of Age: 6-8mcg/kg/day
1-5 Years: 5-6mcg/kg/day
6-12 Years: 4-5mcg/kg/day
>12 Years (Growth/Puberty Incomplete): 2-3mcg/kg/day
Growth/Puberty Complete: 1.7mcg/kg/day

Infants w/ Very Low (<5mcg/dL) or Undetectable Serum T4:
Initial: 50mcg/day

Chronic/Severe Hypothyroidism:
Initial: 25mcg/day
Titrate: Increase by 25mcg increments every 2-4 weeks

DOSE MODIFICATION

Pregnancy

May increase levothyroxine requirements

Elderly

Hypothyroidism:
>50 Years:
Initial: 25-50mcg/day
Titrate: Increase by 12.5-25mcg increments every 6-8 weeks prn
W/ Underlying Cardiac Disease:
Initial: 12.5-25mcg/day
Titrate: Increase by 12.5-25mg increments every 4-6 weeks

Adverse Reactions

Minimize Hyperactivity in Older Children:
Initial: Give 1/4 of full replacement dose
Titrate: Increase on a weekly basis by 1/4 the full recommended replacement dose until the full recommended replacement dose is reached

Other Important Modifications

Hypothyroidism:
W/ Underlying Cardiac Disease:
Infants (Risk for Cardiac Failure):
Initial: Consider lower dose (eg, 25mcg/day)
Titrate: Increase dose in 4-6 weeks prn
<50 Years:
Initial: 25-50mcg/day
Titrate: Increase by 12.5-25mcg increments every 6-8 weeks prn

ADMINISTRATION

Oral route

Take in the am on an empty stomach at least 1/2-1 hr before food
Take at least 4 hrs apart from drugs that are known to interfere w/ its absorption

Pediatrics

Oral route
Administer as a single daily dose, preferably 30-60 min before breakfast
Take at least 4 hrs apart from drugs that are known to interfere w/ its absorption

Unable to Swallow Intact Tab:

1. Crush tab and suspend in small amount (5-10mL or 1-2 tsp) of water
2. Administer using a spoon or dropper
3. Do not store sus for later use
4. Do not use foods that decrease absorption of levothyroxine (eg, soybean infant formula) to administer

HOW SUPPLIED

Tab: 25mcg*, 50mcg*, 75mcg*, 88mcg*, 100mcg*, 112mcg*, 125mcg*, 137mcg*, 150mcg*, 175mcg*, 200mcg*, 300mcg* *scored

CONTRAINDICATIONS

Untreated subclinical (suppressed serum TSH level with normal T3 and T4levels) or overt thyrotoxicosis, acute myocardial infarction (MI), uncorrected adrenal insufficiency.

WARNINGS/PRECAUTIONS

Should not be used in the treatment of male or female infertility unless associated with hypothyroidism. Contraindicated in patients with nontoxic diffuse goiter or nodular thyroid disease, particularly in the elderly or with underlying cardiovascular (CV) disease if serum TSH level is already suppressed; use with caution if TSH level is not suppressed and carefully monitor thyroid function. Has narrow therapeutic index; carefully titrate dose to avoid over- or under-treatment. May decrease bone mineral density (BMD) with long-term use; give minimum dose necessary to achieve desired clinical and biochemical response. Caution with CV disorders and the elderly. If cardiac symptoms develop or worsen, reduce or withhold dose for 1 week and then restart at lower dose. Overtreatment may produce CV effects (eg, increase in HR, increase in cardiac wall thickness, increase in cardiac contractility, precipitation of angina or arrhythmias). Monitor patients with coronary artery disease (CAD) closely during surgical procedures; may precipitate cardiac arrhythmias. Caution in patients with diabetes mellitus (DM). Patients with concomitant adrenal insufficiency should be treated with replacement glucocorticoids prior to therapy.

ADVERSE REACTIONS

Fatigue, increased appetite, weight loss, heat intolerance, headache, hyperactivity, irritability, insomnia, palpitations, arrhythmias, dyspnea, hair loss, menstrual irregularities, pseudotumor cerebri (children), slipped capital femoral epiphysis (children).

DRUG INTERACTIONS

Concurrent sympathomimetics may increase effects of sympathomimetics or thyroid hormone; may increase risk of coronary insufficiency with CAD. Upward dose adjustments may be needed for insulin and oral hypoglycemic agents. May decrease absorption with soybean flour, cottonseed meal, walnuts, and dietary fiber. May increase oral anticoagulant activity; adjust dose of anticoagulant and monitor PT. May decrease levels and effects of digitalis glycosides. Transient reduction in TSH secretion with dopamine/dopamine agonists, glucocorticoids, octreotide. Decreased thyroid hormone secretion with aminoglutethimide, amiodarone, iodide (including iodine-containing radiographic contrast agents), lithium, methimazole, propylthiouracil (PTU), sulfonamides, and tolbutamide. May increase thyroid hormone secretion with amiodarone and iodide. May decrease T4 absorption with antacids (aluminum and magnesium hydroxides), simethicone, bile acid sequestrants (cholestyramine, colestipol), calcium carbonate, cation exchange resins (kayexalate), ferrous sulfate, orlistat, and sucralfate; administer at least 4 hrs apart. May increase serum thyroxine-binding globulin (TBG) concentrations with clofibrate, estrogen-containing oral contraceptives, oral estrogens, heroin/methadone, 5-fluorouracil, mitotane, and tamoxifen. May decrease serum TBG concentrations with androgens/anabolic steroids, asparaginase, glucocorticoids, and slow-release nicotinic acid. May cause protein-binding site displacement with furosemide (>80mg IV), heparin, hydantoins, NSAIDs (fenamates, phenylbutazone), and salicylates (>2g/day). May alter T4 and T3 metabolism with carbamazepine, hydantoins, phenobarbital, and rifampin. May decrease T4 5'-deiodinase activity with amiodarone, β-adrenergic antagonists (eg, propranolol >160mg/day), glucocorticoids (eg, dexamethasone >4mg/day), and PTU. Concurrent use with tricyclic (eg, amitriptyline) and tetracyclic (eg, maprotiline) antidepressants may increase the therapeutic and toxic effects of both drugs. Coadministration with sertraline in patients stabilized on levothyroxine may result in increased levothyroxine requirements. Interferon-α may cause development of antithyroid microsomal antibodies and transient hypothyroidism, hyperthyroidism, or both. Interleukin-2 has been associated with transient painless thyroiditis. Excessive use with growth hormones (eg, somatropin, somatrem) may accelerate epiphyseal closure. Ketamine may produce marked HTN and tachycardia. May reduce uptake of radiographic agents. Decreased theophylline clearance may occur in hypothyroid patients. Altered levels of thyroid hormone and/or TSH levels with choral hydrate, diazepam, ethionamide, lovastatin, metoclopramide, 6-mercaptopurine, nitroprusside, para-aminosalicylate sodium, perphenazine, resorcinol (excessive topical use), and thiazide diuretics.

NURSING CONSIDERATIONS

Assessment: Assess for untreated subclinical or overt thyrotoxicosis, acute MI, uncorrected adrenal insufficiency, CAD, CV disorders, nontoxic diffuse goiter, nodular thyroid disease, DM, hypersensitivity, pregnancy/nursing status, and possible drug interactions. In patients with secondary or tertiary hypothyroidism, assess for additional hypothalamic/pituitary hormone deficiencies. Assess TSH levels. In infants with congenital hypothyroidism, assess for other congenital anomalies.

Monitoring: Monitor for CV effects. In patients on long-term therapy, monitor for signs/symptoms of decreased BMD. In patients with nontoxic diffuse goiter or nodular thyroid disease, monitor for precipitation of thyrotoxicosis. In adults with primary hypothyroidism, perform periodic monitoring of serum TSH levels. In pediatric patients with congenital hypothyroidism, perform periodic monitoring of serum TSH levels and total or free T4 levels. In patients with secondary and tertiary hypothyroidism, perform periodic monitoring of serum free-T4 levels. Refer to PI for TSH and T4 monitoring parameters. Closely monitor PT if coadministered with an oral anticoagulant.

Patient Counseling: Instruct to notify physician if allergic to any foods or medicines, pregnant or planning to become pregnant, breastfeeding or taking any other drugs, including prescriptions and OTC preparations. Instruct to notify physician of any other medical conditions, particularly heart disease, diabetes, clotting disorders, and adrenal or pituitary gland problems. Instruct not to stop or change dose unless directed by physician. Instruct to take on empty stomach, at least 1/2 to 1 hr before eating breakfast. Instruct to notify physician if rapid or irregular heartbeat, chest pain, SOB, leg cramps, headache, or any other unusual medical event occurs. Inform that dose may be increased during pregnancy. Instruct to notify physician or dentist prior to surgery about levothyroxine therapy. Advise that partial hair loss may occur during the 1st few months of therapy, but is usually temporary. Inform that drug should not be used as a primary or adjunctive therapy in a weight control program. Inform that drug should not be administered within 4 hrs of agents such as iron/Ca^{2+} supplements and antacids.

Storage: 20-25°C (68-77°F); excursions permitted to 15-30°C (59-86°F). Store away from heat, moisture, and light.

UNIVASC – moexipril hydrochloride

RX

Class: ACE inhibitor

D/C when pregnancy is detected. Drugs that act directly on the renin-angiotensin system (RAS) can cause injury/death to the developing fetus.

ADULT DOSAGE

Hypertension

Not Receiving Diuretics:
Initial: 7.5mg qd
Titrate: Adjust dose according to BP response
If not adequately controlled, may increase or divide dose
Usual: 7.5-30mg/day given in 1 or 2 divided doses
Max: 60mg/day

PEDIATRIC DOSAGE

Pediatric use may not have been established

DOSE MODIFICATION

Concomitant Medications

Receiving Diuretics:
If possible d/c diuretic 2-3 days prior to therapy to avoid hypotension. If BP is not controlled with moexipril alone, then diuretic therapy may be reinstituted
Initial: 3.75mg

Renal Impairment

CrCl ≤40mL/min/1.73m²:
Initial: 3.75mg qd
Max: 15mg/day

Elderly

Start at lower end of dosing range

ADMINISTRATION

Oral route

Take 1 hr ac

HOW SUPPLIED

Tab: 7.5mg*, 15mg* *scored

CONTRAINDICATIONS

History of ACE inhibitor-associated angioedema. Coadministration with aliskiren in patients with diabetes.

WARNINGS/PRECAUTIONS

Angioedema of the face, extremities, lips, tongue, glottis, and/or larynx reported; d/c and administer appropriate therapy if symptoms develop. Intestinal angioedema reported; monitor for abdominal pain. More reports of angioedema in blacks than nonblacks. Anaphylactoid reactions reported during desensitization with hymenoptera venom, dialysis with high-flux membranes, and LDL apheresis with dextran sulfate absorption. Symptomatic hypotension may occur, most likely with salt and volume depletion; correct depletion prior to therapy. Excessive hypotension associated with oliguria, azotemia, acute renal failure, or death may occur in congestive heart failure (CHF) patients; monitor closely upon initiation and during first 2 weeks of therapy and whenever dose is increased. May cause agranulocytosis and bone marrow depression; monitor WBCs with collagen vascular disease. Rarely, associated with syndrome of cholestatic jaundice, fulminant hepatic necrosis, and death; d/c if jaundice or marked hepatic enzyme elevation occurs. May cause changes in renal function. Increased BUN and SrCr reported in patients with renal artery stenosis and without preexisting renal vascular disease; reduce dose and/or d/c. Hyperkalemia reported; risk factors include diabetes mellitus (DM) and renal insufficiency. Hypotension may occur with major surgery or during anesthesia. Persistent nonproductive cough reported. Dual blockade of the RAS is associated with increased risks of hypotension, hyperkalemia, and changes in renal function (including acute renal failure); closely monitor BP, renal function, and electrolytes with concomitant agents that also affect the RAS. Caution in elderly.

ADVERSE REACTIONS

Cough increased, dizziness, diarrhea, flu syndrome.

DRUG INTERACTIONS

See Contraindications. Avoid with aliskiren in patients with renal impairment (GFR <60mL/min). Hypotension risk and increased BUN and SrCr with diuretics. Increased risk of hyperkalemia with K^+-sparing diuretics (spironolactone, amiloride, triamterene), K^+ supplements, or K^+-containing salt substitutes; use with caution and monitor serum K^+. Increased lithium levels and lithium toxicity symptoms reported; use with caution and monitor lithium levels. Nitritoid reactions (eg, facial flushing, N/V, hypotension) reported with injectable gold (sodium aurothiomalate). NSAIDs, including selective COX-2 inhibitors, may deteriorate renal function. Antihypertensive effect may be attenuated by NSAIDs.

NURSING CONSIDERATIONS

Assessment: Assess for history of ACE inhibitor-associated angioedema, hypersensitivity to the drug, volume/salt depletion, CHF, collagen vascular disease, renal artery stenosis, DM, cerebrovascular disease, hepatic/renal function, pregnancy/nursing status, and possible drug interactions.

Monitoring: Monitor BP, hepatic/renal function, WBCs (collagen vascular disease), and serum K^+ levels. Monitor for head/neck and intestinal angioedema, anaphylactoid reaction, and hypersensitivity reactions.

Patient Counseling: Instruct to d/c use and to report immediately to physician if signs/symptoms of angioedema occur. Inform that lightheadedness may occur, especially during the 1st few days of therapy; instruct to d/c use and to consult physician if fainting occurs. Inform that excessive perspiration, dehydration, and other causes of volume depletion may lead to excessive fall in BP; advise to consult physician if these conditions develop. Instruct not to use K^+ supplements or salt substitutes containing K^+ without consulting physician, and to report any signs/symptoms of infection. Inform of the consequences of exposure during pregnancy and instruct to report pregnancy to physician as soon as possible.

Storage: 20-25°C (68-77°F). Protect from excessive moisture.

UROXATRAL – alfuzosin hydrochloride **RX**

Class: Alpha$_1$-antagonist

ADULT DOSAGE

Benign Prostatic Hypertrophy

10mg qd

PEDIATRIC DOSAGE

Pediatric use may not have been established

ADMINISTRATION

Oral route

Take w/ food and w/ the same meal each day

Do not chew or crush tab

HOW SUPPLIED

Tab, Extended-Release: 10mg

CONTRAINDICATIONS

Moderate or severe hepatic impairment (Child-Pugh categories B and C), concomitant use of potent CYP3A4 inhibitors (eg, ketoconazole, itraconazole, ritonavir).

WARNINGS/PRECAUTIONS

Postural hypotension with or without symptoms (eg, dizziness) may develop within a few hrs after administration; caution with symptomatic hypotension or in those who had a hypotensive response to other medications. Syncope may occur; caution to avoid situations in which injury could result should syncope occur. Prostate carcinoma and BPH frequently coexist and many of their symptoms are similar. D/C if symptoms of angina pectoris appear or worsen. Caution with severe renal impairment, mild hepatic impairment, or congenital/acquired QT prolongation. Intraoperative floppy iris syndrome (IFIS) observed in some patients during cataract surgery. Priapism reported (rare).

ADVERSE REACTIONS

Dizziness, URTI, headache.

DRUG INTERACTIONS

See Contraindications. Avoid use with other α-blockers. May increase risk of hypotension/postural hypotension and syncope with nitrates and other antihypertensives. Caution with medications that prolong the QT interval. Caution with PDE-5 inhibitors; may potentially cause symptomatic hypotension.

NURSING CONSIDERATIONS

Assessment: Assess for hypersensitivity to drug, symptomatic hypotension, history of QT prolongation, hepatic/renal impairment, cataract surgery, and possible drug interactions. Rule out the presence of prostate cancer prior to therapy.

Monitoring: Monitor for postural hypotension, syncope, hypersensitivity reactions, IFIS, QT prolongation, hepatic/renal impairment, and other adverse reactions. Monitor urine flow.

Patient Counseling: Inform about possible occurrence of symptoms related to postural hypotension when beginning therapy; caution about driving, operating machinery, or performing hazardous tasks during this period. Instruct to inform ophthalmologist about use of the product before cataract surgery or other procedures involving the eyes, even if no longer taking the medication. Advise about the possibility of priapism resulting from treatment and to seek immediate medical attention if it occurs.

Storage: 25°C (77°F); excursions permitted to 15-30°C (59-86°F). Protect from light and moisture.

VAGIFEM – estradiol

RX

Class: Estrogen

Estrogens increase the risk of endometrial cancer. Perform adequate diagnostic measures, including endometrial sampling, to rule out malignancy in postmenopausal women with undiagnosed persistent or recurring abnormal genital bleeding. Should not be used for prevention of cardiovascular disease (CVD) or dementia. Increased risk of MI, pulmonary embolism (PE), stroke, invasive breast cancer, and DVT in postmenopausal women (50-79 yrs of age) reported. Increased risk of developing probable dementia in postmenopausal women ≥65 yrs reported. Should be prescribed at the lowest effective dose and for the shortest duration consistent with treatment goals and risks.

ADULT DOSAGE

Atrophic Vaginitis

Due to Menopause:
1 tab intravaginally qd for 2 weeks, followed by 1 tab intravaginally twice weekly; women should generally be started at the 10mcg dose

PEDIATRIC DOSAGE

Pediatric use may not have been established

ADMINISTRATION

Intravaginal route

Use supplied applicator to administer dose
It is advisable to use the same time daily for all applications

HOW SUPPLIED

Tab: 10mcg

CONTRAINDICATIONS

Undiagnosed abnormal genital bleeding, known/suspected/history of breast cancer, known/suspected estrogen-dependent neoplasia, active or history of DVT/PE/arterial thromboembolic disease (eg, stroke, MI), known liver impairment/disease, known protein C, protein S, or antithrombin deficiency, or other known thrombophilic disorders, known/suspected pregnancy.

WARNINGS/PRECAUTIONS

Caution in patients with risk factors for arterial vascular disease and/or venous thromboembolism. If feasible, d/c at least 4-6 weeks before surgery of the type associated with increased risk of thromboembolism, or during periods of prolonged immobilization. May increase risk of gallbladder disease requiring surgery, and ovarian cancer. Consider addition of progestin for women with a uterus or with residual endometriosis post-hysterectomy. May lead to severe hypercalcemia in women with breast cancer and bone metastases; d/c and take appropriate measures if hypercalcemia occurs. Retinal vascular thrombosis reported; if visual abnormalities or migraine occurs, d/c pending exam. If exam reveals papilledema or retinal vascular lesions, d/c permanently. May elevate BP, plasma TGs (with preexisting hypertriglyceridemia), and thyroid-binding globulin levels; d/c if pancreatitis occurs. Caution with history of cholestatic jaundice associated with past estrogen use or with pregnancy; d/c in case of recurrence. May cause fluid retention; caution with cardiac/renal dysfunction. Caution with hypoparathyroidism; hypocalcemia may result. May exacerbate symptoms of angioedema in women with hereditary angioedema. May exacerbate endometriosis, asthma, diabetes mellitus, epilepsy, migraine, porphyria, systemic lupus erythematosus, and hepatic hemangiomas; use with caution. Local abrasion induced by applicator reported, especially in women with severely atrophic vaginal mucosa. May affect certain endocrine and blood components in lab tests.

ADVERSE REACTIONS

Vulvovaginal mycotic infection, vulvovaginal pruritus, back pain, diarrhea.

DRUG INTERACTIONS

CYP3A4 inducers (eg, St. John's wort, phenobarbital, carbamazepine, rifampin) may decrease levels, which may decrease therapeutic effects and/or change uterine bleeding profile. CYP3A4 inhibitors (eg, erythromycin, ketoconazole, ritonavir, grapefruit juice) may increase levels, which may result in side effects. Concomitant thyroid hormone replacement therapy may require increased doses of thyroid replacement therapy.

NURSING CONSIDERATIONS

Assessment: Assess for abnormal vaginal bleeding, presence/history of breast cancer, estrogen-dependent neoplasia, active or history of DVT/PE/arterial thromboembolic disease, liver impairment/disease, thrombophilic disorders, known anaphylactic reaction or angioedema to the drug, pregnancy/nursing status, other conditions where treatment is cautioned, need for progestin therapy, and possible drug interactions.

Monitoring: Monitor for signs/symptoms of CVD, malignant neoplasms, dementia, gallbladder disease, hypercalcemia, visual abnormalities, BP and plasma TG elevations, pancreatitis, cholestatic jaundice, hypothyroidism, fluid retention, and for other adverse events. Perform annual breast exam; schedule mammography based on age, risk factors, and prior mammogram results. Monitor thyroid function in patients on thyroid hormone replacement therapy. Perform adequate diagnostic measures (eg, endometrial sampling) in patients with undiagnosed persistent or recurring genital bleeding. Perform periodic evaluation to determine treatment need.

Patient Counseling: Inform postmenopausal women of the importance of reporting abnormal vaginal bleeding to physician as soon as possible. Inform of possible adverse reactions. Advise to have yearly breast exams by a physician and perform monthly breast self-exams. Instruct on how to use the applicator.

Storage: 25°C (77°F); excursions permitted to 15-30°C (59-86°F). Do not refrigerate.

VALCYTE – valganciclovir hydrochloride — RX

Class: Synthetic guanine derivative nucleoside analogue

Clinical toxicity includes granulocytopenia, anemia, and thrombocytopenia. Carcinogenic, teratogenic, and caused aspermatogenesis in animal studies.

ADULT DOSAGE

Cytomegalovirus Retinitis

Tab:

Treatment in Patients w/ AIDS:

Initial: 900mg bid x 21 days

Maint: 900mg qd following initial treatment, or in patients w/ inactive CMV retinitis

Cytomegalovirus Disease

Tab:

Prevention in Heart or Kidney-Pancreas Transplant:

900mg qd starting w/in 10 days of transplantation until 100 days post-transplantation

Prevention in Kidney Transplant:

900mg qd starting w/in 10 days of transplantation until 200 days post-transplantation

PEDIATRIC DOSAGE

Cytomegalovirus Disease

Tab/Sol:

Prevention in Kidney or Heart Transplant:

4 Months-16 Years:

Once daily dose starting w/in 10 days of transplantation until 100 days post-transplantation is based on BSA and CrCl derived from a modified Schwartz formula; refer to PI for calculation

DOSE MODIFICATION

Renal Impairment

Adults:

CrCl 40-59mL/min:

Initial: 450mg bid

Maint/Prevention: 450mg qd

CrCl 25-39mL/min:

Initial: 450mg qd

Maint/Prevention: 450mg every 2 days

CrCl 10-24mL/min:

Initial: 450mg every 2 days

Maint/Prevention: 450mg 2X/week

CrCl <10mL/min (on Hemodialysis):

Initial: Not recommended for use

Maint/Prevention: Not recommended for use

Elderly

Start at lower end of dosing range

ADMINISTRATION

Oral route

Take w/ food

Tab

Cannot be substituted for ganciclovir capsules on a one-to-one basis

Do not break or crush

Preparation of Oral Sol

1. Measure 91mL of purified water in a graduated cylinder
2. Shake the bottle to loosen the powder and add approx 1/2 the total amount of water for constitution to the bottle and shake the closed bottle well for about 1 min

3. Add the remainder of water and shake the closed bottle well for about 1 minute; this sol contains 50mg of valganciclovir free base per 1mL

Handling

Avoid direct skin or mucous membrane contact w/ broken or crushed tabs, the powder for oral sol, or the constituted oral sol; if contact occurs, wash thoroughly w/ soap and water, and rinse eyes thoroughly w/ plain water

HOW SUPPLIED

Sol: 50mg/mL [88mL deliverable volume]; Tab: 450mg

WARNINGS/PRECAUTIONS

Not for use in liver transplant patients. Safety and efficacy have not been established for prevention of CMV disease in solid organ transplants other than those indicated, prevention of CMV disease in pediatric solid organ transplant patients <4 months of age, or for treatment of congenital CMV disease. Severe leukopenia, neutropenia, pancytopenia, bone marrow aplasia, and aplastic anemia reported. Avoid if absolute neutrophil count (ANC) <500 cells/µL, platelet count <25,000/µL, or Hgb <8g/dL. Cytopenia may occur and may worsen with continued dosing; caution with preexisting cytopenias. May cause inhibition of spermatogenesis in men. May cause suppression of fertility in women. Women of childbearing potential should use effective contraception during and for at least 30 days following treatment. Men should practice barrier contraception during and for at least 90 days following treatment. Acute renal failure may occur in elderly and patients without adequate hydration; maintain adequate hydration in all patients. Caution in elderly and patients with renal impairment. Not recommended for adult patients on hemodialysis (CrCl <10mL/min). Do not substitute tab for ganciclovir caps on a one-to-one basis.

ADVERSE REACTIONS

Diarrhea, N/V, pyrexia, neutropenia, anemia, cough, HTN, constipation, upper respiratory tract infection, tremor, graft rejection, thrombocytopenia, granulocytopenia.

DRUG INTERACTIONS

May increase levels of mycophenolate mofetil metabolites (with renal impairment), zidovudine, and didanosine (monitor for toxicity). Probenecid (monitor for toxicity) and mycophenolate mofetil (with renal impairment) may increase levels. Zidovudine and didanosine may decrease levels. Caution with nephrotoxic drugs, myelosuppressive drugs, or irradiation.

NURSING CONSIDERATIONS

Assessment: Assess for renal impairment, preexisting cytopenia, prior/current irradiation, hydration status, pregnancy/nursing status, and possible drug interactions. Obtain baseline ANC, platelet count, and Hgb.

Monitoring: Monitor for signs/symptoms of hematologic effects (eg, granulocytopenia, anemia, thrombocytopenia, cytopenia), infertility, renal dysfunction, and other adverse reactions. Monitor CBC with differential and platelet counts frequently. Perform ophthalmologic exams at a minimum of every 4-6 weeks during therapy.

Patient Counseling: Advise not to substitute tab for ganciclovir caps on a one-to-one basis. Instruct adults to use tabs, not the oral sol. Inform patients of major toxicities and possible need to adjust dose or d/c. Inform of possible lab abnormalities and the importance of close monitoring of blood counts during therapy. Advise of possible decreased fertility. Instruct women not to use during pregnancy/breastfeeding. Advise women of childbearing potential to use effective contraception during and for at least 30 days following treatment, and men to practice barrier contraception during and for at least 90 days following treatment. Advise that the therapy should be considered a potential carcinogen. Inform that therapy may impair physical/mental ability. Inform that the therapy is not a cure for CMV retinitis and patients may continue to experience progression during or following treatment; advise to have ophthalmologic follow-up exams every 4-6 weeks at minimum while being treated.

Storage: Tab/Dry Powder: 25°C (77°F); excursions permitted to 15-30°C (59-86°F). Constituted Sol: 2-8°C (36-46°F) for no longer than 49 days. Do not freeze.

VALIUM – diazepam CIV

Class: Benzodiazepine

ADULT DOSAGE

Anxiety Disorders

Management of Disorders or for Short-Term Relief of Symptoms:
2-10mg bid-qid

Alcohol Withdrawal

Symptomatic Relief of Acute Withdrawal:
10mg tid or qid for first 24 hrs, then reduce to 5mg tid or qid prn

PEDIATRIC DOSAGE

General Dosing

≥6 Months of Age:
Initial: 1-2.5mg tid or qid
Titrate: Increase gradually prn and as tolerated

Muscle Spasms

Adjunctive Therapy:
2-10mg tid or qid

Convulsive Disorders

Adjunctive Therapy:
2-10mg bid-qid

DOSE MODIFICATION

Elderly/Debilitated

Initial: 2-2.5mg qd or bid
Titrate: Increase gradually prn and as tolerated

ADMINISTRATION

Oral route

HOW SUPPLIED

Tab: 2mg*, 5mg*, 10mg* *scored

CONTRAINDICATIONS

Acute narrow-angle glaucoma, myasthenia gravis, severe respiratory/hepatic insufficiency, sleep apnea syndrome, and in patients <6 months of age.

WARNINGS/PRECAUTIONS

May be used with treated open-angle glaucoma. Periodically reassess usefulness of drug. Not recommended for the treatment of psychotic patients. May increase frequency and/or severity of grand mal seizures and may require an increase in the dose of standard anticonvulsant medication. Abrupt withdrawal may also temporarily increase frequency and/or severity of seizures. May increase risk of congenital malformations and other developmental abnormalities. Caution during labor and delivery. Caution in the severely depressed or with evidence of latent depression or anxiety associated with depression, or suicidal tendencies; protective measures may be necessary. Psychiatric and paradoxical reactions may occur and are more likely in children and the elderly; d/c if these occur. Lower dose is recommended with chronic respiratory insufficiency. Extreme caution with history of alcohol or drug abuse. In debilitated patients, limit dose to smallest effective amount to preclude ataxia or oversedation development. Repeated use for a prolonged time may result in some loss of response to effects. Isolated reports of neutropenia and jaundice reported. Abuse and dependence reported.

ADVERSE REACTIONS

Drowsiness, fatigue, muscle weakness, ataxia.

DRUG INTERACTIONS

Mutually potentiates effects with central acting agents (eg, antipsychotics, anxiolytics/sedatives, MAOIs). Alcohol enhances sedative effects; avoid concomitant use. Slower rate of absorption with antacids. Concomitant use with compounds which inhibit certain hepatic enzymes such as CYP3A and CYP2C19 (eg, cimetidine, ketoconazole, fluvoxamine) may increase and prolong sedation. Decreased metabolic elimination of phenytoin reported.

NURSING CONSIDERATIONS

Assessment: Assess for hypersensitivity to drug, acute narrow-angle glaucoma, myasthenia gravis, severe respiratory/hepatic insufficiency, sleep apnea syndrome, history of seizures, psychosis, depression, history of alcohol/drug abuse, debilitation, pregnancy/nursing status, and possible drug interactions.

Monitoring: Monitor for hypersensitivity reactions, withdrawal symptoms, seizures, psychiatric/paradoxical reactions, respiratory depression, loss of response during prolonged use, abuse, dependence, and other adverse reactions. Monitor CBC and LFTs periodically during long-term therapy.

Patient Counseling: Inform of potential hazard to the fetus during pregnancy; advise to notify physician if nursing, pregnant, or intending to become pregnant during therapy. Inform that medication may produce psychological and physical dependence especially with history of alcohol/drug abuse; advise to consult physician before increasing dose or abruptly discontinuing the drug. Advise against simultaneous ingestion of alcohol and other CNS depressants during therapy. Caution against engaging in hazardous occupations requiring complete mental alertness (eg, operating machinery, driving).

Storage: 15-30°C (59-86°F).

VALTREX — valacyclovir hydrochloride

RX

Class: Nucleoside analogue

ADULT DOSAGE

Herpes Labialis (Cold Sores)

2g q12h for 1 day
Initiate at earliest symptom

Genital Herpes

Initial Episode: 1g bid for 10 days
Most effective when given w/in 48 hrs of onset of signs/symptoms

Recurrent Episodes: 500mg bid for 3 days
Initiate at 1st sign/symptom of episode

Suppressive Therapy:
Normal Immune Function:
1g qd
Alternative if ≤9 Recurrences/Yr: 500mg qd

HIV-1 Infected Patients:
CD4+ Count ≥100 cells/mm³: 500mg bid

Reduction of Transmission:
≤9 Recurrences/Yr: 500mg qd for the source partner

Herpes Zoster

1g tid for 7 days
Initiate at earliest sign/symptom
Most effective if initiated w/in 48 hrs of rash onset

PEDIATRIC DOSAGE

Herpes Labialis (Cold Sores)

≥12 Years:
2g q12h for 1 day
Initiate at earliest symptom

Chickenpox

2-<18 Years:
20mg/kg tid for 5 days
Initiate at earliest sign/symptom
Max: 1g tid

DOSE MODIFICATION

Renal Impairment

Herpes Labialis:
CrCl 30-49mL/min: Reduce dose to 1g q12h for 1 day
CrCl 10-29mL/min: Reduce dose to 500mg q12h for 1 day
CrCl <10mL/min: Reduce dose to 500mg single dose

Genital Herpes (Initial Episode):
CrCl 10-29mL/min: 1g q24h
CrCl <10mL/min: 500mg q24h

Genital Herpes (Recurrent Episode):
CrCl ≤29mL/min: 500mg q24h

Genital Herpes (Suppressive Therapy):
Immunocompetent Patients:
CrCl ≤29mL/min: 500mg q24h
Alternative if ≤9 Recurrences/Yr:
CrCl ≤29mL/min: 500mg q48h

HIV-1 Infected Patients:
CrCl ≤29mL/min: 500mg q24h

Herpes Zoster:
CrCl 30-49mL/min: Reduce dose to 1g q12h
CrCl 10-29mL/min: Reduce dose to 1g q24h
CrCl <10mL/min: Reduce dose to 500mg q24h

Hemodialysis Patients:
Administer dose after hemodialysis

ADMINISTRATION

Oral route

Shake oral sus well before using

Preparation of Oral Sus

Ingredients for Preparation: Valtrex caplets 500mg, cherry flavor, and Suspension Structured Vehicle USP-NF (SSV)
1. Use a pestle and mortar to grind the required number of caplets until a fine powder (5 caplets for 25mg/mL sus; 10 caplets for 50mg/mL sus)
2. Add approx 5mL aliquots of SSV to the mortar and triturate the powder until a paste has been produced

3. Continue to add approx 5mL aliquots of SSV to the mortar, mixing thoroughly between additions, until a concentrated sus is produced, to a minimum total quantity of 20mL SSV and a max total quantity of 40mL SSV for both the 25mg/mL and 50mg/mL sus
4. Transfer the mixture to a suitable 100mL measuring flask
5. Transfer the cherry flavor to the mortar and dissolve in approx 5mL of SSV. Once dissolved, add to the measuring flask
6. Rinse the mortar at least 3X w/ approx 5mL aliquots of SSV, transferring the rinsing to the measuring flask between additions
7. Make the sus to volume (100mL) w/ SSV and shake thoroughly to mix
8. Transfer the sus to an amber glass medicine bottle w/ a child-resistant closure

HOW SUPPLIED

Tab: 500mg, 1g* *scored

WARNINGS/PRECAUTIONS

Thrombotic thrombocytopenic purpura/hemolytic uremic syndrome (TTP/HUS) in immunocompromised patients reported at doses of 8g qd; immediately d/c if signs/symptoms occur. Acute renal failure reported. Maintain adequate hydration. CNS adverse reactions (eg, agitation, hallucinations, confusion, delirium, seizures, encephalopathy) reported in patients with or without reduced renal function and in those with underlying renal disease who received higher than recommended doses for their level of renal function; d/c if these occur. Caution in elderly and with renal impairment.

ADVERSE REACTIONS

Headache, N/V, abdominal pain, dysmenorrhea, arthralgia, nasopharyngitis, fatigue, rash, URTIs, pyrexia, decreased neutrophil counts, diarrhea, elevated ALT/AST.

DRUG INTERACTIONS

Caution with potentially nephrotoxic drugs.

NURSING CONSIDERATIONS

Assessment: Assess for hypersensitivity, immunocompromised state, renal impairment, hydration status, pregnancy/nursing status, and possible drug interactions.

Monitoring: Monitor for signs/symptoms of renal toxicity, TTP/HUS, CNS effects, and other adverse reactions.

Patient Counseling: Advise to maintain adequate hydration. Inform that drug is not a cure for cold sores or genital herpes. For patients with cold sores, instruct to initiate treatment at earliest symptom of a cold sore; inform that treatment should not exceed 1 day (2 doses) and that doses should be taken 12 hrs apart. For patients with genital herpes, instruct to avoid contact with lesions or sexual intercourse when lesions and/or symptoms are present to avoid infecting partner(s), and to use safe sex practice in combination with suppressive therapy. For patients with herpes zoster, advise to initiate treatment as soon as possible after diagnosis. For patients with chickenpox, advise to initiate treatment at the earliest sign/symptom.

Storage: 15-25°C (59-77°F).

VANCOCIN ORAL – vancomycin hydrochloride — RX

Class: Tricyclic glycopeptide antibiotic

ADULT DOSAGE

***Clostridium difficile*-Associated Diarrhea**

Usual: 125mg qid for 10 days

Acute Enterocolitis

Staphylococcal:
500mg-2g/day in 3 or 4 divided doses for 7-10 days

PEDIATRIC DOSAGE

General Dosing

Usual: 40mg/kg/day in 3 or 4 divided doses for 7-10 days
Max: 2g/day

ADMINISTRATION

Oral route

HOW SUPPLIED

Cap: 125mg, 250mg

WARNINGS/PRECAUTIONS

For oral use only; not systemically absorbed. Clinically significant serum concentrations reported in some patients who have taken multiple oral doses of therapy for active CDAD; significant systemic absorption may occur in some patients with inflammatory disorders of the intestinal mucosa. Monitoring of serum concentrations may be appropriate in some instances (eg, in patients with renal insufficiency and/or colitis). Nephrotoxicity reported; increased risk in patients >65 yrs of age. Ototoxicity reported mostly in patients with underlying hearing loss. Serial tests of auditory function may minimize risk of ototoxicity. May result in bacterial resistance if used in the absence of a proven or suspected bacterial infection; take appropriate measures if superinfection develops. Caution in elderly.

ADVERSE REACTIONS

N/V, abdominal pain, hypokalemia, diarrhea, pyrexia, flatulence, urinary tract infection, headache, peripheral edema, back pain, fatigue, nephrotoxicity.

DRUG INTERACTIONS

Monitor serum concentrations if used with an aminoglycoside antibiotic. Increased risk of ototoxicity with concomitant ototoxic agents (eg, aminoglycoside).

NURSING CONSIDERATIONS

Assessment: Assess for inflammatory disorders of the intestinal mucosa, renal insufficiency, colitis, underlying hearing loss, hypersensitivity to the drug, pregnancy/nursing status, and possible drug interactions. Perform culture and susceptibility testing.

Monitoring: Monitor renal function, and for ototoxicity, superinfection, and other adverse reactions. Monitor serum concentrations when appropriate.

Patient Counseling: Counsel that therapy should only be used to treat bacterial, not viral, infections. Instruct to take exactly ud even if patient feels better early in the course of therapy. Inform that skipping doses or not completing the full course of therapy may decrease effectiveness and increase bacterial resistance.

Storage: 15-30°C (59-86°F).

VANCOMYCIN – vancomycin hydrochloride RX

Class: Tricyclic glycopeptide antibiotic

ADULT DOSAGE

General Dosing

Serious/severe infections caused by susceptible strains of methicillin-resistant (β-lactam-resistant) staphylococci, endocarditis (eg, diphtheroid endocarditis, early-onset prosthetic valve endocarditis), septicemia, bone infections, lower respiratory tract infections, skin and skin-structure infections caused by susceptible strains of microorganisms, for penicillin-allergic patients, for patients who cannot receive or have failed to respond to other drugs, and for infections caused by vancomycin-susceptible organisms that are resistant to other antimicrobials
Usual: 2g IV divided either as 500mg q6h or 1g q12h

***Streptococcus viridans/Streptococcus bovis* Endocarditis:**
Use alone or in combination w/ an aminoglycoside
Enterocci Endocarditis:
Use in combination w/ an aminoglycoside

Early-Onset Prosthetic Valve Endocarditis Caused by *Stapylococcus epidermidis* or Diphtheroids:
Use in combination w/ either rifampin, an aminoglycoside, or both

Antibiotic-Associated Pseudomembranous Colitis/Staphylococcal Enterocolitis

Pseudomembranous Colitis Caused by *Clostridium difficile*/Staphylococcal Enterocolitis:
Oral Administration:
Usual: 500-2000mg/day in 3 or 4 divided doses for 7-10 days
Max: 2000mg/day

PEDIATRIC DOSAGE

General Dosing

Usual: 10mg/kg IV q6h

Neonates:
Initial: 15mg/kg
Maint: 10mg/kg q12h for neonates in 1st week of life and q8h thereafter up to 1 month of age

Antibiotic-Associated Pseudomembranous Colitis/Staphylococcal Enterocolitis

Pseudomembranous Colitis Caused by *Clostridium difficile*/Staphylococcal Enterocolitis:
Oral Administration:
Usual: 40mg/kg/day in 3 or 4 divided doses for 7-10 days
Max: 2000mg/day

DOSE MODIFICATION

Renal Impairment

Initial: No less than 15mg/kg, even in mild to moderate renal insufficiency

Dosage per day in mg is about 15X the GFR in mL/min; refer to PI for dosage table in patients w/ impaired renal function

Marked Impairment:

Maint: 250-1000mg once every several days

Functionally Anephric Patients:

Initial: 15mg/kg

Maint: 1.9mg/kg/24h

Anuria:

1000mg every 7-10 days

Elderly

Greater dose reductions than expected may be necessary

Other Important Modifications

Premature Infants: Longer dosing intervals and greater dose reductions may be necessary

Pediatric Patients ≤1 Month of Age: Total daily IV dosage may be lower

ADMINISTRATION

IV/Oral route

PO

May dilute appropriate dose in 1 oz of water

Common flavoring syrup may be added to sol to improve taste

Diluted sol may be administered via NG tube

IV

Intermittent infusion recommended

Administer each dose at no more than 10mg/min, or over a period of at least 60 min, whichever is longer

Flush IV lines between administration of β-lactam antibiotics

Recommended to dilute sol to ≤5mg/mL

Reconstitution:

Reconstitute 500mg vial w/ 10mL, 750mg vial w/ 15mL, or 1g vial w/ 20mL of SWFI

Further dilute reconstituted 500mg vial, 750mg vial or 1g vial w/ 100mL, 150mL or 200mL of compatible IV diluent, respectively

Compatible IV Diluents

D5 inj

0.9% NaCl inj

D5 and 0.9% NaCl inj

Lactated Ringer's inj

Lactated Ringer's and D5 inj

Normosol-M and D5

Isolyte E

HOW SUPPLIED

Inj: 500mg, 750mg, 1g

WARNINGS/PRECAUTIONS

Infusion-related events may occur. Rapid bolus administration may be associated w/ exaggerated hypotension, including shock and rarely cardiac arrest. Ototoxicity reported mostly in patients who have been given excessive doses or w/ an underlying hearing loss. Serial tests of auditory function may minimize risk of ototoxicity. Caution w/ renal insufficiency. *C. difficile*-associated diarrhea (CDAD) reported; may need to d/c if CDAD is suspected or confirmed. Clinically significant serum concentrations reported in some patients who have taken multiple oral doses of therapy for active *C. difficile*-induced pseudomembranous colitis. May result in bacterial resistance w/ prolonged use or use in the absence of a proven or suspected bacterial infection, or a prophylactic indication; take appropriate measures if superinfection develops. Reversible neutropenia reported; periodically monitor leukocyte count w/ prolonged therapy. Thrombophlebitis may occur; administer slowly and rotate venous access sites.

ADVERSE REACTIONS

Infusion-related events, nephrotoxicity, pseudomembranous colitis, ototoxicity, neutropenia, inj-site inflammation, anaphylaxis, drug fever, nausea, drug rash w/ eosinophilia and systemic symptoms.

DRUG INTERACTIONS

Concomitant use of anesthetic agents increased frequency of infusion-related events (eg, hypotension, flushing, erythema); administration as a 60-min infusion prior to anesthetic induction may minimize infusion-related events. Caution w/ concurrent and/or sequential systemic or topical use of other potentially neurotoxic and/or nephrotoxic drugs (eg, amphotericin B, aminoglycosides, bacitracin, polymyxin B, colistin, viomycin, cisplatin). Increased risk of ototoxicity w/ concomitant ototoxic agents (eg, aminoglycoside). Periodically monitor leukocyte count w/ concomitant drugs that may cause neutropenia.

NURSING CONSIDERATIONS

Assessment: Assess for renal impairment, underlying hearing loss, drug hypersensitivity, pregnancy/nursing status, and possible drug interactions. Perform culture and susceptibility testing.

Monitoring: Monitor renal function, and for ototoxicity, CDAD, superinfection, and other adverse reactions. Periodically monitor leukocyte count w/ prolonged therapy. Closely monitor serum concentrations of therapy in pediatric patients.

Patient Counseling: Counsel that therapy should only be used to treat bacterial, not viral, infections. Instruct to take exactly ud even if patient feels better early in the course of therapy. Inform that skipping doses or not completing the full course of therapy may decrease effectiveness and increase bacterial resistance. Inform that diarrhea is a common problem caused by therapy, which usually ends when therapy is discontinued. Instruct to immediately contact physician if watery and bloody stools (w/ or w/o stomach cramps and fever) occur, even as late as ≥2 months after the last dose.

Storage: 20-25°C (68-77°F). Reconstituted Sol w/ SWFI/D5 inj/0.9% NaCl inj: May be refrigerated for 14 days. Further Diluted Sol: May be refrigerated for 96 hrs, depending on diluent used; see Administration.

VANDAZOLE – metronidazole

RX

Class: Nitroimidazole

ADULT DOSAGE

Bacterial Vaginosis

Nonpregnant Women:
Insert 1 applicatorful (approx 5g) intravaginally qhs for 5 days

PEDIATRIC DOSAGE

Bacterial Vaginosis

Post-Menarche/Nonpregnant Females:
Insert 1 applicatorful (approx 5g) intravaginally qhs for 5 days

ADMINISTRATION

Intravaginal route

HOW SUPPLIED

Gel: 0.75% [70g]

CONTRAINDICATIONS

Disulfiram-like reaction to alcohol reported with oral metronidazole use; d/c alcohol consumption during and for ≥3 days after therapy. Psychotic reactions reported with concurrent disulfiram and oral metronidazole in alcoholic patients; avoid in patients who have taken disulfiram within last 2 weeks.

WARNINGS/PRECAUTIONS

Not for ophthalmic, dermal, or oral use. Convulsive seizures, encephalopathy, aseptic meningitis, optic and peripheral neuropathy (characterized by numbness or paresthesia of an extremity) reported with oral or IV metronidazole. Caution with CNS disease; d/c if abnormal neurologic signs appear. May interfere with lab tests (ALT, AST, LDH, triglycerides, and glucose hexokinase); consider postponing lab tests to after treatment. Avoid unnecessary use.

ADVERSE REACTIONS

Fungal infection, headache, pruritus, abdominal pain, nausea, dysmenorrhea.

DRUG INTERACTIONS

See Contraindications. Interactions reported with oral metronidazole. Alcoholic beverages and preparations containing ethanol or propylene glycol should not be consumed during and for ≥3 days after therapy. May potentiate warfarin and other coumarin anticoagulants. Consider monitoring PT, INR, and other coagulation parameters with oral anticoagulants. Caution with lithium and consider monitoring lithium levels; may elevate lithium levels. Cimetidine may prolong half-life and decrease clearance.

NURSING CONSIDERATIONS

Assessment: Assess for hypersensitivity, CNS diseases, vaginal candidiasis, alcohol intake, and possible drug/test interactions.

Monitoring: Monitor for abnormal neurologic signs, psychotic reactions, disulfiram-like reaction, and *Candida* vaginitis.

Patient Counseling: Instruct not to consume alcohol during and for ≥3 days after therapy. Instruct to avoid use if disulfiram was used within the last 2 weeks. Instruct to inform physician if taking oral anticoagulants or lithium. Instruct not to engage in vaginal intercourse or use other vaginal products during therapy. Inform that vaginal fungal infections may occur and may require treatment with an antifungal drug. Advise nursing women to consider d/c milk feeding or pump and discard milk during therapy and for 24 hrs after the last dose. Inform that the contents of the drug may cause burning and irritation of the eye; rinse eyes with cool tap water if accidental contact occurs. Instruct to d/c use and consult physician if vaginal irritation occurs. Instruct that the product is supplied with 5 vaginal applicators and 1 applicator/dose should be used.

Storage: 20-25°C (68-77°F). Avoid exposure to extreme heat or cold. Protect from freezing.

VANOS – fluocinonide

Class: Corticosteroid

RX

ADULT DOSAGE

Inflammatory and Pruritic Manifestations of Corticosteroid-Responsive Dermatoses

Psoriasis/Corticosteroid-Responsive Dermatoses:
Apply a thin layer to affected skin area(s) qd or bid ud

Atopic Dermatitis:
Apply a thin layer to affected skin area(s) qd ud

Max: 60g/week

Limit treatment to 2 consecutive weeks
D/C therapy when control is achieved
Reassess diagnosis if no improvement is seen w/in 2 weeks

PEDIATRIC DOSAGE

Inflammatory and Pruritic Manifestations of Corticosteroid-Responsive Dermatoses

≥12 Years:

Psoriasis/Corticosteroid-Responsive Dermatoses:
Apply a thin layer to affected skin area(s) qd or bid ud

Atopic Dermatitis:
Apply a thin layer to affected skin area(s) qd ud

Max: 60g/week

Limit treatment to 2 consecutive weeks
D/C therapy when control is achieved
Reassess diagnosis if no improvement is seen w/in 2 weeks

ADMINISTRATION
Topical route

HOW SUPPLIED
Cre: 0.1% [30g, 60g, 120g]

WARNINGS/PRECAUTIONS
For dermatologic use only; not for ophthalmic, oral, or intravaginal use. Not for use in rosacea or perioral dermatitis. Do not apply on the face, groin, or axillae. Systemic absorption may produce reversible hypothalamic-pituitary-adrenal (HPA) axis suppression w/ the potential for glucocorticosteroid insufficiency, Cushing's syndrome, hyperglycemia, and unmasking of latent diabetes mellitus (DM). Periodically evaluate for HPA axis suppression and if noted, gradually withdraw treatment, reduce frequency of application, or substitute a less potent steroid. Factors predisposing to HPA axis suppression include use of more potent steroids, use over large surface areas, prolonged use, use under occlusion, use on an altered skin barrier, and use in patients with liver failure. May suppress immune system if used for >2 weeks. Manifestations of adrenal insufficiency may require supplemental systemic corticosteroids. Pediatric patients may be more susceptible to systemic toxicity. Local adverse reactions may be more likely to occur with occlusive use, prolonged use or use of higher potency corticosteroids. Use appropriate antifungal or antibacterial agent if concomitant skin infections are present or develop; if a favorable response does not occur promptly, d/c until infection is controlled. D/C and institute appropriate therapy if irritation develops. Allergic contact dermatitis may occur; confirm by patch testing.

ADVERSE REACTIONS
Headache, application-site burning, nasopharyngitis, nasal congestion.

DRUG INTERACTIONS
Use of >1 corticosteroid-containing product at the same time may increase total systemic absorption.

NURSING CONSIDERATIONS

Assessment: Assess for hypersensitivity to the drug, rosacea, perioral dermatitis, skin infections, liver impairment, pregnancy/nursing status, and possible drug interactions.

Monitoring: Monitor for signs/symptoms of HPA axis suppression, Cushing's syndrome, hyperglycemia, unmasking of latent DM, skin irritation, and other adverse reactions. Monitor for systemic toxicity (eg, adrenal suppression, intracranial HTN) in pediatric patients. Following withdrawal of treatment, monitor for glucocorticosteroid insufficiency. Reassess diagnosis if no improvement is seen w/in 2 weeks.

Patient Counseling: Instruct to use externally and ud. Advise not to use for any disorder other than for which it was prescribed. Instruct to avoid contact w/ eyes and not to use on face, groin, and underarms. Instruct not to bandage, cover, or wrap treated skin, unless directed by physician. Counsel to report any signs of local adverse reactions. Advise that other corticosteroid-containing products should not be used w/o 1st consulting w/ the physician. Instruct to d/c use when control is achieved and to notify physician if no improvement seen w/in 2 weeks. Notify physician if contemplating surgery. Counsel to wash hands following application.

Storage: 15-30°C (59-86°F).

VASOTEC – enalapril maleate

Class: ACE inhibitor

RX

D/C if pregnancy is detected. Drugs that act directly on the renin-angiotensin system (RAS) can cause injury/death to the developing fetus.

ADULT DOSAGE

Hypertension

Not Receiving Diuretics:
Initial: 5mg qd
Titrate: Adjust dose according to BP response
Usual: 10-40mg/day given in single dose or 2 divided doses

May add diuretic if BP not controlled

Receiving Diuretics:
If possible, d/c diuretic 2-3 days prior to therapy. If BP is not controlled w/ enalapril alone, then diuretic therapy may be resumed
Initial: 2.5mg

Heart Failure

Symptomatic CHF in Combination w/ Diuretics and Digitalis:
Initial: 2.5mg qd
Usual: 2.5-20mg bid
Max: 40mg/day in divided doses

Asymptomatic Left Ventricular Dysfunction

Decreasing the Rate of Development of Overt Heart Failure (HF) and the Incidence of Hospitalization for HF in Clinically Stable Patients (Ejection Fraction ≤35%):
Initial: 2.5mg bid
Titrate: Increase as tolerated to 20mg/day (in divided doses)

PEDIATRIC DOSAGE

Hypertension

1 Month-16 Years:
Initial: 0.08mg/kg (up to 5mg) qd
Titrate: Adjust according to BP response
Max: 0.58mg/kg (or 40mg/day)

DOSE MODIFICATION

Renal Impairment

HTN:
CrCl ≤30mL/min:
Initial: 2.5mg qd

Dialysis Patients:
Initial: 2.5mg qd on dialysis days
Titrate: Adjust dose based on BP on nondialysis days

HF:
SrCr >1.6mg/dL:
Initial: 2.5mg/day
Titrate: May increase to 2.5mg bid, then 5mg bid and higher prn, usually at intervals of 4 days or more
Max: 40mg/day

Other Important Modifications

HF:
Hyponatremia (Serum Na^+ <130mEq/L):
Initial: 2.5mg/day
Titrate: May increase to 2.5mg bid, then 5mg bid and higher prn, usually at intervals of 4 days or more
Max: 40mg/day

ADMINISTRATION

Oral route

Preparation of Sus (200mL of a 1.0mg/mL Sus)

1. Add 50mL of Bicitra to a polyethylene terephthalate bottle containing ten 20mg tabs; shake for at least 2 min
2. Let concentrate stand for 60 min, then shake for additional 1 min
3. Add 150mL of Ora-Sweet SF to concentrate and shake sus to disperse ingredients
4. Refrigerate at 2-8°C (36-46°F) for 30 days
5. Shake sus before each use

HOW SUPPLIED

Tab: 2.5mg*, 5mg*, 10mg*, 20mg* *scored

CONTRAINDICATIONS

History of ACE inhibitor-associated angioedema and in patients with hereditary or idiopathic angioedema. Coadministration with aliskiren in patients with diabetes.

WARNINGS/PRECAUTIONS

Head/neck angioedema reported; d/c and administer appropriate therapy if angioedema occurs. Higher incidence of angioedema reported in blacks than nonblacks. Intestinal angioedema reported; monitor for abdominal pain. BP effect that is less in blacks than nonblacks reported. Patients with history of angioedema unrelated to ACE inhibitor therapy may be at increased risk of angioedema during therapy. Anaphylactoid reactions reported during desensitization with hymenoptera venom, dialysis with high-flux membranes, and LDL apheresis with dextran sulfate absorption. Excessive hypotension sometimes associated with oliguria and/or azotemia and rarely with acute renal failure, or death may occur; monitor during first 2 weeks of therapy and whenever dose of the drug and/or diuretic is increased. Consider dose reduction or d/c therapy or diuretic if symptomatic hypotension occurs. Neutropenia or agranulocytosis and bone marrow depression may occur; monitor WBCs in patients with renal disease and collagen vascular disease. Associated with syndrome that starts with cholestatic jaundice and progresses to fulminant hepatic necrosis, and sometimes death; d/c if jaundice or marked elevations of hepatic enzymes develop. Caution with left ventricular outflow obstruction. May cause changes in renal function; may be associated with oliguria and/or progressive azotemia and rarely with acute renal failure or death in severe HF patients whose renal function depends on the renin-angiotensin-aldosterone system. Increases in BUN and SrCr reported with renal artery stenosis; monitor renal function during the 1st few weeks of therapy. Increases in BUN and SrCr reported. Hyperkalemia may occur; caution with diabetes mellitus (DM) and renal insufficiency. Persistent nonproductive cough reported. Hypotension may occur with major surgery or during anesthesia; may be corrected by volume expansion. Avoid in neonates and children with GFR <30mL/min.

ADVERSE REACTIONS

Fatigue, headache, dizziness.

DRUG INTERACTIONS

See Contraindications. Dual blockade of the RAS is associated with increased risk of hypotension, hyperkalemia, and changes in renal function (including acute renal failure); avoid combined use of RAS inhibitors. Closely monitor BP, renal function, and electrolytes with concomitant agents that also affect the RAS. Avoid with aliskiren in patients with renal impairment (GFR <60mL/min). Hypotension risk and increased BUN and SrCr with diuretics. Coadministration with NSAIDs, including selective COX-2 inhibitors, may decrease antihypertensive effect of ACE inhibitors and may further deteriorate renal function. K^+-sparing diuretics, K^+-containing salt substitutes, or K^+ supplements may increase serum K^+ levels; use caution and monitor serum K^+ frequently. Avoid K^+-sparing agents in patients with HF. Antihypertensives that cause renin release (eg, diuretics) may augment antihypertensive effect. Lithium toxicity reported with lithium; monitor serum lithium levels frequently. Nitritoid reactions reported rarely with injectable gold (eg, sodium aurothiomalate).

NURSING CONSIDERATIONS

Assessment: Assess for history of angioedema, hypersensitivity, volume/salt depletion, renal dysfunction/disease, collagen vascular disease, renal artery stenosis, ischemic heart disease, cerebrovascular disease, left ventricular outflow obstruction, DM, pregnancy/nursing status, and possible drug interactions.

Monitoring: Monitor for hypotension, anaphylactoid reactions, angioedema, and other adverse reactions. Monitor BP, renal/hepatic function, and serum K^+ levels. Monitor WBCs periodically in patients with collagen vascular disease and/or renal disease.

Patient Counseling: Inform of pregnancy risks and instruct to notify physician as possible as soon if pregnant/planning to become pregnant; discuss treatment options in women planning to become pregnant. Instruct to d/c therapy and to immediately report signs/symptoms of angioedema. Caution about lightheadedness, especially during the 1st few days of therapy and advise to report to physician. Instruct to d/c and to consult physician if syncope occurs. Caution that excessive perspiration and dehydration may lead to excessive fall in BP; advise to consult with physician. Advise not to use K^+ supplements or salt substitutes containing K^+ without consulting physician. Advise patient to report any indication of infection.

Storage: 25°C (77°F); excursions permitted to 15-30°C (59-86°F). Protect from moisture.

VECTICAL – calcitriol

RX

Class: Vitamin D analogue

ADULT DOSAGE

Plaque Psoriasis

Mild to Moderate:

≥18 Years:

Apply to affected area(s) bid (am and pm)

Max: 200g/week

PEDIATRIC DOSAGE

Pediatric use may not have been established

ADMINISTRATION

Topical route

HOW SUPPLIED

Oint: 3mcg/g [5g, 100g]

WARNINGS/PRECAUTIONS

Not for PO, ophthalmic, or intravaginal use. Hypercalcemia reported; if aberrations in parameters of Ca^{2+} metabolism occur, d/c therapy until these parameters normalize. Increased absorption with occlusive use. Avoid excessive exposure of treated areas to natural or artificial sunlight (eg, tanning booths, sun lamps); avoid or limit phototherapy.

ADVERSE REACTIONS

Lab test abnormality, urine abnormality, psoriasis, hypercalciuria, pruritus, hypercalcemia, skin discomfort.

DRUG INTERACTIONS

Caution with medications known to increase serum Ca^{2+} level (eg, thiazide diuretics), Ca^{2+} supplements, or high doses of vitamin D.

NURSING CONSIDERATIONS

Assessment: Assess for known/suspected Ca^{2+} metabolism disorder, pregnancy/nursing status, and possible drug interactions.

Monitoring: Monitor for hypercalcemia, aberrations in parameters of Ca^{2+} metabolism, and other adverse reactions.

Patient Counseling: Instruct to use ud. Instruct to apply only to areas of the skin affected by psoriasis; advise not to apply to the eyes, lips, or facial skin. Instruct to rub gently into the skin. Advise to notify their physician if adverse reactions occur. Advise to avoid excessive exposure of treated areas to sunlight, tanning booths, sun lamps, or other artificial sunlight and to inform physician about treatment if undergoing phototherapy.

Storage: 20°-25°C (68°-77°F); excursions permitted to 15°-30°C (59°-86°F). Do not freeze or refrigerate.

VELTIN – clindamycin phosphate/tretinoin

RX

Class: Lincosamide derivative/retinoid

ADULT DOSAGE

Acne Vulgaris

Apply pea-sized amount qpm

PEDIATRIC DOSAGE

Acne Vulgaris

≥12 Years:

Apply pea-sized amount qpm

ADMINISTRATION

Topical route

Gently rub the medication to lightly cover the entire affected area

HOW SUPPLIED

Gel: (Clindamycin-Tretinoin) 1.2%-0.025% [30g, 60g]

CONTRAINDICATIONS

Regional enteritis, ulcerative colitis, or history of antibiotic-associated colitis.

WARNINGS/PRECAUTIONS

Not for PO, ophthalmic, or intravaginal use. Avoid the eyes, lips, and mucous membranes. Avoid exposure to sunlight, including sunlamps. Avoid use if sunburn is present. Daily use of sunscreen products and protective apparel are recommended. Weather extremes (eg, wind, cold) may be irritating while under treatment. Clindamycin: Systemic absorption has been demonstrated following topical use. Diarrhea, bloody diarrhea, and colitis (including pseudomembranous colitis) reported; d/c if significant diarrhea occurs. Severe colitis reported following PO or parenteral administration with an onset of up to several weeks following cessation of therapy.

ADVERSE REACTIONS

Local-site reactions (eg, dryness, irritation, exfoliation, erythema).

DRUG INTERACTIONS

Avoid with erythromycin-containing products due to possible antagonism to clindamycin. May enhance action of neuromuscular-blocking agents; use with caution. Antiperistaltic agents (eg, opiates, diphenoxylate with atropine) may prolong and/or worsen severe colitis.

NURSING CONSIDERATIONS

Assessment: Assess for regional enteritis, ulcerative colitis or history of antibiotic-associated colitis, pregnancy/nursing status, and possible drug interactions. Assess use in patients whose occupations require considerable sun exposure.

Monitoring: Monitor for signs/symptoms of diarrhea, bloody diarrhea, colitis, local skin reactions, and other adverse reactions.

Patient Counseling: Instruct to wash face gently with mild soap and water at hs and apply a thin layer over the entire face (excluding the eyes and lips) after patting the skin dry. Advise not to use more than a pea-sized amount and not to apply more than qd (at hs). Advise to avoid exposure to sunlight, sunlamps, UV light, and other medicines that may increase sensitivity to sunlight; instruct to apply sunscreen qam and reapply over the course of the day PRN. Advise that other topical medications with a strong drying effect (eg, abrasive soaps, cleansers) may cause an increase in skin irritation. Inform that medication may cause irritation (eg, erythema, scaling, itching, burning, stinging). Instruct to d/c therapy and contact physician if severe diarrhea or GI discomfort occurs.

Storage: 25°C (77°F); excursions permitted to 15-30°C (59-86°F). Protect from light, heat, and freezing.

VENTOLIN HFA – albuterol sulfate

RX

Class: Beta$_2$-agonist

ADULT DOSAGE

Bronchospasm

Treatment/Prevention:

2 inh q4-6h or 1 inh q4h

Exercise-Induced Bronchospasm

Prevention:

2 inh 15-30 min before exercise

PEDIATRIC DOSAGE

Bronchospasm

Treatment/Prevention:

≥4 Years:

2 inh q4-6h or 1 inh q4h

Exercise-Induced Bronchospasm

Prevention:

≥4 Years:

2 inh 15-30 min before exercise

DOSE MODIFICATION

Elderly

Start at lower end of dosing range

ADMINISTRATION

Oral inh route

Shake well before each spray

Priming

Before using for 1st time, if inhaler has not been used for >2 weeks, or if it has been dropped, prime inhaler by releasing 4 sprays into air, away from face

Refer to PI for further instructions on proper use

HOW SUPPLIED

MDI: 90mcg of albuterol base/inh [60, 200 inhalations]

WARNINGS/PRECAUTIONS

D/C if paradoxical bronchospasm following dosing or if cardiovascular (CV) effects occur. More doses than usual may be a marker of destabilization of asthma and may require reevaluation of the patient and treatment regimen; give special consideration to the possible need for anti-inflammatory treatment (eg, corticosteroids). ECG changes and immediate hypersensitivity reactions, including anaphylaxis, may occur. Fatalities reported with excessive use. Caution with CV disorders (eg, coronary insufficiency, arrhythmias, HTN), convulsive disorders, hyperthyroidism, diabetes mellitus (DM), and in patients unusually responsive to sympathomimetic amines. Large doses of IV albuterol reported to aggravate preexisting DM and ketoacidosis. May cause significant hypokalemia. Caution in elderly.

ADVERSE REACTIONS
Throat irritation, viral respiratory infections, upper respiratory inflammation, cough, musculoskeletal pain.

DRUG INTERACTIONS
Avoid with other short-acting sympathomimetic aerosol bronchodilators; caution with additional adrenergic drugs administered by any route. Use with β-blockers may block pulmonary effects and produce severe bronchospasm in asthmatic patients; avoid concomitant use. If needed, consider cardioselective β-blockers and use with caution. ECG changes and/or hypokalemia caused by non-K^+-sparing diuretics (eg, loop, thiazide diuretics) may be worsened. May decrease serum digoxin levels. Use extreme caution with MAOIs and TCAs, or within 2 weeks of discontinuation of such agents.

NURSING CONSIDERATIONS

Assessment: Assess for history of hypersensitivity to the drug, CV disorders, convulsive disorders, hyperthyroidism, DM, pregnancy/nursing status, and possible drug interactions. Assess use in patients unusually responsive to sympathomimetic amines.

Monitoring: Monitor for paradoxical bronchospasm, deterioration of asthma, CV effects, ECG changes, hypokalemia, immediate hypersensitivity reactions, and other adverse effects. Monitor BP, HR, and blood glucose levels.

Patient Counseling: Counsel not to increase dose/frequency of doses without consulting physician. Advise to seek immediate medical attention if treatment becomes less effective for symptomatic relief, symptoms become worse, and/or there is a need to use the product more frequently than usual. Instruct on how to properly prime, clean, and use inhaler. Instruct to take concurrent inhaled drugs and asthma medications only ud by the physician. Inform of the common adverse effects of treatment. Advise to notify physician if pregnant/nursing. Instruct to avoid spraying in eyes.

Storage: 20-25°C (68-77°F); excursions permitted to 15-30°C (59-86°F). Store with mouthpiece down. Do not puncture or store near heat or open flame.

VERAMYST – fluticasone furoate RX

Class: Corticosteroid

ADULT DOSAGE

Seasonal/Perennial Allergic Rhinitis

Initial: 2 sprays/nostril qd; titrate to minimum effective dose
Maint: 1 spray/nostril qd

PEDIATRIC DOSAGE

Seasonal/Perennial Allergic Rhinitis

2-11 Years:
Initial: 1 spray/nostril qd
Titrate: May increase to 2 sprays/nostril qd if inadequate, then return to initial dose when symptoms are controlled

≥12 Years:
Initial: 2 sprays/nostril qd; titrate to minimum effective dose
Maint: 1 spray/nostril qd

DOSE MODIFICATION
Elderly
Start at lower end of dosing range

ADMINISTRATION
Intranasal route

Avoid spraying in eyes
Shake well before each use
Priming
Shake contents well and release 6 sprays into the air before 1st use
If not used >30 days, or if cap is left off ≥5 days, prime the pump again until a fine mist appears

HOW SUPPLIED
Spray: 27.5mcg/spray [10g]

WARNINGS/PRECAUTIONS
May cause local nasal effects (eg, epistaxis, nasal ulceration, *Candida* infections, nasal septum perforation, impaired wound healing). Avoid with recent nasal ulcers, surgery, or trauma until healing has occurred. Glaucoma and/or cataracts may develop; monitor closely in patients with change in vision, history of increased IOP, glaucoma, and/or cataracts. D/C if hypersensitivity reactions occur. May increase susceptibility to infections; caution with active or quiescent tuberculosis (TB), untreated fungal or bacterial infections, systemic viral or parasitic infections, or

ocular herpes simplex. Avoid exposure to chickenpox and measles. D/C slowly if hypercorticism and adrenal suppression occur. Risk of adrenal insufficiency and withdrawal symptoms when replacing systemic corticosteroids with topical corticosteroids. May reduce growth velocity in pediatric patients. Caution with severe hepatic impairment and elderly patients.

ADVERSE REACTIONS

Headache, epistaxis, pharyngolaryngeal pain, nasal ulceration, back pain, pyrexia, cough.

DRUG INTERACTIONS

Increased exposure with ritonavir; avoid coadministration. Reduced cortisol levels with ketoconazole; caution with ketoconazole or other potent CYP3A4 inhibitors.

NURSING CONSIDERATIONS

Assessment: Assess for drug hypersensitivity, patients who have not been immunized or exposed to infections (eg, measles, chickenpox), active or quiescent TB, untreated fungal/bacterial infection, systemic viral/parasitic infection, ocular herpes simplex, history of increased IOP, glaucoma or cataracts, recent nasal ulcers/surgery/trauma, hepatic impairment, pregnancy/nursing status, and possible drug interactions.

Monitoring: Monitor for acute adrenal insufficiency and withdrawal symptoms when replacing systemic corticosteroid with topical corticosteroid. Monitor for hypercorticism, chickenpox, measles, epistaxis, nasal ulceration, nasal septal perforation, hypoadrenalism (in infants born to a mother who received corticosteroids during pregnancy), suppression of growth velocity in children, vision changes, glaucoma, cataracts, increased IOP, and hypersensitivity reactions. Examine periodically for evidence of nasal *Candida* infections.

Patient Counseling: Inform of possible local nasal effects, cataracts, glaucoma, immunosuppression, and hypersensitivity reactions. Advise not to use with recent nasal ulcers, surgery, or trauma until healing has occurred. Instruct to d/c if hypersensitivity reaction occurs. Instruct to avoid exposure to chickenpox and measles. Instruct to consult physician if symptoms do not improve, the condition worsens, or change in vision occurs. Inform that growth in children may be slowed; counsel to regularly check patient's growth. Advise to avoid spraying into eyes.

Storage: 15-30°C (59-86°F). Store device in upright position with cap in place. Do not freeze or refrigerate. Discard after 120 sprays have been used.

VERAPAMIL INJECTION – verapamil hydrochloride RX

Class: Calcium channel blocker (nondihydropyridine)

ADULT DOSAGE

Paroxysmal Supraventricular Tachycardia

Including those associated w/ accessory bypass tracts

Give as slow IV bolus over at least 2 min under continuous ECG and BP monitoring; individualize interval for subsequent doses
Initial: 5-10mg (0.075-0.15mg/kg)
Repeat: 10mg (0.15mg/kg) 30 min after 1st dose if initial response is inadequate

Atrial Fibrillation/Flutter

Temporary control of rapid ventricular rate except when associated w/ accessory bypass tracts

Give as slow IV bolus over at least 2 min under continuous ECG and BP monitoring; individualize interval for subsequent doses
Initial: 5-10mg (0.075-0.15mg/kg)
Repeat: 10mg (0.15mg/kg) 30 min after 1st dose if initial response is inadequate

PEDIATRIC DOSAGE

Paroxysmal Supraventricular Tachycardia

Including those associated w/ accessory bypass tracts

Give as slow IV bolus over at least 2 min under continuous ECG and BP monitoring; individualize interval for subsequent doses
0-1 Year:
Initial: 0.1-0.2mg/kg
Usual Range: 0.75-2mg
Repeat dose 30 min after 1st dose if initial response is inadequate

1-15 Years:
Initial: 0.1-0.3mg/kg
Max Initial: 5mg
Usual Range: 2-5mg
Repeat dose 30 min after 1st dose if initial response is inadequate
Max: 10mg as single dose

Atrial Fibrillation/Flutter

Temporary control of rapid ventricular rate except when associated w/ accessory bypass tracts
Give as slow IV bolus over at least 2 min under continuous ECG and BP monitoring; individualize interval for subsequent doses
0-1 Year:
Initial: 0.1-0.2mg/kg

Usual Range: 0.75-2mg
Repeat dose 30 min after 1st dose if initial response is inadequate

1-15 Years:
Initial: 0.1-0.3mg/kg
Max Initial: 5mg
Usual Range: 2-5mg
Repeat dose 30 min after 1st dose if initial response is inadequate
Max: 10mg as single dose

DOSE MODIFICATION

Elderly

Give dose over at least 3 min

ADMINISTRATION

IV route

Give as a slow IV inj over at least a 2-min period under continuous ECG and BP monitoring
Do not dilute w/ sodium lactate inj in polyvinyl chloride bags
Avoid admixing verapamil HCl inj w/ albumin, amphotericin B, hydralazine HCl, or trimethoprim w/ sulfamethoxazole
Verapamil HCl inj will precipitate in any solution w/ a pH above 6.0

HOW SUPPLIED

Inj: 2.5mg/mL [2mL, 4mL]

CONTRAINDICATIONS

Severe hypotension or cardiogenic shock, 2nd/3rd-degree atrioventricular (AV) block or sick sinus syndrome (except with functioning ventricular pacemaker), severe congestive heart failure, IV β-blocker (eg, propranolol), A-flutter/fib with an accessory bypass tract, wide-complex ventricular tachycardia.

WARNINGS/PRECAUTIONS

Initiate in a treatment setting with monitoring and resuscitation facilities. May produce transient and asymptomatic decrease in BP below baseline levels which may result in dizziness. May rarely produce 2nd/3rd-degree AV block, bradycardia, and (extreme cases) asystole. Control non-severe or rate related heart failure with digitalis glycosides and diuretics, as appropriate, before therapy. Acute worsening of heart failure may be seen in patients with moderately severe to severe cardiac dysfunction. May require reduction in subsequent doses, or d/c of therapy and institution of appropriate therapy if 2nd/3rd-degree AV block or bundle branch block develops. Avoid multiple doses with significant hepatic/renal failure; if repeated inj are essential, closely monitor BP and PR interval and utilize smaller repeat doses. Cannot be removed by hemodialysis. Caution with Duchenne's muscular dystrophy; may precipitate respiratory muscle failure. Caution and monitor patients with supratentorial tumors during anesthesia induction; may increase intracranial pressure. Caution with neonates/infants; may cause severe hemodynamic side effects (rare).

ADVERSE REACTIONS

Hypotension, bradycardia, severe tachycardia, dizziness, headache.

DRUG INTERACTIONS

See Contraindications. Monitor for AV block or excessive bradycardia with digitalis preparations. May cause exaggerated hypotensive response with oral quinidine, β-blockers, and prazosin. Avoid disopyramide within 48 hrs before or 24 hrs after therapy. May have additive effects reducing myocardial contractility and prolonging AV conduction and repolarization with flecainide. May potentiate depolarizing/nondepolarizing neuromuscular blockers; may need to reduce dose of verapamil and/or dose of the neuromuscular blockers. Caution with highly protein-bound drugs. May increase sensitivity to effects of lithium, and decrease serum lithium levels in patients receiving chronic stable oral lithium; monitor carefully. May increase carbamazepine and cyclosporine levels. Phenobarbital may increase clearance. Rifampin may reduce oral bioavailability. Titrate carefully with inhalation anesthetics to avoid excessive cardiovascular (CV) depression. May cause CV collapse with dantrolene. Hyperkalemia and myocardial depression reported with coadministration of oral therapy and IV dantrolene.

NURSING CONSIDERATIONS

Assessment: Assess for moderately severe to severe cardiac dysfunction, Duchenne's muscular dystrophy, supratentorial tumors, significant hepatic/renal failure, pregnancy/nursing status, and possible drug interactions. Obtain baseline BP.

Monitoring: Monitor for AV block, bradycardia, asystole, acute worsening of heart failure, bundle branch block, precipitation of respiratory muscle failure, and hemodynamic side effects in neonates/infants. Monitor ECG and BP.

Patient Counseling: Inform of risks/benefits of therapy.

Storage: 20-25°C (68-77°F). Protect from light by retaining in package until ready to use.

VERDESO – desonide

Class: Corticosteroid

RX

ADULT DOSAGE

Atopic Dermatitis

Mild to Moderate:
Apply thin layer to affected area(s) bid; dispense smallest amount necessary to adequately cover affected area(s)

Max Duration: 4 consecutive weeks; reassess if no improvement after 4 weeks

D/C when control is achieved

PEDIATRIC DOSAGE

Atopic Dermatitis

≥3 Months of Age:
Mild to Moderate:
Apply thin layer to affected area(s) bid; dispense smallest amount necessary to adequately cover affected area(s)

Max Duration: 4 consecutive weeks; reassess if no improvement after 4 weeks

D/C when control is achieved

ADMINISTRATION

Topical route

Shake can before use
Invert can to dispense foam
In treating areas of the face, dispense foam in hands and gently massage into affected areas until medication disappears; for areas other than the face, foam may be dispensed directly
Avoid w/ occlusive dressings unless directed

HOW SUPPLIED

Foam: 0.05% [100g]

WARNINGS/PRECAUTIONS

May result in systemic absorption and effects, including hypothalamic-pituitary-adrenal (HPA) axis suppression, manifestations of Cushing's syndrome, hyperglycemia, facial swelling, glycosuria, withdrawal syndrome, and growth retardation in children. May suppress immune system if used for >4 weeks. Application over large surface areas, prolonged use, or addition of occlusive dressing may augment systemic absorption. Periodic evaluation of HPA-axis suppression may be required; gradually withdraw, reduce frequency, or substitute a less potent steroid if HPA-axis suppression is noted. Pediatric patients may be more susceptible to systemic toxicity. May cause local skin adverse reactions. D/C and institute appropriate therapy if irritation develops. Institute an appropriate antifungal, antibacterial, or antiviral agent if concomitant skin infections are present or develop; if no prompt favorable response, may need to d/c until infection is controlled. Flammable; avoid fire, flame, and/or smoking during and immediately following application. Cosyntropin (adrenocorticotropic hormone$_{1-24}$) stimulation test may be helpful in evaluating for HPA-axis suppression. Avoid contact with eyes or other mucous membranes. If used during lactation, do not apply on the chest to avoid accidental ingestion by infant. Caution in elderly. Not for oral, ophthalmic, or intravaginal use.

ADVERSE REACTIONS

Upper respiratory tract infection, cough, application-site burning.

DRUG INTERACTIONS

Caution with concomitant topical corticosteroids; may produce cumulative effect.

NURSING CONSIDERATIONS

Assessment: Assess for skin infections, pregnancy/nursing status, and for possible drug interactions.

Monitoring: Monitor for signs/symptoms of HPA-axis suppression, Cushing's syndrome, hyperglycemia, facial swelling, glycosuria, withdrawal syndrome, growth retardation, delayed weight gain, and intracranial HTN in children. Monitor for irritation, concomitant skin infections, and other adverse reactions. Perform periodic monitoring of HPA-axis suppression if medication is used over large BSA, used with occlusive dressing, or with prolonged use of drug. Reassess diagnosis if no improvement is seen within 4 weeks.

Patient Counseling: Instruct to use externally and ud. Advise not to use for any disorder other than that for which it was prescribed. Instruct to avoid contact with eyes or other mucous membranes. Instruct to not bandage, cover, or wrap treated skin area so as to be occlusive unless directed. Counsel to report any signs of local or systemic adverse reactions. Instruct to inform physician about the treatment if surgery is contemplated. Advise to d/c therapy when control is achieved; instruct to contact physician if no improvement seen within 4 weeks. Instruct not to use other corticosteroid-containing products while on medication without consulting the physician. Inform that medication is flammable; avoid fire, flame, or smoking during and immediately after application.

Storage: 20-25°C (68-77°F); excursions permitted between 15-30°C (59-86°F). Do not puncture or incinerate. Do not expose containers to heat, and/or store at temperatures above 49°C (120°F).

VESIcare – solifenacin succinate

RX

Class: Muscarinic antagonist

ADULT DOSAGE

Overactive Bladder

Usual: 5mg qd

Titrate: May increase to 10mg qd if 5mg dose is well tolerated

PEDIATRIC DOSAGE

Pediatric use may not have been established

DOSE MODIFICATION

Concomitant Medications

Potent CYP3A4 Inhibitors:

Max: 5mg qd

Renal Impairment

CrCl <30mL/min:

Max: 5mg qd

Hepatic Impairment

Moderate (Child-Pugh B):

Max: 5mg qd

Moderate (Child-Pugh C): Not recommended

ADMINISTRATION

Oral route

Take w/ water and swallow whole, w/ or w/o food

HOW SUPPLIED

Tab: 5mg, 10mg

CONTRAINDICATIONS

Urinary/gastric retention and uncontrolled narrow-angle glaucoma.

WARNINGS/PRECAUTIONS

Not recommended with severe hepatic impairment (Child-Pugh C). Angioedema of the face, lips, tongue, and/or larynx, and rare anaphylactic reactions reported; d/c and provide appropriate therapy. Risk of urinary retention. Caution with decreased GI motility, controlled narrow-angle glaucoma, renal/hepatic impairment, and history of QT prolongation. CNS anticholinergic effects (eg, headache, confusion, hallucinations, somnolence) reported; may impair mental/physical abilities. Monitor for signs of anticholinergic CNS effects, particularly after beginning treatment or increasing the dose; consider dose reduction or discontinuation if such effects occur.

ADVERSE REACTIONS

Dry mouth, constipation, nausea, dyspepsia, UTI, blurred vision.

DRUG INTERACTIONS

See Dosage. Ketoconazole, a potent CYP3A4 inhibitor, may increase levels. CYP3A4 inducers may decrease concentrations. Caution with medications known to prolong the QT interval.

NURSING CONSIDERATIONS

Assessment: Assess for hypersensitivity to the drug and for any other conditions where treatment is contraindicated or cautioned. Assess for renal/hepatic impairment, pregnancy/nursing status, and possible drug interactions.

Monitoring: Monitor for angioedema, anaphylactic reactions, signs of anticholinergic CNS effects, and other adverse reactions.

Patient Counseling: Inform that constipation may occur; advise to contact physician if severe abdominal pain or constipation for ≥3 days occurs. Inform that blurred vision or CNS anticholinergic effects may occur; advise to exercise caution in decisions to engage in potentially dangerous activities until effects have been determined. Inform that heat prostration (due to decreased sweating) can occur when used in a hot environment. Inform that angioedema may occur and could result in fatal airway obstruction; advise to promptly d/c therapy and seek immediate attention if edema or difficulty breathing develops.

Storage: 25°C (77°F); excursions permitted from 15-30°C (59-86°F).

VFEND — voriconazole

Class: Azole antifungal

RX

ADULT DOSAGE

Aspergillosis

Invasive:
LD: 6mg/kg IV q12h for the first 24 hrs
Maint:
IV: 4mg/kg q12h; may decrease to 3mg/kg q12h if unable to tolerate
PO: 200mg q12h; may increase to 300mg q12h if response is inadequate
Continue IV therapy for at least 7 days

Scedosporiosis and Fusariosis

Serious fungal infections caused by *Scedosporium apiospermum* and *Fusarium* spp. including *Fusarium solani*
LD: 6mg/kg IV q12h for the first 24 hrs
Maint:
IV: 4mg/kg q12h; may decrease to 3mg/kg q12h if unable to tolerate
PO: 200mg q12h; may increase to 300mg q12h if response is inadequate
Continue IV therapy for at least 7 days

***Candida* Infections**

Candidemia (Non-Neutropenic Patients) and Other Deep Tissue *Candida* Infections:
LD: 6mg/kg IV q12h for the first 24 hrs
Maint:
IV: 3-4mg/kg q12h
PO: 200mg q12h

Treat for at least 14 days following resolution of symptoms or last (+) culture, whichever is longer

Esophageal Candidiasis

Maint: 200mg PO q12h
Treat for a minimum of 14 days and for at least 7 days following resolution of symptoms

PEDIATRIC DOSAGE

Fungal Infections

Treatment of invasive aspergillosis; esophageal candidiasis; candidemia in non-neutropenic patients and the following *Candida* infections: disseminated infections in skin and infections in abdomen, kidney, bladder wall, and wounds; serious fungal infections caused by *Scedosporium apiospermum* and *Fusarium* spp. including *Fusarium solani*, in patients intolerant of, or refractory to, other therapy
≥12 Years:
Refer to PI for dosing

DOSE MODIFICATION

Concomitant Medications
Phenytoin/Efavirenz:
Increase maintenance dose of voriconazole

Renal Impairment
Moderate or Severe (CrCl <50mL/min):
Administer oral therapy unless the benefit/risk to the patient justifies the use of IV therapy; monitor SrCr levels closely and consider changing to oral therapy if increases occur

Hepatic Impairment
Mild to Moderate (Child-Pugh Class A and B):
Reduce maint dose by 1/2

Adverse Reactions
If unable to tolerate 300mg PO q12h, reduce oral maint dose by 50mg steps to a minimum of 200mg q12h (or 100mg q12h for adults <40kg)

Other Important Modifications
Adults:
<40kg: Administer 1/2 the oral maint dose; may increase from 100mg q12h to 150mg q12h if response is inadequate

ADMINISTRATION

Oral and IV routes

Oral
Take at least 1 hr before or after a meal
Shake reconstituted sus for approx 10 sec before each use; administer using oral dispenser supplied w/ each pack
Do not mix w/ any other medication or additional flavoring agent

Sus Preparation:
Reconstitute w/ 46mL of water and shake for 1 min

IV
Requires reconstitution to 10mg/mL and subsequent dilution to ≤5mg/mL prior to administration as an infusion, at a max rate of 3mg/kg/hr over 1-2 hrs
Do not administer as an IV bolus inj
Do not infuse concomitantly w/ any blood product or short-term infusion of concentrated electrolytes, even if the 2 infusions are running in separate IV lines/cannulas
May infuse at the same time as other IV sol containing non-concentrated electrolytes or total parenteral nutrition (TPN) through separate lines; for TPN, must administer through a different port if infused through a multiple-lumen catheter

IV Preparation:
Reconstitute w/ 19mL of water for inj to an extractable volume of 20mL containing 10mg/mL of voriconazole
Further dilute required volume of therapy and add to infusion bag/bottle; withdraw and discard at least an equal volume of diluent from infusion bag/bottle to be used
Volume of diluent remaining in the bag or bottle should be such that when 10mg/mL of voriconazole is added, the final concentration is not <0.5mg/mL nor >5mg/mL
Discard partially used vials

Compatible IV Diluents:
9mg/mL (0.9%) NaCl, lactated Ringer's, D5 and lactated Ringer's, D5 and 0.45% NaCl, D5, D5 and 20mEq potassium chloride, 0.45% NaCl, and D5 and 0.9% NaCl

HOW SUPPLIED

Inj: 200mg; Sus: 40mg/mL; Tab: 50mg, 200mg

CONTRAINDICATIONS

Concomitant terfenadine, astemizole, cisapride, pimozide, quinidine, sirolimus, rifampin, carbamazepine, long-acting barbiturates, efavirenz (≥400mg q24h), high-dose ritonavir (400mg q12h), rifabutin, ergot alkaloids (ergotamine, dihydroergotamine), St. John's wort. Low-dose ritonavir (100mg q12h) should be avoided, unless an assessment of benefit/risk justifies the use.

WARNINGS/PRECAUTIONS

Uncommon cases of serious hepatic reactions (eg, clinical hepatitis, cholestasis, fulminant hepatic failure) reported; evaluate LFTs at the start of and during the course of therapy and consider discontinuation if clinical signs and symptoms consistent with liver disease develops. Prolonged visual adverse events (eg, optic neuritis, papilledema) reported; monitor visual function if treatment continues >28 days. May cause fetal harm. Tabs contain lactose; avoid with rare hereditary problems of galactose intolerance, Lapp lactase deficiency, or glucose-galactose malabsorption. May prolong QT interval, and rare cases of arrhythmias, cardiac arrests, and sudden deaths may occur; caution with proarrhythmic conditions. Anaphylactoid-type reactions reported with infusion; consider discontinuing infusion if reactions occur. Correct electrolyte disturbances prior to initiation of therapy. Associated with elevations in LFTs and clinical signs of liver damage. Acute renal failure may occur. Monitor for the development of pancreatitis in patients with risk factors for acute pancreatitis (eg, recent chemotherapy, hematopoietic stem cell transplantation) during treatment. Serious exfoliative cutaneous reactions (eg, Stevens-Johnson syndrome) and photosensitivity skin reaction reported; d/c if exfoliative cutaneous reaction or skin lesion consistent with squamous cell carcinoma or melanoma develops. Fluorosis and periostitis reported with long-term therapy; d/c if skeletal pain and radiologic findings compatible with fluorosis and periostitis develop.

ADVERSE REACTIONS

Visual disturbances, fever, chills, rash, headache, N/V, increased alkaline phosphatase.

DRUG INTERACTIONS

See Contraindications. Avoid with fluconazole and everolimus. Decreased exposure with phenytoin, low-dose ritonavir (100mg q12h), efavirenz, and other non-nucleoside reverse transcriptase inhibitors (NNRTIs). Decrease in AUC with efavirenz (300mg q24h). Increased exposure with fluconazole, oral contraceptives containing ethinyl estradiol and norethindrone, HIV protease inhibitors, delavirdine, and other NNRTIs. Increased exposure of alfentanil, oxycodone, tacrolimus, phenytoin, omeprazole, methadone, fentanyl, NSAIDs, oral contraceptives containing ethinyl estradiol and norethindrone, HIV protease inhibitors, NNRTIs, benzodiazepines, HMG-CoA reductase inhibitors, dihydropyridine calcium channel blockers, sulfonylurea oral hypoglycemics, vinca alkaloids, and everolimus. Increased AUC of efavirenz (300mg q24h) and cyclosporine. Decreased AUC and C_{max} of low-dose ritonavir (100mg q12h). Increased PT with warfarin. Refer to PI for further information on drug interactions.

NURSING CONSIDERATIONS

Assessment: Assess for drug hypersensitivity, proarrhythmic conditions, hereditary problems of galactose intolerance, Lapp lactase deficiency or glucose-galactose malabsorption, hepatic/renal impairment, electrolyte disturbances, pregnancy/nursing status, and possible drug interactions. Obtain fungal cultures to isolate and identify causative organisms.

Monitoring: Monitor for signs/symptoms of hepatotoxicity, arrhythmias, QT prolongation, cardiac arrests, acute renal failure, pancreatitis, serious exfoliative cutaneous reactions, fluorosis, periostitis, and other adverse reactions. Monitor for drug toxicity with hepatic impairment. Monitor renal function and PT or other suitable anticoagulation tests. Monitor visual function (eg, acuity, visual field, color perception) if treatment continues >28 days.

Patient Counseling: Inform of the risks/benefits of therapy. Counsel to take tabs or oral sus at least 1 hr before or pc. Inform of the potential hazards to the fetus if drug is used during pregnancy or if the patient becomes pregnant. Instruct to avoid intense or prolonged exposure to direct sunlight during therapy. Inform women of childbearing potential to use effective contraception during treatment. Inform of the signs and symptoms of hepatic reactions, allergic reactions, vision changes, and serious skin reactions; advise to contact physician if any of these conditions develop.

Storage: Inj: Unreconstituted: 15-30°C (59-86°F). Reconstituted: 2-8°C (36-46°F) for up to 24 hrs. Tab: 15-30°C (59-86°F). Oral Sus: Unreconstituted: 2-8°C (36-46°F) for up to 18 months. Reconstituted: 15-30°C (59-86°F) for up to 14 days. Do not refrigerate or freeze.

VIAGRA – sildenafil citrate

Class: Phosphodiesterase type 5 inhibitor

RX

ADULT DOSAGE

Erectile Dysfunction

Usual: 50mg qd prn 1 hr (recommended) or anywhere from 30 min to 4 hrs before sexual activity

Titrate: May increase to 100mg qd or decrease to 25mg qd, based on effectiveness and tolerance

Max: 100mg qd

PEDIATRIC DOSAGE

Pediatric use may not have been established

DOSE MODIFICATION

Concomitant Medications

Strong CYP3A4 Inhibitors/Erythromycin:

Initial: Consider 25mg qd

α-Blockers:

Patient should be stable on α-blocker therapy prior to initiating treatment

Initial: 25mg qd

Ritonavir:

Usual: 25mg prior to sexual activity

Max: 25mg/48 hrs

Renal Impairment

CrCl <30mL/min:

Initial: Consider 25mg qd

Hepatic Impairment

Initial: Consider 25mg qd

Elderly

Initial: Consider 25mg qd

ADMINISTRATION

Oral route

May be taken w/ or w/o food

HOW SUPPLIED

Tab: 25mg, 50mg, 100mg

CONTRAINDICATIONS

Concomitant use w/ nitric oxide donors (eg, organic nitrates/nitrites) in any form, either taken regularly and/or intermittently.

WARNINGS/PRECAUTIONS

Potential for cardiac risk of sexual activity in patients w/ cardiovascular disease (CVD); do not use in men for whom sexual activity is inadvisable due to underlying cardiovascular status. Has systemic vasodilatory properties that resulted in transient decreases in supine BP in clinical studies. Caution in patients w/ left ventricular outflow obstruction (eg, aortic stenosis, idiopathic hypertrophic subaortic stenosis); severely impaired autonomic control of BP; history of MI, stroke, or life-threatening arrhythmia w/in the last 6 months; resting hypotension (BP <90/50mmHg) or HTN (BP >170/110mmHg); and cardiac failure or coronary artery disease (CAD) causing unstable angina. Prolonged erection >4 hrs and priapism reported; caution w/ anatomical penile deformation (eg, angulation, cavernosal fibrosis, Peyronie's disease), or predispositions to priapism (eg, sickle cell anemia, multiple myeloma, leukemia). Nonarteritic anterior ischemic optic neuropathy (NAION) reported. D/C if sudden loss of vision in 1 or both eyes occurs; may be a sign of NAION. Caution w/ underlying NAION risk factors; increased risk in patients w/ "crowded" optic disc and w/ previous history of NAION. D/C if sudden decrease or loss of hearing occurs. Bleeding events reported. Does not protect against STDs.

ADVERSE REACTIONS

Headache, flushing, dyspepsia, abnormal vision, nasal congestion, back pain, myalgia, nausea, dizziness, rash.

DRUG INTERACTIONS

See Dose Modification and Contraindications. Increased levels w/ CYP3A4 inhibitors (eg, ritonavir, erythromycin, saquinavir); stronger CYP3A4 inhibitors (eg, ketoconazole, itraconazole) may have greater effects. Potential additive BP-lowering effects w/ α-blockers and other antihypertensives (eg, amlodipine). Combination w/ other PDE-5 inhibitors or other ED therapies is not recommended; may further lower BP.

NURSING CONSIDERATIONS

Assessment: Assess for hypersensitivity to drug; history of MI, stroke, or arrhythmia; renal/hepatic impairment; CVD; left ventricular outflow obstruction; impaired autonomic control of BP; resting hypotension or HTN; cardiac failure; CAD; anatomical penile deformation; predisposition to priapism; risk for NAION; potential underlying causes of ED; and for possible drug interactions.

Monitoring: Monitor for prolonged erection, priapism, abnormalities in vision/NAION, decrease/loss of hearing, bleeding, and other adverse reactions.

Patient Counseling: Inform of risks and benefits of therapy. Instruct to notify physician of all prescription/nonprescription medications and supplements currently being taken and inform of the contraindication w/ regular and/or intermittent use of nitric oxide donors (eg, organic nitrates or organic nitrites in any form). Advise patients who experience cardiovascular symptoms (eg, angina pectoris, dizziness, nausea) upon initiation of sexual activity to refrain from further activity and to discuss the episode w/ their physician. Instruct to d/c and seek medical attention if sudden loss of vision in 1 or both eyes or sudden decrease/loss of hearing occurs. Instruct to seek immediate medical assistance if erection persists >4 hrs. Counsel about protective measures necessary to guard against STDs, including HIV.

Storage: 25°C (77°F); excursions permitted to 15-30°C (59-86°F).

VIBATIV – telavancin

RX

Class: Lipoglycopeptide

Increased mortality observed in patients with preexisting moderate/severe renal impairment (CrCl ≤50mL/min) who were treated for hospital-acquired bacterial pneumonia/ventilator-associated bacterial pneumonia (HABP/VABP); consider therapy only when the anticipated benefit outweighs the risk. New onset or worsening renal impairment reported; monitor renal function in all patients. Women of childbearing potential should have a serum pregnancy test prior to administration. Avoid use during pregnancy unless potential benefit to the patient outweighs the potential risk to the fetus. Potential adverse developmental outcomes in humans may occur.

ADULT DOSAGE

Skin and Skin Structure Infections

Complicated Gram-Positive Infections:
10mg/kg IV over 60 min q24h for 7-14 days

Pneumonia

Hospital-Acquired/Ventilator-Associated Bacterial Pneumonia:
Susceptible Isolates of *Staphylococcus aureus*
10mg/kg IV over 60 min q24h for 7-21 days

PEDIATRIC DOSAGE

Pediatric use may not have been established

DOSE MODIFICATION

Renal Impairment

CrCl 30-50mL/min: 7.5mg/kg q24h
CrCl 10-<30mL/min: 10mg/kg q48h

ADMINISTRATION

IV route

Administer IV infusion over 60 min
Do not add additives or other medications to single-use vials or infuse simultaneously through the same IV line

If the same IV line is used for sequential infusion of additional medications, flush the line before and after infusion of therapy with appropriate infusion sol

Preparation

250mg Vial: Reconstitute contents with 15mL of appropriate reconstitution diluent
750mg Vial: Reconstitute contents with 45mL of appropriate reconstitution diluent
For doses of 150-800mg, reconstituted sol must be further diluted in 100-250mL of appropriate infusion sol prior to infusion
Doses <150mg or >800mg should be further diluted in a volume resulting in a final concentration of 0.6-8mg/mL

Appropriate Reconstitution Diluents

5% Dextrose Inj
Sterile Water for Inj
0.9% NaCl Inj

Appropriate Infusion Sol

5% Dextrose Inj
0.9% NaCl Inj
Lactated Ringer's Inj

HOW SUPPLIED

Inj: 250mg, 750mg

CONTRAINDICATIONS

Use of IV unfractionated heparin sodium.

WARNINGS/PRECAUTIONS

Use of telavancin for the treatment of HABP/VABP should be reserved for when alternative treatments are not suitable. Decreased efficacy in patients with cSSSI and preexisting moderate/severe renal impairment (CrCl ≤50mL/min). Renal adverse events were reported more likely to occur in patients with baseline comorbidities known to predispose patients to kidney dysfunction (preexisting renal disease, diabetes mellitus [DM], congestive heart failure [CHF], or HTN). Consider alternative agent if renal toxicity is suspected. Accumulation of the solubilizer hydroxypropyl-β-cyclodextrin may occur in patients with renal dysfunction. May interfere with coagulation tests (eg, PT/INR, activated PTT [aPTT], activated clotting time, coagulation-based factor Xa assay) and urine protein tests; collect blood samples for affected coagulation tests as close as possible prior to the next dose. For patients who require aPTT monitoring while on therapy, a non-phospholipid dependent coagulation test (eg, factor Xa [chromogenic] assay) or an alternative anticoagulant not requiring aPTT monitoring may be considered. Serious and sometimes fatal hypersensitivity reactions, including anaphylactic reactions, may occur after 1st or subsequent doses; d/c at 1st sign of skin rash, or any other signs of hypersensitivity. Caution with known hypersensitivity to vancomycin. Infusion-related reactions (eg, "red man syndrome"-like reactions) may occur with rapid infusion. *Clostridium difficile*-associated diarrhea (CDAD) reported; may need to d/c if CDAD is suspected or confirmed. Use in the absence of a proven or strongly suspected bacterial infection is unlikely to provide benefit and increases the risk of development of drug-resistant bacteria. May result in overgrowth of nonsusceptible organisms; take appropriate measures if superinfection develops. QTc interval prolongation reported; avoid in patients with congenital long QT syndrome, known prolongation of the QTc interval, uncompensated heart failure (HF), or severe left ventricular hypertrophy (LVH). Caution in elderly patients.

ADVERSE REACTIONS

Renal impairment, taste disturbance, N/V, foamy urine, rigors, diarrhea, decreased appetite.

DRUG INTERACTIONS

See Contraindications. Caution with drugs known to prolong the QT interval. Higher renal adverse event rates reported with concomitant medications known to affect kidney function (eg, NSAIDs, ACE inhibitors, loop diuretics).

NURSING CONSIDERATIONS

Assessment: Assess for hypersensitivity to the drug/vancomycin, renal impairment, renal impairment risk (eg, preexisting renal disease, DM, CHF, HTN), congenital long QT syndrome, known prolongation of the QTc interval, uncompensated HF, severe LVH, pregnancy/nursing status, and possible drug interactions. Obtain renal function values.

Monitoring: Monitor for new onset or worsening renal impairment, hypersensitivity reactions, CDAD, development of drug-resistant bacteria, overgrowth of nonsusceptible organisms, superinfection, infusion-related reactions, QTc prolongation, and other adverse reactions. Monitor renal function (eg, SrCr, CrCl) during treatment (at 48- to 72-hr intervals or more frequently, if clinically indicated), and at the end of therapy.

Patient Counseling: Inform women of childbearing potential about the potential risk of fetal harm if drug is used during pregnancy; instruct to have a pregnancy test prior to therapy, to use effective contraceptive methods to prevent pregnancy during treatment if not pregnant, and to notify physician if pregnancy occurs. Encourage pregnant patients to enroll in pregnancy registry. Inform that diarrhea may occur, even as late as ≥2 months after last dose of therapy; instruct to notify physician as soon as possible if watery/bloody stools (with/without stomach cramps and fever) occur. Inform that antibacterial drugs should only be used to treat bacterial, not viral, infections. Instruct to take ud; inform that skipping doses or not completing full course may decrease effectiveness and increase resistance. Counsel about common adverse effects; advise to notify physician if any unusual/known symptom persists or worsens.

Storage: 2-8°C (35-46°F); excursions permitted to ambient temperatures (up to 25°C [77°F]). Avoid excessive heat. Reconstituted/Diluted Sol: Use within 12 hrs when stored at room temperature or use within 7 days when stored under refrigeration at 2-8°C (36-46°F). Diluted sol can also be stored at -30 to -10°C (-22 to 14°F) for up to 32 days.

VIBRAMYCIN – doxycycline **RX**

Class: Tetracyclines

OTHER BRAND NAMES

Vibra-Tabs

ADULT DOSAGE

General Dosing

Treatment of the following infections caused by susceptible microorganisms: Rocky Mountain spotted fever, typhus fever and the typhus group, Q fever, rickettsialpox, tick fevers, respiratory tract infections, lymphogranuloma venereum, psittacosis (ornithosis), trachoma, inclusion conjunctivitis, relapsing fever, chancroid, plague, tularemia, cholera, *Campylobacter fetus* infections, brucellosis, bartonellosis, granuloma inguinale, UTIs, anthrax. Treatment of infections caused by *Escherichia coli*, *Enterobacter aerogenes*, *Shigella* species, or *Acinetobacter* species. Treatment of uncomplicated gonorrhea, yaws, listeriosis, Vincent's infection, actinomycosis, and *Clostridium* species infections when penicillin is contraindicated. Adjunct to amebicides in acute intestinal amebiasis. Adjunctive therapy in severe acne

Initial: 100mg q12h on Day 1
Maint: 100mg/day
More Severe Infections (eg, Chronic UTIs): 100mg q12h

Gonococcal Infections

Uncomplicated:
Except Anorectal Infections in Men:
100mg bid for 7 days or as an alternate single visit dose, 300mg stat followed in 1 hr by a second 300mg dose

Urethral Infections

Uncomplicated:
100mg bid for 7 days

Endocervical Infections

Uncomplicated:
100mg bid for 7 days

Rectal Infections

Uncomplicated:
100mg bid for 7 days

Nongonococcal Urethritis

100mg bid for 7 days

Syphilis

When Penicillin is Contraindicated:

Early Syphilis:
100mg bid for 2 weeks

PEDIATRIC DOSAGE

General Dosing

Treatment of the following infections caused by susceptible microorganisms: Rocky Mountain spotted fever, typhus fever and the typhus group, Q fever, rickettsialpox, tick fevers, respiratory tract infections, lymphogranuloma venereum, psittacosis (ornithosis), trachoma, inclusion conjunctivitis, relapsing fever, chancroid, plague, tularemia, cholera, *Campylobacter fetus* infections, brucellosis, bartonellosis, granuloma inguinale, UTIs, anthrax. Treatment of infections caused by *Escherichia coli*, *Enterobacter aerogenes*, *Shigella* species, or *Acinetobacter* species. Treatment of uncomplicated gonorrhea, yaws, listeriosis, Vincent's infection, actinomycosis, and *Clostridium* species infections when penicillin is contraindicated. Adjunct to amebicides in acute intestinal amebiasis. Adjunctive therapy in severe acne

> 8 Years:
≤100 lbs:
1mg/lb bid on Day 1 then 1mg/lb qd or divided into 2 doses, on subsequent days
More Severe Infections: May use up to 2mg/lb
>100 lbs:
Initial: 100mg q12h on Day 1
Maint: 100mg/day
More Severe Infections (eg, Chronic UTIs): 100mg q12h

Malaria

Prophylaxis of malaria due to *Plasmodium falciparum* in short-term travelers (<4 months) to areas w/ chloroquine and/or pyrimethamine-sulfadoxine resistant strains

>8 Years:
2mg/kg qd
Max: 100mg/day

Begin 1-2 days before travel and continue daily during travel and for 4 weeks after leaving malarious area

Inhalational Anthrax (Postexposure)

<100 lbs:
1mg/lb (2.2mg/kg) bid for 60 days
≥100 lbs:
100mg bid for 60 days

Syphilis of >1-Year Duration:
100mg bid for 4 weeks

Acute Epididymo-Orchitis

100mg bid for at least 10 days

Malaria

Prophylaxis of malaria due to *Plasmodium falciparum* in short-term travelers (<4 months) to areas w/ chloroquine and/or pyrimethamine-sulfadoxine resistant strains

Usual: 100mg qd

Begin 1-2 days before travel and continue daily during travel and for 4 weeks after leaving malarious area

Inhalational Anthrax (Postexposure)

100mg bid for 60 days

Streptococcal Infections

Continue for 10 days

Streptococcal Infections

Continue for 10 days

ADMINISTRATION

Oral route

Administer caps/tabs w/ adequate amount of fluids; if gastric irritation occurs, administer w/ food or milk

HOW SUPPLIED

Cap (Hyclate): 100mg, (Generic) 50mg; Sus (Monohydrate): 25mg/5mL [60mL]; Syrup (Calcium): 50mg/5mL [473mL]; Tab (Hyclate): 100mg

WARNINGS/PRECAUTIONS

May cause permanent teeth discoloration (yellow-gray-brown) if used during tooth development (last 1/2 of pregnancy to 8 yrs of age); avoid use in these age groups for indications other than anthrax. Enamel hypoplasia reported. *Clostridium difficile*-associated diarrhea (CDAD) reported; may need to d/c if CDAD is suspected or confirmed. Associated with intracranial HTN (pseudotumor cerebri); increased risk in women of childbearing age who are overweight or have a history of intracranial HTN. Intracranial pressure can remain elevated for weeks after drug cessation; monitor patients until they stabilize. Possibility of permanent visual loss exists; prompt ophthalmologic evaluation needed if visual disturbance occurs during treatment. May decrease fibula growth rate in prematures or cause fetal harm during pregnancy. May increase BUN. Photosensitivity may occur; d/c at 1st evidence of skin erythema. May result in bacterial resistance if used in the absence of a proven/suspected bacterial infection or a prophylactic indication; take appropriate measures if superinfection develops. When used for malaria prophylaxis, patients may still transmit the infection to mosquitoes outside endemic areas. False elevations of urinary catecholamines may occur due to interference with the fluorescence test. Syrup contains sodium metabisulfite that may cause allergic-type reactions.

ADVERSE REACTIONS

Anorexia, N/V, diarrhea, dysphagia, maculopapular rash, Stevens-Johnson syndrome, toxic epidermal necrolysis, photosensitivity, increased BUN, hypersensitivity reactions, drug rash with eosinophilia and systemic symptoms, hemolytic anemia, thrombocytopenia, neutropenia, eosinophilia.

DRUG INTERACTIONS

Avoid concomitant use with isotretinoin; may also cause pseudotumor cerebri. May depress plasma prothrombin activity; may require downward adjustment of anticoagulant dose. May interfere with bactericidal action of PCN; avoid concurrent use. Bismuth subsalicylate, iron-containing preparations, and antacids containing aluminum, Ca^{2+}, or Mg^{2+} may impair absorption. Barbiturates, carbamazepine, and phenytoin may decrease $T_{1/2}$. Fatal renal toxicity reported with methoxyflurane. May render oral contraceptives less effective.

NURSING CONSIDERATIONS

Assessment: Assess for previous hypersensitivity to any tetracyclines, risk of intracranial HTN, pregnancy/nursing status, and possible drug interactions. Document indications for therapy as well as culture and susceptibility testing results. Perform dark-field exam and blood serology when coexistent syphilis is suspected.

Monitoring: Monitor for signs/symptoms of hypersensitivity reactions, photosensitivity, skin erythema, superinfection, CDAD, intracranial HTN, visual disturbance, and other adverse reactions. In venereal disease with coexistent syphilis, conduct blood serology monthly for at least 4 months. Perform periodic lab evaluation of organ systems, including hematopoietic, renal, and hepatic studies in long-term therapy.

Patient Counseling: Apprise pregnant women of the potential hazard to fetus. Inform that the therapy does not guarantee protection against malaria; instruct to use measures that help avoid contact with mosquitoes. Instruct to avoid excessive sunlight/UV light and to d/c therapy if phototoxicity occurs; advise to consider use of sunscreen or sunblock. Instruct to drink fluids liberally. Inform that drug absorption is reduced when taking bismuth subsalicylate and when taken with food, especially those that contain Ca^{2+}. Inform that drug may increase the incidence of vaginal candidiasis. Instruct to take exactly ud; warn that skipping doses or not completing full course may decrease effectiveness and increase resistance. Counsel that therapy should only be used to treat bacterial, not viral, infections. Inform that diarrhea may be experienced and advise to notify physician as soon as possible if watery and bloody stools (with or without stomach cramps and fever) even as late as ≥2 months after last dose occur.

Storage: (Vibramycin/Vibra-Tabs) <30°C (86°F). (Generic) 20-25°C (68-77°F). Protect from light and moisture.

VICODIN – acetaminophen/hydrocodone bitartrate CII

Class: Opioid analgesic

Associated w/ cases of acute liver failure, at times resulting in liver transplant and death. Most of the cases of liver injury are associated w/ acetaminophen (APAP) use at doses >4000mg/day, and often involve >1 APAP-containing product.

OTHER BRAND NAMES

Vicodin ES, Vicodin HP

ADULT DOSAGE

Moderate to Moderately Severe Pain

Vicodin:
Usual: 1 or 2 tabs q4-6h prn
Max: 8 tabs/day

Vicodin ES/Vicodin HP:
Usual: 1 tab q4-6h prn
Max: 6 tabs/day

PEDIATRIC DOSAGE

Pediatric use may not have been established

DOSE MODIFICATION

Elderly

Start at lower end of dosing range

ADMINISTRATION

Oral route

HOW SUPPLIED

(Hydrocodone/APAP) Tab: (Vicodin) 5mg/300mg*; (Vicodin ES) 7.5mg/300mg*; (Vicodin HP) 10mg/300mg* *scored

WARNINGS/PRECAUTIONS

Increased risk of acute liver failure in patients w/ underlying liver disease. May cause serious skin reactions (eg, acute generalized exanthematous pustulosis, Stevens-Johnson syndrome, toxic epidermal necrolysis); d/c at the 1st appearance of skin rash or any other sign of hypersensitivity. Hypersensitivity and anaphylaxis reported; d/c immediately if signs/symptoms occur. May produce dose-related respiratory depression and irregular/periodic breathing. Respiratory depressant effects and CSF pressure elevation capacity may be markedly exaggerated in the presence of head injury, other intracranial lesions, or a preexisting increased intracranial pressure. May obscure clinical course of acute abdominal conditions and head injuries. Caution w/ hypothyroidism, Addison's disease, prostatic hypertrophy, urethral stricture, severe hepatic/renal impairment, or in the elderly/debilitated. Suppresses cough reflex; caution w/ pulmonary disease and in postoperative use. Lab test interactions may occur. May be habit-forming.

ADVERSE REACTIONS

Acute liver failure, lightheadedness, dizziness, sedation, N/V.

DRUG INTERACTIONS

Increased risk of acute liver failure w/ alcohol. Additive CNS depression w/ other narcotics, antihistamines, antipsychotics, antianxiety agents, or other CNS depressants (eg, alcohol); reduce dose of one or both agents. Concomitant use w/ MAOIs or TCAs may increase the effect of either the antidepressant or hydrocodone.

NURSING CONSIDERATIONS

Assessment: Assess for history of hypersensitivity to drug, level of pain intensity, type of pain, patient's general condition and medical status, renal/hepatic impairment, pregnancy/nursing status, any other conditions where treatment is cautioned, and possible drug interactions.

Monitoring: Monitor for signs/symptoms of hypersensitivity or anaphylaxis, serious skin reactions, acute liver failure, respiratory depression, elevations in CSF pressure, drug abuse/dependence/tolerance, and other adverse reactions. In patients w/ severe hepatic/renal disease, monitor effects w/ serial hepatic and/or renal function tests.

Patient Counseling: Instruct to look for APAP on package labels and not to use >1 APAP-containing product. Instruct to seek medical attention immediately upon ingestion of >4000mg/day of APAP, even if feeling well. Advise to d/c use and contact physician immediately if signs of allergy develop. Inform about signs of serious skin reactions. Inform that drug may impair mental/physical abilities, and to use caution if performing potentially hazardous tasks (eg, driving, operating machinery). Instruct to avoid alcohol and other CNS depressants. Inform that drug may be habit-forming; instruct to take only ud.

Storage: 20-25°C (68-77°F).

VICOPROFEN – hydrocodone bitartrate/ibuprofen CII

Class: Opioid analgesic

OTHER BRAND NAMES

Reprexain

ADULT DOSAGE

Acute Pain

Short-Term (Generally <10 Days) Management:

Use lowest effective dose or longest dosing interval consistent w/ individual treatment goals; adjust based on individual needs

Usual: 1 tab q4-6h prn

Max: 5 tabs/24 hrs

PEDIATRIC DOSAGE

Acute Pain

Short-Term (Generally <10 Days) Management:

≥16 Years:

Use lowest effective dose or longest dosing interval consistent w/ individual treatment goals; adjust based on individual needs

Usual: 1 tab q4-6h prn

Max: 5 tabs/24 hrs

DOSE MODIFICATION

Elderly

Reduce dose

ADMINISTRATION

Oral route

HOW SUPPLIED

(Hydrocodone-Ibuprofen) Tab: (Vicoprofen) 7.5mg-200mg; (Reprexain) 2.5mg-200mg, 5mg-200mg*, 10mg-200mg *scored

CONTRAINDICATIONS

History of asthma, urticaria, or other allergic-type reactions w/ aspirin (ASA) or other NSAIDs. Perioperative pain in the setting of CABG surgery.

WARNINGS/PRECAUTIONS

Not for treatment of osteoarthritis or rheumatoid arthritis. Not for treatment of corticosteroid insufficiency or substitute for corticosteroids; abrupt discontinuation of corticosteroids may lead to disease exacerbation. May diminish utility of fever and inflammation as diagnostic signs in detecting complications of presumed noninfectious, painful conditions. Not recommended w/ advanced renal disease. Ibuprofen: May increase risk of serious cardiovascular (CV) thrombotic events, MI, and stroke; increased risk w/ known CV disease or risk factors for CV disease. May cause serious GI adverse events including inflammation, bleeding, ulceration, and perforation of the stomach and intestine; extreme caution w/ history of ulcer disease or GI bleeding and caution in debilitated patients. May lead to onset of new HTN or worsening of preexisting HTN. Fluid retention and edema reported; caution in patients w/ fluid retention or heart failure (HF). Renal papillary necrosis and other renal injury reported after long-term use; caution w/ impaired renal function, HF, and liver dysfunction. Anaphylactoid reactions may occur; avoid in patients w/ ASA triad. May cause serious skin adverse events (eg, exfoliative dermatitis, Stevens-Johnson syndrome, and toxic epidermal necrolysis); d/c at 1st appearance of skin rash/hypersensitivity. Avoid in late pregnancy; may cause premature closure of ductus arteriosus. Elevations of LFTs and severe hepatic reactions (eg, jaundice, fatal fulminant hepatitis, liver necrosis, hepatic failure) reported; d/c if liver disease or systemic manifestations (eg, eosinophilia, rash) occur. Anemia reported. May inhibit platelet aggregation and prolong bleeding time. Caution w/ preexisting asthma and avoid w/ ASA-sensitive asthma. Aseptic meningitis w/ fever and coma reported. Hydrocodone: May increase risk of misuse, abuse, or diversion. May produce dose-related respiratory depression. Respiratory depressant effects and capacity to elevate CSF pressure may be markedly exaggerated in the presence of head injury, intracranial lesions, or preexisting increased intracranial pressure. May obscure diagnosis/

clinical course of acute abdominal conditions or head injuries. Caution in debilitated patients, severe renal/hepatic impairment, hypothyroidism, Addison's disease, prostatic hypertrophy, or urethral stricture. Suppresses cough reflex; caution when used postoperatively and w/ pulmonary disease.

ADVERSE REACTIONS
Headache, somnolence, dizziness, constipation, dyspepsia, N/V, infection, edema, nervousness, anxiety, pruritus, diarrhea, asthenia, abdominal pain, sweating.

DRUG INTERACTIONS
ASA may increase adverse effects; concomitant administration is not recommended. Use w/ other opioid analgesics, antihistamines, antipsychotics, antianxiety agents, or other CNS depressants (eg, alcohol) may exhibit additive CNS depression; reduce dose of 1 or both agents. Ibuprofen: Increased risk of GI bleeding w/ oral corticosteroids or anticoagulants, smoking, and alcohol. May increase the risk of renal toxicity w/ diuretics and ACE inhibitors. Alterations in platelet function may occur w/ anticoagulants; monitor carefully. May diminish antihypertensive effect of ACE inhibitors. Synergistic effects on GI bleeding w/ warfarin. May decrease natriuretic effect of furosemide and loop/thiazide diuretics; monitor for renal failure. May increase lithium levels; monitor for lithium toxicity. May enhance methotrexate toxicity; caution w/ coadministration. Hydrocodone: Use w/ MAOIs or TCAs may increase the effect of either the antidepressant or hydrocodone. Not recommended for patients taking MAOIs or w/in 14 days of stopping such treatment. May produce paralytic ileus w/ anticholinergics. Caution w/ concurrent agonist/antagonist analgesics (eg, pentazocine, nalbuphine, butorphanol, buprenorphine) use; may reduce analgesic effect of hydrocodone and/or precipitate withdrawal symptoms. May enhance neuromuscular blocking action of skeletal muscle relaxants and increase respiratory depression.

NURSING CONSIDERATIONS

Assessment: Assess for history of asthma, urticaria or allergic-type reactions w/ ASA or NSAIDs, known hypersensitivity to the drug, perioperative pain in setting of CABG surgery, CV disease and its risk factors, HTN, fluid retention or HF, ulcer disease or GI bleeding, coagulation disorders, renal/hepatic impairment, any other conditions where treatment is contraindicated or cautioned, pregnancy/nursing status, and for possible drug interactions. Assess level of pain intensity, type of pain, and patient's general condition and medical status.

Monitoring: Monitor for signs/symptoms of CV thrombotic events, MI, stroke, HTN, fluid retention or edema, drug abuse and dependence, tolerance, respiratory depression, elevations in CSF, GI effects, renal/hepatic effects, anaphylactoid reactions, skin reactions, bronchospasm, aseptic meningitis, and other adverse reactions. If signs/symptoms of anemia develop, evaluate Hgb/Hct. Perform periodic monitoring of CBC and chemistry profile w/ long-term therapy. Monitor for alterations in platelet function w/ coagulation disorders or in those receiving anticoagulants.

Patient Counseling: Caution that drug may impair mental and/or physical abilities required to perform potentially hazardous tasks (eg, operating machinery/driving). Instruct to avoid alcohol and other CNS depressants while on therapy. Warn that drug may be habit-forming; instruct to take only for as long as prescribed, in the amounts prescribed, and no more frequently than prescribed. Instruct to contact physician if CV events, GI effects, unexplained weight gain, or edema occurs. Instruct to immediately d/c therapy and contact physician if signs/symptoms of serious skin reactions or hepatotoxicity develop. Instruct to seek immediate medical attention if signs of anaphylactoid reactions develop. Instruct to report any signs of blurred vision or other eye symptoms. Instruct to avoid use in late pregnancy.

Storage: (Vicoprofen) 25°C (77°F); excursions permitted to 15-30°C (59-86°F). (Reprexain) 20-25°C (68-77°F); excursions permitted to 15-30°C (59-86°F).

VICTOZA – liraglutide (rDNA origin) RX

Class: Glucagon-like peptide-1 receptor agonist

Causes dose-dependent and treatment-duration-dependent thyroid C-cell tumors at clinically relevant exposures in animal studies. It is unknown whether drug causes thyroid C-cell tumors (eg, medullary thyroid carcinoma [MTC]) in humans. Contraindicated in patients w/ a personal or family history of MTC and in patients w/ multiple endocrine neoplasia syndrome type 2 (MEN 2). Counsel patients regarding potential risk for MTC and symptoms of thyroid tumors (eg, mass in the neck, dysphagia, dyspnea, persistent hoarseness). Routine monitoring of serum calcitonin or using thyroid ultrasound is of uncertain value for early detection of MTC.

ADULT DOSAGE

Type 2 Diabetes Mellitus

Initial: 0.6mg SQ qd for 1 week
Titrate: Increase to 1.2mg qd after 1 week; if acceptable glycemic control is not achieved, increase to 1.8mg qd

PEDIATRIC DOSAGE

Pediatric use may not have been established

Missed Dose

If a dose is missed, the once-daily regimen should be resumed w/ the next scheduled dose; if >3 days have elapsed since the last dose, reinitiate at 0.6mg, and titrate ud

DOSE MODIFICATION

Concomitant Medications

Consider reducing dose of concomitant insulin secretagogue or insulin

ADMINISTRATION

SQ route

May be administered qd at any time of the day, independently of meals
Inject into abdomen, thigh, or upper arm
Inj site and timing can be changed w/o dose adjustment

Coadministration w/ Insulin

Administer as separate inj; never mix
May inject in the same body region but the inj should not be adjacent to each other

HOW SUPPLIED

Inj: 6mg/mL [3mL]

CONTRAINDICATIONS

MEN 2, personal or family history of MTC.

WARNINGS/PRECAUTIONS

Not recommended as 1st-line therapy for patients who have inadequate glycemic control on diet and exercise. Not a substitute for insulin; do not use in type 1 DM or for the treatment of diabetic ketoacidosis. Further evaluate patients w/ serum calcitonin elevation or thyroid nodules. Acute pancreatitis, including fatal and nonfatal hemorrhagic or necrotizing pancreatitis, reported; observe for signs/symptoms of pancreatitis after initiation of therapy, d/c promptly if suspected, and do not restart therapy if confirmed. Consider other antidiabetic therapies in patients w/ a history of pancreatitis. Do not share pens between patients, even if the needle is changed; poses a risk for transmission of blood-borne pathogens. Acute renal failure and worsening of chronic renal failure reported; caution when initiating/escalating doses in patients w/ renal impairment. Serious hypersensitivity reactions (eg, anaphylactic reactions, angioedema) reported; d/c if a hypersensitivity reaction occurs. Caution w/ hepatic impairment.

ADVERSE REACTIONS

N/V, diarrhea, constipation, dyspepsia, headache, antibody formation.

DRUG INTERACTIONS

See Dose Modification. Increased risk of hypoglycemia w/ insulin secretagogues (eg, sulfonylureas) or insulin. May affect the absorption of oral medications; use w/ caution.

NURSING CONSIDERATIONS

Assessment: Assess for previous hypersensitivity reactions, MEN 2, personal or family history of MTC, history of pancreatitis, type of DM, diabetic ketoacidosis, renal/hepatic impairment, pregnancy/nursing status, and possible drug interactions.

Monitoring: Monitor for signs and symptoms of thyroid tumor, pancreatitis, serum calcitonin elevation, hypoglycemia, hypersensitivity reactions, and other adverse reactions. Monitor renal function, blood glucose levels, and HbA1c levels.

Patient Counseling: Counsel regarding potential risk of MTC and advise to report symptoms of thyroid tumors (eg, lump in the neck, hoarseness) to physician. Inform of the potential risk of dehydration due to GI adverse reactions and instruct to take precautions to avoid fluid depletion. Inform of the potential risk for pancreatitis and worsening renal function. Instruct to d/c therapy promptly and contact physician if persistent severe abdominal pain and/or symptoms of hypersensitivity reactions occur. Advise not to share pen w/ another person, even if the needle is changed. Counsel on potential risks/benefits of therapy and of alternative modes of therapy, importance of adhering to dietary instructions, regular physical activity, periodic blood glucose monitoring and HbA1c testing, recognition/management of hypo/hyperglycemia, and assessment for diabetes complications. Advise to seek medical advice during periods of stress (eg, fever, trauma, infection), if any unusual symptom develops, or if any known symptom persists or worsens. Instruct not to take an extra dose to make up for a missed dose and to resume as prescribed w/ the next scheduled dose.

Storage: Prior to 1st Use: 2-8°C (36-46°F). Do not freeze and do not use if it has been frozen. After Initial Use: 15-30°C (59-86°F) or 2-8°C (36-46°F) for 30 days. Keep the pen cap on when not in use. Always remove and safely discard the needle after each inj; store pen w/o an inj needle attached. Protect from excessive heat and sunlight.

VIEKIRA PAK – dasabuvir; ombitasvir/paritaprevir/ritonavir RX

Class: CYP3A inhibitor/HCV NS5A inhibitor/HCV non-nucleoside NS5B palm polymerase inhibitor/HCV NS3/4A protease inhibitor

ADULT DOSAGE

Chronic Hepatitis C (Genotype 1)

Usual: 2 tabs (ombitasvir, paritaprevir, ritonavir [RTV]) qd (am) and 1 dasabuvir tab bid (am and pm)

Coadministration w/ RBV:
<75kg: 1000mg/day RBV divided and administered bid w/ food
≥75kg: 1200mg/day RBV divided and administered bid w/ food

Genotype 1a, w/o Cirrhosis:
2 tabs (ombitasvir, paritaprevir, RTV) qd (am) + 1 dasabuvir tab bid + RBV for 12 weeks

Genotype 1a, w/ Cirrhosis:
2 tabs (ombitasvir, paritaprevir, RTV) qd (am) + 1 dasabuvir tab bid + RBV for 24 weeks. 12 week treatment duration may be considered for some patients based on prior treatment history

Genotype 1b, w/o Cirrhosis:
2 tabs (ombitasvir, paritaprevir, RTV) qd (am) and 1 tab (dasabuvir) bid for 12 weeks

Genotype 1b, w/ Cirrhosis:
2 tabs (ombitasvir, paritaprevir, RTV) qd (am) + 1 dasabuvir tab bid + RBV for 12 weeks

Follow the genotype 1a dosing recommendations in patients w/ an unknown genotype 1 subtype or w/ mixed genotype 1 infection

Liver Transplant Recipients w/ Normal Hepatic Function and Mild Fibrosis (Metavir Fibrosis Score ≤2) (Irrespective of HCV Genotype 1 Subtype):
2 tabs (ombitasvir, paritaprevir, RTV) qd (am) and 1 tab (dasabuvir) bid + RBV for 24 weeks. If calcineurin inhibitor used concomitantly, calcineurin inhibitor dosage adjustment is needed

PEDIATRIC DOSAGE

Pediatric use may not have been established

DOSE MODIFICATION

<u>**Hepatic Impairment**</u>

Moderate (Child-Pugh B): Not recommended

ADMINISTRATION

Oral route

Take ombitasvir, paritaprevir, ritonavir tab, and dasabuvir tab w/ a meal w/o regard to fat or calorie content

HOW SUPPLIED

Tab: (Ombitasvir-Paritaprevir-RTV) 12.5mg-75mg-50mg, (Dasabuvir) 250mg

CONTRAINDICATIONS

Severe hepatic impairment. Coadministration w/ drugs that are highly dependent on CYP3A for clearance and for which elevated plasma concentrations are associated w/ serious and/or life-threatening events; coadministration w/ strong inducers of CYP3A and CYP2C8 that may lead to reduced efficacy of therapy; and coadministration w/ strong inhibitors of CYP2C8 that may increase dasabuvir plasma concentrations and the risk of QT prolongation. Coadministration w/ alfuzosin, carbamazepine, phenytoin, phenobarbital, gemfibrozil, rifampin, ergotamine, dihydroergotamine, ergonovine, methylergonovine, ethinyl estradiol containing medications (eg, combined oral contraceptives), St. John's wort, lovastatin, simvastatin, pimozide, efavirenz, sildenafil (when used to treat pulmonary arterial HTN), triazolam, or oral midazolam. When used w/ ribavirin, contraindications to ribavirin also apply to this combination regimen; refer to ribavirin PI.

WARNINGS/PRECAUTIONS

Not recommended for use w/ decompensated liver disease. Elevations of ALT to >5X ULN reported. Perform hepatic lab testing during the first 4 weeks of starting treatment and as clinically indicated thereafter. If ALT is found to be elevated above baseline levels, repeat and monitor closely. Consider discontinuing if ALT levels remain persistently >10X ULN. D/C if ALT elevation is accompanied by signs or symptoms of liver inflammation or increasing conjugated bilirubin, alkaline phosphatase, or INR. If coadministered w/ ribavirin, the warnings and precautions for ribavirin, in particular the pregnancy avoidance warning, apply to this combination regimen; refer to ribavirin PI for a full list of warnings/precautions for ribavirin. Any HCV/HIV-1 coinfected patients being treated should also be on a suppressive antiretroviral drug regimen to reduce the risk of HIV-1 protease inhibitor drug resistance.

ADVERSE REACTIONS

Fatigue, nausea, pruritus, skin reactions, insomnia, asthenia.

DRUG INTERACTIONS

See Contraindications. Not recommended w/ darunavir/RTV, lopinavir/RTV, rilpivirine (qd dosing), and salmeterol. Not recommended w/ voriconazole unless an assessment of the benefit-to-risk ratio justifies the use of voriconazole. Caution and therapeutic monitoring is recommended w/ antiarrhythmics. May increase levels of drugs that are substrates of CYP3A, UGT1A1, breast cancer resistance protein (BCRP), OATP1B1, or OATP1B3. May increase levels of antiarrhythmics, ketoconazole, amlodipine, inhaled/nasal fluticasone, furosemide (C_{max}), rilpivirine, rosuvastatin, pravastatin, cyclosporine, tacrolimus, salmeterol, buprenorphine, norbuprenorphine, and alprazolam. May decrease levels of voriconazole, darunavir (C_{trough}), and omeprazole. Inhibition of P-gp, BCRP, OATP1B1, or OATP1B3 may increase levels of the various components of Viekira Pak. ALT elevation reported more frequently w/ ethinyl estradiol-containing medications (eg, combined oral contraceptives, contraceptive patches, contraceptive vaginal rings); alternative methods of contraception (eg, progestin only contraception, nonhormonal methods) are recommended during therapy; ethinyl estradiol-containing medications can be restarted approx 2 weeks following completion of treatment. Paritaprevir: Atazanavir/RTV (qd dosing), and lopinavir/RTV may increase levels. Paritaprevir/RTV: Strong CYP3A inhibitors may increase levels. Dasabuvir: CYP2C8 inhibitors may increase levels. Refer to PI for further information on drug interactions, including dosing modifications when used w/ certain concomitant therapies.

NURSING CONSIDERATIONS

Assessment: Assess for drug hypersensitivity, decompensated liver disease, hepatic impairment, pregnancy/nursing status, and possible drug interactions.

Monitoring: Monitor for ALT elevation and other adverse reactions. Perform hepatic lab testing during the first 4 weeks of starting treatment and as clinically indicated thereafter. If ALT, is found to be elevated above baseline levels, repeat and monitor closely.

Patient Counseling: Inform to watch for early warning signs of liver inflammation (eg, fatigue, lack of appetite, N/V); instruct to contact physician w/o delay if such symptoms occur. Advise to avoid pregnancy during treatment w/ ribavirin; instruct to notify physician immediately in the event of a pregnancy and inform pregnant patients that there is an Antiretroviral Pregnancy Registry that monitors pregnancy outcomes in women who are HCV/HIV-2 coinfected and taking concomitant antiretrovirals. Inform that therapy may interact w/ some drugs; advise to report to physician the use of any prescription, nonprescription medication or herbal products. Inform that contraceptives containing ethinyl estradiol are contraindicated w/ therapy. Inform that the effect of treatment of HCV infection on transmission is not known, and that appropriate precautions to prevent transmission of the HCV during treatment should be taken. Inform that in case a dose of ombitasvir, paritaprevir, RTV is missed, the prescribed dose can be taken w/in 12 hrs and if dasabuvir dose is missed, the prescribed dose can be taken w/in 6 hrs. Instruct that the missed dose should not be taken if >12 hrs has passed since ombitasvir, paritaprevir, RTV is usually taken or if >6 hrs has passed since dasabuvir is usually taken; inform patient to take the next dose as per the usual dosing schedule. Instruct not to take more than prescribed dose of therapy to make up for a missed dose.

Storage: ≤30°C (86°F).

VIGAMOX — moxifloxacin hydrochloride

RX

Class: Fluoroquinolone

ADULT DOSAGE

Bacterial Conjunctivitis

1 drop in the affected eye tid for 7 days

PEDIATRIC DOSAGE

Bacterial Conjunctivitis

≥1 Year:

1 drop in the affected eye tid for 7 days

ADMINISTRATION
Ocular route

HOW SUPPLIED
Sol: 0.5% [3mL]

WARNINGS/PRECAUTIONS
Not for inj. Do not inject subconjunctivally or introduce directly into the anterior chamber of the eye. Fatal hypersensitivity reactions reported with systemic quinolone therapy. May result in bacterial resistance with prolonged use; take appropriate measures if superinfection develops. Avoid contact lenses when signs and symptoms of bacterial conjunctivitis are present.

ADVERSE REACTIONS
Conjunctivitis, decreased visual acuity, dry eye, keratitis, ocular discomfort/hyperemia, ocular pain/pruritus, subconjunctival hemorrhage, tearing.

NURSING CONSIDERATIONS

Assessment: Assess for proper diagnosis of causative organisms (eg, slit-lamp biomicroscopy, fluorescein staining). Assess for hypersensitivity to other quinolones, and pregnancy/nursing status.

Monitoring: Monitor for signs/symptoms of hypersensitivity or anaphylactic reactions and other adverse reactions. With prolonged therapy, monitor for overgrowth of nonsusceptible organisms (eg, fungi) and for development of superinfection.

Patient Counseling: Instruct not to touch the dropper tip to any surface to avoid contaminating the contents. Instruct to immediately d/c medication and contact physician at the 1st sign of rash or allergic reaction. Instruct not to wear contact lenses if signs and symptoms of bacterial conjunctivitis develop.

Storage: 2-25°C (36-77°F).

VIIBRYD — vilazodone hydrochloride RX

Class: Selective serotonin reuptake inhibitor/5-HT_{1A}-receptor partial agonist

Antidepressants increased the risk of suicidal thoughts and behaviors in patients aged ≤24 yrs in short-term studies. Monitor closely for clinical worsening and for emergence of suicidal thoughts and behaviors.

ADULT DOSAGE

Major Depressive Disorder

Initial: 10mg qd for 7 days
Titrate: Increase to 20mg qd
May increase up to 40mg qd after a minimum of 7 days between dosage increases
Target Dose: 20-40mg qd

Dosing Considerations with MAOIs

Switching to/from an MAOI Antidepressant:
Allow at least 14 days between discontinuation of an MAOI antidepressant and initiation of treatment, and allow at least 14 days after stopping treatment before starting an MAOI antidepressant

PEDIATRIC DOSAGE

Pediatric use may not have been established

DOSE MODIFICATION

Elderly
Start at lower end of dosing range

Concomitant Medications
Strong CYP3A4 Inhibitors (eg, Itraconazole, Clarithromycin, Voriconazole):
Max: 20mg qd; may resume original vilazodone dose level when CYP3A4 inhibitor is discontinued

Strong CYP3A4 Inducers (eg, Carbamazepine, Phenytoin, Rifampin) for >14 Days: Consider increasing vilazodone dose by 2-fold, up to a max of 80mg qd, over 1-2 weeks based on clinical response; gradually reduce vilazodone dosage to its original level over 1-2 weeks if CYP3A4 inducers are discontinued

Discontinuation
Gradually reduce dose whenever possible
Taper down from 40mg qd dose to 20mg qd for 4 days, followed by 10mg qd for 3 days
Taper dose to 10mg qd for 7 days in patients taking 20mg qd

ADMINISTRATION
Oral route

Take w/ food

HOW SUPPLIED
Tab: 10mg, 20mg, 40mg

CONTRAINDICATIONS
Concomitant use of MAOIs, or w/in 14 days of stopping MAOIs (eg, linezolid, IV methylene blue).

WARNINGS/PRECAUTIONS
Serotonin syndrome reported; d/c immediately if symptoms occur and initiate supportive symptomatic treatment. May increase the risk of bleeding events. May precipitate mixed/manic episode in patients w/ bipolar disorder. Avoid abrupt discontinuation. Caution w/ seizure disorder. Pupillary dilation that occurs following use may trigger an angle closure attack in a patient w/ anatomically narrow angles who does not have a patent iridectomy; avoid use in patients w/ untreated anatomically narrow angles. Hyponatremia may occur in association w/ the syndrome of inappropriate antidiuretic hormone secretion; d/c and institute appropriate medical intervention in patients w/ symptomatic hyponatremia. Elderly patients, patients taking diuretics, and those who are volume-depleted may be at greater risk of developing hyponatremia.

ADVERSE REACTIONS
Diarrhea, N/V, headache, dizziness, dry mouth, insomnia, abdominal pain, decreased libido, fatigue, flatulence, somnolence, restlessness.

DRUG INTERACTIONS
See Dose Modification and Contraindications. May cause serotonin syndrome w/ other serotonergic drugs (eg, triptans, TCAs, St. John's wort) and w/ drugs that impair metabolism of serotonin; d/c treatment and any concomitant serotonergic agents immediately if this occurs. Increased risk of bleeding w/ aspirin (ASA), NSAIDs, other antiplatelet drugs, warfarin, and other anticoagulants. Monitor coagulation indices (eg, INR) w/ warfarin when initiating/titrating/discontinuing treatment. Strong CYP3A4 inhibitors may increase exposure. Strong CYP3A4 inducers may decrease exposure. May increase digoxin concentrations; measure digoxin concentrations before initiating concomitant use of vilazodone and continue monitoring and reduce digoxin dose as necessary.

NURSING CONSIDERATIONS

Assessment: Assess for personal/family history of bipolar disorder, mania/hypomania, seizure disorder, untreated anatomically narrow angles, volume depletion, pregnancy/nursing status, and possible drug interactions.

Monitoring: Monitor for clinical worsening and emergence of suicidal thoughts and behaviors (especially during the initial few months of therapy and at times of dosage changes). Monitor for serotonin syndrome, angle-closure glaucoma, bleeding, activation of mania/hypomania, hyponatremia, discontinuation symptoms, and other adverse reactions.

Patient Counseling: Advise patients and caregivers to monitor for clinical worsening and to look for the emergence of suicidality, especially early during treatment and when the dose is adjusted up or down; instruct to report such symptoms to physician. Instruct to take ud. Caution about the risk of serotonin syndrome; instruct to contact physician or report to the emergency room if they experience signs/symptoms of serotonin syndrome. Inform about the increased risk of bleeding w/ ASA, NSAIDs, other antiplatelet drugs, warfarin, or other anticoagulants; advise to inform physician if taking/planning to take any prescription or OTC medications that increase the risk of bleeding. Advise patients and caregivers to observe for signs of activation of mania/hypomania; instruct to report such symptoms to physician. Advise not to abruptly d/c therapy and to discuss any tapering regimen w/ physician. Caution about using the medication if they have a history of seizure disorder. Advise to notify physician if an allergic reaction develops. Advise to inform physician if taking or planning to take any prescription or OTC medications, since there is a potential for interactions.

Storage: 25°C (77°F); excursions permitted to 15-30°C (59-86°F).

VIMOVO – esomeprazole magnesium/naproxen RX

Class: NSAID/proton pump inhibitor

NSAIDs may increase risk of serious cardiovascular (CV) thrombotic events, MI, and stroke; increased risk with duration of use and with cardiovascular disease (CVD) or risk factors for CVD. Contraindicated for the treatment of perioperative pain in the setting of CABG surgery. Increased risk of serious GI adverse events (eg, bleeding, ulceration, stomach/intestinal perforation) that can be fatal and occur anytime during use without warning symptoms; elderly patients are at greater risk.

ADULT DOSAGE

Osteoarthritis

1 tab (375mg-20mg or 500mg-20mg) bid

May also be used to decrease the risk of developing NSAID-associated gastric ulcers

PEDIATRIC DOSAGE

Pediatric use may not have been established

Rheumatoid Arthritis

1 tab (375mg-20mg or 500mg-20mg) bid

May also be used to decrease the risk of developing NSAID-associated gastric ulcers

Ankylosing Spondylitis

1 tab (375mg-20mg or 500mg-20mg) bid

May also be used to decrease the risk of developing NSAID-associated gastric ulcers

DOSE MODIFICATION

Renal Impairment

CrCl <30mL/min: Not recommended

Hepatic Impairment

Mild to Moderate: Closely monitor and consider possible dose reduction based on naproxen component

Severe: Avoid use

Elderly

Use lowest effective dose

ADMINISTRATION

Oral route

Swallow whole w/ liquid; do not split, chew, crush, or dissolve
Take at least 30 min ac

HOW SUPPLIED

Tab, Delayed-Release: (Naproxen-Esomeprazole): 375mg-20mg, 500mg-20mg

CONTRAINDICATIONS

Patients who have experienced asthma, urticaria, or allergic-type reactions after taking aspirin (ASA) or other NSAIDs. Treatment of perioperative pain in the setting of CABG surgery.

WARNINGS/PRECAUTIONS

Use lowest effective dose for the shortest duration possible. Not recommended for initial treatment of acute pain. D/C with active and clinically significant bleeding. Naproxen: May cause HTN or worsen preexisting HTN. Fluid retention and edema reported; caution with HTN, fluid retention, or HF. Caution with history of ulcer disease, GI bleeding, or risk factors for GI bleeding (eg, prolonged NSAID therapy, smoking, poor general health status); d/c if a serious GI event occurs. Caution with history of inflammatory bowel disease (IBD) (ulcerative colitis, Crohn's disease); may exacerbate condition. GI-symptomatic response does not preclude the presence of gastric malignancy. Renal papillary necrosis and other renal injury reported with long-term use. Renal toxicity reported in patients in whom renal prostaglandins have a compensatory role in the maintenance of renal perfusion; increased risk with renal/hepatic impairment, hypovolemia, HF, salt depletion, and in elderly. Not recommended with advanced renal disease or moderate to severe renal impairment; closely monitor renal function if therapy must be initiated. Anaphylactic reactions may occur; avoid with ASA triad. May cause serious skin adverse events (eg, Stevens-Johnson syndrome, toxic epidermal necrolysis); d/c at 1st appearance of skin rash or any sign of hypersensitivity. May cause elevated LFTs or severe hepatic reactions; d/c if liver disease or systemic manifestations occur, or if abnormal LFTs persist/worsen. Caution with chronic alcoholic liver disease and other diseases with decreased/abnormal plasma proteins if high doses are administered; dosage adjustment may be required. Anemia may occur; monitor Hgb/Hct if anemia develops with long-term use. May inhibit platelet aggregation and prolong bleeding time. Caution with asthma and avoid with ASA-sensitive asthma. Avoid use starting at 30 weeks gestation; may cause premature closure of ductus arteriosus. May be associated with a reversible delay in ovulation; not recommended in women who have difficulties conceiving, or undergoing investigation of infertility. Not a substitute for corticosteroids or a treatment for corticosteroid insufficiency. May mask signs of inflammation and fever. Lab test interactions may occur. Esomeprazole: Atrophic gastritis reported with long-term use of omeprazole. Acute interstitial nephritis reported; d/c if this develops. Vitamin B12 deficiency caused by hypo/achlorhydria may occur with long-term use (eg, >3 yrs). May increase risk of *Clostridium difficile*-associated diarrhea (CDAD). May increase risk for osteoporosis-related fractures of the hip, wrist, or spine, especially with high-dose (multiple daily doses) and long-term therapy (≥1 yr). Drug-induced decrease in gastric acidity results in enterochromaffin-like cell hyperplasia and increased chromogranin A (CgA) levels, which may interfere with investigations for neuroendocrine tumors; temporarily d/c treatment at least 14 days before assessing CgA levels and consider repeating test if initial CgA levels are high. Hypomagnesemia reported rarely.

ADVERSE REACTIONS

CV thrombotic events, MI, stroke, GI adverse events, flatulence, diarrhea, nausea, abdominal distension, constipation, dyspepsia, URTI, upper abdominal pain, dizziness, headache.

DRUG INTERACTIONS

May enhance methotrexate (MTX) toxicity; use with caution or consider temporary discontinuation during high-dose MTX administration. Naproxen: Avoid with other naproxen-containing products and other NSAIDs. May be administered with low-dose ASA (≤325mg/day); coadministration with ASA is not generally recommended because of potential of increased adverse effects. Risk of renal toxicity when coadministered with diuretics, ACE inhibitors, or angiotensin II receptor antagonists. Diminished antihypertensive effect of ACE inhibitors, angiotensin II receptor antagonists, and β-blockers (eg, propranolol). Delayed absorption with cholestyramine. Caution with cyclosporine; increased risk of nephrotoxicity. Coadministration may decrease efficacy of thiazides and loop (eg, furosemide) diuretics; monitor for signs of renal failure and diuretic efficacy. May increase lithium levels and reduce renal lithium clearance; monitor for lithium toxicity. Concomitant use with anticoagulants (eg, warfarin, dicumarol, heparin) may result in increased risk of bleeding complications; increased risk of GI bleeding with oral corticosteroids, anticoagulants, antiplatelets (including low-dose ASA), alcohol, and SSRIs; monitor carefully. Potential interaction with albumin-bound drugs (eg, sulfonylureas, sulfonamides, hydantoins). Probenecid increases plasma levels and extends plasma $T_{1/2}$ significantly. Esomeprazole: Concomitant use results in reduced concentrations of the active metabolite of clopidogrel and a reduction in platelet inhibition; avoid concomitant use. Caution with digoxin or other drugs that may cause hypomagnesemia (eg, diuretics). May increase levels of tacrolimus. May reduce absorption of drugs where gastric pH is an important determinant of their bioavailability; ketoconazole, atazanavir, iron salts, erlotinib, and mycophenolate mofetil (MMF) absorption can decrease while digoxin absorption can increase during treatment with omeprazole. Caution in transplant patients receiving MMF. Decreased levels of atazanavir and nelfinavir; coadministration not recommended. Monitor for saquinavir toxicity; consider saquinavir dose reduction. Monitor for increases in INR and PT with warfarin. May inhibit metabolism of CYP2C19 substrates; decreased clearance of diazepam. Exposure may be increased with combined CYP2C19 and 3A4 inhibitor (eg, voriconazole). Increased concentrations of cilostazol; consider dose reduction of cilostazol. Decreased levels with CYP2C19 or 3A4 inducers; avoid with St. John's wort or rifampin.

NURSING CONSIDERATIONS

Assessment: Assess for history of asthma, urticaria, or allergic-type reactions with ASA or other NSAIDs, CVD, risk factors for CVD, HTN, fluid retention, HF, history of ulcer disease, history of/risk factors for GI bleeding, history of IBD, renal/hepatic impairment, coagulation disorders, asthma, decreased/abnormal plasma proteins, tobacco/alcohol use, pregnancy/nursing status, possible drug interactions, or any other conditions where treatment is contraindicated or cautioned. Obtain baseline BP, CBC, and coagulation and chemistry profiles.

Monitoring: Monitor for CV and GI events, active bleeding, anaphylactic reactions, skin reactions, anemia, bone fractures, hypomagnesemia, CDAD, acute interstitial nephritis, vitamin B12 deficiency, and other adverse reactions. Monitor BP, LFTs, renal function, CBC, and coagulation and chemistry profiles. Monitor INR and PT when given with warfarin. Periodically monitor Hgb if initial Hgb ≤10g and receiving long-term therapy. Monitor Mg^{2+} levels prior to and periodically during therapy with prolonged treatment.

Patient Counseling: Instruct to seek medical advice if symptoms of CV events, GI ulceration/bleeding, skin/hypersensitivity reactions, unexplained weight gain or edema, hepatotoxicity, anaphylactic reactions, or hypomagnesemia occur, and for diarrhea that does not improve. Instruct to notify physician if pregnant/nursing, or if patient has a history of asthma or ASA-sensitive asthma. Caution against activities requiring alertness if drowsiness, dizziness, vertigo, or depression occurs.

Storage: 25°C (77°F); excursions permitted to 15-30°C (59-86°F). Protect from moisture.

VIMPAT — lacosamide CV

Class: Sodium channel inactivator

ADULT DOSAGE

Partial Onset Seizures

Monotherapy:
Initial: 100mg bid
Alternative LD: 200mg; follow 12 hrs later by 100mg bid for 1 week
Titrate: Increase by 50mg bid at weekly intervals
Maint: 150-200mg bid

Adjunctive Therapy:
Initial: 50mg bid
Alternative LD: 200mg; follow 12 hrs later by 100mg bid for 1 week

PEDIATRIC DOSAGE

Partial Onset Seizures

≥17 Years:
Monotherapy:
Initial: 100mg bid
Alternative LD: 200mg; follow 12 hrs later by 100mg bid for 1 week
Titrate: Increase by 50mg bid at weekly intervals
Maint: 150-200mg bid

Adjunctive Therapy:
Initial: 50mg bid
Alternative LD: 200mg; follow 12 hrs later by 100mg bid for 1 week

Titrate: Increase by 50mg bid at weekly intervals
Maint: 100-200mg bid
Max Maint: 200mg bid

Use IV when oral administration is temporarily not feasible

Conversions

Convert from Single Antiepileptic to Lacosamide Monotherapy:
Maintain 150-200mg bid for at least 3 days before initiating gradual withdrawal of the concomitant antiepileptic drug over at least 6 weeks

PO to IV Conversion:
Initial total daily IV dosage regimen should equal oral dosage regimen
IV to PO Conversion:
At the end of the IV treatment period, switch to oral lacosamide at the equivalent daily dosage and frequency of IV administration

Titrate: Increase by 50mg bid at weekly intervals
Maint: 100-200mg bid
Max Maint: 200mg bid
Use IV when oral administration is temporarily not feasible

Conversions

Convert from Single Antiepileptic to Lacosamide Monotherapy:
Maintain 150-200mg bid for at least 3 days before initiating gradual withdrawal of the concomitant antiepileptic drug over at least 6 weeks

PO to IV Conversion:
Initial total daily IV dosage regimen should equal oral dosage regimen
IV to PO Conversion:
At the end of the IV treatment period, switch to oral lacosamide at the equivalent daily dosage and frequency of IV administration

DOSE MODIFICATION

Concomitant Medications
Strong CYP3A4 and CYP2C9 Inhibitors w/ Renal/Hepatic Impairment: Dose reduction may be necessary

Renal Impairment
Severe Impairment (CrCl <30mL/min)/ESRD:
Max: 300mg/day
Hemodialysis: Consider dosage supplementation of up to 50% following a 4-hr hemodialysis treatment

Hepatic Impairment
Mild or Moderate Impairment:
Max: 300mg/day
Severe: Not recommended

Discontinuation
Gradually withdraw over at least 1 week

ADMINISTRATION

Oral/IV route

Take w/ or w/o food

Sol
Obtain and use calibrated measuring device

Inj
Infuse over 15-60 min; 30-60 min is preferable when a 15 min administration is not required
May administer IV w/o further dilution or mixed w/ compatible diluents
Diluted sol should not be stored for >4 hrs at room temperature

Compatible IV Diluents
NaCl inj 0.9%
D5 inj
Lactated Ringer's inj

HOW SUPPLIED

Inj: 10mg/mL [20mL]; Sol: 10mg/mL [200mL, 465mL]; Tab: 50mg, 100mg, 150mg, 200mg

WARNINGS/PRECAUTIONS

Administer LD with medical supervision due to increased incidence of CNS adverse reactions. May increase risk of suicidal thoughts or behavior. May cause dizziness and ataxia; may impair physical/mental abilities. Dose-dependent prolongations in PR interval reported. Further PR prolongation is possible when given with other drugs that prolong PR interval. Caution with known conduction problems (eg, atrioventricular block [AV], sick sinus syndrome without pacemaker), Na^+ channelopathies (eg, Brugada syndrome), or with severe cardiac disease (eg, myocardial ischemia, heart failure, structural heart disease); IV infusion may cause bradycardia or AV block. May predispose to atrial arrhythmias, especially in patients with diabetic neuropathy and/or cardiovascular disease (CVD). Syncope or loss of consciousness reported in patients with diabetic neuropathy and those with a history of risk factors for cardiac disease. Withdraw gradually over a minimum of 1 week to minimize potential of increased seizure frequency. Multiorgan hypersensitivity reactions (also known as drug reaction with eosinophilia and systemic symptoms [DRESS]) may occur; d/c and start alternative treatment if suspected. Avoid with severe hepatic impairment. Caution during dose titration in patients with coexisting hepatic/renal impairment and in elderly. (Sol) Contains aspartame, a source of phenylalanine.

ADVERSE REACTIONS

Headache, N/V, diplopia, dizziness, fatigue, blurred vision, somnolence, tremor, nystagmus, vertigo, diarrhea, balance disorder, ataxia, dry mouth, oral hypoesthesia.

DRUG INTERACTIONS

Increased exposure with strong CYP3A4 and CYP2C9 inhibitors in patients with renal or hepatic impairment; dose reduction may be necessary. Caution with medications that prolong PR interval (eg, β-blockers, calcium channel blockers); closely monitor if lacosamide is administered as IV route.

NURSING CONSIDERATIONS

Assessment: Assess for hepatic/renal impairment, history of depression or risk factors for cardiac disease, cardiac conduction problems and/or CVD, diabetic neuropathy, phenylketonuria, pregnancy/nursing status, and possible drug interactions. Obtain baseline ECG in patients with known conduction problems, Na^+ channelopathies, on concomitant medications that prolong PR interval, or with severe cardiac disease.

Monitoring: Monitor for emergence/worsening of depression, suicidal thoughts or behavior and/or any unusual changes in mood or behavior, dizziness, ataxia, PR interval prolongation, syncope or loss of consciousness, DRESS, and other adverse reactions. Obtain an ECG after titration to steady state in patients with known conduction problems, Na^+ channelopathies, on concomitant medications that prolong PR interval, or with severe cardiac disease; closely monitor these patients if administering IV. Closely monitor patients with hepatic/renal impairment during dose titration.

Patient Counseling: Inform of the benefits/risks of therapy. Instruct to take ud. Counsel patients/caregivers/families about increased risk of suicidal thoughts and behavior and of the need to be alert for emergence or worsening of symptoms of depression, any unusual changes in behavior/mood, or the emergence of suicidal thoughts, behavior, or thoughts about self-harm. Instruct to report any behaviors of concern to physician immediately. Inform that dizziness, double vision, abnormal coordination and balance, and somnolence may occur; advise not to engage in hazardous activities (eg, driving/operating complex machinery) until effects of drug are known. Counsel that therapy is associated with ECG changes that may predispose to irregular heartbeat and syncope; if syncope develops, instruct to lay down with raised legs and to contact physician. Instruct to d/c if a serious hypersensitivity reaction is suspected and to promptly report any symptoms of liver toxicity. Advise to notify physician if patient becomes pregnant/intends to become pregnant, or is breastfeeding. Encourage patients to enroll in the North American Antiepileptic Drug Pregnancy Registry if they become pregnant.

Storage: 20-25°C (68-77°F); excursions permitted between 15-30°C (59-86°F). (Inj/Sol) Do not freeze. (Inj) Discard any unused portion. (Sol) Discard any unused portion after 7 weeks of 1st opening bottle.

VIRAMUNE XR – nevirapine RX

Class: Non-nucleoside reverse transcriptase inhibitor

Severe, life-threatening, and in some cases fatal, hepatotoxicity (particularly in the first 18 weeks) and skin reactions (eg, Stevens-Johnson syndrome, toxic epidermal necrolysis, hypersensitivity reactions) reported. Increased risk of hepatotoxicity reported in women and patients with higher $CD4^+$ cell counts, including pregnant women. Hepatic failure reported in patients without HIV taking nevirapine for postexposure prophylaxis (PEP). Use for occupational and non-occupational PEP is contraindicated. D/C therapy and seek medical evaluation immediately if hepatitis, transaminase elevations combined with rash or other systemic symptoms, severe skin rash, or hypersensitivity reactions develop; do not restart therapy. The 14-day lead-in period with 200mg daily dosing must be followed; may decrease the incidence of rash. Monitor intensively during the first 18 weeks of therapy, especially the first 6 weeks.

OTHER BRAND NAMES

Viramune

ADULT DOSAGE

HIV-1 Infection

Combination with Other Antiretrovirals:

Tab (IR):

Initial: 200mg qd for the first 14 days

Maint: 200mg bid

Tab, ER:

Not Currently Taking IR Nevirapine:

Initial: One 200mg IR tab qd for first 14 days

Maint: One 400mg ER tab qd

PEDIATRIC DOSAGE

HIV-1 Infection

Combination with Other Antiretrovirals:

Tab/Oral Sus:

≥15 Days of Age:

Initial: 150mg/m² qd for the first 14 days

Maint: 150mg/m² bid

Max: 400mg/day

Tab, ER:

6-<18 Years:

Switching from IR Tab to ER Tab:
Switch to 400mg ER tab qd without 14-day lead-in period

Initial:
150mg/m^2 IR tab/oral sus qd for first 14 days
Max: 200mg/day
Maint:
BSA 0.58-0.83m^2: Two 100mg ER tabs qd
BSA 0.84-1.16m^2: Three 100mg ER tabs qd
BSA ≥1.17m^2: One 400mg ER tab qd
Max: 400mg/day

DOSE MODIFICATION

Renal Impairment
Requiring Dialysis: Administer additional 200mg IR dose after each dialysis treatment

Hepatic Impairment
Moderate or Severe (Child-Pugh Class B or C): Not recommended for use
Symptomatic Hepatic Event Occurrence: Permanently d/c; do not restart after recovery

Adverse Reactions
Severe Rash/Rash Accompanied by Constitutional Findings: D/C
Mild to Mod Rash Without Constitutional Symptoms During Lead-In Period: Do not initiate XR therapy until rash has resolved; duration of lead-in period should not exceed 28 days, at which point an alternative regimen should be sought

Other Important Modifications
Dose Interruption for >7 Days: Restart using lead-in dosing

ADMINISTRATION

Oral route

Take with or without food

Tab, ER
Swallow whole; do not chew, crush, or divide

Oral Sus
Shake gently prior to administration
Administer the entire measured dose by using an oral dosing syringe or dosing cup

HOW SUPPLIED

[Immediate-Release (IR)] Sus: 50mg/5mL [240mL], Tab: 200mg*; Tab, Extended-Release (ER): 100mg, 400mg *scored

CONTRAINDICATIONS

Moderate or severe (Child-Pugh Class B or C) hepatic impairment. Use as part of occupational and non-occupational PEP regimens.

WARNINGS/PRECAUTIONS

Not recommended for adult females with CD4$^+$ cell counts >250 cells/mm^3 or in adult males with CD4$^+$ cell counts >400 cells/mm^3. Coinfection with hepatitis B or C and/or increased transaminase elevations at the start of therapy may increase risk of later symptomatic events (≥6 weeks after starting therapy) and asymptomatic increases in AST/ALT. Caution with hepatic fibrosis/cirrhosis; monitor for drug-induced toxicity. Rhabdomyolysis reported in some patients with skin and/or liver reactions. Monitor closely if isolated rash of any severity occurs; delay in stopping treatment after the onset of rash may result in a more serious reaction. Do not use as single agent to treat HIV-1 or add on as a sole agent to a failing regimen; resistant virus emerges rapidly when administered as monotherapy. Consider potential for cross-resistance in the choice of new antiretroviral agents to be used in combination with therapy. Take into account the half-lives of the combination antiretroviral drugs when discontinuing the regimen; nevirapine has a long half-life and resistance may develop if antiretrovirals with shorter half-lives are stopped concurrently. Immune reconstitution syndrome, autoimmune disorders (eg, Graves' disease, polymyositis, Guillain-Barre syndrome) in the setting of immune reconstitution, and redistribution/accumulation of body fat reported. Caution in elderly.

ADVERSE REACTIONS

Hepatotoxicity, skin reactions, diarrhea, nausea, headache, fatigue, abdominal pain.

DRUG INTERACTIONS

Avoid with atazanavir, boceprevir, telaprevir, ketoconazole, itraconazole, and rifampin. Not recommended with fosamprenavir (without ritonavir), efavirenz, and St. John's wort or St. John's wort-containing products. May alter levels of other non-nucleoside reverse transcriptase inhibitor (NNRTI) (eg, delavirdine, etravirine, rilpivirine); avoid coadministration. Increased incidence and severity of rash with prednisone during the first 6 weeks of therapy; not recommended to prevent nevirapine-associated rash. May increase levels of 14-OH clarithromycin and rifabutin. May increase levels of antithrombotics (eg, warfarin); monitor anticoagulation levels. May decrease levels of CYP3A/2B6 substrates, clarithromycin, ethinyl estradiol, norethindrone, efavirenz, atazanavir, amprenavir, indinavir, lopinavir, methadone, nelfinavir, boceprevir, telaprevir, antiarrhythmics, anticonvulsants, ketoconazole, itraconazole, calcium channel blockers, cancer chemotherapy, ergot alkaloids, immunosuppressants, motility agents, and opiate agonists. Fluconazole may increase levels and rifampin may decrease levels. Refer to PI for further information when used with certain concomitant therapies.

NURSING CONSIDERATIONS

Assessment: Assess for hepatic fibrosis/cirrhosis, hepatitis B or C coinfection, pregnancy/nursing status, and possible drug interactions. Obtain baseline LFTs. (ER) Assess the ability to swallow tabs in pediatric patients.

Monitoring: Monitor for hepatotoxicity, skin or hypersensitivity reactions, immune reconstitution syndrome, autoimmune disorders, fat redistribution/accumulation, rhabdomyolysis, and other adverse reactions. Perform intensive clinical and lab monitoring, including LFTs, during the first 18 weeks of therapy and frequently throughout treatment. Measure serum transaminases immediately if signs/symptoms of hepatitis, hypersensitivity reactions, and rash develop. Monitor anticoagulation levels with antithrombotics (eg, warfarin).

Patient Counseling: Inform about the risks and benefits of therapy. Inform that severe liver disease/ skin reactions may occur. Counsel about signs/symptoms of hepatotoxicity, skin reactions, and other adverse reactions, and advise to d/c and seek medical evaluation immediately if any occur. Inform to take drug as prescribed. Instruct not to alter the dose without consulting physician. Inform that therapy is not a cure for HIV-1 infection and that illnesses associated with HIV-1 infection, including opportunistic infections, may still occur. Advise to avoid doing things that can spread HIV-1 infection to others (eg, sharing needles or other inj equipment, sharing personal items that can have blood or body fluids on them [toothbrush, razor blades], breastfeeding). Instruct not to have any kind of sex without protection; inform to always practice safe sex by using a latex or polyurethane condom to lower the chance of sexual contact with semen, vaginal secretions, or blood. Advise to notify physician of the use of any other prescription/OTC medication, or herbal products, particularly St. John's wort. Inform women taking therapy that hormonal methods of birth control should not be used as the sole method of contraception. Inform that fat redistribution may occur. Instruct not to take IR tabs/sus and ER tabs at the same time. (ER) Advise that soft remnants of the drug may be seen in stool.

Storage: 25°C (77°F); excursions permitted to 15-30°C (59-86°F).

VIREAD — tenofovir disoproxil fumarate RX

Class: Nucleotide analogue reverse transcriptase inhibitor

Lactic acidosis and severe hepatomegaly with steatosis, including fatal cases, reported with the use of nucleoside analogues in combination with other antiretrovirals. Severe acute exacerbations of hepatitis reported in hepatitis B virus (HBV)-infected patients who have discontinued therapy; closely monitor hepatic function with both clinical and lab follow-up for at least several months. If appropriate, resumption of antihepatitis B therapy may be warranted.

ADULT DOSAGE

HIV-1 Infection

Combination w/ Other Antiretrovirals:
Tab: 300mg qd
Oral Powder: 7.5 scoops qd

Chronic Hepatitis B

Tab: 300mg qd
Oral Powder: 7.5 scoops qd

PEDIATRIC DOSAGE

HIV-1 Infection

Combination w/ Other Antiretrovirals:
≥2 Years:
8mg/kg qd as oral powder or tabs
Max: 300mg qd

Chronic Hepatitis B

≥12 Years:
Tab: 300mg qd
Oral Powder: 7.5 scoops qd

DOSE MODIFICATION

Renal Impairment

CrCl 30-49mL/min: 300mg q48h
CrCl 10-29mL/min: 300mg q72-96h
Hemodialysis: 300mg every 7 days or after a total of about 12 hrs of dialysis; administer following completion of dialysis

ADMINISTRATION

Oral route

Take tabs w/o regard to food

Oral Powder

Measure only w/ the supplied dosing scoop
One level scoop contains 40mg of tenofovir disoproxil fumarate

Mix w/ 2-4 oz of soft food not requiring chewing (eg, applesauce, baby food, yogurt) and administer entire mixture immediately
Do not administer in a liquid

HOW SUPPLIED

Powder: 40mg/g [60g]; Tab: 150mg, 200mg, 250mg, 300mg

WARNINGS/PRECAUTIONS

Obesity and prolonged nucleoside exposure may be risk factors for lactic acidosis and severe hepatomegaly with steatosis. Caution with known risk factors for liver disease. D/C if findings suggestive of lactic acidosis or pronounced hepatotoxicity develop. Renal impairment (eg, acute renal failure, Fanconi syndrome) reported; assess CrCl prior to initiating and as clinically appropriate during therapy. In patients at risk of renal dysfunction, including patients who have previously experienced renal events while receiving adefovir dipivoxil, assess CrCl, serum phosphorus (P), urine glucose, and urine protein prior to initiation and periodically during therapy. Use only in HIV-1 and HBV coinfected patients as part of an appropriate antiretroviral combination regimen. Before initiating therapy, offer HIV-1 antibody testing to all HBV-infected patients and test all patients with HIV-1 for presence of chronic hepatitis B. Decreased bone mineral density (BMD) and increased biochemical markers of bone metabolism reported; consider assessment of BMD for patients with history of pathologic bone fracture or other risk factors for osteoporosis or bone loss. Osteomalacia associated with proximal renal tubulopathy reported; consider hypophosphatemia and osteomalacia secondary to proximal renal tubulopathy in patients at risk of renal dysfunction who present with persistent or worsening bone or muscle symptoms. Redistribution/accumulation of body fat and immune reconstitution syndrome reported. Autoimmune disorders (eg, Graves' disease, polymyositis, Guillain-Barre syndrome) reported in the setting of immune reconstitution and can occur many months after initiation of treatment. Early virological failure and high rates of resistance substitutions reported with certain regimens that only contain 3 nucleoside reverse transcriptase inhibitors; use triple nucleoside regimens with caution. Caution in elderly.

ADVERSE REACTIONS

Lactic acidosis, hepatomegaly with steatosis, N/V, diarrhea, depression, asthenia, headache, pain, rash, abdominal pain, insomnia, pruritus, dizziness, pyrexia.

DRUG INTERACTIONS

Avoid with concurrent or recent use of nephrotoxic agents (eg, high-dose or multiple NSAIDs). Do not coadminister with tenofovir disoproxil fumarate (TDF)-containing products or with adefovir dipivoxil. May increase levels of didanosine; d/c didanosine if didanosine-associated adverse reactions develop. Decreases levels of atazanavir; do not coadminister with atazanavir without ritonavir. Lopinavir/ritonavir, atazanavir with ritonavir, and darunavir with ritonavir may increase levels; d/c treatment if TDF-associated adverse reactions develop. P-glycoprotein and breast cancer resistance protein transporter inhibitors may increase absorption. Coadministration with drugs that reduce renal function or compete for active tubular secretion (eg, cidofovir, acyclovir, valacyclovir, ganciclovir, valganciclovir, aminoglycosides [eg, gentamicin], high-dose or multiple NSAIDs) may increase levels of tenofovir and/or the levels of other renally eliminated drugs. Refer to PI for dosing modifications when used with certain concomitant therapies.

NURSING CONSIDERATIONS

Assessment: Assess for risk factors for lactic acidosis or liver disease, renal dysfunction, pregnancy/nursing status, and possible drug interactions. In patients at risk of renal dysfunction, assess CrCl, serum P, urine glucose, and urine protein. Test for HIV-1 antibody (in HBV-infected patients) and presence of chronic hepatitis B (in patients with HIV-1). Assess BMD in patients with history of pathologic bone fracture or other risk factors for osteoporosis or bone loss.

Monitoring: Monitor for signs/symptoms of lactic acidosis, hepatomegaly with steatosis, hepatotoxicity, renal impairment, bone effects, redistribution/accumulation of body fat, immune reconstitution syndrome (eg, opportunistic infections), autoimmune disorders, and other adverse reactions. Closely monitor hepatic function with both clinical and lab follow-up for at least several months in HBV-infected patients who have discontinued therapy. In patients at risk of renal dysfunction, monitor CrCl, serum P, urine glucose, and urine protein periodically. Periodically monitor weight in pediatric patients to guide dose adjustment.

Patient Counseling: Inform about risks and benefits of therapy. Inform that therapy is not a cure for HIV-1 and patients may continue to experience illness associated with HIV-1 infection (eg, opportunistic infections). Instruct to avoid doing things that can spread HIV or HBV to others (eg, sharing of needles/inj equipment or personal items that can have blood/body fluids on them). Advise to always practice safer sex by using latex or polyurethane condoms. Instruct not to breastfeed. Instruct not to d/c without 1st informing physician. Counsel about the importance of adhering to regular dosing schedule and to avoid missing doses.

Storage: 25°C (77°F); excursions permitted to 15-30°C (59-86°F).

VITEKTA – elvitegravir

RX

Class: HIV-integrase strand transfer inhibitor

ADULT DOSAGE

HIV-1 Infection

In combination w/ an HIV protease inhibitor coadministered w/ ritonavir and other antiretroviral drug(s) in treatment-experienced patients

85mg Dose:

85mg qd + atazanavir 300mg qd + ritonavir 100mg qd

or

85mg qd + lopinavir 400mg bid + ritonavir 100mg bid

150mg Dose:

150mg qd + darunavir 600mg bid + ritonavir 100mg bid

or

150mg qd + fosamprenavir 700mg bid + ritonavir 100mg bid

or

150mg qd + tipranavir 500mg bid + ritonavir 200mg bid

PEDIATRIC DOSAGE

Pediatric use may not have been established

DOSE MODIFICATION

Hepatic Impairment

Severe: Not recommended for use

ADMINISTRATION

Oral route

Take w/ food

HOW SUPPLIED

Tab: 85mg, 150mg

CONTRAINDICATIONS

Refer to the individual monographs for coadministered protease inhibitor and ritonavir.

WARNINGS/PRECAUTIONS

Not recommended for use in patients with severe hepatic impairment. Immune reconstitution syndrome reported. Autoimmune disorders (eg, Graves' disease, polymyositis, Guillain-Barre syndrome) reported in the setting of immune reconstitution and can occur many months after initiation of treatment. Caution in elderly.

ADVERSE REACTIONS

Diarrhea, nausea, headache, hyperbilirubinemia, hematuria, increased serum amylase/creatine kinase/GGT, hypercholesterolemia, hypertriglyceridemia, hyperglycemia, glucosuria, neutropenia.

DRUG INTERACTIONS

Coadministration with HIV-1 protease inhibitors other than ritonavir, atazanavir, lopinavir, darunavir, fosamprenavir, and tipranavir is not recommended. Use with elvitegravir-containing drugs (eg, Stribild) is not recommended. Use in combination with a protease inhibitor and cobicistat is not recommended; may result in suboptimal levels of elvitegravir and/or the protease inhibitor, leading to loss of therapeutic effect and development of resistance. Coadministration with efavirenz, nevirapine, St. John's wort, rifampin, or rifapentine is not recommended; may decrease levels, resulting in loss of therapeutic effect and development of resistance. Coadministration with boceprevir or telaprevir is not recommended; may reduce levels of boceprevir or telaprevir and may alter levels of HIV protease inhibitors, resulting in loss of therapeutic effect and development of resistance. CYP3A inducers may increase the clearance of elvitegravir, as well as ritonavir (RTV). Significantly increases levels with atazanavir/RTV or lopinavir/RTV. Give didanosine at least 1 hr before or 2 hrs after administration. Antacids may lower levels; separate administration by at least 2 hrs. Ketoconazole may increase levels. Coadministration with phenobarbital, phenytoin, carbamazepine, oxcarbazepine, or systemic dexamethasone may decrease levels, which may result in loss of therapeutic effect and in development of resistance; consider alternative anticonvulsants or corticosteroids. Rifabutin or bosentan may decrease levels. May increase levels of ketoconazole, bosentan, rifabutin, or 25-O-desacetylrifabutin. May increase norgestimate and decrease ethinyl estradiol levels; alternative methods of nonhormonal contraception are recommended. Refer to PI for further information on drug interactions, including dose modifications required when used with certain concomitant therapies.

NURSING CONSIDERATIONS

Assessment: Assess for severe hepatic impairment, pregnancy/nursing status, and for possible drug interactions.

Monitoring: Monitor for signs/symptoms of immune reconstitution syndrome, autoimmune disorders, and for other adverse reactions.

Patient Counseling: Advise patients to remain under the care of a healthcare provider during therapy. Inform that drug is not a cure for HIV-1 infection and continuous therapy is necessary to control HIV-1 infection and decrease HIV-related illnesses. Advise to continue to practice safer sex, to use latex or polyurethane condoms, and to not reuse/share needles. Instruct to take ud, on a regular dosing schedule with food, and to avoid missing doses. Inform that therapy may interact with many drugs; advise to notify physician if using any other prescription or nonprescription medication, or herbal product (eg, St. John's wort). Advise to inform physician immediately if any symptoms of infection develop.

Storage: <30°C (86°F).

VIVELLE-DOT – estradiol RX

Class: Estrogen

Estrogens increase the risk of endometrial cancer. Adding a progestin to estrogen therapy reduces the risk of endometrial hyperplasia. Adequate diagnostic measures should be undertaken to rule out malignancy with undiagnosed, persistent, or recurring abnormal genital bleeding. Should not be used for the prevention of cardiovascular (CV) disease or dementia. Increased risk of stroke and deep vein thrombosis (DVT) reported in postmenopausal women (50-79 yrs of age) treated with daily oral conjugated estrogens (CE) alone and when combined with medroxyprogesterone acetate (MPA). Increased risk of pulmonary embolism (PE), MI, and invasive breast cancer reported in postmenopausal women (50-79 yrs of age) treated with daily oral CE combined with MPA. Increased risk of developing probable dementia reported in postmenopausal women ≥65 yrs of age treated with daily CE alone and when combined with MPA. Should be prescribed at the lowest effective dose and for the shortest duration consistent with treatment goals and risks.

ADULT DOSAGE

Menopause

Vasomotor Symptoms/Vulvar and Vaginal Atrophy:
Moderate to Severe:
Initial: 0.0375mg/day 2X/week
Titrate: Dose adjustment should be guided by clinical response. Attempts to taper or d/c therapy should be made at 3- to 6-month intervals

Postmenopausal Osteoporosis

Prevention:
Initial: 0.025mg/day 2X/week

Other Indications

Hypoestrogenism due to hypogonadism, castration, or primary ovarian failure

Conversions

Not Currently on Oral Estrogens/Switching from Another Estradiol Transdermal Therapy: May initiate therapy at once
Currently Taking Oral Estrogens: Initiate therapy 1 week after withdrawal of oral hormone therapy, or sooner if menopausal symptoms reappear in <1 week

PEDIATRIC DOSAGE

Pediatric use may not have been established

ADMINISTRATION

Transdermal route

Apply immediately upon removal from the protective pouch
Apply adhesive side of patch to clean, dry area of the trunk of the body (including abdomen/buttocks); area should not be oily, damaged, or irritated
Do not apply patch to the breasts; avoid application to waistline as tight clothing may rub the system off
Rotate application site w/ an interval of at least 1 week between applications to a particular site
Press the system firmly in place w/ palm of hand for about 10 sec, making sure there is good contact, especially around edges

If the patch falls off, the same system may be reapplied; if it cannot be reapplied, a new system should be applied to another location. Continue original treatment schedule
May be given continuously in patients who do not have an intact uterus or cyclically (eg, 3 weeks on drug followed by 1 week off drug) in patients w/ an intact uterus

HOW SUPPLIED

Patch: 0.025mg/day, 0.0375mg/day, 0.05mg/day, 0.075mg/day, 0.1mg/day [8[s]]

CONTRAINDICATIONS

Undiagnosed abnormal genital bleeding, known/suspected/history of breast cancer, known/suspected estrogen-dependent neoplasia, active/history of DVT/PE, active/history of arterial thromboembolic disease (eg, stroke, MI), known liver impairment or disease, known protein C/protein S/antithrombin deficiency or other known thrombophilic disorders, known/suspected pregnancy.

WARNINGS/PRECAUTIONS

D/C immediately if stroke, DVT, PE, or MI occurs or is suspected. If feasible, d/c at least 4-6 weeks before surgery of the type associated with an increased risk of thromboembolism, or during periods of prolonged immobilization. May increase risk of ovarian cancer, and gallbladder disease requiring surgery. May lead to severe hypercalcemia in patients with breast cancer and bone metastases; d/c and take appropriate measures if hypercalcemia occurs. Retinal vascular thrombosis reported; d/c pending exam if sudden partial/complete loss of vision or sudden onset of proptosis, diplopia, or migraine occurs. D/C permanently if exam reveals papilledema or retinal vascular lesions. May elevate BP and thyroid-binding globulin levels. May elevate plasma TGs leading to pancreatitis in patients with preexisting hypertriglyceridemia; consider discontinuation if pancreatitis occurs. Caution with history of cholestatic jaundice associated with past estrogen use or with pregnancy; d/c in case of recurrence. May cause fluid retention. Caution with hypoparathyroidism as estrogen-induced hypocalcemia may occur. Cases of malignant transformation of residual endometrial implants reported in women treated post-hysterectomy with estrogen therapy alone; consider addition of progestin for patients known to have residual endometriosis post-hysterectomy. Anaphylactic/anaphylactoid reactions, and angioedema involving eye/eyelid, face, larynx, pharynx, tongue, and extremity with or without urticaria requiring medical intervention reported; do not reapply in patients who develop angioedema anytime during the course of treatment. May exacerbate symptoms of angioedema in women with hereditary angioedema. May exacerbate asthma, diabetes mellitus, epilepsy, migraine, porphyria, systemic lupus erythematosus, and hepatic hemangiomas; use with caution. May affect certain endocrine and blood components in lab tests.

ADVERSE REACTIONS

Constipation, dyspepsia, nausea, influenza-like illness, pain, nasopharyngitis, sinusitis, URTI, back pain, headache, depression, insomnia, breast tenderness, intermenstrual bleeding, sinus congestion.

DRUG INTERACTIONS

CYP3A4 inducers (eg, St. John's wort, phenobarbital, carbamazepine) may decrease levels and may decrease therapeutic effects and/or change uterine bleeding profile. CYP3A4 inhibitors (eg, erythromycin, clarithromycin, ketoconazole) may increase levels and may result in side effects. Patients concomitantly receiving thyroid replacement therapy and estrogens may require increased doses of thyroid replacement therapy; monitor thyroid function.

NURSING CONSIDERATIONS

Assessment: Assess for undiagnosed abnormal genital bleeding, presence/history of breast cancer, estrogen-dependent neoplasia, active/history of DVT/PE/arterial thromboembolic disease, liver impairment/disease, thrombophilic disorders, drug hypersensitivity, pregnancy/nursing status, any other conditions where treatment is contraindicated or cautioned, need for progestin therapy, and for possible drug interactions.

Monitoring: Monitor for signs/symptoms of CV disorders, malignant neoplasms, dementia, gallbladder disease, hypercalcemia, visual abnormalities, BP and plasma TG elevations, cholestatic jaundice, fluid retention, anaphylactic/anaphylactoid reactions, angioedema, exacerbation of endometriosis, and other adverse reactions. Perform adequate diagnostic measures (eg, endometrial sampling) to rule out malignancy in case of undiagnosed persistent or recurring genital bleeding. Monitor thyroid function in patients on thyroid replacement therapy. Perform annual breast exam; schedule mammography based on age, risk factors, and prior mammogram results. Periodically reevaluate to determine need for therapy.

Patient Counseling: Inform of the importance of reporting abnormal vaginal bleeding to physician as soon as possible. Inform of possible serious adverse reactions of therapy (eg, CV disorders, malignant neoplasms, probable dementia) and of possible less serious but common adverse reactions (eg, headache, breast pain and tenderness, N/V). Instruct to have yearly breast exams by a physician and to perform monthly breast self-exams.

Storage: 25°C (77°F); do not store unpouched.

VIVITROL – naltrexone

RX

Class: Opioid antagonist

ADULT DOSAGE

Alcohol Dependence

Treatment of Alcohol Dependence in Patients Who are Able to Abstain from Alcohol in an Outpatient Setting Prior to Initiation of Therapy:
Usual: 380mg IM every 4 weeks or once a month

Prior to initiating therapy, an opioid-free duration of a minimum of 7-10 days is recommended

Opioid Dependence

Prevention of Relapse to Opioid Dependence, Following Opioid Detoxification:
Usual: 380mg IM every 4 weeks or once a month

Prior to initiating therapy, an opioid-free duration of a minimum of 7-10 days is recommended

Conversions

Switching from Buprenorphine, Buprenorphine/Naloxone, or Methadone:
Be prepared to manage withdrawal symptomatically w/ nonopioid medications

PEDIATRIC DOSAGE

Pediatric use may not have been established

ADMINISTRATION

IM route

Administer as IM gluteal inj, alternating buttocks for each subsequent inj, using the carton components provided; must not inject using any other needle
Must be prepared and administered by a healthcare provider
Must be suspended only in the diluent supplied in the carton and must be administered only w/ 1 of the administration needles supplied in the carton
For patients w/ a larger amount of subcutaneous tissue overlying the gluteal muscle, may utilize the supplied 2-inch needle w/ needle protection device to help ensure that the injectate reaches the IM mass. For very lean patients, the 1.5-inch needle may be appropriate to prevent the needle contacting the periosteum. Either needle may be used for patients w/ average body habitus. Do not substitute any other components for the components of the carton
Prior to preparation, allow drug to reach room temperature (approx 45 min)
Refer to PI for further preparation and administration instructions

HOW SUPPLIED

Inj, Extended-Release: 380mg

CONTRAINDICATIONS

Concomitant opioid analgesics, current physiologic opioid dependence, acute opioid withdrawal, positive urine screen for opioids, failed naloxone challenge test.

WARNINGS/PRECAUTIONS

Patients may have reduced tolerance to opioids after opioid detoxification; may result in potentially life-threatening opioid intoxication with use of previously tolerated opioid doses. Potential risk to patients attempting to overcome the antagonism by taking opioids; may lead to life-threatening opioid intoxication or fatal overdose. Inj-site reactions reported; inadvertent SQ inj may increase likelihood of severe inj-site reactions. Withdrawal syndrome, severe enough to require hospitalization, may occur when withdrawal is precipitated abruptly by the administration of an opioid antagonist to an opioid-dependent patient. Opioid-dependent patients, including those being treated for alcohol dependence, should be opioid-free before starting treatment to reduce risk of either precipitated withdrawal in patients dependent on opioids or exacerbation of a preexisting subclinical withdrawal syndrome; an opioid-free interval of a minimum of 7-10 days is recommended for patients previously dependent on short-acting opioids. May experience severe manifestations of precipitated withdrawal when being switched from opioid agonist to opioid antagonist therapy; patients transitioning from buprenorphine or methadone may be vulnerable to precipitation of withdrawal symptoms for as long as 2 weeks. A naloxone challenge test may be helpful to determine if patient is opioid-free; however, precipitated withdrawal may occur despite having negative urine toxicology screen or tolerating a naloxone challenge test. Cases of hepatitis, clinically significant liver dysfunction, and transient, asymptomatic hepatic transaminase elevations reported; d/c in the event of symptoms and/or signs of acute hepatitis. Depression and suicidality reported. In emergency situations, suggested plan for pain management is regional analgesia or use of nonopioid analgesics. If opioid therapy is required, monitor continuously in an anesthesia care setting. Cases of eosinophilic pneumonia and hypersensitivity reactions, including anaphylaxis, reported. As with any IM inj, caution with thrombocytopenia or any coagulation disorder (eg, hemophilia, severe hepatic failure). Does not eliminate or diminish alcohol withdrawal symptoms. May cross-react with certain immunoassay methods for the detection of drugs of abuse in urine. Caution with moderate to severe renal impairment.

ADVERSE REACTIONS

N/V, diarrhea, insomnia, depression, inj-site reactions, somnolence, anorexia, muscle cramps, dizziness, syncope, appetite disorder, hepatic enzyme abnormalities, nasopharyngitis, toothache, headache.

DRUG INTERACTIONS

See Contraindications. Antagonizes effects of opioid-containing medicines (eg, cough and cold remedies, antidiarrheals, opioid analgesics).

NURSING CONSIDERATIONS

Assessment: Assess for opioid use, acute opioid withdrawal, thrombocytopenia, coagulation disorders, renal impairment, any other conditions where treatment is contraindicated or cautioned, pregnancy/nursing status, and possible drug interactions. Assess patients, including patients treated for alcohol dependence, for underlying opioid dependence, and for any recent use of opioids. Assess body habitus to assure that needle length is adequate.

Monitoring: Monitor for opioid intoxication/overdose, severe inj-site reactions, precipitation of opioid withdrawal, signs/symptoms of acute hepatitis, depression, suicidality, hypersensitivity reactions, and other adverse reactions.

Patient Counseling: Advise that if they previously used opioids, they may be more sensitive to lower doses of opioids and at risk of accidental overdose if they use opioids when their next dose is due, if they miss a dose, or after treatment is discontinued. Advise that patients will not perceive any effect if they attempt to self-administer heroin or any other opioid drug in small doses while on therapy. Inform that administration of large doses of heroin or any other opioid to try to bypass the blockade may lead to serious injury, coma, or death. Inform that patient may not experience the expected effects from opioid-containing analgesic, antidiarrheal, or antitussive medications. Advise that inj-site reactions may occur and instruct to seek medical attention for worsening skin reactions. Instruct to be off all opioids for a minimum of 7-10 days before starting therapy in order to avoid precipitation of opioid withdrawal. Advise not to take therapy if they have any symptoms of opioid withdrawal. Advise all patients, including those with alcohol dependence, to notify physician of any recent use of opioids or any history of opioid dependence before starting therapy. Inform that drug may cause liver injury; instruct to immediately notify physician if symptoms and/or signs of liver disease develop. Inform the patient, family members, and caregivers that the patient may experience depression while taking therapy and to contact physician if the patient becomes depressed or symptoms of depression are experienced. Instruct to carry documentation to alert medical personnel to therapy. Advise that drug may cause an allergic pneumonia; instruct to immediately notify physician if signs and symptoms of pneumonia develop. Inform that drug may cause nausea, which tends to subside within a few days post-inj. Advise that they may also experience tiredness, headache, vomiting, decreased appetite, painful joints, and muscle cramps. Advise that therapy has been shown to treat alcohol and opioid dependence only when used as part of a treatment program that includes counseling and support. Advise that dizziness may occur; instruct to avoid driving or operating heavy machinery. Advise to notify physician if pregnant or intending to become pregnant during treatment, breastfeeding, or experiencing unusual or significant side effects while on therapy.

Storage: 2-8°C (36-46°F). Do not freeze. Can be stored at ≤25°C (77°F) for no more than 7 days prior administration.

VOLTAREN GEL — diclofenac sodium RX

Class: NSAID

NSAIDs may cause an increased risk of serious cardiovascular (CV) thrombotic events, MI, stroke, and serious GI adverse events including bleeding, ulceration, and perforation of the stomach or intestines, which can be fatal. Patients with cardiovascular disease (CVD) or risk factors for CVD may be at greater risk. Elderly patients are at a greater risk for GI events. Contraindicated for the treatment of perioperative pain in the setting of CABG surgery.

ADULT DOSAGE

Osteoarthritis

Joint Pain:

Lower Extremities:

Apply 4g to affected foot, knee, or ankle qid
Max: 16g/day to any single joint

Upper Extremities:

Apply 2g to affected hand, elbow, or wrist qid
Max: 8g/day to any single joint

Total dose should not exceed 32g/day over all affected joints

PEDIATRIC DOSAGE

Pediatric use may not have been established

ADMINISTRATION

Topical route

Measure onto enclosed dosing card to appropriate 2g or 4g line
Avoid showering or bathing for ≥1 hr after application
Avoid wearing clothing or gloves for ≥10 min after application

HOW SUPPLIED

Gel: 1% [100g]

CONTRAINDICATIONS

History of asthma, urticaria, or allergic-type reactions to aspirin (ASA) or other NSAIDs, setting of CABG surgery.

WARNINGS/PRECAUTIONS

Not evaluated for use on spine, hip, or shoulder. Avoid open wounds, eyes, mucous membranes, external heat, natural or artificial sunlight, and/or occlusive dressings. Caution in patients with prior history of ulcer or GI bleeding. May cause elevations of LFTs; d/c if liver disease develops, systemic manifestations occur, or abnormal liver tests persist or worsen. May lead to onset of new HTN or worsening of preexisting HTN. Fluid retention and edema reported; caution with heart failure (HF). Renal papillary necrosis and other renal injury reported after long-term use. Not recommended for use with advanced renal disease; if therapy must be initiated, monitor renal function. D/C if renal tests persist or worsen. Anaphylactoid reactions may occur. May cause serious skin adverse events (eg, exfoliative dermatitis, Stevens-Johnson syndrome, and toxic epidermal necrolysis). Avoid in late pregnancy; may cause premature closure of ductus arteriosus. Not a substitute for corticosteroids or to treat corticosteroid insufficiency. Use the lowest effective dose for the shortest duration possible. Anemia may occur; with long-term use, monitor Hgb/Hct if signs or symptoms of anemia develop. May inhibit platelet aggregation and prolong bleeding time. Caution with asthma. May diminish utility of diagnostic signs (eg, inflammation, fever) in detecting infectious complications of presumed noninfectious, painful conditions. Caution in elderly.

ADVERSE REACTIONS

Application-site reactions, dermatitis, GI effects.

DRUG INTERACTIONS

May enhance methotrexate toxicity and cyclosporine nephrotoxicity; caution when coadministering. May diminish antihypertensive effect of ACE-inhibitors and impair response of loop diuretics. May reduce natriuretic effect of furosemide and thiazides; monitor for renal failure. May increase lithium levels; monitor for toxicity. Synergistic effects on GI bleeding with anticoagulants (eg, warfarin) reported. Avoid concomitant use with other topical products (eg, topical medications, sunscreens, lot, moisturizers, and cosmetics) on the same skin site; may alter tolerability and absorption. Coadministration with oral NSAIDs or ASA may result in increased adverse effects; concomitant administration with ASA not recommended. Caution with concomitant hepatotoxic drugs (eg, antibiotics, antiepileptics). May increase risk of GI bleeding with oral corticosteroids/anticoagulants, tobacco, or alcohol use.

NURSING CONSIDERATIONS

Assessment: Assess for hypersensitivity to ASA or NSAIDs, history of ulcer or GI bleeding, HTN, fluid retention, congestive HF, asthma, CVD (or risk factors), renal/hepatic impairment, pregnancy/nursing status, and for possible drug interactions. Obtain baseline BP.

Monitoring: Monitor for signs/symptoms of CV events, GI events, HTN, edema, skin reactions, coagulation disorders, and anaphylactoid reactions. Monitor BP, LFTs, CBC, and renal function periodically. Check chemistry profile periodically.

Patient Counseling: Instruct to avoid contact with eyes and mucous membranes; instruct that if contact occurs, to wash with water or saline, and if irritation persists for >1 hr, to call physician. Advise to minimize or avoid exposure of treated areas to natural or artificial sunlight. Instruct to avoid late in pregnancy. Advise to seek medical attention for symptoms of CV events, GI events, hepatotoxicity, unexplained weight gain or edema, skin reactions, or hypersensitivity reactions;

instruct to d/c at 1st appearance of rash/hypersensitivity reactions. Stress the importance of follow-up. Instruct not to apply to open skin wounds, infections, inflammations, or exfoliative dermatitis. Instruct to avoid concomitant use with other topical products. Instruct on how to use the dosing card to measure the proper dose of medication to apply. Instruct on how to correctly measure dose while waiting for a replacement of a lost dosing card.

Storage: 20-25°C (68-77°F). Keep from freezing. Store with dosing card.

VOLTAREN-XR – diclofenac sodium RX

Class: NSAID

NSAIDs may cause an increased risk of serious cardiovascular (CV) thrombotic events, myocardial infarction (MI), stroke, and serious GI adverse events including inflammation, bleeding, ulceration, and perforation of the stomach or intestines, which may be fatal. Contraindicated for the treatment of perioperative pain in the setting of coronary artery bypass graft (CABG) surgery.

ADULT DOSAGE

Osteoarthritis

Usual: 100mg qd

Rheumatoid Arthritis

Usual: 100mg qd-bid

PEDIATRIC DOSAGE

Pediatric use may not have been established

ADMINISTRATION

Oral route

HOW SUPPLIED

Tab, Extended-Release: 100mg

CONTRAINDICATIONS

Aspirin (ASA) or other NSAID allergy that precipitates asthma, urticaria, or allergic-type reactions. Treatment of perioperative pain in the setting of CABG surgery.

WARNINGS/PRECAUTIONS

Use lowest effective dose for the shortest duration possible. Not a substitute for corticosteroids or to treat corticosteroid insufficiency. May lead to onset of new HTN or worsening of preexisting HTN; monitor BP closely. Fluid retention and edema reported; caution with fluid retention or heart failure (HF). Extreme caution with a prior history of ulcer disease, and/or GI bleeding. Caution when initiating treatment in patients with considerable dehydration. Renal papillary necrosis and other renal injury reported after long-term use. Not recommended for use with advanced renal disease; if therapy must be initiated, monitor renal function. Anaphylactoid reactions may occur; avoid in patients with ASA triad. May cause serious skin adverse events (eg, exfoliative dermatitis, Stevens-Johnson syndrome [SJS], toxic epidermal necrolysis). Avoid in late pregnancy; may cause premature closure of ductus arteriosus. May cause elevations of LFTs; d/c if liver disease develops or systemic manifestations occur. Caution in elderly and debilitated patients. Anemia may occur; with long-term use, monitor Hgb/Hct if signs or symptoms of anemia develop. May inhibit platelet aggregation and prolong bleeding time; monitor with coagulation disorders. Caution with asthma and avoid with ASA-sensitive asthma.

ADVERSE REACTIONS

Abdominal pain, constipation, diarrhea, dyspepsia, flatulence, gross bleeding/perforation, heartburn, N/V, GI ulcers, renal function abnormalities, anemia, dizziness, edema, elevated liver enzymes.

DRUG INTERACTIONS

Increased adverse effects with ASA; avoid use. May enhance methotrexate toxicity and increase nephrotoxicity of cyclosporine; caution with coadministration. May diminish antihypertensive effect of ACE inhibitors. Patients taking thiazides and loop diuretics may have impaired response to these therapies. ACE inhibitors and diuretics may precipitate overt renal decompensation. May reduce natriuretic effect of furosemide and thiazides. May increase lithium levels; monitor for toxicity. Synergistic effects with warfarin on GI bleeding. May increase risk of GI bleeding with oral corticosteroids/anticoagulants, tobacco, or alcohol use. Caution with hepatotoxic drugs (eg, antibiotics, antiepileptics). Caution with CYP2C9 inhibitors or inducers (eg, voriconazole, rifampin); dosage adjustment may be warranted.

NURSING CONSIDERATIONS

Assessment: Assess for CV disease or risk factors, fluid retention, edema, conditions affected by platelet function alterations, GI events or risk factors, renal/hepatic function, any other conditions where treatment is contraindicated or cautioned, pregnancy/nursing status, and possible drug interactions. Assess baseline BP, CBC, and chemistry profile.

Monitoring: Monitor for signs/symptoms of GI events, CV thrombotic events, congestive HF, HTN, allergic or skin reactions, hematological effects (eg, anemia, prolongation of bleeding time), renal papillary necrosis or other renal injury/toxicity, hepatotoxicity. Monitor BP, CBC, and chemistry profile periodically.

Patient Counseling: Advise to seek medical attention if signs and symptoms of hepatotoxicity, anaphylactic/anaphylactoid reactions, skin reactions, CV events, GI ulceration or bleeding, weight gain, or edema occur. Inform of pregnancy risks and instruct to avoid use during late pregnancy.

Storage: Protect from moisture. Do not store above 30°C (86°F).

VOTRIENT – pazopanib — RX

Class: Kinase inhibitors

Severe and fatal hepatotoxicity reported; monitor hepatic function and interrupt, reduce, or d/c dosing as recommended.

ADULT DOSAGE

Advanced Renal Cell Carcinoma

Initial: 800mg qd w/o food (≥1 hr ac or 2 hrs pc)
Max: 800mg

Initial Dose Reduction: 400mg
Additional Dose Decrease/Increase: Should be in 200mg steps

Advanced Soft Tissue Sarcoma

Patients Who Have Received Prior Chemotherapy:
Initial: 800mg qd w/o food (≥1 hr ac or 2 hrs pc)
Max: 800mg

Dose Decrease/Increase: Should be in 200mg steps

Missed Dose

If a dose is missed, it should not be taken if it is <12 hrs until the next dose

PEDIATRIC DOSAGE

Pediatric use may not have been established

DOSE MODIFICATION

Hepatic Impairment
Moderate: Consider alternative therapy or reduce dose to 200mg/day
Severe: Not recommended for use

Concomitant Medications
Strong CYP3A4 Inhibitors: Avoid concomitant use; consider an alternate concomitant medication w/ no or minimal potential to inhibit CYP3A4
If coadministration is warranted, reduce pazopanib dose to 400mg; further dose reductions may be needed if adverse effects occur during therapy
Strong CYP3A4 Inducers: Avoid concomitant use; consider an alternate concomitant medication w/ no or minimal enzyme induction potential
Do not use pazopanib if chronic use of strong CYP3A4 inducers cannot be avoided

ADMINISTRATION

Oral route

Do not crush tabs
Take w/o food (≥1 hr ac or 2 hrs pc)

HOW SUPPLIED

Tab: 200mg

WARNINGS/PRECAUTIONS

Patients >65 yrs of age are at greater risk for hepatotoxicity. QT prolongation and torsades de pointes reported. Cardiac dysfunction (eg, decreased left ventricular ejection fraction [LVEF], CHF) reported. Hemorrhagic events reported; avoid w/ history of hemoptysis, cerebral hemorrhage, or clinically significant GI hemorrhage in the past 6 months. Arterial thromboembolic events reported; caution in patients at increased risk for these events or who have had a history of these events and avoid use if an arterial thromboembolic event has occurred w/in the past 6 months. Venous thromboembolic events (VTE) (eg, pulmonary embolism [PE]) and GI perforation/fistula reported. Thrombotic microangiopathy (TMA), including thrombotic thrombocytopenic purpura (TTP) and hemolytic uremic syndrome (HUS), reported; permanently d/c in patients developing TMA. Reversible posterior leukoencephalopathy syndrome (RPLS) reported; permanently d/c in patients developing RPLS. HTN and hypertensive crisis reported; d/c if evidence of hypertensive crisis or if HTN is severe and persistent despite antihypertensive therapy and dose reduction. May impair wound healing; d/c therapy w/ wound dehiscence and ≥7 days prior to scheduled surgery. Hypothyroidism reported. Proteinuria reported; interrupt therapy and reduce dose for 24-hr urine protein ≥3g; d/c for repeat episodes despite dose reductions. Serious infections reported; institute appropriate anti-infective therapy promptly and consider interruption or discontinuation if serious infections develop. May cause serious adverse effects on organ development in pediatric patients; not for use in pediatric patients. May cause fetal harm if used during pregnancy.

ADVERSE REACTIONS

Hepatotoxicity, diarrhea, HTN, hair color changes, N/V, anorexia, fatigue, asthenia, headache, weight/appetite decreased, tumor pain, dysgeusia, dyspnea, musculoskeletal pain, skin hypopigmentation.

DRUG INTERACTIONS

See Dose Modification. Avoid w/ drugs that raise gastric pH (eg, proton pump inhibitors [PPIs]); if such drugs are needed, consider short-acting antacids in place of PPIs and H2 receptor antagonists; separate antacid and pazopanib dosing by several hrs. Do not use in combination w/ other cancer therapy; increased toxicity and mortality reported w/ pemetrexed and lapatinib. Strong CYP3A4 inhibitors (eg, ketoconazole, ritonavir, clarithromycin) may increase concentrations. Avoid grapefruit or grapefruit juice. CYP3A4 inducers (eg, rifampin) may decrease plasma concentrations; consider an alternate concomitant medication w/ no or minimal enzyme induction potential. Avoid use w/ strong inhibitors of P-gp or breast cancer resistance protein (BCRP), and consider alternative concomitant medicinal products w/ no or minimal potential to inhibit P-gp or BCRP. Not recommended w/ agents w/ narrow therapeutic windows that are metabolized by CYP3A4, CYP2D6, or CYP2C8. Simvastatin may increase incidence of ALT elevations; follow pazopanib dosing guidelines or consider alternatives to pazopanib or consider discontinuing simvastatin. Caution in patients taking antiarrhythmics or other medications that may prolong the QT interval.

NURSING CONSIDERATIONS

Assessment: Assess for history of QT interval prolongation, cardiac disease, hepatic impairment, pregnancy/nursing status, and for possible drug interactions. Assess for history of hemoptysis/cerebral hemorrhage, clinically significant GI hemorrhage, or an arterial thromboembolic event in the past 6 months. Assess if patient is planning to undergo any surgical procedure. Assess thyroid function. Obtain baseline BP, LFTs, ECG, electrolytes, and urinalysis. Obtain baseline LVEF in patients at risk of cardiac dysfunction.

Monitoring: Monitor for signs/symptoms of hepatotoxicity, QT prolongation, torsades de pointes, cardiac dysfunction, hemorrhagic events, arterial thromboembolic events, VTE, TMA, TTP, HUS, PE, RPLS, GI perforation or fistula, HTN/hypertensive crisis, impaired wound healing, proteinuria, infections, and other adverse reactions. Monitor BP early after starting treatment and then frequently to ensure BP control. Perform periodic urinalysis w/ follow-up measurement of 24-hr urine protein as clinically indicated. Monitor ECG, thyroid function tests, and serum electrolytes. Monitor LFTs at Weeks 3, 5, 7, and 9, at Months 3 and 4, as clinically indicated, and continue periodic monitoring after Month 4. Periodically monitor LVEF in patients at risk of cardiac dysfunction.

Patient Counseling: Advise the patient to read the FDA-approved patient labeling (Medication Guide). Advise that lab monitoring will be required prior to and while on therapy. Instruct to report any signs/symptoms of liver dysfunction, HTN, CHF, unusual bleeding, arterial thrombosis, new onset of dyspnea, chest pain, localized limb edema, GI perforation/fistula, infection, and worsening of neurologic function consistent w/ RPLS. Advise to d/c treatment ≥7 days prior to a scheduled surgery. Inform that thyroid function testing and urinalysis will be performed during treatment. Advise on how to manage diarrhea and to notify healthcare provider if moderate to severe diarrhea occurs. Advise women of childbearing potential to avoid becoming pregnant during therapy. Advise to inform healthcare provider of all concomitant medications, vitamins, or dietary and herbal supplements. Advise that depigmentation of the hair or skin may occur during treatment.

Storage: 20-25°C (68-77°F); excursions permitted to 15-30°C (59-86°F).

VYTORIN – ezetimibe/simvastatin

RX

Class: Cholesterol absorption inhibitor/HMG-CoA reductase inhibitor

ADULT DOSAGE

Primary Hyperlipidemia/Mixed Hyperlipidemia

Primary (Heterozygous Familial and Nonfamilial) Hyperlipidemia/Mixed Hyperlipidemia:

Reduction of Elevated Total Cholesterol (Total-C), LDL, Apolipoprotein B, TGs, Non-HDL, and to Increase HDL:
Initial: 10mg/10mg or 10mg/20mg qpm
Usual: 10mg/10mg to 10mg/40mg qpm
Titrate: After initiation or titration, analyze lipid levels after ≥2 weeks and adjust dose, if needed

Patients Requiring Larger LDL Reduction (>55%):
Initial: 10mg/40mg qpm

Homozygous Familial Hypercholesterolemia

Adjunct to Other Lipid-Lowering Treatments (eg, LDL Apheresis) or if Such Treatments are Unavailable to Reduce Elevated Total-C and LDL:
10mg/40mg qpm

PEDIATRIC DOSAGE

Pediatric use may not have been established

DOSE MODIFICATION

Concomitant Medications

Lomitapide:

Homozygous Familial Hypercholesterolemia:
Reduce dose by 50% if initiating lomitapide
Max: 10mg/20mg/day (or 10mg/40mg/day for patients who have previously taken simvastatin 80mg/day chronically [eg, for ≥12 months] w/o evidence of muscle toxicity)

Verapamil, Diltiazem, Dronedarone:
Max: 10mg/10mg qd

Amiodarone, Amlodipine, Ranolazine:
Max: 10mg/20mg qd

Bile Acid Sequestrants:
Take either ≥2 hrs before or ≥4 hrs after bile acid sequestrant

Niacin-Containing Products:
Chinese Patients Taking Lipid-Modifying Doses (≥1g/Day Niacin): Caution w/ doses >10mg/20mg/day; do not give 10mg/80mg dose

Renal Impairment

Chronic Kidney Disease (GFR <60mL/min/1.73m^2):
Usual: 10mg/20mg qpm

Other Important Modifications

Restricted Dosing:
Use 10mg/80mg dose only in patients who have been taking 10mg/80mg dose chronically (eg, for ≥12 months) w/o evidence of muscle toxicity

If currently tolerating 10mg/80mg dose and needs to be initiated on drug that is contraindicated or is associated w/ a dose cap for simvastatin, switch to an alternative statin or statin-based regimen w/ less potential for drug-drug interaction

Do not titrate to 10mg/80mg, but place on alternative LDL lowering treatment that provides greater LDL lowering, if unable to achieve LDL goal w/ 10mg/40mg dose

ADMINISTRATION

Oral route

Take qpm w/ or w/o food

HOW SUPPLIED

Tab: (Ezetimibe/Simvastatin) 10mg/10mg, 10mg/20mg, 10mg/40mg, 10mg/80mg

CONTRAINDICATIONS

Concomitant administration of strong CYP3A4 inhibitors (eg, itraconazole, ketoconazole, posaconazole, voriconazole, HIV protease inhibitors, boceprevir, telaprevir, erythromycin, clarithromycin, telithromycin, nefazodone, cobicistat-containing products), gemfibrozil, cyclosporine, or danazol. Active liver disease or unexplained persistent elevations in hepatic transaminases, women who are or may become pregnant, and nursing mothers.

WARNINGS/PRECAUTIONS

Use doses >10mg/20mg w/ caution and close monitoring in patients w/ moderate to severe renal impairment. Myopathy (including immune-mediated necrotizing myopathy [IMNM]) and rhabdomyolysis reported; predisposing factors include advanced age (≥65 yrs of age), female gender, uncontrolled hypothyroidism, and renal impairment. Risk of myopathy, including rhabdomyolysis, is dose related and greater w/ simvastatin 80mg. D/C if markedly elevated CPK levels occur or myopathy is suspected/diagnosed, and temporarily withhold if experiencing an acute or serious condition predisposing to development of renal failure secondary to rhabdomyolysis. Increases in serum transaminases reported. Fatal and nonfatal hepatic failure (rare) reported; promptly interrupt therapy if serious liver injury w/ clinical symptoms and/or hyperbilirubinemia or jaundice occurs and do not restart if no alternate etiology found. Caution w/ history of liver disease, substantial alcohol consumption, and in elderly. Increases in HbA1c and FPG levels reported.

ADVERSE REACTIONS

Headache, increased ALT, myalgia, URTI, diarrhea.

DRUG INTERACTIONS

See Contraindications and Dose Modification. Due to the risk of myopathy/rhabdomyolysis, avoid grapefruit juice and caution w/ fenofibrates (eg, fenofibrate, fenofibric acid), lipid-modifying doses (≥1g/day) of niacin, colchicine, verapamil, diltiazem, dronedarone, lomitapide, amiodarone, amlodipine, and ranolazine. If coadministered w/ a fenofibrate, immediately d/c both agents if myopathy is suspected/diagnosed, and perform gallbladder studies/consider alternative lipid-lowering therapy if cholelithiasis is suspected. Simvastatin: May slightly elevate plasma digoxin concentrations; monitor patients taking digoxin when therapy is initiated. May potentiate effect of coumarin anticoagulants; determine PT before initiation and frequently during therapy. Ezetimibe: Reduced levels w/ cholestyramine; incremental LDL reduction may be reduced. Increased INR reported w/ warfarin.

NURSING CONSIDERATIONS

Assessment: Assess for history of or active liver disease, unexplained persistent hepatic transaminase elevations, predisposing factors for myopathy, renal impairment, alcohol consumption, drug hypersensitivity, any other conditions where treatment is contraindicated or cautioned, pregnancy/nursing status, and possible drug interactions. Assess lipid profile and LFTs.

Monitoring: Monitor for signs/symptoms of myopathy (including IMNM), rhabdomyolysis, liver dysfunction, increases in HbA1c and FPG levels, and other adverse reactions. Monitor lipid profile, and LFTs. Check PT w/ coumarin anticoagulants.

Patient Counseling: Inform of benefits/risks of therapy. Advise to adhere to the National Cholesterol Education Program recommended diet, a regular exercise program, and periodic testing of a fasting lipid panel. Inform about substances that should be avoided during therapy, and advise to discuss all medications, both Rx and OTC, w/ physician. Instruct to report promptly any unexplained muscle pain, tenderness, or weakness, particularly if accompanied by malaise or fever or if these muscle signs/symptoms persist after discontinuation, or any symptoms that may indicate liver injury. Inform patients using the 10mg/80mg dose that the risk of myopathy, including rhabdomyolysis, is increased. Instruct women to use an effective method of birth control to prevent pregnancy while on therapy, to d/c therapy and call physician if pregnant, and not to breastfeed while on therapy.

Storage: 20-25°C (68-77°F).

VYVANSE – lisdexamfetamine dimesylate CII

Class: Sympathomimetic amine

CNS stimulants (amphetamines and methylphenidate-containing products) have a high potential for abuse and dependence. Assess the risk of abuse prior to prescribing and monitor for signs of abuse and dependence while on therapy.

ADULT DOSAGE

Attention-Deficit Hyperactivity Disorder

Initial: 30mg qam
Titrate: May adjust in increments of 10mg or 20mg at approx weekly intervals
Max: 70mg/day

PEDIATRIC DOSAGE

Attention-Deficit Hyperactivity Disorder

≥6 Years:
Initial: 30mg qam
Titrate: May adjust in increments of 10mg or 20mg at weekly intervals
Max: 70mg/day

Binge Eating Disorder

Moderate to Severe:
Initial: 30mg qam
Titrate: Titrate in increments of 20mg at approx weekly intervals
Target Dose: 50-70mg/day
Max: 70mg/day

DOSE MODIFICATION

Renal Impairment

Severe (GFR 15-<30mL/min/1.73m²):
Max: 50mg/day

ESRD (GFR <15mL/min/1.73m²):
Max: 30mg/day

Elderly

Start at lower end of dosing range

ADMINISTRATION

Oral route

Take in am w/ or w/o food; avoid afternoon doses
May swallow caps whole
Do not take anything less than 1 cap/day; do not divide a single cap

Open Caps

May open caps, empty, and mix entire contents w/ yogurt, water, or orange juice; if contents of cap include any compacted powder, may use a spoon to break apart the powder
Mix contents until completely dispersed
Immediately consume entire mixture; do not store
Film containing inactive ingredients may remain in glass/container once mixture is consumed

HOW SUPPLIED

Cap: 10mg, 20mg, 30mg, 40mg, 50mg, 60mg, 70mg

CONTRAINDICATIONS

Concurrent use w/ an MAOI or use w/in 14 days of the last MAOI dose.

WARNINGS/PRECAUTIONS

Not indicated or recommended for weight loss. Sudden death, stroke, and MI reported in adults. Sudden death reported in children and adolescents w/ structural cardiac abnormalities and other serious heart problems. Avoid use in patients w/ known structural cardiac abnormalities, cardiomyopathy, serious heart arrhythmia, coronary artery disease, and other serious heart problems. May cause increase in BP and HR. May exacerbate symptoms of behavior disturbance and thought disorder in patients w/ a preexisting psychotic disorder. May induce a mixed/manic episode in patients w/ bipolar disorder. May cause psychotic or manic symptoms (eg, hallucinations, delusional thinking, mania) in children and adolescents w/o a prior history of psychotic illness or mania; consider discontinuation if symptoms occur. Associated w/ weight loss and slowing of growth rate in pediatric patients. Associated w/ peripheral vasculopathy, including Raynaud's phenomenon; further clinical evaluation (eg, rheumatology referral) may be appropriate for certain patients.

ADVERSE REACTIONS

Decreased appetite, insomnia, upper abdominal pain, irritability, N/V, decreased weight, dry mouth, dizziness, constipation, rash, diarrhea, anxiety, anorexia, jittery feeling, increased HR.

DRUG INTERACTIONS

See Contraindications. Urinary acidifying agents (eg, ascorbic acid) increase urinary excretion and decrease the $T_{1/2}$ of amphetamine, while urinary alkalinizing agents (eg, sodium bicarbonate) decrease urinary excretion and extend the $T_{1/2}$ of amphetamine; adjust dose accordingly.

NURSING CONSIDERATIONS

Assessment: Assess for presence of cardiac disease, risk of abuse, risk factors for developing a manic episode, psychosis, bipolar disorder, hypersensitivity to the drug or amphetamine products, renal impairment, pregnancy/nursing status, and possible drug interactions.

Monitoring: Monitor for potential tachycardia, HTN, exacerbation of preexisting psychosis, psychotic or manic symptoms in children and adolescents, and other adverse reactions. Monitor height and weight in pediatric patients. Further evaluate patients who develop exertional chest pain, unexplained syncope, or arrhythmias. Observe carefully for signs/symptoms of peripheral vasculopathy (eg, digital changes). Monitor for signs of abuse and dependence; periodically reevaluate the need for therapy.

Patient Counseling: Inform about drug abuse/dependence risk. Advise about serious cardiovascular risks; instruct to contact physician immediately if symptoms of cardiac disease develop. Instruct to monitor for elevations of BP and pulse rate. Inform that psychotic or manic symptoms may occur. Instruct parents or caregivers of pediatric patients that therapy may cause slowing of growth, including weight loss. Inform that therapy may impair ability to engage in potentially dangerous activities (eg, operating machinery); instruct patients to assess how the medication affects them before engaging in potentially dangerous activities. Inform about the risk of peripheral vasculopathy, including Raynaud's phenomenon; instruct to report to physician any new numbness, pain, skin color change, or sensitivity to temperature in fingers or toes, and to call physician immediately if any signs of unexplained wounds appear on fingers or toes while on therapy.

Storage: 20-25°C (68-77°F); excursions permitted between 15-30°C (59-86°F).

WelChol – colesevelam hydrochloride RX

Class: Bile acid sequestrant

ADULT DOSAGE

Primary Hyperlipidemia

Reduction of LDL-C in adults w/ primary hyperlipidemia (Fredrickson Type IIa) either alone or in combination w/ a statin

Tab:
Usual: 3 tabs bid or 6 tabs qd

Sus:
Usual: 3.75g qd or 1.875g bid in 4-8 oz of water, fruit juice, or diet soft drinks; stir well and drink

May be dosed at the same time as a statin or dosed apart

Type 2 Diabetes Mellitus

Tab:
Usual: 3 tabs bid or 6 tabs qd

Sus:
Usual: 3.75g qd or 1.875g bid in 4-8 oz of water, fruit juice, or diet soft drinks; stir well and drink

PEDIATRIC DOSAGE

Heterozygous Familial Hypercholesterolemia

Reduction of LDL levels in boys and postmenarchal girls as monotherapy or in combination w/ a statin after an adequate trial of diet therapy

Sus:
10-17 Years:
3.75g qd or 1.875g bid in 4-8 oz of water, fruit juice, or diet soft drinks; stir well and drink

ADMINISTRATION

Oral route

Tab
Take w/ meal and liquid

Sus
Do not take in dry form; take w/ meals

HOW SUPPLIED

Sus: 1.875g, 3.75g [pkt]; Tab: 625mg

CONTRAINDICATIONS

Serum TG concentrations >500mg/dL, history of hypertriglyceridemia-induced pancreatitis or bowel obstruction.

WARNINGS/PRECAUTIONS

Not for treatment of type 1 DM or diabetic ketoacidosis. Analyze lipid levels within 4-6 weeks after initiation. May increase serum TG concentrations; d/c if TG levels >500mg/dL or if hypertriglyceridemia-induced pancreatitis develops. Caution in patients with TG levels >300mg/dL or with susceptibility to deficiencies of vitamin K (eg, malabsorption syndromes, patients on warfarin) or other fat-soluble vitamins. May cause constipation; avoid with gastroparesis, GI motility disorders, those who have had major GI tract surgery, or those at risk for bowel obstruction. (Sus) Contains phenylalanine; caution with phenylketonurics. Always mix with water, fruit juice, or diet soft drinks to avoid esophageal distress; do not take in its dry form. (Tab) Caution in patients with dysphagia or swallowing disorders.

ADVERSE REACTIONS

Asthenia, constipation, dyspepsia, nausea, rhinitis, fatigue, flu syndrome, nasopharyngitis, hypoglycemia, hypertriglyceridemia, headache, influenza, pharyngitis, URTI.

DRUG INTERACTIONS

Greater increase in TG levels may occur with insulin, pioglitazone, or sulfonylureas. May decrease absorption of vitamins A, D, E, and K. May increase seizure activity or decrease phenytoin levels.

May elevate TSH in patients receiving thyroid hormone replacement therapy. May increase levels of metformin extended-release. May decrease levels of cyclosporine, glimepiride, glipizide, glyburide, levothyroxine, olmesartan medoxomil, and oral contraceptives containing ethinyl estradiol and norethindrone. Administer phenytoin, cyclosporine, oral vitamin supplementation, drugs known to have reduced GI absorption when given concomitantly, or drugs that have not been tested for interaction (especially those with narrow therapeutic index) at least 4 hrs prior to colesevelam. Concomitant use with warfarin decreases INR; monitor INR.

NURSING CONSIDERATIONS

Assessment: Assess for history/risk of bowel obstruction, gastroparesis, or other GI motility disorders, history of major GI tract surgery or hypertriglyceridemia-induced pancreatitis, susceptibility to deficiencies of vitamin K or other fat-soluble vitamins, dysphagia or swallowing disorders, pregnancy/nursing status, and possible drug interactions. Obtain baseline lipid parameters (eg, TGs, non-HDL levels). Monitor INR prior to initiation in patients on warfarin therapy.

Monitoring: Monitor for hypertriglyceridemia-induced pancreatitis, hypoglycemia, dysphagia, esophageal obstruction, and other adverse events. Periodically monitor lipid profile (eg, TGs, non-HDL), blood glucose, and coadministered drug levels. Monitor INR frequently in patients on warfarin therapy.

Patient Counseling: Instruct to take with meal and liquid. Instruct to take interacting drugs at least 4 hrs prior to colesevelam. Advise to consume diet that promotes bowel regularity. Instruct to promptly d/c and seek medical attention if severe abdominal pain/constipation or symptoms of acute pancreatitis occur. Instruct patients with primary hyperlipidemia to adhere to the recommended diet of the National Cholesterol Education Program. Instruct patients with type 2 DM to adhere to dietary instructions, regular exercise program, and regular testing of blood glucose. Advise to notify physician if dysphagia or swallowing disorders occur. (Sus) Instruct to empty entire contents of 1 pkt into a glass or cup, then add 4-8 oz of water, fruit juice, or diet-soft drinks before ingesting.

Storage: 25°C (77°F); excursions permitted to 15-30°C (59-86°F). Protect from moisture. (Tab) Brief exposure to 40°C (104°F) does not adversely affect the product.

WELLBUTRIN SR – bupropion hydrochloride RX

Class: Aminoketone

Antidepressants increased the risk of suicidal thoughts and behavior in children, adolescents, and young adults in short-term trials. Monitor closely for worsening, and for emergence of suicidal thoughts and behavior. Advise families and caregivers of the need for close observation and communication with the prescriber. Serious neuropsychiatric reactions reported in patients taking bupropion for smoking cessation; not approved for smoking cessation. (Budeprion SR) Not approved for use in pediatric patients.

OTHER BRAND NAMES

Budeprion SR

ADULT DOSAGE

Major Depressive Disorder

Initial: 150mg/day given as a single daily dose in am
After 3 days, may increase dose to 300mg/day, given as 150mg bid w/ an interval of at least 8 hrs between successive doses
Usual: 300mg/day, given as 150mg bid
Max: May consider 400mg/day, given as 200mg bid, if no clinical improvement after several weeks of treatment at 300mg/day; do not exceed 200mg in any single dose

Periodically reassess the appropriate dose and the need for maint treatment

Dosing Considerations with MAOIs

Switching to/from an MAOI Antidepressant:
Allow at least 14 days between discontinuation of an MAOI and initiation of treatment and allow at least 14 days between discontinuation of treatment and initiation of an MAOI

Use w/ Reversible MAOIs (eg, Linezolid, IV Methylene Blue):
If acceptable alternatives to linezolid or IV methylene blue treatment are not available and

PEDIATRIC DOSAGE

Pediatric use may not have been established

potential benefits of linezolid or IV methylene blue treatment are judged to outweigh risks of hypertensive reactions, bupropion should be stopped promptly, and linezolid or IV methylene blue can be administered
Monitor for 2 weeks or until 24 hrs after the last dose of linezolid or IV methylene blue, whichever comes 1st
May resume bupropion treatment 24 hrs after the last dose of linezolid or IV methylene blue

DOSE MODIFICATION
Renal Impairment
Consider reduced frequency and/or dose
Hepatic Impairment
Wellbutrin SR:
Mild Hepatic Impairment (Child-Pugh Score: 5-6): Consider reducing frequency and/or dose
Moderate to Severe Hepatic Impairment (Child-Pugh Score: 7-15) Max Dose: 100mg/day or 150mg qod
Budeprion SR:
Mild to Moderate Hepatic Cirrhosis: Consider reducing frequency and/or dose
Severe Hepatic Cirrhosis Max Dose: 100mg/day or 150mg qod

ADMINISTRATION
Oral route
Take w/ or w/o food
Swallow whole; do not crush, divide, or chew
Budeprion SR
Avoid hs dosing to minimize insomnia

HOW SUPPLIED
Tab, Sustained-Release (SR): 100mg, 150mg, 200mg; (Budeprion SR) 100mg, 150mg

CONTRAINDICATIONS
Seizure disorder, current/prior diagnosis of bulimia or anorexia nervosa. Use of MAOIs (intended to treat psychiatric disorders) either concomitantly or within 14 days of discontinuing treatment. Treatment within 14 days of discontinuing treatment with an MAOI. Starting treatment in patients being treated with reversible MAOIs (eg, linezolid, IV methylene blue). (Wellbutrin SR) Undergoing abrupt discontinuation of alcohol, benzodiazepines, barbiturates, or antiepileptic drugs. (Budeprion SR) Treated currently with other bupropion products, undergoing abrupt discontinuation of alcohol or sedatives (including benzodiazepines).

WARNINGS/PRECAUTIONS
Dose-related risk of seizures; titrate dose gradually. D/C and do not restart treatment if a seizure occurs. May precipitate a manic, mixed, or hypomanic manic episode; not approved for use in treating bipolar depression. Neuropsychiatric signs and symptoms (eg, delusions, hallucinations, psychosis, concentration disturbance) reported. May result in elevated BP and HTN. D/C treatment if allergic or anaphylactoid/anaphylactic reactions occur. Arthralgia, myalgia, fever with rash, and other serum sickness-like symptoms suggestive of delayed hypersensitivity reported. Caution with renal/hepatic impairment, and in elderly. False (+) urine immunoassay screening tests for amphetamines reported. (Wellbutrin SR) Caution with conditions that may increase risk of seizure. Pupillary dilation that occurs following use may trigger an angle-closure attack in a patient with anatomically narrow angles who does not have a patent iridectomy. (Budeprion SR) Extreme caution with history of seizures, cranial trauma, CNS tumor, or other predisposition(s) toward seizure, and severe hepatic cirrhosis. Agitation, anxiety, and insomnia reported. Altered appetite/weight reported. Caution with recent myocardial infarction and unstable heart disease. (Budeprion SR 100mg) contains tartrazine, which may cause allergic-type reactions (including bronchial asthma) in certain susceptible persons; frequently seen in patients who also have aspirin sensitivity.

ADVERSE REACTIONS
Headache, infection, abdominal pain, dry mouth, N/V, constipation, anorexia, insomnia, dizziness, agitation, anxiety, pharyngitis, sweating, rash, tinnitus.

DRUG INTERACTIONS
See Contraindications. Extreme caution with other drugs that lower seizure threshold (eg, other bupropion products, antipsychotics, antidepressants, theophylline, systemic corticosteroids); use low initial doses and increase the dose gradually. Increased risk of seizure with use of illicit drugs (eg, cocaine), abuse or misuse of prescription drugs (eg, CNS stimulants), use of oral hypoglycemic drugs or insulin, use of anorectic drugs, and excessive use of alcohol, benzodiazepines, sedative/hypnotics, or opiates. Ritonavir, lopinavir, or efavirenz may decrease exposure; may need to increase bupropion dose but not to exceed max dose. Carbamazepine, phenytoin, and phenobarbital may induce metabolism and decrease exposure. May reduce efficacy of drugs that

require metabolic activation by CYP2D6 to be effective (eg, tamoxifen). CNS toxicity reported when coadministered with levodopa or amantadine; use with caution. Minimize or avoid alcohol. Monitor for HTN with nicotine replacement therapy. Potential for drug interactions with CYP2B6 inhibitors/inducers. Increased risk of HTN with MAOIs or other drugs that increase dopaminergic or noradrenergic activity. May increase exposure of CYP2D6 substrates (eg, antidepressants, antipsychotics, β-blockers, and type 1C antiarrhythmics [eg, propafenone, flecainide]); may need to decrease the dose of CYP2D6 substrates, particularly for drugs with a narrow therapeutic index. (Wellbutrin SR) CYP2B6 inhibitors (eg, ticlopidine, clopidogrel) may increase bupropion exposure but decrease hydroxybupropion exposure; may need to adjust dose. If used concomitantly with a CYP inducer, may need to increase the dose of bupropion, but not to exceed the max dose. (Budeprion SR) Paroxetine, sertraline, norfluoxetine, nelfinavir, and fluvoxamine may inhibit hydroxylation. Cimetidine may increase levels of some active metabolites. May increase citalopram levels.

NURSING CONSIDERATIONS

Assessment: Assess for bipolar disorder, hepatic/renal dysfunction, seizure disorders or conditions that may increase risk of seizure, susceptibility to angle-closure glaucoma, hypersensitivity to the drug, and any other conditions where treatment is contraindicated or cautioned, pregnancy/nursing status, and for possible drug interactions. Obtain baseline BP.

Monitoring: Monitor for clinical worsening, suicidality, or unusual changes in behaviors, neuropsychiatric symptoms, suicide risk in smoking cessation treatment, seizures, HTN, activation of mania or hypomania, psychosis and other neuropsychiatric reactions, angle-closure glaucoma, anaphylactoid/anaphylactic reactions, delayed hypersensitivity, and other adverse reactions. Monitor hepatic/renal function, especially in elderly.

Patient Counseling: Inform of benefits/risks of therapy. Advise patients and caregivers of need for close observation for clinical worsening and/or suicidal risks. Educate on the symptoms of hypersensitivity and to d/c if a severe allergic reaction occurs. Instruct to d/c and not restart if a seizure occurs while on therapy. Inform that therapy may impair mental/physical abilities; advise to use caution while operating hazardous machinery/driving. Inform that excessive use or abrupt discontinuation of alcohol or sedatives may alter the seizure threshold; advise to minimize or avoid alcohol use. Instruct to notify physician if taking/planning to take any prescription or OTC medications. Advise not to use therapy in combination with other medicines containing bupropion hydrochloride. Advise to contact physician if pregnancy occurs or is intended during therapy. (Wellbutrin SR) Caution about the risk of angle-closure glaucoma in susceptible patients.

Storage: (Wellbutrin SR) 20-25°C (68-77°F); excursions permitted 15-30°C (59-86°F). Protect from light and moisture. (Budeprion SR) 20-25°C (68-77°F). Dispense in tightly closed, light-resistant container.

WELLBUTRIN XL – bupropion hydrochloride RX

Class: Aminoketone

Antidepressants increased the risk of suicidal thoughts and behavior in children, adolescents, and young adults in short-term trials. Monitor closely for worsening, and for emergence of suicidal thoughts and behaviors. Advise families and caregivers of the need for close observation and communication with the prescriber. Serious neuropsychiatric reactions reported in patients taking bupropion for smoking cessation; not approved for smoking cessation. Observe all patients for neuropsychiatric reactions.

ADULT DOSAGE

Major Depressive Disorder

Initial: 150mg qd in the am
Titrate: May increase to 300mg qd on Day 4
Maint: Reassess periodically to determine need for maint treatment and the appropriate dose

Seasonal Affective Disorder

Initial: 150mg qd in the am
Titrate: May increase to 300mg qd after 7 days
Max: 300mg
Prevention of Seasonal Major Depressive Disorder Episodes Associated w/ Seasonal Affective Disorder:
Initiate in the autumn, prior to the onset of depressive symptoms. Continue through the winter season; taper and d/c in early spring
Treated w/ 300mg/day: Decrease to 150mg qd before discontinuing

PEDIATRIC DOSAGE

Pediatric use may not have been established

Individualize timing of initiation and duration of treatment

Conversions

Switching from Wellbutrin Tab/Wellbutrin SR Tab:
Give same total daily dose when possible

Dosing Considerations with MAOIs

Switching to/from a MAOI Antidepressant:
Allow at least 14 days between discontinuation of an MAOI and initiation of treatment, and allow at least 14 days between discontinuation of treatment and initiation of an MAOI

W/ Other MAOIs (eg, Linezolid, IV Methylene Blue):
Do not start bupropion in a patient being treated w/ linezolid or IV methylene blue
In patients already receiving bupropion, if acceptable alternatives are not available and benefits outweigh risks, d/c bupropion and administer linezolid or IV methylene blue; monitor for 2 weeks or until 24 hrs after the last dose of linezolid or IV methylene blue, whichever comes 1st. May resume bupropion therapy 24 hrs after the last dose of linezolid or IV methylene blue

DOSE MODIFICATION

Renal Impairment

GFR <90mL/min: Consider reducing dose and/or frequency

Hepatic Impairment

Mild (Child-Pugh Score 5-6): Consider reducing dose and/or frequency
Moderate to Severe (Child-Pugh Score 7-15) Max Dose: 150mg qod

Discontinuation

Treated w/ 300mg qd: Decrease to 150mg qd prior to discontinuation

ADMINISTRATION

Oral route
Administer in the am, w/ or w/o food
Swallow whole; do not crush, divide, or chew

HOW SUPPLIED

Tab, ER: 150mg, 300mg

CONTRAINDICATIONS

Seizure disorder, current/prior diagnosis of bulimia or anorexia nervosa. Undergoing abrupt discontinuation of alcohol, benzodiazepines, barbiturates, and antiepileptic drugs. Use of MAOIs (intended to treat psychiatric disorders) either concomitantly or w/in 14 days of discontinuing treatment. Treatment within 14 days of discontinuing treatment with an MAOI. Starting treatment in patients being treated with reversible MAOIs (eg, linezolid, IV methylene blue).

WARNINGS/PRECAUTIONS

Dose-related risk of seizures; increase dose gradually, and do not exceed 300mg qd. D/C and do not restart treatment if a seizure occurs. Caution with conditions that may increase risk of seizure. May result in elevated BP and HTN. May precipitate a manic, mixed, or hypomanic manic episode; not approved for treatment of bipolar depression. Neuropsychiatric signs and symptoms (eg, delusions, hallucinations, psychosis) reported; d/c if these reactions occur. Pupillary dilation that occurs following use may trigger an angle-closure attack in a patient with anatomically narrow angles who does not have a patent iridectomy. Anaphylactoid/anaphylactic reactions reported; d/c treatment if these reactions occur. Erythema multiforme, Stevens-Johnson syndrome, and anaphylactic shock rarely reported. Arthralgia, myalgia, fever with rash, and other symptoms of serum sickness suggestive of delayed hypersensitivity reported. Caution in elderly. False (+) urine immunoassay screening tests for amphetamines reported.

ADVERSE REACTIONS

Headache, infection, dry mouth, nausea, insomnia, dizziness, agitation, tremor, anxiety, constipation, pharyngitis, sweating, tinnitus, diarrhea, anorexia, rash.

DRUG INTERACTIONS

See Contraindications. Extreme caution with drugs that lower seizure threshold (eg, other bupropion products, antipsychotics, antidepressants, theophylline, systemic corticosteroids); use low initial doses and increase the dose gradually. Increased risk of seizure with use of illicit drugs (eg, cocaine), abuse or misuse of prescription drugs (eg, CNS stimulants), use of oral hypoglycemic drugs or insulin, use of anorectic drugs, and excessive use of alcohol, benzodiazepines, sedative/hypnotics, or opiates. Potential for drug interactions with CYP2B6 inhibitors/inducers. CYP2B6 inhibitors (eg, ticlopidine, clopidogrel) may increase bupropion exposure but decrease hydroxybupropion exposure; may need to adjust bupropion dose. Ritonavir, lopinavir, and efavirenz may decrease exposure; may need to increase bupropion dose but not to exceed max dose. Carbamazepine, phenytoin, and phenobarbital may induce metabolism and decrease exposure. If used concomitantly with a CYP inducer, may need to increase bupropion dose, but not to exceed the max dose. May increase exposure of CYP2D6 substrates (eg, antidepressants, antipsychotics, β-blockers, type 1C antiarrhythmics [eg, propafenone, flecainide]); may need to decrease the dose of CYP2D6 substrates, particularly for drugs with a narrow therapeutic index. May reduce efficacy of drugs that require metabolic activation by CYP2D6 to be effective (eg, tamoxifen); may require increased doses of such drugs. CNS toxicity reported when coadministered with levodopa or amantadine; use with caution. Minimize or avoid alcohol. Increased risk of HTN with MAOIs or other drugs that increase dopaminergic or noradrenergic activity. Monitor BP with nicotine replacement therapy.

NURSING CONSIDERATIONS

Assessment: Assess for seizure disorders or conditions that may increase risk of seizure, susceptibility to angle-closure glaucoma, renal/hepatic impairment, hypersensitivity to the drug, any other conditions where treatment is contraindicated or cautioned, pregnancy/nursing status, and possible drug interactions. Obtain baseline BP and screen for risk factors/a history of bipolar disorder.

Monitoring: Monitor for clinical worsening, suicidality, unusual changes in behavior, seizures, activation of mania or hypomania, psychosis and other neuropsychiatric reactions, angle-closure glaucoma, anaphylactoid/anaphylactic reactions, delayed hypersensitivity, and other adverse reactions. Monitor BP periodically. Monitor hepatic/renal function, especially in the elderly.

Patient Counseling: Inform of benefits/risks of therapy and counsel in its appropriate use. Advise patients and caregivers of the need for close observation for clinical worsening and/or suicidal risk. Educate on the symptoms of hypersensitivity and advise to d/c if a severe allergic reaction occurs. Instruct to d/c and not restart if a seizure occurs while on therapy. Inform that excessive use or abrupt discontinuation of alcohol or sedatives may alter the seizure threshold; advise to minimize or avoid alcohol use. Caution about the risk of angle-closure glaucoma in susceptible patients. Advise not to use therapy in combination with other medicines containing bupropion hydrochloride. Inform that therapy may impair mental/physical abilities; advise to use caution while operating hazardous machinery/driving. Instruct to notify physician if taking/planning to take any prescription or OTC medications. Advise to contact physician if pregnancy occurs or is intended during therapy. Communicate with the patient and pediatric healthcare provider regarding the infant's exposure to bupropion through human milk; instruct caregivers to immediately contact the infant's healthcare provider if they note any side effect in the infant that concerns them or is persistent.

Storage: 25°C (77°F); excursions permitted to 15-30°C (59-86°F).

XALATAN – latanoprost RX

Class: Prostaglandin analogue

ADULT DOSAGE

Elevated Intraocular Pressure

Open-Angle Glaucoma/Ocular HTN:
Usual: 1 drop in affected eye(s) qd in pm
Max: Once-daily dosing

PEDIATRIC DOSAGE

Pediatric use may not have been established

DOSE MODIFICATION

Concomitant Medications

Space by at least 5 min if using >1 topical ophthalmic drug

ADMINISTRATION

Ocular route

Continue w/ the next dose as normal if 1 dose is missed

HOW SUPPLIED

Sol: 0.005% [2.5mL]

WARNINGS/PRECAUTIONS

May cause changes to pigmented tissues (eg, increased pigmentation of iris [may be permanent], periorbital tissue/eyelashes [may be reversible]); regularly examine patients who develop noticeably increased iris pigmentation. May gradually change eyelashes and vellus hair in the treated eye. Caution with a history of intraocular inflammation (iritis/uveitis). Macular edema, including cystoid macular edema, reported; caution in aphakic patients, pseudophakic patients with a torn posterior lens capsule, or patients with known risk factors for macular edema. Reactivation of herpes simplex keratitis reported; caution with a history of herpetic keratitis. Avoid with active intraocular inflammation and in cases of active herpes simplex keratitis; inflammation may be exacerbated. Bacterial keratitis associated with the use of multiple-dose containers reported. Contact lenses should be removed prior to administration and may be reinserted 15 min after administration.

ADVERSE REACTIONS

Foreign body sensation, punctate epithelial keratopathy, stinging, itching, burning, conjunctival hyperemia, blurred vision, increased iris pigmentation, excessive tearing, lid discomfort/pain, dry eye, eye pain, lid crusting, lid erythema, URTI/cold/flu.

DRUG INTERACTIONS

Combined use of ≥2 prostaglandins or prostaglandin analogues is not recommended; administration of these prostaglandin drug products more than once daily may decrease the IOP-lowering effect or cause paradoxical IOP elevations. Precipitation occurs when mixed with eye drops containing thimerosal; if such drugs are used, they should be administered at least 5 min apart.

NURSING CONSIDERATIONS

Assessment: Assess for hypersensitivity to drug or benzalkonium chloride, history of or active intraocular inflammation, history of herpetic keratitis, active herpes simplex keratitis, aphakia, pseudophakia with a torn posterior lens capsule, risk factors for macular edema, pregnancy/nursing status, and possible drug interactions.

Monitoring: Monitor for changes to pigmented tissues, eyelash changes, macular edema, herpetic/bacterial keratitis, and other adverse reactions.

Patient Counseling: Inform about the possibility of increased brown pigmentation of the iris, eyelid skin darkening, and eyelash and vellus hair changes in the treated eye. Instruct to avoid allowing the tip of the dispensing container to contact the eye or surrounding structures to avoid contamination. Advise to immediately consult physician about the continued use of treatment if an intercurrent ocular condition (eg, trauma, infection) develops, if undergoing ocular surgery, or if any ocular reactions, particularly conjunctivitis and eyelid reactions, develop. Advise that contact lenses should be removed prior to administration and may be reinserted 15 min after administration. Instruct that if using >1 topical ophthalmic drug, to administer the drugs at least 5 min apart. Inform that if one dose is missed, treatment should continue with the next dose as normal.

Storage: Protect from light. Unopened: 2-8°C (36-46°F). During Shipment to Patient: Up to 40°C (104°F) for a period not exceeding 8 days. Opened: Room temperature up to 25°C (77°F) for 6 weeks.

XANAX – alprazolam CIV

Class: Benzodiazepine

ADULT DOSAGE

Anxiety Disorders

Management of Disorders or Short-Term Relief of Symptoms:
Initial: 0.25-0.5mg tid
Titrate: May increase at intervals of 3-4 days
Max: 4mg/day in divided doses

Panic Disorder

W/ or w/o Agoraphobia:
Initial: 0.5mg tid
Titrate: May increase by ≤1mg/day every 3-4 days; slower titration to doses >4mg/day
Usual: 1-10mg/day

PEDIATRIC DOSAGE

Pediatric use may not have been established

DOSE MODIFICATION

Dose Reduction

May reduce daily dose gradually by ≤0.5mg every 3 days

Hepatic Impairment

Advanced Liver Disease:
Initial: 0.25mg bid-tid
Titrate: May increase gradually prn

Elderly
Initial: 0.25mg bid-tid
Titrate: May increase gradually prn

Other Important Dose Modifications
Debilitated:
Initial: 0.25mg bid-tid
Titrate: May increase gradually prn

ADMINISTRATION
Oral route

HOW SUPPLIED
Tab: 0.25mg*, 0.5mg*, 1mg*, 2mg* *scored

CONTRAINDICATIONS
Acute narrow-angle glaucoma, concomitant ketoconazole or itraconazole.

WARNINGS/PRECAUTIONS
May be used with treated open-angle glaucoma. Increased risk of dependence with doses >4mg/day, treatment for >12 weeks, and in panic disorder patients. Seizures, including status epilepticus, reported with dose reduction or abrupt discontinuation. Early am anxiety and emergence of anxiety symptoms between doses reported; give same total daily dose divided as more frequent administrations. Withdrawal reactions may occur; reduce dose or d/c therapy gradually. May impair mental/physical abilities. May cause fetal harm; avoid use during 1st trimester. Hypomania/mania reported in patients with depression. Caution with severe depression, suicidal ideation/plans, impaired renal/hepatic/pulmonary function, elderly, and debilitated patients. Has a weak uricosuric effect. Decreased systemic elimination rate with alcoholic liver disease/obesity.

ADVERSE REACTIONS
Drowsiness, lightheadedness, fatigue/tiredness, irritability, depression, headache, confusion, insomnia, dry mouth, constipation, diarrhea, N/V, tachycardia/palpitations, blurred vision, nasal congestion.

DRUG INTERACTIONS
See Contraindications. Not recommended with azole antifungals. Avoid with very potent CYP3A inhibitors. Caution with alcohol, other CNS depressants, diltiazem, isoniazid, macrolides (eg, erythromycin, clarithromycin), grapefruit juice, sertraline, paroxetine, ergotamine, cyclosporine, amiodarone, nicardipine, nifedipine, and other CYP3A inhibitors. Additive CNS depressant effects with psychotropics, anticonvulsants, antihistaminics, ethanol, and other drugs that produce CNS depression. Increased digoxin concentrations reported (especially in patients >65 yrs of age); monitor for signs/symptoms of digoxin toxicity. May increase plasma concentrations of imipramine and desipramine. Fluoxetine, fluvoxamine, nefazodone, cimetidine, and oral contraceptives may increase concentrations. CYP3A inducers (eg, carbamazepine), propoxyphene, and smoking may decrease levels. May require dose adjustment or discontinuation with HIV protease inhibitors (eg, ritonavir).

NURSING CONSIDERATIONS

Assessment: Assess for drug hypersensitivity, acute narrow-angle glaucoma, depression, suicidal ideation, renal/hepatic/pulmonary function, debilitation, history of alcohol/substance abuse, history of seizures/epilepsy, pregnancy/nursing status, and possible drug interactions. Assess for risk of dependence among panic disorder patients.

Monitoring: Monitor for dependence, rebound/withdrawal symptoms, early am anxiety and emergence of anxiety symptoms, CNS depression, episodes of hypomania/mania, suicidality, other treatment-emergent symptoms, and adverse reactions. Monitor CBC, urinalysis, and blood chemistry periodically. Periodically reassess usefulness of therapy.

Patient Counseling: Advise to inform physician about any alcohol consumption and medicines taken and if nursing, pregnant, planning to be pregnant, or if pregnancy occurs while on therapy. Advise to avoid alcohol during treatment. Advise not to drive or operate dangerous machinery until becoming familiar with the effects of therapy. Advise not to increase/decrease dose or abruptly d/c therapy without consultation; instruct to follow gradual dosage-tapering schedule. Inform of risks associated with doses >4mg/day.

Storage: 20-25°C (68-77°F).

XANAX XR – alprazolam

CIV

Class: Benzodiazepine

ADULT DOSAGE

Panic Disorder

W/ or w/o Agoraphobia:

Initial: 0.5-1mg qd, preferably in the am
Titrate: May increase at intervals of 3-4 days in increments of ≤1mg/day
Usual: 3-6mg/day; some patients may require doses >6mg/day
Maint: 1-10mg/day

Conversions

Switching from Immediate-Release (IR) Tabs to Extended-Release (ER) Tabs:
Patients who are currently being treated w/ divided doses of IR alprazolam tabs may be switched to ER tabs at the same total daily dose taken qd. If therapeutic response after switching is inadequate, may titrate dose as recommended

PEDIATRIC DOSAGE

Pediatric use may not have been established

DOSE MODIFICATION

Hepatic Impairment

Advanced Liver Disease:
Initial: 0.5mg qd
Titrate: May increase gradually if needed and tolerated

Elderly

Elderly/Debilitated:
Initial: 0.5mg qd
Titrate: May increase gradually if needed and tolerated

Discontinuation

Reduce dose gradually when discontinuing therapy or when decreasing daily dosage. Decrease daily dose by no more than 0.5mg every 3 days; some patients may require an even slower dosage reduction

ADMINISTRATION

Oral route

May be administered qd, preferably in the am
Tabs should be taken intact; do not chew, crush, or break

HOW SUPPLIED

Tab, Extended-Release (ER): 0.5mg, 1mg, 2mg, 3mg

CONTRAINDICATIONS

Acute narrow-angle glaucoma, concomitant ketoconazole or itraconazole.

WARNINGS/PRECAUTIONS

May be used with treated open-angle glaucoma. Increased risk of dependence with doses >4mg/day, treatment for >12 weeks, and in panic disorder patients. Seizures, including status epilepticus, reported with dose reduction or abrupt discontinuation. Early am anxiety/emergence of anxiety symptoms between doses reported. Withdrawal reactions may occur; reduce dose or d/c therapy gradually. May impair mental/physical abilities. May cause fetal harm; avoid use during 1st trimester. Caution with severe depression, suicidal ideation/plans, impaired renal/hepatic/pulmonary function, elderly, and debilitated patients. Hypomania/mania reported in patients with depression. Has a weak uricosuric effect. Decreased systemic elimination rate with alcoholic liver disease/obesity.

ADVERSE REACTIONS

Sedation, somnolence, memory impairment, dysarthria, abnormal coordination, fatigue, depression, constipation, mental impairment, ataxia, dry mouth, nausea, decreased libido, increased/decreased appetite/weight.

DRUG INTERACTIONS

See Contraindications. Not recommended with azole antifungals. Avoid with very potent CYP3A inhibitors. Caution with alcohol, other CNS depressants, diltiazem, isoniazid, macrolides (eg, erythromycin, clarithromycin), grapefruit juice, sertraline, paroxetine, ergotamine, cyclosporine, amiodarone, nicardipine, nifedipine, and other CYP3A inhibitors. Additive CNS depressant effects with psychotropics, anticonvulsants, antihistaminics, ethanol, and other drugs that produce CNS depression. Increased digoxin concentrations reported (especially in patients >65 yrs of age); monitor for signs/symptoms of digoxin toxicity. May increase plasma concentrations of imipramine and desipramine. Fluoxetine, fluvoxamine, nefazodone, cimetidine, and oral contraceptives may increase concentrations. CYP3A inducers (eg, carbamazepine), propoxyphene, and smoking may decrease levels. May require dose adjustment or discontinuation with HIV protease inhibitors (eg, ritonavir).

NURSING CONSIDERATIONS

Assessment: Assess for drug hypersensitivity, acute narrow-angle glaucoma, depression, suicidal ideation, renal/hepatic/pulmonary function, debilitation, history of alcohol/substance abuse, history of seizures/epilepsy, pregnancy/nursing status, and possible drug interactions. Assess for risk of dependence among panic disorder patients.

Monitoring: Monitor for dependence, relapse, rebound or withdrawal symptoms, early am anxiety and emergence of anxiety symptoms, CNS depression, episodes of hypomania/mania, suicidality, other treatment-emergent symptoms, and other adverse reactions. Monitor CBC, urinalysis, and blood chemistry periodically. Periodically reassess usefulness of therapy.

Patient Counseling: Advise to take in the am and not crush or chew tabs. Advise to inform physician about any alcohol consumption and medicines taken and if nursing, pregnant, planning to be pregnant, or if pregnancy occurs while on therapy. Advise to avoid alcohol during treatment. Advise not to drive or operate dangerous machinery until becoming familiar with the effects of the medication. Advise not to increase/decrease dose or abruptly d/c therapy without consultation; instruct to follow gradual dosage-tapering schedule. Inform of risks associated with doses >4mg/day.

Storage: 25°C (77°F); excursions permitted to 15-30°C (59-86°F).

XARELTO – rivaroxaban

RX

Class: Selective factor Xa inhibitor

Premature discontinuation increases the risk of thrombotic events. If therapy is discontinued for a reason other than pathological bleeding or completion of a course of therapy, consider coverage with another anticoagulant. Epidural or spinal hematomas have occurred in patients treated with rivaroxaban who are receiving neuraxial anesthesia or undergoing spinal puncture; long-term or permanent paralysis may result. Use of indwelling epidural catheters, concomitant use of other drugs that affect hemostasis (eg, NSAIDs, platelet inhibitors, other anticoagulants), history of traumatic or repeated epidural or spinal punctures, history of spinal deformity or spinal surgery, or unknown optimal timing between the administration of therapy and neuraxial procedure, may increase the risk of developing epidural or spinal hematomas. Monitor frequently for signs/symptoms of neurological impairment; urgent treatment is necessary if neurological compromise occurs. Consider benefits and risks before neuraxial intervention in patients anticoagulated or to be anticoagulated for thromboprophylaxis.

ADULT DOSAGE

Reduce Risk of Stroke and Systemic Embolism in Nonvalvular Atrial Fibrillation

20mg qd w/ pm meal

Deep Vein Thrombosis/Pulmonary Embolism

Prophylaxis:
Following Hip or Knee Replacement Surgery:
10mg qd
Give initial dose 6-10 hrs after surgery provided that hemostasis has been established

Treatment Duration:
Hip Replacement Surgery: 35 days
Knee Replacement Surgery: 12 days

Treatment:
15mg bid w/ food for the first 21 days, then 20mg qd w/ food, at approx the same time each day

Reduction in Risk of Recurrence Following Initial 6 Months of Treatment:
20mg qd w/ food at approx the same time each day

Conversions

Switching from Warfarin:
D/C warfarin and start therapy as soon as INR is <3.0

Switching to Warfarin:
No clinical trial data available to guide conversion; d/c rivaroxaban and begin both a parenteral anticoagulant and warfarin at the time the next dose of rivaroxaban would have been taken

PEDIATRIC DOSAGE

Pediatric use may not have been established

Switching from Other Anticoagulants:
Start rivaroxaban 0-2 hrs prior to next scheduled pm dose of drug (eg, low molecular weight heparin or non-warfarin oral anticoagulant) and omit administration of other anticoagulant
For continuous IV infusion of unfractionated heparin, stop infusion and start rivaroxaban at the same time

Switching to Other Anticoagulants:
If switching to rapid onset anticoagulant, d/c rivaroxaban and give 1st dose of other anticoagulant (oral or parenteral) at the time that the next dose would have been taken

Missed Dose

Receiving 15mg bid:
Take rivaroxaban immediately to ensure intake of 30mg/day; may take two 15mg tabs at once
Continue w/ regular 15mg bid as recommended on following day

Receiving 20mg, 15mg, or 10mg qd:
Take missed dose immediately

DOSE MODIFICATION

Renal Impairment

Reduction in Risk of Stroke in Nonvalvular Atrial Fibrillation:
CrCl 15-50mL/min: 15mg qd w/ pm meal

Hepatic Impairment

Moderate (Child-Pugh B) and Severe (Child-Pugh C): Avoid use

Other Important Modifications

Surgery/Intervention:
If anticoagulation must be discontinued w/ surgery or other procedures, d/c therapy at least 24 hrs before procedure to reduce the risk of bleeding
Weigh risk of bleeding against urgency of intervention to decide whether procedure should be delayed until 24 hrs after last dose
After procedure, restart therapy as soon as adequate hemostasis has been established

ADMINISTRATION

Oral route
15mg and 20mg tabs should be taken w/ food, while 10mg tabs can be taken w/ or w/o food

Unable to Swallow Whole Tabs
Tabs may be crushed and mixed w/ applesauce immediately prior to use
After administering crushed 15mg or 20mg tabs, immediately follow dose w/ food

Administration via NG Tube/Gastric Feeding Tube
Tabs may be crushed and suspended in 50mL of water after confirming gastric placement of tube
Avoid administration distal to the stomach
After administration of 15mg or 20mg tabs, immediately follow dose w/ enteral feeding

Stability
Crushed tabs are stable in water and applesauce for up to 4 hrs

HOW SUPPLIED

Tab: 10mg, 15mg, 20mg; (Starter Pack) 15mg [42[s]], 20mg [9[s]]

CONTRAINDICATIONS

Active pathological bleeding.

WARNINGS/PRECAUTIONS

May increase risk of bleeding and cause serious or fatal bleeding; risk of thrombotic events should be weighed against risk of bleeding before initiation of treatment. Promptly evaluate any signs/symptoms of blood loss and consider the need for blood replacement; d/c in patients with active pathological hemorrhage. An epidural catheter should not be removed earlier than 18 hrs after last administration of therapy. The next dose should not be administered earlier than 6 hrs after catheter removal. If traumatic puncture occurs, delay administration for 24 hrs. Avoid use in the treatment of DVT/PE, reduction in risk of recurrence of DVT/PE, and for prophylaxis of DVT following hip or knee replacement surgery in patients with CrCl <30mL/min or for nonvalvular A-fib in patients with CrCl <15mL/min. Monitor for signs/symptoms of blood loss in patients with CrCl 30-50mL/min in prophylaxis of DVT following hip or knee replacement surgery. D/C therapy if acute renal failure develops. Avoid with any hepatic disease associated with coagulopathy. Caution in pregnant women due to the potential for pregnancy-related hemorrhage and/or emergent delivery. Not recommended in patients with prosthetic heart valves. Initiation of treatment is not recommended acutely as an alternative to unfractionated heparin in patients with pulmonary embolism (PE) who present with hemodynamic instability or who may receive thrombolysis or pulmonary embolectomy.

ADVERSE REACTIONS

Bleeding events, back pain.

DRUG INTERACTIONS

See Boxed Warning. May result in changes in exposure with inhibitors/inducers of CYP3A4/5, CYP2J2, and P-gp and ATP-binding cassette G2 transporters. Increased exposure with combined P-gp and CYP3A4 inhibitors (eg, ketoconazole, ritonavir, clarithromycin) may increase bleeding risk; avoid with combined P-gp and strong CYP3A4 inhibitors (eg, ketoconazole, itraconazole, lopinavir/ritonavir). Avoid with combined P-gp and strong CYP3A4 inducers (eg, carbamazepine, phenytoin, rifampin); may decrease exposure and efficacy. Concomitant single dose of enoxaparin resulted in an additive effect on anti-factor Xa activity. Concomitant single dose of warfarin resulted in an additive effect on factor Xa inhibition and PT. Concomitant use of other drugs that impair hemostasis (eg, P2Y12 platelet inhibitors, other antithrombotic agents, fibrinolytic therapy, NSAIDs/ASA) increases the risk of bleeding. May increase bleeding time with clopidogrel. Avoid concurrent use with other anticoagulants due to increased bleeding risk unless benefit outweighs risk. Increased exposure and possible increased bleeding risk with combined P-gp and moderate CYP3A4 inhibitors (eg, diltiazem, dronedarone, erythromycin) in renally impaired patients; avoid use in patients with CrCl 15-80mL/min who are receiving concomitant combined P-gp and moderate CYP3A4 inhibitors unless potential benefit justifies risk.

NURSING CONSIDERATIONS

Assessment: Assess for known hypersensitivity, active pathological bleeding, risk factors for developing epidural or spinal hematomas, conditions that may increase risk of bleeding, renal/hepatic impairment, prosthetic heart valves, PE with hemodynamic instability or patients who may receive thrombolysis or pulmonary embolectomy, pregnancy/nursing status, and possible drug interactions.

Monitoring: Monitor for signs/symptoms of bleeding, stroke, thrombotic events, and other adverse reactions. In patients undergoing neuraxial anesthesia or spinal puncture, monitor for epidural or spinal hematomas and neurological impairment. Monitor renal function periodically.

Patient Counseling: Instruct to take only ud. Advise to follow missed dosing instructions. Advise not to d/c without consulting physician. Advise to report any unusual bleeding or bruising. Inform that it may take longer than usual to stop bleeding, and that patients may bruise and/or bleed more easily. Advise patients who had neuraxial anesthesia or spinal puncture to watch for signs and symptoms of spinal/epidural hematoma, especially if concomitantly taking NSAIDs or platelet inhibitors; instruct to contact physician immediately if symptoms occur. Instruct to inform physician about therapy before any invasive procedure. Instruct to inform physicians and dentists if taking, or planning to take, any prescription or OTC drugs or herbals. Advise to inform physician immediately if nursing/pregnant or intending to nurse or become pregnant. Advise pregnant women receiving therapy to immediately report to the physician any bleeding or symptoms of blood loss.

Storage: 25°C (77°F); excursions permitted to 15-30°C (59-86°F).

XELJANZ – tofacitinib

RX

Class: Kinase inhibitors

Increased risk for developing serious infections (eg, active tuberculosis [TB], invasive fungal infections, bacterial/viral infections due to opportunistic pathogens) that may lead to hospitalization or death. Most patients who developed these infections were taking concomitant immunosuppressants (eg, methotrexate [MTX], corticosteroids). If a serious infection develops, interrupt treatment until infection is controlled. Test for latent TB prior to and during therapy; initiate latent TB treatment prior to therapy. Consider risks and benefits prior to initiating therapy in patients with chronic or recurrent infection. Monitor for development of signs and symptoms of infection during and after treatment. Lymphoma and other malignancies reported. Increased rate of Epstein-Barr virus-associated post-transplant lymphoproliferative disorder observed in renal transplant patients with concomitant immunosuppressive medications.

ADULT DOSAGE

Rheumatoid Arthritis

As monotherapy or in combination w/ methotrexate or other nonbiologic disease-modifying antirheumatic drugs for moderately to severely active rheumatoid arthritis in patients who have had an inadequate response or intolerance to methotrexate

Usual: 5mg bid

PEDIATRIC DOSAGE

Pediatric use may not have been established

DOSE MODIFICATION

Concomitant Medications

Potent CYP3A4 Inhibitors: Reduce dose to 5mg qd

≥1 Concomitant Medications Resulting in Both Moderate CYP3A4 Inhibition and Potent CYP2C19 Inhibition: Reduce dose to 5mg qd

Potent CYP3A4 Inducers: Not recommended for use

Renal Impairment

Moderate or Severe: Reduce dose to 5mg qd

Hepatic Impairment

Moderate: Reduce dose to 5mg qd

Severe: Not recommended for use

Adverse Reactions

Lymphopenia:

Absolute Lymphocyte Count <500 cells/mm^3: Do not initiate treatment

Absolute Lymphocyte Count ≥500 cells/mm^3: Maintain dose

Absolute Lymphocyte Count <500 cells/mm^3 (confirmed by repeat testing): D/C treatment

Neutropenia:

Absolute Neutrophil Count (ANC) <1000 cells/mm^3: Do not initiate treatment

ANC >1000 cells/mm^3: Maintain dose

ANC 500-1000 cells/mm^3: For persistent decreases in this range, interrupt dosing until ANC is >1000; when ANC is >1000, resume at 5mg bid

ANC <500 cells/mm^3 (confirmed by repeat testing): D/C treatment

Anemia:

Hgb <9g/dL: Do not initiate treatment

Hgb ≤2g/dL Decrease and ≥9g/dL: Maintain dose

Hgb >2g/dL Decrease or <8g/dL (confirmed by repeat testing): Interrupt administration until Hgb values have normalized

ADMINISTRATION

Oral route

Take w/ or w/o food

HOW SUPPLIED

Tab: 5mg

WARNINGS/PRECAUTIONS

Avoid with active, serious infection, including localized infections. Caution in patients with chronic/recurrent infections, who have been exposed to TB, with history of a serious/opportunistic infection, who have resided in or traveled to areas of endemic TB/mycoses, or with predisposing factors to infection. Viral reactivation, including herpes virus reactivation (eg, herpes zoster), reported; screen for viral hepatitis before starting therapy. Non-melanoma skin cancers reported; periodic skin examination is recommended for patients at increased risk for skin cancer. Consider risks and benefits of treatment in patients with a known malignancy other than a successfully treated non-melanoma skin cancer or when considering continuing treatment in patients who develop a malignancy. GI perforation reported; caution in patients with increased risk for GI perforation (eg, history of diverticulitis). Associated with initial lymphocytosis, neutropenia, increase in lipid parameters, and liver enzyme elevations. Interrupt treatment if drug-induced liver injury is suspected. Use in patients with severe hepatic impairment, absolute lymphocyte count <500 cells/mm^3, absolute neutrophil count (ANC) <1000 cells/mm^3, or Hgb levels <9g/dL is not recommended. D/C if an opportunistic infection or sepsis occurs. Caution in elderly.

ADVERSE REACTIONS

Infections (eg, upper respiratory tract infections, nasopharyngitis), lymphoma, malignancies, diarrhea, headache.

DRUG INTERACTIONS

See Boxed Warning. Avoid with live vaccines. Increased immunosuppression with potent immunosuppressive drugs (eg, azathioprine, tacrolimus, cyclosporine); concurrent use with potent immunosuppressants (eg, azathioprine, cyclosporine) or biologic DMARDs is not recommended. Increased exposure with potent CYP3A4 inhibitors (eg, ketoconazole), and drugs that are both moderate CYP3A4 inhibitors and potent CYP2C19 inhibitors (eg, fluconazole). Decreased exposure resulting in loss of or reduced clinical response to treatment with potent CYP3A4 inducers (eg, rifampin); coadministration is not recommended.

NURSING CONSIDERATIONS

Assessment: Assess for infections (eg, bacteria, fungi, viruses), including latent TB, predisposing factors to infection, active hepatic disease or impairment, known malignancy, risk of GI perforation, pregnancy/nursing status, and possible drug interactions. Obtain baseline absolute lymphocyte count, ANC, and lipid and Hgb levels.

Monitoring: Monitor for TB (active, reactivation, or latent), invasive fungal infections, or bacterial, viral, and other opportunistic infections during and after therapy. Monitor for viral reactivation, lymphoma, malignancy, lymphoproliferative disorders, and GI perforations. Monitor absolute lymphocyte counts every 3 months. Monitor neutrophil counts and Hgb after 4-8 weeks of treatment and every 3 months thereafter. Routinely monitor LFTs. Monitor lipid parameters approximately 4-8 weeks following initiation. Perform periodic skin examination in patients at increased risk of skin cancer.

Patient Counseling: Advise about potential risks/benefits of therapy. Inform that therapy may lower resistance to infection; advise patients not to start taking medication if they have an active infection. Instruct to contact physician immediately if symptoms suggesting an infection appear during treatment to ensure rapid evaluation and appropriate treatment. Inform that medication may increase risk of lymphoma and other cancers; instruct to inform physician of any type of cancer that they have ever had. Inform that certain lab tests may be affected and that blood tests are required before and during treatment. Inform that medication should not be used during pregnancy unless clearly necessary; advise to inform physician right away if pregnant. Advise to enroll in the pregnancy registry for pregnant women who have taken medication during pregnancy.

Storage: 20-25°C (68-77°F).

XELODA – capecitabine **RX**

Class: Fluoropyrimidine carbamate

Altered coagulation parameters and/or bleeding, including death, reported w/ concomitant coumarin-derivative anticoagulants (eg, warfarin, phenprocoumon). Monitor PT and INR frequently in order to adjust anticoagulant dose accordingly. Postmarketing reports showed clinically significant increases in PT and INR in patients who were stabilized on anticoagulants at start of therapy. Age >60 yrs and a diagnosis of cancer independently predispose to an increased risk of coagulopathy.

ADULT DOSAGE

Metastatic Colorectal Cancer

1st-line treatment of metastatic colorectal carcinoma and as a single agent for adjuvant treatment in patients w/ Dukes' C colon cancer who have undergone complete resection of the primary tumor when treatment w/ fluoropyrimidine therapy alone is preferred

Monotherapy:

Usual: 1250mg/m^2 bid for 2 weeks followed by a 1-week rest period, given as 3-week cycles

Adjuvant to Dukes' C Colon Cancer:

Usual: 1250mg/m^2 bid for 2 weeks followed by 1-week rest period, given as 3-week cycles for total of 8 cycles (24 weeks)

Refer to PI for dose calculations based on BSA

Metastatic Breast Cancer

Treatment of metastatic breast cancer in combination w/ docetaxel after failure of prior anthracycline-containing chemotherapy. Monotherapy treatment of metastatic breast cancer in patients resistant to both paclitaxel and anthracycline-containing chemotherapy regimen or resistant to paclitaxel and for whom further anthracycline therapy is not indicated

Monotherapy:

Usual: 1250mg/m^2 bid for 2 weeks followed by a 1-week rest period, given as 3-week cycles

Combination w/ Docetaxel:

Usual: 1250mg/m^2 bid for 2 weeks followed by 1-week rest period, combined w/ docetaxel at 75mg/m^2 as a 1-hr IV infusion every 3 weeks

Premedication:

Start prior to docetaxel administration

Refer to PI for dose calculations based on BSA

PEDIATRIC DOSAGE

Pediatric use may not have been established

DOSE MODIFICATION

Concomitant Medications

Phenytoin and Coumarin-Derivative Anticoagulants: May need to reduce dose of phenytoin and coumarin-derivative anticoagulants

Renal Impairment

Moderate (CrCl 30-50mL/min): Reduce to 75% of starting dose when used as monotherapy or in combination w/ docetaxel (from 1250mg/m^2 to 950mg/m^2 bid)

Adverse Reactions

Toxicity NCIC Grade 2:
1st Appearance: Interrupt until resolved to Grade 0-1, then give 100% of dose
2nd Appearance: Interrupt until resolved to Grade 0-1, then give 75% of dose
3rd Appearance: Interrupt until resolved to Grade 0-1, then give 50% of dose
4th Appearance: D/C treatment permanently

Toxicity NCIC Grade 3:
1st Appearance: Interrupt until resolved to Grade 0-1, then give 75% of dose
2nd Appearance: Interrupt until resolved to Grade 0-1, then give 50% of dose
3rd Appearance: D/C treatment permanently

Toxicity NCIC Grade 4:
1st Appearance: D/C permanently or if physician deems it to be in the best interest to continue, interrupt until resolved to Grade 0-1, then give 50% of dose
Refer to PI for docetaxel dose reductions when used in combination w/ capecitabine

ADMINISTRATION

Oral route

Swallow tabs whole w/ water w/in 30 min pc; do not cut or crush

HOW SUPPLIED

Tab: 150mg, 500mg

CONTRAINDICATIONS

Severe renal impairment (CrCl <30mL/min), known hypersensitivity to 5-fluorouracil (5-FU).

WARNINGS/PRECAUTIONS

May induce diarrhea; give fluid and electrolyte replacement w/ severe diarrhea. Cardiotoxicity (eg, MI/ischemia, angina) observed; may be more common in patients w/ a prior history of coronary artery disease (CAD). Increased risk for acute early-onset of toxicity and severe, life-threatening, or fatal adverse reactions (eg, mucositis, diarrhea, neutropenia, neurotoxicity) in patients w/ certain homozygous or certain compound heterozygous mutations in the dihydropyrimidine dehydrogenase (DPD) gene that results in complete or near complete absence of DPD activity; withhold or permanently d/c therapy based on clinical assessment of the onset, duration, and severity of the observed toxicities. Patients w/ partial DPD activity may also have increased risk of severe, life-threatening, or fatal adverse reactions. Dehydration reported and may cause acute renal failure; patients w/ preexisting compromised renal function are at higher risk. Patients w/ anorexia, asthenia, N/V, or diarrhea may rapidly become dehydrated; monitor during administration and do not restart treatment until patient is rehydrated and any precipitating causes have been corrected or controlled. Caution w/ mild and moderate renal impairment. Severe mucocutaneous reactions (eg, Stevens-Johnson syndrome, toxic epidermal necrolysis) may occur; permanently d/c in patients who experience a severe mucocutaneous reaction possibly attributable to treatment. Hand-and-foot syndrome may occur. Hyperbilirubinemia reported; interrupt therapy if drug-related Grade 3 or 4 elevations in bilirubin occur until the hyperbilirubinemia decreases to ≤3X ULN. Necrotizing enterocolitis, neutropenia, thrombocytopenia, anemia, and decreases in Hgb reported. Avoid w/ baseline neutrophil counts of <1.5 x 10^9/L and/or thrombocyte counts of <100 x 10^9/L. Caution in elderly; patients ≥80 yrs of age may experience greater incidence of Grade 3 or 4 adverse events. Caution w/ mild to moderate hepatic dysfunction due to liver metastases. May cause fetal harm.

ADVERSE REACTIONS

Diarrhea, hand-and-foot syndrome, asthenia, pyrexia, anemia, N/V, fatigue, dermatitis, thrombocytopenia, constipation, taste disturbance, stomatitis, alopecia, abdominal pain, decreased appetite.

DRUG INTERACTIONS

See Boxed Warning and Dose Modification. Higher risk of dehydration w/ known nephrotoxic agents. May increase the mean AUC of S-warfarin. May increase phenytoin levels. Leucovorin may increase levels and toxicity of 5-FU. Caution w/ CYP2C9 substrates.

NURSING CONSIDERATIONS

Assessment: Assess for hypersensitivity to drug or to 5-FU, complete or near complete absence of DPD activity, partial DPD activity, renal/hepatic dysfunction, history of CAD, pregnancy/nursing status, and possible drug interactions. Obtain baseline neutrophil/thrombocyte counts.

Monitoring: Monitor for severe diarrhea, necrotizing enterocolitis, cardiotoxicity, acute early-onset of toxicity, severe/life-threatening/fatal adverse reactions, hand-and-foot syndrome, hyperbilirubinemia, neutropenia, thrombocytopenia, anemia, decreases in Hgb, severe toxicity, dehydration, acute renal failure, severe mucocutaneous reactions, and other adverse reactions. Monitor PT and INR frequently w/ concomitant oral coumarin-derivative anticoagulant therapy.

Patient Counseling: Instruct to d/c therapy and contact physician immediately if moderate/severe toxicity, Grade ≥2 diarrhea/stomatitis, or severe bloody diarrhea w/ severe abdominal pain and fever is experienced. Advise to notify physician if patient has known DPD deficiency; inform that patient is at an increased risk of acute early-onset of toxicity and severe, life-threatening, or fatal adverse reactions if patient has complete or near complete absence of DPD activity. Instruct to d/c therapy immediately in patients experiencing Grade ≥2 dehydration/nausea/vomiting/hand-and-foot syndrome. Instruct to contact physician immediately if fever or infection occurs. Counsel about pregnancy risks; instruct to avoid pregnancy during therapy.

Storage: 25°C (77°F); excursions permitted to 15-30°C (59-86°F). Keep tightly closed.

XERESE – acyclovir/hydrocortisone RX

Class: Anti-infective/corticosteroid

ADULT DOSAGE

Herpes Labialis (Cold Sores)

Early treatment of recurrent herpes labialis to reduce the likelihood of ulcerative cold sores and to shorten the lesion healing time

Apply a quantity sufficient to cover the affected area (including outer margin) 5X/day for 5 days

Initiate therapy as early as possible after the 1st signs/symptoms (eg, during the prodrome or when lesions appear)

PEDIATRIC DOSAGE

Herpes Labialis (Cold Sores)

Early treatment of recurrent herpes labialis to reduce the likelihood of ulcerative cold sores and to shorten the lesion healing time

≥6 Years:
Apply a quantity sufficient to cover the affected area (including outer margin) 5X/day for 5 days

Initiate therapy as early as possible after the 1st signs/symptoms (eg, during the prodrome or when lesions appear)

ADMINISTRATION

Topical route

HOW SUPPLIED

Cre: (Acyclovir-Hydrocortisone) 5%-1% [5g]

WARNINGS/PRECAUTIONS

For cutaneous use only. Do not use in the eye, inside the mouth or nose, or on the genitals. Other orofacial lesions may be difficult to distinguish from a cold sore; monitor for cold sores that fail to heal within 2 weeks. Has a potential for irritation and contact sensitization.

ADVERSE REACTIONS

Application-site reactions (eg, drying/flaking of skin, burning/tingling, erythema, pigmentation changes, inflammation).

NURSING CONSIDERATIONS

Assessment: Assess for type of lesions (eg, bacterial, fungal infections), and pregnancy/nursing status.

Monitoring: Monitor for clinical response, irritation, contact sensitization, and other adverse reactions.

Patient Counseling: Inform that medication is not a cure for cold sores and it is for cutaneous use only for herpes labialis of the lips and around the mouth. Advise not to use in the eye, inside the mouth/nose, or on genitals. Counsel to use ud. Advise to avoid unnecessary rubbing of the affected area to avoid aggravating or transferring the infection. Instruct to seek medical advice when a cold sore fails to heal within 2 weeks. Encourage immunocompromised patients to consult a physician concerning the treatment of any infection.

Storage: 20-25°C (68-77°F); excursions permitted to 15-30°C (59-86°F). Do not freeze.

XGEVA – denosumab

RX

Class: IgG_2 monoclonal antibody

ADULT DOSAGE

Bone Metastasis from Solid Tumors

Prevention of Skeletal-Related Events:
120mg SQ every 4 weeks

Giant Cell Tumor of Bone

Treatment of Tumor that is Unresectable or Where Surgical Resection is Likely to Result in Severe Morbidity:
120mg SQ every 4 weeks with additional 120mg doses on Days 8 and 15 of the 1st month of therapy

Hypercalcemia of Malignancy

Refractory to Bisphosphonate Therapy:
120mg SQ every 4 weeks with additional 120mg doses on Days 8 and 15 of the 1st month of therapy

PEDIATRIC DOSAGE

Giant Cell Tumor of Bone

Treatment of Tumor that is Unresectable or Where Surgical Resection is Likely to Result in Severe Morbidity:
Adolescents (Skeletally Mature):
120mg SQ every 4 weeks with additional 120mg doses on Days 8 and 15 of the 1st month of therapy

ADMINISTRATION
SQ route

Administer in the upper arm, upper thigh, or abdomen
Remove from refrigerator and bring to room temperature (up to 25°C [77°F]) prior to administration; do not warm any other way
Use 27-gauge needle to withdraw and inject entire vial contents
Do not re-enter vial; discard vial after single-use or entry

HOW SUPPLIED
Inj: 120mg/1.7mL

CONTRAINDICATIONS
Hypocalcemia.

WARNINGS/PRECAUTIONS
Do not give with other drugs that contain the same active ingredient (eg, Prolia). Hypersensitivity, including anaphylaxis, reported; initiate appropriate treatment and d/c therapy permanently if an anaphylactic or other clinically significant allergic reaction occurs. May cause severe symptomatic hypocalcemia, and fatal cases reported; increased risk in patients with increasing renal dysfunction, and with inadequate/no Ca^{2+} supplementation. Correct preexisting hypocalcemia prior to treatment, monitor Ca^{2+} levels, and administer Ca^{2+}, Mg^{2+}, and vitamin D as necessary. Osteonecrosis of the jaw (ONJ) may occur; perform an oral exam and appropriate preventive dentistry prior to initiation of therapy and periodically during therapy. Avoid invasive dental procedures during therapy. Atypical femoral fractures reported; evaluate patients with thigh/groin pain to rule out an incomplete femur fracture and consider interruption of therapy. May cause fetal harm.

ADVERSE REACTIONS
Fatigue/asthenia, hypophosphatemia, N/V, dyspnea, diarrhea, hypocalcemia, cough, headache, arthralgia, back pain, pain in extremity, decreased appetite, peripheral edema, anemia, constipation.

DRUG INTERACTIONS
Monitor Ca^{2+} levels more frequently with other drugs that can lower Ca^{2+} levels.

NURSING CONSIDERATIONS

Assessment: Assess for preexisting or risk of hypocalcemia, drug hypersensitivity, pregnancy/nursing status, and possible drug interactions. Perform an oral exam and appropriate preventive dentistry.

Monitoring: Monitor for anaphylactic/hypersensitivity reaction, ONJ, atypical femoral fracture, and other adverse reactions. Monitor Ca^{2+} levels. Perform an oral exam and appropriate preventive dentistry periodically.

Patient Counseling: Advise to contact physician if experiencing symptoms of hypersensitivity reaction, hypocalcemia, ONJ, or atypical femoral fracture; persistent pain or slow healing of the mouth or jaw after dental surgery; or if nursing. Advise of the need for proper oral hygiene and routine dental care, to inform dentist that patient is receiving the drug, and to avoid invasive dental procedures during treatment. Advise females of reproductive potential to use highly effective contraception during therapy, and for at least 5 months after the last dose of the drug; instruct to contact physician if they become pregnant or if a pregnancy is suspected during this time. Advise male patients of potential for fetal exposure to drug if they have unprotected sexual intercourse with a pregnant partner. Advise that denosumab is also marketed as Prolia; instruct to inform physician if taking Prolia.

Storage: 2-8°C (36-46°F). Do not freeze. Once removed from the refrigerator, do not expose to >25°C (77°F) or direct light; use within 14 days. Protect from heat. Avoid vigorous shaking.

XIFAXAN – rifaximin

RX

Class: Semisynthetic rifampin analogue

ADULT DOSAGE

Traveler's Diarrhea

Noninvasive Strains of *Escherichia coli*:
200mg tid for 3 days

Hepatic Encephalopathy

Reduction in Risk of Overt Recurrence:
550mg bid

PEDIATRIC DOSAGE

Traveler's Diarrhea

Noninvasive Strains of *Escherichia coli*:
≥12 Years:
200mg tid for 3 days

ADMINISTRATION

Oral route

Take w/ or w/o food

HOW SUPPLIED

Tab: 200mg, 550mg

WARNINGS/PRECAUTIONS

Should not be used in patients with diarrhea complicated by fever and/or blood in the stool or diarrhea due to pathogens other than *E. coli*. D/C if diarrhea symptoms worsen or persist >24-48 hrs; consider alternative antibiotic therapy. *Clostridium difficile*-associated diarrhea (CDAD) reported; d/c if CDAD suspected or confirmed. May result in bacterial resistance with prolonged use in the absence of proven or strongly suspected bacterial infection or a prophylactic indication. Caution with severe hepatic impairment (Child-Pugh Class C); may increase systemic exposure.

ADVERSE REACTIONS

Flatulence, headache, abdominal pain, rectal tenesmus, nausea, peripheral edema, dizziness, fatigue, ascites, muscle spasms, pruritus, abdominal distention, anemia, cough, depression.

DRUG INTERACTIONS

Caution with P-gp inhibitors (eg, cyclosporine); may increase systemic exposure.

NURSING CONSIDERATIONS

Assessment: If diarrhea is present, assess for causative organisms and assess if diarrhea is complicated by fever or blood in stool. Assess for hepatic function, pregnancy/nursing status, and possible drug interactions.

Monitoring: Monitor for signs/symptoms of a hypersensitivity reaction, CDAD, development of drug-resistant bacteria, worsening of symptoms, and other adverse reactions.

Patient Counseling: If being treated for travelers' diarrhea, instruct to d/c therapy and contact physician if diarrhea persists for >24-48 hrs or worsens. Advise to seek medical care for fever and/or blood in the stool. Inform that watery and bloody stools (with or without stomach cramps and fever) may occur even as late as ≥2 months after last dose; advise to contact physician as soon as possible. Inform that drug only treats bacterial, not viral, infections. Inform that skipping doses or not completing full course of therapy may decrease the effectiveness of treatment and increase resistance. Inform that there is an increase systemic exposure to therapy in patients with severe hepatic impairment (Child-Pugh Class C).

Storage: 20-25°C (68-77°F); excursions permitted to 15-30°C (59-86°F).

XOLAIR – omalizumab

RX

Class: Monoclonal antibody/IgE-blocker

Anaphylaxis, presenting as bronchospasm, hypotension, syncope, urticaria, and/or angioedema of throat or tongue, reported as early as after the 1st dose and beyond 1 yr of therapy; closely observe patients. Inform of the signs/symptoms of anaphylaxis and instruct to seek immediate medical care should symptoms occur.

ADULT DOSAGE

Asthma

Moderate to Severe Persistent Asthma w/ a (+) Skin Test or In Vitro Reactivity to a Perennial Aeroallergen and Inadequately Controlled w/ Inhaled Corticosteroids:
150-375mg SQ every 2 or 4 weeks, based on body weight (kg) and pretreatment serum total IgE level (IU/mL)

Refer to PI for dose determination charts

Chronic Idiopathic Urticaria

Symptomatic Despite H1 Antihistamine Treatment:
150mg or 300mg SQ every 4 weeks

PEDIATRIC DOSAGE

Asthma

Moderate to Severe Persistent Asthma w/ a (+) Skin Test or In Vitro Reactivity to a Perennial Aeroallergen and Inadequately Controlled w/ Inhaled Corticosteroids:
≥12 Years:
150-375mg SQ every 2 or 4 weeks, based on body weight (kg) and pretreatment serum total IgE level (IU/mL)

Refer to PI for dose determination charts

Chronic Idiopathic Urticaria

Symptomatic Despite H1 Antihistamine Treatment:
≥12 Years:
150mg or 300mg SQ every 4 weeks

ADMINISTRATION

SQ route

The inj may take 5-10 sec to administer
Do not administer more than 150mg (contents of one vial) per inj site
150mg inj involves 1 inj (1.2mL total volume inj)
225mg inj involves 2 inj (1.8mL total volume inj)
300mg inj involves 2 inj (2.4mL total volume inj)
375mg inj involves 3 inj (3.0mL total volume inj)

Reconstitution for Single Vial

Before reconstitution, determine the number of vials that will need to be reconstituted
1. Reconstitute w/ sterile water for inj
2. Draw 1.4mL of sterile water for inj into a 3mL syringe equipped w/ a 1 inch, 18-gauge needle
3. Insert the needle and inject the sterile water for inj directly onto the product
4. Gently swirl the upright vial for approx 1 min; do not shake
5. If it takes longer than 20 min to dissolve completely, gently swirl the vial for 5 to 10 sec approx every 5 min until there are no visible gel-like particles in the sol. Do not use if the contents of the vial do not dissolve completely by 40 min
6. Invert the vial for 15 sec in order to allow the sol to drain toward the stopper
7. Using a new 3mL syringe equipped w/ a 1-inch, 18-gauge needle, draw the sol into the syringe
8. Replace the 18-gauge needle w/ a 25-gauge needle for SQ inj

HOW SUPPLIED

Inj: 150mg

WARNINGS/PRECAUTIONS

Not indicated for treatment of other forms of urticaria, relief of acute bronchospasm or status asthmaticus, or other allergic conditions. Administer only in a healthcare setting prepared to manage anaphylaxis and observe patients for an appropriate period after administration. D/C if a severe hypersensitivity reaction occurs. Malignant neoplasms reported. Do not abruptly d/c systemic or inhaled corticosteroids when initiating therapy. Eosinophilic conditions reported; be alert to eosinophilia, vasculitic rash, worsening pulmonary symptoms, cardiac complications, and/or neuropathy, especially upon reduction of oral corticosteroids. Monitor patients at high risk for geohelminth infections (eg, roundworm, hookworm). Signs/symptoms similar to those seen in patients with serum sickness, including arthritis/arthralgia, rash, fever, and lymphadenopathy reported; d/c if these symptoms develop. Serum total IgE levels increase due to formation of Xolair:IgE complexes and may persist for up to 1 yr following discontinuation of therapy; do not use serum total IgE levels obtained <1 yr following discontinuation to reassess dosing regimen for asthma patients.

ADVERSE REACTIONS

Anaphylaxis, inj-site reactions, URTI, sinusitis, headache, nasopharyngitis, pain, fatigue, arthralgia, leg pain, dizziness.

NURSING CONSIDERATIONS

Assessment: Assess for acute bronchospasm or status asthmaticus, malignancies, hypersensitivity reaction to drug or any of its ingredients, risk of geohelminth infections, and pregnancy/nursing status. Obtain baseline body weight and serum IgE levels.

Monitoring: Monitor for anaphylaxis, hypersensitivity reactions, inj-site reactions, malignancies, viral/geohelminth/URTIs, eosinophilia, vasculitic rash, worsening pulmonary symptoms, cardiac complications, neuropathy, arthritis/arthralgia, rash, fever, lymphadenopathy, and other adverse reactions. Periodically reassess need for continued therapy. Monitor body weight, CBC, and IgE levels prn.

Patient Counseling: Instruct to read the medication guide before treatment. Inform of the risk of life-threatening anaphylaxis; instruct to seek immediate medical care if symptoms of anaphylaxis occur. Instruct not to decrease dose of or stop taking any other asthma or CIU medications unless otherwise instructed. Inform that immediate improvement of asthma or CIU symptoms may not be seen after beginning therapy. Encourage pregnant women to enroll in the pregnancy exposure registry.

Storage: 2-8°C (36-46°F). Reconstituted: 2-8°C (36-46°F) for up to 8 hrs, or 4 hrs at room temperature. Protect from direct sunlight.

XOLEGEL — ketoconazole RX

Class: Azole antifungal

ADULT DOSAGE

Seborrheic Dermatitis

Apply qd to affected area for 2 weeks

PEDIATRIC DOSAGE

Seborrheic Dermatitis

≥12 Years:

Apply qd to affected area for 2 weeks

ADMINISTRATION
Topical route

HOW SUPPLIED
Gel: 2% [45g]

WARNINGS/PRECAUTIONS
Not for oral, ophthalmic, or intravaginal use. Flammable; avoid fire, flame, or smoking during and immediately following application. May cause local irritation at application site; d/c if irritation occurs or if disease worsens. If used during lactation and applied to chest, use caution to avoid accidental ingestion by infant. Hepatitis, lowered testosterone, and adrenocorticotropic hormone-induced corticosteroid serum levels reported with orally administered ketoconazole.

ADVERSE REACTIONS
Application-site burning.

DRUG INTERACTIONS
Coadministration of oral ketoconazole with CYP3A4 metabolized HMG-CoA reductase inhibitors (eg, simvastatin, lovastatin, atorvastatin) may increase risk of skeletal muscle toxicity, including rhabdomyolysis.

NURSING CONSIDERATIONS

Assessment: Assess pregnancy/nursing status.

Monitoring: Monitor for irritation and worsening of seborrheic dermatitis.

Patient Counseling: Inform that drug is for external use only. Instruct to use ud and to avoid contact with eyes, nostrils, and mouth. Advise to wash hands after application. Instruct not to use for any disorder other than that for which it has been prescribed. Advise to report any signs of adverse reactions to physician.

Storage: 25°C (77°F); excursions permitted to 15-30°C (59-86°F).

XOPENEX HFA — levalbuterol tartrate RX

Class: Beta$_2$-agonist

ADULT DOSAGE

Bronchospasm

Associated w/ Reversible Obstructive Airway Disease:

2 inh (90mcg) q4-6h

1 inh (45mcg) q4h may be sufficient in some patients

PEDIATRIC DOSAGE

Bronchospasm

Associated w/ Reversible Obstructive Airway Disease:

≥4 Years:

2 inh (90mcg) q4-6h

1 inh (45mcg) q4h may be sufficient in some patients

DOSE MODIFICATION

Elderly

Start at lower end of dosing range

ADMINISTRATION

Oral inh route

Shake well before use
Avoid spraying in the eyes
Wash actuator w/ warm water and air dry thoroughly at least once a week
Discard canister after 200 actuations have been used from the 15g canister and 80 actuations from the 8.4g canister

Priming

Prime inhaler before use for the 1st time or if not used for >3 days by releasing 4 test sprays into the air, away from face

HOW SUPPLIED

MDI: 45mcg/inh [80, 200 inhalations]

WARNINGS/PRECAUTIONS

If a previously effective dose regimen fails to provide the usual response or if more doses than usual are needed, this may be a marker of destabilization of asthma and may require reevaluation of the patient and treatment regimen; anti-inflammatory treatment (eg, corticosteroids) may be needed. D/C if paradoxical bronchospasm occur. ECG changes and immediate hypersensitivity reactions may occur. May need to d/c if cardiovascular (CV) effects occur. Fatalities reported w/ excessive use; do not exceed recommended dose. Caution w/ CV disorders (eg, coronary insufficiency, arrhythmias, HTN), convulsive disorders, hyperthyroidism, or diabetes mellitus (DM), and in patients unusually responsive to sympathomimetic amines. May produce significant hypokalemia. Caution w/ renal impairment.

ADVERSE REACTIONS

Pharyngitis, rhinitis, pain, vomiting, dizziness, asthma, bronchitis.

DRUG INTERACTIONS

Avoid w/ other short-acting sympathomimetic aerosol bronchodilators or epinephrine; caution w/ additional adrenergic drugs administered by any route. Use w/ β-blockers may block pulmonary effects and produce severe bronchospasm in asthmatic patients; avoid concomitant use. If needed, consider cardioselective β-blockers and use w/ caution. ECG changes and/or hypokalemia caused by non-K^+-sparing diuretics (eg, loop or thiazide diuretics) may be worsened; use w/ caution and consider monitoring K^+ levels. May decrease digoxin levels; monitor serum digoxin levels. Use extreme caution w/ MAOIs or TCAs, or w/in 2 weeks of discontinuation of such agents.

NURSING CONSIDERATIONS

Assessment: Assess for history of hypersensitivity to drug or racemic albuterol, CV disorders, convulsive disorders, hyperthyroidism, DM, renal impairment, pregnancy/nursing status, and possible drug interactions. Assess use in patients unusually responsive to sympathomimetic amines.

Monitoring: Monitor for paradoxical bronchospasm, deterioration of asthma, CV effects, ECG changes, hypokalemia, immediate hypersensitivity reactions, and other adverse effects. Monitor BP, HR, and ECG changes.

Patient Counseling: Counsel not to increase dose or frequency of doses w/o consulting physician. Advise to seek immediate medical attention if treatment becomes less effective for symptomatic relief, symptoms become worse, and/or there is a need to use the product more frequently than usual. Inform that drug may cause paradoxical bronchospasm; instruct to d/c if this occurs. Instruct to take concurrent inhaled drugs and other asthma medications only ud. Inform of the common side effects (eg, chest pain, palpitations, rapid HR, tremor, nervousness). Instruct to notify physician if pregnant/nursing. Advise to discard after 200 actuations have been released from the 15g canister or 80 actuations have been released from the 8.4g canister.

Storage: 20-25°C (68-77°F). Store w/ mouthpiece down. Protect from freezing and direct sunlight. Contents under pressure; do not puncture or incinerate. Exposure to temperatures >49°C (120°F) may cause bursting.

XYREM – sodium oxybate **CIII**

Class: CNS depressant

Obtundation and clinically significant respiratory depression occurred at recommended doses; almost all patients in trials were receiving CNS stimulants. Sodium oxybate is the Na^+ salt of gamma hydroxybutyrate (GHB); abuse of GHB, alone or in combination with other CNS depressants, is associated with CNS adverse reactions, including seizure, respiratory depression, decreased level of consciousness, coma, and death. Available only through a restricted distribution program (Xyrem Success Program).

ADULT DOSAGE

Narcolepsy

Treatment of Cataplexy and Excessive Daytime Sleepiness in Narcolepsy:
Initial: 4.5g/night in 2 equally divided doses (2.25g qhs and 2.25g taken 2.5-4 hrs later)
Titrate: Increase by 1.5g/night at weekly intervals (additional 0.75g qhs and 0.75g taken 2.5-4 hrs later)
Effective Dose Range: 6-9g/night
Max: 9g/night

PEDIATRIC DOSAGE

Pediatric use may not have been established

DOSE MODIFICATION

Concomitant Medications

Concomitant Divalproex Sodium:
Patients Already Stabilized on Sodium Oxybate: Reduce nightly dose of sodium oxybate by at least 20% w/ the addition of divalproex sodium
Patients Already Taking Divalproex Sodium: Use lower starting dose of sodium oxybate; monitor patient response and adjust dose accordingly

Hepatic Impairment

Initial: 2.25g/night in 2 equally divided doses (approx 1.13g qhs and 1.13g taken 2.5-4 hrs later)

Elderly

Start at lower end of dosing range

ADMINISTRATION

Oral route

Take 1st dose at least 2 hrs pc and 2nd dose 2.5-4 hrs after 1st dose
Prepare both doses prior to bedtime
Prior to ingestion, dilute each dose w/ approx 1/4 cup (approx 60mL) of water in the empty pharmacy vials provided
Take both doses while in bed and lie down immediately after dosing
Remain in bed following ingestion of the 1st and 2nd doses
May need to set an alarm to awaken for 2nd dose

HOW SUPPLIED

Sol: 0.5g/mL [180mL]

CONTRAINDICATIONS

Concomitant use with sedative hypnotic agents and alcohol. Succinic semialdehyde dehydrogenase deficiency.

WARNINGS/PRECAUTIONS

May impair physical/mental abilities. Evaluate for history of drug abuse and monitor closely for signs of misuse/abuse. May impair respiratory drive, especially in patients with compromised respiratory function. Increased central apneas, oxygen desaturation events, and sleep-related breathing disorders may occur. Sleep-related breathing disorders tend to be more prevalent in obese patients, postmenopausal women not on hormone replacement therapy, and narcolepsy patients. Caution with history of depressive illness and/or suicide attempt; monitor for emergence of depressive symptoms. Confusion, anxiety, and other neuropsychiatric reactions (eg, hallucinations, paranoia) reported; carefully evaluate emergence of confusion, thought disorders, and/or behavior abnormalities. Parasomnias reported; fully evaluate episodes of sleepwalking. Contains high salt content; consider amount of daily Na^+ intake in each dose in patients sensitive to salt intake (eg, heart failure, renal impairment). Caution with hepatic impairment and in elderly.

ADVERSE REACTIONS

Obtundation, respiratory depression, N/V, dizziness, diarrhea, somnolence, enuresis, tremor, attention disturbance, pain, sleep paralysis, paresthesia, disorientation, irritability, hyperhidrosis.

DRUG INTERACTIONS

See Contraindications and Dosage. Other CNS depressants (eg, opioid analgesics, benzodiazepines, sedating antidepressants/antipsychotics/antiepileptic drugs, general anesthetics, muscle relaxants, and/or illicit CNS depressants) may increase risk of respiratory depression, hypotension, profound sedation, syncope, and death; consider dose reduction or discontinuation of ≥1 CNS depressants (including sodium oxybate) if combination therapy is required. Consider interrupting therapy if short-term use of an opioid (eg, post- or perioperative) is required. Concomitant use with divalproex sodium resulted in a 25% mean increase in systemic exposure to sodium oxybate; monitor response closely and adjust dose accordingly if concomitant use is warranted.

NURSING CONSIDERATIONS

Assessment: Assess for succinic semialdehyde dehydrogenase deficiency, alcohol intake, history of drug abuse, compromised respiratory function, history of depressive illness and/or suicide attempt, hepatic impairment, sensitivity to salt intake, pregnancy/nursing status, and possible drug interactions.

Monitoring: Monitor for obtundation, respiratory depression, CNS depression, signs of abuse/misuse, sleep-disordered breathing, depression and suicidality, confusion, anxiety, other neuropsychiatric reactions, parasomnias, and other possible adverse reactions.

Patient Counseling: Inform about the Xyrem Success Program. Instruct to see prescriber frequently (every 3 months) to review therapy. Instruct to store drug in a secure place, out of reach of children/pets. Inform that patients are likely to fall asleep quickly (within 5-15 min) after taking the drug; instruct to remain in bed after taking 1st and 2nd doses. Advise not to drink alcohol or take other sedative hypnotics while on therapy. Inform that therapy can be associated with respiratory depression. Instruct to avoid operating hazardous machinery until patients are reasonably certain that therapy does not affect them adversely and for at least 6 hrs after the 2nd nightly dose. Advise to contact physician if depressed mood, markedly diminished interest or pleasure in usual activities, significant change in weight and/or appetite, psychomotor agitation or retardation, increased fatigue, feelings of guilt or worthlessness, slowed thinking or impaired concentration, or suicidal ideation develops. Inform that sleepwalking may occur; instruct to notify physician if this occurs. Inform patients who are sensitive to salt intake that drug contains a significant amount of Na^+ and they should limit their Na^+ intake.

Storage: 25°C (77°F); excursions permitted to 15-30°C (59-86°F).

XYZAL — levocetirizine dihydrochloride **RX**

Class: H_1-antagonist

ADULT DOSAGE

Seasonal Allergic Rhinitis

Usual: 5mg (1 tab or 2 tsp [10mL]) qpm; some may be adequately controlled by 2.5mg (1/2 tab or 1 tsp [5mL]) qpm

Perennial Allergic Rhinitis

Usual: 5mg (1 tab or 2 tsp [10mL]) qpm; some may be adequately controlled by 2.5mg (1/2 tab or 1 tsp [5mL]) qpm

Chronic Idiopathic Urticaria

Uncomplicated Skin Manifestations:
Usual: 5mg (1 tab or 2 tsp [10mL]) qpm; some may be adequately controlled by 2.5mg (1/2 tab or 1 tsp [5mL]) qpm

PEDIATRIC DOSAGE

Seasonal Allergic Rhinitis

2-5 Years:
Usual/Max: 1.25mg (1/2 tsp [2.5mL]) qpm

6-11 Years:
Usual/Max: 2.5mg (1/2 tab or 1 tsp [5mL]) qpm

≥12 Years:
Usual: 5mg (1 tab or 2 tsp [10mL]) qpm; some may be adequately controlled by 2.5mg qpm

Perennial Allergic Rhinitis

6 Months-5 Yrs:
Usual/Max: 1.25mg (1/2 tsp [2.5mL]) qpm

6-11 Years:
Usual/Max: 2.5mg (1/2 tab or 1 tsp [5mL]) qpm

≥12 Years:
Usual: 5mg (1 tab or 2 tsp [10mL]) qpm; some may be adequately controlled by 2.5mg qpm

Chronic Idiopathic Urticaria

Uncomplicated Skin Manifestations:

6 Months-5 Years:
Usual/Max: 1.25mg (1/2 tsp [2.5mL]) qpm

6-11 Years:
Usual/Max: 2.5mg (1/2 tab or 1 tsp [5mL]) qpm

≥12 Years:
Usual: 5mg (1 tab or 2 tsp [10mL]) qpm; some may be adequately controlled by 2.5mg qpm

DOSE MODIFICATION

Renal Impairment

Mild (CrCl 50-80mL/min): 2.5mg qd
Moderate (CrCl 30-50mL/min): 2.5mg qod
Severe (CrCl 10-30mL/min): 2.5mg twice weekly (administered once every 3-4 days)
ESRD (CrCl <10mL/min): Not recommended

Elderly

Start at lower end of dosing range

ADMINISTRATION

Oral route

Take w/o regard to food

HOW SUPPLIED
Sol: 0.5mg/mL [5 oz]; Tab: 5mg* *scored

CONTRAINDICATIONS
ESRD (CrCl <10mL/min) and patients undergoing hemodialysis, children 6 months-11 yrs of age with renal impairment.

WARNINGS/PRECAUTIONS
Somnolence, fatigue, and asthenia reported. May impair mental/physical abilities. Urinary retention reported; caution with predisposing factors of urinary retention (eg, spinal cord lesion, prostatic hyperplasia). D/C if urinary retention occurs. Caution in elderly.

ADVERSE REACTIONS
Somnolence, nasopharyngitis, fatigue, dry mouth, constipation, diarrhea, cough, pyrexia, pharyngitis, vomiting, otitis media.

DRUG INTERACTIONS
Avoid with alcohol or other CNS depressants; additional reductions in alertness and additional CNS performance impairment may occur. Decreased clearance with theophylline. Increased plasma AUC with ritonavir.

NURSING CONSIDERATIONS

Assessment: Assess for renal impairment, hypersensitivity to the drug, predisposing factors of urinary retention, pregnancy/nursing status, and possible drug interactions.

Monitoring: Monitor for somnolence, fatigue, asthenia, urinary retention, and other adverse reactions.

Patient Counseling: Instruct to use caution when engaging in hazardous occupations requiring complete mental alertness and motor coordination (eg, operating machinery, driving). Instruct to avoid alcohol or other CNS depressants, and to not take more than the recommended dose.

Storage: 20-25°C (68-77°F); excursions permitted to 15-30°C (59-86°F).

YASMIN – drospirenone/ethinyl estradiol — RX

Class: Estrogen/progestogen combination

Cigarette smoking increases the risk of serious cardiovascular (CV) events. Risk increases with age (>35 yrs of age) and with the number of cigarettes smoked. Should not be used by women who are >35 yrs of age and smoke.

OTHER BRAND NAMES
Ocella, Syeda

ADULT DOSAGE

Contraception

1 tab qd at the same time each day for 28 days, then repeat

Start either on 1st day of menses or on 1st Sunday after onset of menses

Conversions

Switching from a Different Birth Control Pill: Start on the same day that a new pack of the previous oral contraceptive would have been started

Switching from a Method Other Than a Birth Control Pill:

Transdermal Patch/Vaginal Ring/Inj: Start when the next application/inj would have been due

Intrauterine Contraceptive/Implant: Start on day of removal

PEDIATRIC DOSAGE

Contraception

Not indicated for use premenarche; refer to adult dosing

DOSE MODIFICATION

Adverse Reactions

GI Disturbances: If vomiting occurs w/in 3-4 hrs after taking tab, may regard as missed dose

ADMINISTRATION
Oral route

Take preferably pm pc or hs w/ some liquid; may be taken w/o regard to meals
Take in the order directed on the package
Use a nonhormonal contraceptive as backup during the first 7 days of initiating therapy

HOW SUPPLIED

Tab: (Drospirenone [DRSP]-Ethinyl Estradiol [EE]) 3mg-0.03mg

CONTRAINDICATIONS

Renal impairment, adrenal insufficiency, high risk of arterial/venous thrombotic disease (eg, smoking if >35 yrs of age, presence/history of DVT/pulmonary embolism, cerebrovascular disease, coronary artery disease, thrombogenic valvular or thrombogenic rhythm diseases of the heart [eg, subacute bacterial endocarditis with valvular disease, or A-fib], inherited/acquired hypercoagulopathies, uncontrolled HTN, diabetes mellitus [DM] with vascular disease, headache with focal neurological symptoms or migraine with/without aura if >35 yrs of age), undiagnosed abnormal uterine bleeding, presence/history of breast or other estrogen/progestin-sensitive cancer, benign/malignant liver tumor, liver disease, pregnancy.

WARNINGS/PRECAUTIONS

Increased risk of VTE and arterial thrombosis (eg, stroke, MI). D/C if an arterial/venous thrombotic event occurs. If feasible, d/c at least 4 weeks before and through 2 weeks after major surgery or other surgeries known to have an elevated risk of thromboembolism. Start therapy no earlier than 4 weeks after delivery in women who do not breastfeed. D/C if there is unexplained loss of vision, proptosis, diplopia, papilledema, or retinal vascular lesions; evaluate for retinal vein thrombosis immediately. Potential for hyperkalemia in high-risk patients; avoid use in patients predisposed to hyperkalemia. May increase risk of cervical cancer or intraepithelial neoplasia, and gallbladder disease. D/C if jaundice develops. Acute or chronic disturbances of liver function may necessitate the discontinuation of combination oral contraceptive (COC) use until markers of liver function return to normal and COC causation has been excluded. Hepatic adenoma and increased risk of hepatocellular carcinoma reported. Cholestasis may occur with history of pregnancy-related cholestasis. Women with a history of COC-related cholestasis may have the condition recur with subsequent COC use. Increased BP reported; d/c if BP rises significantly. May decrease glucose tolerance; monitor prediabetic and diabetic women. Consider alternative contraception with uncontrolled dyslipidemia. May increase risk of pancreatitis with hypertriglyceridemia or family history thereof. May increase frequency/severity of migraine. If new headaches that are recurrent, persistent, or severe develop, evaluate the cause and d/c if indicated. Breakthrough bleeding and spotting may occur; rule out pregnancy or malignancy. May cause post-pill amenorrhea or oligomenorrhea. Administration of oral contraceptives to induce withdrawal bleeding should not be used as a test for pregnancy. Caution with history of depression; d/c if depression recurs to a serious degree. May change results of some lab tests (eg, coagulation factors, lipids, glucose tolerance, binding proteins). May induce/exacerbate angioedema in women with hereditary angioedema. Chloasma may occur; women with a tendency to chloasma should avoid sun exposure or UV radiation. Absorption may not be complete in case of severe vomiting or diarrhea; if vomiting occurs within 3-4 hrs after tab taking, regard this as a missed tab.

ADVERSE REACTIONS

Premenstrual syndrome, headache, migraine, breast pain/tenderness/discomfort, N/V.

DRUG INTERACTIONS

Potential for an increase in serum K^+ concentration in women taking concomitant therapy with other drugs that may increase serum K^+ concentration (eg, ACE inhibitors, ARBs, K^+-sparing diuretics, heparin, aldosterone antagonists); monitor serum K^+ concentration during 1st treatment cycle in women receiving daily, long-term treatment for chronic conditions or diseases with medications that may increase serum K^+ concentration. Drugs or herbal products that induce certain enzymes, including CYP3A4 (eg, phenytoin, bosentan, products containing St. John's wort), may reduce drug effectiveness or increase incidence of breakthrough bleeding; use an alternative method of contraception or a back-up method when enzyme inducers are used, and continue back-up contraception for 28 days after discontinuing the enzyme inducer to ensure contraceptive reliability. Significant changes (increase/decrease) in plasma estrogen and progestin levels reported with HIV/hepatitis C virus protease inhibitors or non-nucleoside reverse transcriptase inhibitors. Pregnancy reported with antibiotics. Atorvastatin increases EE exposure. Ascorbic acid and APAP may increase EE levels. CYP3A4 inhibitors (eg, itraconazole, ketoconazole) may increase hormone levels. May decrease levels of lamotrigine and reduce seizure control; dosage adjustments of lamotrigine may be necessary. May need to increase dose of thyroid hormone in patients on thyroid hormone replacement therapy due to increased thyroid-binding globulin.

NURSING CONSIDERATIONS

Assessment: Assess for renal impairment, abnormal uterine bleeding, adrenal insufficiency, pregnancy/nursing status, any other conditions where treatment is contraindicated or cautioned, and possible drug interactions.

Monitoring: Monitor for bleeding irregularities, venous/arterial thrombotic events, retinal vein thrombosis, jaundice, new/worsening headaches or migraines, depression, and for other adverse reactions. Monitor K^+ levels, thyroid function if receiving thyroid replacement therapy, glucose levels with DM or prediabetes, lipids with dyslipidemia, liver function, and BP in patients with HTN.

Patient Counseling: Counsel that cigarette smoking increases the risk of serious cardiovascular events and to avoid use in women who are >35 yrs old and smoke. Inform that drug does not protect against HIV infection and other STDs. Instruct to take ud. Counsel on what to do if pills are missed or if vomiting occurs within 3-4 hrs after taking tab. Inform that amenorrhea may occur and pregnancy should be ruled out if amenorrhea occurs in ≥2 consecutive cycles. Advise to inform physician of preexisting medical conditions and/or drugs currently being taken. Counsel to use an additional method of contraception when enzyme inducers are used with therapy. Counsel women who start therapy postpartum and have not yet had a period to use an additional method of contraception until drug is taken for 7 consecutive days. Instruct to d/c if pregnancy occurs during treatment.

Storage: (Syeda) 20-25°C (68-77°F). (Yasmin, Ocella) 25°C (77°F); excursions permitted to 15-30°C (59-86°F).

ZALTRAP – ziv-aflibercept RX

Class: Vascular endothelial growth factor (VEGF) inhibitor

Severe and sometimes fatal hemorrhage, including GI hemorrhage, reported in combination with 5-fluorouracil, leucovorin, and irinotecan (FOLFIRI). Monitor for signs and symptoms of GI bleeding and other severe bleeding. Do not administer in patients with severe hemorrhage. Nonfatal/fatal GI perforation may occur; d/c therapy in patients who experience GI perforation. Severe compromised wound healing may occur in combination with FOLFIRI; d/c in patients with compromised wound healing. Suspend for at least 4 weeks prior to elective surgery; do not resume for at least 4 weeks following major surgery and until the surgical wound is fully healed.

ADULT DOSAGE

Metastatic Colorectal Cancer

In combination w/ FOLFIRI for patients w/ cancer that is resistant to or has progressed following an oxaliplatin-containing regimen

Usual: 4mg/kg IV infusion over 1 hr every 2 weeks until disease progression or unacceptable toxicity

Administer prior to any component of the FOLFIRI regimen on day of treatment

PEDIATRIC DOSAGE

Pediatric use may not have been established

DOSE MODIFICATION

Discontinuation

D/C Therapy for:

1. Severe hemorrhage
2. Gastrointestinal perforation
3. Compromised wound healing
4. Fistula formation
5. Hypertensive crisis or hypertensive encephalopathy
6. Arterial thromboembolic events
7. Nephrotic syndrome or thrombotic microangiopathy
8. Reversible posterior leukoencephalopathy syndrome

Temporarily Suspend Therapy:

1. At least 4 weeks prior to elective surgery
2. For recurrent or severe hypertension, until controlled; upon resumption, permanently reduce dose to 2mg/kg
3. For proteinuria of 2g/24 hrs; resume when proteinuria is <2g/24 hrs. For recurrent proteinuria, suspend therapy until proteinuria is <2g/24 hrs and then permanently reduce dose to 2mg/kg

ADMINISTRATION

IV route

Preparation

Do not re-enter the vial after the initial puncture; discard any unused portion left in the vial

Withdraw the prescribed dose and dilute in 0.9% NaCl sol or 5% dextrose sol for inj; final concentration is 0.6-8mg/mL

Use polyvinyl chloride (PVC) infusion bags containing bis (2-ethylhexyl) phthalate (DEHP) or polyolefin infusion bags

Administration

Administer through a 0.2 micron polyethersulfone filter

Do not use filters made of polyvinylidene fluoride or nylon

Do not administer as an IV push or bolus

Do not combine w/ other drugs in the same infusion bag or IV line

Administer using an infusion set made of 1 of the following materials:

1. PVC containing DEHP
2. DEHP-free PVC containing trioctyl-trimellitate

3. Polypropylene
4. Polyethylene-lined PVC
5. Polyurethane

HOW SUPPLIED

Inj: 25mg/mL [4mL, 8mL]

WARNINGS/PRECAUTIONS

D/C if severe hemorrhage develops. For minor surgery (eg, central venous access port placement, biopsy, tooth extraction), may initiate/resume therapy once surgical wound is fully healed. Fistula formation, involving GI and non-GI sites, reported; d/c in patients who develop fistula. Increased risk of Grade 3-4 HTN; treat with appropriate antihypertensives and continue monitoring BP regularly. D/C with hypertensive crisis or hypertensive encephalopathy. Arterial thromboembolic events (ATE) (eg, transient ischemic attack, cerebrovascular accident, angina pectoris); severe proteinuria; nephrotic syndrome; and thrombotic microangiopathy (TMA) reported. D/C if ATE, nephrotic syndrome, or TMA develops. Higher incidence of neutropenic complications (eg, febrile neutropenia, neutropenic infection) reported; delay therapy until neutrophil count is $\geq$1.5 x 10^9/L. Diarrhea and dehydration reported; closely monitor elderly for diarrhea and dehydration. Reversible posterior encephalopathy syndrome (RPLS) reported; confirm diagnosis of RPLS with magnetic resonance imaging and d/c if RPLS develops. Male and female reproductive function and fertility may be compromised during treatment; use highly effective contraception during and up to a minimum of 3 months after the last dose.

ADVERSE REACTIONS

Hemorrhage, GI perforation, compromised wound healing, leukopenia, diarrhea, neutropenia, proteinuria, AST/ALT increased, stomatitis, fatigue, thrombocytopenia, HTN, weight decrease, decreased appetite, epistaxis.

NURSING CONSIDERATIONS

Assessment: Assess for recent surgery, severe hemorrhage, compromised wound healing, HTN, proteinuria, history of ATE, neutropenia, and pregnancy/nursing status. Obtain baseline CBC with differential count.

Monitoring: Monitor for signs/symptoms of bleeding, GI perforation, fistula formation, compromised wound healing, hypertensive crisis/encephalopathy, ATE, nephrotic syndrome, TMA, diarrhea, dehydration, RPLS, and other adverse reactions. Monitor BP every 2 weeks or more frequently as indicated. Monitor proteinuria by urine dipstick analysis and/or urinary protein creatinine ratio (UPCR) for the development or worsening of proteinuria; obtain a 24-hr urine collection in patients with a dipstick of $\geq$2+ for protein or UPCR >1. Monitor CBC with differential count prior to initiation of each cycle.

Patient Counseling: Advise to contact physician if bleeding/symptoms of bleeding, elevated BP/symptoms from HTN, severe diarrhea, vomiting, severe abdominal pain, or fever or other signs of infection occur. Inform of the increased risk of compromised wound healing and instruct not to undergo surgery or procedures, including tooth extractions, without discussing 1st with the physician. Inform of an increased risk of ATE. Inform of the potential risks to the fetus or neonate during pregnancy or nursing; instruct to use highly effective contraception in both males and females during and for at least 3 months following last dose of therapy; advise to immediately contact physician if patient or their partner becomes pregnant during treatment.

Storage: 2-8°C (36-46°F). Keep vials in original carton to protect from light. Diluted Sol: 2-8°C (36-46°F) for up to 24 hrs, or at 20-25°C (68-77°F) for up to 8 hrs.

ZEBETA – bisoprolol fumarate RX

Class: Selective $beta_1$-blocker

ADULT DOSAGE

Hypertension

Initial: 5mg qd

Titrate: May increase to 10mg and then, if necessary, to 20mg qd

PEDIATRIC DOSAGE

Pediatric use may not have been established

DOSE MODIFICATION

Dose Reductions

Patients w/ Bronchospastic Disease:

Initial: 2.5mg qd

Renal Impairment

CrCl <40mL/min:

Initial: 2.5mg qd; use caution w/ dose titration

Hepatic Impairment
Initial: 2.5mg qd; use caution w/ dose titration

ADMINISTRATION
Oral route

HOW SUPPLIED
Tab: 5mg*, 10mg *scored

CONTRAINDICATIONS
Cardiogenic shock, overt cardiac failure, 2nd- or 3rd-degree atrioventricular (AV) block, marked sinus bradycardia.

WARNINGS/PRECAUTIONS
Avoid abrupt withdrawal; exacerbation of angina pectoris, MI, and ventricular arrhythmia in patients with coronary artery disease, and exacerbation of symptoms of hyperthyroidism or precipitation of thyroid storm reported. Reinstitute temporary therapy if withdrawal symptoms occur. May mask manifestations of hypoglycemia or clinical signs of hyperthyroidism (eg, tachycardia). Caution with compensated cardiac failure, diabetes mellitus, bronchospastic disease, and hepatic/renal impairment. May precipitate cardiac failure; d/c at the 1st signs/symptoms of heart failure (HF) or continue therapy while HF is treated with other drugs. Caution with peripheral vascular disease; may precipitate or aggravate symptoms of arterial insufficiency. Caution with history of severe anaphylactic reaction to a variety of allergens; reactivity may increase with repeated challenge.

ADVERSE REACTIONS
Headache, URI, peripheral edema, fatigue, ALT/AST elevation.

DRUG INTERACTIONS
Patients with a history of severe anaphylactic reaction to a variety of allergens taking β-blockers may be unresponsive to usual doses of epinephrine. D/C several days before withdrawal of clonidine. Excessive reduction of sympathetic activity with catecholamine-depleting drugs (eg, reserpine, guanethidine); monitor closely. Avoid with other β-blockers. Caution with myocardial depressants or inhibitors of AV conduction, such as calcium antagonists (eg, verapamil, diltiazem) or antiarrhythmics (eg, disopyramide). Increased risk of bradycardia with digitalis glycosides. Increased clearance with rifampin. Caution with insulin or oral hypoglycemic agents. Reversed effects with bronchodilator therapy. Additive BP lowering effects in mild to moderate HTN with HCTZ.

NURSING CONSIDERATIONS

Assessment: Assess for conditions where treatment is contraindicated or cautioned, pregnancy/nursing status, and possible drug interactions.

Monitoring: Monitor for hypoglycemia, hyperthyroidism, hepatic/renal function, signs/symptoms of HF, withdrawal, and arterial insufficiency. Monitor HR, ECG, CBC with platelet and differential count.

Patient Counseling: Instruct not to interrupt or d/c therapy without consulting physician. Notify physician if difficulty in breathing, signs/symptoms of CHF or excessive bradycardia develop. Educate about signs/symptoms of drug's potential adverse effects. Advise to exercise caution while driving, operating machinery, or engaging in other tasks requiring alertness.

Storage: 20-25°C (68-77°F). Protect from moisture.

ZECUITY – sumatriptan RX

Class: 5-$HT_{1B/1D}$ agonist

ADULT DOSAGE
Migraine
Acute Treatment w/ or w/o Aura:
Usual: Apply 1 patch for 4 hrs or until red light emitting diode light goes off
If headache relief is incomplete, a 2nd patch may be applied ≥2 hrs after activation of the 1st patch to a different site
Max: 1 patch/dose or 2 patches/24 hrs
The safety of using >4 patches in 1 month has not been established

PEDIATRIC DOSAGE
Pediatric use may not have been established

DOSE MODIFICATION
Elderly
Use caution; start at lower end of dosing range

ADMINISTRATION
Transdermal route

Apply to dry intact, non-irritated skin on upper arm or thigh on a site that is relatively hair free and w/o scars, tattoos, abrasions, or other skin conditions; may secure the system w/ medical tape if needed

Do not apply to a previous application site until the site remains erythema free for at least 3 days

Once applied, push the activation button to turn on the red light emitting diode (LED) w/in 15 min

When the LED light turns off, dosing is complete and the system can be removed

After use, fold the system so the adhesive side sticks to itself and safely discard away from children and pets

HOW SUPPLIED

Patch: 6.5mg/4 hrs

CONTRAINDICATIONS

Ischemic coronary artery disease (CAD) (eg, angina pectoris, history of myocardial infarction [MI], documented silent ischemia), coronary artery vasospasm (eg, Prinzmetal's angina), Wolff-Parkinson-White syndrome or arrhythmias associated with other cardiac accessory conduction pathway disorders, history of stroke, transient ischemic attack, history of hemiplegic or basilar migraine, peripheral vascular disease, ischemic bowel disease, uncontrolled HTN, severe hepatic impairment, or allergic contact dermatitis to sumatriptan. Recent (within 24 hrs) use of ergotamine-containing medication, ergot-type medication (eg, dihydroergotamine, methysergide) or another 5-hydroxytryptamine$_1$ agonist. Concurrent administration of an MAO-A inhibitor or recent (within 2 weeks) use of an MAO-A inhibitor.

WARNINGS/PRECAUTIONS

For transdermal use only. Use only if a clear diagnosis of migraine has been established. Reconsider the diagnosis of migraine before giving a 2nd dose if patient does not respond to the 1st dose of therapy. No evidence of benefit for the use of a 2nd transdermal system (TDS) to treat headache recurrence or incomplete headache relief during a migraine attack. Contains metal parts; remove before an MRI procedure. Do not apply in areas near or over electrically-active implantable or body-worn medical devices (eg, implantable cardiac pacemaker, body-worn insulin pump, implantable deep brain stimulator). May lead to allergic contact dermatitis; d/c if suspected. Systemic sensitization or other systemic reactions may develop if other sumatriptan-containing products are taken via other routes (eg, PO, SQ); administer 1st subsequent dose under close medical supervision. May cause coronary artery vasospasm (Prinzmetal's angina) and sensations of tightness, pain, pressure, and heaviness in the chest, throat, neck, and jaw, usually of noncardiac origin. Perform cardiovascular (CV) evaluation in triptan-naive patients who have multiple CV risk factors (eg, increased age, diabetes, HTN, smoking, obesity, strong family history of CAD) before treatment; if negative, consider 1st administration in a medically supervised setting and perform an ECG upon activation of TDS. Consider periodic CV evaluation in intermittent long-term users. Life-threatening cardiac rhythm disturbances (eg, ventricular tachycardia, ventricular fibrillation leading to death) reported; d/c if these occur. Cerebral hemorrhage, subarachnoid hemorrhage, and stroke may occur; exclude other potentially serious neurological conditions prior to therapy in patients not previously diagnosed as migraineurs, and in migraineurs who present with atypical symptoms. May cause noncoronary vasospastic reactions (eg, peripheral vascular ischemia, GI vascular ischemia/infarction, splenic infarction, Raynaud's syndrome). Transient/permanent blindness and significant partial vision loss reported. Overuse may lead to exacerbation of headache; detoxification including drug withdrawal, and treatment of withdrawal symptoms may be necessary. Serotonin syndrome may occur; d/c if suspected. Significant elevation in BP, including hypertensive crisis with acute impairment of organ systems, reported. Anaphylactic/anaphylactoid reactions may occur. Seizures reported; caution in patients with a history of epilepsy or conditions associated with a lowered seizure threshold.

ADVERSE REACTIONS

Application-site reactions (pain, paresthesia, pruritus, warmth, discomfort, irritation, discoloration, vesicles).

DRUG INTERACTIONS

See Contraindications. Serotonin syndrome reported with SSRIs, SNRIs, TCAs, or MAOIs.

NURSING CONSIDERATIONS

Assessment: Assess for cardiovascular disease, HTN, hemiplegic/basilar migraine, ECG changes, and any other conditions where treatment is cautioned or contraindicated, hepatic function, pregnancy/nursing status, and for possible drug interactions. Confirm diagnosis of migraine and exclude other potentially serious neurologic conditions prior to therapy. Perform CV evaluation in patients who have CV risk factors (eg, increased age, diabetes, HTN, smoking, obesity, strong family history of CAD).

Monitoring: Monitor for signs/symptoms of cardiac events, cerebrovascular events, peripheral vascular ischemia, GI vascular ischemia/infarction, serotonin syndrome, allergic contact dermatitis, anaphylactic/anaphylactoid reactions, visual disturbances, HTN, and other adverse reactions. Perform ECG immediately after administration of therapy and monitor CV function in intermittent long-term users. Monitor for medication overuse; exacerbation of headache may occur.

Patient Counseling: Instruct to use TDS ud; instruct not to bathe, shower, or swim while wearing TDS. Inform that most patients experience some skin redness under the TDS upon removal, which usually disappears within 24 hrs. Inform patients that the TDS contains metal parts and must be removed before an MRI procedure. Inform that treatment may cause serious CV adverse reactions (eg, MI or stroke) that may result in hospitalization and even death. Instruct patients to be alert for signs/symptoms of chest pain, SOB, weakness, and slurring of speech; instruct to notify physician if these symptoms and other symptoms of vasospastic reactions occur. Inform patients of the signs and symptoms of allergic contact dermatitis, and instruct to seek medical advice if skin lesions suggestive of allergic contact dermatitis develop. Counsel about the possible drug interactions and the risk of anaphylactic/anaphylactoid reactions. Inform patients that the use of therapy ≥10 days per month may lead to exacerbation of headache; encourage to record headache frequency and drug use. Advise to notify physician if pregnant/nursing or planning to become pregnant. Instruct patients to evaluate their ability to perform complex tasks during migraine attacks and after using therapy.

Storage: 20-25°C (68-77°F); excursions permitted to 15-30°C (59-86°F). Do not refrigerate or freeze. Contains lithium-manganese dioxide batteries; dispose in accordance with state and local regulations.

ZEGERID – omeprazole/sodium bicarbonate — RX

Class: Proton pump inhibitor/antacid

ADULT DOSAGE

Gastroesophageal Reflux Disease

Symptomatic GERD (w/ No Esophageal Erosions):
20mg qd for up to 4 weeks

Erosive Esophagitis (Diagnosed by Endoscopy):
20mg qd for 4-8 weeks
May give up to an additional 4 weeks if no response to 8 weeks of therapy
May consider additional 4- to 8-week courses if there is recurrence of erosive esophagitis or GERD symptoms

Maint of Healing of Erosive Esophagitis:
20mg qd; controlled studies do not extend beyond 12 months

Upper GI Bleeding

Risk Reduction in Critically Ill Patients:
Sus, 40mg/1680mg:
Initial: 40mg, followed by 40mg after 6-8 hrs
Maint: 40mg qd for 14 days

Duodenal Ulcers

Active:
20mg qd for 4-8 weeks

Gastric Ulcers

Active Benign:
40mg qd for 4-8 weeks

PEDIATRIC DOSAGE

Pediatric use may not have been established

DOSE MODIFICATION

Hepatic Impairment
Consider dose reduction, particularly for maint of healing of erosive esophagitis

Other Important Modifications
Asian Population:
Consider dose reduction, particularly for maint of healing of erosive esophagitis

ADMINISTRATION

Oral route

Take on an empty stomach at least 1 hr ac

Cap
Swallow intact w/ water; do not use other liquids
Do not open cap and sprinkle contents into food

Sus

Empty pkt contents into a small cup containing 1-2 tbsp of water; do not use other liquids or foods
Stir well and drink immediately
Refill cup w/ water and drink

Administration Through NG or Orogastric Tube:

Suspend enteral feeding approx 3 hrs before and 1 hr after administration of sus
Constitute the sus w/ approx 20mL of water; do not use other liquids or foods
Stir well and administer immediately
Use an appropriately sized syringe to instill sus in tube
Wash sus through the tube w/ 20mL of water

HOW SUPPLIED

(Omeprazole/Sodium Bicarbonate) Cap: 20mg/1100mg, 40mg/1100mg; Sus: (20mg/1680mg)/pkt, (40mg/1680mg)/pkt

WARNINGS/PRECAUTIONS

Omeprazole: Symptomatic response does not preclude the presence of gastric malignancy. Atrophic gastritis reported with long-term use. Acute interstitial nephritis reported; d/c if this develops. Cyanocobalamin (vitamin B12) deficiency may occur with daily long-term treatment (eg, >3 yrs) with any acid-suppressing medications. May increase risk of *Clostridium difficile*-associated diarrhea (CDAD), especially in hospitalized patients. May increase risk of osteoporosis-related fractures of the hip, wrist, or spine, especially with high-dose and long-term therapy. Use lowest dose and shortest duration appropriate to the condition being treated. Hypomagnesemia reported and may require Mg^{2+} replacement and discontinuation of therapy; consider monitoring Mg^{2+} levels prior to and periodically during therapy with prolonged treatment. Drug-induced decrease in gastric acidity results in enterochromaffin-like cell hyperplasia and increased chromogranin A (CgA) levels, which may interfere with investigations for neuroendocrine tumors; temporarily d/c treatment before assessing CgA levels and consider repeating the test if initial CgA levels are high. Sodium Bicarbonate: Consider the Na^+ content when administering to patients on a Na^+-restricted diet. Caution with Bartter's syndrome, hypokalemia, hypocalcemia, and problems with acid-base balance. Chronic use may lead to systemic alkalosis, and increased Na^+ intake may produce edema and weight increase.

ADVERSE REACTIONS

Agitation, anemia, bradycardia, constipation, rash, tachycardia, diarrhea, fever, thrombocytopenia, hypokalemia, hypomagnesemia, hyperglycemia, atrial fibrillation, HTN, hypotension.

DRUG INTERACTIONS

Monitor for the need to adjust dose of drugs metabolized via CYP450 (eg, cyclosporine, disulfiram, benzodiazepines). Omeprazole: Reduces pharmacological activity of clopidogrel; avoid concomitant use, and consider alternative antiplatelet therapy. Caution with digoxin or drugs that may cause hypomagnesemia (eg, diuretics). May elevate and prolong levels of methotrexate (MTX) and/or its metabolite, possibly leading to MTX toxicities; consider temporary withdrawal of therapy with high-dose MTX. May reduce the absorption of drugs where gastric pH is an important determinant of bioavailability; ketoconazole, atazanavir, iron salts, erlotinib, and mycophenolate mofetil (MMF) absorption may decrease, while digoxin absorption may increase. Monitor when digoxin is taken concomitantly. Caution in transplant patients receiving MMF. May prolong elimination of drugs metabolized by hepatic oxidation (eg, diazepam, warfarin, phenytoin). Increased INR and PT reported with warfarin. Voriconazole (combined inhibitor of CYP2C19 and CYP3A4) may increase levels. May decrease levels of atazanavir and nelfinavir; coadministration not recommended. May increase levels of saquinavir and tacrolimus; consider dose reduction of saquinavir. CYP2C19 or CYP3A4 inducers may decrease levels; avoid with St. John's wort or rifampin. Sodium Bicarbonate: Long-term use of bicarbonate with Ca^{2+} or milk can cause milk-alkali syndrome.

NURSING CONSIDERATIONS

Assessment: Assess for risk of osteoporosis-related fractures, Na^+-restricted diet, Bartter's syndrome, hypokalemia, hypocalcemia, acid-base balance problems, hypersensitivity to the drug, pregnancy/nursing status, and possible drug interactions. Obtain baseline Mg^{2+} levels in patients expected to be on prolonged therapy.

Monitoring: Monitor for signs/symptoms of atrophic gastritis, acute interstitial nephritis, cyanocobalamin deficiency, CDAD, bone fractures, systemic alkalosis, hypersensitivity reactions, and other adverse reactions. Monitor Mg^{2+} levels periodically in patients expected to be on prolonged therapy. Monitor INR and PT when given with warfarin.

Patient Counseling: Inform that different formulations are not bioequivalent; do not substitute one for the other. Inform patients on a Na^+-restricted diet of the Na^+ content in product. Inform that increased Na^+ intake may cause swelling and weight gain; instruct to contact physician if these occur. Inform that the most frequent adverse reactions associated with therapy include headache, abdominal pain, N/V, diarrhea, and flatulence. Advise that harmful effect of therapy on the fetus cannot be ruled out. Advise to use with caution if regularly taking Ca^{2+} supplements. Advise to immediately report and seek care for diarrhea that does not improve and for any cardiovascular/neurological symptoms (eg, palpitations, dizziness, seizures, tetany).

Storage: 25°C (77°F); excursions permitted to 15-30°C (59-86°F). Protect from light and moisture.

ZELBORAF – vemurafenib

RX

Class: Kinase inhibitors

ADULT DOSAGE

Unresectable or Metastatic Melanoma with BRAF V600E Mutation

960mg q12h until disease progression or unacceptable toxicity occurs

PEDIATRIC DOSAGE

Pediatric use may not have been established

DOSE MODIFICATION

Adverse Reactions

D/C if:

Grade 4 adverse reaction, first appearance (if clinically appropriate) or second appearance

QTc prolongation >500ms and increased by >60ms from pretreatment values

Withhold for:

NCI CTCAE Grade 2 or greater adverse reactions

Upon Recovery to Grade 0-1, Restart at a Reduced Dose as Follows:

720mg bid for first appearance of intolerable Grade 2 or Grade 3 adverse reactions

480mg bid for second appearance of Grade 2 (if intolerable) or Grade 3 adverse reactions or for first appearance of Grade 4 adverse reaction (if clinically appropriate)

Do not reduce dose to below 480mg bid

ADMINISTRATION

Oral route

Do not take an additional dose if vomiting occurs after therapy; continue with the next scheduled dose

Take with or without meal

Do not crush or chew

Missed dose can be taken up to 4 hrs prior to next dose

HOW SUPPLIED

Tab: 240mg

WARNINGS/PRECAUTIONS

Not indicated for wild-type BRAF melanoma. Cutaneous malignancies (eg, cutaneous squamous cell carcinoma [SCC], keratoacanthoma, melanoma) and non-cutaneous SCC of the head and neck reported; monitor closely for signs or symptoms of new non-cutaneous SCC or other malignancies. Increased risk of cutaneous SCC in patients ≥65 yrs of age, with prior skin cancer, and chronic sun exposure. May promote malignancies associated with activation of RAS through mutation or other mechanisms. Increased cell proliferation in BRAF wild-type cells can occur with BRAF inhibitors; confirm evidence of BRAF V600E mutation in tumor specimens prior to initiating therapy. Anaphylaxis and serious hypersensitivity/dermatological reactions may occur; d/c permanently if severe hypersensitivity/dermatological reactions occur. QT prolongation leading to an increased risk of ventricular arrhythmias (eg, torsades de pointes) may occur. Do not initiate therapy in patients with uncorrectable electrolyte abnormalities, QT >500 msec, long QT syndrome, or who are taking medicines known to prolong QT interval. Liver injury leading to functional hepatic impairment (eg, coagulopathy or other organ dysfunction) may occur. Uveitis, blurred vision, photophobia, and mild to severe photosensitivity may occur. May cause fetal harm; women of childbearing age and men should use contraception during and for at least 2 months after discontinuation therapy.

ADVERSE REACTIONS

Photosensitivity reaction, alopecia, rash, pruritus, arthralgia, fatigue, peripheral edema, N/V, diarrhea, headache, skin papilloma, hyperkeratosis, pyrexia, myalgia, dysgeusia.

DRUG INTERACTIONS

Strong CYP3A4 inhibitors (eg, ketoconazole, nefazodone, clarithromycin) and inducers (eg, phenytoin, carbamazepine, rifampin) may alter vemurafenib concentrations; avoid concomitant use and replace these drugs with alternative drugs when possible. Not recommended with CYP1A2 substrates with a narrow therapeutic window, due to possibility of increased concentrations of CYP1A2 substrates; if coadministration cannot be avoided, monitor closely for toxicities and consider a dose reduction of concomitant CYP1A2 substrates. Increases in transaminases and bilirubin occurred with concurrent ipilimumab.

NURSING CONSIDERATIONS

Assessment: Assess for BRAF V600E mutation, prior skin cancer, chronic sun exposure, electrolyte abnormality, long QT syndrome, hepatic impairment, pregnancy/nursing status, and possible drug interactions. Perform dermatologic evaluation and obtain baseline ECG, electrolyte levels, and LFTs.

Monitoring: Monitor for development of new primary malignancies, severe dermatologic and hypersensitivity reactions, photosensitivity, uveitis, and other adverse reactions. Perform dermatologic evaluation every 2 months during treatment and for 6 months after discontinuation. Prior to and following treatment initiation or after dose modification of therapy for QTc prolongation, evaluate ECG and electrolytes after 15 days, monthly during the first 3 months, then every 3 months thereafter, or as clinically indicated. Monitor LFTs monthly or as clinically needed.

Patient Counseling: Inform about the potential benefits and risks of treatment. Inform that BRAF V600E mutation assessment is required for patient selection. Inform about the increased risk of developing new primary cutaneous malignancies and advise on the importance of immediately reporting any skin changes. Inform about the risk of QT prolongation, which may result in ventricular arrhythmias; advise on the importance of monitoring ECG and electrolytes during treatment. Inform about the risk of photosensitivity and advise to avoid sun exposure and to wear protective clothing, sunscreen, and lip balm with SPF ≥30 when outdoors. Inform of commonly reported adverse events. Advise of risk of fetal harm; counsel women of childbearing age and men to use contraception during and for at least 2 months after ending therapy. Advise that missed dose can be taken up to 4 hrs prior to next dose.

Storage: 20-25°C (68-77°F); excursions permitted between 15-30°C (59-86°F).

ZENPEP — pancrelipase

Class: Pancreatic enzyme supplement

RX

ADULT DOSAGE

Exocrine Pancreatic Insufficiency

Due to Cystic Fibrosis or Other Conditions:
Start at the lowest recommended dose and increase gradually
Initial: 500 lipase U/kg/meal
Max: 2500 lipase U/kg/meal (or ≤10,000 lipase U/kg/day) or <4000 lipase U/g fat ingested/day

Missed Dose

If a dose is missed, the next dose should be taken w/ the next meal or snack as directed. Doses should not be doubled

PEDIATRIC DOSAGE

Exocrine Pancreatic Insufficiency

Due to Cystic Fibrosis or Other Conditions:
Start at the lowest recommended dose and increase gradually

≤12 Months of Age:
3000 lipase U per 120mL of formula or per breastfeeding immediately prior to each feeding

>12 Months-<4 Years:
Initial: 1000 lipase U/kg/meal
Max: 2500 lipase U/kg/meal (or ≤10,000 lipase U/kg/day) or <4000 lipase U/g fat ingested/day

≥4 Years:
Initial: 500 lipase U/kg/meal
Max: 2500 lipase U/kg/meal (or ≤10,000 lipase U/kg/day) or <4000 lipase U/g fat ingested/day

Missed Dose

If a dose is missed, the next dose should be taken w/ the next meal or snack as directed. Doses should not be doubled

ADMINISTRATION

Oral route

Take during meals or snacks, w/ sufficient fluid
Half of the dose used for meals should be given w/ each snack
Swallow whole; do not crush/chew cap or cap contents
If necessary, the cap contents can be sprinkled on soft acidic foods (eg, applesauce, commercial preparations of bananas or pears)
Contents of the cap may also be given directly to the mouth
Do not mix directly into formula or breast milk

HOW SUPPLIED

Cap, Delayed-Release: (Lipase-Protease-Amylase) 3000 U-10,000 U-14,000 U; 5000 U-17,000 U-24,000 U; 10,000 U-32,000 U-42,000 U; 15,000 U-47,000 U-63,000 U; 20,000 U-63,000 U-84,000 U; 25,000 U-79,000 U-105,000 U; 40,000 U-126,000 U-168,000 U

WARNINGS/PRECAUTIONS

Not interchangeable with other pancrelipase products. Fibrosing colonopathy reported; monitor closely for progression to stricture formation. Colonic strictures have been associated with doses >6000 lipase U/kg/meal in children <12 yrs of age. Caution with doses >2500 lipase U/kg/meal (or >10,000 lipase U/kg/day); use only if these doses are documented to be effective by 3-day fecal fat measures indicating significant improvement. Examine patients receiving >6000 lipase U/kg/meal;

immediately decrease or titrate dose downward to a lower range. Ensure that no drug is retained in the mouth. Should not be crushed or chewed, or mixed in foods with pH >4.5; may disrupt enteric coating of cap, resulting in early release of enzymes, irritation of oral mucosa, and/or loss of enzyme activity. Caution in patients with gout, renal impairment, or hyperuricemia; may increase blood uric acid levels. Risk for transmission of viral diseases. Caution with known allergy to proteins of porcine origin; severe allergic reactions reported.

ADVERSE REACTIONS

GI disorders (eg, abdominal pain, flatulence), headache, cough, weight decreased, early satiety, contusion.

NURSING CONSIDERATIONS

Assessment: Assess for gout, renal impairment, hyperuricemia, allergy to porcine proteins, and pregnancy/nursing status.

Monitoring: Monitor for fibrosing colonopathy, stricture formation, oral mucosa irritation, viral diseases, allergic reactions, and other adverse reactions. Monitor serum uric acid levels.

Patient Counseling: Instruct to take ud, with food and sufficient fluids. Inform that if a dose is missed, take the next dose with the next meal/snack ud; instruct not to double doses. Inform that cap contents can be mixed with soft acidic foods (eg, applesauce), if necessary. Advise to contact physician immediately if allergic reactions develop. Instruct to notify physician if pregnant/breastfeeding or planning to become pregnant/breastfeed during treatment. Instruct to notify physician before initiating treatment if patient has a history of abnormal glucose levels.

Storage: Avoid excessive heat. Protect from moisture. (Original glass container) 20-25°C (68-77°F); brief excursions permitted to 15-40°C (59-104°F). (Repackaged HDPE container) Store up to 30°C (86°F) for up to 6 months; brief excursions permitted to 15-40°C (59-104°F) for up to 30 days.

ZENZEDI — dextroamphetamine sulfate CII

Class: Sympathomimetic amine

High potential for abuse. Prolonged use may lead to drug dependence and must be avoided. Misuse may cause sudden death and serious cardiovascular adverse events.

ADULT DOSAGE

Narcolepsy

Initial: 10mg/day
Titrate: May increase daily dose in increments of 10mg at weekly intervals until optimal response is obtained
Usual: 5-60mg/day in divided doses

Give 1st dose on awakening; additional doses (1 or 2) at intervals of 4-6 hrs

PEDIATRIC DOSAGE

Narcolepsy

Usual: 5-60mg/day in divided doses

Give 1st dose on awakening; additional doses (1 or 2) at intervals of 4-6 hrs

6-12 Years:
Initial: 5mg/day
Titrate: May increase daily dose in increments of 5mg at weekly intervals until optimal response is obtained

≥12 Years:
Initial: 10mg/day
Titrate: May increase daily dose in increments of 10mg at weekly intervals until optimal response is obtained

Attention-Deficit Hyperactivity Disorder

3-5 Years:
Initial: 2.5mg qd
Titrate: May increase daily dose in increments of 2.5mg at weekly intervals until optimal response is obtained

≥6 Years:
Initial: 5mg qd or bid
Titrate: May increase daily dose in increments of 5mg at weekly intervals until optimal response is obtained. Only in rare cases will it be necessary to exceed a total of 40mg/day

Give 1st dose on awakening; additional doses (1 or 2) at intervals of 4-6 hrs

DOSE MODIFICATION

Adverse Reactions

Narcolepsy:

Reduce dose if bothersome adverse reactions appear (eg, insomnia, anorexia)

ADMINISTRATION

Oral route

Avoid late pm doses

HOW SUPPLIED

Tab: 2.5mg, 5mg*, 7.5mg, 10mg*, 15mg, 20mg, 30mg *scored

CONTRAINDICATIONS

Advanced arteriosclerosis, symptomatic cardiovascular disease (CVD), moderate to severe HTN, hyperthyroidism, glaucoma, agitated states, and history of drug abuse. During or within 14 days following MAOI use.

WARNINGS/PRECAUTIONS

Avoid with known serious structural cardiac abnormalities, cardiomyopathy, serious heart rhythm abnormalities, coronary artery disease, or other serious cardiac problems. Sudden death reported in children and adolescents with structural cardiac abnormalities or other serious heart problems. Sudden deaths, stroke, and myocardial infarction (MI) reported in adults. May cause a modest increase in average BP and HR. Promptly perform cardiac evaluation if symptoms of cardiac disease develop. May exacerbate symptoms of behavior disturbance and thought disorder in patients with preexisting psychotic disorder. Caution in patients with comorbid bipolar disorder; may induce mixed/manic episodes. May cause treatment-emergent psychotic or manic symptoms in children and adolescents without prior history of psychotic illness or mania; consider discontinuation if such symptoms occur. Aggressive behavior or hostility reported in children and adolescents with ADHD. May cause long-term suppression of growth in children; may need to interrupt treatment in patients not growing or gaining height or weight as expected. May lower convulsive threshold; d/c if seizures occur. Associated with peripheral vasculopathy, including Raynaud's phenomenon. Difficulties with accommodation and blurring of vision reported. May exacerbate motor and phonic tics, and Tourette's syndrome. May elevate plasma corticosteroid levels and interfere with urinary steroid determinations.

ADVERSE REACTIONS

Palpitations, tachycardia, BP elevation, dizziness, insomnia, euphoria, dyskinesia, tremor, headache, dryness of mouth, diarrhea, constipation, urticaria, impotence, changes in libido.

DRUG INTERACTIONS

See Contraindications. GI acidifying agents (eg, guanethidine, reserpine, glutamic acid HCl) and urinary acidifying agents (eg, ammonium chloride, sodium acid phosphate) lower blood levels and efficacy. Inhibits adrenergic blockers. GI alkalinizing agents (eg, sodium bicarbonate) and urinary alkalinizing agents (eg, acetazolamide, some thiazides) increase blood levels and potentiate actions. May enhance activity of TCAs or sympathomimetic agents. Desipramine or protriptyline and possibly other TCAs cause striking and sustained increases in the concentration of d-amphetamine in the brain; cardiovascular effects can be potentiated. May counteract sedative effects of antihistamines. May antagonize hypotensive effects of antihypertensives. Chlorpromazine and haloperidol blocks dopamine and norepinephrine reuptake, thus inhibiting central stimulant effects. May delay intestinal absorption of ethosuximide, phenobarbital, and phenytoin; coadministration with phenobarbital or phenytoin may produce a synergistic anticonvulsant action. Lithium carbonate may inhibit stimulatory effects. Potentiates analgesic effect of meperidine. Acidifying agents used in methenamine therapy increase urinary excretion and reduce efficacy. Enhances adrenergic effect of norepinephrine. In cases of propoxyphene overdosage, CNS stimulation is potentiated and fatal convulsions can occur. Inhibits hypotensive effect of veratrum alkaloids.

NURSING CONSIDERATIONS

Assessment: Assess for hypersensitivity/idiosyncrasy to sympathomimetic amines, advanced arteriosclerosis, symptomatic CVD, moderate to severe HTN, hyperthyroidism, glaucoma, agitated states, history of drug abuse, tics, Tourette's syndrome, preexisting psychotic disorder, risk for/comorbid bipolar disorder, medical conditions that might be compromised by increases in BP or HR, any other conditions where treatment is cautioned, pregnancy/nursing status, and possible drug interactions.

Monitoring: Monitor for changes in HR and BP, signs/symptoms of cardiac disease, exacerbation of symptoms of behavior disturbance and thought disorder, psychosis, mania, appearance of or worsening of aggressive behavior or hostility, seizures, peripheral vasculopathy (eg, digital changes), visual disturbances, exacerbation of motor and phone tics or Tourette's syndrome, and other adverse reactions. In pediatric patients, monitor growth.

Patient Counseling: Inform about benefits and risks of treatment. Counsel that drug has high potential for abuse. Caution against engaging in potentially hazardous activities (eg, operating machinery/vehicles). Inform about risk of peripheral vasculopathy, including Raynaud's phenomenon. Instruct to report signs/symptoms of peripheral vasculopathy to physician. Instruct to call physician immediately with any signs of unexplained wounds appearing on fingers or toes.

Storage: 20-25°C (68-77°F); excursions permitted to 15-30°C (59-86°F).

ZERBAXA – ceftolozane/tazobactam RX

Class: Beta-lactamase inhibitor/cephalosporin

ADULT DOSAGE

Intra-Abdominal Infections

Complicated Infections:
1.5g (1g/0.5g) q8h for 4-14 days, in conjunction w/ metronidazole 500mg IV q8h

Urinary Tract Infections

Complicated Infections, Including Pyelonephritis:
1.5g (1g/0.5g) q8h for 7 days

PEDIATRIC DOSAGE

Pediatric use may not have been established

DOSE MODIFICATION

Renal Impairment

CrCl 30-50mL/min: 750mg (500mg/250mg) q8h
CrCl 15-29mL/min: 375mg (250mg/125mg) q8h
ESRD on Hemodialysis:
LD: 750mg (500mg/250mg)
Maint: 150mg (100mg/50mg) q8h for remainder of treatment period (on hemodialysis days, administer dose at earliest possible time following completion of dialysis)

ADMINISTRATION

IV route

Infuse over 1 hr
Do not mix w/ other drugs or physically add to sol containing other drugs

Preparation

Constitute vial w/ 10mL of sterile water for inj or 0.9% NaCl for inj (final vol 11.4mL); shake gently to dissolve
Withdraw appropriate volume from reconstituted vial and add to an infusion bag containing 100mL of 0.9% NaCl for inj or D5 inj
Preparation of Doses:
1.5g (1g/0.5g) Dose: Withdraw 11.4mL (entire vial contents)
750mg (500mg/250mg) Dose: Withdraw 5.7mL
375mg (250mg/125mg) Dose: Withdraw 2.9mL
150mg (100mg/50mg) Dose: Withdraw 1.2mL

HOW SUPPLIED

Inj: (Ceftolozane-Tazobactam) 1g-0.5g

WARNINGS/PRECAUTIONS

Serious and occasionally fatal hypersensitivity (anaphylactic) reactions reported; d/c therapy and institute appropriate therapy if an anaphylactic reaction occurs. Caution w/ cephalosporin, penicillin (PCN), or other β-lactam allergy; cross sensitivity may occur. *Clostridium difficile*-associated diarrhea (CDAD) reported; d/c if CDAD is confirmed. Use in the absence of a proven or strongly suspected bacterial infection is unlikely to provide benefit and increases the risk of the development of drug-resistant bacteria. Caution in elderly.

ADVERSE REACTIONS

N/V, headache, diarrhea, pyrexia, constipation, insomnia, hypokalemia.

NURSING CONSIDERATIONS

Assessment: Assess for hypersensitivity/allergy to drug, piperacillin/tazobactam, cephalosporin, PCN, or other β-lactam, renal impairment, pregnancy/nursing status, and possible drug interactions.

Monitoring: Monitor for signs and symptoms of hypersensitivity reactions, CDAD, and other adverse reactions. Monitor CrCl daily in patients w/ changing renal function.

Patient Counseling: Advise that allergic reactions, including serious allergic reactions, may occur and require immediate treatment. Advise that diarrhea is a common problem caused by antibacterial drugs and sometimes, frequent watery or bloody diarrhea may occur and may be a sign of a more serious intestinal infection; if severe watery and bloody diarrhea develops, instruct to contact physician. Inform that therapy should only be used to treat bacterial, not viral, infections. Instruct to take exactly ud even if the patient feels better early in the course of therapy. Inform that skipping doses or not completing the full course of therapy may decrease effectiveness and increase risk of bacterial resistance.

Storage: 2-8°C (36-46°F). Protect from light. Reconstituted Sol: May be held for 1 hr prior to transfer and dilution in a suitable infusion bag upon constitution w/ sterile water for inj or 0.9% NaCl inj. Diluted Sol: May store for 24 hrs at room temperature or for 7 days under refrigeration at 2-8°C (36-46°F). Do not freeze constituted sol or diluted infusion.

ZESTORETIC – hydrochlorothiazide/lisinopril

RX

Class: ACE inhibitor/thiazide diuretic

D/C when pregnancy is detected. Drugs that act directly on the renin-angiotensin system (RAS) can cause injury/death to the developing fetus.

ADULT DOSAGE

Hypertension

BP Uncontrolled w/ Lisinopril/HCTZ Monotherapy:
10mg-12.5mg or 20mg-12.5mg qd, depending on current monotherapy dose
If possible, d/c diuretic 2-3 days prior to therapy. If BP is controlled w/ lisinopril alone, then diuretic therapy may be resumed
Titrate: Base further increases on clinical response
May increase HCTZ dose after 2-3 weeks
May reduce lisinopril dose after addition of diuretic

BP Controlled on HCTZ 25mg qd w/ Hypokalemia: Switch to 10mg-12.5mg qd

Replacement Therapy: May substitute for the titrated individual components

PEDIATRIC DOSAGE

Pediatric use may not have been established

DOSE MODIFICATION

Elderly

Start at lower end of dosing range

ADMINISTRATION

Oral route

HOW SUPPLIED

Tab: (Lisinopril-HCTZ) 10mg-12.5mg, 20mg-12.5mg, 20mg-25mg

CONTRAINDICATIONS

History of ACE inhibitor-associated angioedema, hereditary or idiopathic angioedema, anuria, hypersensitivity to other sulfonamide-derived drugs. Coadministration with aliskiren in patients with diabetes.

WARNINGS/PRECAUTIONS

Not for initial therapy of HTN. Not recommended with severe renal impairment (CrCl ≤30mL/min). Caution in elderly. Lisinopril: Head/neck angioedema reported; promptly d/c and administer appropriate therapy. Higher rate of angioedema in blacks than nonblacks. Intestinal angioedema reported; monitor for abdominal pain. Anaphylactoid reactions reported during desensitization with hymenoptera venom, dialysis with high-flux membranes, and LDL apheresis with dextran sulfate absorption. Excessive hypotension may occur in salt/volume-depleted persons (eg, patients treated vigorously with diuretics or on dialysis). Excessive hypotension, which may be associated with oliguria and/or progressive azotemia, and rarely with acute renal failure and/or death, may occur in patients with severe CHF; monitor closely during first 2 weeks of therapy and whenever dose is increased. Caution with ischemic heart or cerebrovascular disease in whom an excessive fall in BP could result in a MI or cerebrovascular accident. Leukopenia/neutropenia and bone marrow depression may occur. Associated with a syndrome that starts with cholestatic jaundice or hepatitis and progresses to fulminant hepatic necrosis and sometimes death (rare); d/c if jaundice or marked elevations of hepatic enzymes develop. Caution with left ventricular outflow obstruction. May cause changes in renal function; in patients with severe CHF whose renal function is dependent on the RAS system, oliguria and/or progressive azotemia, and (rare) acute renal failure and/or death may occur . May increase BUN and SrCr in patients with renal artery stenosis or with no preexisting renal vascular disease; monitor renal function during the 1st few weeks of therapy in patients with renal artery stenosis. Hyperkalemia and persistent nonproductive cough reported. Hypotension may occur with major surgery or during anesthesia. HCTZ: May cause idiosyncratic reaction, resulting in acute transient myopia and acute angle-closure glaucoma; d/c as rapidly as possible. May precipitate azotemia in patients with renal disease. Caution with hepatic dysfunction or progressive liver disease; may precipitate hepatic coma. Sensitivity reactions may occur. May cause exacerbation or activation of systemic lupus erythematosus (SLE), hyperuricemia or precipitation of frank gout, manifestation of latent diabetes mellitus (DM), hypomagnesemia, and hypercalcemia. Observe for signs of fluid or electrolyte imbalance (hyponatremia, hypochloremic alkalosis, hypokalemia). Hypokalemia may sensitize or exaggerate the response of the heart to toxic effects of digitalis. Enhanced effects in postsympathectomy patients. D/C or withhold if progressive renal impairment becomes evident. D/C before testing for parathyroid function. Increased cholesterol and TG levels reported.

ADVERSE REACTIONS

Dizziness, headache, cough, fatigue, orthostatic effects.

DRUG INTERACTIONS

See Contraindications. NSAIDs, including selective COX-2 inhibitors, may reduce effects of diuretics and ACE inhibitors, and may deteriorate renal function. Increased risk of lithium toxicity; avoid with lithium. Lisinopril: Dual blockade of the RAS is associated with increased risks of hypotension, hyperkalemia, and changes in renal function (including acute renal failure); avoid combined use of RAS inhibitors, or closely monitor BP, renal function, and electrolytes with concomitant agents that also affect the RAS. Avoid with aliskiren in patients with renal impairment (GFR <60mL/min). Hypotension risk, and increased BUN and SrCr with diuretics. Increased risk of hyperkalemia with K^+-sparing diuretics (eg, spironolactone, eplerenone, triamterene, amiloride), K^+ supplements, or K^+-containing salt substitutes; use with caution and monitor serum K^+. Nitritoid reactions reported with injectable gold. HCTZ: Potentiation of orthostatic hypotension may occur with alcohol, barbiturates, or narcotics. Dosage adjustment of antidiabetic drugs (oral agents, insulin) may be required. Additive effect or potentiation with other antihypertensives. Anionic exchange resins (cholestyramine, colestipol) may impair absorption. Corticosteroids and adrenocorticotropic hormone may intensify electrolyte depletion, particularly hypokalemia. May decrease response to pressor amines (eg, norepinephrine). May increase responsiveness to nondepolarizing skeletal muscle relaxants (eg, tubocurarine).

NURSING CONSIDERATIONS

Assessment: Assess for hereditary/idiopathic angioedema, anuria, DM, volume/salt depletion, CHF, ischemic heart or cerebrovascular disease, collagen vascular disease, left ventricular outflow obstruction, SLE, history of ACE inhibitor-associated angioedema, hypersensitivity to drug or sulfonamide-derived drugs, renal/hepatic dysfunction, postsympathectomy status, pregnancy/nursing status, and possible drug interactions.

Monitoring: Monitor for signs/symptoms of angioedema, anaphylactoid/idiosyncratic/hypersensitivity reactions, exacerbation/activation of SLE, hyperuricemia or precipitation of gout, latent DM, fluid/electrolyte imbalance, and other adverse reactions. Monitor BP, renal/hepatic function, serum electrolytes, cholesterol, and TG levels. Consider periodic monitoring of WBCs in patients with collagen vascular disease and renal disease.

Patient Counseling: Inform about fetal risks if taken during pregnancy and discuss treatment options in women planning to become pregnant; instruct to report pregnancy to physician as soon as possible. Instruct to d/c therapy and to immediately report signs/symptoms of angioedema. Instruct to report lightheadedness, especially during the 1st few days of therapy; advise to d/c therapy and consult with a physician if actual syncope occurs. Inform that excessive perspiration, dehydration, and other causes of volume depletion (eg, diarrhea, vomiting) may lead to fall in BP; advise to consult with physician. Advise not to use salt substitutes containing K^+ without consulting physician. Advise to promptly report any indication of infection (eg, sore throat, fever).

Storage: 20-25°C (68-77°F). Protect from excessive light and humidity.

ZESTRIL – lisinopril

RX

Class: ACE inhibitor

D/C when pregnancy is detected. Drugs that act directly on the renin-angiotensin system (RAS) can cause injury/death to the developing fetus.

ADULT DOSAGE

Hypertension

Initial: 10mg qd
Titrate: Adjust dose according to BP response
Usual: 20-40mg qd
Max: 80mg

PEDIATRIC DOSAGE

Hypertension

≥6 Years:
GFR >30mL/min:
Initial: 0.07mg/kg qd (up to 5mg total)

May add a low-dose diuretic if BP is not controlled

Heart Failure

Reduce Signs and Symptoms of Systolic HF: Adjunct w/ Diuretics and (Usually) Digitalis:
Initial: 5mg qd
Titrate: Increase as tolerated
Max: 40mg qd

Diuretic dose may need to be adjusted to help minimize hypovolemia

Acute Myocardial Infarction

Reduction of Mortality in Hemodynamically Stable Patients w/in 24 Hrs of AMI:
5mg w/in 24 hrs of onset of symptoms, followed by 5mg after 24 hrs, 10mg after 48 hrs, and then 10mg qd for at least 6 weeks

Titrate: Adjust dose according to BP response
Max: 0.61mg/kg (up to 40mg) qd

DOSE MODIFICATION

Concomitant Medications

HTN:
Initial Dose w/ Diuretics: 5mg qd

Renal Impairment

CrCl 10-30mL/min: Reduce initial dose to 1/2 the usual recommended dose (eg, HTN, 5mg; systolic HF/AMI, 2.5mg)
Up titrate as tolerated to a max of 40mg qd
Hemodialysis or CrCl <10mL/min:
Initial: 2.5mg qd

Other Important Modifications

HF:
W/ Hyponatremia (Serum Na^+ <130mEq/L):
Initial: 2.5mg qd

Reduction of Mortality in AMI:
Low Systolic BP (SBP) (>100-120mmHg) During First 3 Days After Infarct:
Initial: 2.5mg
Maint: 5mg qd w/ temporary reductions to 2.5mg if needed, if SBP ≤100mmHg occurs
D/C if SBP <90mmHg for >1 hr occurs

ADMINISTRATION

Oral route

HOW SUPPLIED

Tab: 2.5mg, 5mg*, 10mg, 20mg, 30mg, 40mg *scored

CONTRAINDICATIONS

History of ACE inhibitor-associated angioedema, hereditary or idiopathic angioedema. Coadministration with aliskiren in patients with diabetes.

WARNINGS/PRECAUTIONS

Not recommended in pediatric patients with GFR <30mL/min. Head/neck angioedema reported; d/c promptly and administer appropriate therapy. Intestinal angioedema reported; monitor for abdominal pain. Patients with history of angioedema unrelated to ACE inhibitor therapy may be at increased risk of angioedema during therapy. Less effect on BP and more reports of angioedema in blacks than nonblacks. Anaphylactoid reactions reported during desensitization with hymenoptera venom, dialysis with high-flux membranes, and LDL apheresis with dextran sulfate absorption. May cause changes in renal function, including acute renal failure, especially in patients whose renal function depends on the RAS system; consider withholding or discontinuing therapy if a clinically significant decrease in renal function develops. May cause symptomatic hypotension, sometimes complicated by oliguria, progressive azotemia, acute renal failure, or death; closely monitor patients at risk of excessive hypotension during first 2 weeks of treatment and whenever therapy and/or diuretic dose is increased. Symptomatic hypotension may occur in patients with severe aortic stenosis or hypertrophic cardiomyopathy. Increases in BUN and SrCr with renal artery stenosis reported. Hypotension may occur with major surgery or during anesthesia. Hyperkalemia reported. Associated with syndrome that starts with cholestatic jaundice or hepatitis and progresses to fulminant hepatic necrosis, and sometimes death; d/c if jaundice or marked hepatic enzyme elevations occur.

ADVERSE REACTIONS

Dizziness, headache, hypotension, hyperkalemia, syncope, increased creatinine/BUN.

DRUG INTERACTIONS

See Contraindications. Hypotension risk and increased BUN and SrCr with diuretics. Increased hypoglycemic risk with insulin or oral hypoglycemics. NSAIDs, including selective COX-2 inhibitors, may cause deterioration of renal function. Antihypertensive effect may be attenuated by NSAIDs. Dual blockade of the RAS is associated with increased risks of hypotension, hyperkalemia, and changes in renal function (including acute renal failure); avoid combined use of RAS inhibitors, or closely monitor BP, renal function, and electrolytes with concomitant agents that also affect the RAS. Avoid with aliskiren in patients with renal impairment (GFR <60mL/min). Increased risk of hyperkalemia with K^+-sparing diuretics, K^+-containing salt substitutes, or K^+ supplements; monitor serum K^+ periodically. Lithium toxicity reported; monitor serum lithium levels during concurrent use. Nitritoid reactions reported with injectable gold.

NURSING CONSIDERATIONS

Assessment: Assess for hypersensitivity to the drug, history of ACE inhibitor-associated angioedema, hereditary/idiopathic angioedema, risk factors for hyperkalemia, risk for excessive hypotension, severe aortic stenosis or hypertrophic cardiomyopathy, renal impairment, pregnancy/nursing status, and possible drug interactions.

Monitoring: Monitor for angioedema, anaphylactoid reactions, and other adverse reactions. Monitor BP, LFTs, serum K^+, and renal function.

Patient Counseling: Inform of pregnancy risks and discuss treatment options for women planning to become pregnant; instruct to report pregnancy to physician as soon as possible. Instruct to immediately report signs/symptoms of angioedema and to avoid drug until they have consulted with prescribing physician. Instruct to report lightheadedness, especially during 1st few days of therapy; if syncope occurs, advise to d/c therapy until physician is consulted. Advise that excessive perspiration, dehydration, and other causes of volume depletion may lead to excessive fall in BP; instruct to consult with a physician. Advise not to use salt substitutes containing K^+ without consulting physician. Advise diabetic patients treated with oral antidiabetic agents or insulin to closely monitor for hypoglycemia, especially during the 1st month of combined use. Instruct to report promptly any indication of infection, which may be a sign of leukopenia/neutropenia.

Storage: 20-25°C (68-77°F). Protect from moisture, freezing, and excessive heat.

ZETIA — ezetimibe

RX

Class: Cholesterol absorption inhibitor

ADULT DOSAGE

Primary Hyperlipidemia

Heterozygous familial and nonfamilial hyperlipidemia, alone or in combination w/ a statin; mixed hyperlipidemia in combination w/ fenofibrate

10mg qd

Homozygous Familial Hypercholesterolemia

10mg qd in combination w/ atorvastatin or simvastatin

Homozygous Sitosterolemia

10mg qd

PEDIATRIC DOSAGE

Pediatric use may not have been established

DOSE MODIFICATION

Concomitant Medications

Bile Acid Sequestrant:

Give either ≥2 hrs before or ≥4 hrs after bile acid sequestrant

Renal Impairment

Moderate to Severe (GFR <60mL/min):

W/ Simvastatin: Use caution and monitor closely w/ simvastatin doses >20mg

Hepatic Impairment

Moderate to Severe: Use is not recommended

ADMINISTRATION

Oral route

Take w/ or w/o food

HOW SUPPLIED

Tab: 10mg

CONTRAINDICATIONS
Active liver disease or unexplained persistent elevations in hepatic transaminase levels, women who are or may become pregnant, and nursing mothers when used with statins.

WARNINGS/PRECAUTIONS
Not recommended with moderate to severe hepatic impairment. Should be used in accordance with the product labeling for the concurrently administered drug (eg, specific statin or fenofibrate). Liver enzyme elevations reported with statins. Consider withdrawal of therapy and/or statin if an increase in ALT or AST ≥3X ULN persists. Myopathy and rhabdomyolysis reported; immediately d/c therapy and any concomitant statin or fibrate, if myopathy is diagnosed/suspected. Increased risk for skeletal muscle toxicity with higher doses of statin, advanced age (>65 yrs of age), hypothyroidism, renal impairment, depending on the statin used, and concomitant use of other drugs. Caution and close monitoring when used with simvastatin >20mg in patients with moderate to severe renal impairment.

ADVERSE REACTIONS
URTI, diarrhea, arthralgia, sinusitis, pain in extremity.

DRUG INTERACTIONS
Caution with cyclosporine; monitor cyclosporine levels. May increase cholesterol excretion into the bile, leading to cholelithiasis with fibrates; avoid with fibrates (except fenofibrate). Consider alternative lipid-lowering therapy if cholelithiasis occurs with fenofibrate. Decreased levels with cholestyramine; incremental LDL-C reduction may be reduced. Monitor INR levels when used with warfarin.

NURSING CONSIDERATIONS

Assessment: Assess for hepatic impairment, pregnancy/nursing status, and possible drug interactions. Obtain baseline lipid profile (total-C, LDL-C, HDL-C, TG). Assess for conditions where treatment is contraindicated and risk factors for skeletal muscle toxicity. Obtain baseline LFTs (eg, ALT, AST) when used with statin.

Monitoring: Monitor for signs/symptoms of elevated liver enzymes, myopathy, rhabdomyolysis, and other adverse reactions. Perform periodic monitoring of lipid profile. Periodically monitor LFTs during concomitant statin therapy.

Patient Counseling: Advise to adhere to the National Cholesterol Education Program recommended diet, a regular exercise program, and periodic testing of a fasting lipid panel. Counsel about risk of myopathy; instruct to promptly report to the physician if any unexplained muscle pain, tenderness, or weakness occurs. Advise to discuss with physician about all medications, both prescription and OTC, currently being taken. Counsel women of childbearing age to use an effective method of birth control while using added statin therapy and instruct to d/c combination therapy and contact physician if they become pregnant. Instruct breastfeeding women not to take the medication if concomitantly using statins; advise patients who have lipid disorder and are breastfeeding to discuss the options with their physician.

Storage: 25°C (77°F); excursions permitted to 15-30°C (59-86°F). Protect from moisture.

ZIAC – bisoprolol fumarate/hydrochlorothiazide

RX

Class: Selective $beta_1$-blocker/thiazide diuretic

ADULT DOSAGE

Hypertension

Uncontrolled BP on 2.5mg-20mg/day Bisoprolol or Controlled BP on 50mg/day HCTZ w/ Hypokalemia:
Initial: 2.5mg-6.25mg qd
Titrate: May increase at 14-day intervals
Max: 20mg-12.5mg (two 10mg-6.25mg tab) qd, as appropriate

Replacement Therapy:
May substitute for titrated individual components

Cessation of Therapy:
Withdrawal should be achieved gradually over a period of 2 weeks

PEDIATRIC DOSAGE
Pediatric use may not have been established

DOSE MODIFICATION

Renal Impairment
Caution in dosing/titrating

Hepatic Impairment
Caution in dosing/titrating

ADMINISTRATION
Oral route

HOW SUPPLIED
Tab: (Bisoprolol/HCTZ) 2.5mg/6.25mg, 5mg/6.25mg, 10mg/6.25mg

CONTRAINDICATIONS
Cardiogenic shock, overt cardiac failure, 2nd- or 3rd-degree atrioventricular (AV) block, marked sinus bradycardia, anuria, hypersensitivity to sulfonamide-derived drugs.

WARNINGS/PRECAUTIONS
Caution with impaired hepatic function/progressive liver disease. Bisoprolol: Caution with compensated cardiac failure. May precipitate cardiac failure; consider discontinuation at 1st signs/symptoms of heart failure (HF). Exacerbations of angina pectoris, MI, and ventricular arrhythmia with coronary artery disease (CAD) reported upon abrupt discontinuation; caution against interruption or discontinuation without physician's advice. May precipitate or aggravate symptoms of arterial insufficiency with peripheral vascular disease (PVD); exercise caution. Avoid with bronchospastic disease, but may use with caution if unresponsive/intolerant of other antihypertensives. Chronically administered therapy should not be routinely withdrawn prior to major surgery; however, may augment risks of general anesthesia and surgical procedures. Caution with diabetes mellitus (DM); may mask tachycardia occurring with hypoglycemia. May mask hyperthyroidism and precipitate thyroid storm with abrupt discontinuation. HCTZ: May precipitate azotemia with impaired renal function. D/C if progressive renal impairment becomes apparent. May precipitate hepatic coma with hepatic impairment. May cause idiosyncratic reaction, resulting in acute transient myopia and acute angle-closure glaucoma; d/c as rapidly as possible. Monitor for fluid/electrolyte disturbances (eg, hyponatremia, hypochloremic alkalosis, hypokalemia, hypomagnesemia). Decreased Ca^{2+} excretion and altered parathyroid glands, with hypercalcemia and hypophosphatemia, observed on prolonged therapy. Precipitation of hyperuricemia/gout and sensitivity reactions may occur. Photosensitivity reactions and exacerbation/activation of systemic lupus erythematosus (SLE) reported. Enhanced effects in postsympathectomy patient. D/C prior to parathyroid function test.

ADVERSE REACTIONS
Hyperuricemia, dizziness, fatigue, headache, diarrhea.

DRUG INTERACTIONS
May potentiate other antihypertensive agents. Avoid with other β-blockers. Excessive reduction of sympathetic activity with catecholamine-depleting drugs (eg, reserpine, guanethidine); monitor closely. D/C for several days prior to clonidine withdrawal. Caution with myocardial depressants or inhibitors of AV conduction (eg, certain calcium antagonists [particularly phenylalkylamine and benzothiazepine classes], antiarrhythmic agents [eg, disopyramide]). Bisoprolol: Digitalis glycosides may increase risk of bradycardia. Rifampin may increase clearance. May be unresponsive to usual doses of epinephrine. HCTZ: Alcohol, barbiturates, or narcotics may potentiate orthostatic hypotension. Antidiabetic drugs (eg, oral agents, insulin) may require dosage adjustments. Impaired absorption with cholestyramine and colestipol resins. Corticosteroids and adrenocorticotropic hormone may intensify electrolyte depletion, particularly hypokalemia. May decrease response to pressor amines (eg, norepinephrine). May increase response to nondepolarizing skeletal muscle relaxants (eg, tubocurarine). Do not give with lithium; increased risk of lithium toxicity. NSAIDs may reduce diuretic, natriuretic, and antihypertensive effects.

NURSING CONSIDERATIONS

Assessment: Assess for cardiogenic shock, overt/compensated cardiac failure, 2nd- or 3rd-degree AV block, marked sinus bradycardia, anuria, sulfonamide hypersensitivity, CAD, PVD, bronchospastic disease, DM, hyperthyroidism, renal/hepatic impairment, history of sulfonamide/penicillin allergy, parathyroid disease, SLE, pregnancy/nursing status, and possible drug interactions. Obtain baseline serum electrolytes.

Monitoring: Monitor for signs/symptoms of HF, withdrawal, hypoglycemia, hyperthyroidism, renal/hepatic impairment, idiosyncratic reaction, fluid or electrolyte disturbances, precipitation of hyperuricemia or gout, and hypersensitivity reactions. Perform periodic monitoring of serum electrolytes.

Patient Counseling: Instruct not to d/c therapy without physician's supervision, especially in patients with CAD. Advise to consult physician if any difficulty in breathing occurs, or other signs/symptoms of CHF or excessive bradycardia develop. Inform that hypoglycemia may be masked in patients subject to spontaneous hypoglycemia, or diabetic patients receiving insulin or oral hypoglycemic agents; instruct to use with caution. Advise to avoid driving, operating machinery, or engaging in other tasks requiring alertness until reaction to drug is known. Advise that photosensitivity reactions may occur.

Storage: 20-25°C (68-77°F).

ZIANA – clindamycin phosphate/tretinoin

RX

Class: Lincosamide derivative/retinoid

ADULT DOSAGE

Acne Vulgaris

Apply at hs, a pea-sized amount onto 1 fingertip; dot onto the chin, cheeks, nose, and forehead; then gently rub over entire face

PEDIATRIC DOSAGE

Acne Vulgaris

≥12 Years:

Apply at hs, a pea-sized amount onto 1 fingertip; dot onto the chin, cheeks, nose, and forehead; then gently rub over entire face

ADMINISTRATION

Topical route

HOW SUPPLIED

Gel: (Clindamycin-Tretinoin) 1.2%-0.025% [30g, 60g]

CONTRAINDICATIONS

Regional enteritis, ulcerative colitis, or history of antibiotic-associated colitis.

WARNINGS/PRECAUTIONS

Not for oral, ophthalmic, or intravaginal use. Keep away from eyes, mouth, angles of the nose, and mucous membranes. Avoid exposure to sunlight, including sunlamps. Avoid use if sunburn is present. Daily use of sunscreen products and protective apparel are recommended. Weather extremes (eg, wind, cold) may be irritating while under treatment. Clindamycin: Systemic absorption has been demonstrated following topical use. Diarrhea, bloody diarrhea, and colitis (including pseudomembranous colitis) reported; d/c if significant diarrhea occurs. Severe colitis reported following PO or parenteral administration with an onset of up to several weeks following cessation of therapy.

ADVERSE REACTIONS

Nasopharyngitis, local skin reactions (erythema, scaling, itching, burning), GI symptoms.

DRUG INTERACTIONS

Caution with topical medications, medicated/abrasive soaps and cleansers, soaps/cosmetics with strong drying effect, products with high concentrations of alcohol, astringents, spices, or lime because skin irritation may be increased. Avoid with erythromycin-containing products. May enhance action of neuromuscular blocking agents; use with caution. Antiperistaltic agents (eg, opiates, diphenoxylate with atropine) may prolong and/or worsen severe colitis.

NURSING CONSIDERATIONS

Assessment: Assess for regional enteritis, ulcerative colitis, or history of antibiotic-associated colitis, pregnancy/nursing status, and possible drug interactions. Assess use in patients whose occupations require considerable sun exposure.

Monitoring: Monitor for signs/symptoms of diarrhea, bloody diarrhea, colitis, local skin reactions, and other adverse reactions.

Patient Counseling: Instruct to wash face gently with mild soap and warm water at hs and apply a thin layer over the entire face (excluding the eyes and lips) after patting the skin dry. Advise not to use more than recommended amount and not to apply more than qd (at hs). Instruct to apply sunscreen qam and reapply over the course of the day PRN. Advise to avoid exposure to sunlight, sunlamp, UV light, and other medicines that may increase sensitivity to sunlight. Inform that medication may cause irritation (eg, erythema, scaling, itching, burning, stinging). Instruct to d/c therapy and contact physician if severe diarrhea or GI discomfort occurs.

Storage: 25°C (77°F); excursions permitted to 15-30°C (59-86°F). Protect from light and freezing. Keep away from heat. Keep tube tightly closed.

ZIDOVUDINE – zidovudine

RX

Class: Nucleoside reverse transcriptase inhibitor

Associated w/ hematologic toxicity (eg, neutropenia, severe anemia), particularly w/ advanced HIV-1 disease. Symptomatic myopathy associated w/ prolonged use. Lactic acidosis and severe hepatomegaly w/ steatosis, including fatal cases, reported w/ nucleoside analogues; suspend treatment if lactic acidosis or pronounced hepatotoxicity occurs.

OTHER BRAND NAMES

Retrovir

ADULT DOSAGE

Prevention of Maternal-Fetal HIV Transmission

>14 Weeks of Pregnancy:
PO:
100mg 5X/day until start of labor
During Labor and Delivery:
IV:
2mg/kg over 1 hr followed by continuous infusion of 1mg/kg/hr until clamping of umbilical cord

HIV-1 Infection

Combination w/ Other Antiretrovirals:
PO:
300mg bid

IV:
1mg/kg at a constant rate over 1 hr q4h

PEDIATRIC DOSAGE

HIV-1 Infection

Combination w/ Other Antiretrovirals:
4 Weeks-<18 Years:
Weight Based:
4-<9kg: 12mg/kg bid or 8mg/kg tid (24mg/kg/day)
≥9-<30kg: 9mg/kg bid or 6mg/kg tid (18mg/kg/day)
≥30kg: 300mg bid or 200mg tid (600mg/day)

BSA Based:
240mg/m^2 bid or 160mg/m^2 tid (480mg/m^2/day)

Prevention of Maternal-Fetal HIV Transmission

Neonates:
Start w/in 12 hrs after birth and continue through 6 weeks of age
PO: 2mg/kg q6h (8mg/kg/day)
IV: 1.5mg/kg over 30 min q6h (6mg/kg/day)

DOSE MODIFICATION

Renal Impairment

Hemodialysis/Peritoneal Dialysis/CrCl <15mL/min:
PO: 100mg q6-8h
IV: 1mg/kg q6-8h

Adverse Reactions

Significant Anemia (Hgb <7.5g/dL or Reduction >25% of Baseline)/Neutropenia (Granulocyte Count <750 cells/mm^3 or Reduction >50% from Baseline):
May require dose interruption until evidence of marrow recovery occurs
If marrow recovery occurs following dose interruption, may resume dose using adjunctive measures (eg, epoetin alfa), depending on hematologic indices and patient tolerance

ADMINISTRATION

Oral/IV route

Administer IV infusion only until oral therapy can be administered

PO

Take w/ or w/o food

IV

Avoid rapid infusion and bolus inj
Infusion must be diluted prior to administration

Dilution Instructions

1. Remove calculated dose from the 20mL vial and add to D5 inj sol to a concentration ≤4mg/mL
2. Administer diluted sol w/in 8 hrs if stored at 25°C (77°F) or 24 hrs if stored at 2-8°C (36-46°F), to minimize contamination

HOW SUPPLIED

Tab: 300mg; (Retrovir) Cap: 100mg; Inj: 10mg/mL [20mL]; Syrup: 10mg/mL [240mL]

WARNINGS/PRECAUTIONS

Caution w/ granulocyte count <1000 cells/mm^3 or Hgb <9.5g/dL; monitor blood counts frequently in patients w/ poor bone marrow reserve, particularly w/ advanced HIV-1 disease and periodically w/ other HIV-infected patients and w/ asymptomatic/early HIV-1 disease. Vial stoppers for inj contain natural rubber latex which may cause allergic reactions in latex-sensitive individuals. Obesity and prolonged nucleoside exposure may be risk factors for lactic acidosis and severe hepatomegaly w/ steatosis. Caution w/ any known risk factors for liver disease and in elderly. Pancytopenia and immune reconstitution syndrome reported. Autoimmune disorders (eg, Graves' disease, polymyositis, Guillain-Barre syndrome) reported to occur in the setting of immune reconstitution and can occur many months after initiation of treatment. May cause redistribution/accumulation of body fat.

ADVERSE REACTIONS

Hematologic toxicity, myopathy, lactic acidosis, severe hepatomegaly w/ steatosis, headache, N/V, malaise, anorexia, asthenia, constipation, abdominal pain/cramps, arthralgia, chills.

DRUG INTERACTIONS

Avoid w/ stavudine, nucleoside analogues affecting DNA replication (eg, ribavirin), doxorubicin, and other combination products containing zidovudine. Hepatic decompensation may occur in HIV/hepatitis C virus (HCV) coinfected patients receiving interferon alfa w/ or w/o ribavirin; closely monitor for treatment-associated toxicities. May increase risk of hematologic toxicities w/ ganciclovir, interferon alfa, ribavirin, and other bone marrow suppressive or cytotoxic agents.

NURSING CONSIDERATIONS

Assessment: Assess for previous hypersensitivity reaction to the drug, advanced HIV disease, latex sensitivity, risk factors for lactic acidosis/liver disease, bone marrow compromise, renal/hepatic impairment, pregnancy/nursing status, and possible drug interactions. (Oral) Assess ability to swallow cap/tab in children.

Monitoring: Monitor for signs/symptoms of hematologic toxicity, lactic acidosis, hepatomegaly w/ steatosis, myopathy, immune reconstitution syndrome, autoimmune disorders, fat redistribution/ accumulation, and other adverse reactions. Monitor blood counts/hematologic indices periodically and the need for dosage adjustment.

Patient Counseling: Inform that potentially life-threatening hypersensitivity reactions can occur; instruct to immediately contact physician if rash develops. Inform about risk for hematologic toxicities and advise on importance of close blood count monitoring while on therapy. Counsel about the possible occurrence of myopathy and myositis w/ pathological changes during prolonged use and that therapy may cause a rare but serious condition called lactic acidosis w/ liver enlargement (hepatomegaly). Inform that hepatic decompensation has occurred in HIV-1/ HCV coinfected patients receiving combination antiretroviral therapy and interferon alfa w/ or w/o ribavirin. Inform that immune reconstitution syndrome may occur; advise to inform physician immediately of any symptoms of infection. Inform that redistribution/accumulation of body fat may occur. Instruct to report any other adverse events that occur. Instruct not to breastfeed to prevent postnatal transmission. Inform that drug is not a cure for HIV-1 infection and that illness associated w/ HIV-1 may still be experienced. Inform to take all HIV medications exactly as prescribed. Advise to avoid doing things that can spread HIV-1 infection to others; instruct to continue to practice safe sex.

Storage: (Tab) 20-25°C (68-77°F). (Retrovir) 15-25°C (59-77°F). (Cap) Protect from moisture. (Inj) Protect from light. Diluted Sol: Stable for 24 hrs at room temperature and for 48 hrs if refrigerated at 2-8°C (36-46°F).

ZIPSOR – diclofenac potassium RX

Class: NSAID

NSAIDs may increase risk of serious cardiovascular (CV) thrombotic events, MI, and stroke; increased risk w/ duration of use and w/ cardiovascular disease (CVD) or risk factors for CVD. Increased risk of serious GI adverse events (eg, bleeding, ulceration, and stomach/intestinal perforation) that can be fatal and occur anytime during use w/o warning symptoms; elderly patients are at a greater risk. Contraindicated for treatment of perioperative pain in the setting of CABG surgery.

ADULT DOSAGE

Mild to Moderate Pain

Initial: 25mg qid

Use lowest effective dose for the shortest duration of time

PEDIATRIC DOSAGE

Pediatric use may not have been established

DOSE MODIFICATION

Elderly

Start at lower end of dosing range

ADMINISTRATION

Oral route

HOW SUPPLIED

Cap: 25mg

CONTRAINDICATIONS

Asthma, urticaria, or other allergic reactions after taking aspirin (ASA) or other NSAIDs. Hypersensitivity to bovine protein. Treatment of perioperative pain in the setting of CABG surgery.

WARNINGS/PRECAUTIONS

Different formulations of oral diclofenac are not bioequivalent even if the mg strength is the same; not possible to convert dosing from any other formulation of diclofenac. May cause elevations of LFTs, hepatotoxicity, and severe hepatic reactions; d/c if abnormal LFTs persist/worsen, liver disease develops, or systemic manifestations occur. May lead to onset of new HTN or worsening of preexisting HTN. Fluid retention and edema reported; caution w/ fluid retention or heart failure. Caution in patients w/ considerable dehydration. Renal papillary necrosis and other renal injury reported after long-term use. Renal toxicity reported in patients in whom renal prostaglandins have a compensatory role in the maintenance of renal perfusion. Not recommended for use w/ advanced renal disease; if therapy must be initiated, monitor renal function. Anaphylactoid reactions may occur. Contraindicated in ASA triad patients. May cause serious skin adverse events (eg, exfoliative dermatitis, Stevens-Johnson syndrome, toxic epidermal necrolysis); d/c at 1st appearance of skin rash/hypersensitivity. Avoid in late pregnancy; may cause premature closure of ductus arteriosus. Caution in elderly and debilitated. Anemia may occur; w/ long-term use, monitor Hgb/Hct if signs or symptoms of anemia develop. May inhibit platelet aggregation and prolong bleeding time. Caution w/ asthma and avoid w/ ASA-sensitive asthma. May diminish utility of diagnostic signs (eg, inflammation, fever) in detecting complications of presumed noninfectious, painful conditions. Not a substitute for corticosteroids or to treat corticosteroid insufficiency.

ADVERSE REACTIONS

Abdominal pain, constipation, diarrhea, dyspepsia, N/V, dizziness, headache, somnolence, pruritus, increased sweating.

DRUG INTERACTIONS

Increased adverse effects w/ ASA; concomitant use not generally recommended. May increase risk of GI bleeding w/ oral corticosteroids or anticoagulants or tobacco or alcohol use. May impair therapeutic response to ACE inhibitors. May reduce the natriuretic effect of thiazides or loop diuretics; monitor for signs of renal failure and diuretic efficacy. Synergistic effects on GI bleeding w/ warfarin. May increase lithium levels; monitor for lithium toxicity. May enhance methotrexate toxicity; caution when coadministering. May increase nephrotoxicity of cyclosporine; caution when coadministering. Caution w/ coadministration of other drugs that are substrates or inhibitors of CYP2C9. Caution w/ potentially hepatotoxic drugs (eg, acetaminophen [APAP], certain antibiotics, antiepileptics).

NURSING CONSIDERATIONS

Assessment: Assess for history of CABG surgery, asthma and allergic reactions to ASA or other NSAIDs, CVD or risk factors, GI bleeding or risk factors, considerable dehydration, renal/hepatic impairment, coagulation disorders, any other conditions where treatment is contraindicated or cautioned, pregnancy/nursing status, and possible drug interactions. Assess baseline BP, CBC, and chemistry profile.

Monitoring: Monitor for GI/CV events, fluid retention, anaphylactoid/skin reactions, hematological effects, and other adverse reactions. Monitor BP, LFTs, renal function, CBC, and chemistry profile periodically.

Patient Counseling: Advise to seek medical attention if signs and symptoms of CV events, GI ulceration/bleeding, hepatotoxicity, skin reactions, anaphylactoid reactions, weight gain, or edema occur. Instruct to avoid use during late pregnancy. Caution patients to avoid taking unprescribed APAP while on therapy.

Storage: 25°C (77°F); excursions permitted to 15-30°C (59-86°F). Protect from moisture.

ZITHROMAX – azithromycin RX

Class: Macrolide

ADULT DOSAGE

Nongonococcal Urethritis

Sus (Single-Dose 1g Pkt)/Tab:
1g single dose

Nongonococcal Cervicitis

Sus (Single-Dose 1g Pkt)/Tab:
1g single dose

Gonococcal Infections

Gonococcal Urethritis and Cervicitis:
Tab (250mg, 500mg):
2g single dose

Community-Acquired Pneumonia

Inj:
500mg IV qd for at least 2 days, then 500mg PO (two 250mg tabs) qd to complete a 7- to 10-day course

Tab (250mg, 500mg):
500mg single dose on Day 1, then 250mg qd on Days 2-5

PEDIATRIC DOSAGE

Community-Acquired Pneumonia

Inj:
≥16 Years:
500mg IV qd for at least 2 days, then 500mg PO (two 250mg tabs) qd to complete a 7- to 10-day course

Sus (100mg/5mL, 200mg/5mL):
≥6 Months of Age:
10mg/kg single dose on Day 1, then 5mg/kg qd on Days 2-5
Refer to PI for dosage guidelines

Acute Pelvic Inflammatory Disease

Inj:
≥16 Years:
500mg qd IV for 1-2 days, followed by 250mg qd PO to complete a 7-day course

Acute Otitis Media

Sus (100mg/5mL, 200mg/5mL):
≥6 Months of Age:
30mg/kg single dose or 10mg/kg qd for 3 days

Pharyngitis/Tonsillitis

2nd-Line Therapy:
Tab (250mg, 500mg):
500mg single dose on Day 1, then 250mg qd on Days 2-5

Skin and Skin Structure Infections

Uncomplicated:
Tab (250mg, 500mg):
500mg single dose on Day 1, then 250mg qd on Days 2-5

Acute Bacterial Exacerbation of Chronic Bronchitis

Tab (250mg, 500mg):
500mg qd for 3 days or 500mg as a single dose on Day 1, followed by 250mg qd on Days 2-5

Acute Bacterial Sinusitis

Tab (250mg, 500mg):
500mg qd for 3 days

Genital Ulcers

Chancroid:
Tab (250mg, 500mg):
1g single dose

Mycobacterial Infections

Disseminated *Mycobacterium avium* Complex Disease:
Tab (600mg):
Prevention:
1200mg once weekly
Treatment:
600mg/day in combination w/ 15mg/kg/day ethambutol

Acute Pelvic Inflammatory Disease

Inj:
500mg qd IV for 1-2 days, followed by 250mg qd PO to complete a 7-day course

or 10mg/kg single dose on Day 1 followed by 5mg/kg/day on Days 2-5
Refer to PI for dosage guidelines

Pharyngitis/Tonsillitis

2nd Line Therapy:
Sus (100mg/5mL, 200mg/5mL):
≥ 2 Years:
12mg/kg qd for 5 days
Refer to PI for dosage guidelines

ADMINISTRATION
Oral/IV route

Shake sus well before use
Sus/Tab
Take w/ or w/o food
Sus (100mg/5mL, 200mg/5mL)
Reconstitution:
Add 9mL of water to 300mg or 600mg sus bottle, 12mL of water to 900mg sus bottle, or 15mL of water to 1200mg sus bottle
Sus (Single-Dose Pkt)
Do not use to administer doses other than 1000mg
Not for pediatric use
Reconstitution:
Mix entire contents of pkt w/ 2 oz (approx 60mL) of water
Drink entire contents immediately and add an additional 2 oz of water, mix, and drink to ensure complete consumption of dosage
Inj
Infusate concentration and rate of infusion should be either 1mg/mL over 3 hrs or 2mg/mL over 1 hr; avoid higher concentrations
Infuse over at least 60 min
Do not give as bolus or as IM inj
Do not add other IV substances, additives, or other medications or infuse simultaneously through same IV line
Reconstitution:
Reconstitute initial sol w/ 4.8mL of SWFI to 500mg vial using a standard 5mL (non-automated) syringe; each mL of reconstituted sol should contain 100mg azithromycin
Dilute further prior to administration
Refer to Vial-Mate instructions if using this device for reconstitution

Dilution:
Transfer 5mL of the 100mg/mL sol into the appropriate amount of any compatible diluent
Compatible Diluents:
0.9% NaCl, 0.45% NaCl, D5W, Lactated Ringer's Sol, D5 in 0.45% NaCl w/ 20mEq KCl, D5 in Lactated Ringer's Sol, D5 in 0.3% NaCl, D5 in 0.45NaCl, Normosol-M in D5, Normosol-R in D5

HOW SUPPLIED

Inj: 500mg; Sus: 100mg/5mL [15mL], 200mg/5mL [15mL, 22.5mL, 30mL], 1g [pkt]; Tab: 250mg, 500mg, 600mg

CONTRAINDICATIONS

History of cholestatic jaundice/hepatic dysfunction associated w/ prior use of therapy.

WARNINGS/PRECAUTIONS

Serious allergic reactions (eg, angioedema, anaphylaxis) and dermatologic reactions (eg, Stevens Johnson syndrome, toxic epidermal necrolysis) reported; d/c if an allergic reaction occurs and institute appropriate therapy. Allergic symptoms may recur, despite initial successful symptomatic treatment, w/o further therapy exposure. Abnormal liver function, hepatitis, cholestatic jaundice, hepatic necrosis, and hepatic failure reported; d/c immediately if signs and symptoms of hepatitis occur. Prolonged cardiac repolarization and QT interval, imparting a risk of developing cardiac arrhythmia and torsades de pointes reported. Consider risk of QT prolongation that can be fatal for at risk-groups, including patients w/ known QT interval prolongation, history of torsades de pointes, congenital long QT syndrome, bradyarrhythmias, uncompensated heart failure, ongoing proarrhythmic conditions (eg, uncorrected hypokalemia/hypomagnesemia), and clinically significant bradycardia. Elderly may be more susceptible to drug-associated effects on the QT interval. *Clostridium difficile*-associated diarrhea (CDAD) reported; may need to d/c if CDAD is suspected or confirmed. Exacerbation of myasthenia gravis symptoms and new onset of myasthenic syndrome reported. May result in bacterial resistance w/ prolonged use in the absence of proven or suspected bacterial infection, or a prophylactic indication. (Tab [250mg, 500mg]/Sus [100mg/5mL, 200mg/5mL]) Do not use in patients w/ pneumonia who are judged to be inappropriate for oral therapy due to moderate to severe illness or risk factors (eg, cystic fibrosis, nosocomial infections, known/suspected bacteremia, requiring hospitalization, elderly/debilitated patients, or w/ significant underlying health problems that may compromise the ability to respond to their illness [eg, immunodeficiency or functional asplenia]). Should not be relied upon to treat syphilis. (Sus [Single-Dose Pkt]) Should not be relied upon to treat gonorrhea or syphilis. (Inj) Local IV-site reactions reported.

ADVERSE REACTIONS

Diarrhea/loose stools, N/V, abdominal pain. (Tab [600mg]) Hearing impairment, flatulence, headache, abnormal vision. (Inj) Pain at inj site, local inflammation.

DRUG INTERACTIONS

Caution w/ drugs known to prolong the QT interval, Class IA (quinidine, procainamide), and Class III (dofetilide, amiodarone, sotalol) antiarrhythmic agents. Increased levels w/ nelfinavir; closely monitor for known adverse reactions (eg, liver enzyme abnormalities, hearing impairment). May potentiate effects of oral anticoagulants (eg, warfarin); monitor PT. Monitor carefully when coadministered w/ digoxin or phenytoin.

NURSING CONSIDERATIONS

Assessment: Assess for hypersensitivity to drug, history of cholestatic jaundice/hepatic dysfunction associated w/ prior use of therapy, risk for QT prolongation, myasthenia gravis, pregnancy/nursing status, and possible drug interactions. (Tab [250mg, 500mg]/Sus [Single-Dose Pkt]) In patients w/ sexually transmitted urethritis or cervicitis, perform serologic test for syphilis and appropriate testing for gonorrhea at the time of diagnosis. Perform appropriate culture and susceptibility testing. (Tab [250mg, 500mg]/Sus [100mg/5mL, 200mg/5mL]) Assess for pneumonia, cystic fibrosis, nosocomial infections, known/suspected bacteremia, elderly/debilitated patients, underlying health problems that may compromise ability to respond to illness, or if requiring hospitalization.

Monitoring: Monitor for signs/symptoms of serious allergic/dermatologic reactions, hepatotoxicity, CDAD, QT prolongation, new onset of myasthenic syndrome or exacerbation of myasthenia gravis, and other adverse reactions. (Inj) Monitor for local IV-site reactions.

Patient Counseling: Inform that diarrhea may occur and will usually end if therapy is discontinued. Instruct to contact physician as soon as possible if watery and bloody stools (w/ or w/o stomach cramps, fever) develop even as late as 2 or more months after the last dose. (Oral) Inform to d/c therapy immediately and contact physician if any signs of an allergic reaction occur. Instruct not to take the medication simultaneously w/ aluminum- and Mg^{2+}-containing antacids. Counsel that therapy should only be used to treat bacterial, not viral, infections. Instruct to take exactly ud; inform that skipping doses or not completing the full course of therapy may decrease effectiveness of immediate treatment and increase bacterial resistance.

Storage: Tab: (250mg, 500mg) 15-30°C (59-86°F). (600mg) ≤30°C (86°F). Sus (100mg/5mL, 200mg/5mL): Dry Powder: <30°C (86°F). Constituted: 5-30°C (41-86°F); use w/in 10 days. Discard when full dosing is completed. Sus (Single-Dose Pkt): 5-30°C (41-86°F). Inj: Reconstituted Sol: <30°C (86°F) for 24 hrs. Diluted Sol (Final Infusion Sol): ≤30°C (86°F) for 24 hrs or 5°C (41°F) for 7 days.

ZMAX – azithromycin

Class: Macrolide

RX

ADULT DOSAGE

Acute Bacterial Sinusitis

2g single dose

Community-Acquired Pneumonia

2g single dose

PEDIATRIC DOSAGE

Community-Acquired Pneumonia

≥6 Months:

<34kg: 60mg/kg single dose

≥34kg: 2g single dose

ADMINISTRATION

Oral route

Take on an empty stomach, at least 1 hr ac or 2 hrs pc
Constitute w/ 60mL of water; shake well before using
Consume reconstituted sus w/in 12 hrs

Pediatrics

Use a dosing spoon, medicine syringe, or cup for patients <34kg
Discard any remaining sus after dosing in pediatric patients

Additional Treatment After Vomiting

If vomiting occurs w/in 5 min of administration, consider additional antibiotic treatment
If vomiting occurs ≥60 min following therapy, a 2nd dose or alternative treatment is not warranted; in patients w/ delayed gastric emptying, consider alternative therapy

HOW SUPPLIED

Sus, Extended-Release: 2g

CONTRAINDICATIONS

History of cholestatic jaundice/hepatic dysfunction associated with prior use of azithromycin.

WARNINGS/PRECAUTIONS

Serious allergic reactions (eg, angioedema, anaphylaxis, Stevens Johnson syndrome [SJS], toxic epidermal necrolysis [TEN]) reported. Allergic symptoms may recur after initial successful symptomatic treatment without further azithromycin exposure. Abnormal liver function, hepatitis, cholestatic jaundice, hepatic necrosis, and hepatic failure reported, some of which resulted in death; d/c immediately if signs/symptoms of hepatitis occur. *Clostridium difficile*-associated diarrhea (CDAD) reported; d/c if CDAD is confirmed or suspected. Exacerbation of symptoms of myasthenia gravis and new onset of myasthenic syndrome reported. Prolonged cardiac repolarization and QT interval, and torsades de pointes reported; consider the risk of QT prolongation when weighing the risks/benefits for at-risk groups (eg, patients with known QT interval prolongation, history of torsades de pointes, congenital long QT syndrome, bradyarrhythmias or uncompensated heart failure, patients with ongoing proarrhythmic conditions such as uncorrected hypokalemia or hypomagnesemia, clinically significant bradycardia). Caution with GFR <10mL/min; higher incidence of GI adverse events reported. May result in bacterial resistance if used in the absence of a proven/suspected bacterial infection. Consider additional antibiotic if patient vomits within 5 min of administration. Consider alternative therapy if patient vomits between 5 and 60 min after administration, or with delayed gastric emptying. Neither a 2nd dose nor alternative therapy is warranted if patient vomits ≥60 min after administration with normal gastric emptying. Caution in elderly.

ADVERSE REACTIONS

Diarrhea/loose stools, N/V, abdominal pain, rash, headache.

DRUG INTERACTIONS

Caution with drugs known to prolong QT interval, Class IA (quinidine, procainamide), and Class III (dofetilide, amiodarone, sotalol) antiarrhythmic agents. May potentiate effects of oral anticoagulants (eg, warfarin); monitor PT. Monitor carefully with digoxin, ergotamine or dihydroergotamine, cyclosporine, hexobarbital, and phenytoin.

NURSING CONSIDERATIONS

Assessment: Assess for previous hypersensitivity to the drug, erythromycin, or any macrolide/ketolide antibiotic, risk for QT interval prolongation, myasthenia gravis, delayed gastric emptying, history of cholestatic jaundice/hepatic dysfunction associated with prior use of azithromycin, renal/hepatic dysfunction, pregnancy/nursing status, and possible drug interactions. Perform appropriate culture and susceptibility tests prior to treatment.

Monitoring: Monitor for signs/symptoms of allergic/skin reactions, CDAD, GI adverse effects, cardiac repolarization or QT prolongation, torsades de pointes, exacerbation of myasthenia gravis, new onset of myasthenic syndrome, hepatotoxicity, and other adverse reactions.

Patient Counseling: Inform that drug needs time to work and that patient may not feel better right away. Instruct to contact physician if symptoms do not improve in a few days, if any signs of allergic reaction occur, or if watery/bloody stools with or without stomach cramps develop (even as late as ≥2 months after dosing). Instruct to contact physician for further treatment if vomiting occurs within 1st hr of administration. Inform that therapy treats bacterial, not viral (eg, common cold), infections. Instruct to take ud; advise that not taking the complete dose may decrease effectiveness and increase the likelihood of bacterial resistance. Advise to take without regard to antacids containing magnesium hydroxide and/or aluminum hydroxide.

Storage: Dry Powder: ≤30°C (86°F). Reconstituted Sus: 25°C (77°F); excursions permitted to 15-30°C (59-86°F). Do not refrigerate or freeze.

ZOCOR – simvastatin

RX

Class: HMG-CoA reductase inhibitor

ADULT DOSAGE

Hyperlipidemia

Initial: 10mg or 20mg qpm
Range: 5-40mg/day

High Risk for Coronary Heart Disease Events:
Initial: 40mg/day

Lipid determinations should be performed after 4 weeks of therapy and periodically thereafter

Homozygous Familial Hypercholesterolemia

Usual: 40mg/day qpm

Lipid determinations should be performed after 4 weeks of therapy and periodically thereafter

PEDIATRIC DOSAGE

Heterozygous Familial Hypercholesterolemia

10-17 Years (At Least 1 Year Postmenarche):
Initial: 10mg qpm
Range: 10-40mg/day
Titrate: Adjust at ≥4-week intervals
Max: 40mg/day

DOSE MODIFICATION

Concomitant Medications

Verapamil, Diltiazem, or Dronedarone:
Max: 10mg/day

Amiodarone, Amlodipine, or Ranolazine:
Max: 20mg/day

Lomitapide:
Homozygous Familial Hypercholesterolemia:
Reduce dose by 50% if initiating lomitapide
Max: 20mg/day (or 40mg/day for patients who have previously taken simvastatin 80mg/day chronically [eg, ≥12 months] w/o evidence of muscle toxicity)

Niacin-Containing Products:
Chinese Patients Taking Lipid-Modifying Doses (≥1g/day Niacin):
Caution w/ doses >20mg/day; do not give 80mg dose

Renal Impairment

Severe:
Initial: 5mg/day; use caution and monitor closely

Other Important Modifications

Restricted Dosing:
Use 80mg dose only in patients who have been taking simvastatin 80mg chronically (eg, ≥12 months) w/o evidence of muscle toxicity

If currently tolerating 80mg dose and needs to be initiated on a drug that is contraindicated or is associated w/ a dose cap for simvastatin, switch to an alternative statin w/ less potential for drug-drug interaction

In patients unable to achieve LDL goal utilizing the 40mg dose, place on alternative LDL-lowering treatment that provides greater LDL lowering; do not titrate therapy to 80mg dose

ADMINISTRATION

Oral route

HOW SUPPLIED

Tab: 5mg, 10mg, 20mg, 40mg, 80mg

CONTRAINDICATIONS

Concomitant administration of strong CYP3A4 inhibitors (eg, itraconazole, ketoconazole, posaconazole, voriconazole, HIV protease inhibitors, boceprevir, telaprevir, erythromycin, clarithromycin, telithromycin, nefazodone, cobicistat-containing products), gemfibrozil, cyclosporine, or danazol. Active liver disease, which may include unexplained persistent elevations in hepatic transaminases, women who are or may become pregnant, and nursing mothers.

WARNINGS/PRECAUTIONS

Myopathy (including immune-mediated necrotizing myopathy [IMNM]) and rhabdomyolysis reported; predisposing factors include advanced age (≥65 yrs of age), female gender, uncontrolled hypothyroidism, and renal impairment. Risk of myopathy, including rhabdomyolysis, is dose related and greater w/ 80mg doses. D/C if markedly elevated CPK levels occur or myopathy is diagnosed/suspected, and temporarily withhold in any patient experiencing an acute or serious condition predisposing to development of renal failure secondary to rhabdomyolysis. Persistent increases in serum transaminases reported. Fatal and nonfatal hepatic failure (rare) reported; promptly interrupt therapy if serious liver injury w/ clinical symptoms and/or hyperbilirubinemia or jaundice occurs and do not restart if no alternate etiology found. Increases in HbA1c and FPG levels reported. Caution w/ substantial alcohol consumption, history of liver disease, and in the elderly.

ADVERSE REACTIONS

Abdominal pain, headache, myalgia, constipation, nausea, atrial fibrillation, gastritis, diabetes mellitus, insomnia, vertigo, bronchitis, eczema, URTI, UTI(s).

DRUG INTERACTIONS

See Contraindications and Dose Modification. Due to the risk of myopathy/rhabdomyolysis, avoid grapefruit juice and caution w/ fibrates, lipid-modifying doses (≥1g/day) of niacin, colchicine, verapamil, diltiazem, dronedarone, lomitapide, amiodarone, amlodipine, and ranolazine. May slightly elevate digoxin concentrations; monitor patients taking digoxin when therapy is initiated. May potentiate effect of coumarin anticoagulants; determine PT before initiation and frequently during therapy.

NURSING CONSIDERATIONS

Assessment: Assess for history of or active liver disease, unexplained persistent hepatic transaminase elevations, predisposing factors for myopathy, renal impairment, alcohol consumption, drug hypersensitivity, any other conditions where treatment is contraindicated or cautioned, pregnancy/nursing status, and possible drug interactions. Assess lipid profile and LFTs.

Monitoring: Monitor for signs/symptoms of myopathy (including IMNM), rhabdomyolysis, liver dysfunction, increases in HbA1c and FPG levels, and other adverse reactions. Monitor lipid profile, LFTs when clinically indicated, and CPK levels.

Patient Counseling: Inform of benefits/risks of therapy. Advise to adhere to the National Cholesterol Education Program recommended diet, a regular exercise program, and periodic testing of a fasting lipid panel. Inform about substances that should be avoided during therapy, and advise to discuss all medications, both prescription and OTC, w/ physician. Instruct to report promptly any unexplained muscle pain, tenderness, or weakness, particularly if accompanied by malaise or fever or if these muscle signs or symptoms persist after discontinuation, or any symptoms that may indicate liver injury. Inform patients using the 80mg dose that the risk of myopathy, including rhabdomyolysis, is increased. Instruct women of childbearing age to use an effective method of birth control to prevent pregnancy while on therapy, to d/c therapy and call physician if pregnant, and not to breastfeed while on therapy.

Storage: 5-30°C (41-86°F).

ZOLOFT — sertraline hydrochloride

RX

Class: Selective serotonin reuptake inhibitor

Antidepressants increased the risk of suicidal thinking and behavior (suicidality) in children, adolescents, and young adults in short-term studies of major depressive disorder (MDD) and other psychiatric disorders. Monitor and observe closely for clinical worsening, suicidality, or unusual changes in behavior in patients who are started on antidepressant therapy. Not approved for use in pediatric patients except for patients with obsessive-compulsive disorder.

ADULT DOSAGE

Premenstrual Dysphoric Disorder

Initial: 50mg qd throughout menstrual cycle or limited to luteal phase

Titrate: May increase at 50mg increments/cycle up to 150mg/day for throughout menstrual cycle daily dosing, or 100mg/day for luteal phase dosing if not responding

If 100mg/day has been established w/ luteal phase dosing, use a 50mg/day titration step for 3 days at the beginning of each luteal phase dosing period

PEDIATRIC DOSAGE

Obsessive Compulsive Disorder

6-12 Years:

Initial: 25mg qd

13-17 Years:

Initial: 50mg qd

Titrate: Adjust dose at intervals of no <1 week

Max: 200mg/day

Major Depressive Disorder

50mg qd
Max: 200mg/day

Obsessive Compulsive Disorder

50mg qd
Max: 200mg/day

Panic Disorder

Initial: 25mg qd
Titrate: Increase to 50mg qd after 1 week; adjust dose at intervals of no <1 week
Max: 200mg/day

Social Anxiety Disorder

Initial: 25mg qd
Titrate: Increase to 50mg qd after 1 week; adjust dose at intervals of no <1 week
Max: 200mg/day

Post-traumatic Stress Disorder

Initial: 25mg qd
Titrate: Increase to 50mg qd after 1 week; adjust dose at intervals of no <1 week
Max: 200mg/day

Dosing Considerations with MAOIs

Switching to/from an MAOI for Psychiatric Disorders:
Allow at least 14 days between discontinuation of an MAOI and initiation of treatment, and allow at least 14 days between discontinuation of treatment and initiation of an MAOI

Use w/ Other MAOIs (eg, Linezolid, IV Methylene Blue):
If acceptable alternatives are not available and benefits outweigh risks, d/c sertraline and administer linezolid or IV methylene blue; monitor for serotonin syndrome for 2 weeks or until 24 hrs after the last dose of linezolid or IV methylene blue, whichever comes 1st. May resume sertraline therapy 24 hrs after the last dose of linezolid or IV methylene blue

Dosing Considerations with MAOIs

Switching to/from an MAOI for Psychiatric Disorders:
Allow at least 14 days between discontinuation of an MAOI and initiation of treatment, and allow at least 14 days between discontinuation of treatment and initiation of an MAOI

Use w/ Other MAOIs (eg, Linezolid, IV Methylene Blue):
If acceptable alternatives are not available and benefits outweigh risks, d/c sertraline and administer linezolid or IV methylene blue; monitor for serotonin syndrome for 2 weeks or until 24 hrs after the last dose of linezolid or IV methylene blue, whichever comes 1st. May resume sertraline therapy 24 hrs after the last dose of linezolid or IV methylene blue

DOSE MODIFICATION

Adverse Reactions

May consider resuming previously prescribed dose if intolerable symptoms occur following a dose decrease or upon discontinuation of treatment. May continue decreasing the dose subsequently but at a more gradual rate

Hepatic Impairment

Use lower or less frequent dose

Pregnancy

During 3rd Trimester: Consider tapering

ADMINISTRATION

Oral route
Administer qam or qpm

Sol

Must be diluted before use
Mix sol w/ 4 oz of water, ginger ale, lemon/lime soda, lemonade, or orange juice only; do not mix w/ any other liquids
Take dose immediately after mixing

HOW SUPPLIED

Sol: 20mg/mL [60mL]; Tab: 25mg*, 50mg*, 100mg* *scored

CONTRAINDICATIONS

Use of an MAOI for psychiatric disorders either concomitantly or within 14 days of stopping treatment. Treatment within 14 days of stopping an MAOI for psychiatric disorders. Starting treatment in a patient being treated with other MAOIs (eg, linezolid, IV methylene blue). Concomitant use with pimozide. (Sol) Concomitant use with disulfiram.

WARNINGS/PRECAUTIONS

Not approved for treatment of bipolar depression. May precipitate mixed/manic episode in patients at risk for bipolar disorder; screen for risk of bipolar disorder prior to initiating treatment. Serotonin syndrome reported; d/c immediately and initiate supportive symptomatic treatment. Pupillary dilation that occurs following use may trigger an angle-closure attack in a patient with anatomically narrow angles who does not have a patent iridectomy. Activation of mania/hypomania, altered platelet function and/or abnormal lab results, decreased serum uric acid, and weight loss reported. Adverse events reported upon discontinuation, particularly when abrupt; reduce dose gradually whenever possible. May increase the risk of bleeding events. Seizures reported; caution with seizure disorder. Caution with hepatic impairment and diseases/conditions that could affect metabolism or hemodynamic responses. QTc prolongation and torsades de pointes reported; caution in patients with risk factors for QTc prolongation. Hyponatremia may occur; caution in elderly and volume-depleted patients. Consider discontinuation in patients with symptomatic hyponatremia and institute appropriate medical intervention. Caution in 3rd trimester of pregnancy due to risk of serious neonatal complications. False (+) urine immunoassay screening tests for benzodiazepines reported. (Sol) Dropper dispenser contains dry natural rubber; caution with latex sensitivity.

ADVERSE REACTIONS

Ejaculation failure, dry mouth, increased sweating, somnolence, fatigue, tremor, anorexia, dizziness, headache, diarrhea, dyspepsia, nausea, constipation, agitation, insomnia.

DRUG INTERACTIONS

See Dosage and Contraindications. May cause serotonin syndrome with other serotonergic drugs (eg, triptans, TCAs, fentanyl, lithium, tramadol, tryptophan, buspirone, St. John's wort) and with drugs that impair metabolism of serotonin; d/c immediately if this occurs. May cause a shift in plasma concentrations resulting in an adverse effect with other tightly protein bound drugs (eg, warfarin, digitoxin), and conversely adverse effects may result from displacement of sertraline. Increased risk of QTc prolongation and/or ventricular arrhythmias with concomitant use of other drugs that prolong QTc interval (eg, some antipsychotics and antibiotics). Caution with other CNS active drugs. Monitor lithium, phenytoin, and valproate levels with appropriate dose adjustments. May increase levels of drugs metabolized by CYP2D6, especially those with a narrow therapeutic index (eg, TCAs for treatment of MDD, propafenone, flecainide); concomitant use of a drug metabolized by CYP2D6 may require lower doses, and an increase of the coadministered drug may be required when sertraline is withdrawn. Weakness, hyperreflexia, and incoordination reported (rare) with sumatriptan. May induce metabolism of cisapride. Increased risk of bleeding with aspirin (ASA), NSAIDs, warfarin, and other anticoagulants or other drugs known to affect platelet function. Altered anticoagulant effects reported with warfarin; carefully monitor PT when therapy is initiated or stopped. Avoid with alcohol. Increased risk of hyponatremia with diuretics. Cimetidine may increase levels and $T_{1/2}$. May reduce clearance of diazepam and tolbutamide.

NURSING CONSIDERATIONS

Assessment: Assess for presence/risk for bipolar disorder, susceptibility to angle-closure glaucoma, conditions where treatment is contraindicated or cautioned, pregnancy/nursing status, and possible drug interactions.

Monitoring: Monitor for clinical worsening of depression, suicidality, or unusual changes in behavior, serotonin syndrome, hyponatremia, abnormal bleeding, angle-closure glaucoma, activation of mania/hypomania, seizures, QTc prolongation, torsades de pointes, and other adverse reactions. Periodically monitor height and weight of pediatric patients with long-term therapy. Periodically reevaluate long-term usefulness of therapy. Carefully monitor PT when therapy is initiated or stopped with warfarin.

Patient Counseling: Counsel about benefits, risks, and appropriate use of therapy. Encourage families and caregivers to be alert for emergence of unusual changes in behavior, worsening of depression, and suicidal ideation, especially early during treatment and when dose is adjusted up or down; instruct to report symptoms to physician, especially if severe, abrupt in onset, or not part of presenting symptoms. Caution about risk of serotonin syndrome with concomitant triptans, tramadol, or other serotonergic agents. Caution about risk of angle-closure glaucoma. Advise patients to use caution when driving or operating machinery until they learn how they respond to medication. Inform that concomitant use with NSAIDs, ASA, warfarin, and other drugs that affect coagulation may increase the risk of bleeding. Counsel to avoid alcohol and to use caution when using OTC products. Advise to notify physician if pregnant, intending to become pregnant, or if breastfeeding.

Storage: 25°C (77°F); excursions permitted to 15-30°C (59-86°F).

ZOLPIMIST – zolpidem tartrate CIV

Class: Imidazopyridine hypnotic

ADULT DOSAGE

Insomnia

Short-Term Treatment of Insomnia Characterized by Difficulties w/ Sleep Initiation:

Initial: 5mg (women), and either 5mg or 10mg (men), taken qhs

Titrate: May increase to 10mg if the 5mg dose is not effective

Max: 10mg qhs

PEDIATRIC DOSAGE

Pediatric use may not have been established

DOSE MODIFICATION

Concomitant Medications

Use w/ CNS Depressants: May need to adjust dose of zolpidem

Hepatic Impairment

Hepatic Insufficiency:

Usual: 5mg qhs

Elderly

Elderly/Debilitated:

Usual: 5mg qhs

ADMINISTRATION

Oral route

Take immediately before hs w/ at least 7-8 hrs remaining before the planned time of awakening

Must be primed before use for the 1st time

To prime, point the black spray opening away from face and other people and spray 5X

For administration, hold container upright w/ the black spray opening pointed directly into the mouth; fully press down on the pump to make sure a full dose (5mg) is sprayed directly into the mouth over the tongue. If a 10mg dose is prescribed, a 2nd spray should be administered

If not used for at least 14 days, must be primed again w/ 1 spray

Do not take w/ or immediately after a meal

HOW SUPPLIED

Spray: 5mg/actuation [60 actuations]

WARNINGS/PRECAUTIONS

Increased risk of next-day psychomotor impairment if taken with less than a full night of sleep remaining (7-8 hrs). May impair mental/physical abilities. Initiate only after careful evaluation; failure of insomnia to remit after 7-10 days of treatment may indicate presence of a primary psychiatric and/or medical illness. Cases of angioedema involving the tongue, glottis, or larynx reported; do not rechallenge if angioedema develops. Abnormal thinking, behavioral changes, and visual/auditory hallucinations reported. Complex behaviors (eg, sleep-driving) reported; consider discontinuation if a sleep-driving episode occurs. Amnesia, anxiety, and other neuropsychiatric symptoms may occur. Worsening of depression, and suicidal thoughts and actions (including completed suicides) reported in primarily depressed patients; prescribe the least amount of drug that is feasible at a time. Caution with compromised respiratory function; prior to prescribing, consider the risks of respiratory depression, in patients with respiratory impairment (eg, sleep apnea, myasthenia gravis). Withdrawal signs and symptoms reported following rapid dose decrease or abrupt discontinuation; monitor for tolerance, abuse, and dependence.

ADVERSE REACTIONS

Drowsiness, headache, dizziness, allergy, sinusitis, lethargy, drugged feeling, pharyngitis, dry mouth, back pain, diarrhea.

DRUG INTERACTIONS

See Dosage. Increased risk of CNS depression and complex behaviors with other CNS depressants (eg, benzodiazepines, opioids, TCAs, alcohol). Use with other sedative-hypnotics (eg, other zolpidem products) at hs or the middle of the night is not recommended. Increased risk of next-day psychomotor impairment with other CNS depressants or drugs that increase zolpidem levels. May decrease peak levels of imipramine. Additive effect of decreased alertness with imipramine or chlorpromazine. Additive adverse effect on psychomotor performance with chlorpromazine or alcohol. Sertraline and CYP3A inhibitors may increase exposure. Fluoxetine may increase $T_{1/2}$. Rifampin (a CYP3A4 inducer) may reduce exposure, pharmacodynamic effects, and efficacy. Ketoconazole (a potent CYP3A4 inhibitor) may increase pharmacodynamic effects; consider lower dose of zolpidem.

NURSING CONSIDERATIONS

Assessment: Assess for physical and/or psychiatric disorder, depression, compromised respiratory function, sleep apnea, myasthenia gravis, hepatic impairment, history of drug/alcohol addiction or abuse, hypersensitivity to the drug, pregnancy/nursing status, and possible drug interactions.

Monitoring: Monitor for angioedema, emergence of any new behavioral signs/symptoms of concern, respiratory depression, withdrawal signs/symptoms, tolerance, abuse, dependence, and other adverse reactions.

Patient Counseling: Inform about the benefits and risks of treatment. Instruct to take only as prescribed; advise to wait at least 8 hrs after dosing before driving or engaging in other activities requiring full mental alertness. Instruct to contact physician immediately if any adverse reactions (eg, severe anaphylactic/anaphylactoid reactions, sleep-driving, other complex behaviors, suicidal thoughts) develop. Advise not to use the drug if patient drank alcohol that pm or before bed. Instruct patients not to increase the dose and to inform physician if it is believed that the drug does not work.

Storage: 25°C (77°F); excursions permitted to 15-30°C (59-86°F). Store upright. Do not freeze. Avoid prolonged exposure to temperatures >30°C (86°F).

ZOLVIT — acetaminophen/hydrocodone bitartrate CIII

Class: Opioid analgesic

Associated with cases of acute liver failure, at times resulting in liver transplant and death. Most of the cases of liver injury are associated with acetaminophen (APAP) use at doses >4000mg/day, and often involve >1 APAP-containing product.

ADULT DOSAGE

Moderate to Severe Pain

Usual: 2.25 tsp every 4-6 hrs prn
Max: 13.5 tsp/day

PEDIATRIC DOSAGE

Moderate to Severe Pain

12-15kg (2-3 Years):
Usual: 2.8mL every 4-6 hrs
Max Daily Dose: 16.8mL

16-22kg (4-6 Years):
Usual: 3.75mL every 4-6 hrs
Max Daily Dose: 22.5mL

23-31kg (7-9 Years):
Usual: 5.6mL every 4-6 hrs
Max Daily Dose: 33.6mL

32-45kg (10-13 Years):
Usual: 7.5mL
Max Daily Dose: 45mL

≥46kg (≥14 Years):
Usual: 11.25mL
Max Daily Dose: 67.5mL

DOSE MODIFICATION

Elderly

Use caution; start at low end of dosing range

ADMINISTRATION

Oral route

Administer dose accurately; use a calibrated measuring device

HOW SUPPLIED

Sol: (Hydrocodone/APAP) (10mg/300mg)/15mL [16 fl oz]

WARNINGS/PRECAUTIONS

May be habit-forming. Increased risk of acute liver failure in patients with underlying liver disease. May cause serious skin reactions (eg, acute generalized exanthematous pustulosis, Stevens-Johnson syndrome, toxic epidermal necrolysis); d/c at the first appearance of skin rash or any other sign of hypersensitivity. Hypersensitivity and anaphylaxis reported; d/c if signs/symptoms occur. May produce dose-related respiratory depression, and irregular and periodic breathing. Infants may have increased sensitivity to the respiratory depressant effects of opioids; if use is contemplated, administer cautiously, in substantially reduced initial doses, by personnel experienced in administering opioids to infants, with intensive monitoring. Respiratory depressant effects and CSF pressure elevation capacity may be markedly exaggerated in the presence of head injury, other intracranial lesions, or preexisting increased intracranial pressure. May obscure clinical course of head injuries and acute abdominal conditions. Potential for abuse. Caution with hypothyroidism,

Addison's disease, prostatic hypertrophy, urethral stricture, severe hepatic/renal impairment, or in elderly/debilitated. Suppresses cough reflex; caution with pulmonary disease and in postoperative use. Physical dependence and tolerance may develop.

ADVERSE REACTIONS

Acute liver failure, bradycardia, cardiac arrest, anxiety, dizziness, drowsiness, hypoglycemic coma, abdominal pain, constipation, spasm of vesical sphincters, agranulocytosis, hemolytic anemia, skeletal muscle flaccidity, acute airway obstruction, apnea.

DRUG INTERACTIONS

Additive CNS depression with other narcotics, antihistamines, antipsychotics, antianxiety agents, or other CNS depressants (eg, alcohol); reduce dose of one or both agents. Concomitant use with MAOIs or TCAs may increase the effect of either the antidepressant or hydrocodone. Increased risk of acute liver failure with alcohol.

NURSING CONSIDERATIONS

Assessment: Assess for history of hypersensitivity, level of pain intensity, type of pain, patient's general condition and medical status, renal/hepatic impairment, pregnancy/nursing status, any other conditions where treatment is contraindicated or cautioned, and for possible drug interactions.

Monitoring: Monitor for signs/symptoms of hypersensitivity or anaphylaxis, serious skin reactions, respiratory depression, elevations in CSF pressure, drug abuse, tolerance, dependence, and other adverse reactions. In patients with severe hepatic/renal disease, monitor effects with serial hepatic and/or renal function tests.

Patient Counseling: Instruct to look for APAP on package labels and not to use >1 APAP-containing product. Instruct to seek medical attention immediately upon ingestion of >4000mg/day APAP, even if feeling well. Advise to d/c and contact physician if signs of allergy (eg, rash, difficulty breathing) develop. Inform that drug may impair mental/physical abilities; instruct to avoid performing potentially hazardous tasks (eg, driving, operating machinery) while taking the medication. Instruct to avoid alcohol and other CNS depressants. Inform that drug may be habit-forming; instruct to take only ud.

Storage: 20-25°C (68-77°F).

ZONTIVITY — vorapaxar **RX**

Class: Protease-activated receptor-1 (PAR-1) antagonist

Do not use in patients with a history of stroke, transient ischemic attack (TIA), intracranial hemorrhage (ICH), or active pathological bleeding. May increase the risk of bleeding, including ICH and fatal bleeding.

ADULT DOSAGE

Reduction of Thrombotic Cardiovascular Events

In Patients w/ a History of MI or w/ PAD:
1 tab (2.08mg) qd; use w/ ASA and/or clopidogrel according to their indications or standard of care

PEDIATRIC DOSAGE

Pediatric use may not have been established

DOSE MODIFICATION

Hepatic Impairment

Severe: Not recommended for use

ADMINISTRATION

Oral route
Take w/ or w/o food

HOW SUPPLIED

Tab: 2.08mg

CONTRAINDICATIONS

Active pathological bleeding (eg, ICH, peptic ulcer). History of stroke, TIA, or ICH.

WARNINGS/PRECAUTIONS

Increases the risk of bleeding in proportion to the patient's underlying bleeding risk. Suspect bleeding in any patient who is hypotensive and has recently undergone coronary angiography, percutaneous coronary intervention, coronary artery bypass graft surgery, or other surgical procedures. Withholding therapy for a brief period will not be useful in managing an acute bleeding event; has no known treatment to reverse the antiplatelet effect of therapy. Not recommended with severe hepatic impairment.

ADVERSE REACTIONS
Bleeding, anemia.

DRUG INTERACTIONS
May increase risk of bleeding with anticoagulants, fibrinolytic therapy, chronic NSAIDs, SSRIs, and SNRIs; avoid concomitant use of warfarin or other anticoagulants. Avoid concomitant use with strong CYP3A inhibitors (eg, ketoconazole, clarithromycin, ritonavir) or strong CYP3A inducers (eg, rifampin, carbamazepine, St. John's wort).

NURSING CONSIDERATIONS
Assessment: Assess for history of stroke, TIA, or ICH; active pathological bleeding, other risk factors for bleeding, hepatic impairment, pregnancy/nursing status, and for possible drug interactions.

Monitoring: Monitor for signs/symptoms bleeding and other adverse reactions.

Patient Counseling: Inform about the benefits and risks of therapy. Instruct to take exactly ud and not to d/c without discussing it with the prescribing physician. Inform that may bleed and bruise more easily. Advise to report any unanticipated, prolonged, or excessive bleeding, or blood in stool or urine. Instruct to notify physicians or dentists about therapy before any surgery or dental procedure. Advise to inform physician of all medications currently taking/planning to take.

Storage: 20-25°C (68-77°F); excursions permitted to 15-30°C (59-86°F). Protect from moisture.

ZORTRESS — everolimus RX
Class: Macrolide immunosuppressant

Should only be prescribed by physicians experienced in immunosuppressive therapy and management of organ transplant patients. Immunosuppression may lead to increased susceptibility to infection and possible development of malignancies (eg, lymphoma, skin cancer). Increased risk of kidney arterial and venous thrombosis leading to graft loss was reported, mostly w/in the first 30 days post-transplantation. Increased nephrotoxicity may occur in combination w/ standard doses of cyclosporine; reduce dose of cyclosporine to reduce renal dysfunction, and monitor cyclosporine and everolimus whole blood trough concentrations. Increased mortality w/in the first 3 months post-transplantation in heart transplant patients on immunosuppressive regimens w/ or w/o induction therapy; not recommended in heart transplantation.

ADULT DOSAGE
Renal Transplant

Prophylaxis of Organ Rejection in Kidney Transplant:

Initial: 0.75mg bid, in combination w/ basiliximab induction and concurrently w/ reduced dose of cyclosporine; give as soon as possible after transplantation

Initiate oral prednisone once oral medication is tolerated

Titrate: May require dose adjustment based on blood concentrations achieved, tolerability, individual response, change in concomitant medications, and clinical situation; optimal dose adjustments should be based on trough levels obtained 4 or 5 days after a previous dosing change

Recommended Therapeutic Range: 3-8ng/mL (based on LC/MS/MS assay method); if trough level is <3ng/mL, double total daily dose, or if trough level is >8ng/mL on 2 consecutive measures, decrease by 0.25mg bid

Refer to PI for further drug monitoring instructions and for cyclosporine therapeutic drug monitoring parameters

Hepatic Transplant

Prophylaxis of Allograft Rejection w/ a Liver Transplant:

Initial: 1mg bid, in combination w/ reduced dose of tacrolimus; start at least 30 days post-transplant

Titrate: May require dose adjustment based on blood concentrations achieved, tolerability, individual response, change in concomitant

PEDIATRIC DOSAGE
Pediatric use may not have been established

medications, and clinical situation; optimal dose adjustments should be based on trough levels obtained 4 or 5 days after a previous dosing change

Recommended Therapeutic Range: 3-8ng/mL (based on LC/MS/MS assay method); if trough level is <3ng/mL, double total daily dose, or if trough level is >8ng/mL on 2 consecutive measures, decrease by 0.25mg bid

Refer to PI for further drug monitoring instructions and for tacrolimus therapeutic drug monitoring parameters

DOSE MODIFICATION

Hepatic Impairment

Mild (Child-Pugh Class A): Reduce initial daily dose by 1/3 of normal daily dose

Moderate or Severe (Child-Pugh Class B or C): Reduce initial daily dose to 1/2 of the normal daily dose

ADMINISTRATION

Oral route

Do not crush; swallow whole w/ water

Administer consistently approx 12 hrs apart w/ or w/o food and at the same time as cyclosporine or tacrolimus

HOW SUPPLIED

Tab: 0.25mg, 0.5mg, 0.75mg

WARNINGS/PRECAUTIONS

Limit exposure to sunlight and UV light. Prophylaxis for *Pneumocystis jiroveci (carinii)* pneumonia and CMV recommended. Increased risk of hepatic artery thrombosis (HAT), which may lead to graft loss or death; do not give earlier than 30 days after liver transplant. Consider switching to other immunosuppressive therapies if renal function does not improve after dose adjustments or if dysfunction is thought to be drug related. Angioedema, increased risk of delayed wound healing, increased occurrence of wound-related complications, and generalized fluid accumulation reported. Interstitial lung disease (ILD), implying lung intraparenchymal inflammation (pneumonitis) and/or fibrosis of noninfectious etiology reported; resolution may occur upon drug interruption w/ or w/o glucocorticoid therapy. Consider diagnosis of ILD for symptoms of infectious pneumonia that do not respond to antibiotic therapy and in whom non-drug causes have been ruled out. Increased risk of hyperlipidemia and proteinuria w/ higher whole blood trough concentrations; use of anti-lipid therapy may not normalize lipid levels. Reevaluate the risk/benefit of continuing therapy in patients w/ severe refractory hyperlipidemia. Increased risk of polyoma virus infections, including polyoma virus-associated nephropathy (PVAN) and progressive multiple leukoencephalopathy (PML), may occur; consider reductions in immunosuppression if evidence of PVAN or PML develops. Concomitant use w/ cyclosporine may increase risk of thrombotic microangiopathy/TTP/hemolytic uremic syndrome. May increase risk of new-onset diabetes mellitus (DM) after transplant. Azoospermia or oligospermia may be observed. Avoid w/ rare hereditary problems of galactose intolerance (Lapp lactase deficiency, glucose-galactose malabsorption); diarrhea and malabsorption may occur.

ADVERSE REACTIONS

Malignancies, infections, nephrotoxicity, peripheral edema, constipation, HTN, nausea, anemia, hyperlipidemia, diarrhea, pyrexia, hyperkalemia, headache, hypercholesterolemia, leukopenia.

DRUG INTERACTIONS

Caution w/ drugs known to impair renal function. May increase risk of angioedema w/ drugs known to cause angioedema (eg, ACE inhibitors). Monitor for development of rhabdomyolysis w/ HMG-CoA reductase inhibitors and/or fibrates; use of simvastatin and lovastatin are strongly discouraged in patients receiving everolimus w/ cyclosporine. Coadministration w/ strong CYP3A4 inhibitors (eg, ketoconazole, clarithromycin, ritonavir) and strong CYP3A4 inducers (eg, rifampin, rifabutin) is not recommended w/o close monitoring of everolimus whole blood trough concentrations. Avoid w/ live vaccines, grapefruit, and grapefruit juice. Inhibitors of P-gp (eg, digoxin, cyclosporine), moderate inhibitors of CYP3A4 and P-gp (eg, fluconazole, macrolide antibiotics, nicardipine), and verapamil may increase levels. Caution w/ CYP3A4 and CYP2D6 substrates w/ a narrow therapeutic index. Increased levels w/ cyclosporine; dose adjustment may be needed if cyclosporine dose is altered. CYP3A4 inducers (eg, St. John's wort, carbamazepine, phenobarbital) may decrease levels. Combination immunosuppressant therapy should be used w/ caution. May increase octreotide levels.

NURSING CONSIDERATIONS

Assessment: Assess for hereditary problems of galactose intolerance, hepatic impairment, hypersensitivity to the drug or to sirolimus, pregnancy/nursing status, and possible drug interactions. Obtain baseline lipid and glucose levels.

Monitoring: Monitor for infections, angioedema, thrombosis, wound-related complications, fluid accumulation, lymphomas and other malignancies, hyperlipidemia, hepatic impairment, proteinuria, PVAN, HAT, ILD, pneumonitis, and other adverse reactions. Monitor everolimus and cyclosporine or tacrolimus whole blood trough concentrations, lipid profile, blood glucose concentrations, renal function, and hematologic parameters.

Patient Counseling: Counsel to avoid grapefruit and grapefruit juice. Inform of the risk of developing lymphomas and other malignancies, particularly of the skin; instruct to limit exposure to sunlight and UV light. Advise that therapy has been associated w/ an increased risk of kidney arterial and venous thrombosis, resulting in graft loss, usually occurring w/in the first 30 days post-transplantation. Inform of the risks of impaired kidney function w/ concomitant cyclosporine as well as the need for routine blood concentration monitoring for both drugs; advise of the importance of SrCr monitoring. Inform of risk of hyperlipidemia and the importance of lipid profile monitoring. Advise women to avoid pregnancy throughout treatment and for 8 weeks after discontinuation. Instruct to notify physician of all medications and herbal/dietary supplements being taken. Inform that therapy has been associated w/ impaired or delayed wound healing, and fluid accumulation. Inform of increased risk of proteinuria, DM, infections, noninfectious pneumonitis, and angioedema; advise to contact physician if symptoms develop. Instruct to avoid receiving live vaccines.

Storage: 25°C (77°F); excursions permitted to 15-30°C (59-86°F). Protect from light and moisture.

ZOSTAVAX — zoster vaccine live

RX

Class: Vaccine

ADULT DOSAGE

Herpes Zoster

Prevention:

≥50 Years:

Single 0.65mL SQ in deltoid region of upper arm

PEDIATRIC DOSAGE

Pediatric use may not have been established

ADMINISTRATION

SQ route

Inject in deltoid region of upper arm
Do not inject IV or IM

Preparation/Reconstitution

Should be reconstituted immediately upon removal from the freezer
Only use the supplied diluent
Withdraw entire contents of diluent into syringe
To avoid excessive foaming, slowly inject all of diluent in syringe into vial of lyophilized vaccine and gently agitate to mix thoroughly
Withdraw entire contents of reconstituted vaccine into syringe and inject total volume SQ

HOW SUPPLIED

Inj: 19,400 PFU/0.65mL

CONTRAINDICATIONS

History of anaphylactic/anaphylactoid reaction to gelatin or neomycin. Immunosuppression or immunodeficiency, including history of primary or acquired immunodeficiency states, leukemia, lymphoma or other malignant neoplasms affecting the bone marrow or lymphatic system, AIDS or other clinical manifestations of infection with HIV, and those on immunosuppressive therapy. Pregnancy.

WARNINGS/PRECAUTIONS

Avoid pregnancy for 3 months following administration. Serious adverse reactions, including anaphylaxis, reported; have adequate treatment provisions (eg, epinephrine inj [1:1000]) available for immediate use. Transmission of vaccine virus may occur between vaccinees and susceptible contacts. Consider deferral in acute illness (eg, fever) or with active untreated tuberculosis (TB). Duration of protection >4 yrs after vaccination is unknown. May not protect all vaccine recipients.

ADVERSE REACTIONS

Inj-site reactions (erythema, pain, tenderness, swelling, pruritus, warmth), headache.

DRUG INTERACTIONS

See Contraindications. Reduced immune response to zoster vaccine live with pneumococcal vaccine polyvalent; consider administration of the 2 vaccines separated by at least 4 weeks.

NURSING CONSIDERATIONS

Assessment: Assess for acute illness, active untreated TB, history of anaphylactic/anaphylactoid reaction to gelatin, neomycin, or any other component of the vaccine, immunosuppression/immunodeficiency, pregnancy/nursing status, and possible drug interactions.

Monitoring: Monitor for anaphylactic/anaphylactoid reactions and other adverse reactions.

Patient Counseling: Instruct to inform physician about reactions to previous vaccines. Inform of benefits and risks of vaccine, including potential risk of transmitting vaccine virus to susceptible individuals (eg, immunosuppressed/immunodeficient individuals, pregnant women who have not had chickenpox). Instruct to report any adverse reactions or any symptoms of concern to physician.

Storage: Before Reconstitution: -50°C to -15°C (-58°F to 5°F). Use of dry ice may subject the vaccine to temperatures colder than -50°C (-58°F). May store and/or transport at 2-8°C (36-46°F) for up to 72 continuous hrs prior to reconstitution; discard if not used within 72 hrs of removal from -15°C (5°F). Protect from light. Diluent: 20-25°C (68-77°F) or 2-8°C (36-46°F). After Reconstitution: Administer immediately; discard if not used within 30 min. Do not freeze.

ZOSYN – piperacillin/tazobactam RX

Class: Beta-lactamase inhibitor/broad-spectrum penicillin

ADULT DOSAGE

General Dosing

3.375g q6h for 7-10 days

Nosocomial Pneumonia

Initial: 4.5g q6h for 7-14 days plus an aminoglycoside

Aminoglycoside treatment should be continued in patients from whom *Pseudomonas aeruginosa* is isolated

PEDIATRIC DOSAGE

Peritonitis

≤40kg:
2-9 Months of Age: 80mg-10mg/kg q8h
≥9 Months of Age: 100mg-12.5mg/kg q8h

>40kg:
Use adult dose

Appendicitis

≤40kg:
2-9 Months of Age: 80mg-10mg/kg q8h
≥9 Months of Age: 100mg-12.5mg/kg q8h

>40kg:
Use adult dose

DOSE MODIFICATION

Renal Impairment

Adults:

Usual Dosage:
CrCl >40mL/min: 3.375g q6h
CrCl 20-40mL/min: 2.25g q6h
CrCl <20mL/min: 2.25g q8h
Hemodialysis: 2.25g q12h (max: 2.25g q12h)
Administer an additional 0.75g dose following each hemodialysis session on hemodialysis days
Continuous Ambulatory Peritoneal Dialysis: 2.25g q12h

Nosocomial Pneumonia:
CrCl >40mL/min: 4.5g q6h
CrCl 20-40mL/min: 3.375g q6h
CrCl <20mL/min: 2.25g q6h
Hemodialysis: 2.25g q8h (max: 2.25g q8h)
Administer an additional 0.75g dose following each hemodialysis session on hemodialysis days
Continuous Ambulatory Peritoneal Dialysis: 2.25g q8h

Elderly
Start at lower end of dosing range

ADMINISTRATION

IV route. Infuse over 30 min
Do not mixed with other drugs

Compatible Reconstitution Diluents
0.9% NaCl for inj
Sterile water for inj
Dextrose 5%
Bacteriostatic saline/parabens
Bacteriostatic water/parabens
Bacteriostatic saline/benzyl alcohol
Bacteriostatic water/benzyl alcohol

Compatible IV Sol
0.9% NaCl for inj
Sterile water for inj
Dextran 6% in saline

Dextrose 5%
Lactated Ringer's sol

IV Preparation

Use single dose vials immediately after reconstitution
Reconstitute 2.25g, 3.375g, and 4.5g single dose vials with 10mL, 15mL, and 20mL, respectively with a compatible reconstitution diluent
Further dilute reconstituted sol in a compatible IV sol (recommended volume per dose of 50mL to 150mL)
During the infusion it is desirable to discontinue the primary infusion sol
Refer to PI for further preparation/administration instructions and compatibility with aminoglycosides

HOW SUPPLIED

Inj: (Piperacillin-Tazobactam) 2g-0.25g, 3g-0.375g, 4g-0.5g [vial]; 2g-0.25g/50mL, 3g-0.375g/50mL, 4g-0.5g/100mL [Galaxy]. Also available as a Pharmacy Bulk Package.

CONTRAINDICATIONS

History of allergic reactions to cephalosporins.

WARNINGS/PRECAUTIONS

Serious and occasionally fatal hypersensitivity (anaphylactic/anaphylactoid) reactions, including shock, reported; d/c and institute appropriate therapy if an allergic reaction occurs. Serious skin reactions (eg, Stevens-Johnson syndrome, toxic epidermal necrolysis) reported; monitor closely if skin rash occurs and d/c if lesions progress. *Clostridium difficile*-associated diarrhea (CDAD) reported; d/c if CDAD is suspected or confirmed. Bleeding manifestations, sometimes associated with abnormalities of coagulation tests, reported; d/c and institute appropriate therapy if bleeding manifestations occur. Leukopenia/neutropenia may occur and is most frequently associated with prolonged administration. May cause neuromuscular excitability or convulsions with higher than recommended dose, particularly in the presence of renal failure. Caution with restricted salt intake. Monitor electrolytes periodically with low K^+ reserves. May result in bacterial resistance with use in the absence of a proven/suspected bacterial infection. Increased incidence of rash and fever in cystic fibrosis patients reported. Lab test interactions may occur. Caution with renal impairment (CrCl ≤40mL/min). Caution in elderly patients.

ADVERSE REACTIONS

Diarrhea, headache, constipation, N/V, insomnia, rash, fever, dyspepsia, pruritus, oral candidiasis.

DRUG INTERACTIONS

May inactivate aminoglycosides. May decrease serum concentrations of tobramycin; monitor aminoglycoside serum concentrations in patients with end-stage renal disease. Probenecid prolongs $T_{1/2}$; avoid coadministration unless the benefit outweighs the risk. Test coagulation parameters more frequently with high doses of heparin, oral anticoagulants, or other drugs that may affect blood coagulation system or thrombocyte function. Piperacillin: May prolong neuromuscular blockade of vecuronium or any nondepolarizing muscle relaxants. May increase risk of hypokalemia with cytotoxic therapy or diuretics. May reduce methotrexate clearance; monitor methotrexate concentrations and for toxicity.

NURSING CONSIDERATIONS

Assessment: Assess for previous hypersensitivity reaction to PCN, cephalosporins, or other allergens. Assess for history of bleeding disorder, conditions with restricted salt intake, cystic fibrosis, renal impairment, hypokalemia, pregnancy/nursing status, and possible drug interactions.

Monitoring: Monitor hematopoietic function (especially with prolonged therapy [≥21 days]), renal function, and serum electrolytes periodically. Monitor for signs/symptoms of electrolyte imbalance (eg, hypokalemia), hypersensitivity reactions, CDAD, serious skin reactions, leukopenia/neutropenia, bleeding manifestations, and for neuromuscular excitability or convulsions. Monitor for rash and fever in cystic fibrosis patients.

Patient Counseling: Inform about risks/benefits of therapy. Counsel that drug only treats bacterial, not viral, infections. Instruct to take ud; inform that skipping doses or not completing full course may decrease effectiveness and increase resistance. Advise to d/c and notify physician if watery/bloody diarrhea (with or without stomach cramps and fever) even as late as ≥2 months after the last dose, or an allergic reaction occurs. Instruct to notify physician if pregnant/nursing.

Storage: Vial: Prior to Reconstitution: 20-25°C (68-77°F). Reconstituted: Use immediately after reconstitution. Discard any unused portion after 24 hours if stored at 20-25°C (68-77°F) or after 48 hours if stored at 2-8°C (36-46°F). Do not freeze vials after reconstitution. Galaxy Container: ≤-20°C (-4°F). Thawed Sol: 2-8°C (36-46°F) for 14 days, or 20-25°C (68-77°F) for 24 hrs. Do not refreeze.

ZOVIRAX ORAL – acyclovir

RX

Class: Nucleoside analogue

ADULT DOSAGE

Herpes Zoster

800mg q4h, 5X/day for 7-10 days

Genital Herpes

Initial:
200mg q4h, 5X/day for 10 days

Recurrent Disease:
Chronic Suppressive Therapy: 400mg bid up to 12 months
Alternative: 200mg 3-5X/day

Intermittent Therapy:
200mg q4h, 5X/day for 5 days
Initiate at earliest sign/symptom of recurrence

Chickenpox

800mg qid for 5 days
Initiate at earliest sign/symptom

PEDIATRIC DOSAGE

Chickenpox

≥2 Years:
≤40kg: 20mg/kg qid for 5 days
>40kg: 800mg qid for 5 days
Initiate at earliest sign/symptom

DOSE MODIFICATION

Renal Impairment

Genital Herpes (Initial/Intermittent Therapy):
CrCl ≤10mL/min: Reduce dose to 200mg q12h

Genital Herpes (Chronic Suppressive Therapy):
CrCl ≤10mL/min: Reduce dose to 200mg q12h

Herpes Zoster/Chickenpox:
CrCl 10-25mL/min: 800mg q8h
CrCl ≤10mL/min: 800mg q12h

Hemodialysis: Adjust dosing schedule so that an additional dose is administered after each dialysis

ADMINISTRATION

Oral route

Bioequivalence of dosage forms
Sus shown to be bioequivalent to caps
One 800mg tab shown to be bioequivalent to four 200mg caps

HOW SUPPLIED

Cap: 200mg; Sus: 200mg/5mL [473mL]; Tab: 400mg, 800mg

CONTRAINDICATIONS

Hypersensitivity to valacyclovir.

WARNINGS/PRECAUTIONS

Renal failure sometimes resulting in death reported. Thrombotic thrombocytopenic purpura/hemolytic uremic syndrome (TTP/HUS) in immunocompromised patients reported. Maintain adequate hydration. Caution in elderly.

ADVERSE REACTIONS

N/V, diarrhea, malaise.

DRUG INTERACTIONS

Probenecid may increase levels and $T_{1/2}$ of IV formulation. May increase risk of renal impairment and/or CNS symptoms with nephrotoxic agents; use caution.

NURSING CONSIDERATIONS

Assessment: Assess for immunocompromised state, hypersensitivity to valacyclovir, renal impairment, nursing status, and possible drug interactions.

Monitoring: Monitor for signs/symptoms of TTP/HUS. Monitor BUN and SrCr.

Patient Counseling: Instruct to consult physician if experiencing severe or troublesome adverse reactions, if pregnant/intending to become pregnant, or intending to breastfeed. Advise to maintain adequate hydration. Inform that therapy is not a cure for genital herpes; advise to avoid contact with lesions or intercourse when lesions/symptoms are present.

Storage: 15-25°C (59-77°F); protect from moisture.

ZUBSOLV – buprenorphine/naloxone

CIII

Class: Partial opioid agonist/opioid antagonist

ADULT DOSAGE

Opioid Dependence

Used as part of a complete treatment plan to include counseling and psychosocial support

Administer as single daily dose in patients initially inducted using buprenorphine SL tab

One Zubsolv 5.7mg-1.4mg SL tab provides equivalent buprenorphine exposure to one Suboxone 8mg-2mg SL tab

Corresponding Doses From Induction (Buprenorphine) to Maintenance (Zubsolv) Treatment:
One 8mg Buprenorphine Tab:
One 5.7 mg/1.4 mg Zubsolv tab
12mg Buprenorphine (One 8mg and Two 2mg Tabs):
One 8.6 mg/2.1 mg Zubsolv tab
16mg Buprenorphine (Two 8mg Tabs):
One 11.4 mg/2.9 mg Zubsolv tab

Maint:
Target Dose: 11.4mg-2.9mg/day as single daily dose
Titrate: Adjust dose progressively in increments/decrements of 1.4mg-0.36mg or 2.8mg-0.72mg to maintain treatment and suppress opioid withdrawal signs and symptoms
Range: 2.8mg-0.72mg to 17.2mg-4.2mg/day, based on individual needs

Discontinuing Therapy:
Should be made as part of a comprehensive treatment plan

Switching Between Zubsolv and Other Buprenorphine/Naloxone Combination Products:
Dose adjustments may be necessary
Monitor for signs of over-medication or under-dosing (eg, withdrawal)
Corresponding Dosage Strengths when Switching Between Suboxone and Zubsolv:
One 2mg/0.5mg Buprenorphine/Naloxone SL Tab:
One 1.4mg/0.36mg Zubsolv tab
One 8mg/2mg Buprenorphine/Naloxone SL Tab:
One 5.7mg/1.4mg Zubsolv tab
12mg/3mg Buprenorphine/Naloxone (One 8mg/2mg Tab and Two 2mg/0.5mg Tabs):
One 8.6mg/2.1mg Zubsolv tab
16mg/4mg Buprenorphine/Naloxone (Two 8mg/2mg Tabs): One 11.4mg/2.9mg Zubsolv tab

PEDIATRIC DOSAGE

Pediatric use may not have been established

DOSE MODIFICATION

Hepatic Impairment
Severe: Avoid use

Elderly
Start at low end of dosing range

ADMINISTRATION

SL route

Do not cut, chew, or swallow; SL tab should be placed under tongue until dissolved
For dosages requiring more than one SL tab, place all tablets in different places under tongue at same time
Advise patients not to eat or drink anything until tab is completely dissolved

HOW SUPPLIED

Tab, SL: (Buprenorphine-Naloxone) 1.4mg-0.36mg, 5.7mg-1.4mg, 8.6mg-2.1mg, 11.4mg-2.9mg

WARNINGS/PRECAUTIONS

Not appropriate as an analgesic. Hypersensitivity reactions, bronchospasm, angioneurotic edema, and anaphylactic shock reported. May precipitate opioid withdrawal signs and symptoms if administered before the agonist effects of the opioid have subsided. Avoid with severe hepatic impairment; caution in patients with moderate hepatic impairment who have initiated treatment on a buprenorphine product without naloxone. May impair mental/physical abilities. May produce orthostatic hypotension in ambulatory patients. Caution with debilitated patients, myxedema or hypothyroidism, adrenal cortical insufficiency (eg, Addison's disease), CNS depression or coma, toxic psychoses, prostatic hypertrophy, urethral stricture, acute alcoholism, delirium tremens, kyphoscoliosis, and in elderly. Buprenorphine: Potential for abuse. Significant respiratory depression reported; caution with compromised respiratory function. To manage overdose, higher than normal doses and repeated administration of naloxone may be necessary. Accidental pediatric exposure can cause fatal respiratory depression. Chronic use produces physical dependence. Cytolytic hepatitis and hepatitis with jaundice reported. If a hepatic event is suspected, biological and etiological evaluation is recommended; careful discontinuation may be needed depending on the case. Caution with preexisting liver enzyme abnormalities, hepatitis B or C infection, use with other potentially hepatotoxic drugs, and ongoing injecting drug use. Neonatal abstinence syndrome reported when used during pregnancy. May elevate CSF pressure; caution with head injury, intracranial lesions, and other circumstances when CSF pressure may be increased. May produce miosis and changes in consciousness level that may interfere with patient evaluation. May increase intracholedochal pressure; caution with biliary tract dysfunction. May obscure diagnosis or clinical course of patients with acute abdominal conditions.

ADVERSE REACTIONS

Headache, withdrawal syndrome, pain, N/V, insomnia, sweating, constipation, abdominal pain, vasodilation.

DRUG INTERACTIONS

May cause respiratory depression, coma, and death with benzodiazepines or other CNS depressants (eg, alcohol); caution when used concurrently. May cause increased CNS depression with opioid analgesics, general anesthetics, benzodiazepines, phenothiazines, other tranquilizers, sedative/hypnotics, or other CNS depressants (eg, alcohol); consider dose reduction of one or both agents if used concomitantly. Concomitant use with CYP3A4 inhibitors (eg, azole antifungals such as ketoconazole, macrolides such as erythromycin, and HIV protease inhibitors) should be monitored and may require dose reduction of 1 or both agents. Monitor for signs and symptoms of opioid withdrawal with CYP3A4 inducers (eg, efavirenz, phenobarbital, carbamazepine, phenytoin, rifampicin). Monitor dose if non-nucleoside reverse transcriptase inhibitors are added to treatment regimen. Atazanavir and atazanavir/ritonavir may increase levels; monitor and consider dose reduction of buprenorphine.

NURSING CONSIDERATIONS

Assessment: Assess for history of hypersensitivity reactions, debilitation, myxedema, hypothyroidism, acute alcoholism, adrenal cortical insufficiency (eg, Addison's disease), CNS depression or coma, toxic psychoses, prostatic hypertrophy, urethral stricture, delirium tremens, kyphoscoliosis, biliary tract dysfunction, hepatic impairment, compromised respiratory function, hepatitis B or C infection, head injury, intracranial lesions and other circumstances in which CSF pressure may be increased, acute abdominal conditions, pregnancy/nursing status, and possible drug interactions. Perform LFTs prior to therapy.

Monitoring: Monitor for hypersensitivity reactions, signs/symptoms of opioid withdrawal, impaired mental/physical ability, orthostatic hypotension, respiratory depression, drug abuse/dependence, cytolytic hepatitis, hepatitis with jaundice, elevation of CSF pressure, miosis, changes in consciousness levels, and other adverse reactions. Monitor LFTs periodically. Monitor for over-medication as well as withdrawal or other signs of under-dosing when switching between other buprenorphine/naloxone products.

Patient Counseling: Warn about danger of self-administration of benzodiazepines and other CNS depressants, including alcohol, while on therapy. Advise that the drug contains an opioid that can be a target for abuse; instruct to keep tabs in safe place protected from theft and children. Instruct to seek medical attention immediately if a child is exposed to the drug. Caution that drug may impair mental/physical abilities and cause orthostatic hypotension. Advise to take tab qd and not to change dose without consulting physician. Counsel about instructions for missed dose. Inform that treatment can cause dependence and withdrawal syndrome may occur upon discontinuation. Advise patients seeking to d/c treatment with buprenorphine for opioid dependence to work closely with physician on a tapering schedule, and apprise of the potential to relapse to illicit drug use associated with discontinuation of treatment. Advise to report to physician all medications prescribed or currently being used. Advise women regarding possible effects during pregnancy. Advise women who are breastfeeding to monitor the infant for drowsiness and difficulty breathing. Advise to instruct family members that, in event of emergency, the treating physician or staff should be informed that patient is physically dependent on an opioid. Advise to dispose of unused drugs as soon as they are no longer needed by flushing the tabs down the toilet.

Storage: 20-25°C (68-77°F); excursions permitted to 15-30°C (59-86°F).

ZUPLENZ – ondansetron RX

Class: 5-HT_3 receptor antagonist

ADULT DOSAGE

Chemotherapy-Associated Nausea/Vomiting

Prevention of N/V Associated w/ Highly Emetogenic Cancer Chemotherapy (Including Cisplatin ≥50mg/m²):
24mg given successively as three 8mg films administered 30 min before start of single-day chemotherapy

Prevention of N/V Associated w/ Initial and Repeat Courses of Moderately Emetogenic Cancer Chemotherapy:
8mg bid; give 1st dose 30 min before start of chemotherapy, w/ a subsequent dose 8 hrs after 1st dose, then administer 8mg q12h for 1-2 days after completion of chemotherapy

Radiotherapy Associated Nausea/Vomiting

Prevention of N/V Associated w/ Radiotherapy in Patients Receiving Either Total Body Irradiation, Single High-Dose Fraction to the Abdomen, or Daily Fractions to the Abdomen:
Usual: 8mg tid

Total Body Irradiation:
8mg given 1-2 hrs before each fraction of radiotherapy administered each day

Single High-Dose Fraction Radiotherapy to Abdomen:
8mg given 1-2 hrs before radiotherapy, w/ subsequent doses q8h after 1st dose for 1-2 days after completion of radiotherapy

Daily Fractionated Radiotherapy to Abdomen:
8mg given 1-2 hrs before radiotherapy, w/ subsequent doses q8h after 1st dose for each day radiotherapy is given

Postoperative Nausea/Vomiting

Prevention:
16mg given successively as two 8mg films 1 hr before induction of anesthesia

PEDIATRIC DOSAGE

Chemotherapy-Associated Nausea/Vomiting

Prevention of N/V Associated w/ Initial and Repeat Courses of Moderately Emetogenic Cancer Chemotherapy:

4-11 Years:
4mg tid; give 1st dose 30 min before start of chemotherapy, w/ subsequent doses 4 and 8 hrs after 1st dose, then administer q8h for 1-2 days after completion of chemotherapy

≥12 Years:
8mg bid; give 1st dose 30 min before start of chemotherapy, w/ a subsequent dose 8 hrs after 1st dose, then administer 8mg q12h for 1-2 days after completion of chemotherapy

DOSE MODIFICATION

Hepatic Impairment

Severe (Child-Pugh ≥10):
Max: 8mg/day

ADMINISTRATION

Oral route

1. W/ dry hands, fold pouch along the dotted line to expose the tear notch
2. While still folded, tear the pouch carefully along the edge and remove the oral soluble film from pouch
3. Immediately place film on top of the tongue where it dissolves in 4-20 seconds
4. Once oral soluble film is dissolved, swallow w/ or w/o liquid. Allow each film to dissolve completely before administering the next film
5. Wash hands after administration

HOW SUPPLIED
Film, Oral: 4mg, 8mg

CONTRAINDICATIONS
Concomitant use with apomorphine.

WARNINGS/PRECAUTIONS
Hypersensitivity reactions reported in patients hypersensitive to other selective 5-HT_3 receptor antagonists; d/c immediately at the 1st sign of hypersensitivity. ECG changes, including QT interval prolongation and torsades de pointes, reported; avoid in patients with congenital long QT syndrome. Serotonin syndrome reported with 5-HT_3 receptor antagonists; d/c and initiate supportive treatment if symptoms occur. Use in patients following abdominal surgery or with chemotherapy-induced N/V may mask a progressive ileus and/or gastric distension. Does not stimulate gastric/intestinal peristalsis; do not use instead of NG suction.

ADVERSE REACTIONS
Headache, diarrhea, malaise/fatigue, constipation, hypoxia, pyrexia, dizziness, gynecological disorder, anxiety/agitation, urinary retention, pruritus.

DRUG INTERACTIONS
See Contraindications. Potent CYP3A4 inducers (eg, phenytoin, carbamazepine, rifampicin) may significantly increase clearance and decrease blood levels. May reduce analgesic activity of tramadol. Serotonin syndrome reported with concomitant use of other serotonergic drugs (eg, SSRIs, SNRIs, MAOIs, mirtazapine, fentanyl).

NURSING CONSIDERATIONS

Assessment: Assess for previous hypersensitivity to the drug, congenital long QT syndrome, electrolyte abnormalities, congestive heart failure (CHF), bradyarrhythmias, hepatic impairment, pregnancy/nursing status, and possible drug interactions.

Monitoring: Monitor for QT interval prolongation, torsades de pointes, emergence of serotonin syndrome, hypersensitivity reactions, and other adverse reactions. Monitor ECG in patients with electrolyte abnormalities (eg, hypokalemia, hypomagnesemia), CHF, bradyarrhythmias, and in patients taking other medications that lead to QT prolongation. In patients who recently underwent abdominal surgery or in patients with chemotherapy-induced N/V, monitor for masking of a progressive ileus and/or gastric distension.

Patient Counseling: Inform about potential benefits/risks of therapy. Inform that drug may cause serious cardiac arrhythmias; instruct patients to contact physician if they perceive a change in their HR, feel lightheaded, or have a syncopal episode. Inform that chances of developing severe cardiac arrhythmias are higher in patients with a personal/family history of abnormal heart rhythms, in patients taking medications that may cause electrolyte abnormalities, and in patients with hypokalemia or hypomagnesemia. Advise of the possibility of serotonin syndrome with concomitant use of other serotonergic agents; instruct to seek immediate medical attention if changes in mental status, autonomic instability, or neuromuscular symptoms with or without GI symptoms occur. Inform that drug may cause headache, malaise/fatigue, constipation, and diarrhea; instruct to report the use of all medications, especially apomorphine or any drug of the 5-HT_3 antagonist class, to physician. Inform that drug may cause hypersensitivity reactions, some as severe as anaphylaxis and bronchospasm; instruct to report any hypersensitivity reactions to physician. Instruct on how to use drug.

Storage: 20-25°C (68-77°F).

ZYBAN — bupropion hydrochloride RX

Class: Aminoketone

Serious neuropsychiatric reactions reported in patients taking bupropion for smoking cessation. Weigh risks against benefits of use. Antidepressants increased the risk of suicidal thoughts and behavior in children, adolescents, and young adults in short-term trials. Monitor closely for worsening, and emergence of suicidal thoughts and behavior.

ADULT DOSAGE

Smoking Cessation Aid

Initiate treatment while patient is still smoking Patients should set a "target quit date" within the first 2 weeks of treatment
Initial: 150mg qd for first 3 days
Titrate: Increase to 300mg/day, given as 150mg bid with an interval of at least 8 hrs between each dose
Max: 300mg/day

PEDIATRIC DOSAGE

Pediatric use may not have been established

Continue treatment for 7-12 weeks; if patient has not quit smoking after 7-12 weeks, should d/c and reassess treatment plan May consider continuing therapy in patients who successfully quit smoking after 12 weeks of treatment but do not feel ready to d/c treatment; base longer treatment on individual patient benefits/risks	

DOSE MODIFICATION

Concomitant Medications

Reversible MAOIs (eg, Linezolid, IV Methylene Blue):

Do not start bupropion in patients being treated with reversible MAOIs

If acceptable alternatives are not available, d/c bupropion and administer linezolid or IV methylene blue; monitor for 2 weeks or until 24 hrs after the last dose of linezolid or IV methylene blue, whichever comes first. May resume bupropion 24 hrs after the last dose of linezolid or IV methylene blue

Renal Impairment

GFR <90mL/min: Consider reducing dose and/or frequency

Hepatic Impairment

Mild (Child-Pugh Score: 5-6): Consider reducing dose and/or frequency

Moderate to Severe (Child-Pugh Score: 7-15) Max Dose: 150mg qod

Other Important Modifications

Switching to/from an MAOI:

Allow at least 14 days between discontinuation of an MAOI and initiation of treatment and allow at least 14 days between discontinuation of treatment and initiation of an MAOI

ADMINISTRATION

Oral route

Swallow tab whole; do not crush, divide, or chew

Take with or without food

Avoid hs dosing to minimize insomnia

May be used with a nicotine transdermal system

HOW SUPPLIED

Tab, Sustained-Release: 150mg

CONTRAINDICATIONS

Seizure disorder, current/prior diagnosis of bulimia or anorexia nervosa. Undergoing abrupt discontinuation of alcohol, benzodiazepines, barbiturates, and antiepileptic drugs. Use of MAOIs (intended to treat psychiatric disorders) either concomitantly or within 14 days of discontinuing treatment. Treatment within 14 days of discontinuing treatment with an MAOI. Starting treatment in patients being treated with reversible MAOIs (eg, linezolid, IV methylene blue).

WARNINGS/PRECAUTIONS

Dose-related risk of seizures; do not exceed 300mg/day and titrate gradually. D/C and do not restart treatment if a seizure occurs. May result in elevated BP and HTN. May precipitate a manic, mixed, or hypomanic episode; risk appears to be increased in patients with bipolar disorder or who have risk factors for bipolar disorder. Not approved for use in treating bipolar depression. Pupillary dilation that occurs following use may trigger an angle-closure attack in a patient with anatomically narrow angles who does not have a patent iridectomy. D/C if an allergic or anaphylactoid/anaphylactic reaction occurs. Arthralgia, myalgia, fever with rash, and other serum sickness-like symptoms suggestive of delayed hypersensitivity reported. False (+) urine immunoassay screening tests for amphetamines reported. Caution with renal/hepatic impairment and in the elderly.

ADVERSE REACTIONS

Neuropsychiatric reactions, insomnia, rhinitis, dry mouth, dizziness, nausea, disturbed concentration, constipation, anxiety, dream abnormality, arthralgia, nervousness, diarrhea, rash, myalgia.

DRUG INTERACTIONS

See Contraindications. CYP2B6 inhibitors (eg, ticlopidine, clopidogrel) may increase bupropion exposure but decrease hydroxybupropion exposure; may need to adjust bupropion dose. CYP2B6 inducers (eg, ritonavir, lopinavir, efavirenz) may decrease exposure; may need to increase bupropion dose but not to exceed max dose. Carbamazepine, phenytoin, and phenobarbital may induce metabolism and decrease exposure; may be necessary to increase dose of bupropion, but not to exceed max dose if used with a CYP inducer. May increase exposure of CYP2D6 substrates (eg, antidepressants, antipsychotics, β-blockers, Type 1C antiarrhythmics); may need to decrease dose of CYP2D6 substrate, particularly for drugs with a narrow therapeutic index. May reduce efficacy of drugs that require metabolic activation by CYP2D6 to be effective (eg, tamoxifen); may require increased doses of the drug. Extreme caution with other drugs that lower seizure threshold (eg, antipsychotics, theophylline, systemic corticosteroids); use low initial doses and increase gradually. Increased risk of seizure with illicit drugs (eg, cocaine), abuse or misuse of prescription drugs (eg, CNS stimulants), oral hypoglycemic drugs, insulin, anorectic drugs, and excessive use of alcohol, benzodiazepines, sedative/hypnotics, or opiates. CNS toxicity reported with levodopa or amantadine; use with caution. Minimize or avoid alcohol. Increased risk of HTN with MAOIs or other drugs that increase dopaminergic or noradrenergic activity. Monitor for HTN with nicotine replacement therapy. Physiological changes resulting from smoking cessation, with or without bupropion, may alter the pharmacokinetics or pharmacodynamics of certain drugs (eg, theophylline, warfarin, insulin) for which dosage adjustment may be necessary.

NURSING CONSIDERATIONS

Assessment: Assess for bipolar disorder, hepatic/renal dysfunction, susceptibility to angle-closure glaucoma, seizure disorder or conditions that may increase the risk of seizure, hypersensitivity to the drug, any other conditions where treatment is contraindicated or cautioned, pregnancy/nursing status, and possible drug interactions. Assess BP.

Monitoring: Monitor for clinical worsening, suicidality, unusual changes in behavior, seizures, activation of mania or hypomania, neuropsychiatric reactions, angle-closure glaucoma, anaphylactoid/anaphylactic reactions, delayed hypersensitivity, and other adverse reactions. Monitor hepatic/renal function and BP.

Patient Counseling: Inform about benefits/risks of therapy. Advise patients and caregivers to observe for clinical worsening, suicidal risks, and unusual changes in behavior. Inform that quitting smoking may be associated with nicotine withdrawal symptoms or exacerbation of preexisting psychiatric illness. Advise to notify physician immediately if agitation, hostility, depressed mood, changes in thinking or behavior, or suicidal ideation/behavior occurs. Educate on the symptoms of hypersensitivity and to d/c if a severe allergic reaction occurs. Instruct to d/c and not restart if a seizure occurs while on therapy. Inform that excessive use or abrupt discontinuation of alcohol or sedatives may alter the seizure threshold; advise to minimize or avoid alcohol use. Caution about the risk of angle-closure glaucoma. Inform that therapy may impair mental/physical abilities; advise to use caution while operating hazardous machinery/driving. Counsel to notify physician if taking/planning to take any prescription or OTC medications. Advise not to use in combination with any other medications that contain bupropion. Advise to notify physician if pregnant, intending to become pregnant, or if nursing. If taking >150mg/day, instruct to take in 2 doses at least 8 hrs apart, to minimize the risk of seizures. Inform that tab may have an odor.

Storage: 20-25°C (68-77°F); excursions permitted between 15-30°C (59-86°F). Protect from light and moisture.

ZYFLO CR – zileuton RX

Class: 5-lipoxygenase inhibitor

OTHER BRAND NAMES

Zyflo

ADULT DOSAGE

Asthma

Prophylaxis and Chronic Treatment:

Tab:

600mg qid

Tab, ER:

1200mg bid

PEDIATRIC DOSAGE

Asthma

Prophylaxis and Chronic Treatment:

≥12 Years:

Tab:

600mg qid

Tab, ER:

1200mg bid

ADMINISTRATION

Oral route

Tab

May take w/ meals and hs

Tab, ER

Do not chew, cut, or crush

Take w/in 1 hr after am and pm meals

HOW SUPPLIED

Tab: 600mg*; Tab, Extended-Release (ER): 600mg *scored

CONTRAINDICATIONS

Active liver disease or transaminase elevations (≥3X ULN).

WARNINGS/PRECAUTIONS

Not for use in reversal of bronchospasm in acute asthma attacks and status asthmaticus. Elevations of serum ALT/bilirubin may occur; increased risk for ALT elevation in females >65 yrs of age and those with preexisting transaminase elevations. Symptomatic hepatitis with jaundice may develop. D/C and follow transaminase levels until normal if signs of liver dysfunction (eg, right upper quadrant [RUQ] pain, nausea, fatigue) or serum transaminase ≥5X ULN occur. Caution in patients who consume substantial quantities of alcohol and/or have a past history of liver disease. Neuropsychiatric events, including sleep disorders and behavior changes, reported; evaluate risks and benefits of continuing treatment.

ADVERSE REACTIONS

Headache, elevation of ALT/bilirubin, nausea, myalgia, upper respiratory tract infection, sinusitis, pharyngolaryngeal pain, diarrhea.

DRUG INTERACTIONS

May increase theophylline and propranolol concentrations; monitor levels and reduce dose as necessary. Monitor use with other β-blockers. May increase warfarin levels; monitor PT or other coagulation tests and adjust dose appropriately. (Tab) Not recommended for use with terfenadine. Monitor use with certain drugs metabolized by CYP3A4 (eg, dihydropyridine calcium channel blockers, cyclosporine, cisapride, astemizole). (Tab, ER) Monitor use with CYP3A4 inhibitors such as ketoconazole.

NURSING CONSIDERATIONS

Assessment: Assess for active/history of liver disease, acute asthma attacks, status asthmaticus, preexisting transaminase elevation, neuropsychiatric events, alcohol use, previous hypersensitivity, pregnancy/nursing status, and possible drug interactions.

Monitoring: Monitor serum bilirubin level. Monitor serum ALT prior to therapy, once a month for first 3 months, every 2-3 months for remainder of 1st yr, and periodically thereafter. Monitor for signs/symptoms of hepatitis, jaundice, liver dysfunction (eg, RUQ pain, nausea, fatigue), neuropsychiatric events (eg, sleep disorders, behavior changes). Monitor alcohol consumption and worsening of asthma.

Patient Counseling: Inform that drug is indicated for chronic treatment, not for acute episodes, of asthma. Instruct to take regularly as prescribed. Advise not to reduce dose or d/c other antiasthma medications unless instructed. Instruct to notify healthcare provider if signs/symptoms of liver dysfunction or neuropsychiatric events occur. Advise to consult physician before starting or discontinuing any prescription or OTC medications. Counsel about potential for liver damage and need for liver enzyme monitoring on regular basis. (Tab, ER) Instruct to take within 1 hr after am and pm meals. Do not cut, crush, or chew.

Storage: 20-25°C (68-77°F); (Tab, ER) excursions permitted to 15-30°C (59-86°F). Protect from light.

ZYLOPRIM – allopurinol

RX

Class: Xanthine oxidase inhibitor

ADULT DOSAGE

Recurrent Calcium Oxalate Calculi

Management of recurrent calcium oxalate calculi w/ uric acid excretion >800mg/day in males and >750mg/day in females

Uric Acid Excretion >800mg/day in Males and >750mg/day in Females:

Usual: 200-300mg/day in divided doses or as single equivalent

Titrate: Adjusted up or down depending upon the resultant control of the hyperuricosuria based upon subsequent 24-hr urinary urate determinations

Gout

Management of signs and symptoms of primary or secondary gout (acute attacks, tophi, joint destruction, uric acid lithiasis, and/or nephropathy)

Mild Gout:

Usual: 200-300mg/day

Moderately Severe Tophaceous Gout:

Usual: 400-600mg/day

Reduction of Flare-Up of Acute Gouty Attacks:

Initial: 100mg/day

Titrate: Increase by 100mg/week until serum uric acid level is ≤6mg/dL

PEDIATRIC DOSAGE

Secondary Hyperuricemia with Malignancies

<6 Years:

150mg/day

6-10 Years:

300mg/day

Evaluate response after 48 hrs and adjust dose if necessary

Max: 800mg/day

Divide dose if >300mg/day

Uric Acid Nephropathy

Management of elevated serum and urinary uric acid levels in patients w/ leukemia, lymphoma, and malignancies receiving cancer therapy
Usual: 600-800mg/day for 2-3 days w/ high fluid intake
Max: 800mg/day

Divide dose if >300mg/day

Conversions

Conversion from a Uricosuric Agent: Gradually reduce dose of uricosuric agent over several weeks while gradually increasing allopurinol to the required dose

DOSE MODIFICATION
Concomitant Medications
Colchicine/Anti-Inflammatory Agents: While adjusting dose of allopurinol, continue therapy until serum uric acid is normal and no acute gouty attacks occur for months
Renal Impairment
CrCl 10-20mL/min: 200mg/day

CrCl <10mL/min:
Max: 100mg/day

CrCl <3mL/min: Lengthen dosing intervals

ADMINISTRATION
Oral route

Better tolerated if taken following meal
Recommend sufficient fluid intake to yield a daily urinary output of at least 2L; maintain neutral or slightly alkaline urine

HOW SUPPLIED
Tab: 100mg*, 300mg* *scored

WARNINGS/PRECAUTIONS
Not for treatment of asymptomatic hyperuricemia. D/C at 1st appearance of skin rash or other signs which indicate an allergic reaction. Hepatotoxicity, elevated serum alkaline phosphatase/transaminase, and bone marrow suppression reported. Monitor LFTs during early stages of therapy with preexisting liver disease. May impair mental/physical abilities. Acute gouty attacks increase during early stages of therapy reported; give colchicine or anti-inflammatory agents. Maintain sufficient fluid intake to yield a daily urinary output of at least 2L and maintain neutral or slightly alkaline urine. Renal failure reported with hyperuricemia secondary to neoplastic diseases; caution with multiple myeloma and congestive myocardial disease. Caution with renal impairment or concurrent illnesses affecting renal function such as HTN and diabetes mellitus (DM); monitor renal function periodically.

ADVERSE REACTIONS
Acute gout attacks, rash, diarrhea, SGOT/SGPT increase, alkaline phosphatase increase, nausea.

DRUG INTERACTIONS
Inhibits oxidation of mercaptopurine; reduce mercaptopurine or azathioprine to 1/3 or 1/4 of usual dose with concomitant use. Prolongs half-life of dicumarol and chlorpropamide. Decreased effects with uricosuric agents. Increased toxicity with thiazide diuretics; monitor renal function. May increase cyclosporine levels; monitor cyclosporine levels and consider possible adjustment of cyclosporine dose. Increased skin rash with ampicillin and amoxicillin. Enhanced bone marrow suppression with cyclophosphamide and other cytotoxic agents among patients with neoplastic disease, except leukemia.

NURSING CONSIDERATIONS

Assessment: Assess for renal/hepatic function or preexisting disease, concurrent illnesses affecting renal function (eg, HTN, DM, multiple myeloma, congestive myocardial disease), pregnancy/nursing status, and possible drug interactions. Obtain serum uric acid to provide correct dosage and schedule.

Monitoring: Monitor LFTs, serum uric acid, and renal function periodically. Monitor for signs/symptoms of hepatotoxicity, bone marrow depression, renal dysfunction, hypersensitivity/allergic reaction, and other adverse reactions.

Patient Counseling: Advise to seek medical attention immediately at 1st sign of skin rash, painful urination, blood in urine, irritation of eyes, or swelling of the lips/mouth. Inform that optimal benefit may be delayed for 2-6 weeks of therapy. Encourage to increase fluid intake during therapy to prevent renal stones. Counsel not to double the dose at the next scheduled time if a dose is missed. Inform about certain risks associated when used concomitantly with other drugs (eg, dicumarol, sulfinpyrazone, mercaptopurine). Inform that drowsiness may occur and physical/mental abilities may be impaired. Instruct to take after meals to minimize gastric irritation.

Storage: 15-25°C (59-77°F) in dry place. (300mg) Protect from light.

ZYMAXID — gatifloxacin

RX

Class: Fluoroquinolone

ADULT DOSAGE

Bacterial Conjunctivitis

Day 1: 1 drop in the affected eye(s) q2h while awake, up to 8X/day

Days 2-7: 1 drop bid-qid while awake

PEDIATRIC DOSAGE

Bacterial Conjunctivitis

≥1 Year:

Day 1: 1 drop in the affected eye(s) q2h while awake, up to 8X/day

Days 2-7: 1 drop bid-qid while awake

ADMINISTRATION

Ocular route

HOW SUPPLIED

Sol: 0.5% [2.5mL]

WARNINGS/PRECAUTIONS

For ophthalmic use only; should not be introduced directly into the anterior chamber of the eye. Overgrowth of nonsusceptible organisms, including fungi, may result with prolonged use. D/C use and institute alternative therapy if superinfection occurs. Avoid wearing contact lenses if there are signs and symptoms of bacterial conjunctivitis or during the course of therapy.

ADVERSE REACTIONS

Worsening of the conjunctivitis, eye irritation, dysgeusia, eye pain.

NURSING CONSIDERATIONS

Assessment: Assess for conjunctivitis, proper diagnosis of causative organisms (eg, slit-lamp biomicroscopy, fluorescein staining), and pregnancy/nursing status.

Monitoring: Monitor for adverse events and overgrowth of nonsusceptible organisms (eg, fungi) with prolonged therapy.

Patient Counseling: Inform that sol is for ophthalmic use only and should not be introduced directly into the anterior chamber of the eye. Advise not to wear contact lenses if there are signs and symptoms of bacterial conjunctivitis and during course of therapy. Instruct to avoid contaminating the applicator tip with material from the eyes, fingers, or other sources.

Storage: 15-25°C (59-77°F). Protect from freezing.

ZYPREXA — olanzapine

RX

Class: Atypical antipsychotic

Elderly patients with dementia-related psychosis treated with antipsychotic drugs are at an increased risk of death; most deaths appeared to be cardiovascular (eg, heart failure, sudden death) or infectious (eg, pneumonia) in nature. Not approved for the treatment of patients with dementia-related psychosis. When used with fluoxetine, refer to the Boxed Warning section of the PI for Symbyax.

OTHER BRAND NAMES

Zyprexa Zydis

ADULT DOSAGE

Bipolar I Disorder

PO:

Manic or Mixed Episode:

Initial: 10mg or 15mg qd. Adjust dose by increments/decrements of 5mg qd at intervals of not <24 hrs

PEDIATRIC DOSAGE

Schizophrenia

13-17 Years:

PO:

Initial: 2.5mg or 5mg qd

Target Dose: 10mg/day. Adjust dose by increments/decrements of 2.5mg or 5mg

Maint: 5-20mg/day. Periodically reevaluate the long-term usefulness of the drug
Max: 20mg/day

W/ Lithium or Valproate:
Initial: 10mg qd
Max: 20mg/day

Depressive Episodes:
W/ Fluoxetine:
Initial: 5mg w/ 20mg fluoxetine qpm. Adjust dose based on efficacy and tolerability
Usual: 5-12.5mg w/ 20-50mg fluoxetine
Max: 18mg w/ 75mg fluoxetine

Agitation

Acute Agitation Associated w/ Schizophrenia and Bipolar I Mania:
IM:
Usual: 10mg
Range: 2.5-10mg. Assess for orthostatic hypotension prior to subsequent dosing
Max: 3 doses of 10mg 2-4 hrs apart

May initiate PO therapy in a range of 5-20mg/day when clinically appropriate

Depression

Treatment-Resistant Depression:
PO:
W/ Fluoxetine:
Initial: 5mg w/ 20mg fluoxetine qpm. Adjust dose based on efficacy and tolerability
Usual: 5-20mg w/ 20-50mg fluoxetine
Max: 18mg w/ 75mg fluoxetine

Schizophrenia

PO:
Initial: 5-10mg qd
Target Dose: 10mg/day w/in several days. Adjust dose by increments/decrements of 5mg qd at intervals of not <1 week
Max: 20mg/day
Maint: 10-20mg/day. Periodically reevaluate the long-term usefulness of the drug

Max: 20mg/day
Maint: Use lowest dose needed to maintain remission. Periodically reassess the need for maint treatment

Bipolar I Disorder

PO:
Manic or Mixed Episodes:
13-17 Years:
Initial: 2.5mg or 5mg qd
Target Dose: 10mg/day. Adjust dose by increments/decrements of 2.5mg or 5mg
Max: 20mg/day
Maint: Use lowest dose needed to maintain remission. Periodically reassess the need for maint treatment
Depressive Episodes:
W/ Fluoxetine:
10-17 Years:
Initial: 2.5mg w/ 20mg fluoxetine qpm. Adjust dose based on efficacy and tolerability
Max: 12mg w/ 50mg fluoxetine

DOSE MODIFICATION
Hepatic Impairment
Zyprexa and Fluoxetine in Combination: Starting dose of oral olanzapine 2.5-5mg w/ fluoxetine 20mg
Elderly
IM Dosing: 5mg/inj
Other Important Modifications
Debilitated/Predisposed to Hypotensive Reactions/Slower Metabolism/Sensitive to Olanzapine:
Schizophrenia: 5mg as a starting dose
IM Dosing: 2.5mg/inj
Predisposed to Hypotensive Reactions/Slow Metabolizers of Zyprexa or Fluoxetine Combination/Sensitive to Olanzapine:
Zyprexa and Fluoxetine in Combination: Starting dose of oral olanzapine 2.5-5mg w/ fluoxetine 20mg

ADMINISTRATION
Oral/IM routes

Tab, Zydis
Can be taken w/ or w/o food

Inj
Do not administer IV or SQ. Inject slowly, deep into the muscle mass
Dissolve the contents of the vial using 2.1mL of sterile water for inj to provide approx 5mg/mL of olanzapine
Immediately use (w/in 1 hr) after reconstitution

Zydis
After opening sachet, peel back foil on blister

Do not push tab through foil
Upon opening the blister, remove tab and place entire tab in the mouth using dry hands

HOW SUPPLIED

Inj: 10mg; Tab: 2.5mg, 5mg, 7.5mg, 10mg, 15mg, 20mg; Tab, Disintegrating: (Zydis) 5mg, 10mg, 15mg, 20mg

CONTRAINDICATIONS

When used with fluoxetine, refer to the Symbyax monograph. When used with lithium or valproate, refer to the individual monographs.

WARNINGS/PRECAUTIONS

Supervision should accompany therapy in patients at high risk of attempted suicide. Neuroleptic malignant syndrome (NMS) reported; d/c and instill intensive symptomatic treatment and monitoring. Associated with metabolic changes including hyperglycemia, dyslipidemia, and weight gain; may be associated with increased cardiovascular/cerebrovascular risk. Hyperglycemia, in some cases extreme and associated with ketoacidosis or hyperosmolar coma or death, reported; caution in patients with diabetes mellitus or borderline increased blood glucose levels. Dose-related hyperprolactinemia reported. Tardive dyskinesia (TD) may develop; consider discontinuation if signs/symptoms develop unless treatment is required despite the presence of the syndrome. May induce orthostatic hypotension; caution with known cardiovascular disease (CVD), cerebrovascular disease, and conditions that would predispose to hypotension. Leukopenia, neutropenia, and agranulocytosis reported; consider discontinuing at 1st sign of a clinically significant decline in WBC count in the absence of other causative factors. D/C if severe neutropenia (absolute neutrophil count $<1000/mm^3$) develops. May cause esophageal dysmotility and aspiration, and disruption of body temperature regulation. Seizures reported; caution with history of seizures or with conditions that potentially lower the seizure threshold. Not approved for treatment of patients with Alzheimer's disease. May impair mental/physical abilities. Caution in patients with clinically significant prostatic hypertrophy, narrow-angle glaucoma, history of paralytic ileus or related conditions, cardiac patients, and in the elderly.

ADVERSE REACTIONS

Postural hypotension, constipation, dry mouth, weight gain, somnolence, dizziness, personality disorder, akathisia, asthenia, dyspepsia, tremor, increased appetite, abdominal pain, headache, insomnia.

DRUG INTERACTIONS

May potentiate orthostatic hypotension with diazepam and alcohol. Increased clearance with carbamazepine (CYP1A2 inducer), and omeprazole and rifampin (CYP1A2 inducers or glucuronyl transferase inducers). Decreased clearance with fluoxetine (CYP2D6 inhibitor) and fluvoxamine (CYP1A2 inhibitor); consider lower dose of olanzapine with concomitant fluvoxamine. Caution with other centrally acting drugs, alcohol, and drugs whose effects can induce hypotension, bradycardia, or respiratory/CNS depression. May enhance effects of certain antihypertensives. May antagonize effects of levodopa and dopamine agonists. Caution with anticholinergic drugs; may contribute to an elevation in core body temperature. (IM) Not recommended with parenteral benzodiazepines. IM lorazepam may potentiate somnolence. (PO) Decreased levels with activated charcoal.

NURSING CONSIDERATIONS

Assessment: Assess for CVD, cerebrovascular disease, risk of hypotension, history of seizures or conditions that could lower the seizure threshold, prostatic hypertrophy, narrow-angle glaucoma, history of paralytic ileus, hepatic impairment, history of drug abuse, risk factors for leukopenia/neutropenia, pregnancy/nursing status, and possible drug interactions. Assess for dementia-related psychosis and Alzheimer's disease in the elderly. Obtain baseline lipid profile, CBC, and FPG levels.

Monitoring: Monitor for signs/symptoms of NMS, TD, orthostatic hypotension, seizures, disruption of body temperature regulation, hyperprolactinemia, and other adverse reactions. Periodically monitor FPG, lipid levels, CBC, and weight of patient. In patients with clinically significant neutropenia, monitor for fever or other symptoms/signs of infection. Periodically reassess to determine the need for maintenance treatment.

Patient Counseling: Advise of potential benefits and risks of therapy. Counsel about the signs and symptoms of NMS. Inform of potential risk of hyperglycemia-related adverse events. Inform that medication may cause dyslipidemia and weight gain. Inform that medication may cause orthostatic hypotension; instruct to contact physician if dizziness, fast or slow heartbeat, or fainting occurs. Inform that medication may impair judgment, thinking, or motor skills; instruct to use caution when operating hazardous machinery, including automobiles. Instruct to avoid overheating and dehydration and to contact physician if severely ill and have symptoms of dehydration. Instruct to notify physician if taking, planning to take, or have stopped taking any prescription or OTC products, including herbal supplements. Instruct to avoid alcohol. Inform that orally disintegrating tab contains phenylalanine. Advise to notify physician if pregnant or planning to become pregnant during treatment. Advise to avoid breastfeeding during therapy.

Storage: Tab, Zydis, and Inj (Before Reconstitution): 20-25°C (68-77°F); excursions permitted between 15-30°C (59-86°F). Reconstituted Inj: 20-25°C (68-77°F) for up to 1 hr; excursions permitted between 15-30°C (59-86°F). Tab/Zydis: Protect from light and moisture. Inj: Protect from light. Do not freeze.

ZYPREXA RELPREVV – olanzapine

RX

Class: Atypical antipsychotic

Adverse events with signs and symptoms consistent with overdose, in particular, sedation (including coma) and/or delirium reported following inj. Must be administered in a registered healthcare facility with ready access to emergency response services. Observe patient for at least 3 hrs after each inj. Available only through a restricted distribution program called Zyprexa Relprevv Patient Care Program and requires prescriber, healthcare facility, patient, and pharmacy enrollment. Elderly patients with dementia-related psychosis treated with antipsychotic drugs are at an increased risk of death; most deaths appeared to be cardiovascular (eg, heart failure, sudden death) or infectious (eg, pneumonia) in nature. Not approved for the treatment of patients with dementia-related psychosis.

ADULT DOSAGE

Schizophrenia

≥18 Years:
Establish tolerability with PO olanzapine prior to initiating treatment
Usual: 150-300mg IM every 2 weeks or 405mg IM every 4 weeks
Max: 405mg IM every 4 weeks or 300mg IM every 2 weeks

Conversions

10mg/day PO Olanzapine:
Initial: 210mg every 2 weeks or 405mg every 4 weeks for the first 8 weeks
Maint: 150mg every 2 weeks or 300mg every 4 weeks

15mg/day PO Olanzapine:
Initial: 300mg every 2 weeks for the first 8 weeks
Maint: 210mg every 2 weeks or 405mg every 4 weeks

20mg/day PO Olanzapine:
Initial/Maint: 300mg every 2 weeks

PEDIATRIC DOSAGE

Pediatric use may not have been established

DOSE MODIFICATION

Debilitated/Predisposition to Hypotension/Slow Metabolizers/Sensitive to Olanzapine Effects:
Initial: 150mg IM every 4 weeks
Titrate: Increase cautiously; reassess periodically to determine the need for continued treatment

ADMINISTRATION

IM route

Use gloves when reconstituting
Flush with water if contact is made with skin
Must be suspended using only the diluent supplied in the convenience kit

Reconstitution

1. Loosen the powder by lightly tapping the vial
2. Withdraw the pre-determined diluent volume into the syringe
3. Inject the diluent into the powder vial
4. Remove the needle from the vial and engage the needle safety device
5. Pad a hard surface to cushion impact. Tap the vial firmly and repeatedly on the surface until no powder is visible
6. Shake the vial vigorously until the sus appears smooth and is consistent in color and texture. The suspended product will be yellow and opaque
7. If foam forms, let vial stand to allow foam to dissipate
8. If the product is not used right away, it should be shaken vigorously to re-suspend. Reconstituted Zyprexa Relprevv remains stable for up to 24 hrs in the vial

Inj

1. Before administering the inj, confirm there will be someone to accompany the patient after the 3-hr observation period. If this cannot be confirmed, do not give the inj

2. Attach a new safety needle to the syringe
3. Slowly withdraw the desired amount into the syringe
4. Engage the needle safety device and remove needle from syringe
5. For administration, select the 19-gauge, 1.5-inch (38 mm) Hypodermic Needle-Pro needle with needle protection device. For obese patients, a 2-inch (50 mm), 19-gauge or larger needle (not included in convenience kit) may be used. To help prevent clogging, a 19-gauge or larger needle must be used
6. Attach the new safety needle to the syringe prior to injection. Once the sus has been removed from the vial, it should be injected immediately
7. Select and prepare a site for injection in the gluteal area
8. After insertion of the needle into the muscle, aspirate for several sec to ensure that no blood appears. If any blood is drawn into the syringe, discard the syringe and the dose and begin with a new convenience kit. The inj should be performed with steady, continuous pressure
9. Do not massage the inj site
10. Engage the needle safety device

HOW SUPPLIED

Inj, Extended-Release: 210mg, 300mg, 405mg

WARNINGS/PRECAUTIONS

Supervision should accompany therapy in patients at high risk for attempted suicide. Neuroleptic malignant syndrome (NMS) reported; d/c and instill intensive symptomatic treatment and monitoring if NMS occurs. Associated with metabolic changes, including hyperglycemia, dyslipidemia, and weight gain, which may be associated with increased cardiovascular/cerebrovascular risk. Hyperglycemia, in some cases extreme and associated with ketoacidosis or hyperosmolar coma or death, reported; caution in patients with diabetes mellitus (DM) or borderline increased blood glucose levels. Hyperprolactinemia reported. Tardive dyskinesia (TD) may develop; consider discontinuation if signs/symptoms develop unless treatment is required despite the presence of the syndrome. May induce orthostatic hypotension; caution with known cardiovascular disease (CVD), cerebrovascular disease, and conditions that would predispose to hypotension. Leukopenia, neutropenia, and agranulocytosis reported; consider discontinuation at 1st sign of clinically significant decline in WBC in the absence of other causative factors or if severe neutropenia (absolute neutrophil count $<1000/mm^3$) develops. May cause esophageal dysmotility and aspiration, and disruption of body temperature regulation. Seizures reported; caution with history of seizures or with conditions that potentially lower the seizure threshold. Not approved for use in patients with Alzheimer's disease. May impair mental/physical abilities. Caution in patients with clinically significant prostatic hypertrophy, cardiac patients, narrow angle glaucoma, history of paralytic ileus or related conditions, and in the elderly.

ADVERSE REACTIONS

Headache, sedation, diarrhea, cough, back pain, N/V, nasal congestion, dry mouth, nasopharyngitis, weight gain, abdominal pain, somnolence, increased appetite.

DRUG INTERACTIONS

May potentiate orthostatic hypotension with diazepam and alcohol. Increased clearance with carbamazepine (CYP1A2 inducer), and omeprazole and rifampin (CYP1A2 inducers or glucuronyl transferase inducers). Decreased clearance with fluoxetine (CYP2D6 inhibitor) and fluvoxamine (CYP1A2 inhibitor); consider lower dose of olanzapine with concomitant fluvoxamine. Caution with other centrally acting drugs, alcohol, and drugs whose effects can induce hypotension, bradycardia, or respiratory/CNS depression. May enhance effects of certain antihypertensive agents. May antagonize effects of levodopa and dopamine agonists. Caution with anticholinergic drugs; may contribute to an elevation in core body temperature. IM lorazepam may potentiate somnolence. Monitor for excessive sedation and cardiorespiratory depression with parenteral benzodiazepines.

NURSING CONSIDERATIONS

Assessment: Assess for tolerability with PO olanzapine, CVD, cerebrovascular disease, risk of hypotension, history of seizures or conditions that could lower the seizure threshold, prostatic hypertrophy, narrow-angle glaucoma, history of paralytic ileus, risk factors for leukopenia/neutropenia, pregnancy/nursing status, and possible drug interactions. Assess for dementia-related psychosis and Alzheimer's disease in the elderly. Obtain baseline lipid profile, CBC, and FPG levels.

Monitoring: Monitor for sedation and/or delirium for at least 3 hrs post-inj. Monitor for signs/symptoms of NMS, TD, orthostatic hypotension, seizures, disruption of body temperature regulation, hyperprolactinemia, and other adverse reactions. In patients with clinically significant neutropenia, monitor for fever or other symptoms/signs of infection. In high-risk patients, monitor closely for a suicide attempt. Perform periodic monitoring of FPG, lipid levels, and weight of patient. Perform frequent monitoring of CBC in patients with a history of a clinically significant low WBC or drug-induced leukopenia/neutropenia.

Patient Counseling: Advise of potential benefits and risks of therapy. Advise of the risk of post-inj delirium/sedation syndrome following administration; advise not to drive or operate heavy machinery for rest of the day. Counsel about the signs/symptoms of NMS. Inform of potential risk of hyperglycemia-related adverse events. Counsel that medication may cause dyslipidemia and weight gain. Inform that medication may cause orthostatic hypotension; instruct to contact physician if dizziness, fast or slow heartbeat, or fainting occurs. Inform that medication may impair judgment, thinking, or motor skills; instruct to use caution when operating hazardous machinery, including automobiles. Instruct to avoid overheating and dehydration. Instruct to notify physician if taking, planning to take, or have stopped taking any prescription or OTC drugs, including herbal supplements. Instruct to avoid alcohol. Advise to notify physician if pregnant or planning to become pregnant during treatment. Advise to avoid breastfeeding during therapy.

Storage: Room temperature ≤30°C (86°F). Reconstituted Sol: May store at room temperature for 24 hrs. Use immediately once withdrawn into the syringe.

ZYTIGA – abiraterone acetate — RX

Class: Nonsteroidal antiandrogen

ADULT DOSAGE

Metastatic Castration-Resistant Prostate Cancer

1000mg qd w/ prednisone 5mg PO bid

PEDIATRIC DOSAGE

Pediatric use may not have been established

DOSE MODIFICATION

Concomitant Medications

Use w/ Strong CYP3A4 Inducers:

Avoid concomitant strong CYP3A4 inducers

If inducer must be coadministered, increase dosing frequency to bid only during the coadministration period

If inducer is discontinued, reduce dose back to the previous dose and frequency

Hepatic Impairment

Baseline Moderate (Child-Pugh Class B): 250mg qd; use w/ caution

Moderate Impairment w/ ALT and/or AST >5X ULN or Total Bilirubin >3X ULN: D/C use and do not retreat

Severe (Child-Pugh Class C): Not recommended

Adverse Reactions

Hepatotoxicity:

Development During Treatment (ALT and/or AST >5X ULN or Total Bilirubin >3X ULN):

Interrupt treatment

May restart at 750mg qd following return of LFTs to baseline or to AST and ALT ≤2.5X ULN and total bilirubin ≤1.5X ULN

If hepatotoxicity recurs at 750mg qd, may restart retreatment at 500mg qd, following return of LFTs to patient's baseline or to AST and ALT ≤2.5X ULN and total bilirubin ≤1.5X ULN

If hepatotoxicity recurs at 500mg qd, d/c use

ADMINISTRATION

Oral route

No food should be consumed for at least 2 hrs before and 1 hr after the dose is taken

Swallow tab whole w/ water; do not crush or chew

HOW SUPPLIED

Tab: 250mg

CONTRAINDICATIONS

Women who are or may become pregnant.

WARNINGS/PRECAUTIONS

May cause HTN, hypokalemia, and fluid retention; caution w/ history of cardiovascular disease (CVD) or w/ underlying medical conditions that might be compromised by increases in BP, hypokalemia, or fluid retention. Adrenocortical insufficiency reported; use caution and monitor for signs/symptoms, particularly if patients are withdrawn from prednisone, have prednisone dose reductions, or experience unusual stress. Increased dosage of corticosteroids may be indicated before, during, and after stressful situations. Signs/symptoms of adrenocortical insufficiency may be masked by adverse reactions associated w/ mineralocorticoid excess. ALT/AST increases reported; promptly measure serum total bilirubin, AST, and ALT if signs/symptoms of hepatotoxicity develop.

ADVERSE REACTIONS

Fatigue, joint swelling/discomfort, edema, hot flush, diarrhea, vomiting, cough, HTN, dyspnea, UTI, contusion, hypertriglyceridemia, elevated AST/ALT.

DRUG INTERACTIONS

See Dosage. Avoid concomitant strong CYP3A4 inducers (eg, phenytoin, carbamazepine, rifampin). Decreased exposure w/ rifampin. Increased levels of dextromethorphan (CYP2D6 substrate) reported. Avoid coadministration w/ CYP2D6 substrates w/ narrow therapeutic index (eg, thioridazine); if alternative treatments cannot be used, exercise caution and consider dose reduction of the concomitant CYP2D6 substrate. Increased exposure of pioglitazone (CYP2C8 substrate) reported; monitor closely for signs of toxicity related to a CYP2C8 substrate w/ narrow therapeutic index if used concomitantly.

NURSING CONSIDERATIONS

Assessment: Assess for hepatic impairment, history of CVD and underlying medical conditions that might be compromised by increases in BP, hypokalemia, or fluid retention, and for possible drug interactions. Obtain baseline AST, ALT, and bilirubin levels. Control HTN and correct hypokalemia before treatment.

Monitoring: Monitor for HTN, hypokalemia, and fluid retention at least monthly, signs/symptoms of adrenocortical insufficiency, and other adverse reactions. Monitor ALT, AST, and bilirubin levels every 2 weeks for the 1st 3 months (or weekly for the 1st month, then every 2 weeks for the following 2 months in patients w/ baseline moderate hepatic impairment), and monthly thereafter. For patients who resume treatment after development of hepatotoxicity, monitor serum transaminases and bilirubin at a minimum of every 2 weeks for 3 months, and monthly thereafter.

Patient Counseling: Inform that drug is used together w/ prednisone and instruct to take ud and not to interrupt or stop either of these medications w/o consulting a physician. Inform those receiving gonadotropin-releasing hormone agonists to maintain such treatment during therapy. Inform that if a daily dose is missed, take the normal dose the following day, but if >1 daily dose is skipped, advise to consult physician. Counsel about the common side effects (eg, peripheral edema, hypokalemia, HTN, elevated LFTs, UTI). Inform that liver function will be monitored using blood tests. Advise that drug may harm a developing fetus and that women who are pregnant or may be pregnant should not handle the drug w/o protection (eg, gloves). Instruct to use a condom if having sex w/ a pregnant woman, and to use a condom and another effective method of birth control if having sex w/ a woman of childbearing potential; advise that these measures are required during and for 1 week after treatment.

Storage: 20-25°C (68-77°F); excursions permitted from 15-30°C (59-86°F).

ZYVOX – linezolid

Class: Oxazolidinone class antibacterial

RX

ADULT DOSAGE

Pneumonia

Nosocomial/Community-Acquired Pneumonia, Including Concurrent Bacteremia:
600mg q12h for 10-14 consecutive days

Vancomycin-Resistant *Enterococcus faecium* Infections

Including Concurrent Bacteremia:
600mg q12h for 14-28 consecutive days

Skin and Skin Structure Infections

Complicated:
Inj/Sus/Tab:
600mg q12h for 10-14 consecutive days

Uncomplicated:
Sus/Tab:
400mg q12h for 10-14 consecutive days

PEDIATRIC DOSAGE

Skin and Skin Structure Infections

Complicated:
Inj/Sus:
Preterm Neonates <7 Days of Age:
Initial: 10mg/kg q12h
Titrate: Increase to 10mg/kg q8h if clinical response is suboptimal. All neonates should receive 10mg/kg q8h by 7 days of life
Treatment Duration: 10-14 consecutive days
Inj/Sus/Tab:
Birth-11 Years:
10mg/kg q8h for 10-14 consecutive days
≥12 Years:
600mg q12h for 10-14 consecutive days

Uncomplicated:
Sus:
Neonates <7 Days of Age:
Initial: 10mg/kg q12h
Titrate: Increase to 10mg/kg q8h if clinical response is suboptimal. All neonates should receive 10mg/kg q8h by 7 days of life
Treatment Duration: 10-14 consecutive days
Sus/Tab:
<5 Years:
10mg/kg q8h for 10-14 consecutive days
5-11 Years:
10mg/kg q12h for 10-14 consecutive days
≥12 Years:
600mg q12h for 10-14 consecutive days

Pneumonia

Nosocomial/Community-Acquired Pneumonia, Including Concurrent Bacteremia:
Inj/Sus:
Preterm Neonates <7 Days of Age:
Initial: 10mg/kg q12h
Titrate: Increase to 10mg/kg q8h if clinical response is suboptimal. All neonates should receive 10mg/kg q8h by 7 days of life
Treatment Duration: 10-14 consecutive days
Inj/Sus/Tab:
Birth-11 Years:
10mg/kg q8h for 10-14 consecutive days
≥12 Years:
600mg q12h for 10-14 consecutive days

Vancomycin-Resistant *Enterococcus faecium* Infections

Including Concurrent Bacteremia:

Inj/Sus:
Neonates <7 Days of Age:
Initial: 10mg/kg q12h
Titrate: Increase to 10mg/kg q8h if clinical response is suboptimal. All neonates should receive 10mg/kg q8h by 7 days of life
Treatment Duration: 14-28 consecutive days
Inj/Sus/Tab:
Birth-11 Years:
10mg/kg q8h for 14-28 consecutive days
≥12 Years:
600mg q12h for 14-28 consecutive days

ADMINISTRATION
Oral/IV route

May be administered w/o regard to the timing of meals

Inj
Infuse over 30-120 min
Do not use infusion bag in series connections
Do not introduce additives into linezolid inj sol
Compatible IV sol include 0.9% NaCl, D5W, and Lactated Ringer's
Refer to PI for incompatibilities

Sus
Reconstitute w/ 123mL distilled water in 2 portions; shake vigorously after each portion
After constitution, before using, gently mix by inverting the bottle 3-5X
Do not shake
Store reconstituted sus at room temperature; use w/in 21 days

HOW SUPPLIED
Inj: 2mg/mL [100mL, 200mL, 300mL]; Sus: 100mg/5mL [240mL]; Tab: 600mg

CONTRAINDICATIONS
Use of MAOIs A or B (eg, phenelzine, isocarboxazid) either concomitantly or w/in 2 weeks of taking such drugs.

WARNINGS/PRECAUTIONS
Myelosuppression (eg, anemia, leukopenia, pancytopenia, thrombocytopenia) reported; monitor CBC weekly, particularly in those who receive treatment for >2 weeks, w/ preexisting myelosuppression, receiving concomitant drugs that produce bone marrow suppression, or w/ a chronic infection who have received previous or concomitant antibiotic therapy. Consider discontinuation if myelosuppression develops or worsens. Peripheral/optic neuropathies and visual blurring reported; prompt ophthalmic evaluation is recommended if experiencing visual impairment symptoms. Monitor visual function if used for extended periods (≥3 months) or if new visual symptoms develop. Weigh continued use against potential risks if peripheral/optic neuropathy occurs. Do not administer w/ carcinoid syndrome. Not approved and should not be used for the treatment of catheter-related bloodstream infections or catheter-site infections. Not indicated for the treatment of gram-negative infections; initiate specific gram-negative therapy immediately if a concomitant gram-negative pathogen is documented or suspected. *Clostridium difficile*-associated diarrhea (CDAD) reported; may need to d/c if CDAD is suspected or confirmed. Do not administer w/ uncontrolled HTN, pheochromocytoma, or thyrotoxicosis, unless patients are

monitored for potential increases in BP. Lactic acidosis reported; evaluate immediately if recurrent N/V, unexplained acidosis, or a low bicarbonate level develops. Convulsions reported. May result in bacterial resistance if used in the absence of a proven or suspected bacterial infection or a prophylactic indication.

ADVERSE REACTIONS

Diarrhea, headache, N/V, anemia, thrombocytopenia, abnormal Hgb/WBC/neutrophils, serum AST/ALT/alkaline phosphatase/lipase/total bilirubin elevations.

DRUG INTERACTIONS

See Contraindications. Serotonin syndrome reported w/ serotonergic agents, including antidepressants such as SSRIs; do not administer in patients taking serotonin reuptake inhibitors, TCAs, 5-HT_1 receptor agonists (triptans), meperidine, bupropion, or buspirone, unless clinically appropriate and patients are carefully observed for signs/symptoms of serotonin syndrome or neuroleptic malignant syndrome (NMS)-like reactions. If alternatives to linezolid are not available and the potential benefits of linezolid outweigh the risks of serotonin syndrome or NMS-like reactions, promptly d/c the serotonergic antidepressant and administer linezolid; monitor for 2 weeks (5 weeks if fluoxetine was taken) or until 24 hrs after the last dose of linezolid, whichever comes 1st. Do not administer w/ directly and indirectly acting sympathomimetic agents (eg, pseudoephedrine), vasopressive agents (eg, epinephrine, norepinephrine), or dopaminergic agents (eg, dopamine, dobutamine), unless patients are monitored for potential increases in BP. Avoid large amounts of high tyramine-containing foods or beverages. Symptomatic hypoglycemia reported in patients w/ diabetes mellitus (DM) receiving insulin or oral hypoglycemic agents when treated w/ linezolid; may need to decrease dose of insulin or oral hypoglycemic agent, or d/c the oral hypoglycemic agent, insulin, or linezolid, if hypoglycemia occurs.

NURSING CONSIDERATIONS

Assessment: Assess for hypersensitivity to drug, myelosuppression, catheter-related bloodstream/catheter-site infections, uncontrolled HTN, pheochromocytoma, thyrotoxicosis, carcinoid syndrome, pregnancy/nursing status, and possible drug interactions.

Monitoring: Monitor for peripheral/optic neuropathy, CDAD, lactic acidosis, convulsions, and other adverse reactions. Monitor CBC weekly. Monitor visual function if used for extended periods (≥3 months) or if new visual symptoms develop.

Patient Counseling: Counsel that therapy should only be used to treat bacterial, not viral, infections. Instruct to take exactly ud even if the patient feels better early in the course of therapy. Inform that skipping doses or not completing the full course of therapy may decrease effectiveness of treatment and increase bacterial resistance. Instruct to notify physician if patient has a history of HTN or seizures, if taking medications containing pseudoephedrine or phenylpropanolamine (eg, cold remedies, decongestants) or antidepressants, or if experiencing visual changes. Instruct to avoid large quantities of high tyramine-containing foods or beverages. Inform phenylketonurics that oral sus contains phenylalanine. Advise that diarrhea is a common problem caused by therapy that usually ends when therapy is discontinued. Instruct to immediately contact physician if watery and bloody stools (w/ or w/o stomach cramps and fever) occur, even as late as ≥2 months after having taken the last dose. Inform patients, particularly those w/ DM, that hypoglycemia may occur; instruct to contact physician if this occurs.

Storage: 25°C (77°F). Protect from light. (Inj) Keep infusion bags in the overwrap until ready to use. Protect from freezing. (Tab/Sus) Protect from moisture. Constituted Sus: Room temperature. Use w/in 21 days.

Appendix: Reference Tables

Abbreviations, Acronyms, and Symbols

ABBREVIATIONS	DESCRIPTIONS
- (eg, 6-8)	to (eg, 6 to 8)
/	per
<	less than
>	greater than
≤	less than or equal to
≥	greater than or equal to
α	alpha
β	beta
μL	microliter
μm	micrometer
μM	micromolar
μmol	micromole
5-FU	5-fluorouracil
5-HT	5-hydroxytryptamine (serotonin)
aa	of each
ABECB	acute bacterial exacerbation of chronic bronchitis
ac	before meals
ACE inhibitor	angiotensin converting enzyme inhibitor
ACTH	adrenocorticotropic hormone
ad	right ear
ADHD	attention-deficit hyperactivity disorder
A-fib	atrial fibrillation
A-flutter	atrial flutter
AIDS	acquired immunodeficiency syndrome
ALT	alanine transaminase (SGPT)
am or AM	morning
AMI	acute myocardial infarction
ANA	antinuclear antibody
ANC	absolute neutrophil count
APAP	acetaminophen
Apo B	apolipoprotein B
ARB	angiotensin II receptor blocker
as	left ear
ASA	aspirin
AST	aspartate transaminase (SGOT)
au	each ear
AUC	area under the curve

(Continued)

ABBREVIATIONS	DESCRIPTIONS
AV	atrioventricular
bid	twice daily
BMI	body mass index
BP	blood pressure
BPH	benign prostatic hypertrophy
BSA	body surface area
BUN	blood urea nitrogen
Ca^{2+}	calcium
CABG	coronary artery bypass graft
CAD	coronary artery disease
cAMP	cyclic-3',5'-adenosine monophosphate
cap	capsule or gelcap
CAP	community-acquired pneumonia
CBC	complete blood count
CCB	calcium channel blocker
CF	cystic fibrosis
cGMP	cyclic guanosine monophosphate
CHF	congestive heart failure
CK	creatine kinase
Cl^-	chloride
cm	centimeter
C_{max}	peak plasma concentration
CMV	cytomegalovirus
CNS	central nervous system
COMT inhibitor	catechol-O-methyl transferase inhibitor
COPD	chronic obstructive pulmonary disease
COX-2 inhibitor	cyclooxygenase-2 inhibitor
CPK	creatine phosphokinase
CR	controlled-release
CrCl	creatinine clearance
cre	cream
CRF	chronic renal failure
CSF	cerebrospinal fluid
cSSSI	complicated skin and skin structure infection
CTC	common toxicity criteria
CV	cardiovascular
CVA	cerebrovascular accident
CVD	cardiovascular disease
CYP450	cytochrome P450
D5	dextrose 5%

ABBREVIATIONS	DESCRIPTIONS
D5W	dextrose 5% in water
d/c or D/C	discontinue
DHEA	dehydroepiandrosterone
DM	diabetes mellitus
DR	delayed-release
DVT	deep vein thrombosis
ECG	electrocardiogram
EDTA	edetate disodium
EEG	electroencephalogram
eg	for example
EPS	extrapyramidal symptom
ER	extended-release
ESRD	end-stage renal disease
fl oz	fluid ounce
FPG	fasting plasma glucose
FSH	follicle-stimulating hormone
g	gram
G6PD	glucose-6-phosphate dehydrogenase
GABA	gamma-aminobutyric acid
GAD	general anxiety disorder
GERD	gastroesophageal reflux disease
GFR	glomerular filtration rate
GGT	gamma-glutamyl transpeptidase
GI	gastrointestinal
GnRH	gonadotropin-releasing hormone
GVHD	graft-versus-host disease
HbA1c	hemoglobin A1c
hCG	human chorionic gonadotropin
Hct	hematocrit
HCTZ	hydrochlorothiazide
HDL	high-density lipoprotein
HER2	human epidermal growth factor receptor 2
HF	heart failure
Hgb	hemoglobin
HIV	human immunodeficiency virus
HMG-CoA	3-hydroxy-3-methylglutaryl-coenzyme A
HR	heart rate
hr, hrs	hour, hours
hs	bedtime
HSV	herpes simplex virus

(Continued)

ABBREVIATIONS	DESCRIPTIONS
HTN	hypertension
IBD	inflammatory bowel disease
IBS	irritable bowel syndrome
ICH	intracranial hemorrhage
ICP	intracranial pressure
IgG	immunoglobulin G
IM	intramuscular/intramuscularly
INH	isoniazid
inh	inhalation
inj	injection
INR	international normalized ratio
IOP	intraocular pressure
IR	immediate-release
IU*	international unit
IUD	intrauterine device
IV	intravenous/intravenously
K^+	potassium
kg	kilogram
KIU	kallikrein inhibitor unit
L	liter
lb, lbs	pound, pounds
LD	loading dose
LDL	low-density lipoprotein
LFT	liver function test
LH	luteinizing hormone
LHRH	luteinizing-hormone releasing hormone
lot	lotion
loz	lozenge
LVH	left ventricular hypertrophy
M	molar
MAC	*Mycobacterium avium* complex
maint	maintenance
MAOI	monoamine oxidase inhibitor
max	maximum
mcg	microgram
mEq	milli-equivalent
mg	milligram
Mg^{2+}	magnesium
MI	myocardial infarction
min	minute (usually as mL/min)

ABBREVIATIONS	DESCRIPTIONS
mL	milliliter
mm	millimeter
mM	millimolar
MRI	magnetic resonance imaging
MS*	multiple sclerosis
msec	millisecond
MTX	methotrexate
N/A	not applicable or not available
Na^+	sodium
NaCl	sodium chloride
NG	nasogastric
NKA	no known allergies
NMS	neuroleptic malignant syndrome
NPO	nothing by mouth
NSAID	nonsteroidal anti-inflammatory drug
NV or N/V	nausea and vomiting
NYHA Class	New York Heart Association Class
OA	osteoarthritis
OCD	obsessive-compulsive disorder
od	right eye
oint	ointment
os	left eye
OTC	over-the-counter
ou	each eye
oz	ounce
P	phosphorus
PAT	paroxysmal atrial tachycardia
pc	after meals
PCN	penicillin
PCP	*Pneumocystis carinii* pneumonia
PD	Parkinson's disease
PDE-5 inhibitor	phosphodiesterase-5 inhibitor
PE	pulmonary embolism
P-gp	P-glycoprotein
PID	pelvic inflammatory disease
pkt, pkts	packet, packets
pm or PM	evening
po or PO	orally
PONV	postoperative nausea and vomiting

(Continued)

ABBREVIATIONS	DESCRIPTIONS
postop	postoperative/postoperatively
pr	rectally
preop	preoperative/preoperatively
prn or PRN	as needed
PSA	prostate-specific antigen
PSVT	paroxysmal supraventricular tachycardia
PT	prothrombin time
PTSD	post-traumatic stress disorder
PTT	partial thromboplastin time
PTU	propylthiouracil
PUD	peptic ulcer disease
PVD	peripheral vascular disease
q4h, q6h, q8h, etc.	every four hours, every six hours, every eight hours, etc.
qam	once every morning
qd*	once daily
qh	every hour
qhs	every night at bedtime/before retiring
qid	four times daily
qod*	every other day
qpm	once every evening
qs	a sufficient quantity
qs ad	a sufficient quantity to make
RA	rheumatoid arthritis
RAAS	renin-angiotensin-aldosterone system
RAS	renin-angiotensin system
RBC	red blood cell
RDS	respiratory distress syndrome
REM	rapid eye movement
Rx	prescription
SA	sinoatrial
SAH	subarachnoid hemorrhage
SBP	systolic blood pressure
sec	second
SGOT	serum glutamic-oxaloacetic transaminase (AST)
SGPT	serum glutamic-pyruvic transaminase (ALT)
SIADH	syndrome of inappropriate antidiuretic hormone secretion
SJS	Stevens-Johnson syndrome
SL	sublingual/sublingually

ABBREVIATIONS	DESCRIPTIONS
SLE	systemic lupus erythematosus
SNRI	serotonin and norepinephrine reuptake inhibitor
SOB	shortness of breath
sol	solution
SQ, SC	subcutaneous/subcutaneously
SR	sustained-release
SrCr	serum creatinine
SSRI	selective serotonin reuptake inhibitor
SSSI	skin and skin structure infection
STD	sexually transmitted disease
sup or supp	suppository
sus	suspension
SVT	supraventricular tachycardia
$T_{½}$	half-life
T3	triiodothyronine
T4	thyroxine
tab	tablet or caplet
tab, SL	sublingual tablet
TB	tuberculosis
TBG	thyroxine-binding globulin
tbl or tbsp	tablespoonful
TCA	tricyclic antidepressant
TD	tardive dyskinesia
TEN	toxic epidermal necrolysis
TFT	thyroid function test
TG	triglyceride
tid	three times daily
T_{max}	time to maximum concentration
TNF	tumor necrosis factor
total-C	total cholesterol
TPN	total parenteral nutrition
TSH	thyroid-stimulating hormone
tsp	teaspoonful
TTP	thrombotic thrombocytopenic purpura
U*	unit
UC	ulcerative colitis
ud	as directed
ULN	upper limit of normal
URTI/URI	upper respiratory tract infection

(Continued)

ABBREVIATIONS	DESCRIPTIONS
UTI	urinary tract infection
UV	ultraviolet
V_d	volume of distribution
VLDL	very low density lipoprotein
VTE	venous thromboembolism
w/ or W/	with
w/in or W/IN	within
w/o or W/O	without
WBC	white blood cell
WHO	World Health Organization
X	times (eg, >2X ULN)
yr, yrs	year, years

*The Joint Commission cautions use of these abbreviations on orders and medication-related documentation that is handwritten (including free-text computer entry) or on pre-printed forms. Visit www.jointcommission.org for more information.

NORMAL LABORATORY VALUES: BLOOD, PLASMA, AND SERUM

TEST	SPECIMEN	CONVENTIONAL UNITS	SI UNITS
Acetoacetate	Plasma	< 1 mg/dL	< 0.1 mmol/L
Acetylcholinesterase (ACE), RBC	Blood	26.7–49.2 U/g Hb	—
Acid phosphatase	Serum	0.5–5.5 U/L	0–0.9 μkat/L
Activated partial thromboplastin time (aPTT)	Plasma	25–35 sec	—
Adrenocorticotropic hormone (ACTH)	Serum	9–52 pg/mL	2–11 pmol/L
Albumin	Serum	3.5–5.5 g/dL	35–55 g/L
Aldosterone:			
Standing	Serum	7–20 ng/dL	194–554 pmol/L
Supine	Serum	2–5 ng/dL	55–138 pmol/L
Alkaline phosphatase (ALP)	Serum	36–92 U/L	0.5–1.5 μkat/L
$Alpha_1$-antitrypsin (AAT)	Serum	83–199 mg/dL	—
Alpha fetoprotein (AFP)	Serum	0–20 ng/dL	0–20 pg/L
δ-Aminolevulinic acid (ALA)	Serum	15–23 μg/L	1.14–1.75 μmol/L
Aminotransferase, alanine (ALT)	Serum	0–35 U/L	0–0.58 pkat/L
Aminotransferase, aspartate (AST)	Serum	0–35 U/L	0–0.58 pkat/L
Ammonia	Plasma	40–80 μg/dL	23–47 μmol/L
Amylase	Serum	0–130 U/L	0–2.17 μkat/L
Antibodies to extractable nuclear antigen (AENA)	Serum	< 20.0 units	—
Anti–cyclic citrullinated peptide (anti-CCP) antibodies	Serum	≤ 5.0 units	—
Antidiuretic hormone (ADH; arginine vasopressin)	Plasma	< 1.7 pg/mL	< 1.57 pmol/L
Anti–double-stranded DNA (dsDNA) antibodies, IgG	Serum	< 25 IU	—
Antimitochondrial M2 antibodies	Serum	< 0.1 units	—
Antineutrophil cytoplasmic antibodies (cANCA)	Serum	Negative	—
Antinuclear antibodies (ANA)	Serum	≤ 1.0 units	—
Anti–smooth muscle antibodies (ASMA) titer	Serum	≤ 1:80	—
Antistreptolysin O titer	Serum	< 150 units	—
Antithyroid microsomal antibody titer	Serum	< 1:100	—
α_1-Antitrypsin (AAT)	Serum	83–199 mg/dL	15.3–36.6 μmol/L
Apolipoproteins:			
A-I, females	Serum	98–210 mg/dL	0.98–2.1 g/L
A-I, males	Serum	88–180 mg/dL	0.88–1.8 g/L
B-100, females	Serum	44–148 mg/dL	0.44–1.48 g/L
B-100, males	Serum	55–151 mg/dL	0.55–1.51 g/L

(Continued)

TEST	SPECIMEN	CONVENTIONAL UNITS	SI UNITS
Bicarbonate	Serum	23–28 mEq/L	23–28 mmol/L
Bilirubin:			
Direct	Serum	0–0.3 mg/dL	0–5.1 μmol/L
Total	Serum	0.3–1.2 mg/dL	5.1–20.5 μmol/L
Blood volume:			
Plasma, females	Blood	28–43 mL/kg body wt	0.028–0.043 L/kg body wt
Plasma, males	Blood	25–44 mL/kg body wt	0.025–0.044 L/kg body wt
RBCs, females	Blood	20–30 mL/kg body wt	0.02–0.03 L/kg body wt
RBCs, males	Blood	25–35 mL/kg body wt	0.025–0.035 L/kg body wt
Brain (B-type) natriuretic peptide (BNP)	Plasma	< 100 pg/mL	—
Calcitonin, age ≥ 16 yr:			
Females	Serum	< 8 pg/mL	—
Males	Serum	< 16 pg/mL	—
Calcium	Serum	9–10.5 mg/dL	2.2–2.6 mmol/L
Cancer antigen (CA):			
CA 125	Serum	< 35 U/mL	—
CA 15-3	Serum	< 30 U/mL	—
Carbon dioxide (CO_2) content	Serum	23–28 mEq/L	23–28 mmol/L
Carbon dioxide partial pressure (PCO_2)	Blood	35–45 mm Hg	—
Carboxyhemoglobin	Plasma	0.5–5%	—
Carcinoembryonic antigen (CEA)	Serum	< 2 ng/mL	< 2 μg/L
Carotene	Serum	75–300 μg/L	1.4–5.6 μmol/L
CD4:CD8 ratio	Blood	1–4	—
CD4+ T-cell count	Blood	640–1175/μL	0.64–1.18 x 10^9/L
CD8+ T-cell count	Blood	335–875/μL	0.34–0.88 x 10^9/L
Ceruloplasmin	Serum	25–43 mg/dL	250–430 mg/L
Chloride	Serum	98–106 mEq/L	98–106 mmol/L
Cholesterol, desirable level:			
High-density lipoprotein (HDL-C)	Plasma	≥ 40 mg/dL	≥ 1.04 mmol/L
Low-density lipoprotein (LDL-C)	Plasma	≤ 130 mg/dL	≤ 3.36 mmol/L
Total (TC)	Plasma	150–199 mg/dL	3.88–5.15 mmol/L
Coagulation factors:			
Factor I	Plasma	150–300 mg/dL	1.5–3.5 g/L
Factor II	Plasma	60–150% of normal	—
Factor IX	Plasma	60–150% of normal	—
Factor V	Plasma	60–150% of normal	—
Factor VII	Plasma	60–150% of normal	—
Factor VIII	Plasma	60–150% of normal	—
Factor X	Plasma	60–150% of normal	—
Factor XI	Plasma	60–150% of normal	—
Factor XII	Plasma	60–150% of normal	—
Complement:			
C3	Serum	55–120 mg/dL	0.55–1.20 g/L
C4	Serum	20–59 mg/dL	0.20–0.59 g/L
Total	Serum	37–55 U/mL	37–55 kU/L
Copper	Serum	70–155 μg/L	11–24.3 μmol/L

TEST	SPECIMEN	CONVENTIONAL UNITS	SI UNITS
Cortisol:			
1 h after cosyntropin	Serum	> 18 μg/dL and usually ≥ 8 μg/dL above baseline	> 498 nmol/L and usually ≥ 221 nmol/L above baseline
At 5 PM	Serum	3–13 μg/dL	83–359 nmol/L
At 8 AM	Serum	8–20 μg/dL	251–552 nmol/L
After overnight suppression test	Serum	< 5 μg/dL	< 138 nmol/L
C-peptide	Serum	0.9–4.3 ng/mL	297–1419 pmol/L
C-reactive protein (CRP)	Serum	< 0.5 mg/dL	< 0.005 g/L
C-reactive protein, highly sensitive (hsCRP)	Serum	< 1.1 mg/L	< 0.0011 g/L
Creatine kinase (CK)	Serum	30–170 U/L	0.5–2.83 μkat/L
Creatinine	Serum	0.7–1.3 mg/dL	61.9–115 μmol/L
D-Dimer	Plasma	≤ 300 ng/mL	≤ 300 μg/L
Dehydroepiandrosterone sulfate (DHEA-S):			
Females	Plasma	0.6–3.3 mg/mL	1.6–8.9 μmol/L
Males	Plasma	1.3–5.5 mg/mL	3.5–14.9 μmol/L
δ-Aminolevulinic acid (ALA)	Serum	15–23 μg/L	1.14–1.75 μmol/L
11-Deoxycortisol (DOC):			
After metyrapone	Plasma	> 7 μg/dL	> 203 nmol/L
Basal	Plasma	< 5 μg/dL	< 145 nmol/L
D-Xylose level 2 h after ingestion of 25 g of D-xylose	Serum	> 20 mg/dL	> 1.3 nmol/L
Epinephrine, supine	Plasma	< 75 ng/L	< 410 pmol/L
Erythrocyte sedimentation rate (ESR):			
Females	Blood	0–20 mm/h	0–20 mm/h
Males	Blood	0–15 mm/h	0–20 mm/h
Erythropoietin	Serum	4.0–18.5 mIU/mL	4.0–18.5 IU/L
Estradiol, females:			
Day 1–10 of menstrual cycle	Serum	14–27 pg/mL	50–100 pmol/L
Day 11–20 of menstrual cycle	Serum	14–54 pg/mL	50–200 pmol/L
Day 21–30 of menstrual cycle	Serum	19–40 pg/mL	70–150 pmol/L
Estradiol, males	Serum	10–30 pg/mL	37–110 pmol/L
Ferritin	Serum	15–200 ng/mL	15–200 μg/L
α-Fetoprotein (AFP)	Serum	0–20 ng/dL	0–20 pg/L
Fibrinogen	Plasma	150–350 mg/dL	1.5–3.5 g/L
Folate (folic acid):			
RBC	Blood	160–855 ng/mL	362–1937 nmol/L
Serum	Serum	2.5–20 ng/mL	5.7–45.3 nmol/L
Follicle-stimulating hormone (FSH), females:			
Follicular or luteal phase	Serum	5–20 mU/mL	5–20 U/L
Midcycle peak	Serum	30–50 mU/mL	30–50 U/L
Postmenopausal	Serum	> 35 mU/mL	> 35 U/L
Follicle-stimulating hormone (FSH), adult males	Serum	5–15 mU/mL	5–15 U/L
Fructosamine	Plasma	200–285 mol/L	—

(Continued)

TEST	SPECIMEN	CONVENTIONAL UNITS	SI UNITS
Gamma-glutamyl transpeptidase (GGT)	Serum	8–78 U/L	—
Gastrin	Serum	0–180 pg/mL	0–180 ng/L
Globulins:	Serum	2.5–3.5 g/dL	25–35 g/L
α_1-Globulins	Serum	0.2–0.4 g/dL	2–4 g/L
α_2-Globulins	Serum	0.5–0.9 g/dL	5–9 g/L
β-Globulins	Serum	0.6–1.1 g/dL	6–11 g/L
γ-Globulins	Serum	0.7–1.7 g/dL	7–17 g/L
β_2-Microglobulin	Serum	0.7–1.8 μg/mL	—
Glucose:			
2-h postprandial	Plasma	< 140 mg/dL	< 7.8 mmol/L
Fasting	Plasma	70–105 mg/dL	3.9–5.8 mmol/L
Glucose-6-phosphate dehydrogenase (G6PD)	Blood	5–15 U/g Hb	0.32–0.97 mU/mol Hb
γ-Glutamyl transpeptidase (GGT)	Serum	8–78 U/L	—
Growth hormone:			
After oral glucose	Plasma	< 2 ng/mL	< 2 μg/L
In response to provocative stimuli	Plasma	> 7 ng/mL	> 7 μg/L
Haptoglobin	Serum	30–200 mg/dL	300–2000 mg/L
Hematocrit:			
Females	Blood	36–47%	—
Males	Blood	41–51%	—
Hemoglobin:			
Females	Blood	12–16 g/dL	120–160 g/L
Males	Blood	14–17 g/dL	140–170 g/L
Hemoglobin A_{1c}	Blood	4.7–8.5%	—
Hemoglobin electrophoresis, adults:			
Hb A_1	Blood	95–98%	—
Hb A_2	Blood	2–3%	—
Hb C	Blood	0%	—
Hb F	Blood	0.8–2.0%	—
Hb S	Blood	0%	—
Hemoglobin electrophoresis, Hb F in children:			
Neonate	Blood	50–80%	—
1–6 mo	Blood	8%	—
> 6 mo	Blood	1–2%	—
Homocysteine:			
Females	Plasma	0.40–1.89 mg/L	3–14 μmol/L
Males	Plasma	0.54–2.16 mg/L	4–16 μmol/L
Human chorionic gonadotropin (hCG), quantitative	Serum	< 5 mIU/mL	—

TEST	SPECIMEN	CONVENTIONAL UNITS	SI UNITS
Immunoglobulins:			
IgA	Serum	70–300 mg/dL	0.7–3.0 g/L
IgD	Serum	< 8 mg/dL	< 80 mg/L
IgE	Serum	0.01–0.04 mg/dL	0.1–0.4 mg/L
IgG	Serum	640–1430 mg/dL	6.4–14.3 g/L
IgG_1	Serum	280–1020 mg/dL	2.8–10.2 g/L
IgG_2	Serum	60–790 mg/dL	0.6–7.9 g/L
IgG_3	Serum	14–240 mg/dL	0.14–2.4 g/L
IgG_4	Serum	11–330 mg/dL	0.11–3.3 g/L
IgM	Serum	20–140 mg/dL	0.2–1.4 g/L
Insulin, fasting	Serum	1.4–14 μIU/mL	10–104 pmol/L
International normalized ratio (INR):			
Therapeutic range (standard intensity therapy)	Plasma	2.0–3.0	—
Therapeutic range in patients at higher risk (eg, patients with prosthetic heart valves)	Plasma	2.5–3.5	—
Therapeutic range in patients with lupus anticoagulant	Plasma	3.0–3.5	—
Iron	Serum	60–160 μg/dL	11–29 μmol/L
Iron-binding capacity, total (TIBC)	Serum	250–460 μg/dL	45–82 μmol/L
Lactate dehydrogenase (LDH)	Serum	60–160 U/L	1–1.67 μkat/L
Lactic acid, venous	Blood	6–16 mg/dL	0.67–1.8 mmol/L
Lactose tolerance test	Plasma	> 15 mg/dL increase in plasma glucose level	> 0.83 mmol/L increase in plasma glucose level
Lead	Blood	< 40 μg/dL	< 1.9 μmol/L
Leukocyte alkaline phosphatase (LAP) score	Peripheral blood smear	13–130/100/polymorphonuclear (PMN) leukocyte neutrophils and bands	—
Lipase	Serum	< 95 U/L	< 1.58 μkat/L
Lipoprotein (a) [Lp(a)]	Serum	≤ 30 mg/dL	< 1.1 μmol/L
Luteinizing hormone (LH), females:			
Follicular or luteal phase	Serum	5–22 mU/mL	5–22 U/L
Midcycle peak	Serum	30–250 mU/mL	30–250 U/L
Postmenopausal	Serum	> 30 mU/mL	> 30 U/L
Luteinizing hormone, males	Serum	3–15 mU/mL	3–15 U/L
Magnesium	Serum	1.5–2.4 mg/dL	0.62–0.99 mmol/L
Manganese	Serum	0.3–0.9 ng/mL	5.5–16.4 nmol/L
Mean corpuscular hemoglobin (MCH)	Blood	28–32 pg	—
Mean corpuscular hemoglobin concentration (MCHC)	Blood	32–36 g/dL	320–360 g/L
Mean corpuscular volume (MCV)	Blood	80–100 fL	—
Metanephrines, fractionated:			
Metanephrines, free	Plasma	< 0.50 nmol/L	—
Normetanephrines, free	Plasma	< 0.90 nmol/L	—
Methemoglobin	Blood	< 1.0%	—
Methylmalonic acid (MMA)	Serum	150–370 nmol/L	—

(Continued)

TEST	SPECIMEN	CONVENTIONAL UNITS	SI UNITS
Myeloperoxidase (MPO) antibodies	Serum	< 6.0 U/mL	—
Myoglobin:			
Females	Serum	25–58 μg/L	1.4–3.5 nmol/L
Males	Serum	28–72 μg/L	1.6–4.1 nmol/L
Norepinephrine, supine	Plasma	50–440 pg/mL	0.3–2.6 nmol/L
N-Terminal propeptide of BNP (NT-proBNP)	Plasma	< 125 pg/mL	—
5'-Nucleotidase (5'NT)	Serum	4–11.5 U/L	—
Osmolality	Plasma	275–295 mOsm/kg H_2O	275–295 mmol/kg H_2O
Osmotic fragility test	Blood	Increased fragility if hemolysis occurs in > 0.5% NaCl Decreased fragility if hemolysis is incomplete in 0.3% NaCl	—
Oxygen partial pressure (PO_2)	Blood	80–100 mm Hg	—
Parathyroid hormone (PTH)	Serum	10–65 pg/mL	10–65 ng/L
Parathyroid hormone–related peptide (PTHrP)	Plasma	< 2.0 pmol/L	—
Partial thromboplastin time, activated (aPTT)	Plasma	25–35 sec	—
pH	Blood	7.38–7.44	—
Phosphorus, inorganic	Serum	3.0–4.5 mg/dL	0.97–1.45 mmol/L
Platelet count	Blood	150–350 x 10^3/μL	150–350 x 10^9/L
Platelet life span, using chromium-51 (^{51}Cr)	—	8–12 days	—
Porphyrins	Plasma	≤ 1.0 μg/dL	—
Potassium	Serum	3.5–5 mEq/L	3.5–5 mmol/L
Prealbumin (transthyretin)	Serum	18–45 mg/dL	—
Progesterone:			
Follicular phase	Serum	< 1 ng/mL	< 0.03 nmol/L
Luteal phase	Serum	3–30 ng/mL	0.1–0.95 nmol/L
Prolactin:			
Females	Serum	< 20 μg/L	< 870 pmol/L
Males	Serum	< 15 μg/L	< 652 pmol/L
Prostate-specific antigen, total (PSA-T)	Serum	0–4 ng/mL	—
Prostate-specific antigen, ratio of free to total (PSA-F:PSA-T)	Serum	> 0.25	—
Protein C activity	Plasma	67–131%	—
Protein C resistance, activated ratio (APC-R)	Plasma	2.2–2.6	—
Protein S activity	Plasma	82–144%	—
Protein, total	Serum	6–7.8 g/dL	60–78 g/L
Prothrombin time (PT)	Plasma	11–13 sec	—
Pyruvate	Blood	0.08–0.16 mmol/L	—
RBC count	Blood	4.2–5.9 x 10^6 cells/μL	4.2–5.9 x 10^{12} cells/L
RBC survival rate, using ^{51}Cr	Blood	$T_{½}$ = 28 days	—

TEST	SPECIMEN	CONVENTIONAL UNITS	SI UNITS
Renin activity, plasma (PRA), upright, in males and females aged 18–39 yr:			
Sodium-depleted	Plasma	2.9–24 ng/mL/h	—
Sodium-repleted	Plasma	0.6 (or lower)–4.3 ng/mL/h	—
Reticulocyte count:			
Percentage	Blood	0.5–1.5%	—
Absolute	Blood	23–90 x 10^3/μL	23–90 x 10^9/L
Rheumatoid factor (RF)	Serum	< 40 U/mL	< 40 kU/L
Sodium	Serum	136–145 mEq/L	136–145 mmol/L
Testosterone, adults:			
Females	Serum	20–75 ng/dL	0.7–2.6 nmol/L
Males	Serum	300–1200 ng/dL	10–42 nmol/L
Thrombin time	Plasma	18.5–24 sec	—
Thyroid iodine-123 (^{123}I) uptake	—	5–30% of administered dose at 24 h	—
Thyroid-stimulating hormone (TSH)	Serum	0.5–5.0 μIU/mL	0.5–5.0 mIU/L
Thyroxine (T_4):			
Free	Serum	0.9–2.4 ng/dL	12–31 pmol/L
Free index	—	4–11 μg/dL	—
Total	Serum	5–12 μg/dL	64–155 nmol/L
Transferrin	Serum	212–360 mg/dL	2.1–3.6 g/L
Transferrin saturation	Serum	20–50%	—
Triglycerides (desirable level)	Serum	< 250 mg/dL	< 2.82 mmol/L
Triiodothyronine (T_3):			
Uptake	Serum	25–35%	—
Total	Serum	70–195 ng/dL	1.1–3.0 nmol/L
Troponin I	Plasma	< 0.1 ng/mL	< 0.1 μg/L
Troponin T	Serum	≤ 0.03 ng/mL	≤ 0.03 μg/L
Urea nitrogen (BUN)	Serum	8–20 mg/dL	2.9–7.1 mmol/L
Uric acid	Serum	2.5–8 mg/dL	0.15–0.47 mmol/L
Vitamin B_{12}	Serum	200–800 pg/mL	148–590 pmol/L
Vitamin C (ascorbic acid):			
Leukocyte	Blood	< 20 mg/dL	< 1136 μmol/L
Total	Blood	0.4–1.5 mg/dL	23–85 μmol/L
Vitamin D:			
1,25-Dihydroxycholecalciferol (calcitriol)	Serum	25–65 pg/mL	65–169 pmol/L
25-Hydroxycholecalciferol	Serum	15–80 ng/mL	37–200 nmol/L
WBC count	Blood	3.9–10.7 x 10^3 cells/μL	3.9–10.7 x 10^9 cells/L
Zinc	Serum	66–110 μg/dL	10.1–16.8 μmol/L

μkat = microkatal; pkat = picokatal.

From the Merck Manual of Diagnosis and Therapy, edited by Robert Porter. Copyright 2009-2015 by Merck Sharp & Dohme Corp., a subsidiary of Merck & Co., Inc., Whitehouse Station, NJ. Available at: http://www.merckmanuals.com/professional/. Accessed February 2015.

Poison Control Centers

The American Association of Poison Control Centers (AAPCC) uses a single, nationwide emergency number to automatically link callers with their regional poison center. This toll-free number, **800-222-1222**, also works for **teletype lines (TTY)** for the hearing-impaired and **telecommunication devices (TDD)** for individuals who are deaf. The ASPCA/Animal Poison Center is not part of the nationwide system, and has its own emergency number. Within each state, centers are listed alphabetically by city, with their corresponding addresses.

ALABAMA

BIRMINGHAM

Regional Poison Control Center
Children's Hospital of Alabama

1600 7th Ave S
Birmingham AL 35233-1711
www.childrensal.org/rpcc

ALASKA

(PORTLAND, OR)

Oregon Poison Center
Oregon Health & Science University

3181 SW Sam Jackson Park Rd – Suite CB550
Portland OR 97239
oregonpoison.org

ARIZONA

PHOENIX

Banner Good Samaritan Poison and Drug Information Center
Banner Good Samaritan Medical Center

1111 E McDowell
Phoenix AZ 85006
www.bannerpoisoncontrol.com

TUCSON

Arizona Poison & Drug Information Center
Arizona Health Sciences Center

1295 N Martin, Room B308
Tucson AZ 85721
azpoison.com

ARKANSAS

LITTLE ROCK

Arkansas Poison and Drug Information Center
College of Pharmacy – UAMS

4301 W Markham St – MS 522-2
Little Rock AR 72205
www.arpoisoncenter.org

ASPCA/Animal Poison Control Center

1717 S Philo Rd – Suite 36
Urbana IL 61802
Business: 217-337-5030
Emergency: 888-426-4435
(not part of nationwide emergency system)
www.aspca.org/apcc

CALIFORNIA

FRESNO/MADERA

California Poison Control System
Fresno/Madera Division
Children's Hospital Central California

9300 Valley Children's Place – MB 15
Madera CA 93638
www.calpoison.org

SACRAMENTO

California Poison Control System
Sacramento Division
UC Davis Medical Center

2315 Stockton Blvd
Sacramento CA 95817
www.calpoison.org

SAN DIEGO

California Poison Control System
San Diego Division
UC San Diego Medical Center

200 W Arbor Dr
San Diego CA 92103-8925
www.calpoison.org

SAN FRANCISCO

California Poison Control System
San Francisco Division

UCSF Box 1369
San Francisco CA 94143
www.calpoison.org

COLORADO

DENVER

Rocky Mountain Poison & Drug Center

777 Bannock St – MC 0180
Denver CO 80204-4028
www.rmpdc.org

CONNECTICUT

FARMINGTON

Connecticut Poison Control Center
University of Connecticut Health Center

263 Farmington Ave
Farmington CT 06030-5365
poisoncontrol.uchc.edu

DELAWARE

(PHILADELPHIA, PA)

The Poison Control Center
The Children's Hospital of Philadelphia

34th & Civic Center Blvd
Philadelphia PA 19104
www.chop.edu/service/poison-control-center/home.html

DISTRICT OF COLUMBIA

WASHINGTON, DC

National Capital Poison Center

3201 New Mexico Ave NW
Suite 310
Washington DC 20016
www.poison.org

FLORIDA

JACKSONVILLE

Florida/USVI Poison Information Center-Jacksonville

655 W 8th St, Box C23
Jacksonville FL 32209
www.fpicjax.org

(Continued)

MIAMI

Florida Poison Information Center-Miami

Jackson Memorial Hospital/University of Miami Miller School of Medicine
1611 NW 12th Ave (R-131)
Institute Annex, 3rd Floor
Miami FL 33136
www.miamipoison.org

TAMPA

Florida Poison Information Center-Tampa
Tampa General Hospital

PO Box 1289
Tampa FL 33601
www.poisoncentertampa.org

GEORGIA

ATLANTA

Georgia Poison Center
Hughes Spalding Children's Hospital
Grady Health System

50 Hurt Plaza – Suite 600
PO Box 26066
Atlanta GA 30303
www.georgiapoisoncenter.org

HAWAII

(DENVER, CO)

Rocky Mountain Poison & Drug Center

777 Bannock St – MC 0180
Denver CO 80204-4507
www.rmpdc.org

IDAHO

(OMAHA, NE)

Nebraska Regional Poison Center

8401 W Dodge Rd – Suite 115
Omaha NE 68114
www.nebraskapoison.com

ILLINOIS

CHICAGO

Illinois Poison Center

222 S Riverside Plaza – Suite 1900
Chicago IL 60606
www.illinoispoisoncenter.org

INDIANA

INDIANAPOLIS

Indiana Poison Center
IU Methodist Hospital
Indiana University Health

1701 N Senate Blvd, Room B402
Indianapolis IN 46202
www.indianapoison.org

IOWA

SIOUX CITY

Iowa Statewide Poison Control Center

401 Douglas St – Suite 215
Sioux City IA 51101
www.iowapoison.org

KANSAS

KANSAS CITY

The University of Kansas Hospital Poison Control Center
University of Kansas Medical Center

3901 Rainbow Blvd
Room B-400
Kansas City KS 66160-7231
www.kumed.com/poison

KENTUCKY

LOUISVILLE

Kentucky Regional Poison Center

Medical Towers South
234 E Gray St – Suite 847
Louisville KY 40202
www.kosairchildrenshospital.com/poisoncontrol

LOUISIANA

SHREVEPORT

Louisiana Poison Center LSUHSC - Shreveport Department of Emergency Medicine - Section of Clinical Toxicology

1455 Wilkinson St
Shreveport LA 71130
www.lapcc.org

MAINE

PORTLAND

Northern New England Poison Center

22 Bramhall St
Portland ME 04101
www.nnepc.org

MARYLAND

BALTIMORE

Maryland Poison Center
University of Maryland School of Pharmacy

220 Arch St, Office Level 1
Baltimore MD 21201
www.mdpoison.com

(WASHINGTON, DC)

National Capital Poison Center

3201 New Mexico Ave NW
Suite 310
Washington DC 20016
www.poison.org

MASSACHUSETTS

BOSTON

Regional Center for Poison Control and Prevention

300 Longwood Ave
Boston MA 02115
www.maripoisoncenter.com

MICHIGAN

DETROIT

Children's Hospital of Michigan Regional Poison Control Center

4707 St Antoine – Suite 302
Detroit MI 48201
www.mitoxic.org

MINNESOTA

MINNEAPOLIS

Minnesota Poison Control System
Hennepin County Medical Center

701 Park Ave, Mail Code RL
Minneapolis MN 55415
www.mnpoison.org

MISSISSIPPI

JACKSON

Mississippi Poison Control Center
University of Mississippi Medical Center

2500 N State St
Jackson MS 39216
poisoncontrol.umc.edu

MISSOURI

ST. LOUIS

Missouri Regional Poison Center
Cardinal Glennon Children's Medical Center

7980 Clayton Rd – Suite 200
St. Louis MO 63117
www.cardinalglennon.com/Pages/missouri-poison-center.aspx

MONTANA

(DENVER, CO)

Rocky Mountain Poison & Drug Center

777 Bannock St – MC 0180
Denver CO 80204-4028
www.rmpdc.org

NEBRASKA

OMAHA

Nebraska Regional Poison Center

8401 W Dodge Rd – Suite 115
Omaha NE 68114
www.nebraskapoison.com

NEVADA

(DENVER, CO)

Rocky Mountain Poison & Drug Center

777 Bannock St – MC 0180
Denver CO 80204-4028
www.rmpdc.org

NEW HAMPSHIRE

(PORTLAND, ME)

Northern New England Poison Center

22 Bramhall St
Portland ME 04102
www.nnepc.org

NEW JERSEY

NEWARK

New Jersey Poison Information and Education System
University of Medicine and Dentistry at New Jersey

140 Bergen St – PO Box 1709
Newark NJ 07107-170
www.njpies.org

NEW MEXICO

ALBUQUERQUE

New Mexico Poison & Drug Information Center

MSC 09 5080
1 University of New Mexico
Albuquerque NM 87131
nmpoisoncenter.unm.edu

NEW YORK

NEW YORK CITY

New York City Poison Control Center
NYC Bureau of Public Health Labs

455 1st Ave – Room 123
Box 81
New York NY 10016
www.nyc.gov/html/doh/html/environmental/poison-control.shtml

SYRACUSE

Upstate New York Poison Center

750 E Adams St
Syracuse NY 13210
www.upstatepoison.org

NORTH CAROLINA

CHARLOTTE

Carolinas Poison Center
Carolinas Medical Center

PO Box 32861
Charlotte NC 28232
www.ncpoisoncenter.org

NORTH DAKOTA

(MINNEAPOLIS, MN)

Hennepin Regional Poison Center
Hennepin County Medical Center

701 Park Ave, Mail Code RL
Minneapolis MN 55415
www.mnpoison.org

OHIO

CINCINNATI

Cincinnati Drug and Poison Information Center
Regional Poison Control System

3333 Burnett Ave
MLC 9004
Cincinnati OH 45229-9004
www.cincinnatichildrens.org/dpic

COLUMBUS

Central Ohio Poison Center
Nationwide Children's Hospital

700 Children's Dr
Columbus OH 43205
www.bepoisonsmart.com

OKLAHOMA

OKLAHOMA CITY

Oklahoma Poison Control Center
Oklahoma University Health Science Center

940 NE 13th St – Room 3N3510
Oklahoma City OK 73104
www.oklahomapoison.org

OREGON

PORTLAND

Oregon Poison Center
Oregon Health & Science University

3181 SW Sam Jackson Park Rd – CB550
Portland OR 97239
www.oregonpoison.org

PENNSYLVANIA

PHILADELPHIA

The Poison Control Center
Children's Hospital of Philadelphia

34th & Civic Center Blvd
Philadelphia PA 19104
www.chop.edu/service/poison-control-center

PITTSBURGH

Pittsburgh Poison Center

200 Lothrop St
Pittsburgh PA 15213
www.chp.edu/CHP/poisoncenter

RHODE ISLAND

(BOSTON, MA)

Regional Center for Poison Control and Prevention

300 Longwood Ave
IC Smith Building
Boston MA 02115
www.maripoisoncenter.com

(Continued)

SOUTH CAROLINA

COLUMBIA

Palmetto Poison Center
South Carolina College of Pharmacy

University of South Carolina
Columbia SC 29208
www.poison.sc.edu

SOUTH DAKOTA

(MINNEAPOLIS, MN)

Hennepin Regional Poison Center
Hennepin County Medical Center

701 Park Ave, Mail Code RL
Minneapolis MN 55415
www.mnpoison.org

SIOUX FALLS

Sanford Poison Center
Sanford Health USD Medical Center

1305 W 18th St – PO Box 5039
Sioux Falls SD 57117
www.sdpoison.org

TENNESSEE

NASHVILLE

Tennessee Poison Center

501 Oxford House
1161 21st Ave S
Nashville TN 37232-4632
www.tnpoisoncenter.org

TEXAS

AMARILLO

Texas Panhandle Poison Center
Texas Tech University

HSC School of Pharmacy
1501 S Coulter Dr – Suite 105
Amarillo TX 79106
www.poisoncontrol.org

DALLAS

North Texas Poison Center
Parkland Health & Hospital System

5201 Harry Hines Blvd
Dallas TX 75235
www.poisoncontrol.org

EL PASO

West Texas Regional Poison Center
University Medical Center of El Paso

4815 Alameda Ave
El Paso TX 79905
www.poisoncontrol.org

GALVESTON

Southeast Texas Poison Center
The University of Texas Medical Branch

3.112 Trauma Bldg
Galveston TX 77555-1175
www.poisoncontrol.org

SAN ANTONIO

South Texas Poison Center
The University of Texas Health Science Center-San Antonio

7979 Wurzbach Rd, Mail Code 7849
San Antonio TX 78229
www.texaspoison.com

TEMPLE

Central Texas Poison Center
Scott & White Memorial Hospital

2401 S 31st St
Temple TX 76508
www.poisoncontrol.org

UTAH

SALT LAKE CITY

Utah Poison Control Center
University of Utah

30 S 2000 E – Suite 4540
Salt Lake City UT 84112
poisoncontrol.utah.edu

VERMONT

(PORTLAND, ME)

Northern New England Poison Center

22 Bramhall St
Portland ME 04101
www.nnepc.org

VIRGINIA

CHARLOTTESVILLE

Blue Ridge Poison Center

1222 Jefferson Park Ave
PO Box 800774
Charlottesville VA 22908-0774
www.healthsystem.virginia.edu/internet/brpc

RICHMOND

Virginia Poison Center
Medical College of Virginia Hospitals
Virginia Commonwealth University Health System

PO Box 980522
Richmond VA 23298-0522
www.poison.vcu.edu

(WASHINGTON, DC)

National Capital Poison Center

3201 New Mexico Ave NW
Suite 310
Washington DC 20016
www.poison.org

WASHINGTON

SEATTLE

Washington Poison Control Center

155 NE 100th St – Suite 100
Seattle WA 98125-8007
www.wapc.org

WEST VIRGINIA

CHARLESTON

West Virginia Poison Center

3110 MacCorkle Ave SE
Charleston WV 25304
www.wvpoisoncenter.org

WISCONSIN

MILWAUKEE

Wisconsin Poison Center

PO Box 1997, Mail Station C660
Milwaukee WI 53201-1997
www.wisconsinpoison.org

WYOMING

(OMAHA, NE)

Nebraska Regional Poison Center

8401 W Dodge Rd – Suite 115
Omaha NE 68114
www.nebraskapoison.com

ANTIPYRETIC PRODUCTS

BRAND	INGREDIENT(S)/STRENGTH(S)	DOSAGE
ACETAMINOPHENS		
Children's Tylenol Meltaways Chewable Tablets*†	Acetaminophen 80mg	**Peds 11 yrs (72-95 lbs):** 6 tabs q4h. **Peds 9-10 yrs (60-71 lbs):** 5 tabs q4h. **Peds 6-8 yrs (48-59 lbs):** 4 tabs q4h. **Peds 4-5 yrs (36-47 lbs):** 3 tabs q4h. **Peds 2-3 yrs (24-35 lbs):** 2 tabs q4h. **Max:** 5 doses/24h.
Children's Tylenol Oral Suspension*	Acetaminophen 160mg/5mL	**Peds 11 yrs (72-95 lbs):** 3 tsp (15mL) q4h. **Peds 9-10 yrs (60-71 lbs):** 2.5 tsp (12.5mL) q4h. **Peds 6-8 yrs (48-59 lbs):** 2 tsp (10mL) q4h. **Peds 4-5 yrs (36-47 lbs):** 1.5 tsp (7.5mL) q4h. **Peds 2-3 yrs (24-35 lbs):** 1 tsp (5mL) q4h. **Max:** 5 doses/24h.
FeverAll Children's Suppositories	Acetaminophen 120mg	**Peds 3-6 yrs:** 1 supp q4-6h. **Max:** 5 doses/24h.
FeverAll Infants' Suppositories	Acetaminophen 80mg	**Peds 12-36 months:** 1 supp q4-6h. **Max:** 5 doses/24h. **Peds 6-11 months:** 1 supp q6h. **Max:** 4 doses/24h.
FeverAll Jr. Strength Suppositories	Acetaminophen 325mg	**Adults & Peds ≥12 yrs:** 2 supp q4-6h. **Max:** 6 doses/24h. **Peds 6-12 yrs:** 1 supp q4-6h. **Max:** 5 doses/24h.
Infants' Tylenol Oral Suspension*	Acetaminophen 160mg/5mL	**Peds 2-3 yrs (24-35 lbs):** 1 tsp (5mL) q4h. **Max:** 5 doses/24h.
Jr. Tylenol Meltaways Chewable Tablets*†	Acetaminophen 160mg	**Peds 11 yrs (72-95 lbs):** 3 tabs q4h. **Peds 9-10 yrs (60-71 lbs):** 2.5 tabs q4h. **Peds 6-8 yrs (48-59 lbs):** 2 tabs q4h. **Max:** 5 doses/24h.
Little Remedies Children's Fever/Pain Reliever Liquid*	Acetaminophen 160mg/5mL	**Peds 11 yrs (72-95 lbs):** 3 tsp (15mL) q4h. **Peds 9-10 yrs (60-71 lbs):** 2.5 tsp (12.5mL) q4h. **Peds 6-8 yrs (48-59 lbs):** 2 tsp (10mL) q4h. **Peds 4-5 yrs (36-47 lbs):** 1.5 tsp (7.5mL) q4h. **Peds 2-3 yrs (24-35 lbs):** 1 tsp (5mL) q4h. **Max:** 5 doses/24h.
Little Remedies Infant Fever/Pain Reliever Liquid	Acetaminophen 160mg/5mL	**Peds 2-3 yrs (24-35 lbs):** 1 tsp (5mL) q4h. **Max:** 5 doses/24h.
PediaCare Children Fever Reducer/ Pain Reliever Acetaminophen Oral Suspension*	Acetaminophen 160mg/5mL	**Peds 11 yrs (72-95 lbs):** 3 tsp (15mL) q4h. **Peds 9-10 yrs (60-71 lbs):** 2.5 tsp (12.5mL) q4h. **Peds 6-8 yrs (48-59 lbs):** 2 tsp (10mL) q4h. **Peds 4-5 yrs (36-47 lbs):** 1.5 tsp (7.5mL) q4h. **Peds 2-3 yrs (24-35 lbs):** 1 tsp (5mL) q4h. **Max:** 5 doses/24h.
PediaCare Infants Fever Reducer/ Pain Reliever Acetaminophen Oral Suspension*	Acetaminophen 160mg/5mL	**Peds 2-3 yrs (24-35 lbs):** 1 tsp (5mL) q4h. **Max:** 5 doses/24h.
PediaCare Smooth Melts Acetaminophen Fever Reducer/Pain Reliever Chewable Tablets	Acetaminophen 160mg	**Peds 11 yrs (72-95 lbs):** 3 tabs q4h. **Peds 9-10 yrs (60-71 lbs):** 2.5 tabs q4h. **Peds 6-8 yrs (48-59 lbs):** 2 tabs q4h. **Peds 4-5 yrs (36-47 lbs):** 1.5 tabs q4h. **Max:** 5 doses/24h.

(Continued)

BRAND	INGREDIENT(S)/STRENGTH(S)	DOSAGE
ACETAMINOPHENS *(Continued)*		
Triaminic Children's Fever Reducer Pain Reliever Syrup*†	Acetaminophen 160mg/5mL	**Peds 11 yrs (72-95 lbs):** 3 tsp (15mL) q4h. **Peds 9-10 yrs (60-71 lbs):** 2.5 tsp (12.5mL) q4h. **Peds 6-8 yrs (48-59 lbs):** 2 tsp (10mL) q4h. **Peds 4-5 yrs (36-47 lbs):** 1.5 tsp (7.5mL) q4h. **Peds 2-3 yrs (24-35 lbs):** 1 tsp (5mL) q4h. **Max:** 5 doses/24h.
Triaminic Infants' Fever Reducer Pain Reliever Syrup*†	Acetaminophen 160mg/5mL	**Peds 2-3 yrs (24-35 lbs):** 1 tsp (5mL) q4h. **Max:** 5 doses/24h.
Tylenol 8 HR Extended Release Caplets†	Acetaminophen 650mg	**Adults & Peds ≥12 yrs:** 2 tabs q8h. **Max:** 6 tabs/24h.
Tylenol Extra Strength Caplets	Acetaminophen 500mg	**Adults & Peds ≥12 yrs:** 2 tabs q6h. **Max:** 6 tabs/24h.
Tylenol Regular Strength Tablets	Acetaminophen 325mg	**Adults & Peds ≥12 yrs:** 2 tabs q4-6h. **Max:** 10 tabs/24h. **Peds 6-11 yrs:** 1 tab q4-6h. **Max:** 5 tabs/24h.
NONSTEROIDAL ANTI-INFLAMMATORY DRUGS		
Advil Caplets	Ibuprofen 200mg	**Adults & Peds ≥12 yrs:** 1-2 tabs q4-6h. **Max:** 6 tabs/24h.
Advil Film-Coated Caplets	Ibuprofen 200mg	**Adults & Peds ≥12 yrs:** 1-2 tabs q4-6h. **Max:** 6 tabs/24h.
Advil Film-Coated Tablets	Ibuprofen 200mg	**Adults & Peds ≥12 yrs:** 1-2 tabs q4-6h. **Max:** 6 tabs/24h.
Advil Gel Caplets	Ibuprofen 200mg	**Adults & Peds ≥12 yrs:** 1-2 tabs q4-6h. **Max:** 6 tabs/24h.
Advil Liqui-Gels	Ibuprofen 200mg	**Adults & Peds ≥12 yrs:** 1-2 caps q4-6h. **Max:** 6 caps/24h.
Advil Tablets	Ibuprofen 200mg	**Adults & Peds ≥12 yrs:** 1-2 tabs q4-6h. **Max:** 6 tabs/24h.
Aleve Caplets	Naproxen sodium 220mg	**Adults & Peds ≥12 yrs:** 1 tab q8-12h. May take 1 additional tab within 1h of first dose. **Max:** 2 tabs/8-12h or 3 tabs/24h.
Aleve Gelcaps	Naproxen sodium 220mg	**Adults & Peds ≥12 yrs:** 1 tab q8-12h. May take 1 additional tab within 1h of first dose. **Max:** 2 tabs/8-12h or 3 tabs/24h.
Aleve Liquid Gels	Naproxen sodium 220mg	**Adults & Peds ≥12 yrs:** 1 cap q8-12h. May take 1 additional cap within 1h of first dose. **Max:** 2 caps/8-12h or 3 caps/24h.
Aleve Tablets	Naproxen sodium 220mg	**Adults & Peds ≥12 yrs:** 1 tab q8-12h. May take 1 additional tab within 1h of first dose. **Max:** 2 tabs/8-12h or 3 tabs/24h.
Children's Advil Suspension*	Ibuprofen 100mg/5mL	**Peds 11 yrs (72-95 lbs):** 3 tsp (15mL) q6-8h. **Peds 9-10 yrs (60-71 lbs):** 2.5 tsp (12.5mL) q6-8h. **Peds 6-8 yrs (48-59 lbs):** 2 tsp (10mL) q6-8h. **Peds 4-5 yrs (36-47 lbs):** 1.5 tsp (7.5mL) q6-8h. **Peds 2-3 yrs (24-35 lbs):** 1 tsp (5mL) q6-8h. **Max:** 4 doses/24h.

BRAND	INGREDIENT(S)/STRENGTH(S)	DOSAGE
NONSTEROIDAL ANTI-INFLAMMATORY DRUGS *(Continued)*		
Children's Motrin Suspension	Ibuprofen 100mg/5mL	**Peds 11 yrs (72-95 lbs):** 3 tsp (15mL) q6-8h. **Peds 9-10 yrs (60-71 lbs):** 2.5 tsp (12.5mL) q6-8h. **Peds 6-8 yrs (48-59 lbs):** 2 tsp (10mL) q6-8h. **Peds 4-5 yrs (36-47 lbs):** 1.5 tsp (7.5mL) q6-8h. **Peds 2-3 yrs (24-35 lbs):** 1 tsp (5mL) q6-8h. **Max:** 4 doses/24h.
Infants' Advil Concentrated Drops	Ibuprofen 50mg/1.25mL	**Peds 12-23 months (18-23 lbs):** 1.875mL q6-8h. **Peds 6-11 months (12-17 lbs):** 1.25mL q6-8h. **Max:** 4 doses/24h.
Infants' Motrin Concentrated Drops	Ibuprofen 50mg/1.25mL	**Peds 12-23 months (18-23 lbs):** 1.875mL q6-8h. **Peds 6-11 months (12-17 lbs):** 1.25mL q6-8h. **Max:** 4 doses/24h.
Junior Strength Advil Chewable Tablets	Ibuprofen 100mg	**Peds 11 yrs (72-95 lbs):** 3 tabs q6-8h. **Peds 9-10 yrs (60-71 lbs):** 2.5 tabs q6-8h. **Peds 6-8 yrs (48-59 lbs):** 2 tabs q6-8h. **Max:** 4 doses/24h.
Junior Strength Advil Tablets	Ibuprofen 100mg	**Peds 11 yrs (72-95 lbs):** 3 tabs q6-8h. **Peds 6-10 yrs (48-71 lbs):** 2 tabs q6-8h. **Max:** 4 doses/24h.
Motrin IB Caplets	Ibuprofen 200mg	**Adults & Peds ≥12 yrs:** 1-2 tabs q4-6h. **Max:** 6 tabs/24h.
PediaCare Children Pain Reliever/Fever Reducer IB Ibuprofen Oral Suspension	Ibuprofen 100mg/5mL	**Peds 11 yrs (72-95 lbs):** 3 tsp (15mL) q6-8h. **Peds 9-10 yrs (60-71 lbs):** 2.5 tsp (12.5mL) q6-8h. **Peds 6-8 yrs (48-59 lbs):** 2 tsp (10mL) q6-8h. **Peds 4-5 yrs (36-47 lbs):** 1.5 tsp (7.5mL) q6-8h. **Peds 2-3 yrs (24-35 lbs):** 1 tsp (5mL) q6-8h. **Max:** 4 doses/24h.
PediaCare Infants Pain Reliever/Fever Reducer IB Ibuprofen Concentrated Oral Suspension	Ibuprofen 50mg/1.25mL	**Peds 12-23 months (18-23 lbs):** 1.875mL q6-8h. **Peds 6-11 months (12-17 lbs):** 1.25mL q6-8h. **Max:** 4 doses/24h.
SALICYLATES		
PLEASE REFER TO ASPIRIN PRODUCTS TABLE		

*Multiple flavors available.
†Product currently on recall or temporarily unavailable from manufacturer, but generic forms may be available.

Insomnia Products

BRAND	INGREDIENT(S)/STRENGTH(S)	DOSAGE
DIPHENHYDRAMINES		
Compoz Maximum Strength Soft Gel Liquid Capsules	Diphenhydramine HCl 50mg	**Adults & Peds ≥12 yrs:** 1 cap hs prn.
Nytol Extra Strength Tablets	Diphenhydramine HCl 25mg	**Adults & Peds ≥12 yrs:** 1 tab 20-30 minutes before hs.
Nytol QuickCaps	Diphenhydramine HCl 25mg	**Adults & Peds ≥12 yrs:** 2 tabs hs prn.
Simply Sleep Caplets	Diphenhydramine HCl 25mg	**Adults & Peds ≥12 yrs:** 2 tabs hs prn.
Sleepinal Capsules	Diphenhydramine HCl 50mg	**Adults & Peds ≥12 yrs:** 1 cap hs prn.
Sominex Maximum Strength Caplets	Diphenhydramine HCl 50mg	**Adults & Peds ≥12 yrs:** 1 tab hs prn.
Sominex Original Formula Tablets	Diphenhydramine HCl 25mg	**Adults & Peds ≥12 yrs:** 2 tabs hs prn.
Unisom Liquid	Diphenhydramine HCl 50mg/30mL (2 tbsp)	**Adults & Peds ≥12 yrs:** 30mL (2 tbsp) hs prn.
Unisom SleepGels	Diphenhydramine HCl 50mg	**Adults & Peds ≥12 yrs:** 1 cap hs prn.
Unisom QuickMelts	Diphenhydramine HCl 25mg	**Adults & Peds ≥12 yrs:** 2 tabs hs prn.
ZzzQuil LiquiCaps	Diphenhydramine HCl 25mg	**Adults & Peds ≥12 yrs:** 2 caps hs prn. **Max:** 1 dose/24 hrs.
ZzzQuil Liquid	Diphenhydramine HCl 50mg/30mL (2 tbsp)	**Adults & Peds ≥12 yrs:** 30mL (2 tbsp) hs prn. **Max:** 1 dose/24 hrs.
DIPHENHYDRAMINE COMBINATIONS		
Advil PM Caplets	Ibuprofen/Diphenhydramine citrate 200mg-38mg	**Adults & Peds ≥12 yrs:** 2 tabs hs. **Max:** 2 tabs/24 hrs.
Advil PM Liqui-Gels	Ibuprofen/Diphenhydramine HCl 200mg-25mg	**Adults & Peds ≥12 yrs:** 2 caps hs. **Max:** 2 caps/24 hrs.
Aleve PM Caplets	Naproxen sodium/Diphenhydramine HCl 220mg-25mg	**Adults & Peds ≥12 yrs:** 2 tabs hs. **Max:** 2 tabs/24 hrs.
Bayer PM Caplets	Aspirin/Diphenhydramine citrate 500mg-38mg	**Adults & Peds ≥12 yrs:** 2 tabs hs prn.
Excedrin PM Headache Caplets	Acetaminophen/Aspirin/ Diphenhydramine citrate 250mg-250mg-38mg	**Adults & Peds ≥12 yrs:** 2 tabs hs. **Max:** 2 tabs/24 hrs.
Goody's PM Powder	Acetaminophen/Diphenhydramine citrate 500mg-38mg per powder	**Adults & Peds ≥12 yrs:** 2 powders hs prn. **Max:** 4 powders/24 hrs.
Legatrin PM Caplets	Acetaminophen/Diphenhydramine HCl 500mg-50mg	**Adults & Peds ≥12 yrs:** 1 tab hs prn.
Midol PM Caplets	Acetaminophen/Diphenhydramine citrate 500mg-38mg	**Adults & Peds ≥12 yrs:** 2 tabs hs prn.
Motrin PM Caplets	Ibuprofen/Diphenhydramine citrate 200mg-38mg	**Adults & Peds ≥12 yrs:** 2 tabs hs. **Max:** 2 tabs/24 hrs.
Tylenol PM Caplets	Acetaminophen/Diphenhydramine HCl 500mg-25mg	**Adults & Peds ≥12 yrs:** 2 tabs hs. **Max:** 2 tabs/24 hrs.
Unisom PM Pain Caplets	Acetaminophen/Diphenhydramine HCl 325mg-50mg	**Adults & Peds ≥12 yrs:** 1 tab hs. **Max:** 1 tab/24 hrs.
DOXYLAMINES		
Unisom SleepTabs	Doxylamine succinate 25mg	**Adults & Peds ≥12 yrs:** 1 tab 30 minutes before hs.

Smoking Cessation Products

BRAND	INGREDIENT(S)/STRENGTH(S)	DOSAGE
Habitrol Nicotine Transdermal System Patch Step 1	Nicotine 21mg	**Adults:** If smoking >10 cigarettes/day: **Weeks 1 to 4:** Apply one 21mg patch/day. **Weeks 5 to 6:** Apply one 14mg patch/day. **Weeks 7 to 8:** Apply one 7mg patch/day. If smoking <10 cigarettes/day: **Weeks 1 to 6:** Apply one 14mg patch/day. **Weeks 7 to 8:** Apply one 7mg patch/day.
Habitrol Nicotine Transdermal System Patch Step 2	Nicotine 14mg	Refer to Habitrol Nicotine Transdermal System Patch Step 1 dosing.
Habitrol Nicotine Transdermal System Patch Step 3	Nicotine 7mg	Refer to Habitrol Nicotine Transdermal System Patch Step 1 dosing.
NicoDerm CQ Step 1 Clear Patch	Nicotine 21mg	**Adults:** If smoking >10 cigarettes/day: **Weeks 1 to 6:** Apply one 21mg patch/day. **Weeks 7 to 8:** Apply one 14mg patch/day. **Weeks 9 to 10:** Apply one 7mg patch/day. If smoking ≤10 cigarettes/day: **Weeks 1 to 6:** Apply one 14mg patch/day. **Weeks 7 to 8:** Apply one 7mg patch/day.
NicoDerm CQ Step 2 Clear Patch	Nicotine 14mg	Refer to NicoDerm CQ Step 1 Clear Patch dosing.
NicoDerm CQ Step 3 Clear Patch	Nicotine 7mg	Refer to NicoDerm CQ Step 1 Clear Patch dosing.
Nicorette 2mg Gum	Nicotine polacrilex 2mg	**Adults:** If smoking first cigarette >30 minutes after waking up, use 2mg gum. **Weeks 1 to 6:** 1 piece q1-2h. **Weeks 7 to 9:** 1 piece q2-4h. **Weeks 10 to 12:** 1 piece q4-8h. **Max:** 24 pieces/day.
Nicorette 4mg Gum	Nicotine polacrilex 4mg	**Adults:** If smoking first cigarette ≤30 minutes after waking up, use 4mg gum. **Weeks 1 to 6:** 1 piece q1-2h. **Weeks 7 to 9:** 1 piece q2-4h. **Weeks 10 to 12:** 1 piece q4-8h. **Max:** 24 pieces/day.
Nicorette 2mg Lozenge*	Nicotine polacrilex 2mg	**Adults:** If smoking first cigarette >30 minutes after waking up, use 2mg lozenge. **Weeks 1 to 6:** 1 lozenge q1-2h. **Weeks 7 to 9:** 1 lozenge q2-4h. **Weeks 10 to 12:** 1 lozenge q4-8h. **Max:** 5 lozenges/6 hours or 20 lozenges/day.
Nicorette 4mg Lozenge*	Nicotine polacrilex 4mg	**Adults:** If smoking first cigarette ≤30 minutes after waking up, use 4mg lozenge. **Weeks 1 to 6:** 1 lozenge q1-2h. **Weeks 7 to 9:** 1 lozenge q2-4h. **Weeks 10 to 12:** 1 lozenge q4-8h. **Max:** 5 lozenges/6 hours or 20 lozenges/day.
Nicorette 2mg mini Lozenge*	Nicotine polacrilex 2mg	**Adults:** If smoking first cigarette >30 minutes after waking up, use 2mg lozenge. **Weeks 1 to 6:** 1 lozenge q1-2h. **Weeks 7 to 9:** 1 lozenge q2-4h. **Weeks 10 to 12:** 1 lozenge q4-8h. **Max:** 5 lozenges/6 hours or 20 lozenges/day.
Nicorette 4mg mini Lozenge*	Nicotine polacrilex 4mg	**Adults:** If smoking first cigarette ≤30 minutes after waking up, use 4mg lozenge. **Weeks 1 to 6:** 1 lozenge q1-2h. **Weeks 7 to 9:** 1 lozenge q2-4h. **Weeks 10 to 12:** 1 lozenge q4-8h. **Max:** 5 lozenges/6 hours or 20 lozenges/day.

(Continued)

BRAND	INGREDIENT(S)/STRENGTH(S)	DOSAGE
Zonnic 2mg Gum	Nicotine polacrilex 2mg	**Adults:** If smoking first cigarette >30 minutes after waking up, use 2mg gum. **Weeks 1 to 6:** 1 piece q1-2h. **Weeks 7 to 9:** 1 piece q2-4h. **Weeks 10 to 12:** 1 piece q4-8h. **Max:** 24 pieces/day.
Zonnic 4mg Gum	Nicotine polacrilex 4mg	**Adults:** If smoking first cigarette ≤30 minutes after waking up, use 4mg gum. **Weeks 1 to 6:** 1 piece q1-2h. **Weeks 7 to 9:** 1 piece q2-4h. **Weeks 10 to 12:** 1 piece q4-8h. **Max:** 24 pieces/day.

*Product currently on recall or temporarily unavailable from manufacturer.

ANTACID AND HEARTBURN PRODUCTS

BRAND	INGREDIENT(S)/STRENGTH(S)	DOSAGE
ANTACIDS		
Alka-Seltzer Extra Strength Effervescent Tablets	Aspirin/Citric acid/Sodium bicarbonate 500mg-1000mg-1985mg	**Adults ≥60 yrs:** 2 tabs dissolved in 4 oz water q6h. **Max:** 3 tabs/24h. **Adults & Peds ≥12 yrs:** 2 tabs dissolved in 4 oz water q6h. **Max:** 7 tabs/24h.
Alka-Seltzer Gold Effervescent Tablets	Citric acid/Potassium bicarbonate/ Sodium bicarbonate 1000mg-344mg-1050mg	**Adults ≥60 yrs:** 2 tabs dissolved in 4 oz water q4h prn. **Max:** 6 tabs/24h. **Adults & Peds ≥12 yrs:** 2 tabs dissolved in 4 oz water q4h prn. **Max:** 8 tabs/24h. **Peds <12 yrs:** 1 tab dissolved in 4 oz water q4h prn. **Max:** 4 tabs/24h.
Alka-Seltzer Heartburn Relief Effervescent Tablets	Citric acid/Sodium bicarbonate 1000mg-1940mg	**Adults ≥60 yrs:** 2 tabs dissolved in 4 oz water q4h prn. **Max:** 4 tabs/24h. **Adults & Peds ≥12 yrs:** 2 tabs dissolved in 4 oz water q4h prn. **Max:** 8 tabs/24h.
Alka-Seltzer Heartburn ReliefChews Chewable Tablets	Calcium carbonate 750mg	**Adults & Peds ≥12 yrs:** 1-2 tabs q2-4h prn. **Max:** 5 tabs/24h.
Alka-Seltzer Lemon Lime Effervescent Tablets	Aspirin/Citric acid/Sodium bicarbonate 325mg-1000mg-1700mg	**Adults ≥60 yrs:** 2 tabs dissolved in 4 oz water q4h. **Max:** 4 tabs/24h. **Adults & Peds ≥12 yrs:** 2 tabs dissolved in 4 oz water q4h. **Max:** 8 tabs/24h.
Alka-Seltzer Original Effervescent Tablets	Aspirin/Citric acid/Sodium bicarbonate 325mg-1000mg-1916mg	**Adults ≥60 yrs:** 2 tabs dissolved in 4 oz water q4h. **Max:** 4 tabs/24h. **Adults & Peds ≥12 yrs:** 2 tabs dissolved in 4 oz water q4h. **Max:** 8 tabs/24h.
Gaviscon Extra Strength Chewable Tablets	Aluminum hydroxide/Magnesium carbonate 160mg-105mg	**Adults:** 2-4 tabs qid. **Max:** 16 tabs/24h.
Gaviscon Extra Strength Liquid	Aluminum hydroxide/Magnesium carbonate 254mg-237.5mg/5mL	**Adults:** 2-4 tsp (10-20mL) qid. **Max:** 16 tsp (80mL)/24h.
Gaviscon Regular Strength Chewable Tablets	Aluminum hydroxide/Magnesium trisilicate 80mg-14.2mg	**Adults:** 2-4 tabs qid. **Max:** 16 tabs/24h.
Gaviscon Regular Strength Liquid	Aluminum hydroxide/Magnesium carbonate 95mg-358mg/15mL	**Adults:** 1-2 tbl (15-30mL) qid. **Max:** 8 tbl (120mL)/24h.
Maalox Children's Relief Chewable Tablets*	Calcium carbonate 400mg	**Peds 6-11 yrs (48-95 lbs):** 2 tabs prn. **Max:** 6 tabs/24h. **Peds 2-5 yrs (24-47 lbs):** 1 tab prn. **Max:** 3 tabs/24h.
Maalox Regular Strength Chewable Tablets*	Calcium carbonate 600mg	**Adults:** 1-2 tabs prn. **Max:** 12 tabs/24h.
Mylanta Supreme Liquid*	Calcium carbonate/Magnesium hydroxide 400mg-135mg/5mL	**Adults:** 2-4 tsp (10-20mL) between meals and at hs. **Max:** 18 tsp (90mL)/24h.
Mylanta Ultimate Strength Liquid*	Aluminum hydroxide/Magnesium hydroxide 500mg-500mg/5mL	**Adults & Peds ≥12 yrs:** 2-4 tsp (10-20mL) between meals and at hs. **Max:** 9 tsp (45mL)/24h.
Pepto-Bismol Children's Pepto Chewable Tablets	Calcium carbonate 400mg	**Peds 6-11 yrs (48-95 lbs):** 2 tabs prn. **Max:** 6 tabs/24h. **Peds 2-5 yrs (24-47 lbs):** 1 tab prn. **Max:** 3 tabs/24h.
Relief OTC	Calcium carbonate/Potassium bicarbonate/Sodium bicarbonate 273mg-453mg-1055mg/2 oz	**Adults ≥60 yrs:** Up to 4 oz q4h prn. **Max:** 12 oz/24h. **Adults & Peds ≥12 yrs:** Up to 4 oz q4h prn. **Max:** 16 oz/24h.
Rolaids Extra Strength Chewable Tablets	Calcium carbonate/Magnesium hydroxide 675mg-135mg	**Adults:** 2-4 tabs prn. **Max:** 10 tabs/24h.
Rolaids Regular Strength Chewable Tablets	Calcium carbonate/Magnesium hydroxide 550mg-110mg	**Adults:** 2-4 tabs prn. **Max:** 12 tabs/24h.

(Continued)

BRAND	INGREDIENT(S)/STRENGTH(S)	DOSAGE
ANTACIDS *(Continued)*		
Rolaids Regular Strength Liquid	Calcium carbonate/Magnesium hydroxide 550mg-110mg/5mL	**Adults:** 2-4 tsp (10-20mL) prn. **Max:** 12 tsp (60mL)/24h.
Rolaids Ultra Strength Chewable Tablets	Calcium carbonate/Magnesium hydroxide 1000mg-200mg	**Adults:** 2-3 tabs prn. **Max:** 7 tabs/24h.
Rolaids Ultra Strength Liquid	Calcium carbonate/Magnesium hydroxide 1000mg-200mg/5mL	**Adults:** 2-3 tsp (10-15mL) prn. **Max:** 7 tsp (35mL)/24h.
Rolaids Ultra Strength Softchews	Calcium carbonate/Magnesium hydroxide 1330mg-235mg	**Adults:** 2-3 chews prn. **Max:** 5 chews/24h.
Tums Chewy Delights Chewable Tablets	Calcium carbonate 1177mg	**Adults & Peds ≥12 yrs:** 2-3 tabs prn. **Max**[†]: 6 tabs/24h.
Tums Extra Strength 750 Chewable Tablets	Calcium carbonate 750mg	**Adults & Peds ≥12 yrs:** 2-4 tabs prn. **Max**[†]: 10 tabs/24h.
Tums Extra Strength 750 Sugar Free Chewable Tablets	Calcium carbonate 750mg	**Adults & Peds ≥12 yrs:** 2-4 tabs prn. **Max**[†]: 9 tabs/24h.
Tums Freshers Chewable Tablets	Calcium carbonate 500mg	**Adults & Peds ≥12 yrs:** 2-4 tabs prn. **Max**[†]: 15 tabs/24h.
Tums Kids Chewable Tablets	Calcium carbonate 750mg	**Peds >4 yrs (>48 lbs):** 1 tab prn. **Max:** 4 tabs/24h. **Peds 2-4 yrs (24-47 lbs):** ½ tab prn. **Max:** 2 tabs/24h.
Tums Regular Strength Chewable Tablets	Calcium carbonate 500mg	**Adults & Peds ≥12 yrs:** 2-4 tabs prn. **Max**[†]: 15 tabs/24h.
Tums Smoothies Chewable Tablets	Calcium carbonate 750mg	**Adults & Peds ≥12 yrs:** 2-4 tabs prn. **Max**[†]: 10 tabs/24h.
Tums Ultra Strength 1000 Chewable Tablets	Calcium carbonate 1000mg	**Adults & Peds ≥12 yrs:** 2-4 tabs prn. **Max**[†]: 7 tabs/24h.
ANTACIDS/ANTIFLATULENTS		
Alka-Seltzer Heartburn+Gas ReliefChews Chewable Tablets	Calcium carbonate/Simethicone 750mg-80mg	**Adults & Peds ≥12 yrs:** 1-2 tabs q2-4h prn. **Max:** 5 tabs/24h.
Gelusil Chewable Tablets	Aluminum hydroxide/Magnesium hydroxide/Simethicone 200mg-200mg-25mg	**Adults:** 2-4 tabs q1h prn. **Max:** 12 tabs/24h.
Gelusil Liquid	Aluminum hydroxide/Magnesium hydroxide/Simethicone 400mg-400mg-40mg/5mL	**Adults & Peds ≥12 yrs:** 2-4 tsp (10-20mL) between meals and at hs. **Max:** 12 tsp (60mL)/24h.
Maalox Advanced Maximum Strength Chewable Tablets*	Calcium carbonate/Simethicone 1000mg-60mg	**Adults & Peds ≥12 yrs:** 1-2 tabs prn. **Max:** 8 tabs/24h.
Maalox Advanced Maximum Strength Liquid*	Aluminum hydroxide/Magnesium hydroxide/Simethicone 400mg-400mg-40mg/5mL	**Adults & Peds ≥12 yrs:** 2-4 tsp (10-20mL) bid. **Max:** 8 tsp (40mL)/24h.
Maalox Advanced Regular Strength Liquid*	Aluminum hydroxide/Magnesium hydroxide/Simethicone 200mg-200mg-20mg/5mL	**Adults & Peds ≥12 yrs:** 2-4 tsp (10-20mL) qid. **Max:** 16 tsp (80mL)/24h.
Maalox Junior Relief Chewable Tablets*	Calcium carbonate/Simethicone 400mg-24mg	**Peds 6-11 yrs:** 2 tabs prn. **Max:** 6 tabs/24h.
Mylanta Maximum Strength Liquid*	Aluminum hydroxide/Magnesium hydroxide/Simethicone 400mg-400mg-40mg/5mL	**Adults & Peds ≥12 yrs:** 2-4 tsp (10-20mL) between meals and at hs. **Max:** 12 tsp (60mL)/24h.
Mylanta Regular Strength Liquid*	Aluminum hydroxide/Magnesium hydroxide/Simethicone 200mg-200mg-20mg/5mL	**Adults & Peds ≥12 yrs:** 2-4 tsp (10-20mL) between meals and at hs. **Max:** 24 tsp (120mL)/24h.

BRAND	INGREDIENT(S)/STRENGTH(S)	DOSAGE
BISMUTH SUBSALICYLATES		
Maalox Total Relief Maximum Strength Liquid*	Bismuth subsalicylate 525mg/15mL	**Adults & Peds ≥12 yrs:** 2 tbl (30mL) q1h prn. **Max:** 8 tbl (120mL)/24h.
Pepto-Bismol Caplets	Bismuth subsalicylate 262mg	**Adults & Peds ≥12 yrs:** 2 tabs q½-1h prn. **Max:** 8 doses (16 tabs)/24h.
Pepto-Bismol Chewable Tablets	Bismuth subsalicylate 262mg	**Adults & Peds ≥12 yrs:** 2 tabs q½-1h prn. **Max:** 8 doses (16 tabs)/24h.
Pepto-Bismol InstaCool Chewable Tablets	Bismuth subsalicylate 262mg	**Adults & Peds ≥12 yrs:** 2 tabs q½-1h prn. **Max:** 8 doses (16 tabs)/24h.
Pepto-Bismol Liquid	Bismuth subsalicylate 525mg/30mL	**Adults & Peds ≥12 yrs:** 2 tbl (30mL) q½-1h prn. **Max:** 8 doses (16 tbl or 240mL)/24h.
Pepto-Bismol Max Strength Liquid	Bismuth subsalicylate 1050mg/30mL	**Adults & Peds ≥12 yrs:** 2 tbl (30mL) q1h prn. **Max:** 4 doses (8 tbl or 120mL)/24h.
H_2-RECEPTOR ANTAGONISTS		
Pepcid AC Maximum Strength Tablets	Famotidine 20mg	**Adults & Peds ≥12 yrs:** 1 tab prn. **Max:** 2 tabs/24h.
Pepcid AC Original Strength Tablets	Famotidine 10mg	**Adults & Peds ≥12 yrs:** 1 tab prn. **Max:** 2 tabs/24h.
Tagamet HB 200 Tablets	Cimetidine 200mg	**Adults & Peds ≥12 yrs:** 1 tab prn. **Max:** 2 tabs/24h.
Zantac 75 Tablets	Ranitidine 75mg	**Adults & Peds ≥12 yrs:** 1 tab prn. **Max:** 2 tabs/24h.
Zantac 150 Tablets	Ranitidine 150mg	**Adults & Peds ≥12 yrs:** 1 tab prn. **Max:** 2 tabs/24h.
H_2-RECEPTOR ANTAGONISTS/ANTACIDS		
Pepcid Complete Chewable Tablets	Famotidine/Calcium carbonate/ Magnesium hydroxide 10mg-800mg-165mg	**Adults & Peds ≥12 yrs:** 1 tab prn. **Max:** 2 tabs/24h.
PROTON PUMP INHIBITORS		
Nexium 24 HR Capsules	Esomeprazole 20mg	**Adults:** 1 cap qd x 14 days. May repeat 14-day course q4 months.
Prevacid 24 HR Capsules	Lansoprazole 15mg	**Adults:** 1 cap qd x 14 days. May repeat 14-day course q4 months.
Prilosec OTC Tablets	Omeprazole 20mg	**Adults:** 1 tab qd x 14 days. May repeat 14-day course q4 months.
Zegerid OTC Capsules	Omeprazole/Sodium bicarbonate 20mg-1100mg	**Adults:** 1 cap qd x 14 days. May repeat 14-day course q4 months.

*Product currently on recall or temporarily unavailable from manufacturer.
†Please refer to full FDA-approved labeling for information on max dosage during pregnancy.

Antidiarrheal Products

BRAND	INGREDIENT(S)/STRENGTH(S)	DOSAGE*
ABSORBENTS		
Equalactin Chewable Tablets	Calcium Polycarbophil 625mg	**Adults & Peds ≥12 yrs:** 2 tabs qid. **Max:** 8 tabs/24h.† **Peds 6-<12 yrs:** 1 tab qid. **Max:** 4 tabs/24h.† **Peds 3-<6 yrs:** 1 tab qd-bid. **Max:** 2 tabs/24h.†
FiberCon Caplets	Calcium Polycarbophil 625mg	**Adults & Peds ≥12 yrs:** 2 tabs qd. **Max:** Up to qid.‡
Konsyl Fiber Caplets	Calcium Polycarbophil 625mg	**Adults & Peds ≥12 yrs:** 2 tabs qd-qid. **Max:** 8 tabs/24h.‡ **Peds 6-<12 yrs:** 2 tabs qd.‡
ANTIPERISTALTICS		
Imodium A-D Caplets	Loperamide HCl 2mg	**Adults & Peds ≥12 yrs:** 2 tabs after first loose stool; 1 tab after each subsequent loose stool. **Max:** 4 tabs/24h.† **Peds 9-11 yrs (60-95 lbs):** 1 tab after first loose stool; ½ tab after each subsequent loose stool. **Max:** 3 tabs/24h.† **Peds 6-8 yrs (48-59 lbs):** 1 tab after first loose stool; ½ tab after each subsequent loose stool. **Max:** 2 tabs/24h.†
Imodium A-D EZ Chews	Loperamide HCl 2mg	**Adults & Peds ≥12 yrs:** 2 tabs after first loose stool; 1 tab after each subsequent loose stool. **Max:** 4 tabs/24h.† **Peds 9-11 yrs (60-95 lbs):** 1 tab after first loose stool; ½ tab after each subsequent loose stool. **Max:** 3 tabs/24h.† **Peds 6-8 yrs (48-59 lbs):** 1 tab after first loose stool; ½ tab after each subsequent loose stool. **Max:** 2 tabs/24h.†
Imodium A-D Liquid	Loperamide HCl 1mg/7.5mL	**Adults & Peds ≥12 yrs:** 6 tsp (30mL) after first loose stool; 3 tsp (15mL) after each subsequent loose stool. **Max:** 12 tsp (60mL)/24h.† **Peds 9-11 yrs (60-95 lbs):** 3 tsp (15mL) after first loose stool; 1½ tsp (7.5mL) after each subsequent loose stool. **Max:** 9 tsp (45mL)/24h.† **Peds 6-8 yrs (48-59 lbs):** 3 tsp (15mL) after first loose stool; 1½ tsp (7.5mL) after each subsequent loose stool. **Max:** 6 tsp (30mL)/24h.†
Imodium A-D Liquid for Use in Children	Loperamide HCl 1mg/7.5mL	**Adults & Peds ≥12 yrs:** 6 tsp (30mL) after first loose stool; 3 tsp (15mL) after each subsequent loose stool. **Max:** 12 tsp (60mL)/24h.† **Peds 9-11 yrs (60-95 lbs):** 3 tsp (15mL) after first loose stool; 1½ tsp (7.5mL) after each subsequent loose stool. **Max:** 9 tsp (45mL)/24h.† **Peds 6-8 yrs (48-59 lbs):** 3 tsp (15mL) after first loose stool; 1½ tsp (7.5mL) after each subsequent loose stool. **Max:** 6 tsp (30mL)/24h.†
Vaprino A-D Caplets	Loperamide HCl 2mg	**Adults & Peds ≥12 yrs:** 2 tabs after first loose stool; 1 tab after each subsequent loose stool. **Max:** 4 tabs/24h.† **Peds 9-11 yrs (60-95 lbs):** 1 tab after first loose stool; ½ tab after each subsequent loose stool. **Max:** 3 tabs/24h.† **Peds 6-8 yrs (48-59 lbs):** 1 tab after first loose stool; ½ tab after each subsequent loose stool. **Max:** 2 tabs/24h.†
ANTIPERISTALTICS/ANTIFLATULENTS		
Imodium Multi-Symptom Relief Caplets	Loperamide HCl/Simethicone 2mg-125mg	**Adults & Peds ≥12 yrs:** 2 tabs after first loose stool; 1 tab after each subsequent loose stool. **Max:** 4 tabs/24h.† **Peds 9-11 yrs (60-95 lbs):** 1 tab after first loose stool; ½ tab after each subsequent loose stool. **Max:** 3 tabs/24h.† **Peds 6-8 yrs (48-59 lbs):** 1 tab after first loose stool; ½ tab after each subsequent loose stool. **Max:** 2 tabs/24h.†

(Continued)

BRAND	INGREDIENT(S)/STRENGTH(S)	DOSAGE*
ANTIPERISTALTICS/ANTIFLATULENTS *(Continued)*		
Imodium Multi-Symptom Relief Chewable Tablets	Loperamide HCl/Simethicone 2mg-125mg	**Adults & Peds ≥12 yrs:** 2 tabs after first loose stool; 1 tab after each subsequent loose stool. **Max:** 4 tabs/24h.† **Peds 9-11 yrs (60-95 lbs):** 1 tab after first loose stool; ½ tab after each subsequent loose stool. **Max:** 3 tabs/24h.† **Peds 6-8 yrs (48-59 lbs):** 1 tab after first loose stool; ½ tab after each subsequent loose stool. **Max:** 2 tabs/24h.†
BISMUTH SUBSALICYLATES		
Kaopectate Extra Strength Liquid (Peppermint Flavor)	Bismuth Subsalicylate 525mg/15mL	**Adults & Peds ≥12 yrs:** 2 tbl (30mL) q1h prn. **Max:** 4 doses (8 tbl)/24h.†
Kaopectate Liquid (Peppermint Flavor)	Bismuth Subsalicylate 262mg/15mL	**Adults & Peds ≥12 yrs:** 2 tbl (30mL) q1h prn. **Max:** 4 doses (8 tbl)/24h.†
Kaopectate Liquid (Vanilla Flavor; Cherry Flavor)	Bismuth Subsalicylate 262mg/15mL	**Adults & Peds ≥12 yrs:** 2 tbl (30mL) q½-1h prn. **Max:** 8 doses (16 tbl)/24h.†
Pepto Bismol Caplets	Bismuth Subsalicylate 262mg	**Adults & Peds ≥12 yrs:** 2 tabs q½-1h prn. **Max:** 8 doses (16 tabs)/24h.†
Pepto Bismol Chewable Tablets	Bismuth Subsalicylate 262mg	**Adults & Peds ≥12 yrs:** 2 tabs q½-1h prn. **Max:** 8 doses (16 tabs)/24h.†
Pepto Bismol InstaCool Chewable Tablets	Bismuth Subsalicylate 262mg	**Adults & Peds ≥12 yrs:** 2 tabs q½-1h prn. **Max:** 8 doses (16 tabs)/24h.†
Pepto Bismol Liquid	Bismuth Subsalicylate 525mg/30mL	**Adults & Peds ≥12 yrs:** 2 tbl (30mL) q½-1h prn. **Max:** 8 doses (16 tbl)/24h.†
Pepto Bismol Max Strength Liquid	Bismuth Subsalicylate 1050mg/30mL	**Adults & Peds ≥12 yrs:** 2 tbl (30mL) q1h prn. **Max:** 4 doses (8 tbl)/24h.†

*Some medications must be taken with water. Refer to individual product labeling for additional dosing information.

†Do not use for more than 2 days.

‡Do not use for more than 7 days unless directed by a healthcare provider.

ANTIFLATULENT PRODUCTS

BRAND	INGREDIENT(S)/STRENGTH(S)	DOSAGE
ALPHA-GALACTOSIDASES		
Beano Meltaways Tablets	Alpha-galactosidase 300 GALU	**Adults:** Take 1 tab before meals.
Beano Tablets	Alpha-galactosidase enzyme 300 GALU (per 2 tabs)	**Adults:** Take 2-3 tabs before meals.
Beano + Dairy Defense	Alpha-galactosidase 300 GALU/ Lactase enzyme 9000 FCC	**Adults:** Chew 1 tab before meals.
ANTACIDS/ANTIFLATULENTS		
PLEASE REFER TO ANTACID AND HEARTBURN PRODUCTS TABLE		
SIMETHICONE/SIMETHICONE COMBINATIONS		
Gas-X Chewable Tablets	Simethicone 80mg	**Adults:** Chew 1 or 2 tabs prn after meals and at hs. **Max:** 6 tabs/24h.
Gas-X Chewable Tablets Extra Strength	Simethicone 125mg	**Adults:** Chew 1 or 2 tabs prn after meals and at hs. **Max:** 4 tabs/24h.
Gas-X Softgels Extra Strength	Simethicone 125mg	**Adults:** Take 1 or 2 caps prn after meals and at hs. **Max:** 4 caps/24h.
Gas-X Softgels Ultra Strength	Simethicone 180mg	**Adults:** Take 1 or 2 caps prn after meals and at hs. **Max:** 2 caps/24h.
Gas-X Thin Strips Extra Strength	Simethicone 62.5mg	**Adults:** Allow 2-4 strips to dissolve prn after meals and at hs. **Max:** 8 strips/24h.
Infants' Mylicon Drops	Simethicone 20mg/0.3mL	**Peds >2 yrs (>24 lbs):** 0.6mL prn after meals and at hs. **Peds <2 yrs (<24 lbs):** 0.3mL prn after meals and at hs. **Max:** 12 doses/24h.
Little Remedies Gas Relief Drops	Simethicone 20mg/0.3mL	**Peds ≥2 yrs (≥24 lbs):** 0.6mL prn after meals and at hs. **Peds <2 yrs (<24 lbs):** 0.3mL prn after meals and at hs. **Max:** 12 doses/24h.
Mylanta Gas Maximum Strength Chewable Tablets	Simethicone 125mg	**Adults:** Chew 1-2 tabs prn after meals and at hs. **Max:** 4 tabs/24h.
PediaCare Infants Gas Relief Drops	Simethicone 20mg/0.3mL	**Peds ≥2 yrs (≥24 lbs):** 0.6mL prn after meals and at hs. **Peds <2 yrs (<24 lbs):** 0.3mL prn after meals and at hs. **Max:** 12 doses/24h.

Hemorrhoidal Products*

BRAND	INGREDIENT(S)/STRENGTH(S)	DOSAGE†
ANESTHETICS/ANESTHETIC COMBINATIONS		
Americaine Hemorrhoidal Ointment	Benzocaine 20%	**Adults & Peds ≥12 yrs:** Apply externally to affected area up to 6 times a day.
HemAway Cream	Lidocaine/Phenylephrine HCl 5%/0.25%	**Adults & Peds ≥12 yrs:** Apply externally to affected area up to 4 times a day.
Nupercainal Hemorrhoidal Ointment	Dibucaine 1%	**Adults & Peds ≥12 yrs:** Apply externally to affected area up to 3 or 4 times a day.
Preparation H Maximum Strength Pain Relief Cream	Glycerin/Phenylephrine HCl/ Pramoxine HCl/White petrolatum 14.4%/0.25%/1%/15%	**Adults & Peds ≥12 yrs:** Apply externally to affected area up to 4 times a day.
RectiCare Anorectal Cream	Lidocaine 5%	**Adults & Peds ≥12 yrs:** Apply externally to affected area up to 6 times a day.
Tronolane Cream	Pramoxine HCl/Zinc oxide 1%/5%	**Adults & Peds ≥12 yrs:** Apply externally to affected area up to 5 times a day.
Tucks Fast Relief Spray	Pramoxine HCl 1%	**Adults & Peds ≥12 yrs:** Apply externally to affected area up to 5 times a day.
Tucks Hemorrhoidal Ointment	Pramoxine HCl/Zinc oxide/ Mineral oil 1%/12.5%/46.6%	**Adults & Peds ≥12 yrs:** Apply externally to affected area up to 5 times a day.
HYDROCORTISONES		
Preparation H Anti-Itch Cream	Hydrocortisone 1%	**Adults & Peds ≥12 yrs:** Apply externally to affected area not more than tid-qid.
WITCH HAZELS/WITCH HAZEL COMBINATIONS		
Preparation H Cooling Gel	Phenylephrine HCl/Witch hazel 0.25%/50%	**Adults & Peds ≥12 yrs:** Apply externally to affected area up to 4 times a day.
Preparation H Medicated Wipes	Witch hazel 50%	**Adults & Peds ≥12 yrs:** Use externally on affected area up to 6 times a day.
Preparation H Medicated Wipes for Women	Witch hazel 20%	**Adults & Peds ≥12 yrs:** Use externally on affected area up to 6 times a day.
T.N. Dickinson's Hemorrhoidal Pads	Witch hazel 50%	**Adults & Peds ≥12 yrs:** Use externally on affected area up to 6 times a day.
Tucks Medicated Cooling Pads	Witch hazel 50%	**Adults & Peds ≥12 yrs:** Use externally on affected area up to 6 times a day.
MISCELLANEOUS		
Calmol 4 Hemorrhoidal Suppositories	Cocoa butter/Zinc oxide 76%/10%	**Adults & Peds ≥12 yrs:** Insert 1 supp up to 6 times a day.
Preparation H Ointment	Mineral oil/Petrolatum/ Phenylephrine HCl 14%/74.9%/0.25%	**Adults & Peds ≥12 yrs:** Apply to affected area up to 4 times a day.
Preparation H Suppositories	Cocoa butter/Phenylephrine HCl 88.44%/0.25%	**Adults & Peds ≥12 yrs:** Insert 1 supp up to 4 times a day.
Tronolane Suppositories	Hard fat/Phenylephrine HCl 88.7%/0.25%	**Adults & Peds ≥12 yrs:** Insert 1 supp up to 4 times a day.

*Please refer to the *Laxative Products* table for stool softeners or bulk-forming laxatives adjunct therapies.
†Stop use and contact a healthcare provider if condition worsens or does not improve within 7 days.

Laxative Products

BRAND	INGREDIENT(S)/STRENGTH(S)	DOSAGE
BULK-FORMING		
Citrucel Caplets	Methylcellulose 500mg	**Adults & Peds ≥12 yrs:** 2 tabs prn up to 6 times/day. **Max:** 12 tabs/day. **Peds 6-11 yrs:** 1 tab prn up to 6 times/day. **Max:** 6 tabs/day.
Citrucel Orange Powder	Methylcellulose 2g/tbl	**Adults & Peds ≥12 yrs:** 1 tbl prn up to tid. **Peds 6-11 yrs:** 2.5 tsp prn up to tid.
Citrucel Orange Sugar Free Powder	Methylcellulose 2g/tbl	**Adults & Peds ≥12 yrs:** 1 tbl prn up to tid. **Peds 6-11 yrs:** 2 tsp prn up to tid.
Equalactin Chewable Tablets	Calcium polycarbophil 625mg	**Adults & Peds ≥12 yrs:** 2 tabs qid. **Max:** 8 tabs/day. **Peds 6-<12 yrs:** 1 tab qid. **Max:** 4 tabs/day. **Peds 3-<6 yrs:** 1 tab qd-bid. **Max:** 2 tabs/day.
FiberCon Caplets	Calcium polycarbophil 625mg	**Adults & Peds ≥12 yrs:** 2 tabs qd. **Max:** 8 tabs/day.
Konsyl Balance Powder	Psyllium/Inulin 2g-2g/tsp	**Adults & Peds ≥12 yrs:** 1 tsp up to tid. **Peds 7-11 yrs:** ½ tsp up to tid.
Konsyl Easy Mix Powder	Psyllium 4.3g/tsp	**Adults & Peds ≥12 yrs:** 1 tsp qd-tid. **Peds 6-<12 yrs:** ½ tsp qd-tid.
Konsyl Fiber Caplets	Calcium polycarbophil 625mg	**Adults & Peds ≥12 yrs:** 2 tabs qd-qid. **Max:** 8 tabs/day. **Peds 6-<12 yrs:** 2 tabs qd.
Konsyl Naturally Sweetened Powder	Psyllium 3.4g/tsp	**Adults & Peds ≥12 yrs:** 1 tsp qd-tid. **Peds 6-<12 yrs:** ½ tsp qd-tid.
Konsyl Orange Powder	Psyllium 3.4g/tbl	**Adults & Peds ≥12 yrs:** 1 tbl qd-tid. **Peds 6-<12 yrs:** ½ tbl qd-tid.
Konsyl Orange Sugar Free Powder	Psyllium 3.5g/tsp	**Adults & Peds ≥12 yrs:** 1 tsp qd-tid. **Peds 6-<12 yrs:** ½ tsp qd-tid.
Konsyl Original Formula Powder	Psyllium 6g/tsp	**Adults & Peds ≥12 yrs:** 1 tsp qd-tid. **Peds 6-<12 yrs:** ½ tsp qd-tid.
Konsyl Psyllium Capsules	Psyllium 520mg	**Adults & Peds ≥12 yrs:** 5 caps qd-tid.
Metamucil Capsules	Psyllium	**Adults & Peds ≥12 yrs:** 2-5 caps up to qid.
Metamucil Capsules Plus Calcium	Psyllium/Calcium	**Adults & Peds ≥12 yrs:** 2-5 caps up to qid.
Metamucil MultiGrain Wafers	Psyllium	**Adults & Peds ≥12 yrs:** 2 wafers up to tid.
Metamucil Orange Coarse Powder	Psyllium	**Adults & Peds ≥12 yrs:** 1 tsp up to tid.
Metamucil Orange Fiber Therapy Singles	Psyllium 3.4g/packet	**Adults & Peds ≥12 yrs:** 1 packet up to tid. **Peds 6-11 yrs:** ½ packet up to tid.
Metamucil Orange Smooth Powder	Psyllium	**Adults & Peds ≥12 yrs:** 1 tsp up to tid.
Metamucil Orange Smooth Powder Fiber Therapy	Psyllium 3.4g	**Adults & Peds ≥12 yrs:** 1 tbl up to tid. **Peds 6-11 yrs:** ½ tbl up to tid.
Metamucil Orange Sugar Free Fiber Singles	Psyllium	**Adults & Peds ≥12 yrs:** 1 packet up to tid.
Metamucil Orange Sugar Free Fiber Therapy Singles	Psyllium 3.4g	**Adults & Peds ≥12 yrs:** 1 packet up to tid. **Peds 6-11 yrs:** ½ packet up to tid.
Metamucil Orange Sugar Free Smooth Powder Fiber Therapy	Psyllium 3.4g	**Adults & Peds ≥12 yrs:** 1 tsp up to tid. **Peds 6-11 yrs:** ½ tsp up to tid.
Metamucil Original Coarse Powder	Psyllium	**Adults & Peds ≥12 yrs:** 1 tsp up to tid.
Metamucil Sugar Free Smooth Powder (Multi-flavor)	Psyllium	**Adults & Peds ≥12 yrs:** 1 tsp up to tid.

(Continued)

BRAND	INGREDIENT(S)/STRENGTH(S)	DOSAGE
HYPEROSMOTICS		
Fleet Glycerin Suppositories	Glycerin 2g	**Adults & Peds ≥6 yrs:** 1 supp ud.
Fleet Liquid Glycerin Suppositories	Glycerin 5.4g	**Adults & Peds ≥6 yrs:** 1 supp ud.
Fleet Mineral Oil Enema	Mineral oil 100%/118mL	**Adults & Peds ≥12 yrs:** 1 bottle (118mL). **Peds 2-<12 yrs:** ½ bottle (59mL).
Fleet Pedia-Lax Glycerin Suppositories	Glycerin 1g	**Peds 2-<6 yrs:** 1 supp ud.
Fleet Pedia-Lax Liquid Glycerin Suppositories	Glycerin 2.8g	**Peds 2-<6 yrs:** 1 supp ud.
Miralax	Polyethylene glycol 3350, 17g	**Adults & Peds ≥17 yrs:** 1 capful (17g) qd. **Max:** 7 days.
SALINES		
Fleet Enema	Monobasic sodium phosphate/ Dibasic sodium phosphate 19g-7g/118mL	**Adults & Peds ≥12 yrs:** 1 bottle (118mL).
Fleet Enema Extra	Monobasic sodium phosphate/ Dibasic sodium phosphate 19g-7g/197mL	**Adults & Peds ≥12 yrs:** 1 bottle (197mL).
Fleet Pedia-Lax Chewable Tablets	Magnesium hydroxide 400mg	**Peds 6-<12 yrs:** 3-6 tabs qd or in divided doses. **Max:** 6 tabs/day. **Peds 2-<6 yrs:** 1-3 tabs qd or in divided doses. **Max:** 3 tabs/day.
Fleet Pedia-Lax Enema	Monobasic sodium phosphate/ Dibasic sodium phosphate 9.5g-3.5g/59mL	**Peds 5-11 yrs:** 1 bottle (59mL). **Peds 2-<5 yrs:** ½ bottle (29.5mL).
Magnesium Citrate Solution	Magnesium citrate 1.745g/30mL	**Adults & Peds ≥12 yrs:** ½-1 bottle (300mL). **Peds 6-<12 yrs:** ⅓-½ bottle.
Phillips' Caplets	Magnesium 500mg	**Adults & Peds ≥12 yrs:** 2-4 tabs qhs or in divided doses.
Phillips' Chewable Tablets	Magnesium hydroxide 311mg	**Adults & Peds ≥12 yrs:** 8 tabs qhs or in divided doses. **Peds 6-11 yrs:** 4 tabs qhs or in divided doses. **Peds 3-5 yrs:** 2 tabs qhs or in divided doses.
Phillips' Concentrated Milk of Magnesia Liquid	Magnesium hydroxide 2400mg/15mL	**Adults & Peds ≥12 yrs:** 1-2 tbl (15-30mL) qhs or in divided doses.
Phillips' Milk of Magnesia Liquid	Magnesium hydroxide 1200mg/15mL	**Adults & Peds ≥12 yrs:** 2-4 tbl (30-60mL) qhs or in divided doses. **Peds 6-11 yrs:** 1-2 tbl (15-30mL) qhs or in divided doses.
STIMULANTS		
Alophen Tablets	Bisacodyl 5mg	**Adults & Peds ≥12 yrs:** 1-3 tabs qd. **Peds 6-<12 yrs:** 1 tab qd.
Carter's Sodium-Free Tablets	Bisacodyl 5mg	**Adults & Peds ≥12 yrs:** 1-3 tabs (usually 2) qd. **Peds 6-<12 yrs:** 1 tab qd.
Castor Oil	Castor oil 100%	**Adults & Peds ≥12 yrs:** 1-4 tbl (15-60mL) qd. **Peds 2-<12 yrs:** 1-3 tsp (5-15mL) qd.
Correctol Tablets	Bisacodyl 5mg	**Adults & Peds ≥12 yrs:** 1-3 tabs qd. **Peds 6-<12 yrs:** 1 tab qd.
Dulcolax Pink Tablets	Bisacodyl 5mg	**Adults & Peds ≥12 yrs:** 1-3 tabs qd. **Peds 6-<12 yrs:** 1 tab qd.
Dulcolax Suppositories	Bisacodyl 10mg	**Adults & Peds ≥12 yrs:** 1 supp qd. **Peds 6-<12 yrs:** ½ supp qd.
Dulcolax Tablets	Bisacodyl 5mg	**Adults & Peds ≥12 yrs:** 1-3 tabs qd. **Peds 6-<12 yrs:** 1 tab qd.

BRAND	INGREDIENT(S)/STRENGTH(S)	DOSAGE
STIMULANTS *(Continued)*		
Ex-Lax Maximum Strength Pills	Sennosides 25mg	**Adults & Peds ≥12 yrs:** 2 pills qd-bid. **Peds 6-<12 yrs:** 1 pill qd-bid.
Ex-Lax Regular Strength Chocolate Pieces	Sennosides 15mg	**Adults & Peds ≥12 yrs:** 2 pieces qd-bid. **Peds 6-<12 yrs:** 1 piece qd-bid.
Ex-Lax Regular Strength Pills	Sennosides 15mg	**Adults & Peds ≥12 yrs:** 2 pills qd-bid. **Peds 6-<12 yrs:** 1 pill qd-bid.
Fleet Bisacodyl Enema	Bisacodyl 10mg/30mL	**Adults & Peds ≥12 yrs:** 1 bottle (30mL).
Fleet Bisacodyl Tablets	Bisacodyl 5mg	**Adults & Peds ≥12 yrs:** 1-3 tabs qd. **Peds 6-<12 yrs:** 1 tab qd.
Perdiem Overnight Relief Pills	Sennosides 15mg	**Adults & Peds ≥12 yrs:** 2 tabs qd-bid. **Peds 6-<12 yrs:** 1 tab qd-bid.
Senokot Tablets	Sennosides 8.6mg	**Adults & Peds ≥12 yrs:** 2 tabs qd. **Max:** 4 tabs bid. **Peds 6-<12 yrs:** 1 tab qd. **Max:** 2 tabs bid. **Peds 2-<6 yrs:** ½ tab qd. **Max:** 1 tab bid.
SenokotXtra Tablets	Sennosides 17.2mg	**Adults & Peds ≥12 yrs:** 1 tab qd. **Max:** 2 tabs bid. **Peds 6-<12 yrs:** ½ tab qd. **Max:** 1 tab bid.
STIMULANT COMBINATIONS		
Konsyl Senna Prompt Capsules	Psyllium/Sennosides 500mg-9mg	**Adults & Peds ≥12 yrs:** 2-4 caps qd-bid.
Peri-Colace Tablets	Sennosides/Docusate sodium 8.6mg-50mg	**Adults & Peds ≥12 yrs:** 2-4 tabs qhs or in divided doses. **Peds 6-<12 yrs:** 1-2 tabs qhs or in divided doses. **Peds 2-<6 yrs:** up to 1 tab qd.
Senokot-S Tablets	Sennosides/Docusate sodium 8.6mg-50mg	**Adults & Peds ≥12 yrs:** 2 tabs qd. **Max:** 4 tabs bid. **Peds 6-<12 yrs:** 1 tab qd. **Max:** 2 tabs bid. **Peds 2-<6 yrs:** ½ tab qd. **Max:** 1 tab bid.
SURFACTANTS (STOOL SOFTENERS)		
Colace Capsules	Docusate sodium 50mg	**Adults & Peds ≥12 yrs:** 1-6 caps qd or in divided doses. **Peds 2-<12 yrs:** 1-3 caps qd or in divided doses.
Colace Capsules	Docusate sodium 100mg	**Adults & Peds ≥12 yrs:** 1-3 caps qd or in divided doses. **Peds 2-<12 yrs:** 1 cap qd.
Colace Clear Soft Gels	Docusate sodium 50mg	**Adults & Peds ≥12 yrs:** 1-6 caps qd or in divided doses. **Peds 2-<12 yrs:** 1-3 caps qd or in divided doses.
Docusol Kids Mini-Enema	Docusate sodium 100mg	**Peds 2-<12 yrs:** 1 unit qd.
Docusol Mini-Enema	Docusate sodium 283mg	**Adults & Peds ≥12 yrs:** 1-3 units qd.
DulcoEase Pink Softgels	Docusate sodium 100mg	**Adults & Peds ≥12 yrs:** 1-3 caps qd or in divided doses. **Peds 2-<12 yrs:** 1 cap qd.
Dulcolax Stool Softener Capsules	Docusate sodium 100mg	**Adults & Peds ≥12 yrs:** 1-3 caps qd or in divided doses. **Peds 2-<12 yrs:** 1 cap qd.
Fleet Pedia-Lax Liquid Stool Softener	Docusate sodium 50mg/tbl	**Peds 2-<12 yrs:** 1-3 tbl (15-45mL) qd or in divided doses. **Max:** 3 tbl (45mL)/day.
Fleet Sof-Lax Softgels	Docusate sodium 100mg	**Adults & Peds ≥12 yrs:** 1-3 caps qd. **Peds 2-<12 yrs:** 1 cap qd.
Phillips' Stool Softener Liquid Gels	Docusate sodium 100mg	**Adults & Peds ≥12 yrs:** 1-3 caps qd or in divided doses. **Peds 6-<12 yrs:** 1 cap qd.
Surfak Stool Softener Softgels	Docusate calcium 240mg	**Adults & Peds ≥12 yrs:** 1 cap qd.

(Continued)

BRAND	INGREDIENT(S)/STRENGTH(S)	DOSAGE
SURFACTANT COMBINATIONS (STOOL SOFTENERS)		
Docusol Plus Mini-Enema	Docusate sodium/Benzocaine 283mg-20mg	**Adults & Peds ≥12 yrs:** 1-3 units qd.

COUGH-COLD-FLU-ALLERGY PRODUCTS

BRAND NAME	ANALGESIC	ANTIHISTAMINE	COUGH SUPPRESSANT	DECONGESTANT	EXPECTORANT	DOSAGE
ANALGESICS						
Tylenol Cold Sore Throat Liquid	Acetaminophen 500mg/15mL					**Adults & Peds ≥12 yrs:** 2 tbl (30mL) q6h. **Max:** 6 tbl (90mL)/24h.
ANALGESICS + ANTIHISTAMINES						
Coricidin HBP Cold & Flu Tablets	Acetaminophen 325mg	Chlorpheniramine maleate 2mg				**Adults & Peds ≥12 yrs:** 2 tabs q4-6h. **Max:** 12 tabs/24h. **Peds 6-<12 yrs:** 1 tab q4-6h. **Max:** 5 tabs/24h.
ANALGESICS + ANTIHISTAMINES + COUGH SUPPRESSANTS						
Contac Cold + Flu Night Instant Cooling Relief Liquid	Acetaminophen 500mg/15mL	Doxylamine succinate 6.25mg/15mL	Dextromethorphan HBr 15mg/15mL			**Adults & Peds ≥12 yrs:** 2 tbl (30mL) q6h. **Max:** 6 tbl (90mL)/24h.
Coricidin HBP Maximum Strength Flu Tablets	Acetaminophen 500mg	Chlorpheniramine maleate 2mg	Dextromethorphan HBr 15mg			**Adults & Peds ≥12 yrs:** 2 tabs q6h. **Max:** 8 tabs/24h.
Coricidin HBP Nighttime Multi-Symptom Cold Liquid	Acetaminophen 325mg/15mL	Doxylamine succinate 6.25mg/15mL	Dextromethorphan HBr 15mg/15mL			**Adults & Peds ≥12 yrs:** 2 tbl (30mL) q6h. **Max:** 4 doses/24h.
Delsym Night Time Multi-Symptom Liquid*	Acetaminophen 325mg/15mL	Doxylamine succinate 6.25mg/15mL	Dextromethorphan HBr 15mg/15mL			**Adults & Peds ≥12 yrs:** 2 tbl (30mL) q6h. **Max:** 4 doses/24h.
PediaCare Cough & Runny Nose Plus Acetaminophen Liquid	Acetaminophen 160mg/5mL	Chlorpheniramine maleate 1mg/5mL	Dextromethorphan HBr 5mg/5mL			**Peds 6-11 yrs (48-95 lbs):** 2 tsp (10mL) q4h. **Max:** 5 doses/24h.
Vicks Alcohol Free NyQuil Cold & Flu Nighttime Relief Liquid	Acetaminophen 650mg/30mL	Chlorpheniramine maleate 4mg/30mL	Dextromethorphan HBr 30mg/30mL			**Adults & Peds ≥12 yrs:** 2 tbl (30mL) q6h. **Max:** 4 doses/24h.
Vicks NyQuil Cold & Flu Nighttime Relief LiquiCaps	Acetaminophen 325mg	Doxylamine succinate 6.25mg	Dextromethorphan HBr 15mg			**Adults & Peds ≥12 yrs:** 2 caps q6h. **Max:** 4 doses/24h.

(Continued)

BRAND NAME	ANALGESIC	ANTIHISTAMINE	COUGH SUPPRESSANT	DECONGESTANT	EXPECTORANT	DOSAGE
ANALGESICS + ANTIHISTAMINES + COUGH SUPPRESSANTS *(Continued)*						
Vicks NyQuil Cold & Flu Nighttime Relief Liquid	Acetaminophen 650mg/30mL	Doxylamine succinate 12.5mg/30mL	Dextromethorphan HBr 30mg/30mL			**Adults & Peds ≥12 yrs:** 2 tbl (30mL) q6h. **Max:** 4 doses/24h.
ANALGESICS + ANTIHISTAMINES + COUGH SUPPRESSANTS + DECONGESTANTS						
Alka-Seltzer Plus Cold & Cough Formula Effervescent Tablets[†]	Aspirin 325mg	Chlorpheniramine maleate 2mg	Dextromethorphan HBr 10mg	Phenylephrine bitartrate 7.8mg		**Adults & Peds ≥12 yrs:** 2 tabs q4h. **Max:** 8 tabs/24h.
Alka-Seltzer Plus Cold & Cough Formula Liquid Gels	Acetaminophen 325mg	Chlorpheniramine maleate 2mg	Dextromethorphan HBr 10mg	Phenylephrine HCl 5mg		**Adults & Peds ≥12 yrs:** 2 caps q4h. **Max:** 10 caps/24h.
Alka-Seltzer Plus Day & Night Cold & Flu Formula Liquid Gels	Acetaminophen 325mg	Doxylamine succinate 6.25mg (nighttime dose only)	Dextromethorphan HBr 10mg	Phenylephrine HCl 5mg		**Adults & Peds ≥12 yrs:** 2 caps q4h. **Max:** 10 caps/24h.
Alka-Seltzer Plus Day & Night Multi-Symptom Cold Formula Effervescent Tablets[†]	Aspirin 325mg (daytime dose only), 500mg (nighttime dose only)	Doxylamine succinate 6.25mg (nighttime dose only)	Dextromethorphan HBr 10mg	Phenylephrine bitartrate 7.8mg		**Adults & Peds ≥12 yrs:** (Day) 2 tabs q4h; (Night) 2 tabs hs or q4-6h. **Max:** 8 tabs/24h.
Alka-Seltzer Plus-D Multi-Symptom Sinus & Cold Liquid Gels	Acetaminophen 325mg	Chlorpheniramine maleate 2mg	Dextromethorphan HBr 10mg	Pseudoephedrine HCl 30mg		**Adults & Peds ≥12 yrs:** 2 caps q4h. **Max:** 8 caps/24h.
Alka-Seltzer Plus Night Cold Formula Effervescent Tablets[†]	Aspirin 500mg	Doxylamine succinate 6.25mg	Dextromethorphan HBr 10mg	Phenylephrine bitartrate 7.8mg		**Adults & Peds ≥12 yrs:** 2 tabs hs or q4-6h. **Max:** 8 tabs/24h.
Alka-Seltzer Plus Night Cold & Flu Formula Liquid Gels	Acetaminophen 325mg	Doxylamine succinate 6.25mg	Dextromethorphan HBr 10mg	Phenylephrine HCl 5mg		**Adults & Peds ≥12 yrs:** 2 caps q4h. **Max:** 10 caps/24h.
Alka-Seltzer Plus Night Severe Cold + Flu Powder Packets	Acetaminophen 650mg/packet	Doxylamine succinate 12.5mg/packet	Dextromethorphan HBr 20mg/packet	Phenylephrine HCl 10mg/packet		**Adults & Peds ≥12 yrs:** 1 pkt q4h. **Max:** 5 pkts/24h.
Alka-Seltzer Plus Severe Cold & Flu Formula Effervescent Tablets[†]	Acetaminophen 250mg	Chlorpheniramine maleate 2mg	Dextromethorphan HBr 10mg	Phenylephrine HCl 5mg		**Adults & Peds ≥12 yrs:** 2 tabs q4h. **Max:** 8 tabs/24h.
Alka-Seltzer Plus Severe Sinus Congestion Allergy & Cough Liquid Gels	Acetaminophen 325mg	Doxylamine succinate 6.25mg	Dextromethorphan HBr 10mg	Phenylephrine HCl 5mg		**Adults & Peds ≥12 yrs:** 2 caps q4h. **Max:** 10 caps/24h.

BRAND NAME	ANALGESIC	ANTIHISTAMINE	COUGH SUPPRESSANT	DECONGESTANT	EXPECTORANT	DOSAGE
ANALGESICS + ANTIHISTAMINES + COUGH SUPPRESSANTS + DECONGESTANTS *(Continued)*						
PediaCare Flu Plus Acetaminophen Liquid	Acetaminophen 160mg/5mL	Chlorpheniramine maleate 1mg/5mL	Dextromethorphan HBr 5mg/5mL	Phenylephrine HCl 2.5mg/5mL		**Peds 6-11 yrs (48-95 lbs):** 2 tsp (10mL) q4h. **Max:** 5 doses/24h.
PediaCare Multi-Symptom Cold Plus Acetaminophen Liquid	Acetaminophen 160mg/5mL	Chlorpheniramine maleate 1mg/5mL	Dextromethorphan HBr 5mg/5mL	Phenylephrine HCl 2.5mg/5mL		**Peds 6-11 yrs (48-95 lbs):** 2 tsp (10mL) q4h. **Max:** 5 doses/24h.
Theraflu Warming Relief Nighttime Multi-Symptom Cold Caplets*	Acetaminophen 325mg	Chlorpheniramine maleate 2mg	Dextromethorphan HBr 10mg	Phenylephrine HCl 5mg		**Adults & Peds ≥12 yrs:** 2 tabs q4h. **Max:** 12 tabs/24h.
Triaminic Multi-Symptom Fever & Cold Suspension	Acetaminophen 160mg/5mL	Chlorpheniramine maleate 1mg/5mL	Dextromethorphan HBr 5mg/5mL	Phenylephrine HCl 2.5mg/5mL		**Peds 6-<12 yrs:** 2 tsp (10mL) q4h. **Max:** 5 doses/24h.
Tylenol Cold Multi-Symptom Nighttime Liquid	Acetaminophen 325mg/15mL	Doxylamine succinate 6.25mg/15mL	Dextromethorphan HBr 10mg/15mL	Phenylephrine HCl 5mg/15mL		**Adults & Peds ≥12 yrs:** 2 tbl (30mL) q4h. **Max:** 10 tbl (150mL)/24h.
Vicks NyQuil Severe Cold & Flu Caplets	Acetaminophen 325mg	Doxylamine succinate 6.25mg	Dextromethorphan HBr 10mg	Phenylephrine HCl 5mg		**Adults & Peds ≥12 yrs:** 2 tabs q4h. **Max:** 4 doses/24h.
Vicks NyQuil Severe Cold & Flu Liquid	Acetaminophen 650mg/30mL	Doxylamine succinate 12.5mg/30mL	Dextromethorphan HBr 20mg/30mL	Phenylephrine HCl 10mg/30mL		**Adults & Peds ≥12 yrs:** 2 tbl (30mL) q4h. **Max:** 4 doses/24h.
ANALGESICS + ANTIHISTAMINES + COUGH SUPPRESSANTS + EXPECTORANTS						
Coricidin HBP Day & Night Multi-Symptom Cold Softgels/ Tablets	Acetaminophen 500mg (nighttime dose only)	Chlorpheniramine maleate 2mg (nighttime dose only)	Dextromethorphan HBr 10mg (daytime dose), 15mg (nighttime dose)		Guaifenesin 200mg (daytime dose only)	**Adults & Peds ≥12 yrs:** (Day) 1-2 caps q4h. **Max:** 6 caps/12h; (Night) 2 tabs hs and q6h. **Max:** 4 tabs/12h.
ANALGESICS + ANTIHISTAMINES + DECONGESTANTS						
Advil Allergy & Congestion Relief Tablets	Ibuprofen 200mg	Chlorpheniramine maleate 4mg		Phenylephrine HCl 10mg		**Adults & Peds ≥12 yrs:** 1 tab q4h. **Max:** 6 tabs/24h.
Advil Allergy Sinus Caplets	Ibuprofen 200mg	Chlorpheniramine maleate 2mg		Pseudoephedrine HCl 30mg		**Adults & Peds ≥12 yrs:** 1 tab q4-6h. **Max:** 6 tabs/24h.
Alka-Seltzer Plus Cold Formula Effervescent Tablets†‡	Aspirin 325mg	Chlorpheniramine maleate 2mg		Phenylephrine bitartrate 7.8mg		**Adults & Peds ≥12 yrs:** 2 tabs q4h. **Max:** 8 tabs/24h.
Alka-Seltzer Plus Severe Allergy Sinus Congestion & Headache Liquid Gels	Acetaminophen 325mg	Doxylamine succinate 6.25mg		Phenylephrine HCl 5mg		**Adults & Peds ≥12 yrs:** 2 caps q4h. **Max:** 10 caps/24h.

(Continued)

BRAND NAME	ANALGESIC	ANTIHISTAMINE	COUGH SUPPRESSANT	DECONGESTANT	EXPECTORANT	DOSAGE
ANALGESICS + ANTIHISTAMINES + DECONGESTANTS *(Continued)*						
Children's Delsym Cough+ Cold Night Time Liquid	Acetaminophen 325mg/10mL	Diphenhydramine HCl 12.5mg/10mL		Phenylephrine HCl 5mg/10mL		**Adults & Peds ≥12 yrs:** 4 tsp (20mL) q4h. **Max:** 6 doses/24h. **Peds 6-<12 yrs:** 2 tsp (10mL) q4h. **Max:** 5 doses/24h.
Children's Dimetapp Multi-Symptom Cold & Flu Liquid	Acetaminophen 320mg/5mL	Diphenhydramine HCl 12.5mg/5mL		Phenylephrine HCl 5mg/5mL		**Adults & Peds ≥12 yrs:** 4 tsp (20mL) q4h. **Peds 6-<12 yrs:** 2 tsp (10mL) q4h. **Max:** 5 doses/24h.
Children's Mucinex Night Time Multi-Symptom Cold Liquid	Acetaminophen 325mg/10mL	Diphenhydramine HCl 12.5mg/10mL		Phenylephrine HCl 5mg/10mL		**Peds 6-<12 yrs:** 2 tsp (10mL) q4h. **Max:** 5 doses/24h.
Contac Cold + Flu Night Caplets	Acetaminophen 500mg	Chlorpheniramine maleate 2mg		Phenylephrine HCl 5mg		**Adults & Peds ≥12 yrs:** 2 tabs q6h prn. **Max:** 8 tabs/24h.
Delsym Cough+ Cold Night Time Liquid	Acetaminophen 650mg/20mL	Diphenhydramine HCl 25mg/20mL		Phenylephrine HCl 10mg/20mL		**Adults & Peds ≥12 yrs:** 4 tsp (20mL) q4h. **Max:** 6 doses/24h.
Dristan Cold Multi-Symptom Formula Tablets	Acetaminophen 325mg	Chlorpheniramine maleate 2mg		Phenylephrine HCl 5mg		**Adults & Peds ≥12 yrs:** 2 tabs q4h. **Max:** 12 tabs/24h.
Maximum Strength Mucinex Fast-Max Night Time Cold & Flu Caplets	Acetaminophen 325mg	Diphenhydramine HCl 25mg		Phenylephrine HCl 5mg		**Adults & Peds ≥12 yrs:** 2 tabs q4h. **Max:** 12 tabs/24h.
Maximum Strength Mucinex Fast-Max Night Time Cold & Flu Liquid	Acetaminophen 650mg/20mL	Diphenhydramine HCl 25mg/20mL		Phenylephrine HCl 10mg/20mL		**Adults & Peds ≥12 yrs:** 4 tsp (20mL) q4h. **Max:** 6 doses/24h.
Maximum Strength Mucinex Fast-Max Night Time Cold & Flu Packets	Acetaminophen 650mg/packet	Diphenhydramine HCl 25mg/packet		Phenylephrine HCl 10mg/packet		**Adults & Peds ≥12 yrs:** 1 pkt q4h. **Max:** 6 pkts/24h.
Maximum Strength Mucinex Sinus-Max Night Time Congestion & Cough Liquid	Acetaminophen 650mg/20mL	Diphenhydramine HCl 25mg/20mL		Phenylephrine HCl 10mg/20mL		**Adults & Peds ≥12 yrs:** 4 tsp (20mL) q4h. **Max:** 6 doses/24h.
QlearQuil Nighttime Sinus & Congestion LiquiCaps	Acetaminophen 325mg	Doxylamine succinate 6.25mg		Phenylephrine HCl 5mg		**Adults & Peds ≥12 yrs:** 2 caps q4h. **Max:** 4 doses/24h.
Robitussin Peak Cold Nighttime Multi-Symptom Cold CF Liquid	Acetaminophen 640mg/20mL	Diphenhydramine HCl 25mg/20mL		Phenylephrine HCl 10mg/20mL		**Adults & Peds ≥12 yrs:** 4 tsp (20mL) q4h. **Max:** 6 doses/24h.
Sudafed PE Severe Cold Caplets*	Acetaminophen 325mg	Diphenhydramine HCl 12.5mg		Phenylephrine HCl 5mg		**Adults & Peds ≥12 yrs:** 2 tabs q4h. **Max:** 12 tabs/24h.

BRAND NAME	ANALGESIC	ANTIHISTAMINE	COUGH SUPPRESSANT	DECONGESTANT	EXPECTORANT	DOSAGE
ANALGESICS + ANTIHISTAMINES + DECONGESTANTS *(Continued)*						
Theraflu Flu & Sore Throat Powder Packets*	Acetaminophen 650mg/packet	Pheniramine maleate 20mg/packet		Phenylephrine HCl 10mg/packet		**Adults & Peds ≥12 yrs:** 1 pkt q4h. **Max:** 6 pkts/24h.
Theraflu Nighttime Severe Cold & Cough Powder Packets	Acetaminophen 650mg/packet	Diphenhydramine HCl 25mg/packet		Phenylephrine HCl 10mg/packet		**Adults & Peds ≥12 yrs:** 1 pkt q4h. **Max:** 5 pkts/24h.
Theraflu Sinus & Cold Powder Packets*	Acetaminophen 325mg/packet	Pheniramine maleate 20mg/packet		Phenylephrine HCl 10mg/packet		**Adults & Peds ≥12 yrs:** 1 pkt q4h. **Max:** 6 pkts/24h.
Theraflu Sugar-Free Nighttime Severe Cold & Cough Powder Packets*	Acetaminophen 650mg/packet	Diphenhydramine HCl 25mg/packet		Phenylephrine HCl 10mg/packet		**Adults & Peds ≥12 yrs:** 1 pkt q4h. **Max:** 6 pkts/24h.
Theraflu Warming Relief Flu & Sore Throat Syrup*	Acetaminophen 325mg/15mL	Diphenhydramine HCl 12.5mg/15mL		Phenylephrine HCl 5mg/15mL		**Adults & Peds ≥12 yrs:** 2 tbl (30mL) q4h. **Max:** 6 doses (12 tbl or 180mL)/24h.
Theraflu Warming Relief Nighttime Severe Cold & Cough Syrup*	Acetaminophen 325mg/15mL	Diphenhydramine HCl 12.5mg/15mL		Phenylephrine HCl 5mg/15mL		**Adults & Peds ≥12 yrs:** 2 tbl (30mL) q4h. **Max:** 6 doses (12 tbl or 180mL)/24h.
Theraflu Warming Relief Sinus & Cold Syrup*	Acetaminophen 325mg/15mL	Diphenhydramine HCl 12.5mg/15mL		Phenylephrine HCl 5mg/15mL		**Adults & Peds ≥12 yrs:** 2 tbl (30mL) q4h. **Max:** 6 doses (12 tbl or 180mL)/24h.
ANALGESICS + ANTIHISTAMINES + DECONGESTANTS + EXPECTORANTS						
Maximum Strength Mucinex Sinus-Max Day & Night Caplets	Acetaminophen 325mg	Diphenhydramine HCl 25mg (nighttime dose only)		Phenylephrine HCl 5mg	Guaifenesin 200mg (daytime dose only)	**Adults & Peds ≥12 yrs:** 2 tabs q4h. **Max:** 12 tabs/24h.
ANALGESICS + COUGH SUPPRESSANTS						
Delsym Cough+ Soothing Action Lozenges	Menthol 5mg		Dextromethorphan HBr 5mg			**Adults & Peds ≥12 yrs:** 2 lozenges q4h. **Max:** 12 lozenges/24h. **Peds 6-<12 yrs:** 1 lozenge q4h. **Max:** 6 lozenges/24h.

(Continued)

BRAND NAME	ANALGESIC	ANTIHISTAMINE	COUGH SUPPRESSANT	DECONGESTANT	EXPECTORANT	DOSAGE
ANALGESICS + COUGH SUPPRESSANTS *(Continued)*						
PediaCare Cough & Sore Throat Plus Acetaminophen Liquid	Acetaminophen 160mg/5mL		Dextromethorphan HBr 5mg/5mL			**Peds 6-11 yrs (48-95 lbs):** 2 tsp (10mL) q4h. **Max:** 5 doses/24h.
Robitussin Medi-Soothers Cough DM Lozenges	Menthol 5mg		Dextromethorphan HBr 5mg			**Adults & Peds ≥12 yrs:** 2 lozenges q4h. **Max:** 12 lozenges/24h.
Triaminic Cough & Sore Throat Syrup	Acetaminophen 160mg/5mL		Dextromethorphan HBr 5mg/5mL			**Peds 6-<12 yrs:** 2 tsp (10mL) q4h. **Peds 4-<6 yrs:** 1 tsp (5mL) q4h. **Max:** 5 doses/24h.
ANALGESICS + COUGH SUPPRESSANTS + DECONGESTANTS						
Alka-Seltzer Plus Day Non-Drowsy Cold & Flu Formula Liquid Gels	Acetaminophen 325mg		Dextromethorphan HBr 10mg	Phenylephrine HCl 5mg		**Adults & Peds ≥12 yrs:** 2 caps q4h. **Max:** 10 caps/24h.
Alka-Seltzer Plus Severe Sinus Congestion & Cough Liquid Gels	Acetaminophen 325mg		Dextromethorphan HBr 10mg	Phenylephrine HCl 5mg		**Adults & Peds ≥12 yrs:** 2 caps q4h. **Max:** 10 caps/24h.
Robitussin Daytime Cold + Flu Liquid-Filled Capsules	Acetaminophen 325mg		Dextromethorphan HBr 10mg	Phenylephrine HCl 5mg		**Adults & Peds ≥12 yrs:** 2 caps q4h. **Max:** 12 caps/24h.
Sudafed PE Pressure + Pain + Cough Caplets	Acetaminophen 325mg		Dextromethorphan HBr 10mg	Phenylephrine HCl 5mg		**Adults & Peds ≥12 yrs:** 2 tabs q4h. **Max:** 10 tabs/24h.
Theraflu Daytime Severe Cold & Cough Powder Packets	Acetaminophen 650mg/packet		Dextromethorphan HBr 20mg/packet	Phenylephrine HCl 10mg/packet		**Adults & Peds ≥12 yrs:** 1 pkt q4h. **Max:** 5 pkts/24h.
Theraflu Multi-Symptom Severe Cold Powder Packets	Acetaminophen 500mg/packet		Dextromethorphan HBr 20mg/packet	Phenylephrine HCl 10mg/packet		**Adults & Peds ≥12 yrs:** 1 pkt q4h. **Max:** 6 pkts/24h.
Theraflu Warming Relief Daytime Multi-Symptom Cold Caplets*	Acetaminophen 325mg		Dextromethorphan HBr 10mg	Phenylephrine HCl 5mg		**Adults & Peds ≥12 yrs:** 2 tabs q4h. **Max:** 12 tabs/24h.
Theraflu Warming Relief Daytime Severe Cold & Cough Syrup*	Acetaminophen 325mg/15mL		Dextromethorphan HBr 10mg/15mL	Phenylephrine HCl 5mg/15mL		**Adults & Peds ≥12 yrs:** 2 tbl (30mL) q4h. **Max:** 6 doses/24h.
Tylenol Cold Multi-Symptom Caplets	Acetaminophen 325mg		Dextromethorphan HBr 10mg	Phenylephrine HCl 5mg		**Adults & Peds ≥12 yrs:** 2 caps q4h. **Max:** 10 caps/24h.
Tylenol Cold Multi-Symptom Daytime Liquid	Acetaminophen 325mg/15mL		Dextromethorphan HBr 10mg/15mL	Phenylephrine HCl 5mg/15mL		**Adults & Peds ≥12 yrs:** 2 tbl (30mL) q4h. **Max:** 10 tbl (150mL)/24h.

BRAND NAME	ANALGESIC	ANTIHISTAMINE	COUGH SUPPRESSANT	DECONGESTANT	EXPECTORANT	DOSAGE
ANALGESICS + COUGH SUPPRESSANTS + DECONGESTANTS *(Continued)*						
Vicks DayQuil Cold & Flu Multi-Symptom Relief LiquiCaps	Acetaminophen 325mg		Dextromethorphan HBr 10mg	Phenylephrine HCl 5mg		**Adults & Peds ≥12 yrs:** 2 caps q4h. **Max:** 4 doses/24h.
Vicks DayQuil Cold & Flu Multi-Symptom Relief Liquid	Acetaminophen 325mg/15mL		Dextromethorphan HBr 10mg/15mL	Phenylephrine HCl 5mg/15mL		**Adults & Peds ≥12 yrs:** 2 tbl (30mL) q4h. **Peds 6-<12 yrs:** 1 tbl (15mL) q4h. **Max:** 4 doses/24h.
ANALGESICS + COUGH SUPPRESSANTS + DECONGESTANTS + EXPECTORANTS						
Alka-Seltzer Plus Day Severe Cold + Flu Powder Packets	Acetaminophen 500mg/packet		Dextromethorphan HBr 20mg/packet	Phenylephrine HCl 10mg/packet	Guaifenesin 400mg/packet	**Adults & Peds ≥12 yrs:** 1 pkt q4h. **Max:** 6 pkts/24h.
Children's Delsym Cough+ Cold Day Time Liquid	Acetaminophen 325mg/10mL		Dextromethorphan HBr 10mg/10mL	Phenylephrine HCl 5mg/10mL	Guaifenesin 200mg/10mL	**Adults & Peds ≥12 yrs:** 4 tsp (20mL) q4h. **Max:** 6 doses/24h. **Peds 6-<12 yrs:** 2 tsp (10mL) q4h. **Max:** 5 doses/24h.
Children's Mucinex Cold, Cough & Sore Throat Liquid	Acetaminophen 325mg/10mL		Dextromethorphan HBr 10mg/10mL	Phenylephrine HCl 5mg/10mL	Guaifenesin 200mg/10mL	**Peds 6-<12 yrs:** 2 tsp (10mL) q4h. **Max:** 5 doses/24h.
Children's Mucinex Multi-Symptom Cold & Fever Liquid	Acetaminophen 325mg/10mL		Dextromethorphan HBr 10mg/10mL	Phenylephrine HCl 5mg/10mL	Guaifenesin 200mg/10mL	**Peds 6-<12 yrs:** 2 tsp (10mL) q4h. **Max:** 5 doses/24h.
Delsym Cough+ Cold Day Time Liquid	Acetaminophen 650mg/20mL		Dextromethorphan HBr 20mg/20mL	Phenylephrine HCl 10mg/20mL	Guaifenesin 400mg/20mL	**Adults & Peds ≥12 yrs:** 4 tsp (20mL) q4h. **Max:** 6 doses/24h.
Maximum Strength Mucinex Fast-Max Cold, Flu & Sore Throat Caplets	Acetaminophen 325mg		Dextromethorphan HBr 10mg	Phenylephrine HCl 5mg	Guaifenesin 200mg	**Adults & Peds ≥12 yrs:** 2 tabs q4h. **Max:** 12 tabs/24h.
Maximum Strength Mucinex Fast-Max Cold, Flu & Sore Throat Liquid	Acetaminophen 650mg/20mL		Dextromethorphan HBr 20mg/20mL	Phenylephrine HCl 10mg/20mL	Guaifenesin 400mg/20mL	**Adults & Peds ≥12 yrs:** 4 tsp (20mL) q4h. **Max:** 6 doses/24h.
Maximum Strength Mucinex Fast-Max Cold, Flu & Sore Throat Packets	Acetaminophen 650mg/packet		Dextromethorphan HBr 20mg/packet	Phenylephrine HCl 10mg/packet	Guaifenesin 400mg/packet	**Adults & Peds ≥12 yrs:** 1 pkt q4h. **Max:** 6 pkts/24h.
Maximum Strength Mucinex Fast-Max Severe Cold Caplets	Acetaminophen 325mg		Dextromethorphan HBr 10mg	Phenylephrine HCl 5mg	Guaifenesin 200mg	**Adults & Peds ≥12 yrs:** 2 tabs q4h. **Max:** 12 tabs/24h.
Maximum Strength Mucinex Fast-Max Severe Cold Liquid	Acetaminophen 650mg/20mL		Dextromethorphan HBr 20mg/20mL	Phenylephrine HCl 10mg/20mL	Guaifenesin 400mg/20mL	**Adults & Peds ≥12 yrs:** 4 tsp (20mL) q4h. **Max:** 6 doses/24h.

(Continued)

BRAND NAME	ANALGESIC	ANTIHISTAMINE	COUGH SUPPRESSANT	DECONGESTANT	EXPECTORANT	DOSAGE
ANALGESICS + COUGH SUPPRESSANTS + DECONGESTANTS + EXPECTORANTS *(Continued)*						
Maximum Strength Mucinex Fast-Max Severe Cold Packets	Acetaminophen 650mg/packet		Dextromethorphan HBr 20mg/packet	Phenylephrine HCl 10mg/packet	Guaifenesin 400mg/packet	**Adults & Peds ≥12 yrs:** 1 pkt q4h. **Max:** 6 pkts/24h.
Sudafed PE Pressure + Pain + Cold Caplets	Acetaminophen 325mg		Dextromethorphan HBr 10mg	Phenylephrine HCl 5mg	Guaifenesin 100mg	**Adults & Peds ≥12 yrs:** 2 tabs q4h. **Max:** 10 tabs/24h.
Theraflu Max-D Severe Cold & Flu Powder Packets*	Acetaminophen 1000mg/packet		Dextromethorphan HBr 30mg/packet	Pseudoephedrine HCl 60mg/packet	Guaifenesin 400mg/packet	**Adults & Peds ≥12 yrs:** 1 pkt q6h. **Max:** 4 pkts/24h.
Tylenol Cold & Flu Severe Caplets	Acetaminophen 325mg		Dextromethorphan HBr 10mg	Phenylephrine HCl 5mg	Guaifenesin 200mg	**Adults & Peds ≥12 yrs:** 2 tabs q4h. **Max:** 10 tabs/24h.
Tylenol Cold & Flu Severe Warming Liquid	Acetaminophen 325mg/15mL		Dextromethorphan HBr 10mg/15mL	Phenylephrine HCl 5mg/15mL	Guaifenesin 200mg/15mL	**Adults & Peds ≥12 yrs:** 2 tbl (30mL) q4h. **Max:** 10 tbl (150mL)/24h.
Tylenol Cold Multi-Symptom Severe Liquid	Acetaminophen 325mg/15mL		Dextromethorphan HBr 10mg/15mL	Phenylephrine HCl 5mg/15mL	Guaifenesin 200mg/15mL	**Adults & Peds ≥12 yrs:** 2 tbl (30mL) q4h. **Max:** 10 tbl (150mL)/24h.
Vicks DayQuil Severe Cold & Flu Caplets	Acetaminophen 325mg		Dextromethorphan HBr 10mg	Phenylephrine HCl 5mg	Guaifenesin 200mg	**Adults & Peds ≥12 yrs:** 2 tabs q4h. **Max:** 4 doses/24h.
Vicks DayQuil Severe Cold & Flu Liquid	Acetaminophen 325mg/15mL		Dextromethorphan HBr 10mg/15mL	Phenylephrine HCl 5mg/15mL	Guaifenesin 200mg/15mL	**Adults & Peds ≥12 yrs:** 2 tbl (30mL) q4h. **Peds 6-<12 yrs:** 1 tbl (15mL) q4h. **Max:** 4 doses/24h.
ANALGESICS + DECONGESTANTS						
Advil Cold & Sinus Caplets/ Liqui-Gels	Ibuprofen 200mg			Pseudoephedrine HCl 30mg		**Adults & Peds ≥12 yrs:** 1-2 caps q4-6h. **Max:** 6 caps/24h.
Advil Congestion Relief Tablets	Ibuprofen 200mg			Phenylephrine HCl 10mg		**Adults & Peds ≥12 yrs:** 1 tab q4h. **Max:** 6 tabs/24h.
Contac Cold + Flu Day Caplets	Acetaminophen 500mg			Phenylephrine HCl 5mg		**Adults & Peds ≥12 yrs:** 2 tabs q6h. **Max:** 8 tabs/24h.
QlearQuil Daytime Sinus & Congestion LiquiCaps	Acetaminophen 325mg			Phenylephrine HCl 5mg		**Adults & Peds ≥12 yrs:** 2 caps q4h. **Max:** 4 doses/24h.
Sudafed 12 Hour Pressure + Pain Caplets	Naproxen sodium 220mg			Pseudoephedrine HCl 120mg		**Adults & Peds ≥12 yrs:** 1 tab q12h. **Max:** 2 tabs/24h.

BRAND NAME	ANALGESIC	ANTIHISTAMINE	COUGH SUPPRESSANT	DECONGESTANT	EXPECTORANT	DOSAGE
ANALGESICS + DECONGESTANTS *(Continued)*						
Sudafed PE Pressure + Pain Caplets	Acetaminophen 325mg			Phenylephrine HCl 5mg		**Adults & Peds ≥12 yrs:** 2 tabs q4h. **Max:** 10 tabs/24h.
Tylenol Sinus Congestion & Pain Caplets	Acetaminophen 325mg			Phenylephrine HCl 5mg		**Adults & Peds ≥12 yrs:** 2 caps q4h. **Max:** 10 caps/24h.
ANALGESICS + DECONGESTANTS + EXPECTORANTS						
Maximum Strength Mucinex Fast-Max Cold & Sinus Caplets	Acetaminophen 325mg			Phenylephrine HCl 5mg	Guaifenesin 200mg	**Adults & Peds ≥12 yrs:** 2 tabs q4h. **Max:** 12 tabs/24h.
Maximum Strength Mucinex Fast-Max Cold & Sinus Liquid	Acetaminophen 650mg/20mL			Phenylephrine HCl 10mg/20mL	Guaifenesin 400mg/20mL	**Adults & Peds ≥12 yrs:** 4 tsp (20mL) q4h. **Max:** 6 doses/24h.
Maximum Strength Mucinex Sinus-Max Pressure & Pain Caplets	Acetaminophen 325mg			Phenylephrine HCl 5mg	Guaifenesin 200mg	**Adults & Peds ≥12 yrs:** 2 tabs q4h. **Max:** 12 tabs/24h.
Maximum Strength Mucinex Sinus-Max Pressure & Pain Liquid	Acetaminophen 650mg/20mL			Phenylephrine HCl 10mg/20mL	Guaifenesin 400mg/20mL	**Adults & Peds ≥12 yrs:** 4 tsp (20mL) q4h. **Max:** 6 doses/24h.
Maximum Strength Mucinex Sinus-Max Severe Congestion Relief Caplets	Acetaminophen 325mg			Phenylephrine HCl 5mg	Guaifenesin 200mg	**Adults & Peds ≥12 yrs:** 2 tabs q4h. **Max:** 12 tabs/24h.
Maximum Strength Mucinex Sinus-Max Severe Congestion Relief Liquid	Acetaminophen 650mg/20mL			Phenylephrine HCl 10mg/20mL	Guaifenesin 400mg/20mL	**Adults & Peds ≥12 yrs:** 4 tsp (20mL) q4h. **Max:** 6 doses/24h.
Sudafed PE Pressure + Pain + Mucus Caplets	Acetaminophen 325mg			Phenylephrine HCl 5mg	Guaifenesin 200mg	**Adults & Peds ≥12 yrs:** 2 tabs q4h. **Max:** 10 tabs/24h.
Sudafed Triple Action Caplets*	Acetaminophen 325mg			Pseudoephedrine HCl 30mg	Guaifenesin 200mg	**Adults & Peds ≥12 yrs:** 2 tabs q4-6h. **Max:** 8 tabs/24h
Theraflu Warming Relief Cold & Chest Congestion Liquid*	Acetaminophen 325mg/15mL			Phenylephrine HCl 5mg/15mL	Guaifenesin 200mg/15mL	**Adults & Peds ≥12 yrs:** 2 tbl (30mL) q4h. **Max:** 6 doses/24h.
Tylenol Cold Head Congestion Severe Caplets	Acetaminophen 325mg			Phenylephrine HCl 5mg	Guaifenesin 200mg	**Adults & Peds ≥12 yrs:** 2 tabs q4h. **Max:** 10 tabs/24h.

(Continued)

BRAND NAME	ANALGESIC	ANTIHISTAMINE	COUGH SUPPRESSANT	DECONGESTANT	EXPECTORANT	DOSAGE
ANALGESICS + DECONGESTANTS + EXPECTORANTS *(Continued)*						
Tylenol Sinus Congestion & Pain Severe Caplets	Acetaminophen 325mg			Phenylephrine HCl 5mg	Guaifenesin 200mg	**Adults & Peds ≥12 yrs:** 2 tabs q4h. **Max:** 10 tabs/24h.
ANTIHISTAMINES						
Alavert Orally Disintegrating Tablets‡		Loratadine 10mg				**Adults & Peds ≥6 yrs:** 1 tab qd. **Max:** 1 tab/24h.
Benadryl Allergy Dye-Free Liqui-Gels		Diphenhydramine HCl 25mg				**Adults & Peds ≥12 yrs:** 1-2 caps q4-6h. **Peds 6-<12 yrs:** 1 cap q4-6h. **Max:** 6 doses/24h.
Benadryl Allergy Ultratab Tablets		Diphenhydramine HCl 25mg				**Adults & Peds ≥12 yrs:** 1-2 tabs q4-6h. **Peds 6-<12 yrs:** 1 tab q4-6h. **Max:** 6 doses/24h.
Children's Benadryl Allergy Liquid		Diphenhydramine HCl 12.5mg/5mL				**Peds 6-11 yrs:** 1-2 tsp (5-10mL) q4-6h. **Max:** 6 doses/24h.
Children's Benadryl Dye-Free Allergy Liquid*		Diphenhydramine HCl 12.5mg/5mL				**Peds 6-11 yrs:** 1-2 tsp (5-10mL) q4-6h. **Max:** 6 doses/24h.
Children's Claritin Chewables		Loratadine 5mg				**Adults & Peds ≥6 yrs:** 2 tabs qd. **Max:** 2 tabs/24h. **Peds 2-<6 yrs:** 1 tab qd. **Max:** 1 tab/24h.
Children's Claritin Syrup		Loratadine 5mg/5mL				**Adults & Peds ≥6 yrs:** 2 tsp (10mL) qd. **Max:** 2 tsp (10mL)/24h. **Peds 2-<6 yrs:** 1 tsp (5mL) qd. **Max:** 1 tsp (5mL)/24h.
Children's Zyrtec Dissolve Tabs		Cetirizine HCl 10mg				**Adults <65 yrs & Peds ≥6 yrs:** 1 tab qd. **Max:** 1 tab/24h.
Claritin Liqui-Gels		Loratadine 10mg				**Adults & Peds ≥6 yrs:** 1 cap qd. **Max:** 1 cap/24h.
Claritin RediTabs 12-Hour		Loratadine 5mg				**Adults & Peds ≥6 yrs:** 1 tab q12h. **Max:** 2 tabs/24h.

BRAND NAME	ANALGESIC	ANTIHISTAMINE	COUGH SUPPRESSANT	DECONGESTANT	EXPECTORANT	DOSAGE
ANTIHISTAMINES *(Continued)*						
Claritin RediTabs 24-Hour		Loratadine 10mg				**Adults & Peds ≥6 yrs:** 1 tab qd. **Max:** 1 tab/24h.
Claritin Tablets		Loratadine 10mg				**Adults & Peds ≥6 yrs:** 1 tab qd. **Max:** 1 tab/24h.
PediaCare Allergy Liquid‡		Diphenhydramine HCl 12.5mg/5mL				**Peds 6-11 yrs (48-95 lbs):** 1-2 tsp (5-10mL) q4h. **Max:** 6 doses/24h.
PediaCare 24 Hour Allergy Liquid		Cetirizine HCl 5mg/5mL				**Adults ≥65 yrs:** 1 tsp (5mL) qd. **Max:** 1 tsp (5mL)/24h. **Adults <65 yrs & Peds ≥6 yrs:** 1-2 tsp (5-10mL) qd. **Max:** 2 tsp (10mL)/24h. **Peds 2-<6 yrs:** ½-1 tsp (2.5-5mL) qd or ½ tsp (2.5mL) q12h. **Max:** 1 tsp (5mL)/24h.
QlearQuil All Day & All Night 24 Hour Allergy Relief Tablets		Loratadine 10mg				**Adults & Peds ≥6 yrs:** 1 tab qd. **Max:** 1 tab/24h.
QlearQuil Nighttime Allergy Relief Caplets		Diphenhydramine HCl 25mg				**Adults & Peds ≥12 yrs:** 1-2 tabs q4-6h. **Peds 6-<12 yrs:** 1 tab q4-6h. **Max:** 6 doses/24h.
Zyrtec Dissolve Tabs		Cetirizine HCl 10mg				**Adults <65 yrs & Peds ≥6 yrs:** 1 tab qd. **Max:** 1 tab/24h.
Zyrtec Liquid Gels		Cetirizine HCl 10mg				**Adults <65 yrs & Peds ≥6 yrs:** 1 cap qd. **Max:** 1 cap/24h.
Zyrtec Tablets		Cetirizine HCl 10mg				**Adults <65 yrs & Peds ≥6 yrs:** 1 tab qd. **Max:** 1 tab/24h.
ANTIHISTAMINES + COUGH SUPPRESSANTS						
Children's Dimetapp Long Acting Cough Plus Cold Liquid		Chlorpheniramine maleate 2mg/10mL	Dextromethorphan HBr 15mg/10mL			**Adults & Peds ≥12 yrs:** 4 tsp (20mL) q6h. **Peds 6-<12 yrs:** 2 tsp (10mL) q6h. **Max:** 4 doses/24h.

(Continued)

BRAND NAME	ANALGESIC	ANTIHISTAMINE	COUGH SUPPRESSANT	DECONGESTANT	EXPECTORANT	DOSAGE
ANTIHISTAMINES + COUGH SUPPRESSANTS *(Continued)*						
Children's Robitussin Cough & Cold Long-Acting Liquid		Chlorpheniramine maleate 2mg/10mL	Dextromethorphan HBr 15mg/10mL			**Adults & Peds ≥12 yrs:** 4 tsp (20mL) q6h. **Peds 6-<12 yrs:** 2 tsp (10mL) q6h. **Max:** 4 doses/24h.
Coricidin HBP Cough & Cold Tablets		Chlorpheniramine maleate 4mg	Dextromethorphan HBr 30mg			**Adults & Peds ≥12 yrs:** 1 tab q6h. **Max:** 4 tabs/24h.
Robitussin Maximum Strength Nighttime Cough DM Liquid		Doxylamine succinate 12.5mg/10mL	Dextromethorphan HBr 30mg/10mL			**Adults & Peds ≥12 yrs:** 2 tsp (10mL) q6h. **Max:** 4 doses/24h.
Vicks Children's NyQuil Cold & Cough Liquid		Chlorpheniramine maleate 2mg/15mL	Dextromethorphan HBr 15mg/15mL			**Adults & Peds ≥12 yrs:** 2 tbl (30mL) q6h. **Peds 6-11 yrs:** 1 tbl (15mL) q6h. **Max:** 4 doses/24h.
Vicks NyQuil Cough Liquid		Doxylamine succinate 12.5mg/30mL	Dextromethorphan HBr 30mg/30mL			**Adults & Peds ≥12 yrs:** 2 tbl (30mL) q6h. **Max:** 4 doses/24h.
ANTIHISTAMINES + COUGH SUPPRESSANTS + DECONGESTANTS						
Children's Dimetapp Cold & Cough Liquid		Brompheniramine maleate 2mg/10mL	Dextromethorphan HBr 10mg/10mL	Phenylephrine HCl 5mg/10mL		**Adults & Peds ≥12 yrs:** 4 tsp (20mL) q4h. **Peds 6-<12 yrs:** 2 tsp (10mL) q4h. **Max:** 6 doses/24h.
ANTIHISTAMINES + DECONGESTANTS						
Alavert D-12 Hour Extended Release Tablets		Loratadine 5mg		Pseudoephedrine sulfate 120mg		**Adults & Peds ≥12 yrs:** 1 tab q12h. **Max:** 2 tabs/24h.
Allerest PE Tablets		Chlorpheniramine maleate 4mg		Phenylephrine HCl 10mg		**Adults & Peds ≥12 yrs:** 1 tab q4h. **Peds 6-<12 yrs:** ½ tab q4h. **Max:** 6 doses/24h.
Children's Benadryl Allergy Plus Congestion Liquid		Diphenhydramine HCl 12.5mg/5mL		Phenylephrine HCl 5mg/5mL		**Adults & Peds ≥12 yrs:** 2 tsp (10mL) q4h. **Peds 6-11 yrs:** 1 tsp (5mL) q4h. **Max:** 6 doses/24h.
Children's Dimetapp Cold & Allergy Liquid		Brompheniramine maleate 2mg/10mL		Phenylephrine HCl 5mg/10mL		**Adults & Peds ≥12 yrs:** 4 tsp (20mL) q4h. **Peds 6-<12 yrs:** 2 tsp (10mL) q4h. **Max:** 6 doses/24h.
Children's Dimetapp Nighttime Cold & Congestion Liquid		Diphenhydramine HCl 12.5mg/10mL		Phenylephrine HCl 5mg/10mL		**Adults & Peds ≥12 yrs:** 4 tsp (20mL) q4h. **Peds 6-<12 yrs:** 2 tsp (10mL) q4h. **Max:** 6 doses/24h.

BRAND NAME	ANALGESIC	ANTIHISTAMINE	COUGH SUPPRESSANT	DECONGESTANT	EXPECTORANT	DOSAGE
ANTIHISTAMINES + DECONGESTANTS *(Continued)*						
Claritin-D 12 Hour Tablets		Loratadine 5mg		Pseudoephedrine sulfate 120mg		**Adults & Peds ≥12 yrs:** 1 tab q12h. **Max:** 2 tabs/24h.
Claritin-D 24 Hour Tablets		Loratadine 10mg		Pseudoephedrine sulfate 240mg		**Adults & Peds ≥12 yrs:** 1 tab qd. **Max:** 1 tab/24h.
PediaCare Nighttime Multi-Symptom Cold Liquid		Diphenhydramine HCl 6.25mg/5mL		Phenylephrine HCl 2.5mg/5mL		**Peds 6-11 yrs (48-95 lbs):** 2 tsp (10mL) q4h. **Max:** 6 doses/24h.
Sudafed PE Sinus+Allergy Tablets*		Chlorpheniramine maleate 4mg		Phenylephrine HCl 10mg		**Adults & Peds ≥12 yrs:** 1 tab q4h. **Max:** 6 tabs/24h.
Triaminic Night Time Cold & Cough Syrup		Diphenhydramine HCl 6.25mg/5mL		Phenylephrine HCl 2.5mg/5mL		**Peds 6-<12 yrs:** 2 tsp (10mL) q4h. **Max:** 6 doses/24h.
Zyrtec-D Tablets		Cetirizine HCl 5mg		Pseudoephedrine HCl 120mg		**Adults <65 yrs & Peds ≥12 yrs:** 1 tab q12h. **Max:** 2 tabs/24h.
COUGH SUPPRESSANTS						
Children's Delsym 12 Hour Cough Relief Liquid‡			Dextromethorphan HBr 30mg/5mL			**Adults & Peds ≥12 yrs:** 2 tsp (10mL) q12h. **Max:** 4 tsp (20mL)/24h. **Peds 6-<12 yrs:** 1 tsp (5mL) q12h. **Max:** 2 tsp (10mL)/24h. **Peds 4-<6 yrs:** ½ tsp (2.5mL) q12h. **Max:** 1 tsp (5mL)/24h.
Children's Robitussin Cough Long-Acting Liquid			Dextromethorphan HBr 15mg/10mL			**Adults & Peds ≥12 yrs:** 4 tsp (20mL) q6-8h. **Peds 6-<12 yrs:** 2 tsp (10mL) q6-8h. **Max:** 4 doses/24h.
Delsym 12 Hour Cough Relief Liquid‡			Dextromethorphan HBr 30mg/5mL			**Adults & Peds ≥12 yrs:** 2 tsp (10mL) q12h. **Max:** 4 tsp (20mL)/24h. **Peds 6-<12 yrs:** 1 tsp (5mL) q12h. **Max:** 2 tsp (10mL)/24h. **Peds 4-<6 yrs:** ½ tsp (2.5mL) q12h. **Max:** 1 tsp (5mL)/24h.
Robitussin Lingering Cold Long-Acting CoughGels			Dextromethorphan HBr 15mg			**Adults & Peds ≥12 yrs:** 2 caps q6-8h. **Max:** 8 caps/24h.

(Continued)

BRAND NAME	ANALGESIC	ANTIHISTAMINE	COUGH SUPPRESSANT	DECONGESTANT	EXPECTORANT	DOSAGE
COUGH SUPPRESSANTS *(Continued)*						
Robitussin Lingering Cold Long-Acting Cough Liquid			Dextromethorphan HBr 30mg/10mL			**Adults & Peds ≥12 yrs:** 2 tsp (10mL) q6-8h. **Max:** 4 doses/24h.
Vicks DayQuil Cough Liquid			Dextromethorphan HBr 15mg/15mL			**Adults & Peds ≥12 yrs:** 2 tbl (30mL) q6-8h. **Peds 6-<12 yrs:** 1 tbl (15mL) q6-8h. **Max:** 4 doses/24h.
COUGH SUPPRESSANTS + DECONGESTANTS						
Children's Sudafed PE Cold & Cough Liquid			Dextromethorphan HBr 5mg/5mL	Phenylephrine HCl 2.5mg/5mL		**Peds 6-11 yrs:** 2 tsp (10mL) q4h. **Peds 4-5 yrs:** 1 tsp (5mL) q4h. **Max:** 6 doses/24h.
PediaCare Daytime Multi-Symptom Cold Liquid			Dextromethorphan HBr 5mg/5mL	Phenylephrine HCl 2.5mg/5mL		**Peds 6-11 yrs (48-95 lbs):** 2 tsp (10mL) q4h. **Peds 4-5 yrs (36-47 lbs):** 1 tsp (5mL) q4h. **Max:** 6 doses/24h.
Triaminic Day Time Cold & Cough Syrup			Dextromethorphan HBr 5mg/5mL	Phenylephrine HCl 2.5mg/5mL		**Peds 6-<12 yrs:** 2 tsp (10mL) q4h. **Peds 4-<6 yrs:** 1 tsp (5mL) q4h. **Max:** 6 doses/24h.
COUGH SUPPRESSANTS + DECONGESTANTS + EXPECTORANTS						
Children's Mucinex Congestion & Cough Liquid			Dextromethorphan HBr 5mg/5mL	Phenylephrine 2.5mg/5mL	Guaifenesin 100mg/5mL	**Peds 6-<12 yrs:** 2 tsp (10mL) q4h. **Peds 4-<6 yrs:** 1 tsp (5mL) q4h. **Max:** 6 doses/24h.
Children's Mucinex Multi-Symptom Cold Liquid			Dextromethorphan HBr 5mg/5mL	Phenylephrine 2.5mg/5mL	Guaifenesin 100mg/5mL	**Peds 6-<12 yrs:** 2 tsp (10mL) q4h. **Peds 4-<6 yrs:** 1 tsp (5mL) q4h. **Max:** 6 doses/24h.
Children's Robitussin Cough & Cold CF Liquid			Dextromethorphan HBr 10mg/10mL	Phenylephrine HCl 5mg/10mL	Guaifenesin 100mg/10mL	**Adults & Peds ≥12 yrs:** 4 tsp (20mL) q4h. **Peds 6-<12 yrs:** 2 tsp (10mL) q4h. **Max:** 6 doses/24h.
Maximum Strength Mucinex Fast-Max Severe Congestion & Cough Caplets			Dextromethorphan HBr 10mg	Phenylephrine HCl 5mg	Guaifenesin 200mg	**Adults & Peds ≥12 yrs:** 2 tabs q4h. **Max:** 12 tabs/24h.
Maximum Strength Mucinex Fast-Max Severe Congestion & Cough Liquid			Dextromethorphan HBr 20mg/20mL	Phenylephrine HCl 10mg/20mL	Guaifenesin 400mg/20mL	**Adults & Peds ≥12 yrs:** 4 tsp (20mL) q4h. **Max:** 6 doses/24h.

BRAND NAME	ANALGESIC	ANTIHISTAMINE	COUGH SUPPRESSANT	DECONGESTANT	EXPECTORANT	DOSAGE
COUGH SUPPRESSANTS + DECONGESTANTS + EXPECTORANTS *(Continued)*						
Robitussin Peak Cold Maximum Strength Multi-Symptom Cold CF Liquid			Dextromethorphan HBr 20mg/10mL	Phenylephrine HCl 10mg/10mL	Guaifenesin 400mg/10mL	**Adults & Peds ≥12 yrs:** 2 tsp (10mL) q4h. **Max:** 6 doses/24h.
Robitussin Peak Cold Multi-Symptom Cold CF Liquid			Dextromethorphan HBr 20mg/10mL	Phenylephrine HCl 10mg/10mL	Guaifenesin 200mg/10mL	**Adults & Peds ≥12 yrs:** 2 tsp (10mL) q4h. **Max:** 6 doses/24h.
COUGH SUPPRESSANTS + EXPECTORANTS						
Alka-Seltzer Plus Max Cough, Mucus & Congestion Liquid Gels			Dextromethorphan HBr 10mg		Guaifenesin 200mg	**Adults & Peds ≥12 yrs:** 2 caps q4h. **Max:** 12 caps/24h.
Children's Delsym Cough+ Chest Congestion DM Liquid			Dextromethorphan HBr 5mg/5mL		Guaifenesin 100mg/5mL	**Adults & Peds ≥12 yrs:** 2-4 tsp (10-20mL) q4h. **Peds 6-<12 yrs:** 1-2 tsp (5-10mL) q4h. **Peds 4-<6 yrs:** ½-1 tsp (2.5-5mL) q4h. **Max:** 6 doses/24h.
Children's Mucinex Cough Liquid			Dextromethorphan HBr 5mg/5mL		Guaifenesin 100mg/5mL	**Peds 6-<12 yrs:** 1-2 tsp (5-10mL) q4h. **Peds 4-<6 yrs:** ½-1 tsp (2.5-5mL) q4h. **Max:** 6 doses/24h.
Children's Mucinex Cough Mini-Melts			Dextromethorphan HBr 5mg/packet		Guaifenesin 100mg/packet	**Adults & Peds ≥12 yrs:** 2-4 pkts q4h. **Peds 6-<12 yrs:** 1-2 pkts q4h. **Peds 4-<6 yrs:** 1 pkt q4h. **Max:** 6 doses/24h.
Children's Robitussin Cough & Chest Congestion DM Liquid			Dextromethorphan HBr 5mg/5mL		Guaifenesin 100mg/5mL	**Adults & Peds ≥12 yrs:** 2-4 tsp (10-20mL) q4h. **Peds 6-<12 yrs:** 1-2 tsp (5-10mL) q4h. **Max:** 6 doses/24h.
Coricidin HBP Chest Congestion & Cough Softgels			Dextromethorphan HBr 10mg		Guaifenesin 200mg	**Adults & Peds ≥12 yrs:** 1-2 caps q4h. **Max:** 12 caps/24h.
Delsym Cough+ Chest Congestion DM Liquid			Dextromethorphan HBr 20mg/20mL		Guaifenesin 400mg/20mL	**Adults & Peds ≥12 yrs:** 4 tsp (20mL) q4h. **Max:** 6 doses/24h.

(Continued)

BRAND NAME	ANALGESIC	ANTIHISTAMINE	COUGH SUPPRESSANT	DECONGESTANT	EXPECTORANT	DOSAGE
COUGH SUPPRESSANTS + EXPECTORANTS *(Continued)*						
Maximum Strength Mucinex DM Tablets			Dextromethorphan HBr 60mg		Guaifenesin 1200mg	**Adults & Peds ≥12 yrs:** 1 tab q12h. **Max:** 2 tabs/24h.
Maximum Strength Mucinex Fast-Max DM Max Liquid			Dextromethorphan HBr 20mg/20mL		Guaifenesin 400mg/20mL	**Adults & Peds ≥12 yrs:** 4 tsp (20mL) q4h. **Max:** 6 doses/24h.
Mucinex DM Tablets			Dextromethorphan HBr 30mg		Guaifenesin 600mg	**Adults & Peds ≥12 yrs:** 1-2 tabs q12h. **Max:** 4 tabs/24h
PediaCare Cough & Congestion Liquid			Dextromethorphan HBr 5mg/5mL		Guaifenesin 100mg/5mL	**Peds 6-11 yrs (48-95 lbs):** 1-2 tsp (5-10mL). **Peds 4-6 yrs (36-47 lbs):** ½-1 tsp (2.5-5mL). **Max:** 6 doses/24h.
Robitussin Maximum Strength Cough + Chest Congestion DM Liquid-Filled Capsules			Dextromethorphan HBr 10mg		Guaifenesin 200mg	**Adults & Peds ≥12 yrs:** 2 caps q4h. **Max:** 12 caps/24h.
Robitussin Peak Cold Cough + Chest Congestion DM Liquid			Dextromethorphan HBr 20mg/10mL		Guaifenesin 200mg/10mL	**Adults & Peds ≥12 yrs:** 2 tsp (10mL) q4h. **Max:** 6 doses/24h.
Robitussin Peak Cold Maximum Strength Cough + Chest Congestion DM Liquid			Dextromethorphan HBr 20mg/10mL		Guaifenesin 400mg/10mL	**Adults & Peds ≥12 yrs:** 2 tsp (10mL) q4h. **Max:** 6 doses/24h.
Robitussin Peak Cold Sugar-Free Cough + Chest Congestion DM Liquid			Dextromethorphan HBr 20mg/10mL		Guaifenesin 200mg/10mL	**Adults & Peds ≥12 yrs:** 2 tsp (10mL) q4h. **Max:** 6 doses/24h.
Triaminic Cough & Congestion Syrup			Dextromethorphan HBr 5mg/5mL		Guaifenesin 100mg/5mL	**Peds 6-<12 yrs:** 1-2 tsp (5-10mL) q4h. **Peds 4-<6 yrs:** ½-1 tsp (2.5-5mL) q4h. **Max:** 6 doses/24h.
Vicks DayQuil Mucus Control DM Liquid			Dextromethorphan HBr 10mg/15mL		Guaifenesin 200mg/15mL	**Adults & Peds ≥12 yrs:** 2 tbl (30mL) q4h. **Peds 6-<12 yrs:** 1 tbl (15mL) q4h. **Max:** 6 doses/24h.
DECONGESTANTS§						
Children's Sudafed Nasal Decongestant Liquid				Pseudoephedrine HCl 15mg/5mL		**Peds 6-11 yrs:** 2 tsp (10mL) q4-6h. **Peds 4-5 yrs:** 1 tsp (5mL) q4-6h. **Max:** 4 doses/24h.

BRAND NAME	ANALGESIC	ANTIHISTAMINE	COUGH SUPPRESSANT	DECONGESTANT	EXPECTORANT	DOSAGE
DECONGESTANTS[§] *(Continued)*						
Children's Sudafed PE Nasal Decongestant Liquid				Phenylephrine HCl 2.5mg/5mL		**Peds 6-11 yrs:** 2 tsp (10mL) q4h. **Peds 4-5 yrs:** 1 tsp (5mL) q4h. **Max:** 6 doses/24h.
Sudafed 12 Hour Tablets				Pseudoephedrine HCl 120mg		**Adults & Peds ≥12 yrs:** 1 tab q12h. **Max:** 2 tabs/24h.
Sudafed 24 Hour Tablets				Pseudoephedrine HCl 240mg		**Adults & Peds ≥12 yrs:** 1 tab/24h. **Max:** 1 tab/24h.
Sudafed Congestion Tablets				Pseudoephedrine HCl 30mg		**Adults & Peds ≥12 yrs:** 2 tabs q4-6h. **Max:** 8 tabs/24h. **Peds 6-11 yrs:** 1 tab q4-6h. **Max:** 4 tabs/24h.
Sudafed PE Congestion Tablets				Phenylephrine HCl 10mg		**Adults & Peds ≥12 yrs:** 1 tab q4h. **Max:** 6 tabs/24h.
DECONGESTANTS + EXPECTORANTS						
Children's Mucinex Stuffy Nose & Cold Liquid				Phenylephrine HCl 2.5mg/5mL	Guaifenesin 100mg/5mL	**Peds 6-<12 yrs:** 2 tsp (10mL) q4h. **Peds 4-<6 yrs:** 1 tsp (5mL) q4h. **Max:** 6 doses/24h.
Maximum Strength Mucinex D Tablets				Pseudoephedrine HCl 120mg	Guaifenesin 1200mg	**Adults & Peds ≥12 yrs:** 1 tab q12h. **Max:** 2 tabs/24h.
Mucinex D Tablets				Pseudoephedrine HCl 60mg	Guaifenesin 600mg	**Adults & Peds ≥12 yrs:** 2 tabs q12h. **Max:** 4 tabs/24h.
Sudafed PE Non-Drying Sinus Caplets*				Phenylephrine HCl 5mg	Guaifenesin 200mg	**Adults & Peds ≥12 yrs:** 2 tabs q4h. **Max:** 12 tabs/24h.
EXPECTORANTS						
Children's Mucinex Chest Congestion Liquid					Guaifenesin 100mg/5mL	**Peds 6-<12 yrs:** 1-2 tsp (5-10mL) q4h. **Peds 4-<6 yrs:** ½-1 tsp (2.5-5mL) q4h. **Max:** 6 doses/24h.

(Continued)

BRAND NAME	ANALGESIC	ANTIHISTAMINE	COUGH SUPPRESSANT	DECONGESTANT	EXPECTORANT	DOSAGE
EXPECTORANTS *(Continued)*						
Children's Mucinex Chest Congestion Mini-Melts					Guaifenesin 100mg/packet	**Adults & Peds ≥12 yrs:** 2-4 pkts q4h. **Peds 6-<12 yrs:** 1-2 pkts q4h. **Peds 4-<6 yrs:** 1 pkt q4h. **Max:** 6 doses/24h.
Maximum Strength Mucinex Tablets					Guaifenesin 1200mg	**Adults & Peds ≥12 yrs:** 1 tab q12h. **Max:** 2 tabs/24h.
Mucinex Tablets					Guaifenesin 600mg	**Adults & Peds ≥12 yrs:** 1-2 tabs q12h. **Max:** 4 tabs/24h.
Robitussin Mucus + Chest Congestion Liquid					Guaifenesin 200mg/10mL	**Adults & Peds ≥12 yrs:** 2-4 tsp (10-20mL) q4h. **Max:** 6 doses/24h.
MISCELLANEOUS[¶]						
Vicks BabyRub Soothing Ointment						**Peds ≥3 months:** Gently massage on the chest, neck, and back to help soothe and comfort.
Vicks VapoDrops[‡]						**Adults & Peds ≥5 yrs:** 3 drops (cherry) or 2 drops (menthol) in the mouth.
Vicks VapoRub Ointment						**Adults & Peds ≥2 yrs:** Rub on chest and throat. **Max:** 3-4 times/24h.
Vicks VapoSteam (For use in a hot steam vaporizer)						**Adults & Peds ≥2 yrs:** 1 tbl per quart of water or 1½ tsp per pint of water. **Max:** 3 times/24h.

*Product currently on recall or temporarily unavailable from manufacturer, but generic forms may be available.

[†]Fully dissolve tablets in 4 oz of water.

[‡]Multiple flavors available.

[§]Refer to *Nasal Preparations* table for additional decongestants.

[¶]Refer to packaging for ingredients.

Nasal Preparations

BRAND	INGREDIENT(S)/STRENGTH(S)	DOSAGE
TOPICAL NASAL DECONGESTANTS		
Afrin NoDrip Extra Moisturizing Pump Mist	Oxymetazoline HCl 0.05%	**Adults & Peds ≥6 yrs:** 2-3 sprays per nostril not more than q10-12h. **Max:** 2 doses q24h.*
Afrin NoDrip Original Pump Mist	Oxymetazoline HCl 0.05%	**Adults & Peds ≥6 yrs:** 2-3 sprays per nostril not more than q10-12h. **Max:** 2 doses q24h.*
Afrin NoDrip Severe Congestion Pump Mist	Oxymetazoline HCl 0.05%	**Adults & Peds ≥6 yrs:** 2-3 sprays per nostril not more than q10-12h. **Max:** 2 doses q24h.*
Afrin NoDrip Sinus Pump Mist	Oxymetazoline HCl 0.05%	**Adults & Peds ≥6 yrs:** 2-3 sprays per nostril not more than q10-12h. **Max:** 2 doses q24h.*
Afrin Original Nasal Spray	Oxymetazoline HCl 0.05%	**Adults & Peds ≥6 yrs:** 2-3 sprays per nostril not more than q10-12h. **Max:** 2 doses q24h.*
Afrin Original Pump Mist	Oxymetazoline HCl 0.05%	**Adults & Peds ≥6 yrs:** 2-3 sprays per nostril not more than q10-12h. **Max:** 2 doses q24h.*
Afrin Severe Congestion Nasal Spray	Oxymetazoline HCl 0.05%	**Adults & Peds ≥6 yrs:** 2-3 sprays per nostril not more than q10-12h. **Max:** 2 doses q24h.*
Afrin Sinus Nasal Spray	Oxymetazoline HCl 0.05%	**Adults & Peds ≥6 yrs:** 2-3 sprays per nostril not more than q10-12h. **Max:** 2 doses q24h.*
Benzedrex Inhaler	Propylhexedrine 250mg	**Adults & Peds ≥6 yrs:** 2 inhalations per nostril not more than q2h.*
Dristan 12-Hr Nasal Spray	Oxymetazoline HCl 0.05%	**Adults & Peds ≥12 yrs:** 2-3 sprays per nostril not more than q10-12h. **Max:** 2 doses q24h.*
Little Remedies Decongestant Nose Drops	Phenylephrine HCl 0.125%	**Peds 2-<6 yrs:** 2-3 drops per nostril not more than q4h.*
Mucinex Sinus-Max Full Force Nasal Spray	Oxymetazoline HCl 0.05%	**Adults & Peds ≥6 yrs:** 2-3 sprays per nostril not more than q10-12h. **Max:** 2 doses q24h.*
Mucinex Sinus-Max Moisture Smart Nasal Spray	Oxymetazoline HCl 0.05%	**Adults & Peds ≥6 yrs:** 2-3 sprays per nostril not more than q10-12h. **Max:** 2 doses q24h.*
NeilMed Sinu Inhaler	Levmetamfetamine 50mg	**Adults & Peds ≥12 yrs:** 2 inhalations per nostril not more than q2h.† **Peds 6-<12 yrs:** 1 inhalation per nostril not more than q2h.†
NeilMed SinuFrin Nasal Spray	Oxymetazoline HCl 0.05%	**Adults & Peds ≥6 yrs:** 2 sprays per nostril not more than q10-12h. **Max:** 2 doses q24h.*
NeilMed SinuFrin Plus Moisturizing Gel	Oxymetazoline HCl 0.05%	**Adults & Peds ≥6 yrs:** 2 sprays per nostril not more than q10-12h. **Max:** 2 doses q24h.*
Neo-Synephrine Cold & Sinus Extra Strength Nasal Spray	Phenylephrine HCl 1%	**Adults & Peds ≥12 yrs:** 2-3 sprays per nostril not more than q4h.*
Neo-Synephrine Cold & Sinus Mild Strength Nasal Spray	Phenylephrine HCl 0.25%	**Adults & Peds ≥6 yrs:** 2-3 sprays per nostril not more than q4h.*
Neo-Synephrine Cold & Sinus Regular Strength Nasal Spray	Phenylephrine HCl 0.5%	**Adults & Peds ≥12 yrs:** 2-3 sprays per nostril not more than q4h.*
Nostrilla Original Fast Relief Nasal Spray	Oxymetazoline HCl 0.05%	**Adults & Peds ≥6 yrs:** 2-3 sprays per nostril not more than q10-12h. **Max:** 2 doses q24h.*
Privine Nasal Drops	Naphazoline HCl 0.05%	**Adults & Peds ≥12 yrs:** 1-2 drops per nostril not more than q6h.*

(Continued)

BRAND	INGREDIENT(S)/STRENGTH(S)	DOSAGE
TOPICAL NASAL DECONGESTANTS *(Continued)*		
QlearQuil 12 Hour Nasal Decongestant Moisturizing Nasal Spray	Oxymetazoline HCl 0.05%	**Adults & Peds ≥6 yrs:** 2-3 sprays per nostril not more than q10-12h. **Max:** 2 doses q24h.*
Vicks Sinex 12-Hour Decongestant Nasal Spray	Oxymetazoline HCl 0.05%	**Adults & Peds ≥6 yrs:** 2-3 sprays per nostril not more than q10-12h. **Max:** 2 doses q24h.*
Vicks Sinex 12-Hour Decongestant UltraFine Mist Moisturizing Nasal Spray	Oxymetazoline HCl 0.05%	**Adults & Peds ≥6 yrs:** 2-3 sprays per nostril not more than q10-12h. **Max:** 2 doses q24h.*
Vicks Sinex 12-Hour Decongestant UltraFine Mist Nasal Spray	Oxymetazoline HCl 0.05%	**Adults & Peds ≥6 yrs:** 2-3 sprays per nostril not more than q10-12h. **Max:** 2 doses q24h.*
Zicam Extreme Congestion Relief Nasal Gel	Oxymetazoline HCl 0.05%	**Adults & Peds ≥6 yrs:** 2-3 sprays per nostril not more than q10-12h. **Max:** 2 doses q24h.*
Zicam Intense Sinus Relief Nasal Gel	Oxymetazoline HCl 0.05%	**Adults & Peds ≥6 yrs:** 2-3 sprays per nostril not more than q10-12h. **Max:** 2 doses q24h.*
TOPICAL NASAL MOISTURIZERS		
Ayr Allergy & Sinus Hypertonic Saline Nasal Mist	Sodium chloride 2.65%‡	**Adults & Peds ≥6 yrs:** 2 sprays per nostril bid-tid prn.
Ayr Saline Nasal Drops	Sodium chloride 0.65%	**Adults & Peds:** 2-6 drops per nostril prn.
Ayr Saline Nasal Gel	Sodium chloride‡	**Adults & Peds:** Apply around nostrils and under nose during the day and hs prn.
Ayr Saline Nasal Gel No-Drip Sinus Spray	Sodium chloride‡	**Adults & Peds:** 1 spray per nostril prn.
Ayr Saline Nasal Mist	Sodium chloride 0.65%‡	**Adults & Peds:** Use ud.
Ayr Saline Nasal Neti Rinse Kit	Sodium chloride‡	**Adults & Peds ≥6 yrs:** Use qd-bid or ud.
Ayr Saline Nasal Rinse Kit & Refills	Sodium chloride‡	**Adults & Peds ≥6 yrs:** Use qd-bid or ud.
Baby Ayr Saline Nose Spray/ Drops	Sodium chloride 0.65%‡	**Peds:** 2-6 drops/sprays per nostril.
Little Remedies Saline Spray/ Drops	Sodium chloride‡	**Adults & Peds:** 2-6 drops/sprays per nostril prn or ud.
Little Remedies Sterile Saline Nasal Mist	Sodium chloride	**Adults & Peds:** 1-3 short sprays per nostril.
Little Remedies Stuffy Nose Kit	Sodium chloride‡	**Adults & Peds:** 2-6 drops/sprays per nostril prn or ud.
NeilMed NasaMist Extra Strength Nasal Spray	Sodium chloride 2.7%	**Adults & Peds ≥6 months:** Spray into each nostril prn.
NeilMed NasaMist Nasal Spray	Sodium chloride	**Adults & Peds ≥1 yr:** Use ud.
NeilMed NasoGel Spray	Sodium chloride‡	**Adults & Peds:** 1-2 sprays per nostril q4-6h.
Ocean Complete Sinus Rinse	Sodium chloride‡	**Adults & Peds:** Use ud.
Ocean Gel Nasal Moisturizer	Purified water, Glycerin, Carbomer 940, Trolamine, Hyaluronan, Methylparaben, Propylparaben	**Adults & Peds:** Apply to affected areas in and around the nose prn.
Ocean for Kids Saline Nasal Spray	Sodium chloride 0.65%‡	**Peds:** 2 sprays/drops per nostril prn.
Ocean Saline Nasal Spray	Sodium chloride 0.65%‡	**Adults & Peds:** 2 sprays/drops per nostril prn.
Simply Saline Allergy & Sinus Relief	Sodium chloride‡	**Adults:** Spray into each nostril prn.
Simply Saline Baby Nasal Moisturizer plus Aloe Vera	Sodium chloride‡	**Peds:** Apply around the nose prn.

BRAND	INGREDIENT(S)/STRENGTH(S)	DOSAGE
TOPICAL NASAL MOISTURIZERS *(Continued)*		
Simply Saline Baby Nasal Relief	Sodium chloride 0.9%‡	**Peds:** Spray into each nostril prn.
Simply Saline Baby Swabs	Sodium chloride‡	**Peds:** Apply in nostrils prn.
Simply Saline Extra Strength Nighttime Formula plus Eucalyptus	Sodium chloride‡	**Adults & Peds ≥2 yrs:** Spray into each nostril hs prn.
Simply Saline Nasal Relief	Sodium chloride 0.9%‡	**Adults & Peds:** Spray into each nostril prn.
Simply Saline Neti Pot Kit	Sodium chloride‡	**Adults & Peds ≥5 yrs:** Use qd-bid or ud.
MISCELLANEOUS		
Nasacort Allergy 24HR Nasal Spray	Triamcinolone acetonide 55mcg	**Adults & Peds ≥12 yrs:** 2 sprays per nostril qd; reduce to 1 spray per nostril qd if symptoms improve. **Peds 6-<12 yrs:** 1-2 sprays per nostril qd; reduce to 1 spray per nostril qd if symptoms improve. **Peds 2-<6 yrs:** 1 spray per nostril qd.
NasalCrom Nasal Allergy Spray	Cromolyn sodium 5.2mg	**Adults & Peds ≥2 yrs:** 1 spray per nostril q4-6h. **Max:** 6 doses q24h.
Similasan Nasal Allergy Relief Nasal Mist	*Cardiospermum* 6X, *Galphimia glauca* 6X, *Luffa operculata* 6X, *Sabadilla* 6X	**Adults & Peds:** 1-3 sprays per nostril prn.
Similasan Sinus Relief Nasal Mist	Kalium bichromicum 6X, *Luffa operculata* 6X, *Sabadilla* 6X	**Adults & Peds:** 1-3 sprays per nostril prn.
Simply Saline Children's Cold Formula plus Moisturizers Nasal Mist	*Luffa operculata* 6X, *Sabadilla* 6X	**Adults & Peds ≥2 yrs:** Use prn.†
Simply Saline Cold Formula plus Menthol Nasal Mist	*Luffa operculata* 6X, *Sabadilla* 6X	**Adults & Peds ≥2 yrs:** Use prn.†
SinoFresh Nasal & Sinus Care Nasal Spray	*Eucalyptus globulus* 20X, Kalium bichromicum 30X	**Adults & Peds ≥12 yrs:** 1-2 sprays per nostril in the morning and evening.
Zicam Allergy Relief Nasal Gel	*Luffa operculata* (4X, 12X, 30X), *Galphimia glauca* (12X, 30X), Histaminum hydrochloricum (12X, 30X, 200X), *Sulphur* (12X, 30X, 200X)	**Adults & Peds ≥12 yrs:** 1 pump per nostril q4h.
Zicam Cold Remedy Nasal Spray	*Galphimia glauca* 4X, *Luffa operculata* 4X, *Sabadilla* 4X	**Adults and Peds ≥12 yrs:** 2 pumps per nostril q3h. **Max:** 5 doses q24h.†

*Do not use for more than 3 days.

†Do not use for more than 7 days.

‡This product contains multiple ingredients. Please check product label for a complete list of ingredients.

Aspirin Products

BRAND	INGREDIENT(S)/STRENGTH(S)	DOSAGE
SALICYLATES		
Bayer Advanced Aspirin Extra Strength Tablets	Aspirin 500mg	**Adults & Peds ≥12 yrs:** 1-2 tabs q4-6h. **Max:** 8 tabs/24h.
Bayer Aspirin Extra Strength Caplets	Aspirin 500mg	**Adults & Peds ≥12 yrs:** 1-2 tabs q4-6h. **Max:** 8 tabs/24h.
Bayer Aspirin Safety Coated Caplets	Aspirin 325mg	**Adults & Peds ≥12 yrs:** 1-2 tabs q4h. **Max:** 12 tabs/24h.
Bayer Genuine Aspirin Tablets	Aspirin 325mg	**Adults & Peds ≥12 yrs:** 1-2 tabs q4h or 3 tabs q6h. **Max:** 12 tabs/24h.
Bayer Low Dose Aspirin Chewable Tablets*	Aspirin 81mg	**Adults & Peds ≥12 yrs:** 4-8 tabs q4h. **Max:** 48 tabs/24h.
Bayer Low Dose Aspirin Safety Coated Tablets	Aspirin 81mg	**Adults & Peds ≥12 yrs:** 4-8 tabs q4h. **Max:** 48 tabs/24h.
Ecotrin Low Strength Tablets	Aspirin 81mg	**Adults & Peds ≥12 yrs:** 4-8 tabs q4h prn. **Max:** 48 tabs/24h.
Ecotrin Regular Strength Tablets	Aspirin 325mg	**Adults & Peds ≥12 yrs:** 1-2 tabs q4h prn. **Max:** 12 tabs/24h.
St. Joseph Aspirin Chewable Tablets	Aspirin 81mg	**Adults & Peds ≥12 yrs:** 4-8 tabs q4h. **Max:** 48 tabs/24h.
St. Joseph Rapid Dissolving Melts	Aspirin 81mg	**Adults & Peds ≥12 yrs:** 4-8 tabs q4h. **Max:** 48 tabs/24h.
St. Joseph Regular Strength Safety Coated Tablets	Aspirin 325mg	**Adults & Peds ≥12 yrs:** 1-2 tabs q4h prn. **Max:** 12 tabs/24h.
St. Joseph Safety Coated Low Dose Tablets	Aspirin 81mg	**Adults & Peds ≥12 yrs:** 4-8 tabs q4h. **Max:** 48 tabs/24h.
UrgentRx Critical Care Aspirin To-Go Powder	Aspirin 325mg	**Adults & Peds ≥12 yrs:** Place 1-2 powders on tongue q4-6h prn. Swallow with or without water. **Max:** 8 powders/24h.
SALICYLATES, BUFFERED		
Alka-Seltzer Extra Strength Effervescent Tablets	Aspirin/Citric acid/Sodium bicarbonate 500mg-1000mg-1985mg	**Adults ≥60 yrs:** 2 tabs dissolved in 4 oz water q6h. **Max:** 3 tabs/24h. **Adults & Peds ≥12 yrs:** 2 tabs dissolved in 4 oz water q6h. **Max:** 7 tabs/24h.
Alka-Seltzer Lemon Lime Effervescent Tablets	Aspirin/Citric acid/Sodium bicarbonate 325mg-1000mg-1700mg	**Adults ≥60 yrs:** 2 tabs dissolved in 4 oz water q4h. **Max:** 4 tabs/24h. **Adults & Peds ≥12 yrs:** 2 tabs dissolved in 4 oz water q4h. **Max:** 8 tabs/24h.
Alka-Seltzer Original Effervescent Tablets	Aspirin/Citric acid/Sodium bicarbonate 325mg-1000mg-1916mg	**Adults ≥60 yrs:** 2 tabs dissolved in 4 oz water q4h. **Max:** 4 tabs/24h. **Adults & Peds ≥12 yrs:** 2 tabs dissolved in 4 oz water q4h. **Max:** 8 tabs/24h.
Bayer Aspirin Extra Strength Plus Caplets	Aspirin 500mg buffered with Calcium carbonate	**Adults & Peds ≥12 yrs:** 1-2 tabs q4-6h. **Max:** 8 tabs/24h.
Bayer Women's Low Dose Aspirin Caplets	Aspirin 81mg buffered with Calcium carbonate 777mg	**Adults & Peds ≥12 yrs:** 4-8 tabs q4h. **Max:** 10 tabs/24h.
Bufferin Tablets	Aspirin 325mg buffered with Calcium carbonate/Magnesium carbonate/Magnesium oxide	**Adults & Peds ≥12 yrs:** 2 tabs q4h prn. **Max:** 12 tabs/24h.
SALICYLATE COMBINATIONS		
Anacin Caplets	Aspirin/Caffeine 400mg-32mg	**Adults & Peds ≥12 yrs:** 2 tabs q6h. **Max:** 8 tabs/24h.

(Continued)

BRAND	INGREDIENT(S)/STRENGTH(S)	DOSAGE
SALICYLATE COMBINATIONS *(Continued)*		
Anacin Max Strength Tablets	Aspirin/Caffeine 500mg-32mg	**Adults & Peds ≥12 yrs:** 2 tabs q6h. **Max:** 8 tabs/24h.
Anacin Tablets	Aspirin/Caffeine 400mg-32mg	**Adults & Peds ≥12 yrs:** 2 tabs q6h. **Max:** 8 tabs/24h.
Bayer Back & Body Extra Strength Caplets	Aspirin/Caffeine 500mg-32.5mg	**Adults & Peds ≥12 yrs:** 2 tabs q6h. **Max:** 8 tabs/24h.
Bayer Headache Relief Caplets	Aspirin/Caffeine 500mg-32.5mg	**Adults & Peds ≥12 yrs:** 2 tabs q6h. **Max:** 8 tabs/24h.
Bayer Migraine Formula Caplets	Aspirin/Acetaminophen/Caffeine 250mg-250mg-65mg	**Adults:** 2 tabs qd. **Max:** 2 tabs/24h.
BC Arthritis Strength Powder	Aspirin/Caffeine 1000mg-65mg per powder	**Adults & Peds ≥12 yrs:** Place 1 powder on tongue q6h prn. May stir powder into glass of water. **Max:** 4 powders/24h.
BC Powder*	Aspirin/Caffeine 845mg-65mg per powder	**Adults & Peds ≥12 yrs:** Place 1 powder on tongue q6h prn. May stir powder into glass of water. **Max:** 4 powders/24h.
Excedrin Extra Strength Caplets	Acetaminophen/Aspirin/Caffeine 250mg-250mg-65mg	**Adults & Peds ≥12 yrs:** 2 tabs q6h. **Max:** 8 tabs/24h.
Excedrin Migraine Caplets	Acetaminophen/Aspirin/Caffeine 250mg-250mg-65mg	**Adults:** 2 tabs prn. **Max:** 2 tabs/24h.
Goody's Back & Body Pain Powder	Acetaminophen/Aspirin 325mg-500mg	**Adults & Peds ≥12 yrs:** Place 1 powder on tongue q6h prn. May stir powder into glass of water. **Max:** 4 powders/24h.
Goody's Cool Orange Extra Strength Headache Powder	Acetaminophen/Aspirin/Caffeine 325mg-500mg-65mg	**Adults & Peds ≥12 yrs:** Place 1 powder on tongue q6h prn. May stir powder into glass of water. **Max:** 4 powders/24h.
Goody's Extra Strength Caplets	Acetaminophen/Aspirin/Caffeine 250mg-250mg-65mg	**Adults & Peds ≥12 yrs:** 2 tabs q6h. **Max:** 8 tabs/24h.
Goody's Extra Strength Headache Powder	Acetaminophen/Aspirin/Caffeine 260mg-520mg-32.5mg	**Adults & Peds ≥12 yrs:** Place 1 powder on tongue q6h prn. May stir powder into glass of water. **Max:** 4 powders/24h.
UrgentRx Ache & Pain Relief To-Go Powder	Aspirin/Caffeine 650mg-60mg	**Adults & Peds ≥12 yrs:** Place 1 powder on tongue q4-6h prn. Swallow with or without water. **Max:** 4 powders/24h.
SALICYLATES/SLEEP AIDS		
Bayer PM Caplets	Aspirin/Diphenhydramine citrate 500mg-38mg	**Adults & Peds ≥12 yrs:** 2 tabs hs prn.
Excedrin PM Headache Caplets	Acetaminophen/Aspirin/Diphenhydramine citrate 250mg-250mg-38mg	**Adults and Peds ≥12 yrs:** 2 tabs hs. **Max:** 2 tabs/24h.

*Multiple flavors available.

Commonly Used Herbal Products

NAME	ACCEPTED USES	UNPROVEN USES	INTERACTIONS
Aloe vera	**Topical:** Herpes simplex, resolution of psoriatic plaques, reduce desquamation, erythema, and infiltration **Oral:** Constipation	**Topical:** Burns, frostbite, sunburn, wound healing **Oral:** Diabetes, ulcerative colitis, hyperlipidemia	Antidiabetics, digoxin, diuretics, sevoflurane, stimulant laxatives, warfarin, decreased absorption of oral medications
Black cohosh	Menopausal symptoms (eg, hot flashes)	Labor induction, osteoporosis	Atorvastatin, cisplatin, drugs metabolized by the liver (CYP2D6 substrates), hepatotoxic drugs
Black psyllium	Constipation, hypercholesterolemia	Cancer, diabetes, diarrhea, irritable bowel syndrome	Antidiabetics, carbamazepine, digoxin, lithium
Capsicum	**Topical:** Pain, fibromyalgia, prurigo nodularis **Intranasal:** Cluster headache, perennial rhinitis (nonallergic, noninfectious)	**Oral:** Dyspepsia, peptic ulcers, swallowing dysfunction **Intranasal:** Migraine headaches, sinonasal polyposis, allergic rhinitis	Cocaine, ACE inhibitors, anticoagulants, antiplatelets, theophylline, coca
Chamomile	Colic, dyspepsia, oral mucositis	Restlessness, insomnia, menstrual cramps, diarrhea, fibromyalgia	Benzodiazepines, CNS depressants, contraceptives, drugs metabolized by the liver (CYP1A2, CYP3A4, CYP2C9, CYP2D6 substrates), estrogens, tamoxifen, warfarin
Cranberry	Urinary tract infections	Benign prostatic hyperplasia, urine deodorant	Drugs metabolized by the liver (CYP2C9 substrates), warfarin
Echinacea	**Oral:** Common cold, vaginal candidiasis	**Oral:** Influenza **Topical:** Superficial wounds, burns	Caffeine, drugs metabolized by the liver (CYP1A2, CYP3A4 substrates), etoposide, immunosuppressants, midazolam, warfarin
Eucalyptus	Bronchitis	Asthma, upper respiratory tract inflammation, wounds, burns, congestion, ulcers, acne, bleeding gums, bladder disease, diabetes, fever, flu, loss of appetite, arthritis pain, liver/gallbladder problems	Drugs metabolized by the liver (CYP1A2, CYP2C19, CYP2C9, CYP3A4 substrates), antidiabetics, herbs that contain hepatotoxic pyrrolizidine alkaloids
Evening primrose oil	Osteoporosis	Mastalgia, rheumatoid arthritis, Sjogren's syndrome, chronic fatigue syndrome	Anesthesia, anticoagulants, antiplatelets, phenothiazines
Feverfew	Migraine headaches	Fever, menstrual irregularities, arthritis, psoriasis, allergies, asthma, dizziness, nausea, vomiting, earache, cancer, common cold	Drugs metabolized by the liver (CYP1A2, CYP2C19, CYP2C9, CYP3A4 substrates), anticoagulants, antiplatelets
Flaxseed	Diabetes, hypercholesterolemia, systemic lupus erythematosus nephritis	Breast cancer, cardiovascular disease, colorectal cancer, constipation, endometrial cancer, lung cancer, mastalgia, prostate cancer, menopausal symptoms	Acetaminophen, antibiotics, anticoagulants, antiplatelets, antidiabetics, estrogens, furosemide, ketoprofen, metoprolol, decreased absorption of oral medications

(Continued)

NAME	ACCEPTED USES	UNPROVEN USES	INTERACTIONS
Garlic	**Oral:** Atherosclerosis, gastric cancer, hypertension, tick bites **Topical:** Tinea corporis (ringworm), tinea cruris (jock itch), tinea pedis (athlete's foot)	**Oral:** Benign prostatic hyperplasia, common cold, preeclampsia, prostate cancer **Topical:** Corns, warts	Anticoagulants, antiplatelets, contraceptives, cyclosporine, drugs metabolized by the liver (CYP2E1, CYP3A4 substrates), isoniazid, non-nucleoside reverse transcriptase inhibitors, saquinavir, warfarin
Ginger	Dysmenorrhea, morning sickness, osteoarthritis, postoperative nausea and vomiting, vertigo	Chemotherapy-induced nausea and vomiting, migraine headache, myalgia, rheumatoid arthritis	Anticoagulants, antiplatelets, antidiabetics, calcium channel blockers, phenprocoumon, warfarin
Ginkgo	Age-related memory impairment, anxiety, cognitive function, dementia, diabetic retinopathy, glaucoma, peripheral vascular disease, premenstrual syndrome, schizophrenia, vertigo	Age-related macular degeneration, anxiety, ADHD, colorectal cancer, fibromyalgia, hearing loss, ovarian cancer, radiation exposure, Raynaud's syndrome, stroke, vitiligo	Alprazolam, anticoagulants, antiplatelets, anticonvulsants, antidiabetics, buspirone, drugs metabolized by the liver (CYP1A2, CYP2C19, CYP2C9, CYP2D6, CYP3A4 substrates), efavirenz, fluoxetine, hydrochlorothiazide, ibuprofen, omeprazole, seizure threshold-lowering drugs, trazodone, St John's wort, warfarin
Ginseng	Diabetes, respiratory tract infections	ADHD, breast cancer	Antidiabetics, immunosuppressants, monoamine oxidase inhibitors, warfarin
Licorice	**Oral:** Dyspepsia **Topical:** Atopic dermatitis	**IV:** Hepatitis **Oral:** Hypercholesterolemia, irritable bowel syndrome, muscle cramps, peptic ulcers **Topical:** Bleeding, psoriasis	Cardiac glycoside-containing herbs (eg, digitalis), stimulant laxative herbs (eg, aloe), antihypertensives, cisplatin, corticosteroids, drugs metabolized by the liver (CYP2B6, CYP2C9, CYP3A4 substrates), digoxin, diuretics, estrogens, ethacrynic acid, furosemide, midazolam, warfarin, grapefruit juice, salt
Milk thistle	Diabetes, dyspepsia, menopausal symptoms	Alcohol-related liver disease, *Amanita* mushroom poisoning, hepatitis B or C, prostate cancer, toxin-induced liver damage	Antidiabetics, drugs metabolized by the liver (CYP2C9, CYP3A4, CYP2D6 substrates), estrogens, drugs that undergo glucuronidation (eg, metronidazole), HMG-CoA reductase inhibitors ("statins"), sirolimus, tamoxifen
Peppermint	**Rectal:** Barium enema-related colonic spasm **Oral:** Dyspepsia, irritable bowel syndrome **Topical:** Tension headache	**Topical:** Postherpetic neuralgia	Antacids, cyclosporine, drugs metabolized by the liver (CYP1A2, CYP2C19, CYP2C9, CYP3A4 substrates), H_2-blockers, proton pump inhibitors
Saw palmetto	Benign prostatic hyperplasia	Androgenic alopecia, prostate cancer, prostatitis and chronic pelvic pain syndrome	Anticoagulants, antiplatelets, contraceptives, estrogens
Senna	Constipation, bowel preparation	Hemorrhoids, irritable bowel syndrome, weight loss	Contraceptive drugs, digoxin, diuretics, estrogens, warfarin, horsetail, licorice, stimulant laxatives

NAME	ACCEPTED USES	UNPROVEN USES	INTERACTIONS
St. John's wort	Depression, menopausal symptoms, somatization disorder, wound healing	Obsessive-compulsive disorder, premenstrual syndrome, seasonal affective disorder	Numerous medications
Valerian	Insomnia	Anxiety, dysmenorrhea, dyssomnia, stress	Alcohol, alprazolam, drugs metabolized by the liver (CYP3A4 substrates), benzodiazepines, CNS depressants, herbs and supplements with sedative properties

Source: Jellin JM, Gregory PJ, et al. Natural Medicines Comprehensive Database. www.naturaldatabase.com. Accessed February 4, 2015.

ANGINA TREATMENT OPTIONS

GENERIC (BRAND)	HOW SUPPLIED	DOSAGE	RENAL/HEPATIC DOSAGE ADJUSTMENT
BETA BLOCKERS			
Atenolol (Tenormin)	**Tab:** 25mg, 50mg, 100mg	**Initial:** 50mg qd. **Titrate:** May increase to 100mg qd after 1 week. **Max:** 200mg qd.	Renal
Metoprolol succinate (Toprol-XL)	**Tab, ER:** 25mg, 50mg, 100mg, 200mg	**Initial:** 100mg qd. **Titrate:** May gradually increase weekly until optimum response is achieved or there is pronounced slowing of HR. **Max:** 400mg/day. Reduce dose gradually over 1-2 weeks if to be d/c.	Hepatic
Metoprolol tartrate (Lopressor)	**Tab:** (Lopressor) 50mg, 100mg, (generic) 25mg, 50mg, 100mg	**Initial:** 100mg/day in 2 divided doses. **Titrate:** May gradually increase weekly until optimum response is achieved or there is pronounced slowing of HR. **Effective Range:** 100-400mg/day. **Max:** 400mg/day. Reduce dose gradually over 1-2 weeks if to be d/c.	Hepatic
Nadolol (Corgard)	**Tab:** 20mg, 40mg, 80mg	**Initial:** 40mg qd. **Titrate:** May gradually increase in 40-80mg increments at 3- to 7-day intervals until optimum response is achieved or there is pronounced slowing of HR. **Maint: Usual:** 40 or 80mg qd. Doses up to 160 or 240mg qd may be needed. **Max:** 240mg/day. Reduce dose gradually over 1-2 weeks if to be d/c.	Renal
Propranolol HCl	**Sol:** 20mg/5mL, 40mg/5mL; **Tab:** 10mg, 20mg, 40mg, 60mg, 80mg	80-320mg/day given bid-qid. Reduce dose gradually over several weeks if to be d/c.	
Propranolol HCl (Inderal LA)	**Cap, ER:** 60mg, 80mg, 120mg, 160mg	**Initial:** 80mg qd. **Titrate:** May gradually increase at 3- to 7-day intervals until optimum response is achieved. **Maint:** 160mg qd. **Max:** 320mg/day. Reduce dose gradually over a few weeks if to be d/c.	
CALCIUM CHANNEL BLOCKERS (DIHYDROPYRIDINES)			
Amlodipine besylate (Norvasc)	**Tab:** 2.5mg, 5mg, 10mg	**Usual:** 5-10mg qd.	Hepatic
Nicardipine	**Cap:** 20mg, 30mg	**Initial:** 20mg tid. **Titrate:** Allow at least 3 days before increasing dose. **Effective Range:** 20-40mg tid.	Renal/Hepatic
Nifedipine (Procardia XL)	**Tab, ER:** 30mg, 60mg, 90mg	**Initial:** 30 or 60mg qd. **Titrate:** Increase over a 1- to 2-week period (usual), but may proceed more rapidly if symptoms warrant. **Max:** 120mg/day.	
CALCIUM CHANNEL BLOCKERS (NON-DIHYDROPYRIDINES)			
Diltiazem HCl (Cardizem CD, Cartia XT)	**Cap, ER:** (Cardizem CD/ Cartia XT) 120mg, 180mg, 240mg, 300mg; (Cardizem CD) 360mg	**Initial:** 120mg or 180mg qd. **Titrate:** Increase over a 1- to 2-week period when necessary. **Max:** 480mg qd.	
Diltiazem HCl (Cardizem LA)	**Tab, ER:** 120mg, 180mg, 240mg, 300mg, 360mg, 420mg	**Initial:** 180mg qd (am or hs). **Titrate:** Increase at 1- to 2-week intervals if adequate response is not achieved. **Max:** 360mg.	

(Continued)

GENERIC (BRAND)	HOW SUPPLIED	DOSAGE	RENAL/HEPATIC DOSAGE ADJUSTMENT
CALCIUM CHANNEL BLOCKERS (NON-DIHYDROPYRIDINES) *(Continued)*			
Diltiazem HCl (Cardizem)	**Tab:** (Cardizem) 30mg, 60mg, 120mg; (generic) 30mg, 60mg, 90mg, 120mg	**Initial:** 30mg qid (before meals and hs). **Titrate:** Increase gradually (given in divided doses tid-qid) at 1- to 2-day intervals until optimum response obtained. **Usual:** 180-360mg/day.	
Diltiazem HCl (Taztia XT, Tiazac)	**Cap, ER:** (Taztia XT) 120mg, 180mg, 240mg, 300mg, 360mg; (Tiazac) 120mg, 180mg, 240mg, 300mg, 360mg, 420mg	**Initial:** 120-180mg qd. **Titrate:** Increase over 1-2 weeks when necessary. **Max:** 540mg qd.	
Verapamil HCl (Calan)	**Tab:** 40mg, 80mg, 120mg	**Usual:** 80-120mg tid. Upward titration should be based on therapeutic efficacy and safety evaluated approximately 8 hrs after dosing. **Titrate:** May increase daily (eg, patients with unstable angina) or weekly, until optimum response is obtained.	Hepatic
Verapamil HCl (Covera-HS)	**Tab, ER:** 180mg, 240mg	**Initial:** 180mg qhs. **Titrate:** If inadequate response with 180mg, increase to 240mg qhs, then 360mg (two 180mg tab) qhs, then 480mg (two 240mg tab) qhs.	Hepatic
CALCIUM CHANNEL BLOCKERS/HMG COA REDUCTASE INHIBITORS			
Amlodipine besylate-Atorvastatin calcium (Caduet)	**Tab:** 2.5-10mg, 2.5-20mg, 2.5-40mg, 5-10mg, 5-20mg, 5-40mg, 5-80mg, 10-10mg, 10-20mg, 10-40mg, 10-80mg	**Initial:** 5-10mg or 5-20mg qd. **Max:** 10-80mg qd.	Hepatic
COAGULATION MODIFIERS			
Abciximab (ReoPro)	**Inj:** 2mg/mL	0.25mg/kg IV bolus followed by 10mcg/min infusion for 18-24 hrs, concluding 1 hr after PCI.	
Bivalirudin (Angiomax)	**Inj:** 250mg	Give with ASA (300-325mg/day). **Patients Without HIT/HITTS:** 0.75mg/kg IV bolus, then 1.75mg/kg/hr infusion for the duration of the PCI/PTCA procedure. An activated clotting time should be performed 5 min after the bolus dose and an additional 0.3mg/kg bolus should be given if needed. **Patients With HIT/HITTS:** 0.75mg/kg IV bolus, then 1.75mg/kg/hr infusion for the duration of the procedure. **Ongoing Treatment Post-Procedure:** Continuation of infusion following PCI/PTCA for up to 4 hrs post-procedure is optional. After 4 hrs, an additional infusion may be initiated at a rate of 0.2mg/kg/hr (low-rate infusion), for up to 20 hrs, if needed.	Renal
Clopidogrel bisulfate (Plavix)	**Tab:** 75mg, 300mg	**LD:** 300mg. **Maint:** 75mg qd. Initiate ASA (75-325mg qd) and continue in combination with clopidogrel.	

GENERIC (BRAND)	HOW SUPPLIED	DOSAGE	RENAL/HEPATIC DOSAGE ADJUSTMENT
COAGULATION MODIFIERS *(Continued)*			
Dalteparin sodium (Fragmin)	**Inj:** (Syringe) 2500 IU/0.2mL, 5000 IU/0.2mL, 7500 IU/0.3mL, 10,000 IU/0.4mL, 10,000 IU/1mL, 12,500 IU/0.5mL, 15,000 IU/0.6mL, 18,000 IU/0.72mL; (MDV) 95,000 IU/3.8mL, 95,000 IU/9.5mL	**Prophylaxis of Ischemic Complications in Unstable Angina:** 120 IU/kg q12h with PO ASA (75-165mg qd) until clinically stabilized. **Usual Duration:** 5-8 days. **Max:** 10,000 IU q12h.	Renal
Enoxaparin (Lovenox)	**Inj:** [100mg/mL] (Prefilled Syringe) 30mg/0.3mL, 40mg/0.4mL; (Graduated Prefilled Syringe) 60mg/0.6mL, 80mg/0.8mL, 100mg/mL; (MDV) 300mg/3mL; [150mg/mL] (Graduated Prefilled Syringe) 120mg/0.8mL, 150mg/mL	1mg/kg SQ q12h with PO ASA (100-325mg qd) until clinically stabilized. **Usual Duration:** 2-8 days (up to 12.5 days in clinical trials).	Renal
Prasugrel (Effient)	**Tab:** 5mg, 10mg	**LD:** 60mg. **Maint:** 10mg qd with ASA (75-325mg/day). **<60kg:** Consider lowering the maintenance dose to 5mg qd.	
Ticagrelor (Brilinta)	**Tab:** 90mg	**LD:** 180mg with ASA (usually 325mg). **Maint:** 90mg bid with ASA (75-100mg/day).	
VASODILATORS			
Isosorbide dinitrate (Dilatrate-SR)	**Cap, ER:** 40mg	40mg bid; separate doses by 6 hrs. **Max:** 160mg/day. Allow a dose-free interval of >18 hrs.	
Isosorbide mononitrate (Imdur)	**Tab, ER:** 30mg, 60mg, 120mg	**Initial:** 30mg (given as single tab or as ½ of a 60mg tab) or 60mg (given as single tab) qam on arising. **Titrate:** May increase to 120mg (given as single tab or as two 60mg tabs) qam after several days. Rarely, 240mg qam may be required.	
Isosorbide mononitrate (Monoket)	**Tab:** 10mg, 20mg	20mg bid (give doses 7 hrs apart). **Small Stature Patients: Initial:** 5mg (½ of a 10mg tab). **Titrate:** Increase to ≥10mg by 2nd or 3rd day.	
Nitroglycerin (Nitrolingual)	**Spray:** 400mcg/spray	**Acute Relief:** 1 or 2 sprays at the onset of attack onto or under the tongue. **Max:** 3 sprays/15 min. If chest pain persists, prompt medical attention is recommended. **Prophylaxis:** May be used 5-10 min prior to engaging in activities that might precipitate an acute attack.	

(Continued)

GENERIC (BRAND)	HOW SUPPLIED	DOSAGE	RENAL/HEPATIC DOSAGE ADJUSTMENT
VASODILATORS *(Continued)*			
Nitroglycerin (Nitromist)	**Spray:** 400mcg/spray	**Acute Relief:** 1 or 2 sprays at the onset of attack onto or under the tongue. May repeat every 5 min PRN. If 2 sprays are used initially, may only administer 1 more spray after 5 min. **Max:** 3 sprays/15 min. If chest pain persists after a total of 3 sprays, prompt medical attention is recommended. **Prophylaxis:** May be used 5-10 min before engaging in activities that might precipitate an acute attack.	
Nitroglycerin (Minitran, Nitro-Dur)	**Patch:** (Minitran) 0.1mg/hr, 0.2mg/hr, 0.4mg/hr, 0.6mg/hr; (Nitro-Dur) 0.1mg/hr, 0.2mg/hr, 0.3mg/hr, 0.4mg/hr, 0.6mg/hr, 0.8mg/hr	**Initial:** 0.2-0.4mg/hr patch for 12-14 hrs/day. Remove patch for 10-12 hrs/day.	
Nitroglycerin (Nitrostat)	**Tab, SL:** 0.3mg, 0.4mg, 0.6mg	**Acute Relief:** 1 tab SL or in buccal pouch at onset of attack. May repeat every 5 min until relief is obtained. If pain persists after a total of 3 tabs in 15 min, or if pain is different than typically experienced, prompt medical attention is recommended. **Prophylaxis:** May be used 5-10 min prior to engaging in activities that might precipitate an acute attack.	
Nitroglycerin (Nitro-Bid)	**Oint:** 2%	**Initial:** ½-inch (7.5mg) bid (one in the am and one 6 hrs later). **Titrate:** May increase to 1 inch bid, then to 2 inches bid. Allow a dose-free interval of 10-12 hrs.	
Nitroglycerin in 5% Dextrose	**Inj:** 100mcg/mL, 200mcg/mL, 400mcg/mL	**Initial:** 5mcg/min IV. **Titrate:** Increase by 5mcg/min at intervals of 3-5 min. If no response at 20mcg/min, may use increments of 10 and even 20mcg/min. Once some hemodynamic response is observed, dosage increments should be smaller and less frequent.	
MISCELLANEOUS			
Ranolazine (Ranexa)	**Tab, ER:** 500mg, 1000mg	**Initial:** 500mg bid. **Titrate:** May increase to 1000mg bid, PRN, based on clinical symptoms. **Max:** 1000mg bid.	

Refer to full FDA-approved labeling for additional product information.

Abbreviations: ASA = aspirin; HIT/HITTS = heparin-induced thrombocytopenia/heparin-induced thrombocytopenia and thrombosis syndrome; PCI = percutaneous coronary intervention; PTCA = percutaneous transluminal coronary angioplasty.

CHOLESTEROL-LOWERING AGENTS

GENERIC (BRAND)	HOW SUPPLIED (MG)*	USUAL DOSAGE RANGE†	T-CHOL (% DECREASE)	LDL (% DECREASE)	HDL (% INCREASE)	TG (% DECREASE)
HMG-COA REDUCTASE INHIBITORS (STATINS)						
Atorvastatin (Lipitor)	**Tab:** 10, 20, 40, 80	10-80mg/day	29 to 45	39 to 60	5 to 9	19 to 37
Fluvastatin (Lescol)	**Cap:** 20, 40	20-80mg/day	17 to 27	22 to 36	3 to 6	12 to 18
Fluvastatin (Lescol XL)	**Tab, ER:** 80	80mg/day	25	35	7	19
Lovastatin (Altoprev)	**Tab, ER:** 20, 40, 60	20-60mg/day	17.9 to 29.2	23.8 to 40.8	9.4 to 13.1	9.9 to 25.1
Lovastatin	**Tab:** 10, 20, 40	10-80mg/day	17 to 29	24 to 40	6.6 to 9.5	10 to 19
Pitavastatin (Livalo)	**Tab:** 1, 2, 4	1-4mg/day	23 to 31	32 to 43	5 to 8	15 to 19
Pravastatin (Pravachol)	**Tab:** 20, 40, 80	40-80mg/day	16 to 27	22 to 37	2 to 12	11 to 24
Pravastatin	**Tab:** 10, 20, 40, 80	40-80mg/day	16 to 27	22 to 37	2 to 12	11 to 24
Rosuvastatin (Crestor)	**Tab:** 5, 10, 20, 40	5-40mg/day	33 to 46	45 to 63	8 to 14	10 to 35
Simvastatin (Zocor)	**Tab:** 5, 10, 20, 40, 80	5-40mg/day	19 to 36	26 to 47	8 to 16	12 to 33
FIBRATES‡						
Fenofibrate (Antara)	**Cap:** 30, 90	30-90mg/day	16.8 to 22.4	20.1 to 31.4	9.8 to 14.6	23.5 to 35.9
Fenofibrate (Fenoglide)	**Tab:** 40, 120	40-120mg/day	16.8 to 22.4	20.1 to 31.4	9.8 to 14.6	23.5 to 35.9
Fenofibrate (Lipofen)	**Cap:** 50, 150	50-150mg/day	16.8 to 22.4	20.1 to 31.4	9.8 to 14.6	23.5 to 35.9
Fenofibrate (Lofibra)	**Tab:** 54, 160; **Cap:** 67, 134, 200	54-160mg/day, 67-200mg/day	16.8 to 22.4	20.1 to 31.4	9.8 to 14.6	23.5 to 35.9
Fenofibrate (Tricor)	**Tab:** 48, 145	48-145mg/day	16.8 to 22.4	20.1 to 31.4	9.8 to 14.6	23.5 to 35.9
Fenofibrate (Triglide)	**Tab:** 50, 160	50-160mg/day	16.8 to 22.4	20.1 to 31.4	9.8 to 14.6	23.5 to 35.9
Fenofibric acid (Fibricor)	**Tab:** 35, 105	35-105mg/day	16.8 to 22.4	20.1 to 31.4	9.8 to 14.6	23.5 to 35.9
Fenofibric acid (Trilipix)	**Cap, DR:** 45, 135	45-135mg/day	16.8 to 22.4	20.1 to 31.4	9.8 to 14.6	23.5 to 35.9
Gemfibrozil (Lopid)	**Tab:** 600	1200mg/day in divided doses	Moderate reduction	4.1	12.6	Significant reduction

(Continued)

GENERIC (BRAND)	HOW SUPPLIED (MG)*	USUAL DOSAGE RANGE†	T-CHOL (% DECREASE)	LDL (% DECREASE)	HDL (% INCREASE)	TG (% DECREASE)
BILE-ACID SEQUESTRANTS						
Cholestyramine (Prevalite)	**Powder for Oral Suspension:** 4g/packet or level scoopful	2-6 packets or level scoopfuls (8-24g)/day	7.2	10.4	N/A	N/A
Colesevelam HCl (Welchol)	**Tab:** 625; **Powder for Oral Suspension:** 3.75g packet, 1.875g packet	3750mg/day	7	15	3	+10
Colestipol HCl (Colestid)	**Granules for Suspension:** 5g/packet or level scoopful; **Tab:** 1000	**Granules for Suspension:** 1-6 packets or level scoopfuls/ day; **Tab:** 2-16g/day	N/A	N/A	N/A	N/A
CHOLESTEROL ABSORPTION INHIBITORS						
Ezetimibe (Zetia)	**Tab:** 10	10mg/day	13	18	1	8
NICOTINIC ACID DERIVATIVES						
Niacin, ER (Niaspan)	**Tab, ER:** 500, 750, 1000	1000-2000mg/ day	3 to 10	5 to 14	18 to 22	13 to 28
LIPID-REGULATING AGENTS						
Icosapent Ethyl (Vascepa)	**Cap:** 1000	4g/day	7	5	4	27
Omega-3-Acid Ethyl Esters (Lovaza)	**Cap:** 1000	4g/day	9.7	+44.5	9.1	44.9
Omega-3-Acid Ethyl Esters A (Omtryg)	**Cap:** 1200	4 cap/day	9.7	+44.5	9.1	44.9
COMBINATIONS						
Amlodipine/ Atorvastatin (Caduet)	**Tab:** 2.5/10, 2.5/20, 2.5/40, 5/10, 5/20, 5/40, 5/80, 10/10, 10/20, 10/40, 10/80	5/10mg – 10/80mg/day	N/A	32.3 to 48.0	N/A	N/A
Ezetimibe/ Atorvastatin (Liptruzet)	**Tab:** 10/10, 10/20, 10/40, 10/80	10/10mg – 10/80mg/day	38 to 46	53 to 61	5 to 9	30 to 40
Ezetimibe/ Simvastatin (Vytorin)	**Tab:** 10/10, 10/20, 10/40, 10/80	10/10mg – 10/40mg/day	31 to 43	45 to 60	6 to 10	23 to 31
Niacin, ER/ Lovastatin (Advicor)	**Tab, ER:** 500/20, 750/20, 1000/20, 1000/40	1000/20mg – 2000/40mg/day	N/A	30 to 42	20 to 30	32 to 44
Niacin, ER/ Simvastatin (Simcor)	**Tab, ER:** 500/20, 500/40, 750/20, 1000/20, 1000/40	1000/20mg – 2000/40mg/day	1.6 to 11.1	5.1 to 14.3	15.4 to 29.0	22.8 to 38.0

GENERIC (BRAND)	HOW SUPPLIED (MG)*	USUAL DOSAGE RANGE†	T-CHOL (% DECREASE)	LDL (% DECREASE)	HDL (% INCREASE)	TG (% DECREASE)
COMBINATIONS *(Continued)*						
Sitagliptin/ Simvastatin (Juvisync)	**Tab:** 50/10, 50/20, 50/40, 100/10, 100/20, 100/40	50/10mg – 100/40mg/day	23 to 31	29 to 41	8 to 13	15 to 28

Abbreviations: DR = delayed-release; ER = extended-release; N/A = not applicable.

*Unless otherwise indicated.

† Usual Dosage Range shown is for adults and may need to be adjusted to individual patient needs. For specific dosing and administration information including pediatric, geriatric, and renal/hepatic impairment dosing, please refer to the individual monograph listing or the FDA-approved labeling. According to NCEP-ATP III guidelines, lipid-altering agents should be used in addition to a diet restricted in saturated fat and cholesterol only when the response to diet and other nonpharmacological measures has been inadequate.

‡ Refer to the FDA-approved labeling for the lipid parameter changes observed for the treatment of hypertriglyceridemia; LDL increases reported.

Major Contraindications (refer to the FDA-approved labeling for a complete list of warnings and precautions):

Statins: Active liver disease or unexplained persistent elevations of hepatic transaminase levels; women who are pregnant or may become pregnant; nursing mothers.

Fibrates: Severe renal dysfunction (including patients receiving dialysis), active liver disease, gallbladder disease, nursing mothers.

Bile-acid sequestrants: History of bowel obstruction; serum triglycerides >500mg/dL; history of hypertriglyceridemia-induced pancreatitis.

Cholesterol absorption inhibitors: Statin contraindications apply when used with a statin: active liver disease or unexplained persistent elevations in hepatic transaminase levels, women who are pregnant or may become pregnant, nursing mothers.

Nicotinic acid derivatives: Active liver disease or unexplained persistent elevations in hepatic transaminases; active peptic ulcer disease; arterial bleeding.

Combinations: Refer to individual therapeutic class contraindications.

Heart Failure Treatment Options

GENERIC (BRAND)	HOW SUPPLIED	DOSAGE	RENAL/HEPATIC DOSAGE ADJUSTMENT
ACE INHIBITORS			
Captopril	**Tab:** 12.5mg, 25mg, 50mg, 100mg	**Initial:** 25mg tid. **Usual:** 50-100mg tid. **Max:** 450mg/day.	Renal
Enalapril maleate (Vasotec)	**Tab:** 2.5mg, 5mg, 10mg, 20mg	**Initial:** 2.5mg qd. **Usual:** 2.5-20mg bid. **Max:** 40mg/day in divided doses.	Renal
Fosinopril sodium	**Tab:** 10mg, 20mg, 40mg	**Initial:** 10mg qd. **Usual:** 20-40mg qd. **Max:** 40mg qd.	Renal
Lisinopril (Prinivil)	**Tab:** 5mg, 10mg, 20mg	**Initial:** 5mg qd. **Usual:** 5-20mg qd.	Renal
Lisinopril (Zestril)	**Tab:** 2.5mg, 5mg, 10mg, 20mg, 30mg, 40mg	**Initial:** 5mg qd. **Usual:** 5-40mg qd. **Max:** 40mg/day.	Renal
Quinapril (Accupril)	**Tab:** 5mg, 10mg, 20mg, 40mg	**Initial:** 5mg bid. **Usual:** 20-40mg/day given in 2 equally divided doses.	Renal
Ramipril (Altace)	**Cap:** 1.25mg, 2.5mg, 5mg, 10mg	**Post-MI: Initial:** 2.5mg bid (switch to 1.25mg bid if hypotensive). **Titrate:** Increase (if tolerated) to target dose of 5mg bid at 3-week intervals after 1 week of initial dose.	Renal
Trandolapril (Mavik)	**Tab:** 1mg, 2mg, 4mg	**Post-MI: Initial:** 1mg qd. **Titrate:** Increase (as tolerated) to target dose of 4mg qd; if not tolerated, continue with the greatest tolerated dose.	Renal/Hepatic
ALDOSTERONE BLOCKERS			
Eplerenone (Inspra)	**Tab:** 25mg, 50mg	**Post-MI: Initial:** 25mg qd. **Titrate:** Increase to 50mg qd, preferably within 4 weeks as tolerated.	
ALPHA/BETA BLOCKERS			
Carvedilol (Coreg)	**Tab:** 3.125mg, 6.25mg, 12.5mg, 25mg	**Initial:** 3.125mg bid for 2 weeks. **Titrate:** May double dose over successive intervals of at least 2 weeks up to 25mg bid as tolerated. Maintain on lower doses if higher doses not tolerated. **Max:** 50mg bid if >85kg with mild-moderate HF. Reduce dose if HR <55 beats/min.	
Carvedilol phosphate (Coreg CR)	**Cap, ER:** 10mg, 20mg, 40mg, 80mg	**Initial:** 10mg qd for 2 weeks. **Titrate:** May double dose over successive intervals of at least 2 weeks up to 80mg qd as tolerated. Maintain on lower doses if higher doses not tolerated. Reduce dose if HR <55 beats/min.	
ANGIOTENSIN II RECEPTOR ANTAGONISTS			
Candesartan cilexetil (Atacand)	**Tab:** 4mg, 8mg, 16mg, 32mg	**Initial:** 4mg qd. **Titrate:** Double the dose at 2-week intervals, as tolerated, to the target dose of 32mg qd.	
Valsartan (Diovan)	**Tab:** 40mg, 80mg, 160mg, 320mg	**Initial:** 40mg bid. **Titrate:** May increase to 80mg or 160mg bid (use highest dose tolerated). Consider dose reduction of concomitant diuretics. **Max:** 320mg/day in divided doses.	
BETA BLOCKERS			
Metoprolol succinate (Toprol-XL)	**Tab, ER:** 25mg, 50mg, 100mg, 200mg	**Initial:** (NYHA Class II HF) 25mg qd or (Severe HF) 12.5mg qd for 2 weeks. **Titrate:** Double dose every 2 weeks to the highest dose level tolerated. **Max:** 200mg. Reduce dose if experiencing symptomatic bradycardia.	Hepatic

(Continued)

GENERIC (BRAND)	HOW SUPPLIED	DOSAGE	RENAL/HEPATIC DOSAGE ADJUSTMENT
DIURETICS (POTASSIUM SPARING)			
Spironolactone (Aldactone)	**Tab:** 25mg, 50mg, 100mg	**Initial:** 25mg qd. **Titrate:** If tolerated, may increase to 50mg qd as clinically indicated. May reduce to 25mg qod if not tolerated.	
VASODILATORS			
Isosorbide dinitrate-Hydralazine HCl (Bidil)	**Tab:** 20mg-37.5mg	**Initial:** 1 tab tid. **Titrate:** Increase to a maximum of 2 tabs tid, if tolerated. **Intolerable Side Effects:** May decrease to as little as ½ tab tid. Titrate up as soon as side effects subside.	
Nitroglycerin in 5% Dextrose	**Inj:** 100mcg/mL, 200mcg/mL, 400mcg/mL	**Initial:** 5mcg/min IV. **Titrate:** Increase by 5mcg/min at intervals of 3-5 min. If no response at 20mcg/min, may use increments of 10 and even 20mcg/min. Once some hemodynamic response is observed, dosage increments should be smaller and less frequent.	
MISCELLANEOUS			
Digoxin (Lanoxin)	**Inj:** (Lanoxin) 250mcg/mL, (Lanoxin Pediatric)* 100mcg/mL; **Sol:** (generic) 50mcg/mL; **Tab:** (Lanoxin) 62.5mcg, 125mcg, 187.5mcg, 250mcg	**LD:** (Sol) 10-15mcg/kg PO. (Inj, Tab) Administer ½ the total LD initially, then ¼ the LD q6-8h, twice. (Inj) 8-12 mcg/kg IV, (Tab) 10-15mcg/kg PO. **Maint:** (Sol) 3-4.5mcg/kg qd PO. **Initial:** (Inj) 2.4-3.6mcg/kg qd IV, (Tab) 3.4-5.1mcg/kg qd PO. **Titrate:** (Inj, Tab) May increase every 2 weeks based on response, serum drug levels, and toxicity.	Renal
Milrinone lactate	**Inj:** 1mg/mL	**LD:** 50mcg/kg IV given slowly over 10 min. **Maint: Continuous IV Infusion: Minimum:** 0.59mg/kg/day at 0.375mcg/kg/min. **Standard:** 0.77mg/kg/day at 0.5mcg/kg/min. **Titrate:** Adjust to desired response. **Max:** 1.13mg/kg/day at 0.75mcg/kg/min.	Renal
Nesiritide (Natrecor)	**Inj:** 1.5mg	2mcg/kg IV bolus over 60 sec, then 0.01mcg/kg/min continuous IV infusion.	

Refer to full FDA-approved labeling for additional information.

Abbreviations: ER = extended-release; HF = heart failure; MI = myocardial infarction.

*Please refer to complete monograph for full dosing information, including pediatric dosing.

HYPERTENSION TREATMENT OPTIONS

GENERIC (BRAND)	HOW SUPPLIED	ADULT DOSAGE	PEDIATRIC DOSAGE
ACE INHIBITORS			
Benazepril HCl (Lotensin)	**Tab:** 5mg, 10mg, 20mg, 40mg	**Initial:** 10mg qd or 5mg qd if on diuretic. **Maint:** 20-40mg/day given qd or bid. **Max:** 80mg/day.	**≥6 Yrs: Initial:** 0.2mg/kg qd. **Max:** 0.6mg/kg or 40mg/day.
Captopril	**Tab:** 12.5mg*, 25mg*, 50mg*, 100mg*	**Initial:** 25mg bid or tid. **Titrate:** May increase to 50mg bid or tid after 1 or 2 wks. **Usual:** 25-150mg bid or tid. **Max:** 450mg/day.	
Enalapril (Epaned)	**Sol:** 1mg/mL [150mL]	**Initial:** 5mg qd or 2.5mg qd if on diuretics. **Titrate:** Increase dose prn. **Max:** 40mg/day.	**>1 Month: Initial:** 0.08mg/kg (up to 5mg) qd. **Max:** 0.58mg/kg or 40mg/day.
Enalapril maleate (Vasotec)	**Tab:** 2.5mg*, 5mg*, 10mg*, 20mg*	**Initial:** 5mg qd or 2.5mg qd if on diuretic. **Usual:** 10-40mg/day given qd or bid.	**1 Month-16 Yrs: HTN: Initial:** 0.08mg/kg (up to 5mg) qd. **Max:** 0.58mg/kg or 40mg/day.
Enalaprilat	**Inj:** 1.25mg/mL [1mL, 2mL]	**Usual:** 1.25mg IV over 5 min q6h for ≤48 hrs. **Max:** 20mg/day. **Concomitant Diuretic: Initial:** 0.625mg over 5 min; may repeat after 1 hr. **Maint:** Additional 1.25mg dose q6h.	
Fosinopril sodium	**Tab:** 10mg*, 20mg, 40mg	**Initial:** 10mg qd. **Usual:** 20-40mg qd. **Max:** 80mg/day.	**>50kg:** 5-10mg qd.
Lisinopril (Prinivil, Zestril)	**Tab:** (Prinivil) 5mg*, 10mg*, 20mg*; (Zestril) 2.5mg, 5mg*, 10mg, 20mg, 30mg, 40mg	**Initial:** 10mg qd or 5mg qd if on diuretic. **Usual:** 20-40mg qd. **Max:** 80mg/day.	**≥6 Yrs: Initial:** 0.07mg/kg qd (up to 5mg). **Max:** 0.61mg/kg or 40mg.
Moexipril HCl (Univasc)	**Tab:** 7.5mg*, 15mg*	**Initial:** 7.5mg qd 1 hr ac or 3.75mg qd if on diuretic. **Usual:** 7.5-30mg/day given qd or bid. **Max:** 60mg/day.	
Perindopril erbumine (Aceon)	**Tab:** 2mg*, 4mg*, 8mg*	**Initial:** 4mg qd. **Maint:** 4-8mg/day given qd or bid. **Max:** 16mg/day.	
Quinapril HCl (Accupril)	**Tab:** 5mg*, 10mg, 20mg, 40mg	**Initial:** 10-20mg qd or 5mg qd if on diuretic. **Titrate:** According to BP at 2-wk intervals. **Usual:** 20-80mg/day given qd or bid.	
Ramipril (Altace)	**Cap:** 1.25mg, 2.5mg, 5mg, 10mg	**Initial:** 2.5mg qd. **Maint:** 2.5-20mg/day given qd or bid.	
Trandolapril (Mavik)	**Tab:** 1mg*, 2mg, 4mg	**Initial:** 1mg qd in nonblack patients; 2mg qd in black patients or 0.5mg qd if on diuretic. **Titrate:** According to BP at 1-wk intervals. **Usual:** 2-4mg qd. **Max:** 8mg/day.	
ACE INHIBITORS-CALCIUM CHANNEL BLOCKERS			
Amlodipine besylate-Benazepril HCl (Lotrel)	**Cap:** (Amlodipine-Benazepril) 2.5mg-10mg, 5mg-10mg, 5mg-20mg, 5mg-40mg, 10mg-20mg, 10mg-40mg	**Initial:** 2.5mg-10mg qd. **Titrate:** May increase up to 10mg-40mg qd if BP remains uncontrolled.	

(Continued)

GENERIC (BRAND)	HOW SUPPLIED	ADULT DOSAGE	PEDIATRIC DOSAGE
ACE INHIBITORS-CALCIUM CHANNEL BLOCKERS *(Continued)*			
Perindopril arginine-Amlodipine (Prestalia)	**Tab:** (Perindopril-Amlodipine) 3.5mg-2.5mg, 7mg-5mg, 14mg-10mg	**Initial:** 3.5mg-2.5mg qd. **Titrate:** Adjust based on BP at 7- to 14-day intervals. **Max:** 14mg-10mg qd.	
Trandolapril-Verapamil HCl (Tarka)	**Tab, ER:** (Trandolapril-Verapamil ER) 2mg-180mg, 1mg-240mg, 2mg-240mg, 4mg-240mg	Combination may be substituted for same component doses.	
ACE INHIBITORS-THIAZIDE DIURETICS			
Captopril-HCTZ	**Tab:** (Captopril-HCTZ) 25mg-15mg*, 25mg-25mg*, 50mg-15mg*, 50mg-25mg*	**Initial:** 25mg-15mg qd 1 hr ac. **Titrate:** Adjust at 6-wk intervals, unless situation demands more rapid adjustment. **Max:** 150mg captopril and 50mg HCTZ per day.	
Enalapril maleate-HCTZ (Vaseretic)	**Tab:** (Enalapril-HCTZ) 5mg-12.5mg, 10mg-25mg; (Vaseretic) 10mg-25mg*	**Not Controlled with Enalapril or HCTZ Monotherapy: Initial:** 5mg-12.5mg or 10mg-25mg qd. **Titrate:** May increase after 2-3 wks. **Max:** 20mg enalapril and 50mg HCTZ per day.	
Fosinopril sodium-HCTZ	**Tab:** (Fosinopril-HCTZ) 10mg-12.5mg, 20mg-12.5mg*	**Not Controlled with Fosinopril or HCTZ Monotherapy:** 10mg-12.5mg tab or 20mg-12.5mg tab qd.	
Lisinopril-HCTZ (Zestoretic)	**Tab:** (Lisinopril-HCTZ) 10mg-12.5mg, 20mg-12.5mg, 20mg-25mg	**Not Controlled with Lisinopril or HCTZ Monotherapy: Initial:** 10mg-12.5mg or 20mg-12.5mg qd, depending on current monotherapy dose. **Titrate:** May increase after 2-3 wks.	
Moexipril HCl-HCTZ (Uniretic)	**Tab:** (Moexipril-HCTZ) 7.5mg-12.5mg*, 15mg-12.5mg*, 15mg-25mg*	**Not Controlled with Moexipril or HCTZ Monotherapy: Initial:** 7.5mg-12.5mg, 15mg-12.5mg, or 15mg-25mg qd 1 hr ac. **Titrate:** May increase after 2-3 wks. **Max:** 30mg moexipril and 50mg HCTZ per day.	
Quinapril HCl-HCTZ (Accuretic)	**Tab:** (Quinapril-HCTZ) 10mg-12.5mg*, 20mg-12.5mg*, 20mg-25mg	**Not Controlled with Quinapril Monotherapy: Initial:** 10mg-12.5mg or 20mg-12.5mg qd. **Titrate:** May increase after 2-3 wks.	
ALDOSTERONE BLOCKERS			
Eplerenone (Inspra)	**Tab:** 25mg, 50mg	**Initial:** 50mg qd. **Titrate:** May increase to 50mg bid. **Max:** 100mg/day.	
ALPHA ADRENERGIC AGONISTS			
Clonidine (Catapres, Catapres-TTS)	**Patch, ER (TTS):** (TTS-1) 0.1mg, (TTS-2) 0.2mg, (TTS-3) 0.3mg; **Tab:** 0.1mg, 0.2mg, 0.3mg	(Patch) **Initial:** 0.1mg/24 hrs patch wkly. **Titrate:** May increase after 1-2 wks. **Max:** 0.6mg/24 hrs. (Tab) **Initial:** 0.1mg bid. **Titrate:** May increase by 0.1mg/day wkly. **Usual:** 0.2-0.6mg/day in divided doses. **Max:** 2.4mg/day.	

GENERIC (BRAND)	HOW SUPPLIED	ADULT DOSAGE	PEDIATRIC DOSAGE
ALPHA ADRENERGIC AGONISTS-THIAZIDE DIURETICS			
Clonidine HCl-Chlorthalidone (Clorpres)	**Tab:** (Clonidine-Chlorthalidone) 0.1mg-15mg*, 0.2mg-15mg*, 0.3mg-15mg*	0.1mg-15mg tab qd-bid. **Max:** 0.6mg-30mg/day.	
ALPHA/BETA BLOCKERS			
Carvedilol (Coreg, Coreg CR)	**Cap, ER:** 10mg, 20mg, 40mg, 80mg; **Tab:** 3.125mg, 6.25mg, 12.5mg, 25mg	(Cap, ER) **Initial:** 20mg qd. **Titrate:** May double dose every 7-14 days. **Max:** 80mg/day. (Tab) **Initial:** 6.25mg bid. **Titrate:** May double dose every 7-14 days. **Max:** 50mg/day.	
Labetalol HCl	**Inj:** 5mg/mL [20mL, 40mL]; **Tab:** 100mg*, 200mg*, 300mg	(Inj) **Repeated Inj: Initial:** 20mg over 2 min. **Titrate:** May give additional 40mg or 80mg at 10-min intervals until desired BP achieved or total of 300mg is injected. **Slow Continuous Infusion:** 200mg (1mg/mL) at 2mg/min. **Alternate:** 200mg (2mg/3mL) at 3mL/min. **Effective Dose Range:** 50-200mg. **Max:** 300mg. (Tab) **Initial:** 100mg bid. **Titrate:** After 2-3 days, may increase in increments of 100mg bid every 2-3 days. **Maint:** 200-400mg bid. **Severe:** 1200-2400mg/day given bid.	
ALPHA$_1$ RECEPTOR BLOCKERS (QUINAZOLINE)			
Doxazosin mesylate (Cardura)	**Tab:** 1mg*, 2mg*, 4mg*, 8mg*	**Initial:** 1mg qd (am or pm). **Titrate:** May increase to 2mg and if necessary to 4mg, 8mg, and 16mg qd.	
Prazosin HCl (Minipress)	**Cap:** 1mg, 2mg, 5mg	**Initial:** 1mg bid-tid. **Titrate:** May slowly increase to 20mg/day in divided doses. **Usual:** 6-15mg/day in divided doses.	
Terazosin HCl	**Cap:** 1mg, 2mg, 5mg, 10mg	**Initial:** 1mg hs. **Usual:** 1-5mg qd. Slowly increase dose or use bid regimen if substantially diminished response at 24 hrs. **Max:** 40mg/day.	
ANGIOTENSIN II RECEPTOR ANTAGONISTS			
Azilsartan medoxomil (Edarbi)	**Tab:** 40mg, 80mg	**Usual:** 80mg qd. **With High Dose Diuretics: Initial:** 40mg qd.	
Candesartan cilexetil (Atacand)	**Tab:** 4mg*, 8mg*, 16mg*, 32mg*	**Monotherapy without Volume Depletion: Initial:** 16mg qd. **Usual:** 8-32mg/day given qd or bid.	Administer qd or divide into 2 equal doses. **6-<17 Yrs: >50kg: Initial:** 8-16mg. **Usual:** 4-32mg/day. **<50kg: Initial:** 4-8mg. **Usual:** 2-16mg/day. **1-<6 Yrs: Initial:** (PO Sus) 0.20mg/kg. **Usual:** 0.05-0.4mg/kg/day.

(Continued)

GENERIC (BRAND)	HOW SUPPLIED	ADULT DOSAGE	PEDIATRIC DOSAGE
ANGIOTENSIN II RECEPTOR ANTAGONISTS *(Continued)*			
Eprosartan mesylate (Teveten)	**Tab:** 400mg, 600mg	**Initial (Monotherapy and Not Volume-Depleted):** 600mg qd. **Usual:** 400-800mg/day given qd-bid. May give bid using same total daily dose or consider dose increase if effect is inadequate. **Max:** 800mg/day.	
Irbesartan (Avapro)	**Tab:** 75mg, 150mg, 300mg	**Initial:** 150mg qd. **Titrate:** May increase to 300mg qd. **Max:** 300mg qd.	
Losartan potassium (Cozaar)	**Tab:** 25mg, 50mg, 100mg	**Initial:** 50mg qd. **Usual:** 25-100mg/day given qd or bid.	**≥6 Yrs: Initial:** 0.7mg/kg qd (up to 50mg total). **Max:** 1.4mg/kg/day or 100mg/day.
Olmesartan medoxomil (Benicar)	**Tab:** 5mg, 20mg, 40mg	**Initial:** 20mg qd. **Titrate:** May increase to 40mg qd after 2 wks.	**6-16 Yrs: ≥35kg: Initial:** 20mg qd. **Titrate:** May increase to 40mg qd after 2 wks. **Max:** 40mg qd. **20-<35kg: Initial:** 10mg qd. **Titrate:** May increase to 20mg qd after 2 wks. **Max:** 20mg qd.
Telmisartan (Micardis)	**Tab:** 20mg, 40mg, 80mg	**Initial:** 40mg qd. **Usual:** 20-80mg/day.	
Valsartan (Diovan)	**Tab:** 40mg*, 80mg, 160mg, 320mg	**Initial:** 80mg or 160mg qd. **Max:** 320mg/day.	**6-16 Yrs: Initial:** 1.3mg/kg qd (up to 40mg total). **Max:** 2.7mg/kg (up to 160mg) qd.
ANGIOTENSIN II RECEPTOR ANTAGONISTS-CALCIUM CHANNEL BLOCKERS-THIAZIDE DIURETICS			
Amlodipine-Valsartan-HCTZ (Exforge HCT)	**Tab:** (Amlodipine-Valsartan-HCTZ) 5mg-160mg-12.5mg, 5mg-160mg-25mg, 10mg-160mg-12.5mg, 10mg-160mg-25mg, 10mg-320mg-25mg	**Usual:** Dose qd. May increase after 2 wks. **Max:** 10mg-320mg-25mg qd.	
Olmesartan medoxomil-Amlodipine besylate-HCTZ (Tribenzor)	**Tab:** (Olmesartan-Amlodipine-HCTZ) 20mg-5mg-12.5mg, 40mg-5mg-12.5mg, 40mg-5mg-25mg, 40mg-10mg-12.5mg, 40mg-10mg-25mg	**Usual:** Dose qd. May increase after 2 wks. **Max:** 40mg-10mg-25mg qd.	
ANGIOTENSIN II RECEPTOR ANTAGONISTS-THIAZIDE DIURETICS			
Azilsartan medoxomil-Chlorthalidone (Edarbyclor)	**Tab:** (Azilsartan-Chlorthalidone) 40mg-12.5mg, 40mg-25mg	**Initial:** 40mg-12.5mg qd. **Titrate:** May increase to 40mg-25mg after 2-4 wks. **Max:** 40mg-25mg.	
Candesartan cilexetil-HCTZ (Atacand HCT)	**Tab:** (Candesartan-HCTZ) 16mg-12.5mg*, 32mg-12.5mg*, 32mg-25mg*	**Not Controlled on 25mg HCTZ qd or Controlled on 25mg HCTZ qd with Hypokalemia:** 16mg-12.5mg qd. **Not Controlled on 32mg Candesartan qd:** 32mg-12.5mg qd, and then 32mg-25mg qd.	
Eprosartan mesylate-HCTZ (Teveten HCT)	**Tab:** (Eprosartan-HCTZ) 600mg-12.5mg, 600mg-25mg	**Usual (Not Volume-Depleted):** 600mg-12.5mg qd. **Titrate:** May increase to 600mg-25mg qd. **Max:** 600mg-25mg qd.	

GENERIC (BRAND)	HOW SUPPLIED	ADULT DOSAGE	PEDIATRIC DOSAGE
ANGIOTENSIN II RECEPTOR ANTAGONISTS-THIAZIDE DIURETICS *(Continued)*			
Irbesartan-HCTZ (Avalide)	**Tab:** (Irbesartan-HCTZ) 150mg-12.5mg, 300mg-12.5mg	**Initial:** 150mg-12.5mg qd. **Titrate:** May increase after 1-2 wks. **Max:** 300mg-25mg qd.	
Losartan potassium-HCTZ (Hyzaar)	**Tab:** (Losartan-HCTZ) 50mg-12.5mg, 100mg-12.5mg, 100mg-25mg	**Usual:** 50mg-12.5mg qd. **Max:** 100mg-25mg qd.	
Olmesartan medoxomil-HCTZ (Benicar HCT)	**Tab:** (Olmesartan-HCTZ) 20mg-12.5mg, 40mg-12.5mg, 40mg-25mg	**Usual:** 1 tab qd. **Titrate:** May adjust at intervals of 2-4 wks. **Max:** 1 tab/day.	
Telmisartan-HCTZ (Micardis HCT)	**Tab:** (Telmisartan-HCTZ) 40mg-12.5mg, 80mg-12.5mg, 80mg-25mg	**Not Controlled on 80mg Telmisartan or Controlled on 25mg/day HCTZ with Hypokalemia: Initial:** 80mg-12.5mg tab qd. **Not Controlled on 25mg/day of HCTZ: Initial:** 80mg-12.5mg qd or 80mg-25mg tab qd. **Titrate/Max:** Increase to 160mg-25mg after 2-4 wks.	
Valsartan-HCTZ (Diovan HCT)	**Tab:** (Valsartan-HCTZ) 80mg-12.5mg, 160mg-12.5mg, 160mg-25mg, 320mg-12.5mg, 320mg-25mg	**Initial:** 160mg-12.5mg qd. **Titrate:** May increase after 1-2 wks. **Max:** 320mg-25mg qd.	
BETA BLOCKERS			
Acebutolol HCl (Sectral)	**Cap:** 200mg, 400mg	**Mild-Moderate: Initial:** 400mg/day, given qd-bid. **Usual:** 200-800mg/day. **Severe/Inadequate Control:** 1200mg/day, given bid.	
Atenolol (Tenormin)	**Tab:** 25mg, 50mg*, 100mg	**Initial:** 50mg qd. **Titrate:** May increase to 100mg qd after 1-2 wks. **Max:** 100mg qd.	
Betaxolol	**Tab:** 10mg*, 20mg	**Initial:** 10mg qd. **Titrate:** May increase to 20mg qd after 7-14 days. **Max:** 20mg/day.†	
Bisoprolol fumarate (Zebeta)	**Tab:** 5mg*, 10mg	**Initial:** 5mg qd. **Titrate:** May increase to 10mg and then, if necessary, to 20mg qd.	
Metoprolol succinate (Toprol-XL)	**Tab, ER:** 25mg*, 50mg*, 100mg*, 200mg*	**Initial:** 25-100mg qd. **Titrate:** May increase at wkly (or longer) intervals. **Max:** 400mg/day.	**≥6 Yrs: Initial:** 1mg/kg qd up to 50mg qd. **Max:** 2mg/kg (up to 200mg) qd.
Metoprolol tartrate (Lopressor)	**Tab:** (Generic) 25mg*, 50mg*, 100mg*; (Lopressor) 50mg*, 100mg*	**Initial:** 100mg/day qd or in divided doses. **Titrate:** May increase at wkly (or longer) intervals. **Effective Range:** 100-450mg/day. **Max:** 450mg/day.	
Nadolol (Corgard)	**Tab:** 20mg*, 40mg*, 80mg*	**Initial:** 40mg qd. **Titrate:** May gradually increase in 40-80mg increments. **Maint: Usual:** 40 or 80mg qd. Doses up to 240 or 320mg qd may be needed.	

(Continued)

GENERIC (BRAND)	HOW SUPPLIED	ADULT DOSAGE	PEDIATRIC DOSAGE
BETA BLOCKERS *(Continued)*			
Nebivolol (Bystolic)	**Tab:** 2.5mg, 5mg, 10mg, 20mg	**Initial:** 5mg qd. **Titrate:** May increase at 2-wk intervals. **Max:** 40mg.	
Penbutolol sulfate (Levatol)	**Tab:** 20mg*	**Initial/Maint:** 20mg qd.	
Pindolol	**Tab:** 5mg*, 10mg*	**Initial:** 5mg bid. **Titrate:** May adjust dose in increments of 10mg/day at 3- to 4-wk intervals. **Max:** 60mg/day.	
Propranolol HCl	**Sol:** 20mg/5mL, 40mg/5mL [500mL]; **Tab:** 10mg*, 20mg*, 40mg*, 60mg*, 80mg*	**Initial:** 40mg bid. **Usual Maint:** 120-240mg/day. In some instances, 640mg/day may be required.	
Propranolol HCl (Inderal LA)	**Cap, ER:** 60mg, 80mg, 120mg, 160mg	**Initial:** 80mg qd. **Titrate:** May increase to 120mg qd or higher. **Maint:** 120-160mg qd. 640mg/day may be required.	
Propranolol HCl (Innopran XL)	**Cap, ER:** 80mg, 120mg	**Initial:** 80mg qhs. **Titrate:** May increase to 120mg qhs.	
Timolol maleate	**Tab:** 5mg, 10mg*, 20mg*	**Initial:** 10mg bid. **Maint:** 20-40mg/day. Wait at least 7 days between dose increases. **Max:** 60mg/day given bid.	
BETA BLOCKERS-THIAZIDE DIURETICS			
Atenolol-Chlorthalidone (Tenoretic)	**Tab:** (Atenolol-Chlorthalidone) 50mg-25mg*, 100mg-25mg	**Initial:** 50mg-25mg tab qd. **Titrate:** May increase to 100mg-25mg tab qd.	
Bisoprolol fumarate-HCTZ (Ziac)	**Tab:** (Bisoprolol-HCTZ) 2.5mg-6.25mg, 5mg-6.25mg, 10mg-6.25mg	**Not Controlled on 2.5-20mg/day Bisoprolol or Controlled on 50mg/day HCTZ with Hypokalemia: Initial:** 2.5mg-6.25mg qd. **Titrate:** May increase at 14-day intervals. **Max:** 20mg-12.5mg (two 10mg-6.25mg tabs) qd.	
Metoprolol succinate-HCTZ (Dutoprol)	**Tab:** (Metoprolol ER-HCTZ) 25mg-12.5mg, 50mg-12.5mg, 100mg-12.5mg*	**Initial:** 25mg-12.5mg qd. **Titrate:** Every 2 wks. **Max:** 200mg-25mg (two 100mg-12.5mg tabs) qd.	
Metoprolol tartrate-HCTZ (Lopressor HCT)	**Tab:** (Metoprolol-HCTZ) 50mg-25mg*, 100mg-25mg*, 100mg-50mg*; (Lopressor HCT) 50mg-25mg*, 100mg-25mg*, 100mg-50mg*	**Combination Therapy: Metoprolol:** 100-200mg/day given qd or in divided doses. **HCTZ:** 25-50mg/day given qd or in divided doses. **Max:** 50mg/day.	
Nadolol-Bendroflumethiazide (Corzide)	**Tab:** (Nadolol-Bendroflumethiazide) 40mg-5mg*, 80mg-5mg*	**Initial:** 40mg-5mg qd. **Titrate:** May increase to 80mg-5mg qd.	
Propranolol HCl-HCTZ	**Tab:** (Propranolol-HCTZ) 40mg-25mg*, 80mg-25mg*	**Usual:** 1 tab bid. **Max:** 160mg-50mg/day.	

GENERIC (BRAND)	HOW SUPPLIED	ADULT DOSAGE	PEDIATRIC DOSAGE
CALCIUM CHANNEL BLOCKERS (DIHYDROPYRIDINE)			
Amlodipine besylate (Norvasc)	**Tab:** 2.5mg, 5mg, 10mg	**Initial:** 5mg qd. **Titrate:** 7- to 14-day intervals. If clinically warranted, titrate more rapidly. **Max:** 10mg qd.	**6-17 Yrs: Usual:** 2.5-5mg qd. **Max:** 5mg qd.
Clevidipine (Cleviprex)	**Inj:** 0.5mg/mL [50mL, 100mL, 250mL]	**Initial:** 1-2mg/hr. **Titrate:** May double dose at 90-sec intervals initially. As BP approaches goal, interval should be lengthened to every 5-10 min. **Maint:** 4-6mg/hr. **Max:** 16mg/hr.	
Felodipine	**Tab, ER:** 2.5mg, 5mg, 10mg	**Initial:** 5mg qd. **Titrate:** May decrease to 2.5mg qd or increase to 10mg qd at intervals of not <2 wks. **Range:** 2.5-10mg qd.	
Isradipine	**Cap:** 2.5mg, 5mg	**Initial:** 2.5mg bid. **Titrate:** May adjust in increments of 5mg/day at 2- to 4-wk intervals. **Max:** 20mg/day.	
Nicardipine HCl	**Cap:** 20mg, 30mg	**Initial:** 20mg tid. **Titrate:** Allow at least 3 days before increasing dose. **Usual:** 20-40mg tid.	
Nicardipine HCl (Cardene IV)	**Inj:** 2.5mg/mL [10mL], 0.1mg/mL [200mL], 0.2mg/mL [200mL]	**Patients Not Receiving PO Nicardipine: Initial:** 5mg/hr IV infusion. **Titrate:** May increase by 2.5mg/hr every 5 min (for rapid titration) to 15 min (for gradual titration). **Max:** 15mg/hr.	
Nicardipine HCl (Cardene SR)	**Cap, SR:** 30mg, 45mg, 60mg	**Initial:** 30mg bid. **Effective Range:** 30-60mg bid.	
Nifedipine (Nifedical XL, Procardia XL)	**Tab, ER:** (Nifedical XL) 30mg, 60mg; (Procardia XL) 30mg, 60mg, 90mg	**Initial:** 30 or 60mg qd. **Titrate: Usual:** 7- to 14-day period. May proceed more rapidly if needed. **Max:** 120mg/day.	
Nisoldipine (Sular)	**Tab, ER:** 8.5mg, 17mg, 34mg	**Initial:** 17mg qd. **Titrate:** May increase by 8.5mg/wk or longer intervals. **Maint:** 17-34mg qd. **Max:** 34mg qd.	
CALCIUM CHANNEL BLOCKERS (DIHYDROPYRIDINE)-ANGIOTENSIN II RECEPTOR ANTAGONISTS			
Amlodipine-Olmesartan medoxomil (Azor)	**Tab:** (Amlodipine-Olmesartan) 5mg-20mg, 5mg-40mg, 10mg-20mg, 10mg-40mg	**Initial:** 5mg-20mg qd. **Titrate:** May increase dose after 1-2 wks. **Max:** 10mg-40mg qd.	
Amlodipine-Valsartan (Exforge)	**Tab:** (Amlodipine-Valsartan) 5mg-160mg, 10mg-160mg, 5mg-320mg, 10mg-320mg	**Initial:** 5mg-160mg qd. **Titrate:** May increase after 1-2 wks. **Max:** 10mg-320mg qd.	
Telmisartan-Amlodipine (Twynsta)	**Tab:** (Telmisartan-Amlodipine) 40mg-5mg, 40mg-10mg, 80mg-5mg, 80mg-10mg	**Initial:** 40mg-5mg qd or 80mg-5mg qd. **Titrate:** May be increased after at least 2 wks. **Max:** 80mg-10mg qd.	

(Continued)

GENERIC (BRAND)	HOW SUPPLIED	ADULT DOSAGE	PEDIATRIC DOSAGE
CALCIUM CHANNEL BLOCKERS (DIHYDROPYRIDINE)-HMG COA REDUCTASE INHIBITORS			
Amlodipine besylate-Atorvastatin calcium (Caduet)	**Tab:** (Amlodipine-Atorvastatin) 2.5mg-10mg, 2.5mg-20mg, 2.5mg-40mg, 5mg-10mg, 5mg-20mg, 5mg-40mg, 5mg-80mg, 10mg-10mg, 10mg-20mg, 10mg-40mg, 10mg-80mg	**Amlodipine: Initial:** 5mg qd. **Titrate:** Adjust generally every 7-14 days. **Max:** 10mg qd. **Atorvastatin: Initial:** 10mg or 20mg qd (or 40mg qd for LDL reduction >45%). **Titrate:** Analyze lipids within 2-4 wks and adjust accordingly. **Usual:** 10-80mg qd.	**Amlodipine: 6-17 Yrs: Usual:** 2.5-5mg qd. **Max:** 5mg qd. **Atorvastatin: 10-17 Yrs: Initial:** 10mg/day. **Titrate:** Adjust at intervals of ≥4 wks. **Max:** 20mg/day.
CALCIUM CHANNEL BLOCKERS (DIHYDROPYRIDINE)-RENIN INHIBITORS			
Aliskiren-Amlodipine (Tekamlo)	**Tab:** (Aliskiren-Amlodipine) 150mg-5mg, 150mg-10mg, 300mg-5mg, 300mg-10mg	**Initial:** 150mg-5mg qd. **Titrate:** May increase after 2-4 wks. **Max:** 300mg-10mg qd.	
CALCIUM CHANNEL BLOCKERS (DIHYDROPYRIDINE)-RENIN INHIBITORS-THIAZIDE DIURETICS			
Aliskiren-Amlodipine-HCTZ (Amturnide)	**Tab:** (Aliskiren-Amlodipine-HCTZ) 150mg-5mg-12.5mg, 300mg-5mg-12.5mg, 300mg-5mg-25mg, 300mg-10mg-12.5mg, 300mg-10mg-25mg	**Usual:** Dose qd. **Titrate:** May increase after 2 wks. **Max:** 300mg-10mg-25mg.	
CALCIUM CHANNEL BLOCKERS (NON-DIHYDROPYRIDINE)			
Diltiazem HCl (Cardizem CD, Cardizem LA, Cartia XT)	**Cap, ER:** (Cardizem CD, Cartia XT) 120mg, 180mg, 240mg, 300mg, (Cardizem CD) 360mg; **Tab, ER:** (Cardizem LA) 120mg, 180mg, 240mg, 300mg, 360mg, 420mg	(Cardizem CD, Cartia XT) **Initial (Monotherapy):** 180-240mg qd. **Usual:** 240-360mg qd. **Max:** 480mg qd. (Cardizem LA) **Initial (Monotherapy):** 180-240mg qd (am or hs). **Range:** 120-540mg qd. **Max:** 540mg/day.	
Diltiazem HCl (Taztia XT, Tiazac)	**Cap, ER:** (Taztia XT) 120mg, 180mg, 240mg, 300mg, 360mg; (Tiazac) 120mg, 180mg, 240mg, 300mg, 360mg, 420mg	**Initial (Monotherapy):** 120-240mg qd. **Usual Range:** 120-540mg qd. **Max:** 540mg qd.	
Verapamil HCl (Calan)	**Tab:** 40mg, 80mg*, 120mg*	**Initial (Monotherapy):** 80mg tid (240mg/day). **Max:** 360mg/day.	
Verapamil HCl (Calan SR)	**Tab, ER:** 120mg, 180mg*, 240mg*	**Initial:** 180mg qam. **Titrate:** May increase to 240mg qam, then 180mg bid (am and pm) or 240mg qam plus 120mg qpm, then 240mg q12h.	
Verapamil HCl (Covera-HS)	**Tab, ER:** 180mg, 240mg	**Initial:** 180mg qhs. **Titrate:** May increase to 240mg qhs, then 360mg (two 180mg tabs) qhs, then 480mg (two 240mg tabs) qhs.	
Verapamil HCl (Verelan)	**Cap, SR:** 120mg, 180mg, 240mg, 360mg	**Usual:** 240mg qam.	

GENERIC (BRAND)	HOW SUPPLIED	ADULT DOSAGE	PEDIATRIC DOSAGE
CALCIUM CHANNEL BLOCKERS (NON-DIHYDROPYRIDINE) *(Continued)*			
Verapamil HCl (Verelan PM)	**Cap, ER:** 100mg, 200mg, 300mg	**Usual:** 200mg qhs.	
LOOP DIURETICS			
Furosemide (Lasix)	**Sol:** (Generic) 10mg/mL [60mL, 120mL], 40mg/5mL [500mL]; **Tab:** (Generic) 20mg, 40mg*, 80mg*; (Lasix) 20mg, 40mg*, 80mg	**Initial:** 40mg bid.	
Torsemide (Demadex)	**Inj:** (Generic) 10mg/mL [2mL, 5mL]; **Tab:** (Demadex) 5mg*, 10mg*, 20mg*, 100mg*	**Initial:** 5mg qd. **Titrate:** May increase to 10mg qd after 4-6 wks.	
POTASSIUM-SPARING DIURETICS			
Amiloride HCl (Midamor)	**Tab:** 5mg	**Initial:** 5mg qd. **Titrate:** May increase to 10mg/day.	
Spironolactone (Aldactone)	**Tab:** 25mg, 50mg*, 100mg*	**Initial:** 50-100mg/day given qd or in divided doses for at least 2 wks.	
POTASSIUM-SPARING DIURETICS-THIAZIDE DIURETICS			
Amiloride HCl-HCTZ	**Tab:** (Amiloride-HCTZ) 5mg-50mg*	**Initial:** 1 tab/day. **Titrate:** May increase to 2 tabs/day if necessary. **Max:** 2 tabs/day.	
Spironolactone-HCTZ (Aldactazide)	**Tab:** (Spironolactone-HCTZ) 25mg-25mg, 50mg-50mg*	**Usual:** 50-100mg of each component as single dose or in divided doses.	
Triamterene-HCTZ (Dyazide)	**Cap:** (Triamterene-HCTZ) 37.5mg-25mg	1-2 caps qd.	
Triamterene-HCTZ (Maxzide, Maxzide-25)	**Tab:** (Triamterene-HCTZ) (Maxzide) 75mg-50mg*, (Maxzide-25) 37.5mg-25mg*	(Maxzide-25) 1-2 tabs qd, given as a single dose; (Maxzide) 1 tab qd.	
QUINAZOLINE DIURETICS			
Metolazone (Zaroxolyn)	**Tab:** 2.5mg, 5mg	2.5-5mg qd.	
RENIN INHIBITORS			
Aliskiren (Tekturna)	**Tab:** 150mg, 300mg	**Initial:** 150mg qd. **Titrate:** May increase to 300mg qd. **Max:** 300mg/day.	
RENIN INHIBITORS-THIAZIDE DIURETICS			
Aliskiren-HCTZ (Tekturna HCT)	**Tab:** (Aliskiren-HCTZ) 150mg-12.5mg, 150mg-25mg, 300mg-12.5mg, 300mg-25mg	**Add-On/Initial Therapy:** Initiate with 150mg-12.5mg qd. **Titrate:** May increase after 2-4 wks. **Max:** 300mg-25mg qd.	
THIAZIDE DIURETICS			
Chlorothiazide (Diuril)	**Sus:** (Diuril) 250mg/5mL [237mL]; **Tab:** (Generic) 250mg*, 500mg*	**Initial:** 0.5-1g/day given qd or in divided doses. **Max:** 2g/day in divided doses.	**Usual:** 10-20mg/kg/day given qd-bid. **Max: 2-12 Yrs:** 1g/day. **≤2 Yrs:** 375mg/day. **<6 Months:** Up to 30mg/kg/day given bid.

(Continued)

GENERIC (BRAND)	HOW SUPPLIED	ADULT DOSAGE	PEDIATRIC DOSAGE
THIAZIDE DIURETICS *(Continued)*			
Chlorthalidone (Thalitone)	**Tab:** (Generic) 25mg, 50mg*; (Thalitone) 15mg	(Thalitone) **Initial:** 15mg qd. **Titrate:** May increase to 30mg qd, then to 45-50mg qd. **Maint:** May be lower than initial. (Generic) **Initial:** 25mg qd. **Titrate:** May increase to 50mg qd, then to 100mg qd. **Max:** 100mg qd. **Maint:** May be lower than initial.	
Hydrochlorothiazide	**Tab:** 12.5mg, 25mg*, 50mg*	**Initial:** 25mg qd. **Titrate:** May increase to 50mg/day given qd or in 2 divided doses.	1-2mg/kg/day given qd or in 2 divided doses. **Max: 2-12 Yrs:** 100mg/day. **Infants up to 2 Yrs:** 37.5mg/day. **<6 Months:** Up to 3mg/kg/day given in 2 divided doses may be required.
Hydrochlorothiazide (Microzide)	**Cap:** 12.5mg	**Initial:** 12.5mg qd. **Max:** 50mg/day.	
Indapamide	**Tab:** 1.25mg, 2.5mg	**Initial:** 1.25mg qam. **Titrate:** May increase to 2.5mg qd after 4 wks, then to 5mg qd after additional 4 wks.	
Methyclothiazide	**Tab:** 5mg*	**Usual:** 2.5-5mg qd.	
VASODILATORS			
Hydralazine HCl	**Inj:** 20mg/mL; **Tab:** 10mg, 25mg, 50mg, 100mg	(Tab) **Initial:** 10mg qid for the first 2-4 days. **Titrate:** Increase to 25mg qid for the rest of the 1st wk, then increase to 50mg qid for 2nd and subsequent wks. **Resistant Patients:** ≤300mg/day. (Inj) **Usual:** 20-40mg only when drug cannot be given PO.	(Tab) **Initial:** 0.75mg/kg/day given qid. **Titrate:** Increase gradually over 3-4 wks. **Max:** 7.5mg/kg/day or 200mg/day. (Inj) **Usual:** 1.7-3.5mg/kg divided in 4-6 doses only when drug cannot be given PO.

Refer to full FDA-approved labeling for additional information.

*Scored.

†Doses >20mg have not shown a statistically significant additional antihypertensive effect, but the 40mg dose has been studied and is well tolerated.

Abbreviations: ACE = angiotensin-converting enzyme; ER = extended-release; HCTZ = hydrochlorothiazide; SR = sustained-release.

ACNE MANAGEMENT

GENERIC (BRAND)	HOW SUPPLIED	DOSAGE
SYSTEMIC AGENTS		
Isotretinoin (Absorica)	**Cap:** 10mg, 20mg, 25mg, 30mg, 35mg, 40mg	**Adults & Peds ≥12 yrs:** 0.5-1mg/kg/day given in 2 divided doses for 15-20 wks. **Max:** 2mg/kg/day.
Isotretinoin (Amnesteem, Claravis)	**Cap:** (Amnesteem) 10mg, 20mg, 40mg; (Claravis) 10mg, 20mg, 30mg, 40mg	**Adults & Peds ≥12 yrs:** 0.5-1mg/kg/day given in 2 divided doses for 15-20 wks. **Max:** 2mg/kg/day.
Minocycline HCl (Solodyn)	**Tab, Extended-Release:** 55mg, 65mg, 80mg, 105mg, 115mg	**Adults & Peds ≥12 yrs:** 1mg/kg qd for 12 wks.
TOPICAL AGENTS		
Adapalene (Differin)	**Cre:** 0.1%	**Adults & Peds ≥12 yrs:** Apply a thin layer to affected area qpm.
	Gel: 0.1%, 0.3%	**Adults & Peds ≥12 yrs:** Apply a thin layer to affected area qhs after washing.
	Lot: 0.1%	**Adults & Peds ≥12 yrs:** Apply a thin layer to cover the entire face and other affected area qd after washing.
Azelaic acid (Azelex)	**Cre:** 20%	**Adults & Peds ≥12 yrs:** Wash and dry skin. Massage gently but thoroughly into affected area bid (am and pm).
Benzoyl peroxide (BenzEFoam, BenzEFoam Ultra)	(BenzEFoam) **Foam:** 5.3%	**Adults & Peds ≥12 yrs:** Rub into affected area qd or ud until completely absorbed. **Facial Acne:** Use a dollop the size of a marble. **Back/Chest Acne:** Use a dollop the size of a whole walnut.
	(BenzEFoam Ultra) **Foam:** 9.8%	**Adults & Peds ≥12 yrs:** Rub into affected area qd, then bid-tid prn or ud until completely absorbed. Rinse off after 2 min.
Benzoyl peroxide (NeoBenz Micro SD, NeoBenz Micro Wash)	(SD) **Cre:** 5.5%	**Adults & Peds ≥12 yrs:** Apply to affected area qd-bid.
	(Wash) **Sol:** 7%	
Benzoyl peroxide	**Gel:** 2.5%, 5%, 10%	**Adults & Peds ≥12 yrs: (2.5%) Initial:** Apply to affected area qd for 1 week, then bid. **(5%, 10%)** May be initiated in patients demonstrating accommodation to 2.5% gel.
Clindamycin phosphate (Evoclin)	**Foam:** 1%	**Adults & Peds ≥12 yrs:** Apply to affected area qd.
Clindamycin phosphate (Cleocin T)	**Gel:** 1%	**Adults & Peds ≥12 yrs:** Apply thin layer to affected area bid.
	Lot: 1%	
	Sol: 1%	
Clindamycin phosphate (Clindagel)	**Gel:** 1%	**Adults & Peds ≥12 yrs:** Apply thin layer to affected area qd.
Dapsone (Aczone)	**Gel:** 5%	**Adults & Peds ≥12 yrs:** Apply pea-sized amount to affected area bid.
Erythromycin (Akne-Mycin)	**Oint:** 2%	**Adults:** Apply to affected area bid (am and pm).
Erythromycin	**Gel:** 2%	**Adults:** Wash and dry skin. Apply a thin layer to affected area qd-bid. Do not rub in; spread lightly.
	Pledgets: 2%	**Adults:** Wash and dry skin. Rub pledget or apply sol to affected area bid (am and pm).
	Sol: 2%	
Gentamicin sulfate	**Cre:** 0.1%	**Adults & Peds >1 yr:** Apply small amount to affected area tid-qid.
	Oint: 0.1%	

(Continued)

GENERIC (BRAND)	HOW SUPPLIED	DOSAGE
TOPICAL AGENTS *(Continued)*		
Tazarotene (Fabior)	**Foam:** 0.1%	**Adults & Peds ≥12 yrs:** Wash and dry skin. Apply thin layer to affected area of face and/or upper trunk qpm. Massage into skin.
Tazarotene (Tazorac)	**Cre:** 0.1%	**Adults & Peds ≥12 yrs:** Wash and dry skin. Apply thin layer to affected area qpm.
	Gel: 0.1%	
Tretinoin (Atralin)	**Gel:** 0.05%	**Adults & Peds ≥10 yrs:** Apply thin layer to affected area qhs.
Tretinoin (Avita)	**Cre:** 0.025%	**Adults:** Apply thin layer to affected area qpm.
	Gel: 0.025%	
Tretinoin (Retin-A)	**Cre:** 0.025%, 0.05%, 0.1%	**Adults:** Apply thin layer to affected area qhs.
	Gel: 0.01%, 0.025%	
Tretinoin (Retin-A Micro)	**Gel:** 0.04%, 0.08%, 0.1%	**Adults & Peds ≥12 yrs:** Apply thin layer to affected area qpm.
Tretinoin (Tretin-X)	**Cre:** 0.025%, 0.0375%, 0.05%, 0.075%, 0.1%	**Adults & Peds ≥12 yrs:** Apply thin layer to affected area qhs.
COMBINATION PRODUCTS, TOPICAL		
Adapalene-Benzoyl peroxide (Epiduo)	**Gel:** 0.1%-2.5%	**Adults & Peds ≥9 yrs:** Apply pea-sized amount to affected area of face and/or trunk qd after washing.
Benzoyl peroxide-Clindamycin phosphate (Acanya)	**Gel:** 2.5%-1.2%	**Adults & Peds ≥12 yrs:** Apply pea-sized amount to face qd.
Benzoyl peroxide-Clindamycin phosphate (BenzaClin)	**Gel:** 5%-1%	**Adults & Peds ≥12 yrs:** Wash and dry skin. Apply to affected area bid or ud.
Benzoyl peroxide-Clindamycin phosphate (Duac)	**Gel:** 5%-1.2%	**Adults & Peds ≥12 yrs:** Wash and dry skin. Apply thin layer to face qpm or ud.
Benzoyl peroxide-Erythromycin (Benzamycin)	**Gel:** 5%-3%	**Adults & Peds ≥12 yrs:** Wash and dry skin. Apply to affected area bid or ud.
Clindamycin phosphate-Tretinoin (Veltin)	**Gel:** 1.2%-0.025%	**Adults & Peds ≥12 yrs:** Apply pea-sized amount lightly covering the entire affected area qpm.
Clindamycin phosphate-Tretinoin (Ziana)	**Gel:** 1.2%-0.025%	**Adults & Peds ≥12 yrs:** Apply pea-sized amount onto 1 fingertip, dot onto chin, cheeks, nose, and forehead, then gently rub over entire face qhs.
Hydrocortisone acetate-Iodoquinol (Alcortin-A)	**Gel:** 2%-1%	**Adults & Peds ≥12 yrs:** Apply to affected area tid-qid or ud.
Sodium sulfacetamide (Klaron)	**Lot:** 10%	**Adults & Peds ≥12 yrs:** Apply thin layer to affected area bid.
Sodium sulfacetamide-Sulfur (Avar Cleanser, Avar Cleansing Pads, Avar LS Cleanser, Avar LS Cleansing Pads, Avar-e Cream, Avar-e Green Cream, Avar-e LS Cream)	**Pads:** (Avar Cleansing Pads) 9.5%-5%; (Avar LS Cleansing Pads) 10%-2%	**Adults & Peds ≥12 yrs:** Wash affected area qd-bid or ud.
	Cre: (Avar-e Cream, Avar-e Green Cream) 10%-5%; (Avar-e LS Cream) 10%-2%	**Adults & Peds ≥12 yrs:** Cleanse affected area. Apply a thin layer to affected area qd-tid or ud. Massage into skin.
	Sol: (Avar Cleanser) 10%-5%; (Avar LS Cleanser) 10%-2%	**Adults & Peds ≥12 yrs:** Wash affected area qd-bid or ud.
Sodium sulfacetamide-Sulfur (Sumadan)	**Wash:** 9%-4.5%	**Adults & Peds ≥12 yrs:** Apply to affected area qd-bid or ud.

GENERIC (BRAND)	HOW SUPPLIED	DOSAGE
COMBINATION PRODUCTS, TOPICAL *(Continued)*		
Sodium sulfacetamide-Sulfur	**Lot:** 10%-5%	**Adults & Peds ≥12 yrs:** Apply thin layer to affected area with light massaging qd-tid or ud.
Refer to full FDA-approved labeling for additional information.		

Psoriasis Management: Systemic Therapies

GENERIC (BRAND)	HOW SUPPLIED	ADULT DOSAGE
ANTIMETABOLITES		
Methotrexate (Otrexup, Rasuvo, Rheumatrex, Trexall)*	**Inj:** (Generic) 25mg/mL, 1g/vial, (Otrexup) 7.5mg/0.4mL, 10mg/0.4mL, 15mg/0.4mL, 20mg/0.4mL, 25mg/0.4mL, (Rasuvo) 7.5mg/0.15mL, 10mg/0.20mL, 12.5mg/0.25mL, 15mg/0.30mL, 17.5mg/0.35mL, 20mg/0.40mL, 22.5mg/0.45mL, 25mg/0.50mL, 27.5mg/0.55mL, 30mg/0.60mL **Tab:** 2.5mg, (Trexall) 5mg, 7.5mg, 10mg, 15mg	**Initial:** 10-25mg PO/IM/SQ/IV as a single weekly dose, or 2.5mg PO q12h for 3 doses. **Titrate:** May adjust gradually to achieve optimal response. **Max:** 30mg/wk.
IMMUNOSUPPRESSIVES		
Cyclosporine (Gengraf, Neoral)	**Cap:** 25mg, 100mg **Sol:** 100mg/mL	**Initial:** 1.25mg/kg bid for ≥4 wks. **Titrate:** May increase by 0.5mg/kg/day at 2-wk intervals, as tolerated. **Max:** 4mg/kg/day.
MONOCLONAL ANTIBODIES		
Ustekinumab (Stelara)	**Inj:** 45mg/0.5mL, 90mg/mL	**SQ: >100kg:** 90mg initially and 4 wks later, 90mg q12wks. **≤100kg:** 45mg initially and 4 wks later, 45mg q12wks.
MONOCLONAL ANTIBODIES/IL-17A ANTAGONISTS		
Secukinumab (Cosentyx)	**Inj:** 150mg/mL, 150mg/vial	**SQ:** 300mg at 0, 1, 2, 3, and 4 wks, followed by 300mg q4wks. A dose of 150mg may be acceptable for some patients.
MONOCLONAL ANTIBODIES/TNF BLOCKERS		
Adalimumab (Humira)	**Inj:** 20mg/0.4mL, 40mg/0.8mL	**SQ:** 80mg initial dose, followed by 40mg every other wk starting 1 wk after the initial dose.
Infliximab (Remicade)	**Inj:** 100mg/vial	Infuse over ≥2 hrs. **IV: Induction:** 5mg/kg at 0, 2, and 6 wks. **Maint:** 5mg/kg q8wks.
PSORALENS		
Methoxsalen† (8-Mop, Oxsoralen-Ultra)	**Cap:** 10mg	Take 2 hrs before UVA exposure with some food or milk. **<30kg:** 10mg; **30-50kg:** 20mg; **51-65kg:** 30mg; **66-80kg:** 40mg; **81-90kg:** 50mg; **91-115kg:** 60mg; **>115kg:** 70mg. **Titrate:** May increase by 10mg after 15th treatment under certain conditions ud. **Max:** No more than once qod.
RETINOIDS		
Acitretin (Soriatane)*	**Cap:** 10mg, 17.5mg, 25mg	**Initial:** 25-50mg/day as a single dose with the main meal. **Maint:** 25-50mg/day.
TNF-BLOCKING AGENTS		
Etanercept (Enbrel)	**Inj:** 25mg, 50mg	**SQ: Initial:** 50mg twice weekly for 3 months. **Maint:** 50mg once weekly.

Refer to full FDA-approved labeling for additional information.
*Contraindicated in pregnancy.
†Oxsoralen-Ultra and 8-Mop should not be used interchangeably.

INSULIN FORMULATIONS

TYPE OF INSULIN	BRAND	CLASS (Rx/OTC)	ONSET*	PEAK*	DURATION*
Rapid-acting					
Insulin glulisine	Apidra	Rx	15 mins	0.5-1.5 hrs	3-5 hrs
Insulin lispro	Humalog	Rx	15 mins	0.5-1.5 hrs	3-5 hrs
Insulin aspart	NovoLog	Rx	15 mins	0.5-1.5 hrs	3-5 hrs
Short-acting					
Regular insulin	Humulin R†	OTC	30-60 mins	2-4 hrs	5-8 hrs
	Novolin R	OTC	30-60 mins	2-4 hrs	5-8 hrs
Intermediate-acting					
NPH	Humulin N	OTC	1-3 hrs	8 hrs	12-16 hrs
	Novolin N	OTC	1-3 hrs	8 hrs	12-16 hrs
Long-acting					
Insulin glargine	Lantus	Rx	1 hr	Peakless	20-26 hrs
Insulin detemir	Levemir	Rx	1 hr	Peakless	20-26 hrs
Combinations					
NPH (70%)/regular insulin (30%)	Humulin 70/30	OTC	30-60 mins	Varies	10-16 hrs
NPH (70%)/regular insulin (30%)	Novolin 70/30	OTC	30-60 mins	Varies	10-16 hrs
Insulin aspart protamine (70%)/ insulin aspart (30%)	NovoLog Mix 70/30	Rx	5-15 mins	Varies	10-16 hrs
Insulin lispro protamine (50%)/ insulin lispro (50%)	Humalog Mix50/50	Rx	10-15 mins	Varies	10-16 hrs
Insulin lispro protamine (75%)/ insulin lispro (25%)	Humalog Mix75/25	Rx	10-15 mins	Varies	10-16 hrs

Refer to full FDA-approved labeling for detailed information.

*Onset, peak, and duration will vary among patients and dosage should be determined by the healthcare professional familiar with the patient's metabolic needs, eating habits, and other lifestyle variables.

†Also available as 500 U/mL (Rx only) for insulin-resistant patients (rapid onset [within 30 mins]; up to 24-hr duration).

Source: Types of Insulin. National Diabetes Information Clearinghouse (NDIC) website. http://diabetes.niddk.nih.gov/dm/pubs/medicines_ez/insert_C.aspx. Updated February 16, 2012. Accessed February 5, 2015.

ORAL ANTIDIABETIC AGENTS

BRAND (GENERIC)	HOW SUPPLIED	INITIAL* & (MAX) DOSAGE	USUAL DOSAGE RANGE*	PROPERTIES
BIGUANIDES				
Fortamet[†] (Metformin HCl)	**Tab, ER:** 500mg, 1000mg	500-1000mg qd with evening meal (2500mg/day)	500mg-2500mg/day	**Mechanism:** Activates AMP-Kinase **Action(s):** Hepatic glucose production ↓, intestinal glucose absorption ↓, insulin action ↑ **Advantages:** No weight gain, no hypoglycemia, reduction in cardiovascular events and mortality **Disadvantages:** GI side effects (diarrhea, abdominal cramping), lactic acidosis (rare), vitamin B12 deficiency
Glumetza[†] (Metformin HCl)	**Tab, ER:** 500mg, 1000mg	**Metformin-Naive:** 500mg qd with evening meal (2000mg/day)	500mg-2000mg/day	
Glucophage[†], **Riomet**[†] (Metformin HCl)	**Tab:** 500mg, 850mg, 1000mg **Sol:** 500mg/5mL	500mg bid or 850mg qd with meals (2550mg/day)	850mg-2000mg/day	
Glucophage XR[†] (Metformin HCl)	**Tab, ER:** 500mg, 750mg	500mg qd with evening meal (2000mg/day)	500mg-2000mg qd or divided doses	
BILE-ACID SEQUESTRANTS				
Welchol (Colesevelam HCl)	**Tab:** 625mg; **Sus:** 1.875g, 3.75g [pkt]	**Tab:** 1875mg bid or 3750mg qd with meal and liquid; **Sus:** 1.875g pkt bid or 3.75g pkt qd with meal	3750mg/day	**Mechanism:** Binds bile acids/cholesterol **Action(s):** Unknown **Advantages:** No hypoglycemia, LDL cholesterol ↓ **Disadvantages:** Constipation, triglycerides ↑, may interfere with absorption of other medications, may decrease absorption of fat-soluble vitamins
DIPEPTIDYL PEPTIDASE-4 INHIBITORS				
Tradjenta (Linagliptin)	**Tab:** 5mg	5mg qd	5mg/day	**Mechanism:** Inhibits DPP-4 activity, prolongs survival of endogenously released incretin hormones **Action(s):** Active GLP-1 concentration ↑, active GIP concentration ↑, insulin secretion ↑, glucagon secretion ↓ **Advantages:** No hypoglycemia, weight "neutrality" **Disadvantages:** Occasional reports of urticaria/angioedema, cases of pancreatitis observed, nasopharyngitis, headache, upper respiratory tract infection, long-term safety unknown
Onglyza (Saxagliptin)	**Tab:** 2.5mg, 5mg	2.5-5mg qd	2.5-5mg/day	
Januvia (Sitagliptin)	**Tab:** 25mg, 50mg, 100mg	100mg qd	100mg/day	
GLUCOSIDASE INHIBITORS				
Precose (Acarbose)	**Tab:** 25mg, 50mg, 100mg	25mg tid at start of each meal, or qd to minimize GI side effects (**≤60kg:** 50mg tid, **>60kg:** 100mg tid)	50-100mg tid	**Mechanism:** Inhibits intestinal α-glucosidase **Action(s):** Delayed glucose absorption **Advantages:** Nonsystemic medication, postprandial glucose ↓ **Disadvantages:** GI side effects (gas, flatulence, diarrhea), dosing frequency
Glyset (Miglitol)	**Tab:** 25mg, 50mg, 100mg	25mg tid at start of each meal, or qd to minimize GI effects (300mg/day)	50-100mg tid	

(Continued)

BRAND (GENERIC)	HOW SUPPLIED	INITIAL* & (MAX) DOSAGE	USUAL DOSAGE RANGE*	PROPERTIES
MEGLITINIDES				
Starlix (Nateglinide)	**Tab:** 60mg, 120mg	120mg tid 1-30 min before meals	120mg tid	**Mechanism:** Closes KATP channels on β-cell plasma membranes **Action(s):** Insulin secretion ↑ **Advantages:** Accentuated effects around meal ingestion **Disadvantages:** Hypoglycemia, weight gain, upper respiratory tract infections, may blunt myocardial ischemic preconditioning, dosing frequency
Prandin (Repaglinide)	**Tab:** 0.5mg, 1mg, 2mg	0.5-2mg within 30 min before each meal (16mg/day)	0.5-4mg with each meal	
SODIUM-GLUCOSE COTRANSPORTER 2 INHIBITORS				
Invokana (Canagliflozin)	**Tab:** 100mg, 300mg	100mg qd before the first meal (300mg/day)	100-300mg qd	**Mechanism:** Inhibits sodium-glucose cotransporter 2 in the proximal renal tubules **Action(s):** Urinary glucose excretion ↑ **Advantages:** No weight gain **Disadvantages:** BP ↓, impairment in renal function, hyperkalemia, genital mycotic infections, LDL ↑
Farxiga (Dapagliflozin)	**Tab:** 5mg, 10mg	5mg qd in the am (10mg/day)	5-10mg qd	
Jardiance (Empagliflozin)	**Tab:** 10mg, 25mg	10mg qd in the morning (25mg/day)	10-25mg/day	
SULFONYLUREAS				
(Chlorpropamide)	**Tab:** 100mg, 250mg	250mg qd with breakfast (750mg/day)	<100-500mg qd; most patients controlled with 250mg qd	**Mechanism:** Stimulates the release of insulin from the pancreas **Action(s):** Insulin secretion ↑ **Advantages:** Generally well tolerated **Disadvantages:** Relatively glucose-independent stimulation of insulin secretion; GI effects; hypoglycemia; weight gain; ↑ risk of cardiovascular mortality; low "durability"
Amaryl (Glimepiride)	**Tab:** 1mg, 2mg, 4mg	1-2mg qd with breakfast or first main meal (8mg/day)	1-8mg/day	
Glucotrol (Glipizide)	**Tab:** 5mg, 10mg	5mg qd 30 min before breakfast (40mg/day)	5-40mg qd; divided doses if >15mg/day	
Glucotrol XL (Glipizide)	**Tab, ER:** 2.5mg, 5mg, 10mg	5mg qd with breakfast (20mg/day)	5-10mg/day	
Diabeta (Glyburide)	**Tab:** 1.25mg, 2.5mg, 5mg	2.5-5mg qd with breakfast or first main meal (20mg/day)	1.25-20mg/day in single or divided doses	
Glynase PresTab (Glyburide, micronized)	**Tab:** 1.5mg, 3mg, 6mg	1.5-3mg qd with breakfast or first main meal (12mg/day)	0.75-12mg/day in single or divided doses	
(Tolazamide)	**Tab:** 250mg, 500mg	100-250mg qd with breakfast or first main meal (1000mg/day)	100-1000mg/day; divided doses if >500mg/day	
(Tolbutamide)	**Tab:** 500mg	1000-2000mg qd in single or divided doses (3000mg/day)	250-3000mg/day in single or divided doses	

BRAND (GENERIC)	HOW SUPPLIED	INITIAL* & (MAX) DOSAGE	USUAL DOSAGE RANGE*	PROPERTIES
THIAZOLIDINEDIONES				
Actos‡ (Pioglitazone)	**Tab:** 15mg, 30mg, 45mg	15-30mg qd (45mg/day)	15-45mg/day	**Mechanism:** Activates the nuclear transcription factor PPAR-γ **Action(s):** Peripheral insulin sensitivity ↑ **Advantages:** No hypoglycemia, HDL cholesterol ↑; (Actos) triglycerides ↓ **Disadvantages:** Weight gain, edema, heart failure, bone fractures; (Avandia) LDL cholesterol ↑, MI ↑
Avandia‡ (Rosiglitazone maleate)	**Tab:** 2mg, 4mg, 8mg	2mg bid or 4mg qd (8mg/day)	4-8mg/day	
COMBINATIONS				
Invokamet† (Canagliflozin/ Metformin HCl)	**Tab:** 50mg/500mg, 50mg/1000mg, 150mg/500mg, 150mg/1000mg	Individualize initial dose based on patient's current regimen (300mg/2000mg/day)		
Xigduo XR† (Dapagliflozin/ Metformin HCl)	**Tab, ER:** 5mg/500mg, 5mg/1000mg, 10mg/500mg, 10mg/1000mg	Individualize initial dose based on patient's current treatment (10mg/2000mg/day)		
Glyxambi (Empagliflozin/ Linagliptin)	**Tab:** 10mg/5mg, 25mg/5mg	10mg/5mg qd in the morning	10mg/5mg-25mg/5mg qd	
(Glipizide/ Metformin HCl)†	**Tab:** 2.5mg/250mg, 2.5mg/500mg, 5mg/500mg	2.5mg/250mg qd or 2.5mg/500mg bid with meals (20mg/2000mg/day)	2.5mg/250mg qd-5mg/500mg bid	
Glucovance† (Glyburide/ Metformin HCl)	**Tab:** 1.25mg/250mg, 2.5mg/500mg, 5mg/500mg	1.25mg/250mg qd or bid with meals (20mg/2000mg/day)	1.25mg/250mg qd-5mg/500mg bid	
Jentadueto† (Linagliptin/ Metformin HCl)	**Tab:** 2.5mg/500mg, 2.5mg/850mg, 2.5mg/1000mg	2.5mg/500mg bid with meals (5mg/2000mg/day)	2.5mg/500mg-2.5mg/1000mg bid	
Duetact‡ (Pioglitazone/ Glimepiride)	**Tab:** 30mg/2mg, 30mg/4mg	30mg/2mg or 30mg/4mg qd with first meal (45mg/8mg/day)	30mg/2mg-30mg/4mg/day	
Actoplus Met†‡ (Pioglitazone/ Metformin HCl)	**Tab:** 15mg/500mg, 15mg/850mg	15mg/500mg bid or 15mg/850mg qd with meal (45mg/2550mg/day)	15/500mg bid-15/850mg qd	
Actoplus Met XR†‡ (Pioglitazone/ Metformin HCl)	**Tab, ER:** 15mg/1000mg, 30mg/1000mg	15mg/1000mg or 30mg/1000mg qd with meal (45mg/2000mg/day)	15mg/1000mg-30mg/1000mg/day	
PrandiMet† (Repaglinide/ Metformin HCl)	**Tab:** 1mg/500mg, 2mg/500mg	1mg/500mg bid 15-30 min before meals (10mg/2500/day or 4mg/1000mg/meal)	1mg/500mg-2mg/500mg bid or tid	

(Continued)

BRAND (GENERIC)	HOW SUPPLIED	INITIAL* & (MAX) DOSAGE	USUAL DOSAGE RANGE*	PROPERTIES
COMBINATIONS *(Continued)*				
Avandaryl‡ (Rosiglitazone maleate/ Glimepiride)	**Tab:** 4mg/1mg, 4mg/2mg, 4mg/4mg, 8mg/2mg, 8mg/4mg	4mg/1mg qd or 4mg/2mg qd with first meal (8mg/4mg/day)	4mg/1mg-4mg/2mg qd	
Avandamet†‡ (Rosiglitazone maleate/ Metformin HCl)	**Tab:** 2mg/500mg, 4mg/500mg, 2mg/1000mg, 4mg/1000mg	2mg/500mg qd or bid with meals (8mg/2000mg/day)	2mg/500mg-4mg/1000mg/day in divided doses	
Kombiglyze XR† (Saxagliptin/ Metformin HCl)	**Tab, ER:** 5mg/500mg, 5mg/1000mg, 2.5/1000mg	5mg/500mg or 2.5mg/1000mg qd with evening meal (5mg/2000mg/day)	5mg/500mg-2.5/1000mg qd	
Janumet† (Sitagliptin/ Metformin HCl)	**Tab:** 50mg/500mg, 50mg/1000mg	50mg/500mg or 50mg/1000mg bid with meals (100mg/2000mg/day)	50mg/500mg-50mg/1000mg bid	
Janumet XR† (Sitagliptin/ Metformin HCl)	**Tab:** 100mg/1000mg, 50mg/500mg, 50mg/1000mg	50mg/1000mg or 100mg/1000mg qd with meals (100mg/2000mg/day)	50mg/1000mg-100mg/1000mg qd	

*Usual dosage ranges are derived from FDA-approved labeling. There is no fixed dosage regimen for the management of diabetes mellitus with any hypoglycemic agent. The initial and maintenance dosing should be conservative, depending on the patient's individual needs, especially in elderly, debilitated, or malnourished patients, and with impaired renal or hepatic function. Management of type 2 diabetes should include blood glucose and HbA1c monitoring, nutritional counseling, exercise, and weight reduction as needed. For more detailed information, refer to the individual monograph listings or FDA-approved labeling.

†**BOXED WARNING:** Products containing metformin may cause lactic acidosis due to metformin accumulation. Refer to package insert for more details.

‡**BOXED WARNING:** Products containing thiazolidinediones, including pioglitazone or rosiglitazone, may cause or exacerbate congestive heart failure in some patients. Refer to package insert for more details regarding this warning.

Crohn's Disease Treatments

GENERIC	BRAND	HOW SUPPLIED	ADULT DOSAGE	PEDIATRIC DOSAGE
CORTICOSTEROIDS				
Betamethasone sodium phosphate-Betamethasone acetate	Celestone Soluspan	**Inj:** 3mg-3mg/mL [5mL, multidose]	**Initial:** 0.25-9mg/day IM.*	**Initial:** 0.02-0.3mg/kg/day in 3 or 4 divided doses IM.*
Budesonide	Entocort EC	**Cap:** 3mg	**Usual:** 9mg qam for up to 8 wks. **Recurring Episodes:** Repeat therapy for 8 wks. **Maint:** 6mg qd for up to 3 months, then taper to complete cessation.	
Dexamethasone	Generic	**Sol:** 0.5mg/5mL, 1mg/mL; **Tab:** 0.5mg†, 0.75mg†, 1mg†, 1.5mg†, 2mg†, 4mg†, 6mg†	**Initial:** 0.75-9mg/day.*	**Initial:** 0.02-0.3mg/kg/day in 3 or 4 divided doses.*
	Generic	**Inj:** 4mg/mL [1mL, 5mL, 30mL], 10mg/mL [1mL]	**Initial:** 0.5-9mg/day IV/IM.*	
Hydrocortisone	Cortef	**Tab:** 5mg†, 10mg†, 20mg†	**Initial:** 20-240mg/day.*	**Initial:** 20-240mg/day.*
	Solu-Cortef	**Inj:** 100mg, 250mg, 500mg, 1000mg	**Initial:** 100-500mg IV/IM. May repeat dose at 2-, 4-, or 6-hr intervals. High-dose therapy should continue only until patient is stabilized, usually not beyond 48-72 hrs.*	**Initial:** 0.56-8mg/kg/day IV/IM in 3 or 4 divided doses.*
Methylprednisolone	Depo-Medrol	**Inj:** 20mg/mL, 40mg/mL, 80mg/mL	**Initial:** 4-120mg IM.*	**Initial:** 0.11-1.6mg/kg/day.*
	Medrol	**Tab:** 2mg†, 4mg†, 8mg†, 16mg†, 32mg†; (Dose-Pak) 4mg† [21s]	**Initial:** 4-48mg/day.* Refer to PI for detailed information for ADT.	**Initial:** 4-48mg/day.* Refer to PI for detailed information for ADT.
	Solu-Medrol	**Inj:** 40mg, 125mg, 500mg, 1g, 2g	**Initial:** 10-40mg IV/IM inj or IV infusion. **High-Dose Therapy:** 30mg/kg IV over at least 30 min. May repeat dose q4-6h for 48 hrs. High-dose therapy should continue only until patient is stabilized, usually not beyond 48-72 hrs.*	**Initial:** 0.11-1.6mg/kg/day in 3 or 4 divided doses.*
Prednisolone	Flo-Pred	**Sus:** 15mg/5mL [37mL, 52mL, 65mL]	**Initial:** 5-60mg/day.*	**Initial:** 0.14-2mg/kg/day in 3 or 4 divided doses.*
	Orapred	**Sol:** 15mg/5mL [20mL, 237mL]; **Tab, Disintegrating:** 10mg, 15mg, 30mg	**(Sol) Initial:** 5-60mg/day. **(Tab, Disintegrating) Initial:** 10-60mg/day.*	**Initial:** 0.14-2mg/kg/day in 3 or 4 divided doses.*
	Pediapred	**Sol:** 5mg/5mL [120mL]	**Initial:** 5-60mg/day.*	**Initial:** 0.14-2mg/kg/day in 3 or 4 divided doses.*

(Continued)

GENERIC	BRAND	HOW SUPPLIED	ADULT DOSAGE	PEDIATRIC DOSAGE
CORTICOSTEROIDS *(Continued)*				
Prednisolone *(Continued)*	Generic	**Syrup:** 15mg/5mL [240mL, 480mL]; **Tab:** 5mg†	**Initial:** 5-60mg/day.* **(Tab)** Refer to PI for detailed information for ADT.	**Initial:** 5-60mg/day.* **(Tab)** Refer to PI for detailed information for ADT.
Prednisone	Rayos	**Tab, Delayed-Release:** 1mg, 2mg, 5mg	**Initial:** 5-60mg/day.*	**Initial:** 5-60mg/day.*
	Generic	**Sol:** 5mg/mL [30mL], 5mg/5mL [120mL, 500mL]; **Tab:** 1mg†, 2.5mg†, 5mg†, 10mg†, 20mg†, 50mg†	**Initial:** 5-60mg/day.* Refer to PI for detailed information for ADT.	**Initial:** 5-60mg/day.* Refer to PI for detailed information for ADT.
Triamcinolone	Kenalog-40	**Inj:** 40mg/mL [1mL, 5mL, 10mL]	**Initial:** 2.5-100mg/day.*	**Initial:** 0.11-1.6mg/kg/day in 3 or 4 divided doses.*
MONOCLONAL ANTIBODIES				
Adalimumab	Humira	**Inj:** 20mg/0.4mL, 40mg/0.8mL	**Initial:** 160mg SQ on Day 1 (given as four 40mg inj in 1 day or as two 40mg inj/day for 2 consecutive days); then 80mg after 2 wks (Day 15). **Maint:** 40mg every other wk beginning wk 4 (Day 29).	
Certolizumab pegol	Cimzia	**Inj:** 200mg/mL	**Initial:** 400mg (given as 2 SQ inj of 200mg) initially and at wks 2 and 4. **Maint:** 400mg q4wks.	
Infliximab	Remicade	**Inj:** 100mg/20mL	**Induction:** 5mg/kg IV at 0, 2, and 6 wks. **Maint:** 5mg/kg q8wks. **Patients Who Initially Respond but Lose Their Response:** May increase to 10mg/kg. Refer to PI for administration and preparation instructions.	**≥6 yrs: Induction:** 5mg/kg IV at 0, 2, and 6 wks. **Maint:** 5mg/kg q8wks. Refer to PI for administration and preparation instructions.
Natalizumab	Tysabri	**Inj:** 300mg/15mL	300mg IV infusion over 1 hr q4wks.	
Vedolizumab	Entyvio	**Inj:** 300mg/20mL	300mg IV over 30 min at 0, 2, and 6 wks. **Maint:** 300mg q8wks.	

Refer to full FDA-approved labeling for additional information.

Abbreviation: ADT = alternate day therapy.

*Maintenance dose should be determined by decreasing initial dose in small decrements to lowest effective dose. Withdraw gradually after long-term therapy.

†Scored.

H_2 Antagonists and PPIs Comparison*

	DRUG	HOW SUPPLIED	INDICATIONS								
			Heartburn	Gastric Ulcer	GERD	Esophagitis	Zollinger-Ellison	*Helicobacter pylori*	NSAID Induced[†]	Upper GI Bleeding[‡]	Duodenal Ulcer
H_2 ANTAGONISTS	**CIMETIDINE**										
	Generic	**Sol:** 300mg/5mL **Tab:** 200mg, 300mg, 400mg, 800mg		X	X	X	X				X
	FAMOTIDINE										
	Pepcid	**Inj:** 10mg/mL (Generic) **Sus:** 40mg/5mL **Tab:** 20mg, 40mg		X	X	X	X				X
	NIZATIDINE										
	Axid	**Cap:** 150mg, 300mg (Generic) **Sol:** 15mg/mL	X	X	X	X					X
	RANITIDINE										
	Zantac	**Inj**[§]**:** 25mg/mL					X				X
		Cap: 150mg, 300mg (Generic) **Syrup:** 15mg/1mL **Tab:** 150mg, 300mg	X	X	X	X	X				X
PPIs	**DEXLANSOPRAZOLE**										
	Dexilant	**Cap, DR:** 30mg, 60mg	X		X	X					
	ESOMEPRAZOLE										
	Nexium	**Cap, DR:** 20mg, 40mg **Sus, DR:** 2.5mg, 5mg, 10mg, 20mg, 40mg (granules/pkt)	X		X	X	X	X	X		X
	Nexium I.V.	**Inj**[¶]**:** 20mg, 40mg			X	X					X
	LANSOPRAZOLE										
	Prevacid	**Cap, DR:** 15mg, 30mg **Tab, Disintegrating:** 15mg, 30mg	X	X	X	X	X	X	X		X
	Prevpac	**Cap:** (Amoxicillin) 500mg **Tab:** (Clarithromycin) 500mg **Cap, DR:** (Lansoprazole) 30mg						X			X

(Continued)

PPIs *(Continued)*

DRUG	HOW SUPPLIED	Heartburn	Gastric Ulcer	GERD	Esophagitis	Zollinger-Ellison	*Helicobacter pylori*	NSAID Induced†	Upper GI Bleeding‡	Duodenal Ulcer
OMEPRAZOLE										
Prilosec	**Cap, DR:** 10mg, 20mg, 40mg **Sus, DR:** 2.5mg, 10mg (granules/pkt)	X	X	X	X	X	X			X
Zegerid	**Cap:** (Omeprazole-Sodium bicarbonate) 20mg-1100mg, 40mg-1100mg **Pow:** 20mg-1680mg/pkt, 40mg-1680mg/pkt	X	X	X	X				X (40mg-1680mg)	X
PANTOPRAZOLE										
Protonix	**Tab, DR:** 20mg, 40mg **Sus, DR:** 40mg (granules/pkt)	X		X	X	X				
Protonix I.V.	**Inj:** 40mg			X	X	X				
RABEPRAZOLE										
Aciphex	**Cap, DR:** 5mg, 10mg **Tab, DR:** 20mg	X		X		X	X			X

Refer to full FDA-approved labeling for additional information.

Abbreviations: DR = delayed-release; GERD = gastroesophageal reflux disease; GI = gastrointestinal; NSAID = nonsteroidal anti-inflammatory drug; PPI = proton pump inhibitor.

*Rx products only. For OTC products, refer to the *Antacid and Heartburn Products* table.

†Prevention of NSAID-induced gastric ulcers.

‡Prevention of upper GI bleeding in critically ill patients.

§May also be used as an alternative to oral dosage form for short-term use in patients unable to take oral medications.

¶Also indicated for risk reduction of rebleeding of gastric/duodenal ulcers following therapeutic endoscopy.

Ulcerative Colitis Treatments

GENERIC	BRAND	HOW SUPPLIED	ADULT DOSAGE	PEDIATRIC DOSAGE
AMINOSALICYLATES				
Balsalazide disodium	Colazal	**Cap:** 750mg	3 caps tid for up to 8 wks (or 12 wks if needed). May open cap and sprinkle on applesauce.	**5-17 yrs:** 1 or 3 caps tid for up to 8 wks. May open cap and sprinkle on applesauce.
	Giazo	**Tab:** 1.1g	**Male:** 3 tabs bid for up to 8 wks.	
Mesalamine	Apriso	**Cap, ER:** 0.375g	4 caps qam. Avoid with antacids.	
	Asacol	**Tab, DR:** 400mg	2 tabs tid for 6 wks. **Maint:** 1600mg/day in divided doses.*	**5-17 yrs: 54-90kg:** 27-44mg/kg/day up to 2400mg/day. **33-<54kg:** 37-61mg/kg/day up to 2000mg/day. **17-<33kg:** 36-71mg/kg/day up to 1200mg/day.*
	Asacol HD	**Tab, DR:** 800mg	2 tabs tid for 6 wks.*	
	Delzicol	**Cap, DR:** 400mg	2 tabs tid for 6 wks. **Maint:** 1600mg/day in divided doses.	**≥12 yrs: 54-90kg:** 27-44mg/kg/day up to 2400mg/day. **33-<54kg:** 37-61mg/kg/day up to 2000mg/day. **17-<33kg:** 36-71mg/kg/day up to 1200mg/day.
	Lialda	**Tab, DR:** 1.2g	**Induction:** 2-4 tabs qd with a meal. **Maint:** 2 tabs qd with a meal.	
	Pentasa	**Cap, CR:** 250mg, 500mg	1000mg qid for up to 8 wks.	
	SF Rowasa	**Rect Sus:** 4g/60mL	1 instillation (4g) qhs for 3-6 weeks. Retain for 8 hrs.	
Olsalazine sodium	Dipentum	**Cap:** 250mg	1000mg/day in 2 divided doses.	
Sulfasalazine	Azulfidine	**Tab:** 500mg[†]	**Initial:** 3-4g/day in evenly divided doses with dose intervals ≤8 hrs. May initiate at 1-2g/day to reduce GI intolerance. **Maint:** 2g/day.	**≥6 yrs: Initial:** 40-60mg/kg/day divided into 3-6 doses. **Maint:** 30mg/kg/day divided into 4 doses.
	Azulfidine EN-tabs	**Tab, DR:** 500mg		
CORTICOSTEROIDS				
Betamethasone sodium phosphate-Betamethasone acetate	Celestone Soluspan	**Inj:** 3mg-3mg/mL [5mL, multidose]	**Initial:** 0.25-9mg/day IM.[‡]	**Initial:** 0.02-0.3mg/kg/day in 3 or 4 divided doses IM.[‡]
Budesonide	Uceris	**Tab, ER:** 9mg	9mg qam for up to 8 wks.	
		Rectal Foam: 2mg/metered dose	1 metered dose rectally bid for 2 wks followed by 1 metered dose rectally qd for 4 wks.	

(Continued)

GENERIC	BRAND	HOW SUPPLIED	ADULT DOSAGE	PEDIATRIC DOSAGE
CORTICOSTEROIDS *(Continued)*				
Dexamethasone	Generic	**Elixir:** 0.5mg/5mL; **Sol:** 0.5mg/5mL, 1mg/mL; **Tab:** 0.5mg†, 0.75mg†, 1mg†, 1.5mg†, 2mg†, 4mg†, 6mg†	**Initial:** 0.75-9mg/day.‡	**Initial:** 0.02-0.3mg/kg/day in 3 or 4 divided doses.‡
	Generic	**Inj:** 4mg/mL [1mL, 5mL, 30mL], 10mg/mL [1mL]	**Initial:** 0.5-9mg/day IV/IM.‡	
Hydrocortisone	Anusol-HC	**Sup:** 25mg	**Nonspecific Proctitis:** 1 sup rectally bid for 2 wks. **More Severe Cases:** 1 sup rectally tid or 2 sup rectally bid. **Factitial Proctitis:** Use up to 6-8 wks.	
	Colocort	**Rect Sus:** 100mg/60mL	1 instillation (100mg) qhs for 21 days or until remission. Retain for ≥1 hr, preferably all night.	
	Cortef	**Tab:** 5mg†, 10mg†, 20mg†	**Initial:** 20-240mg/day.‡	**Initial:** 20-240mg/day.‡
	Proctocort	**Sup:** 30mg	**Nonspecific Proctitis:** 1 sup rectally bid for 2 wks. **More Severe Cases:** 1 sup rectally tid or 2 sup rectally bid. **Factitial Proctitis:** Use up to 6-8 wks.	
	Solu-Cortef	**Inj:** 100mg, 250mg, 500mg, 1000mg	**Initial:** 100-500mg IV/IM. May repeat dose at 2-, 4-, or 6-hr intervals. High-dose therapy should continue only until patient is stabilized, usually not beyond 48-72 hrs.‡	**Initial:** 0.56-8mg/kg/day IV/IM in 3 or 4 divided doses.‡
Methylprednisolone	Depo-Medrol	**Inj:** 20mg/mL, 40mg/mL, 80mg/mL	**Initial:** 4-120mg IM.‡	**Initial:** 0.11-1.6mg/kg/day.‡
	Medrol	**Tab:** 2mg†, 4mg†, 8mg†, 16mg†, 32mg†; (Dose-Pak) 4mg† [21s]	**Initial:** 4-48mg/day.‡ Refer to PI for detailed information for ADT.	**Initial:** 4-48mg/day.‡ Refer to PI for detailed information for ADT.
	Solu-Medrol	**Inj:** 40mg, 125mg, 500mg, 1g, 2g	**Initial:** 10-40mg IV/IM inj or IV infusion. **High-Dose Therapy:** 30mg/kg IV over at least 30 min. May repeat dose q4-6h for 48 hrs. High-dose therapy should continue only until patient is stabilized, usually not beyond 48-72 hrs.‡	**Initial:** 0.11-1.6mg/kg/day in 3 or 4 divided doses.‡

GENERIC	BRAND	HOW SUPPLIED	ADULT DOSAGE	PEDIATRIC DOSAGE
CORTICOSTEROIDS *(Continued)*				
Prednisolone	Flo-Pred	**Sus:** 15mg/5mL [37mL, 52mL, 65mL]	**Initial:** 5-60mg/day.‡	**Initial:** 0.14-2mg/kg/day in 3 or 4 divided doses.‡
	Orapred	**Sol:** 15mg/5mL [20mL, 237mL]; **Tab, Disintegrating:** 10mg, 15mg, 30mg	(Sol) **Initial:** 5-60mg/day. (Tab, Disintegrating) **Initial:** 10-60mg/day.‡	**Initial:** 0.14-2mg/kg/day in 3 or 4 divided doses.‡
	Pediapred	**Sol:** 5mg/5mL [120mL]	**Initial:** 5-60mg/day.‡	**Initial:** 0.14-2mg/kg/day in 3 or 4 divided doses.‡
	Generic	**Syrup:** 15mg/5mL [240mL, 480mL]; **Tab:** 5mg†	**Initial:** 5-60mg/day.‡ (Tab) Refer to PI for detailed information for ADT.	**Initial:** 5-60mg/day.‡ (Tab) Refer to PI for detailed information for ADT.
Prednisone	Rayos	**Tab, DR:** 1mg, 2mg, 5mg	**Initial:** 5-60mg/day.‡	**Initial:** 5-60mg/day.‡
	Generic	**Sol:** 5mg/mL [30mL], 5mg/5mL [120mL, 500mL]; **Tab:** 1mg†, 2.5mg†, 5mg†, 10mg†, 20mg†, 50mg†	**Initial:** 5-60mg/day.‡ Refer to PI for detailed information for ADT.	**Initial:** 5-60mg/day.‡ Refer to PI for detailed information for ADT.
Triamcinolone	Kenalog-40	**Inj:** 40mg/mL [1mL, 5mL, 10mL]	**Initial:** 2.5-100mg/day.‡	**Initial:** 0.11-1.6mg/kg/day in 3 or 4 divided doses.‡
MONOCLONAL ANTIBODIES				
Adalimumab	Humira	**Inj:** 20mg/0.4mL, 40mg/0.8mL	**Initial:** 160mg SQ on Day 1 (given as four 40mg inj in 1 day or as two 40mg inj/day for 2 consecutive days); then 80mg after 2 wks (Day 15). **Maint:** 40mg every other wk beginning Wk 4 (Day 29). Continue only with evidence of clinical remission by 8 wks (Day 57) of therapy.	
Golimumab	Simponi	**Inj:** 50mg/0.5mL, 100mg/mL	**Induction:** 200mg SQ at Week 0, then 100mg at Week 2. **Maint:** 100mg q4wks. Refer to PI for administration and preparation instructions.	
Infliximab	Remicade	**Inj:** 100mg/20mL	**Induction:** 5mg/kg IV at 0, 2, and 6 wks. **Maint:** 5mg/kg q8wks. Refer to PI for administration and preparation instructions.	**≥6 yrs: Induction:** 5mg/kg IV at 0, 2, and 6 wks. **Maint:** 5mg/kg q8wks. Refer to PI for administration and preparation instructions.

(Continued)

GENERIC	BRAND	HOW SUPPLIED	ADULT DOSAGE	PEDIATRIC DOSAGE
MONOCLONAL ANTIBODIES *(Continued)*				
Vedolizumab	Entyvio	**Inj:** 300mg/20mL	300mg IV over 30 min at 0, 2, and 6 wks. **Maint:** 300mg q8wks.	

Refer to full FDA-approved labeling for additional information.

Abbreviations: ADT = alternate day therapy; CR = controlled-release; DR = delayed-release; ER = extended-release.

*Do not use two 400mg tabs and one 800mg tab interchangeably.

†Scored.

‡Maintenance dose should be determined by decreasing initial dose in small decrements to lowest effective dose. Withdraw gradually after long-term therapy.

ANTIVIRALS TREATMENT COMPARISON

GENERIC (BRAND)	HOW SUPPLIED	INDICATIONS							
		HIV	HBV	HCV	Genital Herpes	Herpes Zoster	Herpes Labialis	CMV Retinitis	Influenza
ADAMANTANES									
Rimantadine HCl (Flumadine)	**Tab:** 100mg								✓-A
BIOLOGICAL RESPONSE MODIFIERS									
Interferon alfa-2b (Intron A)	**Inj:** (Powder) 10 MIU, 18 MIU, 50 MIU; (Vial) 18 MIU, 25 MIU		✓	✓					
CCR5 ANTAGONISTS									
Maraviroc (Selzentry)	**Tab:** 150mg, 300mg	✓							
CYP3A INHIBITORS									
Cobicistat (Tybost)	**Tab:** 150mg	✓							
DOPAMINE RECEPTOR AGONISTS									
Amantadine HCl	**Cap:** 100mg; **Syr:** 50mg/5mL [473mL]; **Tab:** 100mg								✓-A
FUSION INHIBITORS									
Enfuvirtide (Fuzeon)	**Inj:** 90mg/mL [108mg]	✓							
GUANOSINE NUCLEOSIDE ANALOGUES									
Entecavir (Baraclude)	**Sol:** 0.05mg/mL [210mL]; **Tab:** 0.5mg, 1mg		✓						
HIV-INTEGRASE STRAND TRANSFER INHIBITORS									
Dolutegravir (Tivicay)	**Tab:** 50mg	✓							
Elvitegravir (Vitekta)	**Tab:** 85mg, 150mg	✓							
Raltegravir (Isentress)	**Sus Powder:** 100mg/pkt; **Tab:** 400mg; **Tab, Chewable:** 25mg, 100mg	✓							
NEURAMINIDASE INHIBITORS									
Oseltamivir phosphate (Tamiflu)	**Cap:** 30mg, 45mg, 75mg; **Sus:** 6mg/mL [60mL]								✓
Peramivir (Rapivab)	**Inj:** 10mg/mL								✓
Zanamivir (Relenza)	**Powder, Inh:** 5mg/inh								✓-A,B

(Continued)

GENERIC (BRAND)	HOW SUPPLIED	INDICATIONS: HIV	HBV	HCV	Genital Herpes	Herpes Zoster	Herpes Labialis	CMV Retinitis	Influenza
NON-NUCLEOSIDE REVERSE TRANSCRIPTASE INHIBITORS									
Delavirdine mesylate (Rescriptor)	**Tab:** 100mg, 200mg	✓							
Efavirenz (Sustiva)	**Cap:** 50mg, 200mg; **Tab:** 600mg	✓							
Etravirine (Intelence)	**Tab:** 25mg, 100mg, 200mg	✓							
Nevirapine (Viramune, Viramune XR)	**Sus:** 50mg/5mL [240mL]; **Tab:** 200mg; **Tab, ER:** 100mg, 400mg	✓							
Rilpivirine (Edurant)	**Tab:** 25mg	✓							
NUCLEOSIDE ANALOGUES									
Acyclovir (Zovirax Oral)	**Cap:** 200mg; **Sus:** 200mg/5mL [473mL]; **Tab:** 400mg, 800mg				✓	✓			
Acyclovir (Zovirax Cream)	**Cre:** 5% [5g]						✓		
Acyclovir (Zovirax Ointment)	**Oint:** 5% [15g, 30g]				✓				
Acyclovir sodium	**Inj:** 50mg/mL				✓	✓			
Famciclovir (Famvir)	**Tab:** 125mg, 250mg, 500mg				✓	✓	✓		
Ganciclovir sodium (Cytovene)	**Inj:** 500mg/10mL							✓	
Penciclovir (Denavir)	**Cre:** 1% [1.5g, 5g]						✓		
Ribavirin (Copegus)	**Tab:** 200mg			✓					
Ribavirin (Rebetol)	**Cap:** 200mg; **Sol:** 40mg/mL [100mL]			✓					
Ribavirin (Ribasphere Capsules)	**Cap:** 200mg			✓					
Ribavirin (Ribasphere Tablets)	**Tab:** 200mg, 400mg, 600mg			✓					
Valacyclovir HCl (Valtrex)	**Tab:** 500mg, 1000mg				✓	✓	✓		
Valganciclovir HCl (Valcyte)	**Sol:** 50mg/mL [88mL]; **Tab:** 450mg							✓	

GENERIC (BRAND)	HOW SUPPLIED	INDICATIONS							
		HIV	HBV	HCV	Genital Herpes	Herpes Zoster	Herpes Labialis	CMV Retinitis	Influenza
NUCLEOSIDE REVERSE TRANSCRIPTASE INHIBITORS									
Abacavir sulfate (Ziagen)	**Sol:** 20mg/mL [240mL]; **Tab:** 300mg	✓							
Didanosine (Videx, Videx EC)	**Cap, DR:** (Videx EC) 125mg, 200mg, 250mg, 400mg; **Sol:** (Videx) 10mg/mL [2g, 4g]	✓							
Emtricitabine (Emtriva)	**Cap:** 200mg; **Sol:** 10mg/mL [170mL]	✓							
Lamivudine (Epivir)	**Sol:** 10mg/mL [240mL]; **Tab:** 150mg, 300mg	✓							
Lamivudine (Epivir-HBV)	**Sol:** 5mg/mL [240mL]; **Tab:** 100mg		✓						
Stavudine (Zerit)	**Cap:** 15mg, 20mg, 30mg, 40mg; **Sol:** 1mg/mL [200mL]	✓							
Telbivudine (Tyzeka)	**Tab:** 600mg; **Sol:** 100mg/5mL [300mL]		✓						
Zidovudine (Retrovir)	**Cap:** 100mg; **Inj:** 10mg/mL; **Syrup:** 10mg/mL [240mL]; **Tab:** 300mg	✓							
NUCLEOTIDE ANALOGUE INHIBITORS									
Sofosbuvir (Sovaldi)	**Tab:** 400mg			✓					
NUCLEOTIDE ANALOGUE REVERSE TRANSCRIPTASE INHIBITORS									
Adefovir dipivoxil (Hepsera)	**Tab:** 10mg		✓						
Tenofovir disoproxil fumarate (Viread)	**Powder:** 40mg/g [60g]; **Tab:** 150mg, 200mg, 250mg, 300mg	✓	✓						
PEGYLATED VIRUS PROLIFERATION INHIBITORS									
Peginterferon alfa-2a (Pegasys)	**Inj:** 135mcg/0.5mL, 180mcg/0.5mL, 180mcg/mL		✓	✓					
Peginterferon alfa-2b (PegIntron)	**Inj:** 50mcg/0.5mL, 80mcg/0.5mL, 120mcg/0.5mL, 150mcg/0.5mL			✓					

(Continued)

GENERIC (BRAND)	HOW SUPPLIED	INDICATIONS							
		HIV	HBV	HCV	Genital Herpes	Herpes Zoster	Herpes Labialis	CMV Retinitis	Influenza
PROTEASE INHIBITORS									
Atazanavir (Reyataz)	**Cap:** 150mg, 200mg, 300mg; **Powder:** 50mg/pkt	✓							
Boceprevir (Victrelis)	**Cap:** 200mg			✓					
Darunavir (Prezista)	**Sus:** 100mg/mL [200mL]; **Tab:** 75mg, 150mg, 600mg, 800mg	✓							
Fosamprenavir calcium (Lexiva)	**Sus:** 50mg/mL [225mL]; **Tab:** 700mg	✓							
Indinavir sulfate (Crixivan)	**Cap:** 200mg, 400mg	✓							
Nelfinavir mesylate (Viracept)	**Powder:** 50mg/g [144g]; **Tab:** 250g, 625mg	✓							
Ritonavir (Norvir)	**Cap, Tab:** 100mg; **Sol:** 80mg/mL [240mL]	✓							
Saquinavir mesylate (Invirase)	**Cap:** 200mg; **Tab:** 500mg	✓							
Simeprevir (Olysio)	**Cap:** 150mg			✓					
Tipranavir (Aptivus)	**Cap:** 250mg; **Sol:** 100mg/mL [95mL]	✓							
PYROPHOSPHATE BINDING INHIBITORS									
Foscarnet sodium (Foscavir)	**Inj:** 24mg/mL							✓	

Refer to full FDA-approved labeling for additional information.

Abbreviations: CMV = cytomegalovirus; HBV = hepatitis B virus; HCV = hepatitis C virus; HIV = human immunodeficiency virus.

Oral Antibiotics Treatment Comparison

GENERIC (BRAND)	HOW SUPPLIED	INDICATIONS																						
		ABECB	AECB	Bone & Joint	CAP	Endocarditis	GI	Intra-Ab	LRTI	URTI	Lyme Disease	MAC	Meningitis	Oph	Otitis Media	PCP	Septicemia	Sinusitis	SSSI	SSTI	TB	UTI	UGI	Gyn
CEPHALOSPORINS																								
1st Generation																								
Cefadroxil	**Cap:** 500mg; **Susp:** 250mg/5mL, 500mg/5mL; **Tab:** 1g									X									X			X		
Cephalexin (Keflex)	**Cap:** 250mg, 500mg, 750mg; **Susp:** 125mg/5mL, 250mg/5mL; **Tab:** 250mg, 500mg			X					X	X					X				X			X	X	
2nd Generation																								
Cefaclor	**Cap:** 250mg, 500mg; **Susp:** 125mg/5mL, 187mg/5mL, 250mg/5mL, 375mg/5mL								X	X					X				X			X		
Cefaclor ER	**Tab, ER:** 500mg	X							X	X									X					
Cefprozil	**Susp:** 125mg/5mL, 250mg/5mL; **Tab:** 250mg, 500mg	X							X	X					X			X	X					
Cefuroxime axetil (Ceftin)	**Susp:** 125mg/5mL, 250mg/5mL; **Tab:** 250mg, 500mg	X (Tab)							X (Tab)	X	X (Tab)				X			X (Tab)	X			X (Tab)	X (Tab)	X (Tab)

(Continued)

GENERIC (BRAND)	HOW SUPPLIED	INDICATIONS																						
		ABECB	AECB	Bone & Joint	CAP	Endocarditis	GI	Intra-Ab	LRTI	URTI	Lyme Disease	MAC	Meningitis	Oph	Otitis Media	PCP	Septicemia	Sinusitis	SSSI	SSTI	TB	UTI	UGI	Gyn
CEPHALOSPORINS *(Continued)*																								
3rd Generation																								
Cefdinir	**Cap:** 300mg; **Susp:** 125mg/5mL, 250mg/5mL		X		X					X					X			X	X					
Cefditoren pivoxil (Spectracef)	**Tab:** 200mg, 400mg	X			X					X									X					
Cefixime (Suprax)	**Cap:** 400mg; **Susp:** 100mg/5mL, 200mg/5mL, 500mg/5mL; **Tab:** 400mg; **Tab, Chew:** 100mg, 150mg, 200mg		X							X					X							X	X	X
Cefpodoxime proxetil	**Susp:** 50mg/5mL, 100mg/5mL; **Tab:** 100mg, 200mg	X			X					X					X			X	X			X	X	X
Ceftibuten (Cedax)	**Cap:** 400mg; **Susp:** 90mg/5mL, 180mg/5mL	X								X					X									
FLUOROQUINOLONES																								
Ciprofloxacin (Cipro)	**Susp:** 250mg/5mL, 500mg/5mL; **Tab:** 250mg, 500mg			X			X	X	X									X	X			X	X	X
Ciprofloxacin (Cipro XR)	**Tab, ER:** 500mg, 1000mg																					X		
Gemifloxacin mesylate (Factive)	**Tab:** 320mg	X			X																			

GENERIC (BRAND)	HOW SUPPLIED	INDICATIONS																						
		ABECB	AECB	Bone & Joint	CAP	Endocarditis	GI	Intra-Ab	LRTI	URTI	Lyme Disease	MAC	Meningitis	Oph	Otitis Media	PCP	Septicemia	Sinusitis	SSSI	SSTI	TB	UTI	UGI	Gyn
FLUOROQUINOLONES *(Continued)*																								
Levofloxacin (Levaquin)	**Sol:** 25mg/mL; **Tab:** 250mg, 500mg, 750mg	X			X				X									X	X			X	X	
Moxifloxacin HCl (Avelox)	**Tab:** 400mg	X			X			X										X	X					
Ofloxacin	**Tab:** 200mg, 300mg, 400mg	X			X														X			X	X	X
MACROLIDES																								
Azithromycin (Zithromax)	**Susp:** 100mg/5mL, 200mg/5mL; **Tab:** 250mg, 500mg	X			X					X					X			X	X				X	X
Azithromycin (Zithromax)	**Susp:** 1g/pkt; **Tab:** 600mg											X											X	X
Azithromycin (Zmax)	**Susp, ER:** 2g (27mg/mL)				X													X						
Clarithromycin (Biaxin)	**Susp:** 125mg/5mL, 250mg/5mL; **Tab:** 250mg, 500mg	X			X		X (Tab)			X		X			X			X	X					
Clarithromycin (Biaxin XL)	**Tab, ER:** 500mg	X			X													X						
Erythromycin (ERYC)	**Cap, DR:** 250mg						X		X	X				X					X			X	X	X
Erythromycin (Ery-Tab)	**Tab, DR:** 250mg, 333mg, 500mg						X		X	X				X					X			X	X	X
Erythromycin (PCE)	**Tab:** 333mg, 500mg						X		X	X				X					X			X	X	X
Erythromycin base	**Tab:** 250mg, 500mg						X		X	X				X					X			X	X	X

(Continued)

GENERIC (BRAND)	HOW SUPPLIED	INDICATIONS																						
		ABECB	AECB	Bone & Joint	CAP	Endocarditis	GI	Intra-Ab	LRTI	URTI	Lyme Disease	MAC	Meningitis	Oph	Otitis Media	PCP	Septicemia	Sinusitis	SSSI	SSTI	TB	UTI	UGI	Gyn
MACROLIDES *(Continued)*																								
Erythromycin ethylsuccinate (E.E.S.)	**Susp:** 200mg/5mL; **Tab:** 400mg						X		X	X				X					X			X	X	X
Erythromycin ethylsuccinate (EryPed)	**Susp:** 200mg/5mL, 400mg/5mL						X		X	X				X					X			X	X	X
Erythromycin ethylsuccinate-Sulfisoxazole acetyl	**Susp:** 200-600mg/5mL														X									
Erythromycin stearate (Erythrocin)	**Tab:** 250mg						X		X	X				X					X			X	X	X
Fidaxomicin (Dificid)	**Tab:** 200mg						X																	
PENICILLINS																								
Amoxicillin	**Cap:** 250mg, 500mg; **Susp:** 125mg/5mL, 200mg/5mL, 250mg/5mL, 400mg/5mL; **Tab:** 500mg, 875mg; **Tab, Chew:** 125mg, 250mg						X		X	X									X				X	

GENERIC (BRAND)	HOW SUPPLIED	INDICATIONS																						
		ABECB	AECB	Bone & Joint	CAP	Endocarditis	GI	Intra-Ab	LRTI	URTI	Lyme Disease	MAC	Meningitis	Oph	Otitis Media	PCP	Septicemia	Sinusitis	SSSI	SSTI	TB	UTI	UGI	Gyn
PENICILLINS *(Continued)*																								
Amoxicillin (Moxatag)	**Tab, ER:** 775mg									X														
Amoxicillin-Clavulanate potassium (Augmentin)	**Susp:** 125-31.25mg/5mL, 200-28.5mg/5mL, 250-62.5mg/5mL, 400-57mg/5mL; **Tab:** 250-125mg, 500-125mg, 875-125mg; **Tab, Chew:** 125-31.25mg, 200-28.5mg, 250-62.5mg, 400-57mg								X						X			X	X			X		
Amoxicillin-Clavulanate potassium (Augmentin XR)	**Tab, ER:** 1000-62.5mg				X													X						
Amoxicillin-Clavulanate potassium	**Susp:** 600-42.9mg/5mL														X									
Ampicillin	**Cap:** 250mg, 500mg; **Susp:** 125mg/5mL, 250mg/5mL						X		X	X			X										X	
Penicillin V potassium (Penicillin VK)	**Susp:** 125mg/5mL, 250mg/5mL; **Tab:** 250mg, 500mg								X	X										X				

(Continued)

GENERIC (BRAND)	HOW SUPPLIED	INDICATIONS																						
		ABECB	AECB	Bone & Joint	CAP	Endocarditis	GI	Intra-Ab	LRTI	URTI	Lyme Disease	MAC	Meningitis	Oph	Otitis Media	PCP	Septicemia	Sinusitis	SSSI	SSTI	TB	UTI	UGI	Gyn
TETRACYCLINES																								
Demeclocycline HCl	**Tab:** 150mg, 300mg						X		X	X				X					X			X	X	X
Doxycycline (Vibramycin)	**Cap:** 100mg; **Susp:** 25mg/5mL; **Syrup:** 50mg/5mL; **Tab:** 100mg						X		X	X				X					X			X	X	X
Doxycycline hyclate (Doryx)	**Tab, DR:** 75mg, 100mg, 150mg, 200mg						X		X	X				X					X			X	X	X
Doxycycline monohydrate (Monodox)	**Cap:** 50mg, 75mg, 100mg						X		X	X				X					X			X	X	X
Minocycline HCl (Dynacin)	**Tab:** 50mg, 75mg, 100mg						X		X	X				X					X			X	X	X
Minocycline HCl (Minocin)	**Cap:** 50mg, 75mg, 100mg						X		X	X				X					X			X	X	X
Tetracycline HCl	**Cap:** 250mg, 500mg						X		X	X				X						X		X	X	X
MISCELLANEOUS																								
Clindamycin (Cleocin, Cleocin Pediatric)	**Cap:** 75mg, 150mg, 300mg; **Sol:** 75mg/5mL							X	X	X							X			X			X	X
Fosfomycin tromethamine (Monurol)	**Powder:** 3g/sachet																					X		
Isoniazid-Pyrazinamide-Rifampin (Rifater)	**Tab:** 50-300-120mg																				X			

GENERIC (BRAND)	HOW SUPPLIED	INDICATIONS																						
		ABECB	AECB	Bone & Joint	CAP	Endocarditis	GI	Intra-Ab	LRTI	URTI	Lyme Disease	MAC	Meningitis	Oph	Otitis Media	PCP	Septicemia	Sinusitis	SSSI	SSTI	TB	UTI	UGI	Gyn
MISCELLANEOUS *(Continued)*																								
Isoniazid-Rifampin (Rifamate)	**Cap:** 150-300mg																				X			
Linezolid (Zyvox)	**Susp:** 100mg/5mL; **Tab:** 600mg				X				X										X					
Metronidazole (Flagyl)	**Cap:** 375mg; **Tab:** 250mg, 500mg			X		X	X	X	X				X				X		X					X
Nitrofurantoin (Furadantin)	**Susp:** 25mg/5mL																					X		
Nitrofurantoin macrocrystals (Macrodantin)	**Cap:** 25mg, 50mg, 100mg																					X		
Nitrofurantoin macrocrystals and Nitrofurantoin monohydrate (Macrobid)	**Cap:** 100mg																					X		
Rifampin (Rifadin)	**Cap:** 150mg, 300mg																				X			
Rifapentine (Priftin)	**Tab:** 150mg																				X			
Sulfamethoxazole-Trimethoprim (Bactrim, Bactrim DS, Sulfatrim)	**Susp:** 200-40mg/5mL; **Tab:** 400-80mg, 800-160mg		X				X								X	X						X		

(Continued)

GENERIC (BRAND)	HOW SUPPLIED	INDICATIONS																						
		ABECB	AECB	Bone & Joint	CAP	Endocarditis	GI	Intra-Ab	LRTI	URTI	Lyme Disease	MAC	Meningitis	Oph	Otitis Media	PCP	Septicemia	Sinusitis	SSSI	SSTI	TB	UTI	UGI	Gyn
MISCELLANEOUS *(Continued)*																								
Tedizolid phosphate (Sivextro)	**Tab:** 150mg																		X					
Telithromycin (Ketek)	**Tab:** 300mg, 400mg				X																			
Trimethoprim	**Tab:** 100mg, 200mg																					X		
Trimethoprim HCl (Primsol)	**Sol:** 50mg/5mL														X							X		
Vancomycin HCl (Vancocin)	**Cap:** 125mg, 250mg						X																	

Refer to full FDA-approved labeling for additional information.

Abbreviations:
ABECB = acute bacterial exacerbation of chronic bronchitis
AECB = acute exacerbation of chronic bronchitis
CAP = community-acquired pneumonia
GI = gastrointestinal
LRTI = lower respiratory tract infection
MAC = *Mycobacterium avium* complex
PCP = *Pneumocystis jiroveci* pneumonia
SSSI = skin and skin structure infection
SSTI = skin and soft tissue infection
TB = tuberculosis
UGI = urogenital infection
URTI = upper respiratory tract infection
UTI = urinary tract infection

ORAL AND SYSTEMIC ANTIFUNGALS

GENERIC (BRAND)	INDICATIONS	DOSAGE FORM	ADDITIONAL COMMENTS
Amphotericin B	• Aspergillosis • Cryptococcosis • North American blastomycosis • Systemic candidiasis • Coccidioidomycosis • Histoplasmosis • Zygomycosis • Sporotrichosis • Infections due to *Conidiobolus* and *Basidiobolus* species • Leishmaniasis	**Inj:** 50mg	**BW:** Used primarily to treat progressive and potentially life-threatening fungal infections. Doses greater than 1.5mg/kg should not be given. Verify product's name and dosage preadministration and use caution to prevent inadvertent overdosage that may result in cardiopulmonary arrest. • Administer by slow IV infusion.
Amphotericin B lipid complex (Abelcet)	• Fungal infections in patients refractory to or intolerant of conventional amphotericin B therapy	**Inj:** 5mg/mL	• If the infusion time exceeds 2 hrs, mix the contents by shaking the infusion bag every 2 hrs. • Administer IV.
Amphotericin B lipid complex (Amphotec)	• Aspergillosis in patients with renal impairment, unacceptable toxicity, or previous failure to amphotericin B deoxycholate	**Inj:** 50mg, 100mg	• Infusion time may be shortened to a minimum of 2 hrs if no evidence of intolerance or infusion-related reactions. • If patient experiences acute reactions or cannot tolerate the infusion volume, the infusion time may be extended. • Administer IV.
Amphotericin B liposome (AmBisome)	• Infections due to *Aspergillus*, *Candida*, and/or *Cryptococcus* species refractory to amphotericin B deoxycholate or where renal impairment or unacceptable toxicity precludes the use of amphotericin B deoxycholate • Visceral leishmaniasis • Empirical therapy for presumed fungal infections in febrile neutropenic patients • Cryptococcal meningitis in HIV-infected patients	**Inj:** 50mg	• AmBisome should be administered by IV infusion using a controlled infusion device over a period of approximately 120 minutes. • May reduce infusion time to 60 minutes in patients whom treatment is well tolerated, or may increase infusion duration if the patient experiences discomfort during infusion. • Administer IV.
Anidulafungin (Eraxis)	• Candidemia and other forms of *Candida* infections • Esophageal candidiasis	**Inj:** 50mg, 100mg	• The rate of infusion should not exceed 1.1mg/min. • Administer IV.
Caspofungin acetate (Cancidas)	• Candidemia • Intra-abdominal abscesses, peritonitis, and pleural space infections due to *Candida* • Esophageal candidiasis • Aspergillosis in patients who are refractory to or intolerant of other therapies • Empirical therapy for presumed fungal infections in febrile neutropenic patients	**Inj:** 50mg, 70mg	• Maximum LD and daily maintenance dose should not exceed 70mg, regardless of the patient's calculated dose. • Administer by slow IV infusion over approximately 1 hr.
Clotrimazole	• Oropharyngeal candidiasis • Prevention of oropharyngeal candidiasis in immunocompromised conditions	**Loz:** 10mg	• Not indicated for treatment of systemic mycoses, including systemic candidiasis.

(Continued)

GENERIC (BRAND)	INDICATIONS	DOSAGE FORM	ADDITIONAL COMMENTS
Fluconazole (Diflucan)	• Vaginal (oral route only), oropharyngeal, and esophageal candidiasis • UTIs and peritonitis caused by *Candida* • Systemic *Candida* infections, including candidemia, disseminated candidiasis, and pneumonia • Cryptococcal meningitis • Prevention of candidiasis in patients undergoing bone marrow transplantation who are receiving chemotherapy and/or radiation therapy	**Inj:** 200mg/100mL, 400mg/200mL; **Sus:** 10mg/mL, 40mg/mL; **Tab:** 50mg, 100mg, 150mg, 200mg	• The IV infusion of fluconazole should be administered at a maximum rate of approximately 200mg/hr as a continuous infusion.
Flucytosine (Ancobon)	• Septicemia, endocarditis, and UTIs caused by *Candida* • Meningitis and pulmonary infection caused by *Cryptococcus*	**Cap:** 250mg, 500mg	**BW:** Use with extreme caution in patients with impaired renal function; monitor hematologic, renal, and hepatic status. • Ancobon should be used in combination with amphotericin B for the treatment of systemic candidiasis and cryptococcosis because of the emergence of resistance to Ancobon.
Griseofulvin (Grifulvin V)	• Tinea capitis • Tinea corporis • Tinea pedis • Tinea unguium • Tinea barbae • Tinea cruris	**Sus:** 125mg/5mL; **Tab:** 250mg, 500mg	• Periodic monitoring of organ system function, including renal, hepatic, and hematopoietic, should be done. • Medication must be continued until the infecting organism is completely eradicated as indicated by appropriate clinical or laboratory examination.
Griseofulvin (Gris-PEG)	• Tinea capitis • Tinea corporis • Tinea pedis • Tinea unguium • Tinea barbae • Tinea cruris	**Tab:** 125mg, 250mg	• Periodic monitoring of organ system function, including renal, hepatic, and hematopoietic, should be done. • Medication must be continued until the infecting organism is completely eradicated as indicated by appropriate clinical or laboratory examination.
Itraconazole (Sporanox)	• Blastomycosis (pulmonary/extrapulmonary) • Histoplasmosis (eg, chronic cavitary pulmonary disease and disseminated, nonmeningeal) • Aspergillosis (pulmonary/extrapulmonary) if refractory to or intolerant of amphotericin B therapy • Onychomycosis of the toenail and fingernail in nonimmunocompromised patients	**Cap:** 100mg	**BW:** Sporanox should not be administered for the treatment of onychomycosis in patients with evidence of ventricular dysfunction. Coadministration of methadone, disopyramide, dofetilide, dronedarone, quinidine, ergot alkaloids, irinotecan, lurasidone, oral midazolam, pimozide, triazolam, felodipine, nisoldipine, ranolazine, eplerenone, cisapride, lovastatin, simvastatin and, in subjects with renal or hepatic impairment, colchicine, is contraindicated. • Sporanox Capsules is a different preparation than Oral Solution; these should not be used interchangeably. • Take with a full meal.

GENERIC (BRAND)	INDICATIONS	DOSAGE FORM	ADDITIONAL COMMENTS
Itraconazole (Sporanox)	• Oropharyngeal and esophageal candidiasis	**Sol:** 10mg/mL	**BW:** If signs or symptoms of congestive heart failure occur during administration of Sporanox Oral Solution, continued use should be reassessed. Coadministration of methadone, disopyramide, dofetilide, dronedarone, quinidine, ergot alkaloids, irinotecan, lurasidone, oral midazolam, pimozide, triazolam, felodipine, nisoldipine, ranolazine, eplerenone, cisapride, lovastatin, simvastatin and, in subjects with renal or hepatic impairment, colchicine, is contraindicated. • Sporanox Capsules is a different preparation than Oral Solution; these should not be used interchangeably.
Ketoconazole	Treatment of the following systemic fungal infections in patients who have failed/are intolerant to other therapies: • Blastomycosis • Coccidioidomycosis • Histoplasmosis • Chromomycosis • Paracoccidioidomycosis	**Tab:** 200mg	**BW:** Oral use of ketoconazole has been associated with hepatic toxicity. Coadministration of dofetilide, quinidine, pimozide, and cisapride is contraindicated. • Tablets should not be used for treatment of fungal meningitis.
Micafungin sodium (Mycamine)	• Candidemia • Acute disseminated candidiasis • *Candida* peritonitis and abscesses • Esophageal candidiasis • Prevention of *Candida* infection in patients undergoing hematopoietic stem cell transplantation	**Inj:** 50mg, 100mg	• LD is not required. • Infuse IV over 1 hour.
Miconazole (Oravig)	• Oropharyngeal candidiasis	**Tab, Buccal:** 50mg	• Oravig should not be crushed, chewed, or swallowed.
Nystatin	**Sus:** • Oral candidiasis **Tab:** • Non-esophageal mucous membrane GI candidiasis	**Sus:** 100,000 U/mL; **Tab:** 500,000 U	• Not indicated for treatment of systemic mycoses.
Posaconazole (Noxafil)	• Prevention of *Aspergillus* and *Candida* infections **Sus:** • Oropharyngeal candidiasis, including oropharyngeal candidiasis refractory to itraconazole and/or fluconazole	**Inj:** 18mg/mL; **Sus:** 40mg/mL; **Tab, DR:** 100mg	• DR tablet and oral suspension are not interchangeable. • DR tablet should be swallowed whole, and not be divided, crushed, or chewed. It should be taken with food. • Each dose of Noxafil Oral Suspension should be administered during or immediately (ie, within 20 minutes) following a full meal. In patients who cannot eat a full meal, administer with a liquid nutritional supplement or an acidic carbonated beverage. • Administer injection via central venous line over 90 minutes. If central venous catheter is not available, may administer through a peripheral venous catheter over 30 minutes.

(Continued)

GENERIC (BRAND)	INDICATIONS	DOSAGE FORM	ADDITIONAL COMMENTS
Terbinafine HCl (Lamisil)	**Granules:** • Tinea capitis **Tab:** • Onychomycosis of the toenail or fingernail	**Granules:** 125mg/pkt, 187.5mg/pkt; **Tab:** 250mg	• (Tab) Prior to initiating treatment, appropriate nail specimens for laboratory testing (potassium hydroxide preparation, fungal culture, or nail biopsy) should be obtained to confirm the diagnosis of onychomycosis.
Voriconazole (Vfend)	• Aspergillosis • Esophageal candidiasis • Candidemia in non-neutropenic patients • Disseminated infections in skin and infections in abdomen, kidney, bladder wall, and wounds caused by *Candida* • Fungal infections caused by *Scedosporium apiospermum* and *Fusarium* spp. including *Fusarium solani,* in patients intolerant of, or refractory to, other therapy	**Inj:** 200mg; **Sus:** 40mg/mL; **Tab:** 50mg, 200mg	• Vfend Tablets or Oral Suspension should be taken at least 1 hour before or after a meal. • Vfend IV for Injection requires reconstitution to 10mg/mL and subsequent dilution to 5mg/mL or less prior to administration as an infusion, at a maximum rate of 3mg/kg per hour over 1 to 2 hours. • Do not administer as an IV bolus injection.

Refer to full FDA-approved labeling for additional information.

Abbreviations: BW = Boxed Warning; DR = Delayed-Release.

SYSTEMIC ANTIBIOTICS TREATMENT COMPARISON

GENERIC (BRAND)	HOW SUPPLIED	INDICATIONS																	
		AECB	Bone & Joint Inf	CAP	Endocarditis	GI Inf	Gyn Inf	Intra-Ab Inf	LRTI	URTI	Meningitis	Otitis Media	PCP	Septicemia	Sinusitis	SSSI	SSTI	TB	UTI
AMINOGLYCOSIDES																			
Amikacin sulfate	**Inj:** 250mg/mL		X					X	X	X	X			X			X		X
Gentamicin sulfate	**Inj:** 10mg/mL, 40mg/mL; **Isotonic Inj:** 60mg, 80mg, 100mg, 120mg		X			X			X	X	X			X			X		X
Streptomycin	**Inj:** 1g				X				X		X							X	X
Tobramycin	**Inj:** 10mg/mL, 40mg/mL		X					X	X		X			X		X			X
CARBAPENEMS																			
Cilastatin-Imipenem (Primaxin IV)	**Inj:** 250-250mg, 500-500mg		X		X		X	X	X					X		X			X
Doripenem (Doribax)	**Inj:** 250mg, 500mg							X											X
Ertapenem (Invanz)	**Inj:** 1g			X			X	X								X			X
Meropenem (Merrem IV)	**Inj:** 500mg, 1g							X			X					X			
CEPHALOSPORINS																			
1st Generation																			
Cefazolin	**Inj:** 500mg, 1g		X		X				X	X				X		X			X
2nd Generation																			
Cefotetan	**Inj:** 1g, 2g		X				X	X	X					X		X			X
Cefoxitin	**Inj:** 1g, 2g		X				X	X	X					X		X			X
Cefuroxime (Zinacef)	**Inj:** 750mg, 1.5g*		X				X		X		X			X		X			X

(Continued)

GENERIC (BRAND)	HOW SUPPLIED	INDICATIONS																	
		AECB	Bone & Joint Inf	CAP	Endocarditis	GI Inf	Gyn Inf	Intra-Ab Inf	LRTI	URTI	Meningitis	Otitis Media	PCP	Septicemia	Sinusitis	SSSI	SSTI	TB	UTI
CEPHALOSPORINS *(Continued)*																			
3rd Generation																			
Cefotaxime (Claforan)	**Inj:** 500mg, 1g, 2g*		X				X	X	X		X			X		X			X
Ceftazidime (Fortaz)	**Inj:** 500mg, 1g, 2g*		X				X	X	X		X			X		X			X
Ceftazidime (Tazicef)	**Inj:** 1g, 2g*		X				X	X	X		X			X		X			X
Ceftazidime-Avibactam (Avycaz)	**Inj:** 2-0.5g							X											X
Ceftriaxone sodium (Rocephin)	**Inj:** 250mg, 500mg, 1g, 2g		X				X	X	X		X	X		X		X			X
4th Generation																			
Cefepime HCl (Maxipime)	**Inj:** 500mg, 1g, 2g							X	X							X			X
5th Generation																			
Ceftaroline fosamil (Teflaro)	**Inj:** 400mg, 600mg			X												X			
FLUOROQUINOLONES																			
Ciprofloxacin (Cipro IV)	**Inj:** 200mg/100mL, 400mg/200mL		X					X	X						X	X			X
Levofloxacin (Levaquin)	**Inj:** 5mg/mL	X		X					X						X	X			X
Moxifloxacin HCl (Avelox)	**Inj:** 400mg/250mL	X		X				X							X	X			
MACROLIDES																			
Azithromycin (Zithromax)	**Inj:** 500mg			X			X												

GENERIC (BRAND)	HOW SUPPLIED	INDICATIONS																	
		AECB	Bone & Joint Inf	CAP	Endocarditis	GI Inf	Gyn Inf	Intra-Ab Inf	LRTI	URTI	Meningitis	Otitis Media	PCP	Septicemia	Sinusitis	SSSI	SSTI	TB	UTI
MACROLIDES *(Continued)*																			
Erythromycin lactobionate (Erythrocin)	**Inj:** 500mg						X		X	X						X			
MONOBACTAMS																			
Aztreonam (Azactam)	**Inj:** 1g, 2g, 1g/50mL, 2g/50mL						X	X	X					X		X			X
PENICILLINS																			
Ampicillin sodium	**Inj:** 125mg, 250mg, 500mg, 1g, 2g*				X	X			X	X	X			X					X
Ampicillin sodium-Sulbactam sodium (Unasyn)	**Inj:** 1-0.5g, 2-1g*						X	X								X			
Penicillin G benzathine-Penicillin G procaine (Bicillin C-R)	**Inj:** 600,000-600,000 U/2mL								X	X		X					X		
Penicillin G benzathine-Penicillin G procaine (Bicillin C-R 900/300)	**Inj:** 900,000-300,000 U/2mL								X	X		X					X		
Penicillin G benzathine (Bicillin L-A)	**Inj:** 600,000 U/mL, 1,200,000 U/2mL, 2,400,000 U/4mL									X									
Penicillin G benzathine (Permapen)	**Inj:** 600,000 U/mL									X									
Penicillin G potassium (Pfizerpen)	**Inj:** 5 MU, 20 MU				X				X		X			X					

(Continued)

GENERIC (BRAND)	HOW SUPPLIED	INDICATIONS																	
		AECB	Bone & Joint Inf	CAP	Endocarditis	GI Inf	Gyn Inf	Intra-Ab Inf	LRTI	URTI	Meningitis	Otitis Media	PCP	Septicemia	Sinusitis	SSSI	SSTI	TB	UTI
PENICILLINS *(Continued)*																			
Piperacillin-Tazobactam (Zosyn)	**Inj:** 2-0.25g/50mL, 3-0.375g/50mL, 4-0.5g/100mL, 2-0.25g, 3-0.375g, 4-0.5g*			X			X	X	X							X			
Ticarcillin disodium-Clavulanate potassium (Timentin)	**Inj:** 3g-100mg, 3g-100mg/100mL*		X				X	X	X					X		X			X
TETRACYCLINES																			
Doxycycline (Doxy 100)	**Inj:** 100mg					X			X	X									X
Minocycline (Minocin)	**Inj:** 100mg					X	X		X	X	X					X			X
MISCELLANEOUS																			
Clindamycin (Cleocin Phosphate)	**Inj:** 150mg/mL, 300mg/50mL, 600mg/50mL, 900mg/50mL*		X				X	X	X					X		X			
Dalbavancin (Dalvance)	**Inj:** 500mg															X			
Dalfopristin-Quinupristin (Synercid)	**Inj:** 350-150mg															X			
Daptomycin (Cubicin)	**Inj:** 500mg				X											X			
Linezolid (Zyvox)	**Inj:** 2mg/mL			X					X							X			
Metronidazole	**Inj:** 500mg/100mL		X		X		X	X	X		X			X		X			
Oritavancin (Orbactiv)	**Inj:** 400mg/50mL															X			
Rifampin (Rifadin)	**Inj:** 600mg																	X	

GENERIC (BRAND)	HOW SUPPLIED	INDICATIONS																	
		AECB	Bone & Joint Inf	CAP	Endocarditis	GI Inf	Gyn Inf	Intra-Ab Inf	LRTI	URTI	Meningitis	Otitis Media	PCP	Septicemia	Sinusitis	SSSI	SSTI	TB	UTI
MISCELLANEOUS *(Continued)*																			
Sulfamethoxazole-Trimethoprim	**Inj:** 80-16mg/mL					X							X						X
Tedizolid phosphate (Sivextro)	**Inj:** 200mg															X			
Telavancin (Vibativ)	**Inj:** 250mg, 750mg								X							X			
Tigecycline (Tygacil)	**Inj:** 50mg/5mL, 50mg/10mL			X				X								X			
Vancomycin HCl	**Inj:** 500mg, 750mg, 1g		X		X				X					X		X			

Refer to full FDA-approved labeling for additional information.

*Also available as a Pharmacy Bulk Package.

Abbreviations:
AECB = acute exacerbations of chronic bronchitis
CAP = community-acquired pneumonia
GI = gastrointestinal
LRTI = lower respiratory tract infection
PCP = *Pneumocystis jiroveci* pneumonia
SSSI = skin and skin structure infection
SSTI = skin and soft tissue infection
TB = tuberculosis
URTI = upper respiratory tract infection
UTI = urinary tract infection

Arthritis Treatment Comparison

GENERIC (BRAND)	HOW SUPPLIED	AS	GA	JIA	JRA	OA	OA of Knee	PsA	RA
CHELATING AGENTS									
Penicillamine (Cuprimine)	**Cap:** 250mg								✓
Penicillamine (Depen)	**Tab:** 250mg								✓
CYCLIC POLYPEPTIDE IMMUNOSUPPRESSANTS									
Cyclosporine (Gengraf, Neoral)	**Cap:** 25mg, 100mg; **Sol:** 100mg/mL								✓
CYCLOOXYGENASE-2 INHIBITORS									
Celecoxib (Celebrex)	**Cap:** 50mg, 100mg, 200mg, 400mg	✓			✓	✓			✓
DIHYDROFOLIC ACID REDUCTASE INHIBITORS									
Methotrexate (Rasuvo)	**Inj:** 50mg/mL			✓					✓
Methotrexate (Rheumatrex)	**Inj:** 25mg/mL; **Tab:** 2.5mg				✓				✓
Methotrexate (Trexall)	**Tab:** 5mg, 7.5mg, 10mg, 15mg				✓				✓
INTERLEUKIN RECEPTOR ANTAGONISTS									
Anakinra (Kineret)	**Inj:** 100mg/0.67mL								✓
Tocilizumab (Actemra)	**Inj:** 20mg/mL, 162mg/0.9mL			✓					✓
GOLD COMPOUNDS									
Auranofin (Ridaura)	**Cap:** 3mg								✓
HYALURONAN AND DERIVATIVES									
Hyaluronan (Orthovisc)	**Inj:** 30mg/2mL						✓		
Sodium hyaluronate (Euflexxa)	**Inj:** 1%						✓		
Sodium hyaluronate (Hyalgan)	**Inj:** 10mg/mL						✓		
Sodium hyaluronate (Supartz)	**Inj:** 25mg/2.5mL						✓		
HYLAN POLYMERS									
Hylan G-F 20 (Synvisc, Synvisc One)	**Inj:** 8mg/mL						✓		
KINASE INHIBITORS									
Tofacitinib (Xeljanz)	**Tab:** 5mg								✓
MONOCLONAL ANTIBODIES									
Ustekinumab (Stelara)	**Inj:** 45mg/0.5mL, 90mg/mL							✓	
MONOCLONAL ANTIBODIES/CD20-BLOCKERS									
Rituximab (Rituxan)	**Inj:** 100mg/10mL, 500mg/50mL								✓

(Continued)

GENERIC (BRAND)	HOW SUPPLIED	AS	GA	JIA	JRA	OA	OA of Knee	PsA	RA
MONOCLONAL ANTIBODIES/TNF-BLOCKERS									
Adalimumab (Humira)	**Inj:** 10mg/0.2mL, 20mg/0.4mL, 40mg/0.8mL	✓		✓				✓	✓
Golimumab (Simponi)	**Inj:** 50mg/0.5mL, 100mg/mL	✓						✓	✓
Golimumab (Simponi Aria)	**Inj:** 50mg/4mL								✓
Infliximab (Remicade)	**Inj:** 100mg	✓						✓	✓
NON-STEROIDAL ANTI-INFLAMMATORY DRUGS (NSAIDs)									
Diclofenac (Zorvolex)	**Cap:** 18mg, 35mg					✓			
Diclofenac potassium (Cataflam)	**Tab:** 50mg					✓			✓
Diclofenac sodium	**Tab, DR:** 25mg, 50mg, 75mg	✓				✓			✓
Diclofenac sodium (Pennsaid)	**Sol:** 1.5%, 2%						✓		
Diclofenac sodium (Voltaren Gel)	**Gel:** 1%					✓	✓		
Diclofenac sodium (Voltaren-XR)	**Tab, ER:** 100mg					✓			✓
Diflunisal	**Tab:** 500mg					✓			✓
Etodolac	**Cap:** 200mg, 300mg; **Tab:** 400mg, 500mg					✓			✓
Etodolac Extended-Release	**Tab, ER:** 400mg, 500mg, 600mg				✓	✓			✓
Fenoprofen calcium (Nalfon)	**Cap:** 200mg, 400mg; **Tab:** 600mg					✓			✓
Ibuprofen	**Tab:** 400mg, 600mg, 800mg; **Susp:** 100mg/5mL					✓			✓
Indomethacin	**Cap:** 25mg, 50mg	✓	✓			✓			✓
Indomethacin (Indocin)	**Sup:** 50mg; **Susp:** 25mg/5mL	✓	✓			✓			✓
Indomethacin Extended-Release	**Cap, ER:** 75mg	✓				✓			✓
Ketoprofen	**Cap:** 50mg, 75mg					✓			✓
Ketoprofen Extended-Release	**Cap, ER:** 100mg, 150mg, 200mg					✓			✓
Meloxicam (Mobic)	**Susp:** 7.5mg/5mL; **Tab:** 7.5mg, 15mg				✓	✓			✓
Nabumetone	**Tab:** 500mg, 750mg					✓			✓
Naproxen (Naprosyn, EC-Naprosyn)	**Susp:** 125mg/mL; **Tab:** 250mg, 375mg, 500mg; **Tab, DR:** 375mg, 500mg	✓			✓*	✓			✓

GENERIC (BRAND)	HOW SUPPLIED	AS	GA	JIA	JRA	OA	OA of Knee	PsA	RA
NON-STEROIDAL ANTI-INFLAMMATORY DRUGS (NSAIDs) *(Continued)*									
Naproxen sodium (Anaprox, Anaprox DS)	**Tab:** 275mg, 550mg	✓				✓			✓
Naproxen sodium (Naprelan)	**Tab, CR:** 375mg, 500mg, 750mg	✓				✓			✓
Oxaprozin (Daypro)	**Tab:** 600mg				✓	✓			✓
Piroxicam (Feldene)	**Cap:** 10mg, 20mg					✓			✓
Sulindac	**Tab:** 150mg, 200mg	✓	✓			✓			✓
Tolmetin	**Cap:** 400mg; **Tab:** 200mg, 600mg				✓	✓			✓
PHOSPHODIESTERASE-4 INHIBITORS									
Apremilast (Otezla)	**Tab:** 10mg, 20mg, 30mg							✓	
PURINE ANTAGONIST ANTIMETABOLITES									
Azathioprine (Azasan)	**Tab:** 75mg, 100mg								✓
Azathioprine (Imuran)	**Tab:** 50mg								✓
PYRIMIDINE SYNTHESIS INHIBITORS									
Leflunomide (Arava)	**Tab:** 10mg, 20mg, 100mg								✓
QUININE DERIVATIVES									
Hydroxychloroquine sulfate (Plaquenil)	**Tab:** 200mg								✓
SELECTIVE COSTIMULATION MODULATORS									
Abatacept (Orencia)	**Inj:** 125mg/mL, 250mg			✓					✓
5-AMINOSALICYLIC ACID DERIVATIVES/SULFAPYRIDINES									
Sulfasalazine (Azulfidine EN-tabs)	**Tab, DR:** 500mg				✓				✓
TNF-RECEPTOR BLOCKERS									
Certolizumab pegol (Cimzia)	**Inj:** 200mg/mL	✓						✓	✓
Etanercept (Enbrel)	**Inj:** 25mg, 50mg	✓		✓				✓	✓
COMBINATION PRODUCTS									
NSAIDs/H_2-RECEPTOR ANTAGONISTS									
Ibuprofen/Famotidine (Duexis)	**Tab:** 800mg/26.6mg					✓			✓
NSAIDs/PROTON PUMP INHIBITORS									
Naproxen/Esomeprazole magnesium (Vimovo)	**Tab, DR:** 375mg/20mg, 500mg/20mg	✓				✓			✓

(Continued)

GENERIC (BRAND)	HOW SUPPLIED	AS	GA	JIA	JRA	OA	OA of Knee	PsA	RA
COMBINATION PRODUCTS *(Continued)*									
NSAIDs/PROSTAGLANDIN ANALOGUES									
Diclofenac sodium/ Misoprostol (Arthrotec)	**Tab:** 50mg/200mcg, 75mg/200mcg					✓			✓

Refer to full FDA-approved labeling for additional information.

*Susp only.

Abbreviations: AS = ankylosing spondylitis; DR = delayed-release; ER = extended-release; GA = gouty arthritis; JIA = juvenile idiopathic arthritis; JRA = juvenile rheumatoid arthritis; OA = osteoarthritis; PsA = psoriatic arthritis; RA = rheumatoid arthritis.

Osteoporosis Agents

GENERIC (BRAND)	HOW SUPPLIED	DOSAGE	SPECIAL INSTRUCTIONS
BISPHOSPHONATES AND COMBINATIONS			
Alendronate sodium (Binosto)	**Tab, Effervescent:** 70mg	**Osteoporosis: Treatment:** 70mg once weekly. **Increase Bone Mass in Men with Osteoporosis:** 70mg once weekly.	Take at least 30 min before 1st food, drink (other than plain water), or medication of day with plain water only. Dissolve tabs in 4 oz room temperature plain water and wait at least 5 min after the effervescence stops. Stir the solution for about 10 sec and ingest. Do not lie down for at least 30 min and until after 1st food of day.
Alendronate sodium (Fosamax)	**Sol:** (Generic) 70mg [75mL]; **Tab:** (Generic) 5mg, 10mg, 35mg, 40mg, 70mg; (Fosamax) 70mg	**Osteoporosis: Treatment:** 70mg once weekly or 10mg qd. **Prevention:** 35mg once weekly or 5mg qd. **Increase Bone Mass in Men with Osteoporosis:** 70mg once weekly or 10mg qd. **Glucocorticoid-Induced:** 5mg qd; 10mg qd for postmenopausal women not on estrogen.	Take at least 30 min before 1st food, drink (other than plain water), or medication of day with plain water only. Take tabs with 6-8 oz water or 2 oz with oral sol. Do not lie down for at least 30 min and until after 1st food of day.
Alendronate sodium/ Cholecalciferol (Fosamax Plus D)	**Tab:** (Alendronate-Cholecalciferol) 70mg-2800 IU, 70mg-5600 IU	**Osteoporosis: Treatment:** 1 tab (70mg-2800 IU or 70mg-5600 IU) once weekly. **Usual:** 70mg-5600 IU once weekly. **Increase Bone Mass in Men with Osteoporosis:** 1 tab (70mg-2800 IU or 70mg-5600 IU) once weekly. **Usual:** 70mg-5600 IU once weekly.	Take at least 30 min before 1st food, drink (other than plain water), or medication of day. Take with 6-8 oz water. Do not lie down for at least 30 min and until after 1st food of day.
Ibandronate sodium (Boniva)	**Inj:** 3mg/3mL; **Tab:** 150mg	**Osteoporosis: Treatment: Inj:** 3mg IV over 15-30 sec every 3 months. **Prevention/Treatment: PO:** 150mg once monthly.	**PO:** Take at least 60 min before 1st food, drink (other than plain water), medication, or supplement of day. Swallow whole with 6-8 oz plain water while standing or sitting upright. Do not lie down for 60 min after dose.
Risedronate sodium (Actonel)	**Tab:** 5mg, 30mg, 35mg, 75mg, 150mg	**Osteoporosis: Prevention/ Treatment:** 5mg qd or 35mg once weekly or 150mg once monthly or 75mg on 2 consecutive days each month. **Increase Bone Mass in Men with Osteoporosis:** 35mg once weekly. **Glucocorticoid-Induced: Prevention/ Treatment:** 5mg qd.	Take at least 30 min before 1st food, drink (other than plain water), medication, or supplement of day. Take with 6-8 oz plain water in an upright position. Do not lie down for 30 min after dose.
Risedronate sodium (Atelvia)	**Tab, Delayed-Release:** 35mg	**Osteoporosis: Treatment:** 35mg once weekly.	Take in am immediately after breakfast. Swallow whole with 4 oz of plain water. Do not lie down for 30 min after dose. Do not chew, cut, or crush tabs.

(Continued)

GENERIC (BRAND)	HOW SUPPLIED	DOSAGE	SPECIAL INSTRUCTIONS
BISPHOSPHONATES AND COMBINATIONS *(Continued)*			
Zoledronic acid (Reclast)	**Inj:** 5mg/100mL	**Osteoporosis: Treatment:** 5mg IV over ≥15 min once a year. **Prevention:** 5mg IV over ≥15 min once every 2 years. **Increase Bone Mass in Men with Osteoporosis:** 5mg IV over ≥15 min once a year. **Glucocorticoid-Induced: Prevention/Treatment:** 5mg IV over ≥15 min once a year.*	Flush IV line with 10mL normal saline after infusion. Administration of acetaminophen after Reclast may decrease acute-phase reaction symptoms.
HORMONE THERAPY†‡			
Conjugated estrogens (Premarin Tabs)	**Tab:** 0.3mg, 0.45mg, 0.625mg, 0.9mg, 1.25mg	**Osteoporosis: Prevention: Initial:** 0.3mg qd continuously or cyclically (eg, 25 days on, 5 days off). Reevaluate periodically.	
Conjugated estrogens (CEs)/ Medroxyprogesterone acetate (MPA) (Premphase)	**Tab:** (CEs) 0.625mg and (CEs-MPA) 0.625mg-5mg	**Osteoporosis: Prevention:** 1 CE tab qd on Days 1-14 and 1 CE-MPA tab qd on Days 15-28. Reevaluate periodically.	
Conjugated estrogens (CEs)/ Medroxyprogesterone acetate (MPA) (Prempro)	**Tab:** (CEs-MPA) 0.3mg-1.5mg, 0.45mg-1.5mg, 0.625mg-2.5mg, 0.625mg-5mg	**Osteoporosis: Prevention:** 1 tab qd. Reevaluate periodically.	
Estradiol (Alora)	**Patch:** 0.025mg/day, 0.05mg/day, 0.075mg/day, 0.1mg/day	**Osteoporosis: Prevention:** 0.025mg/day twice weekly. May increase depending on bone mineral density and adverse events. Reevaluate periodically.	Apply to lower abdomen, upper quadrant of buttock, or outer aspect of hip; avoid breasts and waistline. Rotate application sites. Allow 1 week between applications to same site.
Estradiol (Climara)	**Patch:** 0.025mg/day, 0.0375mg/day, 0.05mg/day, 0.06mg/day, 0.075mg/day, 0.1mg/day	**Osteoporosis: Prevention:** 0.025mg/day once weekly. Reevaluate periodically.	Apply to lower abdomen or upper quadrant of buttock; avoid breasts and waistline. Rotate application sites. Allow 1 week between applications to same site.
Estradiol (Estrace)	**Tab:** 0.5mg§, 1mg§, 2mg§	**Osteoporosis: Prevention:** Lowest effective dose has not been determined. Reevaluate periodically.	
Estradiol (Estraderm)	**Patch:** 0.05mg/day, 0.1mg/day	**Osteoporosis: Prevention: Initial:** 0.05mg/day twice weekly. May give continuously in patients without intact uterus. May give cyclically (eg, 3 weeks on, 1 week off) in patients with intact uterus. Reevaluate periodically.	Apply to trunk of body (including buttocks and abdomen); avoid breasts and waistline. Rotate application sites. Allow 1 week between applications to same site.
Estradiol (Menostar)	**Patch:** 14mcg/day	**Osteoporosis: Prevention:** Apply 1 patch weekly. Reevaluate periodically.	Apply to lower abdomen or upper quadrant of buttock; avoid breasts and waistline. Rotate application sites. Allow 1 week between applications to same site.

GENERIC (BRAND)	HOW SUPPLIED	DOSAGE	SPECIAL INSTRUCTIONS
HORMONE THERAPY†† *(Continued)*			
Estradiol (Vivelle-Dot)	**Patch:** 0.025mg/day, 0.0375mg/day, 0.05mg/day, 0.075mg/day, 0.1mg/day	**Osteoporosis: Prevention:** **Initial:** 0.025mg/day twice weekly. May give continuously in patients without intact uterus. May give cyclically (eg, 3 weeks on, 1 week off) in patients with intact uterus. Reevaluate periodically.	Apply to trunk of body (including abdomen or buttocks); avoid breasts and waistline. Rotate application sites. Allow 1 week between applications to same site.
Estradiol/ Levonorgestrel (Climara Pro)	**Patch:** (Estradiol-Levonorgestrel) 0.045mg-0.015mg/day	**Osteoporosis: Prevention:** Apply 1 patch weekly. Reevaluate periodically.	Apply to lower abdomen or upper quadrant of the buttock; avoid breasts and waistline. Rotate application sites. Allow 1 week between applications to same site.
Estradiol/ Norethindrone (Activella)	**Tab:** (Estradiol-Norethindrone) 1mg-0.5mg, 0.5mg-0.1mg	**Osteoporosis: Prevention:** 1 tab qd. Reevaluate periodically.	
Estradiol/ Norgestimate (Prefest)	**Tab:** (Estradiol) 1mg and (Estradiol-Norgestimate) 1mg-0.09mg	**Osteoporosis: Prevention:** 1 estradiol (peach color) tab for 3 days followed by 1 estradiol-norgestimate (white color) tab for 3 days. Repeat regimen continuously. Reevaluate periodically.	
Estropipate	**Tab:** 0.75mg§, 1.5mg§, 3mg§	**Osteoporosis: Prevention:** 0.75mg qd for 25 days of a 31-day cycle per month.	
Ethinyl Estradiol/ Norethindrone (Femhrt)	**Tab:** (Ethinyl Estradiol-Norethindrone) 2.5mcg-0.5mg, 5mcg-1mg	**Osteoporosis: Prevention:** 1 tab qd. Reevaluate periodically.	
MISCELLANEOUS			
Calcitonin-Salmon (Fortical)	**Nasal Spray:** 200 IU/actuation	**Osteoporosis (>5 yrs Postmenopause): Treatment:** 200 IU qd intranasally. Alternate nostrils daily.	Patients should take supplemental calcium and vitamin D.
Calcitonin-Salmon (Miacalcin)	**Inj:** 200 IU/mL; **Nasal Spray:** 200 IU/actuation	**Osteoporosis (>5 yrs Postmenopause): Treatment:** (Inj) 100 IU IM/SQ qd. If >2mL, use IM and multiple inj sites. (Spray) 200 IU qd intranasally. Alternate nostrils daily.	Patients should take supplemental calcium and vitamin D.
Denosumab (Prolia)	**Inj:** 60mg/mL	**Osteoporosis: Treatment:** 60mg as a single SQ inj once every 6 months. **Increase Bone Mass in Men with Osteoporosis:** 60mg as a single SQ inj once every 6 months.	Administer in the upper arm, upper thigh, or abdomen. All patients should receive calcium 1000mg and at least 400 IU vitamin D qd.

(Continued)

GENERIC (BRAND)	HOW SUPPLIED	DOSAGE	SPECIAL INSTRUCTIONS
MISCELLANEOUS *(Continued)*			
Raloxifene HCl[†] (Evista)	**Tab:** 60mg	**Osteoporosis: Prevention/ Treatment:** 60mg qd.	Calcium and vitamin D supplementation is recommended.
Teriparatide[†] (Forteo)	**Inj:** 250mcg/mL	**Osteoporosis: Treatment/ Increase Bone Mass in Men/Glucocorticoid-Induced:** 20mcg SQ qd into thigh or abdominal wall. Use of the drug for >2 years during a patient's lifetime is not recommended.	Administer initially under circumstances where patient can sit or lie down if symptoms of orthostatic hypotension occur. Discard pen after 28 days.

Refer to full FDA-approved labeling for additional information.

*Patients on Reclast must be adequately supplemented with calcium and vitamin D if dietary intake is not sufficient. An average of at least 1200mg calcium and 800-1000 IU vitamin D daily is recommended.

† Check FDA-approved labeling for important Boxed Warnings.

‡ When prescribing solely for the prevention of postmenopausal osteoporosis, therapy should be considered only for women at significant risk for osteoporosis; non-estrogen medications should be carefully considered.

§ Scored.

Alzheimer's Disease Agents

GENERIC (BRAND)	HOW SUPPLIED	ADULT DOSAGE	SPECIAL INSTRUCTIONS
Donepezil HCl (Aricept)	**Tab:** 5mg, 10mg, 23mg; **Tab, Disintegrating:** 5mg, 10mg	**Mild-Moderate: Initial:** 5mg qhs. **Usual:** 5-10mg qhs. **Titrate:** May increase to 10mg after 4-6 weeks. **Moderate-Severe: Initial:** 5mg qhs. **Usual:** 10-23mg qhs. **Titrate:** May increase to 10mg after 4-6 weeks, then to 23mg after ≥3 months.	• Monitor for vagotonic effects on sinoatrial and atrioventricular nodes, syncopal episodes, diarrhea, N/V, active/occult GI bleeding, weight loss, bladder outflow obstruction, and generalized convulsions. • Do not split or crush 23mg tablet.
Ergoloid mesylates	**Tab:** 1mg	1mg tid.	• Monitor for transient nausea and gastric disturbances. • Monitor for relief of signs and symptoms.
Galantamine HBr (Razadyne, Razadyne ER)	(Razadyne) **Sol:** 4mg/mL [100mL]; **Tab:** 4mg, 8mg, 12mg; (Razadyne ER) **Cap, ER:** 8mg, 16mg, 24mg	(Sol, Tab) **Initial:** 4mg bid (8mg/day) with am and pm meals. **Titrate:** Increase to initial maint dose of 8mg bid (16mg/day) after a minimum of 4 weeks, then increase to 12mg bid (24mg/day) after a minimum of 4 weeks. Restart at the lowest dose and increase to current dose if therapy is interrupted for more than 3 days. (Cap, ER) **Initial:** 8mg qd with am meal. **Titrate:** Increase to initial maint dose of 16mg qd after a minimum of 4 weeks, then increase to 24mg qd after a minimum of 4 weeks.	• Monitor for GI bleeding, cardiac conduction abnormalities, bladder outflow obstruction, and convulsions. • Not recommended for patients with severe renal/hepatic impairment. • Dose adjustment required for moderate renal/hepatic impairment.
Memantine HCl (Namenda, Namenda XR)	(Namenda) **Sol:** 2mg/mL [360mL]; **Tab:** 5mg, 10mg; (Namenda XR) **Cap, ER:** 7mg, 14mg, 21mg, 28mg	(Sol, Tab) **Initial:** 5mg qd. **Titrate:** Increase in 5mg increments to 10mg/day (5mg bid), 15mg/day (5mg and 10mg as separate doses), and 20mg/day (10mg bid) at ≥1-week intervals. Dosage shown to be effective in controlled clinical trials is 20mg/day. (Cap, ER) **Initial:** 7mg qd. **Titrate:** Increase in 7mg increments to 28mg qd at ≥1-week intervals. **Max/Target Dose:** 28mg qd.	• Monitor renal/hepatic function. • Do not divide or crush Namenda XR; capsules may be opened and sprinkled on applesauce. • Administer oral solution with dosing device and do not mix with any other liquid. • Dose adjustment required in severe renal insufficiency.

(Continued)

GENERIC (BRAND)	HOW SUPPLIED	ADULT DOSAGE	SPECIAL INSTRUCTIONS
Rivastigmine tartrate (Exelon)	**Cap:** 1.5mg, 3mg, 4.5mg, 6mg; **Patch:** 4.6mg/24 hrs, 9.5mg/24 hrs, 13.3mg/24 hrs; **Sol:** 2mg/mL [120mL]	(PO) **Initial:** 1.5mg bid. **Titrate:** May increase to 3mg bid after a minimum of 2 weeks, if 1.5mg bid is well tolerated. Subsequent increases to 4.5mg bid and 6mg bid should be attempted after a minimum of 2 weeks at the previous dose. **Max:** 12mg/day (6mg bid). **Interruption of Treatment: Intolerance:** D/C therapy for several doses and then restart at same or next lower dose level. **≤3 Days Interruption:** Restart with same or lower dose. **>3 Days Interruption:** Restart with 1.5mg bid and titrate as above. (Patch) **Initial:** Apply 4.6mg/24 hrs patch qd to skin. **Titrate:** Increase dose only after a minimum of 4 weeks at the previous dose, and only if the previous dose is well tolerated. **Effective Dose: Mild-Moderate:** 9.5mg/24 hrs qd or 13.3mg/24 hrs qd. **Severe:** 13.3mg/24 hrs qd. **Max:** 13.3mg/24 hrs. Replace with a new patch q24h. **Interruption of Treatment: ≤3 Days Interruption:** Restart with same or lower strength patch. **>3 Days Interruption:** Restart with 4.6mg/24 hrs patch and titrate as above.	• Monitor for signs/symptoms of active or occult GI bleeding, extrapyramidal symptoms, urinary obstruction, seizures, and GI adverse events. • (Patch) Monitor for skin reactions. • (PO) Administer with meals in divided doses in am and pm. • Dose adjustment required for moderate to severe renal insufficiency (PO only), mild to moderate hepatic insufficiency, or low body weight.

Refer to full FDA-approved labeling for additional information.
Abbreviation: ER = extended-release.

ANTIPARKINSON AGENTS

GENERIC (BRAND)	HOW SUPPLIED	ADULT DOSAGE	SIDE EFFECTS
Amantadine HCl	**Cap, Tab:** 100mg; **Sol:** 50mg/5mL	**Parkinsonism: Usual:** 100mg bid. **Serious Associated Illness/Concomitant High-Dose Antiparkinson Agent: Initial:** 100mg qd. **Titrate:** May increase to 100mg bid after 1 to several weeks. **Max:** 400mg/day. **Drug-Induced Extrapyramidal Reactions: Usual:** 100mg bid. **Max:** 300mg/day.*	Nausea, dizziness, insomnia, depression, anxiety and irritability, hallucinations, confusion, anorexia, dry mouth, constipation, ataxia, livedo reticularis, peripheral edema, orthostatic hypotension, headache, somnolence, nervousness, dream abnormality, agitation, dry nose, diarrhea, fatigue
Apomorphine HCl (Apokyn)	**Inj:** 10mg/mL	**Test Dose/Initial:** 0.2mL (2mg) SQ; assess efficacy/tolerability. See PI for details. **Max:** 0.6mL (6mg)/dose. **Renal Impairment: Test Dose/Initial:** 0.1mL (1mg).	Yawning, dyskinesia, nausea, vomiting, somnolence, dizziness, rhinorrhea, hallucinations, edema, chest pain, increased sweating
Benztropine mesylate (Cogentin)	**Inj:** 1mg/mL; (Generic) **Tab:** 0.5mg, 1mg, 2mg	Initiate with a low dose. **Titrate:** May increase every 5-6 days by 0.5mg. **Max:** 6mg/day. **Postencephalitic/Idiopathic Parkinsonism: Usual:** 1-2mg/day. **Range:** 0.5-6mg/day. **Idiopathic Parkinsonism: Initial:** 0.5-1mg PO or IV/IM qhs. **Postencephalitic Parkinsonism: Initial:** 2mg/day PO or IV/IM given in 1 or more doses. **Highly Sensitive Patients: Initial:** 0.5mg PO or IV/IM qhs; increase as necessary. **Drug-Induced Extrapyramidal Disorders: Usual:** 1-4mg PO or IV/IM qd or bid. Give 1-2mg bid or tid for transient extrapyramidal disorders that develop soon after initiation of neuroleptic drugs; d/c and reevaluate necessity after 1 or 2 weeks. May reinstitute therapy if disorders recur.	Tachycardia, paralytic ileus, constipation, vomiting, nausea, dry mouth, confusion, blurred vision, urinary retention, heat stroke, hyperthermia, fever
Bromocriptine mesylate (Parlodel)	**Tab, Snap:** 2.5mg†; **Cap:** 5mg	**Initial:** ½ SnapTab bid. **Titrate:** May increase by 2.5mg/day q2-4 weeks. **Max:** 100mg/day. Take with food. Assess need for medication at 2-week intervals.	Dizziness, insomnia, hallucinations, dyskinesia, visual disturbance, nausea, confusion, drowsiness, vomiting, abdominal pain, hypotension, constipation
Carbidopa (Lodosyn)	**Tab:** 25mg†	**With Sinemet or Levodopa:** Determine dose by careful titration. Most patients respond to a 1:10 proportion of carbidopa and levodopa, provided carbidopa dose is ≥70mg/day. **Max:** 200mg/day. Consider amount of carbidopa in Sinemet when calculating dose. See PI for detailed dosing information.	Dyskinesia (choreiform, dystonic, and other involuntary movements), nausea; check PI for a more comprehensive list of adverse reactions
Carbidopa/Levodopa (Duopa)	**Sus:** (Carbidopa-Levodopa) 4.63mg-20mg/mL	Prior to initiation of therapy, convert patient from all other forms of levodopa to oral IR carbidopa-levodopa (1:4 ratio). See PI for details. **Max:** 2g of levodopa component (eg, 1 cassette/day) over 16 hrs.	Complication of device insertion, nausea, depression, peripheral edema, hypertension, upper respiratory tract infection, oropharyngeal pain, incision site erythema

(Continued)

GENERIC (BRAND)	HOW SUPPLIED	ADULT DOSAGE	SIDE EFFECTS
Carbidopa/Levodopa (Parcopa)	**Tab, Disintegrating:** (Carbidopa-Levodopa) 10mg-100mg†, 25mg-100mg†, 25mg-250mg†	**25mg-100mg Tab: Initial:** 1 tab tid. **Titrate:** Increase by 1 tab qd or qod up to 8 tabs/day. **10mg-100mg Tab: Initial:** 1 tab tid-qid. **Titrate:** Increase by 1 tab qd or qod up to 8 tabs/day. **Maint:** 70-100mg/day carbidopa required. **Max:** 200mg/day carbidopa. **Conversion from Levodopa:** See PI.	Dyskinesia (choreiform, dystonic, and other involuntary movements), nausea; check PI for a more comprehensive list of adverse reactions
Carbidopa/Levodopa (Rytary)	**Cap, ER:** (Carbidopa-Levodopa) 23.75mg-95mg, 36.25mg-145mg, 48.75mg-195mg, 61.25mg-245mg	**Levodopa Naive: Initial:** 23.75mg-95mg tid for the first 3 days. On 4th day of treatment, may increase to 36.25mg-145mg tid. **Titrate:** May increase up to 97.5mg-390mg tid to 5X/day. **Max:** 612.5mg-2450mg/day. **Conversion to ER Caps:** See PI.	Nausea, dizziness, headache, insomnia, abnormal dreams, dry mouth, dyskinesia, anxiety, constipation, vomiting, orthostatic hypotension
Carbidopa/Levodopa (Sinemet, Sinemet CR)	**Tab:** (Carbidopa-Levodopa) 10mg-100mg, 25mg-100mg, 25mg-250mg; **Tab, ER:** 25mg-100mg, 50mg-200mg	(Tab) **25mg-100mg Tab: Initial:** 1 tab tid. **Titrate:** Increase by 1 tab qd or qod up to 8 tabs/day. **10mg-100mg Tab: Initial:** 1 tab tid-qid. **Titrate:** May increase by 1 tab qd or qod up to 8 tabs/day. **Maint:** 70-100mg/day carbidopa required. **Max:** 200mg/day carbidopa. **Conversion from Levodopa:** See PI. (Tab, ER) **No Prior Levodopa Use: Initial:** One 50mg-200mg tab bid at intervals ≥6 hrs. **Titrate:** Increase or decrease dose or interval accordingly. Adjust dose at interval of ≥3 days. **Usual:** 400-1600mg/day levodopa, given in 4- to 8-hr intervals while awake. **Conversion to ER Tabs:** See PI.	Dyskinesia (choreiform, dystonic, and other involuntary movements), nausea; check PI for a more comprehensive list of adverse reactions
Carbidopa/Levodopa/ Entacapone (Stalevo)	**Tab:** (Carbidopa-Levodopa-Entacapone): Stalevo 50: 12.5mg-50mg-200mg; Stalevo 75: 18.75mg-75mg-200mg; Stalevo 100: 25mg-100mg-200mg; Stalevo 125: 31.25mg-125mg-200mg; Stalevo 150: 37.5mg-150mg-200mg; Stalevo 200: 50mg-200mg-200mg	**Currently Taking Carbidopa/Levodopa and Entacapone:** May switch directly to corresponding strength of Stalevo with same amounts of carbidopa/levodopa. **Currently Taking Carbidopa/Levodopa Without Entacapone:** First, titrate individually with carbidopa/levodopa product and entacapone product, then transfer to corresponding dose once stabilized. **Max:** 8 tabs/day (Stalevo 50, 75, 100, 125, 150); 6 tabs/day (Stalevo 200).	Dyskinesia, urine discoloration, diarrhea, nausea, hyperkinesia, vomiting, dry mouth; check PI for a more comprehensive list of adverse reactions
Diphenhydramine HCl Injection	**Inj:** 50mg/mL	**Usual:** 10-50mg IV at ≤25mg/min or deep IM. May use 100mg IM if needed. **Max:** 400mg/day.	Sedation, sleepiness, dizziness, disturbed coordination, epigastric distress, thickening of bronchial secretions
Entacapone (Comtan)	**Tab:** 200mg	**Usual:** 200mg administered concomitantly with each levodopa/carbidopa dose. **Max:** 1600mg/day. Withdraw slowly for discontinuation.	Dyskinesia, hyperkinesia, hypokinesia, dizziness, nausea, diarrhea, abdominal pain, constipation, urine discoloration, fatigue
Hyoscyamine sulfate (Levbid, Levsin)	(Levbid) **Tab, ER:** 0.375mg. (Levsin) **Tab:** 0.125mg; **Tab, SL:** 0.125mg	**Levbid:** 0.375-0.75mg q12h. **Max:** 1.5mg/24 hrs. Do not crush or chew. **Levsin:** 0.125-0.25mg q4h or prn. **Max:** 1.5mg/24 hrs. May chew or swallow SL tab.	Dry mouth, urinary hesitancy and retention, blurred vision, tachycardia, mydriasis, increased ocular tension, loss of taste, headache, nervousness, drowsiness, weakness, fatigue, dizziness, nausea, vomiting

GENERIC (BRAND)	HOW SUPPLIED	ADULT DOSAGE	SIDE EFFECTS
Pramipexole dihydrochloride (Mirapex)	**Tab:** 0.125mg, 0.25mg†, 0.5mg†, 0.75mg, 1mg†, 1.5mg†	**Initial:** 0.125mg tid. **Titrate:** May increase not more frequently than every 5-7 days (eg, Week 2: 0.25mg tid; Week 3: 0.5mg tid; Week 4: 0.75mg tid; Week 5: 1mg tid; Week 6: 1.25mg tid; Week 7: 1.5mg tid). **Maint:** 0.5-1.5mg tid. **Max:** 1.5mg tid.*	Nausea, dizziness, somnolence, constipation, asthenia, hallucinations, vision abnormalities, general and peripheral edema, insomnia, confusion, amnesia, hypesthesia
Pramipexole dihydrochloride (Mirapex ER)	**Tab, ER:** 0.375mg, 0.75mg, 1.5mg, 2.25mg, 3mg, 3.75mg, 4.5mg	**Initial:** 0.375mg qd. **Titrate:** May increase not more frequently than every 5-7 days, first to 0.75mg/day and then by 0.75mg increments based on efficacy and tolerability. **Max:** 4.5mg/day. **Switching from IR to ER:** May switch overnight from IR to ER tabs at same daily dose.*	Somnolence, nausea, constipation, dizziness, fatigue, hallucinations, dry mouth, muscle spasms, peripheral edema, dyskinesia, headache, anorexia
Rasagiline mesylate (Azilect)	**Tab:** 0.5mg, 1mg	**Monotherapy:** 1mg qd. **Adjunctive Therapy: Initial:** 0.5mg qd. **Titrate:** May increase to 1mg qd. Adjust dose of levodopa with concomitant use. **Concomitant Ciprofloxacin or Other CYP1A2 Inhibitors/Mild Hepatic Impairment:** 0.5mg qd.	Headache, accidental injury, arthralgia, depression, fall, flu syndrome, dyskinesia, nausea, weight loss, constipation, postural hypotension, vomiting, dry mouth, rash, somnolence
Rivastigmine (Exelon)	**Cap:** 1.5mg, 3mg, 4.5mg, 6mg; **Patch:** 4.6mg/24 hrs, 9.5mg/24 hrs, 13.3mg/24 hrs; **Sol:** 2mg/mL	(Cap, Sol) **Usual:** 1.5-6mg bid. **Initial:** 1.5mg bid with meals in am and pm. **Titrate:** May subsequently increase to 3mg bid and further to 4.5mg bid and 6mg bid with a minimum of 4 weeks at each dose, based on tolerability. (Patch) **Usual:** 9.5mg/24 hrs or 13.3mg/24 hrs qd. **Initial:** Apply 4.6mg/24 hrs patch qd to clean, dry, hairless, intact skin. **Titrate:** Increase dose only after a minimum of 4 weeks, if well tolerated. Continue effective dose of 9.5mg/24 hrs for as long as therapeutic benefit persists. **Max:** 13.3mg/24 hrs.	Nausea, vomiting, anorexia, dizziness, diarrhea, tremor
Ropinirole (Requip, Requip XL)	**Tab:** 0.25mg, 0.5mg, 1mg, 2mg, 3mg, 4mg, 5mg; **Tab, ER:** 2mg, 4mg, 6mg, 8mg, 12mg	**Initial:** 0.25mg tid. **Titrate:** May increase weekly by 0.25mg tid (0.75mg/day) for 4 weeks. After Week 4, may increase weekly by 1.5mg/day up to 9mg/day, then by 3mg/day weekly to 24mg/day. **Max:** 24mg/day. **Withdrawal:** Decrease dose to bid for 4 days, then qd for 3 days. (Tab, ER) **Initial:** 2mg qd for 1-2 weeks. Swallow whole. **Titrate:** May increase at ≥1-week intervals by 2mg/day. **Max:** 24mg/day. **Switching from IR to ER:** Closely match total daily IR dose with initial ER dose. See PI for detailed information.	Dyskinesia, hallucinations, somnolence, vomiting, headache, constipation, dyspepsia, abdominal pain, pharyngitis, UTI, increased sweating, asthenia, edema, fatigue, syncope, orthostatic symptoms, dizziness, nausea, viral infection, confusion, abnormal vision

(Continued)

GENERIC (BRAND)	HOW SUPPLIED	ADULT DOSAGE	SIDE EFFECTS
Rotigotine (Neupro)	**Patch:** 1mg/24 hrs, 2mg/24 hrs, 3mg/24 hrs, 4mg/24 hrs, 6mg/24 hrs, 8mg/24 hrs	**Early-Stage:** Initial: 2mg/24 hrs. **Titrate:** May increase weekly by 2mg/24 hrs based on response and tolerability. **Lowest Effective Dose:** 4mg/24 hrs. **Max:** 6mg/24 hrs. **Advanced-Stage: Initial:** 4mg/24 hrs. **Titrate:** May increase weekly by 2mg/24 hrs based on response and tolerability. **Usual:** 8mg/24 hrs.	Nausea, vomiting, somnolence, application-site reactions, dizziness, anorexia, hyperhidrosis, insomnia
Selegiline HCl (Zelapar)	**Tab, Disintegrating:** 1.25mg	**Initial:** 1.25mg qd before breakfast for ≥6 weeks. Take without liquid. **Titrate:** After 6 weeks, may increase to 2.5mg qd if the desired benefit is not achieved and patient can tolerate it. **Max:** 2.5mg/day.	Nausea, dizziness, pain, headache, insomnia, rhinitis, skin disorders, dyskinesia, back pain, dyspepsia, stomatitis, constipation, hallucinations, pharyngitis, rash
Selegiline HCl (Eldepryl)	**Cap:** 5mg; (Generic) **Tab:** 5mg	5mg bid at breakfast and lunch. **Max:** 10mg/day. May attempt to reduce levodopa/carbidopa by 10-30% after 2-3 days of therapy. May reduce further with continued therapy.	Nausea, dizziness, lightheadedness, fainting, abdominal pain, confusion, hallucinations, dry mouth
Tolcapone (Tasmar)	**Tab:** 100mg	**Initial:** 100mg tid. Use 200mg tid only if clinical benefit is justified. May need to decrease levodopa dose.	Dyskinesia, nausea, sleep disorder, dystonia, excessive dreaming, anorexia, muscle cramps, orthostatic complaints, somnolence, diarrhea, confusion, dizziness, headache, hallucination, vomiting, constipation, fatigue, upper respiratory tract infection, falling, increased sweating, UTI, xerostomia, abdominal pain, urine discoloration, hepatotoxicity (including liver failure)
Trihexyphenidyl HCl	**Sol:** 2mg/5mL; **Tab:** 2mg[†], 5mg[†]	**Idiopathic Parkinsonism:** 1mg on Day 1. **Titrate:** May increase by 2mg increments at intervals of 3-5 days, until 6-10mg/day is given. **Postencephalitic Patients:** May require 12-15mg/day. **Drug-Induced Parkinsonism: Initial:** 1mg. **Titrate:** If extrapyramidal manifestations not controlled in a few hrs, increase dose until control is achieved. **Usual:** 5-15mg/day. **Concomitant Levodopa or Other Parasympathetic Inhibitors:** See PI.	Dry mouth, blurred vision, dizziness, nausea, nervousness, constipation, drowsiness, urinary hesitancy/retention, tachycardia, pupil dilation, increased intraocular pressure, vomiting, weakness, headache

Refer to full FDA-approved labeling for additional information.

Abbreviations: ER = extended-release; IR = immediate-release; SL = sublingual.

*Refer to FDA-approved labeling for dosing instructions in renally compromised patients.

[†]Scored.

Opioid Products

GENERIC	BRAND	DEA SCHEDULE	DOSAGE FORMS	ADDITIONAL COMMENTS
MILD TO MODERATELY SEVERE PAIN				
Codeine sulfate		Schedule II	**Tab:** 15mg, 30mg, 60mg; **Sol:** 30mg/5mL	• **BW:** Death related to ultra-rapid metabolism of codeine to morphine • Pregnancy category C, caution in nursing
Codeine phosphate/Acetaminophen		Schedule V	**Sol:** 12mg-120mg/5mL	• **BW:** Hepatotoxicity; death related to ultra-rapid metabolism of codeine to morphine • Pregnancy category C, not for use in nursing
		Schedule III	**Tab:** 15mg-300mg	
	Tylenol #3	Schedule III	**Tab:** 30mg-300mg	
	Tylenol #4	Schedule III	**Tab:** 60mg-300mg	
MODERATE TO MODERATELY SEVERE PAIN				
Dihydrocodeine bitartrate/ Acetaminophen/Caffeine	Trezix	Schedule III	**Cap:** 16mg-320.5mg-30mg	• **BW:** Death related to ultra-rapid metabolism of codeine to morphine; hepatotoxicity • Pregnancy category C, not for use in nursing
Dihydrocodeine bitartrate/Aspirin/ Caffeine	Synalgos-DC	Schedule III	**Cap:** 16mg-356.4mg-30mg	• **BW:** Death related to ultra-rapid metabolism of codeine to morphine • Safety not known in pregnancy, not for use in nursing
Hydrocodone bitartrate/ Acetaminophen	Norco	Schedule II	**Tab:** 5mg-325mg, 7.5mg-325mg, 10mg-325mg	• **BW:** Hepatotoxicity • Pregnancy category C, not for use in nursing
	Vicodin		**Tab:** 5mg-300mg	
	Vicodin ES		**Tab:** 7.5mg-300mg	
	Vicodin HP		**Tab:** 10mg-300mg	
Hydrocodone bitartrate/Ibuprofen	Reprexain	Schedule II	**Tab:** 2.5mg-200mg, 5mg-200mg, 10mg-200mg	• Pregnancy category C, not for use in nursing
	Vicoprofen		**Tab:** 7.5-200mg	

(Continued)

GENERIC	BRAND	DEA SCHEDULE	DOSAGE FORMS	ADDITIONAL COMMENTS
MODERATE TO MODERATELY SEVERE PAIN *(Continued)*				
Oxycodone HCl/Acetaminophen	Percocet	Schedule II	**Tab:** 2.5mg-325mg, 5mg-325mg, 7.5mg-325mg, 10mg-325mg	• **BW:** Hepatotoxicity • Pregnancy category C, not for use in nursing
	Roxicet		**Tab:** 5mg-325mg; **Sol:** 5mg-325mg/5mL	
Oxycodone HCl/Aspirin	Percodan	Schedule II	**Tab:** 4.8355mg-325mg	• Pregnancy category B (oxycodone) and D (aspirin), not for use in nursing
Tramadol HCl	Conzip	Schedule IV	**Cap, ER:** 100mg, 200mg, 300mg	• Pregnancy category C, not for use in nursing
	Ultram		**Tab:** 50mg	
	Ultram ER		**Tab, ER:** 100mg, 200mg, 300mg	
Tramadol HCl/Acetaminophen	Ultracet	Schedule IV	**Tab:** 37.5mg-325mg	• **BW:** Hepatotoxicity • Pregnancy category C, not for use in nursing
MODERATE TO SEVERE OR CHRONIC PAIN				
Buprenorphine	Butrans	Schedule III	**Patch:** 5mcg/hr, 7mcg/hr, 10mcg/hr, 15mcg/hr, 20mcg/hr	• **BW:** Addiction, abuse, and misuse; life-threatening respiratory depression; accidental exposure; neonatal opioid withdrawal syndrome • Pregnancy category C, not for use in nursing
Fentanyl	Duragesic	Schedule II	**Patch:** 12mcg/hr, 25mcg/hr, 50mcg/hr, 75mcg/hr, 100mcg/hr	• **BW:** Addiction, abuse, and misuse; life-threatening respiratory depression; accidental exposure; neonatal opioid withdrawal syndrome; CYP3A4 interaction; exposure to heat • Pregnancy category C, not for use in nursing
Hydrocodone bitartrate	Hysingla ER	Schedule II	**Tab, ER:** 20mg, 30mg, 40mg, 60mg, 80mg, 100mg, 120mg	• **BW:** Addiction, abuse, and misuse; life-threatening respiratory depression; accidental ingestion; neonatal opioid withdrawal syndrome; CYP3A4 interaction; (Zohydro ER) interaction with alcohol • Pregnancy category C, not for use in nursing
	Zohydro ER		**Cap, ER:** 10mg, 15mg, 20mg, 30mg, 40mg, 50mg	

GENERIC	BRAND	DEA SCHEDULE	DOSAGE FORMS	ADDITIONAL COMMENTS
MODERATE TO SEVERE OR CHRONIC PAIN *(Continued)*				
Hydromorphone HCl	Dilaudid, Dilaudid-HP	Schedule II	**Tab:** 2mg, 4mg, 8mg; **Sol:** 1mg/mL; **Inj:** 1mg/mL, 2mg/mL, 4mg/mL; **HP: Inj:** 10mg/mL [1mL, 5mL, 50mL], 250mg (sterile, lyophilized powder)	• **BW:** Risk of respiratory depression, abuse, and medication errors; Dilaudid-HP injection is for use in opioid-tolerant patients only • Pregnancy category C, not for use in nursing
	Exalgo		**Tab, ER:** 8mg, 12mg, 16mg, 32mg	• **BW:** Addiction, abuse, and misuse; life-threatening respiratory depression; accidental ingestion; neonatal opioid withdrawal syndrome • Pregnancy category C, not for use in nursing
Levorphanol tartrate		Schedule II	**Tab:** 2mg	• Pregnancy category C, not for use in nursing
Meperidine HCl		Schedule II	**Inj:** 10mg/mL; **Sol:** 50mg/5mL	• (Oral) Pregnancy category C, not for use in nursing; (Inj) Safety not known in pregnancy and nursing
	Demerol		**Tab:** 50mg, 100mg; **Inj:** 25mg/mL, 50mg/mL, 75mg/mL, 100mg/mL	
Methadone HCl		Schedule II	**Inj:** 10mg/mL	• **BW:** Life-threatening QT prolongation; conditions for distribution and use for opioid addiction treatment • Pregnancy category C, not for use in nursing
			Sol: 5mg/5mL, 10mg/5mL; **Sol, Concentrated:** 10mg/mL	• **BW:** Addiction, abuse, and misuse; life-threatening respiratory depression; accidental ingestion; life-threatening QT prolongation; neonatal opioid withdrawal syndrome; conditions for distribution and use for opioid addiction treatment • Pregnancy category C, caution in nursing
	Dolophine		**Tab:** 5mg, 10mg	
Morphine sulfate/Naltrexone HCl	Embeda	Schedule II	**Cap, ER:** 20mg-0.8mg, 30mg-1.2mg, 50mg-2mg, 60mg-2.4mg, 80mg-3.2mg, 100mg-4mg	• **BW:** Addiction, abuse, and misuse; life-threatening respiratory depression; accidental ingestion; neonatal opioid withdrawal syndrome; interaction with alcohol • Pregnancy category C, not for use in nursing

(Continued)

GENERIC	BRAND	DEA SCHEDULE	DOSAGE FORMS	ADDITIONAL COMMENTS
MODERATE TO SEVERE OR CHRONIC PAIN *(Continued)*				
Morphine sulfate		Schedule II	**Tab:** 15mg, 30mg; **Sol:** 10mg/5mL, 20mg/5mL, 100mg/5mL; **Inj:** 2mg/mL, 4mg/mL, 5mg/mL, 8mg/mL, 10mg/mL, 15mg/mL, 25mg/mL, 50mg/mL	• **BW:** (Sol) Risk of medication errors and accidental ingestion; 100mg/5mL dosage is indicated for opioid-tolerant patients only • Pregnancy category C, not for use in nursing; (25mg/mL, 50mg/mL) Safety not known in nursing
	Astramorph/PF		**Inj:** 0.5mg/mL, 1mg/mL	• **BW:** Risk of severe adverse reactions with epidural or intrathecal route; observe patients in an equipped and staffed environment for at least 24 hrs after initial dose • Pregnancy category C, safety not known in nursing
	Avinza		**Cap, ER:** 30mg, 45mg, 60mg, 75mg, 90mg, 120mg	• **BW:** Addiction, abuse, and misuse; life-threatening respiratory depression; accidental ingestion; neonatal opioid withdrawal syndrome; interaction with alcohol • Pregnancy category C, not for use in nursing
	Duramorph		**Inj:** 0.5mg/mL, 1mg/mL	• **BW:** Risk of severe adverse reactions with epidural or intrathecal route; observe patients in an equipped and staffed environment for at least 24 hrs after initial dose • Pregnancy category C, safety not known in nursing
	Infumorph		**Inj:** 10mg/mL (200mg/20mL), 25mg/mL (500mg/20mL)	• **BW:** Not recommended for single-dose IV, IM, or SQ administration. Risk of severe adverse reactions; observe patients in an equipped and staffed environment for at least 24 hrs after initial (single) test dose, and as appropriate, for the 1st several days after catheter implantation. Improper or erroneous substitution of Infumorph for Duramorph is likely to result in serious overdosage. Naloxone injection and resuscitative equipment should be available in case of life-threatening or intolerable side effects whenever therapy is initiated or any manipulation of the reservoir system takes place • Pregnancy category C, safety not known in nursing
	Kadian		**Cap, ER:** 10mg, 20mg, 30mg, 40mg, 50mg, 60mg, 70mg, 80mg, 100mg, 130mg, 150mg, 200mg	• **BW:** Addiction, abuse, and misuse; life-threatening respiratory depression; accidental ingestion; neonatal opioid withdrawal syndrome; interaction with alcohol • Pregnancy category C, not for use in nursing
	MS Contin		**Tab, ER:** 15mg, 30mg, 60mg, 100mg, 200mg	• **BW:** Addiction, abuse, and misuse; life-threatening respiratory depression; accidental ingestion; neonatal opioid withdrawal syndrome • Pregnancy category C, not for use in nursing

GENERIC	BRAND	DEA SCHEDULE	DOSAGE FORMS	ADDITIONAL COMMENTS
MODERATE TO SEVERE OR CHRONIC PAIN *(Continued)*				
Oxycodone HCl		Schedule II	**Cap:** 5mg; **Sol:** 1mg/mL, 20mg/mL; **Tab:** 10mg, 20mg	• **BW:** (Sol) Risk of medication errors and accidental ingestion; 100mg/5mL dosage is indicated for opioid-tolerant patients only • Pregnancy category B, not for use in nursing
	Oxecta		**Tab:** 5mg, 7.5mg	• Pregnancy category B, not for use in nursing
	Roxicodone		**Tab:** 5mg, 15mg, 30mg	
	OxyContin		**Tab, ER:** 10mg, 15mg, 20mg, 30mg, 40mg, 60mg, 80mg	• **BW:** Addiction, abuse, and misuse; life-threatening respiratory depression; accidental ingestion; neonatal opioid withdrawal syndrome; CYP3A4 interaction • Pregnancy category C, not for use in nursing
Oxycodone HCl/Acetaminophen	Xartemis XR	Schedule II	**Tab, ER:** 7.5mg-325mg	• **BW:** Addiction, abuse, and misuse; life-threatening respiratory depression; accidental exposure; neonatal opioid withdrawal syndrome; hepatotoxicity • Pregnancy category C, not for use in nursing
Oxymorphone HCl	Opana	Schedule II	**Inj:** 1mg/mL; **Tab:** 5mg, 10mg	• Pregnancy category C, caution in nursing
	Opana ER		**Tab, ER:** 5mg, 7.5mg, 10mg, 15mg, 20mg, 30mg, 40mg	• **BW:** Addiction, abuse, and misuse; life-threatening respiratory depression; accidental ingestion; neonatal opioid withdrawal syndrome; interaction with alcohol • Pregnancy category C, caution in nursing
Tapentadol	Nucynta	Schedule II	**Tab:** 50mg, 75mg, 100mg	• **BW:** (Nucynta ER) Addiction, abuse, and misuse; life-threatening respiratory depression; accidental ingestion; neonatal opioid withdrawal syndrome; interaction with alcohol • Pregnancy category C, not for use in nursing
	Nucynta ER		**Tab, ER:** 50mg, 100mg, 150mg, 200mg, 250mg	

(Continued)

GENERIC	BRAND	DEA SCHEDULE	DOSAGE FORMS	ADDITIONAL COMMENTS
BREAKTHROUGH PAIN				
Fentanyl	Abstral	Schedule II	**Tab, SL:** 100mcg, 200mcg, 300mcg, 400mcg, 600mcg, 800mcg	• **BW:** Risk of respiratory depression, medication errors, and abuse potential • Pregnancy category C, not for use in nursing
	Fentora		**Tab, Buccal:** 100mcg, 200mcg, 400mcg, 600mcg, 800mcg	
	Lazanda		**Spr, Nasal:** 100mcg/spr, 400mcg/spr	
	Subsys		**Spr, SL:** 100mcg/spr, 200mcg/spr, 400mcg/spr, 600mcg/spr, 800mcg/spr, 1200mcg/spr, 1600mcg/spr	
Fentanyl citrate	Actiq	Schedule II	**Loz:** 200mcg, 400mcg, 600mcg, 800mcg, 1200mcg, 1600mcg	• **BW:** Risk of respiratory depression, medication errors, and abuse potential • Pregnancy category C, not for use in nursing

Refer to full FDA-approved labeling for more detailed dosing.

Abbreviations: BW = boxed warning; ER = extended-release; SL = sublingual.

ORAL ANTICONVULSANTS

GENERIC (BRAND)	USUAL ADULT DOSAGE*	THERAPEUTIC SERUM LEVELS	INDICATIONS: SEIZURE DISORDERS						INDICATIONS
			ABSENCE	AKINETIC	LENNOX-GASTAUT SYNDROME	MYOCLONIC	PARTIAL	TONIC-CLONIC	NEUROPATHIC PAIN
BARBITURATES									
Phenobarbital[†]	60-200mg/day	N/A					X		
Primidone (Mysoline)	750-2000mg/day	5-12mcg/mL					X	X	
BENZODIAZEPINES									
Clobazam (Onfi)	10-40mg/day	N/A			X				
Clonazepam (Klonopin)	1.5-20mg/day	N/A	X	X	X	X			
Clorazepate dipotassium (Tranxene T-Tab)	22.5-90mg/day	N/A					X		
Diazepam (Valium)[‡]	4-40mg/day	N/A							
HYDANTOINS									
Ethotoin (Peganone)	2000-3000mg/day	N/A					X	X	
Phenytoin (Dilantin, Dilantin-125, Dilantin Infatabs, Phenytek)	300-600mg/day (Sus: 375-625mg/day)	10-20mcg/mL					X	X	
SUCCINIMIDES									
Ethosuximide (Zarontin)	500-1500mg/day	40-100mcg/mL	X						
Methsuximide (Celontin)	300-1200mg/day	N/A	X						
MISCELLANEOUS									
Carbamazepine (Carbatrol, Tegretol, Tegretol XR)	Epilepsy: 800-1200mg/day Trigeminal Neuralgia: 400-800mg/day	4-12mcg/mL					X	X	X
Divalproex sodium[§] (Depakote, Depakote ER, Depakote Sprinkle Capsules)	10-60mg/kg/day	50-100mcg/mL	X				X		

(Continued)

GENERIC (BRAND)	USUAL ADULT DOSAGE*	THERAPEUTIC SERUM LEVELS	INDICATIONS						
			SEIZURE DISORDERS						NEUROPATHIC PAIN
			ABSENCE	AKINETIC	LENNOX-GASTAUT SYNDROME	MYOCLONIC	PARTIAL	TONIC-CLONIC	
MISCELLANEOUS *(Continued)*									
Valproic acid[§] (Depakene, Stavzor)	10-60mg/kg/day	50-100mcg/mL	X				X		
Eslicarbazepine (Aptiom)	800-1200mg/day	N/A					X		
Ezogabine (Potiga)	600-1200mg/day	N/A					X		
Felbamate[¶] (Felbatol)	2400-3600mg/day	N/A			X		X		
Gabapentin (Neurontin)	Epilepsy: 900-1800mg/day Postherpetic Neuralgia: 1800-3600mg/day	N/A					X		X
Lacosamide (Vimpat)	200-400mg/day	N/A					X		
Lamotrigine (Lamictal, Lamictal ODT, Lamictal XR)	100-500mg/day (Lamictal XR: 200-600mg/day)	N/A			X (IR, ODT)		X	X	
Levetiracetam (Keppra, Keppra XR)	1000-3000mg/day	N/A				X (IR)	X	X (IR)	
Oxcarbazepine (Oxtellar XR, Trileptal)	1200-2400mg/day	N/A					X		
Pregabalin (Lyrica)	Epilepsy: 150-600mg/day Neuropathic Pain Associated with Diabetic Peripheral Neuropathy/Postherpetic Neuralgia: 150-300mg/day	N/A					X		X
Rufinamide (Banzel)	400-3200mg/day	N/A			X				
Tiagabine HCl (Gabitril)	4-56mg/day	N/A					X		

GENERIC (BRAND)	USUAL ADULT DOSAGE*	THERAPEUTIC SERUM LEVELS	INDICATIONS						
			SEIZURE DISORDERS						NEUROPATHIC PAIN
			ABSENCE	AKINETIC	LENNOX-GASTAUT SYNDROME	MYOCLONIC	PARTIAL	TONIC-CLONIC	
MISCELLANEOUS *(Continued)*									
Topiramate (Qudexy XR, Topamax, Topamax Sprinkle, Trokendi XR)	200-400mg/day	N/A			X		X	X	
Vigabatrin (Sabril)	3g/day	N/A					X		
Zonisamide (Zonegran)	100-400mg/day	N/A					X		

Abbreviation: N/A = not applicable.

*Refer to complete monograph for full dosing information, including pediatric dosing.

†Phenobarbital is also indicated in generalized seizures.

‡Oral Valium may be used adjunctively in convulsive disorders, although it has not proved useful as the sole therapy.

§Divalproex sodium and valproic acid are also indicated as adjuncts in multiple seizure types.

¶For severe epilepsy refractory to other treatment where the risk of aplastic anemia and/or liver failure is deemed acceptable. Fully advise patient and obtain written, informed consent before treatment. Closely monitor patient.

MENTAL HEALTH TREATMENT OPTIONS

GENERIC (BRAND)	HOW SUPPLIED	INDICATIONS														
		BIPOLAR DISORDER (MAINTENANCE)	BIPOLAR, MANIC EPISODES	BIPOLAR, MIXED EPISODES	BIPOLAR, DEPRESSIVE EPISODES	DEPRESSION	SCHIZOPHRENIA	ANXIETY	OCD	PANIC DISORDER	PTSD	PMDD	IRRITABILITY ASSOCIATED W/ AUTISTIC DISORDER	PSYCHOSIS	RLS
BENZISOXAZOLE DERIVATIVES																
Iloperidone (Fanapt)	**Tab:** 1mg, 2mg, 4mg, 6mg, 8mg, 10mg, 12mg						✓								
Paliperidone (Invega)	**Tab, ER:** 1.5mg, 3mg, 6mg, 9mg						✓								
Paliperidone palmitate (Invega Sustenna)	**Inj, ER:** 39mg, 78mg, 117mg, 156mg, 234mg						✓								
Risperidone (Risperdal Consta)	**Inj:** 12.5mg, 25mg, 37.5mg, 50mg	✓*					✓								
Risperidone (Risperdal, Risperdal M-Tab)	**Sol:** 1mg/mL; **Tab:** 0.25mg, 0.5mg, 1mg, 2mg, 3mg, 4mg; **Tab, Disintegrating:** 0.25mg, 0.5mg, 1mg, 2mg, 3mg, 4mg		✓*	✓*			✓						✓		
Ziprasidone (Geodon)	**Cap:** 20mg, 40mg, 60mg, 80mg; **Inj:** 20mg/mL	✓* (PO)	✓ (PO)	✓ (PO)			✓								

(Continued)

GENERIC (BRAND)	HOW SUPPLIED	INDICATIONS													
		BIPOLAR DISORDER (MAINTENANCE)	BIPOLAR, MANIC EPISODES	BIPOLAR, MIXED EPISODES	BIPOLAR, DEPRESSIVE EPISODES	DEPRESSION	SCHIZOPHRENIA	ANXIETY	OCD	PANIC DISORDER	PTSD	PMDD	IRRITABILITY ASSOCIATED W/ AUTISTIC DISORDER	PSYCHOSIS	RLS
BENZODIAZEPINES															
Alprazolam	**Tab, Disintegrating:** 0.25mg, 0.5mg, 1mg, 2mg							✓		✓					
Alprazolam (Xanax)	**Tab:** 0.25mg, 0.5mg, 1mg, 2mg							✓		✓					
Alprazolam (Xanax XR)	**Tab, ER:** 0.5mg, 1mg, 2mg, 3mg									✓					
Chlordiazepoxide HCl (Librium)	**Cap:** 5mg, 10mg, 25mg							✓							
Clonazepam (Klonopin)	**Tab:** 0.5mg, 1mg, 2mg; **Tab, Disintegrating:** (ODT) 0.125mg, 0.25mg, 0.5mg, 1mg, 2mg									✓					
Clorazepate dipotassium (Tranxene T-Tabs)	**Tab:** 3.75mg, 7.5mg, 15mg							✓							
Diazepam (Valium)	**Tab:** 2mg, 5mg, 10mg							✓							
Lorazepam (Ativan)	**Sol:** 2mg/mL; **Tab:** 0.5mg, 1mg, 2mg							✓							

GENERIC (BRAND)	HOW SUPPLIED	INDICATIONS													
		BIPOLAR DISORDER (MAINTENANCE)	BIPOLAR, MANIC EPISODES	BIPOLAR, MIXED EPISODES	BIPOLAR, DEPRESSIVE EPISODES	DEPRESSION	SCHIZOPHRENIA	ANXIETY	OCD	PANIC DISORDER	PTSD	PMDD	IRRITABILITY ASSOCIATED W/ AUTISTIC DISORDER	PSYCHOSIS	RLS
BENZODIAZEPINES *(Continued)*															
Midazolam HCl	**Inj:** 1mg/mL, 5mg/mL; **Syrup:** 2mg/mL							✓							
BENZISOTHIAZOL DERIVATIVES															
Lurasidone HCl (Latuda)	**Tab:** 20mg, 40mg, 60mg, 80mg, 120mg				✓*		✓								
DIBENZAPINE DERIVATIVES															
Asenapine (Saphris)	**Tab, SL:** 5mg, 10mg		✓*	✓*			✓								
Clozapine (Clozaril, Fazaclo, Versacloz)	**Sus:** 50mg/mL; **Tab:** 25mg, 50mg, 100mg, 200mg; **Tab, Disintegrating:** 12.5mg, 25mg, 100mg, 150mg, 200mg						✓								
Loxapine (Adasuve)†	**Powder, Inhalation:** 10mg						✓								

(Continued)

GENERIC (BRAND)	HOW SUPPLIED	INDICATIONS													
		BIPOLAR DISORDER (MAINTENANCE)	BIPOLAR, MANIC EPISODES	BIPOLAR, MIXED EPISODES	BIPOLAR, DEPRESSIVE EPISODES	DEPRESSION	SCHIZOPHRENIA	ANXIETY	OCD	PANIC DISORDER	PTSD	PMDD	IRRITABILITY ASSOCIATED W/ AUTISTIC DISORDER	PSYCHOSIS	RLS
DIBENZAPINE DERIVATIVES *(Continued)*															
Quetiapine fumarate (Seroquel)	**Tab:** 25mg, 50mg, 100mg, 200mg, 300mg, 400mg	✓*	✓*		✓		✓								
Quetiapine fumarate (Seroquel XR)	**Tab, ER:** 50mg, 150mg, 200mg, 300mg, 400mg	✓*	✓*	✓*	✓	✓*	✓								
Olanzapine (Zyprexa, Zyprexa Zydis, Zyprexa IntraMuscular)	**Inj**†:10mg; **Tab:** 2.5mg, 5mg, 7.5mg, 10mg, 15mg, 20mg; **Tab, Disintegrating:** 5mg, 10mg, 15mg, 20mg	✓ (PO)	✓* (PO)	✓* (PO)	✓* (PO)	✓* (PO)	✓ (PO)								
Olanzapine (Zyprexa Relprevv)	**Inj, ER:** 210mg, 300mg, 405mg						✓								
DOPAMINE RECEPTOR AGONISTS															
Pramipexole dihydrochloride (Mirapex)	**Tab:** 0.125mg, 0.25mg, 0.5mg, 0.75mg, 1mg, 1.5mg														✓

GENERIC (BRAND)	HOW SUPPLIED	INDICATIONS													
		BIPOLAR DISORDER (MAINTENANCE)	BIPOLAR, MANIC EPISODES	BIPOLAR, MIXED EPISODES	BIPOLAR, DEPRESSIVE EPISODES	DEPRESSION	SCHIZOPHRENIA	ANXIETY	OCD	PANIC DISORDER	PTSD	PMDD	IRRITABILITY ASSOCIATED W/ AUTISTIC DISORDER	PSYCHOSIS	RLS
DOPAMINE RECEPTOR AGONISTS *(Continued)*															
Ropinirole (Requip)	**Tab:** 0.25mg, 0.5mg, 1mg, 2mg, 3mg, 4mg, 5mg														✓
Rotigotine (Neupro)	**Patch, ER:** 1mg/24 hrs, 2mg/24 hrs, 3mg/24 hrs, 4mg/24 hrs, 6mg/24 hrs, 8mg/24 hrs														✓
DOPAMINE/NOREPINEPHRINE REUPTAKE INHIBITORS															
Bupropion HBr (Aplenzin)	**Tab, ER:** 174mg, 348mg, 522mg					✓									
Bupropion HCl (Forfivo XL)	**Tab, ER:** 450mg					✓									
Bupropion HCl (Wellbutrin, Wellbutrin SR, Wellbutrin XL)	**Tab:** 75mg, 100mg; **Tab, SR:** 100mg, 150mg, 200mg; **Tab, ER:** 150mg, 300mg					✓									
MONOAMINE OXIDASE INHIBITORS															
Isocarboxazid (Marplan)	**Tab:** 10mg					✓									

(Continued)

GENERIC (BRAND)	HOW SUPPLIED	INDICATIONS													
		BIPOLAR DISORDER (MAINTENANCE)	BIPOLAR, MANIC EPISODES	BIPOLAR, MIXED EPISODES	BIPOLAR, DEPRESSIVE EPISODES	DEPRESSION	SCHIZOPHRENIA	ANXIETY	OCD	PANIC DISORDER	PTSD	PMDD	IRRITABILITY ASSOCIATED W/ AUTISTIC DISORDER	PSYCHOSIS	RLS
MONOAMINE OXIDASE INHIBITORS *(Continued)*															
Phenelzine sulfate (Nardil)	**Tab:** 15mg					✓									
Selegiline (Emsam)	**Patch:** 6mg/24 hrs, 9mg/24 hrs, 12mg/24 hrs					✓									
Tranylcypromine sulfate (Parnate)	**Tab:** 10mg					✓									
PARTIAL $D_2/5HT_{1A}$ AGONISTS/$5HT_{2A}$ ANTAGONISTS															
Aripiprazole (Abilify, Abilify Discmelt)	**Inj**†: 7.5mg/mL; **Sol:** 1mg/mL; **Tab:** 2mg, 5mg, 10mg, 15mg, 20mg, 30mg; **Tab, Disintegrating:** 10mg, 15mg	✓*	✓*	✓*		✓*	✓						✓		
Aripiprazole (Abilify Maintena)	**Inj, ER:** 300mg, 400mg						✓								
PHENOTHIAZINES															
Chlorpromazine HCl	**Inj:** 25mg/mL; **Tab:** 10mg, 25mg, 50mg, 100mg, 200mg						✓							✓ (PO)	
Fluphenazine decanoate	**Inj:** 25mg/mL						✓								

GENERIC (BRAND)	HOW SUPPLIED	INDICATIONS													
		BIPOLAR DISORDER (MAINTENANCE)	BIPOLAR, MANIC EPISODES	BIPOLAR, MIXED EPISODES	BIPOLAR, DEPRESSIVE EPISODES	DEPRESSION	SCHIZOPHRENIA	ANXIETY	OCD	PANIC DISORDER	PTSD	PMDD	IRRITABILITY ASSOCIATED W/ AUTISTIC DISORDER	PSYCHOSIS	RLS
PHENOTHIAZINES *(Continued)*															
Fluphenazine HCl	**Elixir:** 2.5mg/5mL; **Inj:** 2.5mg/mL; **Sol, Concentrated:** 5mg/mL; **Tab:** 1mg, 2.5mg, 5mg, 10mg													✓	
Perphenazine	**Tab:** 2mg, 4mg, 8mg, 16mg						✓								
Thioridazine HCl	**Tab:** 10mg, 25mg, 50mg, 100mg						✓								
Trifluoperazine HCl	**Tab:** 1mg, 2mg, 5mg, 10mg						✓	✓							
SEROTONIN/NOREPINEPHRINE REUPTAKE INHIBITORS															
Desvenlafaxine (Khedezla)	**Tab, ER:** 50mg, 100mg					✓									
Desvenlafaxine (Pristiq)	**Tab, ER:** 50mg, 100mg					✓									
Duloxetine (Cymbalta)	**Cap, DR:** 20mg, 30mg, 60mg					✓		✓							
Levomilnacipran (Fetzima)	**Cap, ER:** 20mg, 40mg, 80mg, 120mg					✓									

(Continued)

GENERIC (BRAND)	HOW SUPPLIED	INDICATIONS													
		BIPOLAR DISORDER (MAINTENANCE)	BIPOLAR, MANIC EPISODES	BIPOLAR, MIXED EPISODES	BIPOLAR, DEPRESSIVE EPISODES	DEPRESSION	SCHIZOPHRENIA	ANXIETY	OCD	PANIC DISORDER	PTSD	PMDD	IRRITABILITY ASSOCIATED W/ AUTISTIC DISORDER	PSYCHOSIS	RLS
SEROTONIN/NOREPINEPHRINE REUPTAKE INHIBITORS *(Continued)*															
Nefazodone HCl	**Tab:** 50mg, 100mg, 150mg, 200mg, 250mg					✓									
Venlafaxine HCl	**Tab:** 25mg, 37.5mg, 50mg, 75mg, 100mg; **Tab, ER:** 37.5mg, 75mg, 150mg, 225mg					✓		✓ (ER)							
Venlafaxine HCl (Effexor XR)	**Cap, ER:** 37.5mg, 75mg, 150mg					✓		✓		✓					
SELECTIVE SEROTONIN REUPTAKE INHIBITORS/5HT$_{1A}$ PARTIAL AGONISTS															
Vilazodone HCl (Viibryd)	**Tab:** 10mg, 20mg, 40mg					✓									
SELECTIVE SEROTONIN REUPTAKE INHIBITORS AND COMBINATIONS															
Citalopram HBr (Celexa)	**Sol:** 10mg/5mL; **Tab:** 10mg, 20mg, 40mg					✓									
Escitalopram oxalate (Lexapro)	**Sol:** 5mg/5mL; **Tab:** 5mg, 10mg, 20mg					✓		✓							
Fluoxetine	**Sol:** 20mg/5mL; **Tab:** 10mg, 20mg, 60mg				✓* (10mg, 20mg Tab)	✓			✓	✓					
Fluoxetine (Prozac)	**Cap:** 10mg, 20mg, 40mg				✓*	✓*			✓	✓					

GENERIC (BRAND)	HOW SUPPLIED	INDICATIONS														
		BIPOLAR DISORDER (MAINTENANCE)	BIPOLAR, MANIC EPISODES	BIPOLAR, MIXED EPISODES	BIPOLAR, DEPRESSIVE EPISODES	DEPRESSION	SCHIZOPHRENIA	ANXIETY	OCD	PANIC DISORDER	PTSD	PMDD	IRRITABILITY ASSOCIATED W/ AUTISTIC DISORDER	PSYCHOSIS	RLS
SELECTIVE SEROTONIN REUPTAKE INHIBITORS AND COMBINATIONS *(Continued)*																
Fluoxetine (Prozac Weekly)	**Cap, DR:** 90mg				✓*	✓*			✓	✓					
Fluoxetine HCl (Sarafem)	**Cap:** 10mg, 20mg; **Tab:** 10mg, 15mg, 20mg											✓			
Fluoxetine-Olanzapine (Symbyax)	**Cap:** 25-3mg, 25-6mg, 50-6mg, 25-12mg, 50-12mg				✓	✓									
Fluvoxamine maleate	**Tab:** 25mg, 50mg, 100mg								✓						
Fluvoxamine maleate (Luvox CR)	**Cap, ER:** 100mg, 150mg								✓						
Paroxetine HCl (Paxil)	**Sus:** 10mg/5mL; **Tab:** 10mg, 20mg, 30mg, 40mg					✓		✓	✓	✓	✓				
Paroxetine HCl (Paxil CR)	**Tab, Controlled-Release:** 12.5mg, 25mg, 37.5mg					✓		✓		✓		✓			

(Continued)

GENERIC (BRAND)	HOW SUPPLIED	INDICATIONS													
		BIPOLAR DISORDER (MAINTENANCE)	BIPOLAR, MANIC EPISODES	BIPOLAR, MIXED EPISODES	BIPOLAR, DEPRESSIVE EPISODES	DEPRESSION	SCHIZOPHRENIA	ANXIETY	OCD	PANIC DISORDER	PTSD	PMDD	IRRITABILITY ASSOCIATED W/ AUTISTIC DISORDER	PSYCHOSIS	RLS
SELECTIVE SEROTONIN REUPTAKE INHIBITORS AND COMBINATIONS *(Continued)*															
Paroxetine mesylate (Pexeva)	**Tab:** 10mg, 20mg, 30mg, 40mg					✓		✓	✓	✓					
Sertraline HCl (Zoloft)	**Sol:** 20mg/mL; **Tab:** 25mg, 50mg, 100mg					✓		✓	✓	✓	✓	✓			
TETRACYCLIC ANTIDEPRESSANTS															
Maprotiline HCl	**Tab:** 25mg, 50mg, 75mg					✓		✓							
Mirtazapine (Remeron, Remeron SolTab)	**Tab:** 7.5mg, 15mg, 30mg, 45mg; **Tab, Disintegrating:** 15mg, 30mg, 45mg					✓									
THIOXANTHENE DERIVATIVES															
Thiothixene	**Cap:** 1mg, 2mg, 5mg, 10mg						✓								
TRICYCLIC ANTIDEPRESSANTS AND COMBINATIONS															
Amitriptyline HCl	**Tab:** 10mg, 25mg, 50mg, 75mg, 100mg, 150mg					✓									
Amitriptyline HCl-Chlordiazepoxide	**Tab:** 12.5-5mg, 25-10mg					✓		✓							

GENERIC (BRAND)	HOW SUPPLIED	INDICATIONS													
		BIPOLAR DISORDER (MAINTENANCE)	BIPOLAR, MANIC EPISODES	BIPOLAR, MIXED EPISODES	BIPOLAR, DEPRESSIVE EPISODES	DEPRESSION	SCHIZOPHRENIA	ANXIETY	OCD	PANIC DISORDER	PTSD	PMDD	IRRITABILITY ASSOCIATED W/ AUTISTIC DISORDER	PSYCHOSIS	RLS
TRICYCLIC ANTIDEPRESSANTS AND COMBINATIONS *(Continued)*															
Amitriptyline HCl-Perphenazine	**Tab:** 10-2mg, 10-4mg, 25-2mg, 25-4mg, 50-4mg					✓	✓	✓							
Amoxapine	**Tab:** 25mg, 50mg, 100mg, 150mg					✓									
Desipramine HCl (Norpramin)	**Tab:** 10mg, 25mg, 50mg, 75mg, 100mg, 150mg					✓									
Doxepin HCl	**Cap:** 10mg, 25mg, 50mg, 75mg, 100mg, 150mg; **Sol:** 10mg/mL					✓		✓							
Imipramine HCl (Tofranil)	**Tab:** 10mg, 25mg, 50mg					✓									
Imipramine pamoate (Tofranil-PM)	**Cap:** 75mg, 100mg, 125mg, 150mg					✓									
Nortriptyline HCl (Pamelor)	**Cap:** 10mg, 25mg, 50mg, 75mg; **Sol:** 10mg/5mL					✓									

(Continued)

GENERIC (BRAND)	HOW SUPPLIED	INDICATIONS													
		BIPOLAR DISORDER (MAINTENANCE)	BIPOLAR, MANIC EPISODES	BIPOLAR, MIXED EPISODES	BIPOLAR, DEPRESSIVE EPISODES	DEPRESSION	SCHIZOPHRENIA	ANXIETY	OCD	PANIC DISORDER	PTSD	PMDD	IRRITABILITY ASSOCIATED W/ AUTISTIC DISORDER	PSYCHOSIS	RLS
TRICYCLIC ANTIDEPRESSANTS AND COMBINATIONS *(Continued)*															
Protriptyline HCl (Vivactil)	**Tab:** 5mg, 10mg					✓									
Trimipramine maleate (Surmontil)	**Cap:** 25mg, 50mg, 100mg					✓									
VALPROATE COMPOUNDS															
Divalproex sodium (Depakote)	**Tab, DR:** 125mg, 250mg, 500mg		✓												
Divalproex sodium (Depakote ER)	**Tab, ER:** 250mg, 500mg		✓	✓											
MISCELLANEOUS															
Buspirone HCl	**Tab:** 5mg, 7.5mg, 10mg, 15mg, 30mg							✓							
Carbamazepine (Equetro)	**Cap, ER:** 100mg, 200mg, 300mg		✓	✓											
Gabapentin enacarbil (Horizant)	**Tab, ER:** 300mg, 600mg														✓

GENERIC (BRAND)	HOW SUPPLIED	INDICATIONS													
		BIPOLAR DISORDER (MAINTENANCE)	BIPOLAR, MANIC EPISODES	BIPOLAR, MIXED EPISODES	BIPOLAR, DEPRESSIVE EPISODES	DEPRESSION	SCHIZOPHRENIA	ANXIETY	OCD	PANIC DISORDER	PTSD	PMDD	IRRITABILITY ASSOCIATED W/ AUTISTIC DISORDER	PSYCHOSIS	RLS
MISCELLANEOUS *(Continued)*															
Lamotrigine (Lamictal, Lamictal ODT)	**Tab, Chewable:** 2mg, 5mg, 25mg; **Tab:** 25mg, 100mg, 150mg, 200mg; **Tab, Disintegrating:** (ODT) 25mg, 50mg, 100mg, 200mg	✓													
Lithium carbonate	**Cap:** 150mg, 300mg, 600mg; **Sol:** 8mEq/5mL; **Tab:** 300mg	✓	✓												
Lithium carbonate (Lithobid)	**Tab, ER:** 300mg, 450mg	✓	✓												
Trazodone HCl	**Tab:** 50mg, 100mg, 150mg, 300mg					✓									
Trazodone HCl (Oleptro)	**Tab, ER:** 150mg, 300mg					✓									
Valproic acid (Stavzor)	**Cap, DR:** 125mg, 250mg, 500mg		✓												

(Continued)

GENERIC (BRAND)	HOW SUPPLIED	INDICATIONS													
		BIPOLAR DISORDER (MAINTENANCE)	BIPOLAR, MANIC EPISODES	BIPOLAR, MIXED EPISODES	BIPOLAR, DEPRESSIVE EPISODES	DEPRESSION	SCHIZOPHRENIA	ANXIETY	OCD	PANIC DISORDER	PTSD	PMDD	IRRITABILITY ASSOCIATED W/ AUTISTIC DISORDER	PSYCHOSIS	RLS
MISCELLANEOUS *(Continued)*															
Vortioxetine (Brintellix)	**Tab:** 5mg, 10mg, 15mg, 20mg					✓									

Refer to full FDA-approved labeling for additional information.

*Has indication to be used as adjunctive therapy or in combination with other drug.

†Has indication to be used for agitation associated with schizophrenia or bipolar disorder.

Abbreviations: ER = extended-release; DR = delayed-release; OCD = obsessive-compulsive disorder; PTSD = post-traumatic stress disorder; PMDD = premenstrual dysphoric disorder; RLS = restless legs syndrome.

Asthma and COPD Management

GENERIC (BRAND)	DOSAGE FORM	ADULT DOSAGE	PEDIATRIC DOSAGE
β_2-AGONISTS, LONG-ACTING			
Arformoterol tartrate (Brovana)*	**Sol, Inh:** 15mcg/2mL	15mcg bid (am/pm) via nebulizer. **Max:** 30mcg/day.	
Formoterol fumarate (Foradil Aerolizer)†	**Cap, Inh:** 12mcg	1 cap (inh) q12h. **Max:** 24mcg/day.	**Asthma: ≥5 yrs:** 1 cap (inh) q12h. **Max:** 24mcg/day.
Formoterol fumarate (Perforomist)*	**Sol, Inh:** 20mcg/2mL	2mL q12h via nebulizer. **Max:** 40mcg/day.	
Indacaterol (Arcapta Neohaler)*	**Cap, Inh:** 75mcg	1 cap (inh) daily. **Max:** 1 cap/day.	
Olodaterol (Striverdi Respimat)*	**MDI:** 2.5mcg/inh	2 inh qd. **Max:** 2 inh/24 hrs.	
Salmeterol xinafoate (Serevent Diskus)†	**DPI:** 50mcg/inh	1 inh bid (am/pm q12h).	**Asthma: ≥4 yrs:** 1 inh bid (am/pm q12h).
β_2-AGONISTS, SHORT-ACTING			
Albuterol sulfate	**Sol, Inh:** 0.083%, 0.5%	**Usual/Max:** 2.5mg tid-qid via nebulizer over 5-15 min.	**2-12 yrs: Initial:** 0.1-0.15mg/kg/dose. **Max:** 2.5mg tid-qid by nebulization.
	Syr: 2mg/5mL	2mg or 4mg tid-qid. **Max:** 8mg qid.	**>14 yrs:** 2mg or 4mg tid-qid. **Max:** 8mg qid. **6-14 yrs:** 2mg tid-qid. **Max:** 24mg/day. **2-5 yrs: Initial:** 0.1mg/kg tid (not to exceed 2mg tid). **Titrate:** May increase to 0.2mg/kg tid. **Max:** 4mg tid.
	Tab: 2mg‡, 4mg‡	2mg or 4mg tid-qid. **Max:** 8mg qid.	**>12 yrs:** 2mg or 4mg tid-qid. **Max:** 8mg qid. **6-12 yrs:** 2mg tid-qid. **Max:** 24mg/day.
	Tab, ER: 4mg, 8mg	4-8mg q12h. **Max:** 32mg/day.	**>12 yrs:** 4-8mg q12h. **Max:** 32mg/day. **6-12 yrs:** 4mg q12h. **Max:** 24mg/day.
Albuterol sulfate (AccuNeb)	**Sol, Inh:** 0.63mg/3mL, 1.25mg/3mL		**2-12 yrs:** 0.63mg or 1.25mg tid-qid prn via nebulizer over 5-15 min.
Albuterol sulfate (ProAir HFA, Proventil HFA, Ventolin HFA)	**MDI:** 90mcg/inh	2 inh q4-6h or 1 inh q4h.	**≥4 yrs:** 2 inh q4-6h or 1 inh q4h.
Levalbuterol HCl (Xopenex)	**Sol, Inh:** 1.25mg/0.5mL, 0.31mg/3mL, 0.63mg/3mL, 1.25mg/3mL	0.63-1.25mg tid (q6-8h) via nebulizer.	**≥12 yrs:** 0.63-1.25mg tid (q6-8h) via nebulizer. **6-11 yrs:** 0.31mg tid via nebulizer. **Max:** 0.63mg tid.
Levalbuterol tartrate (Xopenex HFA)	**MDI:** 45mcg/inh	1-2 inh q4-6h.	**≥4 yrs:** 1-2 inh q4-6h.
Metaproterenol sulfate	**Syrup:** 10mg/5mL; **Tab:** 10mg‡, 20mg‡	20mg tid-qid.	**>9 yrs or >60 lbs:** 20mg tid-qid. **6-9 yrs or <60 lbs:** 10mg tid-qid. **<6 yrs:** (Syrup) 1.3-2.6mg/kg/day.
Pirbuterol acetate (Maxair Autohaler)	**MDI:** 200mcg/inh	1-2 inh q4-6h. **Max:** 12 inh/day.	**≥12 yrs:** 1-2 inh q4-6h. **Max:** 12 inh/day.

(Continued)

GENERIC (BRAND)	DOSAGE FORM	ADULT DOSAGE	PEDIATRIC DOSAGE
β_2-AGONISTS, SHORT-ACTING *(Continued)*			
Terbutaline sulfate	**Tab:** 2.5mg, 5mg	2.5-5mg q6h tid. **Max:** 15mg/day.	**12-15 yrs:** 2.5mg tid. **Max:** 7.5mg/day.
	Inj: 1mg/mL	0.25mg SQ into the lateral deltoid area. May repeat dose in 15-30 min if no improvement. **Max:** 0.5mg/4 hrs.	**≥12 yrs:** 0.25mg SQ into the lateral deltoid area. May repeat dose in 15-30 min if no improvement. **Max:** 0.5mg/4 hrs.
ANTICHOLINERGICS			
Aclidinium bromide (Tudorza Pressair)*	**MDI:** 400mcg/inh	1 inh bid.	
Ipratropium bromide (Atrovent HFA)*	**MDI:** 17mcg/inh	**Initial:** 2 inh qid. May take additional inh prn. **Max:** 12 inh/day.	
Tiotropium bromide (Spiriva HandiHaler)*	**Cap, Inh:** 18mcg	2 inh of contents of 1 cap qd.	
Tiotropium bromide (Spiriva Respimat)*	**MDI:** 2.5mcg/inh	2 inh qd. **Max:** 2 inh/24 hrs.	
Umeclidinium (Incruse Ellipta)*	**DPI:** 62.5mcg/inh	1 inh qd. **Max:** 1 inh/24 hrs	
COMBINATION AGENTS			
Budesonide/Formoterol fumarate dihydrate (Symbicort)†	**MDI:** (Budesonide-Formoterol) 80mcg-4.5mcg/inh, 160mcg-4.5mcg/inh	**Asthma: Initial:** 2 inh bid (am/pm q12h). Starting dose is based on asthma severity. **Max:** 160mcg-4.5mcg bid. **COPD:** 2 inh of 160mcg-4.5mcg bid.	**Asthma: ≥12 yrs:** 2 inh bid (am/pm q12h). Starting dose is based on asthma severity. **Max:** 160mcg-4.5mcg bid.
Fluticasone propionate/ Salmeterol (Advair Diskus)†	**DPI:** (Fluticasone-Salmeterol) 100mcg-50mcg/inh, 250mcg-50mcg/inh, 500mcg-50mcg/inh	**Asthma:** 1 inh bid (am/pm q12h). Starting dose is based on asthma severity. **Max:** 500mcg-50mcg bid. **COPD:** 1 inh of 250mcg-50mcg bid (am/pm q12h).	**Asthma: ≥12 yrs:** 1 inh bid (am/pm q12h). Starting dose is based on asthma severity. **Max:** 500mcg-50mcg bid. **4-11 yrs:** 1 inh of 100mcg-50mcg bid (am/pm q12h).
Fluticasone propionate/ Salmeterol (Advair HFA)	**MDI:** (Fluticasone-Salmeterol) 45mcg-21mcg/inh, 115mcg-21mcg/inh, 230mcg-21mcg/inh	**Initial:** 2 inh bid (am/pm q12h). Starting dose is based on asthma severity. **Max:** 2 inh of 230mcg-21mcg bid.	**≥12 yrs: Initial:** 2 inh bid (am/pm q12h). Starting dose is based on asthma severity. **Max:** 2 inh of 230mcg-21mcg bid.
Fluticasone furoate-Vilanterol (Breo Ellipta)*	**Powder, Inh:** (Fluticasone-Vilanterol) 100mcg-25mcg	1 inh qd. **Max:** 1 inh/day.	
Ipratropium bromide/ Albuterol sulfate (Combivent)*	**MDI:** (Ipratropium-Albuterol) 18mcg-90mcg/inh	2 inh qid. May take additional inh prn. **Max:** 12 inh/day.	
Ipratropium bromide/ Albuterol (Combivent Respimat)*	**MDI:** (Ipratropium-Albuterol) 20mcg-100mcg/inh	1 inh qid. May take additional inh prn. **Max:** 6 inh/day.	
Ipratropium bromide/ Albuterol sulfate (Duoneb)*	**Sol, Inh:** (Ipratropium-Albuterol) 0.5mg-3mg/3mL	3mL qid via nebulizer with up to 2 additional 3mL doses/day prn.	

GENERIC (BRAND)	DOSAGE FORM	ADULT DOSAGE	PEDIATRIC DOSAGE
COMBINATION AGENTS *(Continued)*			
Mometasone furoate/ Formoterol fumarate dihydrate (Dulera)	**MDI:** (Mometasone-Formoterol) 100mcg-5mcg/inh, 200mcg-5mcg/inh	**Previous Inhaled Medium-Dose Corticosteroids: Initial:** 2 inh of 100mcg-5mcg bid. **Max:** 400mcg-20mcg/day. **Previous Inhaled High-Dose Corticosteroids: Initial:** 2 inh of 200mcg-5mcg bid. **Max:** 800mcg-20mcg/day.	**≥12 yrs: Previous Inhaled Medium-Dose Corticosteroids: Initial:** 2 inh of 100mcg-5mcg bid. **Max:** 400mcg-20mcg/day. **Previous Inhaled High-Dose Corticosteroids: Initial:** 2 inh of 200mcg-5mcg bid. **Max:** 800mcg-20mcg/day.
Umeclidinium/Vilanterol (Anoro Ellipta)*	**Powder, Inh:** (Umeclidinium-Vilanterol) 62.5mcg-25mcg	1 inh qd. **Max:** 1 inh/day	
CORTICOSTEROIDS			
Beclomethasone dipropionate (QVAR)	**MDI:** 40mcg/inh, 80mcg/inh	**Previous Bronchodilators Alone: Initial:** 40-80mcg bid. **Max:** 320mcg bid. **Previous Inhaled Corticosteroids: Initial:** 40-160mcg bid. **Max:** 320mcg bid.	**≥12 yrs:** Refer to adult dosing. **5-11 yrs: Previous Bronchodilators Alone/ Inhaled Corticosteroids: Initial:** 40mcg bid. **Max:** 80mcg bid.
Budesonide (Pulmicort Flexhaler)	**DPI:** 90mcg/inh, 180mcg/inh	**Initial:** 180-360mcg bid. **Max:** 720mcg bid.	**6-17 yrs: Initial:** 180-360mcg bid. **Max:** 360mcg bid.
Budesonide (Pulmicort Respules)	**Sus, Inh:** 0.25mg/2mL, 0.5mg/2mL, 1mg/2mL		**12 mths-8 yrs: Previous Bronchodilators: Initial:** 0.5mg/day given qd or bid. **Max:** 0.5mg/day. **Previous Inhaled Corticosteroids: Initial:** 0.5mg/day given qd or bid. **Max:** 1mg/day. **Previous Oral Corticosteroids: Initial:** 1mg/day given qd or bid. **Max:** 1mg/day.
Ciclesonide (Alvesco)	**MDI:** 80mcg/inh, 160mcg/inh	**Previous Bronchodilator Alone: Initial:** 80mcg bid. **Max:** 160mcg bid. **Previous Inhaled Corticosteroids: Initial:** 80mcg bid. **Max:** 320mcg bid. **Previous Oral Corticosteroids: Initial/Max:** 320mcg bid.	**≥12 yrs:** Refer to adult dosing.
Flunisolide (Aerospan)	**MDI:** 80mcg/inh	**Initial:** 160mcg bid. **Max:** 320mcg bid.	**≥12 yrs: Initial:** 160mcg bid. **Max:** 320mcg bid. **6-11 yrs: Initial:** 80mcg bid. **Max:** 160mcg bid.
Fluticasone furoate (Arnuity Ellipta)	**DPI:** 100mcg/inh, 200mcg/inh	1 inh qd. **Max:** 1 inh/24 hrs.	**≥12 yrs:** 1 inh qd. **Max:** 1 inh/24 hrs.
Fluticasone propionate (Flovent Diskus)	**DPI:** 50mcg/inh, 100mcg/inh, 250mcg/inh	**Previous Bronchodilators Alone: Initial:** 100mcg bid. **Max:** 500mcg bid. **Previous Inhaled Corticosteroids: Initial:** 100-250mcg bid. **Max:** 500mcg bid. **Previous Oral Corticosteroids: Initial:** 500-1000mcg bid. **Max:** 1000mcg bid.	**≥12 yrs:** Refer to adult dosing. **4-11 yrs: Initial:** 50mcg bid. **Max:** 100mcg bid.

(Continued)

GENERIC (BRAND)	DOSAGE FORM	ADULT DOSAGE	PEDIATRIC DOSAGE
CORTICOSTEROIDS *(Continued)*			
Fluticasone propionate (Flovent HFA)	**MDI:** 44mcg/inh, 110mcg/inh, 220mcg/inh	**Previous Bronchodilators Alone: Initial:** 88mcg bid. **Max:** 440mcg bid. **Previous Inhaled Corticosteroids: Initial:** 88-220mcg bid. **Max:** 440mcg bid. **Previous Oral Corticosteroids: Initial:** 440mcg bid. **Max:** 880mcg bid.	**≥12 yrs:** Refer to adult dosing. **4-11 yrs: Initial/Max:** 88mcg bid.
Mometasone furoate (Asmanex Twisthaler)	**DPI:** 110mcg/inh, 220mcg/inh	**Previous Bronchodilators Alone/Inhaled Corticosteroids: Initial:** 220mcg qpm. **Max:** 440mcg/day. **Previous Oral Corticosteroids: Initial:** 440mcg bid. **Max:** 880mcg/day.	**≥12 yrs:** Refer to adult dosing. **4-11 yrs: Initial/Max:** 110mcg/day qpm.
LEUKOTRIENE MODIFIERS			
Montelukast sodium (Singulair)	**Granules:** 4mg; **Tab:** 10mg; **Tab, Chewable:** 4mg, 5mg	10mg qpm.	**≥15 yrs:** 10mg qpm. **6-14 yrs:** 5mg chewable tab qpm. **2-5 yrs:** 4mg chewable tab or 4mg oral granules pkt qpm. **12-23 mths:** 4mg oral granules pkt qpm.
Zafirlukast (Accolate)	**Tab:** 10mg, 20mg	20mg bid. Take at least 1 hr before or 2 hrs after meals.	Take at least 1 hr before or 2 hrs after meals. **≥12 yrs:** 20mg bid. **5-11 yrs:** 10mg bid.
Zileuton (Zyflo, Zyflo CR)	(Zyflo) **Tab:** 600mg‡	**Tab:** 600mg qid. Take with meals and at hs.	**≥12 yrs: Tab:** 600mg qid. Take with meals and at hs.
	(Zyflo CR) **Tab, ER:** 600mg	1200mg bid. Take within 1 hr after am and pm meals.	**≥12 yrs:** 1200mg bid. Take within 1 hr after am and pm meals.
MAST CELL STABILIZERS			
Cromolyn sodium	**Sol, Inh:** 20mg/2mL	20mg nebulized qid.	**≥2 yrs:** 20mg nebulized qid.
METHYLXANTHINES			
Theophylline anhydrous (Elixophyllin)§	**Elixir:** 80mg/15mL	**16-60 yrs: Initial:** 300mg/day divided q6-8h. **After 3 Days if Tolerated:** 400mg/day divided q6-8h. **After 3 More Days if Tolerated:** 600mg/day divided q6-8h.	**1-15 yrs: >45kg:** Refer to adult dosing. **<45kg: Initial:** 12-14mg/kg/day divided q4-6h. **Max:** 300mg/day. **After 3 Days if Tolerated:** 16mg/kg/day divided q4-6h. **Max:** 400mg/day. **After 3 More Days if Tolerated:** 20mg/kg/day divided q4-6h. **Max:** 600mg/day. See PI for infant dose.
Theophylline anhydrous (Theo-24)§	**Cap, ER:** 100mg, 200mg, 300mg, 400mg	**16-60 yrs: Initial:** 300-400mg/day q24h. **After 3 Days if Tolerated:** 400-600mg/day q24h. **After 3 More Days if Tolerated and Needed:** Doses >600mg should be titrated according to blood levels (see PI).	**12-15 yrs: >45kg:** Refer to adult dosing. **<45kg: Initial:** 12-14mg/kg/day q24h. **Max:** 300mg/day. **After 3 Days if Tolerated:** 16mg/kg/day q24h. **Max:** 400mg/day. **After 3 More Days if Tolerated and Needed:** 20mg/kg/day q24h. **Max:** 600mg/day.
Theophylline anhydrous§	**Tab, ER:** 400mg‡, 600mg‡		

GENERIC (BRAND)	DOSAGE FORM	ADULT DOSAGE	PEDIATRIC DOSAGE
MONOCLONAL ANTIBODIES/IgE-BLOCKERS			
Omalizumab (Xolair)	**Inj:** 150mg/5mL	150-375mg SQ q2 or 4 wks. Determine dose and dosing frequency by serum total IgE level measured before the start of treatment, and body weight. See PI for dose determination charts.	**≥12 yrs:** 150-375mg SQ q2 or 4 wks. Determine dose and dosing frequency by serum total IgE level measured before the start of treatment, and body weight. See PI for dose determination charts.
PHOSPHODIESTERASE-4 INHIBITORS			
Roflumilast (Daliresp)*	**Tab:** 500mcg	500mcg qd.	
SYSTEMIC CORTICOSTEROIDS			
Methylprednisolone (Medrol)	**Tab:** 2mg‡, 4mg‡, 8mg‡, 16mg‡, 32mg‡	**Initial:** 4-48mg/day. Dosage must be individualized based on the disease state and patient response.	
Prednisolone	**Sol:** 15mg/5mL; **Tab:** 5mg‡	**Initial:** 5-60mg/day. Dosage must be individualized based on the disease state and patient response.	
Prednisone	**Sol:** 5mg/5mL, 5mg/mL; **Tab:** 1mg‡, 2.5mg‡, 5mg‡, 10mg‡, 20mg‡, 50mg‡		

Refer to full FDA-approved labeling for additional information.

Abbreviations: DPI = dry-powder inhaler; ER = extended-released; MDI = metered-dose inhaler.

*Indicated for COPD only.

†Indicated for asthma and COPD.

‡Scored.

§The dose of theophylline must be individualized based on peak serum theophylline concentrations.

Adapted from *Expert Panel Report 3 (EPR-3): Guidelines for the Diagnosis and Management of Asthma – Summary Report 2007.* NIH Publication No 08-5846, October 2007.

Erectile Dysfunction Agents

GENERIC (BRAND)	HOW SUPPLIED	DOSAGE
PROSTAGLANDINS		
Alprostadil (Edex, Caverject, Caverject Impulse)	**Inj:** (Edex) 10mcg, 20mcg, 40mcg; (Caverject) 5mcg, 10mcg, 20mcg, 40mcg; (Caverject Impulse) 10mcg, 20mcg	Use lowest possible effective dose. Patient must stay in physician's office until complete detumescence occurs. If there is no response, give next higher dose within 1 hr. If there is a response, allow 1-day interval before the next dose. Reduce dose if erection lasts >1 hr. **Vasculogenic, Psychogenic, or Mixed Etiology: Initial:** 2.5mcg. **Titration: Partial Response to 2.5mcg:** Increase to 5mcg and then in increments of 5-10mcg, depending upon response, until erection of 1 hr max duration. **No Response to 2.5mcg:** Increase 2nd dose to 7.5mcg followed by increments of 5-10mcg. **Pure Neurogenic Etiology (Spinal Cord Injury): Initial:** 1.25mcg. **Titration:** Increase to 2.5mcg, then to 5mcg, and then by 5mcg increments until erection of 1 hr max duration. **Maint:** Give no more than 3 doses/week; allow at least 24 hrs between doses. (Edex) **Dose Range:** 1-40mcg. Give inj over 5- to 10-sec interval. (Caverject, Caverject Impulse) **Max:** 60mcg/dose.
Alprostadil (Muse)	**Supp, Urethral:** 125mcg, 250mcg, 500mcg, 1000mcg	**Initial:** 125-250mcg. **Titration:** Increase or decrease dose based on individual response. **Max:** 2 administrations/24 hrs.
PHOSPHODIESTERASE INHIBITORS		
Avanafil (Stendra)	**Tab:** 50mg, 100mg, 200mg	**Initial:** 100mg prn as early as 15 min prior to sexual activity. **Titration:** Increase to 200mg or decrease to 50mg based on efficacy/tolerability. **Max Frequency:** 1 dose/day. **Max Dose:** 200mg.
Sildenafil (Viagra)	**Tab:** 25mg, 50mg, 100mg	**Usual:** 50mg prn 1 hr prior to sexual activity. May be taken ½-4 hrs prior to sexual activity. **Titration:** Increase to 100mg or decrease to 25mg based on efficacy/tolerability. **Max Frequency:** 1 dose/day. **Max Dose:** 100mg.
Tadalafil (Cialis)	**Tab:** 2.5mg, 5mg, 10mg, 20mg	**PRN Use: Initial:** 10mg prior to sexual activity. **Titration:** Increase to 20mg or decrease to 5mg based on efficacy/tolerability. **Max Frequency:** 1 dose/day. **QD Use: Initial:** 2.5mg qd. **Titration:** Increase to 5mg qd based on efficacy/tolerability.
Vardenafil (Levitra)	**Tab:** 2.5mg, 5mg, 10mg, 20mg	**Initial:** 10mg prn 1 hr prior to sexual activity. **Titration:** Increase to 20mg or decrease to 5mg based on efficacy/tolerability. **Max Frequency:** 1 dose/day. **Max Dose:** 20mg.
Vardenafil (Staxyn)	**Tab, Disintegrating:** 10mg	10mg prn 1 hr prior to sexual activity. **Max:** 1 dose/day. Place on tongue to disintegrate. Take without liquid.

Refer to full FDA-approved labeling for additional information.

Benign Prostatic Hypertrophy Agents

GENERIC	BRAND	HOW SUPPLIED	DOSAGE	DOSING CONSIDERATIONS
ALPHA-BLOCKERS				
Alfuzosin	Uroxatral	**Tab, ER:** 10mg	**Usual:** 10mg qd.	• Take dose with the same meal each day. Swallow whole. • **Moderate or Severe Hepatic Impairment/ Concomitant Potent CYP3A4 Inhibitors:** Contraindicated.
Doxazosin	Cardura	**Tab:** 1mg, 2mg, 4mg, 8mg	**Initial:** 1mg qd. **Max:** 8mg qd.	• Stepwise titration in 1- to 2-week intervals, if needed.
	Cardura XL	**Tab, ER:** 4mg, 8mg	**Initial:** 4mg qd. **Max:** 8mg qd.	• Take with breakfast. Swallow whole. • Titrate in 3- to 4-week intervals, if needed.
Silodosin	Rapaflo	**Cap:** 4mg, 8mg	**Usual:** 8mg qd.	• Take with food. • **Moderate Renal Impairment (CrCl 30-50mL/min):** 4mg qd. • **Severe Renal Impairment (CrCl <30mL/min)/Severe Hepatic Impairment:** Contraindicated. • Carefully open and sprinkle the powder inside of capsule on a tablespoon of applesauce if difficult to swallow.
Tamsulosin	Flomax	**Cap:** 0.4mg	**Usual:** 0.4mg qd. **Max:** 0.8mg qd.	• Take dose 30 min after the same meal each day. • Titrate after 2-4 weeks if needed. • Restart at 0.4mg dose if therapy is interrupted. • **Concomitant Strong CYP3A4 Inhibitors:** Avoid use.
Terazosin	Generic	**Cap:** 1mg, 2mg, 5mg, 10mg	**Initial:** 1mg qhs. **Usual:** 10mg qd. **Max:** 20mg/day.	• Increase stepwise as needed. • Restart at initial dose if therapy is interrupted.
5-ALPHA REDUCTASE INHIBITORS				
Dutasteride	Avodart	**Cap:** 0.5mg	**Usual:** 0.5mg qd.	• Swallow whole. May take with or without food. • May be administered with tamsulosin.
Finasteride	Proscar	**Tab:** 5mg	**Usual:** 5mg qd.	• May take with or without food. • May be administered with doxazosin.
PHOSPHODIESTERASE-5 INHIBITORS				
Tadalafil	Cialis	**Tab:** 2.5mg, 5mg, 10mg, 20mg	**Usual:** 5mg qd.	• Take dose at approximately the same time every day. • **CrCl 30-50mL/min:** 2.5mg is recommended. • **CrCl <30mL/min or on Hemodialysis:** Not recommended for once daily use. • Not recommended for use in combination with alpha-blockers for benign prostatic hypertrophy. • **Severe Hepatic Impairment:** Not recommended.
COMBINATIONS				
Dutasteride/ Tamsulosin	Jalyn	**Cap:** 0.5mg/0.4mg	**Usual:** 1 cap qd.	• Swallow whole. • Take dose 30 min after the same meal each day. • **Concomitant Strong CYP3A4 Inhibitors:** Avoid use.

Refer to full FDA-approved labeling for additional information.

Abbreviation: ER = extended-release.

OVERACTIVE BLADDER AGENTS

GENERIC	BRAND	HOW SUPPLIED	DOSAGE	COMMENTS
MUSCARINIC ANTAGONISTS				
Darifenacin	Enablex	**Tab, ER:** 7.5mg, 15mg	**Initial:** 7.5mg qd. **Max:** 15mg qd.	Swallow whole. **Moderate Hepatic Impairment/ Concomitant Potent CYP3A4 Inhibitors:** Do not exceed 7.5mg/day. **Severe Hepatic Impairment:** Avoid use.
Fesoterodine	Toviaz	**Tab, ER:** 4mg, 8mg	**Initial:** 4mg qd. **Max:** 8mg qd.	Swallow whole. **Severe Renal Impairment (CrCl <30mL/min)/ Concomitant Potent CYP3A4 Inhibitors:** Do not exceed 4mg/day. **Severe Hepatic Impairment:** Avoid use.
Oxybutynin*	Generic	**Syrup:** 5mg/5mL; **Tab:** 5mg	**Usual:** 5mg bid-tid. **Max:** 5mg qid.	**Elderly:** A lower starting dose of 2.5mg bid-tid is recommended. **Pediatrics >5 yrs:** 5mg bid. **Max:** 5mg tid.
	Ditropan XL	**Tab, ER:** 5mg, 10mg, 15mg	**Initial:** 5mg or 10mg qd. **Max:** 30mg/day.	Swallow whole. Increase dose by 5mg weekly if needed. **Pediatrics ≥6 yrs:** 5mg qd. **Max:** 20mg/day.
	Gelnique	**Gel:** 3% (28mg/pump), 10% (1g/pkt)	Apply to dry, intact skin on abdomen, upper arms/ shoulders, or thighs. **3%:** 3 pumps qd. **10%:** 1 pkt qd.	Rotate application sites.
	Oxytrol	**Patch:** 3.9mg/day	Apply 1 patch to dry, intact skin on abdomen, hip, or buttock twice weekly (every 3-4 days).	Rotate application sites (avoid using the same site within 7 days).
Solifenacin	Vesicare	**Tab:** 5mg, 10mg	**Usual:** 5mg qd. **Max:** 10mg qd.	Swallow whole. **Severe Renal Impairment (CrCl <30mL/min)/ Moderate Hepatic Impairment/ Concomitant Potent CYP3A4 Inhibitors:** Do not exceed 5mg/day. **Severe Hepatic Impairment:** Avoid use.
Tolterodine	Detrol	**Tab:** 1mg, 2mg	**Initial:** 2mg bid.	Decrease dose to 1mg bid if needed. **Significant Hepatic or Renal Dysfunction/ Concomitant Potent CYP3A4 Inhibitors:** 1mg bid.
	Detrol LA	**Cap, ER:** 2mg, 4mg	**Usual:** 4mg qd.	Swallow whole. Decrease dose to 2mg qd if needed. **Mild-Moderate Hepatic Impairment/Severe Renal Impairment (CrCl 10-30mL/min)/ Concomitant Potent CYP3A4 Inhibitors:** 2mg qd. **Severe Hepatic Impairment/ CrCl <10mL/min:** Avoid use.

(Continued)

GENERIC	BRAND	HOW SUPPLIED	DOSAGE	COMMENTS
MUSCARINIC ANTAGONISTS *(Continued)*				
Trospium	Sanctura	**Tab:** 20mg	**Usual:** 20mg bid.	Take 1 hr before meals or on empty stomach. **Severe Renal Impairment (CrCl <30mL/min):** 20mg qhs. **Elderly ≥75 yrs:** May titrate down to 20mg qd based on tolerability.
	Sanctura XR	**Cap, ER:** 60mg	**Usual:** 60mg qam.	Take on empty stomach 1 hr before a meal. **Severe Renal Impairment (CrCl <30mL/min):** Avoid use.
MISCELLANEOUS				
Mirabegron	Myrbetriq	**Tab, ER:** 25mg, 50mg	**Initial:** 25mg qd. **Max:** 50mg qd.	Take with or without food. Swallow whole. **Severe Renal Impairment (CrCl 15-29mL/min)/ Moderate Hepatic Impairment:** Do not exceed 25mg/day. **End-Stage Renal Disease/Severe Hepatic Impairment:** Avoid use.
OnabotulinumtoxinA	Botox	**Inj:** (sterile powder) 100 U, 200 U	**Usual:** 100 U. **Max:** 100 U.	Recommended dilution is 100 U/10mL with 0.9% non-preserved saline solution.

Abbreviation: ER = extended-release.

*Oxytrol for women (oxybutynin) patch is available as an OTC product for overactive bladder.

DRUGS THAT SHOULD NOT BE CRUSHED

Listed below are various slow-release as well as enteric-coated products that should not be crushed or chewed. Slow-release (sr) represents products that are controlled-release, extended-release, long-acting, or timed-release. Enteric-coated (ec) represents products that are delayed release.

In general, capsules containing slow-release or enteric-coated particles may be opened and their contents administered on a spoonful of soft food. Instruct patients not to chew particles, though. (Patients should, in fact, be discouraged from chewing any medication unless it is specifically formulated for that purpose.)

This list should not be considered all-inclusive. Generic and alternate brands of some products may exist. Tablets intended for sublingual or buccal administration (not included in this list) should be administered only as intended, in an intact form.

DRUG	MANUFACTURER	FORM
Aciphex	Eisai	ec
Actoplus Met XR	Takeda	sr
Adalat CC	Bayer HealthCare	sr
Adderall XR	Shire U.S.	sr
Adenovirus Type 4 and Type 7 Vaccine	Teva Women's Health, Inc.	ec
Advicor	AbbVie Inc.	sr
Afeditab CR	Watson	sr
Aggrenox	Boehringer Ingelheim	sr
Aleve-D Cold & Sinus	Bayer HealthCare	sr
Aleve-D Sinus & Headache	Bayer HealthCare	sr
Allegra-D 12 Hour	sanofi-aventis	sr
Allegra-D 24 Hour	sanofi-aventis	sr
Alophen	Numark	ec
Altoprev	Watson	sr
Ambien CR	sanofi-aventis	sr
Ampyra ER	Acorda Therapeutics	sr
Amrix	Cephalon	sr
Aplenzin	sanofi-aventis	sr
Apriso	Salix	sr
Arthrotec	Pfizer	ec
Asacol	Procter & Gamble	ec
Asacol HD	Procter & Gamble	ec
Astagraf XL	Astellas	sr
Augmentin XR	GlaxoSmithKline	sr
Avinza	King	sr
Azulfidine EN-tabs	Pfizer	ec
Bayer Aspirin Regimen	Bayer HealthCare	ec
Biaxin XL	AbbVie Inc.	sr
Bontril Slow-Release	Valeant	sr
Budeprion SR	Teva	sr
Calan SR	Pfizer	sr
Campral	Forest	ec
Carbatrol	Shire U.S.	sr
Cardene SR	EKR Therapeutics	sr
Cardizem CD	Biovail	sr
Cardizem LA	AbbVie Inc.	sr
Cardura XL	Pfizer	sr
Cartia XT	Actavis	sr
Chlor-Trimeton Allergy	Schering Plough	sr
Cipro XR	Schering Plough	sr
Clarinex-D 12 Hour	Schering Plough	sr
Clarinex-D 24 Hour	Schering Plough	sr
Claritin-D 12 Hour	Schering	sr
Claritin-D 24 Hour	Schering	sr
Cometriq	Exelixis, Inc.	sr
Concerta	Ortho-McNeil-Janssen	sr
Coreg CR	GlaxoSmithKline	sr
Covera-HS	Pfizer	sr
Creon	AbbVie Inc.	ec
Cymbalta	Eli Lilly	ec
Dairycare	Plainview	ec
Deconex DM	Poly	sr
Delzicol	Warner Chilcott	ec
Depakote	AbbVie Inc.	ec
Depakote ER	AbbVie Inc.	sr
Depakote Sprinkles	AbbVie Inc.	ec
Detrol LA	Pfizer	sr
Dexedrine Spansules	GlaxoSmithKline	sr
Dexilant	Takeda	sr
Diamox Sequels	Duramed	sr
Diclegis	Duchesnay USA	sr
Dilacor XR	Watson	sr
Dilantin	Pfizer	sr
Dilantin Kapseals	Pfizer	sr
Dilatrate-SR	UCB	sr
Diltia XT	Watson	sr
Dilt-CD	Apotex	sr
Ditropan XL	Ortho-McNeil Janssen	sr
Donnatal Extentabs	PBM	sr

(Continued)

DRUG	MANUFACTURER	FORM
Doryx	Mayne	ec
Duavee	Wyeth	ec
Dulcolax	Boehringer Ingelheim	ec
EC Naprosyn	Genentech	ec
Ecotrin 81 mg	GlaxoSmithKline	ec
Ecotrin 325 mg	GlaxoSmithKline	ec
Effexor-XR	Wyeth	sr
Embeda	King	sr
Enablex	Novartis Consumer	sr
Entocort EC	Prometheus	ec
Equetro	Validus	sr
ERYC	Mayne	sr
Ery-Tab	AbbVie Inc.	ec
Exalgo	Mallinckrodt	sr
Ferro-Sequels	Inverness Medical	sr
Fetzima	Forest	sr
Flagyl ER	Pfizer	sr
Fleet Bisacodyl	Fleet, C.B.	ec
Focalin XR	Novartis	sr
Folitab 500	Rising	sr
Forfivo XL	IntelGenx	sr
Fortamet	Shionogi Pharma	sr
Fulyzaq	Salix	ec
Fumatinic	Laser	sr
Galzin	Gate	ec
Gilphex TR	Gil	sr
Glucophage XR	Bristol-Myers Squibb	sr
Glucotrol XL	Pfizer	sr
Glumetza	Depomed	sr
Hemax	Pronova	sr
Horizant	GlaxoSmithKline	sr
Imbruvica	Pharmacyclics	ec
Inderal LA	Akrimax	sr
Innopran XL	GlaxoSmithKline	sr
Intuniv	Shire	sr
Invega	Ortho-McNeil-Janssen	sr
Janumet XR	Merck Sharp & Dohme Corp.	sr
Kadian	Actavis	sr
Kapvay ER	Shionogi	sr
Keppra XR	UCB	sr
Khedezla ER	Par	sr
Klor-Con 8	Upsher-Smith	sr
Klor-Con 10	Upsher-Smith	sr
Klor-Con M10*	Upsher-Smith	sr
Klor-Con M15*	Upsher-Smith	sr
Klor-Con M20*	Upsher-Smith	sr
Kombiglyze XR	BMS/AstraZeneca	sr
K-Tab	AbbVie Inc.	sr
Lamictal XR	GlaxoSmithKline	sr
Lescol XL	Novartis	sr
Levbid	Meda	sr
Lialda	Shire	ec
Liptruzet	Merck	ec
Lithobid	Noven Therapeutics	sr
Luvox CR	Jazz Pharmaceuticals	sr
Mag64	Rising	ec
MagDelay	Major	ec
Mag-Tab SR	Niche	sr
Maxifed	MCR American	sr
Maxifed DM	MCR American	sr
Maxifed DMX	MCR American	sr
Maxifed-G	MCR American	sr
Menopause Relief Trio	Mason Vitamins	sr
Mestinon Timespan	Valeant	sr
Metadate CD	UCB	sr
Metadate ER	UCB	sr
Methylin ER	Mallinckrodt	sr
Micro-K	Ther-Rx	sr
Micro-K 10	Ther-Rx	sr
Mild-C	Carlson, J.R.	sr
Mirapex ER	Boehringer Ingelheim	sr
Moxatag	Victory	sr
MS Contin	Purdue	sr
Mucinex	Reckitt Benckiser	sr
Mucinex D	Reckitt Benckiser	sr
Mucinex DM	Reckitt Benckiser	sr
Myfortic	Novartis	ec
Myrbetriq	Astellas	sr
Namenda XR	Forest	sr
Namzaric	Forest	sr
Naprelan	Victory	sr
Nexium	AstraZeneca	ec
Niaspan	AbbVie Inc.	sr
Nifediac CC	Teva	sr
Nifedical XL	Teva	sr
Nitro-Time	Time-Cap	sr
Norel SR	U.S. Pharmaceutical	sr
Norpace CR	Pfizer	sr
Nucynta ER	Janssen	sr
Oleptro	LaboPharm	sr
Olysio	Janssen	ec

DRUG	MANUFACTURER	FORM
Opana ER	Endo	sr
Opsumit	Actelion	ec
Oracea	Galderma	ec
Orenitram	United Therapeutics Corp.	sr
Oxtellar XR	Supernus	sr
Oxycontin	Purdue	sr
Pancreaze	Ortho-McNeil-Janssen	ec
Paser	Jacobus	ec
Paxil CR	GlaxoSmithKline	sr
PCE Dispertab	Arbor	sr
Pentasa	Shire U.S.	sr
Pentoxil	Upsher-Smith	sr
Phenytek	Mylan	sr
Poly Hist Forte	Poly	sr
Poly-Vent	Poly	sr
Prevacid	Takeda	ec
Prilosec	AstraZeneca	ec
Prilosec OTC	Procter & Gamble	sr
Pristiq	Wyeth	sr
Procardia XL	Pfizer	sr
Protonix	Wyeth	ec
Prozac Weekly	Eli Lilly	ec
Qsymia	Vivus	sr
Qudexy XR	Upsher-Smith	sr
Ranexa	Gilead	sr
Rayos	Horizon	ec
Razadyne ER	Ortho-McNeil-Janssen	sr
Requip XL	GlaxoSmithKline	sr
Rescon-Jr	Capellon	sr
Ritalin LA	Novartis	sr
Ritalin-SR	Novartis	sr
Rodex Forte	Legere	sr
Rytary	Impax	sr
Rythmol SR	GlaxoSmithKline	sr
SAM-e	Pharmavite	ec
Sanctura XR	Allergan	sr
Seroquel XR	AstraZeneca	sr
Simcor	AbbVie Inc.	sr
Sinemet CR	Bristol-Myers Squibb	sr
Sitavig	Farmea	ec
Slo-Niacin	Upsher-Smith	sr
Slow Fe	Novartis Consumer	sr
Slow-Mag	Purdue	ec
Solodyn	Medicis	sr
St. Joseph Pain Reliever	McNeil Consumer	ec
Stavzor	Noven	ec
Sudafed 12 hour	McNeil Consumer	sr
Sudafed 24 hour	McNeil Consumer	sr
Sular	Shionogi Pharma	sr
Sulfazine EC	Qualitest	ec
Symax Duotab	Capellon	sr
Symax-SR	Capellon	sr
Tafinlar	GlaxoSmithKline	ec
Tarka	AbbVie Inc.	sr
Taztia XT	Watson	sr
Tecfidera	biogen	ec
Tegretol-XR	Novartis	sr
Theo-24	UCB	sr
Tiazac	Forest	sr
Toprol XL[†]	AstraZeneca	sr
Totalday	National Vitamin	sr
Toviaz	Pfizer	sr
Trental	sanofi-aventis	sr
Treximet	GlaxoSmithKline	ec
Trilipix	AbbVie Inc.	ec
Trokendi XR	Supernus	sr
Tussicaps	Mallinckrodt	sr
Tylenol Arthritis	McNeil Consumer	sr
Uceris	Santarus, Inc.	sr
Ultram ER	Valeant	sr
Urocit-K	Mission	sr
Uroxatral	sanofi-aventis	sr
Verelan	UCB	sr
Verelan PM	UCB	sr
Videx EC	Bristol-Myers Squibb	ec
Vimovo	AstraZeneca	ec
Voltaren-XR	Novartis	sr
Vospire ER	Dava	sr
Votrient	GlaxoSmithKline	ec
Wellbutrin SR	GlaxoSmithKline	sr
Wellbutrin XL	GlaxoSmithKline	sr
Wobenzym N	Marlyn	ec
Xanax XR	Pfizer	sr
Xartemis XR	Mallinckrodt	sr
Xigduo XR	AstraZeneca	sr
Zenpep	Eurand	ec
Zohydro ER	Zogenix	sr
Zyban	GlaxoSmithKline	sr
Zyflo CR	Cornerstone	sr
Zyrtec-D	McNeil Consumer	sr

*May split in half or dissolve in water.

[†]May divide tablet.

Drugs That Should Not Be Used in Pregnancy

Abiraterone acetate
Acetohydroxamic acid
Acitretin
Ambrisentan
Amlodipine besylate/Atorvastatin calcium
Anastrozole
Aspirin
Atorvastatin calcium
Atorvastatin/Ezetimibe
Aveed
Benzphetamine hydrochloride
Bexarotene
Bicalutamide
Boceprevir
Bosentan
Caffeine
Cetrorelix acetate
Chenodiol
Cholecalciferol
Choriogonadotropin alfa
Chorionic gonadotropin
Clomiphene citrate
Danazol
Degarelix
Denosumab
Desogestrel/Ethinyl estradiol
Diclofenac sodium/Misoprostol
Dihydroergotamine mesylate
Dronedarone
Drospirenone/Ethinyl estradiol
Dutasteride
Dutasteride/Tamsulosin hydrochloride
Enzalutamide
Ergotamine tartrate
Estazolam
Estradiol
Estradiol valerate
Estradiol/Norethindrone acetate
Estrogens, Conjugated, Synthetic B
Estropipate
Ethinyl estradiol
Ethinyl estradiol/Ethynodiol diacetate
Ethinyl estradiol/Etonogestrel
Ethinyl estradiol/Ferrous fumarate/Norethindrone acetate
Ethinyl estradiol/Levonorgestrel
Ethinyl estradiol/Norelgestromin
Ethinyl estradiol/Norethindrone
Ethinyl estradiol/Norgestimate
Ethinyl estradiol/Norgestrel
Exemestane
Ezetimibe/Simvastatin
Finasteride
Fluorouracil
Fluoxymesterone
Fluvastatin sodium
Follitropin alfa
Follitropin beta
Ganirelix acetate
Genistein aglycone
Goserelin acetate
Histrelin acetate
Iodine I 131 tositumomab
Isotretinoin
Leflunomide
Lenalidomide
Letrozole
Leuprolide acetate
Leuprolide acetate/Norethindrone acetate
Levonorgestrel
Lomitapide
Lorcaserin hydrochloride
Lovastatin
Lovastatin/Niacin
Lutropin alfa
Macitentan
Medroxyprogesterone acetate
Megestrol acetate
Menotropins
Mequinol/Tretinoin
Mestranol/Norethindrone
Methotrexate
Methyltestosterone
Mifepristone
Miglustat
Minivelle
Misoprostol
Mitomycin
Nafarelin acetate
Niacin/Simvastatin
Norethindrone
Orlistat
Ospemifene
Oxandrolone
Phendimetrazine tartrate
Phentermine hydrochloride
Phentermine/Topiramate
Pitavastatin
Pomalidomide
Pravastatin sodium
Radium Ra 223 dichloride
Raloxifene hydrochloride
Rasuvo
Ribavirin
Riociguat
Rosuvastatin calcium
Simeprevir
Simvastatin
Simvastatin/Sitagliptin
Sofosbuvir
Tazarotene
Telaprevir
Temazepam
Teriflunomide
Tesamorelin
Testosterone
Testosterone cypionate
Testosterone enanthate
Thalidomide
Triazolam
Triptorelin pamoate
Ulipristal acetate
Urofollitropin
Vitamin A palmitate
Vogelxo
Warfarin sodium
Zinc bisglycinate

PREGNANCY CATEGORY X

Studies in animals or humans, or investigational or postmarketing reports, have demonstrated fetal risk, which clearly outweighs any possible benefit to the patient.

FDA-APPROVED NEW DRUG PRODUCTS

BRAND	GENERIC	INDICATION
Akynzeo	netupitant and palonosetron	To treat nausea and vomiting in patients undergoing cancer chemotherapy.
Avycaz	ceftazidime-avibactam	To treat adults with complicated intra-abdominal infections (cIAI), in combination with metronidazole, and complicated urinary tract infections (cUTI), including kidney infections (pyelonephritis), who have limited or no alternative treatment options.
Beleodaq	belinostat	To treat patients with peripheral T-cell lymphoma (PTCL).
Belsomra	suvorexant	To treat difficulty in falling and staying asleep (insomnia).
Blincyto	blinatumomab	To treat patients with Philadelphia chromosome-negative precursor B-cell acute lymphoblastic leukemia (B-cell ALL).
Cerdelga	eliglustat	For the long-term treatment of adult patients with the Type 1 form of Gaucher disease.
Cosentyx	secukinumab	To treat adults with moderate-to-severe plaque psoriasis.
Cresemba	isavuconazonium sulfate	To treat adults with invasive aspergillosis and invasive mucormycosis.
Cyramza	ramucirumab	To treat patients with advanced stomach cancer or gastroesophageal junction adenocarcinoma.
Dalvance	dalbavancin	To treat adults with skin infections.
Entyvio	vedolizumab	To treat adult patients with moderate to severe ulcerative colitis and adult patients with moderate to severe Crohn's disease.
Esbriet	pirfenidone	For the treatment of idiopathic pulmonary fibrosis (IPF).
Farydak	panobinostat	To treat patients with multiple myeloma.
Harvoni	ledipasvir/sofosbuvir	To treat chronic hepatitis C virus (HCV) genotype 1 infection.
Ibrance	palbociclib	To treat advanced (metastatic) breast cancer.
Impavido	miltefosine	To treat a tropical disease called leishmaniasis.
Jardiance	empagliflozin	To improve glycemic control in adults with type 2 diabetes.
Jublia	efinaconazole	To treat mild to moderate onychomycosis (fungal infection).
Kerydin	tavaborole	For the topical treatment of onychomycosis of the toenails.
Keytruda	pembrolizumab	For treatment of patients with advanced or unresectable melanoma who are no longer responding to other drugs.
Lenvima	lenvatinib	To treat patients with progressive, differentiated thyroid cancer (DTC) whose disease progressed despite receiving radioactive iodine therapy (radioactive iodine refractory disease).
Lumason	sulfur hexafluoride lipid microsphere	For patients whose ultrasound image of the heart (echocardiograms) are hard to see with ultrasound waves.
Lynparza	olaparib	To treat advanced ovarian cancer.
Movantik	naloxegol	To treat opioid-induced constipation in adults with chronic non-cancer pain.
Myalept	metreleptin for injection	To treat the complications of leptin deficiency.
Natpara	parathyroid hormone	To control hypocalcemia (low blood calcium levels) in patients with hypoparathyroidism.
Neuraceq	florbetaben F 18 injection	For Positron Emission Tomography (PET) imaging of the brain.
Northera	droxidopa	To treat neurogenic orthostatic hypotension (NOH).
Ofev	nintedanib	For the treatment of idiopathic pulmonary fibrosis (IPF).

(Continued)

BRAND	GENERIC	INDICATION
Opdivo	nivolumab	To treat patients with unresectable (cannot be removed by surgery) or metastatic (advanced) melanoma who no longer respond to other drugs.
Orbactiv	oritavancin	To treat adults with skin infections.
Otezla	apremilast	To treat adults with active psoriatic arthritis (PsA).
Plegridy	peginterferon beta-1a	For the treatment of patients with relapsing forms of multiple sclerosis.
Rapivab	peramivir	To treat influenza infection in adults.
Savaysa	edoxaban	To reduce the risk of stroke and dangerous blood clots (systemic embolism) in patients with atrial fibrillation that is not caused by a heart valve problem.
Sivextro (injection); Sivextro (tablet)	tedizolid phosphate	To treat adults with skin infections.
Striverdi Respimat	olodaterol	To treat chronic obstructive pulmonary disease.
Sylvant	siltuximab	To treat patients with multicentric Castleman's disease (MCD), a rare disorder similar to lymphoma (cancer of the lymph nodes).
Tanzeum	albiglutide	To improve glycemic control, along with diet and exercise, in adults with type 2 diabetes.
Trulicity	dulaglutide	To treat adults with type 2 diabetes.
Viekira Pak	(ombitasvir, paritaprevir and ritonavir tablets co-packaged with dasabuvir tablets)	To treat patients with chronic hepatitis C virus (HCV) genotype 1 infection, including those with a type of advanced liver disease called cirrhosis.
Vimizim	elosulfase alfa	Treatment for Mucopolysaccharidosis Type IVA (Morquio A syndrome).
Xtoro	finafloxacin otic suspension	To treat acute otitis externa, commonly known as swimmer's ear.
Zerbaxa	ceftolozane/tazobactam	To treat adults with complicated intra-abdominal infections (cIAI) and complicated urinary tract infections (cUTI).
Zontivity	vorapaxar	To reduce the risk of heart attacks and stroke in high-risk patients.
Zydelig	idelalisib	To treat patients with three types of blood cancers.
Zykadia	ceritinib	To treat patients with a certain type of late-stage (metastatic) non-small cell lung cancer (NSCLC).

Note: This list is not comprehensive and only includes new molecular entities that have not been approved by the FDA previously, either as a single ingredient drug or as part of a combination product. For a complete list, please refer to the FDA website, www.accessdata.fda.gov/scripts/cder/drugsatfda/index.cfm?fuseaction=Reports.ReportsMenu.

ISMP's List of Confused Drug Names

This list has been reproduced with permission from the Institute for Safe Medication Practices (ISMP), and includes ISMP's most current updates, which are completed through April 2014.

DRUG NAME	CONFUSED DRUG NAME
Abelcet	amphotericin B
Accupril	Aciphex
aceta**ZOLAMIDE**	aceto**HEXAMIDE**
acetic acid for irrigation	glacial acetic acid
aceto**HEXAMIDE**	aceta**ZOLAMIDE**
Aciphex	Accupril
Aciphex	Aricept
Activase	Cathflo Activase
Activase	TNKase
Actonel	Actos
Actos	Actonel
Adacel (Tdap)	Daptacel (DTaP)
Adderall	Inderal
Adderall	Adderall XR
Adderall XR	Adderall
ado-trastuzumab emtansine	trastuzumab
Advair	Advicor
Advicor	Advair
Advicor	Altocor
Afrin (oxymetazoline)	Afrin (saline)
Afrin (saline)	Afrin (oxymetazoline)
Aggrastat	argatroban
Aldara	Alora
Alkeran	Leukeran
Alkeran	Myleran
Allegra (fexofenadine)	Allegra Anti-Itch Cream (diphenhydr**AMINE**/allantoin)
Allegra	Viagra
Allegra Anti-Itch Cream (diphenhydr**AMINE**/allantoin)	Allegra (fexofenadine)
Alora	Aldara
ALPRAZolam	**LOR**azepam
Altocor	Advicor
amantadine	amiodarone
Amaryl	Reminyl
Ambisome	amphotericin B
Amicar	Omacor
Amikin	Kineret
a**MIL**oride	am**LODIP**ine
amiodarone	amantadine
am**LODIP**ine	a**MIL**oride
amphotericin B	Abelcet
amphotericin B	Ambisome
Anacin	Anacin-3
Anacin-3	Anacin
antacid	Atacand
Antivert	Axert
Anzemet	Avandamet
Apidra	Spiriva
Apresoline	Priscoline
argatroban	Aggrastat
argatroban	Orgaran
Aricept	Aciphex
Aricept	Azilect
ARIPiprazole	proton pump inhibitors
ARIPiprazole	**RABE**prazole

DRUG NAME	CONFUSED DRUG NAME
Arista AH (absorbable hemostatic agent)	Arixtra
Arixtra	Arista AH (absorbable hemostatic agent)
Asacol	Os-Cal
Atacand	antacid
atomoxetine	atorvastatin
atorvastatin	atomoxetine
Atrovent	Natru-Vent
Avandamet	Anzemet
Avandia	Prandin
Avandia	Coumadin
AVINza	**INV**anz
AVINza	Evista
Axert	Antivert
aza**CITID**ine	aza**THIO**prine
aza**THIO**prine	aza**CITID**ine
Azilect	Aricept
B & O (belladonna and opium)	Beano
BabyBIG	HBIG (hepatitis B immune globulin)
Bayhep-B	Bayrab
Bayhep-B	Bayrho-D
Bayrab	Bayhep-B
Bayrab	Bayrho-D
Bayrho-D	Bayhep-B
Bayrho-D	Bayrab
Beano	B & O (belladonna and opium)
Benadryl	benazepril
benazepril	Benadryl
Benicar	Mevacor
Betadine (with povidone-iodine)	Betadine (without povidone-iodine)
Betadine (without povidone-iodine)	Betadine (with povidone-iodine)
Bextra	Zetia
Bicillin C-R	Bicillin L-A
Bicillin L-A	Bicillin C-R
Bicitra	Polycitra
Bidex	Videx
Brethine	Methergine
Bio-T-Gel	T-Gel
Brevibloc	Brevital
Brevital	Brevibloc
bu**PROP**ion	bus**PIR**one
bus**PIR**one	bu**PROP**ion
Capadex [non-US product]	Kapidex
Capex	Kapidex
Carac	Kuric
captopril	carvedilol
car**BAM**azepine	**OX**carbazepine
CARBOplatin	**CIS**platin
Cardene	Cardizem

(Continued)

Brand names always start with an uppercase letter. Some brand names incorporate tall man letters in initial characters and may not be readily recognized as brand names. Brand name products appear in black; generic/other products appear in **color**.

DRUG NAME	CONFUSED DRUG NAME
Cardizem	Cardene
Cardura	Coumadin
carvedilol	captopril
Casodex	Kapidex
Cathflo Activase	Activase
Cedax	Cidex
ce**FAZ**olin	cef**TRIAX**one
cef**TRIAX**one	ce**FAZ**olin
Cele**BREX**	Cele**XA**
Cele**BREX**	Cerebyx
Cele**XA**	Zy**PREXA**
Cele**XA**	Cele**BREX**
Cele**XA**	Cerebyx
Cerebyx	Cele**BREX**
Cerebyx	Cele**XA**
cetirizine	sertraline
cetirizine	stavudine
chlordiaze**POXIDE**	chlorpro**MAZINE**
chlorpro**MAZINE**	chlordiaze**POXIDE**
chlorpro**MAZINE**	chlorpro**PAMIDE**
chlorpro**PAMIDE**	chlorpro**MAZINE**
Cidex	Cedax
CISplatin	**CARBO**platin
Claritin (loratadine)	Claritin Eye (ketotifen fumarate)
Claritin-D	Claritin-D 24
Claritin-D 24	Claritin-D
Claritin Eye (ketotifen fumarate)	Claritin (loratadine)
Clindesse	Clindets
Clindets	Clindesse
clobazam	clonaze**PAM**
clomi**PHENE**	clomi**PRAMINE**
clomi**PRAMINE**	clomi**PHENE**
clonaze**PAM**	clobazam
clonaze**PAM**	clo**NID**ine
clonaze**PAM**	**LOR**azepam
clo**NID**ine	clonaze**PAM**
clo**NID**ine	Klono**PIN**
Clozaril	Colazal
coagulation factor IX (recombinant)	factor IX complex, vapor heated
codeine	Lodine
Colace	Cozaar
Colazal	Clozaril
colchicine	Cortrosyn
Comvax	Recombivax HB
Cortrosyn	colchicine
Coumadin	Avandia
Coumadin	Cardura
Cozaar	Colace
Cozaar	Zocor
cyclophosphamide	cyclo**SPORINE**
cyclo**SERINE**	cyclo**SPORINE**
cyclo**SPORINE**	cyclophosphamide
cyclo**SPORINE**	cyclo**SERINE**
Cymbalta	Symbyax
DACTINomycin	**DAPTO**mycin
Daptacel (DTaP)	Adacel (Tdap)
DAPTOmycin	**DACTIN**omycin

DRUG NAME	CONFUSED DRUG NAME
Darvocet	Percocet
Darvon	Diovan
DAUNOrubicin	**DAUNO**rubicin citrate liposomal
DAUNOrubicin	**DOXO**rubicin
DAUNOrubicin	**IDA**rubicin
DAUNOrubicin citrate liposomal	**DAUNO**rubicin
Denavir	indinavir
Depakote	Depakote ER
Depakote ER	Depakote
Depo-Medrol	Solu-**MEDROL**
Depo-Provera	Depo-subQ provera 104
Depo-subQ provera 104	Depo-Provera
desipramine	disopyramide
dexmethylphenidate	methadone
Diabinese	Diamox
Diabeta	Zebeta
Diamox	Diabinese
Diflucan	Diprivan
Dilacor XR	Pilocar
Dilaudid	Dilaudid-5
Dilaudid-5	Dilaudid
dimenhy**DRINATE**	diphenhydr**AMINE**
diphenhydr**AMINE**	dimenhy**DRINATE**
Dioval	Diovan
Diovan	Dioval
Diovan	Zyban
Diovan	Darvon
Diprivan	Diflucan
Diprivan	Ditropan
disopyramide	desipramine
Ditropan	Diprivan
DOBUTamine	**DOP**amine
DOPamine	**DOBUT**amine
Doribax	Zovirax
Doxil	Paxil
DOXOrubicin	**DAUNO**rubicin
DOXOrubicin	**DOXO**rubicin liposomal
DOXOrubicin	**IDA**rubicin
DOXOrubicin liposomal	**DOXO**rubicin
Dulcolax (bisacodyl)	Dulcolax (docusate sodium)
Dulcolax (docusate sodium)	Dulcolax (bisacodyl)
DULoxetine	**FLU**oxetine
Durasal	Durezol
Durezol	Durasal
Duricef	Ultracet
Dynacin	Dynacirc
Dynacirc	Dynacin
edetate calcium disodium	edetate disodium
edetate disodium	edetate calcium disodium
Effexor	Effexor XR
Effexor XR	Enablex
Effexor XR	Effexor
Enablex	Effexor XR
Enbrel	Levbid
Engerix-B adult	Engerix-B pediatric/ adolescent
Engerix-B pediatric/ adolescent	Engerix-B adult
Enjuvia	Januvia
e**PHED**rine	**EPINEPH**rine

Brand names always start with an uppercase letter. Some brand names incorporate tall man letters in initial characters and may not be readily recognized as brand names. Brand name products appear in black; generic/other products appear in **color**.

DRUG NAME	CONFUSED DRUG NAME
EPINEPHrine	e**PHED**rine
epirubicin	eribulin
eribulin	epirubicin
Estratest	Estratest HS
Estratest HS	Estratest
ethambutol	Ethmozine
ethaverine [non-US name]	etravirine
Ethmozine	ethambutol
etravirine	ethaverine [non-US name]
Evista	**AVIN**za
factor IX complex, vapor heated	coagulation factor IX (recombinant)
Fanapt	Xanax
Fastin (phentermine)	Fastin (dietary supplement)
Fastin (dietary supplement)	Fastin (phentermine)
Femara	Femhrt
Femhrt	Femara
fenta**NYL**	**SUF**entanil
Fioricet	Fiorinal
Fiorinal	Fioricet
flavox**ATE**	fluvoxa**MINE**
Flonase	Flovent
Floranex	Florinef
Florastor	Florinef
Florinef	Floranex
Florinef	Florastor
Flovent	Flonase
flumazenil	influenza virus vaccine
FLUoxetine	**PAR**oxetine
FLUoxetine	**DUL**oxetine
FLUoxetine	Loxitane
fluvoxa**MINE**	flavox**ATE**
Folex	Foltx
folic acid	folinic acid (leucovorin calcium)
folinic acid (leucovorin calcium)	folic acid
Foltx	Folex
fomepizole	omeprazole
Foradil	Fortical
Foradil	Toradol
Fortical	Foradil
gentamicin	gentian violet
gentian violet	gentamicin
glacial acetic acid	acetic acid for irrigation
glipi**ZIDE**	gly**BURIDE**
Glucotrol	Glycotrol
gly**BURIDE**	glipi**ZIDE**
Glycotrol	Glucotrol
Granulex	Regranex
guai**FEN**esin	guan**FACINE**
guan**FACINE**	guai**FEN**esin
HBIG (hepatitis B immune globulin)	BabyBIG
Healon	Hyalgan
heparin	Hespan
Hespan	heparin
HMG-CoA reductase inhibitors ("statins")	nystatin
Huma**LOG**	Humu**LIN**
Huma**LOG**	Novo**LOG**
Huma**LOG** Mix 75/25	Humu**LIN** 70/30
Humapen Memoir (for use with Huma**LOG**)	Humira Pen
Humira Pen	Humapen Memoir (for use with Huma**LOG**)
Humu**LIN**	Novo**LIN**
Humu**LIN**	Huma**LOG**
Humu**LIN** 70/30	Huma**LOG** Mix 75/25
Humu**LIN** R U-100	Humu**LIN** R U-500
Humu**LIN** R U-500	Humu**LIN** R U-100
Hyalgan	Healon
hydr**ALAZINE**	hydr**OXY**zine
Hydrea	Lyrica
HYDROcodone	oxy**CODONE**
Hydrogesic	hydr**OXY**zine
HYDROmorphone	morphine
hydroxychloroquine	hydroxyurea
hydroxyurea	hydroxychloroquine
hydr**OXY**zine	Hydrogesic
hydr**OXY**zine	hydr**ALAZINE**
IDArubicin	**DAUNO**rubicin
IDArubicin	**DOXO**rubicin
Inderal	Adderall
indinavir	Denavir
in**FLIX**imab	ri**TUX**imab
influenza virus vaccine	flumazenil
influenza virus vaccine	tuberculin purified protein derivative (PPD)
Inspra	Spiriva
Intuniv	Invega
INVanz	**AVIN**za
Invega	Intuniv
iodine	Lodine
Isordil	Plendil
ISOtretinoin	tretinoin
Jantoven	Janumet
Jantoven	Januvia
Janumet	Jantoven
Janumet	Januvia
Janumet	Sinemet
Januvia	Enjuvia
Januvia	Jantoven
Januvia	Janumet
K-Phos Neutral	Neutra-Phos-K
Kaopectate (bismuth subsalicylate)	Kaopectate (docusate calcium)
Kaopectate (docusate calcium)	Kaopectate (bismuth subsalicylate)
Kadian	Kapidex
Kaletra	Keppra
Kapidex	Capadex [non-US product]
Kapidex	Capex
Kapidex	Casodex
Kapidex	Kadian
Keflex	Keppra
Keppra	Kaletra
Keppra	Keflex
Ketalar	ketorolac
ketorolac	Ketalar
ketorolac	methadone
Kineret	Amikin
Klono**PIN**	clo**NID**ine
Kuric	Carac
Kwell	Qwell

(Continued)

Brand names always start with an uppercase letter. Some brand names incorporate tall man letters in initial characters and may not be readily recognized as brand names. Brand name products appear in black; generic/other products appear in **color**.

DRUG NAME	CONFUSED DRUG NAME
La**MIC**tal	Lam**ISIL**
Lam**ISIL**	La**MIC**tal
lami**VUD**ine	lamo**TRI**gine
lamo**TRI**gine	lami**VUD**ine
lamo**TRI**gine	lev**ETIRA**cetam
lamo**TRI**gine	levothyroxine
Lanoxin	levothyroxine
Lanoxin	naloxone
lanthanum carbonate	lithium carbonate
Lantus	Latuda
Lantus	Lente
Lariam	Levaquin
Lasix	Luvox
Latuda	Lantus
Lente	Lantus
Letairis	Letaris [non-US product]
Letaris [non-US product]	Letairis
leucovorin calcium	Leukeran
leucovorin calcium	levoleucovorin
Leukeran	Alkeran
Leukeran	Myleran
Leukeran	leucovorin calcium
Levaquin	Lariam
Levbid	Enbrel
lev**ETIRA**cetam	lamo**TRI**gine
Levemir	Lovenox
lev**ETIRA**cetam	lev**OCARN**itine
lev**ETIRA**cetam	levofloxacin
lev**OCARN**itine	lev**ETIRA**cetam
levofloxacin	lev**ETIRA**cetam
levoleucovorin	leucovorin calcium
levothyroxine	lamo**TRI**gine
levothyroxine	Lanoxin
levothyroxine	liothyronine
Lexapro	Loxitane
Lexiva	Pexeva
liothyronine	levothyroxine
Lipitor	Loniten
Lipitor	Zyr**TEC**
lithium	Ultram
lithium carbonate	lanthanum carbonate
Lodine	codeine
Lodine	iodine
Loniten	Lipitor
Lopressor	Lyrica
LORazepam	**ALPRAZ**olam
LORazepam	clonaze**PAM**
LORazepam	Lovaza
Lotronex	Protonix
Lovaza	**LOR**azepam
Lovenox	Levemir
Loxitane	Lexapro
Loxitane	**FLU**oxetine
Loxitane	Soriatane
Lunesta	Neulasta
Lupron Depot-3 Month	Lupron Depot-Ped
Lupron Depot-Ped	Lupron Depot-3 Month
Luvox	Lasix
Lyrica	Hydrea
Lyrica	Lopressor
Maalox	Maalox Total Stomach Relief

DRUG NAME	CONFUSED DRUG NAME
Maalox Total Stomach Relief	Maalox
Matulane	Materna
Materna	Matulane
Maxzide	Microzide
Menactra	Menomune
Menomune	Menactra
Mephyton	methadone
Metadate	methadone
Metadate CD	Metadate ER
Metadate ER	Metadate CD
Metadate ER	methadone
met**FORMIN**	metro**NIDAZOLE**
methadone	dexmethylphenidate
methadone	ketorolac
methadone	Mephyton
methadone	Metadate
methadone	Metadate ER
methadone	methylphenidate
methadone	metolazone
methadone	metoprolol
Methergine	Brethine
methimazole	metolazone
methylphenidate	methadone
metolazone	methadone
metolazone	methimazole
metoprolol	methadone
metoprolol succinate	metoprolol tartrate
metoprolol tartrate	metoprolol succinate
metro**NIDAZOLE**	met**FORMIN**
Mevacor	Benicar
Micronase	Microzide
Microzide	Maxzide
Microzide	Micronase
midodrine	Midrin
Midrin	midodrine
mifepristone	misoprostol
Miralax	Mirapex
Mirapex	Miralax
misoprostol	mifepristone
mito**MY**cin	mito**XANTRONE**
mito**XANTRONE**	mito**MY**cin
morphine	**HYDRO**morphone
morphine - non-concentrated oral liquid	morphine - oral liquid concentrate
morphine - oral liquid concentrate	morphine - non-concentrated oral liquid
Motrin	Neurontin
MS Contin	Oxy**CONTIN**
Mucinex	Mucomyst
Mucinex D	Mucinex DM
Mucinex DM	Mucinex D
Mucomyst	Mucinex
Myleran	Alkeran
Myleran	Leukeran
nalbuphine	naloxone
naloxone	Lanoxin
naloxone	nalbuphine
Narcan	Norcuron
Natru-Vent	Atrovent
Navane	Norvasc

Brand names always start with an uppercase letter. Some brand names incorporate tall man letters in initial characters and may not be readily recognized as brand names. Brand name products appear in black; generic/other products appear in **color**.

DRUG NAME	CONFUSED DRUG NAME
Neo-Synephrine (oxymetazoline)	Neo-Synephrine (phenylephrine)
Neo-Synephrine (phenylephrine)	Neo-Synephrine (oxymetazoline)
Neulasta	Lunesta
Neulasta	Neumega
Neulasta	Nuedexta
Neumega	Neupogen
Neumega	Neulasta
Neupogen	Neumega
Neurontin	Motrin
Neurontin	Noroxin
Neutra-Phos-K	K-Phos Neutral
Nex**AVAR**	Nex**IUM**
Nex**IUM**	Nex**AVAR**
ni**CAR**dipine	**NIFE**dipine
NIFEdipine	ni**CAR**dipine
NIFEdipine	ni**MOD**ipine
ni**MOD**ipine	**NIFE**dipine
Norcuron	Narcan
Normodyne	Norpramin
Noroxin	Neurontin
Norpramin	Normodyne
Norvasc	Navane
Novo**LIN**	Humu**LIN**
Novo**LIN**	Novo**LOG**
Novo**LIN** 70/30	Novo**LOG** Mix 70/30
Novo**LOG**	Huma**LOG**
Novo**LOG**	Novo**LIN**
Novo**LOG** FLEXPEN	Novo**LOG** Mix 70/30 FLEXPEN
Novo**LOG** Mix 70/30 FLEXPEN	Novo**LOG** FLEXPEN
Novo**LOG** Mix 70/30	Novo**LIN** 70/30
Nuedexta	Neulasta
nystatin	HMG-CoA reductase inhibitors ("statins")
Occlusal-HP	Ocuflox
Ocuflox	Occlusal-HP
OLANZapine	**QUE**tiapine
Omacor	Amicar
omeprazole	fomepizole
opium tincture	paregoric (camphorated tincture of opium)
Oracea	Orencia
Orencia	Oracea
Orgaran	argatroban
Ortho Tri-Cyclen	Ortho Tri-Cyclen LO
Ortho Tri-Cyclen LO	Ortho Tri-Cyclen
Os-Cal	Asacol
oxaprozin	**OX**carbazepine
OXcarbazepine	oxaprozin
OXcarbazepine	car**BAM**azepine
oxy**CODONE**	**HYDRO**codone
oxy**CODONE**	Oxy**CONTIN**
Oxy**CONTIN**	MS Contin
Oxy**CONTIN**	oxy**CODONE**
PACLitaxel	**PACL**itaxel protein-bound particles
PACLitaxel protein-bound particles	**PACL**itaxel
Pamelor	Panlor DC
Pamelor	Tambocor
Panlor DC	Pamelor

DRUG NAME	CONFUSED DRUG NAME
paregoric (camphorated tincture of opium)	opium tincture
PARoxetine	**FLU**oxetine
PARoxetine	piroxicam
Patanol	Platinol
Pavulon	Peptavlon
Paxil	Doxil
Paxil	Taxol
Paxil	Plavix
pazopanib	ponatinib
PEMEtrexed	**PRALA**trexate
penicillin	penicillamine
penicillamine	penicillin
Peptavlon	Pavulon
Percocet	Darvocet
Percocet	Procet
Pexeva	Lexiva
PENTobarbital	**PHEN**obarbital
PHENobarbital	**PENT**obarbital
Pilocar	Dilacor XR
piroxicam	**PAR**oxetine
Platinol	Patanol
Plavix	Paxil
Plavix	Pradax [Non-US Product]
Plavix	Pradaxa
Plendil	Isordil
pneumococcal 7-valent vaccine	pneumococcal polyvalent vaccine
pneumococcal polyvalent vaccine	pneumococcal 7-valent vaccine
Polycitra	Bicitra
ponatinib	pazopanib
potassium acetate	sodium acetate
PRALAtrexate	**PEME**trexed
Pradax [Non-US Product]	Plavix
Pradaxa	Plavix
Prandin	Avandia
Precare	Precose
Precose	Precare
predniso**LONE**	predni**SONE**
predni**SONE**	predniso**LONE**
Prenexa	Ranexa
Pri**LOSEC**	Pristiq
Pri**LOSEC**	**PRO**zac
Priscoline	Apresoline
Pristiq	Pri**LOSEC**
probenecid	Procanbid
Procan SR	Procanbid
Procanbid	probenecid
Procanbid	Procan SR
Procardia XL	Protain XL
Procet	Percocet
Prograf	**PRO**zac
propylthiouracil	Purinethol
Proscar	Provera
Protain XL	Procardia XL
protamine	Protonix
proton pump inhibitors	**ARIP**iprazole
Protonix	Lotronex
Protonix	protamine
Provera	Proscar
Provera	**PRO**zac

(Continued)

Brand names always start with an uppercase letter. Some brand names incorporate tall man letters in initial characters and may not be readily recognized as brand names. Brand name products appear in black; generic/other products appear in **color**.

DRUG NAME	CONFUSED DRUG NAME
PROzac	Prograf
PROzac	Pri**LOSEC**
PROzac	Provera
Purinethol	propylthiouracil
Pyridium	pyridoxine
pyridoxine	Pyridium
QUEtiapine	**OLANZ**apine
qui**NID**ine	qui**NINE**
qui**NINE**	qui**NID**ine
Qwell	Kwell
RABEprazole	**ARIP**iprazole
Ranexa	Prenexa
Rapaflo	Rapamune
Rapamune	Rapaflo
Razadyne	Rozerem
Recombivax HB	Comvax
Regranex	Granulex
Reminyl	Robinul
Reminyl	Amaryl
Renagel	Renvela
Renvela	Renagel
Reprexain	Zy**PREXA**
Restoril	Risper**DAL**
Retrovir	ritonavir
Rifadin	Rifater
Rifamate	rifampin
rifampin	Rifamate
rifampin	rifaximin
Rifater	Rifadin
rifaximin	rifampin
Risper**DAL**	Restoril
risperi**DONE**	r**OPINIR**ole
Ritalin	ritodrine
Ritalin LA	Ritalin SR
Ritalin SR	Ritalin LA
ritodrine	Ritalin
ritonavir	Retrovir
ri**TUX**imab	in**FLIX**imab
Robinul	Reminyl
r**OPINIR**ole	risperi**DONE**
Roxanol	Roxicodone Intensol
Roxanol	Roxicet
Roxicet	Roxanol
Roxicodone Intensol	Roxanol
Rozerem	Razadyne
Salagen	selegiline
Sand**IMMUNE**	Sando**STATIN**
Sando**STATIN**	Sand**IMMUNE**
saquinavir	**SINE**quan
saquinavir (free base)	saquinavir mesylate
saquinavir mesylate	saquinavir (free base)
Sarafem	Serophene
selegiline	Salagen
Serophene	Sarafem
SEROquel	**SERO**quel XR
SEROquel	Serzone
SEROquel	**SINE**quan
SEROquel XR	**SERO**quel
sertraline	cetirizine
sertraline	Soriatane
Serzone	**SERO**quel
silodosin	sirolimus

DRUG NAME	CONFUSED DRUG NAME
Sinemet	Janumet
SINEquan	saquinavir
SINEquan	**SERO**quel
SINEquan	Singulair
SINEquan	Zonegran
Singulair	**SINE**quan
sirolimus	silodosin
sita**GLIP**tin	**SUMA**triptan
sodium acetate	potassium acetate
Solu-**CORTEF**	Solu-**MEDROL**
Solu-**MEDROL**	Depo-Medrol
Solu-**MEDROL**	Solu-**CORTEF**
Sonata	Soriatane
Soriatane	Loxitane
Soriatane	sertraline
Soriatane	Sonata
sotalol	Sudafed
Spiriva	Apidra
Spiriva	Inspra
stavudine	cetirizine
Sudafed	sotalol
Sudafed	Sudafed PE
Sudafed PE	Sudafed
SUFentanil	fenta**NYL**
sulf**ADIAZINE**	sulfa**SALA**zine
sulf**ADIAZINE**	sulfi**SOXAZOLE**
sulfa**SALA**zine	sulf**ADIAZINE**
sulfi**SOXAZOLE**	sulf**ADIAZINE**
SUMAtriptan	sita**GLIP**tin
SUMAtriptan	**ZOLM**itriptan
Symbyax	Cymbalta
T-Gel	Bio-T-Gel
Tambocor	Pamelor
Taxol	Taxotere
Taxol	Paxil
Taxotere	Taxol
TEGretol	**TEG**retol XR
TEGretol	Tequin
TEGretol	**TREN**tal
TEGretol XR	**TEG**retol
Tenex	Xanax
Tequin	**TEG**retol
Tequin	Ticlid
Testoderm TTS	Testoderm
Testoderm TTS	Testoderm with Adhesive
Testoderm with Adhesive	Testoderm
Testoderm with Adhesive	Testoderm TTS
Testoderm	Testoderm TTS
Testoderm	Testoderm with Adhesive
tetanus diphtheria toxoid (Td)	tuberculin purified protein derivative (PPD)
Thalomid	Thiamine
Thiamine	Thalomid
tia**GAB**ine	ti**ZAN**idine
Tiazac	Ziac
Ticlid	Tequin
ti**ZAN**idine	tia**GAB**ine
TNKase	Activase
TNKase	t-PA
Tobradex	Tobrex
Tobrex	Tobradex
TOLAZamide	**TOLBUT**amide

Brand names always start with an uppercase letter. Some brand names incorporate tall man letters in initial characters and may not be readily recognized as brand names. Brand name products appear in black; generic/other products appear in **color**.

DRUG NAME	CONFUSED DRUG NAME
TOLBUTamide	**TOLAZ**amide
Topamax	Toprol-XL
Toprol-XL	Topamax
Toradol	Foradil
t-PA	TNKase
Tracleer	Tricor
tra**MAD**ol	tra**ZOD**one
trastuzumab	ado-trastuzumab emtansine
tra**ZOD**one	tra**MAD**ol
TRENtal	**TEG**retol
tretinoin	**ISO**tretinoin
Tricor	Tracleer
tromethamine	Trophamine
Trophamine	tromethamine
tuberculin purified protein derivative (PPD)	influenza virus vaccine
tuberculin purified protein derivative (PPD)	tetanus diphtheria toxoid (Td)
Tylenol	Tylenol PM
Tylenol PM	Tylenol
Ultracet	Duricef
Ultram	lithium
val**ACY**clovir	val**GAN**ciclovir
Valcyte	Valtrex
val**GAN**ciclovir	val**ACY**clovir
Valtrex	Valcyte
Varivax	VZIG (varicella-zoster immune globulin)
Vesanoid	Vesicare
Vesicare	Vesanoid
Vexol	Vosol
Viagra	Allegra
Videx	Bidex
vin**BLAS**tine	vin**CRIS**tine
vin**CRIS**tine	vin**BLAS**tine
Viokase	Viokase 8
Viokase 8	Viokase
Vioxx	Zyvox
Viracept	Viramune
Viramune	Viracept
Viramune (nevirapine)	Viramune (herbal product)
Viramune (herbal product)	Viramune (nevirapine)
Vosol	Vexol
VZIG (varicella-zoster immune globulin)	Varivax
Wellbutrin SR	Wellbutrin XL
Wellbutrin XL	Wellbutrin SR
Xanax	Fanapt
Xanax	Tenex
Xanax	Zantac
Xeloda	Xenical
Xenical	Xeloda
Yasmin	Yaz
Yaz	Yasmin
Zantac	Xanax
Zantac	Zyr**TEC**
Zavesca (escitalopram) [non-US product]	Zavesca (miglustat)
Zavesca (miglustat)	Zavesca (escitalopram) [non-US product]
Zebeta	Diabeta
Zebeta	Zetia

DRUG NAME	CONFUSED DRUG NAME
Zegerid	Zestril
Zelapar (Zydis formulation)	Zy**PREXA** Zydis
Zerit	Zyr**TEC**
Zestril	Zegerid
Zestril	Zetia
Zestril	Zy**PREXA**
Zetia	Bextra
Zetia	Zebeta
Zetia	Zestril
Ziac	Tiazac
Zocor	Cozaar
Zocor	Zyr**TEC**
ZOLMitriptan	**SUMA**triptan
zolpidem	Zyloprim
Zonegran	**SINE**quan
Zostrix	Zovirax
Zovirax	Doribax
Zovirax	Zyvox
Zovirax	Zostrix
Zyban	Diovan
Zyloprim	zolpidem
Zy**PREXA**	Cele**XA**
Zy**PREXA**	Reprexain
Zy**PREXA**	Zestril
Zy**PREXA**	Zyr**TEC**
Zy**PREXA** Zydis	Zelapar (Zydis formulation)
Zyr**TEC**	Lipitor
Zyr**TEC**	Zantac
Zyr**TEC**	Zerit
Zyr**TEC**	Zocor
Zyr**TEC**	Zy**PREXA**
Zyr**TEC**	Zyr**TEC**-D
Zyr**TEC** (cetirizine)	Zyr**TEC** Itchy Eye Drops (ketotifen fumarate)
Zyr**TEC**-D	Zyr**TEC**
Zyr**TEC** Itchy Eye Drops (ketotifen fumarate)	Zyr**TEC** (cetirizine)
Zyvox	Vioxx
Zyvox	Zovirax

Brand names always start with an uppercase letter. Some brand names incorporate tall man letters in initial characters and may not be readily recognized as brand names. Brand name products appear in black; generic/other products appear in **color**.

Brand/Generic Index

BRAND/GENERIC INDEX

This index includes the brand and generic names of each drug in the Concise Drug Monographs section. The main monograph names are fully capitalized (eg, ALBUTEROL) and generic names begin with initial caps (eg, Abacavir sulfate). Any brand name associated with an entry is listed under the product.

A

D

F

G

H

M

N

O

P

Q

R

U

V

Therapeutic Class Index

THERAPEUTIC CLASS INDEX

Organized alphabetically, this index includes the therapeutic class of each drug in the Concise Drug Monographs section. Therapeutic class headings are based on information provided in the drug monographs. The drug entries listed under each bold therapeutic class are organized alphabetically by brand name or monograph title (shown in capitalized letters), followed by the generic name in parentheses.

A

Q

R

S

V

W

X

Notes

Notes

Notes

Notes

Notes

Notes

Notes

Notes

Visual Identification Guide

VISUAL IDENTIFICATION GUIDE*

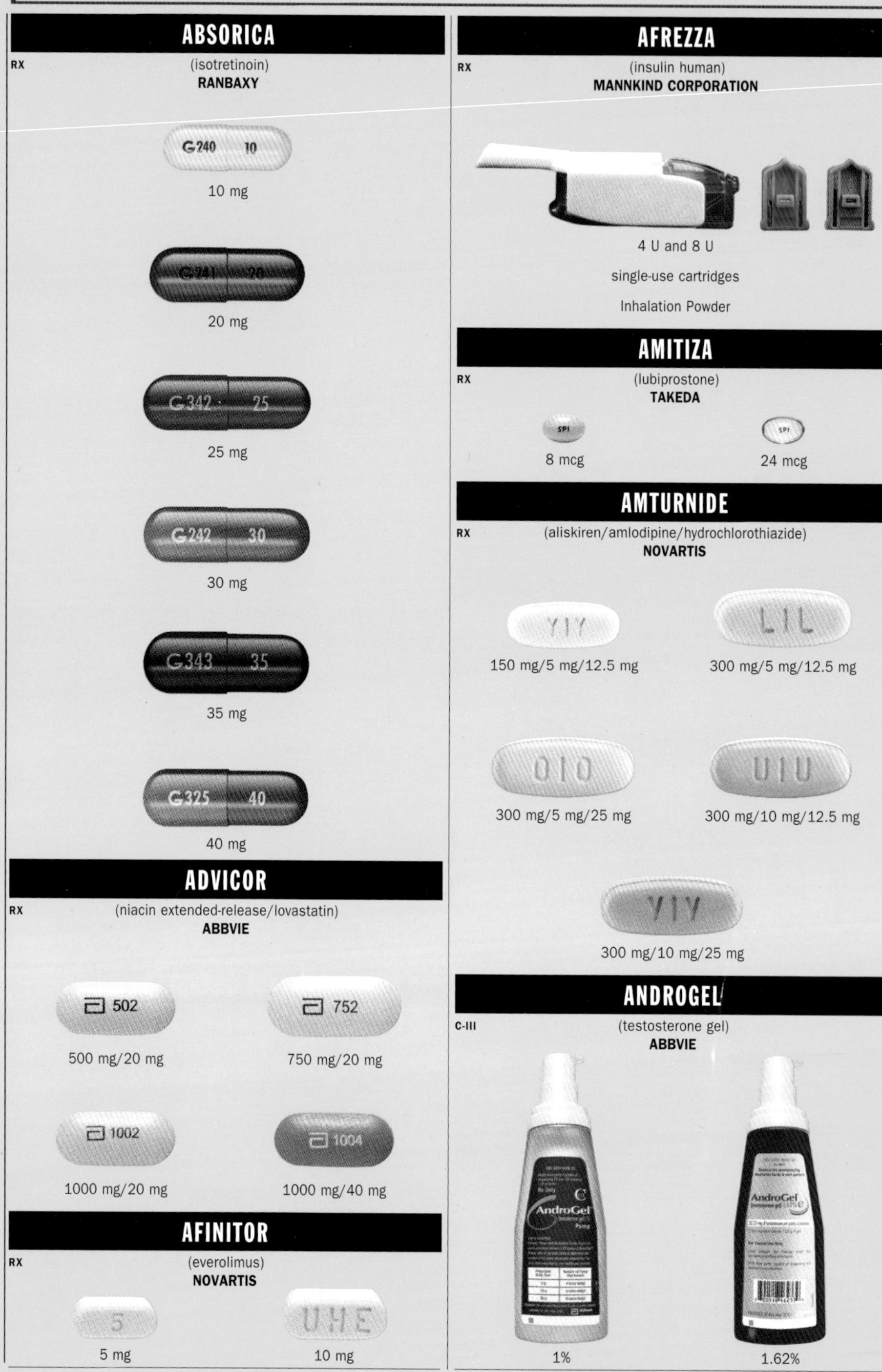

ABSORICA

RX (isotretinoin)
RANBAXY

10 mg

20 mg

25 mg

30 mg

35 mg

40 mg

ADVICOR

RX (niacin extended-release/lovastatin)
ABBVIE

500 mg/20 mg

750 mg/20 mg

1000 mg/20 mg

1000 mg/40 mg

AFINITOR

RX (everolimus)
NOVARTIS

5 mg

10 mg

AFREZZA

RX (insulin human)
MANNKIND CORPORATION

4 U and 8 U

single-use cartridges

Inhalation Powder

AMITIZA

RX (lubiprostone)
TAKEDA

8 mcg

24 mcg

AMTURNIDE

RX (aliskiren/amlodipine/hydrochlorothiazide)
NOVARTIS

150 mg/5 mg/12.5 mg

300 mg/5 mg/12.5 mg

300 mg/5 mg/25 mg

300 mg/10 mg/12.5 mg

300 mg/10 mg/25 mg

ANDROGEL

C-III (testosterone gel)
ABBVIE

1%

1.62%

*Other dosage forms and strengths may be available and this list is not inclusive of all drugs in this book.

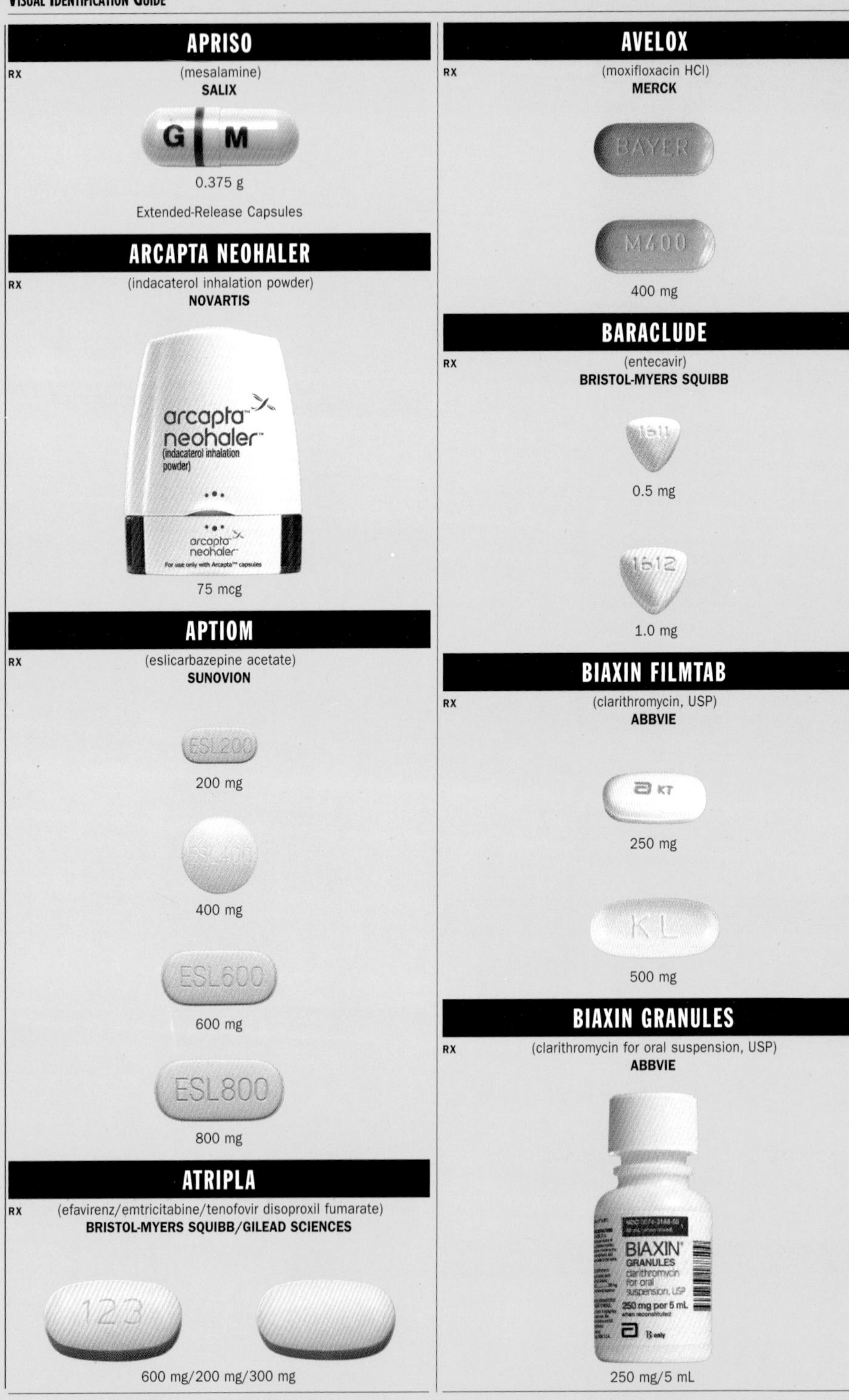

APRISO

RX

(mesalamine)

SALIX

0.375 g

Extended-Release Capsules

ARCAPTA NEOHALER

RX

(indacaterol inhalation powder)

NOVARTIS

75 mcg

APTIOM

RX

(eslicarbazepine acetate)

SUNOVION

200 mg

400 mg

600 mg

800 mg

ATRIPLA

RX

(efavirenz/emtricitabine/tenofovir disoproxil fumarate)

BRISTOL-MYERS SQUIBB/GILEAD SCIENCES

600 mg/200 mg/300 mg

AVELOX

RX

(moxifloxacin HCl)

MERCK

400 mg

BARACLUDE

RX

(entecavir)

BRISTOL-MYERS SQUIBB

0.5 mg

1.0 mg

BIAXIN FILMTAB

RX

(clarithromycin, USP)

ABBVIE

250 mg

500 mg

BIAXIN GRANULES

RX

(clarithromycin for oral suspension, USP)

ABBVIE

250 mg/5 mL

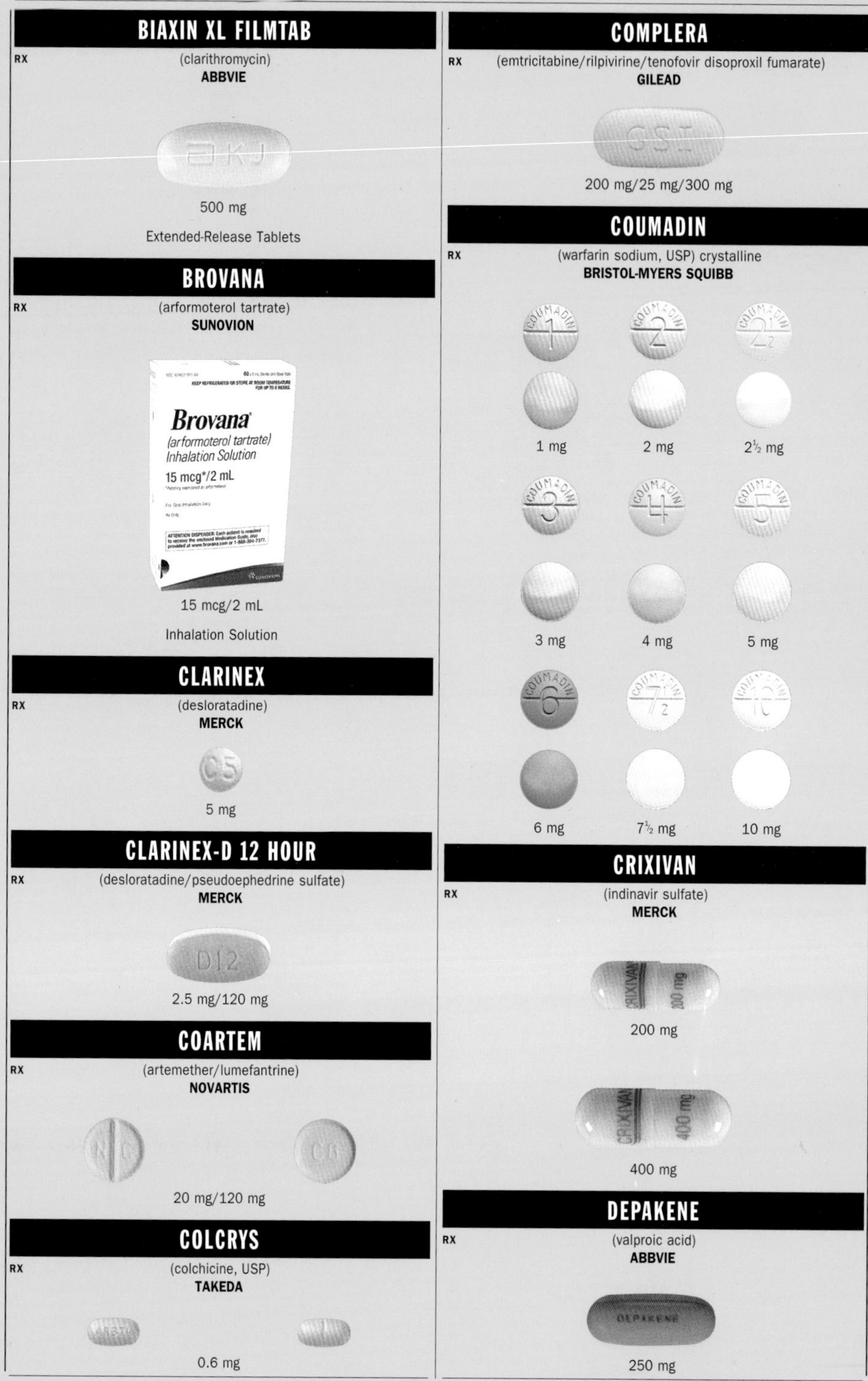
BIAXIN XL FILMTAB
RX
(clarithromycin)
ABBVIE
500 mg
Extended-Release Tablets
BROVANA
RX
(arformoterol tartrate)
SUNOVION
Brovana
(arformoterol tartrate)
Inhalation Solution
15 mcg*/2 mL
15 mcg/2 mL
Inhalation Solution
CLARINEX
RX
(desloratadine)
MERCK
C5
5 mg
CLARINEX-D 12 HOUR
RX
(desloratadine/pseudoephedrine sulfate)
MERCK
D12
2.5 mg/120 mg
COARTEM
RX
(artemether/lumefantrine)
NOVARTIS
20 mg/120 mg
COLCRYS
RX
(colchicine, USP)
TAKEDA
0.6 mg
COMPLERA
RX
(emtricitabine/rilpivirine/tenofovir disoproxil fumarate)
GILEAD
200 mg/25 mg/300 mg
COUMADIN
RX
(warfarin sodium, USP) crystalline
BRISTOL-MYERS SQUIBB
1 mg
2 mg
2½ mg
3 mg
4 mg
5 mg
6 mg
7½ mg
10 mg
CRIXIVAN
RX
(indinavir sulfate)
MERCK
CRIXIVAN 200 mg
200 mg
CRIXIVAN 400 mg
400 mg
DEPAKENE
RX
(valproic acid)
ABBVIE
DEPAKENE
250 mg

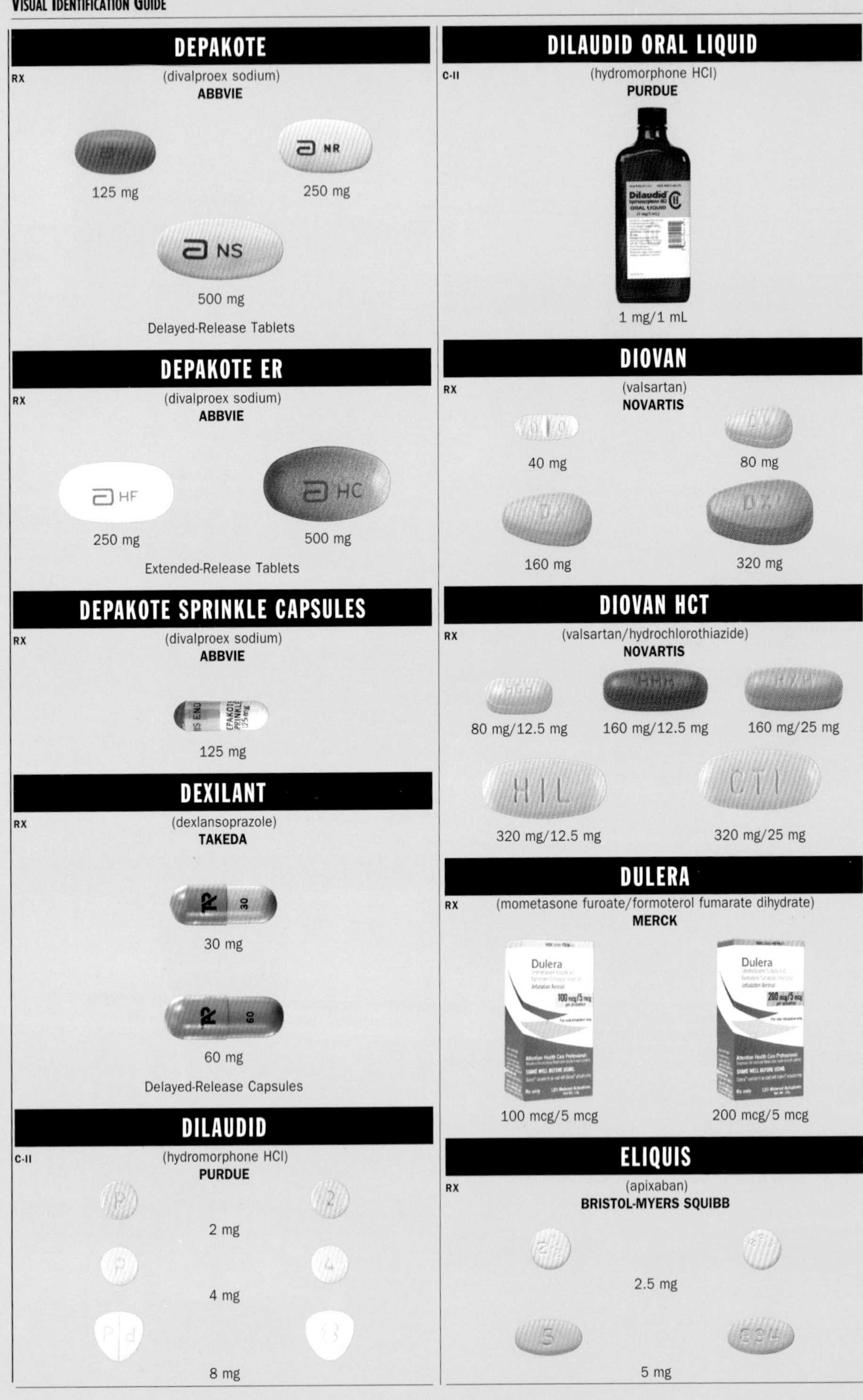
DEPAKOTE
RX
(divalproex sodium)
ABBVIE
125 mg
250 mg
500 mg
Delayed-Release Tablets
DEPAKOTE ER
RX
(divalproex sodium)
ABBVIE
250 mg
500 mg
Extended-Release Tablets
DEPAKOTE SPRINKLE CAPSULES
RX
(divalproex sodium)
ABBVIE
125 mg
DEXILANT
RX
(dexlansoprazole)
TAKEDA
30 mg
60 mg
Delayed-Release Capsules
DILAUDID
C-II
(hydromorphone HCl)
PURDUE
2 mg
4 mg
8 mg
DILAUDID ORAL LIQUID
C-II
(hydromorphone HCl)
PURDUE
1 mg/1 mL
DIOVAN
RX
(valsartan)
NOVARTIS
40 mg
80 mg
160 mg
320 mg
DIOVAN HCT
RX
(valsartan/hydrochlorothiazide)
NOVARTIS
80 mg/12.5 mg
160 mg/12.5 mg
160 mg/25 mg
320 mg/12.5 mg
320 mg/25 mg
DULERA
RX
(mometasone furoate/formoterol fumarate dihydrate)
MERCK
100 mcg/5 mcg
200 mcg/5 mcg
ELIQUIS
RX
(apixaban)
BRISTOL-MYERS SQUIBB
2.5 mg
5 mg

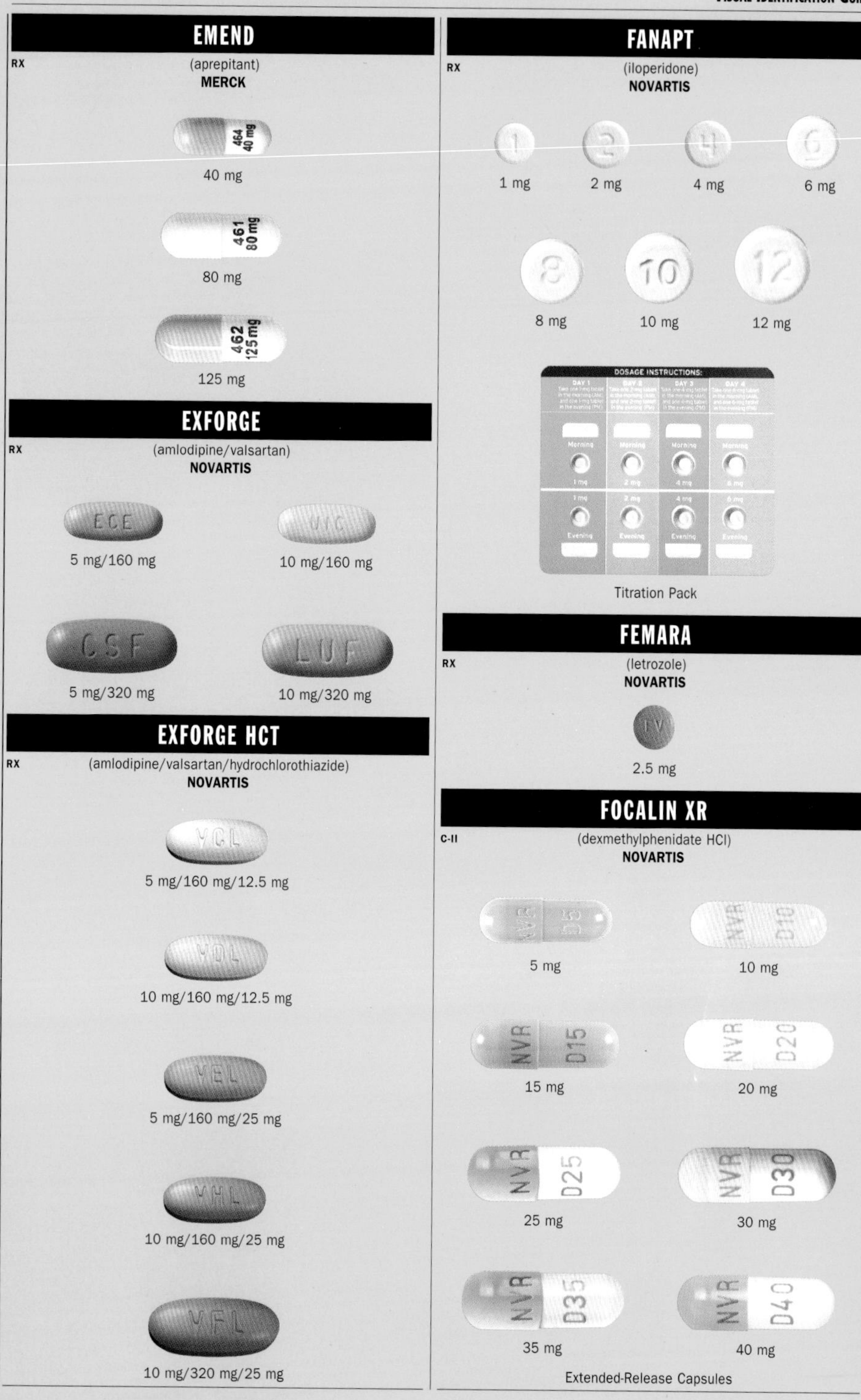
EMEND
RX
(aprepitant)
MERCK
464 40 mg
40 mg
461 80 mg
80 mg
462 125 mg
125 mg
EXFORGE
RX
(amlodipine/valsartan)
NOVARTIS
ECE
5 mg/160 mg
10 mg/160 mg
CSF
5 mg/320 mg
LUF
10 mg/320 mg
EXFORGE HCT
RX
(amlodipine/valsartan/hydrochlorothiazide)
NOVARTIS
VCL
5 mg/160 mg/12.5 mg
VDL
10 mg/160 mg/12.5 mg
VEL
5 mg/160 mg/25 mg
VHL
10 mg/160 mg/25 mg
VFL
10 mg/320 mg/25 mg
FANAPT
RX
(iloperidone)
NOVARTIS
1 mg
2 mg
4 mg
6 mg
8 mg
10 mg
12 mg
DOSAGE INSTRUCTIONS:
Titration Pack
FEMARA
RX
(letrozole)
NOVARTIS
2.5 mg
FOCALIN XR
C-II
(dexmethylphenidate HCl)
NOVARTIS
5 mg
NVR D10
10 mg
NVR D15
15 mg
NVR D20
20 mg
NVR D25
25 mg
NVR D30
30 mg
NVR D35
35 mg
NVR D40
40 mg
Extended-Release Capsules

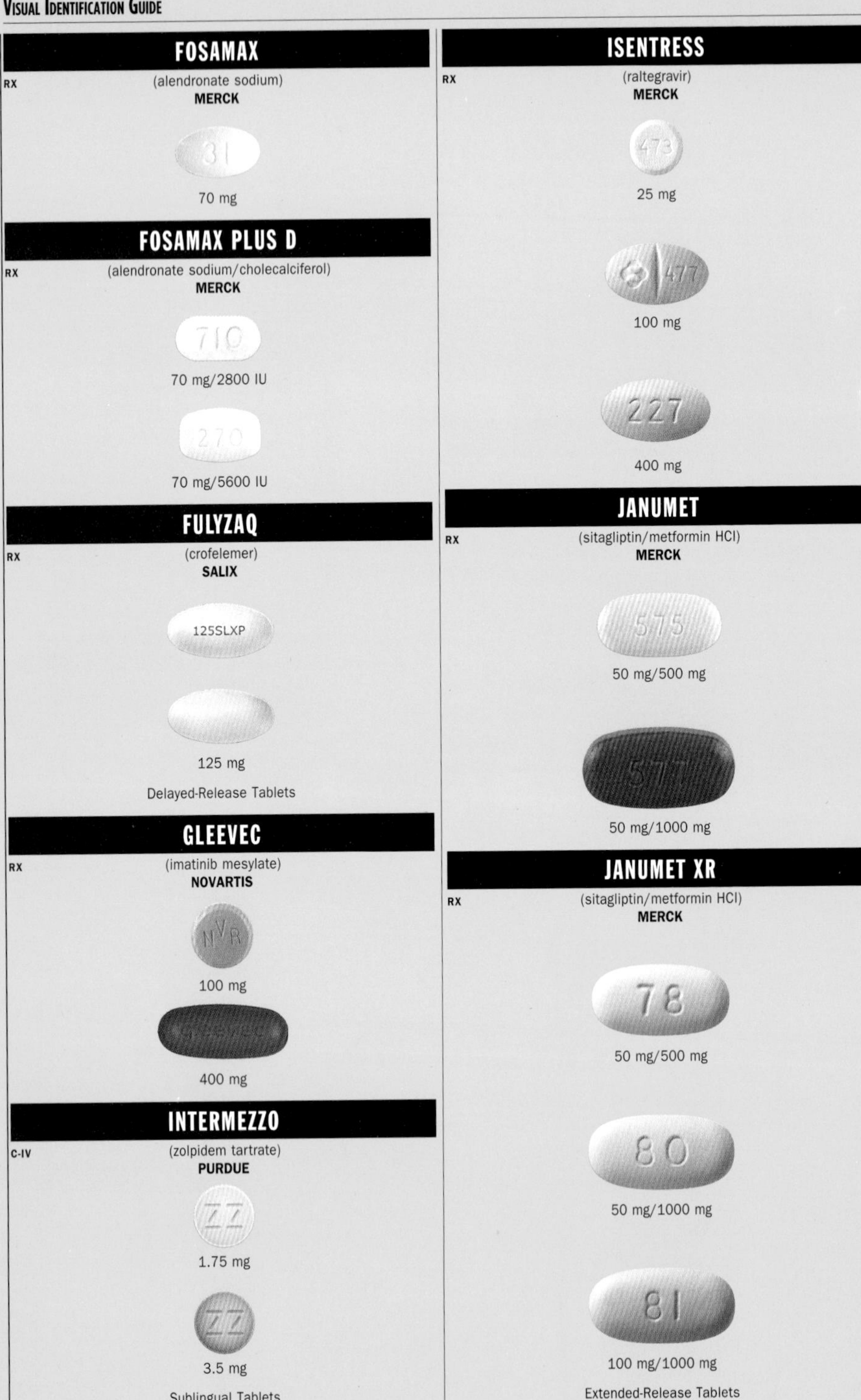
FOSAMAX
RX
(alendronate sodium)
MERCK
31
70 mg
FOSAMAX PLUS D
RX
(alendronate sodium/cholecalciferol)
MERCK
710
70 mg/2800 IU
270
70 mg/5600 IU
FULYZAQ
RX
(crofelemer)
SALIX
125SLXP
125 mg
Delayed-Release Tablets
GLEEVEC
RX
(imatinib mesylate)
NOVARTIS
NVR
100 mg
400 mg
INTERMEZZO
C-IV
(zolpidem tartrate)
PURDUE
ZZ
1.75 mg
ZZ
3.5 mg
Sublingual Tablets
ISENTRESS
RX
(raltegravir)
MERCK
473
25 mg
477
100 mg
227
400 mg
JANUMET
RX
(sitagliptin/metformin HCl)
MERCK
575
50 mg/500 mg
577
50 mg/1000 mg
JANUMET XR
RX
(sitagliptin/metformin HCl)
MERCK
78
50 mg/500 mg
80
50 mg/1000 mg
81
100 mg/1000 mg
Extended-Release Tablets

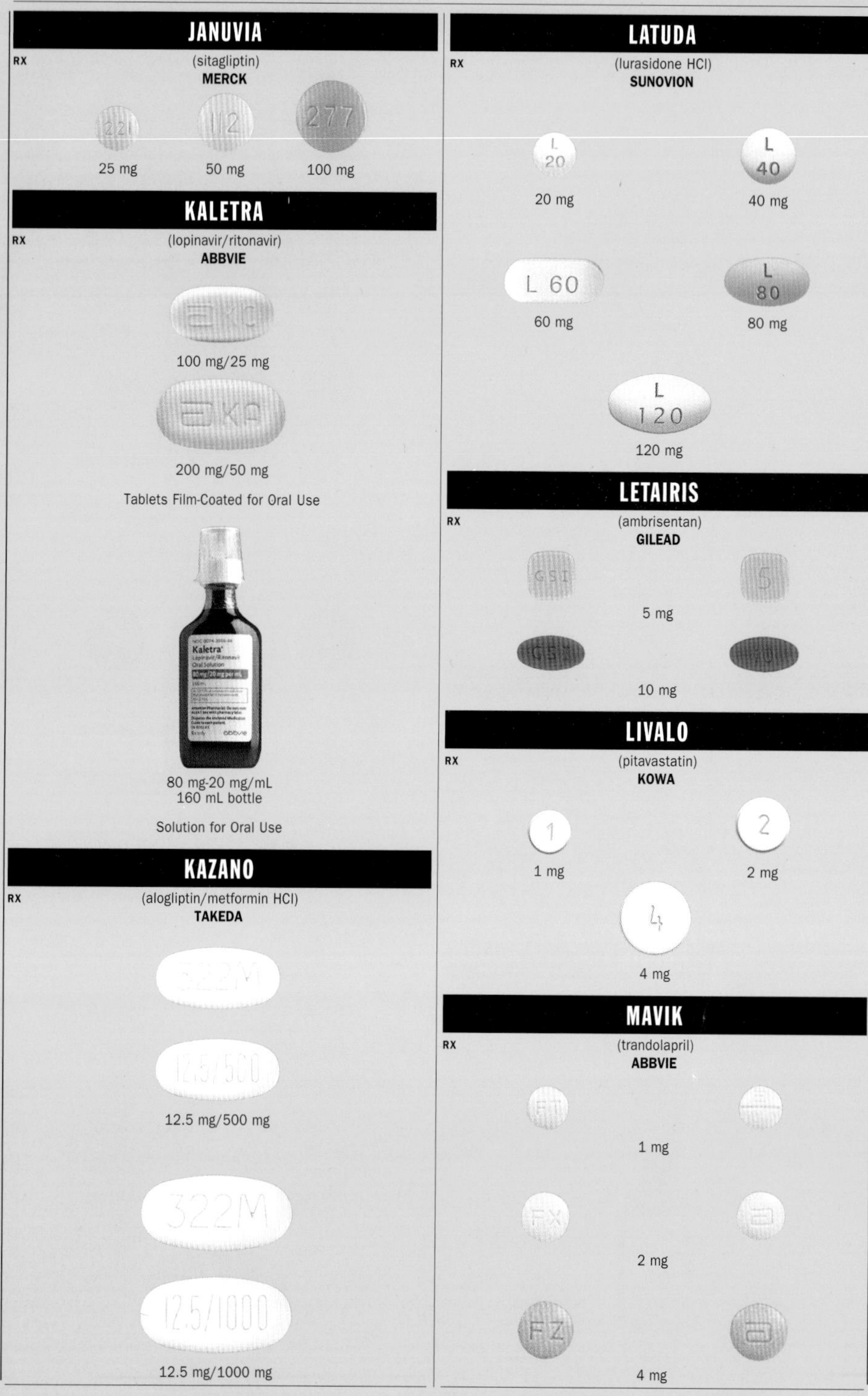

JANUVIA

RX

(sitagliptin)

MERCK

25 mg | 50 mg | 100 mg

KALETRA

RX

(lopinavir/ritonavir)

ABBVIE

100 mg/25 mg

200 mg/50 mg

Tablets Film-Coated for Oral Use

80 mg-20 mg/mL
160 mL bottle

Solution for Oral Use

KAZANO

RX

(alogliptin/metformin HCl)

TAKEDA

12.5 mg/500 mg

12.5 mg/1000 mg

LATUDA

RX

(lurasidone HCl)

SUNOVION

20 mg | 40 mg

60 mg | 80 mg

120 mg

LETAIRIS

RX

(ambrisentan)

GILEAD

5 mg

10 mg

LIVALO

RX

(pitavastatin)

KOWA

1 mg | 2 mg

4 mg

MAVIK

RX

(trandolapril)

ABBVIE

1 mg

2 mg

4 mg

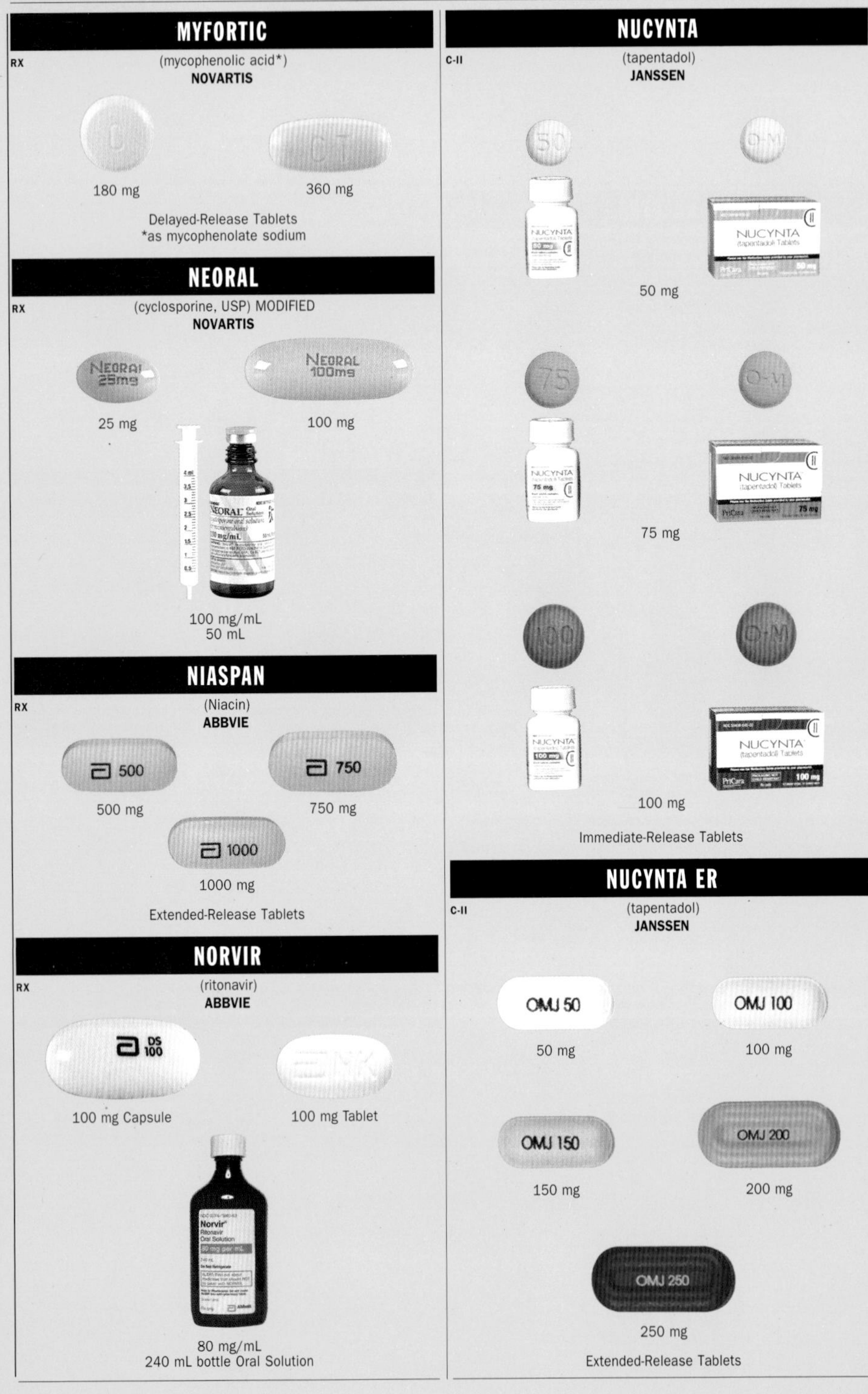
MYFORTIC
RX
(mycophenolic acid*)
NOVARTIS
180 mg
360 mg
Delayed-Release Tablets
*as mycophenolate sodium
NEORAL
RX
(cyclosporine, USP) MODIFIED
NOVARTIS
NEORAL 25mg
NEORAL 100mg
25 mg
100 mg
100 mg/mL
50 mL
NIASPAN
RX
(Niacin)
ABBVIE
500
750
1000
500 mg
750 mg
1000 mg
Extended-Release Tablets
NORVIR
RX
(ritonavir)
ABBVIE
DS 100
100 mg Capsule
100 mg Tablet
Norvir
Ritonavir
Oral Solution
80 mg/mL
240 mL bottle Oral Solution
NUCYNTA
C-II
(tapentadol)
JANSSEN
NUCYNTA
50 mg
75 mg
100 mg
Immediate-Release Tablets
NUCYNTA ER
C-II
(tapentadol)
JANSSEN
OMJ 50
OMJ 100
50 mg
100 mg
OMJ 150
OMJ 200
150 mg
200 mg
OMJ 250
250 mg
Extended-Release Tablets

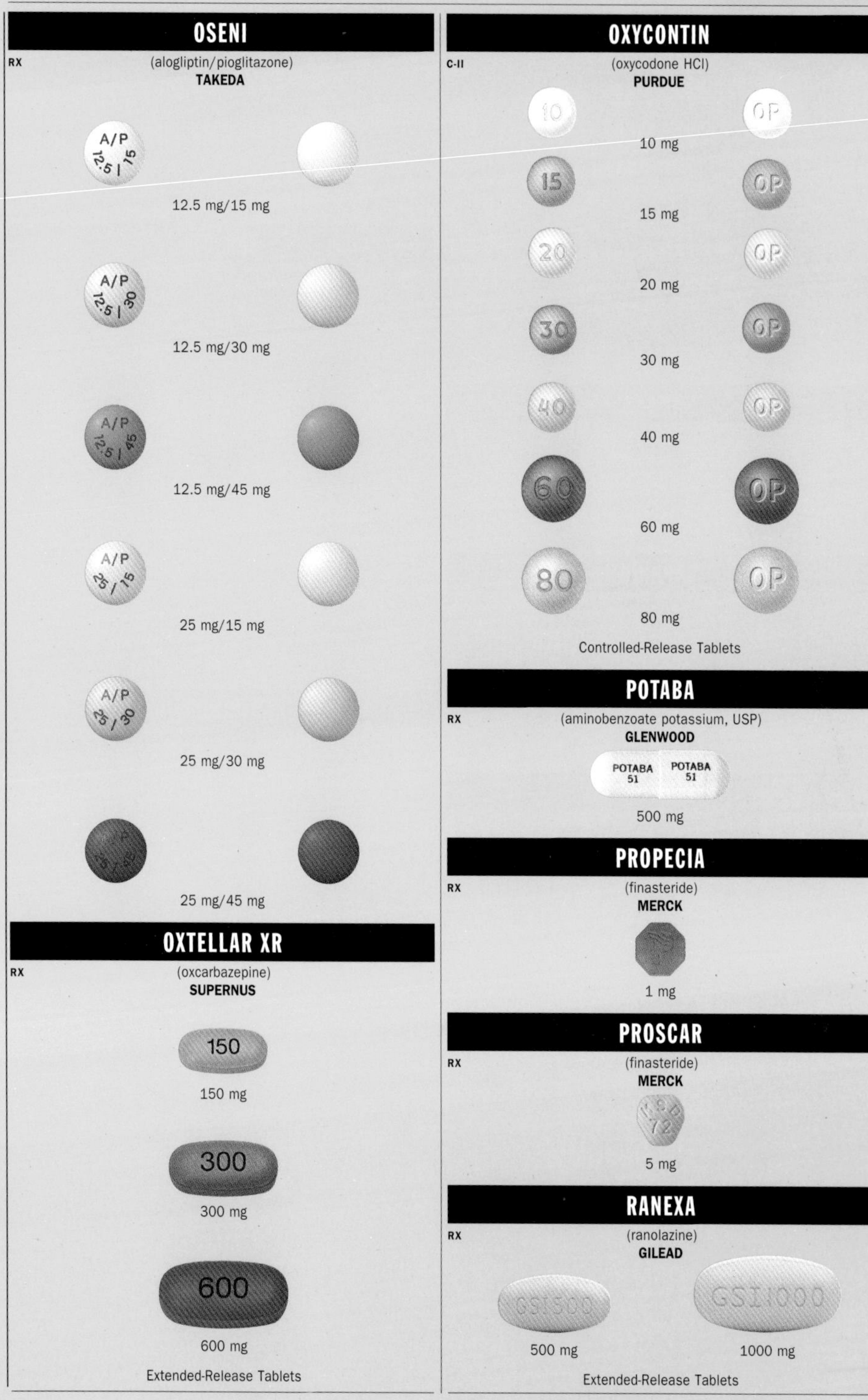
OSENI
RX
(alogliptin/pioglitazone)
TAKEDA
A/P 12.5 / 15
12.5 mg/15 mg
A/P 12.5 / 30
12.5 mg/30 mg
A/P 12.5 / 45
12.5 mg/45 mg
A/P 25 / 15
25 mg/15 mg
A/P 25 / 30
25 mg/30 mg
25 mg/45 mg
OXTELLAR XR
RX
(oxcarbazepine)
SUPERNUS
150
150 mg
300
300 mg
600
600 mg
Extended-Release Tablets
OXYCONTIN
C-II
(oxycodone HCl)
PURDUE
10
OP
10 mg
15
OP
15 mg
20
OP
20 mg
30
OP
30 mg
40
OP
40 mg
60
OP
60 mg
80
OP
80 mg
Controlled-Release Tablets
POTABA
RX
(aminobenzoate potassium, USP)
GLENWOOD
POTABA 51
POTABA 51
500 mg
PROPECIA
RX
(finasteride)
MERCK
1 mg
PROSCAR
RX
(finasteride)
MERCK
MSD 72
5 mg
RANEXA
RX
(ranolazine)
GILEAD
GSI500
GSI1000
500 mg
1000 mg
Extended-Release Tablets

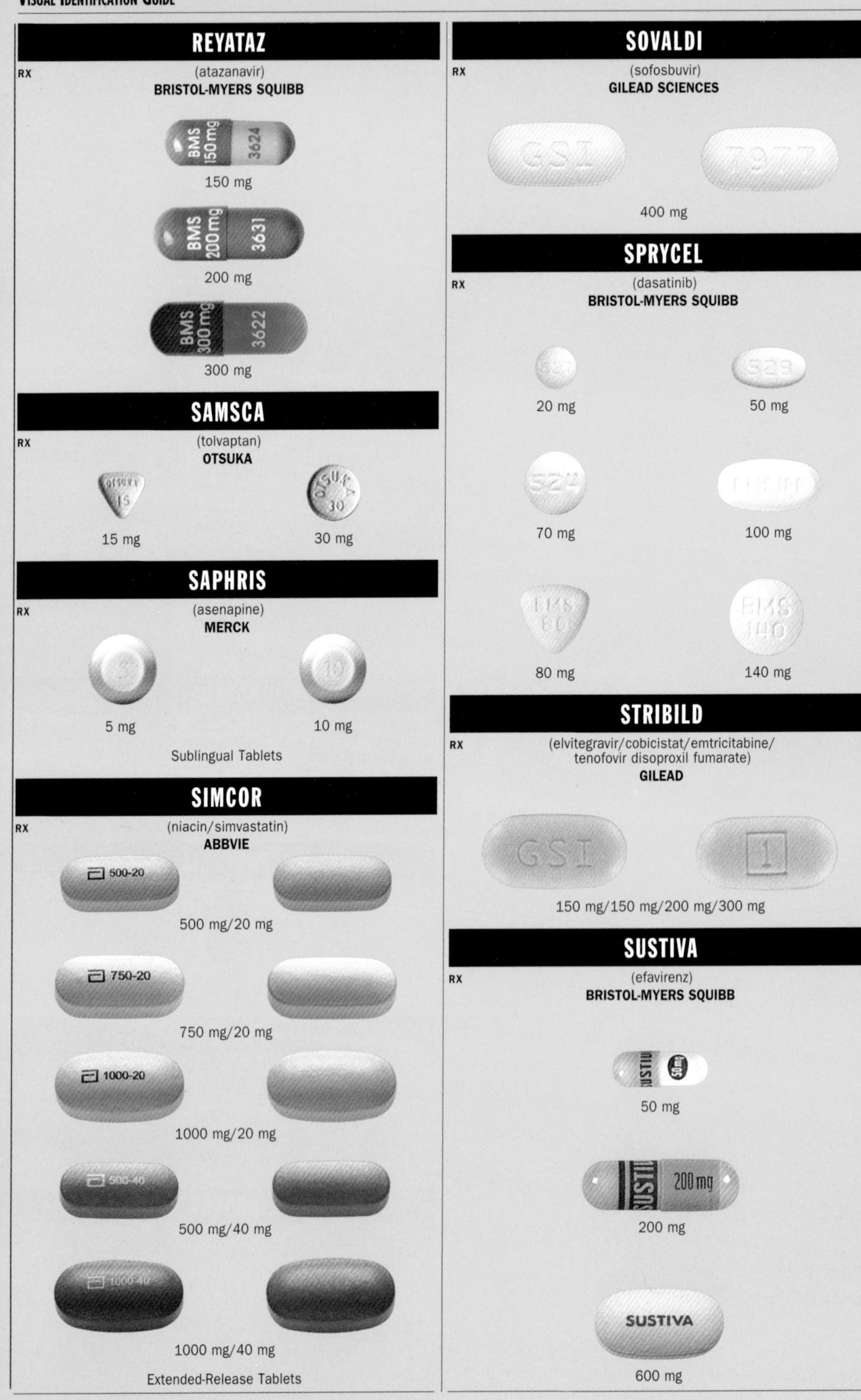
REYATAZ
RX
(atazanavir)
BRISTOL-MYERS SQUIBB
BMS 150 mg 3624
150 mg
BMS 200 mg 3631
200 mg
BMS 300 mg 3622
300 mg
SAMSCA
RX
(tolvaptan)
OTSUKA
OTSUKA 15
15 mg
OTSUKA 30
30 mg
SAPHRIS
RX
(asenapine)
MERCK
5 mg
10 mg
Sublingual Tablets
SIMCOR
RX
(niacin/simvastatin)
ABBVIE
500-20
500 mg/20 mg
750-20
750 mg/20 mg
1000-20
1000 mg/20 mg
500-40
500 mg/40 mg
1000-40
1000 mg/40 mg
Extended-Release Tablets
SOVALDI
RX
(sofosbuvir)
GILEAD SCIENCES
GSI
7977
400 mg
SPRYCEL
RX
(dasatinib)
BRISTOL-MYERS SQUIBB
20 mg
50 mg
524
70 mg
100 mg
BMS 80
80 mg
BMS 140
140 mg
STRIBILD
RX
(elvitegravir/cobicistat/emtricitabine/
tenofovir disoproxil fumarate)
GILEAD
GSI
1
150 mg/150 mg/200 mg/300 mg
SUSTIVA
RX
(efavirenz)
BRISTOL-MYERS SQUIBB
50 mg
50 mg
SUSTIVA 200 mg
200 mg
SUSTIVA
600 mg

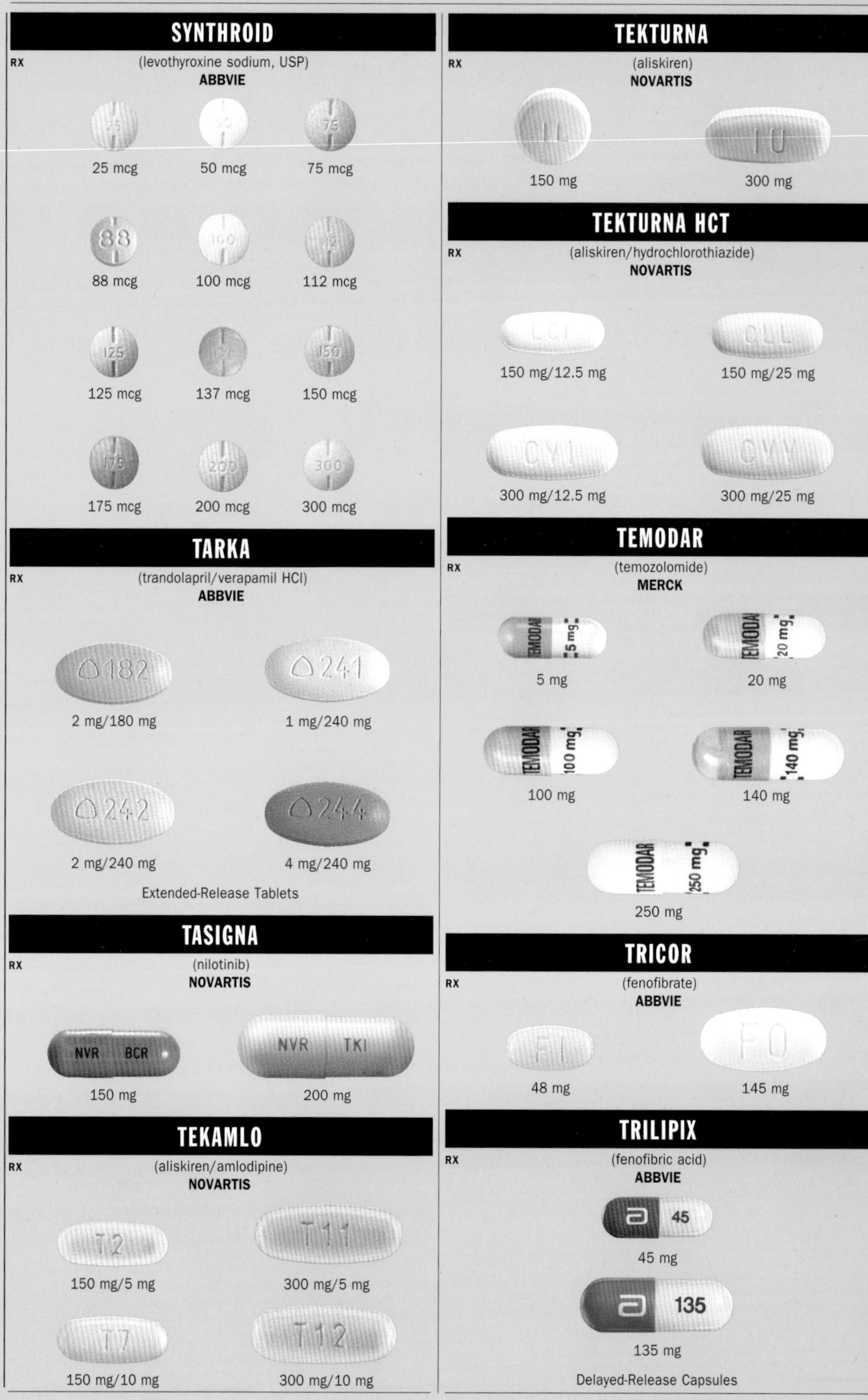
SYNTHROID
RX
(levothyroxine sodium, USP)
ABBVIE
25 mcg
50 mcg
75 mcg
88
88 mcg
100 mcg
112 mcg
125 mcg
137 mcg
150 mcg
175 mcg
200 mcg
300 mcg
TARKA
RX
(trandolapril/verapamil HCl)
ABBVIE
182
2 mg/180 mg
241
1 mg/240 mg
242
2 mg/240 mg
244
4 mg/240 mg
Extended-Release Tablets
TASIGNA
RX
(nilotinib)
NOVARTIS
NVR BCR
150 mg
NVR TKI
200 mg
TEKAMLO
RX
(aliskiren/amlodipine)
NOVARTIS
T2
150 mg/5 mg
T11
300 mg/5 mg
T7
150 mg/10 mg
T12
300 mg/10 mg
TEKTURNA
RX
(aliskiren)
NOVARTIS
150 mg
300 mg
TEKTURNA HCT
RX
(aliskiren/hydrochlorothiazide)
NOVARTIS
150 mg/12.5 mg
150 mg/25 mg
300 mg/12.5 mg
300 mg/25 mg
TEMODAR
RX
(temozolomide)
MERCK
TEMODAR 5 mg
5 mg
TEMODAR 20 mg
20 mg
TEMODAR 100 mg
100 mg
TEMODAR 140 mg
140 mg
TEMODAR 250 mg
250 mg
TRICOR
RX
(fenofibrate)
ABBVIE
48 mg
145 mg
TRILIPIX
RX
(fenofibric acid)
ABBVIE
45
45 mg
135
135 mg
Delayed-Release Capsules

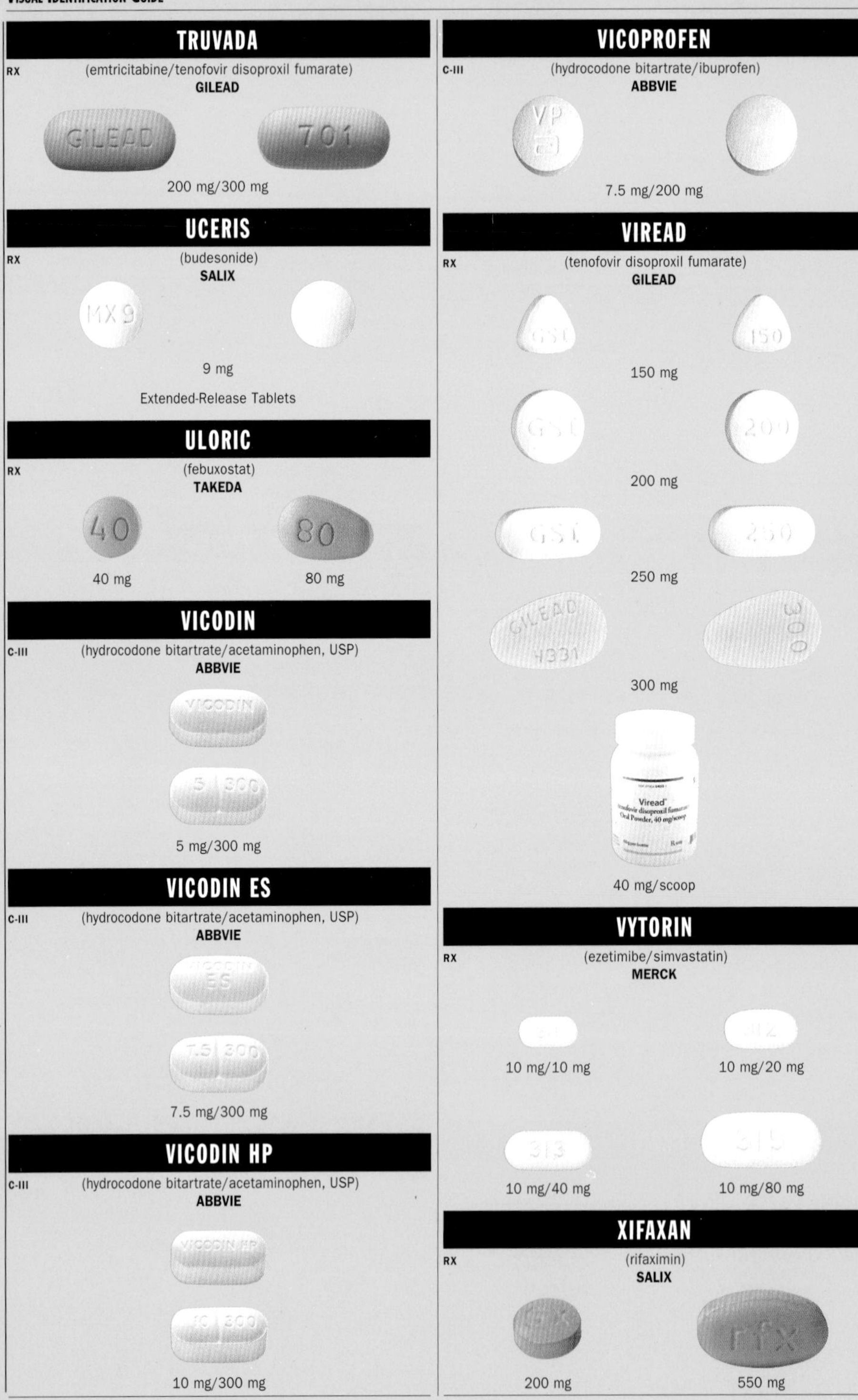

TRUVADA
RX (emtricitabine/tenofovir disoproxil fumarate)
GILEAD

200 mg/300 mg

UCERIS
RX (budesonide)
SALIX

9 mg

Extended-Release Tablets

ULORIC
RX (febuxostat)
TAKEDA

40 mg | 80 mg

VICODIN
C-III (hydrocodone bitartrate/acetaminophen, USP)
ABBVIE

5 mg/300 mg

VICODIN ES
C-III (hydrocodone bitartrate/acetaminophen, USP)
ABBVIE

7.5 mg/300 mg

VICODIN HP
C-III (hydrocodone bitartrate/acetaminophen, USP)
ABBVIE

10 mg/300 mg

VICOPROFEN
C-III (hydrocodone bitartrate/ibuprofen)
ABBVIE

7.5 mg/200 mg

VIREAD
RX (tenofovir disoproxil fumarate)
GILEAD

150 mg

200 mg

250 mg

300 mg

40 mg/scoop

VYTORIN
RX (ezetimibe/simvastatin)
MERCK

10 mg/10 mg | 10 mg/20 mg

10 mg/40 mg | 10 mg/80 mg

XIFAXAN
RX (rifaximin)
SALIX

200 mg | 550 mg